Essentials of
Maternity Nursing

Essentials of Maternity Nursing

IRENE M. BOBAK, R.N., M.S.

Professor, San Francisco State University,
San Francisco, California

MARGARET DUNCAN JENSEN, R.N., M.S.

Professor, San Jose State University,
San Jose, California

with 948 illustrations

The C. V. Mosby Company

ST. LOUIS TORONTO 1984

To the following members of our families

Marianne K. Zalar
Albert B. Bobak
Irene L. Bobak
Stephen J. Bobak
Veronica Bobak
Sister Mary Eleanor, V.S.C.
Doreen E. Duncan
Russ Duncan
John F. Duncan
Marjory Jensen
Carlo Jensen

who by virtue of their belief in us prompted the courage and motivation to complete this textbook.

Irene M. Bobak
Margaret Duncan Jensen

MOSBY

A TRADITION OF PUBLISHING EXCELLENCE

Editor: Alison Miller
Assistant editor: Susan R. Epstein
Manuscript editor: Mary Wright
Design: Diane Beasley
Production: Margaret B. Bridenbaugh, Judith England

Printed in the United States of America

The C.V. Mosby Company
11830 Westline Industrial Drive, St. Louis, Missouri 63146

Library of Congress Cataloging in Publication Data

Bobak, Irene M.
Essentials of maternity nursing.

Bibliography: p.
Includes index.
1. Obstetrical nursing. I. Jensen, Margaret Duncan.
II. Title. [DNLM: 1. Obstetrical nursing.
2. Perinatology—Nursing texts. WY 157 B663e]
RG951.B66 1984 610.73'678 83-19518
ISBN 0-8016-2486-X

C/D/D 9 8 7 6 5 4 3 2 02/A/246

Contributors

JEANNE DeJOSEPH, R.N., C.N.M., Ph.D.

Assistant Director of Nursing,
Perinatal and Critical Care Transport,
Stanford University Hospital, Stanford, California;
Lecturer, Department of Family, Community, and Preventative Medicine, Stanford University Hospital and Medical Center, Stanford, California;
Assistant Clinical Professor, Department of Physiological Nursing, University of California, San Francisco; Affiliated Faculty Member, Center for Research on Women, Stanford, University, Palo Alto, California

JOAN EDELSTEIN, R.N., P.N.P., M.S.N., M.P.H.

Dr. P.H. Candidate—University of California, Berkeley; Assistant Professor,
San Jose State University,
San Jose, California

CHERYL HARRIS, R.N., B.S.

Staff Nurse,
Neonatal Intensive Care Unit,
Childrens Mercy Hospital,
Kansas City, Missouri

BEVERLY HORN, R.N., Ph.D.

Associate Professor,
School of Nursing,
University of Washington,
Seattle

BARBARA PETREE, R.N., M.A.

Clinical Nursing Coordinator,
Delivery Room,
Stanford University Hospital,
Stanford, California

CELESTE PHILLIPS, R.N., Ed.D.

Director of Nursing Education,
Cabrillo College,
Aptos, California

SUSAN TUCKER, R.N., B.S.N., P.H.N.

Assistant Director of Nursing,
Kaiser-Permanente Medical Center,
Panorama City, California

LUCILLE WHALEY, R.N., B.S., M.S.

Professor,
San Jose State University,
San Jose, California; Ed.D. Candidate,
University of Southern California,
Los Angeles

BONNIE WORTHINGTON-ROBERTS, Ph.D.

Professor, Director of Nutritional Sciences
and Chief Nutritionist,
Child Development Center,
University of Washington,
Seattle

MARIANNE K. ZALAR, R.N., Ed.D.

Assistant Director of Nursing,
Department of Nursing Research,
Stanford University Hospital and Medical Center,
Stanford, California;
Associate Clinical Professor,
Department of Family Health Care Nursing,
University of California,
San Francisco

Preface

Writing a single textbook to meet the varied needs of today's maternity students, educators, and practitioners is indeed a challenging, if not impossible, task. We have been gratified by the response to and acceptance of our other text, *Maternity Care: The Nurse and the Family,* and through the years have received and welcomed many helpful comments from readers. Although a great many maternity nurses and students have found our text to be a definitive guide and resource, other users have expressed their desire for a text focused on the basics of providing safe, family-centered maternity care. *Essentials of Maternity Nursing* has been written and designed with the particular needs of this group of students, educators, and practitioners in mind.

Philosophy

Philosophically, *Essentials of Maternity Nursing* reflects our belief that maternity nursing is a scientifically based problem-solving process. The five-step nursing process—assessment, nursing diagnosis, planning, implementation, and evaluation of nursing care—provides not only the underlying theory for practice in this text, but also its organizing framework. To support the integration of the nursing process in the text, readers will find numerous tables, charts, and nursing care plans that highlight clinical assessments, therapeutic strategies and interventions, and evaluative criteria. Inherent in our philosophy of the maternity nursing process is the belief that its steps or stages move toward goals for holistic care. The goals for a mother are a safe, satisfying pregnancy, a normal birth, and a healthy infant; the goals for the infant are a healthy intrauterine existence and adjustment to extrauterine life; the goals for the family and significant others are a childbirth experience promoting parenting for the child, the personal growth of all involved individuals, and participation in future health maintenance and promotion activities.

Organization and Coverage

Essentials of Maternity Nursing presents a survey of maternity nursing that addresses in some depth those conditions of importance to the student or practicing nurse. Those conditions rarely encountered in practice have been briefly addressed with a minimum of detailed information. The overriding guiding principle to the selection and coverage of information has been to present information that is current, accurate, theoretically sound, and *essential* to the delivery of safe, comprehensive, and holistic care to mothers, fetuses/neonates, and families by nurses who assume varying roles.

The organization of the text reflects this emphasis on essential information. Content related to the normal maternity cycle is presented first and comprises most of the text. The last unit deals with high-risk childbearing families. Each unit is organized so that the initial chapters discuss the biologic and psychosocial content necessary for implementation of the nursing process. Learning how to make accurate clinical assessments, interpret findings, and understand the significance of signs and symptoms are of paramount importance to the maternity nurse. Therefore carefully developed, measurable, evaluative criteria provide the nurse with guidelines for continuous evaluation of the effectiveness of nursing care. The evaluation serves as a basis for adapting care plans to changing conditions.

Unit One, "Introduction to Maternity Care," provides the theoretical base for family-centered, holistic maternity nursing. Present day issues and trends are reviewed within a historic perspective of maternity nursing. In addition, chapters on nursing process, the nurse-client relationship, and related ethical and legal aspects provide an overview of the maternity nursing practice arena.

Unit Two, "Basic Concepts of Reproduction," presents the basic concepts of human sexuality and reproduction. The biologic and psychosocial aspects of reproduction are emphasized as a foundation for care before, during, and after pregnancy. The family, its structure, and its supportive roles are explored as well as biologic inheritance and reproductive planning and their influence on the family decision-making process and childbearing responsibilities.

Unit Three, "Prenatal Period," follows the progression of a normal pregnancy. Nursing care during pregnancy requires knowledge of fetal development as well as an understanding of maternal and family adaptations to the biopsychosocial realities of pregnancy. Separate chapters on maternal and fetal nutrition and preparation for parenting reflect the growing body of knowledge and importance of the nurse's role in these vital areas.

Unit Four, "The Birth Period," begins with the essential factors that influence the outcome of childbirth, followed by the nursing care of the maternity client and her support persons during labor and birth. The nursing process provides the format for care and is specific for the four stages of labor. Subsequent chapters discuss the nursing role as related to fetal monitoring and the pharmacologic control of discomfort. A chapter on alternative birthing centers focuses on the needs of clinicians in these settings.

Unit Five, "Nursing Care of the Normal Newborn," uses the nursing process as the basis for care. Content includes biologic and behavioral characteristics of the healthy neonate at term, relevant nursing assessments and diagnoses, and the planning, implementation, and evaluation of nursing care. A chapter on the nutritional needs for the first year of life assists the nurse in providing care of the neonate and anticipatory guidance to parents.

Unit Six, "Nursing Care During the Postpartum Period," is devoted to nursing care of the new mother and her family. Discussions of maternal physiology and the psychologic impact of parenthood on the mother and other family members provide the basis for selection of nursing strategies appropriate for individualized care.

Unit Seven, "High-Risk Mother and Neonate," describes populations at high risk and the necessary alterations in the plans of care for the high-risk childbearing family. Selected risk factors are presented in a biopsychosocial dysfunction framework. This format facilitates a conceptual approach to common symptoms and therapies (preventive, curative, rehabilitative) as well as the study of the distinctive characteristics of specific disorders. Wherever possible, the mother and fetus/neonate are discussed as a unit, e.g., the childbearing cycle complicated by diabetes mellitus. Separate chapters deal with issues such as loss and grief, adolescent parenthood, and sociocultural risk factors.

In-Text Learning Aids

Written in a clear, readable style and logical in its organization, *Essentials of Maternity Nursing* has been designed with the specific needs of the learner in mind. Concise chapter outlines open every chapter, affording the reader an opportunity to review a chapter's contents and coverage at a glance. Hundreds of photographs, illustrations, tables, and charts enhance and support the text and provide quick reference information. A two-color format has been incorporated in the design of the text to enhance reader usability.

The 14 appendices are in reality an information resource pool for students and practitioners alike. The extensive glossary contains definitions of major obstetric and nursing terms introduced in the text. The thorough and complete index is an invaluable aid in assisting readers in finding information logically and quickly.

Teaching-Learning Package

To facilitate the teaching-learning process and help instructors and students in using the text to its fullest potential, three supplements are offered: an instructor's manual, a test bank manual, and an overhead transparency set.

1. The "Instructor's Manual" (by Judith H. Isbell and Janice E. Webb) includes 41 chapters, each keyed to one chapter in the text. Each chapter includes the goals for learning, evaluative criteria (cognitive, affective, and psychomotor objectives), a list of key terms introduced in the chapter, a topical lecture outline, and suggestions for clinically based activities. The appendix expands on the resources found in the text and contains information about instructional materials and audiovisual aids.
2. The "Test Bank" includes over 1,000 questions. The questions are directly related to the student learning objectives and include multiple choice, fill-in-the-blank, and essay questions. Answer key and rationales for the questions are also included.
3. An overhead transparency set includes 50 two-color illustrations from this new text.

■ ■ ■

We are fully aware of the increasingly important contribution men are making to the nursing profession as well as the growing number of women entering the medical profession. We hope this trend will continue. The construction of the English language, however, sometimes makes it awkward to totally eliminate the feminine and masculine pronouns. Therefore, to present material clearly and smoothly we have generally used the feminine pronoun to refer to the nurse.

Over the years we have received many comments and suggestions regarding our maternity nursing texts. Some of these comments provided the impetus for writing *Essentials of Maternity Nursing,* and we have incorporated many of these suggestions in the organization and development of this text. We welcome comments from instructors, students, and practitioners who use this text so that we may continue to be responsive to the needs of the profession.

Irene M. Bobak
Margaret Duncan Jensen

Acknowledgments

We wish to thank everyone whose comments and suggestions prompted this collaborative effort and the reviewers who provided valuable criticism of the manuscript: Sheldon B. Korones, M.D., Anna McHargue, M.D., Susan Virden, Mary Byrne, Shirley Cashio, Beverly Gaglione, Celeste Phillips, Rosie Steffen, Janice Webb, Annette Worthy, and Jack Kundin, M.D.

To the staffs of Stanford University Medical Center, Stanford, California; Kaiser-Permanente Hospital and Santa Clara Valley Medical Center, Santa Clara, California; St. Luke's Hospital, Kansas City, Missouri; and Jewish Hospital and Barnes Hospital, St. Louis, Missouri, we offer thanks for their shared expertise and photographs.

We would like to thank the following photographers: Judith Bamber, San Jose, California; Jacqueline Capra, Santa Cruz, California; Joan Edelstein, San Jose, California; Linda Maxwell, San Francisco, California; Nanci Newell, Fountain Valley, California; Marjorie Pyle, of Lifecircle, Costa Mesa, California; Linda Rae Rose, San Francisco, California, and the many nurses, both students and practitioners, who appeared in the photographs.

Several families outside of our own have made unique contributions to the original photographic illustrations in this text. Their names, listed alphabetically, are Elaine Chan and daughter, Chris and Renee Cowing and son, Mr. and Mrs. A. Cox and daughters, C. Michael and Romaine Davie and infant, Patricia Dillon and daughters, Keith and Susan Dole and infant, Terrence and Donna Farley and daughters, Janet Farish, Delores Foster and infant, Mr. and Mrs. Goodkind, Dr. and Sallie Goertz and infant, Jeff and Virginia Graham and infant, Bob and Carol Graviano and infant, Michael and Sylvia Herrick and children, Barbara J. Hager, Imanil family, Mr. and Mrs. Klobe, Violet Lee and family, Mr. McKinley and grandchild, Peter and Janis Omlansky and sons, Gloria Perez and infant, John and Mary Lynn Rather, Mr. and Mrs. Riffle and son, Norma Romano, Mr. and Mrs. Walker, Leslie Watts, Kevin and Debra Williams-Weaver and infant, and Mrs. and Mrs. Wulff.

We are indebted to our typists Shirley Knutzen, Kristi Pritchard, and Margarita Bobak for their willing and tireless efforts. This edition contains new artwork by George Wassilchenko, Oral Roberts University, Tulsa, Oklahoma, whose precise, detailed anatomic drawings have made a substantial contribution to facilitating the study of complex theory. We look forward to a continuing association with this outstanding medical illustrator. Special words of gratitude are extended to Suzi Epstein, Alison Miller, and Mary Gleason at The C.V. Mosby Company, St. Louis, Missouri, for their encouragement, inspiration, and assistance in the preparation and production of this text. We acknowledge the assistance of our families, both concrete and supportive, and we thank each other for the stimulation, support, and mutual respect generated by this collaboration.

Irene M. Bobak
Margaret Duncan Jensen

Contents

UNIT ONE
Introduction to Maternity Care

1 Issues and Trends in maternity nursing, 2
2 Maternity Nursing Today, 8
3 Maternity Nursing Process, 16
4 Maternity Nurse-Client Relationships, 25
5 Legal and Ethical Aspects of Maternity Nursing, 39

UNIT TWO
Basic Concepts of Reproduction

6 Anatomy and Physiology of Reproduction, 50
7 Psychosocial Aspects of Reproduction, 102
8 Cultural Aspects of Maternity Nursing, 114
9 The Family, 128
10 Genetics, 141
11 Fertility, 158
12 Infertility, 163
13 Control of Fertility, 186

UNIT THREE
Prenatal Period

14 From Conception to Birth, 206
15 Anatomic and Physiologic Adaptations to Pregnancy, 221
16 Family Responses to Pregnancy, 252
17 Nursing Care During the Prenatal Period, 267
18 Maternal and Fetal Nutrition, 314
19 Preparation for Parenting, 341

UNIT FOUR
The Birth Period

20 Essential Factors of Labor, 362
21 First Stage of Labor, 394
22 Second Stage of Labor, 418
23 Third and Fourth Stages of Labor, 450
24 Fetal Monitoring, 468
25 Pharmacologic Control of Discomfort During the Birth Period, 500
26 Alternative Settings for Childbirth, 529

UNIT FIVE
Nursing Care of the Normal Newborn

27 Biologic and Behavioral Characteristics of the Newborn, 554
28 Nursing Assessment and Diagnosis of the Newborn, 574
29 Planning, Implementing, and Evaluating Care of the Newborn, 615
30 Newborn Nutrition and Feeding, 650

UNIT SIX
Nursing Care During the Postpartum Period

31 Maternal Physiology and Nursing Care, 686
32 Family Responses to the Birth of a Child and Nursing Care, 707

UNIT SEVEN
High-Risk Mother and Neonate

33 Introduction to the High-Risk Mother and Neonate, 738
34 Loss and Grief, 765
35 Complications of Pregnancy, 779
36 Major Complications Coincident with Pregnancy, 826
37 Complications During Birth, 873
38 Adolescent Parenthood, 937
39 Psychosocial Risk Factors, 950
40 Neonates with Hyperbilirubinemia and Congenital Disorders, 958
41 Other Medical and Surgical Conditions, 982

APPENDIXES, 1003

GLOSSARY, 1048

Detailed Contents

UNIT ONE

Introduction to Maternity Care

1 **Issues and Trends in Maternity Nursing,** 2
- Maternity nursing issues, 3
- Maternity nursing trends, 4
  - Education, 4
  - Practice, 5
  - Role, 6

2 **Maternity Nursing Today,** 8
- Beliefs, 8
- Nature and scope, 9
  - Preventive activities, 9
  - Curative activities, 9
  - Rehabilitative activities, 10
- Maternity client, 10
  - Statistical picture, 11
- Maternity nurse, 12
  - Technician, 12
  - Teacher and counselor, 12
  - Advocate, 12
  - Manager, 12
  - Researcher, 12
  - Expanding roles, 13
    - Obstetric-gynecologic nurse practitioner, 13
    - Nurse-midwife, 13
- Summary, 15

3 **Maternity Nursing Process,** 16
- Assessment, 18
  - Interview, 18
    - Reason for client's request for care, 18
    - Biographic data, 18
    - Medical history, 18
    - Reproductive history, 18
    - Family history, 19
    - Review of biopsychosocial systems, 19
  - Physical examination, 19
    - Observation, 19
    - Palpation, 19
    - Percussion, 20
    - Auscultation, 20
    - Laboratory tests, 20
- Formulating the nursing diagnosis, 20
- Planning, 21
- Implementation, 21
- Evaluation, 22
- Recording data, 22
  - Nursing care plan, 22
    - Flow sheets, 22
    - Discharge summary, 22
  - Problem-oriented record, 22
    - Data base, 23
    - Problem list, 23
    - Initial plan, 23
    - Progress notes, 23
- Summary, 24

4 **Maternity Nurse-Client Relationships,** 25
- Essential factors, 25
  - Communication, 25
    - Techniques, 26
    - Language, 27
    - Space, 27
    - Touch, 28
    - Voice, 28
    - Eye contact, 29
    - Time, 29
  - Self-awareness, 29
    - Concept of social role, 30
    - Self-concept, 30
    - Values clarification, 31
  - Decision-making process, 33
  - Personal characteristics, 34
    - Trust, 34
    - Empathy, 34
    - Setting mutual goals, 35
- Process of nurse-client relationship, 35
  - Preparatory phase, 35
  - Initiation phase, 36
  - Consolidation and growth phase, 36
  - Termination phase, 37
- Summary, 37

5 **Legal and Ethical Aspects of Maternity Nursing,** 39
- General legal concepts, 39
  - Accountability, 39
  - Standards of care, 40
  - Statutory law, 40
  - Common law of torts, 40
  - Reasonably prudent nurse, 40
  - Floating, 40

Negligence, 40
Charting, 41
Informed consent, 41
Maternal rights, 41
Insurance, 41
Nurse-midwives, 42
Legal and ethical concepts for preconceptional clients, 42
Sexual counseling, 42
Sterilization, 42
Genetic counseling, 42
In vitro fertilization and embyro transplantation, 42
Artificial insemination, 43
Prenatal diagnosis, 43
Mass screening, 43
Amniocentesis, 43
Fetal research, 44
Home births, 44
Ethical and legal issues of abortion, 44
Congressional amendment, 45
Court cases, 45
Ethical considerations, 45
Fetal rights, 46
Legal concepts during labor and delivery, 46
Fetal monitors, 46
Anesthetics, 46
Maternal complications, 46
Stillborn infants, 46
Legal issues in the postpartum unit, 47
Summary, 47

UNIT TWO
Basic Concepts of Reproduction

6 **Anatomy and Physiology of Reproduction,** 50
Female reproductive system, 54
External structures, 54
Pelvic floor and perineum, 56
Internal genitalia, 59
Fallopian tubes, 59
Ureters, 62
Uterus, 62
Vagina, 68
Ovaries: female gonads, 68
Abdominal wall, 68
Anatomy of the bony pelvis, 69
Breasts, 71
Anatomy, 72
Physiology, 74
Male reproductive system, 76
Overview of reproductive system structures throughout the life span, 76
External genitalia, 77
Mons pubis, 77
Penis, 77
Scrotum, 78
Internal genitalia, 79
Testes: male gonads, 79
Canal system, 81
Accessory reproductive tract glands, 82
Semen, 82
Menstrual cycle, 83
Menstrual myths, 83
Historical perspective, 83
Hypothalamus and pituitary, 85
Hypothalamic-pituitary cycle, 86
Ovarian cycle, 86
Endometrial cycle, 87
Cervical changes, 88
Puberty, 88
Prostaglandins, 92
Role in reproductive functions, 92
Primary dysmenorrhea, 92
Physiologic response to sexual stimulation, 93
Four-phase response cycle, 93
Excitement phase: women, 93
Excitement phase: men, 93
Plateau phase: women, 93
Plateau phase: men, 93
Orgasmic phase: women, 93
Orgasmic phase: men, 93
Resolution phase: women, 93
Resolution phase: men, 100
Biphasic response, 100
Phase 1: vasocongestive reaction, 100
Phase 2: reflex clonic muscular contractions, 100
Clinical significance, 100
Multiple orgasm, 100
Simultaneous orgasm, 100
Clitoral vs. vaginal orgasm, 100
Variations in orgasmic patterns, 100
Summary, 101

7 **Psychosocial Aspects of Reproduction,** 102
Childhood, 102
Gender identity, 103
Gender preference, 103
Identification with parent of same sex, 103
Sex role standards, 103
Clinical considerations, 104
Adolescence, 105
Early adolescence (ages 12 to 15 years), 107
Middle adolescence (ages 15 to 18 years), 107
Late adolescence (ages 18 to 20 years), 108
Clinical considerations, 108
Adult sexuality, 109
Young adulthood, 109
Middle and late adulthood, 111
Clinical considerations, 112

8 **Cultural Aspects of Maternity Nursing,** 114
Definitions, 115
Reproduction in various cultures, 115
Childhood preparation for parenthood, 116

Prenatal care and expected behaviors of parents and family, 116
Diet, 117
Clothing, 118
Activity and rest, 118
Sexual activity, 118
Emotional response, 119
Labor and delivery, 119
Postpartal care, 120
Maintenance of a state of balance, 120
Pollution state, 121
Parental, familial, and societal reactions to childbearing, 122
The American family, 122
Cultural variations, 122
Fertility and infertility, 124
Family planning and contraception, 124
Implications for nursing, 125

9 The Family, 128

Structure, 129
Nuclear family, 129
Extended family, 131
Expanded family, 132
Communal family, 132
Single-parent family, 132
Family dynamics and functions, 133
Psychosocial development, 133
Cognitive development, 134
Sensorimotor stage (birth to 2 years), 134
Preoperational stage (2 to 7 years), 135
Concrete operations stage (7 to 11 years), 135
Formal operations stage (12 to 18 years), 135
Personality development, 135
Trust vs. mistrust (birth to 1 year), 135
Autonomy vs. shame and doubt (1 to 3 years), 135
Initiative vs. guilt (3 to 6 years), 136
Industry vs. inferiority (6 to 12 years), 136
Identity vs. identity confusion (12 to 18 years), 136
Intimacy vs. isolation (early adulthood), 136
Generativity vs. self-absorption (young and middle adulthood), 136
Ego integrity vs. despair (old age), 136
Family and crisis, 136
Perception of an event, 137
Coping mechanisms, 138
Support systems, 138
Summary, 138

10 Genetics, 141

Biologic basis of inheritance, 141
Chromosomes, 141
Cell division, 143
Gametogenesis, 144
Genes in families, 145
Disorders caused by a single gene, 145
Autosomal-dominant inheritance, 146
Autosomal-recessive inheritance, 146
X-linked inheritance, 146
Chromosomal aberrations, 147
Disorders of cell division, 148
Nondisjunction, 148
Translocation, 148
Disorders caused by chromosomal aberrations, 149
Autosomal aberrations, 149
Aberrations of sex chromosomes, 149
Multifactorial inheritance, 150
Detection of genetic disease, 152
Preconceptional detection, 152
Prenatal detection, 152
Amniocentesis, 152
Ultrasonography, 152
Roentgenography, 152
Fetoscopy (amnioscopy), 153
Postdelivery detection, 153
Biochemical tests, 153
Cytologic studies, 154
Dermatoglyphics, 154
Other postdelivery diagnostic studies, 154
Genetic counseling, 155
Clients, 155
Goals of counseling, 155
Counseling process, 155
Counseling services, 155
Role of the nurse, 155

11 Fertility, 158

Factors essential to normal fertility, 158
Profile of a fertile woman: assessment data, 159
History of menstrual cycle, 159
Physical examination, 159
Laboratory tests, 160
Profile of a fertile man: assessment data, 161
Other factors contributing to fertility, 161
Age, 161
Length of exposure, 161
Intercourse, 161
Health promotion, 161

12 Infertility, 163

Investigation of infertility, 163
Religious factors leading to infertility problems, 164
Use of marijuana (a cannabinoid), 164
General nursing care, 164
Investigation of female infertility, 165
Factors implicated in female infertility, 165
Identification of infertility factors, 166
Fertility tests and examinations, 166
Therapy for female infertility, 177
Congenital or developmental factors, 177
Ovulation, 177
Tubal (peritoneal) factors, 178
Endometriosis, 178
Uterine factors, 179
Vaginal-cervical factors, 179

In vitro fertilization, 180
Investigation of male infertility, 181
Factors implicated in male infertility, 181
Identification of infertility factors, 182
Therapy for male infertility, 182
Artificial insemination, 182
The emotional crisis of infertility: implications for nursing action, 183
Summary of nursing actions, 184

13 **Control of Fertility,** 186
Methods of control of fertility, 187
Natural family planning (biologic periodic abstinence), 188
Rhythm or calendar method, 188
Basal body temperature, 189
Cervical mucus method, 190
Sympto-thermal method, 190
Fertility awareness method, 192
Oral hormonal therapy, 192
Mode of action, 192
Combined oral hormone therapy, 192
Injectable medication, 195
Intrauterine device, 196
Procedure for insertion of the IUD: client preparation, 197
Diaphragm with spermicide, 198
Procedure for insertion and follow-up, 198
Cervical cap, 199
The 48-hr contraceptive, 199
Vaginal spermicides, 199
Male contraception, 199
Condom, 199
Other methods of male contraception, 200
Nursing actions, 201
Evaluative criteria, 201
Assessment, 202
Planning and implementation, 202
Evaluation, 202

UNIT THREE
Prenatal Period

14 **From Conception to Birth,** 206
Conception, 206
Developmental stages, 207
Ovum, 207
Embryo, 207
Fetus, 208
Gestational time units, 208
Implantation (nidation), 210
The decidua, 211
Placentation, 212
Fetal membranes, 212
Umbilical cord, 212
Placenta, 213
Placental physiology, 213
Placental transfer, 215
Placental variations, 215
Amniotic fluid, 215
Embryonic development and fetal maturation, 216
Cardiovascular system, 216
Hematopoietic system, 217
Respiratory system, 217
Renal system, 217
Neurologic system, 218
Fetal neuromuscular behavior, 218
Gastrointestinal system, 218
Metabolism, 218
Meconium, 219
Hepatic system, 219
Endocrine system, 219
Reproductive system, 219
Female genital development and function, 219
Male genital development and function, 219
Immune system, 220
Viability, 220

15 **Anatomic and Physiologic Adaptations to Pregnancy,** 221
Female reproductive system: external structures, 222
Female reproductive system: internal genitalia, 223
Ovaries and fallopian tubes, 223
Uterus, 223
Enlargement, 223
Arrangement of muscle fibers, 224
Shape and consistency, 224
Position, 224
Contractility, 225
Auscultation of intrauterine sounds, 225
Uterine blood flow, 225
Isthmus, 225
Posture, 225
Implications for nursing actions, 225
Cervix, 226
Vagina and vulva, 227
Implications for nursing actions, 227
Breasts, 228
Implications for nursing actions, 228
Cardiovascular system, 228
Anatomic changes: cardiac size and position, 229
Auscultatory changes, 229
Changes in hemodynamics, 230
Hematologic changes: changes in blood constituents, 232
Vascular headache, 232
Implications for nursing actions, 232
Respiratory system, 233
Anatomic changes, 233
Pulmonary function, 234
Basal metabolism rate, 234
Acid-base balance, 234
Implications for nursing actions, 234
Kidneys and renal function: an overview, 235
Urinary system, 235
Anatomic changes, 235

Renal pelves and ureters, 235
Implications for nursing actions, 235
Bladder and urethra, 235
Renal function changes, 236
Renal plasma flow, 236
Glomerular filtration rate, 236
Fluid and electrolyte balance, 236
Implications for nursing actions, 237
Nutrient, including glucose, excretion, 237
Proteinuria, 237
Skin changes, 238
Pigmentation, 238
Striae gravidarum, 238
Vascular abnormalities: spider angiomas, palmar erythema, and epulis, 238
Oily skin and acne, 239
Hirsutism, 239
Fingernail changes, 239
Implications for nursing actions, 239
Changes in the musculoskeletal system, 239
Implications for nursing actions, 239
Neurologic changes, 240
Implications for nursing actions, 240
Gastrointestinal changes, 240
Mouth, 240
Teeth, 240
Appetite, 241
Esophagus and stomach, 241
Small intestine, 241
Colon, 241
Gallbladder, 241
Liver, 241
Abdominal pain, 242
Implications for nursing actions, 242
Endrocrine changes, 242
Pituitary gland, 242
Fetoplacental hormone production, 245
Ovary, 246
Thyroid gland, 246
Parathyroid glands, 246
Adrenal glands, 247
Pancreas, 247

16 **Family Responses to Pregnancy,** 252
Mother-to-be, 252
Maternal tasks, 253
First trimester, 253
Second trimester, 254
Third trimester, 254
Body image, 255
Ambivalence about pregnancy, 256
Stress and anxiety, 256
Behavior, 256
Dependence vs. independence, 256
Sexual concerns, 257
Adult responsibilities, 257
Birth process, 257
The child, 258
Father-to-be, 258
Couvade, 258
Paternal tasks, 258
First trimester, 259
Second trimester, 260
Third trimester, 261
Siblings, 263
Grandparents, 265
Summary, 265

17 **Nursing Care During the Prenatal Period,** 267
Definitions, 268
Assessment, 269
Diagnosis of pregnancy, 269
Presumptive signs and symptoms, 269
Probable signs and symptoms, 274
Positive signs, 275
Laboratory tests, 277
Duration of pregnancy and estimated date of confinement, 277
Fetal gestational age and health status, 281
Ultrasonography, 281
Amniocentesis, 281
Maternal urinary or plasma estriol level, 282
Fetal heart rate, 282
Fetal movement, 283
Radiography, 283
Amnioscopy, 283
Maternal and family need for psychosocial care, 283
Nursing role, 283
Assessment: gravidas, 284
Assessment: family, 284
Prenatal examination procedures, 285
Clean-catch urine specimen, 285
Pelvic examination, 285
Papanicolaou smear, 285
Gonorrheal culture, 287
Herpes simplex, types 1 and 2, culture, 287
Vaginal discharges, 287
Maternal urinary estriol determinations, 287
Amniocentesis, 287
Nursing diagnoses in the prenatal period, 291
Planning, 291
Initial contact with woman and family, 291
Protocol for care, 291
Collection of specimens, 291
First prenatal visit, 292
Protocol for care: comprehensive examination, 292
Subsequent visits, 296
Implementation, 297
Goals, 297
Nursing actions, 298
Instruction regarding danger signals, 298
Childbirth and parenthood education, 299
Nutritional counseling, 299
Frequent questions, 299
Discomforts of pregnancy, 301
Sexual counseling during pregnancy, 302

Symptomatology of impending labor, 309
Evaluation, 310

18 Maternal and Fetal Nutrition, 314
Physiologic adjustments and the basis for nutrition needs in pregnancy, 315
Tissue growth, 315
The placenta, 315
Blood volume and constituents, 315
Functional alterations, 316
Alimentary canal, 316
Respiratory system, 316
Renal function, 316
Hormonal effects, 316
Weight gain during pregnancy, 316
Deviations in weight and weight gain, 316
Nutrient needs, 320
Energy, 320
Tissue deposition, 320
Metabolic needs, 320
Activity, 320
Protein, 320
Major minerals, 321
Iron, 321
Calcium, 321
Sodium, 322
Fat-soluble vitamins, 322
Vitamin A, 322
Vitamin D, 322
Vitamin E, 322
Water-soluble vitamins, 322
Folic acid, 322
Pyridoxine (vitamin B_6), 322
Thiamin (vitamin B_1), 322
Riboflavin (vitamin B_2), 323
Cobalamin (vitamin B_{12}), 323
Ascorbic acid (vitamin C), 323
Trace minerals, 323
Zinc, 323
Flourine, 323
Nutritional supplements: their role in pregnancy, 323
Nutrition risk factors in pregnancy, 325
Risk factors at the onset of pregnancy, 325
Adolescence, 325
Frequent pregnancies, 325
Poor reproductive history, 325
Economic deprivation, 325
Bizarre food patterns, 326
Vegetarian diets, 326
Smoking, drug addition, and alcoholism, 326
Chronic systemic diseases, 326
Prepregnant weight, 326
Risk factors in pregnancy, 326
Anemia of pregnancy, 326
Pregancy-induced hypertension, 326
Inadequate weight gain, 326
Excessive weight gain, 326
Demands of lactation, 327
Guidelines for management, 327
Nutrition assessment, 327
History, 327
Physical examination, 327
Biochemical tests, 327
Dietary assessment, 329
Nutrition counseling, 331
Referral for additional services, 336
Summary of nursing care: maternal and fetal nutrition, 336
Goals for care, 336
Assessment and analysis, 338
Examples of nursing diagnoses, 338
Plan and implementation, 338
Evaluation, 340

19 Preparation for Parenting, 341
Parent education, 341
Early pregnancy classes, 341
Midpregnancy classes, 342
Late pregnancy classes, 342
After-birth classes, 342
Childbirth preparation, 344
Historical overview, 344
Effectiveness of methods, 346
Psychophysical components, 346
Psychologic components, 346
Intellectual components, 346
Methods of childbirth preparation, 346
Dick-Read method: childbirth without fear, 347
Lamaze (PPM) method, 347
Bradley method, 348
Breathing techniques, 348
Cervical dilatation to 3 cm, 348
Cervical dilatation of 4 to 7 cm, 348
Cervical dilatation of 8 to 10 cm, 348
Explusion breathing, 349
Childbirth exercises, 350
Exercises for the pelvic floor (Kegel exercise), 350
Pain in childbirth, 352
Causes of pain in labor, 352
Reactions to pain, 352
Nursing actions, 353
Preparation for becoming a grandparent, 355
Assessment and planning, 356
Intervention, 356
Evaluation, 357
Conclusion, 357
Organizations involved in parent education, 357

UNIT FOUR
The Birth Period

20 Essential Factors of Labor, 362
Essential factors in labor: basis for assessment, 362
The passenger, 363
Fetal head, 363

Shoulders and pelvic girdle, 366
Fetal lie, 366
Presentation, 367
Attitude, 367
Position, 369
The passageway, 369
Pelvis, 370
Soft tissues, 379
The powers, 379
Uterine contractions, 380
Voluntary bearing-down efforts, 382
Implications for nursing care, 382
The placenta, 382
Psychologic response, 382
Techniques for assessment, 382
Abdominal palpation, 382
Auscultation, 384
Vaginal examination, 384
Effacement of the cervix, 385
Dilatation of the cervix, 385
Station, 386
Conventional x-ray films, 386
Computed tomography, 386
Ultrasonography, 388
Process of labor, 388
Changes preliminary to onset of labor (prodromal labor), 388
Onset of labor, 388
Mechanism of labor, 388
Phases of the mechanism of labor in vertex presentation, 388
Persistent occiput posterior or occiput transverse position, 392
Duration of labor, 392
First stage of labor, 392
Second stage of labor, 392
Third stage of labor, 392
Fourth stage of labor, 392

21 First Stage of Labor, 394

Assessment: review of client's history, 395
Initial assessment, 395
Is she in labor? 395
How far has she progressed? 395
Have the membranes ruptured? 397
Are there complications that may require treatment? 397
What is her psychologic response to the beginning of labor? 397
Progress in labor, 398
Cervical dilatation and descent, 398
Uterine contractions, 398
Characteristics, 398
Assessing uterine contractions, 398
Rupture of membranes and amniotic fluid, 401
Tests for rupture of membranes, 401
Assessment of amniotic fluid, 401
Complications, 402
Stress in labor, 402
Fetal stress, 402
Monitoring techniques, 402
Maternal stress, 403
Paternal stress, 403
Nursing diagnoses, 404
Planning, 404
Implementation, 404
Procedures, 404
Preparation of the vulva: the "mini-prep," 405
Enema, 405
Intravenous therapy, 405
Assisting the physician with vaginal examinations, 406
Emergency procedures, 407
Prolapsed cord, 407
Fetal distress or abnormal FHR pattern, 407
Uterine contractions, 407
Motherhood with dignity, 409
Admission to the labor unit, 409
Intake and output, 410
Maternal position during labor, 411
Comfort measures, 411
General hygiene, 414
Atmosphere of the labor and delivery area, 414
Touch, 414
Pain and its relief, 414
Fatherhood with dignity, 414
Birth process as seen through father's eyes, 415
Father in labor suite, 415
Supporting the father during labor, 416
Preparation for delivery, 416
Evaluation, 417

22 Second Stage of Labor, 418

Mechanism of delivery, 419
Delivery of head, 419
Delivery of shoulders, 420
Delivery of body and extremities, 420
Nursing care of mother and fetus, 421
Goals, 421
Assessment, 421
Examples of nursing diagnoses, 421
Plan, 421
Implementation, 421
Maternal position, 421
Bearing-down efforts, 421
Amnesia, 425
Fetal heart rate, 425
Coach, 425
Care for delivery, 425
Nursing care of the newborn, 439
Goals, 439
Assessment, 439
Examples of nursing diagnoses, 439
Plan and implementation, 440
Parent-child relationships, 446

Emergency childbirth: when the nurse assists the mother to give birth, 447
Emergency birth of fetus in vertex presentation, 447
Unusual occurrences during and after birth, 448
Lateral Sims' position for delivery, 448
Shoulder dystocia, 448
Prebirth passage of meconium with fetus in vertex presentation, 448
Tight nuchal cord, 449
Maternal postdelivery hemorrhage, 449
Emergency birth of fetus in breech presentation, 449
Birth and management of preterm infant, 449

23 Third and Fourth Stages of Labor, 450
Third stage, 450
Separation and delivery of placenta, 450
Assessment for placental separation, 450
Immediate care of mother, 451
General assessment of mother, 451
Assessment of the birth canal, 452
Factors associated with uterine atony, 452
Pharmacologic stimulation of uterine contractions after delivery of placenta, 452
Nursing diagnoses, 453
Plan and implementation, 453
Fourth stage, 453
Maternal recovery, 453
Goals of care, 453
Assessment, 454
Nursing diagnoses, 454
Plan and implementation, 454
Neonatal adjustment to extrauterine existence, 462
Evaluative criteria for care during four stages of labor, 464

24 Fetal Monitoring, 468
History, 468
Objectives, 470
Physiologic basis of monitoring, 470
Uteroplacental and fetal circulation, 470
Factors affecting circulation, 470
Fetal heart rate regulation, 471
Instrumentation for monitoring, 471
External mode of monitoring, 471
Fetal heart rate, 471
Uterine activity: tocotransducer, 475
Internal mode of monitoring, 476
Fetal heart rate: spiral electrode, 476
Uterine activity: intrauterine catheter, 478
Pattern recognition, 479
Display of fetal heart rate and uterine activity on chart paper, 480
Base-line fetal heart rate, 480
Tachycardia and bradycardia, 480
Variability, 480
Periodic changes, 485
Prolonged decelerations, 485
Uterine activity monitoring, 485
Increased uterine activity, 490
Fetal distress, 491
Fetal blood sampling, 491
Nursing care, 491
Prepared childbirth, 492
Monitor care, 493
Charting, 493
Legal aspects, 493
Antepartum testing, 496
Nonstress testing/fetal activity determination, 496
Oxytocin challenge test, 496
Daily fetal movement count, 498

25 Pharmacologic Control of Discomfort During the Birth Period, 500
Introduction, 500
Goals of care, 500
Informed consent, 501
Choices of pharmacologic control of discomfort during birth period, 501
Origin of discomfort during labor, 501
Definitions, 501
Intravenous and intramuscular routes of administration of medications, 504
Intravenous route, 504
Intramuscular route, 504
General nursing care, 504
Pharmacologic analgesia and anesthesia, 508
Combination anesthesia for cesarean birth, 524
Intraspinal narcotic method, 524
Nonpharmacologic, noninvasive relief of discomfort, 528
Transcutaneous electrical nerve stimulation (TENS), 528

26 Alternative Settings for Childbirth, 529
Historical perspective, 529
Impetus of consumerism, 531
Family-centered care, 531
Birth choices, 532
Birthing rooms, 532
Alternative birth centers, 534
High-risk factors excluding admission to the alternative birth center, 536
High-risk factors developing after admission requiring transfer to labor and delivery, 538
Freestanding birth centers, 538
Nurse-midwifery, 541
Cesarean birth, 541
Home birth, 542
Advantages, 543
Disadvantages, 543
Contraindications, 548
Family's preparation for home birth, 548
Choice and the nurse, 549

UNIT FIVE
Nursing Care of the Normal Newborn

27 Biologic and Behavioral Characteristics of the Newborn, 554

Biologic characteristics, 555
Cardiovascular system, 555
Hematopoietic system, 558
Respiratory system, 558
Renal system and water balance, 559
Digestive system, 560
Hepatic system, 561
Physiologic hyperbilirubinemia, 561
Breast milk jaundice, 562
Immunity, 562
IgG, 562
IgM, 562
IgA, 562
Neurologic system, 563
Integumentary system, 563
Thermogenesis, 566
Heat production, 566
Heat loss, 566
Temperature regulation, 566
Cold stress, 566
Reproductive system, 567
Behavioral characteristics, 567
Sensory behaviors, 567
Vision, 568
Hearing, 568
Touch, 568
Taste, 568
Smell, 568
Sleeping and waking behaviors, 569
Sleep-wake cycles, 570
Social behaviors, 571
Feeding behaviors, 571
Elimination behaviors, 572

28 Nursing Assessment and Diagnosis of the Newborn, 574

Facilities and personnel, 574
Assessment, 576
Physical assessment, 576
Neurologic assessment, 594
Behavioral assessment, 602
Brazelton Neonatal Behavioral Assessment Scale, 602
Factors influencing behavior of the newborn, 610
Assessment strategies and tools for normal newborn: first day (2 to 24 hours), 610
Respirations, 610
Temperature, 611
Cardiovascular system, 611
Integumentary system, 611
Cord and circumcised penis, 612
Defecation, 612
Urination, 612
Physical assessment, 613
Neurologic assessment, 613
Behavioral assessment, 613
Newborn nutrition, 613
Parenthood, 613
Summary of assessment strategies and tools for normal newborn: days 2 to 14, 613
Summary of assessment strategies and tools for normal newborn: days 15 to 28 (first well-baby visit), 613
Nursing diagnoses, 614
Planning, 614

29 Planning, Implementing, and Evaluating Care of the Newborn, 615

Plan and implementation, 616
General care of the neonate, 616
Maintenance of respirations and adequate oxygen supply, 616
Maintenance of neonate's temperature, 616
Positioning and holding the infant, 619
Cleansing infant, 620
Umbilical cord care, 621
Diaper rash, 621
Clothing the infant, 621
Care of infant's linens, 624
Circumcision, 625
Historic perspective, 625
Current views, 625
Parental decision, 627
The procedure, 627
Care of the newly circumcised penis, 628
Care of the uncircumcised penis, 628
Anticipatory guidance of parents: before discharge from hospital, 628
Anticipatory guidance of parents: at first well-baby visit, 630
Procedures, 630
Monitoring and recording of infant responses, 630
Heat support: controlling the environment, 630
Overhead radiant heater, 630
Servo-Control incubator, 631
Warming the hypothermic infant, 632
Suctioning the newborn, 632
Upper airway aspiration: mouth and nose, 632
Midairway (nasopharynx, oropharynx) and stomach aspiration, 632
Mouth-to-mouth resuscitation, 633
Cardiopulmonary resuscitation, 635
Positioning the newborn, 636
Oxygen therapy, 636
Hypoxemia, 636
Regulating oxygen dosage, 636
Methods of oxygen administration, 637
Heel stick, 637
Intramuscular injection, 637
Therapy for hyperbilirubinemia, 641

Phototherapy, 641
Restraining neonate, 643
Mummy, 643
Extremity restraints, 645
Towel support, 645
Restraint without appliance, 645
Assisting with collection of blood specimen: venipuncture, 645
Using urine specimen collectors, 645
Birth certificate, 646
Evaluative criteria for nursing actions, 647
Normal newborn: first day of life, 647
Days 2 to 14, 647
Days 15 to 28, 648

30 **Newborn Nutrition and Feeding,** 650
Infant development and its relationship to feeding, 651
Physical growth, 651
Physiologic development, 651
Neuromuscular development, 651
Psychosocial development, 652
Nutrient needs of infants, 652
Calories, 654
Protein and amino acids, 654
Fats, 654
Carbohydrates, 655
Water, 655
Vitamins, 656
Minerals, 656
Breast feeding, 657
Maternal nutritional needs, 660
Impact of maternal diet on milk composition, 660
Composition of human milk, 660
Counseling the breast-feeding mother, 662
Preparation, 662
The technique, 663
Duration of breast feeding, 666
Care of breasts, 667
Common problems and how to avoid them, 667
Engorged breasts, 667
Sore nipples, 667
Plugged ducts, 668
Infection, 668
Leaking, 668
Failure to thrive in the breast-feeding infant, 668
Relactation and induced lactation, 669
Breast pumping, 671
Formula feeding, 671
Types of commercial formulas, 671
Evaporated milk formulas, 671
Goat's milk, 671
Soy formulas, 671
Special formulas, 672
Preparation of commercial formulas, 672
Skim milk, 672
Bottle-feeding techniques, 672
Common problems, 673
Introduction of solids, 673
Selected problems, 675
Overweight and obesity, 675
Atherosclerosis, 676
Hypertension, 676
General guidelines for feeding the normal infant, 676
Initial oral feeding, 676
First 6 months, 677
After 6 months, 677
Nutritional screening and assessment of infants, 677
Children at nutritional risk, 679
Nutritional intervention in clinical practice, 681

UNIT SIX
Nursing Care During the Postpartum Period

31 **Maternal Physiology and Nursing Care,** 686
Physiologic changes, 686
Vascular system, 686
Reproductive system, 687
Urinary system, 688
Vital signs, 689
Endocrine system, 689
Gastrointestinal system, 689
Abdominal musculature, 689
Postpartum care, 689
Assessment, 690
Initial assessment, 690
Subsequent assessment, 692
Child care activities and response to birth of child, 695
Examples of nursing diagnoses, 695
Planning, 695
Implementation, 695
Goals, 695
Nursing actions, 695
Evaluation, 705

32 **Family Responses to the Birth of a Child and Nursing Care,** 707
Part 1: Family responses, 707
Parenthood, 707
Components, 707
Parent-child attachment, 708
Contact and attachment, 710
Process of assuming parental role: reality phase, 711
Parental tasks, 713
Stages of development of parental role, 713
Siblings, 718
Grandparents, 719
Factors influencing parental responses, 719
Physical condition of mother, 719
Physical condition of infant, 720
Parental expectations, 720
Parental age, 720

Social and economic conditions, 722
Interference with personal aspirations, 722
Sensory impairment, 722
Part 2: Nursing care, 723
Assessment of parental responses, 723
Assessment strategies, 724
Assessment tools, 725
Examples of nursing diagnoses, 729
Planning and implementation, 730
Evaluation, 733

UNIT SEVEN
High-Risk Mother and Neonate

33 **Introduction to the High-Risk Mother and Neonate,** 738
Definition and scope of the problem, 738
Risk factors, 739
Maternal factors, 740
Paternal factors, 740
Fetal factors, 740
Neonatal factors, 740
Goals for care, 743
Regionalization of health care services, 745
Maternal health problems, 745
Statistical profile, 745
Fetal and neonatal health problems, 746
Statistical profile, 746
Fetal death, 746
Neonatal death, 746
Perinatal death rate, 746
Infant mortality, 746
General care of the infant at risk, 747
Nursing the neonate with respiratory distress, 747
Goals of care, 747
Assessment and analysis, 747
Example of nursing diagnosis, 747
Plan and implementation, 747
Evaluation, 749
Oxygen therapy, 749
Temperature support and regulation, 750
Goals of care, 750
Assessment and analysis, 750
Example of nursing diagnosis, 751
Plan and implementation, 751
Evaluation, 751
Nutrition and elimination, 751
General considerations, 751
Nutritional requisites, 752
Weight and fluid loss, 752
Formula and feeding schedules, 753
Goals of care, 753
Assessment and analysis, 754
Examples of nursing diagnoses, 754
Plan and implementation, 754
Evaluation, 754
Nasogastric tube feeding, 754
Monitoring parenteral fluid administration, 757
Total parenteral nutrition, 759
Emotional aspects of care, 761
Neonate's emotional needs, 761
Supportive care, 761
Postmortem care: stillbirth, 762
Definition of fetal death, 762
Parents and family, 762
Care of the child, 763
Legal requirements for filing certificate of death (California), 763

34 **Loss and Grief,** 765
The grieving process, 765
Shock and disbelief, 766
Developing awareness and acute mourning, 766
Resolution or acceptance, 766
Pathologic mourning, 766
Loss, grief, and maternity nursing, 766
General goals of care, 766
Assessment, 766
Examples of nursing diagnoses, 766
Plan and implementation, 767
Evaluation, 767
Psychosocial role of nurse in care of parents after birth of child with disorder, 767
Mourning loss of perfect child, 767
Early mother-child relationship, 767
Continuing parent-child relationship, 767
Families' grief reactions, 768
Immediate diagnosis and management of child, 768
Clinical evaluation and diagnosis of causes, 768
Long-term management of child, 768
Redefinition of parental role and social network, 769
Premature labor and delivery: psychologic aspects, 769
Reactions to premature delivery, 769
Giving birth too early, 770
Mother-child relationship, 770
Goals of care, 770
Spontaneous abortion and ectopic pregnancy: psychologic aspects, 773
Fetal death: psychologic aspects, 774
Intranatal fetal death: psychologic aspects, 776
The nurse, 776
The parents, 776
Response of family members, 778
Sibling reaction to birth of a high-risk infant, 778
Grandparents of high-risk infant, 778

35 **Complications of Pregnancy,** 779
Hemorrhagic disorders, 780
Early pregnancy, 780
Spontaneous abortion, 780
Recurrent abortion, 780
Etiology, 780
Management, 780
Incompetent cervix, 781
Other categories of spontaneous abortion, 781

Clinical classification, 781
Clinical findings, 781
Diagnosis, 782
Prevention, 782
Management, 783
Prognosis, 783
Summary of nursing actions, 783
Ectopic pregnancy, 784
Etiology, 785
Clinical classification, 785
Clinical findings, 785
Diagnosis, 785
Prevention, 786
Management, 786
Prognosis, 787
Summary of nursing actions, 787
Hydatidiform mole, 787
Etiology, 787
Clinical classification, 787
Clinical findings and diagnosis, 787
Prevention, 788
Management, 788
Prognosis, 789
Summary of nursing actions, 789
Late pregnancy, 789
Premature separation of placenta, 789
Incidence, 789
Etiology, 789
Clinical manifestations and differential diagnosis, 789
Complications, 790
Therapy, 792
Prognosis, 792
Summary of nursing actions, 792
Placenta previa, 792
Etiology, 792
Pathology, 792
Clinical manifestations and differential diagnosis, 793
Clinical classification, 793
Prevention, 793
Management, 793
Prognosis, 796
Summary of nursing actions, 796
Clotting disorders in pregnancy, 796
Normal clotting, 796
Clotting problems, 797
Summary of nursing actions, 799
Idiopathic thrombocytopenic purpura, 800
Hemophilia, 800
Management of hemorrhagic shock, 800
Physiologic mechanisms, 800
Assessment and interventions, 801
Hazards of therapy, 802
Postdelivery hemorrhage, 802
Etiology, 802
Clinical findings and differential diagnosis, 803
Specific problems, 803
Uterine atony, 803
Lacerations of the birth canal, 803
Retained placenta, 805
Inversion of uterus, 806
Subinvolution of uterus, 807
Postdelivery anterior pituitary necrosis, 807
Neonatal hematologic conditions, 807
Hematologic status: anemia and polycythemia, 807
Anemia, 807
Polycythemia, 807
Summary of nursing actions, 807
Neonatal hypovolemic shock, 808
Summary of nursing actions, 809
Hypertensive states in pregnancy, 809
Pregnancy-induced hypertension, 809
Incidence, 809
Maternal and fetal morbidity and mortality, 810
Definitions, 810
Preeclampsia, 811
Eclampsia, 811
Etiology, 811
Pathologic findings, 812
Medical diagnosis, 812
Maternal prognosis, 813
Fetal prognosis, 813
Management, 813
Mild preeclampsia, 813
Moderate to severe preeclampsia, 814
Hypertensive cardiovascular disease, 823
Differential diagnosis, 824
Prognosis, 824
Medical and nursing management, 824

36 Major Complications Coincident with Pregnancy, 826
Infection, 827
Prenatal infection, 827
Suggested symptomatic management for woman with genital herpes, 827
Assessment for syphilis, 827
Postnatal infection, 832
Puerperal infection, 832
Mastitis, 833
Urinary tract infections, 833
Vaginal infections, 833
Trichomonas vaginitis, 834
Monilial vaginitis, 834
Simple vaginitis, 834
Vaginal douche procedure, 835
Bacteremic shock, 835
Summary of nursing actions: infections, 836
Goals of care, 836
Evaluation, 837
Neonatal sepsis, 837
Clinical findings, 837
Incidence, 837
Prognosis, 837
Sequelae, 837
Modes of transmission, 837

General nursing care, 837
Rubella, 838
Herpesvirus type 2 infection, 838
Prognosis, 839
Gonorrhea, 839
Prognosis, 839
Syphilis, 839
Clinical findings, 839
Diagnosis, 840
Medical management, 840
Prognosis and sequelae, 841
Chlamydial disease, 841
Cytomegalovirus infection, 841
Acquired immune deficiency syndrome (AIDS), 841
Oral thrush, 842
Summary of nursing actions: neonatal infection, 842
Goals of care, 842
Examples of nursing diagnosis, 844
Evaluation, 844
Endocrine and metabolic disorders, 844
Diabetes mellitus, 844
Definitions, 844
Significance, 844
Incidence, 844
Pathogenesis, 844
Classification, 845
Normal pregnancy: maternal metabolic adaptations, 845
Gestational diabetes mellitus (type I, class A), 845
Insulin-dependent diabetes mellitus (type II and all other classes), 846
Effects of diabetes on pregnancy, 846
Prognosis, 847
Goals of management, 848
Management, 848
Summary of nursing actions: the diabetic mother, 853
Effects of diabetes on the embryo-fetus-neonate, 853
Neonatal hypoglycemia, 863
Neonatal hypocalcemia, 863
Definition, 863
Clinical manifestations, 864
Infants at risk, 864
Summary of nursing actions: neonatal hypocalcemia, 864
Hyperemesis gravidarum, 865
Definition, 865
Clincial manifestations, 866
Summary of nursing actions: hyperemesis gravidarum, 866
Goals of care, 866
Evaluation, 866
Hyperthyroidism, 866
Heart disease, 867
Effects of pregnancy on heart disease, 867
Effects of heart disease on pregnancy, 867
Symptoms, 867
Diagnosis, 867
Classification, 868
Medical management, 868
Class I, 868
Class II, 868
Class III, 868
Class IV, 868
Nursing actions, 868
Prenatal care, 869
Natal care, 869
Postdelivery care, 870
Evaluation, 871

37 Complications During Birth, 873
Dystocia, 874
Definition and classification, 874
Pelvic dystocia, 874
Inlet contracture, 875
Midpelvic contracture, 875
Outlet contracture, 875
Soft tissue dystocia, 875
Dystocia of fetal origin, 875
Fetopelvic disproportion, 876
Uterine dystocia, 879
Primary uterine inertia, 879
Secondary uterine inertia, 882
Complications of uterine dysfunction, 882
Nursing care of dystocia, 884
Assessment, 884
Examples of nursing diagnoses, 884
Plan and implementation, 884
Evaluation, 886
Therapies for dystocia, 886
Trial of labor, 886
Stimulation of labor, 886
Obstetric operations, 890
Episiotomy, 890
Forceps delivery, 890
Vacuum extraction, 892
Cesarean delivery, 893
Goal, 893
Maternal indications, 893
Fetal indications, 893
Types of cesarean procedures, 893
Postmortem cesarean delivery, 895
Prognosis after cesarean delivery, 895
Nursing care, 895
Target population, 895
Prenatal period: preparation for cesarean birth, 896
Natal period: care in hospital, 899
Infant birth trauma, 905
Classification or birth traumas, 906
Goals for care, 906
Soft tissue injuries, 906
Skeletal injuries, 906
Nervous system injuries, 907

Preterm birth, 909
Prognosis for infants, 909
Obstetric management of premature labor, 910
Prevention, 910
Suppression of uterine activity (labor), 910
Outpatient management, 910
In-hospital suppression of preterm labor, 910
Pharmacologic stimulation of fetal lung maturity, 912
Care during irreversible or acceptable preterm labor and delivery, 912
Postpartum care, 912
Care of preterm infants, 912
Definitions, 912
Physiologic basis for problems, 915
Nursing care, 915
Admission to nursery, 915
Classifications, 915
Environmental support, 915
Transfer from community (hospital or home) to regional neonatal care center, 915
Examination for gestational age, 918
Nursing actions, 922
Complications of prematurity, 925
Respiratory distress syndrome, 925
Prematurity and oxygen toxicity, 926
Neonatal necrotizing enterocolitis, 927
Prognosis for preterm infants, 927
Base-line examination, 927
Favorable evaluative criteria, 928
Psychologic aspects of preterm labor and delivery of a preterm infant, 928
Child abuse and neglect, 928
Baptism, 929
Evaluation, 929
Multiple pregnancy, 930
Maternal problems, 932
Fetal problems, 933
Diagnosis, 933
Management, 933
Prenatal care, 933
Natal care, 933
Puerperal care, 934

38 Adolescent Parenthood, 937
Adolescent mother, 937
Trends, 937
Factors, 937
Pregnancy at risk, 937
Dynamics, 938
Adolescent developmental tasks, 939
Developmental tasks of pregnancy, 940
Developmental tasks of parenthood, 942
Nursing care, 943
Adolescent clinics, 943
Characteristics of personnel, 943
Prenatal period, 943
Labor period, 945
Postdelivery period, 945
Adolescent father, 947
Trends, 947
Factors, 947
Nursing care, 947

39 Psychosocial Risk Factors, 950
Childbearing psychosis, 950
Manic-depressive psychosis, 950
Schizophrenia, 951
Drug dependence, 951
Fetal alcohol syndrome, 952
Narcotic drug dependence, 953
Poverty, 956
Reproductive experience, 956
Complications, 956
Prenatal care, 956

40 Neonates with Hyperbilirubinemia and Congenital Disorders, 958
Hyperbilirubinemia, 958
Definitions, 958
Kernicterus, 959
Pathosis, 959
Symptomatology, 960
Summary of nursing actions: hyperbilirubinemia, 960
Goals of care, 960
Example of nursing diagnosis, 960
Evaluation, 960
Isoimmune hemolytic disease of the newborn (erythroblastosis fetalis, Rh or ABO incompatibility), 960
RBC antigenicity, 960
Rh incompatibility, 960
Therapy for hyperbilirubinemia, 964
Exchange transfusion, 964
Intrauterine fetal transfusion, 966
Umbilical catheterization, 966
Congenital anomalies, 966
Assessment of perinatal signs and factors, 967
Amount of amniotic fluid, 967
Respiratory tract, 967
Neurologic system, 967
Cardiovascular system, 967
Gastrointestinal tract, 970
Urogenital tract, 970
General preoperative and postoperative care, 970
Most common surgical emergencies, 971
Diaphragmatic hernia, 971
Tracheoesophageal anomalies, 971
Omphalocele, 972
Intestinal obstruction, 973
Imperforate anus, 974
Common malformations, 975
Meningomyelocele, 975
Congenital hydrocephalus, 975
Anencephaly and microcephaly, 976
Cleft-lip or palate, 976
Musculoskeletal problems, 977

Genitourinary tract anomalies, 978
Teratoma, 980
Disorders not apparent at birth, 980
Diethylstilbestrol, 981

41 Other Medical and Surgical Conditions, 982
Medical problems complicating pregnancy, 983
Anemia, 983
Iron deficiency anemia, 983
Folic acid deficiency anemia, 983
Sickle cell hemoglobinopathy, 984
Thalassemia, 984
Urinary problems, 984
Urinary tract infection, 984
Glomerulonephritis, 985
Nephroureterolithiasis, 985
Pulmonary complications, 985
Bronchial asthma, 985
Adult respiratory distress syndrome, 986
Pulmonary embolus, 986
Aspiration pneumonia, 986
Gastrointestinal problems, 987
Hyperemesis gravidarum (pernicious vomiting of pregnancy), 987
Peptic ulcer, 987
Cholelithiasis and cholecystitis, 987
Ulcerative colitis, 987
Dermatologic problems, 987
Neurologic disorders, 987
Epilepsy, 987
Multiple sclerosis, 988
Myasthenia gravis, 988
Disseminated lupus erythematosus, 988
Nursing management of medical complications, 988
Surgical conditions coincident with pregnancy, 988
Appendicitis, 989
Management, 989
Prognosis, 989
Gynecologic problems, 989
Abdominal hernias, 989
Carcinoma of the breast, 989
Intestinal obstruction, 990
Varices and hemorrhoids, 990
Nursing management of surgical conditions coincident with pregnancy, 990
Surgical interruption of pregnancy, 990
Early abortion, 992
Potential complications, 994
Second- and third-trimester abortions, 994
Nurse's role, 995
Surgical termination of fertility, 996
Motivation for sterilization, 996
Laws and regulations, 996
Sterilization procedures, 997
Female sterilization, 997
Timing of female sterilization, 997
Tubal occlusion, 997
Hysterectomy, 999
Male sterilization: vasectomy, 999
Nurse's role, 999
Counselor, 999
Preoperative preparation, 1000
Postoperative care, 1000
Discharge planning, 1000

Appendixes

A The Pregnant Patient's Bill of Rights, 1003
B Statements on Maternity Care and on Parent and Newborn Interaction, 1005
C Community Resources, 1007
D Nursing Magazines and Publications, 1011
E Nurse-Midwife Education, 1013
F Conversion Tables and Equivalents, 1015
G Standard Laboratory Values: Pregnant and Nonpregnant Women, 1018
H Human Fetotoxic Chemical Agents, 1022
I Standard Laboratory Values in the Neonatal Period, 1025
J Relationship of Drugs to Breast Milk and Effect on Infant, 1029
K Recommended Schedule for Active Immunization of Normal Infants and Children, 1038
L Brazelton Scale, 1039
M Birth and Death Certificates, 1045
N Standards of Care for Maternal-Child Nursing, 1047

Glossary, 1048

Tables

4.1 Communication—space, voice, touch and eye contact—and common violations, 28
4.2 Example of value clarification process implemented by a nursing student, 33
4.3 Examples of client noncompliance, 35
6.1 Female and male homologues: external genitalia, 51
6.2 Female and male homologues: internal structures, 51
6.3 Composition of semen, 82
6.4 Hypothalamic-pituitary-gonadal axis, 88
6.5 Effects of estrogens on target organs and tissues, 89
6.6 Effects of progesterone on target organs and tissues, 89
6.7 Effects of prolactin on target organs and tissues, 90
6.8 Stages of sexual development: female, 91
6.9 Stages of sexual development: male, 91
6.10 Female sexual response cycle, 94
6.11 Male sexual response cycle, 96
7.1 Childhood sexual development, 104

Tables

- **7.2** Adolescent sexual development, 106
- **7.3** Adult sexual development, 110
- **9.1** Summary of cognitive and personality development, 134
- **10.1** Common autosomal aberrations, 150
- **10.2** Common sex chromosome abnormalities, 151
- **10.3** Inherited component in some common disorders, 151
- **11.1** Markers (signs and symptoms) of the phases of the menstrual cycle, 159
- **12.1** Factors associated with fertility and infertility, 165
- **12.2** Tests and examinations for fertility, 166
- **12.3** Behavior associated with infertility, 184
- **13.1** Estimated annual deaths associated with fertility control and no control per 100,000 fertile women, 187
- **13.2** Risk factors and degree of associated risk by age for users of oral contraceptives, 187
- **13.3** Contraceptive methods and pregnancies per 100 women, 187
- **13.4** Contraceptives in common use, their modes of action, and female/male involvement, 200
- **13.5** Contraceptive techniques or appliances to block fertility, in common use, 201
- **14.1** Comparison of gestational time units, 208
- **15.1** Comparison of uterine measurements for nonpregnant and pregnant at 40 wk, 223
- **15.2** Regional increases in blood flow during pregnancy, 230
- **15.3** Cardiovascular system: maternal adaptations and implications for nursing, 233
- **15.4** Hormonal factors in pregnancy, 242
- **15.5** Summary: fetoplacental growth and development by calendar months, and maternal response, 247
- **17.1** Parity and gravidity using five-digit and two-digit systems, 269
- **17.2** Summary of signs and symptoms of pregnancy, 270
- **17.3** Symptoms and signs of pregnancy in order of appearance, 271
- **17.4** Differential assessment of signs and symptoms of pregnancy, 271
- **17.5** Comparison of fundal heights, 280
- **17.6** Summary of biochemical monitoring techniques, 283
- **17.7** Typical amniotic fluid increase during pregnancy, 287
- **17.8** Summary of laboratory tests in prenatal period, 296
- **17.9** Correlation of fetal weight and biparietal diameter, 297
- **17.10** Discomforts related to maternal adaptations to pregnancy, 303
- **17.11** Assessment during pregnancy with evaluative criteria, 310
- **18.1** Standard and deviations from standard weight (<85% and >120%) for 17- to 24-year-old nonpregnant women, 318

Tables

- **18.2** Recommended daily dietary allowances of some selected nutrients for pregnancy and lactation, 320
- **18.3** Nutrient needs of pregnancy, 324
- **18.4** Physical assessment of nutritional status, 328
- **18.5** Characteristics of some cultural food patterns, 329
- **18.6** Daily food plan for pregnancy and lactation, 332
- **18.7** Sample menus, 335
- **18.8** Modified food guide for vegetarian diets, 336
- **18.9** Vegetarian food guide, 337
- **18.10** Pregnancy protocol for nutrition counseling, 339
- **19.1** Summary of support measures, 354
- **20.1** Fetal lie and position, 371
- **20.2** Obstetric measurements, 376
- **20.3** Comparison of pelvic types, 379
- **20.4** Stages of labor and comparison of mean durations for nulliparas and multiparas, 392
- **21.1** Comparison of labors, 396
- **21.2** Maternal progress in first stage of labor within normal limits, 396
- **21.3** Minimal reassessment of progress of first stage of labor, 399
- **23.1** Physical assessment of the mother during fourth stage, 454
- **23.2** Evaluation criteria for care during labor, 463
- **24.1** External and internal modes of monitoring, 471
- **24.2** Tachycardia and bradycardia, 481
- **24.3** Increased and decreased variability, 483
- **24.4** Acceleration and early deceleration, 485
- **24.5** Late deceleration vs. variable deceleration, 487
- **24.6** Uterine activity information and signal source, 490
- **25.1** Comparison of general surgical client and obstetric client, 504
- **25.2** Four general categories of pharmacologic analgesia and anesthesia, 508
- **25.3** Pharmacologic control of discomfort during the birth period and the nursing process, 509
- **25.4** Comparison of modalities for obstetric analgesia, 523
- **27.1** Cardiovascular changes at birth, 557
- **27.2** Sleeping and waking states, 569
- **28.1** Physical assessment of newborn, 576
- **28.2** Assessment of newborn's reflexes, 594
- **28.3** Behavioral evaluation, 603
- **30.1** Digestion in infancy, 652
- **30.2** Neuromuscular and psychosocial development: birth to 3 months, 653
- **30.3** Recomended dietary allowances for infants, 653
- **30.4** Suggested supplements for infants, 656
- **30.5** Supplemental fluorine dosage schedule (mg/day), 657

Tables

30.6 Recommended daily dietary allowances for lactation, 661

30.7 Nutrient content of human milk and cow's milk, 662

30.8 Common problems and their solutions, 667

30.9 Guide for formula feeding, 673

30.10 Suggested ages for introduction of semisolid foods and table foods, 674

30.11 Guidelines for population groups in community nutrition: infants and children, 682

31.1 Hormonal reduction after delivery, 689

31.2 Clinical significance of key factors from prenatal and natal periods and associated nursing actions, 691

31.3 Evaluative criteria, area assessed, and normal findings, 698

32.1 Age-related pregnancy problems, 721

32.2 Evaluation criteria: parent-child relationships, 732

33.1 Immaturity and resultant problems, 741

33.2 Factors that place the pregnancy and fetus-neonate at high risk, 742

33.3 Goals for care, 744

35.1 Assessing abortion, 782

35.2 Types of spontaneous abortion and usual management, 783

35.3 Summary of findings: abruptio placentae and placenta previa, 790

35.4 Blood clotting factors, 797

35.5 Coagulation tests, 798

35.6 Symptoms of shock, 801

35.7 Differential diagnosis of essential hypertension and preeclampsia, 810

35.8 Protein readings, 811

Tables

35.9 Pharmacologic control of hypertension and its sequelae in pregnancy and labor, 816

35.10 Assessing deep tendon reflexes (DTRs), 820

35.11 Drugs and equipment for preventive treatment of convulsions of eclampsia, 822

36.1 Maternal infections: effects on pregnancy and fetus or neonate, 828

36.2 Summary: maternal response to fetal glucose demands and her changing insulin requirements, 847

36.3 Blood test for diabetes mellitus in pregnancy, 849

36.4 Differentiation of hypoglycemia, ketoacidosis, and hyperglycemic hyperosmolar nonketotic coma (HHNK), 851

36.5 Patient care guidelines: diabetic teaching, 856

37.1 Bishop's scale for assessing candidates for induction of labor, 887

37.2 Oxytocin administration, 888

37.3 Elaboration of neuromuscular maturity scales, 920

37.4 Care of the preterm infant: goals, physiologic problems, and nursing actions—assessment and implementation, 922

38.1 Ages at which mothers expect children to accomplish specific behaviors, 946

39.1 Nursing care of the addicted infant, 953

41.1 Interruption of pregnancy: basis for counseling, 991

41.2 Comparison of prostaglandin and 20% saline solution abortion procedures, 995

41.3 Surgical sterilization procedures: basis for counseling, 997

41.4 Summary of sterilization methods: basis for counseling, 1000

Essentials of Maternity Nursing

Introduction to Maternity Care

1 Issues and Trends in Maternity Nursing

2 Maternity Nursing Today

3 Maternity Nursing Process

4 Maternity Nurse–Client Relationships

5 Legal and Ethical Aspects of Maternity Nursing

UNIT ONE

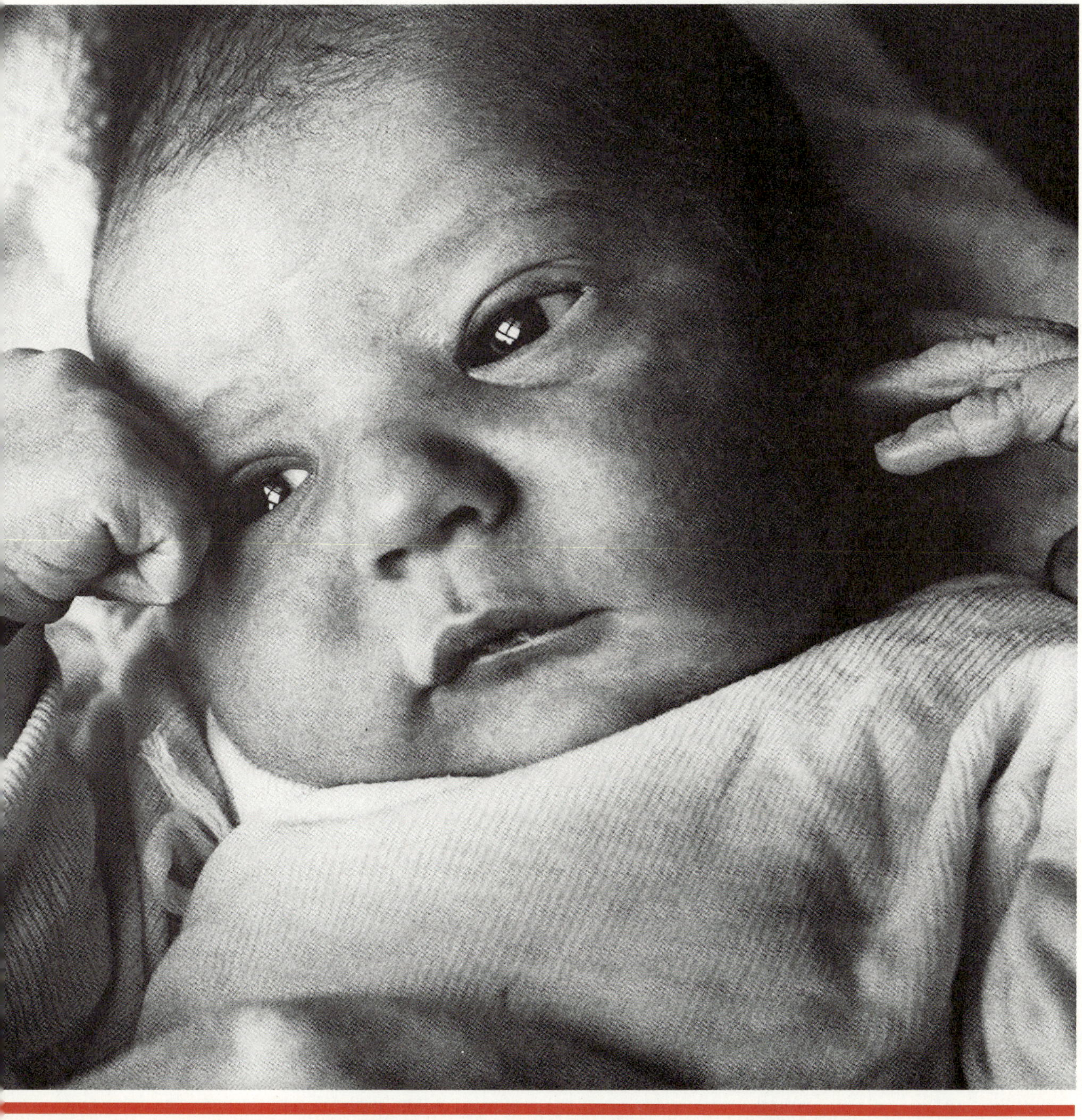

Robert Maust

1

Issues and Trends in Maternity Nursing

- Maternity Nursing Issues
- Maternity Nursing Trends
  - Education
  - Practice
  - Role

To understand some of the issues and trends in maternity care today, one must look at what has occurred in the past. From the beginning of time the birth of a baby was a very significant event. It was important to the woman giving birth and to the people around her. It was of vital importance to the tribe because it meant the continuation of their community. It was accompanied by fear because the death of the mother or the baby was a likely occurrence. It was surrounded by mystery because having a baby was something only a woman could do. The role of the man in reproduction was not really understood until comparatively recent times. After the invention of the microscope it became possible to visualize sperm and to speculate on their role in reproduction.

The practices of women during pregnancy and birth have always been an integral part of the social fabric of a society. They mirror the culture and mores of a people. Looking at prenatal care through the years, for example, one can observe changes in the way health care has been perceived. When we were a tribal people, women viewed pregnancy as a normal event. Wise women in the tribe would oversee the progression of pregnancy. Herbal remedies such as teas and poultices were prescribed to facilitate conception as well as to prevent it. During the pregnancy, special herbal preparations were used to attempt to ensure a good outcome. The spiritual aspects of care were very important as reflected by the use of magic and the incantations surrounding pregnancy and birth.

Over time, observations of the process and care needed during pregnancy, labor, and birth led to an organized body of knowledge. The knowledge was accumulated by the wise women of the tribe, the forerunners of midwives, and passed as oral tradition from mother to daughter much as the knowledge of hunting was passed from father to son. No written record of childbearing practices exists from the earliest times, although it has been suggested that some of our current beliefs and superstitions are remnants of those times.

Wertz and Wertz (1977) have chronicled childbirth practices in colonial America. Birth was a social event that was the exclusive responsibility of women. Midwives assisted women in giving birth and a woman's friends and neighbors participated in the event as her support both during the birth and in the critical days afterward during the "lying-in" period.

During the eighteenth century perinatal mortality decreased, probably as a result of improved nutrition and better general health in the colonies. Also during that century physicians gradually replaced midwives as birth attendants, although the role of women in bringing comfort and aid to other women during childbirth continued. Through the growing knowledge of asepsis and the use of forceps and anesthesia, physicians who had been trained in Europe sought to improve the natural processes of birth and thereby reduce death and debilitation from childbirth.

Birth in the United States, even more than in Europe, has become a medical event as the primary birth attendant shifted from wise woman/midwife to physician. The setting where birth occurs in the United States has also changed from a *borning room,* a small room usually located near the chimney of the family's home, to the bedroom or kitchen, to the hospital. Although most births in the United States occur in the hospital today, a growing number occur in the home or in freestanding birth centers.

Today attitudes and beliefs about pregnancy and childbirth are shaped by many influences. It is important to understand that childbirth does not occur in a vacuum. It reflects the status of women, men, and families in a society, as well as economic, political, social, religious and medical values. One can observe the interplay of these social forces and the effect they have on the choices women, men, and families make about pregnancy and birth.

Another concept that is important in planning care for the obstetric client relates to the individual's definition of health. A woman may make contact with the health care system because of a concern related to reproduction, but the care of that woman should always be viewed by care givers in the context of the woman's general well-being.

Nurses are now expected to take increasingly active parts in the social, political, and economic aspects of providing holistic health care to the childbearing family.

Maternity Nursing Issues

There are three areas of concern for the maternity nurse: practice, role in relation to other health care providers, and responsibility to society. In nurses' *practice,* family-centered care is stressed. The care of the pregnant woman is learned in the context of the family. Nursing students study the stressors, positive and negative, of a new family member on each member of the support system that the woman defines as her family. Maternity nurses believe that care extends beyond physical care to a consideration of other needs as well. Nurses are expected to use a holistic approach in the application of the nursing process with the family. In this way, nursing care is family centered. But is the practice truly family centered? To answer this question, one must speculate on what care might look like if the focus were shifted and the family made the decisions. When would prenatal care begin? How often would prenatal visits occur and what might they include? When would preparations for labor, delivery, and parenting begin and how would they fit into the prenatal preparation the family had selected? Who would the care provider be for all phases of the childbearing cycle? Who would assist the family to make choices that promote health, as that family defined health? Where would birth occur, and how would the family be educated to make their choices around the birth experience? If families chose to deliver their babies in a hospital, how might the routine change if the family were the locus for decision making? Would we still see sitz baths and clean beds by 9 AM? How can the needs of the formal health care setting, such as clinics, physician/certified nurse-midwife/nurse-practitioner offices, and hospitals, be reconciled with the needs and choices of families? And what is the role of the maternity nurse? The student is invited to consider these questions thoughtfully. The answers will probably differ, depending on the group of people for whom care is provided. The way to find the answers is to ask the families, ask the care providers, explore the realities of the setting, and propose a plan. The individual nurse's ability to develop such a plan may be limited by the nurse's knowledge, skills, or commitment to such a process. However, in whatever setting or role the nurse finds herself, the nurse can ask the families what they need and be aware and flexible in the way she thinks about and provides nursing care.

The nurse's *role* with other health care providers, notably physicians, is another issue for the maternity nurse. Both nurses and physicians have areas of expertise in providing care to families. Each group can bring unique knowledge and a set of skills to the family. Both groups can make significant contributions to perinatal outcome. And yet, nurse-physician relationships are often difficult. Nurses do not always act as if they believe that providing care for childbearing families is a team effort. In job satisfaction surveys, nurses report that dealing with physicians' attitudes is often a ''dissatisfier'' in their jobs. Many physicians do not realize that nurses' perceptions of the role of the maternity nurse have changed. Maternity nurses view their role as more autonomous, with an emphasis on interdependence with the physician. Most physicians have been educated to view the maternity nurse's role as dependent. This collision of values between physicians and nurses can cause conflict that is not in the best interest of the families for whom both groups are committed to care. Maternity nurses have a responsibility to deal with this conflict by educating physicians as well as the public about their roles, their education, and the skills they bring to the family. The registered nurse–physician relationship must be based on mutual respect for the person and his or her practice while recognizing the differences in the roles.

Maternity nurses must also support each other; that is, nurses must share nursing knowledge and skills with each other. Maternity nurses must learn to confront each other assertively on nursing practice issues, to celebrate excellence, and to remedy deficiencies. Maternity nurses must promote actively the practice of maternity nursing by being clear and straightforward about what that practice includes. The ability to communicate skillfully is vital if nurses are to educate physicians and support each other.

The maternity nurse's *responsibility* extends to the concerns of the larger society: the consumer movement, technologic advances, ethics, economics, and politics.

The consumer movement has had an impact on maternity care. As consumers of health care, some women and their partners have begun to demand more participation in that care (see p. 10).

Advances in technology related to the birth process have raised several issues. The development of the silicon chip has revolutionized information processing and storage as well as monitoring capabilities. Some speculate that the new technology will revolutionize nurses' lives and practice much as the industrial revolution did. The nurses' challenge will be to humanize that technology while working with childbearing families.

Ethical issues have become increasingly problematic, related both to technology and to social pressures. For example, in the intensive care of the neonate, the development of more sophisticated machines for diagnosis and treatment has posed ethical questions about the quality of life, the rights of babies, parents, and providers, and the responsibility of the nurse. Issues of in vitro fertilization, genetic manipulation, and fetal surgery have enormous ethical implications. Social and political pressures about the rights of the fetus and the rights and responsibilities of society have crystallized in the abortion issue.

The economic situation may have a profound effect on practitioners as well as on women seeking care. Staffing patterns in health care facilities and third-party reimbursement have a direct impact on the services the maternity nurse is able to provide to families. A woman's economic status affects her health at the time of conception, her care-seeking behaviors, and the resources available to her.

The political climate influences maternity care because of allocation of resources based on federal, state, and local priority setting. Some political issues that affect the field of maternity nursing include abortion, family planning, programs for prenatal care, prenatal education, and nutritional supplements for mothers and babies, child care centers, job training, Head Start programs, and social and family services.

Maternity nurses have a responsibility to become aware of and involved in these issues that affect families. Maternity nurses have a role in relation (1) to practice at the bedside in the hospital and the home, (2) to health care colleagues, and (3) to society at large. As private citizens, each individual can add support to or defeat legislation related to families by voting, lobbying, writing to congressional representatives, and so forth. Concerns of families in the 1980s will continue to be issues for the future. The challenge to maternity nurses is to respond and to make a difference.

Maternity Nursing Trends

Trends in maternity nursing can be viewed from three perspectives: education, practice, and role.

EDUCATION

Nurses are educated to care for the childbearing family. It is no longer enough to study the physiology of pregnancy, the mechanisms of labor, and the processes of birth and involution. These are important, but they are only part of the responsibilities of nursing care. The focus is on the *family*. Physiology is studied in perspective. The woman's preparation for childbearing begins when she herself is a fetus. What she brings to a pregnancy is a sum of her own genetic inheritance, her nurturance, both physical and psychologic, her attitudes, and her health practices. Because of the importance of all these factors to the outcome of pregnancy, each is emphasized in nursing education. Nurses learn to assess a woman's physical status, to ask questions that provide a picture of what a woman brings to the pregnancy. Health assessment includes questions related to childhood diseases, menarche, menstrual history, and medical, surgical, and family history. These data provide a base for an assessment of physiologic status. Nurses are educated to elicit information referred to as psychosocial: information about relationships, feelings, attitudes, and beliefs. The woman is asked about the date of her last menstrual period and her reaction to being pregnant. Examples of questions include the following: "What would you like your childbearing experience to be like?" "What kinds of changes will this baby make in your life?" "When you think about yourself as a mother, what do you see yourself doing?" "When you think about your mate as a parent, what do you see your mate doing?" These types of questions illustrate another facet of the role of the maternity nurse, that of preparing the woman and her mate for many of the activities of parenting.

Education for providing maternity care has expanded to include other people whom the woman has identified as her family; for example, the central role of the woman's mate is recognized. In the prenatal, intrapartal, and postpartal periods, maternity nurses are educated to seek information about the pregnant woman's mate or other support person she has chosen. Even though students may initially feel uncomfortable about "prying" into intrafamily relationships and issues, the type of noninvasive assessment that this book will help you to develop can be a great help as you support the family.

Other family members are considered in the assessment and care of the childbearing family because the importance of the birth of a new family member to others in that family is recognized. Children and other adults also need support to make the physical and psychologic adjustments to an infant.

PRACTICE

The practice of maternity nursing is related to the community, the setting, and the nurse. Historically, the survival of a community depended on good perinatal outcomes. Because of the significance of the event to the community, birth customs developed. In one community it may be the custom to give birth at home; in another to give birth in a hospital is the norm. The practice of maternity nursing in these two communities would be different. The expected behaviors of physicians and maternity nurses change with the community values. Are physicians viewed as consultants to the pregnant woman, as partners in care, or as decision makers with absolute authority and responsibility? Do pregnant women expect nurses to have a role in their care or merely to follow their physicians' orders?

Trends in the practice of maternity nursing include accommodation to expanding technology, elaboration of the practice of teaching and consultation to the family, and reaffirmation of a support function.

Technology has influenced the medical care of the pregnant woman. Ultrasound has provided a method of evaluating the fetal size, dating pregnancy, and detecting certain anomalies. Amniocentesis can provide information about the maturity of the fetal lungs, some genetic abnormalities, and the sex of the fetus. New drugs to suppress labor have been developed. Electronic fetal monitoring allows health care providers to assess the well-being of the fetus late in pregnancy with nonstress and contraction stress testing and during labor. In some settings fetal scalp pH is tested and hemodynamic monitoring of the laboring woman is available. Nurses now practice the science as well as the art of maternity care. It has been difficult for some nurses to respond to these changes. For example, during the 1960s electronic fetal monitoring began to be used in several settings. Of course, babies had always been monitored by nurses, midwives, and physicians who had used their eyes to observe, their ears to listen to the baby with a fetoscope and to listen to the mother's responses, and their hands to feel the uterine contractions. Then came the electronic monitors. Many nurses felt intimidated by the machines and uncertain of nursing practice with the monitors. Some nurses are still intimidated by them! Change is inevitable and will always remain a challenge to nursing care.

Consumers are also change agents in maternity care. In many places pregnant women and their families choose to participate fully in their care and make their own choices about that care. The health care industry, including those who practice in its settings, has slowly and in some cases grudgingly accommodated to the wishes of the woman and her partner. In communities where consumers have choices about health care providers and settings, consumers are making their choices known by taking their business where they can get their needs met.

Consumers are also responsible for instituting changes within hospitals. Alternatives in the place to give birth exist in many hospitals today as a result of consumer desires. Women may choose to labor and deliver in the traditional setting in a labor room, in an alternative birth center in the hospital, or in a birth room.

It is now a common practice to offer rooming-in to mothers who wish to have their babies with them at all times. Whether babies are breast or bottle fed, the current practice is to feed them when they are hungry, rather than employing the "gas tank" theory for feeding. The gas tank theory says that since it takes a baby approximately 4 hours to empty the stomach the baby should then be fed every 4 hours! More providers are accepting the idea that babies know what they need and want and when. A change in practice that illustrates the acceptance of the theory that babies know what they need is the change in the procedure for breast feeding infants. Each baby used to be weighed before being taken to the mother for breast feeding. The baby would then be reweighed on return to the nursery so that everyone "knew" how much the baby had received from the mother's breast. If the baby did not receive "enough" according to the nurse's (or physician's) definition, the baby would be fed with glucose water to "make up" the difference.

Arrangements for sibling visitation represent another consumer push. Some hospitals now encourage the new baby's brothers and sisters to visit before the mother brings the new family member home. In many places visiting hours have become more liberal, and those who may visit the new mother now extend beyond the husband. It is interesting but not really surprising that this liberalization of hospital policy has not been accompanied by an increased rate of infection as had been predicted.

Although the impetus for change has come primarily from consumers, some nurses and physicians (privately or professionally) have supported these changes. They have acted as advocates for the parents and their choices.

A significant trend in the last 20 years is the inclusion of the baby's father in the choices and the decision making during the childbearing year. Just as it was difficult for some nurses to make the transition to electronic monitors, the need to include the father or other support person of the woman's choosing was hard for many nurses and physicians. When the father came in as support person and coach, it took time for many nurses to recognize the new role as support to the family. Some physicians as well as nurses still have difficulty with the level of involvement of fathers in the birth process. Others encourage increased participation in the prenatal visits and classes, labor support, and even in parts of the birth such as cutting the baby's umbilical cord. In some hospitals, fathers are encouraged to be present and actively involved in the birth, whether in a traditional or an alternative setting or when the mother must have a cesarean birth.

Today maternity nurses function as teachers and counselors to the childbearing family. Maternity nurses have extensive knowledge about nutrition, exercise, and other health information related to childbearing. Nurses counsel about options in maternity care and facilitate parents' decision making. The decisions are multiple, including whether or when to become pregnant, scheduling of prenatal care, options in childbirth practices, and feeding the newborn. Through the teaching and counseling roles, the nurse is also providing support. Support can be offered in many ways: with the hands as the nurse touches the woman (during physical examination or back massage); to the mate (offering a cup of coffee); or through coordination of services of other health team members (social workers, nutritionists). Support has been a traditional part of the practice of maternity nursing and will continue to be one of nurses' significant contributions to the care of the childbearing family.

The way individual nurses practice nursing is shaped in part by the legislation, policies of the agency, and standards of care. Each individual nurse brings individual beliefs and values to the setting and those individuals can help to shape the way nursing is practiced even in traditional settings. Nursing practice in those settings can range from traditional to innovative while still remaining safe and appropriate.

Other external forces also affect the practice of maternity nursing. The importance of economics cannot be ignored. The economic status of families during hard times affects the choices they make (e.g., deciding to become parents) as well as what resources are available (e.g., for contraception or for inoculations for the children). The economic situation affects health care in silent ways such as the availability of transportation for people to obtain health care or to buy nutritious foods. It is informative to trace economic and societal trends and observe the effect they have had and will continue to have on the practice of nursing.

ROLE

One of the more visible changes is the expanded role of the nurse, represented by the certified nurse-midwife (CNM), the family nurse-practitioner (FNP), clinical nurse specialists, and the women's health care specialist (see p. 13). These expanded roles present options for the individual nurse's professional and personal growth. Changes have also occurred in the traditional role of the nurse at the bedside in the hospital or in the home and in outpatient settings. Today care givers often have more responsibility in the management of uncomplicated pregnancy. In the hospital setting this role expansion is reflected in greater accountability for the management of labor and care of the woman following delivery. Accountability is the key. For example, very experienced labor room nurses frequently have made care decisions in uncomplicated labors for the timing of the medications ordered for the woman. Nurses document observations and other nursing actions in progress notes. Documentation is a vehicle for the nurse to take credit (or blame) for nursing decisions. That level of accountability, while not universal, is an encouraging trend in nursing practice that will affect the way the public, other health care professionals, and maternity nurses themselves view the role of the nurse.

Other trends in the role of the nurse are equally exciting. Historically, nurses have chosen the role of educator or administrator, and more recently, of researcher. Nurses have viewed those roles as ''less than'' that of the bedside clinical nurse. A change in the attitude, although small, is an encouraging trend. When different choices within nursing are valued, the nursing profession as a whole is strengthened. Then options exist within nursing that capitalize on nurses' varied talents.

As a group, nurses are developing political ''savvy'' and choosing to participate in the legislative process. Nurses have a unique perspective of the health care needs of people and the delivery of health care. This perspective is valuable when legislation is drafted.

Involvement in the legislative process and support for each other blend into another role, that of advocate for families and for other nurses. The nurse's role as an advocate for the childbearing family can be complex. Nurses can strive to carry out the parents' wishes. However, nurses are also advocates for the unborn child. Sometimes that can put them in a difficult position. For example, a woman and her mate may make a choice that is not in the best interest of the child (e.g., their use of hard drugs [heroin] during pregnancy), or they may refuse to seek medical intervention in the presence of a serious complication. What is the role of the advocate in those and similar circumstances? Nurses are also community members. As nurses, individuals have the privilege and responsibility of information; as community members, nurses have a stake in the outcome of pregnancy. Complex situations require thoughtful decisions of nurses who are family advocates. Nurses must challenge assumptions and make informed choices only after weighing alternatives.

The nurse's role as advocate also extends to that of advocate for each other. It does not help other nurses or nursing as a whole to make comments, gossip, or participate in ''running down'' nursing colleagues. A more helpful approach is to share observations and participate in discussion to solve the problem mutually.

The nursing care of childbearing families is exciting and challenging. Education prepares the nurse for practice that can be expressed in a variety of roles. A central question for nursing students to ask now is, ''How do we get from here to there?''

References and Readings

Bermosk, L., and Porter, S.: Women's health and human wholeness, New York, 1979, Appleton-Century-Crofts.

Chaska, N.: The nursing profession: views through the mist, New York, 1978, McGraw-Hill Book Co.

Chinn, P., editor: Women's health, Adv. Nurs. Sci., vol. 3, no. 2, Jan. 1981.

Chodorow, N.: The reproduction of mothering, Berkeley, Calif., 1978, University of California Press.

Edlund, B., and McKenzie, C.: Symposium on women's health issues, Nurs. Clin. North Am. **17**:111-185, March 1982.

Ehrenreich, B., and English, D.: For her own good, New York, 1979, Anchor Press/Doubleday.

Kaplan, A., and Bean, J., editors: Beyond sex role stereotypes, Boston, 1976, Little, Brown & Co.

May, I.: Spiritual midwifery, Tennessee, 1975, The Book Publishing Company.

Sandelowski, M.: Women, health, and choice, Englewood Cliffs, N.J., 1981, Prentice-Hall, Inc.

Schneir, M.: Feminism: the essential historical writings, New York, 1972, Vintage.

Sheehy, G.: Passages, New York, 1976, E.P. Dutton & Co., Inc.

Stimpson, C., editor: The labor of women: work and family, Signs **4**(4): Summer 1979.

Stone, M.: Ancient mirrors of womanhood, vols. 1 and 2, New York: 1979, New Sibylline Books.

Wertz, R., and Wertz, D.: Lying-in: a history of childbirth in America, New York, 1977, The Free Press/Macmillan.

2

Maternity Nursing Today

- Beliefs
- Nature and Scope
  - Preventive activities
  - Curative activities
  - Rehabilitative activities
- Maternity Client
  - Statistical picture
- Maternity Nurse
  - Technician
  - Teacher and counselor
  - Advocate
  - Manager
  - Researcher
  - Expanding roles
    - Obstetric-gynecologic nurse practitioner
    - Nurse-midwife
- Summary

Maternity nursing today is a complex health service. Its nursing activities range across the health-illness continuum from promotion of health to client rehabilitation. What prompts nurses to provide this service—what are their beliefs? What types of services are offered? Who are the users or consumers of this care? Who provides the care? This chapter is devoted to a discussion of these questions.

Beliefs

Every culture develops beliefs or convictions that give direction to the form or structure of its institutions. Nursing is one of many social institutions in our culture. Nurses have certain beliefs that act as a source for the structure and functions of nursing.* For example, nurses believe that nursing is concerned with a holistic view of human beings and ''an occupational force for social good.'' This means that the nurse treats the total person and by doing so returns that individual to society more able to function in an independent and socially responsive way. This holds true whether nurses are engaged in medical-surgical nursing or maternity nursing. Maternity nursing has as its source the beliefs common to all nursing and specific beliefs that have a direct reference to the childbearing family. The specific beliefs outlined below give guidance to the development of health services on a national and local level and to the selection of pertinent nursing strategies for maternity clients, their offspring, and their families.

1. *Childbearing is a normal physiologic function*. For most women and their children, pregnancy and birth represent a physically and emotionally safe process. With this belief as a guide to action, ambulatory care of women during prenatal and postnatal periods has been established (see Chapter 17). Classes are offered in the community to prepare couples for childbirth and parenthood (see Chapter 19). Early discharge of mother and infant within 24 to 48 hours after delivery with follow-up by home care nurses is becoming a common hospital practice.

2. *Childbearing is family centered*. The family is now recognized by nursing and medical groups as the major support system for the pregnant woman and her infant. Efforts are being made to include the family in all aspects of maternity care since childbearing is a normal part of family life. In addition to the traditional

*For a more detailed discussion of beliefs about nursing see Styles, M.: On nursing: toward a new endowment, St. Louis, 1982, The C.V. Mosby Co.

hospital or home settings for birth, other types of birth centers are being developed. These combine the safety features associated with hospital care with a more homelike atmosphere. Close contact between the parents and their child is emphasized. Most hospitals have liberalized visiting hours and some are open to sibling visitors as well as to grandparents (see Chapter 26).

3. *Continuity of care is essential to the health of the pregnant woman and her infant.* The health history the woman brings to pregnancy affects the outcome. Therefore maternity nurses are involved in health promotion among potential parents in the school age population (see Chapter 38). The total response of the pregnant woman to the developing embryo/fetus means significant deviations in any of her body systems and is reflected in the maternal-fetal-placental unit. Deviations in body systems may arise at any point in the maternity cycle and are not always predictable. This knowledge has led to the development of protocols for care spanning the prenatal, natal, and postnatal periods of pregnancy. All societies recognize the importance of parental care and socialization of children and design "models" for parents to follow. Psychosocial stress can occur if parents find these models difficult to emulate. Therefore repeated assessments of a client's perceptions of self and parental responsibilities, coping mechanisms, and support systems are necessary (see Chapter 16). Categories of clients who are at risk have been developed to alert their caretakers to the possible need to adapt routines of care to their specific needs (see Chapter 33).

4. *Children have a right to be "well-born" and to be provided with opportunities to realize their potential.* The rapidly developing embryo/fetus is vulnerable to many types of stress and the newborn is dependent on others for safety, shelter, feeding, and stimulation. Examples of nursing strategies that may be credited to this belief are arranging for prenatal testing of the pregnant woman for blood type and concurrent infections such as syphilis (see p. 827), establishing protocols for assessment of fetal well-being during labor (see p. 399), immediate evaluation of the newborn after delivery (see p. 439), teaching parents child care activities (see p. 616), and supporting legislation relating to rights of children (see Appendix B).

5. *Parenthood is a responsible role to be assumed voluntarily.* Parenthood is not a role to be undertaken without thought for the consequences since it has such profound effects on the adult and child involved. Ideally every child should be a wanted child and every parent a parent because he or she desires it. The availability of different methods of birth control to increasingly large numbers of people means this ideal is a possibility. Nurses engage in discussions of responsible sexuality with teenagers or instruct clients in the use of birth control measures because of these beliefs (see Chapters 8 and 13).

The beliefs discussed above are subscribed to by professional groups of nurses. Each nurse will have personal beliefs about childbearing and the role the nurse will play in it. It is helpful to write these beliefs down and use them as a basis for discussions with peers and instructors. Personal beliefs can either support or undermine professional beliefs. Nurses need to be aware of this potential source of conflict.

Nature and Scope

Maternity nursing involves activities that can be designated as preventive, curative, or rehabilitative in nature. It spans the lifetime of an individual from preconceptional planning of children through pregnancy and birth and the early adjustment of the family to a newborn child and may be carried out in the home, clinic, or hospital.

PREVENTIVE ACTIVITIES

The preventive aspects of maternity care include health promotion and prevention of disease states. Efforts are made to increase and strengthen the individual's ability to withstand the stress of everyday living. The nursing actions associated with these efforts represent many of the nurses' independent functions. They occur wherever nurse and client meet whether the client is directly under the care of a physician or not. The nurse who teaches good nutrition, personal hygiene, and beneficial exercises to a pregnant woman is promoting the health of the woman and her developing fetus. The nurse who encourages a teenager to seek care for pregnancy or who discusses sexual adjustment with pregnant couples is acting to prevent possible complications.

CURATIVE ACTIVITIES

The early detection of physical and emotional disabilities in the mother or infant and initiation of corrective measures are essential components of maternity nursing. The check points in prenatal evaluation correspond to the times during pregnancy when difficulties are known to occur. Women with diseases complicating pregnancy, for example, medical conditions such as nephritis or cardiac impairment, or with conditions peculiar to pregnancy, such as hypertensive states, may be confined to a hospital for continuous evaluation and treatment. Cesarean birth may be chosen to safeguard a mother or child.

REHABILITATIVE ACTIVITIES

Rehabilitative activities are directed toward returning an individual to her previous state with an equal or greater ability to function. The care given a pregnant teenager illustrates the rehabilitative aspects of maternity care. Through the physical and emotional support provided these young people, nurses hope they will be able to complete their development toward responsible adulthood. Nurses have provided the impetus toward founding teenage clinics, high school programs for pregnant teenagers, and follow-up care to help teenagers give their children the mothering needed.

The nursing activities—preventive, curative, and rehabilitative—often overlap as nurses give care to any one client. The nurse responsible for the care of a premature infant in a neonatal intensive care unit makes continuous assessments of the infant's condition and modifies care to maintain an optimal state (curative). She promotes his future welfare by educating his parents regarding his care (preventive). She rehabilitates the infant by ''weaning'' him from intensive care until he can be cared for as a healthy newborn.

The enlarged scope and nature of the care offered the pregnant woman and her family have made necessary a collaborative approach to the delivery of the service. Nurses, physicians, nutritionists, and other health professionals work with the woman for mutual assessment of maternal and infant needs, formulation of goals for their health maintenance or attainment, effective use of therapies based on clinical assessment of their needs, and rehabilitative treatment to prevent maternal and infant disability and to assist them in realizing their potentials. No one group of health practitioners possesses either the competence or the time to act as the sole dispenser of health care—full utilization of all groups is needed.

Maternity Client

Who are the individuals who now or in the future will use the nursing services maternity nurses have to offer? Potentially all sexually mature persons are candidates for reproductive care. They come from all racial, ethnic, economic, and social groups. Approximately 70% are white and 30% are nonwhite. They or their forebears were nativeborn Indians or Eskimos or came to this continent mainly from Europe, Africa, or Asia. Their age groups will vary from fetus and neonate, to the adolescent, to the young adult, and to individuals approaching middle age. Many, both male and female, will seek assistance concerning methods of contraception, and approximately 15% of all couples of childbearing age will seek help for infertility problems.

Three million, six hundred thousand women, ranging in age from 12 to 52 years, give birth each year. Some of them will have the support of family, husbands, parents, children, and friends. Others will be alone. Some will be overjoyed by their pregnancies; others will be angry, defensive, or apathetic about their state. Most will be physically healthy; others, at least 500,000 a year, will be designated as *high risk* for either maternal, fetal, or familial reasons. Some of this latter group through ignorance of American concepts of health care will not seek medical attention until their or their infant's life is threatened.

An increasing number of the consumers of our health services are well informed (Stainton, 1981):

> Knowledgeable consumers no longer comply with the power base of professionals and wish to be participants in the experience of their family members. The childbirth experience is perceived to be one of the most significant events in the life of an adult. Parents wish to have their children born in an environment which welcomes them, provides safe *and* satisfying care and promotes the early bonding to their infant among the family members.

Consumers are eager to participate as partners with the health professional in their own care. The maternity nurse is in a key position to affect consumer-oriented care by promoting and safeguarding the health of the maternity client.

Most maternity clients do not fit into the sick role as it is defined in our society. This definition includes sets of expectations about client's behavior. Clients are expected to take a dependent role, accede to hospital regulations and rules, and be relieved of normal role responsibilities because of illness. The care and treatment afforded are not to be based on external power and prestige but given without consideration for color, race, or creed. Suffering and pain are to be expected and accepted stoically. The average pregnant woman is, however, well, not sick. She is ambulatory, attends an office or a clinic for most of her care, is hospitalized for only a few days, and participates in her own care and in the care of her child within 24 hours after delivery. Yet her needs and those of her family require nursing and medical management that can be described as intensive, critical, long term, and rehabilitative. The conflict inherent in the role of the maternity client is one of the challenges of maternity nursing.

STATISTICAL PICTURE

The *fertility rate* is the number of births per 1000 women between the ages of 15 and 44 years (inclusive) calculated on a yearly basis. It is a more accurate means of comparing different population groups than the birthrate. The National Center for Health Statistics (1982) noted the fertility rate in 1980 was 68.4 births per 1000 women of childbearing age. The fertility rate among American women rose by 2% in 1980 to its highest level in 7 years but probably declined 1% in 1981. The *birthrate,* the number of live births per 1000 population was 15.9 babies/1000 persons in 1980. It rose by 2% overall in 1980 and probably held steady in 1981. The largest increase in the birthrate was among women aged 30 to 34, who had 2.7% more babies. Rates of first births for women in their early 30s climbed by 60% between 1975 and 1980, continuing a trend of postponed childbearing among women who have established careers.

A total of 665,747 babies, or 18.4% of those born in 1980, were born to unwed women. This was an increase of 11.4% from 1979. A third of the increase was the result of new methods of calculation. If the method had not changed, the 1980 rate would have been 645,000 births, up 7.9% from 1979. The increase in the rate of childbearing among unmarried women was attributed to "the substantial rise in the rate for unmarried white women," which rose by 18.1% while the rate for unwed black women fell slightly.

The sharpest rise in births to unmarried women occurred in the 20- to 24-year-old age range, while the rate declined slightly for 15- to 19-year old women. While 9.4% of all white births, compared to 55% of all black births, were to unmarried women, the actual increase in out of wedlock births was 5% higher for white births.

Infant mortality is usually expressed as the number of deaths per 1000 live births and is the ratio between the number of deaths of infants before their first birthday during any given year and the number of live births occurring in the same year. The United States is experiencing a slow but continuing downward trend in infant mortality dating from 1964. That year new public health programs that affected the health of mothers and children received support from federal, state, and local funds. Maternal and infant care projects provided prenatal care and infant care for high-risk mothers and infants through the first year of life. The children and youth projects extended pediatric care from birth to 21 years of age. Family planning services increased with support from the Maternal and Child Health Service, Office of Economic Opportunity, and the Family Planning Service and Population Research Act of 1970. The development of intensive care units for the newborn and of regional perinatal centers increased.

Despite these efforts, mortality for different segments of the population and differing socioeconomic groups still shows inequities. Naeye (1979) reports that perinatal mortality for blacks in the United States was 47% higher than for whites during the period from 1959 to 1966. For those same years, mortality for black infants in the United States was three times as high as for white infants. Infant neonatal mortality has been a traditional indicator of environmental influences. In the 1960s, professionals, local communities, and state and federal governmental agencies identified factors that cause a higher mortality for the poor and designed programs to combat the problems. The major contributing factor to a higher mortality for the poor was inadequate nutrition. Another factor was the lack of prenatal care because the poor did not realize the importance of early and continuous prenatal care, they could not afford care, private providers limited or excluded them from their practice, and impersonal treatment was delivered in overcrowded public clinics.

Contraceptive techniques are preventing many unwanted pregnancies; however, a large number of people are still not reached (Barnes, 1978). More than 3.5 million low- and marginal-income women and almost 2.5 million sexually active adolescents still lack family planning services, and even among married couples more than 20% of all births continue to be unwanted or mistimed.

A maternal death is the death of a woman from any cause during pregnancy or within 42 days of the termination of pregnancy, irrespective of the duration or site of the pregnancy. *Maternal mortality* measures the number of maternal deaths per 100,000 live births. The rate remained relatively static between 1916 and 1929. By the end of the 1920s a downward trend became apparent, and by approximately 1936 the rate of decline in maternal morality became rapid. Within 9 years (1936 to 1945) the rate was cut by almost two thirds. A combination of factors stimulated this decline: availability of sulfa drugs for the control of infections, availability of blood and blood substitutes for treatment of hemorrhage, and formation of hospital and community committees to investigate causes and circumstances of each maternal death and assign responsibility.

The rate of decline in maternal mortality further accelerated after World War II as antibiotics became available and hospitalization for deliveries increased. By 1949 the rate was 90.3 maternal deaths per 100,000 live births. Between 1957 and 1964 the rate of decline slowed. After 1964 the downward trend again became evident until 1972, when maternal mortality stood at

18.8 per 100,000. This rate reflects the decrease in maternal deaths from abortion as states legalized the abortion procedure and safer techniques were employed.

There continue to be differences between white and nonwhite maternal mortality. Currently mortality for nonwhite women approximates the figure for white women in 1954. The young and poor members of any racial group also represent a population vulnerable to maternity complications and maternal death. Many women still do not receive adequate prenatal care, and many women categorized as high risk are still without specialized treatment. Only 61.6% of black women and 79.1% of white women were receiving prenatal care during the first trimester. Almost 20% of women under the age of 15 years received no prenatal care or delayed prenatal care. This delay in prenatal care and the large number of black low–birth weight infants may have resulted in the finding that black infants were twice as likely to receive low Apgar scores at 1 and 5 minutes as white infants. The percentage of black low–birth weight infants was twice as high as the percentage of white low–birth weight infants. More equal distribution and utilization of health resources to all citizens will be necessary to effect a beneficial change within these categories.

Maternity Nurse

The maternity nurse functions in a variety of roles to bring comprehensive health care to individuals during the childbearing years. As a *clinician* the nurse acts as technician, teacher and counselor, advocate, manager, and researcher.

TECHNICIAN

Technical skills include assessment of health status, deriving nursing diagnoses from the collected data, setting up environments that afford safety and comfort to clients and others, initiating therapeutically based nursing measures and evaluating their effectiveness, and being aware of the implications of efficient use of time, energy, and materials both for the client and the nurse.

The nursing profession has developed standards for nursing practice that provide criteria for evaluating the degree of competence attained. A competent nurse inspires confidence in clients, and this confidence is an important part of the supportive care clients require. The following excerpt from a letter written by the husband of a woman, 8 months pregnant, who was admitted to the hospital with a massive vaginal hemorrhage illustrates this concept:

> We would like to thank all those who helped my wife and myself during this difficult time . . . . The nurses were particularly helpful. They were skilled in the emergency care they gave my wife and at all times were kind to her and to myself. We felt we were in safe hands, it was very reassuring.

TEACHER AND COUNSELOR

Maternity nursing emphasizes the preventive aspects of health care. Much of this is accomplished through teaching and counseling clients. As a teacher or counselor the nurse's interventions are directed toward assisting clients in acquiring knowledge that will help them make the best possible decisions for the care of themselves or their children. The nurse provides a nonjudgmental environment in which these decisions can take place and helps clients evaluate their efforts realistically. The nurse acts as a role model for the technical care of clients or their infants and with supportive teaching can assist even the most anxious or unknowledgeable client to learn how to provide safe care.

ADVOCATE

As health care becomes more complex there is a need for someone to act as a liaison or advocate between the client and the other personnel or health agencies. The maternity nurse encourages clients to be aware of their health care rights and responsibilities. The nurse is committed to a holistic view of health care and therefore often knows more about clients than do other health workers. The nurse is in a good position to explain, interpret, defend, or protect clients' rights. As an advocate, the nurse attempts to modify health services on a local or national level so they reflect a humanitarian approach to health care.

MANAGER

Nurse managers act to coordinate and facilitate the many services required in health care of clients. Team leaders or charge nurses are examples of nurse managers since they direct the care of groups of clients and nursing personnel. They need to be knowledgeable concerning client care and able to communicate effectively with various types of health workers.

RESEARCHER

Research has had a valuable effect on shaping nursing practice and developing ideas for further inquiry that will keep our future practice alive. All nurses have the responsibility of adding new knowledge through descriptive studies, the validation of knowledge utilizing research design, and publication of results in professional literature. The idea of scientific research in nursing is as old as Florence Nightingale. She admonished nurses to develop the habit of systematically making and recording correct observations and then contemplating their meaning. Observations should not be for curious facts but rather as the only means for discovering and verifying knowledge useful for saving lives.

Nurses need to evaluate the effectiveness of established methods of clinical nursing by measuring the outcomes in the health status of clients.

To assist the nurse with these new responsibilities, courses in research techniques are offered as part of a nurse's preparatory program or as inservice or continuing education for practicing nurses. Many health agencies are establishing nursing research divisions. These are staffed by nurse researchers who work with the nurse clinician to help translate clinical problems into nursing research problems. They provide assistance for writing a research proposal, collecting and analyzing data, and implementing findings in nursing practice.

EXPANDING ROLES

The increasing health care needs of the public have necessitated an expansion in the responsibilities nurses have assumed and resulted in the development of new nursing roles.

Obstetric-gynecologic nurse practitioner. In 1979 the American College of Obstetrics and Gynecology (ACOG) and the Nurses' Association of the American College of Obstetrics and Gynecology (NAACOG) jointly defined the obstetric-gynecologic nurse practitioner as follows:

> A registered nurse who has satisfactorily completed a formal and accredited Obstetric-Gynecologic Nurse Practitioner educational program. The Obstetric-Gynecologic Nurse Practitioner will thus have been provided with special knowledge and skills in health maintenance, disease prevention, psychosocial and physical assessment, and management of health-illness needs in the primary care of women. This care is predominantly provided in an ambulatory setting. The Obstetric-Gynecologic Nurse Practitioner will provide such care interdependently with the physician and other members of the health care team.

Nursing activities of the obstetric-gynecologic nurse practitioner include the following:

1. Secure and complete health, psychosocial, and obstetric-gynecologic history, and record findings in a systematic, accurate, and succinct form.
2. Perform complete screening and physical examination techniques with specific emphasis on evaluation of the breasts, abdomen, and pelvis, visualization of the cervix, Papanicolaou smear, cervical culture, and a bimanual vaginal and rectovaginal examination (Fig. 2.1).
3. Perform, order, and interpret routine laboratory tests.
4. Develop a health maintenance plan, including health education, disease prevention, and general anticipatory guidance.
5. Provide periodic health supervision of healthy, nonpregnant, and asymptomatic women for health maintenance.
6. Provide clinical management within medical protocols for women with uncomplicated gynecologic illness.
7. Provide assessment, education, and management for family planning.
8. Provide ambulatory prenatal care with attention to both maternal and fetal health for women with uncomplicated pregnancies.
9. Provide ambulatory postnatal care for women who have had an uncomplicated pregnancy with attention to the mother-infant relationship while not assuming primary care of the infant.
10. Provide health education and counseling, including the psychosocial dimensions, in the areas of nutrition, sexuality, childbearing, parenting, and family life.
11. Arrange referrals as needed to other members of the health care team.

In 1981 the NAACOG Certification Cooperation (NCC) instituted a certification program for the in-hospital obstetric nurse and for the obstetric-gynecologic nurse practitioner (Nurses' Association of the American College of Obstetrics and Gynecology, 1982). This program requires a candidate to meet eligibility criteria based on educational and/or practice requirements and to successfully complete a 200-item multiple choice examination. Nurses who achieve certification are entitled to use RNC (registered nurse certified) after their name. Beginning with the 1983 examination, all nurses taking the examination for the Ob/Gyn Nurse Practitioner certification will be required to be graduates from a nurse-practitioner program acceptable to the NCC. Also, beginning in 1983 a neonatal nurse clinician/practitioner certification examination will be offered.

Nurse-midwife. Certified nurse-midwives are registered nurses who have additional knowledge and skill gained through an organized program of study and clinical experience recognized by the American College of Nurse Midwives (ACNM). (See Appendix E for a list of nurse-midwife programs.) Certification for entry into

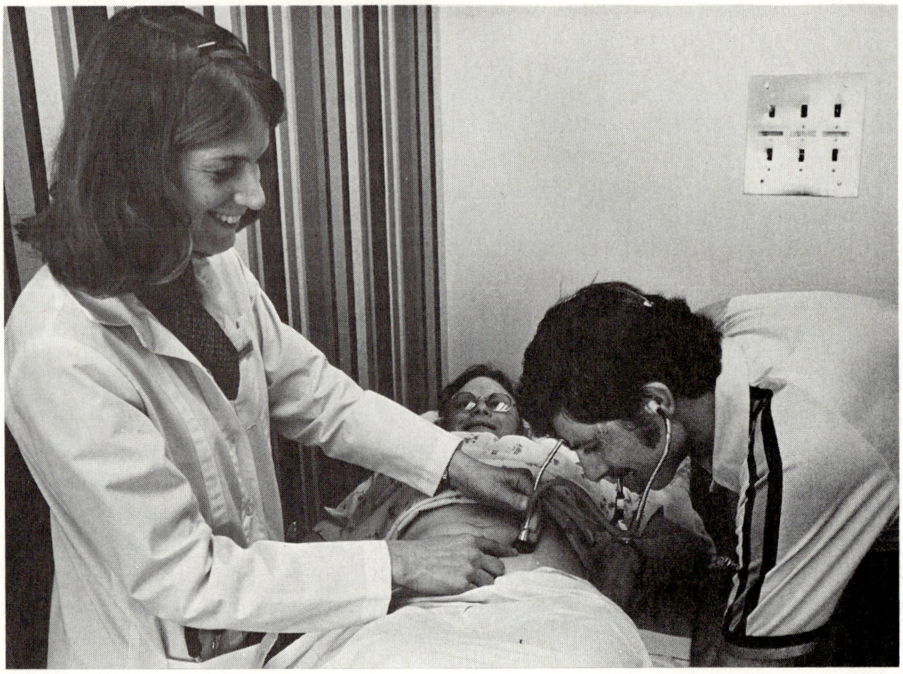

Fig. 2.1
Obstetric-gynecologic nurse-practitioner performs prenatal physical examinations. (Courtesy Stanford University Hospital.)

practice includes successful passage of a 6-hr essay examination and meeting other ACNM criteria. If certified as a nurse-midwife, individuals are able to use the designation CNM after their names. They are able to perform the tasks and care for the client in the same way as obstetric-gynecologic nurse practitioners, but their primary focus is in the area of management and care of mothers and babies throughout the maternity cycle (including delivery), so long as maternal progress meets criteria accepted as normal. The nurse-widwife is prepared to teach, interpret, and provide support as an integral part of services.

Many studies have shown client satisfaction in utilizing the nurse-midwife's service. Nurse-midwives' clients required less medication and had fewer low-forcep deliveries.

The issue of who should deliver the low-risk client does not arise out of clients' nonacceptance of the nurse-midwife or because of questionable competency but rather because legislative controls limit the practice. Some states have not yet changed their laws or codes to legitimize the nurse-midwife's practice and third-party payers such as Blue Cross do not cover the services.

In 1970 the American College of Obstetricians and Gynecologists (ACOG), the NAACOG, and the ACNM issued a joint statement that in "medically directed teams, qualified nurse-midwives may assume responsibility for the complete care and management of uncomplicated maternity patients." This position has opened the door to the increased use of nurse-midwives in North America. In a number of states in the United States that have not permitted the full functioning of these nurses, legislative bills are pending that will provide the necessary license to practice.

The professional role of the midwife as defined by the World Health Organization (1976) and amended by the Working Party on Midwifery Training in European Countries is as follows:

> A midwife is a person who is qualified to practice midwifery. She is trained to give the necessary care and advice to women during pregnancy, labor and the postnatal period, to conduct normal deliveries on her own responsibility and to care for the newly born infant. At all times she must be able to recognize the warning signs of abnormal or potentially abnormal conditions which necessitate referral to a doctor and to carry out emergency measures in the absence of a doctor. She may practice in hospitals, health units or domiciliary services. In any one of these situations she has an important task in health education with the family and the community.

Summary

Maternity care is a direct service to women and their families during childbearing and the childbearing phases of the life cycle. This service now provides care that is preventive, curative, and rehabilitative in nature. The maternity nurse assumes both traditional and new roles as she carries out the increased responsibilities such care engenders.

References and Readings

American Nurses' Association: Standards of maternal and child health nursing practice, Kansas City, Mo., 1973, The Association.

Barnard, K.: Infants at risk. Paper presented at the 1978 ANA Convention, Hawaii, 1978.

Barnard, K., and Neal, M.: Maternal-child nursing research: review of the past and strategies for the future, Nurs. Res. **26:**193, May-June 1977.

Barnes, F.E.F.: Ambulatory maternal health care and family planning services, Washington, D.C., 1978, American Public Health Association.

Beebe, J.E.: NERCEN. A prototype of regional education efforts in nurse-midwifery (education exchange), J.O.G.N. Nurs. **25**(3):22, 1980.

Bibb, B.N.: The effectiveness of nonphysician as providers of family planning services, J.O.G.N. Nurs. **88:**137, 1979.

Brook, C.: Social, economic and biologic correlates of infant mortality in city neighborhoods, J. Health Soc. Behav. **21**(1), March 1980.

Burst, H.: The American College of Nurse Midwives. A professional organization, J. Nurs. Midwife. **25**(1), Jan.-Feb. 1980.

Charles, A.G., et al.: Obstetric and psychoprophylactic preparation for childbirth, Am. J. Obstet. Gynecol. **131:**44, 1978.

Committee to Study Extended Roles for Nurses: Extending the scope of nursing practice: report to the Secretary of Health, Education, and Welfare, Nurs. Outlook **20:**46, 1972.

Doering, et al.: Modeling the quality of women's birth experience, J. Health Soc. Behav. **21**(1), March 1980.

Dillon, T.F.: Midwifery, Am. J. Obstet. Gynecol. **130:**917, 1978.

Edgil, A.: Moral problems in nursing practice, J.O.G.N. Nurs. **12**(3):210, 1983.

Everett, M.: Group work in the prenatal clinic, Health Soc. Work **5**(1), Feb. 1980.

Garfinkel, J., and Pratt, M.: Infant, maternal, and childhood mortality in the United States, 1968-1973, Washington, D.C., 1975, U.S. Department of Health, Education, and Welfare, Public Health Service, Health Services Administration, Bureau of Community Health Services.

Gruis, M.: Beyond maternity: postpartum concerns of mothers, M.C.N. **77:**182, May-June 1977.

Haire, D.: Improving the outcome of pregnancy through increased utilization of midwives, J.O.G.N. Nurs. **26**(11):5, 1981.

Hilliard, M.E.: New horizons in maternity care, Nurs. Outlook **15:**33, 1967.

Hunt, E.P.: Infant mortality and poverty areas, Wel. Rev. **5:**1, Aug.-Sept. 1967.

Manisoff, M.: Impact of family planning nurse practitioners, J.O.G.N. Nurs. **8**(2):73, March-April, 1979.

March of Dimes Birth Defects Foundation: Toward improving the outcome of pregnancy, recommendations for the regional development of maternal and perinatal health services, White Plains, N.Y., 1977, The Foundation.

Nurses' Association of the American College of Obstetrics and Gynecology: Standards for obstetric, gynecologic and neonatal nursing. The Nurses' Association of the American College of Obstetricians and Gynecologists, ed. 2, 1981.

Nurses' Association of the American College of Obstetrics and Gynecology: Certification's role in nursing (part 1), NAACOG Newsletter, vol. 9, no. 3, May/June 1982.

Naeye, R.L.: Causes of fetal and neonatal mortality by race in a selected U.S. population, Am. J. Pub. Health **69:**857, 1979.

Olsen, L.: Portrait of nurse-midwifery patients in a private practice, J. Nurs. Midwife. **24**(4) :10, July-Aug. 1979.

Roush, R.: The development of midwifery—male and female, yesterday and today, J.O.G.N. Nurs. **24**(3):27, May-June 1979.

Slatin, M.: Why mothers bypass prenatal care, Am. J. Nurs. **71:**1388, 1971.

Sprague, H.A., and Taylor, J.R.: The health impact of maternity and infant care programs. Report of Michigan Public Health Service, 1979.

Stainton, M.C.: Parent-infant interaction: putting theory into nursing practice, Calgary, Alta., 1981, The University of Calgary, Faculty of Nursing.

U.S. Department of Health, Education, and Welfare, Public Health Service, Health Services Administration: The maternity and infant care projects, Washington, D.C., 1975, The Department.

U.S. National Center for Health Statistics, U.S. Department of Commerce, Bureau of the Census, 1982.

World Health Organization: Improvement in infant and perinatal mortality in the United States, 1965-1973, Washington D.C., 1976, U.S. Department of Health, Education, and Welfare.

World Health Organization: Technical report series no. 331, Geneva, 1976, The Organization.

World Health Organization: Population statistics, household and family characteristics, March 1977, Washington, D.C., 1977, U.S. Department of Commerce, Bureau of the Census.

World Health Organization: The obstetric-gynecologic nurse practitioner, ACOG and NAACOG, Geneva, 1979, The Organization.

3

Maternity Nursing Process

- Assessment
  - Interview
    - Reason for client's request for care
    - Biographic data
    - Medical history
    - Reproductive history
    - Family history
    - Review of biopsychosocial systems
  - Physical examination
    - Observation
    - Palpation
    - Percussion
    - Auscultation
    - Laboratory tests
- Formulating the Nursing Diagnosis
- Planning
- Implementation
- Evaluation
- Recording Data
  - Nursing care plan
    - Flow sheets
    - Discharge summary
  - Problem-oriented record
    - Data base
    - Problem list
    - Initial plan
    - Progress notes
- Summary

Maternity nursing, in common with other branches of nursing, is a scientifically based, problem-solving process. If one examines the terms *scientifically based, problem solving,* and *process,* the implications of the above definition for maternity nursing become apparent.

Individuals *solve problems* in a number of ways: by intuition, by using traditional solutions, or by trial and error. Although these approaches have been used in maternity nursing, they are no longer adequate. Modern maternity nursing is very complex, based as it is on rapidly expanding fields of knowledge. Maternity nurses are performing more and more independent functions as nursing responsibilities are added, and maternity clients expect to participate as partners in their own care. These fundamental changes in the nature of maternity care have necessitated the use of a more precise and rational method of problem solving—the *scientific method.* Problem solving in maternity nursing now consists of five phases: assessment or data collection, formulation of a nursing diagnosis, planning, implementation, and evaluation of care.

A *process* by definition has a beginning and is constantly evolving as the condition progresses systematically from one stage to another toward an end point or goal. The word "process" is used in various contexts in medicine and nursing. Nurses speak of the inflammatory process, labor process, and developmental process. In nursing, the word "process" is also used in conjunction with problem solving, that is, the problem-solving process. The *nursing process* therefore has a *beginning* when individuals or groups of individuals seek assistance for an actual or potential health problem. It *progresses systematically* through the stages of assessing → diagnosing → planning → implementing → evaluating toward the *goal* of preventing illness, promoting and maintaining health, curing disease, or rehabilitating clients (Fig. 3.1).

The maternity nursing process follows this same pattern. Maternity nurses work within a specific area of health—the reproductive aspects of human sexuality. Therefore client problems and goals reflect this specific-

Fig. 3.1
Steps in the nursing process. (From Gordon, M.: Nurs. Clin. North Am. **14**[3]:492, 1979.)

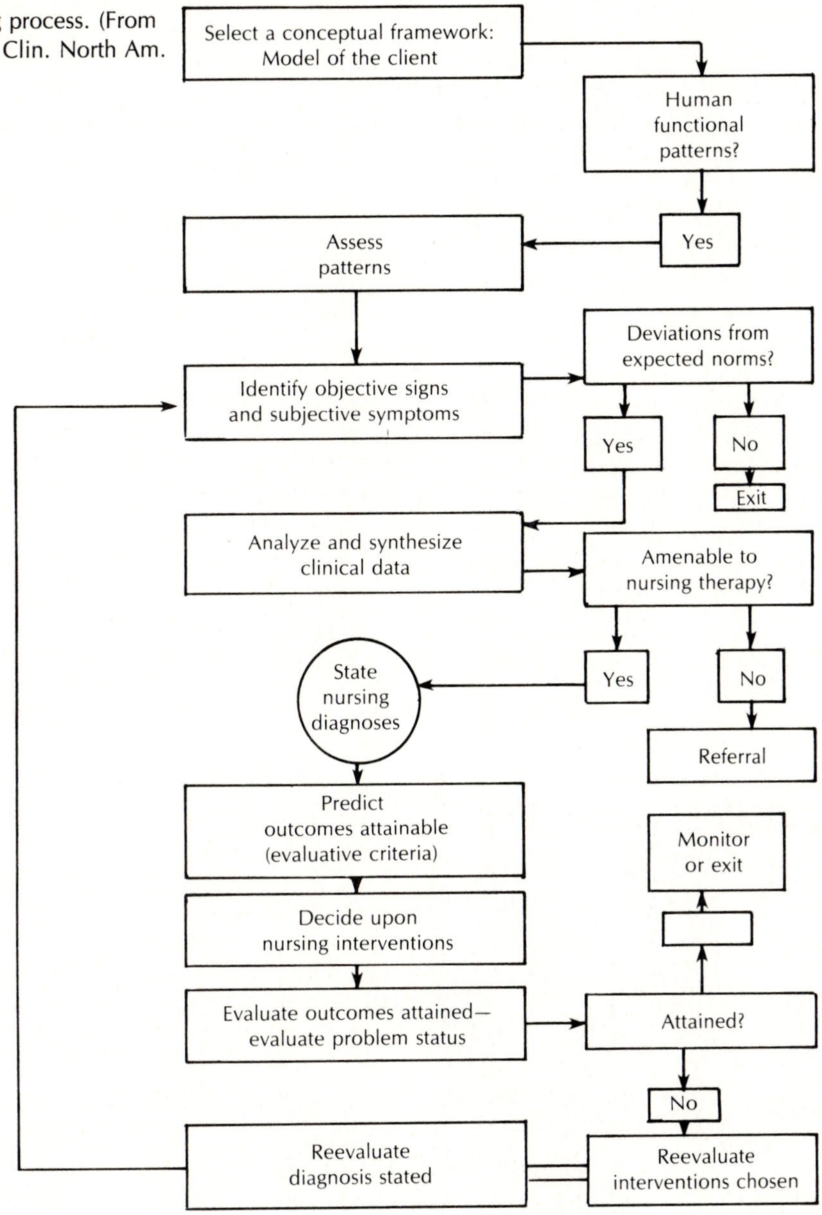

ity. For example, the maternity client may seek assistance for problems relating to family planning, pregnancy, or child care activities. The goals for care of the childbearing family are stated as follows:

1. *For the mother:* a safe and satisfying pregnancy, a normal birth, and a healthy infant
2. *For the infant:* an uncomplicated intrauterine existence and a satisfactory adjustment to extrauterine existence
3. *For the family:* a childbirth experience that promotes loving and concerned parenting for the child and enhances the personal growth of all individuals involved
4. *For the family:* a model of health care that promotes participation in future health maintenance

For ease of discussion the five stages of the maternity nursing process, that is, assessment, diagnosis, planning, implementation, and evaluation are reviewed separately. In reality all five stages may overlap or occur at the same time. They are interrelated and interdependent.

Assessment

An essential first step in the nursing process is the collection of sufficient data to serve as a basis for formulating nursing diagnoses. The primary source of data is the maternity client. The client provides information about her reasons for seeking health care, her medical and reproductive history, and her present health status. Other data sources are the client's health records and reports. The client's family and friends may provide information if this is acceptable to the client. If the client is a newborn, the parents act as the primary sources of information.

The data will include information from the biologic and psychosocial systems. Some of the data will be *subjective,* that is, information supplied by the client. Other data obtained by physical examination or laboratory tests will be *objective* (see Table 17.6). The data constitutes the client's health history. It is obtained through the interview, physical examination, and laboratory tests.

Fig. 3.2
Record keeping done concurrently with care.

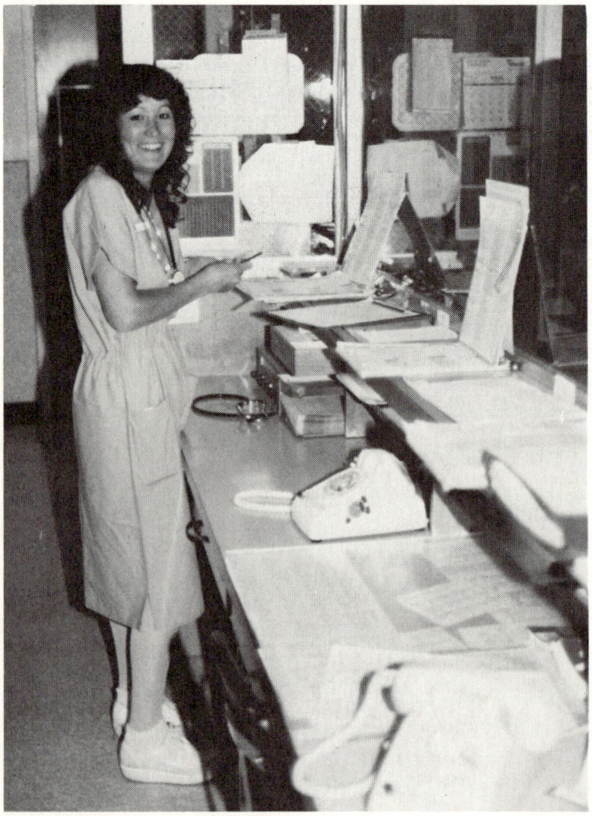

INTERVIEW

The interview is planned, purposeful communication that focuses on specific content. The initial assessment interview is usually the first contact between nurse and client; therefore at this time the nurse and client need to begin the process of establishing a therapeutic relationship. (See Chapter 4 for discussion of this process.)

The interview provides information about the client's biopsychosocial status. Although the format for interviewing or recording the client's health history will differ with agencies, the information obtained will include the following:

1. Reason for client's request for care
2. Biographic data
3. Medical history
4. Reproductive history
5. Family history
6. Review of psychosocial and biologic systems

Reason for client's request for care. The client's description of the purpose for the request for care is quoted verbatim in the record. For example, "I think I am pregnant," or "My legs get so swollen I can hardly walk." This statement does not constitute a diagnosis since the client's condition has to be confirmed by the nurse or physician before any care is instituted. The interviewer alerts other personnel to the "priority of need" as seen by the client by recording the chief purpose of a visit in the client's own words.

Biographic data. Biographic data includes the client's full name, address, phone number, and the same information about the nearest relative or friend to be called in case of emergency. Other information includes age, occupation, marital status, insurance coverage, and Social Security number.

This information is usually given freely, but the recorder may note inconsistency or evasiveness. Such reactions may indicate a need to reconfirm the information later. Some of this data, for example, a maternal age of 14 years or 45 years, will have a direct influence on the type of care planned for the client.

Medical history. The present health status of the client is assessed. Any past or current health problems are noted on the record. For example, it is important for the practitioner to know a pregnant woman is a diabetic or that the woman was exposed to rubella infection early in pregnancy, since either of these conditions can have an adverse effect on the developing fetus.

Reproductive history. The interviewer will record such information as the woman's menstrual history, sexual activity, and previous pregnancies and their outcomes. The information is basic to planning therapy for infertility or the choice of contraceptive measures. The conduct of a present pregnancy is predicated on the reports of previous pregnancies. For example, if a woman has a history of rapid labors she will be instructed to report to the nurse when her labor contractions begin. She will be admitted to the labor unit for close monitoring during labor at an earlier stage in the labor process than a woman who has had labors of average duration.

Family history. The family history provides information about the client's immediate family, parents, siblings, spouse, or children to identify familial, genetic, or environmental disorders or conditions that could have a bearing on the present health status of the client. For example, multiple ovulation resulting in twins is carried genetically by daughters of mothers of twins; if the client's mother had pregnancy-induced hypertension, the client may have a predisposition to develop this hypertensive condition during her pregnancy; or a sibling may have Down's syndrome, so the client's offspring would be carefully assessed for evidence of this condition.

Review of biopsychosocial systems

Biologic system. During the interview the client is questioned about physical symptoms. Most of the subjective data pertaining to the biologic system, however, is obtained during the physical examination. For example, while examining a woman's legs for the presence of edema, the practitioner would question the woman about any edema she has noticed, when it occurred, and what relieved it. Supplemental nutritional data may be obtained during the interview or by questionnaire before the physical examination is done (see Chapter 18).

Psychosocial system. The information collected as psychosocial data includes the following: the client's developmental age, a woman's acceptance or rejection of her pregnancy, the expectations of the woman and her family of what constitutes health care, situational factors (e.g., family's culture and socioeconomic status, availability of health resources) that may prove supportive or nonsupportive, and patterns of coping and interacting used by the client and her family that can act as assets or liabilities in her care.

Assessment of the psychosocial status of a client is often more difficult and complicated than that involved in assessing the physical health of the mother and fetus. It requires skill in communication and the ability to establish a trusting relationship. All persons possess areas of openness and privacy and at times resent the questioning of a stranger. For example, in assessing a family for the kind of support family members will provide a mother and her newborn, we need to know the following: Who can be supportive to this woman and her unborn baby at this time? What kinds of support are available? What changes might be attempted to produce the needed support now or in the future? What preparation is being made for the care of the infant once born? The nurse has to be tactful in obtaining this information. Some of the data will be obtained through direct questions during interviews and other data from (1) *observing* and noting relationships, attitudes, and stress responses; (2) *listening* to conversations about community and family involvements or hopes and aspirations; and (3) *being aware* of matters such as what persons have missed appointments or refused to utilize existing health care facilities. Nurses begin to collect this data during the initial interview. However, as nurse and client work together more data is revealed. Nurses can expect changes in the woman's outlook as pregnancy advances and the reality of parenthood comes closer.

PHYSICAL EXAMINATION

The physical examination includes an assessment of general body systems as well as the reproductive system. The response of the maternal organism to pregnancy involves all systems. The initial physical examination provides base lines for assessing whether the changes noted as pregnancy progresses are within the normal range (see Fig. 6.12). The examination begins with determining the client's temperature, pulse, respiration, and blood pressure. The examiner uses a formalized sequence of assessment (cephalocaudal) to prevent omitting any key information. The techniques used are observation, palpation, percussion, and auscultation. As the examination proceeds the examiner continues to question the client about pertinent symptoms.

Observation. The general inspection of the client begins with the first meeting and continues through the interview and physical examination. This provides an overall impression of the client's health status. The observations made are noted in the client's record. They include the following (Malasanos, 1981):

> apparent age; sex; race; body type (constitution), stature, and symmetry; weight and nutritional status; posture and motor activity; mental status; speech; general skin condition; apparent state of health and signs of distress or disorder. These are factors that are not limited to a single system of the body but are instead parameters for the total or whole person—the general appearance, head to toe.

Specific observations are made concerning the various body parts, for example, the os of the cervix changes from a circular opening in the woman who has never delivered an infant to one that has a slitlike appearance in the woman who has delivered one or more infants.

Palpation. By applying light pressure with the fingers over a body surface, the examiner can determine the condition of parts below the surface. For example, the examiner is able to determine the part of the fetus that will deliver first by palpating the uterus (see Fig. 20.24).

Percussion. The size, density, and position of an internal organ can be determined by tapping a part of the body with short sharp blows of the finger. The sound that is made changes in pitch as the fingers move from solid to less solid areas. The size and location of the woman's heart are checked in this way. The nurse uses this technique to assess fullness of the urinary bladder during labor.

Auscultation. Sounds produced within the body can be heard with the unaided ear or by using an instrument. The fetal heartbeat can be heard as early as the twentieth week of pregnancy by using a fetoscope (see Fig. 17.2).

Laboratory tests. Laboratory tests are used to establish base line data and to monitor the health of the mother and fetus. Examples of laboratory tests used in the assessment of the pregnant woman and her fetus are routine urinalysis to detect the presence of protein and sonography to estimate fetal age.

Formulating the Nursing Diagnosis

Once the data has been collected the information that pertains to a particular area is grouped together or categorized.* By doing this it becomes easier to distinguish problems. For example, does the problem relate to a family or to a previous pregnancy? By categorizing the data into separate areas, such as reproductive history or personal profile, it becomes easier to distinguish problems that are independent or interrelated. The data below illustrates this.

Physical Examination	Personal Profile
Assessment confirms pregnancy of 20 weeks duration, mother's health excellent.	Client states husband will be stationed overseas at time of delivery.

The data under Physical Examination would lead to continuing the assessment and care routine to normal pregnancy. The data under Personal Profile, however, would prompt nurse and client to explore what other supportive people could be present at the delivery. These sets of data indicate differing client needs. Another example from a client's history is as follows:

Biographic Data	Personal Profile
Recently divorced, living by self with children ages 2, 4, and 5 years. Home 1 mile beyond bus line, no other transportation.	Client missed appointment.

In the above instance the nurse would work with the apparent interrelatedness of the categories of data to assist with solving the client's inability to comply with prenatal care.

After the data have been categorized the findings can be compared to norms of what should or could be and conclusions drawn about the significance of similarities or differences (Bailey and Claus, 1975). If nurses feel their conclusions indicate significant differences from the norm, they infer that a client may have a health problem that they can assist in solving. For example, in the following situation the nurse compares the findings with the norm:

■ Anna P. brings her 4-week-old son to the clinic because he has a rash on his buttocks. Anna is 18, living with her husband, also 18 years, in his family home. The nurse observes Anna handling the infant as she undresses him. She does not look at her baby's face or talk to him. She drags the T-shirt over his head with rough, jerky movements. When she is removing the diaper he defecates. She grimaces and holds her nose and wipes him roughly with another diaper. She tells him to "shush" when he cries.

Norm	Present Findings
By 4 weeks mother maintains eye contact and talks to infant. Is reasonably skilled in child care activities.	Avoids eye contact; no loving talk; handles child roughly; is upset with child's excretions.
Accepts feces odor of own child as normal.	
Uses gentle touch, comforts child when hurt or frightened.	

By comparing the *norm* with *what actually is* the nurse can identify the client's problem, in this case, "alterations in parenting." In other words the nurse makes a nursing diagnosis. Nursing diagnoses are concise statements describing a potential or actual state of a client, "which nurses by virtue of their education and experience are capable and licensed to treat" (Campbell, 1978).

Once a nursing diagnosis has been made it needs to

*Format used for nursing diagnoses from Kim, M., and Moritz, D., editors: Proceedings of the 3rd and 4th National Conferences, Classification of Nursing Diagnoses, New York, 1981, McGraw-Hill Book Co.

be validated by the client. The validation is essential if nurse and client are to work together to resolve a client's problem. The problem may be overt or covert, existing or potential. If more than one problem is present, the nurse ranks the problems in order of importance.

The following example illustrates this phase of the nursing process, that is, analysis of data leading to a nursing diagnosis and validation of the diagnosis with the client:

■ Mary L., a 20-year-old, delivered her first child 24 hours ago. The nurse assigned to Mary's care is making rounds to assist her clients with feeding their infants. She finds Mary flushed, the muscles of her face and hands tensed. Her baby cries and stiffens his body every time she puts him to breast. The nurse infers that Mary, a new mother, is highly anxious about her inability to breast feed her infant and her anxiety has been picked up by her infant. The nurse puts her arm around Mary's shoulders and says, "Sometimes it is hard to get babies to start breast feeding. It can make you anxious and worried." Mary started crying and said, "I'll never be able to do it and he'll starve."

Pertinent data: first baby, infant 24 hours old, mother's appearance (face flushed, muscles tense), infant tensing and crying when held to breast.

Nursing diagnoses:

1. Disturbance in self-concept because of inability to breast feed and provide nourishment for her baby
2. Potential problem with infant's nutritional intake

Validation: Mother confirms the nurse's statement

Knowledge base: The nurse's knowledge includes the following:

1. Maternal milk supply comes in 48 to 72 hours after delivery
2. Infant has fluid reserve up to 10% of birth weight
3. Some infants need assistance in learning how to suckle
4. Mother's anxiety is contagious; her tense hands convey feelings to infant
5. Infant's behavior, tensing body, is normal in a newborn when frustrated
6. The let-down reflex can be inhibited by maternal anxiety
7. The long-term nutritional intake of the infant depends on a relaxed mother and child

Nursing diagnoses, statements concerning client problems, generate nursing actions. The nurse incorporates the nursing actions into a plan for nursing care.

Planning

Determining the *goal* for nursing actions is an essential part of any nursing plan. If it is feasible, the goal for therapy is devised mutually by nurse and client. On some occasions this is not possible (the client is a newborn or unconscious), and the nurse must assume responsibility for clarifying the objectives of care. Once the goal has been established the nurse needs to state the criteria used to measure progress toward a goal. The criteria are stated objectively and specifically as possible so they can be used as evaluative criteria.

For example, one of the *goals* for successful transition of the neonate from intrauterine to extrauterine existence is that the neonate establishes and maintains respirations. The *evaluative criteria* used are as follows: airway is open and respirations stabilized at 40 to 60 breaths/min; breathing is quiet (no grunting or wheezing); chest and abdomen rise and fall in synchronized motion with no sternal retraction; and color indicates adequate oxygenation.

Implementation

Nursing actions used to attain the goals of care include activities from three main areas: assessment strategies, therapeutic measures, and educational measures.

Assessment strategies are used to continue the process of data collection; for example, the nurse continues to assess a woman's blood pressure every time she comes for prenatal evaluation. By doing so the nurse confirms the woman's continued healthy state, or should the woman's blood pressure rise significantly the nurse could institute therapy to control the condition. Assessment strategies are used to confirm progress toward the goal as well as accumulate additional data as a basis for modification of the care plan.

Therapeutic measures are those measures a nurse uses to provide for treatment of a condition or for comfort. For example, if a woman develops a breast abscess the nurse would administer the antibiotic medication prescribed by the woman's physician and fit her with a supportive brassiere to lessen the discomfort.

Educational measures include nursing activities that prevent complications or promote a healthy state through consumer education. These measures also provide clients with the reasons or rationale for a particular nursing intervention. Clients who understand why nurses are doing certain things tend to be more cooperative in participating in their own care and assuming responsibilities.

Nursing actions are *selected* on the basis of anticipated effectiveness, the amount of risk involved for the client, and the availability of health resources, facilities, and personnel. Nursing actions are *instituted* on the basis of priority. For example, to encourage the attachment process between mother and child (goal), the newborn infant is given to the mother to hold (therapeutic measure). Suddenly the nurse notes that the infant is becoming dusky in color and his respirations are grunting in nature. Based on this evaluation (assessment strategy = new nursing diagnosis), the nurse's goal is now to reestablish and maintain respirations. The infant is placed in a warmed environment and resuscitation is initiated (therapeutic measures). The rationale for these actions is shared with the mother, and she is kept informed on her infant's progress (educational measures).

Evaluation

Evaluation on an ongoing basis is essential if nursing actions are to be relevant to the client's changing physical and psychologic status. The evaluative criteria can be used to assess progress toward, as well as attainment of, the goal (see Table 17.11).

Recording Data

Communication, both written and verbal, among health team members is essential to provide holistic care for maternity clients. In the past much of the information about a client that served as a basis for individualizing care was passed verbally from one group of health workers to the next. Often the information became distorted or lost. Cooperative planning between health professionals and between health professional and client was minimal, fragmented, and rarely recorded. The disjointed nature of providing "total" care is exemplified in the traditional format of client record. Each professional recorded his or her findings in a separate section of the record. The information provided by nurses was limited; such statements as "a good day" or "slept well" were frequently noted. Although nurses were held responsible for the care given, the "nurses' notes" provided little incentive for them to initiate nursing care based on the nursing process. Today many health care facilities have instituted a form of the nursing care plan or problem-oriented records.

NURSING CARE PLAN

The nursing care plan reflects the nursing process. There is space for recording collection of data, predicted outcomes, and nursing intervention. Certain difficulties with the use of nursing care plans have become evident in maternity care. To be effective, nursing care plans must be kept up-to-date. This consistent review and revision can be very time consuming. The nursing care plan is often part of the Kardex and as such is written in pencil and not considered part of the client's permanent record. Successful or unsuccessful nursing strategies are therefore not available for future review. In some areas, for example, the postdelivery unit for normal pregnancy, the similarity of the details of care for all clients, and the rapid turnover of clients may result in a stereotyping of plans for care. Nursing care may become routine, rather than individualized for a particular client.

Flow sheets. Flow sheets used in conjunction with the nurse's narrative notes are an excellent way to follow the course of a health or disease process. They may be used to record the results of monitoring potential problems, for example, fluctuations in blood pressure; they may be used for rapidly changing states as during progress in labor; or they may be used for expected changes in postdelivery recovery of the mother or growth of the infant, for example, the postpartum record or nursery record. Flow sheets can be used in lieu of narrative progress notes, but a summary of change, stability, or progress should appear periodically in narrative form. The flow sheet readily reveals relationships between many variables and indicates the client's progress at a glance.

Discharge summary. The focus is on providing for continuity of care and an overall assessment of accomplishments of hospitalization or care given. The summary should include proposed follow-up, and any prescribed regimen should be spelled out in detail. Consultations are requested in reference to a specific problem, but it is essential that the consultant is aware of all the client's problems so as to avoid treatment out of context.

PROBLEM-ORIENTED RECORD

The problem-oriented record (POR), a method of improving client care through a system of compiling and using medical-related data, was devised by Weed (1969, 1970). It is essentially a problem-solving process. The management of care is based on a succinct list of client problems derived from a data base. By prior identification of client problems, no one problem is treated out of context or in direct opposition to other problems. The components of the POR are the data base, problem list, initial plan, and progress notes. These components are analogous to the components in the nursing process.

Data base. The data base encompasses the sum total of all information gathered about any one client on admission. Included in the data base are the client's history, present medical and nursing history, personal and psychosocial history, family history, physical examination and review of systems, laboratory findings, and client profile. The client profile is a brief narrative about the client's life-style and that of the family. The data base is akin to the assessment phase or data collection phase of the nursing process.

Problem list. The information collected must be scrutinized and condensed to synthesize a problem list. Conclusions as to the nature of problems are supported by the information accumulated in the data base. The data base continues to grow as more information is added, and it is out of the data base that problems continue to emerge. Deriving a problem list resembles the process of formulating nursing diagnoses.

Initial plan. The initial plan contains the proposed actions to be taken in relation to the problem. It establishes the need for further data and type of therapy to be used (see box). This portion of the POR incorporates parts of both the diagnostic phase and the implementation phase of the nursing process. The format used in recording the initial and subsequent plans is divided into four sections: subjective data, objective data, assessment, and plan. The acronym SOAP has proved a useful reminder of the four sections. *Subjective* refers to the problem from the client's point of view. *Objective* data includes findings by an examiner and laboratory data. The *assessment* is the conclusion that one reaches after analyzing the subjective and objective findings. Assessment may connote progression or regression in relation to the problem. The *plan* signifies in detail the course to be followed regarding the problem. This aspect is written as a threefold plan containing three elements: diagnostic plans, therapeutic plans, and plans for client education. In this text these three elements are called assessment strategies, therapeutic measures, and educational measures.

Initial Plan for Problem 3: Nausea and Vomiting*

S Comes on early in morning on rising and late in afternoon. Cannot face making dinner. Embarrassed at work by nausea.

O
1. Pregnancy of 8 weeks' duration.
2. No history of flu or contact with persons with stomach upsets.
3. Bouts daily and intermittent.
4. Temperature normal.
5. Pulse: 80/min.
6. Blood pressure: 110/80.
7. No proteinuria or glycosuria.

A Nausea and vomiting associated with early pregnancy.

P Instruct woman concerning following:
1. Probable cause: normal response to pregnancy; may be expected to last about 4 more weeks (educational measure).
2. Diet: small frequent feedings, some carbohydrates (e.g., crackers and milk) before rising and as afternoon snack (therapeutic measure).
3. Motion: Discuss ways of rising slowly to minimize sudden hypotension (therapeutic measure).
4. Telephone progress report in 1 week's time (assessment strategy).

*Excerpt from client's prenatal record.

Progress notes. Progress notes constitute the follow-up phase of the problem-oriented record. Progress notes include narrative notes, the flow sheet, and the discharge summary. Each narrative note refers directly to a problem and is titled accordingly. The format is the same as the initial plan. The narrative note describes the progress of the client in relation to a specific problem and represents the evaluative phase of the nursing process (see box). Flow sheets are used in the same manner as in other records. The general format for the discharge summary is problem oriented and includes all problems listed on the problem list.

Progress Notes for Problem 3: Nausea and Vomiting*

S No nausea for 10 days; feels well.
O 1. Pregnancy of 14 weeks' duration.
2. Appearance healthy; skin: good turgor.
3. Temperature: 96.6° F (37° C).
4. Pulse: 78/min.
5. Blood pressure: 105/80.
6. No proteinuria or glycosuria.
A Recovered from nausea and vomiting of early pregnancy (problem resolved).
P No further actions needed.

*Excerpt from client's prenatal record.

The problem-oriented system acts as a tool for quality control of medical and nursing care since documentary proof regarding client problems is now readily available. Health personnel become directly accountable to the client for the quality of care rendered.

Summary

The maternity nursing process is a scientifically based, problem solving process. It involves assessment of the client's biopsychosocial system, formulation of nursing diagnoses, planning and implementing nursing therapy, and evaluation of the results of therapy and of the process itself. All pertinent information obtained at each contact with the client must be recorded in such a way as to ensure that each member of the health team can contribute to continuity of client care.

Maternity clients represent typical consumers of health care services in that they are now more aware of what constitutes quality health care and more likely to demand greater accountability of the health care team. Concurrent with this attitude toward accountability, in certain states clients have the right to full and complete disclosure of the medical records documenting their care.

References and Readings

Ademoware, A.S., and Meyers, E.: Use of the problem-oriented record by nursing care for high-risk antepartum patients, J.O.G.N. Nurs. **6**:17, 1977.
Bailey, J., and Claus, K.: Decision making in nursing, St. Louis, 1975, The C.V. Mosby Co.
Bower, F.: The process of planning nursing care, ed. 3, St. Louis, 1981, The C.V. Mosby Co.
Bower, F., and Bevis, E.: Fundamentals of nursing practice, St. Louis, 1979, The C.V. Mosby Co.
Campbell, C.: Nursing diagnosis and intervention in nursing practice, New York, 1978, John Wiley & Sons, Inc.
Connolly, M.L.: Organize your workday—for more effective discharge planning, Nurs. '81, **2**(7):44, 1981.
Dossey, B., and Guzzetta, C.: Nursing diagnoses, Nurs. '81, **2**(6):34, 1981.
Field, L.: The implementation of nursing diagnosis in clinical practice, Nurs. Clin. North Am. **14**:497, Sept. 1979.
Ford, J.A., et al: Applied decision making for nurses, St. Louis, 1979, the C.V. Mosby Co.
Kim, M., and Moritz, D., editors: Proceedings of the 3rd and 4th National Conferences, Classification of Nursing Diagnoses, New York, 1981, McGraw-Hill Book Co.
Malasanos, L., et al.: Health assessments, St. Louis, 1981, The C.V. Mosby Co.
Matson, H.N.: Values, how and where, Nurs. Dig., p. 46, Sept. 1974.
Popkess, S.: Diagnosing your patient's strengths, Nurs. '81 **2**(7):34, 1981.
Price, M.: Nursing diagnosis: making a concept come alive. Am. J. Nurs. **80**:668, April 1980.
Shoemaker, J.: How nursing diagnosis helps focus your care, R.N., p. 42, Aug. 1979.
Vasey, E.K.: Writing your patients' care plan efficiently, NSG **9**(4):64-71, 1979.
Weed, L.: Medical records, medical education, and patient care, Chicago, 1969, Year Book Medical Publishers, Inc.
Weed, L.: Medical records, medical education and patient care: the P-O record as a basic tool, Chicago, 1970, Year Book Medical Publishers, Inc.
Wiley, L.: The nursing care plan. A communication system that really works, Nurs. '78, **8**:28, 1978.

4

Maternity Nurse-Client Relationships

- Essential Factors
  - Communication
    - Techniques
    - Language
    - Space
    - Touch
    - Voice
    - Eye contact
    - Time
  - Self-awareness
    - Concept of social role
    - Self-concept
    - Values clarification
  - Decision-making process
  - Personal characteristics
    - Trust
    - Empathy
    - Setting mutual goals
- Process of Nurse-Client Relationship
  - Preparatory phase
  - Initiation phase
  - Consolidation and growth phase
  - Termination phase
- Summary

Developing a relationship between nurse and client is a dynamic process. The interpersonal relationship is characterized by growth between individuals who respect each other's differences and uniqueness. It requires openness with each other and genuine respect.

The interpersonal relationship that takes place between nurse and client, the nurse-client relationship, is a process in that it has a goal and evolves sequentially through phases toward that goal. The goal is to better the health of the client through assisting the client with learning, coping, and adapting. The phases of the process are the preparatory phase, initiation phase, consolidation and growth phase, and termination phase. Each phase accomplishes certain tasks and builds on a previous phase or phases.

As professional people with interpersonal skills, nurses act as leaders to begin and maintain nurse-client relationships. To do this the nurse needs to develop skill in communicating, more awareness of how personal values affect nursing performance, and ability to make and help others make logical decisions. In addition to possessing these skills, research demonstrates that the nurse who is most successful in interpersonal relationships is one with certain characteristics; that is, the nurse is able to establish a trust relationship, empathize with a client, and develop mutually acceptable goals and therapy for care. These skills and abilities are essential factors to the process of nurse-client relationships.

Essential Factors

COMMUNICATION

Communication is central to the nurse-client relationship. The communication process includes verbal and written messages as well as nonverbal behavior. Every aspect of our lives conveys information about ourselves to others. For example, such different entities as the way persons dress, their behavior and speech patterns, where they were born, their church affiliations, and their choice of magazines are interpreted by an onlooker and value judgments made. Every culture sets up an entire repertoire of communication patterns, most of which are acquired by members of that culture as a result of mingling with various social groups and informally learning these patterns. The failure on the part of a stranger to the culture to recognize these communication patterns and operate within their context can lead to misunderstandings and the inability to carry on meaningful exchanges.

Techniques. Certain communication techniques have proven successful as tools for strengthening therapeutic relationships. To become skilled in their use requires considerable practice. At first they may seem cumbersome or obvious. However, gradually they become part of the nurse's communication pattern and as such are useful in establishing the *meaning* of what one hears or says.

1. *Listening* is an active not a passive activity. It takes effort to hear what another says, interpret, and analyze its meaning. The nurse has to concentrate on the speaker, not herself or himself. Sometimes something a client says will trigger ideas or remind the nurse of a problem. Only practice will help the nurse cope with these interruptions to true listening. Listening is a sign of respect for another and acts as a powerful reinforcer.

2. *Broad opening statements* give the client an opportunity to select the topic for discussion. "What" questions can be helpful; for example, "What are you thinking about?" or "What were you able to do about . . . ?" "Why" questions tend to make a client defensive; for example, "Why did you miss last week's appointment?" Closed questions that can be answered "yes" or "no" are avoided if the nurse is trying to find out what something means to a client. To gather biographic data the nurse would ask, "Are you single, married, or divorced?" A simple "yes" or "no" to these questions is sufficient. If the nurse is trying to discover the meaning to the client of being married or not, a question such as, "It is hard to be on your own just now; how are you managing?" would be more effective.

3. *Focusing* assists the client in identifying and expanding an area of importance. The nurse can encourage the client to describe how she perceives an event or to compare a present response with a similar one experienced in the past. The nurse can also bring the primary problem into focus by developing a time frame for a sequence of events. The following example illustrates this technique:

Patricia L., aged 14 years, came to the nurse in the clinic because she thought she was pregnant. During the interview with the nurse, Patricia gave a rambling report about how she loved her boyfriend, about her parents' angry divorce, and how they blamed everything on her. The nurse said, "Let me see if I can get the time worked out. Your parents got a divorce and you feel they blame you. You have a loving boyfriend, you had intercourse and now you feel you are pregnant. Let's talk about the possibility of your being pregnant first and then we will go back to the others."

The nurse needs to be sensitive to a client's reluctance to discuss certain ideas or feelings and respect the need for privacy. When the bond between the nurse and client is stronger, the nurse can return to the topic.

4. *Clarification* occurs when the nurse attempts to elicit the *meaning* of what the client is saying. Often the client will find it difficult to express emotional responses in other than a hesitant or fragmentary manner. The nurse needs to help the client clarify feelings as a first step in the client's recognition of the correlation between thought and action. Statements such as "Did you mean. . .?" or "I can't quite follow you. Are you saying. . . ?" are helpful.

5. *Restating* is the repetition of a client's main thought or concern. Restating focuses attention on a thought that may otherwise be treated as trivial. It indicates also that the nurse is listening attentively as the following example shows:

Marie talked to the nurse about her concerns over taking care of the baby. She said she had no experience with children as she had been an only child. Her mother found the care of one child enough and hadn't had any more. Marie said she was like her mother in so many ways, people often thought they were sisters. She wanted the home care nurse to come and check on how she was doing.

The nurse commented, "You said you were like your mother *(restating)*. Did you mean you were like your mother in finding the care of a baby difficult *(clarification)*?"

6. *Validation* of what is said and its meaning to the client conveys the nurse's understanding of not only content but also the feelings the client has about what is being said. If the nurse can reflect this accurately the client senses the nurse's empathy, interest, and respect.

Client: I hate having to wear maternity clothes. It makes it so obvious you are pregnant. People treat you so differently, as though you weren't attractive anymore, just a dowdy old housewife.

Nurse: It is hard to see one's figure change—hard to get used to—it can make a person feel quite different about herself *(validation)*.

The information the nurse gains from interviews or discussions with clients forms an important part of the data used to plan nursing care. The professional nurse assumes responsibility for obtaining data that is both pertinent and verifiable. The techniques discussed above assist the nurse to attain this end.

Other aspects of communication can affect the quality of the data nurses obtain from clients and add to or detract from the effectiveness of the interpersonal relationship; these include the *language* used, the way *space* is used, and the meaning attributed to *touch, voice,* and *time*.

Language. The social or lay language of any culture contains elements that are known and recognized by all who speak it. Each subgroup, however, develops a language of its own. Subgroups may be determined by ethnic origin, age, or profession. The nurse speaks a number of languages. A professional language is learned as part of being initiated into the nursing group. For transactions between colleagues, a professional language provides for a precise, meaningful exchange of information. Between nurse and client it can serve the same purpose if the client has the requisite background. If the client has not been schooled in medical terminology, use of the professional language may mean that the nurse is unable to translate medical ideas into the social language familiar to another individual. Many clients in maternity nursing will not have attended prenatal classes so the nurse will have to translate terms such as dilation and effacement of the cervix or involution of the uterus. The nurse working with teenagers in a family planning clinic needs to be aware of the social terms used for sexual intercourse, because some people do not know and do not use the medical terms for genital organs. Unless the information given is couched in familiar language and feedback for mutual understanding is sought *(validation)*, much of what is said is either unclear or lost.

Various ethnic groups in the United States use their own language in the greater part of their daily living, and their knowledge of English may be limited. After being in North America for a few years, a hybrid language develops that is part original language and part English; frequently the terms relating to medical care become part of the graft. In a prenatal clinic in a predominantly Mexican-American community, the pamphlets relating to care were written in Castillian Spanish. Unfortunately the people spoke a mixture of Spanish and English (''Spanglish'' as one nurse described it), and the information was therefore still not available to them.

Language may also be used defensively. Nurses who maintain a joking relationship with clients regardless of the client's condition and thereby call forth a similar response on the part of clients may be acting to defend themselves against the hurt and weight of involvement in the pain of others. Using language as a defense mechanism is often an unconscious act, the nurse is unaware of why she or he behaves in such a manner.

Space. Various cultural groups use space in well-defined ways, for example, research has shown that middle-class Americans use the space between communicators in specific ways. There are definite distances used to connote varying interpersonal relationships, and the voice range and tone, the topic discussed, and the body language employed are specific for each range (Table 4.1).

Such findings have many implications for nursing. Nursing activities, particularly those of the intrusive type, are carried out within the intimate distance, indicating personal involvement. At times the nurse uses the cultural connotation of space as an advantage as this report illustrates:

> I observed R.A., the nurse in the delivery area, instruct a woman how to bear down with a contraction. R.A. placed her face close to that of the woman, spoke softly and gently, and had the full attention and cooperation of the woman, who appeared trusting of this comforting and protective person.

At other times the nurse does not wish to convey other than professional concern and therefore uses various techniques to indicate the impersonal nature of the activity. For example, when performing a vaginal examination, the nurse gives the purpose of the procedure before beginning and then uses a definite body set; the face becomes impassive and preoccupied, the touch firm but gentle and precise, and the eyes directed away from the client's eyes. This body set accomplishes two objectives. It permits the nurse to concentrate thought processes on what is being palpated by eliminating distracting stimuli. By breaking eye contact with the client, the nurse moves the action from an intimate to an impersonal space range.

Frequently the nurse consciously or unconsciously violates the norms of distance to prevent true communication with clients. The nurse pauses at the doorway and calls, ''How goes it?'' The reply is usually noncommmittal. An individual is unable to discuss personal matters in a public distance range and may feel frustrated at being placed in this unsuitable position.

Another example of the use of space is the procedure adopted in a physician's or midwife's office. Once an examination is completed, the woman is given time to dress and is then seated in a chair by the practitioner's desk. The pattern of intimate distance is broken and one of personal distance established, wherein personal matters may be discussed in a soft voice while maintaining eye contact. A feeling that the practitioner has a warm and friendly interest in the client as well as a professional one, is conveyed.

Another aspect of space is the idea of territoriality.

Table 4.1
Communication—Space, Voice, Touch and Eye Contact—and Common Violations

Topic	Space	Tone of Voice
Secret or sensitive information exchanged with client (e.g., positive VDRL); comforting parents whose infant has a defect; emotional reponses of parents as they hold and admire child and express their love for child or each other	Intimate (3-18 in) Message: I accept you; I want to help you; I love you	Low, soft murmur
Report of health status; coaching during labor; assisting with feeding an infant; explanations of care; reports to other staff	Personal (1½-4 ft) Message: concern, warmth, friendliness	Soft, clear, concise
Small group teaching of health care topics; discussions with parents in shared accommodation	Social (4-12 ft) Message: I like you; let us share this time	Louder, more definite, more formal
Lecture topics: sanitation, health insurance, positions during labor	Public (over 12 ft) Message: I have information for you	Loud, clear; may be used dramatically

This has been called *personal space.* It moves with the individual, with the body as its center. Violations of this personal space arouse defensive reponses, either covert or overt. Formerly the allocation of space in a delivery room was illustrative of this. The pregnant woman, nurse, and physician had their appointed spots, and if others moved into these areas, they were subtly or openly asked to move. The nurse's territory consisted of the head of the delivery table, the worktable, and the cupboards. The physician's territory was the area at the foot of the delivery table bounded by the instrument table and sterile solution basin. The receiving crib for the infant was the nurse's territory unless medical intervention was necessary, in which case it was shared by the physician and the nurse.

When the father was introduced into the delivery room, decisions had to be made as to just what territory he was to occupy. It could not be on the periphery (the traditional neutral area into which most observers are placed), since the goal was to promote a closeness between father-to-be and mother-to-be. In most units the father is seated near the head of the table and is expected to remain there. Freedom to move about is not often permitted. All these space assignments may have a rational basis, but once assigned they become territories to be defended.

A third aspect of space is the way it is utilized. In North America the outer areas of a room are traditionally used for sitting, leaving the center clear for activity. The pattern is found in clinic waiting rooms. From a psychologic point of view, grouping of chairs or even single chairs would better answer the client's need to group together or to be alone, but the normative pattern persists. If clients change the chair arrangement of their own accord, the personnel often become uneasy and make comments regarding the liberties some will take—the message against nonconformity has been communicated.

Touch. Touch is an important component of communication. On a social level people use touch to convey various messages about liking or disliking another person. Most people respect a firm handshake but are angered by a crushing one. People may hug friends but are offended if strangers press against them in an elevator. In person-to-person contacts with clients nurses can touch therapeutically as a technique to indicate caring; as an assessment technique, for example, palpating the uterus; and as a part of nursing interventions such as bathing clients or giving injections. If mothers are observed caring for their firstborn, they begin by using a tentative fingertip touch and as they become more secure in their role, they use the whole hand to support or manipulate the infant. Nurses teach parents safe methods to hold their infants that give the child a feeling of security (See Fig. 29.4). Touch can transcend cultural barriers. Even though the nurse may not speak a client's language she can express concern through holding the client's hand or stroking her brow. The importance of touch as nonverbal communication means the nurse has to be aware of how touch may indicate distaste for another. Nurses may avoid touching people they dislike or touch them as little as possible. When giving them nursing care the hand is held stiffly instead of curving or abrasive pressure is used rather than a caress. The recipients readily interpret the message, "I am distasteful to this person, she does not wish to be near me." These messages can interfere with the therapy being given.

Voice. Tone or rate, rhythm, and intensity of the voice are other critical elements in communicating with other persons: parents croon to their infants, mothers and fathers talk in high-pitched voices when alerting a

Touch and Eye Contact	Common Violations
Nurse establishes eye contact with client; sits close to client in *en face* position; touches client (e.g., put arm around shoulder); parents stroke, caress, kiss infant or each other	Condition of infant reported while standing at foot of mother's bed; sensitive information given out in loud voice during report at change of shift; healthy infants separated from parents before intimacy can take place
Eye contact maintained; nurse leans toward client; client discusses care with family; touch is with relaxed hand, gentle sure movements	Walks away from client while giving instructions; hurried, abrupt movements; voice loud, can be overheard by other clients, scolding tone; touch jerky, with flat of hand, poking with fingertips, grasps too firmly
May stand or sit; eye contact maintained while talking; body gestures expansive, more formalized	Mumbling explanations; talking to one of a group only; gestures too unrestrained, "comes on too strong"; shouts instructions, greetings
Gestures exaggerated to be seen (e.g., arms flung out); eye contact moves over whole audience	Using models, etc., that can be seen only by those in the front row; ignoring questions; staff shouting to each other in hospital corridors

newborn, and a nurse repeats instructions in a calm, gentle tone. These uses of voice tone convey love and acceptance. Conversely, talking loudly or mumbling, speaking rapidly or hesitantly, convey negative messages. Nurses sometimes speak loudly to clients who do not speak English; unfortunately, not only do they not help the client comprehend, but they appear angry as well as incomprehensible to the client.

Eye contact. Eye contact is considered an important factor in establishing parent-child relationships (see Chapter 32). It also has cultural connotations. Some ethnic groups expect eye contact on first meeting another and during conversations. If eye contact is avoided, an uneasiness develops. The avoidance may be interpreted in a number of ways; for example, "She's not telling me the truth" or "I'm not worth being looked at." Other ethnic groups may avert their eyes when introduced as a token of respect or avoid looking at a new baby if unable to touch the baby also (evil eye). As nurses we need to clarify our concepts of eye contact and validate the concepts with members of differing ethnic groups.

Touch, tone of voice, eye contact, and space, if used thoughtfully, can do much to promote a nurse-client relationship (Table 4.1).

Time. Another element in nonverbal commmunication is time, its meaning and use. Many aspects of North American culture are related to time. Appointments are made at definite times, and although a little leeway is allowed, the person is expected to be on time and, conversely, does not expect to be kept waiting. To be kept waiting is interpreted as a slight, as an indication that one is of an inferior status. This can be particularly enraging if individuals suspect that there may be reasons to assume others are downgrading their status. Frequently one sees such reactions in government-sponsored health clinics, where clients suspect that the personnel are looking down on them as charity cases.

Clients who do not keep appointments are assumed to be shiftless and unconcerned. One of us (M.J.) visited an Indian village on the west coast of British Columbia to carry out a previously planned immunization program. Only a few older residents were found there; the others had left because the salmon were running. No offenses were intended—one project could wait; the other could not. Being guided by the timing of natural events rather than by hours, days, weeks, months, or any other division of time seems incomprehensible to many North Americans. Communication can break down on such provocation.

Nurses are becoming increasingly conscious of the significance of communication behaviors in establishing relationships with clients and members of the health team. An important first step in becoming skilled in interpersonal communication is to be able to recognize one's own thoughts and feelings—to become more self-aware.

SELF-AWARENESS

"Why did I say that?" and "Why did I do that?" are questions that all of us ask ourselves. Part of the answer to such questions lies in becoming aware of the effect values have on actions. Values as defined by Uustal (1978) as "general guides to behavior, standards of conduct that one endorses and tries to live up to or maintain." For example, nurses say it is important for the nurse to institute therapeutic nurse-client relationships. Nurses value this ability and believe the nurse has a responsibility for becoming skilled in the interpersonal process. Other values that act as bases for one's actions are obscure. Individuals are not conscious of their presence yet the values of which persons are unaware shape actions as directly as do conscious values. Many of the values that individuals hold consciously or unconsciously and that influence actions stem from concepts of *social roles* and of *the self*. A brief review of these two concepts follows and then there is an examination of a process of increasing self-awareness.

Concept of social role. Social roles may be defined as socially prescribed patterns for behavior. Persons who share common attitudes and beliefs and assume responsibilities for certain tasks are performing a social role. These roles are learned in the process of social interaction, which begins at birth and continues throughout life. An individual's concept of a role (role expectations) governs how he expects others to act and how he expects to act. Every society sets up cultural norms for essential roles that serve as models for individuals to emulate in developing their personalized versions.

Awareness of a role comes from myriad sources. Individuals use all their senses (hearing, seeing, touching, tasting, and smelling) as well as their cognitive powers (assessing, planning, and evaluating). Once a person is committed to the idea of a role, it is incorporated into the self, and *values* are assigned to it.

The concept of certain social roles becomes stereotyped to such a degree that only minor modifications in attitudes, beliefs, and responsibilities are permitted. The traditional role of mother falls into this category. In the traditional role the mother is expected to behave in a motherly fashion, that is, willingly give children love, attention, and support, even though she is simultaneously acting as career woman, lover, or wife. A nurse who expects a woman to function in the traditional role of mother can be upset if her client does not live up to the nurse's expectations. Individuals come to value their concepts of social roles (role expectation) and resist attempts to change them. When expectations are similar, nurse-client interaction can flow smoothly. When expectations are not similar, stress arises, and the differing role expectations can act as a source of conflict between nurse and client. As a result the nurse may consciously or unconsciously withhold supportive care, for example, be abrupt in contacts, avoid touching the client, or teach the client as little as possible. The following incident is illustrative of this:

> Laura P., a new mother, was a senior partner in a law firm. She announced she would be returning to work immediately and had hired a nurse to care for the baby. She did not appear for the informal discussion on baby care held in the ward lounge. When her nurse was questioned as to why L.P. had not come, the nurse replied, "I did not tell her about it. I figured she's not interested. She's not going to be looking after the baby."

In this instance the nurse assumed the mother was not interested in her new baby because the mother did not conform to stereotyped mother-role behavior. The nurse's value judgment about the behavior prevented the nurse from functioning adequately in her role as a nurse.

At times the value nurses place on certain aspects of a role can prove of great benefit to a client. The following incident as reported by a student is an example:

> One of the infants in west nursery developed suspicious lesions on its face. The mother had a history of herpes simplex II. The baby was roomed-in with the mother. All infants in the nursery were considered as potentially infected and isolated in the "B" room. The incoming babies were admitted to "A" room. I realized maintaining medical asepsis was vital to the babies' well-being and knew the problem would be enforcement. During report I noticed two doctors coming from "B" room and going into "A" room without changing gowns or scrubbing. I took it upon myself to confront this "traffic" and afterwards set up a routine for everyone to follow. I found it nerve *wracking* to stop doctors but realized the implications for the babies.

The student accepted the responsibility of acting as an advocate for her clients because she felt strongly (valued) that being an advocate was an important component of the nursing role.

The concept of a life role, with the various responsibilities and relationships it entails, is not a static one. Change is inevitable as new life situations occur. If the initial adaptation results in a satisfactory outcome, subsequent alteration in role structure comes with less stress. The individual can trust his ability to adjust, modify, or enlarge his role commitments; the foundation for growth in the role has been established. The maternity nurse is in a unique position to assist women and men to adapt to the role of parent. Teaching classes such as preparation for parenthood during the prenatal period, encouraging participation by the father during birth, and instructing parents in the care of the newborn are examples of strategies the maternity nurse uses. As parents become proficient in the role, a favorable *self-concept* ensues.

Self-concept. The *self* has been variously defined since studies of the self began in the late 1800s. It still defies precise definition although it is recognized as the core of an individual's personality. Through the *self* each person perceives and evaluates the world. The idea of the self develops slowly; the infant begins the process by defining the physical boundaries of his self as he manipulates his body. As children grow older they begin to act as they observe others acting. They play at social roles, either *sexual* (e.g., mother, father) or *mastery* (e.g., grocery man, teacher), and thereby practice role behaviors. This process of role taking continues throughout life. In some instances the process of role taking is formalized; the role taker becomes a student (nursing student). In other instances the actual role is assumed without a concerted social effort to prepare the participants. Until recently parenthood came into this latter category.

A central component in the self-concept each of us possesses is *body image*.

Body image. Body image can be defined as a subjective picture of one's physical appearance derived from one's own observations and by noting the response of others. This picture is constantly changing as new perceptions and experiences occur. The adolescent becomes particularly conscious of his physical body as the body undergoes rapid change. Value judgments made about physical size, hair styles, and skin can be a source of pleasure or pain to the young person. The pregnant woman's body also reflects rapid change, and for some women this change can be disturbing to them.

Another important component of self-concept is self-esteem.

Self-esteem. Over the years an individual gradually becomes *a self* that is distinct from others. This self can be admired by the individual (''I am proud of myself'') or by others (''You are the best father in the world''). Conversely the self can be disliked by the individual (''I am not worth your interest'') or by others (''She is a poor mother''). The liking or disliking of the self is called self-esteem. Self-esteem develops as persons attempt to master social roles. If individuals play out social roles well, they are applauded (rewarded) by people important to them (significant others) and as a result develop *high self-esteem*. If their efforts are not considered successful, the significant others may ignore them, criticize them, blame them. As a result of these responses the person develops *low self-esteem*. Sullivan (1963) called this process ''learning about the self from the mirror of other people.'' How an individual views himself (self-esteem) conditions responses to his world. Some persons feel masterful, others are afraid. Some develop methods of coping with crisis, others ''go to pieces'' if their daily routines are interrupted. Some become part of a social group that acts as a support system, others remain alone.

There are happenings in the lives of all of us that have great meaning to us personally. Assuming the role of parent is one of these important times; it will have an effect on us and others for all our lives. It can be called a crucial life experience. How individuals function during this time has an important effect on self-esteem. Persons need to share these times with others who care and to be helped by the nurturing of others in the environment. Clients often turn to nurses to help them develop the behaviors, attitudes, and responsibilities that are part of the role of parent. Low self-esteem has an important impact on maternity nursing. Research has indicated that low feelings of self-esteem may be determining factors in a person's use of health facilities, particularly those relative to preventive care. Much effort in maternity care is directed to the early detection of abnormalities, as well as to health maintenance. Regardless of the source of events that serve to lower feelings of self-worth, nursing must attempt to counteract such feelings to be successful in the delivery of health services.

Values clarification. Decision making wherever or whenever it occurs is based on *values* regardless of ''how objective the criteria and whether the process is conscious or unconscious'' (Hawley and Hawley, 1975). Since decision making is a key component in the nursing process, nurses need to become aware of the values (perceptions, beliefs, biases) that can add to or detract from their efforts to make decisions congruent with therapeutic goals.

As noted earlier, personal values arise as individuals concern themselves with establishing self-identity and attaining chosen life roles. Certain areas of life are ''value rich.'' These include health, personal habits, male-female roles, sex, love, family, friends, and religion. While other areas such as money and politics are also value laden, the first set is of particular importance to maternity nursing. It is within these realms that much of maternity nursing takes place. For example, the family is encouraged to take as great a part in the care process as possible.

Obviously not all persons will hold the same values. Varying social and ethnic groups hold values particular to a given set of persons and even members of the same family can hold differing values. Nurses hold values that are both personal and professional. The professional values are derived as an individual becomes part of a professional group and subscribes to and supports the standards of the group (e.g., American Nurses' Association nursing standards). The more the values are in agreement, the fewer the possibilities of value conflict. To expect perfect harmony between sets of values is unrealistic and each nurse needs to recognize value conflict when it occurs and how to go about resolving it. The first step in this process is values clarification. The results of values clarification for the individual have been shown to increase self-esteem and foster belief in personal control over personal life. While individuals may change their value systems as a result of values clarification, that is not the goal. The goal is to become clearer about values held and the effect values have on performance. It is an aspect of increased self-awareness. Uustal (1978) adapted the process of values clarification for nursing. Three major activities are involved in the process. They are choosing, prizing, and acting.

Choosing: Making choices about our values after consideration of alternatives.

Example: I've thought and thought about going back to school just now, and I've come to the conclusion that I need to be with the kids at their ages. I have to put first things first. I talked it over with John and he agrees. I can always go back to school later. After all, the kids will only be young once.

Prizing: Assigning a "value" to values, arranging our values in rank order, and acknowledging them publicly when appropriate.

Example: Some principles I feel very strongly about, others I can adjust to circumstances. I try to let others know how I feel about certain things so they are forewarned about how I'll react if they try to make me change.

Acting: Behaving in a manner that is consistent with the individual's values. Through repetitious actions, a pattern of behavior can be discerned.

Example: I could have said nothing about giving Mrs. S. the Tylenol instead of Darvon. They are both stock drugs so they wouldn't be missed and physically they wouldn't hurt her, but I felt I had to be honest and report the error or I couldn't stand myself. In some things such as medications, even small differences could have adverse effects. I feel better that I acted according to my beliefs.

In the three examples cited above the individuals were making decisions and acting on the basis of professed values (principles, beliefs). Values clarification is part of everyday living. However, it can be used in a formal sense to assist in recognizing the effect values have on action. The following example illustrates how a student used the values clarification process after a conflict in nurse-client values prevented her from providing therapeutic care:

One of my clients was M.M. Before beginning her care I reviewed her record and found the following history. "She was 20 years old and unmarried. She had an abortion at 16, another at 17, and a baby at 19 and kept her baby. She was going to keep the baby from this pregnancy also." My reaction was one of shock. I felt resentment toward her and felt uncomfortable knowing I would have to interact with her. I remembered all I'd read and talked about unwed mothers and so decided to accept this challenge and not let my feelings get in the way. My feelings stem from the fact that as a result of a strict Catholic upbringing, I am fiercely against abortions and consider them an act of murder. Also, I was adopted, so I am extra sensitive to the fact that unwed girls are not giving their babies up for adoption, but rather bringing them home to an incomplete family.

After getting home I reflected on my behavior toward M.M. I failed in reaching my goal. I talked to M.M. very little, only when it was necessary. When I did talk to her, I kept it brief in order to be able to ignore her situation. I also did not want to find anything out about her home situation—if she had an adequate income or a significant other for emotional support, for fear of what I would learn. When I did ask her about contraception in the future, she said she had never used any and felt there was no need for it. It tore me apart inside to even think that she may possibly bring more children into her insufficient family. In essence, I wanted as little to do with her as possible.

I now realize how much my personal views prevented me from performing therapeutic nursing care. I definitely want to work on this one, but I do know it will be difficult to overcome."

In an effort to work through the value conflicts the student sorted the data as follows:

Conflict

My values	Clients' values as assumed by the nurse
Abortion as morally wrong	Abortion is an acceptable means of birth control
Family should consist of a wedded mother and father with children	Family without a father is alright
Methods of birth control (other than abortion) should be used if a person is sexually active, to prevent birth of children	Birth control other than abortion not necessary

As a result of the conflict in values, the nurse had the following responses:

1. Shock and disbelief but desire to give good care
2. Inability to set up therapeutic nurse-client relationship
   "I talked to M.M. very little, only when it was necessary." "In essence, I wanted as little to do with her as possible."
3. Inadequate collection of data
   "When I did talk to her, I kept it brief in order to be able to ignore her situation."

   "I also did not want to find anything out about her home situation—if she had an adequate income or a significant other for emotional support, for fear of what I would learn."

   "When I did ask her about contraception in the future, she said she had never used any (abortion?) and felt there was no need for it."
4. Feeling of guilt and anxiety over care given to client
   "I now realize how much my personal views prevented me from performing therapeutic nursing care."

Table 4.2
Example of Value Clarification Process Implemented by a Nursing Student

Choosing Values	Prizing	Acting
Abortion morally wrong	Part of my religious and moral beliefs	Would request another client assignment giving reasons for my request Would not assist with abortion procedure If client asked for information would find client another resource person (for legally accepted actions, see Chapter 5)
Sexually active adults need to assume responsible attitude toward possible pregnancy (use acceptable [not abortion] birth control measure)	Part of my belief about being a responsible citizen	Would include teaching and counseling about family planning in my care
Different family definitions in our society; for every child, a caring adult, social and economic support, and a place in society would be my goals	With reading and discussion enlarged my view of family; still feel mother, father, and children family the best but can "see" other forms now	Could work with single parents; am going to act as volunteer this summer at "Center for Life" where counseling is given to pregnant women, emphasizing adoption but also working on other support system if adoption alternative not chosen

5. Desire to change
   "I definitely want to work on this one, but I do know it will be difficult to overcome."

Once the data had been organized the student used the values clarification process to help her with growth in the professional role. Table 4.2 illustrates how this student accomplished clarification of her values.

DECISION-MAKING PROCESS

Many of the individuals who seek nurses' help will be concerned about making major *decisions* that will affect themselves and others for the rest of their lives. For example, the sexually mature adult will make such decisions as whether to have intercourse, whether to become pregnant, whether to sustain a pregnancy or abort the fetus, whether to become a parent or give up a child for adoption, and whether to utilize health facilities and the health supervision of professionals. The decisions noted above are not made in a vacuum; all the values, beliefs, and attitudes of the individuals are factors in the decision-making process. For some persons, decisions are made with much thought for the consequences and are based on carefully gathered information. For others, decisions are made without thought for the future or are based on ignorance, prejudice, or myth.

Nurses may assist clients with decision making in a number of ways:

1. The nurse can help the client collect sufficient valid data on which to base decisions. The nurse can provide information that is more advanced and technical than is generally accessible to either the well-informed lay public or those who show little understanding of the birth process. In addition to being able to provide information the nurse is able to tell the client about the clinical significance of the data relating to the health of the client, fetus, or newborn. The nurse also acts to refer clients to other resources for information she is unable to provide. For example, the nurse refers families to specialists for genetic counseling. The nurse's knowledge of inheritable disorders prompts this action (see Chapter 10).

2. The nurse can also help the client to consider alternative actions. The nurse can review with the client the risks and consequences of each action and the responsibilities each choice involves. The nurse makes an effort to discuss a number of alternatives with the client so that the client does not feel trapped into making decisions not of benefit to her. If possible, choices are introduced early. For example, the method of infant feeding is introduced by the twentieth week of pregnancy so the parents have ample time to discuss the advantages and disadvantages of breast and bottle feeding for their infant and themselves.

3. The nurse can assist the client or family to set up relevant criteria for evaluating the outcomes of their actions. Nurse and client can mutually consider reasonable standards for the client's own behavior or that of her family and eventually their newborn child. Rigid adherence to impossible standards can be destructive of the self-concept as there is a tendency to consider the standards as correct and appropriate and the individual's performance a failure. Such a response to a change in expectations may be seen as a result of incidents occurring during labor:

Janice and Peter O. had attended prenatal classes and were planning a "natural birth" without analgesia or anesthesia. Everything progressed as planned until just before delivery. The fetal heart rate slowed to 90 (normal rate: 120 to 160) and the physician decided to use outlet forceps to hasten the infant's birth. Anesthesia was used to numb the vagina and perineum, forceps applied, the infant delivered. The cord was wrapped three times around the infant's neck and was considered the probable cause of the slowing of the heart rate. In spite of the fact that Janice could not have foreseen or controlled the event, she and Peter were depressed by her inability to deliver their infant as planned.

Nurses teaching prenatal or other classes need to discuss what can happen in reality. Role playing "what if . . . . ." can be used as an effective learning technique.

4. The more clients are involved actively in their care, the more they become committed to complying with appropriate therapy. Participation in decisions that have an effect on an individual's welfare prompts a feeling of control of one's destiny, and self-esteem is increased. Therefore when possible, the *locus* or place of decision making is with the client. It has to be recognized by the client that once the client assumes responsibility for a decision, accountability for the outcome rests with the client. If a decision is considered to be detrimental to the well-being of the mother or child, every effort is made to have the client modify the decision; for example:

Sarah H., an uncontrolled diabetic, pregnant with her third child, living with her parents, repeatedly missed appointments at the clinic. The nurse phoned each time to encourage her to come and tried to emphasize the need for consistent monitoring of her condition. She maintained "it was too much bother." At 36 weeks she delivered a stillborn child.

In this instance the mother made the decision not to attend the clinic (the *locus* of decision making was with the client), and the outcome of the pregnancy rested with her.

In some instances the professional care giver, because of knowledge and expertise, assumes responsibility for decisions. The nursing care of critically ill infants illustrates the decision-making responsibilities of the nurse-clinician. The nurse assumes accountability for decisions because the *locus* of decision making is with the care giver.

PERSONAL CHARACTERISTICS

Certain personal characteristics of the nurse have a positive effect on the nurse-client relationship. As noted earlier, these characteristics include skill in verbal and nonverbal behavior and awareness of attitudes and feelings behind responses to the client and her family. In addition, the nurse's ability to trust and be trusted, to empathize, and to work with the client toward mutually acceptable goals facilitates the interpersonal process.

Trust. In this age of complex medical care clients take much of what is done for them "on trust." If individuals can trust each other they feel secure. Travelkee (1971) has defined trust as "the assured belief that other individuals are capable of assisting in times of distress and will probably do so."

In the context of nursing, what behaviors prompt a client to trust? Clients described some of the behaviors as follows:

"The baby began to choke, the nurse quickly picked him up, turned him over and suctioned out his mouth. When he recovered she cuddled him until he relaxed. She was very *skillful.*"

"She always hangs up my clothes carefully, doesn't leave them in a heap on the chair. She is *careful of my belongings* so I figure she will be *careful of me.*"

"She came round to see if I were sleeping. I couldn't, for thinking about my baby (born with a cleft palate). She said she'd come back after settling the others. When she *came back,* she brought me some hot milk and sat and talked. I remembered my *mother* and how she used to *comfort* me."

"You can *rely* on her for information you ask about—if she doesn't know she'll find out. I *checked out* what she told me and it was right. She *didn't get angry* when I told her what I had done."

Certain descriptive terms occur again and again when people are asked to describe someone they would trust; for example, consistent, reliable, genuine, sincerely interested, accepting. Although nurses can give care without trusting or being trusted, the level of care tends to be more mechanical and limited largely to physical aspects.

Empathy. Empathy, the ability "to sense the client's private world as *if it* were your own but without losing the *'as if'* quality" (Rodgers, 1961), is an important component of the intrapersonal process. Empathy includes an individual's sensitivity to another's thoughts and feelings, an ability to communicate this awareness and yet retain one's own identification. Sympathy is different from empathy. Sympathy implies a feeling *for* another person while empathy implies gettng *inside* another person and feeling what that person is feeling. For example, two nurses expressed their responses to a mother who had lost her first-born infant; the first was sympathetic and the second empathetic:

"I feel so sorry for her. My sister lost a baby and I thought she (the sister) would never get over it. She acted much the same as Mrs. P. I told Mrs. P. about my sister and what helped her."

"I sensed in her (the client) an awful loneliness. I said to her 'How lonely it must feel when you lose your baby.' She nodded and said, 'I never realized what a feeling of desolation I would have. I miss her so terribly.' I made a point of being with her when the babies came out for feeding. Sometimes she talked, other times she cried and sometimes we just sat quietly together."

The uniqueness of each individual precludes our complete understanding of another; yet the potential for understanding grows with life experiences and with increased self-awareness. The ability "to walk in another's shoes" is a great asset for the nurse.

Setting mutual goals. Determining what nursing care is needed for a particular client is largely the responsibility of the nurse. However, the extent to which the client accepts the therapy and complies with the recommended health regimen is essential to the success of the undertaking. In former days there was a tendency on the part of medical and nursing personnel to dictate the form of therapy and the client's behavior. Research indicates that today clients are much more independent and there are a variety of reasons that prompt noncompliance with a recommended health regimen (Table 4.3).

One of the ways the nurse can increase compliance with therapy is to review the goals for care and discuss the actions (behaviorally stated) the client would need to undertake to reach the goals. At that time client difficulties can be discussed and innovative ways of solving problems often result. Involving clients in the care process increases their awareness of their responsibility for health.

Another effective approach is to ensure the client's understanding of therapy. Reviewing rationale for care may involve obtaining an interpreter, and a review of the client's anxiety level may mean teaching or counseling has to be repeated.

The atmosphere in which care is provided can be instrumental in the success of therapy. Making clinics and hospitals more homelike can have a beneficial effect as the following incident indicates:

In a small rural community the nurses in the maternity clinic were concerned about the inadequate diets of their clients. To improve the clients' diets they instituted "coffee klatches" at the clinic; nurses and clients contributed refreshments. Only healthful drinks were served (e.g., milk, fruit juice) and the food was prepared using natural ingredients. The women swapped recipes along with other helpful knowledge about pregnancy and child rearing. The health workers considered the venture to be one of the most successful in their health program.

During the process of therapy, nurse and client need to make periodic checks of mutuality. At times, because of pressure of work, it is easy to resume old patterns of relationships (i.e., the all-knowing nurse and the dependent client), so an effort has to be made to maintain a partnership. Client and nurse share accountability for successful health care; therefore each needs to participate in a responsible way.

Table 4.3
Examples of Client Noncompliance

Example	Reason for Noncompliance
I didn't take the iron pills; they made me constipated so I felt if they did that they couldn't be helping me	Lack of knowledge or understanding of therapy
Client sent home and told to be on strict bed rest with bathroom privileges only; client has 4 children under 6 yr, no help, husband at work 6 AM to 7 PM	Inability to comply with therapy because home responsibilities made bed rest impossible
Client was advised she was underweight and anemic; a special diet and iron supplement were ordered	Client did not comply as she was a firm believer in macrobiotic diets; therapy not accepted because of conflict of values

Process of Nurse-Client Relationship

Much of nursing takes place during interactions between two individuals, the client and the nurse. These interactions may be described as ones in which one person has "the intent of promoting the growth, development, maturity, improved functioning, and improved coping with the life of the other" (Rodgers, 1961). The process of developing a relationship is the same regardless of the time frame (short or long term) in which it takes place. All relationships have a preparatory phase, an initiation phase, a consolidation and growth phase, and a termination phase.

PREPARATORY PHASE

Portions of the preparatory phase begin long before nurses come in contact with a particular client. The areas previously reviewed (i.e., communication, self-awareness, decision making, and personal qualities) are essential factors in the nurse-client relationship. Becoming skilled in these areas is done partly in preparation for client contact. However, becoming increasingly skilled in nurse-client relationships continues throughout one's career.

Before the first meeting with a client, the nurse gathers as much data as possible and plans the first interaction. (Students may find it helpful to role play approaches to clients using a videotape and then review the results with their peers and instructor.) An example of preparation for the first contact with the client is the nursing actions taken when a woman in labor is expected for admission to the labor unit. The nurse reviews the client's record and notes information such as the following: client's name, age, obstetric history, estimated date of confinement (delivery), pulse rate, blood pressure, weight gain, results of urinalysis, VDRL, any allergies, any physical problems during prenatal period (e.g., vaginal bleeding), desired method of feeding infant, desire for infant circumcision or not, fetal heart rate (FHR) area of maximal density, fetal presentation, attendance at prenatal preparation classes, and any social problems (e.g., no support person available). By completing the review the nurse is alerted to any possible problems the client may expect and is ready to personalize the first meeting (e.g., call her by name).

INITIATION PHASE

The first meeting of client and nurse tends to set the stage for future contacts. The nurse attempts to establish a climate of trust, open communication, mutual understanding, and acceptance. The dialogue begins with an exchange of names. The client determines which name reference she prefers, Mrs., Ms., Miss, or given name. With the adolescent client, using a given name tends to set them at ease, but older clients may view this practice as presumptuous.

During the first meeting the nurse elicits the biographic and physical data as noted under "Interview" on p. 18. In addition to gathering and compiling this data the nurse has additional tasks to complete:

1. The nurse must establish a contract for care and for the nurse and client participation in that care. For example, for the client admitted in labor, the nurse reviews with the client what type of care the client will be receiving, who will be giving the care, whether or not the client is to be confined to bed, how to use call bells, explanations of facilities that are in the room (e.g., fetal monitor), and what part the client and her support person will play in her care. For example, the husband may be prepared to act as support person for his wife during labor.

   In establishing a contract for care the nurse might introduce the topic by saying, "Let me tell you what to expect. . . ." and then later, "Let's go over how you and your husband can help. . . ." and finish by telling the client how long the nurse will be acting as her chief nurse.

   The contract is not a formal contract in the legal sense but by discussing expectations of nurse and client functions, conflict can be minimized and the client's sense of security increased.
2. The nurse must review the issue of confidentiality with the client. For example, in some instances a client does not wish her obstetric history reviewed openly with the husband. She may have had an infant out of wedlock or a therapeutic abortion that her husband is not aware of. The knowledge is relevant to her obstetric care but otherwise such information is treated confidentially.
3. The nurse must elicit information about support persons the woman wishes to include in her pregnancy and the extent to which they will participate in her care. For example, even today some hospitals do not permit husbands to be present at delivery. The client and her husband need to be aware of such a policy so that if necessary they can make other plans for care.

During the first meeting nurse and client lay the groundwork for the individualized plan of care for the client. The development of the plan comes during the next phase, the consolidation and growth phase.

CONSOLIDATION AND GROWTH PHASE

Throughout the consolidation and growth phase the nurse and client clarify goals, plan care, and put the plans into action. It is a phase based on mutual trust, growing insight into the reasons behind behaviors, and working together for the benefit of the client. A certain amount of client dependency may be observed during this phase, and as long as it does not interfere with client actions it serves to cement a relationship. It is as though the client were saying, "If I need you, I know you will be here." As the nurse establishes a "safe" environment the client becomes free to express anxieties or doubts openly, knowing she will be heard by an understanding person. Dependency acts as a basis for future independent action as the client develops a feeling of self-esteem and respect for her own judgment.

Most of the care given to clients takes place during the consolidation and growth phase of the interpersonal relationship; for example:

1. Client problems are discussed and stressors identified.
2. Methods used by the client and her family to cope with present or potential crises are evaluated and, if necessary, alternatives suggested.
3. Family and community support systems are explored and plans for assistance in the care of other children as well as the new baby can be made.

The nurse functions in a variety of roles—clinician,

teacher, counselor, and manager. She also uses her abilities to communicate and problem solve. Gradually both client and nurse reveal more of their true feelings and perceptions and share their concepts of the purposes of therapy and the responsibilities of client and professional worker. Part of the nurse's functions will relate to the process of evaluation of client progress and consequent restructuring of plans. Although in the first meeting with the client the nurse indicates when the relationship will end, discussion of the termination phase of the nurse-client relationship is repeated so that both are ready for the termination phase when it occurs.

TERMINATION PHASE

The termination phase acts as a summary for all that has gone before. Nurse and client review the goals that they accomplished and plan for future health care.

Because of the nature of maternity care the termination phase may occur at any time during the course of pregnancy. For example, the nurse-client relationship established during the prenatal period is interrupted when the client goes to the hospital for delivery and immediate recovery care, is reestablished when the client returns for later postnatal care, and then eventually is terminated when postnatal care is completed. An intense nurse-client relationship is usually set up during labor and delivery. Sometimes if the nurse feels she was not able to terminate the relationship satisfactorily she will visit the client in the postnatal unit to accomplish the termination. A nurse from the labor unit described such a visit as follows:

> I visited Sheila A. today. She was so upset about having to have some analgesia during labor. I wanted her to know just how well she actually did. I didn't want her to feel she had failed. We had a long talk. I think she really felt better about herself.

The nurse on the postpartum unit has only a slightly longer time to establish a relationship with a client. The last morning a client is in the hospital is usually devoted to the termination phase. The nurse plans time to review again such areas as health maintenance for the infant, family planning for the couple, and the community resources available for continued support.

The termination phase of the nurse-client relationship leaves a final impression of the health care system with the client. A positive impression can affect the client's future health maintenance. Satisfied clients are more likely to return for health care that is preventive rather than just curative.

Summary

Nurse-client relationships are at the heart of nursing service. They are repeated time and again throughout the nurse's professional career. Although all human relationships have characteristics in common, the nurse-client relationship is instigated by the nurse for the benefit of the client. Nurse-client relationships take place wherever nurse and client meet and may be of long or short duration. The nurse employs professional skills in communication and decision making to facilitate the process. The nurse's responsive dimensions, trust, empathetic understanding, and readiness to work with a client are necessary ingredients of the nurse's role in therapeutic relationships. The nurse's self-awareness is basic to the genuine acceptance of others. All nurses can benefit from asking themselves such questions as the following (Stuart and Sundeen, 1979):

- Do I label clients with the stereotype of a group?
- Is my need to be liked so great that I become angry or hurt when a client is rude, hostile, or uncooperative?
- Am I afraid of the responsibility I must assume for the relationship and do I therefore limit my independent functions?
- Do I cover feelings of inferiority with a front of superiority?
- Do I require sympathy, warmth, and protection so much that I err by being too sympathetic or too protective toward clients?
- Do I fear closeness so much that I am indifferent, rejecting, or cold?
- Do I need to feel important and keep clients dependent on me?

References and Readings

Ford, J.A., et al.: Applied decision making for nurses, St. Louis, 1979, The C.V. Mosby Co.

Gardner, K.G.: Supportive nursing: a critical review of the literature, J. Psych. Nurs. **17:**10, 1979.

Hamachek, D.: Encounters with the self, New York, 1971, Holt, Rinehart & Winston, Inc.

Hawley, R.C., and Hawley, I.L.: Human values in the classroom, a handbook for teachers, New York, 1975, Hart Publishing Co.

Hays, S., and Larson, K.: Interacting with patients, New York, 1964, Macmillan Publishing Co., Inc.

Hines, J.: Only five minutes—nurse-patient communications, M.C.N. **5:**240, July/Aug. 1980.

Jourard, S.: The transparent self, New York, 1971, Litton Educational Publishing, Inc.

Kalisch, B.: What is empathy? Am. J. Nurs. **73:**1548, 1973.

Kesler, A.R.: Pitfalls to avoid in interviewing outpatients, Nurs. '77 **7:**70, 1977.

Kron, T.: How we communicate nonverbally with patients, Can. Nurse **68:**23, 1972.

Luft, J.: Of human interaction, Palo Alto, Calif., 1969, National Press Books.
Rodgers, C.: On becoming a person, Boston, 1961, Houghton & Mifflin Co.
Satir, V.: Peoplemaking, Palo Alto, Calif., 1972, Science and Behavior Books.
Simon, S.B., Howe, L.W., and Kirchenbaum, H.: Value clarification: a handbook of practical strategies for teachers and students, rev. ed., New York, 1978, Hart Publishing Co., Inc.
Stuart, G., and Sundeen, S.: Principles and practice of psychiatric nursing, St. Louis, 1979, The C.V. Mosby Co.
Sullivan, H.S.: The interpersonal theory of psychiatry, New York, 1963, W.W. Norton & Co., Inc., Publishers.
Sundeen, S., et al.: Nurse-client interaction, St. Louis, 1981, The C.V. Mosby Co.
Tildes, V.P., and Gustafson, L.: Termination in the student-patient relationship: use of a teaching tool, J. Nurs. Ed. **18**:9, 1979.
Topf, M.: A behavioral checking for estimating the development of communication skills, J. Nurs. Educ. **8**:29, 1969.
Travelkee, J.: Interpersonal aspects of nursing, Philadelphia, 1971, The F.A. Davis Co.
Uustal, D.B.: Values clarification in nursing application to practice Am. J. Nurs. **78**:2058, 1978.
Walke, M.: When a patient needs to unburden his feelings, Am. J. Nurs., **77**:1164, July 1977.

5

Legal and Ethical Aspects of Maternity Nursing

- General Legal Concepts
  - Accountability
  - Standards of care
  - Statutory law
  - Common law of torts
  - Reasonably prudent nurse
  - Floating
  - Negligence
  - Charting
  - Informed consent
  - Maternal rights
  - Insurance
  - Nurse-midwives
- Legal and Ethical Concepts for Preconceptional Clients
  - Sexual counseling
  - Sterilization
  - Genetic counseling
  - In vitro fertilization and embryo transplantation
  - Artificial insemination
  - Prenatal diagnosis
  - Mass screening
    - Anniocentesis
  - Fetal research
  - Home births
- Ethical and Legal Issues of Abortion
  - Congressional amendment
  - Court cases
  - Ethical considerations
  - Fetal rights
- Legal Concepts During Labor and Delivery
  - Fetal monitors
  - Anesthetics
  - Maternal complications
  - Stillborn infants
- Legal Issues in the Postpartum Unit
- Summary

A woman who places herself in the care of a maternity nurse has the right to safe and competent nursing care. The maternity nurse is responsible for knowledge about nursing assessments and appropriate nursing intervention for maternity clients. The nurse assumes ethical obligations for providing the best possible nursing care for the client.

Maternity nurses should understand the legal aspects of maternity care. According to Ladimer (1975), legal actions involving obstetric and gynecologic clients are fourth in incidence of all malpractice suits. Hakanson (1980) suggests that this area of practice is considered at such high risk for malpractice suits because there are two potential claimants: the pregnant woman and the infant in utero. This chapter will review some of the ethical and legal issues that confront maternity nurses.

General Legal Concepts

Law, as applied to nursing, is designed to perform several functions for nurses. The law helps to relate nurses' roles to those of other health professionals. It helps to define boundaries for independent nursing actions and provides a framework for judging nursing care of maternity clients as either legally acceptable or unacceptable. Nurse practice acts define the scope of nursing in broad general terms. To understand the influence of law on the practice of nursing, nurses should understand several basic legal concepts.

ACCOUNTABILITY

The nurse of today is legally accountable for her/his actions. In the past, when the nurse was viewed as a secondary-level health care provider, the hospital and the physician were considered to be the primary accountable parties. Now that health care has become more complex and nurses have assumed a more independent role as health care providers, they are considered to be accountable for their own actions. Once the nurse-client relationship is established, the nurse is legally accountable to the client for nursing care and, within certain limits, for the client's well-being.

If the quality of care given by other members of the health care team is less than appropriate, the nurse has ethical as well as legal obligations to report the problem through established channels. For example, if a nurse discovers that another nurse is not performing duties according to hospital policy, the problem should be referred to the head nurse for solution. Every nurse has ethical, legal, and moral responsibilities toward society that cannot be denied in the practice of the nursing arts.

STANDARDS OF CARE

Standards of care are definitions of appropriate nursing care, as outlined by nursing educators, nursing professional organizations, and the facility that employs the nurse. For example, the Nurses' Association of the American College of Obstetrics and Gynecology (NAACOG) has defined standards of care for nurses involved in maternity care. Maternity nurses should be familiar with the standards of care relevant to their area of practice.

If a nurse does not adhere to the standards of care, a breach of duty may occur, with consequences possibly including professional penalties or loss of license, or the client may initiate a malpractice lawsuit with the nurse named as defendant. A breach of duty occurs when the nurse (1) fails to act, (2) has the authority to act but performs the authorized act in an improper manner, or (3) performs an unauthorized act.

STATUTORY LAW

Legislated definitions of nursing practice are one type of statutory law. Although these laws vary from state to state, essentially all nursing practice acts delineate the boundaries for nurse practice by describing educational requisites, setting licensure requirements, and defining standards of care expected of nurses who practice in that state. These laws, which are stated in broad general terms, are designed to exercise legal controls over the profession.

COMMON LAW OF TORTS

Common law comprises decisions made by judges in individual cases. A *tort* is a wrongful act, intentional or nonintentional, that results in injury, loss, or damage and that causes the injured party to seek redress in civil courts against the person who inflicted the injury, such as a nurse. During the trial, the jury decides whether the defendant (nurse) performed to the standard of care of the profession. Usually the law is designed not to punish the defendant (nurse) who committed the wrongful act but rather to financially compensate the injured party.

REASONABLY PRUDENT NURSE

In any given situation the nurse must exercise that degree of care that a *reasonably* prudent nurse would exercise under similar circumstances. Nurses who perform in highly specialized areas of care are expected to perform as a well-educated nurse in that specialty would perform. For example, if a nurse is caring for a woman in labor who has a fetal monitor in place, the nurse must be able to recognize ominous fetal heart rate patterns and take appropriate action to prevent harm to the infant.

In highly specialized areas, such as labor and delivery, specific technical training is required to educate the nurse. A thorough orientation program and continuing education courses should be provided by the employing institution. Any nurse employed in this setting should attend these courses and have this additional training documented in a personnel file.

FLOATING

Due to economic pressures, many hospitals require nurses to "float" from their normal area of practice to another section of the hospital. For example, a nurse who usually is employed as a medical-surgical nurse may be assigned to care for maternity clients. The nurse who is required to float to an area with which she/he is not familiar should inform the supervising nurse of the lack of qualification (if that is the case). The nurse should also request and receive orientation to the new area (Creighton, 1982).

NEGLIGENCE

Negligence is a failure of the professional person to act within accepted standards of the profession at all times. In a malpractice lawsuit initiated by a nurse's client who suspects that the nurse performed care in a negligent manner, the following steps must be proven: (1) the nurse's duty to the client, (2) a failure to carry out that duty, (3) an injury sustained by the client, and (4) proximate cause—a causal relationship is established between the breach of duty and the client's injury. If a nurse acts in a negligent manner, the nurse risks implication as a defendant in a malpractice lawsuit. The award of monetary damages in these cases is intended to compensate the injured person and, where possible, to restore the original state of well-being that existed before the injury.

One example of negligence within the context of maternity nursing involved a woman who began premature labor. During the first 1½ hours, the nurses neglected to notify either a house physician or the attending obstetrician. When delivery became imminent, the nurses rushed the mother to the delivery suite. The delivery was unattended by an obstetrician, pediatrician, or nurse. This care was unacceptable given the fact that the delivery was considered high risk because of prematurity. Although the infant later developed neurologic problems, legal action was not initiated by the parents. The nurses and the institution could have been found liable by the courts if the parents had brought suit.

Various other incidents have been the subject of malpractice litigation. Errors in the administration of medications are among the most common. Within the context of maternity nursing, lawsuits have been initiated when the identities of newborns have been mistaken at the time of discharge because of a failure to check name bands. The legal importance of fetal monitoring cannot be stressed enough. These examples illustrate the legal responsibilities of nurses to practice nursing in a competent manner.

Over the past few years, malpractice suits have become more numerous, and the monetary awards have increased (Regan, 1981). The public has become more aware of legal rights. Nursing has become more complex with increased possibilities for error. Although nurses must certainly consider the legal aspects of nursing care, the most important concern should be to deliver accurate, safe nursing care for the client's benefit.

CHARTING

The legal significance of full and accurate charting by the nurse cannot be overemphasized. Many malpractice suits have been decided on the basis of information (or lack of information) contained in the nurse's record. The best way for a nurse to prove that a certain task was performed is by written documentation in nursing progress notes. There is legal significance attached to nursing observations of a client's condition at a particular time.

The items a nurse charts, nursing actions not documented, as well as how the written notes are prepared are all important factors when considered from a legal perspective (Bergerson, 1982). A nurse should chart nursing observations, nursing intervention, and the results of nursing care. Entries should be made frequently with summary comments at the conclusion of a nursing shift. Since a nurse cannot rely on memory to recall specific actions in a given situation, the importance of careful charting acquires additional legal significance (Bergerson, 1982).

INFORMED CONSENT

A legally effective consent must provide the following elements: (1) It must be given voluntarily, without coercion. (2) The client must be given information about the procedure, its benefits and risks, and any alternative procedures and their consequences. (3) The client must have all questions answered to her/his satisfaction. (4) The person giving consent must be legally competent to give consent, that is, legally an adult and mentally competent. If a client refuses to give consent for treatment, the physician or nurse must explain the risks of refusal and ask the client to sign a form stating that therapy was refused, even though the client is aware that refusal may prove detrimental to health or life. *If there is a language difference between the person who is attempting to gain consent and the person giving it, the consent must be obtained through an interpreter.*

MATERNAL RIGHTS

A recent innovation in maternity care is provided by "The Pregnant Patient's Bill of Rights," by Doris B. Haire (see Appendix A). Although not legally recognized, this document states that the pregnant woman deserves as much information as possible about the effects of any drugs or treatment on herself or her infant, since she or her baby may suffer from any adverse sequelae to the drugs or treatment she receives. The general public is aware that although the Food and Drug Administration may approve a particular drug and a physician may then prescribe it, that drug may not be safe for every woman or baby. Furthermore, the "Bill of Rights" argues that a woman has the right to have a support person accompany her through labor and delivery.

INSURANCE

Nurses should carry professional liability insurance for their protection. Even if an institution provides insurance coverage for its employees, this coverage generally applies only while the nurse is on duty and acting within the scope of assigned duties at the institution. In the event of malpractice during other times in the nurse's professional practice, the nurse would not be covered by the employer's policy. Legal expenses for a nurse to prove innocence in a malpractice suit can be exorbitant. There have also been instances of a hospital losing a malpractice suit and then suing the nurse responsible. Reasonably priced insurance policies are available to nurses and are generally considered to be well worth the expense.

NURSE-MIDWIVES

In the United States, most nurse-midwives function not as independent practitioners but rather as part of a health care team directed by a physician. Whether a nurse-midwife can practice is determined by licensure within the legal jurisdiction in which the nurse-midwife is employed. Nurse-midwives are trained to perform normal deliveries and to give care to mothers and infants at the time of delivery as well as during prenatal and postnatal periods. The nurse-midwife can provide care for mothers throughout a *normal* pregnancy, labor, and delivery. If abnormalities should be discovered, clients then must be transferred to the care of a physician.

Legal and Ethical Concepts for Preconceptional Clients

SEXUAL COUNSELING

Discussion of sexual matters has become more open during recent years. This frankness has led to a rise in the number of self-styled sexuality counselors, some of whom are charlatans. Sexual counseling should be done by trained sexuality counselors who are skilled in helping people with sexual problems. There are currently few statutes that regulate this field. Any person who receives counseling on sexual matters has the right to privacy and confidentiality.

STERILIZATION

Both men and women are candidates for sterilization, but for the purpose of this discussion, only female sterilization will be considered. Sterilization is only occasionally essential for health reasons; hence most sterilization operations are elective. For voluntary sterilization the woman must give her informed consent. The explanations given to obtain this consent must explain the major alternatives to sterilization, including the principal benefits and risks involved. The psychologic risks should be mentioned as well. Most individuals who later regret having made the decision to be sterilized are those who are young, made their decision during a period of stress, or made the decision on the advice of a physician without allowing time to carefully consider all aspects of the procedure.

In June 1982, the Connecticut Supreme Court ruled in favor of a woman who sued her physician for "wrongful conception." The woman became pregnant after sterilization proved ineffective. She was awarded monetary damages not only to help in raising the child but also for the stress of going through an unwanted pregnancy.

At least 300,000 sterilizations are performed in North America each year. Hospitals that are supported entirely by taxation funds cannot refuse to perform sterilizations. However, there are "conscience" clauses that allow physicians, nurses, and institutions (other than tax-supported ones) to refuse to perfrom sterilizations on moral, religious, or medical judgment grounds.

GENETIC COUNSELING

A nurse may be the first health care provider to identify a possible genetic problem such as a couple who are consanguineous (blood relatives) or a woman at risk (e.g., a woman who has had more than two spontaneous abortions or has produced an infant with a defect). In such a situation the nurse is responsible for knowing where genetic resources are available to facilitate referrals (Thompson and Thompson, 1981).

Genetic counseling is often given to a couple after the birth of an infant with a defect. Before counseling sessions are held, an accurate diagnosis should be made. The purpose of counseling is to enable the couple to understand the recurrence risk and the possibilities for conceiving other affected children. Based on that information, the couple decides whether or not to have additional children. Complete accuracy in genetic counseling is of paramount importance, and therefore nurses who are not trained in genetic counseling (on a graduate level) risk legal consequences if they choose to do genetic counseling without appropriate training.

Parents who receive genetic counseling have a right to privacy concerning these matters. However, there is an ethical question raised if a parent is found to be the carrier of a lethal disease trait regarding who should inform other potential carriers in the extended family. The parents may be unwilling to inform these individuals because of guilt or embarrassment, even though they do have an ethical obligation to notify their relatives. If the physician notifies other family members without receiving consent from the parents, the physician may breach the laws concerning privileged information.

IN VITRO FERTILIZATION AND EMBRYO TRANSPLANTATION

One of the most recent ethical dilemmas brought to focus by modern obstetrics is the issue of in vitro fertilization with subsequent embryo transplantation, known in the vernacular as test-tube babies. In 1978 Steptoe's work resulted in the first successful live birth in which this method of conception was employed. Since then, there have been many other successful cases.

In March 1979 the ethics advisory board recommended to the Secretary of the Department of Health, Education and Welfare that in vitro fertilization and embryo transplantation be considered not only ethically acceptable but also an inevitable treatment for infertility. There were several questions raised concerning the possible disrespect for human life; for example, problems might arise regarding the fertilized eggs that were discarded. Steinfels (1979) suggests that the developing eggs could be discarded at 14 days or less after fertilization, since normal uterine implantation would (or would not) have occurred by that time.

One question is whether or not the personnel and agency where the procedure is performed are legally liable for defects if the child conceived by this method is born with physical or mental handicaps. Because of the ethical issues of working with fertilized human eggs as experimental tissue, only minimal medical research has been done. Therefore it is unknown what legal risks this technique may carry (Culliton, 1978).

The issue of in vitro fertilization is certainly legally, morally, and ethically significant. As the use of this technique proliferates, questions will probably increase.

ARTIFICIAL INSEMINATION

Numerous legal problems stem from the practice of artificial insemination. There are two types: insemination of the wife with her husband's sperm (i.e., AIH [artificial insemination husband]) to fertilize her egg within her reproductive tract and artificial insemination of the woman with a donor's sperm (i.e., AID [artificial insemination donor]). AID will be considered here because it alone has serious legal questions. The probability of an increase in the use of AID is significant as adoptions become increasingly difficult to arrange. The primary indications for AID are male infertility and genetic problems.

Five people are involved in artificial insemination with a donor's sperm: the husband, wife, donor, physician, and resultant child. Several questions have been raised by Richardson (1975):

1. Is the child conceived illegitimate?
2. Does AID constitute criminal adultery or adultery that could lead to divorce on those grounds?
3. Could the donor be held liable for rape if the woman denies she gave consent?
4. Does the child produced as a result of AID have legal claims to the donor's estate if the donor leaves his estate to his children?
5. What are the AID child's rights to his mother's husband's estate?

Legal obligations can be met by ensuring that the husband, wife, and donor all give written informed consent for the procedure. It is recommended that the donor not know the identity of the husband and wife and vice versa and that the physician be given permission to select the donor. The consent may also include a clause to remove liability from the physician should the infant be abnormal. The best way to ensure that the AID child is legitimate is for the couple to adopt him formally. However, many states are considering legislation giving such a child automatic rights as a legitimate heir to the husband and wife. Legislation must be carefully drawn to prevent children produced by AID from initiating legal action against the physician, according to Edwards (1973). The basis for these suits includes withholding information from these children concerning the donor's identity, thereby preventing the child from claiming natural rights as the donor's child.

PRENATAL DIAGNOSIS

Recent advances in medical knowledge have produced several prenatal diagnostic techniques that are used to decrease the incidence of infants with specific birth defects. Maternity nurses should be aware of these tests and be reminded of the legal significance of accuracy.

MASS SCREENING

Screening specific groups of people for specific genetic defects involves drawing blood samples for testing to determine if a couple is at risk for producing an infant with that defect. For example, drawing blood samples from Ashkenazic Jewish persons can determine potential parents who carry the Tay-Sachs gene. Sampling members of the black race can screen for carriers of sickle cell anemia. The information obtained through screening techniques can help potential parents determine whether or not they wish to produce a child. All results of screening procedures are reported to the person who has undergone the test. The legal significance of accuracy cannot be overstressed.

Amniocentesis. Laboratory studies can be performed on samples of amniotic fluid obtained through a needle-syringe aspiration technique called amniocentesis. The routine use of this procedure for all mothers at risk is rapidly becoming available. More than 200 hereditary diseases can now be diagnosed through the use of this technique. There are categories of women who are at risk, including women over 35 years of age, those who have produced a child with Down's syndrome, those who have a history of specific genetic disease, those who have undergone fetal irradiation, or those who have elevated toxoplasmosis titers. Amniocentesis is reasonably safe for the mother and carries less than a 2% risk of injury to the fetus. The mother should be informed of the risks and benefits of the procedure when she is asked to sign the consent form.

Amniocentesis and subsequent abortion of affected fetuses can help reduce the incidence of birth defects. Naturally, accuracy in these tests is also important from a legal standpoint. If a mother is told that her fetus is normal and she later delivers an infant with a disease which could have been detected by amniocentesis, the physician who performed the amniocentesis and the laboratory that performed the tests could be held accountable.

Some physicians will not perform an amniocentesis unless the parents agree to an abortion if an abnormal fetus is detected. Milunsky (1974) disagrees with this practice. He believes that in such an instance, the physician imposes his philosophy on the parents; Milunsky argues that they have a right to know if their infant is normal. In a study by Golbers and co-workers (1979), based on 3000 high-risk cases in which amniocentesis was done, 95% of the studies showed fetal normalcy. Milunsky further suggested that it is the physician's duty to inform high-risk parents of the availability of, risks of, and indications for amniocentesis and to refer them elsewhere if personal beliefs prevent the physician from doing the procedure.

A case involving amniocentesis with ethical overtones was recently reported by Abert and associates (1978). A couple had produced one child with Hurler's syndrome, and although they desired other children, they did not want another one affected with the condition. During a subsequent pregnancy, studies performed at 18 weeks showed twin fetuses. Amniocentesis revealed that twin 1 was affected with Hurler's syndrome, while twin 2 was not. The parents decided to abort both fetuses, but asked whether there was any way to selectively abort the affected twin only. After the risks were explained, the physicians performed an intracardiac puncture of the affected twin, with the result that the fetal heart stopped. Twin 2 was delivered at 33 weeks' gestation without problems.

Amniocentesis may be used to determine fetal gestational age in cases in which early elective delivery is indicated, such as with Rh sensitization. The lecithin/sphingomyelin (L/S) ratio in amniotic fluid is an index of fetal lung maturity. If the L/S ratio shows immature fetal lungs, an obstetrician might delay the elective delivery of an immature infant with the potential for developing respiratory distress syndrome (RDS).

In summary, prenatal diagnosis is filled with difficulties through errors of omission or commission. Accuracy in performing the tests, appropriate action after the results are known, and confidentiality regarding results are important legal precepts relating to prenatal diagnosis.

FETAL RESEARCH

Research should not be permitted on fetuses if the investigators offer to perform the abortion to obtain the fetus for research. A Massachusetts law prohibits researchers from offering free abortions to women in exchange for fetuses to be used as research subjects, including some still in utero. Interesting questions regarding fetal research and abortion have been posed by Hirsch (1975). May women who plan to have abortions consent to experimentation on the fetus in utero? Does the woman have a legal right to the disposition of fetal remains? Can an aborted fetus be kept alive for experimental purposes? These and numerous other questions require careful legal scrutiny.

HOME BIRTHS

Many health professionals are reluctant to attend home births because they fear a malpractice action if problems arise. If acceptable steps have been taken to screen for possible problems and to provide for back-up medical facilities in the event of difficulties, Annas (1978) suggests it is highly unlikely that a malpractice suit would be successful. Many hospitals have made an effort to humanize deliveries, with use of birthing rooms and the like, in an attempt to provide family-centered maternity care.

Ethical and Legal Issues of Abortion

''Pro-life'' and ''pro-choice'' public groups have dramatically focused ethical and legal attention on the issue of abortion. Maternity nurses may be involved in the ethical dilemmas presented by this controversial issue, from a personal as well as a professional perspective. In order for a nurse to provide service to a client seeking an abortion, the nurse must understand her/his personal ethical position on abortion (Thompson and Thompson, 1981). A review of legal proceedings and court cases is presented to give the nurse information about the legal aspects of this issue.

As a result of the U.S. Supreme Court decision of January 1973 (reaffirmed in June 1983) abortion is legal anywhere in the United States. In a momentous seven-to-two decision, the Court declared the following:

1. During the first trimester, the state cannot bar any

woman from obtaining an abortion from a licensed physician.

2. In the second trimester, the state can regulate the performance of an abortion if such regulation relates to protection of the woman's health.
3. In the third trimester, the state can regulate and even prohibit abortions, except those deemed necessary to protect the woman's life and health, and the state may impose safeguards for the fetus.

The essence of the Court's decision is that existing state abortion control laws were found to be unconstitutional on the basis that they invaded the privacy of the mother. One of the major problems with the decision is that the Court did not decide the issue of when life begins. The Court reasoned that since physicians, theologians, and philosophers were unable to decide this issue, neither could the judiciary. However, the Court did define viability as that point of development when the fetus can survive outside the uterus (perhaps with artificial aid), at about 22 to 23 weeks' gestation. The decision also included the concept that the fetus is not a person, for purposes of protection under the Fourteenth Amendment, and that neither the woman's spouse nor the father of the fetus has any rights to prevent an abortion.

The Supreme Court decision did not provide for abortion on demand; the physician still has the right and the obligation to exercise professional judgment. Moreover, the decision did not mention pregnant minors. In some states, however, minors can obtain an abortion without the consent of their parents.

Provisions termed *conscience clauses* are found in most state laws. These stipulations allow physicians, institutions, and hospital personnel to refuse to assist in abortions if participation is against their moral, ethical, or religious principles, without fear of reprisal. Recent court decisions continue to uphold these conscience clauses. Nonetheless, public hospitals (city, county, and state) must permit their facilities to be used for abortions, since they are supported by public funds.

CONGRESSIONAL AMENDMENT

In December 1978, Congress passed the Hyde Amendment, which severely restricted the use of federal funds for abortions. This law allowed Medicaid funds to be used for abortions under three conditions only: (1) the woman's life is endangered by carrying the fetus to term; (2) two physicians have determined that the pregnancy would cause severe and long-lasting physical damage to the woman; or (3) the pregnancy was a result of rape or incest and was reported promptly to a law enforcement or public health agency. In response to this law, a class action suit was filed in federal court, but the law's constitutionality was upheld. In July 1980, the U.S. Supreme Court upheld the Hyde Amendment.

COURT CASES

In two prominent abortion cases, a primary dispute was the determination of the point at which an aborted fetus becomes a separate individual. Is this at the time it is separated from the mother (but still physically in utero) or when it is physically outside the mother's body? After summarizing these two cases, Wecht (1975) offered suggestions for physicians who perform abortions to terminate a late pregnancy. First, there should be documentation of any signs of fetal life either before or after delivery, especially at the point at which the fetus is considered a person, and second, emergency resuscitation should be initiated for any live-born fetus as defined in the state's statutes. Wecht further surmises that prosecutors could conceivably attempt indirect control over therapeutic abortions by producing fear in physicians about possible manslaughter or murder charges. He believes that the Supreme Court should further clarify its ruling.

ETHICAL CONSIDERATIONS

From an ethical standpoint, abortion is essentially the removal of the woman's support from the fetus, leading to loss of fetal survival, since it cannot sustain its own life without the mother. Bok (1978) suggests that if an abortion is performed after the diagnosis of a fetal defect, then the parents have consented to remove support from that particular fetus. This raises the issue of abortion for the fetus's own sake.

Camenisch (1976) concludes that one does not have the right to inflict the pain and tragic consequences of certain detectable serious diseases on an innocent infant. In his view this argument for abortion is not offered as a mask for other motives such as the economic and psychologic difficulties parents of such an infant would face, but rather to alleviate the suffering of the child. By this reasoning, the fetus receives "nothingness" rather than abnormality, and therefore no suffering because of its own malformations. He further suggests that if we could, we should choose health, normalcy, and lack of suffering for ourselves, so why not for another? If a damaged fetus is aborted, there would be more room and resources for a normal one. This line of thought does raise the questions of what is normal and healthy and who should make that decision.

It is difficult to summarize the abortion controversy, but basically the pro-choice proponents believe that the mother's rights take precedence and that abortion should be allowed to grant the mother freedom of choice and privacy. Many pro-choice proponents believe that abortions should be used only as a last resort, with contraception and adoption being other alternatives. Most pro-life advocates believe that the fetus is human from the moment of conception and as such should be protected from abortion, which ends life.

FETAL RIGHTS

Legally, from the time of conception, a fetus can inherit property and be the beneficiary of a trust. If a child is born alive and then dies of prenatal injuries, a wrongful death action may be brought, in most states, regardless of gestational duration. Even preconception injuries to the mother are grounds for suit by subsequent children for their resulting injuries.

Some courts have upheld fetal rights in utero. In a case in which the mother, a Jehovah's Witness, refused a blood transfusion, the court ordered the transfusion because the infant might otherwise have died. Legally, a fetus is not considered a person until it is born, but in the case of Smith vs. Brennan, reported by Ament (1974), "justice requires that the principle be recognized that a child has a legal right to begin life with a sound mind and body."

Legal Concepts During Labor and Delivery

Nurses who are involved in the care of women in labor have numerous legal responsibilities to these women. They must be knowledgeable about fetal monitoring and the proper actions to take in maternal, fetal, and neonatal emergencies. In addition, nurses have a legal obligation to inform the attending physician of their observations of the mother in labor.

FETAL MONITORS

Fetal monitors are now widely used in labor and delivery units. The nurse is responsible for applying the monitoring equipment to the client, operating the equipment, and assessing the tracings for possible complications. Any signs indicating problems should be reported to the physician immediately. There are guidelines for monitoring fetal heart rates defined by the American College of Obstetrics and Gynecology (ACOG) (Wiley, 1976). Wiley further suggests that the fetal heart rate records should be saved since they might prove to be vital evidence in a malpractice lawsuit.

If an alarm system is available on the monitoring device, the nurse should not deactivate the alarm for convenience. If the alarm is turned off and the woman subsequently develops a problem that is undetected as a result, the nurse could be held accountable for deactivating the alarm.

ANESTHETICS

During labor and delivery, anesthetics may be given for the mother's comfort, even though there are risks to the mother and infant. Nurse-anesthetists must be aware of correct procedures for administering anesthetics and nursing attendants must also strive to ensure the woman's safety.

General anesthetic risks to the infant should be considered, since all inhalant or intravenous anesthetic drugs promptly cross the placenta. The infant should be carefully observed after delivery if a general anesthetic is used, since these drugs may have severe depressant effects on the infant.

MATERNAL COMPLICATIONS

Numerous maternal complications may occur during the period of labor and delivery. Ideally, a woman should not be left unattended during labor, and frequent physical assessment of her condition should be made and recorded by the nurse. If the proper standard of care is not followed and the woman develops a complication, a case for negligence could be made.

If nurses detect signs of fetal distress, such as meconium staining of the amniotic fluid or a prolapsed cord, they must notify the physician immediately and prepare for emergency treatment. If a cesarean delivery is likely, all details relevant to the operation should be completed, such as noting the woman's condition, observance of sterile technique, and counting of sponges.

STILLBORN INFANTS

When an infant is born dead, there must be careful documentation of the events surrounding the delivery. Even though the birth of a stillborn infant is disquieting, the nurse must carefully chart the events as they occur. The physician may order that the infant be examined for congenital anomalies by means of x-ray and laboratory studies, including chromosome studies when possible. Even though a nurse may find such examinations repugnant, she should assist as necessary since the information may help to determine the cause of fetal death as well as provide information for genetic counseling. Legal problems could arise if proper procedures are not followed.

Legal Issues in the Postpartum Unit

Nursing care of new mothers involves legal obligations. If a woman convulses or hemorrhages, the nurse must notify the physician as well as take appropriate supportive action. Suits have been initiated because of postdelivery infections. If a woman can prove that incorrect technique was the cause of her infection, she may have a legal claim to negligence. If a woman is discharged early from the hospital and later develops a problem, she may sue the physician claiming *abandonment* because of the untimely discharge.

Summary

A wide variety of ethical and legal issues arise in the multifaceted field of maternity care. This chapter has presented a review of current legal attitudes toward several of the issues a nurse may encounter in the care of the maternity client and her infant. Perinatal nursing is a rapidly developing subspecialty, and the continued emergence of nurse-midwifery will probably be a trend of the future. Not only does genetics present legal problems today, but more legal issues will probably arise in the years to come. The abortion issue remains controversial and probably always will. Legal aspects of maternity nursing are essential knowledge for all nurses who plan to care for new mothers and their infants.

References and Readings

Aberg, A.F., et al.: Cardiac puncture of fetus with Hurler's disease avoiding abortion of unaffected co-twin (letter), Lancet **2**:990, Nov. 1978.

Ament, M.: The right to be well-born, Leg. Aspects Med. Pract. **2**:24, Nov./Dec. 1974.

Annas, G.J.: Homebirth: autonomy vs. safety, Hastings Cent. Rep. **8**:19, Aug. 1978.

Benjamin, M., and Curtis, J.: Ethics in nursing, London, 1981, Oxford University Press.

Bergerson, S.R.: Charting with a jury in mind, Nursing Life, pp. 30-33, July/Aug. 1982.

Bok, S.: Ethical problems of abortion, Hastings Cent. Rep. **8**:19, Aug. 1978.

Camenisch, P.F.: Abortion: for the fetus' own sake, Hastings Cent. Rep. **6**:38, April 1976.

Creighton, H.: Law every nurse should know, ed. 4, Philadelphia, 1981, W.B. Saunders Co.

Creighton, H.: Liability of nurse floated to another unit, Nsg. Management **13**(3):54, Mar. 1982.

Culliton, B.E.: Ethics Advisory Board confronts conception in the test tube, Science **202**:4364, Oct. 1978.

Edwards, R.G.: The problem of compensation for antenatal injuries, Nature **246**:54, Nov. 1973.

Golbers, M.S., et al.: Prenatal genetic diagnosis in 3000 amniocenteses, N. Engl. J. Med. **300**,1979.

Hakanson, E.Y.: Reducing the risk involved in providing medical care for women, Malpractice Digest, St. Paul Fire and Marine, July/Aug. 1980.

Hirsch, H.L.: Legal guidelines for the performance of abortions, Am. J. Obstet. Gynecol. **122**:679, 1975.

Ladimer, I.: Risks in the practice of modern obstetrics: a legal point of view. In Aladjem, S., editor: Risks in the practice of modern obstetrics, ed. 2, St. Louis, 1975, The C.V. Mosby Co.

Milunsky, A.: Prenatal diagnosis of genetic abnormalities, Clin. Perinatol. **1**:25, 1974.

Murchison, I., Nichols, T.S., and Hanson, R.: Legal accountability in the nursing process, ed. 2, St. Louis, 1982, The C.V. Mosby Co.

Regan, W.A.: Nursing malpractice: a giant leap in damages, R.N., Dec. 1981.

Richardson, D.W.: Artificial insemination in the human. In Emery, A.E.H., editor: Modern trends in human genetics, London, 1975, Butterworth and Co.

Steinfels, M.: In vitro fertilization: "ethically acceptable" research, Hastings Cent. Rep. **9**:5, June 1979.

Thompson, J.B., and Thompson, H.O.: Ethics in nursing, New York, 1981, Macmillan Publishing Co., Inc.

Wecht, C.H.: A comparison of two abortion-related legal inquiries, Legal Aspects Med. Pract. **3**:26, 1975.

Wiley, J.: The nurse's legal responsibility in obstetric monitoring, J.O.G.N. Nurs. Sept./Oct. 1976.

Basic Concepts of Reproduction

6 Anatomy and Physiology of Reproduction

7 Psychosocial Aspects of Reproduction

8 Cultural Aspects of Maternity Nursing

9 The Family

10 Genetics

11 Fertility

12 Infertility

13 Control of Fertility

UNIT TWO

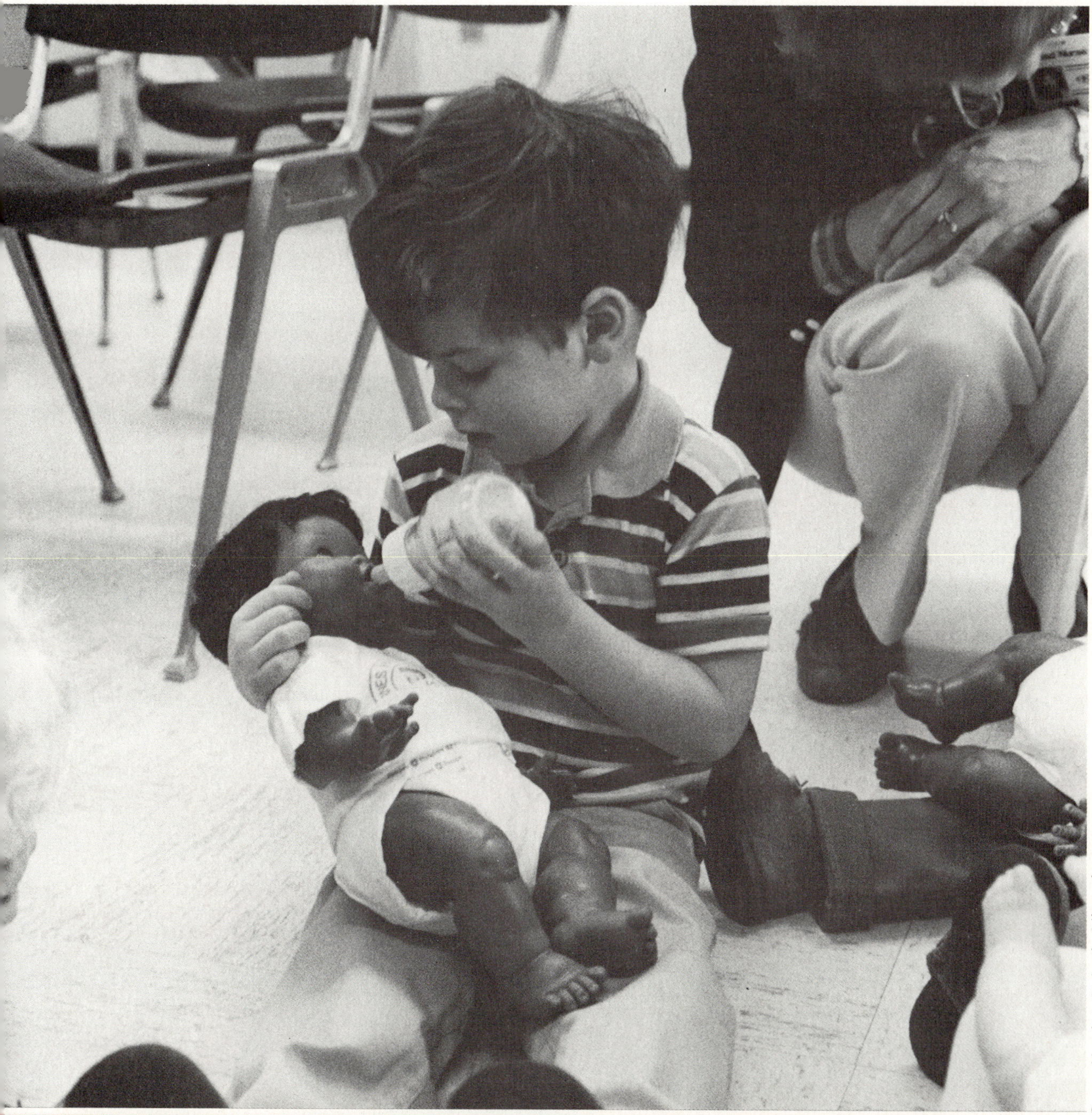

Barnes Hospital, St. Louis, Missouri

6
Anatomy and Physiology of Reproduction

- **Female Reproductive System**
  - External structures
    - Pelvic floor and perineum
  - Internal genitalia
    - Fallopian tubes
    - Ureters
    - Uterus
    - Vagina
    - Ovaries: female gonads
    - Abdominal wall
    - Anatomy of the bony pelvis
  - Breasts
    - Anatomy
    - Physiology
- **Male Reproductive System**
  - Overview of reproductive system structures throughout the life span
  - External genitalia
    - Mons pubis
    - Penis
    - Scrotum
  - Internal genitalia
    - Testes: male gonads
    - Canal system
    - Accessory reproductive tract glands
    - Semen
- **Menstrual Cycle**
  - Menstrual myths
  - Historical perspective
  - Hypothalamus and pituitary
  - Hypothalamic-pituitary cycle
  - Ovarian cycle
  - Endometrial cycle
  - Cervical changes
- **Puberty**
- **Prostaglandins**
  - Role in reproductive functions
  - Primary dysmenorrhea
- **Physiologic Response to Sexual Stimulation**
  - Four-phase response cycle
    - Excitement phase: women
    - Excitement phase: men
    - Plateau phase: women
    - Plateau phase: men
    - Orgasmic phase: women
    - Orgasmic phase: men
    - Resolution phase: women
    - Resolution phase: men
  - Biphasic response
    - Phase 1: vasocongestive reaction
    - Phase 2: reflex clonic muscular contractions
  - Clinical significance
    - Multiple orgasm
    - Simultaneous orgasm
    - Clitoral vs. vaginal orgasm
    - Variations in orgasmic patterns
  - Summary

The maternity nurse shares in an experience as old as humanity—the emergence of new life. The nurse brings to that experience a rich heritage of skills and technology, as well as greater freedom to apply that heritage than ever before. Maternity nursing provides opportunity to care for and care about the childbearing family. The maternity nurse begins with a sound knowledge of the basic components of life and its continuity: the anatomic structures and their functions in conception, pregnancy, and birth. Knowledge of the anatomy and physiology of those structures, both female and male, involved in reproduction is basic to planning for, implementing, and evaluating nursing care of the obstetric client and her family.

Although the female and male reproductive systems differ markedly in appearance, their structures are homologous (having the same embryonic origin) (Tables 6.1 and 6.2; Figs. 6.1 and 6.2.). Each structure performs a vital role in the continuation of the human species and the generation and maintenance of secondary sexual characteristics. Through hormonal influences the genitals, pelvis, and breasts acquire the unique adaptations necessary to childbearing. Both female and male reproductive systems consist of the following four principal components:

1. External genitalia
2. A pair of primary sex glands (gonads)
3. Ducts leading from the gonads to the body's exterior
4. Secondary (accessory) sex glands

In the normal course of events, life begins and is sustained for 9 months within the protective environment of the female. Therefore the female organs will be considered first, beginning with the external genital structures.

The female's external and internal reproductive structures are targets for estrogens throughout her life span and they atrophy (reduce in size) with age and/or a drop in estrogen production. An extensive and complex innervation and very generous blood supply support the functions of these structures. The comparative size, shape, and color vary extensively from woman to woman depending on her heredity, age, race, and number of children she has borne.

Table 6.1
Female and Male Homologues: External Genitalia

Female	Male
Glans clitoris	Glans penis
Prepuce (identifiable only by microscopic histologic examination)	Prepuce (foreskin)
Corpus clitoris	Shaft (body)
Vestibule	Penile urethra
Labia minora	Penoscrotal raphe (seam that closes urethra)
Entire urethra	Prostatic urethra
Labia majora	Scrotum

Table 6.2
Female and Male Homologues: Internal Structures*

Female		Male
Bartholin's glands		Cowper's glands
Paraurethral glands		Prostate gland
Fallopian tubes Uterus Upper four fifths of vagina	Müllerian ducts	Appendix testis Utricle (prostatic)
Ovary		Testis
Scattered vestigial (trace) remnants	Mesonephric ducts	Epididymis, vas deferens, seminal vesicles, ejaculatory duct

*In the genetic *female,* the *Müllerian* embryonic tissue should develop fully, while the mesonephric embryonic tissue should disappear. In the genetic *male,* the structures of *mesonephric* origin should develop fully, while the Müllerian embryonic tissue should disappear.

Clinical significance: Drugs taken by the mother affect certain embryonic tissue; for example, diethylstilbestrol (DES) affects all structures of the Müllerian system leading to the syndrome called "DES daughter." In the male if the Müllerian system does not degenerate, or in the female if the mesonephric system does not degenerate, various forms of abnormalities occur, for example, pseudohermaphroditism.

Fig. 6.1
Homologues of external genitalia.

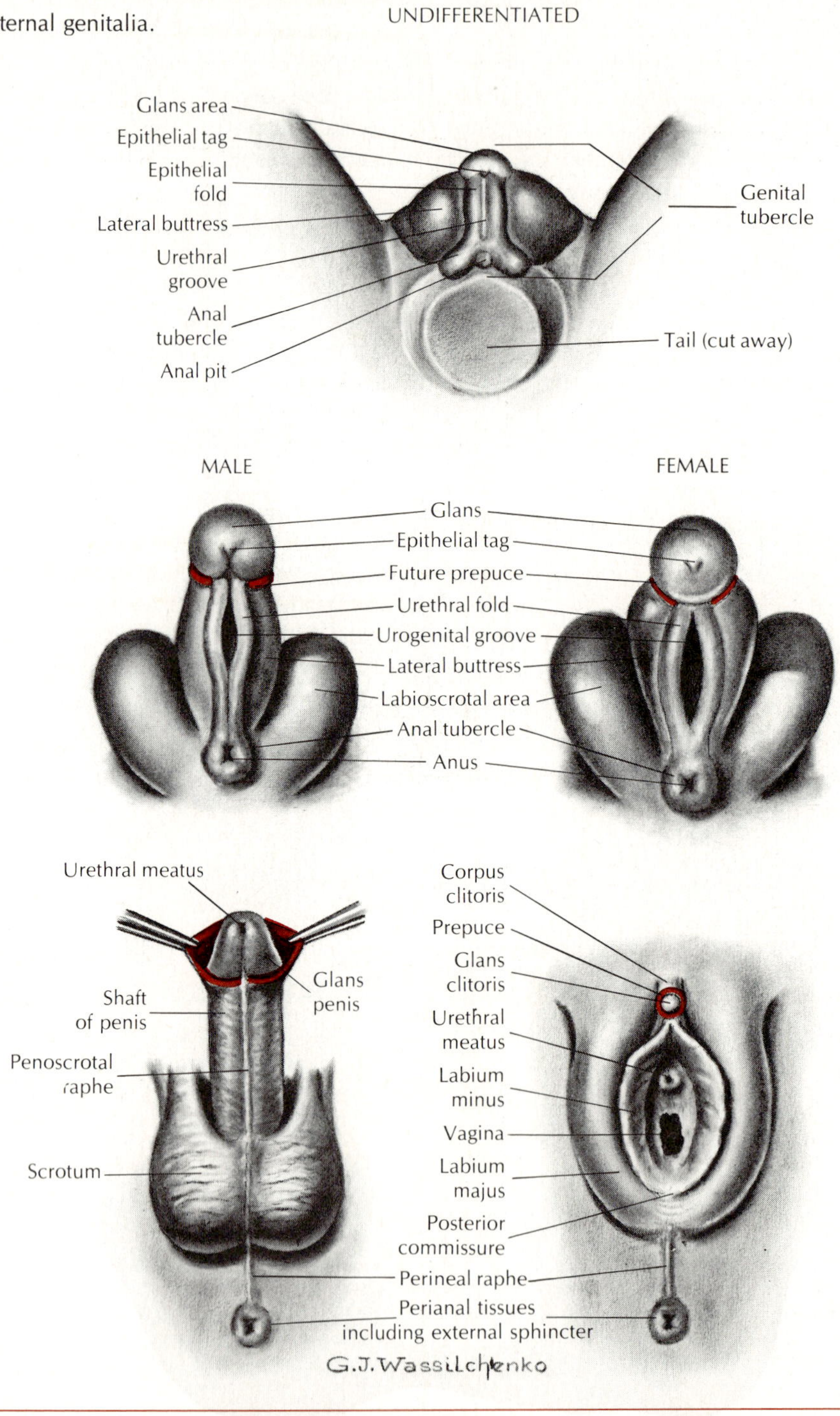
UNDIFFERENTIATED
Glans area
Epithelial tag
Epithelial fold
Lateral buttress
Urethral groove
Anal tubercle
Anal pit
Genital tubercle
Tail (cut away)
MALE
FEMALE
Glans
Epithelial tag
Future prepuce
Urethral fold
Urogenital groove
Lateral buttress
Labioscrotal area
Anal tubercle
Anus
Urethral meatus
Shaft of penis
Glans penis
Penoscrotal raphe
Scrotum
Corpus clitoris
Prepuce
Glans clitoris
Urethral meatus
Labium minus
Vagina
Labium majus
Posterior commissure
Perineal raphe
Perianal tissues including external sphincter
G.J.Wassilchenko

Fig. 6.2
Homologues of internal genitalia.

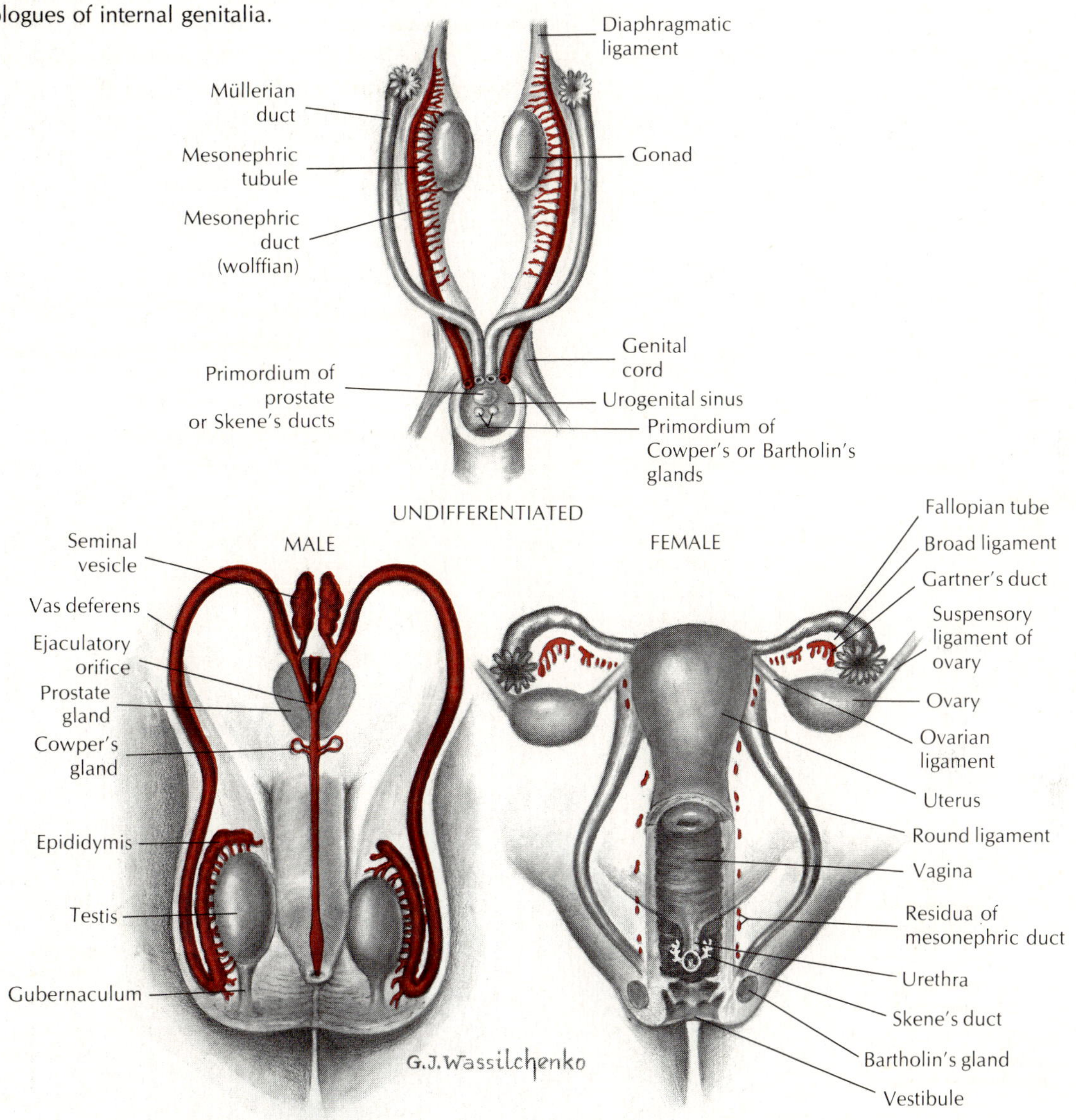

Female Reproductive System

EXTERNAL STRUCTURES

Following are the external female genitalia (vulva, pudenda) (Fig. 6.3):

1. Mons veneris (mons pubis)
2. Labia majora (sing., labium majus) and minora (sing., labium minus)
3. Clitoris
4. Vestibule
    a. Urinary meatus, or urethral orifice
    b. Lesser vestibular, paraurethral, or Skene's glands
    c. Hymen and vaginal introitus, or orifice
    d. Greater vestibular, vulvovaginal, or Bartholin's glands
5. Fourchet
6. Perineum

The *mons veneris,* or *mons pubis,* is the rounded, soft fullness of subcutaneous fatty tissue and loose connective tissue over the symphysis pubis. The loose connective tissue permits considerable edema formation in this area. This information is useful when assessing degree of fluid retention when the woman suffers pregnancy-induced hypertension (PIH). It contains many sebaceous (oil) glands and develops coarse, dark, curly hair at pubarche, about 1 to 2 years before the onset of the menses. Menarache occurs on the average at 13 years of age. Typically, the pattern of hair growth (the escutcheon) in 75% of women is a triangle shape with the base along the top of the symphysis pubis, while the escutcheon in males is more diamond shaped. In 25% of women, pubic hair extends upward toward the umbilicus along the linea alba. Characteristics of pubic hair vary from sparse and fine among Oriental women to thick, coarse, and curly among black women. The functions of the mons are to play a role in sensuality and to protect the symphysis pubis during coitus.

Labia majora are two rounded lengthwise folds of skin-covered fat and connective tissue that merge with the mons. They extend from the mons downward around the labia minora, ending in the perineum in the

Fig. 6.3
External female genitalia.

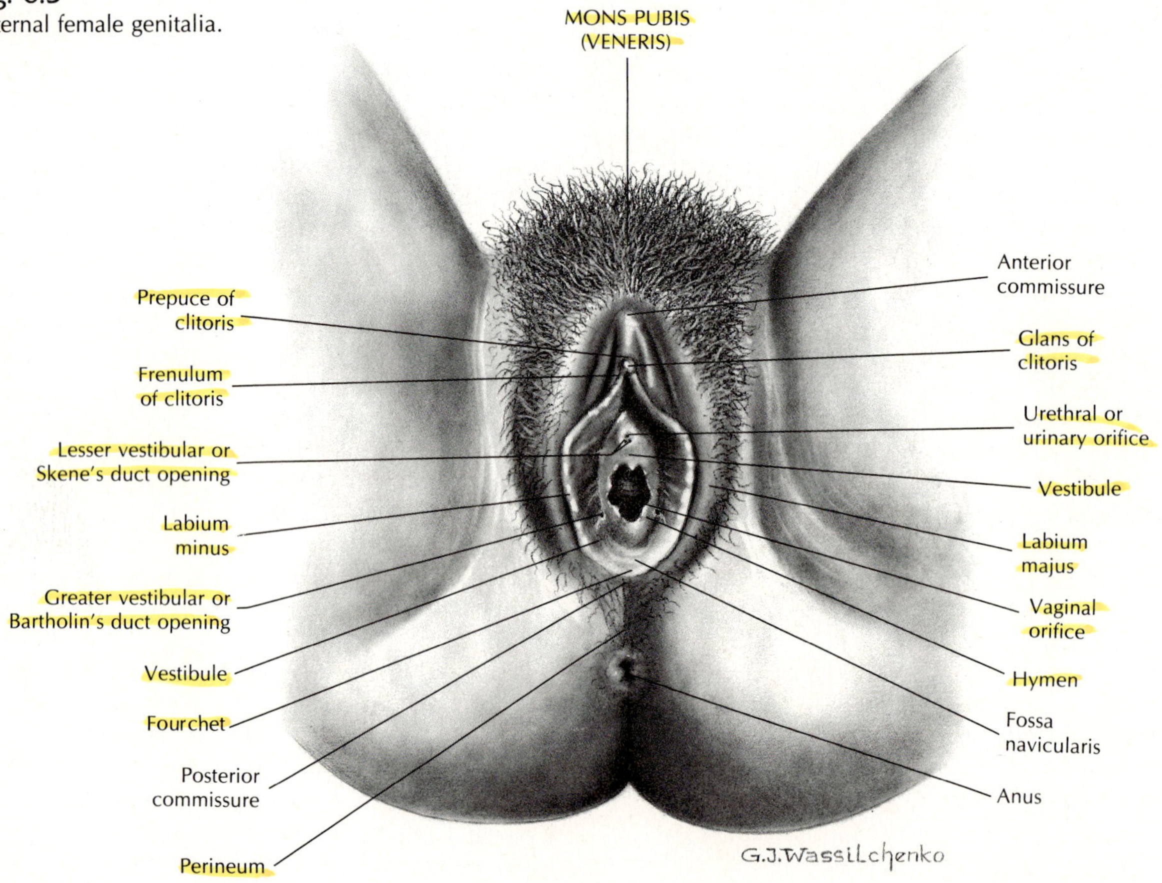

midline, and act as protection for the labia minora, urinary meatus, and vaginal introitus. In the nulliparous woman,* the labia majora come together in the midline, obscuring the vaginal introitus. Some labial separation and even gaping of the vaginal introitus follow childbirth and perineal or vaginal injury.

On their lateral surfaces, the labial skin is thick, usually pigmented darker than the surrounding tissues, and covered with coarse hair (similar to that of the mons) that thins out toward the perineum. The medial (inner) surfaces of the labia majora are smooth, thick, and without hair. They contain an abundant supply of sebaceous glands and sweat glands and are highly vascular. Varicose veins in the labia may occur and become prominent when the woman is obese or stands for long periods of time or during pregnancy. Obstetric or sexual injury to this area of extensive vascularization may result in hematomas (collections of blood in a small area).

The lymphatic system is extensive and serves many structures in the pelvic area. This is the reason for the extensive and rapid spread of reproductive tract malignancies.

The extreme sensitivity of the labia majora to touch, pain, and temperature is due to the extensive network of nerves. Innervation of the anterior one third of the labia is from L1 (lumbar 1), while the posterior two thirds is supplied mainly from S3 (sacral 3). Because of their nerve network the functions of the labia majora include sensual arousal.

The pair of round ligaments from the uterus inserts into the anterior portion of the labia majora.

The *labia minora,* located between the labia majora, are narrow, lengthwise folds of hairless skin extending downward from beneath the clitoris and merging with the fourchet. While the lateral and anterior aspects of the labia are usually pigmented, their medial surfaces are similar to vaginal mucosa, that is, pink and moist. Their rich vascularity gives them a reddish color and permits marked turgescence (swelling) of the labia minora with emotional or physical stimulation. The numerous sebaceous glands that open onto the skin surface are subject to cyst formation. A rich nerve supply makes them very sensitive. While the heightened sensitivity of the labia minora adds to their erotic function, any irritation in the area, such as vulvovaginitis, is very uncomfortable. The glands in the labia minora also serve to lubricate the vulva. The space between the labia minora is called the vestibule.

The *clitoris* is a short, cylindric, erectile organ fixed just beneath the arch of the pubis; the visible portion is about 6 × 6 mm or less in the unaroused state. The tip of the clitoral body is called the glans and is more sensitive than its shaft. In healthy women the length of the clitoral body varies from 2 mm to 1 cm, and the width is usually estimated at 4 to 5 mm. When sexually aroused, the glans and shaft increase in size.

Its rich vascularity and innervation make the clitoris highly sensitive to temperature, touch, and pressure sensation. The clitoris contains more nerve endings than does its male homologue, the glans penis. Its main function is to stimulate and elevate levels of sexual tension.

Sebaceous glands of the clitoris secrete smegma, a fatty substance with a distinctive odor, that serves as a pheromone (an organic compound that provides communication with other members of the same species to elicit a certain response, which in this case is erotic stimulation of the human male). The term *clitoris* comes from a Greek word meaning "key" because the clitoris was seen as the key to female sexuality.

Near their anterior junction, the right and left labia minora separate into medial and lateral portions. The lateral portions unite above the clitoris to form its prepuce, a hoodlike covering; the medial portions unite below the clitoris to form its frenulum. Sometimes the prepuce covers the clitoris. As a result, this area has the appearance of an opening that can be mistaken for the urethral meatus if the nurse does not identify vulvar structures carefully. Attempts to insert a catheter into this sensitive area can cause considerable discomfort.

The *vestibule* is an ovoid or boat-shaped area formed between the labia minora, clitoris, and fourchet. The vestibule contains the openings to the urethra, paraurethral (lesser vestibular, Skene's) glands, the vagina, and the paravaginal (greater vestibular, vulvovaginal, or Bartholin's) glands. The thin, almost mucosal, surface of the vestibule is easily irritated by chemicals (feminine deodorant sprays, bubble bath salts), heat, discharges, and friction (tight jeans).

Although not a true part of the reproductive system, the *urinary (urethral) meatus* (Fig. 6.4) is considered here because of its closeness and relationship to the vulva. The meatus is a pink or reddened opening of varying shapes, often with slightly puckered margins. The meatus marks the terminal, or distal, part of the urethra. It is usually located about 2.5 cm below the clitoris.

The *lesser vestibular* (paraurethral, Skene's) *glands* are short tubular structures that are situated posterolaterally just inside the urethral meatus, at about the 5 and 7 o'clock positions around the meatus (Fig. 6.4). They produce a small amount of mucus and are especially susceptible to gonorrheal infection.

The *hymen* (Fig. 6.5) is a partial, rarely complete, elastic but tough mucosa-covered fold around the *vagi-*

*Woman who has never carried a pregnancy to viability (24 weeks).

Fig. 6.4
Structure of female urethra.

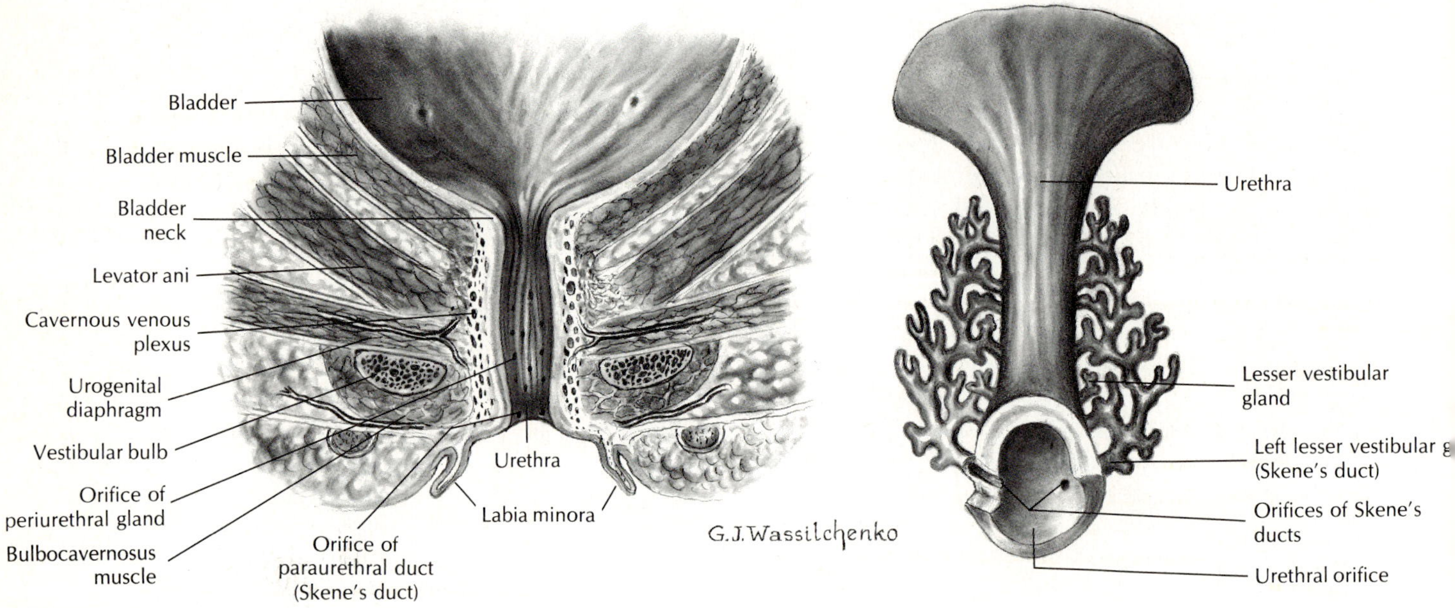

nal introitus. In virginal females, the hymen may be an impediment to vaginal examination, insertion of internal menstrual tampons, or coitus. The hymen may be elastic and allow distention, or it may be torn easily. Occasionally the hymen covers the orifice completely, resulting in an imperforate hymen that prevents passage of menstrual flow, instrumentation (e.g., with a speculum), or coitus. A hymenotomy may be necessary in some cases. After instrumentation, use of tampons, coitus, or vaginal delivery, residual tags of the hymen (hymenal caruncles or carunculae myrtiformes) may be seen.

One common myth is that one can tell by the condition of the hymen whether or not a female is a virgin. Sexually active and even parous females may have intact hymens. For other women the hymen may be torn during strenuous physical work or exercise, masturbation, or use of tampons. Some cultural groups cleanse the infant girl so vigorously, the hymen is torn, leaving only vaginal tags in its place. Therefore the "test for virginity"—evidence of bleeding following sexual intercourse—is an unreliable criterion.

The *greater vestibular* (vulvovaginal, Bartholin's) *glands* are two compound glands at the base of the labia majora, one on either side of the vaginal orifice. Each gland is drained by several ducts, about 1.5 cm long. Each opens into the groove between the hymen and the labia minora. Usually the gland openings are not visible or palpable. The glands secrete a small amount of clear, viscid mucus, especially during coitus. The alkaline pH of the mucus is supportive of sperm. These glands are susceptible to gonorrheal infection and to abscess and cyst formation.

The *fourchet* is a thin, flat, transverse fold of tissue formed where the tapering labia majora and minora merge in the midline below the vaginal orifice. A small depression, the fossa navicularis, lies between the fourchet and the hymen. The perineum, fourchet, and fossa navicularis, richly vascular areas, are subject to laceration or are purposely incised to enlarge the opening (episiotomy) during vaginal delivery (see discussion of episiotomy, Chapter 37).

The *perineum* is the skin-covered muscular area between the vaginal introitus and the anus. The perineum forms the base of the perineal body (see below). The terms *vulva* and *perineum* occasionally but inaccurately are used interchangeably.

Pelvic floor and perineum. The pelvic floor and perineum are composed of the pelvic diaphragm, the urogenital diaphragm or triangle, and the muscles of the external genitalia and anus (Figs. 6.4, 6.6, and 6.7).

The *upper pelvic diaphragm,* composed of muscles and their fascia and ligaments, extends across the lowest part of the pelvic cavity like a hammock. The larg-

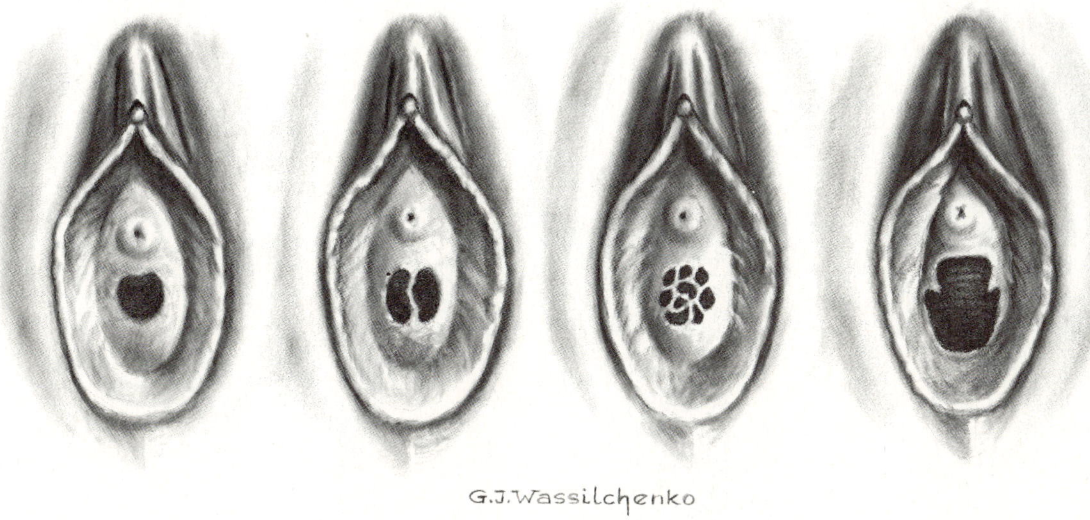

Fig. 6.5
Hymens.

est and most significant portion of the diaphragm is formed by the pair of broad, thin *levator ani muscles* that extend sheetlike between the ischial spines and coccyx, and the sacrum. The levator ani group of muscles is made up of three muscle pairs: puborectalis, iliococcygeus, and pubococcygeus muscles. The pubococcygeus muscle is particularly significant for women. Its importance lies not only in sexual sensory function (see discussion of sexual response cycle, p. 93), but also in bladder control and during labor for controlling perineal relaxation and expulsion of the fetus during birth.

The second paired muscles of the upper pelvic diaphragm are the closely joined *coccygeus muscles*. These muscles extend from the ischial spines to the coccyx and lower sacrum. The several parts of the pelvic diaphragm provide a slinglike support to abdominal and pelvic viscera.

The strength and resilience of this sling are derived from the way in which the layered parts of this sling are interwoven and interlaced. The layers are not fixed; that is, they slide over each other. This unique arrangement not only strengthens its supportive capacity but also allows for dilation of the vagina during the birth process and its closure after delivery and assists with constriction of the urethra, vagina, and anal canal that pass through the diaphragm.

The *urogenital (lower pelvic) diaphragm* is located in the hollow of the pubic arch and consists of the *transverse perineal muscles*. The transverse perineal muscles originate at the ischial tuberosities and insert into the perineal body. The strong muscle fibers provide support to the anal canal during defecation and to the lower vagina during delivery. The deep transverse perineal muscles join to form a central seam or raphe. Some of their fibers encircle the urinary meatus and vaginal sphincters.

The *perineum* is located below the upper and lower pelvic diaphragm. Its muscles and fascia reinforce the strength of the pelvic diaphragm and aid in constricting the urinary, vaginal, and anal openings. The *bulbocavernosus muscle* (sphincter vaginae; Fig. 6.7) fibers originate in the perineal body and surround the vaginal opening as the muscle fibers pass forward to insert into the pubis.

The *ischiocavernosus muscles* originate in the tuberosities of the ischium and continue at an angle to insert next to the bulbocavernosus muscles. These muscle fibers contract to cause erection of the clitoris.

Anal sphincter muscle fibers originate at the coccyx, separate to pass on either side of the anus, fuse, and then insert into the transverse perineal muscles.

The bulbocavernosus, transverse perineal, and anal sphincter muscle fibers can be strengthened through Kegel exercises (see p. 309).

Fig. 6.6
A, Muscles and fascia of urogenital diaphragm. **B,** Pubococcygeus muscle. **C,** Pubic bone.

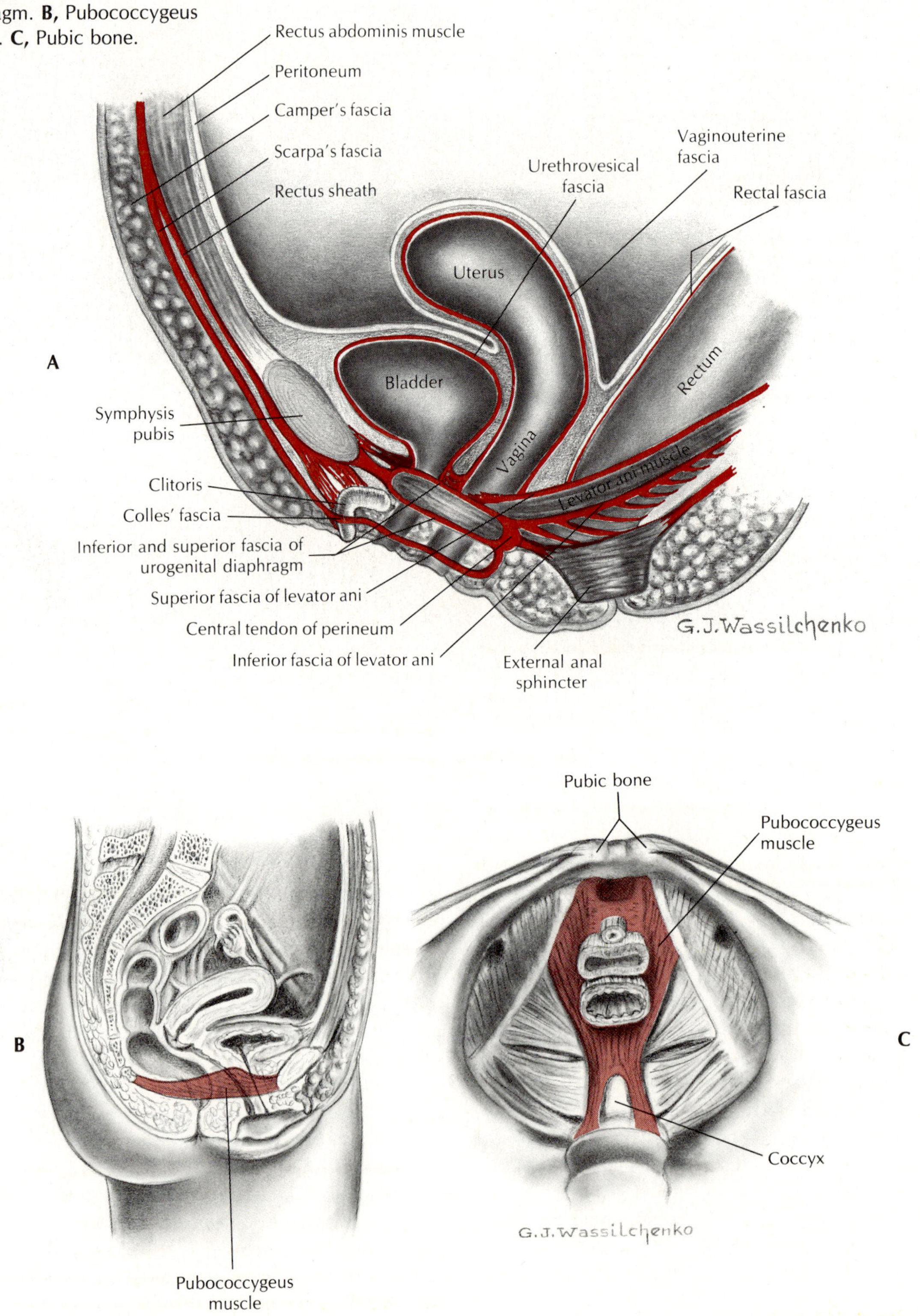

Fig. 6.7
Internal female reproductive tract and supporting structures.

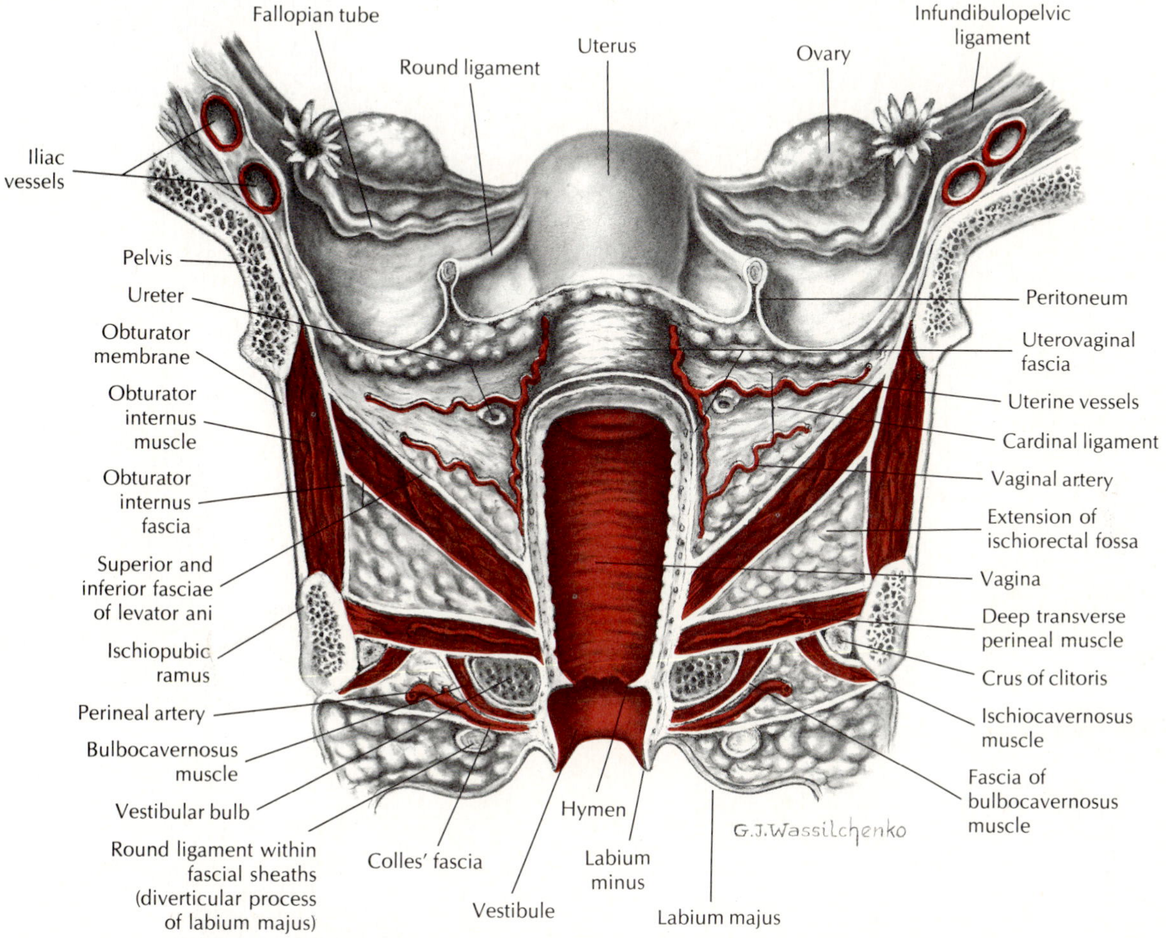

The *perineal body,* the wedge-shaped mass between the vaginal and anal openings, serves as an anchor point for the muscles, fascia, and ligaments of the upper and lower pelvic diaphragms. The skin-covered base of the body is known as the perineum.* The perineal body, about 4 cm wide by 4 cm deep, is continuous with the septum between the rectum and vagina. This tissue is flattened and stretched as the fetus moves through the birth canal. Occasionally the perineal body is lacerated or surgically cut (episiotomy) during delivery. Appropriate surgical repair is necessary to reestablish support to the pelvic structures.

Knowledge of the anatomy and physiology of the pelvic floor and perineum provides a basis for understanding and implementing appropriate nursing actions in relation to voluntary sphincter control during urination, coitus, and defecation and the normal mechanism of labor and delivery. In addition, the student has the information necessary to understand and utilize knowledge regarding the etiology, management, and prevention of disorders such as uterine prolapse and urinary stress incontinence.

*The perineum is sometimes defined as including all the muscles, fascia, and ligaments of the upper (pelvic) and lower (urogenital) diaphragms.

INTERNAL GENITALIA

Fallopian tubes. The paired fallopian (uterine) tubes (Figs. 6.8 to 6.10) measure about 12 cm in length. Each tube has an outer coat of peritoneum, a middle, thin muscular coat, and an inner mucosa. The smooth muscle fibers are arranged in an inner circular and an outer longitudinal layer. The mucosal lining consists of columnar cells some of which are ciliated and others of which are secretory.

Fig. 6.8
Uterus and adnexa posterior view.

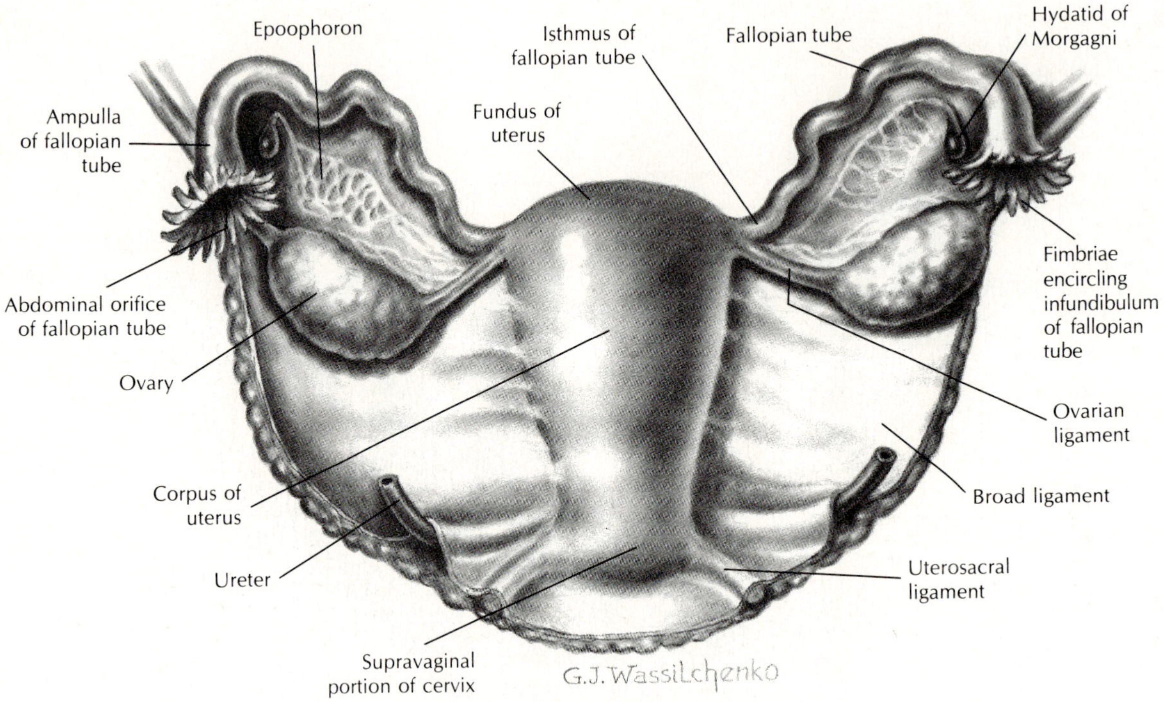

Fig. 6.9
Cross section of uterus, adnexa, and upper vagina.

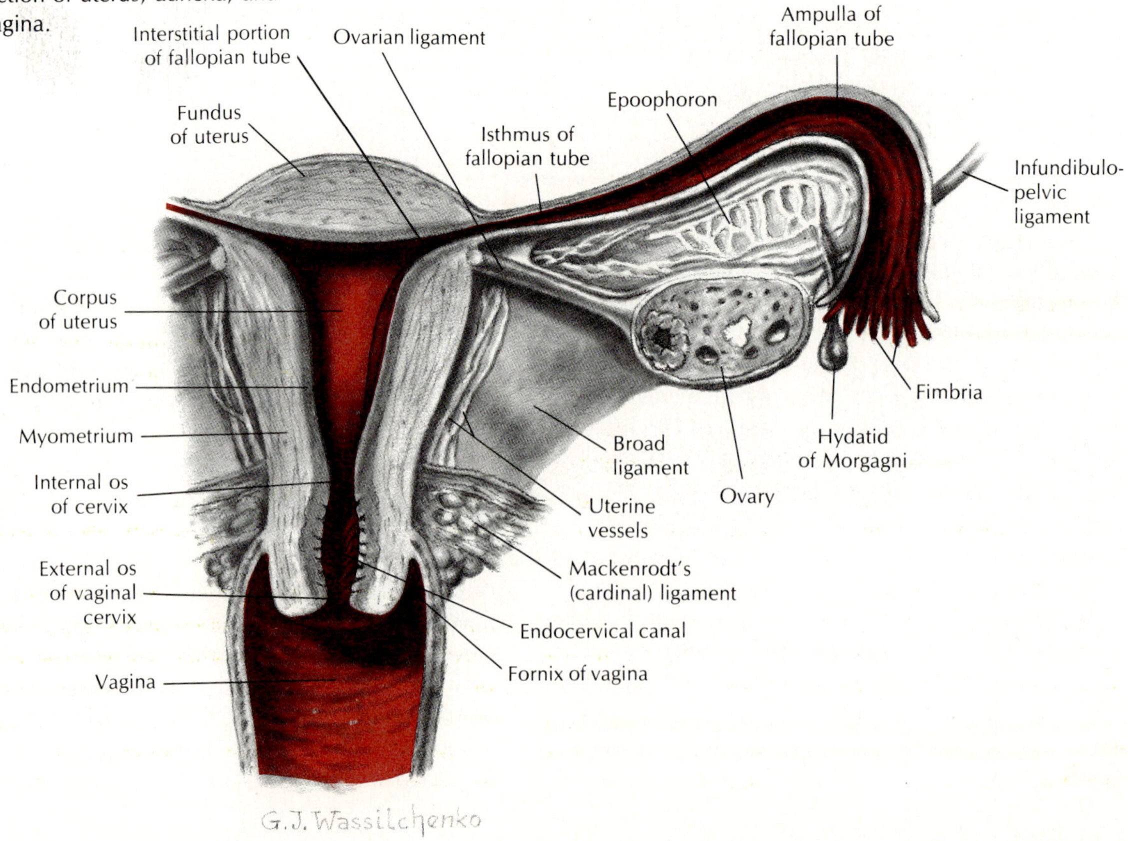

Fig. 6.10
Midsagittal view of female pelvic organs, with woman lying supine.

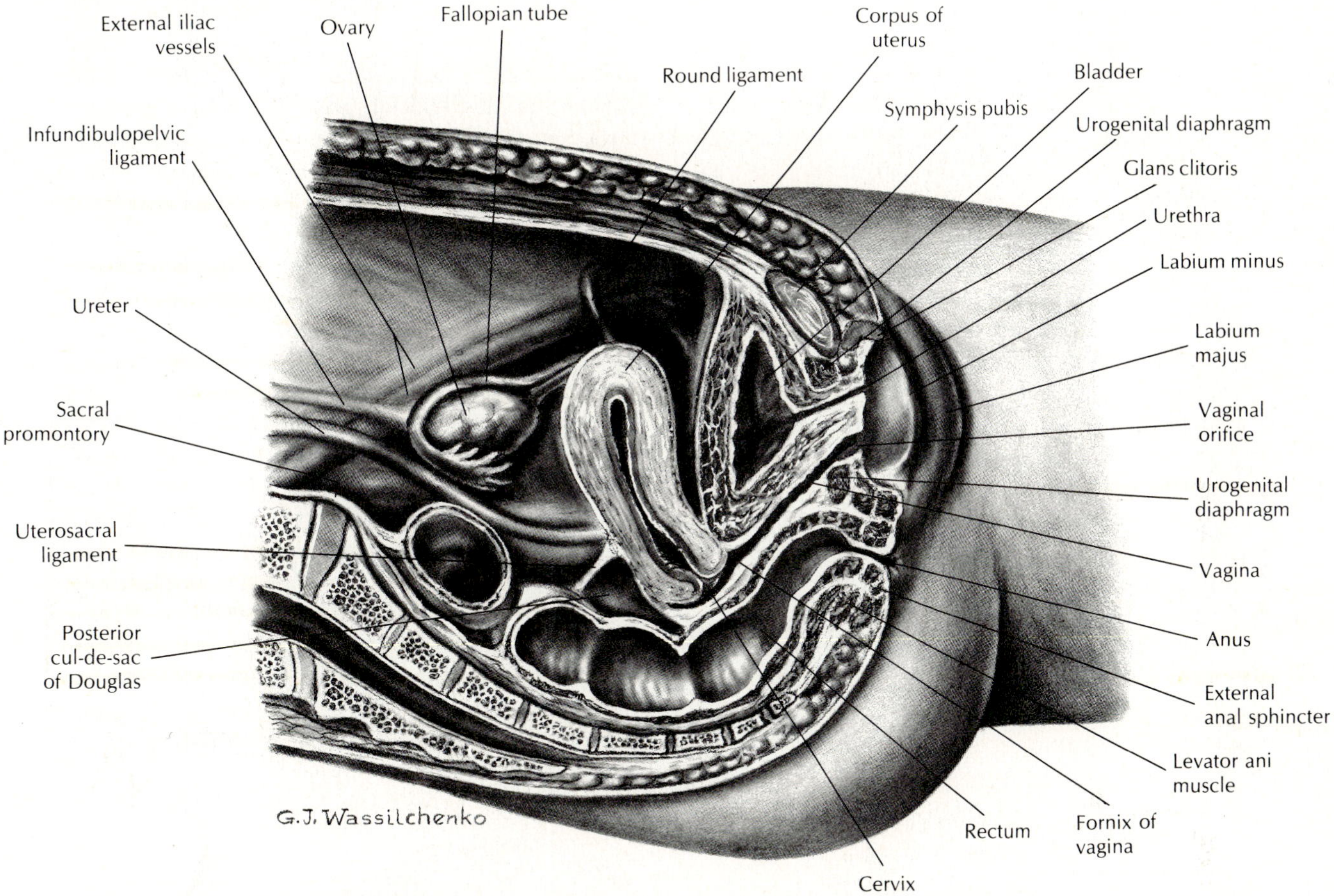

The structure of the fallopian tube changes along its length. Four distinctive segments can be identified: (1) the infundibulum, (2) the ampulla, (3) the isthmus, and (4) the interstitial part. The *infundibulum* is the most distal portion. Its funnel or trumpet-shaped opening is encircled with fimbriae. The infundibulum has been described as a ruffled petunia or a sea anemone. The fimbriae become swollen, almost erectile, at ovulation. The function of these fingerlike projections is to pull the ovum into the tube with wavelike beckoning motions. Infertility to some degree occurs if the fimbriae are cut off or diseased (as from pelvic inflammatory disease).

The *ampulla* makes up the distal and middle segment of the tube. It is in the ampulla that the sperm and ovum meet, where fertilization occurs.

The *isthmus* is proximal to the ampulla. It is small and firm, much like the round ligament. Because it looks and feels like the round ligament, care must be taken during tubal surgery to avoid confusing the two structures.

The *interstitial* (or intramural) portion passes through the myometrium between the fundus and the body of the uterus and has the smallest lumen. Before the fertilized ovum can pass through this lumen or tunnel, measuring less then 1 mm in diameter, it has to discard its crown of granulosa cells.

The ovum is propelled along the tube partially by the cilia but primarily by the peristaltic movements of the muscular coat, toward the uterine cavity. Peristaltic motion is influenced by estrogen and prostaglandins. Peristaltic activity of the fallopian tubes and the secretory function of their mucosal lining are greatest at the time of ovulation. The columnar cells secrete a nutrient to sustain the ovum while it is in the tube. The mucosa is thinnest at the time of menstruation.

Special clinical significance. Each tube and its mucosa are continuous with that of the uterus and the vagina. Therefore infection can spread by direct extension from the vaginal orifice into the peritoneal cavity. Gonorrheal infection of the fallopian tubes is a major cause of infertility if it is not treated early and intensively with antibiotics. Gonorrhea spreads by direct extension and produces a purulent discharge that glues the mucosal surfaces together, closing the tube. Scar formation occurs with healing. The tube may be permanently blocked from scar tissue, resulting in sterility, or partially blocked, resulting in ectopic pregnancy (see p. 784) because the path of the fertilized egg is blocked from entering the uterine cavity.

Ureters. Although the ureters are not part of the reproductive tract, they are discussed here because of their close anatomic proximity (Figs. 6.8 and 6.10). As the ureters leave the kidney, they pass just behind the ovarian blood vessels close to the fallopian tubes and in front of the uterine blood vessels. The closeness of these structures is important, especially during surgery. Surgical procedures (e.g., tubal ligation) in this area could result in injury to the ureters. If bleeding from an ovarian or uterine artery must be stopped by clamping, the ureter may be accidentally injured or clamped.

Uterus. The uterus is normally in the midline and is fully movable, symmetric in shape, and nontender, smooth, and firm to the touch. The degree of firmness varies with several factors; for example, it is spongier during the secretory phase of the menstrual cycle, softer during pregnancy, and firmer after menopause.

Structure

Shape, size, and divisions. The uterus is a flattened, hollow, muscular, thick-walled organ that looks somewhat like an upside-down pear (Fig. 6.9). Its length, width, and thickness vary, averaging about 7.5 cm × 3.5 cm × 2 cm (3 × 1½ × ¾ in). In the adult woman who has never been pregnant, the uterus weighs 60 g (2 oz).

The uterus has three parts: the *fundus*, the upper, rounded prominence above the insertion of the fallopian tubes; the *corpus*, or main portion, encircling the intrauterine cavity; and the *isthmus*, the slightly constricted portion that joins the corpus to the cervix and is known as the lower uterine segment during pregnancy.

Uterine wall. The wall of the uterus is made up of three layers: the endometrium, the myometrium, and a partial outer layer of parietal peritoneum (Fig. 6.9).

The highly vascular *endometrium* is a lining of mucous membrane composed of three layers: a compact surface layer, a spongy middle layer of loose connective tissue, and a dense inner layer that attaches the endometrium to the myometrium. During menstruation

Fig. 6.11
Schematic arrangement of directions of muscle fibers of three layers of myometrium. Note that uterine muscle fibers are continuous with supportive ligaments of uterus.

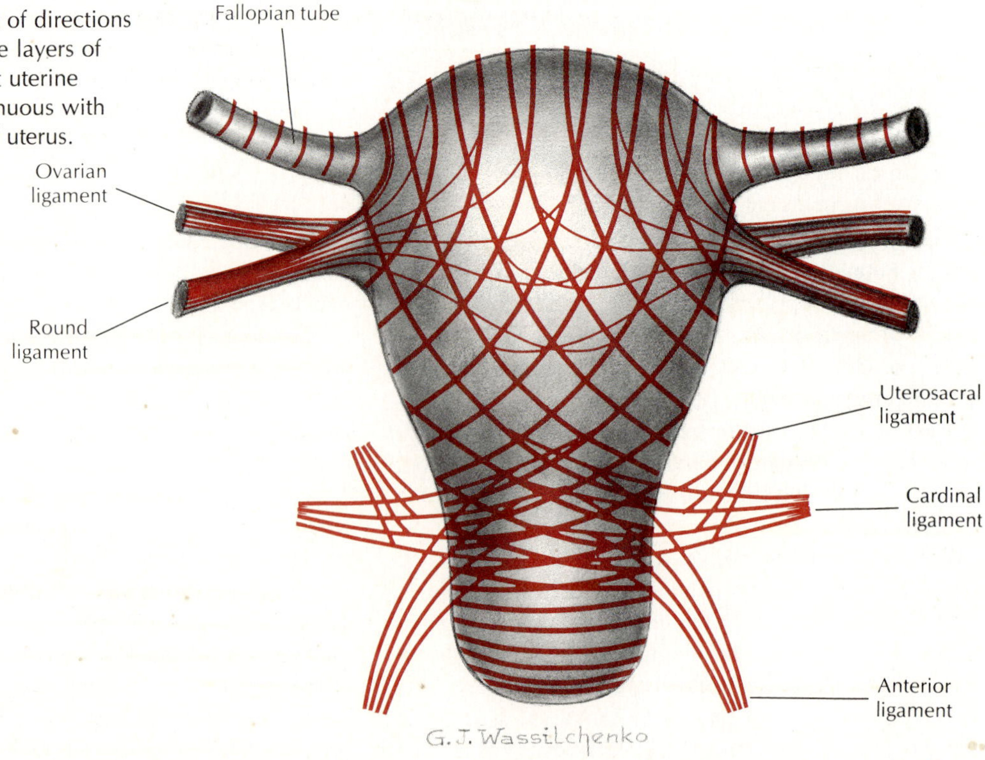

and following delivery, the compact surface and middle spongy layers slough off. Just after menstrual flow ends, the endometrium is 0.5 mm thick; near the end of the endometrial cycle, just before menstruation begins again, it is about 5.0 mm (less than ¼ in) thick.

Layers of smooth muscle fibers that extend in three directions (longitudinal, transverse, and oblique) make up the thick *myometrium* (Fig. 6.11). The smooth muscle fibers interlace with elastic and connective tissues and blood vessels throughout the uterine wall and blend with the dense inner layer of the endometrium. The myometrium is particularly thick in the fundus, thins out as it nears the isthmus, and is thinnest in the cervix.

The *outer* myometrial layer, found mostly in the fundus, is made up of longitudinal fibers, and is therefore well suited for expelling the fetus during the birth process. In the thick *middle* myometrial layer, the interlaced muscle fibers form a figure-of-eight pattern encircling large blood vessels. Contraction of the middle layer produces a hemostatic action. Only a few circular fibers of the *inner* myometrial layer are found in the fundus. Most of the circular fibers are concentrated in the cornua, the place where the fallopian tubes join the uterine body, and around the internal os. The sphincter action of this layer prevents the regurgitation of menstrual blood out of the fallopian tubes during menstruation. Their sphincter action around the internal cervical os helps to retain the uterine contents during pregnancy. Injury to this sphincter can weaken the internal os and result in an incompetent internal cervical os (see Chapter 35).

For clarity and interest, each muscle layer and its function were described individually. It must be remembered that the myometrium works as a whole. The structure of the myometrium, which gives strength and elasticity, presents an example of adaptation to function:

1. To thin out, pull up, and open the cervix and to push the fetus out of the uterus, the fundus must contract with the most force.
2. Contraction of interlacing smooth muscle fibers that surround the blood vessels controls blood loss after abortion and childbirth. Because of their ability to close off (ligate) blood vessels between them, the smooth muscle fibers of the uterus are referred to as the *living ligature*.

Muscle fibers of the uterine myometrium are continuous with the muscle layers in the fallopian tubes and vagina and with muscle fibers in the ovarian, round, and cardinal ligaments; they are minimally continuous with those in the uterosacral ligaments.

The *parietal peritoneum,* a serous membrane, coats all the uterine corpus except for the lower one fourth of the anterior surface, where the bladder is attached, and the cervix. Because parietal peritoneum does not completely cover this organ, it is possible for diagnostic tests and surgery involving the uterus to be performed without entering the abdominal cavity.

Cervix. The lowermost portion of the uterus is the cervix, or neck (Fig. 6.9). The attachment site of the uterine cervix to the vaginal vault divides the cervix into the longer supravaginal (above the vagina) portion and the shorter vaginal portion. The length of the cervix is about 2.5 to 3.0 cm, of which about 1 cm protrudes into the vagina in the nongravid woman.

The cervix is composed primarily of fibrous connective tissue with some muscle fibers and elastic tissue. The cervix of the nulliparous woman is a rounded, almost conical, rather firm, spindle-shaped body approximately 2 to 2.5 cm in external diameter. The narrowed opening between the uterine cavity and the endocervical (canal inside the cervix that connects the uterine cavity with the vagina) canal is the internal os. The narrowed opening between the endocervix and the vagina is the external os. The external cervical os is a small circular opening in women who have not borne children. Childbirth injury changes the circular os to a small transverse opening dividing the cervix into an anterior and a posterior lip (Fig. 6.12).

When the woman is not ovulating or pregnant, the

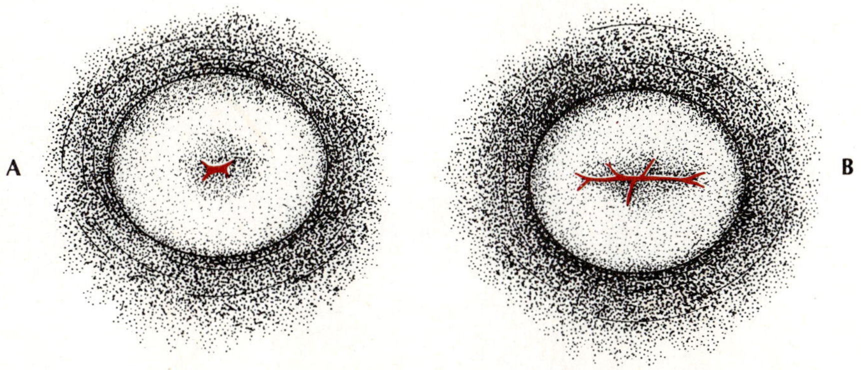

Fig. 6.12
External cervical os as seen through speculum. **A,** Nonparous cervix. **B,** Parous cervix.

Fig. 6.13
Squamo-columnar junction.

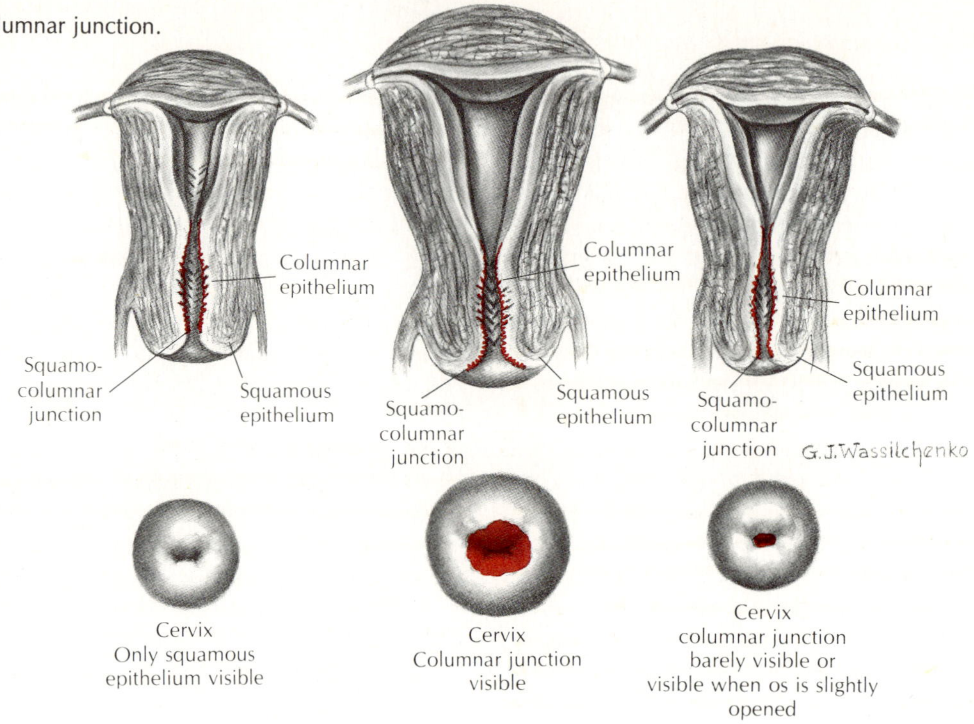

Fig. 6.14
Uterine positions.

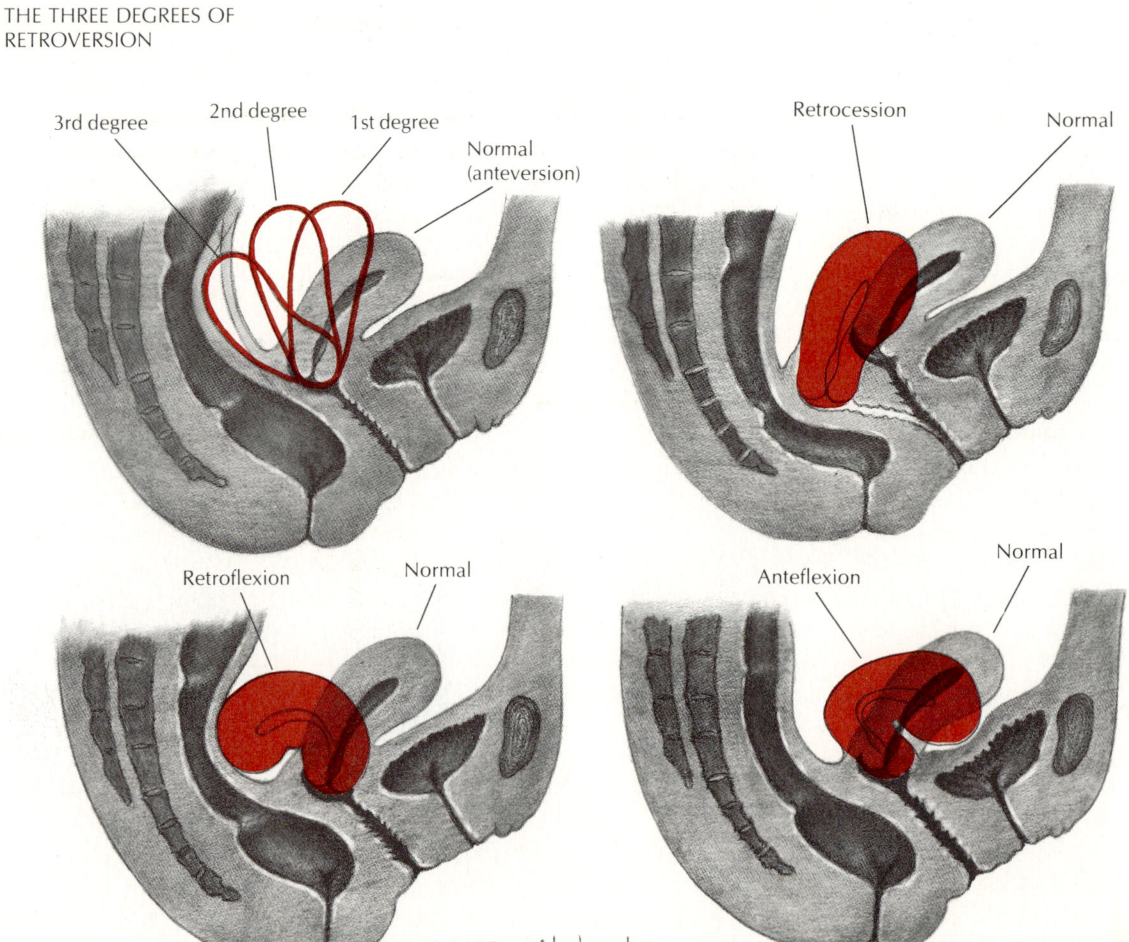

tip of the cervix feels firm much like the end of one's nose, with a dimple in the center. The dimple marks the site of the external os.

The most significant characteristic of the cervix is its ability to stretch during vaginal childbirth. Several factors contribute to cervical elasticity: high connective tissue and elastic fiber content, numerous infoldings in the endocervical lining, and a muscle fiber content of about 10%.

Canals. There are two cavities within the uterus known as the uterine and cervical canals (Fig. 6.9). The uterine canal in the nonpregnant state is compressed by thick muscular walls so that it is only a potential space, flat and triangular in shape. The base of the triangle is formed by the fundus. The fallopian tubes open into either end of the base. The apex of the triangle points downward and forms the internal os (opening) of the cervical canal.

The endocervical canal with its many infoldings has a surface layer of tall, columnar, mucus-producing cells. *Columnar epithelium* is beefy red in color, deeper, and rougher looking in texture than the epithelial outer covering of the cervix. After menarche (the start of menstruation) *squamous epithelium* covers the outside of the cervix (ectocervix). This external covering of flat cells gives a glistening pink color to the cervix. A pale pink color is seen if the woman is anemic or menopausal; a deeper bluish red color is seen when the woman is ovulating or pregnant. A reddened (hyperemic) cervix may indicate inflammation.

The two types of epithelium meet at the *squamocolumnar junction* (Fig. 6.13). This junction line is usually just inside the external cervical os but may be found on the ectocervix in some women. The squamocolumnar junction is the most frequent site of neoplastic cellular changes. Therefore cells for cytologic study, the Papanicolaou smear, are scraped from this junction.

The columnar epithelial cells produce odorless and nonirritating mucus in response to ovarian endocrine hormones---estrogen and progesterone. (See discussion of cervical mucus characteristics and functions, Chapters 11 and 12).

Uterine location. Between birth and puberty the uterus descends gradually into the true pelvis from the lower abdomen. After puberty, the uterus is located in the true pelvis behind the symphysis pubis and urinary bladder and in front of the rectum. During menopause, the uterus begins a process of involution resulting in a decrease in size and a location deep in the pelvis.

Uterine position. For the majority of normal women, with the urinary bladder empty, the uterus is anteverted (tipped forward) and slightly anteflexed (bent forward), with the corpus lying over the top of the posterior wall of the bladder. The cervix is directed downward and backward toward the tip of the sacrum so that it is usually at approximately a right angle to the plane of the vagina. For other women the uterus may be in the midposition or tipped backward (retroverted) (Fig. 6.14).

A full bladder pushes the uterus back toward the rectum, while a full rectum moves the uterus forward against the bladder. Uterine position also changes depending on the woman's position (e.g., lying supine, prone, on her side, or standing), her age, and pregnancy.

The free mobility permits the uterus to rise slightly during the sexual response cycle so that the cervix is placed in a position to increase the likelihood of fertilization. However, the free mobility of the uterus may also lead to malpositions of this organ. The uterus that is bent more than usual so that the fundus is closer to the cervix is said to be anteflexed, or retroflexed (Fig. 6.14).

Uterine support. The uterus is supported by ligaments and by muscles of the pelvic floor, including the perineal body. A total of 10 ligaments stabilize the uterus within the pelvic cavity: four paired ligaments (broad, round, uterosacral, and cardinal) and two single ligaments (anterior and posterior).

The paired *broad ligaments* (Figs. 6.8 and 6.9) are double folds of parietal peritoneum that extend winglike from the sides of the uterus to the pelvic walls. These ligaments divide the pelvic cavity into anterior and posterior components. In the upper portion of the broad ligaments are suspended the fallopian tubes, ovaries, round ligaments, and ovarian ligaments. This upper portion consists of loose connective tissue that does *not* influence uterine position.

The two *round ligaments* (Fig. 6.7) are composed of smooth muscle and connective tissue. The round ligaments extend from the upper outer angles formed where the fallopian tubes join the uterine corpus (at the cornua), through the inguinal canals, and ending in the labia majora. In the nonpregnant state it is a lax cord; in pregnancy it is stretched and increases in diameter (see discussion of discomforts of pregnancy, p. 307).

The single *anterior* (uterovesical or pubocervical) *ligament* is a continuation of parietal peritoneum that forms the anterior fold of the broad ligament, extending from the anterior surface of the supravaginal cervix of the uterus to the posterior surface of the bladder. The pouch formed by the fold of peritoneum is less deep than the posterior pouch.*

The denser connective tissue of the lower portion of the broad ligaments is sometimes known as the *cardinal, transverse,* or *Mackenrodt's ligaments* (Fig. 6.9).

---

*This feature is of significance for low-segment cesarean incision (Chapter 37).

The uterine blood vessels and the ureters are enclosed within the cardinal ligaments where they are connected to the lateral margin of the uterus. The cardinal ligaments form the upper portion of the posterior ligament.

The single *posterior* (or rectovaginal) *ligament* is a continuation of parietal peritoneum (posterior fold of broad ligament) extending from the posterior surface of the uterus to the rectum. The posterior ligament forms the deep rectouterine pouch also known as the *cul-de-sac of Douglas* (Fig. 6.10).

This pouch is the lowest part of the abdominal cavity so that blood, pus, or other drainage collects here. The pouch can be reached through the posterior vaginal fornix. Passage of a scope through the posterior vaginal fornix into the cul-de-sac permits visualization of the cul-de-sac for any evidence of inflammation, purulent drainage, ectopic pregnancy, ovarian cysts, or bleeding is known as culdotomy. Passage of a scope to obtain a sample of discharge is known as culdocentesis.

The two *uterosacral ligaments* (Figs. 6.8 and 6.10) are cordlike folds of peritoneum extending from the supravaginal cervical portion of the uterus to the fascia over the second and third sacral vertebrae passing on each side of the rectum. These ligaments hold the uterus in position by maintaining traction on the cervix.

In summary the main uterine supports are the ligaments surrounding the supravaginal cervix:

1. Anterior (pubocervical)
2. Cardinal (transverse, Mackenrodt's)
3. Posterior (rectovaginal)
4. Uterosacral

When uterine support structures, ligaments, and muscles weaken, the uterus descends into the vaginal vault (prolapse of the uterus).

Uterine lymphatics. The lymphatics of the uterus are extensive. They are contained in three networks: at the base of the endometrium, within the myometrium, and just under the peritoneal coat of the uterus. There are *no* lymphatics in the more superficial layers of the endometrium. Lymphatic drainage occurs mainly at the isthmus along the uterine vessels. Near the uterine fundus, drainage joins that of the ovarian and tubal lymphatics to the nodes around the aorta. The lymphatic drainage from lesions of the cervix may quickly seed tumor cells to the ureteral nodes, lateral sacral nodes, and nodes of the sacral promontory. Some lymphatics may drain into femoral, iliac, and hypogastric nodes.

Uterine blood supply. The abdominal aorta divides at about the level of the umbilicus and forms the two iliac arteries. Each iliac artery divides to form two arteries, the major one of which is the hypogastric artery. The uterine arteries branch off from the hypogastric arteries. The closeness of the uterus to the aorta ensures an ample blood supply to meet the needs of the growing uterus and conceptus.

In addition, the ovarian artery, a direct subdivision of the aorta, first supplies the ovary with blood and then proceeds to join the uterine artery, thus further adding to the blood supply (Fig. 6.15).

In the nonpregnant state the uterine blood vessels are coiled and tortuous. With advancing pregnancy and an enlarging uterus, these blood vessels straighten out. The uterine veins follow along the arteries and empty into the internal iliac veins.

Innervation of the uterus. The internal genitalia have a rich supply of afferent and efferent autonomic nerves, both motor and sensory.

Motor nerves. Parasympathetic fibers from the sacral nerves are probably responsible for producing vasodilation and inhibiting muscular contraction. Efferent sympathetic motor nerves arise from the ganglia of T5 (thoracic 5) to T10, come together over the sacrum, and reach the uterus through ganglia that lie near the base of the uterosacral ligaments. These efferent sympathetic motor nerves are believed to cause vasoconstriction and muscular contraction. The autonomic nerves just described (parasympathetic fibers and efferent sympathetic motor) regulate the action of the uterus, but the uterus has an intrinsic motility (i.e., it can contract and relax even if the nerves to it are cut). This means that even if a woman suffers an accident that injures the spinal cord at or above T5, she may still be able to have uterine contractions sufficient to deliver an infant vaginally.

Sensory nerves. Sensory fibers, carrying pain sensation from the uterus, come together in the paracervical areas and proceed upward to pass just below the division (bifurcation) of the aorta, and then travel into the spinal cord at the level of T11 and T12. Because of this arrangement, pain that originates in the ovary or in the ureters may mimic pain that originates in the uterus, any of which may be felt in the flank and down to the inguinal and vulvar areas.

As in other hollow viscera, the stimuli from the uterus and tubes that result in pain are stretching and ischemia. This characteristic of hollow viscera is best illustrated by contrasting the responses to cervical biopsy and to stretching of the internal cervical os. Minimal discomfort may be expected from a biopsy of the cervix; however, stretching of the internal cervical os is often painful enough to necessitate anesthesia. If the fallopian tube is twisted in such a way as to interfere with its blood supply, severe pain will be experienced. Stretching or direct chemical irritation of peritoneal surfaces (e.g., from inflammation or collection of purulent drainage or blood) results in pain. Chemical irritation that results from the presence of a blood clot is thought to be caused by the chemical *serotonin* that is released during the clotting process.

Functions. The three functions of the uterus are essential for the survival of the species but not for the

Fig. 6.15
A, Pelvic blood supply. **B,** Blood supply of perineum and uterus.

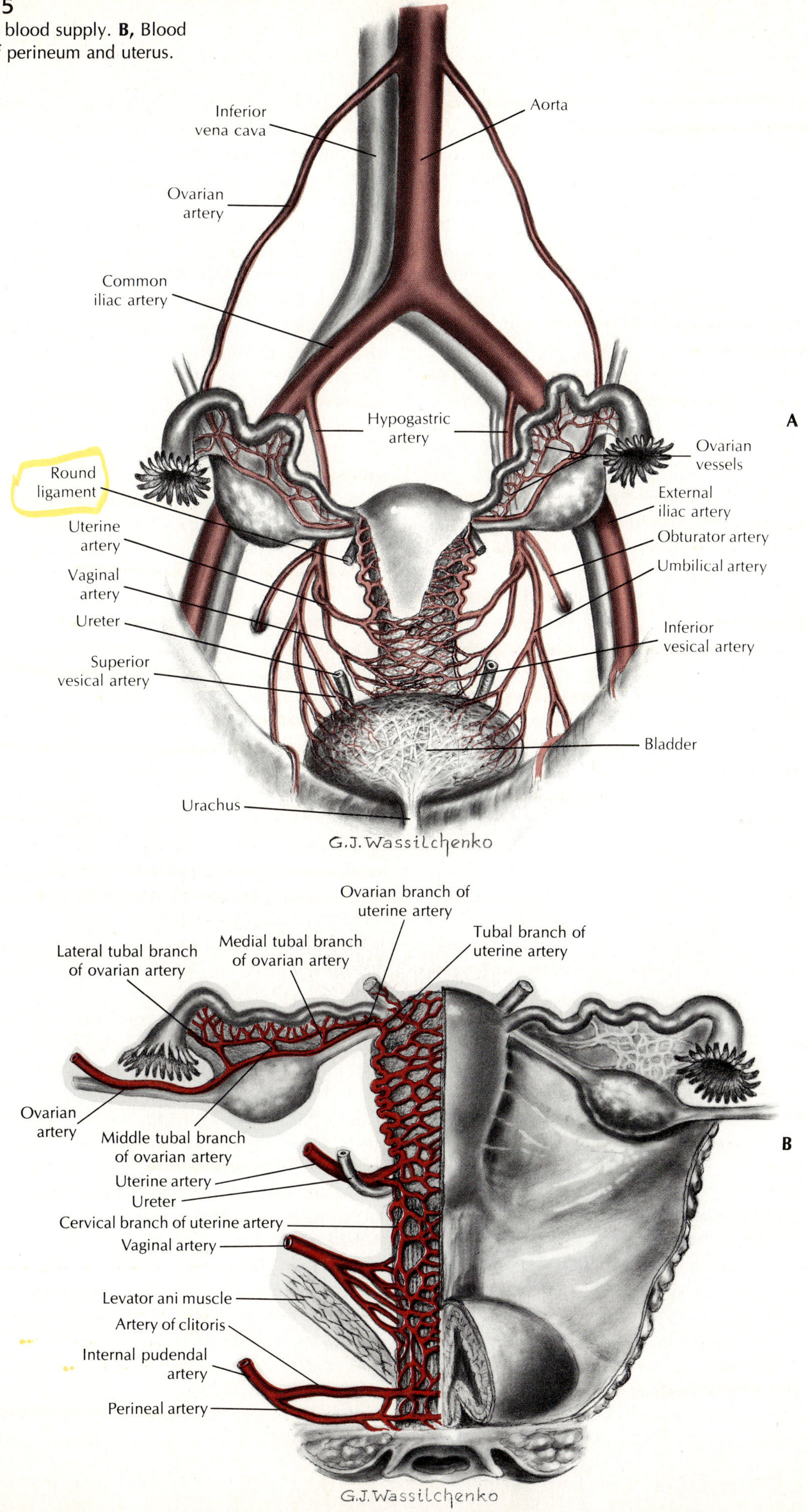

Inferior vena cava
Aorta
Ovarian artery
Common iliac artery
Hypogastric artery
A
Ovarian vessels
Round ligament
External iliac artery
Uterine artery
Obturator artery
Vaginal artery
Umbilical artery
Ureter
Inferior vesical artery
Superior vesical artery
Bladder
Urachus
G.J.Wassilchenko
Ovarian branch of uterine artery
Medial tubal branch of ovarian artery
Tubal branch of uterine artery
Lateral tubal branch of ovarian artery
Ovarian artery
Middle tubal branch of ovarian artery
B
Uterine artery
Ureter
Cervical branch of uterine artery
Vaginal artery
Levator ani muscle
Artery of clitoris
Internal pudendal artery
Perineal artery
G.J.Wassilchenko

individual: cyclic menstruation with rejuvenation of the endometrium, pregnancy, and labor.

Vagina

Location and support. The vagina is a tubular structure located in front of the rectum and behind the bladder and urethra. The vagina extends from the introitus, the external opening in the vestibule between the labia minora of the vulva, to the cervix. When the woman is standing, the vagina slants backward and upward. It is supported mainly by its attachments to the pelvic floor musculature and fascia.

Structure. The vagina is a thin-walled, collapsible tube that is capable of great distention. Because of the way the cervix protrudes into the uppermost portion of the vagina, the length of the anterior wall of the vagina is only about 7 to 8 cm while that of the posterior wall is about 10 cm. The recesses formed all around the protruding cervix are called fornices: right, left, anterior, and posterior. The posterior fornix is deeper than the other three.

The smooth muscle walls are lined with glandular mucous membrane. During the reproductive years, this mucosa is arranged in transverse folds called rugae.

The vaginal mucosa responds promptly to estrogen and progesterone stimulation. Cells are lost from the mucosa, especially during the menstrual cycle and pregnancy. Cells scraped from the vaginal mucosa can be used to estimate steroid sex hormone levels.

Innervation. The vagina is relatively insensitive. There is some innervation from the pudendal and hemorrhoidal nerves to the lowest one third. Because of this minimal innervation and no special nerve endings, the vagina is the source of very little sensation during sexual excitement and coitus and less pain during the second stage of labor than if this tissue were well supplied with nerve endings. The nerve supply is mainly autonomic. Sensations arising in the vagina terminate at the level of S2, S3, and S4.

Blood supply. The copious blood supply to the vagina is derived from the descending branches of the uterine artery, the middle hemorrhoidal artery, and the internal pudendal arteries. The venous return of vaginal blood is through the pudendal, external hemorrhoidal, and uterine veins.

Lymphatics. The lymphatics of the upper vagina drain to the rectovaginal septal, presacral, external iliac, and hypogastric nodes. The lower vaginal lymphatics are directed to the superficial inguinal nodes. The spread of vaginal infection and malignant disease follows these routes.

Vaginal fluid. Vaginal fluid is derived from the lower or upper genital tract. The continuous flow of fluid from the vagina maintains relative cleanliness of the vagina. Therefore, vaginal douching in normal circumstances is not necessary. Vaginal fluid may also contain bacteria, parasites, or neoplastic cells. A spread of vaginal mucus from the posterior vaginal fornix and a scraping from the squamocolumnar junction of the cervix, fixed in ethyl ether and alcohol and then treated with trichrome nucleocytoplasmic stain, constitute the Papanicolaou (Pap) smear used throughout the world for gynecologic cancer detection.

Ovaries: female gonads

Location and support. One ovary is located on each side of the uterus, below and behind the uterine tubes. The ovaries are held in place by two ligaments, the *mesovarian* portions of the uterine broad ligament, which suspend them from the lateral pelvic side walls at about the level of the anterosuperior iliac crest, and the *ovarian* ligaments (Fig. 6.8), which anchor them to the uterus. The ovaries are movable with palpation.

Structure. The ovaries are similar in origin (homologous) to the testes in the male. Each ovary is composed of two layers around a central zone (Fig. 6.16). Each ovary resembles a large almond in size and shape. Each is whitish and rounded but flattened, weighes about 3 g, and measures approximately 3 × 2 × 1 cm. At the time of ovulation, ovarian size may double temporarily. The oval-shaped ovaries are firm in consistency and slightly tender. The surface of the ovary is smooth before menarche. After sexual maturity, scarring from repeated ruptures of follicles and ovulation roughens the nodular surface.

Blood supply and lymphatics. Ovarian arteries carry a rich blood supply from the aorta to the ovaries. The left ovarian vein empties into the left renal vein, but the right drains into the inferior vena cava. The ovarian lymphatics drain into the iliac and periaortic nodes.

Innervation. The nerve supply to the ovary is through T10 to L1, together with fibers of the pelvic sympathetic nervous system.

Functions. The two functions of the ovary are ovulation and hormone production. At birth the normal female's ovaries contain countless thousands of primordial (primitive) ova. At intervals during the productive life (generally monthly), one or more ova mature and undergo ovulation. The ovary is also the major site of production of steroid sex hormones (estrogens, progesterone, and androgens) in amounts required for normal female growth, development, and function.

Abdominal wall. The abdominal wall consists of an outer layer of skin, a layer of subcutaneous fat, and a layer of muscles and their fascia. The thickness of subcutaneous fat varies with the person's nutritional state. The thickness and tone of the muscular layer vary with individual heredity and exercise.

Four pairs of muscles make up the muscular layers of the abdominal wall: three pairs of thin, flat lateral

Fig. 6.16
Cross section of ovary.

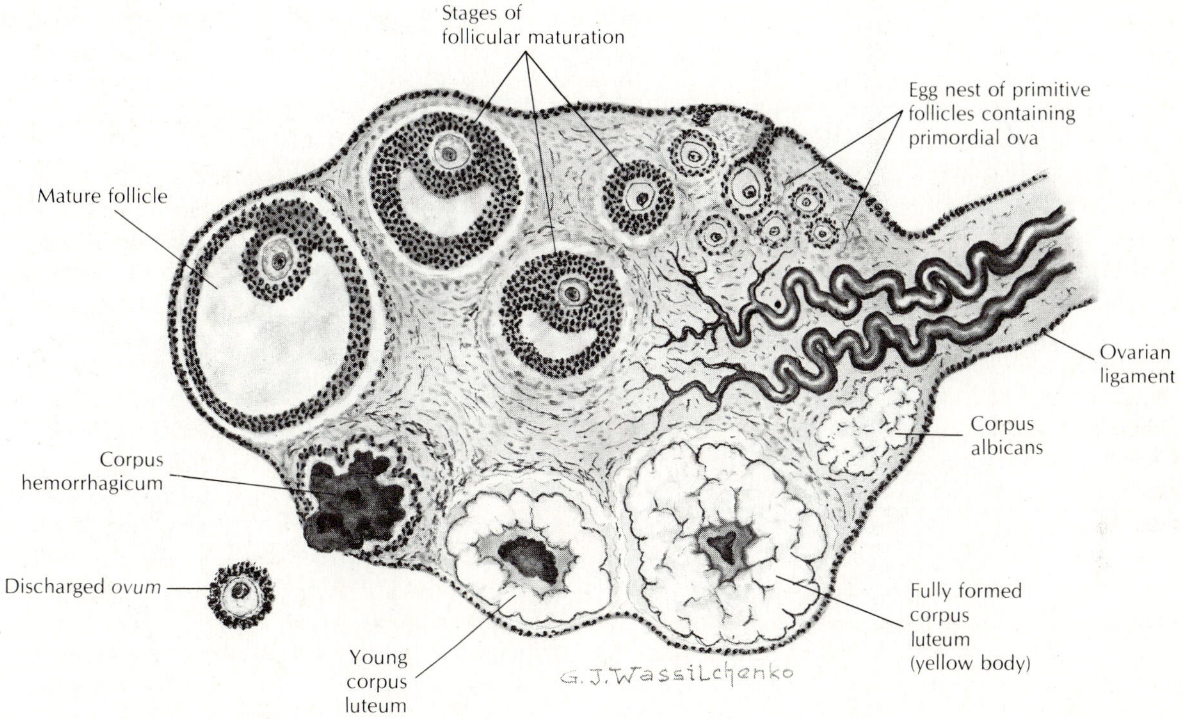

muscles and one pair of thicker central muscles, the *recti abdominis* (Fig. 6.6). On either side of the midline, the recti (Latin, straight) abdominis attach to the lower costal border and to the pubis. A thick sheet of fascia covers the recti anteriorly and a narrow band of fascia joins the pair in the midline. In the nonpregnant state the skin overlying this band of fascia in the midline appears slightly lighter in color than the surrounding skin (linea alba). If this narrow band of fascial tissue is separated as can occur because of marked obesity or greatly enlarged uterus during pregnancy, the lateral muscles contract and pull apart the strained recti abdominis, resulting in a condition called diastasis (Greek, simple separation) of the recti abdominis (see Chapter 31).

Landmarks or reference points of the abdomen are described below:

1. Lower sternal border or lower border of the breast bone. This is the uppermost marker for the abdomen.
2. Xiphoid, or ensiform (sword-shaped), process attached to the lower border of the sternum.
3. Costal border, the lower margins of the rib cage.
4. Umbilicus, the scar marking the site of attachment to the umbilical cord. This scar is a depression in the midline roughly half way between the lower sternal border and the pubic crest. The person's height and weight influence the scar's position.
5. Iliac crest, the upper margin of the ilium. The upper and foremost projection of the ilium is the anterior superior iliac spine.
6. Pubic crest. Located in the midline, the pubic crest includes the upper border of the pubic bones and the symphysis pubis. This is the lowermost marker for the abdomen.

Anatomy of the bony pelvis. Maternity care emphasizes the study of the pelvis from the perspective of its role in childbearing—its component parts and size and those bony relationships that are of special importance in accommodating a growing fetus throughout pregnancy and during the birth process.

Discussion of this important structure is divided for easier study and application of knowledge. The anatomy of the pelvis is included here. Expected changes in the pelvis as it adapts to pregnacy and related discomforts are presented in Chapter 15. The mechanics of labor are influenced by the relationship between a mother's pelvis and her fetus. Therefore the measurements of the pelvis, techniques of assessment, and the fetal skull are explained in Chapter 20.

Fig. 6.17
Adult female pelvis, showing origin of parts from separate embryonic bones.

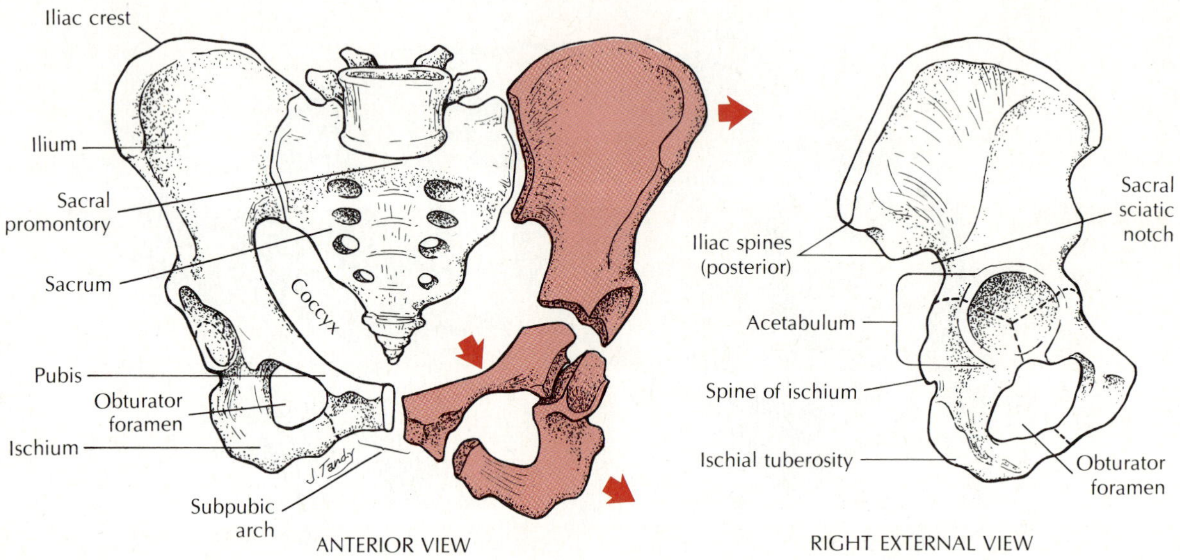

Bony pelvis. During birth, the fetus must pass through the bony passage formed by the pelvis (Fig. 6.17). The pelvis is a bony ring that is supported by the lower extremities and that in turn bears the weight of the trunk and upper body. The pelvis is made up of the following four bones: the right and left innominate bones, each of which is made up of the right or left pubic bone, ilium, and ischium, which fuse after puberty; the sacrum; and the coccyx. The two innominate bones (hip bones) form the sides and front of the bony passage, and the sacrum and coccyx form the back.

Below the ilium is the *ischium,* a heavy bone terminating posteriorly in the rounded protuberances known as the *ischial tuberosities.* The tuberosities bear the body's weight in the sitting position.

The sharp projections, the *ischial spines,* project from the posterior border of the ischium into the pelvic cavity. The spines, which may be blunt or prominent, have obstetric importance for two reasons:

1. The distance between the two ischial spines is the narrowest diameter of the pelvic cavity. Optimal characteristics for vaginal delivery are discussed on p. 374.
2. They serve as the landmark to determine the degree of descent of the fetus during labor (see station, p. 386).

The *pubis,* forming the front portion of the pelvic cavity, is located beneath the mons. In the midline, the two pubic bones are joined by strong ligaments and a thick cartilage to form the joint called the symphysis pubis. The descending rami (ramus [sing.] branch or arm) form the subpubic arch. In the female, the angle formed by the arch optimally measures slightly more than 90 degrees (see p. 375).

The *sacrum* is formed by five fused vertebrae. The upper anterior portion of the body of the first sacral vertebra, the promontory, forms the posterior margin of the pelvic brim. The promontory is a landmark of an important obstetric measurement (see p. 373). In some cases the coccyx may be of significance in labor (see p. 375). The coccyx (tailbone), composed of three to five fused vertebrae, articulates with the sacrum. The coccyx projects downward and forward from the lower border of the sacrum.

The pelvis is divided into two sections, the shallow upper basin, or false pelvis, and the deeper lower, or true, pelvis (Fig. 6.18). The *false pelvis* lies above the linea terminalis (brim, inlet) and varies considerably in size in different women. It supports the enlarged uterus but has no specific obstetric significance.

The *true pelvis,* consisting of the brim, or inlet, and the area below, is of great importance in obstetrics because it must be adequate in size and shape to permit passage of the fetus. The cavity of the true pelvis resembles an irregularly curved canal (Fig. 6.19) with unequal anterior and posterior surfaces. These surfaces

Fig. 6.18
Female pelvis: False pelvis is shallow basin above inlet; true pelvis is deeper cavity below inlet.

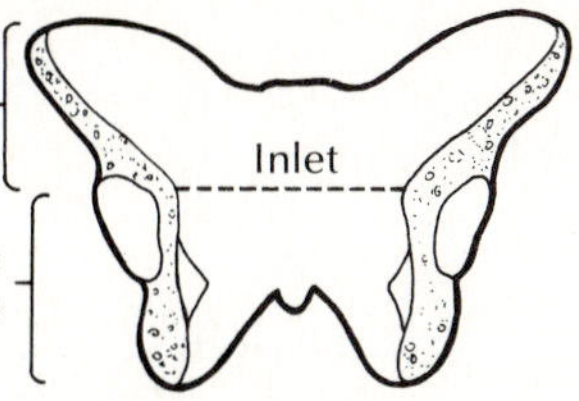

Fig. 6.19
Female pelvis: cavity of true pelvis is an irregularly curved canal.

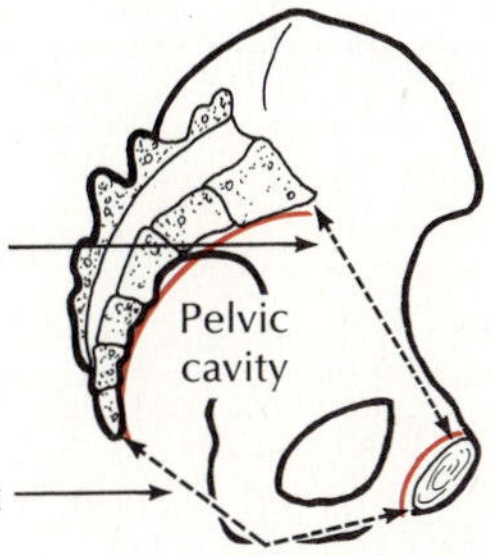

correspond to the length of the symphysis (4.5 cm) and the length of the sacrum (12 cm). Because of its irregular shape, the canal is studied at different levels or planes. These planes include those of the *inlet,* the *mid pelvis,* and the *outlet.* The diameters of these planes (see p. 373) determine whether vaginal delivery is possible and the manner by which the fetus may pass through the birth canal (see discussion of mechanism of labor, p. 388).

In studying the bony pelvis, the following structures and *landmarks* are especially important:

1. Iliac crest and superior, anterior iliac spine
2. Sacral promontory
3. Sacrum
4. Coccyx
5. Sacrosciatic notch
6. Ischial spines
7. Side walls
8. Subpubic arch
9. Symphysis pubis
10. Ischial tuberosities

Pelvic variations. Age, sex, and race are responsible for the greatest variations in pelvic shape and size. There is considerable change in the pelvis during growth and development. Pelvic ossification is complete at about 20 years of age or slightly later. Smaller people have smaller, lighter bones than larger people. Moreover, the male pelvis in all population groups is heavier, deeper, and more angular, and the pelvic cavity is less spacious, than in the female (Fig. 6.20). Some loss of strength was traded for an adequate birth canal in the female. As a consequence the internal contours of the woman's pelvis are rounder and the diameters of the pelvic canal are significantly greater than those of the man. The male and female pelves are compared in Fig. 6.20.

BREASTS

The breasts are paired mammary glands located between the second and sixth ribs (Fig. 6.21). About two thirds of the breast overlies the pectoralis major muscle, between the sternum and mid axillary line, with an extension to the axilla referred to as the tail of Spence. The lower one third of the breast overlies the serratus anterior muscle. The breasts are attached to the muscles by connective tissue or fascia.

The breasts of healthy mature women are approximately symmetric in size and shape but are often not absolutely equal. The breasts of women who have never given birth to a child are usually shaped like half cones or hemispheres. Their size and shape vary depending on the woman's age, heredity, and nutrition. However, the contour should be smooth with no retractions, dimpling or masses. If a woman has nursed at some time, her breasts may be pendulous. Proper breast support

Fig. 6.20
Contrast of female and male pelves.

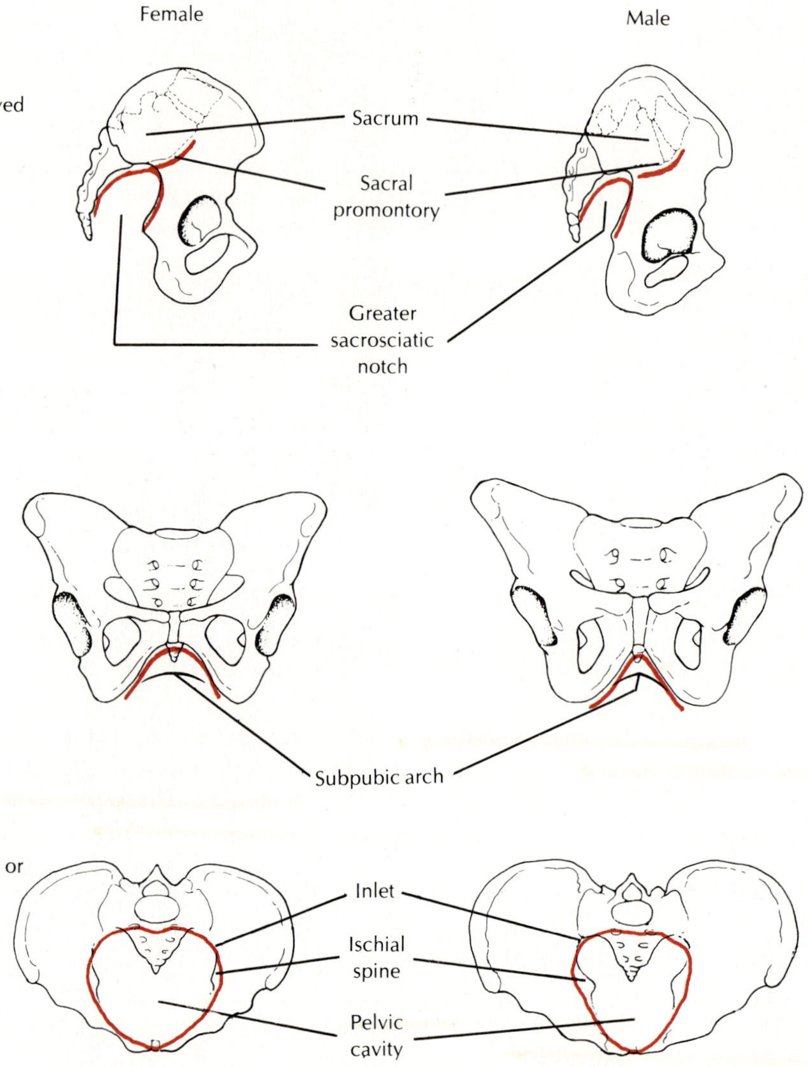

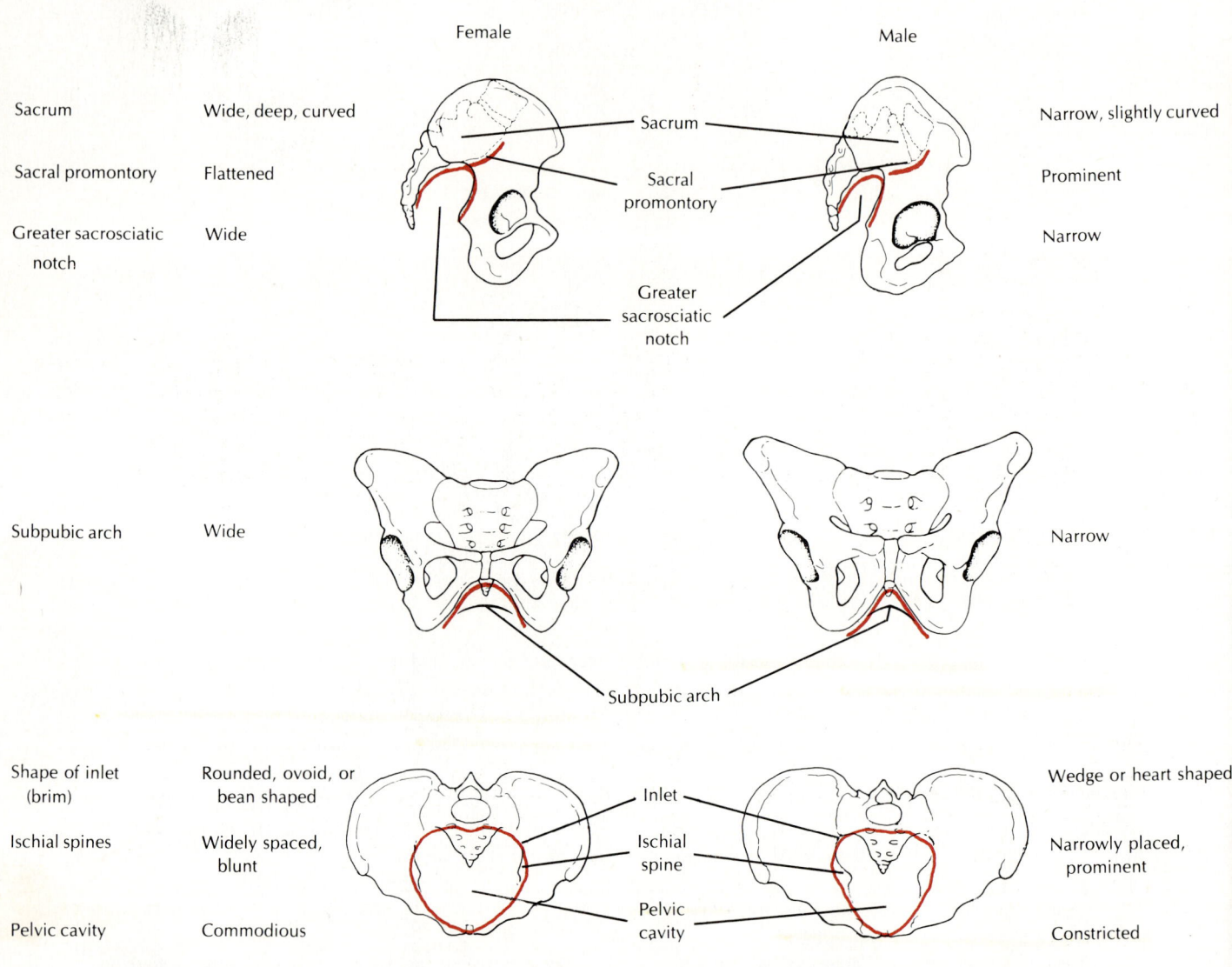

	Female	Male
Sacrum	Wide, deep, curved	Narrow, slightly curved
Sacral promontory	Flattened	Prominent
Greater sacrosciatic notch	Wide	Narrow
Subpubic arch	Wide	Narrow
Shape of inlet (brim)	Rounded, ovoid, or bean shaped	Wedge or heart shaped
Ischial spines	Widely spaced, blunt	Narrowly placed, prominent
Pelvic cavity	Commodious	Constricted

during pregnancy and lactation and certain exercises help to restore the tone of breast tissue after lactation ends.

Anatomy. True glandular tissue is called *parenchyma;* supporting tissues, the fat and fibrous connective tissue, are called *stroma.* It is the relative amount of stroma that determines the size and consistency of the breast.

Each mammary gland is made up of 15 to 20 lobes, which are then divided into lobules. Lobules are clusters of acini (Fig. 6.22). An acinus is a saclike terminal part of a compound gland emptying through a narrow lumen or duct. In discussions of mammary glands, the correct anatomic term (acinus) is often used interchangeably with alveolus. The acini are lined with epithelial cells that secrete colostrum and milk. Just below the epithelium is the myoepithelium (myo, muscle), which contracts to expel milk from the acini.

The ducts from the clusters of acini that form the lobules merge to form larger ducts draining the lobes. Ducts from the lobes converge in a single nipple (papilla) that is surrounded by an areola. Just as the ducts converge, they dilate to form common lactiferous sinuses, which are also called ampullae. The lactiferous sinuses serve as milk reservoirs. Many tiny ducts drain the ampullae and exit in the nipple.

Fig. 6.21
Position and structure of mammary gland.

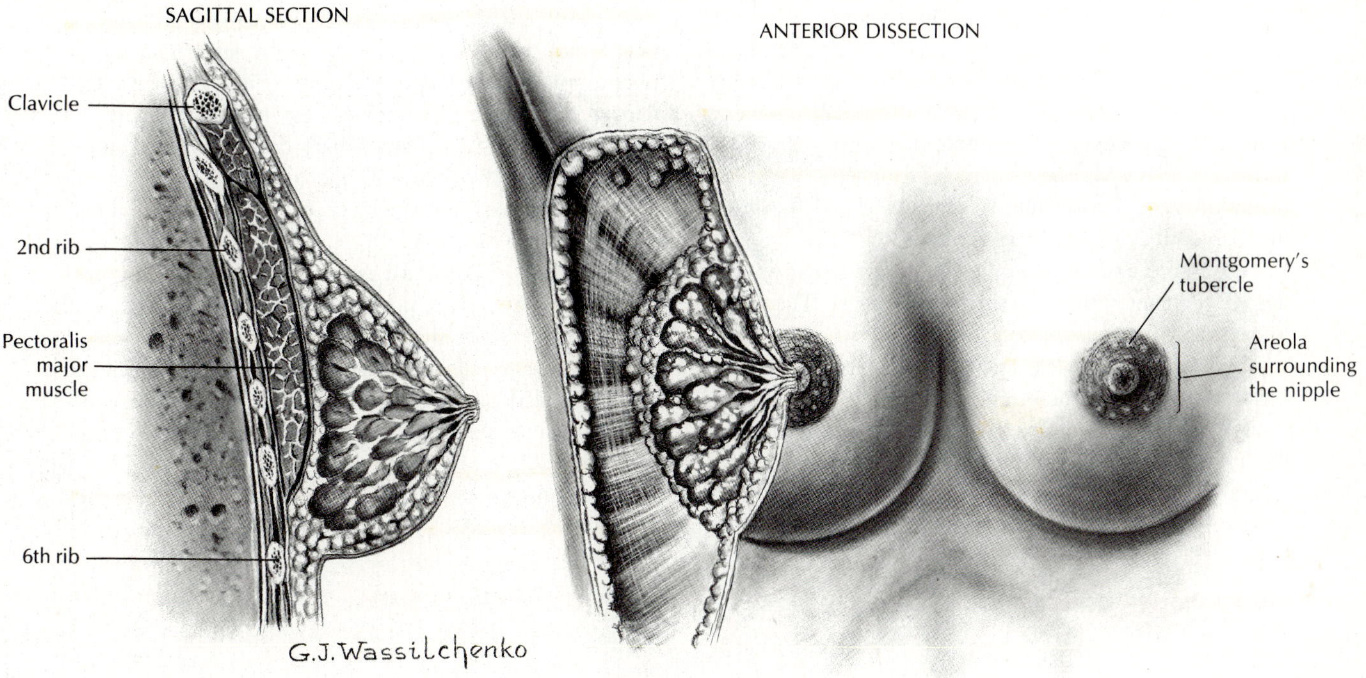

Fig. 6.22
Milk-producing structures and ducts in human breast (simplified cross section).

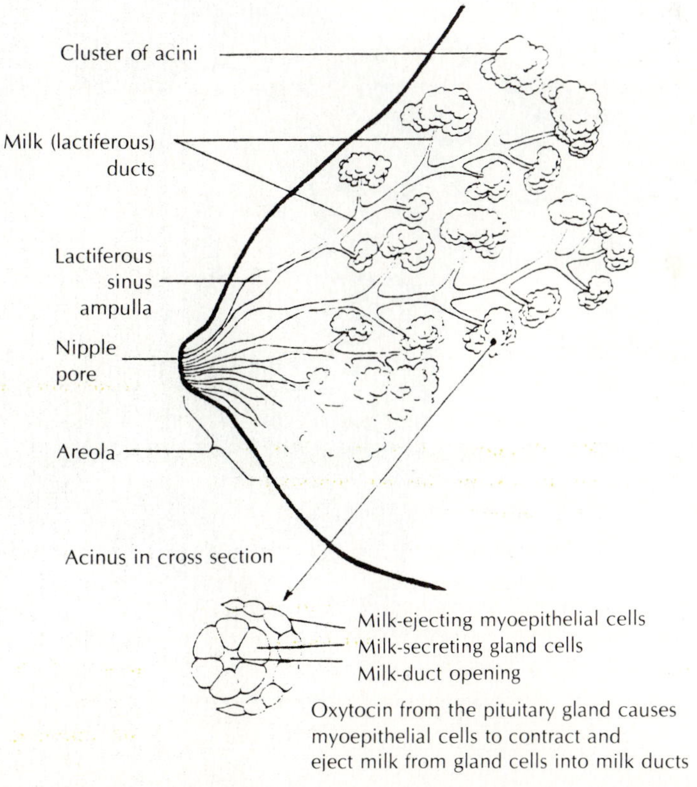

The glandular structures and ducts are surrounded by protective fatty tissue and are separated and supported by fibrous suspensory Cooper's ligaments. Cooper's ligaments provide support to the mammary glands while permitting their mobility on the chest wall.

The round nipple is usually slightly elevated above the breast. On each breast the nipple projects slightly upward and laterally. It contains 15 to 20 openings from lactiferous ducts. The nipple (mammary papilla) is surrounded by fibromuscular tissue and covered by wrinkled skin. Except during pregnancy and lactation, there is no discharge from the nipple.

The nipple and surrounding areola are usually more deeply pigmented than the skin of the breast. The rough appearance of the areola is caused by sebaceous glands, the glands of Montgomery (Fig. 6.21) directly beneath the skin. These glands secrete a fatty substance that is thought to lubricate the nipple. Smooth muscle fibers in the areola contract to stiffen the nipple to make it easier to grasp by the nursing child.

The vascular supply to the mammary gland is abundant. In the nonpregnant state the skin does not have an obvious vascular pattern. The normal skin is smooth without tightness or shininess.

The skin covering the breasts contains an extensive superficial lymphatic network that serves the entire chest wall and is continuous with the superficial lymphatics of the neck and abdomen (Fig. 6.23). In the deeper portions of the breasts, the lymphatics form a rich network as well. The primary deep lymphatic pathway drains laterally toward the axillae. Therefore regional metastasis from cancer of the breast is most likely to occur here first.

Physiology. The breast is a target organ for the endocrine system. The hormone levels throughout the woman's life span determine its physical and microscopic characteristics. Breast growth and development are stimulated primarily by secretions from the hypothalamus, anterior pituitary, and ovaries in the presence of normal levels of insulin and thyroid hormone.

Development and growth. Engorgement of the breasts of all newborn infants, female or male, in response to

Fig. 6.23
Mammary gland: lymphatic drainage.

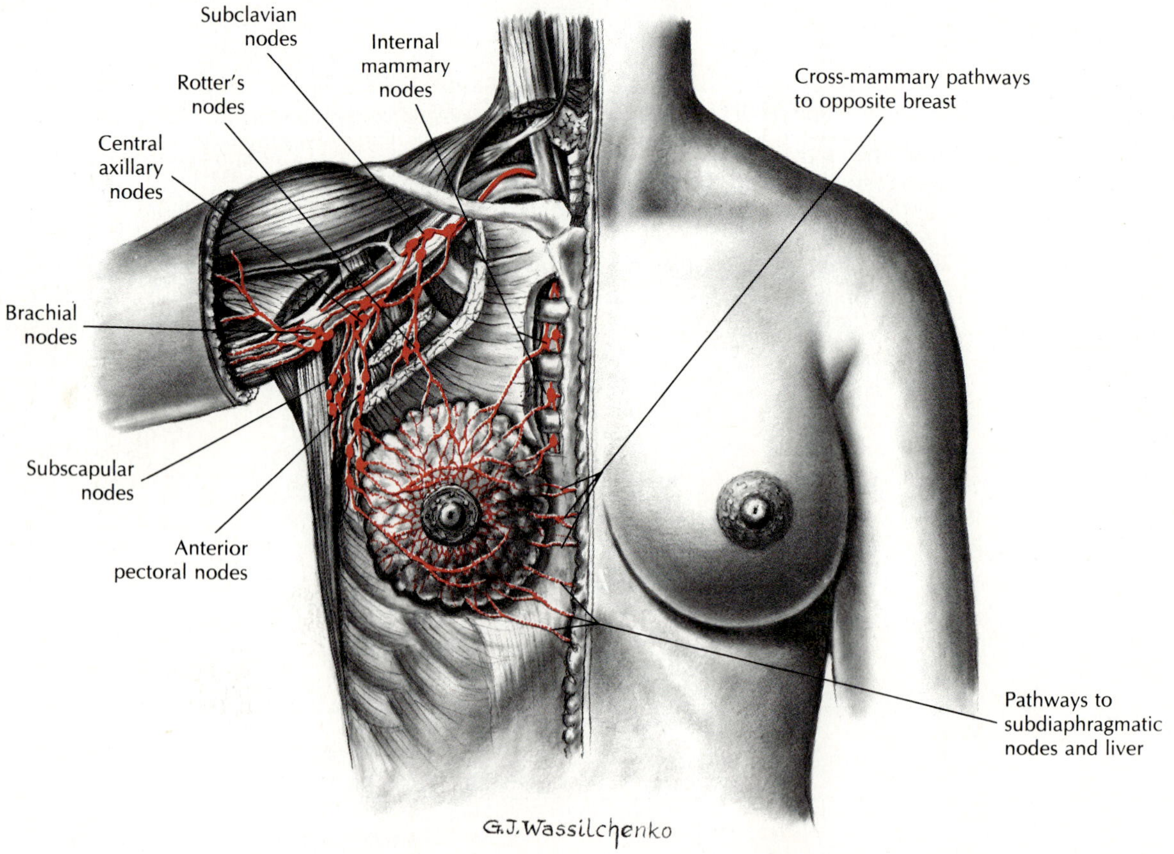

Fig. 6.24
Mammary gland: influence of estrogen and progesterone stimulation.

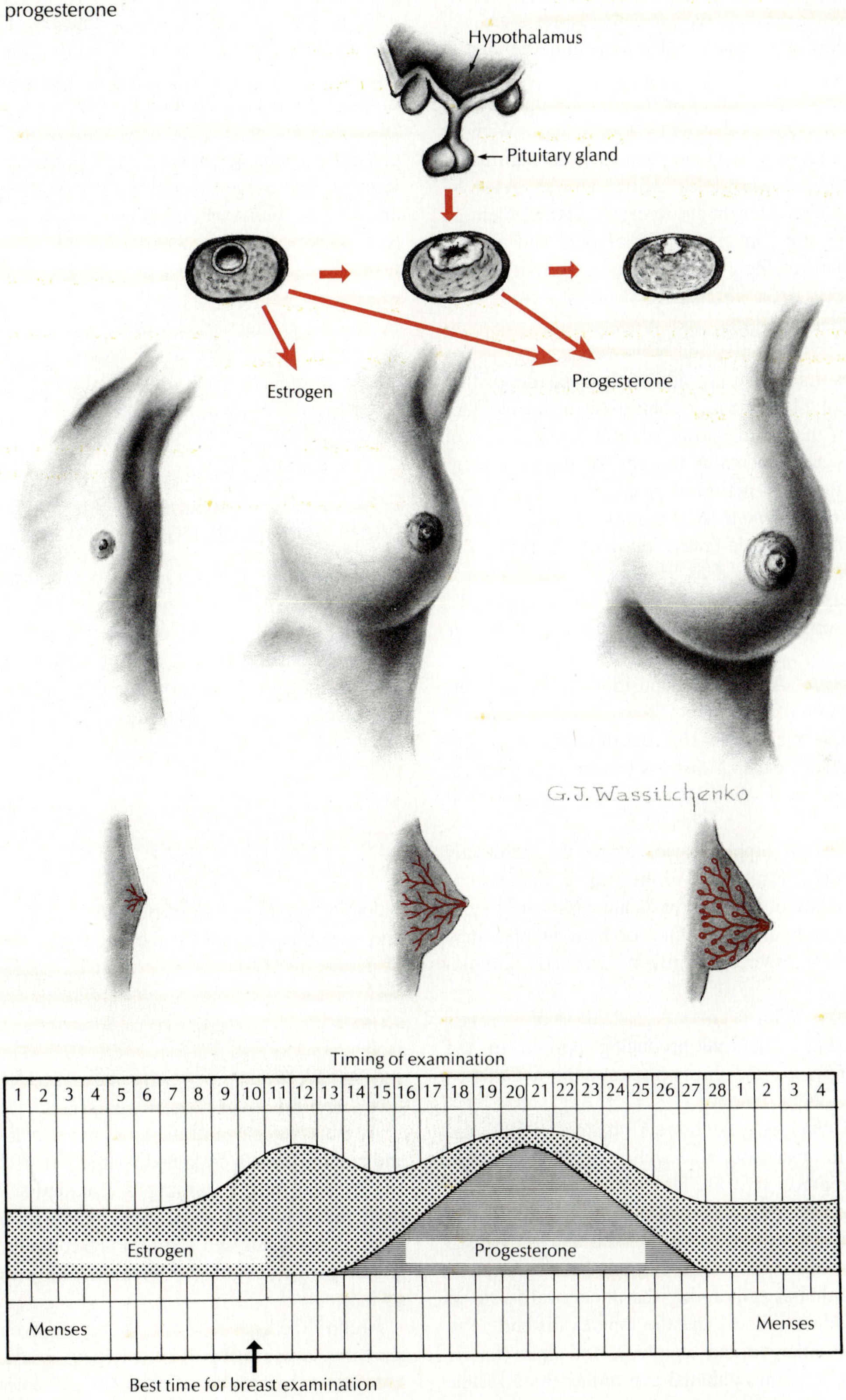

circulating maternal hormones is not uncommon. In a few infants slight secretion, which persists for about 7 days, may be noticed. This milklike secretion, or "witch's milk," starts about 2 to 3 days after birth. All neonatal breast phenomena subside within the first 3 weeks of life.

Estrogen is the primary hormone in early puberty because early cycles tend to be anovulatory. Without ovulation, progesterone is not available in significant amounts. Estrogen stimulates growth of the breast by inducing fat deposition in the breasts, development of stromal tissue (i.e., increase in its amount and elasticity) and growth of the extensive ductile system. Estrogen also increases the vascularity of breast tissue.

After ovulation begins and progesterone levels increase, gland tissue, specifically the lobules and acinar structures, matures. During adolescence fat deposition and growth of fibrous tissue contribute to the increase in the size of the gland. However, full development of the breast is achieved after the end of the first pregnancy or in the early period of lactation.

Stages of development. A summary of stages of development of the female breast follows (Fig. 6.24):

First stage. At about 8 to 9 years the gonadotropin levels increase in serum and urine. Mammary buds, domelike elevations of the areolar tissue, appear by age 12.

Second stage. A gradual deposition of fat and the growth of glandular elements change the contour of the breasts to cone shape. This development may progress unilaterally, causing distress to some adolescents, who are concerned about the uneven sizes of their breasts.

Third stage. The nipple projects above the areola and becomes erectile in response to thermal or tactile stimulation. By adulthood both breasts are reasonably symmetric in contour and size. One or both nipples may flatten or invert rather than project (evert) on stimulation.

Fourth stage. With decreased production of estrogen after menopause, the milk-producing portion of the breasts retrogresses and the breasts assume a flattened rather than globular contour.

Menstrual changes. The breasts change in size and nodularity in response to cyclic ovarian changes throughout reproductive life. Increasing levels of both estrogen and progesterone in the 3 to 4 days before menstruation increase vascularity of the breasts, induce growth of the ducts and acini, and promote water retention. The epithelial cells lining the ducts proliferate in number, the ducts dilate, and the lobules distend. The acini become enlarged and secretory, and lipid (fat) is deposited within their epithelial cell lining. As a result, breast swelling, tenderness, and discomfort are common symptoms just before the onset of menstruation. After menstruation, cellular proliferation begins to regress, acini begin to decease in size, and retained water is lost.

After undergoing numerous changes in response to the ovarian cycle, the proliferation and involution (regression) are not uniform throughout the breast. In time after repeated hormonal stimulation, small persistent areas of nodulations may develop. This normal physiologic change must be remembered when examining breast tissue. Nodules may develop just before and during menstruation, when the breast is most active. The physiologic alterations in breast size and activity reach their minimal level about 5 to 7 days after menstruation stops. Therefore it is easiest to detect pathologic changes at this time.

Routine assessment of the breast and maternal adaptations to pregnancy are discussed on pp. 228 and 693; lactation is discussed in Chapter 30.

Male Reproductive System

For the male, puberty occurs between the ages of 12 and 16 years. In this maturation process, the endocrine system plays a key role in the development of the genitalia and secondary sex characteristics. A brief overview of the pattern of growth and development of male reproductive system structures over the life span follows.

OVERVIEW OF REPRODUCTIVE SYSTEM STRUCTURES THROUGHOUT THE LIFE SPAN

Just before the onset of puberty, the hair on the scrotum is similar to that on the abdomen. With the onset of puberty, sparse, downy, straight hair appears at the base of the penis; scrotal skin reddens, the testes and scrotum enlarge, but the penis does not enlarge yet. As maturation continues, the pubic hair (mons) darkens and spreads over the entire pubic area, facial hair appears, and the prostatic gland enlarges.

At the completion of puberty, pigmentation of penile and scrotal skin is darkened, pubic hair is long, dense, coarse, and curly, forming a diamond-shaped pattern from the umbilicus to the anus. Growth and development of the testes and scrotum are complete. The penis is enlarged in length and breadth. The penile shaft has no hair.

Around the age of 50 years, the male enters the climacteric, some atrophy of genitalia gradually occurs, and pubic hair thins. The penis becomes somewhat flabby. Emotional changes may be attributed to the climacteric.

EXTERNAL GENITALIA

The structures that make up the external genitalia are the mons pubis, the penis, and the scrotal sac.

Mons pubis. At maturity, pubic hair is long, dense, coarse, and curly, forming a diamond-shaped pattern from the umbilicus to the anus.

Penis. The penis, an organ of copulation and urination, consists of the shaft or body and the glans. The shaft of this external male reproductive organ, which enters the vagina during coitus, is composed of three cylindric layers of erectile tissue, two lateral *corpora cavernosa* and a *corpus spongiosum*, which contains the urethra. These corpora terminate distally in the smooth, sensitive *glans penis*, which is the counterpart of the female glans clitoris. Skin and fascia loosely envelop the penis to permit enlargement during erection.

The glans is the enlarged end of the penis that contains many sensitive nerve endings and a urethral meatus at the tip (usually). The *prepuce* (foreskin), an extended fold of skin, covers the glans in uncircumcised males.* In the neonate, the foreskin is not retractable and may not be retractable for 4 to 6 months or even as long as 13 years. It is easily retractable in the adolescent and the adult. With sexual arousal, neurocirculatory factors cause considerable increase in blood flow to the erectile tissue of the corpora, and enlargement and erection of the penis occur.

The *urethra* is an exiting passageway for both urine and semen (Fig. 6.25). The urethra consists of four anatomic segments: the *prostatic*, or posterior, segment is encircled by the prostate gland and houses the ejaculatory ducts that connect the seminal vesicles with the urethra. The next segment is known as the *membranous* urethra and is located within the perineum. Cowper's glands are located on either side of the membra-

*If the urinary meatus is not situated on the tip of the penis, as in hypospadias and epispadias, early correction of the defect is important. These males definitely should *not* be circumcised because the foreskin may be needed later for constructing the portion of the urethra that is missing.

Fig. 6.25
Anatomy of urethra and penis.

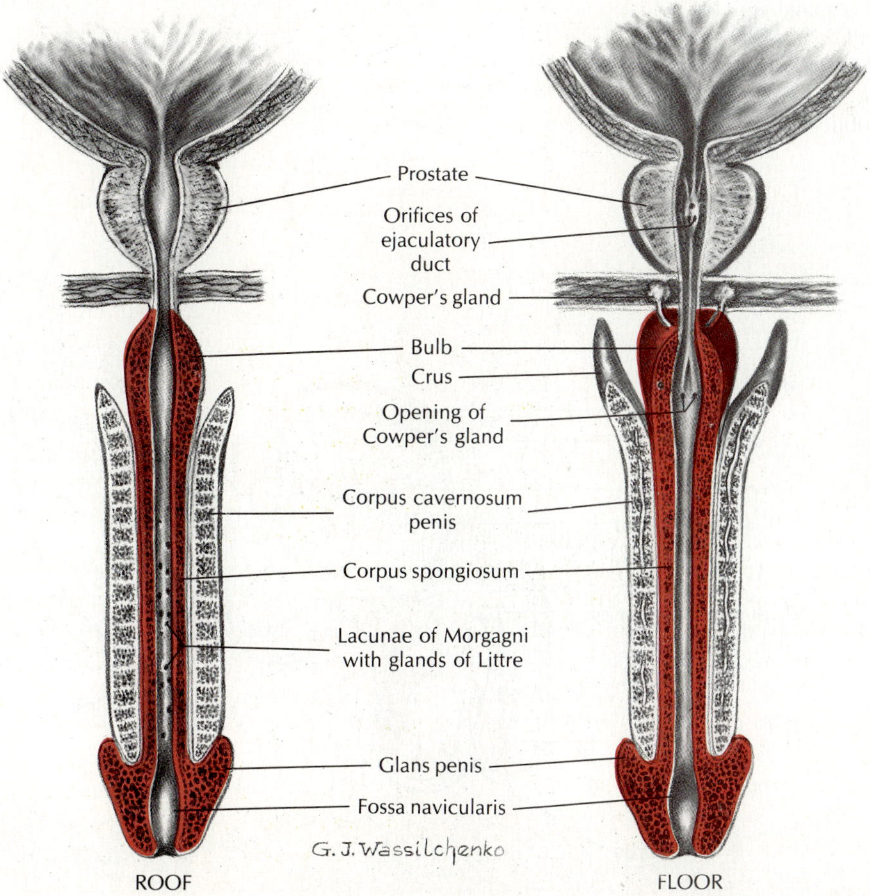

nous urethra. The *bulbous* urethra is found in the region of the bulb of the urethra. The longest portion, the *penile* urethra, extends the entire length of the male organ.

Located especially in the roof of the penile urethra are many small, branched tubular glands known as glands of Littre. The glands of Littre open into small recesses, or niches, called lacunae (lakes) of Morgagni. These lacunae and glands are of clinical significance because they often become chronically infected following urethritis. Chronic infection leads to recurrent urethral discharges containing infectious microorganisms (e.g., gonococci), resulting in reinfection of the man himself and of his sexual partners.

Scrotum. The *scrotum,* a wrinkled, pouchlike fullness of skin, muscles, and fascia, is divided internally by a septum, and each compartment normally contains one *testis,* one *epididymis,* and one *vas deferens* (seminal duct). The left side of the scrotum hangs somewhat lower (about 1 cm) than the right. Six separate layers of tissue make up the scrotal sac. The skin is abundantly supplied with sebaceous and sweat glands and is sparsely covered with hair. Under the skin is found the cremaster fascia and thin smooth muscle layer. Contraction and relaxation of this smooth muscle result in retraction of the testes to protect them from external trauma and cold. During hot external (environmental) or internal (fever) temperature, the cremaster muscle relaxes, dropping the testes away from the body. Conversely, cold external temperature stimulates contraction of the cremaster muscle to bring the testes close to the body.

The purpose of this mobility is to maintain the testes within an optimal temperature range for the production and viability of spermatozoa. Hot tubbing, tight underwear (jockey shorts) and pants, and long-term sitting (long-distance truck drivers) present too hot an external environment or prevent testicular mobility so that spermatogenesis and spermatozoa are jeopardized and relative infertility is likely to occur.

Fig. 6.26
Fascial planes of male lower genitourinary tract. **A,** Transverse section of penis. **B,** Relationship of bladder, prostate, seminal vesicles, penis, urethra, and scrotal contents. (Adapted from Smith, D.R.: General urology, Los Altos, Calif., 1975, Lange Medical Publications.)

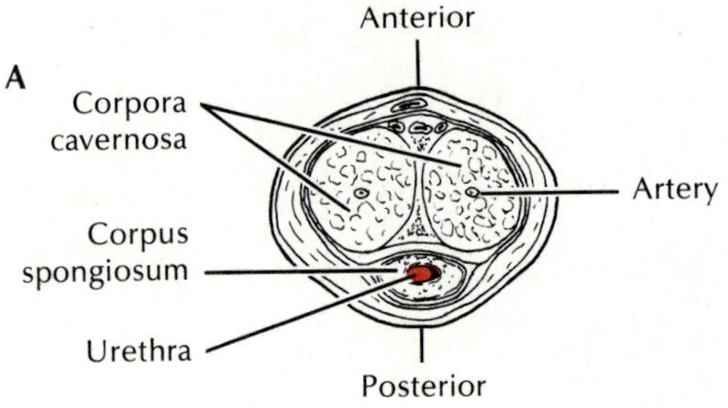

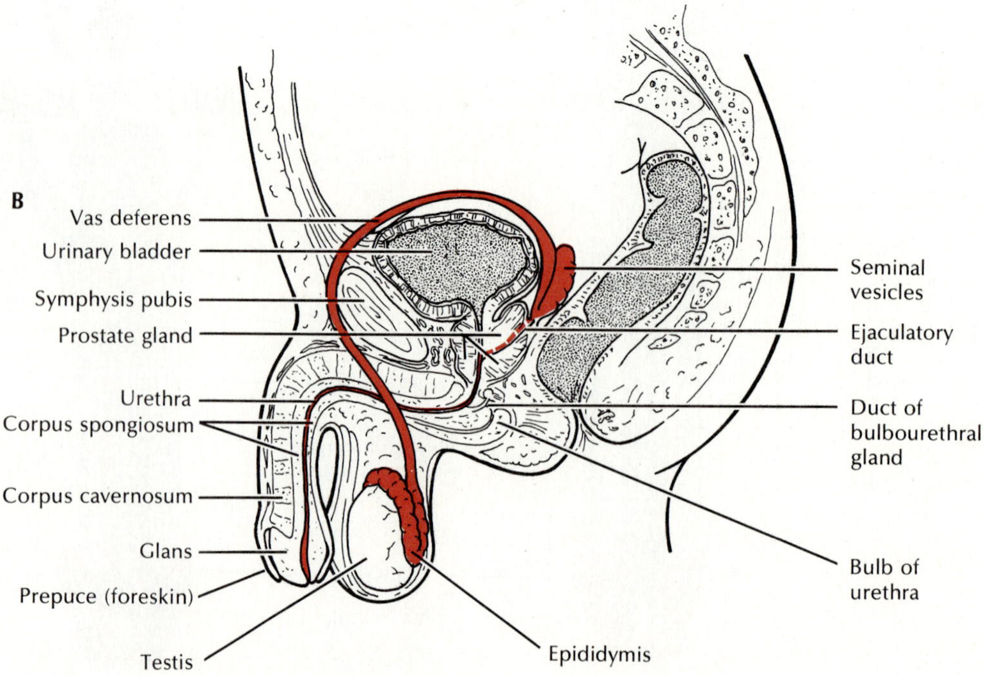

INTERNAL GENITALIA

Internal structures include the following (Figs. 6.26 and 6.27):

1. Testes: male gonads
2. Canal system
3. Accessory reproductive tract glands
   a. Seminal vesicles
   b. Prostate glands
   c. Bulbourethral glands
4. Semen

Testes: male gonads. By the end of the seventh lunar month of fetal life, the testes descend through the inguinal canal. At term birth one or both of the oval-shaped testes may still be within the inguinal canals with final descent occurring in the early postnatal period. The factors responsible for descent from the abdominal cavity into the scrotal sac are not fully understood. Maternal and fetal hormones along with numerous mechanical forces have been considered. When testes fail to descend completely into the scrotal sac, the developmental defect is referred to as cryptorchidism (*crypt,* from the Greek, meaning hidden, covered, occult; *orchi,* from the Greek, meaning testis); surgical repair is called orchiopexy. The testes must be within the scrotum for spermatogenesis to occur.

Testicular functioning. The two principal functions of

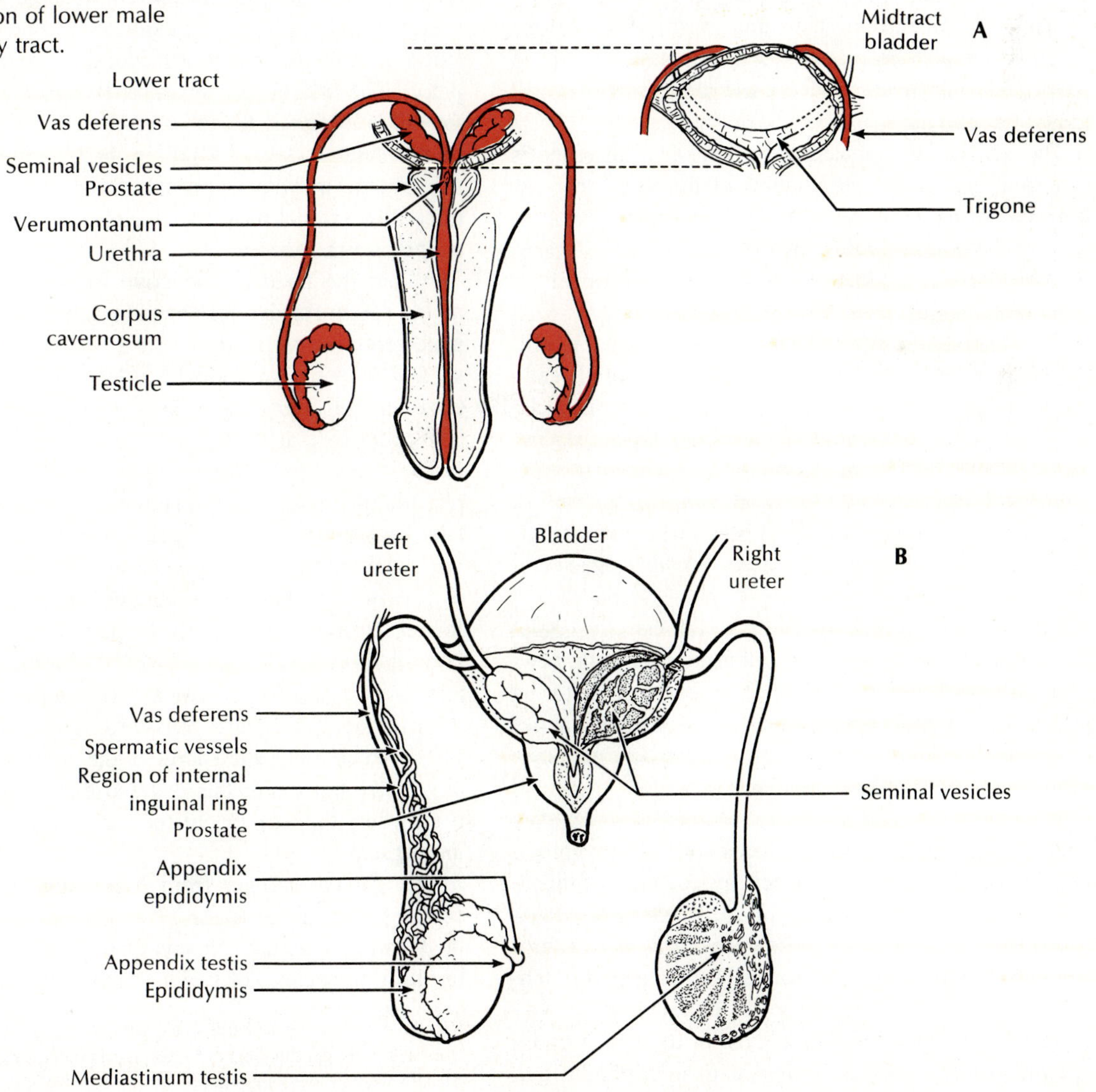

Fig. 6.27
A, Frontal section of lower male genitourinary tract. **B,** Enlarged frontal section of lower male genitourinary tract.

the testes are spermatogenesis and hormone production. White fibrous tissue surrounds each testis and divides it into several lobules. Within each lobule are one to three long (about 75 cm), narrow, coiled *seminiferous tubules* and clusters of *interstitial cells* (Leydig's cells). Spermatids attach to the germinal epithelium (Sertoli's cells) within the seminiferous tubules and develop into spermatozoa. The interstitial cells are large connective or supportive tissue (stromal) cells responsible for the production of testosterone. Testosterone is an androgen, or masculinizing hormone. Normal male growth and development of secondary male sexual characteristics, accessory organs such as the prostate, seminal vesicles, and adult male sexual behaviors are largely dependent on androgenic hormones, principally testosterone (Table 6.4).

Testosterone also has a role in regulating metabolism. This androgen stimulates protein anabolism (construction), which results in greater growth and development of skeletal muscles and bone. Testosterone functions in fluid and electrolyte metabolism; that is, it promotes renal tubular sodium and water retention and potassium excretion.

The normal adult male production of testosterone is 4 to 9 mg/24 hr. Slight amounts of this and other androgens normally are secreted by the ovaries in women and by the adrenal cortex in men and women. Traces of estrogenic hormones are also produced by either Leydig's or closely associated Sertoli's cells.

The anterior pituitary gland in males produces follicle-stimulating hormone (FSH) and interstitial cell–stimulating hormone (ICSH) (luteinizing hormone [LH] in the female). FSH causes more rapid sperm production by the tubules, and ICSH stimulates Leydig's (interstitial) cells, increasing testosterone secretion. A feedback mechanism from the testes to the anterior pituitary aids in the control of steroid sex hormone secretion.

Spermatogenesis. Primitive sex cells (spermatogonia) are present in the seminiferous tubules of the male newborn. During puberty these cells undergo a maturing process called *spermatogenesis*. This process is a series of meiotic divisions in which one primary spermatocyte divides into two secondary spermatocytes, each of which redivides, ultimately producing four spermatids (sperm cells). Meiosis also reduces the full, or diploid, number of chromosomes carried by each spermatid to the half, or haploid, number of 23. Twenty-two chromosomes are autosomes; one is either an X or a Y chromosome. Spermatogenesis normally continues throughout a man's lifetime (see Chapters 10 and 14).

Sperm. One of the smallest cells in the human body, spermatozoa have been compared to microscopic tadpoles in shape. Sperm have characteristic parts identified as the head, neck, middle piece, and tail. The flattened, oval-shaped *head* is a compact package of chromosomes (cell nucleus) that makes up the bulk of the sperm. Human sperm are unusually heterogeneous in size and shape because the amount of cytoplasm left in the head varies and the size of cavities (vacuoles) within the nucleus differs from sperm to sperm. (Fig. 6.28).

The head is covered by a cap specialized to penetrate an ovum. The cap (acrosome) contains enzymes (e.g., hyaluronidase) that are capable of dissolving the gelatin-like covering of the ovum. The gelatinous covering of the egg includes the cumulus and corona radiata. The enzymes from many acrosome-topped sperm are required to disperse this covering.

The *neck* houses a centriole and connects the head to the cylindric *middle piece* that contains mitochondria around a central helix. An oxidation process in the mitochondria (small granules present in all cells) generates energy for the whipping motion of the tail. The elongated, lashlike *tail* has a principal piece and a short end piece. The whipping motion in the principal piece of the tail is from side to side (two-dimensional) while that of the short end of the tail is three-dimensional. The side-to-side movement propels the sperm forward; the three-dimensional movement causes the sperm to rotate as they swim forward.

Within the male reproductive tract the resting nonmotile sperm survive for several months. Within the female reproductive tract, sperm may remain motile for up to 7 days but are thought to lose their ability to fertilize an egg after only 3 days. Only motile sperm are able to fertilize an egg.

The entire spermatozoon is encased within a cytoplasmic membrane. The membrane, or outer coat, contains antigens.* These antigens may be responsible for the specificity of the interaction between sperm and ova. However, these same antigens may be responsible for one form of infertility (see pp. 172 and 180).

Sperm just leaving the testes are not fertile. Their maturation process continues as sperm are moved through the epididymis. Peristaltic contractions of the vas deferens move the sperm to the ampulla (most distal, dilated portion of the vas) and the ejaculatory duct, from where they are ejaculated through the urethra during orgasm.

The ejaculate ranges from 3 to 5 ml in volume and contains from about 60 to 120 million sperm per milliliter. In any ejaculate, many sperm are not capable of fertilization because of various factors such as immatur-

*This is mentioned here because antigens (any protein that is foreign to a person causes that person to develop antibodies) in this coat can cause a woman to develop antibodies against the man's sperm. This results in infertility (see pp. 172 and 180).

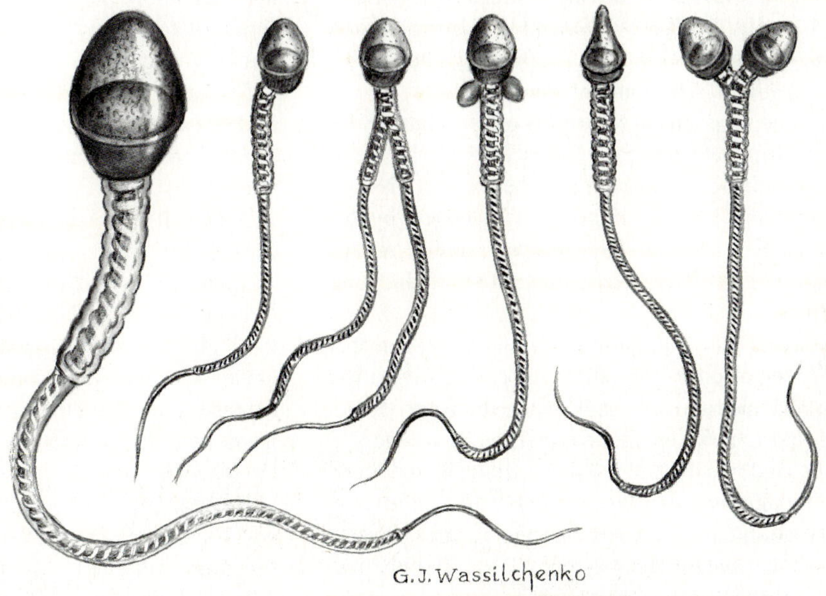

Fig. 6.28
Sperm: normal and abnormal.

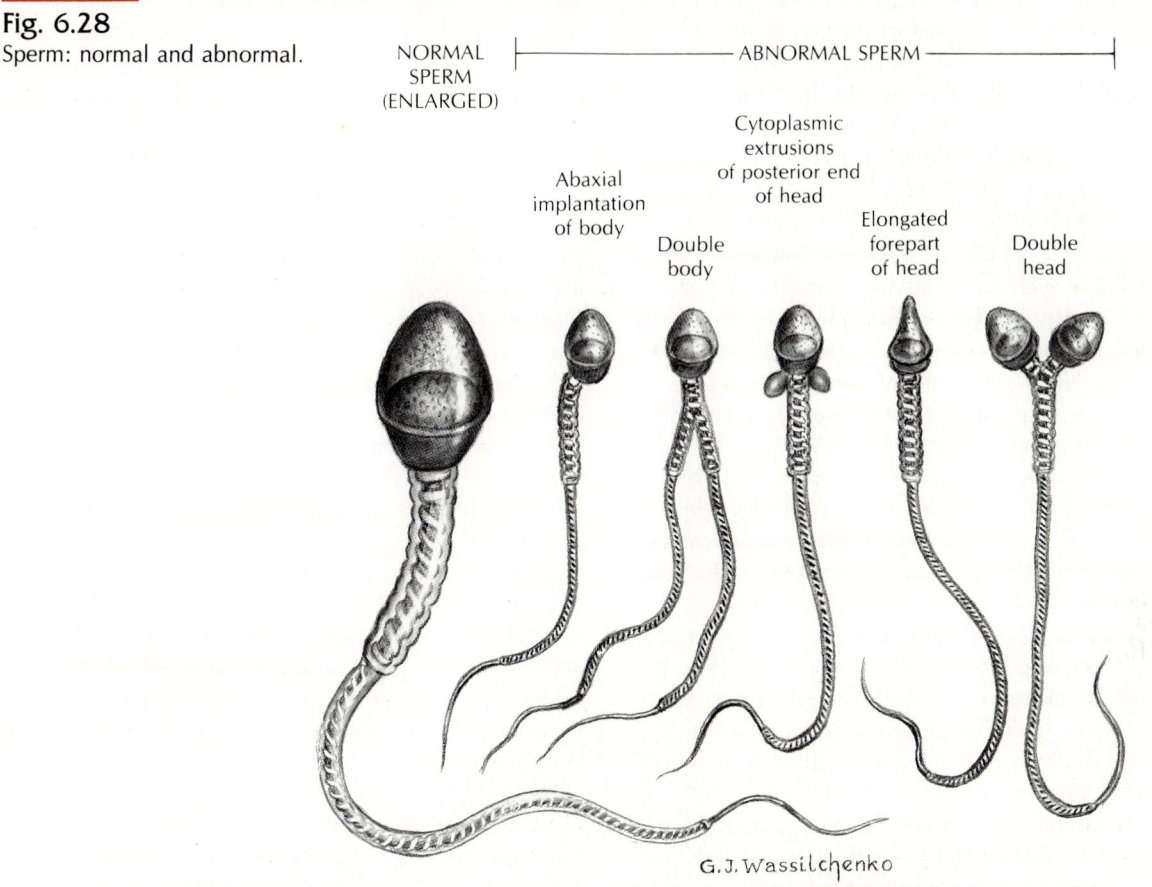

ity, abnormal development, and aging. The healthiest, most vigorous sperm only can reach the fallopian tubes.

After sperm are deposited, usually near the cervical os, several will penetrate the cervical mucus if the mucus is receptive (see p. 170) and rapidly enter the uterine cavity. Some sperm will reach the fallopian tubes within *5 minutes* after sperm are deposited in the vagina. Uterine contractions may assist the sperm's rapid transport. If the cervical mucus is favorable, sperm trapped within it are released to be transported into the uterus and fallopian tubes at a steady rate for 2 to 3 days. Progesterone makes the cervical mucus unreceptive and unsupportive to sperm. Because of this effect, the woman who is in the luteal phase of the menstrual cycle (see p. 86) or who is taking oral contraceptives containing progestin (see p. 192) is relatively infertile; that is, it is unlikely that sperm will be able to migrate into the uterine cavity.

Capacitation is the final step in sperm maturation. It is the physiologic change that removes the protective covering from sperm. Capacitation must be completed before fertilization can occur.

Canal system. Each testis has one tightly coiled tube, about 6 m (20 ft) in length. The tube, the *epididymis,* lies along the top and side of each testis. Seminiferous tubules are continuous with the epididymis, which in turn connects to the vas deferens. The epididymides are storage sites for maturing spermatozoa and produce a small part of the seminal fluid (semen).

The *vas deferens* (vas refers to a vessel; deferens means to carry off), or ductus deferens, is a tube extending from each epididymis to join the duct from a seminal vesicle to form a comon duct, the ejaculatory duct. The vas deferens ascends from the scrotum and passes through the inguinal canal into the abdominal cavity within a structure known as the spermatic cord. In addition to the vas deferens, the spermatic cord contains blood vessels, lymphatics, and nerves. Once within the abdominal cavity, each vas deferens passes along the top and down the posterior surface of the bladder, where, together with the duct from the seminal vesicle, it forms the ejaculatory duct. The two *ejaculatory ducts* pass through the prostate gland and open into the prostatic urethra. The *urethra* (see p. 77) completes the canal system. For sperm to exit the body, they must travel the full length of the canal system in succession: seminiferous tubules, epididymides (pl.), vasa deferentia (pl.), ejaculatory ducts, and the urethra. For this reason, vasectomy, a surgical procedure that interrupts this canal system, results in sterility (for a discussion of male sterilization, see Chapter 41).

Accessory reproductive tract glands. The *seminal vesicles* are pouchlike structures located along the lower posterior surface of the bladder, anterior to the rectum. These vesicles secrete a thick, yellowish, viscous (sticky) liquid with the following characteristics. Seminal fluid is rich in fructose, a simple sugar that provides energy for sperm mobility following ejaculation. Seminal secretion also contains prostaglandins (see p. 92) to a concentration of 55 μg/ml of ejaculate. Prostaglandins stimulate uterine contractility, which increases rate of sperm migration to the oviduct. Nearly one third of the volume of semen is secreted by the seminal vesicles. Adequate levels of testosterone are essential to sustain normal secretory activity of the seminal vesicles.

The *prostate* is a fibromuscular glandular organ that surrounds the posterior (prostatic) urethra. This chestnut-shaped gland measures about 4 cm in diameter. It occupies a space between the musculofascial urogenital diaphragm and the bladder. The prostate is separated from the rectum by a thin layer of tissue. Palpation during rectal examination reveals that the normal prostate bulges into the rectum about 1 cm or less. The prostate produces a thin alkaline vehicle for the spermatozoa released at the time of ejaculation. This alkaline substance constitutes more than half the seminal fluid, protecting the sperm from the acid environment of the male urethra and female vagina and enhancing the sperm's motility. Slight acidity depresses sperm motility; stronger acidity kills sperm. Sperm motility is best in a neutral or slightly alkaline pH environment.

Aging often causes enlargement of the prostate, with consequent constriction of the urethra and resultant urinary retention. Surgical removal of the prostate gland (prostatectomy) may be necessary to relieve this condition.

Prostatic function also depends on an adequate level of testosterone. Without testicular secretion, both the seminal vesicles and the prostate stop functioning and atrophy.

A pair of *bulbourethral, or Cowper's, glands* are located below the prostate, one at either side of the membranous urethra. These glands resemble peas in both size and shape. A 2.5 cm duct connects each bulbourethral gland with the penile urethra. The bulbourethral glands also secrete an alkaline fluid into the semen as a defense against urethral and vaginal acidity. Secretion from the bulbourethral glands accounts for about 5% of the ejaculate.

Semen. The components of semen derive from several sources. Each component of semen and its origin, function, and percent of total volume are presented in Table 6.3. Sperm are stored primarily in the epididymi-

Table 6.3
Composition of Semen

Origin	Component	Functions	Percent of ejaculate
Testes and epididymides	Some fluid	Vehicle for sperm transport	Under 5%*
	Sperm (hundreds of millions)	Fertilization of ova to perpetuate species	
Seminal vesicles	Seminal fluid containing:		30%
	Fructose	Energy source	
	Prostaglandins	Increase motility of uterus	
	Thick mucus	Vehicle for sperm transport	
	Coagulation protein	Entrap sperm	
Prostate gland	Prostatic secretion containing:		60%
	Alkaline fluid	Support and enhance sperm motility	
	Thin mucus	Vehicle for sperm transport	
	Fibrinolysin	Liquefies semen 10 minutes after ejaculation, to release sperm	
	Citrate, acid phosphatase, spermine, spermidine, zinc, magnesium		
	Immunoglobulins (IgG and IgA)		
Bulbourethral glands	Alkaline fluid	Support and enhance sperm motility	Under 5%
	Fibrinolysin	Assist in liquefying semen to release entraped sperm	

*Vasectomy affects only the production of this portion of the ejaculate so that there is no noticeable change in volume, even after sperm are no longer available for transport through the remaining canal system.

des. At the time of ejaculation, 3 to 5 ml of semen containing secretions from the prostate, seminal vesicles,* and bulbourethral glands, as well as about 60 to 120 million spermatozoa per milliliter, is released.

After ejaculation, semen coagulates quickly, but within 15 to 20 minutes, it liquefies. Spontaneous liquefaction is the result of its fructose content and an enzyme, fibrinolysin, which is one component of the prostatic fluid. Liquefaction unclumps the spermatozoa so that motility is possible.

Many factors influence male fertility, the most important of which are the number of sperm released at ejaculation and their size and shape. Sperm capable of fertilization are uniform in size and shape. Millions of sperm seem to be required for fertilization to occur (see p. 206), even though a single sperm actually fertilizes the ovum. If the sperm count drops to less than 20 million/ml of semen, the male is considered infertile (see p. 181).

• • •

Females experience two important cyclic phenomena—the menstrual cycle and the sexual response cycle. A description of the way the woman's body participates in these cyclic changes follows.

Menstrual Cycle

MENSTRUAL MYTHS

An awareness of some myths about menstruation and their cultural origins is necessary to use the nursing process effectively with both female and male clients. The belief systems held by researchers may also influence the research methodology used and the way results are interpreted, presented in the literature, and used by society in general (i.e., people tend to color things the way they want to see them).

Many myths have their origin in the mystery that surrounded the woman, her hidden reproductive organs, and her uniqueness in adding new members to society. As a consequence, a vast store of folklore, fancies, and superstitions evolved. Before the eighteenth century, the relationship of the menstrual cycle to reproduction was obscure. Menstrual flow was believed to be the elimination of poisons that had accumulated in the woman. The discovery of the fallopian tubes did nothing to clear up this misconception. At first the fallopian tubes were seen as chimneys through which vile humors were vented.

Because of their recurring nature, menstrual cycles were thought to be under the control of the moon. Before the discovery of ovulation in humans, it was thought that an egg was produced during menstruation only when fruitful intercourse had occurred. Not until the nineteenth century was knowledge available about the existence of the human egg, ovulation, and ovarian functioning. As new knowledge emerged, a few facts were added to the accumulated body of folklore.

The most common myths in existence today can be sorted out under the following headings:

1. During menstruation, the woman is vulnerable and therefore needs to be protected.
2. The menstruating woman can pose a danger.
3. Menstrual blood has been viewed as possessing healing powers, as an aphrodisiac, or as capable of bestowing fertility.

The menstruating woman is seen as being vulnerable to physical and psychologic stress. Recall some of the myths you may have heard; for example, "Don't wash your hair," "Don't take a bath," "Watch out, you'll catch cold," "That's too heavy for you to carry now." Review what you remember about the onset of your menarche or that of other adolescent females. (See discussion of onset of menstruation, p. 88.) Recall what you had been told before onset and what was said by your family and peers when they learned of your menarche.

Historical literature contains many references to dangers attributed to menstrual women. Should a menstruating woman walk through a farmer's fields, the crops would not grow and the flowers would wilt; if she tried to bake bread, the dough would not rise. The danger also exists for her husband so that physical contact, especially sexual intercourse, was and in some places still is prohibited. In many cultures the menstruating woman is kept in a separate menstrual hut or in separate quarters. Following a ritualized "cleansing," the woman returns to her place in her family.

As late as the second half of this century, the many behavioral changes falsely attributed to women during their menstrual cycles has been used to argue why it would be unwise to have a woman for president of the United States, for example.

HISTORICAL PERSPECTIVE

During this century there have been significant additions to the knowledge of the biophysical and emotional aspects of the menstrual cycle. The endometrial cycle was described in 1907, the ovarian cycle in 1914, the activity of estrogen in 1923, and progesterone in 1929.

*Semen comes from the Latin meaning "place of origin." It was once thought that sperm originated and were stored in the seminal vesicles. Vesicle comes from the Latin, meaning "oval-shaped bladder."

Fig. 6.29
Hormonal control of menstrual cycle.

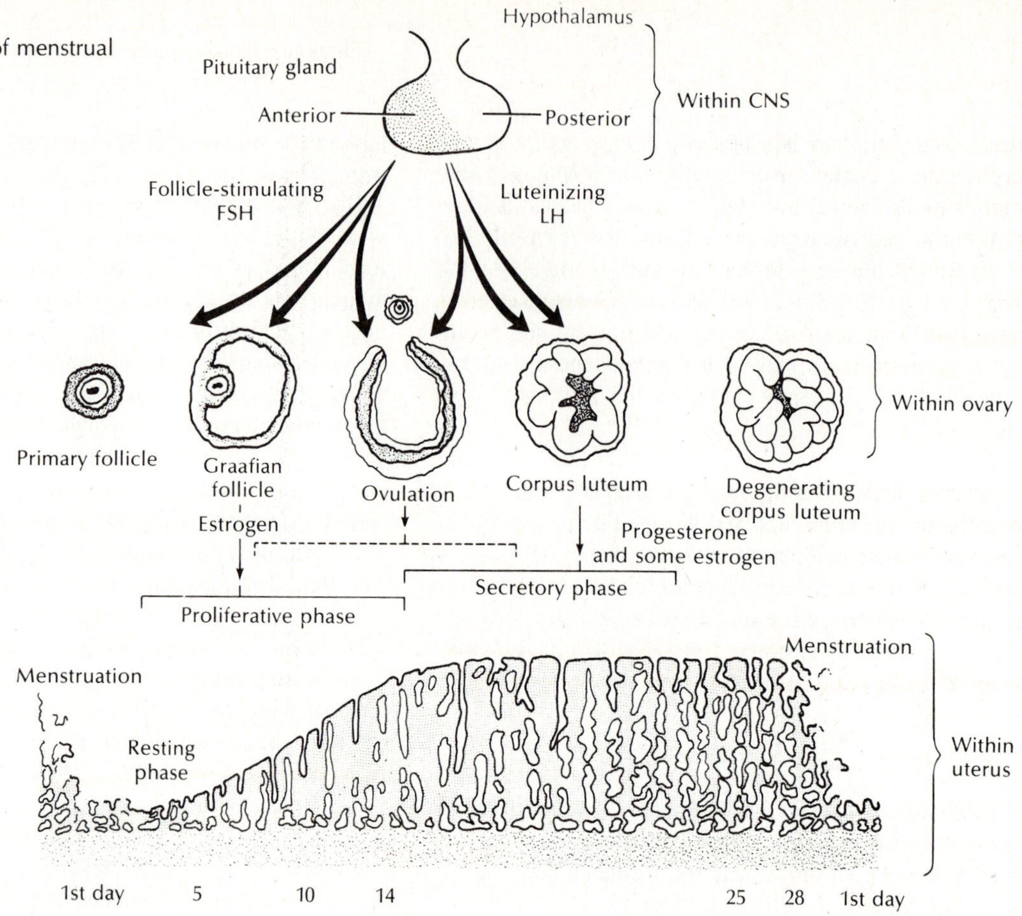

Fig. 6.30
Sequence of events leading to amenorrhea because of stressful emotional stimuli. Other factors that could lead to amenorrhea or alter the interval between cycles include internal stimuli such as illness, excessive fatigue, or excessive weight and external stimuli from environmental temperature and high altitude.

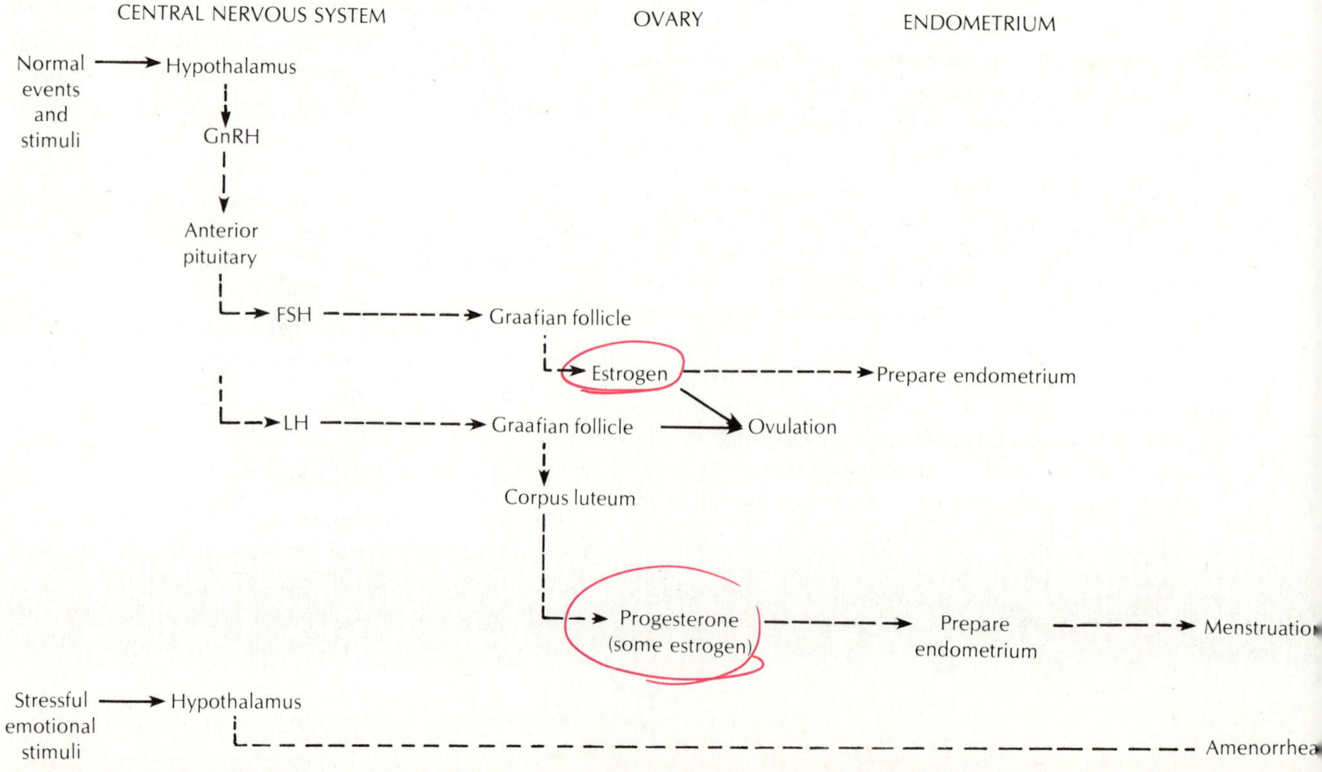

Since then, pituitary hormones have been purified and hypothalamic control over the pituitary gland has been studied extensively.

The pituitary gland, formerly called the master gland, is controlled by secretions from the hypothalamus. In turn, the hypothalamus is under the feedback control of hormones from the ovaries and testes. Hormonal control over the menstrual cycle is illustrated in Fig. 6.29.

HYPOTHALAMUS AND PITUITARY

Neurons from several portions of the brain terminate in the hypothalamus. The cell bodies of secretory neurons are located within the median eminence (middle portion) of the hypothalamus while the nerve endings lie close to capillary loops slightly above the pituitary portal (circulatory) system. Thus the circulation picks up the hypothalamic neurohormones and carries them to the anterior pituitary, which normally responds to each specific releasing or inhibiting neurohormone "command."

One releasing hormone, gonadotropin-releasing hormone (GnRH)* causes the synthesis and release of both follicle-stimulating hormone (FSH) and luteinizing hormone (LH)† from the anterior pituitary gland. See boxes for effects of FSH and LH on female and male gonads. Emotional stress communicated to the hypothalamus can depress the formation and release of GnRH, preventing the release of FSH and LH. As a result, ovulation does not occur, progesterone is not produced, and amenorrhea results (Fig. 6.30).

The hypothalamic-pituitary-gonad interaction in the male is shown in Fig. 6.31.

---

*Until recently, it was believed that there were two releasing hormones: one for FSH and one for LH.

†LH is identical to interstitial cell–stimulating hormone (ICSH).

Fig. 6.31
Feedback mechanism between hypothalamic-pituitary axis and gonads is similar to that in female.

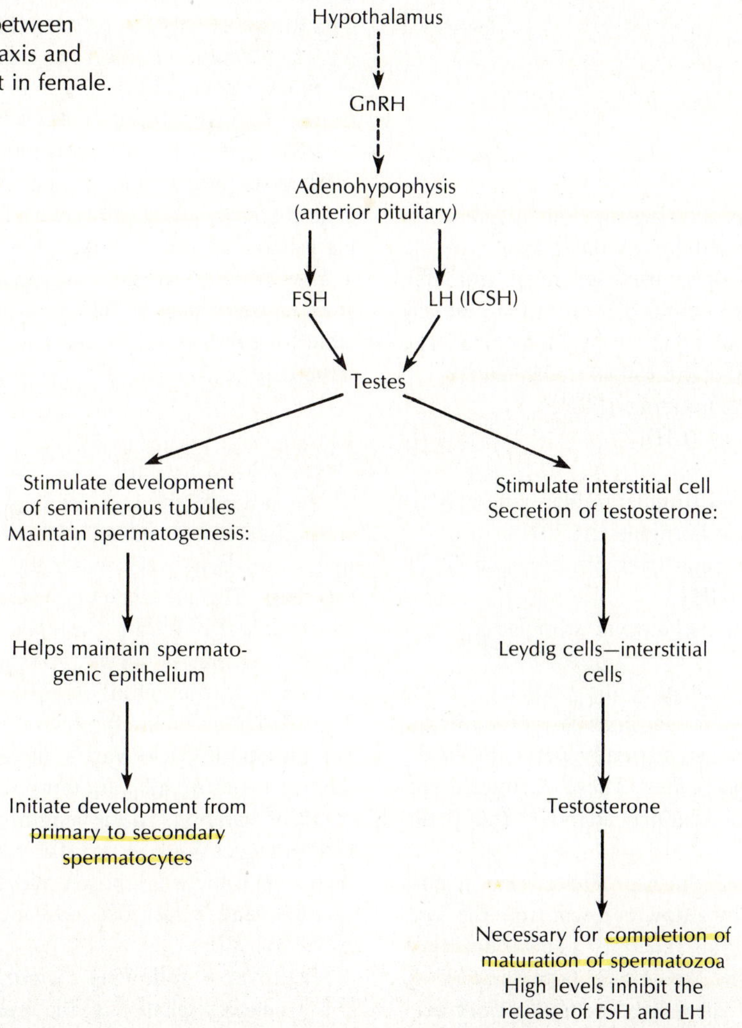

Follicle-stimulating Hormone (FSH)

Female Ovary	Male Testis
Growth and maturation of graafian follicles and preparation of these cells so that they can respond to LH	Development of seminiferous tubules and stimulation of Sertoli's cells

Luteinizing Hormone (LH)

Female Ovary	Male Testis
Works with FSH to stimulate estrogen secretion. Along with a surge of LH, estrogen stimulates ovulation, then luteinizes the follicle to form the corpus luteum. The corpus luteum produces progesterone and estrogen.	Stimulates Leydig's cells to produce androgens (e.g., testosterone).

The *adenohypophysis*, the *anterior and middle lobes of the pituitary*, is formed by an invagination of the embryonic oropharynx. It is then separated from the oral cavity to lie near the neural portion of the pituitary in a small indentation of bone, the sella turcica. The adenohypophysis produces the following hormones:

1. Follicle-stimulating hormone (FSH)
2. Luteinizing hormone (LH)
3. Prolactin
4. Thyrotropin (thyroid stimulating hormone [TSH])
5. Adrenocorticotropic hormone (ACTH)
6. and 7. Alpha- and beta-lipotropin hormone (LPH)
8. Growth hormone (GH)
9. Alpha- and beta-melanocyte–stimulating hormones (MSH)

In the normal middle lobe of the pituitary can be found high levels of beta-endorphins and encephalins. Endorphins and encephalins, naturally occurring in the body, have analgesic properties. These chemicals currently are receiving considerable attention and publicity.

The *posterior pituitary*, the *neurohypophysis*, is nonglandular. It is formed by a down growth from the forebrain. The neurohypophysis functions as a storage place for oxytocin (pitocin) and antidiuretic hormone (ADH), which are produced by specialized neurosecretory cells in the hypothalamus. ADH is also called vasopressin. (See discussion of renal system p. 235 for functions of ADH.) These neurosecretory cells in the hypothalamus are neurons that are modified so that ganules carrying oxytocin and vasopressin are transported down the axons to the posterior lobe of the pituitary, where the hormones are stored until released. Oxytocin is responsible for increasing the contractility of the uterine muscles during labor and delivery and for enhancing milk ejection in the mammary glands during lactation. Oxytocin will be discussed along with labor (see p. 887) and lactation (see p. 658).

It is generally assumed that the menstrual cycle represents a complex sequence of cyclic hypothalamic-pituitary stimulation and ovarian response that renews the endometrium each cycle for implantation and nutrition of a fertilized egg.

HYPOTHALAMIC-PITUITARY CYCLE

Toward the end of the normal menstrual cycle, blood levels of estrogen and progesterone fall. Low blood levels of these ovarian hormones stimulate the hypothalamus to secrete GnRH, which in turn stimulates anterior pituitary secretion of FSH. FSH stimulates development of ovarian graafian follicles and their production of estrogen. Estrogen levels begin to fall and hypothalamic GnRH triggers the anterior pituitary release of LH. A marked surge of LH and a smaller peak of estrogen precede the expulsion of the ovum from the graafian follicle by about 24 to 36 hours.

Low concentrations of estrogen and high concentrations of androgens in the normal adult male are responsible for the noncyclic male pattern of gonadotropin release (Fig. 6.31).

OVARIAN CYCLE

The primary graafian follicles contain immature oocytes. Before ovulation, from 1 to 30 follicles begin to mature in each ovary under the influence of FSH and estrogen. The preovulatory surge of LH affects a selected follicle. Within the chosen follicle, the oocyte matures, ovulation occurs, and the empty follicle begins its transformation into the corpus luteum (yellow body). This *follicular phase* (preovulatory phase) of the ovarian menstrual cycle varies in length from woman to woman. Almost all variations in cycle length are the result of varations in the length of the follicular phase. On rare occasions (1 in 100 menstrual cycles), more than one follicle is chosen and more than one oocyte matures and undergoes ovulation (see discussion of twins, p. 930).

The events following *ovulation*, the *luteal phase* (postovulatory phase) of the ovarian menstrual cycle, usually require 14 days (range of 13 to 15 days). Eight days after ovulation, the corpus luteum reaches its peak of functional activity, secreting both of the steroids, estrogen and progesterone. Coincident with this time of peak luteal functioning, the fertilized egg is implanted in the endometrium. If no implantation occurs, the corpus luteum regresses, and steroid levels drop. Two weeks after ovulation, if fertilization and implantation do not occur, uterine endometrium is shed through menstruation.

After ovulation, estrogen levels drop. For 90% of women, only a small amount of *withdrawal bleeding* occurs so that is goes unnoticed. In 10% of women, there is sufficient bleeding for it to be visible, resulting in what is known as *midcycle bleeding*.

ENDOMETRIAL CYCLE

The endometrium responds to fluctuating levels of ovarian steroids. The endometrium consists of three layers. The basal layer intermingles with the myometrium. The other two functional layers undergo cyclic changes and are shed in menstrual flow.

When labeled according to phases in the endometrial cycle, the *menstrual phase* extends over the first 5 days when the two functional layers (the compact and spongy layers) are shed. The resting, or *repair,* phase (the early proliferative phase) includes days 4 through 7. The most rapid growth of the functional layers occurs between days 5 to 7 and the day of ovulation and is known as the *proliferative phase*. In a 28-day cycle, ovulation occurs on day 14 (range of 13 to 15 days). The *secretory phase* spans days 15 through 28; the last 3 days before menstruation make up the *ischemic phase* (stage of regression). In Fig. 6.32, the phases are presented in linear fashion.

The endometrium has different characteristics at different times during the cycle depending on the levels of estrogen and progesterone. Therefore the endometrium can be "dated" (the phase of the cycle can be determined) and the presence and level of estrogen and progesterone can be measured. If the levels of hormones are too low or too high, the endometrium would reflect this (see discussion of infertility, p. 172).

The first day of menstrual discharge has been designated as *day 1* of the cycle. The average duration of menstrual flow is 5 days (range of 3 to 6 days), and the average blood loss is approximately 50 ml (range of 20 to 80 ml), but there is great variation. During menstruation, the average daily loss of iron is 0.5 to 1 mg. If the woman's usual blood loss is over 80 ml, she will most likely need iron supplementation to prevent secondary anemia.

For about 50% of women, menstrual blood does not appear to clot. The menstrual blood clots within the uterus, but the clot is liquefied before it is discharged from the uterus. If the discharge leaves the uterus too rapidly, liquefaction may not be complete so that clots will appear in the vagina. Uterine discharge includes mucus and epithelial cells in addition to blood.

Ovulation occurs about 14 days before the start of the next menstrual flow, for example, day 10 of a 24-day cycle, day 14 of a 28-day cycle, or day 18 of a 32-day cycle.

The endometrial surface is completely restored in approximately 4 days or slightly before the menstrual flow stops. From this point on, an eightfold to tenfold thickening occurs, with a leveling off of growth at ovulation. During the proliferative phase, the glands are tubular or columnar in shape. About 3 to 4 days before ovulation, vascularity to the endometrium increases. Endometrial growth during proliferation is dependent on estrogen produced by ovarian follicles before ovulation.

After ovulation, the graafian follicle develops into the corpus luteum. The corpus luteum produces estrogen and large amounts of progesterone. Progesterone causes the blood vessels in the endometrium to dilate and assume a spiral or corkscrew shape. Endometrial glands elongate, become more active, and secrete a glycogen-containing fluid. The endometrium reaches the thickness of heavy, soft velvet and becomes luxuriant with blood and glandular secretions, a suitable protective and nutritive bed for a fertilized ovum. In the fully matured secretory endometrium, three strata are noted: the two functional layers, the superficial or compact layer and

Fig. 6.32
Endometrial cycle phases in a 28-day ovulatory menstrual cycle.

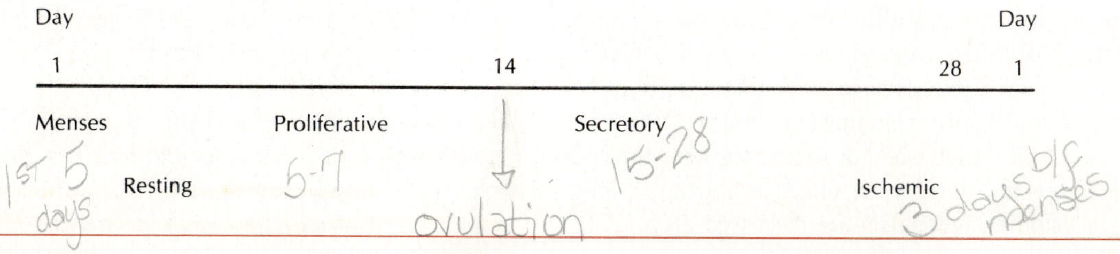

Table 6.4
Hypothalamic-Pituitary-Gonadal Axis

Female	Male
Hypothalamus	
Anterior Pituitary	**Anterior Pituitary**
FSH LH Prolactin (luteotropin [LTH])	FSH LH (ICSH)
Excreted via kidneys as urinary gonadotropins	
Target: ovary 1. Cytogenic function (ova) 2. Endocrine secretory function a. Estrogen (estrone, estriol, estradiol); target structures: breasts (stroma/ducts), bones, sodium/water balance, fallopian tubes, uterus, vagina, pelvic girdle, fat deposit b. Progesterone; target structures: breasts (glands), uterus, vagina, increased BBT	Target: testis 1. Cytogenic function (sperm) 2. Endocrine secretory function a. Testosterone (androgen); target structures: testis, facial hair, larynx, increased bone growth, increased muscle mass, mineral/water balance, seminal vesicles, prostate gland, epididymis, penis, shoulder girdle b. Some estrogen (?)
Metabolized in the liver and excreted via kidneys	
1. Estradiol 2. Pregnanediol*	1. Androgens 2. 17-ketosteroids (two fifths from testes; three fifths from adrenal glands)

*No 17-ketosteroids; in female, all produced in adrenal glands.

an intermediate or spongy layer; and the basal or inner, inactive layer.

If fertilization does not occur, about 3 days before menstruation begins, the corpus luteum degenerates with subsequent withdrawal of estrogen and progesterone. Vasospasm of the spiral arteries occurs. This vasoconstriction results in ischemia, necrosis, and sloughing off of the upper two layers of the endometrium. Near the end of the secretory phase, just before the start of menstrual flow, regeneration begins from the retained basal layer. Rebuilding the endometrium from the basal layer upward is responsible for its healing and rejuvenation without scar formation. Further discussion about the ability of the endometrium to heal without scarring after repeated menstrual cycles and repeated childbirth is discussed in Chapter 31.

CERVICAL CHANGES

Changes also occur within the cells of the lining of the cervix and in the characteristics of cervical mucus. These changes will be addressed along with the symptothermal (natural family planning) method, p. 190.

The available methods for detecting the time of ovulation for the purpose of either achieving a pregnancy or avoiding pregnancy are discussed on p. 171.

Puberty

Puberty marks a period of development between childhood and maturity. ***Menarche*** refers to the cyclic discharge of menstrual blood *(menstruation, menses)* and is a step from prepuberty to postpuberty. In the female, ovulation and the production of viable ova (gametes) do not occur for a year or two after the menarche.

The causes of the onset of puberty are as yet unknown. Various theories have been elaborated as explanations. Frisch and co-workers (1974) theorized that menarche may be triggered when a critical weight is achieved for the girl's height. In support of this theory a steady decline in the age at menarche has been noted to correlate with an observed trend in increased height. Others argue that better health and nutrition determine the time of the onset of puberty. In the United States, for example, the average age at menarche in 1900 was 14.3 years; in 1960 it was 12.7 years with a normal range from 11 to 16 years. For the past 2 decades adult height is not increasing nor is menarche occurring earlier, indicating that there is probably an ultimate limit.

Although young girls secrete small, rather constant amounts of estrogen, a marked increase occurs between 8 and 11 years of age, and this increase, along with

Table 6.5
Effects of Estrogens on Target Organs and Tissues

Target Organ/Tissue	Effect
Basal layer of vaginal epithelium	Thickened mucosa Development of rugae (folds)
Endocervical glandular cells	Cervical mucus that is clear, watery, stretchable, high in sodium chloride so that a fernlike pattern is seen when the mucus is allowed to dry; facilitates sperm transport
Endometrium and myometrium	Growth of cells by hypertrophy and hyperplasia
Breasts	Growth of mammary ductal system resulting in increased size of breasts
Central nervous system Anterior hypothalamus and adenohypophysis	Inhibit synthesis of FSH, prolactin; stimulate brief surge of LH; affect temperature regulatory center so that BBT drops
Metabolism and bony skelton	Favors bone formation over bone absorption Female body build: narrower shoulders, wider hips, sites of fat deposition, increase in carrying angle of the arms, gynecoid bony pelvis
Hematologic system	Decreased plasma cholesterol (when compared to males, in females there is a lower incidence of atherosclerosis and coronary heart disease before menopause) Decreased strength in capillary walls when estrogen falls so that just before and during menses, females may have spontaneous nosebleeds
Androgenic target organs—prostate gland in male	Decreased rate of growth, therefore used in therapy for prostatic cancer; a side effect, however, is decreased libido and erectile problems (impotency)

Table 6.6
Effects of Progesterone on Target Organs and Tissues

Target Organ/Tissue	Effect
Endometrium, that has been previously primed by estrogen	Secretory phase of endometrial menstrual cycle
Endocervical glandular cells	Thick, sticky mucus that does not form a fernlike pattern when dried; nonreceptive to sperm
Myometrium	Decreased irritability with sustained tonic vs. clonic contraction pattern
Breasts	Stimulates development of acini (alveoli)
Central nervous system Hypothalamus	Increases BBT; increases respirations so carbon dioxide tension in blood decreases
Metabolism	Loss of sodium; breakdown of proteins; is *not* responsible for premenstrual edema

maturation of the hypothalamic-pituitary-gonadal axis results in menstruation.

Initially, periods are irregular, unpredictable, painless, and anovulatory in the majority of young girls. After 1 or more years, a hypothalamic-pituitary rhythm develops, and enough cyclic estrogen is produced in the ovary to cause a number of graafian follicles to mature. Approximately 14 days before the next menstrual period, a rise in FSH accompanies a surge of LH from the anterior pituitary and ovulation (extrusion of the ovum) occurs.

Ovulatory periods tend to be regular, monitored by progesterone. Although not universal, ovulatory periods may be associated with slight uterine cramping (dysmenorrhea), which may be an effect of progesterone or of prostaglandins or both. This discomfort is rarely serious, is readily relieved by simple analgesics, and when viewed from one perspective, may be reassuring to the girl and her parents as an indication of normal ovulatory function.

Although pregnancy may occur in exceptional cases of true precocious puberty, most pregnancies in very young girls occur well after the normally timed menarche. *However, all girls would benefit from knowing that pregnancy can occur at any time after the onset of menses.*

Summaries of the hypothalamic-pituitary-gonadal axis and its effects on the development of female and male characteristics are presented in Table 6.4. Summaries of the effects of estrogen and of progesterone on target organs and tissues are given in Tables 6.5 and 6.6. The effects of prolactin on target organs are discussed in Table 6.7. Summaries of the stages of sexual development of the female and of the male are presented in Tables 6.8 and 6.9. The changes in the female reproductive system over the life span are illustrated in Fig. 6.33.

Table 6.7
Effects of Prolactin on Target Organs and Tissues

Female	Male
In ovary, helps LH to luteinize ruptured follicle; primary function: regulation of lactation *after* mammary gland is prepared by actions of insulin, estrogens, progestins, growth hormone, corticosteroids; Emotional stress stimulates hypothalamus to release an inhibiting hormone to suppress lactation (see Chapter 31)	In testis, potentiates effect of LH on Leydig's cells; acts with testosterone to produce male secondary sexual characteristics; too high levels (from pituitary tumors) lead to erectile problems (impotence)

Fig. 6.33
Summary of changes in female reproductive system over life span. (Courtesy Merrill-National Laboratories. Division of Richardson-Merrill, Inc., Cincinnati.)

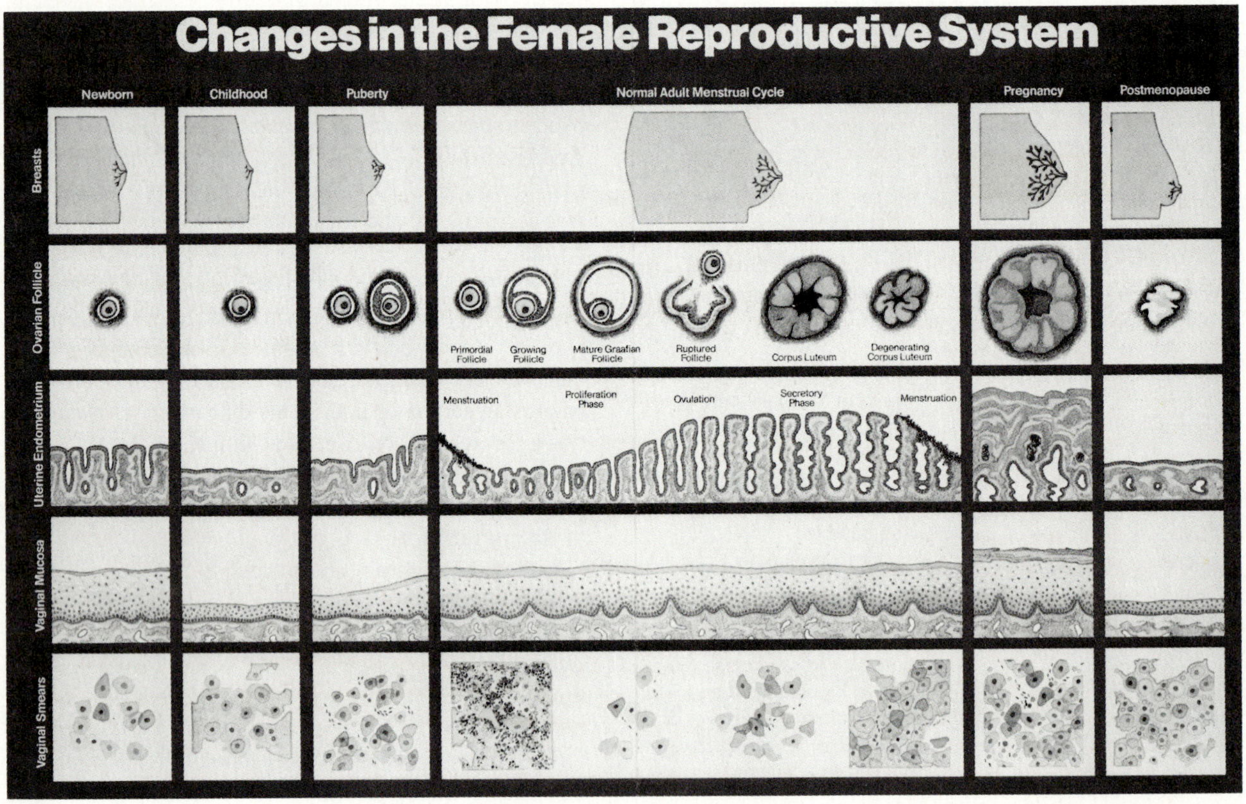

Table 6.8
Stages of Sexual Development: Female*

Age	Stages
0-12	I. Preadolescent. Female pelvic contour evident, breasts flat, labia majora smooth and minora are poorly developed, hymenal opening small or absent, mucous membranes dry and red, vaginal cells lack glycogen.
8-13	II. *Breasts:* Elevation of nipple, small mound beneath areola, which is enlarging and begins pigmentation. *Labia majora* become thickened, more prominent and wrinkled, *labia minora* easily identified due to increased size along with clitoris, urethral opening more prominent, mucous membranes moist and pink, some glycogen present in vaginal cells. *Hair:* First appears on mons and then on labia majora about time of menarche, still scanty, soft and straight. *Skin:* Increased activity of sebaceous and merocrine sweat glands and initial function of apocrine glands in axilla and vulva begin.
9-14	III. Rapid growth peak is passed, menarche most often at this stage and invariably follows the peak of growth acceleration. *Breasts:* Areola and nipple further enlarge and pigmentation more evident, continued increase in glandular size. *Labia minora* well developed and vaginal cells have increased glycogen content, mucous membranes increasingly more pale. *Hair* in pubic region thicker, coarser, often curly (considerable normal variation including a few girls with early stage II at menarche). *Skin:* Further increased activity of sebaceous and sweat glands with beginning of *acne* in some girls; adult body odor.
12-15	IV. *Breasts:* Projection of areola above breast plane and areolar (Montgomery) glands apparent (this development is absent in about 20% of normal girls). Glands easily palpable. *Labia:* Both majora and minora assume adult structure, glycogen content of vaginal cells begins cyclic characteristics. *Hair* in pubic area more abundant, axillary hair present (rarely present at stage II, often present at stage III).
12-17	V. *Breasts:* Mature histologic morphology, nipple enlarged and erect, areolar (Montgomery's) glands well developed, globular shape. *Hair* in pubic area more abundant and may spread to thighs (in about 10% of women it assumes "male" distribution with extension toward umbilicus). Facial hair increased often in form of slight mustache. *Skin:* Increased sebaceous gland activity and increased severity of *acne* if present before.

*Reproduced with permission from Lowrey, G.H.: Growth and development of children, ed. 7. Copyright © 1978 by Year Book Medical Publishers, Inc., Chicago.

Table 6.9
Stages of Sexual Development: Male*

Age	Stages
0-14	I. Preadolescent
10-14	II. Increasing size of *testes* and *penis* is evident (testis length reaches 2.0 cm or more). Scrotum integument is thinner and assumes an increased pendulous appearance. *Hair:* First appearance of pubic hair in area at base of penis. *Skin:* Increased activity of sebaceous and apocrine sweat glands and initial function of apocrine glands on axilla and scrotal area begin.
11-15	III. Rapid growth peak is passed, nocturnal emissions begin. *Testes and penis:* Further increase in size and pigmentation apparent. Leydig's cells (interstitial) first appear at stage II, are now prominent in testes. *Hair:* In pubic area more abundant and present on scrotum, still scanty and fine textured, axillary hair begins. *Breasts:* Button-type hypertrophy in 70% of boys at stages I and III. *Larynx:* Changes in voice due to laryngeal growth begin. *Skin:* Increasing activity of sebaceous and sweat glands with beginning of *acne*, adult body odor.
12-16	IV. *Testes:* Further increase in size, length 4.0 cm or greater, increase in size of *penis* greatest at stages III and IV. *Hair:* Pubic hair thicker and coarser and in most ascends toward umbilicus in typical male pattern, axillary hair increases, facial hair increases over lip and upper cheeks. *Larynx:* Voice deepens. *Skin:* Increasing pigmentation of scrotum and penis, *acne* often more severe. *Breasts:* Previous hypertrophy decreased or absent.
13-17	V. *Testes* Length greater than 4.5 cm. *Hair:* Pubic hair thick, curly, heavily pigmented, extend to thighs and toward umbilicus. Adult distribution and increase in body hair (chest, shoulders, thighs, etc.) continue for more than another 10 years. Baldness, if present, may begin. *Skin:* Acne may persist and increase. *Larynx:* Adult character of voice.

*Reproduced with permission from Lowrey, G.H.: Growth and development of children, ed. 7. Copyright © 1978 by Year Book Medical Publishers, Inc., Chicago.

Prostaglandins

Prostaglandins (PGs) are oxygenated fatty acids now classified as hormones. The different kinds of PGs are distinguished by letters (PGE, PGF), numbers (PGE_2), and letters of the Greek alphabet ($PGF_{2\alpha}$).

PGs are produced in most organs of the body but most notably by the prostate and the endometrium. Therefore semen and menstrual blood are potent prostaglandin sources. PGs are metabolized quickly by most tissues and are biologically active in minute amounts in the cardiovascular, gastrointestinal, respiratory, urogenital, and nervous systems. They also exert a marked effect on metabolism, particularly on glycolysis. Prostaglandins play an important role in many physiologic, pathologic, and pharmacologic reactions. $PGF_{2\alpha}$, PGE_1, and PGE_2, are most frequently used in reproductive medicine.

ROLE IN REPRODUCTIVE FUNCTIONS

Prostaglandins affect smooth muscle contractility and modulation of hormonal activity. Indirect evidence supports PGs' effects on the following events:

1. Ovulation
2. Fertility
3. Cervical and cervical mucus changes that affect receptivity to sperm
4. Tubal and uterine motility
5. Sloughing of endometrium (menstruation)
6. Onset of abortion, spontaneous and induced
7. Onset of labor, term and preterm

PGs may play a key role in ovulation. If PG levels do not rise along with the surge of LH, the ovum remains trapped within the graafian follicle. Following ovulation, PGs may influence production of estrogen and progesterone by the corpus luteum.

The introduction of PGs into the vagina or into the uterine cavity (from ejaculated semen) increases the motility of uterine musculature, which may assist the transport of sperm through the uterus and into the oviduct.

High concentrations of PGs in the semen (about 55 μg/ml) may be necessary for normal fertility (see p. 181) in males.

PGs produced by the woman cause regression (return to an earlier state) of the corpus luteum, regression of the endometrium, and sloughing of the endometrium that results in menstruation.

PGs increase myometrial response to oxytocic stimulation, enhance uterine contractions, and cause cervical dilation. They may be one factor in the initiation or maintenance of labor or both. In addition, prostaglandins may be involved in the following pathologic states: male infertility, dysmenorrhea, hypertensive states, preeclampsia-eclampsia, and anaphylactic shock. Further discussion of PGs relevant to abortion may be found on p. 991; for a discussion of PGs' role in pregnancy and childbirth, see Chapter 37.

After exerting their biologic actions, newly synthesized prostaglandins are rapidly metabolized by tissues in such organs as the lungs, kidneys, and liver.

PRIMARY DYSMENORRHEA

Primary dysmenorrhea (dys, painful; menorrhea, normal menstrual flow) is painful menstruation that occurs in the absence of pelvic pathologic findings. Anovulatory cycles are not accompanied by dysmenorrhea so that it does not occur during the 6 to 12 months following the onset of menarche.

Symptoms of primary dysmenorrhea (premenstrual tension plus uterine cramping and occasionally backache, dizziness, vomiting and diarrhea) are associated with a functioning corpus luteum. Spasmodic pain starts with the menstrual flow and lasts 1 to 3 days. Intense myometrial contractions lead to uterine ischemia (decreased blood flow) that results in pain. Pregnancy increases vascularity and blood flow to the uterus so that, following pregnancy, intense uterine contractions may no longer lead to ischemia.

PGs have been implicated in primary dysmenorrhea. Significantly elevated $PGF_{2\alpha}$ has been detected in the endometrium and menstrual fluid of women with primary dysmenorrhea. Dysmenorrhea can be produced by administration of $PGF_{2\alpha}$. The symptoms can be relieved by drugs that inhibit production of PGs. Although most of the nonsteroid antiprostaglandin drugs have been recognized for the treatment of primary dysmenorrhea, cautious short-term use of mefenamic acid (Ponstel), ibuprofen (Motrin), maproxen (Anaprox), or indomethacin (Indocin) in selected cases is reasonable, although the physician must accept the responsibility for prescribing these anti-inflammatory–analgesic drugs, as yet unapproved by the Food and Drug Administration. Drug therapy is started with the onset of menstrual flow and continued for 3 days.

Drugs that prevent ovulation, the conventional birth control pills, do not constitute specific therapy for dysmenorrhea, but they are effective for some women.

Finally, but of equal importance, is to provide the woman with reassurance and a listening ear. Personal attention, a caring atmosphere, and accurate information help to dispel insecurity and fear, which exaggerate the pain and interfere with therapy.

Physiologic Response to Sexual Stimulation

Anatomic and reproductive differences notwithstanding women and men are more alike than different in their physiologic response to sexual excitement and orgasm.* For example, the glans clitoris and the glans penis are homologues with the same number of nerve endings (see Fig. 6.1 and Table 6.1). This explains why the clitoris is so sensitive to sexual stimulation. Not only is there little difference between female and male sexual response, but also it is now accepted that the physical response is essentially the same whether the source of stimulation is coitus, fantasy, or mechanical or manual masturbation.

Currently there are two theories to explain the physiologic response to sexual stimulation. The first and most widely used theory is the four-phase response cycle described by Masters and Johnson. The second is Helen Kaplan's biphasic sexual response cycle.

FOUR-PHASE RESPONSE CYCLE

Physiologically, sexual response, according to Masters and Johnson (1966), can be analyzed in terms of two processes: vasocongestion and myotonia.

1. *Vasocongestion*. Sexual stimulation results in reflex dilation of penile blood vessels (erection) and circumvaginal blood vessels (lubrication), causing engorgement and distention of the genitalia. Venous congestion is localized primarily in the genitalia, but it also occurs to a lesser degree in the breasts and other parts of the body.
2. *Myotonia*. Arousal is characterized by increased muscular tension resulting in voluntary and involuntary rhythmic contractions. Examples of sexually stimulated myotonia are pelvic thrusting, facial grimacing, and spasms of the hands and feet (carpopedal spasms).

The response cycle is arbitrarily divided into four phases: excitement phase, plateau phase, orgasmic phase, and resolution phase. One moves through the four phases progressively, and there is no sharp dividing line between any two phases. However, there are specific bodily changes that take place in sequence. The time, intensity, and duration for cyclic completion also vary for individuals and situations.

The following descriptions and drawings of the female and male pelves show the major body changes during the four phases of the response cycle. (For a description of total body response, refer to Tables 6.10 and 6.11).

Excitement phase: women. The first observable reaction to sexual stimulation is vaginal lubrication, which has the biologic function of preparing the vagina for penile penetration. The inner two thirds of the vaginal barrel lengthens and distends. The cervix and fundus are pulled upward.

The external genitalia become congested and darker in color. The clitoris increases in diameter and in tumescence (vascular congestion and swelling) (Fig. 6.34).

Excitement phase: men. The first observable reaction to sexual stimulation is erection of the penis (increase in length and diameter). The scrotal skin becomes congested and thick. The testes elevate because of contraction of the cremasteric musculature (Fig. 6.35).

Plateau phase: women. The wall of the outer one third of the vagina becomes greatly engorged, along with the labia minora, forming the "orgasmic platform." The clitoris retracts under the clitoral hood to protect the clitoris from intense, direct stimulation (Fig. 6.36).

Plateau phase: men. Preorgasmic emission of two or three drops of mucoid substance is released from Cowper's glands. The testes continue to elevate until they are situated close to the body to facilitate ejaculatory pressure (Fig. 6.37).

Orgasmic phase: women. Strong, rhythmic (every 0.8 second), muscular contractions occur in the orgasmic platform (Fig. 6.38). The number of contractions ranges from 3 to 15. The uterus also contracts rhythmically.

This phase may be subjectively described as follows:

Stage 1: sensation of "suspension," followed by "intense sensual awareness, clitorally oriented and radiating upward into the pelvis"

Stage 2: "suffusion of warmth" especially in the pelvic area

Stage 3: "pelvic throbbing" located in the vaginal and lower pelvis

Orgasmic phase: men. Testes are held at maximal elevation (Fig. 6.39). Rhythmic contractions of the penis and rectal sphincter occur at 18-sec intervals.

This phase may be subjectively described as follows:

Stage 1: point of "inevitability," which occurs just before ejaculation and lasts 2 or 3 seconds; awareness of presence of fluid in the urethra

Stage 2: ejaculation with rhythmic contractions capable of expelling semen up to 60 cm (24 in)

Resolution phase: women. Blood returns from the engorged walls of vagina, and the labia majora and minora rapidly return to their unexcited state. The clitoris rapidly returns from under the hood; however, return to

Text continued on p. 100.

*See Chapter 7 for a discussion of the psychosocial components of human sexuality.

Table 6.10
Female Sexual Response Cycle*

	I. Excitement Phase (several minutes to hours)	II. Plateau Phase (30 sec to 3 min)	III. Orgasmic Phase (3-15 sec)	IV. Resolution Phase (10-15 min; if no orgasm, ½-1 day)
Skin	No change	Sexual flush inconstant except in fair-skinned; pink mottling on abdomen, spreads to breasts, neck, face, often to arms, thighs, and buttocks—looks like measles rash	No change (flush at its peak)	Fine perspiration, mostly on flush areas: flush disappears in reverse order
Breasts	Nipple erection in two thirds of subjects	Flush: mottling coalesces to form a red papillary rash	No change (venous tree pattern stands out sharply; breasts may become tremulous)	Return to normal in reverse order of appearance in ½ hr or more
	Venous congestion	Size: increase one fourth over normal, especially in breasts that have not been nursed		
	Areolar enlargement	Areolae: enlarge; impinge on nipples so they seem to disappear		
Clitoris	Glans: half of subjects, no change visible, but with colposcope, enlargement always observed; half of subjects, glans diameter always increased twofold or more	Retraction: shaft withdraws deep into swollen prepuce; just before orgasm, it is difficult to visualize; may relax and retract several times if phase II is unduly prolonged	No change (shaft movements continue throughout if thrusting maintained)	Shaft returns to normal position in 5-10 sec; full detumescence in 5-30 min (if no orgasm, clitoris remains engorged for several hours)
	Shaft: variable increase in diameter: elongation occurs in only 10% of subjects	Intrapreputial movement with thrusting; movements synchronized with thrusting due to traction on labia minora and prepuce		
Labia majora	Nullipara: thin down; elevated; flattened against perineum	Nullipara: totally disappear (may reswell if phase II unduly prolonged)	No change	Nullipara: *increase* to normal size in 1 or 2 min or less
	Multipara: rapid congestion and edema; increases to 2 or 3 times normal size	Multipara: become so enlarged and edematous, they "hang like folds of a heavy curtain"		Multipara: *decrease* to normal size in 10-15 min
Labia minora	Color change: to bright pink in nullipara and red in multipara	Color change: suddenly turn bright red in nullipara, burgundy red in multipara; signifies onset of phase II; orgasm will then always follow within 3 min if stimulation is continued	Firm proximal areas contract with contractions of lower third	Returns to pink, blotchy color in 2 min or less; total resolution of color and size in 5 min (decoloration, clitoral return, and detumescence of lower third all occur as rapidly as loss of erection in men)
	Size: increase 2 or 3 times over normal; prepuce often much more; proximal portion firms, adding up to 1.9 cm to functional vaginal sidewalls	Size: enlarged labia gap widely to form vestibular funnel into vaginal orifice		

Bartholin's glands	No change	A few drops of mucoid secretion form; aid in lubricating vestibule (insufficient to lubricate vagina)	No change	No change
Vagina	Vaginal transudate: appears 10-30 sec after onset of arousal; drops of clear fluid coalesce to form a well-lubricated vaginal barrel (aids in buffering acidity of vagina to neutral pH required by sperm)	Copious transudate continues to form; quantity of transudate generally increased only by prolonging preorgasm stimulation (increased flow occurs during premenstrual period)	No change (transudate provides maximal degree of lubrication)	Some transudate collects on floor of upper two thirds formed by its posterior wall (in supine position); ejaculate deposited in this area, forming seminal pool
	Color change: mucosa turns patchy purple	Color change; uniform dark purple mucosa		
Upper two thirds	Balloons; dilates convulsively as uterus moves up, pulling anterior vaginal wall with it; fornices lengthen; rugae flatten	Further ballooning creates diameter of 6.25-7.5 cm; then wall relaxes in slow, tensionless manner	No change; fully ballooned out and motionless	Cervical descent: descends to seminal pool in 3 or 4 min
Lower third	Dilation of vaginal lumen to 2.5-3.1 cm occurs; congestion of walls proceeds gradually, increasing in rate as phase II approaches	Maximum distention reached rapidly; contracts lumen of lower third and upper labia to half or more its diameter in phase I; contraction around penis allows thrusting traction on clitoral shaft via labia and prepuce	3-15 contractions of lower third and proximal labia minora at ¾-sec intervals	Congestion disappears in seconds (if no orgasm, congestion persists for 20-30 min)
Uterus	Ascent; moves into false pelvis late in phase I	Contractions: strong, sustained contractions begin late in phase II; have same rhythm as contractions late in labor, lasting 2 + min	Contractions throughout orgasm; strongest with pregnancy and masturbation	Descent: slowly returns to normal
	Cervix: passively elevated with uterus (no evidence of any cervical secretions during entire cycle)	Cervix: slight swelling; patchy purple (instant; related to chronic cervicitis)		Cervix: color and size return to normal in 4 min; patulous for 10 min
Others	Fourchet: color changes throughout cycle as in labia minora	Perineal body: spasmodic tightening with involuntary elevation of perineum Hyperventilation and carpopedal spasms: both are usually present, the latter less frequently and only in female-supine postion	Irregular spasms continue Rectum: rhythmic contractions inconstant; more apt to occur with masturbation than coitus External urethral sphincter; occasional contraction, no urine loss	All reactions cease abruptly or within a few seconds

*Adapted by permission of Random House, Inc., from *The Nature and Evolution of Female Sexuality*, by Mary Jane Sherfy. Copyright © 1966, 1972 by Mary Jane Sherfy.

Table 6.11
Male Sexual Response Cycle*

	I. Excitement Phase (several minutes to hours)	II. Plateau Phase (30 sec to 3 min)	III. Orgasmic Phase (3-15 sec)	IV. Resolution Phase (10-15 min; if no orgasm, ½-1 day)
Skin	No change	Sexual flush: inconsistently appears; maculopapular rash originates on abdomen and spreads to anterior chest wall, face and neck and can include shoulders and forearms	Well-developed flush	Flush disappears in reverse order of appearance; inconsistently appearing film of perspiration on soles of feet and palms of hands
Penis	Erection within (0-30 sec, caused by vasocongestion of erectile bodies of corpus cavernosa of shaft; loss of erection may occur with introduction of asexual stimulus, loud noise	Increase in size of glans and diameter of penile shaft; inconsistent deepening of coronal and glans coloration	Ejaculation: 3 or 4 contractions of vasa, seminal vesicles, prostate, and urethra at 0.8-sec intervals; followed by minor contractions with increasing intervals	Erection: partial involution in 5-10 sec with variable refractory period; full detumescence in 5-30 min
Scrotum and testes	Tightening and lifting of scrotal sac and partial elevation of testes toward perineum	50% increase in size of testes over unstimulated state due to vasocongestion and flattening of testes against perineum, signaling impending ejaculation	No change	Decrease to baseline size due to loss of vasocongestion; testicular and scrotal descent within 5-30 min after orgasm; involution may take several hours if there is no orgasmic release
Cowper's glands	No change	2 or 3 drops of mucoid fluid that contain viable sperm	No change	No change
Other	Breasts: inconsistent nipple erection	Myotonia: semispastic contractions of facial, abdominal, and intercostal muscles Tachycardia: up to 175 beats/min Blood pressure: rise in systolic, 20-80 mm Hg; in diastolic, 10-40 mm Hg Respiration: increased	Loss of voluntary muscular control Rectum: rhythmic contractions of sphincter Up to 180 beats/min 40-100 mm Hg systolic; 20-50 mm Hg diastolic Up to 40 respirations/min Ejaculatory spurt: 30-50 cm at age 18, decreasing with age to seepage at 70	Return to baseline state in 5-10 min

*Table prepared by Virginia A. Sadock, M.D., after Masters and Johnson data. From Sadock, B.J., Kaplan, H., and Freeman, A.: The sexual experience, Baltimore, 1976, The Williams & Wilkins Co.

Fig. 6.34
Excitement phase. (From Fogel, C.I., and Woods, N.F.: Health care of women: A nursing perspective, St. Louis, 1981, The C.V. Mosby Co.)

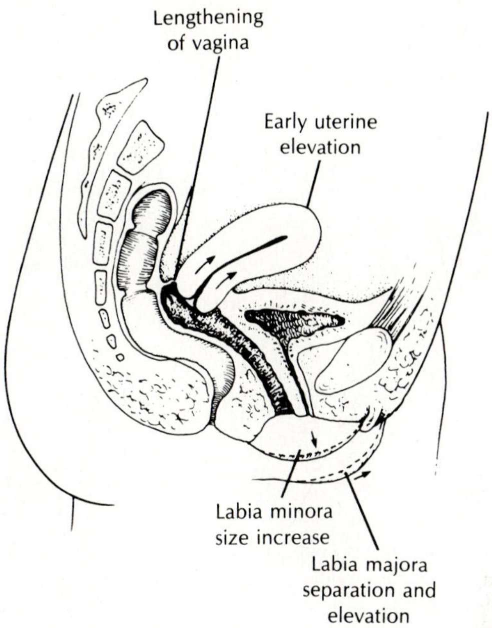

Fig. 6.35
Male pelvic organs during excitement phase. (From Masters, W.H., and Johnson, V.E.: Human sexual response, Boston, 1966, Little, Brown & Co.)

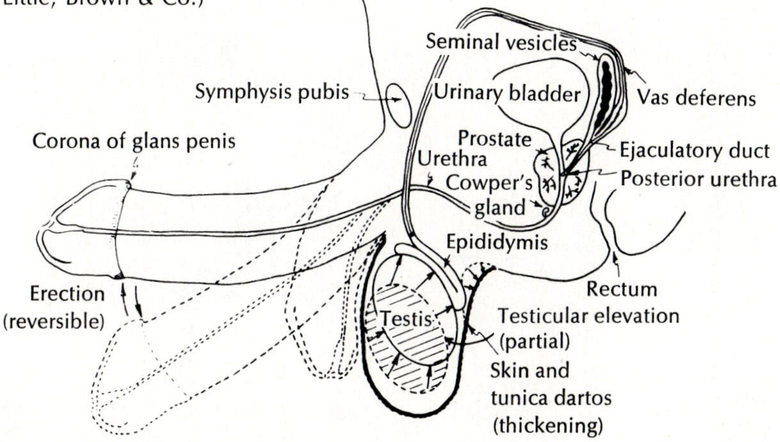

Fig. 6.36
Plateau phase. (From Fogel, C.I., and Woods, N.F.: Health care of women: a nursing perspective, St. Louis, 1981, The C.V. Mosby Co.)

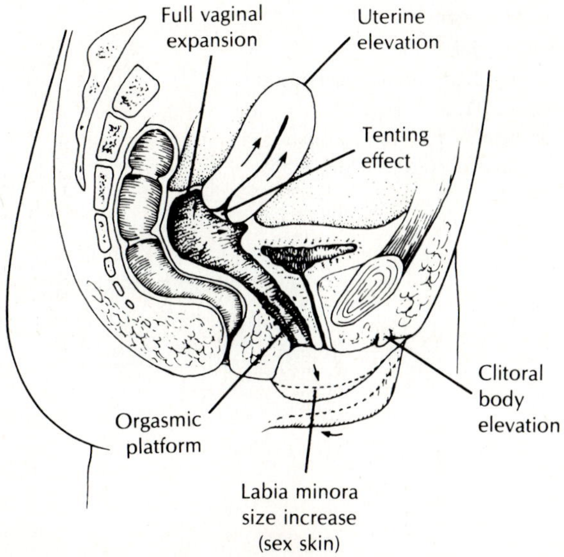

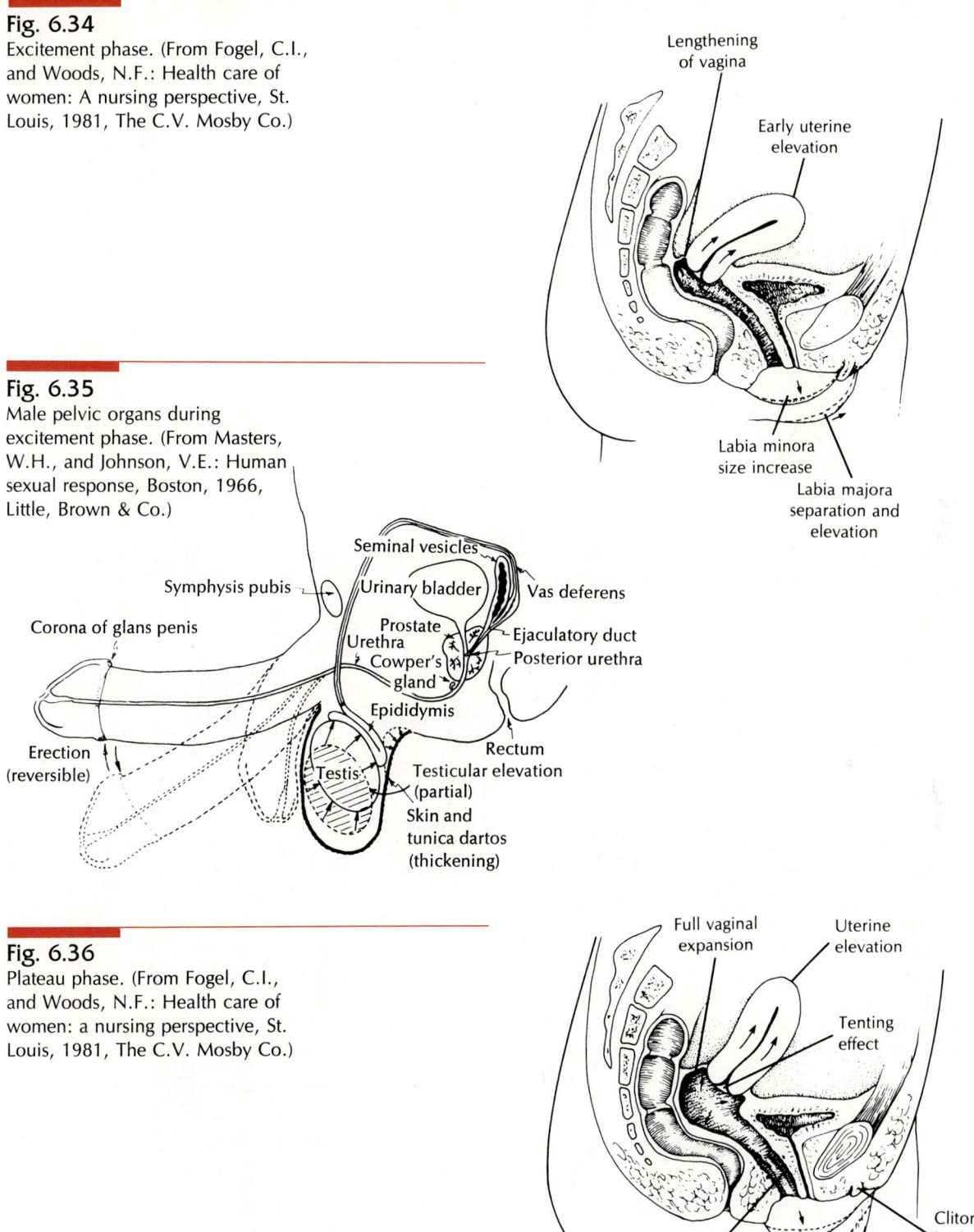

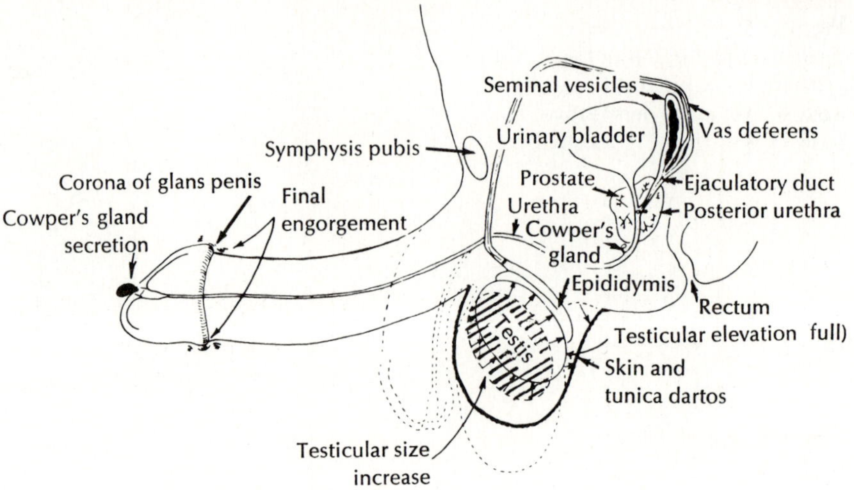

Fig. 6.37
Male pelvic organs during plateau phase. (From Masters, W.H., and Johnson, V.E.: Human sexual response, Boston, 1966, Little, Brown & Co.)

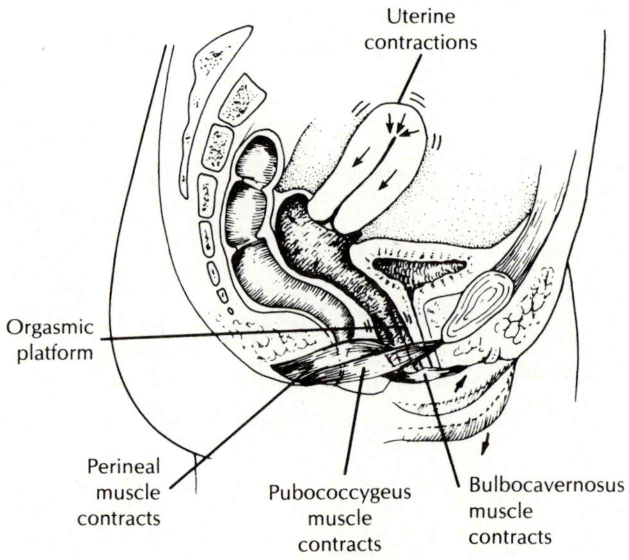

Fig. 6.38
Orgasm phase. (From Fogel, C.I., and Woods, N.F.: Health care of women: a nursing perspective, St. Louis, 1981, The C.V. Mosby Co.)

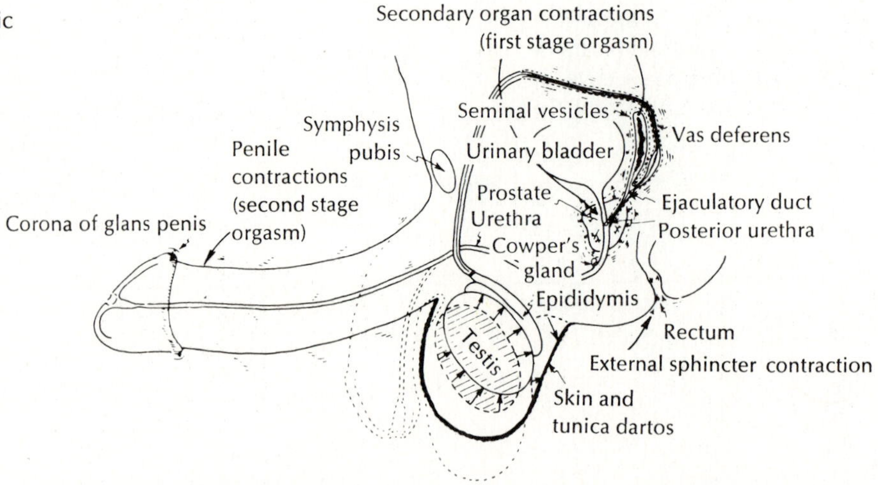

Fig. 6.39
Male pelvic organs during orgasmic phase. (From Masters, W.H., and Johnson, V.E.: Human sexual response, Boston, 1966, Little, Brown & Co.)

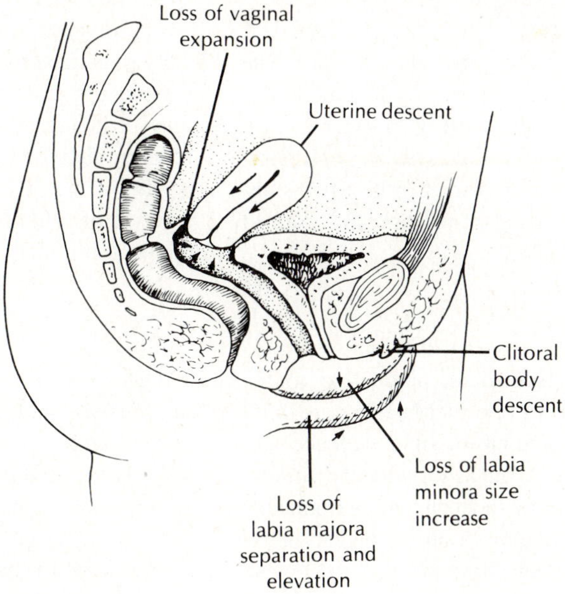

Fig. 6.40
Resolution phase. (From Fogel, C.I., and Woods, N.F.: Health care of women: a nursing perspective, St. Louis, 1981, The C.V. Mosby Co.)

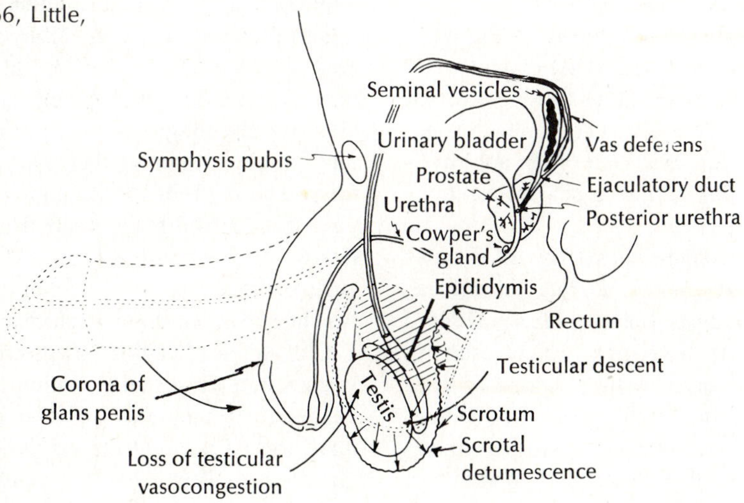

Fig. 6.41
Male pelvic organs during resolution phase. (From Masters, W.H., and Johnson, V.E.: Human sexual response, Boston, 1966, Little, Brown & Co.)

normal size may take longer. Uterus descends, and cervix dips into seminal pool (Fig. 6.40).

Resolution phase: men. In the first stage of the resolution phase 50% of erection is lost rather rapidly. The second stage can last much longer, depending on the maintenance of physical condition (Fig. 6.41).

The *refractory* period is the time necessary to complete the cycle again. The time varies from a few minutes to a few days, depending on the age and state of physical and emotional health.

BIPHASIC RESPONSE

Kaplan (1974) has presented an alternative to the four-phase sexual response cycle of Masters and Johnson. She believes clinical and physiologic evidence suggests that sexual response is biphasic, with the following two distinct and relatively independent components:

1. Genital vasocongestive reaction—produces vaginal lubrication and swelling in the female and penile erection in the male
2. Reflex clonic muscular contractions—constitute orgasm in both sexes

Phase 1: vasocongestive reaction. Erection in the male is local vasocongestive response. During erection the corpora cavernosa become engorged with blood. Special valves in the penile veins are closed by reflex action, preventing loss of blood. This mechanism is regulated by the parasympathetic division of the autonomic nervous system, which controls the diameter and valves of the penile blood vessels, thus causing erection or loss of erection. Once erection has occurred, excitement can be maintained for some time. Men are physically capable of losing and regaining several erections during love play.

Kaplan calls the vasocongestive reaction in females the ''lubrication-swelling'' phase. During this phase, dilation of the circumvaginal venous plexus causes a transudate on the walls of the vagina, which results in lubrication. The tissues become the ''orgasmic platform'' (analogous to erection in the male). In addition, the uterus becomes engorged and begins to rise slightly out of the pelvic cavity so that the cervix is placed in a position to increase the likelihood of fertilization.

Phase 2: reflex clonic muscular contractions. The visceral aspects of the ejaculatory reflex are under control of the sympathetic division of the autonomic nervous system, as opposed to the parasympathetic division that is involved with erection. Male orgasm has two phases: emission and ejaculation. Emission comprises contractions of the vasa deferentia, the prostate, the seminal vesicles, and the internal part of the urethra. Masters and Johnson (1966) have called the subjective response to emission ''ejaculatory inevitability.'' Ejaculation is the external mechanism that causes spurts of semen to be forced outward from the penis.

The biphasic nature of the response cycle is dramatically explained by the impact of aging on the refractory period. For example, a man's frequency of ejaculation may be reduced, but his ability to have erections may remain relatively the same.

The woman, like the man, has orgasm consisting of a series of reflex, involuntary rhythmic contractions of the orgasmic platform.

CLINICAL SIGNIFICANCE

There are four important findings from the research of Masters and Johnson that have significance for nurses working with pregnant women and their families. These findings concern (1) multiple orgasm, (2) simultaneous orgasm, (3) clitoral vs. vaginal orgasm, and (4) variations in orgasmic patterns.

Multiple orgasm. Since women never physically have a refractory period, they are capable of having one orgasm after another until exhausted. Multiple orgasms are most frequently reported by women in their late thirties and early forties. Some women have also reported being multiply orgasmic for the first time during the second trimester of pregnancy. The reason is that because of the increased vasocongestion of pregnancy, total completion of the resolution phase never occurs.

Simultaneous orgasm. Many couples have considered simultaneous orgasm the ultimate goal of sexual bliss. The findings of Masters and Johnson and of others show the illogic of such goals, because many couples progress through the response cycle at different rates. The myth of the desirability of simultaneous orgasm has harmed many relationships because of the dificulty of achieving this goal. Although possible, simultaneous orgasm is the exception rather than the rule and is achieved when the woman reaches orgasm easily.

Clitoral vs. vaginal orgasm. Freud taught that women transfer sexual sensation from the clitoris to the vagina when they reach psychosexual maturity. A clitoral orgasm was considered therefore to be an immature orgasm. This belief existed until Masters and Johnson demonstrated that an orgasm is a total body response to sexual stimulation, with the most intense response located in the pelvic area. The response is essentially the same regardless of whether it is experienced through coitus, masturbation, or mechanical stimulation. The clitoris is defined as the ''transmitter and conductor'' of erotic sensation. Hite (1976) reported that 30% of the women in her sample of 3000 were orgasmic during intercourse without additional clitoral stimulation.

Variations in orgasmic patterns. There are many

response patterns for both women and men. These patterns vary in both intensity and duration.

SUMMARY

Knowledge of the normal sexual response cycle provides the foundation for sexual counseling during pregnancy and the postdelivery period. The four phases described by Masters and Johnson show that sexual response, from the excitement phase through the resolution phase, is a continuous process and can be altered by such conditions as pregnancy. Kaplan's biphasic framework is useful for planning interventions or making referrals to a sex therapist because of the distinct nature of the biphasic framework.

References and Readings

Anthony, C.P., and Thibodeau, G.A.: Textbook of anatomy and physiology, ed. 10, St. Louis, 1979, The C.V. Mosby Co.

Benson, R.: Handbook of obstetrics and gynecology, ed. 6, Los Altos, Calif., 1977, Lange Medical Publications.

Brenner, W.E.: The place of prostaglandins in modern obstetrics. In Aladjem, S., editor: Risks in the practice of modern obstetrics, ed. 2, St. Louis, 1975, The C.V. Mosby Co.

Frisch, R.E.: A method of prediction of age of menarche from height and weight at ages 9 through 13 years, Pediatrics **5**:384, 1974.

Hellman, L.M., and Pritchard, J.A.: Williams' obstetrics, ed. 15, New York, 1976, Appleton-Century-Crofts.

Hite, S.: The Hite report: a nationwide study on female sexuality, New York, 1976, Macmillian Publishing Co.

Kaplan, H.S.: The new sex therapy, New York, 1974, Brunner Mazel.

Lowrey, G.: Growth and development of children, ed. 4, Chicago, 1978, Year Book Medical Publisher.

Masters, W.H., and Johnson, V.E.: Human sexual response, Boston, 1966, Little, Brown and Co.

Page, E.W., Villee, C.A., and Villee, D.B.: Human reproduction: essentials of reproductive and perinatal medicine, ed. 3, Philadelphia, 1981, W.B. Saunders Co.

Sadock, B.J., Kaplan, H.I., and Freedman, M.: The sexual experience, Baltimore, 1976, The Williams & Wilkins Co.

Sherfey, M.J.: The nature and evolution of female sexuality, New York, 1972, Random House.

7

Psychosocial Aspects of Reproduction

- Childhood
  - Gender identity
  - Gender preference
  - Identification with parent of same sex
  - Sex role standards
  - Clinical considerations
- Adolescence
  - Early adolescence (ages 12 to 15 years)
  - Middle adolescence (ages 15 to 18 years)
  - Late adolescence (ages 18 to 20 years)
  - Clinical considerations
- Adult Sexuality
  - Young adulthood
  - Middle and late adulthood
  - Clinical considerations

Sexual identity begins at conception. At that time, through the chance combination of an ovum and a sperm, a person's biologic sex is determined. Thereafter, intrauterine and extrauterine environmental influences play their part in the realization of each human's sexual potential.

This potential pervades the whole of a person's life; it is more than a sum of isolated physical acts. It functions as a purposeful force in human nature and is observable in everyday life in endless variations. It may find expression in the love of parent for child and child for parent, of friend for friend, or of woman for man and man for woman. It can be the source of pleasure or pain, fulfillment or deprivation, and sharing or exploitation. Recognition of the power of such drives has prompted each culture throughout history to develop social codes, religious dogmas, or legal restraints that delineate the sex role models and patterns to follow in the process of achieving adult sexuality.

Childhood

We are born into a sexually oriented world and from birth onward assume socially defined sexual roles. The roles reflect the basic pattern prescribed by the society and are learned informally as a result of being part of a social group. The process of sexual identity begins at an early age and continues as a series of developmental tasks throughout the person's life span. Newman and Newman (1975) described four of the essential tasks to be accomplished in childhood as follows:

Dimension	Sex-role Outcome
Learning the gender label	I am a "boy" I am a "girl"
Establishing the sex preference	I like being a boy; I'd rather be a boy than a girl I like being a girl; I'd rather be a girl than a boy
Identifying with the same sex parent	I want to be like "Daddy" I want to be like "Mommy"
Acquiring the sex role standards	Males are "independent," "achievement oriented," "assertive" Females are "interpersonal," "nurturant," "docile"*

In addition, Newman and Newman (1975) state:

> The outcome of the process for an individual child depends greatly on the characteristics of his parents, the child's own capacities and preferences, and the cultural and familial values placed on one gender or the other. It should be obvious that a strong, positive identification with the appropriate sex, regardless of the specific standards associated with that sex, is essential for the development of self-esteem and for the elaboration of peer group relationships.*

*From Newman, B., and Newman, R.: Development through life: a psychosocial approach, Homewood, Ill., 1975, Dorsey Press, p. 111.

GENDER IDENTITY

Efforts to determine the emphasis to be placed on biologic rather than environmental contributions to one's gender identity have generated much controversy and research. Although some studies indicate that there are certain different biologic responses in male and female newborns and suggest differences in the infants' responses to the environment and readiness for various learning experiences, other studies reveal the importance of gender labeling on the eventual acceptance of gender identity. Infants whose sex was uncertain at birth accepted the sex role assigned by their parents and identified with that role (Maccoby, 1966). From the child's perspective, knowing oneself as either a boy or a girl begins before full realization of the implications of sexual identity. It is largely accomplished by acceptance of parental labeling, for example, "Be a good boy," "That's my girl," and "This is our big boy." By 2 or 3 years of age a child can correctly identify his or her own sex.

GENDER PREFERENCE

Gender preference implies not only a knowledge of one's gender and the appropriate sex role but also a liking for it. The process of developing gender preference involves three main elements: (1) success in the role, (2) liking the same-sex parent, and (3) reinforcement from family, ethnic group, and social institutions as to the value of the role (Newman and Newman, 1975). As with other attitudes, fluctuations in preference can and do occur as persons are confronted with situations in which one sex role either enhances or hinders personal goals. Deep-seated sex preferences on the part of parents can affect initial parent-child relationships if the child is of the undesired sex. The parenting lag that results can last a day or a lifetime as the parents act to resolve or not resolve the conflicting emotions. Certain ethnic groups have welcoming rituals for one sex and not for the other. These seemingly innocuous societal and personal preferences eventually lead a person to make value judgments about the worthiness of his or her own sex and consequently increase or diminish self-esteem.

IDENTIFICATION WITH PARENT OF SAME SEX

Identification with the parent of the same sex results in the child's internalization of the values, attitudes, and ideals of the parent of the same sex. The exact method by which the process of identification is accomplished is not yet known. However, the child does perceive actual physical and psychologic similarities and is told about similarities by others. The adoption of the same-sex parent's behaviors may be motivated by fear of loss of the love of the important person or by awareness of that person's power to control rewards, such as in a situation in which the parent's expectations of the child's sex role behaviors are not fulfilled. Behaviors of influential persons may also be imitated and eventually taken over and considered one's own. For a girl to forego identification with her father, she must love her mother sufficiently to form a positive identification with her. A boy needs to relinquish his early identification with his mother and form a strong commitment to his father.

SEX ROLE STANDARDS

Sex role standards refer to the various behaviors, attitudes, and attributes that differentiate the roles. Even the 2 year-old child is exposed to this conditioning by means of the clothing, kinds of toys, and activities selected by parents, which reflect their expectations of sex role standards.

Much is learned by observing the behaviors of mothers, fathers, and siblings. The child formulates a concept of who should perform what tasks, who provides the comforting, who provides the active play, and who takes care when there is sickness.

In our society adjectives used to describe a female predominantly express a mothering capacity, that is, "gentle, loving, submissive, patient, warm, and concerned." These qualities suit a person whose central reason for being is assumed to be the care and nurturing of the young and, by extension, any persons who need such care. Those adjectives used to describe the male, namely, "dominant, aggressive, impatient, objective, and ambitious," portray a person capable of independent, decisive actions with qualities needed in the marketplace and the basis for career orientation.

In reality, persons of both sexes possess these qualities in common, some personalities leaning more to the socially defined concept of either male or female and others having no clear demarcation of roles. These latter persons, termed *androgynous personalities*, utilize those qualities most needed at the moment without feeling guilty over usurping another's role. A male nursing student made the following comment during a discussion of mothering:

> It is not a case of one or the other, it is what the time calls forth. The most nurturing behavior of "mothering," if you want to call it that, that I've ever seen was in Vietnam when a man was trying to get a wounded friend out of range of fire. He protected him, covering him with his own body, gave him his food and water. No "mother" could have shown more devotion.

Table 7.1
Childhood Sexual Development*

Age	Behavior	Function
Infancy (birth to 18 mo)	Oral exploration, sucking, mouthing; explores own body	Erotic attachments and pleasures achieved from self-stimulation are forerunners of future development
	Quality and quantity of touch by caretaker; color of clothes, blankets, room; style of clothes	Beginning of formation of core gender identity
	Mothers look at and talk to girls more than boys and respond to girls' irritability more quickly; boys are touched, held, rocked, and kissed more as infants	Parental acceptance of general societal roles for males and females
	Boys: erections in first few days of life; girls: vaginal lubrication	Reflex response, not yet eroticized
Early childhood (18 mo to 3 yr)	Act of releasing contents of bowel and bladder is source of enjoyment	Learns to associate genitalia with privacy, and cleanliness or dirt
	Phallic exhibitionistic period (discovers genitalia and finds they can bring pleasure)	Beginning of lifelong association between sexual feelings and genitalia
	Sporadic investigation of playmate's genitalia; sex play probably more homosexual than heterosexual	Knowledge seeking; experimental, imitative, exploratory play, precursor to future sociosexual encounters
Middle childhood (3-5 yr)	Observes relationship between parents (kiss, hug, talk to each other)	Works through beginning relationships with parent of opposite sex; much of warmth the child experiences from close relationships with parents is later transferred to relationships with persons of opposite sex
	Self-exploration and self-manipulation	Learns erotic potential
Late childhood (5-11 yr)	Transition from home environment to school	Develops meaningful relationships with peers of same sex; solidifies sexual identity with homosocial relationships
	Begins to read; watches movies and television	Latent erotic inquiry develops; moral categories are learned
	Learns "dirty" words	Cognitive and affective meanings of words and symbols are not understood and possibly may be distorted by child
	May be labeled as "tomboy" or "sissy"	Early gender distinction; learns early that male role is more important than female role

*Adapted by Marianne Zalar from Sadock, B.J., Kaplan, H.D., and Freedman, A.M.: The sexual experience, Baltimore, 1976, The Williams & Wilkins Co.

By the time puberty occurs the person has completed most of the developmental tasks of early childhood. Acceptance of childhood sexual identity will have consequences for self-esteem, peer relations, and selection of skills and interest. The concomitant development of moral standards such as honesty and fidelity results in a linkage between sexual identity (role) and moral commitments. Feelings of self-acceptance or guilt can be generated by either upholding or violating standards in these spheres.

Table 7.1 describes the sex-related behaviors of infancy, early childhood, and late childhood. In addition, the function for each behavior is given. As the reader will see from this table and the following two tables, human sexuality is a developmental process throughout the life cycle.

CLINICAL CONSIDERATIONS

The exploratory sexual behaviors of children provide the foundation for adult sexuality. The feelings children develop about themselves as persons in general and as sexual persons in particular are directly related to their own experiences with their bodies and the attitudes and values they derive from many sources. For example, McNab (1976) found a strong correlation between scores of parents and children on a sex attitude test.

Sex play is one of the most important ways children learn about their bodies. Sex play is defined by Kinsey and co-workers (1948, 1953) as "actual genital play." Four categories of sex play are listed as follows:

1. Same-sex comparisons: comparison of size and shape. It is important to stress that prepubescent homosexual behaviors do not necessarily lead to

adult homosexuality. Example: "Let me see yours and I'll let you see mine."

2. Coital play: when a boy lies on top of a girl. The activities are largely experimental, imitative, and exploratory. Example: Momma and Papa.
3. Self-exploration and self-manipulation: most common forms of sex play. Fondling of the penis and manual stimulation of the clitoris are most common. Example: playing with oneself.
4. Exhibitionism: showing and handling genitalia in public, especially in the presence of companions.

Most children engage in sex play activities only sporadically, especially when these activities are ignored by adults. For example, one out of four boys who had engaged in sex play had done so only during 1 year, and some had participated in such play only once before puberty (Kinsey and co-workers, 1948). Kinsey and co-workers (1948, 1953) found that 9 years of age was the peak age for girls, when 14% engaged in some form of sex play. For boys the peak was 12 years of age, when 39% were similarly involved.

Nurses and parents must be careful not to ascribe adult motives to the sexual behaviors of children. Katchadourian and Lunde (1972) stated: "It is particularly important not to label the sex play of children as deviant or perverse, no matter what it entails. To do so would be like calling a child who believes in ghosts and fairies delusional or mentally ill."

Kolodny and co-workers (1979) cautioned nurses that contradictory messages about one's body (parental encouragement to be aware of one's body but to exclude the genitalia from awareness) are among the earliest recognizable common determinants of adult sexual problems. For example, parents tell their children to "wash behind their ears" and then remind them to "wash down there." Parents and many health professionals respond to their own insecurities about sex when confronted by the overt but innocent sexuality of children.

A knowledgeable maternity nurse has many opportunities to help young parents provide age-appropriate sex education. For example, the nurse can help an anxious pregnant mother role play telling her 4-year-old child about where babies come from.

Adolescence

It is not until adolescence that the socially and parentally defined sex role is openly questioned. In recent years changes in the conceptualization of what constitutes male and female roles have had great impact on teenagers as they grope for standards consonant with their peer group's attitudes and parental expectations.

Adolescence, the transitional period between childhood and adulthood, is considered to begin with puberty. However, the onset of puberty varies in timing for each person, and the clue that puberty has begun may lie in any number of behaviors. Sometimes it is a sudden growth spurt and clumsiness that heralds the beginning of change. At other times moodiness, tearfulness, or withdrawal is suddenly noticeable in a previously serene youngster. For example, one mother related, "My daughter (aged 12) asked my where I had put her baby teeth. When I replied that I had thrown them away, she burst into tears and cried that I didn't think much of her to throw away something so precious." (See also Chapters 7 and 38 for discussions of adolescence.)

Menstruation can be the first indication of puberty, as one woman reported:

> The three of us had a routine we followed whenever our mother was away from the house. We trooped into the living room and marched over the tops of the sofa and chairs and piano. Then we rushed outside to walk astraddle the high fence separating us from the neighbors. One Sunday I slipped on the fence and hurt myself. I noticed I was bleeding, but because what I was doing was forbidden, I didn't say anything to my mother but put my panty in the laundry. On Monday night, Mother asked me about it. I told her about falling on the fence. After she examined me for injuries she said, "You are not hurt, I think you have started to menstruate." I remember being amazed that I hadn't thought of it. My sister (1 year older) was furious that she hadn't started before I did and wouldn't speak to me for a week. I waited eagerly for the next month and proof. Looking back, it seems such a childish way to start being a woman.

Erikson (1959) has described this stage of development as one with the major task of achieving identity rather than one characterized by identity confusion. It is now recognized that rather than being a single stage the process proceeds in sequential fashion through three phases. These phases—early, middle, and late adolescence—place a characteristic stamp on the manner of accomplishing the developmental tasks. These tasks may be defined as follows (adapted from Havighurst, 1972):

1. *Achieving new and more mature relations with age mates of both sexes*. A satisfactory social adjustment is achieved through social activities and experimentation with the peer group. Here adolescents learn to behave as adults as they create, on a small scale, the society of their elders. The influence of the peer group increasingly takes precedence over that of the family.
2. *Achieving a masculine or feminine social role*. Although sex is biologically determined, the mas-

culine and feminine roles are culturally established behavior sets that must be learned.

3. *Accepting one's physique and using one's body effectively*. The body image is well established by about 15 years of age. The adolescent must cope with normal but rapid changes in physical appearance and concomitant alterations in functional capacity. Deviations from the "norm" are a source of stress and may or may not be incorporated into the adolescent's body image.

4. *Achieving emotional independence of parents and other adults*. The movement away from depen-

Table 7.2
Adolescent Sexual Development*

Age	Behavior	Function
Early adolescence (12-15 yr)	Talking; being given greater autonomy and less direct adult supervision	Enlargement of the testing of superego formation
	Greater involvement in and importance of peer groups, especially same sex (homosocial peer involvement); social recognition of sexual interest even if premature in terms of biologic development	Reflects commitment to anticipated roles
	Masturbation, necking, petting, and especially heterosexual intercourse	Frequently generates feelings of anxiety and guilt
	Boys	Directly linked to sexual pleasure
	Capacity to ejaculate; first orgasm within 2 years of puberty for all but a few boys	
	Pattern of masturbation initiated	Leads to independent commitment to sexuality (i.e., capacity to engage in sexual activity without social or emotional attachments); exploring of biologic capacities
	Active fantasy life	Helps reinforce commitments to heterosexual behavior
	Girls	
	Menstruation	Serves as direct reminder that intercourse can result in pregnancy
	Masturbation to orgasm rare at this age	
	Homosocial peer involvement	Reflects a commitment to anticipated roles as girlfriend, wife, and mother
Middle adolescence (15-18 yr)	Rating and dating system becomes central aspect of adolescent society	Heterosociality becomes fairly normative in terms of both adult and youth culture expectations
	Masturbation, especially for boys, is an important sexual outlet	Represents way station in transition from infantile to adult sexuality and from narcissism to object relatedness
	Sociosexual activity colored by homosocial attachments (activity involves sharing stories about scoring, going steady, etc.)	Role confirmation
	Petting, genital involvement without coitus; when there is coital involvement, relationships are usually not serious and do not generate numerous repetitions	Associated with involvement in peer social life (i.e., general popularity, frequency of dating, number of partners dated)
Late adolescence (18-20 yr)	Premarital intercourse virtually normative	Period of maximal interpersonal and intrapsychic sexual self-consciousness
	Beginning of superficial problems of sexual competence (i.e., secondary impotence, premature ejaculation, penis size, failure to achieve orgasm)	One's sexual status is a matter of public concern
	Unresolved problems of relating erotic to sentimental (residual of good girl vs. bad girl syndrome, masturbation)	
	Girl's anxieties about unintended pregnancy and concern for effect on her reputation if relationship does not culminate in marriage	

*Adapted by Marianne Zalar from Sadock, B.J., Kaplan, H.D., and Freedman, A.M.: The sexual experience, Baltimore, 1976, The Williams & Wilkins Co.

dence on parents that was begun during the school years is completed in this period of development. Successful accomplishment results in affection and respect for one's parents without a childish dependence on them.

5. *Establishing a life-style that is personally and socially satisfying.* This includes the choice of a career, as well as contemplation of sexual relationships, marriage, family interdependence, and parenthood.
6. *Acquiring a set of values and an ethical system as a guide to socially responsible behavior.* This includes assuming responsibility for one's behavior and recognizing the effect one's behavior may have on another's welfare.

Table 7.2 outlines the sexual behaviors and sexual functions of early, middle, and late adolescence.

EARLY ADOLESCENCE (AGES 12 TO 15 YEARS)

In terms of cognitive powers early adolescent thought represents a mixture of two stages, the concrete operational stage and the beginning of the formal operational stage. Although there is a greater capacity for logical reasoning, it is still based largely on concrete evidence rather than on abstract thought. Some adolescents never reach the final level of cognition (the ability to deal with abstractions), whereas others move smoothly through the intervening period. As a result of this mixed ability, young adolescents tend to view the world about them only in relation to the effect it has on *them.* As their capacity for abstract thought increases, they become intensely interested in themselves, their thoughts, ideas, and fantasies, and what effect they are having on others. As a result they are introspective, self-conscious, and easily hurt by imagined or real slights. Their feeling that everyone is looking critically at them results in a demand for privacy. The slamming of the bedroom door, the "NO ADMITTANCE" signs put on retreats, and the long periods of self-enforced isolation from the family are typical of this phase.

An increase in height and the appearance of secondary sex characteristics cause adolescents to spend much time thinking about their bodies and comparing their physiques with those of others. Girls are interested in their developing breasts and often want to wear brassieres before they are needed. They tend to idealize body structure and feel depressed when their skin, hair, and legs do not compare favorably with the "ideal."

This is the time of intense relationships with members of one's sex, and these relationships are used primarily for support and mutual understanding. Young adolescents have endless face-to-face and telephone conversations with each other about hypothetical activities; for example, "If Peter speaks to me, I will say . . . ." By doing so they weigh alternatives, assess risks, evaluate results, and in fact practice the problem-solving approach.

Parents are still in control, and the young adolescent is aware of his vulnerability and need for dependence. However, parents and siblings notice a beginning of the critical appraisal to which they will be increasingly subjected. The adolescent becomes aware of the status of the family in the community and is anxious that his family measure up to certain standards.

Vocational choice is not a source of conflict. The young adolescent's choice is often unrealistic or idealistic. Young adolescents fantasize about what they are able to do, and although their increasing cognitive powers make them accept this as daydreaming, they are defensive about their abilities. They do like to work for money and often take newspaper routes or act as babysitters.

MIDDLE ADOLESCENCE (AGES 15 TO 18 YEARS)

Middle adolescence marks the time when adolescents vacillate between acting as responsible adults and acting as dependent children. Their ability to step into the adult role, even if briefly, increases their resentment about being considered children. They are very critical of parents, and the parents' appearance, behavior, dress, and social manners are all subjected to intense scrutiny and disparagement. Siblings are considered a nuisance, and the adolescent sees himself as being treated unfairly in terms of other members of the family. An adult outside the family group, for example, a nurse, a physician, a coach, or a school counselor, may be taken as a role model.

There is a definite movement away from the family and increased participation in the adult world—middle adolescents become advocates of various ideologies and enjoy debating the merits of current ideas. Many show evidence of potential leadership as they engage in developing their cognitive skills. Rebellion is usually couched in verbal terms rather than physical ones and is more destructive than constructive. Running away is a common phenomenon for adolescents between the ages of 15 and 18 years as an attempt to solve problems and to prove they are not children.

Almost all adolescents have reached their growth peak by mid adolescence. Many aspects of the body have attained a semblance of what they will be. For example, in boys the development of the lower jaws alters the contour of the face from the round, childish one to that of the adult. There is a general acceptance of their bodies on the part of both boys and girls, although this acceptance is tempered with a desire to look otherwise. As a result, the interest in their bodies is expressed in efforts to improve themselves. Grooming, makeup, and the right clothes become incredibly important. Stabilizing the body image is very important in developing a sense of identity. Adolescents of this age can now remember that they looked the same a year ago.

Peer relationships now dominate over family ones, and there is a change from relationships with members of the same sex to heterosexual relationships. Most conflicts with parents reflect this change, and communication patterns that were once open may become closed.

Role experimentation becomes a central process. Vocational choice is related to the middle adolescents' concern about obtaining the life-style they desire. The settled occupations of their parents and parents' friends may be seen as too confining and limiting to their activities. They want to engage in something new, different, and monetarily rewarding.

LATE ADOLESCENCE (AGES 18 TO 20 YEARS)

The cognitive development of boys and girls in late adolescence reflects the decentering of thought and production of a life plan, as described by Elkind (1968) and Piaget (1950). This occurs as the adolescent boy or girl moves from being an idealistic reformer to an achiever. Adolescents finally realize that criticism alone will not bring about changes and that ideals must be linked to a commitment and work. They become self-supporting or begin their professional education.

Most late adolescents have achieved a stable body image, and the agonizing over this or that real or fancied disability is largely over. Their relationships are still peer centered, but they realize that with the changes in locale necessitated by job or education these early friendships may end and be replaced by others.

Late adolescents are more tolerant of their families, in part perhaps because they sense the ending of the intense dependency relationship. If, on the whole, parents have permitted growth through role experimentation and through support of the need for increasng independence, the conflicts of parent and child seem to fade. On the other hand, the now self-supporting person may feel totally alienated and break all family ties.

The choice of career pattern is reasonably set. Whatever it may be, it will establish the adult life-style. Although young women are now assuming the right to choose careers rather than early marriage, the majority still suspend the final shaping of a career until after commitments to parenthood are fulfilled.

CLINICAL CONSIDERATIONS

Adolescence is a period of rapid change. In addition to other physical, social, and emotional changes that reflect the developmental tasks of adolescence, heightened sexual awareness becomes a salient issue. This heightened sexual awareness brings to the surface myths about masturbation, concerns about possible homosexuality, and concerns about the presence, frequency, and content of sexual fantasies and dreams.

Adolescents are surrounded by mixed messages. Parents, religious groups, teachers, health professionals, and others tell them to refrain from sexual contact, to control sexual impulses, and to keep away from temptation, although many of these same adults are asking the adolescents to refrain from activities they themselves openly practice. At the same time books, movies, music, and advertisements are laden with sexually stimulating messages.

Questions about whether and when to be sexually active and whether one needs to have sex to be popular, confusion about love and how one expresses love, and concerns about sexual adequacy become a major part of the lives of adolescents. Pajama parties and locker room discussions are often the only outlet the adolescent has to discuss some of these concerns and to obtain information and a great deal of misinformation about sex.

Adolescents are hesitant to talk to adults, especially parents, because the adult often discounts or invalidates their feelings. For example, when the adolescent talks about being in love the adult often responds with a condescending smile, a pat on the shoulder, and an expression such as, "My dear, what do you know about love at your young age?" Some parents are threatened by their adolescent's budding sexuality. They deal with their own uncertainty about sex by ignoring the reality of adolescent sexuality or by becoming hostile and punishing.

Sexual fantasies and dreams can be frightening for the young adolescent. A dream about being petted by one's handsome mathematics teacher or a fantasy about fondling the breasts of the prettiest girl in the class can result in feelings of guilt and shame. Fantasies about members of one's own sex can be even more frightening, especially if the adolescent has not begun dating. Memories of early same-sex explorations compound the adolescent's fear of becoming homosexual. At the same time it is important to note that some adult homosexuals report awareness of their homosexuality as early as adolescence. It is important for nurses working with adolescents to be aware of this aspect of adolescent life and to reassure the adolescent that he does not have to act on the fantasy or dream.

Masturbatory activity increases during adolescence. Kinsey and co-workers (1948, 1953) reported that by the age of 15 years, 82% of boys and 20% of girls had masturbated to orgasm. Although masturbation is now considered a normal release of sexual tension and a mechanism for learning about one's own sexuality, there are still many myths that masturbation causes acne, insanity, and a host of other mental and physical afflictions. When counseling the adolescent about masturbation, the nurse must refrain from making moral judgments but at the same time must recognize and respect religious and cultural attitudes regarding masturbation.

Not all adolescents are sexually active; however, the number having intercourse is increasing. In 1972 Kantner and Zelnik reported that 14% of girls had had coitus by 15 years of age, 21% by 16, 27% by 17, 37% by 18, and 46% by 19. In 1977 Zelnik and Kantner found the prevalence of sexual experience among adolescent girls had increased by 30% above their previous survey performed 5 years earlier. By 19 years of age, 55% of unmarried adolescent girls had experienced sexual intercourse. By 1978 the number of sexually active 19-year-olds had increased to 70% according to statistics from the Alan Guttmacher Institute.

An increased incidence of adolescent pregnancy and the increased number of adolescents with sexually transmitted diseases make sex education and sex counseling a major task for nurses working with adolescents. Adolescents need to know that their sexual feelings are normal and that they do not have to act on these feelings. They need to have accurate information about masturbation, contraception, pregnancy, venereal disease, and their bodies in order to become sexually responsible adults.

Health professionals need to be knowledgeable and comfortable with their own sexuality to work effectively with adolescents. Glossing over important issues and making broad generalizations about sexual concerns can be more confusing than helpful.

Adult Sexuality

Prior to the twentieth century, sex was seen as negative and sinful but necessary for procreation. Marriage was seen as the prerequisite to sexual relations. Reliable contraceptives were not available; therefore sexually active women were very vulnerable to becoming pregnant during the childbearing years.

The double standard was functionally necessary. Sexually active single women became pregnant and had unwanted babies that were a financial burden to society. Women therefore were given the responsibility to control sexual interactions. Men, on the other hand, were encouraged to express their sexuality freely. Men "sowed their wild oats" and women "saved themselves for marriage." These ideals, although functional for population control, were a burden for both men and women. Women were expected to be asexual until marriage and then learn about their sexuality from their husbands. Men were expected to be responsible not only for their own sexuality but for the sexuality of their wives as well. It is not surprising, therefore, that sexual dissatisfaction and a host of sexual dysfunctional problems resulted from relationships based on the double standard.

The change in attitudes toward sex that occurred between 1915 and 1965 laid the foundation for changes in sexual behavior that followed. By the mid-1970s candor replaced guilt and pretense. Hypocrisy and guilt about sex, sexual feelings, and sexual behavior were waning, but confusion and contradictions remained.

Some scholars do not concur that a sexual revolution is underway. One authority says that some Americans are going in a more permissive direction that does not represent a sudden change but rather a broadening of our concepts of masculinity and femininity. Old codes are relaxing, allowing people more freedom to choose their own patterns of behavior. Contraception separating coitus from childbearing leaves both sexes free of the question of parenthood in their sexual expression.

As one result of the change in sexual expression, the incidence of sexually transmitted diseases rose rapidly. The most common of these, syphilis and gonorrhea, are susceptible to antibiotic therapy. However, the increasing incidence of herpes simplex II, a viral sexually transmitted disease of the genital area, and the acquired immune disease syndrome (AIDS) may cause a change in future sexual behavior. At the present time there is no cure for the diseases. Adults are expressing considerable anxiety about the prospect of having an incurable disease and are concerned about how it may affect future sexual relationships as well as their own health. (See Chapter 36 for further details.)

Table 7.3 outlines the sexual behaviors and sexual functions of early, middle, and late adulthood and old age.

YOUNG ADULTHOOD

The tasks of sexual development for the young adult described below include maintaining a long-term commitment to a sexual relationship, practicing responsible reproductive health care, and making rational decisions about childbearing.

1. *Commitment to a relationship* is strengthened by the need to give and receive pleasure. Commitments vary in length and type. For example, some couples remain monogamous throughout their

Table 7.3
Adult Sexual Development*

Age	Behavior	Function
Early adulthood (23-30 yr)	Formal engagement and marriage	Sexual access legitimized and regularized; as sexual access ceases to be a problem, more attention focused on activity
	Sexual dysfunction problems become more meaningfully symptomatic	Problems with gender competence, regularization of sexual access plus sheer density of interaction may result in declining eroticism especially for men
	Pregnancy and child rearing	Many pressures (fatigue, economic, time, occupational) contribute to decreased eroticism
	Beginning of extramarital affairs	More common among men of low socioeconomic class because of weaker commitment to occupational success and resulting loss of homosocial masculinity
Middle adulthood (30-46 yr)	Rates of marital intercourse decline	Maximal involvement in careers, family, and child rearing
	Men's interest in marital competence decreases	Much of decline caused by (1) de-eroticization of wife-mother role and (2) husband's alternative attachments
	Women's interest in marital competence increases	Commitment to the sensual and away from continuing confirmation of emotional attachment
	Period of rising extramarital activity	For men, homosocial validation of masculinity; for women, justification
Late adulthood (46-65 yr)	Imperative to continue sexual activity	Harder for either sex to continue to function because of long sexual abstinence
	Loss of sexual partner through death or illness	Frequently have guilt feelings about sexual fantasies
	Performance problems (particularly erectile difficulties)	Source of anxiety
	Menopause	Can be freedom from pregnancy worries and also source of concern in youth-oriented society
Old age (65 + yr)	Sexual feelings still experienced although desire and ability have decreased somewhat	Result in guilt feelings because of cultural taboo against sexuality among aged persons

*Adapted by Marianne Zalar from Sadock, B.J., Kaplan, H.D., and Freedman, A.M.: The sexual experience, Baltimore, 1976, The Williams & Wilkins Co.

marriage. Others have open marriages, in which the couple agrees that one or both may participate in other sexual encounters. Some couples remain in relationships without formal marriage. Relationships can be terminated by divorce or death. Finally, serial monogamy is practiced by many people in the United States. Serial monogamy is characterized by repeated marriages and divorces. The person is married to only one person at a time but is married a number of times throughout his or her life.

2. *Responsible reproductive health care* is characterized by women having a Papanicolaou smear at prescribed intervals and both men and women avoiding sexually transmitted diseases.
3. *Rational decisions about childbearing* are important to ensure that every child is a wanted child. The couple is responsible for using a reliable contraceptive technique when pregnancy is not desired. Unwanted pregnancies and multiple abortions represent an irresponsible disregard for life and personal well-being. Unwanted children often become the targets of abuse and neglect.

There are a variety of sexual orientations and forms of sexual expression open to adults. Heterosexuality, homosexuality, and bisexuality are the three major sexual orientations. Heterosexuals express a sexual preference for a person of the opposite sex, homosexuals prefer sexual partners of the same sex, and bisexuals relate sexually to both sexes. The most common forms of sexual expression include vaginal-penile intercourse, anal intercourse, orogenital intercourse, self-stimulation, and mutual masturbation. These are all valid forms of sexual expression and are practiced according to personal preferences.

In a culture characterized by a rapid increase in

knowledge and technology, many persons still are misinformed about human sexuality. McCary (1973) has listed 100 of the most common fallacies about human sexuality that plague the country today. Listed below are 19 of these myths about reproduction and birth control*:

1. There is an absolutely safe period for sexual intercourse, in which coitus cannot cause impregnation.
2. A couple must have simultaneous climaxes if conception is to take place.
3. A woman can become pregnant only through coitus or artificial insemination.
4. Urination by the woman after coitus or having sexual intercourse in a standing position will prevent pregnancy.
5. Abortion, whether legal or criminal, is always dangerous.
6. Frigid women, prostitutes, and promiscuous women are not as likely to conceive as women whose sexual response or activity is more normal.
7. There must be two acts of sexual intercourse to produce twins, three for triplets, and so on.
8. Sperm from one testis will produce males, and sperm from the other testis will produce females; or the ova from one ovary will produce males, and the ova from the other ovary will produce females.
9. Having only one testis reduces a man's ability to father a child.
10. The woman determines the sex of the child.
11. A woman's diet during pregnancy has a bearing on the sex of the child.
12. The sex of a child to be conceived is a matter of pure chance, and nothing can be done to change the odds.
13. A fetus sleeps during the day and is awake at night (and kicks).
14. An infant born after 7 months has a better chance of survival than one born after 8 months.
15. An unborn child can be "marked."
16. "Virginal birth" (parthenogenesis) does not occur in humans or animals.
17. Taking oral contraceptives will delay a woman's menopause.
18. Humans and infrahuman animals can crossbreed.
19. A breast-feeding mother cannot become pregnant again as long as she continues to nurse her baby (even if she supplements some feedings).

*From McCary's human sexualtiy, ed. 3, by James Leslie McCary. Copyright 1978 by Litton Educational Publishing, Inc. Reprinted by permission of D. Van Nostrand Co.

MIDDLE AND LATE ADULTHOOD

The sexual developmental tasks of middle and late adulthood focus primarily on adapting to the physical and emotional changes in sexual performance caused by the aging process. The childbearing years are coming to an end. This is a relief for many couples because the threat of pregnancy can be removed from their lovemaking activities. Others may mourn the loss of the choice for another child.

The fear of growing older in a youth-oriented society can be a source of depression and anxiety. Bodily changes, lower hormone production, and menopause all contribute to anxiety and depression.

The research of Masters and Johnson (1966) has shown that aging does not decrease libido or the capacity to be orgasmic. Men and women are capable of sexual activity well into old age. Disinterest and abstinence are more probably caused by loss of a partner, boredom, ill health, or cultural attitudes about the appropriateness of sex in old age rather than being caused by the ability of the older person to perform sexually.

Many older persons do not understand the impact of aging on their physical response to sexual stimulation. They perceive these changes as an indication to terminate sexual activity rather than merely as a need to make minor adaptations. For example, lubrication for women is slower and decreased in amount, and erection is slower and erectile firmness is decreased. Love play will probably need to be extended, with more direct genital stimulation, to produce lubrication and erection. Women have a shortened orgasmic phase and men's need to ejaculate decreases, resulting in decreased force and volume of ejaculation. These physiologic changes require adaptations in sexual behavior and not cessation of sexual activity.

Mims and Swenson (1980) have stated:

> Sexual fulfillment throughout adulthood and into old age is not only possible but likely. The feeling that older people are not interested in sex (except if they are abnormal—the "dirty old man" syndrome) is largely caused by our inability to imagine our parents or our grandparents as sexually active people. The greatest danger of such attitudes is that they tend to comprise a "self-fulfilling prophecy": if people believe that sexual interest ceases with advancing age, they will find that it does cease. Or, if sexual interest persists, people may believe themselves to be abnormal, sinful, or psychologically sick.

CLINICAL CONSIDERATIONS

Early pregnancy detection is one of the most significant technologic advances in twentieth-century health care delivery. Its contribution to responsible sexuality may be demonstrated by the following paradigm: wanted vs. unwanted pregnancy and positive vs. negative pregnancy test results.

When the pregnancy is wanted and the results are positive, the woman can be directed to early prenatal care. If the pregnancy is wanted and the test is negative, the couple can be referred to a fertility clinic. If, on the other hand, the pregnancy is unwanted and the test is positive, the woman can be referred for early abortion counseling. Finally, when the pregnancy is unwanted and the test is negative, the woman or couple can be directed to a family planning clinic for contraceptive counseling.

The role of sex educator is an important role for nurses working with families during the childbearing and child-rearing years. Parents often need assistance with the sex education of their children. Frequently adults are misinformed about many aspects of reproduction and how their own bodies function. Therefore parents need to have accurate sex information in order to teach their children to be healthy and responsible sexual beings.

In addition to providing assistance with childhood and adult sexuality, the nurse can help prepare clients for the sexual problems and changes occurring with age. Many nurses have not been aware of the importance of sex education for older persons because of the myth that the elderly are no longer interested in sex.

Sexual dysfunctional problems often begin after children are born. The mother especially may become so involved with child rearing that her relationship with her husband suffers. At the same time the husband may be actively involved in career establishment, thereby depleting his energies at home. The nurse needs to be aware of how the demands of parenting can adversely affect the marital relationship. Simple counseling provided during these early years may prevent serious marital problems in later years.

The older woman, in particular, who has been able to gracefully move into old age and who continues to recognize herself as a sexual being is probably better able to accept the sexuality of the young. The pregnancy of a daughter then may be accepted as a continuation of her own sexuality rather than as a threat or reminder of her lost youth.

A knowledgeable, nonjudgmental nurse who recognizes personal sexual biases can contribute a great deal to the sexual health of young families. The nurse can recognize potential problems within the marriage and either intervene or refer the couple for further counseling.

References and Readings

Bardwick, J.: The psychology of women, New York, 1971, Harper & Row, Publishers.

Brown, F.: Sexual problems of the adolescent girl, Pediatr. Clin. North Am. **19:**759, 1972.

Clark, A.L., and Hale, P.W.: Sex during and after pregnancy, Am. J. Nurs. **73:**1430, 1974.

Claytor, S.B.: Coitus during pregnancy, Med. Asp. Hum. Sex. **8:**39, July 1974.

Colman, A.D., and Colman, L.: Pregnancy: the psychological experience, New York, 1973, The Seabury Press.

Cronenwett, L., and Newmark, L.: Fathers' responses to childbirth, Nurs. Res. **23:**210, May-June 1974.

Daniel, W.A.: Adolescents in health and dsease, St. Louis, 1977, The C.V. Mosby Co.

Deutsch, H.: The psychology of women, vol. 2, New York, 1945, Bantam Books.

Edwards, M.: Communications: dimensions in childbirth education, Pacific Grove, Calif., 1973, M. Edwards.

Elkind, D.: Cognitive development in adolescence. In Adams, J.F., editor: Understanding adolescence, Boston, 1968, Allyn & Bacon.

Erikson, E.: Identity and the life cycle; selected papers. In Psychological issues, New York, 1959, International Universities Press.

Fattich, A., Leach, W., and Wilkinson, C.: Fatal air embolism in pregnancy resulting from orogenital sex play, Forensic Sci. **2:**247, May 1973.

Gagnon, J.H.: Human sexualities, Glenview, Ill., 1977, Scott, Foresman and Co.

Goldstein, B.: Human sexuality, New York, 1976, McGraw-Hill Book Co.

Goodlin, R.C., Keller, D.W., and Raffin, M.: Orgasm during late pregnancy—possible deleterious effects, Obstet. Gynecol. **38:**916 1971.

Havighurst, R.J.: Developmental tasks and education, ed. 3, New York, 1972, David McKay Co.

Hazell, L.D.: Common sense childbirth, Berkeley, Calif., 1976, Windhover Press.

Human sexuality feature section, M.C.N. **1:**165, 1976.

Jessner, L., Weigert, E., and Foy, J.L.: The development of parental attitudes during pregnancy. In Anthony, E.J., and Benedek, T., editors: Parenthood: its psychology and psychopathology, Boston, 1970, Little, Brown & Co.

Kantner, J.F., and Zelnik, M.: Sexual experience of young unmarried women in the United States, Fam. Plann. Perspect. **4:**9, 1972.

Katchadourian, H.A., and Lunde, D.T.: Fundamentals of human sexuality, New York, 1972, Holt, Rinehart & Winston.

Kinsey, A.C., et al.: Sexual behavior in human male, Philadelphia, 1948, W.B. Saunders Co.

Kinsey, A.C., et al.: Sexual behavior in human female, Philadelphia, 1953, W.B. Saundrs Co.

Kolodny, R.C., el al.: Textbook of human sexuality for nurses, Boston, 1979, Little, Brown & Co.

Lang, R.: Birth book, Palo Alto, Calif., 1972, Genesis Press.

Maccoby, E.R., editor: The development of sex differences, Stanford, Calif., 1966, Stanford University Press.

Maccoby, E.E., and Jacklin, C.: The psychology of sex differences, Stanford, Calif., 1974, Stanford University Press.

Masters, W.H., and Johnson, V.E.: Human sexual response, Boston, 1966, Little, Brown & Co.

McCary, J.L.: Human sexuality, ed. 2, New York, 1973, Van Nostrand Reinhold Co.

McNab, W.L.: Sexual attitude development in children and the parent's role, J. Sch. Health **46:**537, 1976.

Mead, M.: Male and female, New York, 1949, William Morrow & Co.

Mims, F.H., and Swenson, M.: Sexuality: a nursing perspective, New York, 1980, McGraw-Hill Book Co.

Mouey, J., and Ehrhardt, A.A.: Man and woman, boy and girl: the differentiation and demorphism of gender identity from conception to maturity, Baltimore, 1972, The Johns Hopkins University Press.

Newman, B., and Newman, R.: Development through life: a psychosocial approach, Homewood, Ill., 1975, Dorsey Press.

Piaget, J.: The psychology of intelligence, Boston, 1950, Routledge & Kegan Paul.

Piaget, J.: Intellectual evolution from adolescence to adulthood, Hum. Dev. **15:**1012, 1972.

Piaget, J., and Inhelder, B.: The psychology of the child, New York, 1969, Basic Books, Inc., Publishers.

Rainwater, L.: And the poor have children, J. Marriage Family **26:**457, 1964.

Sadock, B.J., Kaplan, H.I., and Freedman, A.M.: The sexual experience, Baltimore, 1976, The Williams & Wilkins Co.

The Sex Information and Education Council of the United States: Sexual relations during pregnancy and the postdelivery period (study guide no. 6), New York, 1967, SIECUS Publications.

Solberg, D.A., Butler, J., and Wagner, N.M.: Sexual behavior in pregnancy, N. Engl. J. Med. **288:**1098, 1973.

Witters, W., and Witters, P.: Drugs and sex, New York, 1975, Macmillan Publishing Co., Inc.

Woods, N.F.: Uterine tension and fetal heart rate during maternal orgasm, Obstet. Gynecol. **39:**125, 1972.

Woods, N.F.: Sexual activity during pregnancy, N. Engl. J. Med. **289:**379, 1973.

Woods, N.F.: Human sexuality in health and illness, ed. 2, St. Louis, 1979, The C.V. Mosby Co.

Zelnik, M., and Kantner, J.F.: Sexual and contraceptive experience of young unmarried women in the United States, 1976 and 1971, Fam. Plann. Perspect. **9:**55, 1977.

8

Cultural Aspects of Maternity Nursing

- Definitions
- Reproduction in Various Cultures
- Childhood Preparation for Parenthood
- Prenatal Care and Expected Behaviors of Parents and Family
  - Diet
  - Clothing
  - Activity and rest
  - Sexual activity
  - Emotional response
- Labor and Delivery
- Postpartal Care
  - Maintenance of a state of balance
  - Pollution state
- Parental, Familial, and Societal Reactions to Childbearing
  - The American family
  - Cultural variations
- Fertility and Infertility
- Family Planning and Contraception
- Implications for Nursing

Culturally sensitive nursing care is stressed by nursing leaders today (Aamodt, 1978; Kay, 1982; Leininger, 1977). Becoming knowledgeable about, and sensitive to, beliefs, values, and practices concerning childbearing in our multicultural society poses a unique challenge for nursing. Nurses are becoming increasingly aware of the need to focus on cultural variations in childbearing because of cultural pluralism in the United States and the rapid expansion of international nursing. Every community, social, or ethnic group has its culture, and individuals behave within the context of that culture.

Griffith (1982, pp. 181-182) stated that childbearing concepts focus on four components of a cultural system: (1) the moral and value system; (2) the kinship system; (3) the knowledge and belief system; and (4) the ceremonial and ritual system. This chapter, of course, cannot completely describe the entire cultural system of each group to whom reference is made. Furthermore, the cultural characteristics of pregnant women from all existing subcultural groups in the United States and abroad are not exhaustively analyzed. The paucity of data on cross-cultural perspectives on maternity care hinders one from achieving a complete analysis. Merely listing the various practices and beliefs of cultural groups would be of little value to maternity nurses. Since cultural values and practices undergo change, nurses must continually enhance their knowledge of the major cultural underpinnings of their clients' health beliefs and adapt this knowledge accordingly in their nursing care. Some events in childbearing are more important illustrations of a particular culture than others. The events depicted in this chapter were selected from the literature as examples of the concepts being explored and are taken out of their social context. It is hoped that nurses reading these descriptions will be motivated to explore more fully the cultural meaning of childbearing for their clients. To understand presentations in this chapter, the following terms need to be defined: culture, subculture, acculturation, ethnocentrism, and cultural relativism.

Definitions

Culture has many definitions. Spradley (1981, p. 6) defined culture as the "acquired knowledge people use to interpret experience and generate behavior." Each cultural group passes this knowledge to its members from generation to generation. Cultural knowledge includes beliefs and values about each facet of life from birth to death. A person's world view results from his or her cultural knowledge and provides rules for interaction with others, with nature, and with the supernatural (Powers, 1982). These rules have been tested over time and relate to food, language, religion, art, health, and healing practices, kinship relationships, and all other systems of behavior.

Subculture refers to a group existing within a larger cultural system that retains characteristics of its own; individuals identify themselves as members of the group. A subculture may be an ethnic group or a group organized in other ways. For example, there is a subculture of nursing and a subculture of medicine.

Acculturation refers to those changes that take place when individuals from different cultures have contact with each other and change takes place in one or both groups. Persons may retain some of their own culture and also reformulate cultural elements. Acculturation is contrasted with assimilation in which a cultural group loses its identity and becomes a part of the dominant culture. The group is no longer recognizable as a separate entity when it is assimilated. Persons who are acculturated have retained the cultural practices that they find useful and also accept some of the practices of the group with whom they are in contact. In acculturation, there is also a synthesis of some cultural elements, with new practices being formed. An example of acculturation involves food practices of ethnic groups in the United States. Pizza is of Italian origin, accepted by many other groups, and multiple variations are introduced by others as well. The original recipe for pizza has been adapted by every other group.

Each subgroup and subculture has rich and complex traditions with regard to health practices that have proven effective over time. These traditions vary from group to group. Furthermore, since no two members of a group are identical, nurses must always recognize that a wide range of diversity may exist within a group. Assessment of beliefs and practices of a group and individuals within the group is essential for the health care provider striving to plan culturally sensitive health care.

Ethnocentrism means "being centered in one's own ethnic or cultural system, judging the world in general by the standards established in that particular system" (Downs, 1971, p. 15). Socialization into the profession of nursing occurs within the framework of the Western health care system, which places great emphasis on the biomedical model and which, in the United States, is based primarily on the white, middle-class value system. The biomedical model views pregnancy and childbirth as phenomena with inherent risks, most appropriately managed through scientific knowledge and technology. The nurse encountering behavior in women incongruent with these models, may become perplexed and make judgments that label the women's behavior as inappropriate and in conflict with good health practices. If the Western health care system provides the only standards for judging, the behavior of the nurse is termed ethnocentric.

Cultural relativism, the opposite of ethnocentrism, means learning about and applying the standards of another person's culture to activities within that culture. To be culturally relativistic means that the nurse recognizes that people from different cultural backgrounds actually see the same objects and situations differently. There are reasons why persons behave in the way they do, and these reasons are for the most part culturally determined. For example, the nurse caring for a woman in labor usually offers juice for nourishment and ice water to prevent dehydration and to provide comfort. If the woman is from a culture that organizes concepts of health around the balance of heat and cold and views labor and delivery as causing a loss of heat, cold fluids would be steadfastly refused.

Cultural relativism does not mean that the nurse must accept the beliefs and values of another culture. Rather, it means that the nurse recognizes that the behavior of others may be based on a system of logic quite different from the one she uses, such as in the example of fluids given during labor. For culturally relativistic nursing care, the nurse acknowledges different belief and value systems and incorporates knowledge of them and sensitivity to them in the nursing care plan of each client. Cultural relativism is an affirmation of the uniqueness and value of every culture.

Reproduction in Various Cultures

Childbearing represents one facet of health that is related to all aspects of a woman's life. While most cultures do not view pregnancy and childbirth as an illness state, it is considered a time of heightened susceptibility to dangerous elements. Stern and co-workers (1980, p. 68) noted that ". . . pregnant women seek security measures and court benevolent gods with ritualized behavior, whether anointing their abdomens with herbal oils in an African village or practicing daily yoga in California." Perception of the time of greatest vulnerability varies cross-culturally, with some groups placing greatest emphasis on the prenatal stage and others on labor and delivery or the puerperium. Western health care culture places the greatest emphasis on the prenatal and labor and delivery stages and least emphasis on the postpartal stage.

Childbearing in all cultures is replete with norms and behavioral expectations for each stage of the perinatal cycle. All relate to each culture's view of how one maintains health and prevents illness. Foster (1979) noted that the concept of humoral pathology is common to many belief systems. Humoral pathology was first documented in ancient Babylonia (Kay, 1982) and included qualitites of heat and cold, and moisture and dryness. The balance of these intrinsic body qualities must be maintained or illness occurs. Latin American folk practices (Foster, 1979) and southern United States practices reflect theories of balance and harmony among opposing forces. Although Chinese yin and yang is a highly complex system that is not the same as the humoral system, the concepts of balance and harmony, especially of heat and cold, are prominent (Campbell and Chang, 1973). Kay (1982) also referred to extrinsic factors that influence balance and harmony of the intrinsic factors, heat and cold. The extrinsic factors included air and water, food and drink, sleep and wakefulness, movement, exercise and rest, evacuation and retention, and passions of the spirits, or emotions. Thus for pregnant women of many cultures, maintenance of health during childbearing implies a balance and harmony in each individual's relationship to her physical, social, and spiritual environment.

Childhood Preparation for Parenthood

In most cultures parenthood is revered, and in many cultures, grandparenthood is even more highly revered (Gallo, et al., 1980; Morey and Gilliam, 1974). A desire to achieve these high-status positions results from socialization for adult roles. Meleis and Sorrell (1981) identified pregnancy for the Arab woman as her greatest opportunity to actualize her potential, and she has been prepared for this role since childhood. Stern (1981) also said that for the Filipino woman, the role of motherhood has been internalized since childhood.

The importance of children within the family is well documented for many cultures. Farris (1978) and Wright (1982) described American Indian families as child centered. Spanish-speaking groups in the United States place a high value on children (Clark, 1970; Dorsey and Jackson, 1976; Enriquez, 1982). Blacks (Carrington, 1978) and Southeast Asians (Hollingsworth, et al., 1980) inculcate a desire for children.

A common way to prepare children for their future parenting role is through sibling care taking (Weisner and Gallimore, 1977). Sibling care taking involves older children from either the nuclear or extended family caring for younger children. Older children are used to provide role flexibility for mothers and for the development of care-taking skills by children (Weisner and Gallimore, 1977, p. 180). Stereotyped sex roles, so important in many cultures, are maintained when children assume child care responsibilities for younger members in the family (Clark, 1978; Leyn, 1978; Munroe and Munroe, 1975; Parken, 1978; Sodetani-Shibata, 1981).

Prenatal Care and Expected Behaviors of Parents and Family

Prenatal care as we know it is a phenomenon of Western medicine. The Western biomedical model of care encourages women to seek prenatal care as early as possible in their pregnancy by visiting a physician or clinic. The initial visit followed by monthly and then weekly visits is usually routine and follows a systematic time sequence. Monitoring of weight and blood pressure, testing of blood and urine, teaching specific information about diet, rest, and activity, and preparation for childbirth are common components of prenatal care.

The above model is not only unfamiliar but frequently seems very strange to many groups. Even when the prenatal care described is familiar, some practices may conflict with a subcultural group's beliefs and practices. Because of these and other factors, such as lack of money, lack of transportation, and poor communication on the part of health care providers, many groups do not participate in the prenatal care system, and their behavior may be misinterpreted by nurses as uncaring, lazy, or ignorant. For example, Muecke (1976) pointed out that the Northern Thai do not focus on the prenatal period at all, only on the childbirth and postpartum periods. According to their beliefs, they personally perceive themselves as having little influence on pregnancy until the time of birth. For them spiritual influences, apart from human beings, control what occurs before birth. Western prenatal care, which does not deal with the spiritual influences, appears irrelevant.

My own research (Horn, 1982) with a group of Northwest Coast Indians elicited the strongly held belief that visible preparation for the coming infant was frequently associated with the infant's death. Women could identify many instances when preparation such as buying infant clothes or preparing a crib was followed by the death of the infant. A high infant mortality rate supported this belief. Another group not favoring preparation by the mother before birth is the Arab-American population. Meleis and Sorrell (1981) stressed that the Egyptian Arab mothers do not have a layette or room set aside for newborns at the time of birth. They believe that planning ahead has the potential of defying God's will. Also, planning ahead only to have those plans not materialize can be disappointing. Women on the Caribbean island of St. Kitt prefer not discussing the coming infant, mentioning its name, or referring to it directly until it is christened (Gussler, 1982). Until the time of christening, spirits of the dead would come and make the infant ill or kill it. This same concern for the dead spirits' influence was expressed by the Muckleshoot, who kept a candle burning to keep the spirits from coming to get the baby. Kendall (1979) described the pregnant Iranian woman's grandmother who prepared a complete set of clothing for her expected grandchild during the sixth or seventh month of pregnancy. Included within the set of clothing, however, was a triangular scarf with beads, amulets, and shells to ward off the evil eye and thus protect the unborn infant.

A concern for modesty is also a deterrent for prenatal care for many persons. Exposing one's body parts, especially to a man, is a major violation of modesty. Puerto Ricans (Parken, 1978), Mexicans (Kay, 1982; Zepeda, 1982), and Japanese (Bernstein and Kidd, 1982) expressed great concern over body exposure. Arab women also value modesty (Meleis and Sorrell, 1981). Besides being fully clothed, the Arab woman is expected to manifest modesty through diffidence, shyness, and showing bashfulness when interacting with men and strangers. For many women invasive procedures such as vaginal examinations may be so threatening that they cannot be discussed, even with one's own husband. Thus a midwife rather than a male physician is preferred by many. Besides the above groups, recent immigrants such as Southeast Asians prefer a midwife (Gallo et al., 1980; Hollingsworth et al., 1980).

For numerous cultural groups, a physician is deemed appropriate only in times of illness. A physician, then, is certainly not appropriate when pregnancy is considered a normal process and the woman is in a state of wellness. Even when problems with pregnancy develop according to beliefs of Western medicine, they may not be perceived as problems, but rather considered normal. Muecke (1976) noted that Thai women did not perceive weakness, fainting spells, palpitations, tremors, and diarrhea as abnormal. Many Muckleshoot women perceived puffiness of the hands, eyes, and feet and frequent headaches as quite normal (Horn, 1982).

Although pregnancy is considered normal by many, certain practices are expected of women of all cultures to ensure a good outcome. There are prescriptions that tell women what to do and proscriptions that establish taboos. The purposes of these practices are to (1) prevent maternal illness from a pregnancy-induced imbalanced state, (2) protect the vulnerable infant, and (3) protect other persons from illness caused by a woman in a state of imbalance. Prescriptions and proscriptions discussed in this chapter are related to dietary practices, clothing, activity and rest, sexual activity, and emotional response.

DIET

Women in most cultures are encouraged to eat a normal diet, whatever that may be. For the nurse, it is important to know what constitutes a normal diet for each ethnic group. For example, Southeast Asian women have rice and fish as basic foods, with supplements of vegetables, poultry, meats, eggs, and fruit depending on the season and family wealth. Fresh milk products are generally not consumed. This is true for the Filipino woman as well (Stern, 1981). Among Chinese-Americans, herbal teas, such as ginseng, may be used as a tonic in early pregnancy, and to strengthen the womb during the seventh and eighth month (Campbell and Chang, 1973; Dunn, 1978). Chung (1977) refers to the use of ginseng tea as a dietary supplement by Chinese mothers, but these same women refuse iron supplements supplied by Western medicine because they believe their bones will harden and they will have a difficult delivery.

Food taboos are more common than food prescriptions. Vietnamese women are to avoid "unclean" foods such as beef, dog, rat, and snake meat (Hollingsworth et al., 1980). Japanese women are cautioned against hot, spicy, and salty food, as are Filipino women. Filipino women are to avoid sweet foods because they may cause a big baby and a difficult delivery (Affonso, 1978), whereas Japanese women are encouraged to gain as much weight as they are comfortable with, believing that a large weight gain is good for the baby (Bernstein and Kidd, 1982). Blacks in the southern United States, as well as Guatemalans, Mexicans, and Mexican-Americans, should not eat acid foods or fresh fruits and vegetables (Kay, 1982). According to Snow (1974) red meat should be avoided by blacks because it is too strong and virile a food.

Food taboos often follow the principles of imitative magic, in which physical characteristics of food eaten by the mother may be transmitted to the child. Filipinos avoid eating prunes (Affonso, 1978) and Chinese avoid eating soy sauce (Campbell and Chang, 1973), in both instances to prevent a dark-skinned infant. Birthmarks and their pigmentation are often associated with the shape and color of the food eaten, such as the strawberry mark (Carrington, 1978). Campbell and Chang (1973) reported that some Chinese mothers shun shellfish during the first trimester, believing it is responsible for allergies in the later life of the child. Filipino mothers said that they were not to eat squid during pregnancy for fear that the mother's insides would become tangled and the baby's cord would tie around its neck (Affonso, 1978).

Food cravings during pregnancy are considered normal by many cultures, but the specific kinds of cravings may be culturally specific (Carring, 1978; Obeyesekere, 1963). In most cultures women crave acceptable foods, such as chicken, fish, and greens among blacks (Carrington, 1978) or fruits, nuts, bird meat, and taro among the Gadsup (Leininger, 1979). Satisfaction of food cravings is considered vital for culturally specific reasons. For example, Obeyesekere (1963) described the foods craved by Sinhalese women as being extremely difficult to obtain. Sinhalese women had a very low status in their society and were unable to express their anger about it or ever to demand anything for themselves. Their demand for foods difficult to obtain was interpreted as the only time hostility toward their role as women was acceptable. and Sinhalese men were required to obtain the food even at great cost to themselves. Affonso (1978) noted that the Filipino culture believes cravings should be satisfied to prevent the premature arrival of the infant.

Women in some cultures desire nonnutritive substances such as laundry starch, clay, and dirt. Eating of these substances is called pica. Kay (1982) described Mexican/American women eating clay. All of these substances—laundry starch, clay, and dirt—were used by black women (Carrington, 1978). A longitudinal study reported that 40% of pregnant women in Mississippi ate clay (Vermeer and Frate, 1975). One Canadian Ojibwa woman who had had five children stated that with each pregnancy she craved and ate large quantities of "clean" dirt.

Certain ethnic groups have been identified as having a greater incidence of pica than others. Lackey (1978) studied black and white women and found that women in both groups ate substances such as clay and starch, although the percentage of black women was higher. Causes of pica have been attributed to a variety of reasons and may be engaged in by children as well as pregnant women. Pica may be a psychologic response of someone needing attention, a truly cultural phenomenon, a response to hunger, or the body's response to needed nutrients. There is scientific controversy about whether the iron deficiency seen in persons with pica is the cause or the effect of the anemia. Whatever the reason, according to Leiderman and co-workers (1977), a documented sequela is increased iron deficiency anemia because of interference with absorption of necessary nutrients when clay is eaten.

Nutritional information given by Western health care providers may be a source of conflict for many cultural groups. The conflict is frequently not known by the health care providers unless they have an understanding of dietary beliefs and practices of the persons for whom they are caring. Stern (1981) found that Filipino-Americans rarely attempted to explain their dietary beliefs to maternity nurses and obstetricians. They would concur politely with dietary instructions and then return home to follow their traditional diet. When food habits are considered by the nurse, however, it is important to remember that dietary patterns, although ingrained, actually change rapidly, sometimes within one generation, and an individual food history is an important adjunct to knowledge of cultural food ways.

CLOTHING

In most cultural groups there is no prescribed clothing for pregnancy. Modesty is an expectation for many (Clark, 1970; Meleis and Sorrell, 1981). Spanish-speaking people of the Southwest wear a cord beneath the breast and knotted over the umbilicus. This cord, called a muneco, is thought to prevent morning sickness and ensure a safe delivery (Brown, 1976). Amulets, medals, and beads may be worn to ward off evil spirits.

ACTIVITY AND REST

Norms that regulate physical activity of mothers during pregnancy vary tremendously. Many groups (Carrington, 1978; Horn, 1982; Stringfellow, 1978) encourage women to be active, to walk, and to carry on normal although not strenuous activities. This will cause the baby to be healthy and not too large. On the other hand, the Filipino woman is cautioned that any activity is dangerous, and others willingly take over her work (Affonso, 1978; Stern, 1981). The belief among Filipinos is that inactivity constitutes a protection for mother and child. The mother is encouraged to simply produce the succeeding generation. Health care providers could misinterpret this behavior as laziness or noncompliance with the health regimen desired in prenatal care. Again, it is very important for the nurse to find out the meaning of activity and rest for each culture.

SEXUAL ACTIVITY

In most cultures sexual activity is not prohibited until toward the end of pregnancy. Among blacks sexual relations are viewed as natural since pregnancy is a state of wellness (Carrington, 1978). Mexican-Americans view sexual activity as necessary to keep the birth canal lubricated (Kay, 1982). On the other hand, Vietnamese have definite proscriptions about sexual intercourse, requiring abstinence as early as the sixth month (Hollingsworth et al., 1980; Stringfellow, 1978). Sexual taboos are more frequent after delivery and will be discussed later.

EMOTIONAL RESPONSE

Virtually all cultures emphasize the importance of a socially harmonious and agreeable environment. Absence of stressful relationships is important for a successful outcome for mother and baby. Harmony with other persons must be fostered. Visits from extended family members may be required to demonstrate continued pleasant and noncontroversial relationships. If dissonance exists in any relationship with others, it is usually dealt with in culturally prescribed ways. For example, an informant on the Muckleshoot reservation described how she became ill after eating chili at a drive-in. Chili is a food to avoid during pregnancy because of its spiciness. The pregnant woman's mother had specifically warned her about eating chili. Disharmony had been produced in two areas—physiologic and social—by eating a proscribed food and by not following her mother's admonitions. To remedy the situation and to reestablish harmony, the pregnant woman attended a Shaker prayer service. She prayed for herself and was ''brushed off''; that is, a church member symbolically brushed the problem away by touching her shoulder lightly. She believed she had now regained a state of physiologic and social harmony.

Imitative magic functions in other proscriptions in addition to food. Mexicans advise against pregnant women witnessing an eclipse of the moon believing it may cause a cleft palate in the infant. Exposure to an earthquake may result in premature delivery or miscarriage. A breech may occur if the earthquake was exceptionally strong (Clark, 1970, p. 21). Snow (1974) noted that among blacks, a pregnant woman must not ridicule someone with an affliction for fear that her child might be born with that same handicap. A mother should not hate a person lest her child resemble that person, and dental work should not be done while pregnant since it may cause a baby to have a harelip. Carrington (1978) described a widely held folk belief in many cultures that includes refraining from raising one's arm above one's head and refraining from tying knots, so that the umbilical cord does not wrap around the baby's neck and become knotted.

Labor and Delivery

Although the biologic process of labor and delivery is the same for all cultures, it is managed differently and surrounded by different attitudes in different cultures. The initiation of labor begins the birthing process. In the United States today, childbirth may take place in a hospital, birthing center, or the home. The most common site is the hospital. There is increasing acceptance of the more natural childbirth approaches, including conversion of major hospital facilities to resemble a home atmosphere. When this exists, fathers, other family members, and friends of the parents may be participants in the event of childbirth. A review of the literature indicates that cross-cultural concerns about hospital deliveries occur in relation to (1) who is present during labor and delivery, (2) the position assumed during delivery, and (3) management of pain.

Today, hospitals encourage the father's presence during labor and delivery. If he is not able to be there, another significant person may be present. In several cultures the father may be available, but his presence with the mother may not be appropriate, and he may resist involvement at this time. His behavior could be misconstrued by the nursing staff as lack of concern, caring, or interest on his part. Griffith (1982) identified the importance of the affectional bond between a Mexican woman and her mother and sisters or other female relatives in regard to home-related activities such as childbearing. This is true for many other groups as well, and the presence of another woman or women is highly desired. If the childbearing occurs in the hospital, it is imperative that some woman is present for assistance. Southeast Asians (Hollingsworth et al., 1980); blacks (Carrington, 1978; Johnson and Snow, 1978), and American Indians (Farris, 1978; Horn, 1982) are some of the major cultural groups indicating a preference for a woman's assistance during childbearing. Pillsbury (1978) noted that the Chinese husband is not allowed in the delivery room, lest he become polluted by the woman's blood. In India all attendants at birth are women, with men totally excluded (Flint, 1982). On the other hand, in Guatemala, a husband may assist his wife and the midwife during delivery (Cosminsky, 1982). During the labor process of the Navajo in the Southwestern United States, individuals passing by the hogan are encouraged to enter and provide support for the mother (Newton, 1972). Because of the wide variation in who is the preferred person or persons, it is critical for the nurse to determine from the woman and her family what persons are wanted during labor and delivery.

In American hospitals, the lithotomy position continues to be most frequently used in delivery. In the recent past women were not given a choice of position for delivery. Bauwens and Anderson (1978) attributed an increase in home births among all Americans to loss of control and to medical interference. These two factors may cause a great deal of conflict for women whose practices and beliefs are different from those of the hospital. With the advent of birthing rooms, beds are now constructed in such a manner that alternatives exist. In hospitals where midwives attend Southeast Asian women, a woman is frequently allowed to assume the position normal for her, and this is often the squatting position. Gordon and co-workers (1980) recommend providing a large white pad beside the bed for the woman to squat on. Acceptance by hospital personnel of the mother's choice of position for delivery will greatly decrease cultural conflict for many women.

Expression and control of pain are also culturally prescribed. In most hospitals today, analgesia and anesthesia are used in childbirth. Contrary to a myth of the past, delivery of women in traditional societies was not without pain (Stanton, 1979). How persons perceive and respond to pain varies cross-culturally, however. Psychic control of pain is demonstrated by many cultural groups, and use of medications is generally decried. For example, Mormons have a special rule not to behave badly and not to cry out during labor and delivery. The Mormon woman must remember that she is of pioneer stock and should behave as a strong woman (Stark, 1982). Indochinese women will walk around during labor and not ask for medications. These women exert great self-control, to the point that the nurse may not recognize an impending delivery (Hollingsworth et al., 1980). Black women frequently find comfort in having another woman such as a mother or sister pray with them during the discomfort of labor. Meleis and Sorrell (1981) describe the pain tolerance of Arab women as seeming quite low and expressed quite verbally. Arab women moan, cry out, and scream during labor. Yet few will accept anesthesia because of fear of danger with these options.

In addition to the concerns described, food may be an issue during labor. Warm teas are used by many cultural groups to counteract the effects of heat loss during labor and delivery. Personal communications from Cambodian women who have been in the United States for 2 years or less indicated that they would consume a special meal consisting of fried meat and rice several hours before delivery. If they went to the hospital early in labor, they were concerned that this kind of meal would not be available to them but thought that they might eat it before they left home.

Postpartal Care

The greatest conflict between Western and non-Western beliefs and practices in childbearing occurs in the postpartal period. If a woman delivers in the hospital, she and her family are directly confronted with culturally related problems that are not as easily resolved as those encountered in the prenatal and labor and delivery stages. Moreover, nurses caring for these mothers may view the women's behavior as totally incomprehensible since it deviates so dramatically from Western health care givers' expectations.

The behavior patterns for many cultures include a period of seclusion for women lasting from 7 to 40 days with a minimum of activity allowed for mothers. These practices are based on two beliefs previously mentioned in this chapter: that delivery has upset the balance of the mother's body and that the mother, infant, and those caring for them are in a state of pollution.

MAINTENANCE OF A STATE OF BALANCE

Cultures that subscribe to a belief in the necessity of body balance believe that the body has lost a great deal of heat during the labor and delivery process and that the mother is therefore subject to a number of potential illnesses. Thus certain practices must be followed to restore the balance of heat and cold. Adherents of both humoral and yin and yang theories have prescriptions and proscriptions for restoration of balance of heat and cold (Currier, 1978).

Food is one way in which heat can be restored and cold diminished. The classic Chinese diet (Campbell and Chang, 1973) represents an effort to decrease yin forces, which are cold. Included are an abundance of hot foods. The quality of heat and cold cannot always be measured by actual temperature. The essence of cold might be in a food even if the food is heated. Pillsbury (1978) noted that some foods are considered cold because they are grown in the damp earth or in watery places. Green vegetables, fruits, meats, and fish are frequently considered cold foods. For Asians, rice, eggs, and chicken soup are foods high in the quality of hotness and should be eaten frequently. For many cultures, chicken surpasses all other foods as a desirable hot food. Chicken soup is also believed important in the production of a nursing mother's milk. It is quite obvious that many, if not most, of the foods served on hospital trays, such as meats, vegetables, fruits, and fruit juices, are considered cold. These will probably not be eaten by many Asian, Southeast Asian, and Spanish-speaking women.

In addition to food, contact with air and wind is proscribed by Asians, Filipinos, Mexican-Americans, and southern blacks. Cold must be prevented from entering the body, to counteract further imbalance. Air is considered cold, whatever the temperature, and thus windows and doors must be kept closed. The Chinese belief that a woman's pores are open for 30 days after delivering a baby coincides with the period in which they believe the mother has an excess of cold (Campbell and Chang, 1973; Pillsbury, 1978). Air conditioners are a source of fear for women in the hospital. Fans are to be avoided. New mothers will keep themselves totally covered with blankets despite how hot the temperature of the room may be.

Water is considered cold at all times, even if it is heated. Therefore not bathing for a period of time is a widely held belief. Some mothers will take all kinds of measures to avoid the daily shower but will not directly refuse, complying by going to the shower room, turning on the water, and remaining in such a position that the water will not touch them. Pillsbury (1978) noted that Chinese women who have been westernized in so many ways still adhere to the postpartal practice of avoiding water. They must not wash themselves, their dishes, or their clothes. To the Chinese and other Asians, contact with water, considered cold, causes wind to enter the body and will result in future years in asthma, arthritis, and chronic aches and pains. However, if a hot substance is added to boiled water, it may counteract the coldness. For example, the chicken in soup is so powerful that the cold quality of the water with which it is made is counteracted. Ginger added to very hot water that has been boiled may cause the same effect. It is obvious then, that ice water, used frequently in hospitals, is forbidden.

POLLUTION STATE

In addition to an imbalance of hot and cold, several cultures consider that the mother and infant are in a state of pollution after delivery. A certain time must elapse and certain rituals must be performed before purity is restored. A state of seclusion is frequently compulsory, during which time the mother is encouraged to limit her activities. This is in contrast to the hospital practice of early ambulation following delivery, early infant care responsibilities, and early discharge from the hospital. Mexican-Americans may observe *la cuarentina* for 40 days after the birth of babies (Clark, 1970). For the Chinese mother, going out during the first month after birth will offend the gods because dirty birth blood remains throughout the month (Pillsbury, 1978). The Filipino mother (Stern et al., 1980) is frequently misunderstood as lazy and not caring when she refuses to do what is requested in the hospital and at home. Recently, in a personal communication from a group of Cambodian women, concern was expressed about how they will manage after the baby is born because they do not have an extended family to assist during the required time of seclusion and limited activity. The fear of subsequent illness, especially arthritis, in later years is very real to them. Homemaker services are not available to them because according to the Western view, they are able bodied and assistance could not be justified. Their hope for the future is based on the belief that counteracting the bad effects of not carrying out cultural prescriptions for the postpartal period can only be accomplished by going through a follow-up pregnancy correctly. Their chances of doing future pregnancies "correctly" is remote, however. The cultural quandary for these women is very clear!

Snow (1974) described the view of southern blacks that blood is a pollutant that carries contaminants from the body. Southern blacks and others feel that an adequate lochia flow is essential and going outside in the wind or air could thicken and halt the flow of blood, extending the time of pollution. Some Filipino mothers may remain bedfast for 2 weeks, after which time a special bath is taken to further remove the debris of pregnancy believed to be found in perspiration. "Roasting" or sitting on a slotted chair over a small fire, according to Stern and co-workers (1980), is practiced by Filipinos in the most remote provinces only. The purpose of this was to hasten the healing process, much like perineal heat lamps used in recent times.

A recent example of acculturated behavior was given to the author (Horn, 1982). Following the birth of her first child, a Greek-American mother followed the ancient proscription of participation in church activities for 40 days postpartum. While her husband attended the church wedding of a friend, this woman did her weekly shopping at the local supermarket. In most cultural groups sexual relations are prohibited until after the seclusion period and sometimes throughout lactation.

Some cultural groups have unique practices. For example, the women of Northern Thailand bind their wrists with string. The purpose of wrist binding is to prevent the loss of soul, which may lead to wind disease, a specific complex of symptoms indicating a state of humoral imbalance characterized by weakness, nausea, and hypersensitivity to odors (Kundstadter, 1978). Northern Thai women giving birth will most likely have their wrists bound and would be extremely frightened and upset if the strings were removed.

The above examples indicate that, from the time of delivery to a certain designated time afterward, mothers in many cultures are considered highly susceptible to ensuing illness, either immediately or at an unspecified time in the future. Further, their state of pollution requires that only certain persons contact them during the specified time they remain in seclusion. Most of their activities are carried on by others, usually members of the extended family or friends. The end of the time of seclusion is often marked by a ceremony and includes ritual cleansing of the woman, child, and place of seclusion (Brownlee, 1978). It is important for nurses to understand these factors, assist women in carrying out their beliefs and practices insofar as is possible, and assist them with necessary adjustments when their expectations are not feasible.

Parental, Familial, and Societal Reactions to Childbearing

Childbearing has significance for parents, extended family, and each society as a whole. Complex meanings that vary cross-culturally underlie each aspect of the process from conception until there is recognition of attainment of adult status for each individual. Unless one has been enculturated into a specific group, the real significance of that group's approach may elude even the most culturally sensitive nurse. Understanding in depth may be gained only through long and intensive living with, and exposure to, a group. Just as the previous selections were not comprehensive descriptions of the values, beliefs, or practices of any single group during pregnancy, labor and delivery, and the postpartal period, the following descriptions were simply chosen to indicate some of the rich variations that exist among people.

Before descriptions of subcultural groups, a review of the dominant American culture's reactions to childbearing is appropriate. I am including what is most commonly viewed as the dominant white American culture, but the astute nurse can readily describe variations within this culture also.

THE AMERICAN FAMILY

American culture is focused around a nuclear family that includes married parents and children. Extended family relationships are recognized as existing, but their influence varies. Geographic distance among family members is frequent, and telephone calls, letters, and occasional visits bridge the distances between the nuclear family and uncles, aunts, and grandparents. However, each nuclear family is considered a self-sufficient unit and ultimately responsible for its own functioning, especially child rearing.

Children in the American family are desirable. Parents, however, do not define themselves in terms of being parents only, and if a couple cannot, or chooses not to, have children, they are accepted as being whole persons and not incomplete in some way. Some value is also placed on delaying the arrival of the first child until the married couple has adjusted to one another and until they are financially able to begin a family. The desirable number of children in the American family is small, usually two or three.

Infants are immediately accepted as members of the society in which they are born. Children are considered as individuals with certain rights. They are not considered miniature adults, and some of the behaviors they engage in are not in preparation for adulthood. Play is valued for its own sake. On the other hand, early independence is encouraged. Toilet training is begun early, sometimes as early as 6 months of age. Parents are the primary disciplinarians, and this function remains in the nuclear family during the entire childhood. Parents may resent interference in the discipline of their child by others, even if the other person is a grandparent, aunt, or uncle. Discipline does exist in the school system, but it is viewed as a temporary extension of the parents' right to discipline.

Parents are the major caretakers, with the mother assuming primary responsibility. Johnston (1980) points out that in the United States parenting is often not seen as intrinsically rewarding and enjoyable, but rather as a series of difficult, hygienic, and unrewarding activities. Children are enjoyed only when parental activities result in a child that gains weight, learns to walk and talk, or is toilet trained. Although recently father and mother are sharing more responsibility for care, in early infancy the father is often working and the mother remains at home to care for the infant. Other caretakers are used, but they are usually not kin and may be babysitters or day care persons. These caretakers are paid for their services with money, usually by the hour.

Differences in the dominant culture of the United States and other cultures in general are reflected in how roles of parents are expressed and how children are viewed. The following highlights describe some cultures' major differences in (1) the meaning of pregnancy to parents, (2) incorporation of a child into the society, and (3) child rearing.

CULTURAL VARIATIONS

In contrast to the dominant American value system, for some cultures becoming a parent is the major way individuals define themselves as whole persons. For Mormons, the highest place in heaven can only be reached through marriage and childbearing. The greater the number of children, the higher the place in heaven (Stark, 1982). The Navajo woman's role is defined to a large extent in reproductive terms (Wright, 1982). For many blacks, pregnancy is necessary for a man and a woman to be seen as whole persons (Carrington, 1978). The Puerto Rican couple have their first child as soon as possible to indicate to themselves and the community that the husband is virile and the woman fertile (Murillo-Rohde, 1978). Among the Gadsup (Leininger, 1979) a woman becomes a woman and a man a man when each is married and has at least one child. For Mexican-Americans, childbearing is a privilege and obligation of married women and they should have children as often as they can (Enriquez, 1982). Thus for many cultural groups, parenthood is an ascribed status and for women there is no social role without a family.

Recognition of the infant not only as a member of a nuclear family but also of the extended family and the society as a whole is culturally constituted. With Filipinos, the sanctity of the baby's arrival is established through visiting of older relatives (Stern, 1980), and solidarity with the extended family is recognized. When this underlying reason is not understood by nurses, the crowds of visitors to the newborn may seem unnecessary and exasperating! The baptismal ceremony of Mexican-Americans establishes a bond between the child and godparents that is unique in the development of mutural rights and responsibilities. In Japan, 34 days after birth, parents bring the child to the Shinto shrine to integrate the newborn into the community (Bernstein and Kidd, 1982). In Samoan families the infant is introduced to the society when the mother and infant return from the hospital. A large party is held, with an abundance of food and gifts (Clark, 1978).

One of the ways in which societies deal with incorporation into the group is the manner in which the umbilical cord is handled. In the United States, the cord is normally kept uncovered, allowed to dry and fall off, and then destroyed. In many cultures a sympathetic union persists between a person and his cord even though the physical connection has been severed (Perry, 1982). In Japan the umbilical cord is carefully wrapped, placed in a box or envelope, kept in a safe place in the home, and finally, placed in the coffin of the person at death. Wherever the person goes, his real home is where the umbilical cord is (Bernstein and Kidd, 1982). Some American Indian groups (personal communication [Makah mother], Horn, 1974) place the cord in a highly decorated leather pouch and leave the pouch in the home of birth. This symbolizes belonging to the group forever.

A problem identified by American nurses is the initial familial response to the newborn based on its sex. Preference for a male child exists in several cultures, and obvious disappointment ensues when the newborn is female. The Arab woman defines herself as a woman not only by her ability to conceive and produce a healthy infant but also by her ability to produce a male infant (Meleis and Sorrell, 1981). The importance of male progeny is also emphasized among Southeast Asians. A vital point for nurses to remember is that initial disappointment demonstrated by the parents and extended family does not mean rejection of the female child. The female infant will be cared for and loved as much as the male infant. The display of disappointment when the infant is not male is culturally prescribed, and the behavior of the family would be considered inappropriate if they did not demonstrate this reaction.

Infant care is carried out in a variety of ways and has different aims for various groups. For the Japanese, mothering remains a source of social status for the mother and requires almost selfless devotion to her child (Bernstein and Kidd, 1978). Japanese mothers try to satisfy a baby at all times, not allowing the infant to cry more than a few seconds. The mother holds the baby almost constantly and there is close skin-to-skin contact. Through this close physical intimacy, the infant develops a sense of dependence on the mother that is fostered throughout childhood. The Japanese mother does not have the assistance of in-laws and lives in a nuclear family. Because of strong parental sex role differentiation, the mother gives most of the early parenting.

Among Filipinos, the extended family assume most of the infant care responsibilities for the first month and a great deal of the care in the ensuing months. In-laws and friends who have had children spend a great deal of time teaching both mother and father about infant and child care.

In many American Indian groups the responsibility of the kin group to raise the child is commonly understood (Farris, 1978). Aunts and grandmothers are considered additional mothers. Grandparents teach the mother how care is given. Among Indians, a child is highly respected, and a permissive upbringing exists. Toilet training does not occur until a child is ready. All extended family members have rights and definite duties to perform. Women teach girls, and men teach boys. Grandparents give advice and spiritual guidance.

Among Southeast Asians, the extended family is the basic unit and shares responsibility for child rearing (SantoPietro, 1981). During the period of confinement, infants are cared for by other female members of the family and not the mother. Most Southeast Asians believe that the soul resides in the baby's head and touching the head may disturb the soul, so they are very careful not to touch the baby on the top of the head (Leyn, 1978; SantoPietro, 1981). In Vietnamese families the grandmother is the major caretaker (Grosso, 1981). Enriquez (1982) pointed out that the differences in childrearing behavior between Mexican-Americans and Anglo-Americans are really the fusion of Mexican and American practices.

These variations in societies' and families' responses to the newborn infant and child simply touch on a few major differences. There are innumerable others that influence how the infant and child are viewed and socialized. The contrast between the dominant culture of the United States with the illustrations given influences how nurses perceive and teach about infant care. Recognition by the nurse that infants and children are reared by adults in a variety of cultural frames of reference is a basic step in intercultural understanding.

Fertility and Infertility

When the ability to procreate is the norm used to recognize individuals in a culture as whole and complete persons, infertility becomes a tragedy. For example, in Samoa sterility is serious enough to be a cause for divorce (Clark, 1978). The person without children in Samoa is pitied. According to Brownlee (1978, p. 202), in many cultures a woman's inability to conceive may be due to her sins, to evil spirits, or to the fact that she is an inadequate person. The virility of a man in some cultures remains in question until he demonstrates his ability to reproduce by having at least one child.

If a culturally defined cause for sterility is determined, there is usually a culturally proposed solution for the problem. These proposed solutions may or may not be effective. For example, Vietnamese men thought sterility was caused by loss of sperm or spermatorrhea during wet dreams at night or through daytime discharge (Coughlin, 1965). Tonics consisting of licorice, aconite, and ginseng might be used to counteract the effect. Certain foods such as cereal were to be eaten, and substances such as alcohol were to be avoided.

In most cultures, infertility is usually blamed on the woman. If infertility is believed to be caused by a misplaced uterus, methods are used to replace it. A Samoan woman may go to a bush doctor who will massage the uterus with oil and attempt to put it back in place (Clark, 1978, p. 165). For Mexican-American women and others who subscribe to heat/cold balance and imbalance theories, barrenness is considered having a "cold womb" (Clark, 1970). The cold womb may be heated through external and internal means. Clark (1970, p. 170) described two ways used by Mexican-American women. A barren woman was required to sit over a washtub of hot water to which rosemary was added. The vapors would warm the womb. Another way to counteract the cold was to build up body heat over a period of 3 days, by avoiding cold foods and water, using a belladonna plaster over the sacral area, and ingesting cathartic pills and hot chocolate.

Family Planning and Contraception

Cross-cultural information about contraceptive practices is limited. Before modern times, probably the most effective contraception resulted from sexual taboos. Postpartal taboos previously mentioned were generally very effective. Kay (1982) pointed out that the Mexican-Americans she studied continued to place a 40-day restriction on sexual intercourse after childbirth.

In the past American Indians used herbs as oral contraceptives (Vogel, 1973). Information about these herbs was useful in the development of today's oral contraceptives. Some American Indian groups today favor the use of contraceptives, but some also believe that they are against God's will. Although the Japanese were one of the earliest cultural groups to accept the use of birth control and abortion (Okamoto, 1978), Japanese couples are reluctant to use contraception until they have borne one child (Bernstein and Kidd, 1982).

Some subcultural groups in the United States and in third-world countries believe that the great emphasis placed on family planning is based on the desire of the white middle class to limit minority groups. Darity and Turner (1972) reported that there was a significant group of black Americans wary of family planning methods.

The religion of some groups does not permit the use of contraception. The Catholic Church does not allow contraception. Affonso (1978) studied Filipinos who were predominantly Catholic. In her survey two thirds of the women thought that it would be all right to use contraceptives. Mormons prohibit birth control not as an evil in itself but as an impediment to meeting one's spiritual obligations (Stark, 1982). Samoans represent a variety of religions, but for them contraceptive practices are not highly valued (Clark, 1978). Rather, priority is placed on demonstration of male and female fertility through childbirth.

The ability to control fertility is based on an understanding of the menstrual cycle. According to Scott (1978) a majority of Bahamians, Cubans, Haitians, and Puerto Ricans believed the function of menstruation to be that of ridding the person of unclean waste or unnecessary blood. A large number of Bahamians believed that menstruating means a person is healthy. Less bleeding means that something is wrong. Snow's research (1974, p. 82) among blacks in parts of the western and northern United States also indicates the prevalent belief in impure blood.

If the belief that menstrual flow indicates health or lack of it, anything that would interfere with menstruation would be considered undesirable. The pill, which often reduces the amount and duration of menstrual-like flow, is considered dangerous to one's health. The IUD often affects the cycle and is also considered dangerous.

Family planning and contraception have posed numerous problems for nurses working with persons whose belief systems place a high value on having children and having them in large numbers. Nevertheless, many persons with these belief systems are interested in learning about contraception and will listen to explanations if they include respect for another's values. According to Dougherty (1972), health care innovations are accepted or rejected depending on how they fit with the client's cultural pattern.

Implications for Nursing

Cross-cultural variations in childbearing occur with respect to interpersonal relationships, family and kinship relationships, and folk practices. Clients have a right to expect that their cultural needs relative to childbearing will be met, as well as their physiologic and psychologic needs. Childbearing beliefs and practices for each culture are embedded in the entire social system of that culture and can only truly be understood as they relate to the economic, religious, kinship, and political structures of each group. To expect that the nurse will have this kind of knowledge for each cultural group is unrealistic. How, then, can information presented in this chapter be utilized effectively by the nurse?

Stern (1981, p. 50) presents a model for improving communication between Filipino-American and Western health care providers. Identified in this model are barriers in communication that exist on three levels: approach, custom, and language. Such a model, if generalized to other cultures as well as Filipino, is useful for nurses.

Approach includes numerous factors one considers in interpersonal relationships. The American approach to most issues in health care is to address the problem directly. With many cultures (Clark, 1970; Stern, 1981) engaging in small talk is vital before a serious discussion. Commenting on flowers or pictures and having tea or a cold drink are considered showing respect. To begin talking to an expectant mother about the need for prenatal care before commenting on the other children, the pretty chair, or the lovely, or not so lovely, day might set up an atmosphere of distrust. For women such as Southeast Asians and Mexican-Americans, who prefer a care giver of the same sex, it is critical that the initial encounter be with a woman. Spradley (1981, p. 93) stated: "show respect for clients . . . be patient, it takes time to build trust and effect cultural change."

Custom includes practices and behaviors identified in the cultures described in this chapter. Understanding that there is a cultural reason for all behaviors and making a sincere effort to ascertain the person's rationale for behavior is an important step in establishing trust. The clients themselves may be the most helpful in assisting the nurse to understand their cultural logic. The literature for each group may describe customs and their underlying rationale, but individual differences must be acknowledged. Assessment of health beliefs and practices is essential for the health care professional who is striving to achieve a holistic approach to care (O'Brien, 1982). For the client, adherence to a particular cultural custom provides a sense of constancy with one's cultural heritage.

Language is an important factor in the United States with the constant stream of immigrants and also for persons who are not immigrants but speak another language. For example, for many Spanish-speaking people, Spanish is their first language, with English a second language. Stern (1981) emphasized the use of clear, jargon-free English. An interpreter, either a family member or a member of the same cultural group, may be used as well. When using an interpreter, it is important to address questions and responses to the client and not the interpreter.

The most important asset for the nurse interested in working effectively in maternal and child care cross-culturally is to have an attitude of cultural relativism and a desire to know as much about each culture as possible. Informant and client interviewing as well as the literature about each culture and subculture can augment the basic posture of respect and understanding expressed by the culturally relativistic nurse.

Kleinman and co-workers (1978) refer to the individual's explanatory model for illness. Cultural explanatory models exist for each facet of the childbearing process as well. The cultural construction of clinical reality may be ascertained by asking a few key questions. The following questions are not exhaustive but only serve to indicate the kind of questions used to elicit cultural explanations:

1. What do you think you should do to keep healthy during pregnancy?
2. What are those things you can do or not do to affect your health and the health of your baby?
3. Who are the persons you want with you during your labor and delivery?

4. What are considered abnormal signs during pregnancy?
5. What things or actions are important for you to do after the baby is born?
6. What do you expect from the nurse or nurses caring for you?
7. What are ways that the nurse might help you?

A nurse cannot be expected to know all there is to know about every culture and subculture, as well as their many life-styles. Understanding one's own culture is necessary to come to a better realization of why we behave as we do. Understanding clients' cultures, through interview, study, contact, and a demonstrated sincere interest, is invaluable and enables nurses to render culturally sensitive and relevant nursing care.

References and Readings

Aamodt, A. A.: Culture. In Clark, A., editor: Culture/childbearing/health professionals, Philadelphia, 1978, F.A. Davis Co.

Affonso, D.D.: The Filipino American. In Clark, A., editor: Culture/childbearing/health professionals, Philadelphia, 1978, F.A. Davis Co.

Bauwens, E.E., and Anderson, S.: Home births: a reaction to hospital environmental stressors. In Bauwens, E.E., editor: The anthropology of health, St. Louis, 1978, The C.V. Mosby Co.

Bernstein, J.L., and Kidd, Y.A.: Childbearing in Japan. In Kay, M.A., editor: Anthropology of human birth, Philadelphia, 1982, F.A. Davis Co.

Brown, M.S.: A cross-cultural look at pregnancy, labor and delivery, Obstet. Gynecol. Nurs. **5:**35, 1976.

Brownlee, A.T.: Community, culture and care, St. Louis, 1978, The C.V. Mosby Co.

Campbell, T., and Chang, B.: Health care of the Chinese in America, Nurs. Outlook **21:**245, 1973.

Carrington, B.W.: The Afro-American. In Clark, A.L., editor: Culture/childbearing/health professionals, Philadelphia, 1978, F.A. Davis Co.

Chung, J.J.: Understanding the Oriental maternity patient, Nurs. Clin. North Am. **12:**67, 1977.

Clark, A.L., and Howland, I.H.: The American Samoan. In Clark, A.L., editor: Culture/childbearing/health professionals, Philadelphia, 1978, F.A. Davis Co.

Clark, M.: Health in the Mexican-American culture: a community study, Berkeley, Calif., 1970, University of California Press.

Cosminsky, S.: Knowledge and body concepts of Guatemalan midwives. In Kay, M.A., editor: Anthropology of human birth, Philadelphia, 1982, F.A. Davis Co.

Coughlin, R.: Pregnancy and birth in Vietnam. In Hart, D., Rajadhon, P.A., and Coughlin, R., editors: Southeast Asian birth customs, three studies in human reproduction, New Haven, Conn., 1965, Human Relations Area Files.

Currier, R.L.: The hot-cold syndrome and symbolic balance in Mexican and Spanish-American folk medicine. In Martinez, R.A., editor: Hispanic culture and health care: fact, fiction, folklore, St. Louis, 1978, The C.V. Mosby Co.

Darity, W.A., and Turner, C.B.: Family planning, race consciousness and the fear of genocide, Am. J. Pub. Health **62:**1454, 1972.

Dorsey, P.R., and Jackson, H.Q.: Cultural traditions: the Latino/Chicano perspective. In Branch, M.F., and Paxton, P.R., editors: Providing safe nursing care for ethnic people of color, New York, 1976, Appleton-Century-Crofts.

Dougherty, M.C.: A cultural approach to the nurse's role in health-care planning, Nurs. Forum **11:**310, 1972.

Downs, J.F.: Cultures in crisis, Beverly Hills, Calif., 1971, Glencoe Press.

Dunn, F.L.: Medical care in the Chinese communities of peninsular Malaysia. In Kleinman, A., et al., editors: Culture and healing in Asian societies, Cambridge, Mass., 1978, Schenkman Publishing Co.

Enriquez, M.G.: Studying maternal-infant attachment: a Mexican-American example. In Kay, M.A., editor: Anthropology of human birth, Philadelphia, 1982, F.A. Davis Co.

Farris, L.: The American Indian. In Clark, A.L., editor: Culture/childbearing/health professionals, Philadelphia, 1978, F.A. Davis Co.

Flint, M.: Lockmi: an Indian midwife. In Kay, M.A., editor: Anthropology of human birth, Philadelphia, 1982, F.A. Davis Co.

Foster, G.M.: Humoral traces in United States folk medicine, Med. Anthropol. newsletter **10:**17, 1979.

Gallo, A.M., Edwards, J., and Vessey, J.: Little refugees with big needs, R.N. **43:**45, 1980.

Gordon, V.C., Matousek, I.M., and Lang, T.A.: Southeast Asian refugees: life in America, Am. J. Nurs. **80:**2031, 1980.

Griffith, S.: Childbearing and the concept of culture, J.O.G.N. Nurs. **11:**181, 1982.

Grosso, C., et al.: The Vietnamese American family . . . and grandma makes three, M.C.N. **6:**177, 1981.

Gussler, J.: Poor mothers and modern medicine in St. Kitts. In Kay, M.A., editor: Anthropology of human birth, Philadelphia, 1982, F.A. Davis Co.

Hollingsworth, A.O., Brown, L.P., and Brooten, D.A.: The refugees and childbearing: what to expect, R.N. **43:**45, 1980.

Horn, B.M.: Northwest coast Indians: the Muckleshoot. In Kay, M.A., editor: Anthropology of human birth, Philadelphia, 1982, F.A. Davis Co.

Johnson, S.M., and Snow, L.F.: The profile of some unplanned pregnancies. In Bauwens, E.E., editor: The anthropology of health, St. Louis, 1978, The C.V. Mosby Co.

Johnston, M.: Cultural variations in professional and parenting patterns, J.O.G.N. Nurs. **9:**9, 1980.

Kay, M.A., editor: Anthropology of human birth, Philadelphia, 1982, F.A. Davis Co.

Kendall, K.: Maternal and child care in an Iranian village. In Leininger, M., editor: Transcultural nursing '79, New York, 1979, Masson Publishing Co.

Kleinman, A., Eisenberg, L., and Good, B.: Clinical lessons from anthropologic and cross-cultural research, Ann. Intern. Med. **88:**251, 1978.

Kundstadter, P.: Do cultural differences make any difference? Choice points in medical systems available in Northwestern Thailand. In Kleinman, A., et al., editors: Culture and healing in Asian societies, Cambridge, Mass., 1978, Schenkman Publishing Co.

Lackey, C.J.: Pica—a nutritional anthropology concern. In Bauwens, E.E., editor: The anthropology of health, St. Louis, 1978, The C.V. Mosby Co.

Leiderman, P.H., Tulkin, S.R., and Rosenfeld, A.: Culture and infancy, New York, 1977, Academic Press, Inc.

Leininger, M.: Cultural diversities of health and nursing care, Nurs. Clin. North Am. **12:**5, 1977.

Leininger, M.: The Gadsup of New Guinea and early child-caring behaviors with nursing implications. In Leininger, M., editor: Transcultural nursing '79, New York, 1979, Masson Publishing Co.

Leyn, R.B.: The challenge of caring for child refugees from Southeast Asia, Am. J. Matern. Child Nurs. **3:**178, 1978.

Meleis, A.F., and Sorrell, L.: Arab American women and their birth experiences, M.C.N. **6:**171, 1981.

Minturn, L., and Lambert, W.W.: Mothers of six cultures, New York, 1964, John Wiley & Sons.

Morey, S., and Gilliam, O., editors: Respect for life, New York, 1974, Myrin Institute Books.

Moser, M.B.: Seri: from conception through infancy. In Kay, M.A., editor: Anthropology of human birth, Philadelphia, 1982, F.A. Davis Co.

Muecke, M.A.: Health care systems as socializing agents: childbearing the North Thai and Western ways, Soc. Sci. Med. **10:**377, 1976.

Munroe, R.L., and Munroe, R.H.: Cross-cultural human development, Monterey, Calif., 1975, Brooks/Cole Publishing Co.

Murillo-Rohde, I.: The Puerto Rican. Part II. In Clark, A., editor: Culture/childbearing/health professionals, Philadelphia, 1978, F.A. Davis Co.

Newton, N.: Childbearing in broad perspective: pregnancy, birth and the newborn baby, Boston, 1972, Delacorte Press.

Obeyesekere, G.: Pregnancy cravings (dola-duka) in relation to social structure and personality in a Sinhalese village, Am. Anthropol. **65:**323, 1963.

O'Brien, M.E.: Pragmatic survivalism behavior patterns affecting low-level wellness among minority group members, Adv. Nurs. Sci. **4:**13, 1982.

Okamoto, N.J.: The Japanese American. In Clark, A., editor: Culture/childbearing/health professionals, Philadelphia, 1978, F.A. Davis Co.

Parken, M.: Culture and preventive health care, J.O.G.N. Nurs. **7:**40, 1978.

Perry, D.S.: The umbilical cord: transcultural care and customs, J. Nurs. Midwife. **27:**25, 1982.

Pillsbury, B.L.K.: "Doing the month": confinement and convalescence of Chinese women after childbirth, Soc. Sci. Med. **12:**11, 1978.

Powers, B.A.: The use of orthodox and Black-American folk medicine, Adv. Nurs. Sci. **4:**35, 1982.

SantoPietro, M.C.: How to get through to a refugee patient, R.N. **44:**43, 1981.

Scott, C.S.: The theoretical significance of a sense of well-being for the delivery of gynecological health care. In Bauwens, E.E., editor: The anthropology of health, St. Louis, 1978, The C.V. Mosby Co.

Snow, L.: Folk medical beliefs and their implications for care of patients, Ann. Intern. Med. **81:**82, 1974.

Sodetani-Shibata, A.E.: The Japanese American. In Clark, A.L., editor: Culture and childrearing, Philadelphia, 1981, F.A. Davis Co.

Spradley, B.W.: Community health nursing, Boston, 1981, Little, Brown & Co.

Spradley, J.P.: The ethnographic interview, New York, 1979, Holt, Rinehart & Winston.

Stanton, M.E.: The myth of "natural" childbirth, the practices of people in traditional cultures, J. Nurs. Midwife. **24:**25, 1979.

Stark, S.: Mormon childbearing. In Kay, M.A., editor: Anthropology of human birth, Philadelphia, 1982, F.A. Davis Co.

Stern, P.N.: Solving problems of cross-cultural health teaching: the Filipino childbearing family, Image **13:**47, 1981.

Stern, P.N., Tilden, V.P., and Maxwell, E.K.: Culturally-induced stress during childbearing: the Filipino-American experience, Issues in Health Care of Women **2:**67, 1980.

Stringfellow, L.: The Vietnamese. In Clark, A., editor: Culture/childbearing/health professionals, Philadelphia, 1978, F.A. Davis Co.

Vermeer, D.E., and Frate, D.A.: Geophagy in a Mississippi county, Ann. Assoc. Am. Geographers **65:**414, 1975.

Vogel, G.: American Indian medicine, New York, 1973, Ballantine Books.

Weisner, T.S., and Gallimore, R.: My brother's keeper: child and sibling caretaking, Curr. Anthropol. **18:**169, 1977.

Wright, A.: Attitudes toward childbearing and menstruation among the Navajo. In Kay, M.A., editor: Anthropology of human birth, Philadelphia, 1982, F.A. Davis Co.

Zepeda, M.: Selected maternal infant care practices of Spanish-speaking women, J.O.G.N. Nurs. **11:**371, 1982.

9

The Family

- **Structure**
  - Nuclear family
  - Extended family
  - Expanded family
  - Communal family
  - Single-parent family
- **Family Dynamics and Functions**
- **Psychosocial Development**
  - Cognitive development
    - Sensorimotor stage (birth to 2 years)
    - Preoperational stage (2 to 7 years)
    - Concrete operations stage (7 to 11 years)
    - Formal operations stage (12 to 18 years)
  - Personality Development
    - Trust vs. mistrust (birth to 1 year)
    - Autonomy vs. shame and doubt (1 to 3 years)
    - Initiative vs. guilt (3 to 6 years)
    - Industry vs. inferiority (6 to 12 years)
    - Identity vs. identity confusion (12 to 18 years)
    - Intimacy vs. isolation (early adulthood)
    - Generativity vs. self-absorption (young and middle adulthood)
    - Ego integrity vs. despair (old age)
- **Family and Crisis**
  - Perception of an event
  - Coping mechanisms
  - Support systems
- **Summary**

Every society sets up organized patterns or institutions to ensure the introduction and socialization of new individuals and support for those individuals responsible for this vital function. The family represents one of these institutions and, in spite of the stresses and strains to which it now is subject, remains one of the most potent sources of support. It is recognized as the fundamental social unit because most people have more contact with this social group than with any other.

Families are striking in the variability and complexity of their family styles and may be defined in many ways. A sociologist, Burgess (1926), defined the family as a group of interacting personalities not bound necessarily by legal agreements. The family exists as long as the interactions continue. When individuals are asked to define a family, quite different definitions emerge.

- "God and me, Mommie, Daddy and J R, Nana and Grandpa, Grandma and Grandpa, and Great Nana—people who love you and you have fun together." Stacie (age 5)
- "A family is where everybody shares and cares for each other. A family is where there is love in the home. A family is where they go on vacations together. A family is where everybody shares with the work." Robert (age 15)
- "People sharing and striving together toward goals; caring and hurting for each other, and always unconditionally loving each other." Kristi (age 29, mother of two)

Regardless of how the family is defined the family unit is incomplete without the presence of an adult (Fig. 9.1). From an adult's perspective, the family can comprise persons of any age or sex bound by a blood or love relationship or both. From the child's perspective, the family is a set of relationships between his dependent self and one or more protective adults.

Because the family acts as a primary force in generating support for the pregnant woman, knowledge of this unit forms an essential part of the data basic to the nursing care plan. The nurse not only must identify the family but also must be aware of family dynamics in order to plan for the day-to-day care of families and to predict certain future events that may necessitate a modification of the care.

Fig. 9.1
Family configurations. Presence of an adult is basic to a family.

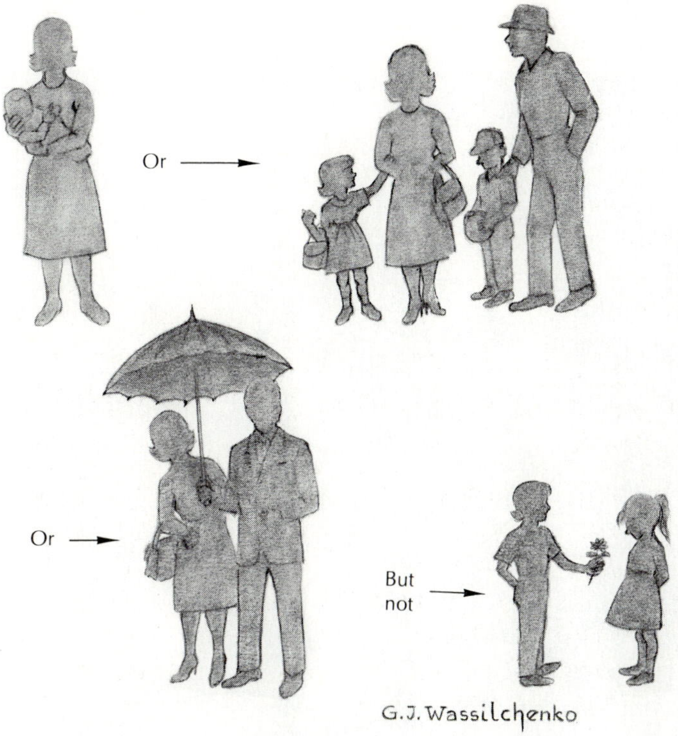

The family may be viewed from a number of perspectives, for example, family structure, family dynamics, growth of its members, and the ways the family deals with stress or crisis.

Structure

Identifying families by structure can provide insight into stresses that families may experience as they differ from the normative structure dictated by society.

NUCLEAR FAMILY

The nuclear family is the one that is considered "normal" in contemporary Western society, and in spite of all the talk of new life-styles it still represents 73% of all households (U.S. National Center for Health Statistics, 1982). This family group lives apart from either the husband's or wife's family of orientation. Parsons and Bales (1955) defined the nuclear family as follows:

> The members of the nuclear family, consisting of parents and their still dependent children, ordinarily occupy a separate dwelling not shared with members of the family of orientation of either spouse, and . . . this household is in the typical case economically independent, subsisting in the first instance from the occupational earnings of the husband-father.

The definition quoted above still represents the structure of most nuclear families; however, the percentage of two wage earners has risen dramatically over the last decade. In 1979 no fewer than 59.1% of married women with children aged 6 to 17 were in the labor force. According to Harris (1982) what caused the change was that by the early 1960s families were "finding it increasingly difficult to achieve or hold onto middle class standards of consumption for themselves and their children." The parents in this family are expected to play complementary roles of husband-wife and father-mother in giving emotional and physical support to each other and the offspring to accomplish family goals. Ideally this family institution provides for the care and socialization of children and social control for its members and is flexible enough to survive in an industrial world. Such a family can be perceived as "existing to fulfill the cultural dictates of its society as that society seeks to perpetuate itself," and in times of crisis the family can become an area for social change. The family is held together not so much by structure as by strong social bonds.

Fig. 9.2
Nuclear family in the 1920s.

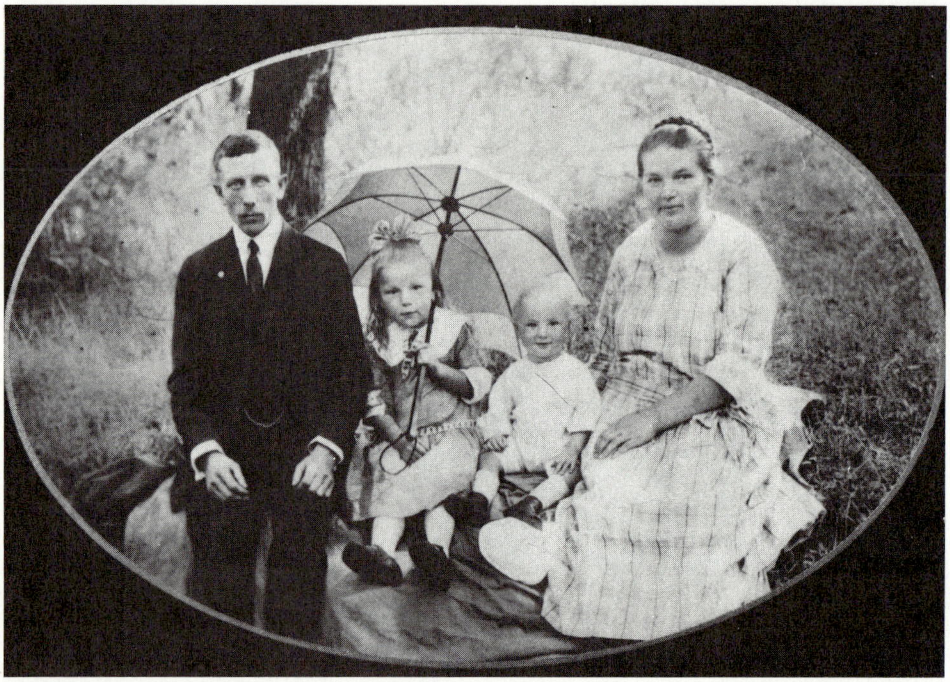

Fig. 9.3
Nuclear family in the 1980s.

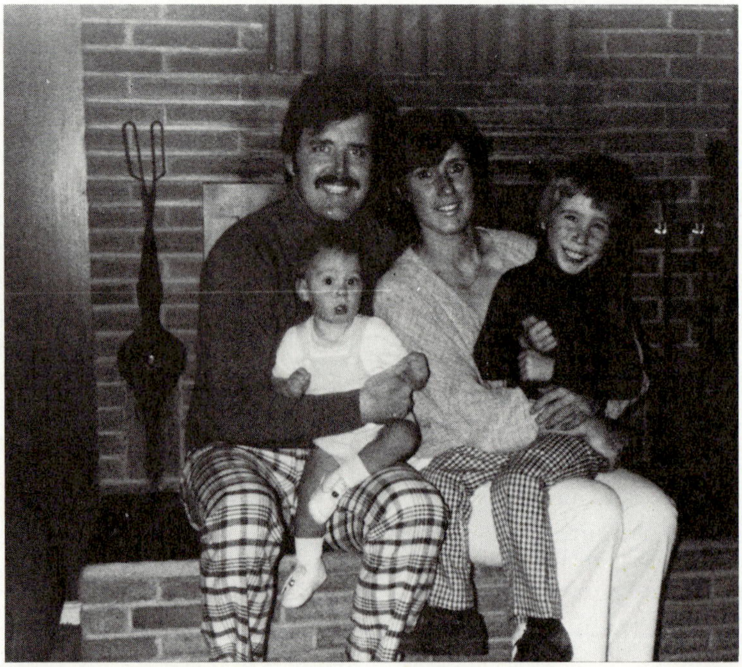

Fig. 9.4
A family develops by adding new members.

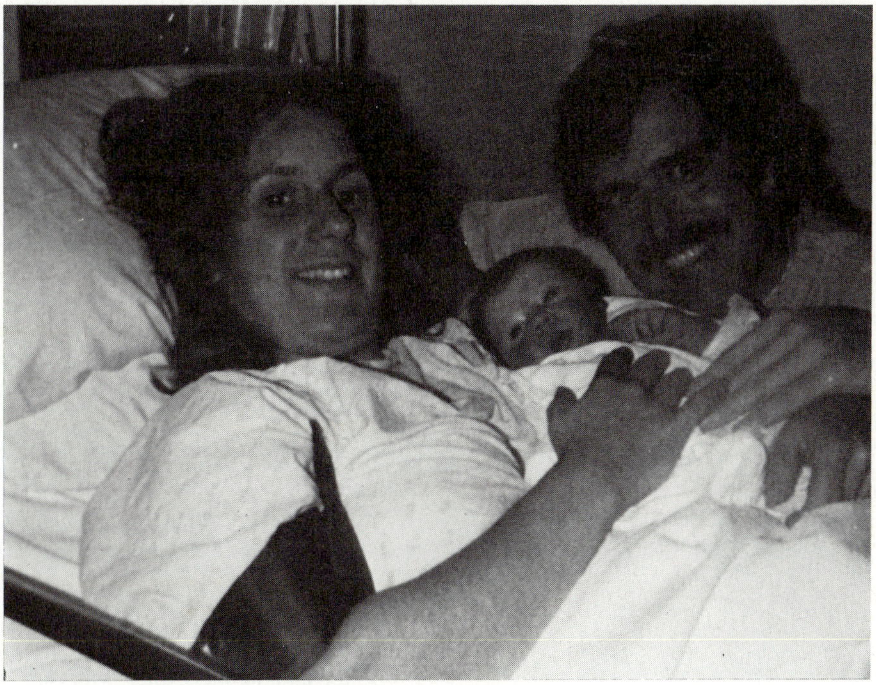

The nuclear family has been described as isolated, but there is increasing evidence that kinship ties to previous family structures are not broken. Frequently, sons and daughters, although established in their own nuclear family, remain in the same community as their families of orientation, and visiting relatives is part of their social life. The increased mobility of all segments of the population means that grandparents, sisters, uncles, cousins, and other relatives can be more readily available to the isolated family. One often hears new mothers say, "My mother is going to fly in to help me for a week or so." Friends and social groups (church, work) also provide support for the nuclear family and act in the role of absent families.

EXTENDED FAMILY

By definition the extended family includes three generations, is family centered, and through its kinship network provides supportive functions to all members. This family structure acts to prescribe the responsibilities and actions of family members. Some individuals regard the extended family as impeding the free mobility necessary in an industrialized society with its economic demands.

Fig. 9.5
An extended family.

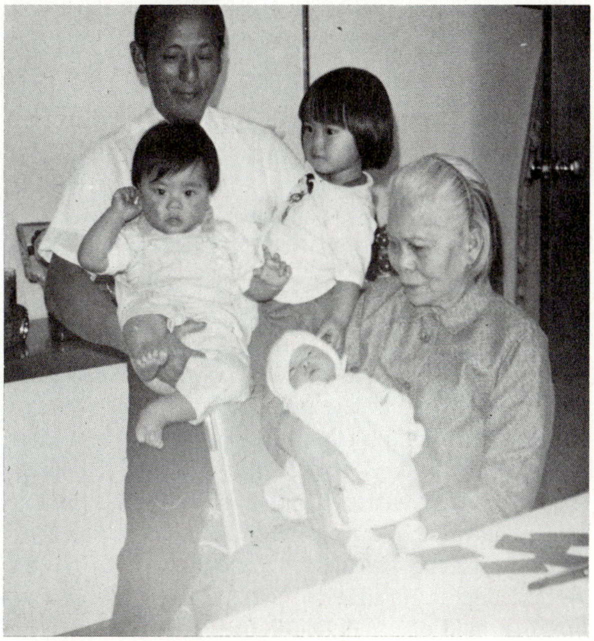

With the influx of new citizens from southeast Asia, the Caribbean, and Mexico, the extended family is again playing an important function. Until these peoples are assimilated, their family groups provide the primary source of identity through maintaining language and cultural identification, economic support through families "taking in" needy relatives and sharing food, shelter, and jobs, and emotional support through maintaining kinship ties.

Persons who have experienced such a family grouping may chafe at the bonds it creates but, when they leave, regret the absence of a wider sense of acceptance and recognition such a family provides. In changing to a more socially functional group, individuals from such "old-fashioned" families may need help in viewing the social structure as an alternative family to which they can legitimately turn for help and sustenance in times of stress. As pointed out by Anderson and Carter (1974): "Other institutions, such as social welfare services that provide income maintenance, health care, emotional support, and day care, have grown up to specialize in functions previously fulfilled by the extended family."

EXPANDED FAMILY

The expanded family resembles the extended family and the commune family. It consists of varying age groups, kinship groups, or unrelated family members that have become a part of the household. Boulding (1972) uses the term *expanded* to stress the similarities "between the biologically related extended family and the household as a voluntary association."

COMMUNAL FAMILY

Communal family groupings vary within the societal context, from the highly formalized structure of the Amish community in Lancaster County, Pa., to loosely knit groups such as are found in the Santa Cruz Mountains near Boulder Creek, Calif. These communities of persons are formed for specific ideologic or societal purposes and frequently are considered an alternative life-style for individuals feeling alienated from a predominantly economically oriented society. Some communes consist of nuclear groups living in an extended or expanded family community and are envisioned as persisting over time. Others may provide temporary shelter for single-parent families or may be a mixture of dual-parent and single-parent families. In some communes all parents participate in care-taking activities for all the children. In many of these groups the combination is a fluid one; individuals and families are free to come and go as their needs dictate. Just what the outcome of such communities will be with regard to the children is yet to be determined. For the groups that lack some permanence, the difficulties associated with the highly mobile nuclear family in seeking stability and continuity in social contacts may be perpetuated. Those communes composed solely of young adults and their children may be reproducing the ghettolike aspects of suburbia, with its limited contacts with diversified age, cultural, and economic groups.

SINGLE-PARENT FAMILY

The single-parent family is becoming an increasingly recognized structure in our society. The 1980 U.S. Census reveals that altogether 23.4% of all children aged 17 or under live in a family with a single parent, another relative, or a nonrelative. This was the situation for 17.3% of white children and 57.8% of black children. As many as 85% of babies born to young unmarried mothers were kept by their mothers, and another 7% were given to other family members, leaving only 8% for adoption. Of these single parents, 95% are women, most commonly under 25 years of age and in a low-income bracket. Of the group with children under 6 years of age, almost 55% of the single parents are working; and in the group with school-aged children, about 65% are working mothers.

The single-parent family may result from loss of a spouse by death, divorce, separation, or desertion; from the out-of-wedlock birth of a child; or from the adoption of a child. Whatever its cause, the single-parent family tends to be a vulnerable grouping economically and socially and, unless buttressed by a concerned society, may provide an unstable and deprived environment for the growth potential of children. Various researchers (e.g., Hetherington and co-workers, 1977) have commented on specific effects on children; for example, nutrition is often haphazard, communication and overt displays of affection are curtailed, and discipline is inconsistent. For many of the adults involved it represents a lonely existence in which decision making and other family tasks depend on a single adult. Public policy is beginning to reflect recognition of the facts that a pluralistic society necessarily produces pluralistic forms of the family and that high levels of marital instability are probably to be expected in modern society. As with individuals who have broken away from the support of extended families, these adults may need help in learning how to use community resources in developing or maintaining a satisfactory family life.

For other adults the single-parent family is a chosen life-style that provides a free and open system for development of parents and children. In these families, decision making and communication are seen as joint commitments between parent and child, and the parent-child relationship is considered a major source of life fulfillment.

Family Dynamics and Functions

Families work cooperatively to accomplish family goals and functions by family members assuming appropriate social roles. Social roles are learned in the family, the first social group, and are learned in pairs, for example, mother-father, parent-child, and brother-sister. A social role does not exist by itself but is designed to mesh with that of a role partner. By pairing roles social interactions can take place in an orderly, predictable manner—the roles are said to be *complementary*. Some families maintain a traditional pairing of roles, whereas other families have changed the behavior patterns to suit a change in family life-style. The process by which paired roles are brought into a new alignment is known as *negotiation*. The process of negotiation is essential if family equilibrium is to be maintained.

Over time the family develops protocols for *problem solving*, particularly with reference to decisions deemed important to the family, for example, having a baby, buying a house, sending only sons to college. The criteria used in making decisions are based on family values and attitudes concerning the appropriateness of the behavior of its various members and the moral, social, political, and economic events of the wider social system. The *power* to make critical decisions is conferred on a family member through tradition or negotiation. This power may be overt or covert and reflects the family's concepts of male or female dominance and cultural practices, social customs, and community norms.

Throughout everyday interactions the family, that changing, growing entity made up of individuals, develops and uses its own patterns of verbal and nonverbal *communication*. These patterns give insight into the feeling exchange within a family and act as reliable indicators of interpersonal functioning. Family members not only react to the communication or actions of other family members but interpret and define them. For example, a crying baby usually elicits care-taking activities on the part of the mother; however, she may interpret the crying as the baby's saying that she is not a good mother.

In assessing family dynamics nurses examine not only what is happening (the process) and who is doing what to whom (the praxis) but also the sense of feeling, or how people perceive what is being done, what it means to them, and how this meaning is expressed. Nurses cannot take family actions always at face value.

As the family progresses through its life cycle, beginning with the commitment of two individuals to share a life and ending with the dissolution of the family through death or other separations, it carries out certain *functions* for the well-being of its members. Although certain functions are relegated or emphasized more in one phase of the family's life cycle than another (e.g., the care and socialization of children are part of the childbearing and child-rearing phase of the cycle), many of the functions persist as critical for the continuing survival and progress of the family.

The family provides for the *nurturing* of the newborn and the gradual socialization of the growing child. It is the source of first relationships with others. The relationships children form with parents (or parenting persons) are the earliest and closest and persist throughout a lifetime. For better or for worse, parent-child relationships influence concepts of self-worth and the ability to form later relationships. The family and parents also interpret and mediate the child's perceptions of the complex outside world. The family provides the growing child with an identity that possesses both a past and a sense of the future.

The family from the time it is formed sets up boundaries between itself and the outside. Individuals are very conscious of those who are considered members of their family and those who rank as outsiders, those who do not have kinship status. Some families isolate themselves from the community. Others have a wide community network to help in times of stress. Although boundaries exist for every family, family members also set up channels (1) through which they mediate with external forces and attempt to protect the family from disturbances and (2) to ensure that the family receives its share of social resources.

Ideally the family provides a safe intimate environment for the biopsychosocial development of children and its adult members.

Psychosocial Development

Family members act as the first significant others for the child's cognitive and personality development (Table 9.1). As the child matures and ventures into the wider world, peer, educational, and other social groups provide environments that may promote or retard an individual's potential development. Concomitant with cognitive and personality development is the development of a person's sexuality. These spheres of development along with physical growth are interdependent processes that progress in an orderly manner to culmi-

Table 9.1
Summary of Cognitive and Personality Development

Stage	Significant Others	Cognitive Development	Personality Development
Infancy (birth to toddlerhood)	Maternal person	Sensorimotor: reflex → repetition → imitation	Trust vs. mistrust
	+		
Early childhood (2-7 yr)	Parental persons and other family members	Preoperational, direct experience (seeing, hearing, feeling) within a well-defined world	Initiative vs. guilt
	+		
Middle childhood (7-12 yr)	Neighborhood and school	Concrete thinking (not abstract), humanized (limited inductive reasoning)	Industry vs. inferiority
	+		
Adolescence (12-18 yr)	Peer groups and models of leadership	Formal thinking (deductive and abstract reasoning) may be limited up to 15 yr	Identity vs. identity confusion
	+		
Early adulthood	Partners in friendship, sex, competition, and cooperation	Formal thinking includes problem solving and separation of fantasy and fact	Intimacy and solidarity vs. isolation
	+		
Young and middle adulthood	Divided labor and shared household	Formal thinking includes problem solving and separation of fantasy and fact	Generativity vs. self-absorption
	+		
Later adulthood	Humankind, family, and friends	Formal thinking includes problem solving and separation of fantasy and fact	Ego integrity vs. despair

nate in the ultimate maturity, physical and psychologic, of an individual.

Cognitive and personality development are reviewed briefly in this chapter. See Chapter 6 for the physical components of sexuality and Chapter 7 for the psychosocial components.

COGNITIVE DEVELOPMENT

Cognition is the process by which an individual recognizes, accumulates, and organizes the knowledge of his world and uses that knowledge to solve problems and change behavior. The process begins with the *perception* or recognition of an event as a problem. Then the person searches his *memory* to see if the problem is similar to any past experience. Next he *generates ideas* as to a possible solution and finally he *evaluates* the accuracy of his choice. Obviously the richer the source of ideas, concepts, and past experiences used in successful resolution of problems, the greater the odds are for success in resolving present difficulties. Both a person's native ability and the quality of his environment are decisive factors in cognitive development.

Piaget (1950), a Swiss scientist, developed theories concerning how adult thought develops. He contends that two mental activities, *organization* and *adaptation,* continue throughout life. Adaptation derives from two complementary processes: *assimilation,* which is the absorption of new information interpreted in terms of existing structures, and *accommodation,* which is the changing of existing structure to fit new information. According to Piaget, cognitive development progresses in an orderly and sequential manner through four stages. The process is one of gradual evolution, with each stage building on the specific attainments of the previous one.

Sensorimotor stage (birth to 2 years). Reflex activity dominates the beginning of the sensorimotor stage and then gives way to repetitive and finally to imitative behavior. Any problem solving is the result of trial and error; however, a sense of "what causes what" begins to emerge. Discovery can be exciting as the child becomes aware of his own body as well as other familiar objects. Language begins, although it is limited to simple or double words, for example, "mine" or "me too." By the end of this period, an object can exist without being present. As a result, hide-and-seek is no longer frightening but becomes a pleasurable game.

However, the very young child may experience the absense of his mother for the birth of a sibling as an absolute loss. Hence, some hospitals are making efforts to reunite the mother and the older children as soon as possible after the birth to minimize the separation anxiety and the alienation experienced by the toddler (see Chapter 32).

Preoperational stage (2 to 7 years). During the preoperational stage the child is very self-centered or egocentric. As Whaley and Wong (1979) express it: "They are unable to see things from any perspective other than their own; they cannot see another's point of view, nor can they see any reason to do so." They live in a well-defined world made up of what they see, hear, or otherwise experience. Their thought processes are immature. Characteristically, children are "centered" in that they see one aspect of a situation but are unable to take any other factors into account. They are unaware of the transition process between one static state (the beginning) and another static state (the end). Also, their immature thinking does not involve reversibility. In problem solving adults often retrace their steps to see if their thinking has been logical, or they are able to see similarity in dissimilar-appearing objects by reversing their properties. By contrast, a child sees what he sees. Gradually his language becomes more complex, and single words progress to multiples and then to sentences. Children grow dramatically through direct experience and through an increasing ability to use symbolic communication.

Behavior appears to assume *cyclic trends* of equilibrium and disequilibrium. Awareness of these patterns can help parents assist siblings to assume new roles with the birth of a new brother or sister. For example, this age group (2 to 7 years) reacts in many different ways to the birth of a sibling. One 3-year-old child encouraged his mother to put the new baby "out with the garbage because we've seen enough of her." The 6- or 7-year-old child may respond by wanting to act like a second mother and boasting about the new baby to friends and teachers.

Concrete operations stage (7 to 11 years). The concrete operations stage is characterized by a gradual increase in problem-solving ability. The method of reasoning used is inductive, and solutions to problems are not based on abstractions but are derived from what has been perceived and categorized. The "social self" appears; these children are no longer exclusively egocentric but can relate to the feelings and thoughts of others. They are usually very responsive to the birth of a brother or sister. Since their world has horizons beyond the family boundaries, competition for parental interest is not so intense. They can assume care-taking activities and will take responsibility for the safety of younger children. Birth of handicapped siblings can be very traumatic to them because they cannot use logical reasoning to explain the event. These children need to be included with the parents in counseling efforts.

Some adolescents still operate in this concrete, limited, but humanized sphere, at least until the age of 15 years. This must be kept in mind when helping them adjust to being pregnant. They are unable to view the tasks and responsibilities of parenthood beyond the present and immediate future, although they may like the idea of a baby (see Chapter 38).

Formal operations stage (12 to 18 years). Although the progress may be erratic and sometimes stormy, by the end of the formal operations stage, individuals can consider hypotheses and analyze scientifically. They can deduce conclusions from a set of observations, consider alternatives, and assess risks. In short, they are capable of reasoning logically by using abstractions and assuming responsibility for the actions generated as solutions to their problems.

Piaget noted that formal thinking involves two major dimensions: the use of propositional logic, that is, the ability to think about a problem, and by doing so rearrange aspects of it until clarity is realized; and the ability to separate fantasy from fact.

PERSONALITY DEVELOPMENT

Personality development is a lifelong process that occurs as an individual interacts with his environment. Erikson's theory of personality development (1967) views the process as one occurring in stages, with each stage dependent on the one before and each stage focusing on a central problem. These problems are envisioned as conflicts between opposites, for example, trust vs. mistrust. As each conflict is resolved or mastered to a greater or lesser degree, the individual is ready to move to the next level. Unresolved conflicts can hamper a person's further development and may persist as residuals throughout life.

Trust vs. mistrust (birth to 1 year). The development of basic trust comes in response to being loved and cared for by a giving and concerned adult. This is a period of "taking in" for the infant; he needs nurturing, security, and a feeling of continuity (see Chapter 27). If such care makes up the bulk of his experiences, trust takes precedence over mistrust, and a sense of trust will be reflected in his responses to others for the rest of his life.

Autonomy vs. shame and doubt (1 to 3 years). The development of a sense of autonomy comes with the gradual unfolding of the child's control of his own body, his self, and persons in his environment. If those who provide for this care applaud his efforts toward self-control and increasing his motor skills and, conversely, accept with minimal comment his failure, feelings of self-doubt and shame will not negate the good feelings about himself. Success brings a beginning of internalized controls and a sense of power to function.

Initiative vs. guilt (3 to 6 years). The stage of initiative vs. guilt ushers in an active exploratory phase in the child's development. He learns much from his world by playing games and asking endless questions. He shows more evidence of being guided by an inner conscience: the "parent" has been increasingly internalized. This is a time for fears and phobias. The child's developmental tasks revolve around directing his efforts toward purposeful activity and achieving a balance between *daring* and *caution*.

Industry vs. inferiority (6 to 12 years). During the period of industry vs. inferiority, the child develops a sense of being a productive worker. He needs opportunities to complete activities and be rewarded for his efforts. Introduction to formalized schooling begins, and success or failure in this respect can set the stage for later career choice. Social conditioning is more relative to male and female roles.

Identity vs. identity confusion (12 to 18 years). The period of adolescence comes after a period of relative calm. In this transition period between childhood and adulthood, the adolescent has certain tasks to perform with reference to establishing sexual roles, selecting an occupation, becoming independent of the family, and acquiring a social rather than an egocentric response to individuals and the wider society. He must also accept a new body image that includes the ability to reproduce. Successful mastery of these tasks helps the adolescent develop a sense of self and identity that both he and society can accept. With this sense comes the ability for devotion and fidelity. Without it the individual knows not "who he is" or "where he is going" and identity confusion persists.

Intimacy vs. isolation (early adulthood). Once a person has a sense of identity he can move toward intimate relationships with others. This can be expressed on a personal level as friendship, sexual intimacy, or the intimacy of parent-child relationships. On a social level love of fellow human beings is expressed in concern for the welfare of others not part of one's primary group. Without this sense of freedom to love and be loved, an individual is isolated and a sense of alienation from family, friends, and society may occur.

Generativity vs. self-absorption (young and middle adulthood). It is during the period of generativity vs. self-absorption that individuals are much concerned with creating the next generation and providing the necessary nurturing and care taking that the next generation requires. Preparation for assuming the role of parent, participating in the birth of children, and adapting to the reality of parenthood are the tasks many assume. Others may become surrogate parents in a myriad of ways: adopting children, being friends to adolescents, teaching, or nursing. Whatever form this involvement of the self with others takes, it acts to regulate self-absorption with its consequent narrowing and turning inward of the personality. With growth of the personality as it seeks balance between commitment to self and commitment to others comes a sense of productiveness and fulfillment.

Ego integrity vs. despair (old age). Emphasis on maintaining productivity and involvement in the welfare of others is increasing the satisfaction of those in the old age group. (In the United States old age arbitrarily begins at 65 years.) However, eventually there are limitations imposed by physical and mental ability, and the sphere of activity is curtailed. As individuals are confronted with this curtailment, acceptance must be balanced against despair. Wisdom and a sense of satisfaction with what has been accomplished come to those who are successful in the search for personal meaning.

Family and Crisis

No family exists in a nonstress environment whether the stress arises internally or externally to the family system. Although many families cope with stress, the situation may become acute and take on the characteristics of a crisis. Crisis may be defined as a disturbance of habit, a disruption in a family's or an individual's usual means of maintaining control over a situation. If faced with a crisis, the family or individual attempts to resolve the crisis using customary values and behaviors.

Caplan (1959), one of the developers of crisis intervention, maintains that the successful resolution of a crisis very often depends on the client's support system. A client's support system may include his family, his friends, or significant others and his environment. If, for example, a client's support system is strong, only minimal intervention may be necessary to resolve the crisis situation and assist the client's recovery. If the client's support system is not strong, disorganization may occur and the client may not recover.

One of the goals of crisis intervention is that a client will learn new ways of dealing with conflict or problems. Although the client may have sought help for one specific problem, the strategies learned may be applied to future problems.

Aguilera and Messick (1978) have devised a stratagem for assessing a family's or an individual's potential or actual response to a crisis (Fig. 9.6). They maintain

Fig. 9.6
Paradigm of effect of balancing factors in stressful event. (From Aguilera, D., and Messick, J.: Crisis intervention: theory and methodology, ed. 4, St. Louis, 1982, The C.V. Mosby Co.)

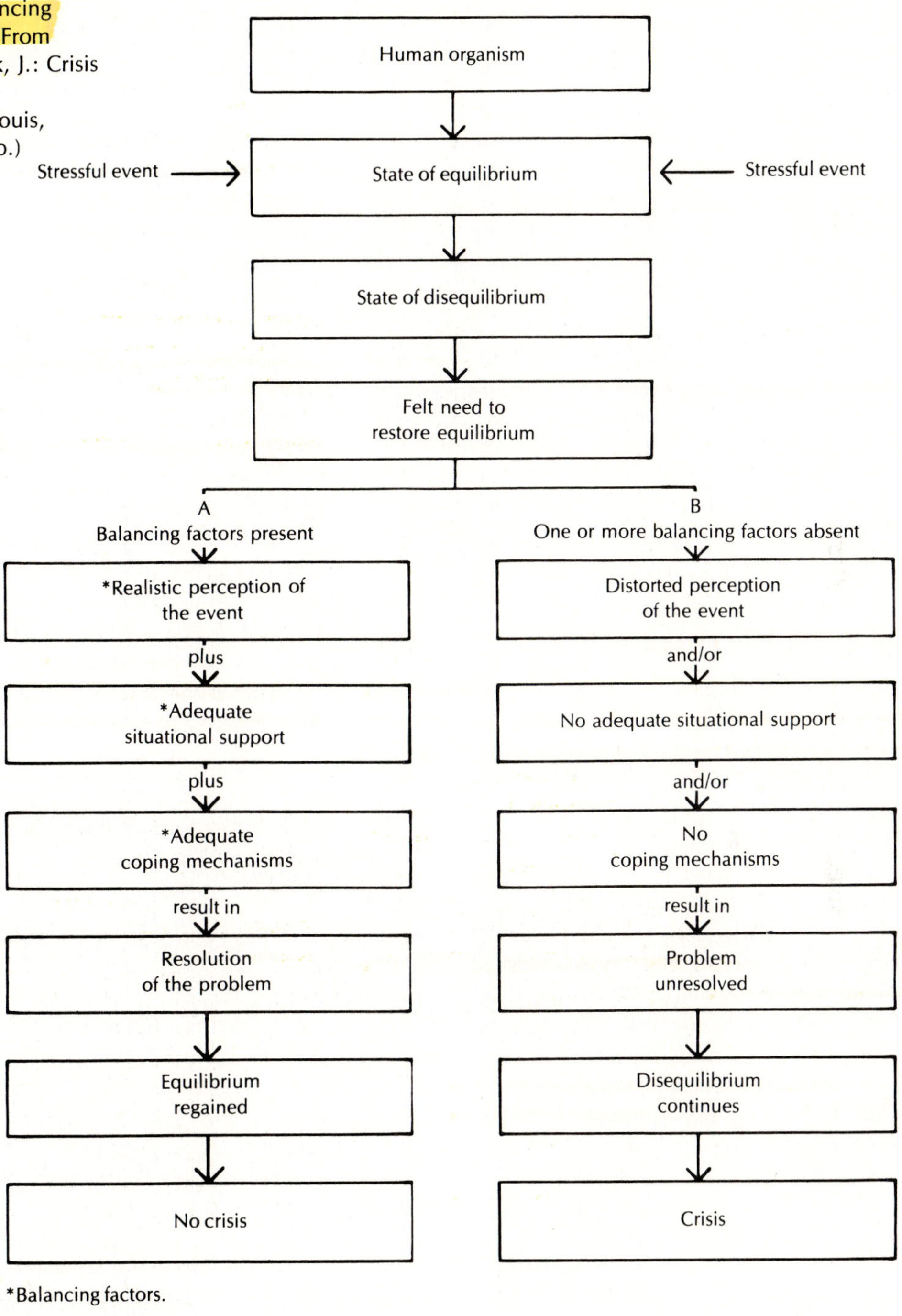

that there are three key areas or components to investigate: the client's perception of the crisis event, the client's coping mechanisms, and the client's support system. The interplay between these three areas is critical for the outcome or resolution of a problem. A brief discussion of each of the three areas follows.

PERCEPTION OF AN EVENT

What one person considers a crisis may or may not be perceived as a crisis by someone else. Such factors as *age* and *previous experience* can alter perception; for example, an event viewed as a crisis by an adolescent may not be seen as a crisis by a 30-year-old individual.

Emotional states, anxiety, or hostility may color a person's perception of a happening. The highly anxious young mother of a first-born child may become disorganized by her infant's crying while a mother of four may accept the crying as a normal annoyance but nothing to worry about. Previous experience may also be a factor in determining what event is considered a crisis. For example, women who experience hunger and who have little understanding of nutrition accept their daily prenatal diet without questioning the fact that it is lacking in essential nutrients that safeguard their health and that of the developing child.

Nursing intervention relative to a client's perception of a crisis-provoking event may be limited to helping the client state "what the problem is." If, however, the event can have a negative effect on the client, the infant, or the family, more intervention is indicated. For example, for the women with inadequate prenatal diets, the nurse would need to include efforts to teach the fundamentals of nutrition as well as to utilize community resources to provide the necessary nutrients.

COPING MECHANISMS

Coping mechanisms may be defined as patterns of behavior that persons or families have developed for dealing with threats to their sense of well-being. The infant learns that by crying his mother comes and attends to his needs. Crying acts as a coping mechanism for the baby. As individuals grow older, coping behavior becomes more complex and habitual. For some individuals a characteristic response to a perceived threat may be to "charge ahead" while others "beat a hasty retreat." Such habitual responses may be incorporated into the unconscious, and it may require considerable effort to bring such responses into conscious focus to enable persons to change or adapt them. Nurses may use the values clarification process with clients (as well as with themselves) to increase self-awareness. Nurses have developed parent education programs to provide women and men with mechanisms to cope with the stress of labor and to provide parents with knowledge of their infants' needs and child care activities so that they are better able to cope with the changing needs of a growing child.

SUPPORT SYSTEMS

Support systems refer to the support that people may expect from others in their environment during a time of crisis. These others as noted earlier include members of the immediate family, friends, and neighbors. In times of stress, those persons closest to an individual become necessary to one's well-being. An example of this occurred after the delivery of an apparently normal infant. The father and mother were excited and happy and were waiting to hear the baby's first cry. When the baby did not cry, the parents became noticeably upset. The health team initiated resuscitation measures for the baby, and their attention, interest, and concern were focused on the infant. The parents seemed to huddle together in their response to the threat of losing their infant. The husband clasped his wife's hand and shoulder as they murmured to each other. Then the mother was observed to reach out and take a fold of the nurse's uniform in her fingers, thus establishing a link from the father and mother through the nurse to the baby. When queried about her actions later, the mother remarked, "We needed to be in touch with him; it was all we could do to help."

Other persons who function as support systems are health personnel, or "community caretakers" (Caplan, 1959). Community caretakers are persons located in the various agencies that represent the organized health resources of a community. Because these individuals are knowledgeable and experienced, they may be able to assist those unable to handle crises on their own or with the help of family and friends. The assistance may take the form of being supportive (i.e., teaching or counseling) or of knowing the procedures for enlisting the help of other community agencies.

Summary

The family represents a primary social group that both influences and is influenced by other persons and institutions. Regardless of the form it assumes or the society in which the family is found, it possesses enduring characteristics that have far-reaching personal and societal effects. Birth of children represents one of the most important events in the life of a family. Birth and the subsequent care of the children require parental intellectual and psychologic maturity and account for periods of crisis in a family.

Maternity nurses come in intimate contact with the family. They are present at the birth of children (i.e., the growth period of the family) and can provide support for the adults as they undertake active parenting roles. Nurses' knowledge of human psychosocial development assists them in helping parents view their children in a reasonable context and establishes appropriate criteria for children's behavior. Nurses' knowledge of the family's reactions to crisis prompts a more rational assessment of the family's ability to withstand stress. The maternity nurse may use this unique relationship with a family to promote birth as a family-centered happening with great potential for growth of all participating persons.

References and Readings

Aguilera, D., and Messick, J.: Crisis intervention: theory and methodology, ed. 3, St. Louis, 1978, The C.V. Mosby Co.

Aldous, J.: Family careers and developmental change in families, New York, 1978, John Wiley & Sons.

Anderson, R., and Carter, J.: Human behavior in the social environment, Chicago, 1974, Aldine Publishing Co.

Aries, P.: Centuries of childhood, London, 1962, Jonathan Cape.

Bibb, B.: The effectiveness of non-physicians as providers of family planning services, J.O.G.N. Nurs. **8**(3):137, 1979.

Bobak, I.: Self-image: a universal concern of women becoming mothers, C.N.A. Bull. **9**:7, April 1969.

Bolton, F.: The pregnant adolescent: problems of premature parenthood, Beverly Hills, Calif., 1980, Sage Publications.

Boulding, E.: The family as an agent of social change, The Futurist **6**:186, Oct. 1972.

Bower, F., and Jacobson, M.: Family theories: frameworks for nursing practice. In Archer, S., and Fleshman, R., editors: Community health nursing: patterns and practice, Scituate, Mass., 1978, Duxbury Press.

Bronfenbrenner, U.: The changing American family. Presentation at the meeting of the Society for Research in Child Development. In Hetherington, E., and Parke, E., editors: Contemporary reading in child psychology, New York, 1977, McGraw-Hill Book Co.

Burgess, E.W.: The family as a unit of interacting personalities, The Family **7**:3, March 1926.

Caplan, G.: Concepts of mental health and consultation, Washington, D.C., 1959, Childrens Bureau, U.S. Department of Health, Education and Welfare.

Corfman, E.: Introduction and overview. NIMH Science Monograph 1, Rockville, Md., 1982, National Institute of Mental Health, Division of Scientific and Public Information.

Dougherty, S.A.: Single adoptive mothers and their children, Social Work **23**:311, July 1978.

Duhl, F.R.: Grief. Paper presented to the Ohio League for Nursing Convention, Columbus, Ohio, 1964.

Duvall, E.R.: Family development, ed. 2, Philadelphia, 1978, J.B. Lippincott Co.

Dyer, W.: Working with groups. In Reinhardt, A., and Quinn, M., editors: Family-centered community nursing, St. Louis, 1973, The C.V. Mosby Co.

Erikson, E.: Identity and the life cycle; selected papers. In Psychological issues, New York, 1959, International Universities Press.

Erikson, E.: Childhood and society, ed. 2, New York, 1967, W.W. Norton & Co.

Erikson, E.: Identity: youth and crisis, New York, 1968, W.W. Norton & Co.

Fromer, M.: Community health care and the nursing process, St. Louis, 1979, The C.V. Mosby Co.

Goode, W.J.: The family, Englewood Cliffs, N.J., 1964, Prentice-Hall, Inc.

Harris, M.: American now: The anthropology of a changing culture, New York, 1982, Simon & Schuster.

Hays, W.: Theorists and theoretical frameworks identified by sociologists, J. Marriage Family, p. 50, Feb. 1977.

Hearn, G., editor: The general systems approach: contributions toward a holistic conception of social work, New York, 1969, Council of Social Work Education.

Heiss, J.: Family roles and interaction, Chicago, 1968, Rand McNally & Co.

Hetherington, E., Cox, M., and Cox, R.: Beyond father absence: conceptualization of effects of divorce. In Hetherington, E., and Parke, R., editors: Contemporary readings in child psychology, New York, 1977, McGraw-Hill Book Co.

Hill, R.: Interdisciplinary workshop on marriage and family research, Marriage and Family Living **13**:13, Feb. 1951.

Hill, R., and Hansen, D.: The identification of conceptual frameworks used in family study, Marriage and Family Living **22**:311, Nov. 1960.

Household and family characteristics. Bureau of the Census, Current Population Reports Series P-20, no. 366, Washington, D.C., Sept. 1981, U.S. Government Printing Office.

Johnston, M.: Cultural variations in professional and parenting patterns, J.O.G.N. Nurs., vol. 9, Jan.-Feb. 1980.

Jourard, S.: The transparent self, New York, 1964, Van Nostrand Reinhold Co.

Kanter, R.M.: Communes, Psychology Today **4**:2, July 1970.

Kübler-Ross, E.: On death and dying, New York, 1969, Macmillan Publishing Co., Inc.

LaRossa, R.: Conflict and power in marriage. Expecting the first child, Beverly Hills, Calif., 1977, Sage Publications.

Leininger, M.: About interdisciplinary health education for the future, Nurs. Outlook **19**:791, 1971.

Lenero-Otero, L.: Beyond the nuclear family. Model of cross-cultural perspectives, Beverly Hills, Calif., 1977, Sage Publications.

Lindeman, E.: Symptomatology and management of acute grief, AM. J. Psychol. **101**:141, 1944.

Lovell, M., et al.: Combating myth: a conceptual framework for analyzing the stress of motherhood, Adv. Nurs. Sci. **1**(4), July 1979.

Lowrey, G.H.: Growth and development of children, Chicago, 1978, Year Book Medical Publishers.

Luft, J.: Group processes: an introduction to group dynamics, ed. 2, Palo Alto, Calif., 1970, National Press Books.

Lysought, J.: An abstract for action: National Commission for the Study of Nursing and Nursing Education, New York, 1971, McGraw-Hill Book Co.

Malinowski, B.: The dynamics of cultural change, New Haven, Conn., 1945, Yale University Press.

Marital status and living arrangements, Bureau of the Census, Current Population Reports Series P-20, no. 365, Washington, D.C., Oct. 1981, U.S. Government Printing Office.

Mead, G.H.: Mind, self and society, Chicago, 1934, The University of Chicago Press.

Mead, M.: Understanding cultural patterns, Nurs. Outlook **4**:260, 1956.

Meglen, M., and Burst, H.: Nurse-midwives make a difference, Nurs. Outlook **22**:386, 1974.

Money income and poverty status of families and persons, Bureau of the Census, Current Population Reports Series P-60, no. 127, Washington, D.C., Aug. 1981, U.S. Government Printing Office.

Morris, N., Hatch, M., and Chapman, S.: Alienation: a deterrent to well-child supervision, Am. J. Pub. Health **56**:874, 1966.

Newman, B., and Newman, R.: Development through life, Homewood, Ill., 1975, The Dorsey Press.

Nye, F.I., et al.: Role structure and analysis of the family. Library of social research, vol. 24, Beverly Hills, Calif. 1976, Sage Publications.

Otto, H.: A framework for assessing family strengths. In

Reinhardt, M., and Quinn, A., editors: Family-centered community nursing, St. Louis, 1980, The C.V. Mosby Co.
Parsons, T., and Bales, R.: Family socialization and interaction, New York, 1955, The Free Press.
Perkins, M.R.: Does availability of health services ensure their use, Nurs. Outlook **22:**496, 1974.
Phillips, C., and Anzalone, J.: Fathering: participation in labor and birth, St. Louis, 1982, The C.V. Mosby Co.
Piaget, J.: The psychology of intelligence, London, 1950, Routledge and Kegan Paul Ltd.
Rose, A.: Human behaviors and social processes: an interactional approach, Boston, 1962, Houghton Mifflin Co.
Ross, A.S., Kagan, J., and Hareven, T.K., editors: The family, New York, 1978, W.W. Norton & Co.
Rubin, R.: Cognitive style in pregnancy, Am. J. Nurs. **70:**502, 1970.
Satir, V.: Conjoint family therapy, Palo Alto, Calif., 1967, Science & Behavior Books.
Schulman, S., and Smith, A.: The concept of health among Spanish-speaking villagers of New Mexico and Colorado, J. Health Hum. Behav. **4:**226, Winter 1963.
Schvaneveldt, J.: The international framework in the study of the family. In Nye, F.A., and Bernardo, F.M., editors: Emerging conceptual frameworks in family analysis, New York, 1966, MacMillan Publishing Co., Inc.
Smoyak, S.: Cultural incongruence: the effect on nurses' perception, Nurs. Forum **7:**234, 1968.
Stinnett, N., and Birdsong, C.W.: The family and alternate life styles, Chicago, 1978, Nelson-Hall Co.
Stryker, S.: Symbolic interaction as an approach to family research, Marriage and Family Living **21:**111, May 1959.
Sugerman, M.: Toward really improving the outcome of pregnancy. What you can do, Birth Fam. J. **6:**2, Summer 1979.
U.S. National Center for Health Statistics, U.S. Department of Commerce, Bureau of the Census, Washington, D.C., 1982, The Center.
Whaley, L., and Wong, D.: Nursing care of infants and children, St. Louis, 1979, The C.V. Mosby Co.
Williams, F.: Intervention in maturational crisis. In Hall, J., and Weaver, J.B., editors: Nursing of families in crisis, Philadelphia, 1974, J.B. Lippincott Co.

10

Genetics

- Biologic Basis of Inheritance
  - Chromosomes
  - Cell division
    - Gametogenesis
- Genes in Families
  - Disorders caused by a single gene
    - Autosomal-dominant inheritance
    - Autosomal-recessive inheritance
    - X-linked inheritance
- Chromosomal Aberrations
  - Disorders of cell division
    - Nondisjunction
    - Translocation
  - Disorders caused by chromosomal aberrations
    - Autosomal aberrations
    - Aberrations of sex chromosomes
- Multifactorial Inheritance

  Detection of Genetic Disease
  - Preconceptional detection
  - Prenatal detection
    - Amniocentesis
    - Ultrasonography
    - Roentgenography
    - Fetoscopy (amnioscopy)
  - Postdelivery detection
    - Biochemical tests
    - Cytologic studies
    - Dermatoglyphics
    - Other postdelivery diagnostic studies
- Genetic Counseling
  - Clients
  - Goals of counseling
  - Counseling process
    - Counseling services
  - Role of the nurse

Biologic Basis of Inheritance

The biologic and behavioral characteristics of each human being are determined by the action of thousands of minute particles of hereditary material, the *genes*. The genes are composed of tiny segments of *deoxyribonucleic acid (DNA)*, which enables them to duplicate themselves exactly during cell division. Each body cell contains two sets of genes arranged in a line to form larger structures, the *chromosomes*, within the cell nucleus. Each cell nucleus contains two sets of chromosomes consisting of two matching sets of genes, one set obtained from each parent during the process of fertilization (see p. 145). When a pair of genes are alike and produce the same effect they are called *homozygous*; when they are not alike and produce different effects they are said to be *heterozygous* (Fig. 10.1).

Sometimes a gene will change, causing a *mutation*. Mutations can occur for no apparent reason or can be produced by some process (e.g., radiation or drugs). They can take the form of a change in a chromosome or, more frequently, a change in a gene. Mutations are a rare occurrence, but when a mutation takes place the new gene is passed on unchanged to future generations.

CHROMOSOMES

Chromosomes cannot be seen except under a microscope. For analysis they are stained, magnified, and photographed; then each individual chromosome is cut out and arranged in a *karyotype* according to size and shape. They appear as structures with either an X or a Y shape. Fig. 10.2 illustrates the chromosomes in a body cell.

The hoped-for and expected outcome of every wanted pregnancy is a normal infant, but delivery of a normal infant depends on numerous factors, both hereditary and environmental. Probably all human characteristics have a genetic component. Some diseases are produced through the action of a single gene or the combined action of many genes inherited from the parents; others are the result of the action of the environ-

Fig. 10.1
Genes on a pair of chromosomes illustrating like and unlike gene pairs. (From Whaley, L.F.: Understanding inherited disorders, St. Louis, 1974, The C.V. Mosby Co.)

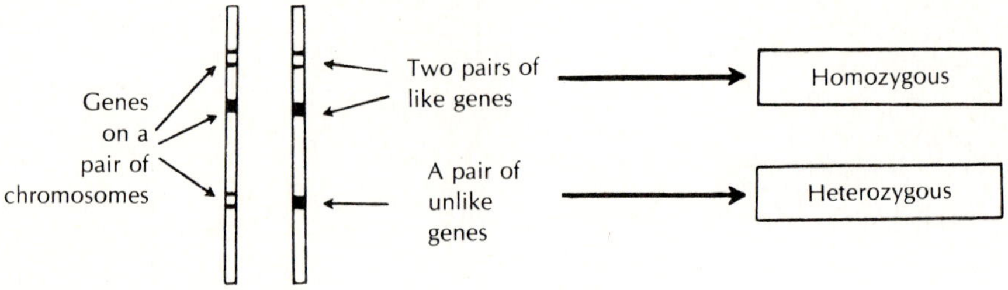

Fig. 10.2
Male chromosomes during cell division. **A,** Example of photomicrograph. **B,** Chromosomes arranged in karyotype. (From Whaley, L.F.: Understanding inherited disorders, St. Louis, 1974, The C.V. Mosby Co.)

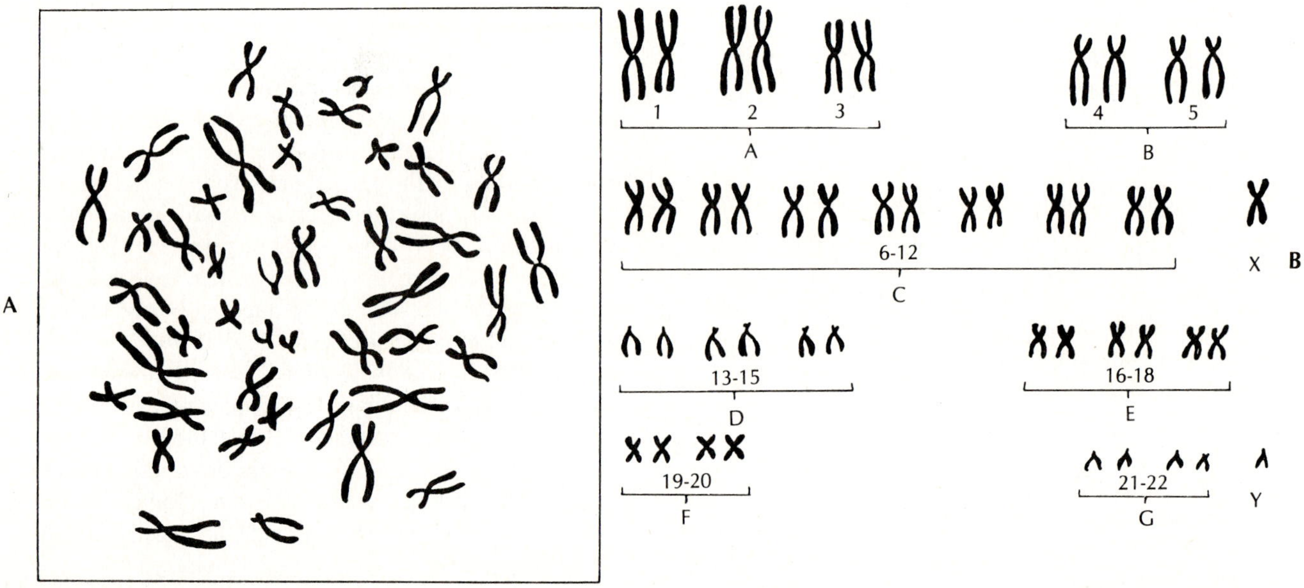

ment on the genes. Sometimes the genetic component is obvious; other times it is hidden. Many disorders are apparent at birth; others do not become apparent for days, weeks, months, or even years. A disease or disorder that can be passed from generation to generation is termed *genetic* or *hereditary*. A *congenital* disorder is one that is present at birth and can be caused by genetic factors, environmental factors, or both.

Genetic disorders can be divided into three broad categories:

1. Diseases that are caused by a *single gene* and occur in families according to the basic patterns of inheritance (see p. 145). Examples include cystic fibrosis, hemophilia, and achondroplastic dwarfism.
2. Disorders caused by *chromosomal aberrations*, in which there is a change in a chromosome (see p. 147). Examples are Down's, Turner's, Klinefelter's, and cri du chat syndromes.
3. Common conditions that are *multifactorial*. These may be the result of many genes *(polygenic)* or a combination of both genetic and environmental factors. Examples include diabetes mellitus, pyloric stenosis, and common birth defects.

To provide accurate and meaningful nursing care in the identification, treatment, and prevention of disease in which there is a genetic element, nurses need an understanding of basic genetic concepts and the ways in which hereditary factors interact with the constantly changing environment. This includes knowledge of the biologic basis of heredity, basic laws of inheritance, and some understanding of the way in which genes produce their effect in the individual.

The normal chromosomal number in the body (so-

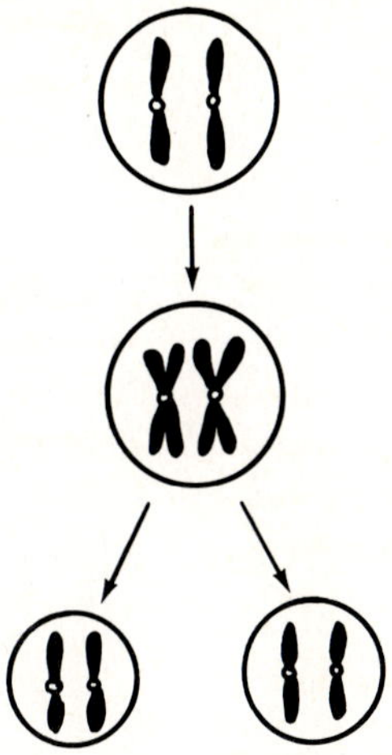

Fig. 10.3
Mitosis in somatic cell. (From Whaley, L.F., and Wong, D.L.: Nursing care of infants and children, St. Louis, 1979, The C.V. Mosby Co.)

Fig. 10.4
Process of meiosis. A premeiotic germ cell with two sets of chromosomes forms four germ cells, each with single set of chromosomes. Two alternative arrangements of chromosome pairs on first meiotic spindle are diagrammed. (From Sandberg, E.C.: Synopsis of obstetrics, ed. 10, St. Louis, 1978, The C.V. Mosby Co.)

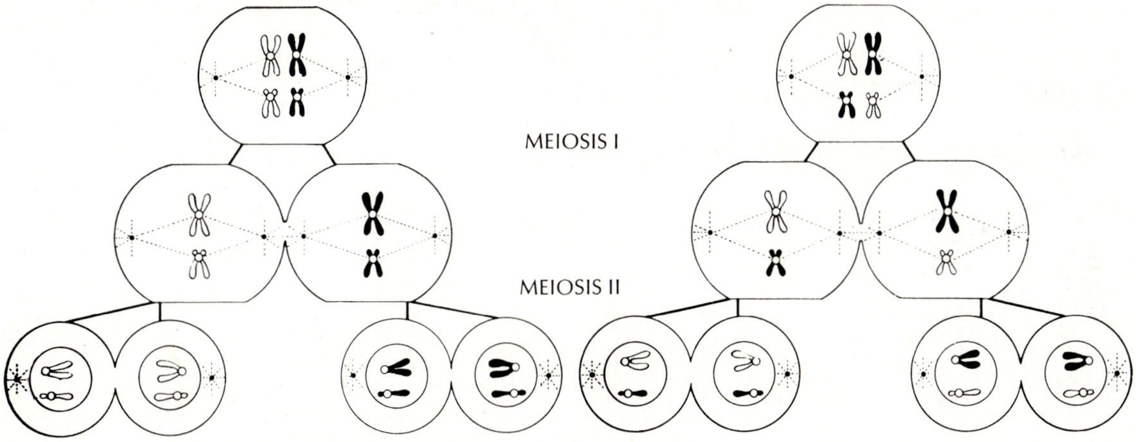

matic) cells of humans is 46. This number consists of 22 pairs of *autosomes* plus one pair of *sex chromosomes,* the X (female) and Y (male) chromosomes. Both sex chromosomes are alike in the female (XX) but are different in the male (XY). The reproductive cells contain only one set of chromosomes, or half the total number contained in body cells; that is, 11 autosomes and 1 sex chromosome. In female cells the sex chromosome is always an X; the male cell may contain either X or Y. The way in which the cells divide and distribute their chromosomes is basic to the understanding of heredity.

CELL DIVISION

Somatic cells divide by the process of *mitosis,* in which the cell, including the chromosomes, divides and is distributed equally to the two newly formed cells. Each new cell contains the same number of chromosomes as the original cell. This is sometimes called *equational division* (Fig. 10.3).

The process of cell division in the reproductive cells *(germ cells, gametes)* is such that the total number of chromosomes is reduced by half. Formation of germ cells, or *gametogenesis,* takes place in the male and female gonads by the processes of *meiosis* and *reduction division.* Meiotic division consists of two divisions, one following the other. In the *first* division the pairs of chromosomes are randomly separated from each other to form two nonidentical cells containing 23 chromosomes. In the *second* meiotic division the individual chromosomes split to form two identical cells, each with the same number of chromosomes (23) (Fig. 10.4). When the male and female gametes, the ovum and sperm, unite at fertilization, the original number (46) is restored and cell division in the fertilized cell continues by the process of mitosis.

Gametogenesis. Gametogenesis takes place by meiotic division, but the process by which the mature ovum is formed *(oogenesis)* differs in several ways from formation of mature sperm *(spermatogenesis)*. Meiosis in the male gonad is a continuous process that begins about the time of puberty and extends until old age. A primitive germ cell (spermatogonia) matures to form a *primary spermatocyte,* which divides to form two *secondary spermatocytes,* each with half the original chromosomes. These subsequently divide equally to form the spermatids, which gradually change to form active, motile *spermatozoa* (Fig. 10.5,*A*).

Unlike spermatogenesis, the process of meiosis in the ovaries is not a continuous process. Oogenesis begins during intrauterine life, and the female gametes have already enlarged and developed into *primary oocytes* at the time of birth. These primary oocytes (approximately 500,000 in number) have begun the first meiotic division but remain at this stage until, one at a time each month, they are released from the oocyte. When the primary oocyte divides, there is unequal division of the

Fig. 10.5
Gametogenesis. **A,** Spermatogenesis produces four gametes. **B,** Oogenesis results in only one ovum. (From Whaley, L.F., and Wong, D.L.: Nursing care of infants and children, St. Louis, 1979, The C.V. Mosby Co.)

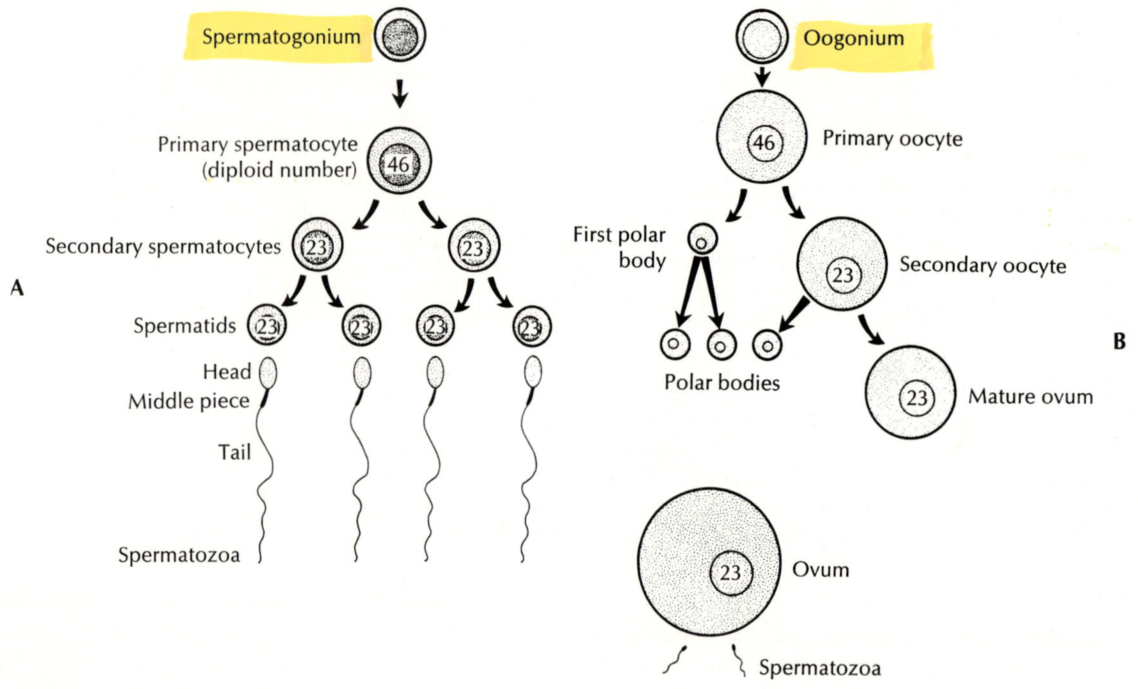

Fig. 10.6
Fertilization. **A,** Ovum fertilized by X-bearing sperm to form female zygote. **B,** Ovum fertilized by Y-bearing sperm to form male zygote. (From Whaley, L.F., and Wong, D.L.: Nursing care of infants and children, St. Louis, 1979, The C.V. Mosby Co.)

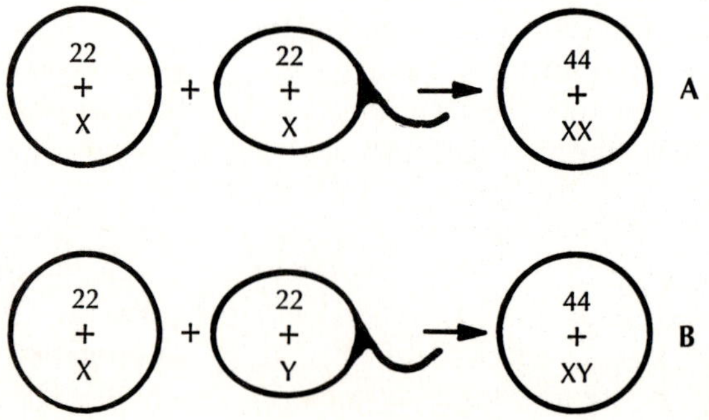

cellular contents. Although the chromosome number is reduced to half the original number and equally divided between the two cells, there is unequal distribution of the cytoplasm. The result is one large *secondary oocyte* containing the bulk of the cellular contents and a small, nonfunctioning *first polar body*. The second meiotic division begins at ovulation when the secondary oocyte divides to form a large *ovum* and a *second polar body*. The ovum does not complete the second meiotic division until triggered by the entrance of the sperm at fertilization. The polar bodies, unable to support reproduction, soon disintegrate (Fig. 10.5,*B*).

The number of chromosomes is restored at the time of fertilization when the sperm with its 23 chromosomes unites with the ovum with an equal number to form a new organism, the *zygote,* with 46 chromosomes (Fig. 10.6).

Genes in Families

The genes are predictable in the way they separate during division and combine during fertilization. It is these processes that explain the way in which genes are passed from one generation to the next and form the basis for the common principles of genetics, or Mendel's laws. Knowledge of these principles is essential to an understanding of heredity.

the principle of dominance Not all genes have equal strength. When each gene of a pair produces a different effect, one gene may be stronger and hide the effect of the other. The trait that is observed in the individual (and the stronger gene that produces the effect) is called *dominant;* the gene that is weaker and not seen is called *recessive*.

the principle of segregation The paired chromosomes, bearing genes derived from each parent, are separated when gametes are formed during meiosis. Each gene segregates in pure form, and chance alone determines which gene (the one from the mother or the one from the father) will travel to a specific gamete.

the principle of independent assortment The members of one pair of genes are distributed in the gametes in random fashion unrelated to any of the other pairs.

DISORDERS CAUSED BY A SINGLE GENE

Conditions caused by a single gene are passed from one generation to the next according to the patterns just described. For any given trait the individual has two genes, one gene contributed by each parent at the time of conception. Fig. 10.7 illustrates the possible outcomes of mating between parents with three different types of gene combinations. A trait determined by a gene on an autosome (a nonsex chromosome) is referred to as an *autosomal* trait; a trait determined by a gene borne on one of the sex chromosomes is said to be *sex linked*. Since the sex-linked diseases are caused

Fig. 10.7
Possible offspring in three types of matings. **A,** Homozygous dominant parent and homozygous recessive parent. Children all heterozygous, displaying dominant trait. **B,** Heterozygous parent and homozygous recessive parent. Children 50% heterozygous display dominant trait; 50% homozygous display recessive trait. **C,** Both parents heterozygous. Children 25% homozygous show dominant trait; 25% homozygous display recessive trait; 50% heterozygous display dominant trait. NOTE: Mating between homozygous dominant parent and heterozygous parent produces 50% homozygous and 50% heterozygous children all of which display dominant trait: reverse of **B.** (From Whaley, L.F., and Wong, D.L.: Nursing care of infants and children, St. Louis, 1979, The C.V. Mosby Co.)

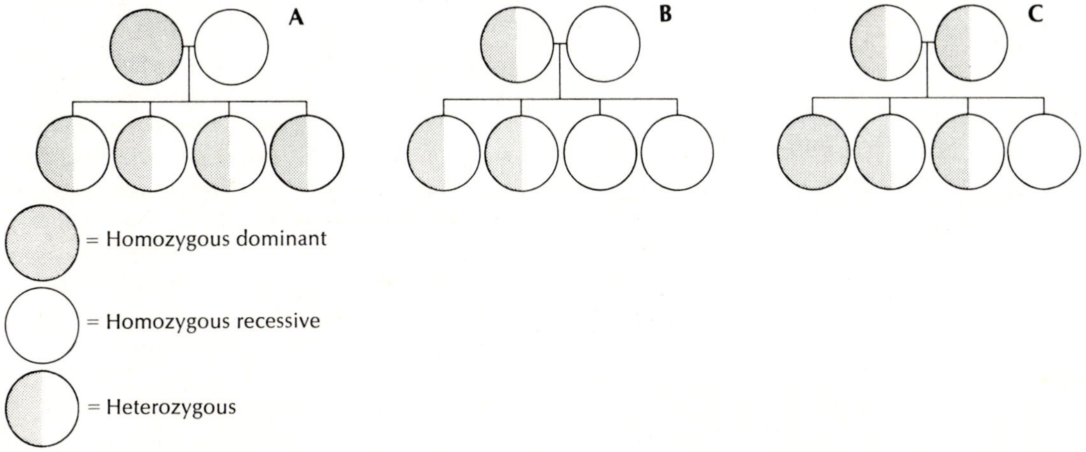

Fig. 10.8
Punnett square illustrating sex differences in offspring ratios in X-linked recessive inheritance. O = Recessive allele on X chromosome. (From Whaley, L.F.: Understanding inherited disorders, St. Louis, 1974, The C.V. Mosby Co.)

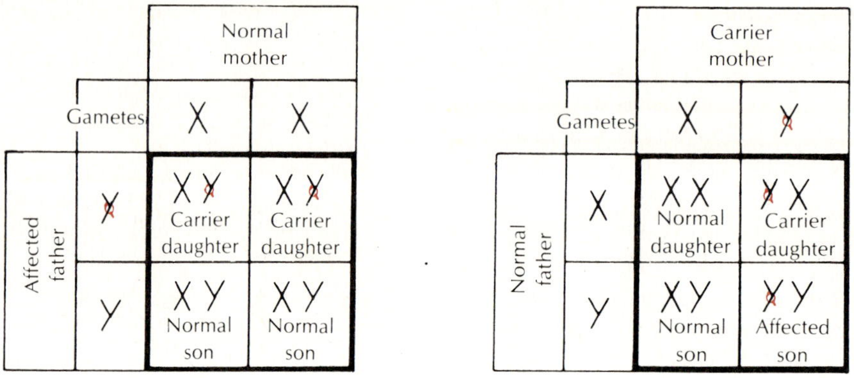

by genes borne on the X chromosome, the more accurate term *X linked* is given to these disorders.

The various inheritance patterns and their characteristics are briefly described below. Since there are 44 autosomes and only 2 sex chromosomes, the majority of disorders are caused by a single gene on an autosome. X-linked inherited disorders vary according to the sex of the person with the defective gene. Females, with two X chromosomes, have two genes for a trait and therefore X-linked genes in the female act like genes on autosomes. It is in the male, with only one X chromosome, that a gene on the X chromosome acts differently.

Autosomal-dominant inheritance. Disorders caused by a dominant gene on an autosome are those in which the abnormal trait dominates and the normal gene is recessive. Whenever the gene is present it appears in the individual. The following are characteristics of a disorder caused by a dominant gene on an autosome (Whaley, 1974):

1. Males and females are affected with equal frequency.
2. Affected individuals will have an affected parent (unless the condition is caused by a fresh mutation).
3. Half the children of a heterozygous affected parent will be affected.
4. Normal children of affected parents will have normal children.
5. Traits can be traced through previous generations (positive family history).

Examples of disorders caused by autosomal-dominant inheritance are polydactyly, achondroplasia, osteogenesis imperfecta, and Marfan's syndrome.

Autosomal-recessive inheritance. Persons with an autosomal-recessive disorder will always be homozygous for that trait. The trait does not appear in the heterozygous parents, although each will pass the defective recessive gene to the offspring. Characteristics of autosomal-recessive disorders (Whaley, 1974) are summarized as follows:

1. Males and females are affected with equal frequency.
2. Affected individuals will have unaffected parents who are heterozygous for the trait.
3. One fourth of the children of two unaffected heterozygous parents will be affected.
4. Affected individuals married to unaffected individuals will have normal children, all of whom will be carriers.
5. There is usually no evidence of the trait in previous generations (negative family history).

Some autosomal-recessive disorders are cystic fibrosis, phenylketonuria (PKU), galactosemia, sickle cell anemia, Tay-Sachs disease, and albinism.

X-linked inheritance. The outstanding characteristic of X-linked disorders is that the defective genes on the X chromosome have no similar gene on the Y chromosome. Consequently, traits (both dominant and recessive) determined by the X-linked genes are *always* expressed in the male. One of the most significant aspects of X-linked inheritance is the lack of father-to-son transmission, since the father gives his one X chromosome to his female offspring.

X-linked dominant disorders. There are few disorders that are known to be inherited as X-linked dominant, probably because they superficially resemble the autosomal-dominant inheritance pattern. Briefly summa-

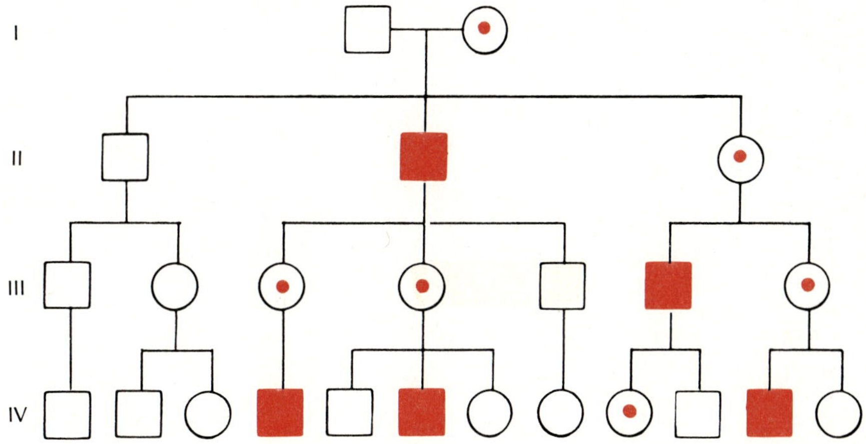

Fig. 10.9
X-linked recessive inheritance pattern. ⊙ = carrier female; ■ = affected male. (From Whaley, L.F.: Understanding inherited disorders, St. Louis, 1974, The C.V. Mosby Co.)

rized, characteristics of X-linked dominant inheritance (Whaley, 1974) are as follows:

1. Affected individuals will have an affected parent.
2. All the daughters but none of the sons of an affected male will be affected.
3. Half the sons and half the daughters of an affected female will be affected.
4. Normal children of an affected parent will have normal offspring.
5. The inheritance pattern shows a positive family history of the disorder.

Hypophosphatemic (vitamin D–resistant) rickets is an example of a disorder thought to be caused by X-linked dominant inheritance.

X-linked recessive disorders. A number of serious conditions caused by a recessive gene on an X chromosome have been identified. The gene behaves as any recessive gene; that is, when its effect is opposed by a normal dominant gene, as it is in the female, the trait is not observed in the individual. However, in the male the recessive gene on the X chromosome always produces an effect. Fig. 10.8 illustrates the manner in which the X-linked gene is transmitted to the offspring, and Fig. 10.9 is an example of the pattern of X-linked inheritance in a family. Characteristics of X-linked recessive inheritance (Whaley, 1974) are as follows:

1. Affected individuals are principally males.
2. Affected individuals will have unaffected parents (except in the rare possibility that the father is affected and the mother is a carrier).
3. All the female children of an affected male will be carriers of the trait.
4. Unaffected male children of an affected male cannot transmit the disorder.
5. Sons of an affected male are unaffected.
6. Daughters of an affected male are carriers.
7. The unaffected male children of a carrier female do not transmit the disorder.

Examples of X-linked recessive disorders are hemophilia and Duchenne muscular dystrophy.

Chromosomal Aberrations

An aberration is defined as a deviation from the normal or typical. Aberrations of chromosomes are deviations in either chromosomal number or structure. A structural defect involves the loss, addition, or rearrangement of the genes on a chromosome or the exchange of genes between chromosomes. The most notable of the structural abnormalities are (1) the *cri du chat syndrome,* in which there is loss of a portion of a group B chromosome and (2) the *translocation phenomenon,* in which two chromosomes (one from each of two different groups) become attached and therefore act as one chromosome.

Abnormalities in chromosomal number result from the gain or loss of an entire chromosome during the process of cell division. Numeric alterations in pairs of chromosomes during cell division will cause unequal distribution of chromosomes to the resulting cells. These abnormal numbers are referred to by the suffix "-somy." A cell that contains 45 chromosomes, one less than the basic number (46), is called a *monosomy* because one chromosomal pair has but a single member. Cells that have three chromosomes instead of a normal pair are termed *trisomies,* and the total chromosomal count of the cell is 47.

Fig. 10.10
Mechanism of maldistribution of chromosomes during meiosis in ovum and fertilization with normal sperm. **A,** During first meiotic division. **B,** During second meiotic division. Only one mature ovum is formed, but all ova are illustrated to better visualize four possible gametes and consequences of fertilization. (Adapted from Whaley, L.F.: Understanding inherited disorders, St. Louis, 1974, The C.V. Mosby Co.)

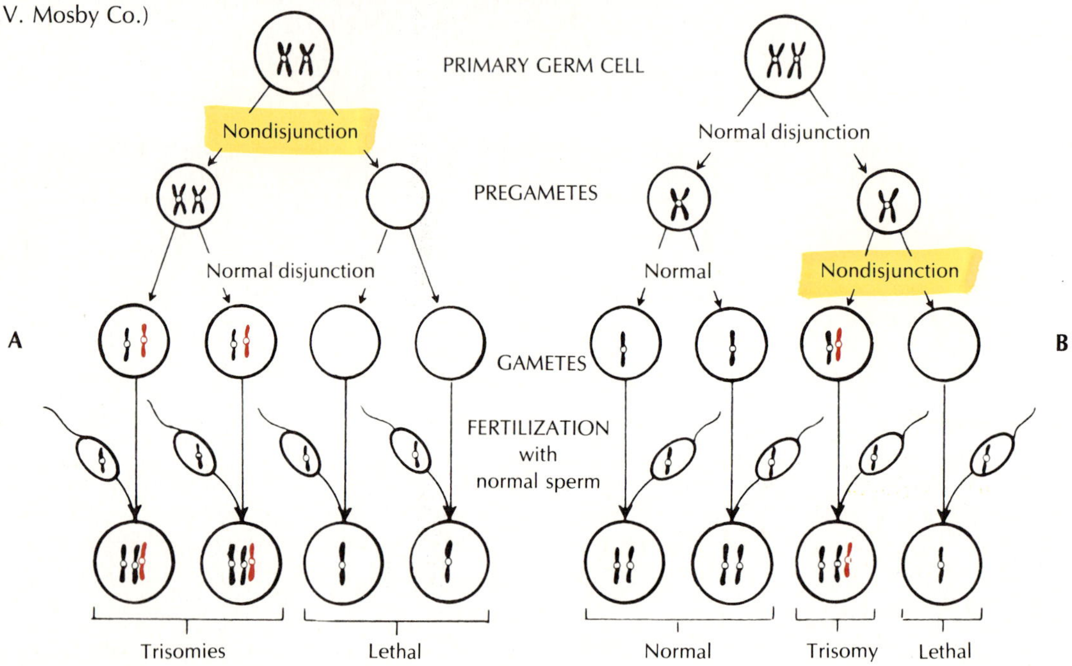

DISORDERS OF CELL DIVISION

The majority of variations in chromosomal number are caused by failure of the chromosome to separate during cell division. This is known as *nondisjunction*. Less frequently, two chromosomes become attached, or *translocated*.

Nondisjunction. When the chromosome fails to separate, the resulting cells contain an uneven number of chromosomes: one cell contains an extra chromosome, the other is minus a chromosome. The ratio of trisomic, normal, or monosomic gametes depends on whether the disjunction occurs during the first or second meiotic divisions (Fig. 10.10).

There is a marked relationship between the incidence of trisomic births and advancing parental age regardless of the number of pregnancies. The largest percentage of cases are related to the age of the mother, and the number of affected infants increases with the increased age of the mother. Paternal influence levels off at 45 years of age. A possible explanation is that whereas the male continuously produces fresh sperm during his lifetime, the total number of primitive ova is present in the female at birth, and thus they are at risk for damage by a variety of external influences as well as the effect of the aging process.

Nondisjunction can also occur during early cell division following fertilization in the zygote. The chromosomal number of the resulting cell lines and their ratio depend, again, on whether the nondisjunction takes place at the first division or a later division. Nondisjunction during later divisions can result in a mixture of normal and trisomic cells called *mosaicism*. The extent to which there is abnormal development in mosaicism depends on the type and amount of tissues that are affected. This can vary from near normal to a full-blown syndrome.

Translocation. Translocation is a more complex chromosomal abnormality than nondisjunction; it occurs when one chromosome becomes attached to another to create one large double chromosome. This occurs most frequently between a group D and a group G chromosome or between two group G chromosomes. The normal person who carries a translocated chromosome has a full amount of genetic material with a chromosome count of only 45. Since the chromosomes are attached, they behave as one chromosome during the process of

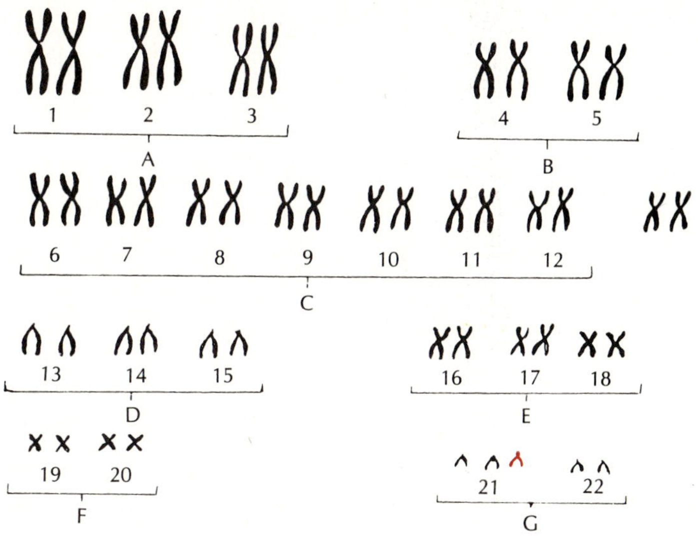

Fig. 10.11
Model of a female karyotype with trisomy of the 21(G) chromosome group (47,XX,21+). (From Whaley, L.F.: Understanding inherited disorders, St. Louis, 1974, The C.V. Mosby Co.)

division. Therefore the abnormal chromosome can be passed on to future generations.

DISORDERS CAUSED BY CHROMOSOMAL ABERRATIONS

The most common chromosomal abnormalities are the trisomies, which can affect any of the cell pairs, including the sex chromosomes.

Autosomal aberrations. Abnormalities of both structure and number can produce defective development that is easily identified in the newborn. The one seen with greatest frequency is trisomy 21, or Down's syndrome, which results from duplication of the number 21 group G chromosome (Fig. 10.11). The incidence is relatively high, approximately 1 in 500 live births. However, the incidence is strongly related to the age of the mother. In mothers less than 35 years of age the ratio of infants born with Down's syndrome is between 1:1000 and 1:2000. For mothers between 35 and 40 years of age, the incidence rises to 1:300. Beyond a maternal age of 40 years there is a marked increase to between 1:30 and 1:50.

The majority of cases of Down's syndrome (95%) are attributed to nondisjunction during prefertilization division in the gametes. A small percentage of cases (5%) are the result of a translocation in which the chromosome 21 becomes attached to either a group D or another group G chromosome.

Other trisomies are encountered less often. Trisomies of chromosomes 13 and 18 are seen occasionally, but the defects are more serious and the prognosis less favorable. The characteristics of the three viable autosomal trisomies and the cri-du-chat syndrome, the most commonly occurring structural anomaly, are outlined in Table 10.1.

Aberrations of sex chromosomes. A number of abnormalities of sex chromosomes are known and involve trisomies or other multiples of sex chromosomes. The only monosomy known to be compatible with life is the XO monosomy, or Turner's syndrome. The presence of at least one X chromosome appears to be essential to life. The possible outcomes of nondisjunction of the sex chromosomes are shown in Fig. 10.12. The characteristics are described in Table 10.2.

There is decidedly less disability in persons who have multiple sex chromosomes when compared to the disabilities encountered in persons with multiple autosomes. This is attributed to a characteristic peculiar to the X chromosome: *X inactivation*. In all body cells only one X chromosome is biologically active. The other (or others) is in some way inactivated or "switched off" during early divisions of the zygote and remains so throughout life. Therefore both males and females possess only one active X chromosome. The inactivated X chromosome is easily observed under the microscope as a condensed, dark-staining mass lying at the periphery of the cell nucleus in 20% to 50% of body cells. This is known as the *sex chromatin,* or *Barr body*. The number of chromatin bodies is one less than the total number of X chromosomes in that cell nucleus. Consequently, cells of females normally contain one Barr body and are thus chromatin positive; normal males, with no inactivated X chromosome, are chromatin negative. The sex chromatin can also appear in polymorphonuclear leukocytes as a drumsticklike mass attached to one of the nuclear lobes of the cell (Fig. 10.13).

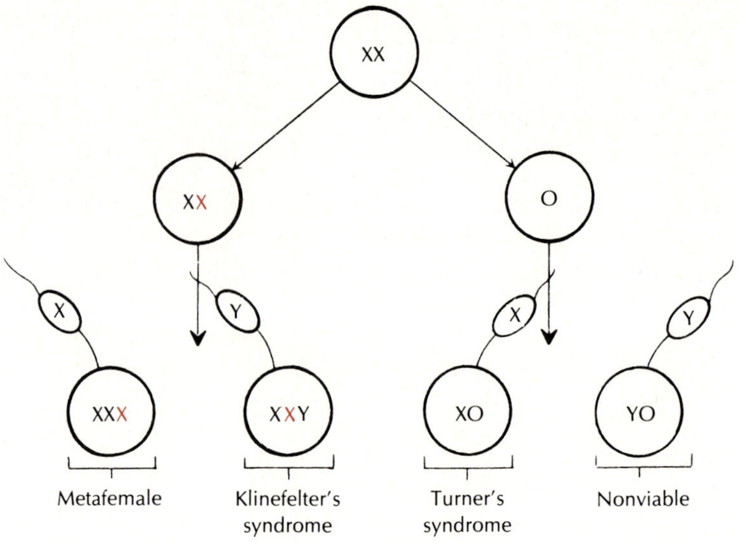

Fig. 10.12
Nondisjunction of X chromosomes in ovum fertilized by normal sperm to produce more common sex chromosomal aberrations. (From Whaley, L.F.: Understanding inherited disorders, St. Louis, 1974, The C.V. Mosby Co.)

Table 10.1
Common Autosomal Aberrations

Syndrome	Chromosomal Abnormality and Nomenclature	Average Incidence	Major Clinical Manifestations
Cri du chat	Deletion of short arm of a B (no. 5) chromosome—46,XY,5p−		Distinctive weak, high-pitched mewlike cry resembling the cry of a cat; small head; hypertelorism; failure to thrive; severe mental retardation—profound with age
Trisomy 13 (Patau's)	Trisomy of a group D (no. 13) chromosome—47,XY,13+	1/15,000	Multiple anomalies, including cleft lip and palate (frequently bilateral); ear malformations; microphthalmia; polydactyly; eye defects; mental retardation; early death
Trisomy 18 (Edwards')	Trisomy of a group E (no. 18) chromosome—47,XY,18+	1/5000	Deformed and low-set ears; micrognathia; rocker-bottom feet; overlapping (index over third) fingers; prominent occiput; hypertelorism; failure to thrive and early death; mental retardation
Trisomy 21 (Down's)	Trisomy of a group G (no. 21) chromosome—47,XY,21 + (trisomy); 46XY,D−G−, (DqGq)+ (translocation); 46,XY/ 47,XY, 21+(mosaic)	1/500	Brachycephaly with flat occiput; inner epicanthal folds; small ears, nose, and mouth with protruding tongue; muscular hypotonia; broad, short hands with stubby fingers and transverse palmar crease; broad stubby feet with wide space between big and second toes; mental retardation; variable life expectancy

From Whaley, L.F., and Wong, D.L.: Nursing care of infants and children, St. Louis, 1979, The C.V. Mosby Co.

Multifactorial Inheritance

The largest category of conditions in which genetic factors play a large role includes those that are multifactorial in their causation, that is, those disorders in which genes and environment interact to produce a disease or structural defect. No inheritance pattern can be identified in these cases, although there is an increased risk of recurrence in families in which cases are known.

Another term used to describe common diseases and disorders is *polygenic* (which literally means many genes). Polygenic refers to those genes that individually do not produce a large effect but several minor genes in combination produce a large effect in the individual.

Relatives have more genes in common and the closer the relationship, the greater will be the number of

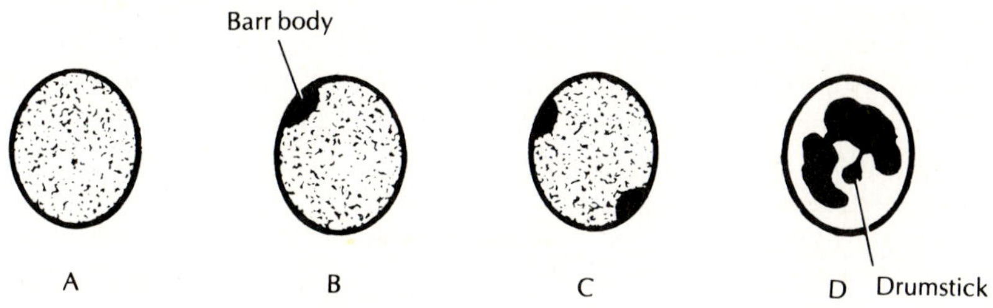

Fig. 10.13
Sex chromatin, or Barr body. **A,** No sex chromatin is found in normal male somatic cells. **B,** One Barr body is normal in female somatic cells. **C,** Two Barr bodies are found in cells with three X chromosomes (XXX or XXXY). **D,** "Drumstick" is found in many polymorphonuclear leukocytes of normal female. (From Whaley, L.F.: Understanding inherited disorders, St. Louis, 1974, The C.V. Mosby Co.)

Table 10.2
Common Sex Chromosome Abnormalities

Syndrome	Chromosomal Description	Body Type	X Chromosome	Y Chromosome	Clinical Manifestations
Turner's	45,X	Female	0	0	Short stature; webbed neck; low posterior hairline; shield-shaped chest with widely spaced nipples; sterile; lymphedema of hands and feet in infant
Triple X (super female)	47,XXX (can also be 48,XXXX or 49,XXXXX)	Female	+ 1 or more	0	Normal female characteristics; usually mentally retarded; mental deficiency in others; fertile
XYY male	47,XYY (can also be 48,XYYY or mosaic)	Male	0	+ 1 per Y	Usually normal sexual development; tendency to be tall with long head; poor coordination; may demonstrate aberrant behavior
Klinefelter's	47,XXY (48,XXYY, 48,XXXY, 49,XXXXY, etc. mosaics)	Male	+ 1 or more (1 per X)	+ 1 per Y	Tall with long legs; hypogenitalism; sterile; may have deficient male secondary sexual characteristics; may demonstrate aberrant behavior

From Whaley, L.F., and Wong, D.L.: Nursing care of infants and children, St. Louis, 1979, The C.V. Mosby Co.

shared genes. First-degree relatives (parent, child, sibling) will have half their genes in common; second-degree relatives (grandparent, grandchild, uncle, aunt, etc.) have one fourth of their genes in common, and so on. If there is more than one affected member in a family, the greater is the number of harmful genes the members have in common.

Conditions that are multifactorial include a variety of structural defects such as cleft lip, cleft palate, congenital dislocated hip, congenital heart defects, pyloric stenosis, and the neural tube defects such as myelomeningocele and hydrocephalus. Diseases that fall into this category are diabetes mellitus, psoriasis, schizophrenia, peptic ulcers, hypertension, and ischemic heart disease. Table 10.3 compares the incidence of some common conditions in the general population and in first-degree relatives who have the disorder.

Table 10.3
Inherited Component in Some Common Disorders

	Incidence	
Condition	**General Population**	**First-Degree Relatives**
Cleft lip and palate	1/750	1/20
Clubfoot	1/1000	1/40
Congenital dislocated hip	1/1400	1/20
Congenital heart disease	1/128	1/27
Juvenile diabetes mellitus	1/500	1/15
Pyloric stenosis	3/1000	1/15
Schizophrenia	1/100	1/10

Adapted from Whaley, L.F., and Wong, D.L.: Nursing care of infants and children, ed. 2, St. Louis, 1983, The C.V. Mosby Co.

Detection of Genetic Disease

The increase in the incidence and survival of persons with a genetic disorder together with the increasing number of disorders recognized through advances in biochemistry and cytology has made detection of genetic disease an important aspect of both prevention and treatment of genetic disorders. Early detection of the presence of a disease promotes prompt therapy and thus reduces the impact of many diseases. Heterozygote detection provides families with information regarding the likelihood of a genetic defect in their offspring. Special prenatal examination can detect the presence of a genetic disorder in the fetus. Both mandatory and voluntary screening procedures have been implemented to detect disease in infants or heterozygotes and in families or populations at risk.

PRECONCEPTIONAL DETECTION

Many persons or families are eager to know whether or not they carry a defective gene. These persons are usually members of a population with a high risk for a disease (e.g., sickle cell disease in blacks and Tay-Sachs disease in Ashkenazic Jews) or those in whose family there is a genetic disorder and who plan to marry or start a pregnancy. With the increasing number of techniques available for detecting the presence of a genetic disease, more and more persons are seeking this information as a basis for family planning. In fact, mass screening for numerous defects may eventually become routine just as is the present widespread screening of infants for phenylketonuria (PKU).

PRENATAL DETECTION

Prenatal detection of genetic disease has assumed an important role in obstetric care during recent years. Several intrauterine techniques are employed to detect the presence of a genetic defect before the birth of a child. Of these the one method that has demonstrated a high degree of accuracy and safety is *amniocentesis* (or more specifically, genetic amniocentesis). Perfection of the technique has made it a relatively common diagnostic tool. Other diagnostic methods include ultrasonography, roentgenography, and direct fetoscopy.

Amniocentesis. Diagnosis of disorders in the fetus during pregnancy can be done by amniocentesis. Amniocentesis consists of removing some of the amniotic fluid by way of a needle inserted into the uterus through the mother's abdomen. Ideally the procedure is performed between the fourteenth and sixteenth weeks of gestation. The placenta is located by radiography or ultrasonography to avoid trauma from the needle to the placenta with resultant bleeding (Fig. 10.14), and fluid removal is done with the woman under local anesthesia. The fluid containing fetal urine, secretions, and cells shed from the respiratory tract and the skin is centrifuged. The cells are separated from the fluid where they can then be studied and analyzed depending on the purpose for the examination. For example, cells may be examined to determine the sex of the fetus or a possible chromosomal abnormality. The amniotic fluid can be tested for the presence of Rh antibodies, infection, or a variety of metabolic by-products.

Indications for amniocentesis are the following:

1. Pregnant women 40 years of age and older
2. Couples who already have borne one child with a detectable genetic disorder
3. Couples who are heterozygous for a recessive disorder (approximately 80 biochemical defects can be detected)
4. To determine the presence of an X-linked disorder in a male fetus when the mother is a known or suspected carrier
5. Couples in which one member is a chromosomal mosaic or possesses a translocated chromosome
6. When one or both parents are affected with a genetic disorder

Amniocentesis is performed to determine the management of the pregnancy. Since there is some element of risk (although very small), the procedure is usually carried out only if an elective abortion will be performed if the fetus is found to be affected. However, even if parents are opposed to abortion, some prefer to know in advance if their unborn child has a defect. Prior knowledge allows time to prepare emotionally and to mobilize necessary family and community support before the child is born.

Ultrasonography. Ultrasonography is an easily accomplished test that involves the passage of high-frequency sound waves through the uterine area to determine pelvic measurements, locate the placenta, and observe the fetal outline. This is routinely performed before amniocentesis. Some skeletal abnormalities, such as anencephaly, microcephaly, and hydrocephaly, and the presence of multiple fetuses can be detected by this technique. Ultrasonography is noninvasive and painless to the client.

Roentgenography. Bone abnormalities can be detected by simple x-ray studies, although the bone structure is at a very early stage of development at about 16 weeks' gestation. Most bone defects are not apparent until a later stage. A special x-ray technique, termed *amniography* or *fetography*, involves injecting a con-

Fig. 10.14
A, Amniocentesis and laboratory utilization of amniotic fluid aspirant. **B,** 1a, 2a, 3, 4, 5, and 6 are front views with arrows indicating appropriate sites for amniocentesis varying with placental position. 1b and 2b are side views. (From Whaley, L.F.: Understanding inherited disorders, St. Louis, 1974, The C.V. Mosby Co.)

A

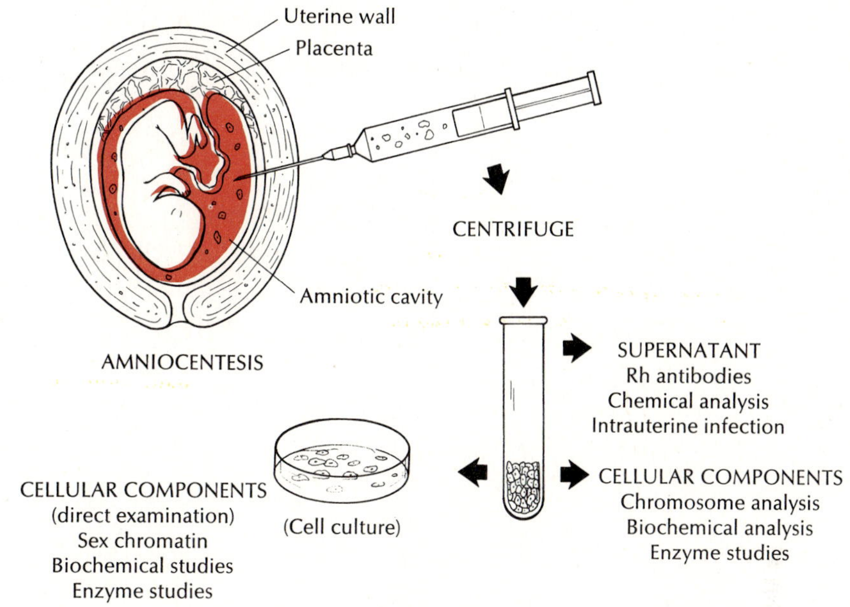

B

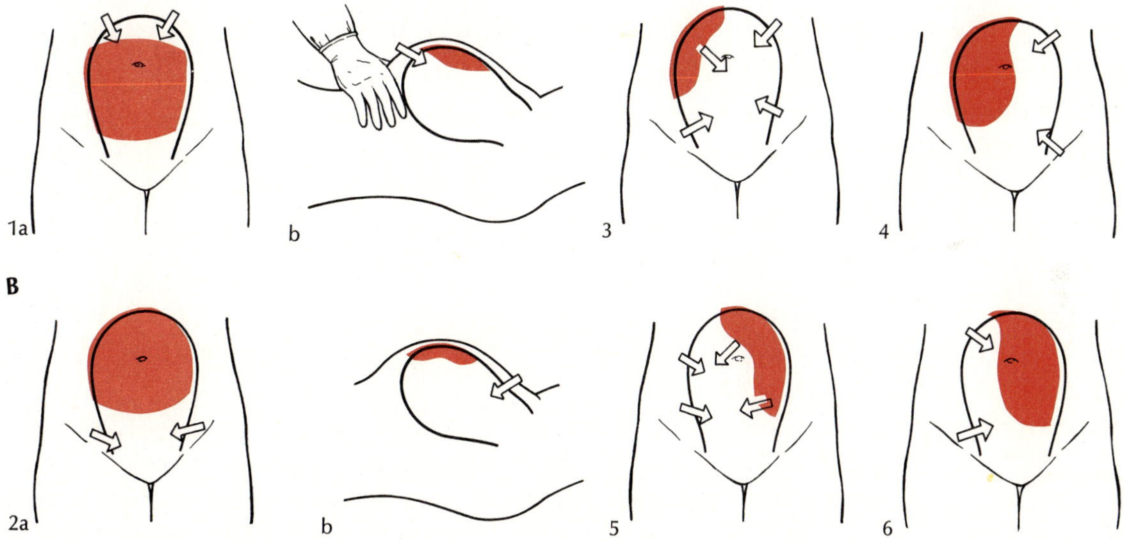

trast medium into the amniotic fluid. The medium adheres to fetal skin to produce a clear fetal outline on the x-ray film.

Fetoscopy (amnioscopy). A direct view of the fetus is possible by way of a tiny telescope-like instrument the size of a large hypodermic needle. It is introduced into the uterus through the abdominal wall with the woman under local anesthesia. This method is not used extensively at this time because there is a risk of causing premature labor. The fetoscope is more often used to obtain fetal blood samples for analysis.

POSTDELIVERY DETECTION

Most diagnostic procedures for detection of genetic disorders can be carried out after birth at any time from the postnatal period through adulthood. The number and variety of these tests are too extensive to include here; therefore only those employed most frequently in the newborn period will be discussed.

Biochemical tests. The most widespread use of postdelivery testing for genetic disease is the routine screening of newborn infants for PKU, hypothyroidism, and

Fig. 10.15
A, Dermatoglyphics on palms and fingertips with nomenclature. **B,** Mean position of most triradii in children up to 4 yr of age. **C,** Examples of flexion creases on palm. *Left,* normal; *center,* simian line; *right,* Sydney line. (**C** from Whaley, L.F.: Understanding inherited disorders, St. Louis, 1974, The C.V. Mosby Co.)

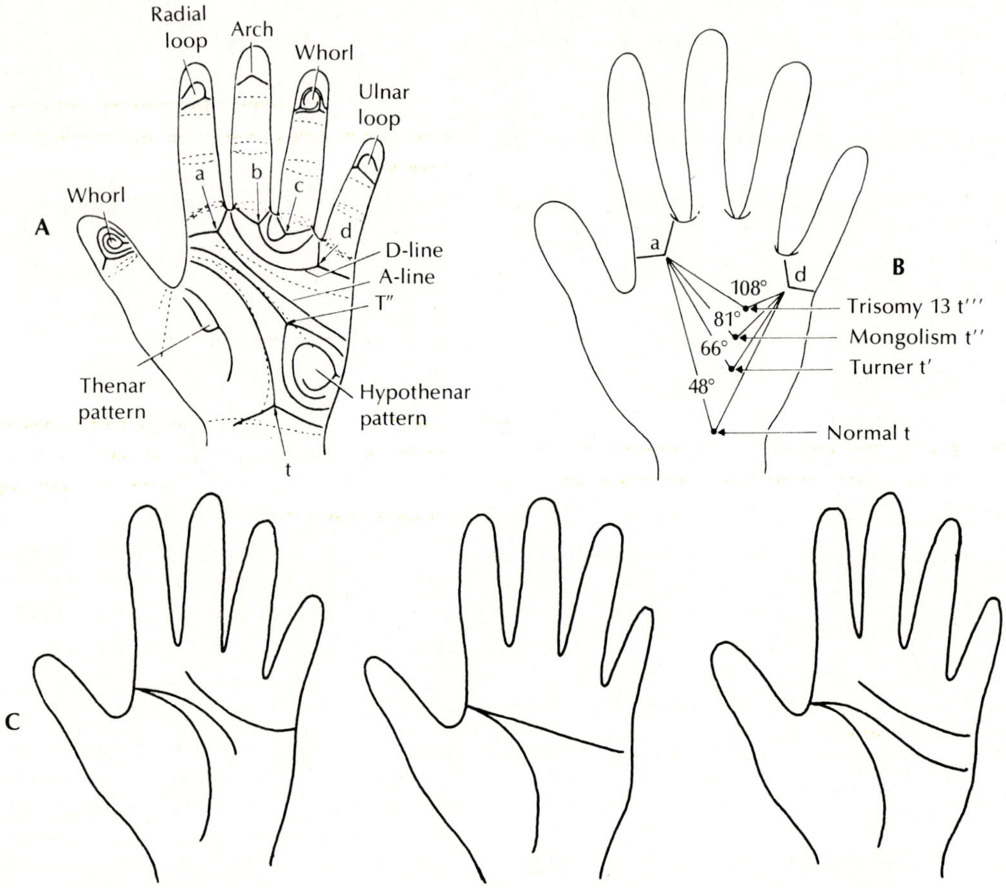

galactosemia, which is mandatory in most of the United States. Numerous other tests are now available to detect suspected defects in the newborn (see Chapter 28).

Cytologic studies. Occasionally an infant is born whose clinical appearance suggests a chromosomal abnormality. In such cases microscopic examination of the infant's cells are sometimes carried out to confirm or rule out a tentative diagnosis. It may require examination of the cells stained and viewed under a microscope. These stains can be prepared from any cells in the body. The most easily obtained and therefore the most frequently used are mucosal cells scraped from the inside of the cheek, placed on a glass slide, prepared, and stained (buccal smear). Preparation of a karyotype (see p. 141) requires that the cells be in the process of division; therefore they are grown in a culture medium. The most commonly used cells are those obtained from bone marrow, skin, or peripheral blood.

Dermatoglyphics. The pattern formed by dermal ridges early in development is largely genetically determined by many genes on many chromosomes. Therefore addition or deletion of genetic material will produce alterations in the loops, swirls, and arches of the finger and toe prints, in the palm lines, and in the flexion creases on palms of the hands and soles of the feet (Fig 10.15, *A*). Characteristic dermatoglyphic patterns have been noted in almost all the chromosomal abnormalities (Fig 10.15, *B*). Characteristic palm creases have also been noted in a significant number of children with rubella syndrome and leukemia. The Sydney line (Fig. 10.15, *C*) has been observed more frequently in children with rubella syndrome than in children in a control group.

Other postdelivery diagnostic studies. Many other diagnostic studies may be performed in the neonatal period to detect or rule out genetic defects, for example, x-ray studies for a variety of structural defects of bone and for gastrointestinal, renal, and neurologic disorders. The presence of a symptom known to be associated with a hereditary disease alerts the health professional to the need for further testing and assessment. For example, meconium ileus in the newborn is often the first manifestation of cystic fibrosis, the most frequently occurring genetic disease.

Genetic Counseling

Rapid expansion in the identification, understanding, and diagnosis of genetic disease has been accompanied by effective medical or surgical therapies in a small number of cases; however, for the majority of genetic conditions therapeutic or preventive measures are nonexistent or disappointingly limited. Consequently, providing families, through health professionals, with genetic information and services is at present the best means for reducing the number of children born with genetic defects.

CLIENTS

The reasons that persons seek genetic counseling are varied. The persons may or may not be affected themselves. Persons seeking counseling commonly fall into the following categories:

1. Persons who want to know if they have a genetic disease or if they are carriers of a genetic disease
2. Persons who are concerned whether they are at risk for producing a child with a specific genetic disease
3. Persons who are planning parenthood and who want to know the prognosis and treatment of a genetic disease affecting one or both partners
4. Persons seeking help in making a decision about prenatal diagnosis, selective abortion, artificial insemination by donor, or adoption
5. Persons seeking help for a child affected with a genetic disease
6. Persons referred to counseling by other health professionals

GOALS OF COUNSELING

There are three major goals of genetic counseling. The *first* is to provide families with accurate information regarding recurrence risks when a member of the family has a disorder that might be genetically determined. The risk in their particular situation should be presented in language the clients can understand and should be placed in the proper perspective in relation to the risk for any other person in the population. The *second* goal of genetic counseling is to alert health professionals to the possibility of a genetic disease in a family. This increases the likelihood that the disease will be detected and treatment initiated earlier. Clues to this possibility are the presence of an affected sibling or parent or environmental factors that may have been operating during a pregnancy. The *third* goal of genetic counseling is to reduce the numbers of children affected with a hereditary condition by prenatal detection of a disorder, heterozygote testing in families and populations at risk, and providing information about recurrence risks as a basis for family planning in families at risk.

COUNSELING PROCESS

Counseling is a process of communication involving a mutual exchange of ideas and opinions that provides the basis for mutual problem solving. The counseling process begins with an accurate diagnosis and a careful, detailed family history. The correct diagnosis is essential, because there are a number of diseases that have similar manifestations but different modes of inheritance. It is the function of the genetic counselor to apply a thorough understanding of genetic principles and multifactorial inheritance to the diagnosis and the information obtained from the history and arrive at the risks related to this particular case. The risks are determined by the mode of inheritance. The counselor explains the risk estimates to clients without making recommendations or decisions and avoids allowing personal biases to interfere.

Counseling services. The most efficient counseling facilities are associated with the larger universities and major medical centers where support services are available (e.g., biochemical and cytology laboratories). A number of specialized groups provide clinics and services for persons with a specific genetic disorder such as cystic fibrosis, muscular dystrophy, hemophilia, and diabetes. Maternity nurses should become familiar with persons who provide genetic counseling and places where counseling services are available to clients in their area of practice.

ROLE OF THE NURSE

All nurses, and particularly those involved in the care of mothers and children, should have some understanding of genetic theory and the nature of the more common genetic disorders. With this knowledge they are more likely to recognize clues that indicate a genetically related problem. They are then able to assist families in obtaining appropriate counseling services.

The nurse is usually the person who prepares clients for diagnostic tests and assists with the procedures. The family and persons directly involved need to know the purpose of each test, what they can expect, and what they can do to make the process easier. They may be concerned about whether or not the test will be painful, if they will be required to undress, and if they can be accompanied by a family member. Nurses can do a great deal to reduce their fears and to supply support and reassurance.

Nurses should be able to interpret and reinforce accurately the information given to the client by the genetic counselor. Since most clients do not have an adequate knowledge of genetics and human biology, the complex concepts of cell division, segregation, and recombination are often difficult to understand. However, most persons have an adequate understanding of games of chance and have had experience with flipping coins, lotteries, and various other games based on probabilities. These are effective devices for illustrating single-gene disorders; weather forecasts and horse-racing handicaps are excellent examples for estimates of risks for multifactorial disorders.

The most important concept that must be emphasized to families is that each pregnancy is *an independent event*. For example, in single-gene disorders in which the risk factor is one in four that the child will be affected, the risk remains the same no matter how many affected children are already in the family. It is not uncommon for families to maintain the belief that the presence of one affected child assures that the next three will be free of the disease. The risk is one in four for *each* pregnancy. It is the same concept as the chance of a child being either a boy or a girl. In each pregnancy the odds are 50-50 regardless of how many children of one sex have been born to a couple.

Probably the most important of all nursing functions is providing emotional support to the family during all aspects of the counseling process. Clients react to the threat of a genetic disorder in their families in a variety of ways. Responses may include all stress reactions, such as apathy, denial, anger, hostility, fear, embarrassment, grief, and loss of self-esteem. Guilt and self-blame are universal reactions.

Nurses are sympathetic listeners and are able to do much to ease the stresses surrounding the impact of a genetic diagnosis. A great deal can be accomplished by allowing the clients to express openly their feelings about their genetic problem. Simple explanations of the way in which cells divide and the remote chance that both parents happened to have the same "bad" genes is often enough to relieve the feelings of guilt in some clients. However, the type of disability associated with a specific disorder may affect persons in different ways. One family may risk having a child with a disorder that produces a minor defect or even an early death but will not risk having a child with a lifelong physical or mental disability.

Nurses, too, have feelings and opinions about certain genetic disorders and whether or not clients should risk having an affected child. It is often difficult for them to avoid giving the clients the impression that they should make a particular decision. Families and individuals need education, guidance, and support throughout the counseling process. They should be given the facts and possible consequences and all the assistance they need in problem solving, but the final decision regarding a course of action must be their own.

References and Readings

Afriat, C.I., and Schifrin, B.S.: Antepartum fetal evaluation. In McNall, L.K., and Galeener, J.T., editors: Current practice in obstetric and gynecologic nursing, vol. II, St. Louis, 1978, The C.V. Mosby Co.

Athey, P.A., and Hadlock, F.P.: Ultrasound in obstetrics and gynecology, St. Louis, 1981, The C.V. Mosby Co.

Bocian, M.E., and Kaback, M.M.: Crisis counseling: the newborn infant with a chromosomal anomaly, Pediatr. Clin. North Am. **25**:643, 1979.

Bogdanovic, S.: Prenatal detection of Down's syndrome, J.O.G.N. Nurs. **4**:35, 1975.

Childs, B.: Genetic screening. In Roman, H.L., Campbell, A., and Sandler, L.M., editors: Annual review of genetics, Palo Alto, Calif., 1975, Annual reviews.

Clow, C.L., et al.: On the application of knowledge to the patient with genetic disease, Prog. Med. Genet. **9**:159, 1973.

Ferguson-Smith, M.A.: Chromosome abnormalities. II. Sex chromosome defects. In McKusick, V.A., and Claiborn, R., editors: Medical genetics, New York, 1973, H.P. Publishing Co.

Ferrer, T.L.: Counseling patients with genetic abnormalities, Nurs. Clin. North Am. **10**:293, 1975.

Fraser, F.C.: Genetic counseling, Am. J. Hum. Genet. **26**:636, 1974.

Hirschhorn, K.: Chromosome abnormalities. I. Autosomal defects. In McKusick, V.A., and Claiborne, R., editors: Medical genetics, New York, 1973, H.P. Publishing Co.

Holtzman, N.A.: Newborn screening for inborn errors of metabolism, Pediatr. Clin. North Am. **25**:411, 1979.

Infant screening for inborn errors or metabolism, Nutr. Today **9**:105, Nov.-Dec. 1974.

Jackson, L.G.: Heterozygote detection for autosomal recessive genetic diseases, Clin. Pediatr. **13**:307, 1974.

Justice, P., and Smith, G.F.: Phenylketonuria, Am. J. Nurs. **75**:1303, Aug. 1975.

Kabak, M.M.: Medical genetics: an overview, Pediatr. Clin. North Am. **25**:395, 1979.

Kelly, P.T.: Dealing with dilemma: a manual for genetic counselors, New York, 1977, Springer-Verlag.

Lamberg, L.: Genetic screening: learning what you never wanted to know, Today's Health **54**:30, 1976.

Leonard, D.O., Chase, G.A., and Childs, B.: Genetic counseling: a consumer's view, N. Engl. J. Med. **287**:433, 1972.

Macintyre, M.N.: Problems and limitations of prenatal genetic evaluation. In Aladjem, S., editor: Risks in the practice of modern obstetrics, ed. 2, St. Louis, 1975, The C.V. Mosby Co.

Malter, S.: Genetic counseling, Nurs. Forum **16:**26, 1977.

Miles, J.H., and Kaback, M.M.: Prenatal diagnosis of hereditary disorders, Pediatr. Clin. North Am. **25:**593, 1979.

Milunsky, A.: Know your genes, New York, 1979, Avon Books.

Nitowsky, H.M., and Legum, C.P.: Genetic counseling: general principles and clinical applications, Adv. Pediatr. **18:**13, 1971.

Paris Conference: Standardization in human cytogenetics. Birth defects: original article series, vol. VIII, no. 7, 1971, The National Foundation.

Pearn, J.H.: Patients' subjective interpretation of risks in genetic counseling, J. Med. Genet. **10:**129, 1973.

Sahin, S.T.: The multifaceted role of the nurse as genetic counselor, M.C.N. **1:**211, 1976.

Tishler, C.L.: The psychological aspects of genetic counseling, Am. J. Nurs. **81:**733, 1981.

Valentine, G.H.: The reproductive counseling process, Clin. Pediatr. **16:**233, 1977.

Whaley, L.F.: Understanding inherited disorders, St. Louis, 1974, The C.V. Mosby Co.

Whaley, L.F.: Genetic counseling in maternity nursing. In McNall, L.K., and Galeener, J.T., editors: Current practice in obstetric and gynecologic nursing, vol. I, St. Louis, 1976, The C.V. Mosby Co.

Whaley, L.F.: Genetic counseling. In Curry, J.B., and Peppe, K.K., editors: Mental retardation: nursing approaches to care, St. Louis, 1978, The C.V. Mosby Co.

Wilson, M.G.: Genetic counseling, Curr. Probl. Pediatr. **5:**1, 1975.

11
Fertility

- Factors Essential to Normal Fertility
- Profile of a Fertile Woman: Assessment Data
  - History of menstrual cycle
  - Physical examination
  - Laboratory tests
- Profile of a Fertile Man: Assessment Data
- Other Factors Contributing to Fertility
  - Age
  - Length of exposure
  - Intercourse
  - Health promotion

Fertility is defined as the normal fertilization of the ovum, normal implantation of the zygote, and normal growth and development of the embryo/fetus to the point of viability.

Factors Essential to Normal Fertility

Fertility depends on a number of closely interrelated and timed events. Acquiring knowledge of the factors basic to fertility is an essential step to effective counseling of people who need information or reinforcement of facts relative to planning for pregnancy; avoiding pregnancy; etiology, tests for, and management of infertility; sterility; and voluntary sterilization. This chapter focuses on factors that are essential to fertility. It then details information about correlates of the normally functioning reproductive system of the sexually mature adult. Guidelines are provided to assist the nurse in giving appropriate information to people regarding fertility.

The following factors or conditions are essential to fertility:

1. Hypothalamus-pituitary-gonadal axis must function normally in both the man and in the woman.
2. An ovum must be released from a mature ovarian follicle.
3. The ovum must enter the fallopian tube promptly after ovulation.*
4. Cervical mucus must be receptive and supportive to spermatozoa.
5. The uterine endometrium must be adequately prepared to receive the fertilized ovum.†
6. Spermatozoa must be of normal structure, adequate in number, and ejaculated into the anatomically normal female reproductive tract.‡
7. Spermatozoa must migrate into the fallopian tube, where fertilization of the ovum normally occurs.‡
8. The fertilized ovum must find its way down the fallopian tube into the endometrial cavity to implant into the hormone-prepared endometrium 7 to 10 days after ovulation.*
9. Normal development of the conceptus must occur until viability has been reached (minimum of 24 to 28 weeks' gestation) and delivery is accomplished.§

---

*If the ovum does not enter the fallopian tube promptly, an ectopic (outside the intrauterine cavity) pregnancy may occur. This complication is mentioned in the section about complications later in this text.

†Pregnancies have occurred when the endometrium is inadequately prepared, but these pregnancies are usually associated with less than optimal outcome, that is, complications such as placenta previa, small babies, and lost pregnancies.

‡See discussion of in vitro fertilization as treatment for infertility, p. 180. It is recognized that semen deposited on the vulva (not inside the vagina) can also result in pregnancy.

§"Normal development" refers to those events that permit the pregnancy to continue. In this definition of fertility, the couple (woman) who has a problem with repeated spontaneous abortions without carrying any pregnancy to viability requires therapy for infertility. The fact that a child is born after viability has been reached but has a congenital malformation does not result in the need for therapy for infertility. This women (couple) may need to be referred for genetic counseling, however.

Profile of a Fertile Woman: Assessment Data

HISTORY OF MENSTRUAL CYCLE

The function of the hypothalamus-pituitary-gonadal axis in the woman is evidenced by the responses of the target organs (p. 85). These cyclic responses, seen in both physical and emotional changes, can be observed and felt by the woman (Table 11.1). A careful history of the menstrual pattern of the fertile woman reveals the following data:

1. All primary and secondary sexual characteristics and menarche are present by the age of 17.
2. The menstrual cycle is regular, occurring every 28 days on the average for the mature woman, but the range is from 24 to 32 days. The average duration of menstrual flow is 5 days, and the average blood loss is approximately 70 ml, but some variations are still within normal range.
3. The objective signs such as changes in the basal body temperature (BBT), breasts, and cervix correlate with the appropriate phase of the menstrual cycle (Table 11.1).
4. The subjective symptoms, such as discomfort in the breasts and abdomen, and behavioral changes correlate with the appropriate phase of the menstrual cycle (Table 11.1).

In Table 11.1, the approximate time of occurrence of the various signs and symptoms that mark the phases of the menstrual cycle is presented. For precise timing of events, refer to Chapter 6.

PHYSICAL EXAMINATION

Physical examination of a sexually mature women with a normally functioning reproductive system reveals the following data:

1. General appearance indicates good nutritional state, for example, condition of hair and nails; weight is within normal limits (see Table 18.4).
2. Breast glandular tissue has undergone development (p. 71); there is no nipple discharge.
3. External and internal genitalia, including escutcheon, are within normal limits (p. 54). General distribution of body hair is consistent with female secondary sexual characteristics.
4. Examination of cervical mucus reveals changes characteristic of the phase of the menstrual cycle.
5. Thyroid gland is not palpable; there is no exophthalmos.
6. There is no evidence of infection: nonpalpable

Table 11.1
Markers (Signs and Symptoms) of the Phases of the Menstrual Cycle

Marker	Preovulation	Ovulation	At Least 2 Days Post Ovulation up to Menses
Objective signs			
BBT	36.2-36.3° C (97.2-97.4° F)	24-36 hrs before BBT drops 0.2-0.3° F; 24-48 hr after, BBT rises 0.7-0.8° F	≥36.7° C (98° F)
Respiration			Hyperventilation with decrease in alveolar P_{CO_2}
Heart rate			Increased slightly
Breasts	Time of least hormonal effect and smallest breast size	Increased nipple erectility; increased areolar pigmentation	Increased nodularity; enlarged
Bleeding	Menstruation (days 1-5)	Midcycle spotting	
Cervix (Fig. 11.1) Mucus characteristics	"Dry" (no mucus) progressing to clear, opaque, watery, slippery mucus and increasing spinnbarkeit; increasing numbers of vaginal and cervical cells and lymphocytes	Abundant, thin, clear (egg white) mucus with spinnbarkeit (4 cm [often up to 10 cm]) that dries in a fern pattern (arborization)	Cloudy, sticky, impenetrable to sperm; dries in granular pattern
Mucus pH	About 7.0	7.5	
Os	Gradual, progressive widening	Open, with mucus seen spilling out	Gradual closing of os
Color of exocervix	Pink	Hyperemic (red)	Gradual return to pink
Body	Firm to touch (like tip of nose)	Soft (like earlobe)	Gradual return to firm

Continued.

Table 11.1—cont'd
Markers (Signs and Symptoms) of the Phases of the Menstrual Cycle

Marker	Preovulation	Ovulation	At Least 2 Days Post Ovulation up to Menses
Subjective signs			
Physical discomfort			
Breasts			Heaviness, fullness; enlarged, tender*
Abdomen	Dysmenorrhea: uterine cramping; nausea, vomiting, and diarrhea; dizziness	Intermenstrual pain (mittelschmerz) occurs 1.7 days after peak of cervical mucus and 2.5 days before increase in BBT	Premenstrual syndrome: backaches; feeling of increasing pelvic fullness
General	Increased weight; feeling of heaviness		Headache†; acne
Affective changes‡			
Moods	Some depression may persist from premenses	Sense of well-being	Premenstrual syndrome (PMS): increased irritability, passivity, depression
Libido		Increased sexual desire	
Energy levels			Spurt of energy, followed by fatigue
Other changes			
Fallopian tubes		Motility greatest	Motility least
Vagina		Epithelium thickens (cornifies); increased number of cell layers	Increased number of precornified cells, mucous shreds, and cells
Myometrium	Vascularity increased with hypertrophy and hyperplasia		
Ovary	Increases in size and nodularity	Returns to usual size; nodularity becomes less noticeable to palpation	

*Sociocultural influences may affect symptoms reported by women. Breast tenderness is rarely reported by Japanese women.
†Headaches reported with greater frequency by Nigerian women.
‡NOTE: Literature usually attributes negative premenstrual symptoms to biology while good moods and rational behavior are not. When men and women are compared in activity patterns, mood changes, and symptoms, similar variability has been found in *both* men and women even though the changes in women are given more attention by society.

lymph nodes, absence of skin lesions, absence of inflammation of vagina or abnormal vaginal discharge.

LABORATORY TESTS

Laboratory tests are appropriate to rule out any condition that could jeopardize a pregnancy if a pregnancy occurs, as well as to identify a condition that may be contributing to a person's infertility. The performance of the laboratory tests and a discussion with the client about the findings open another channel of communication between client and care giver. This presents another opportunity for the health care team to teach good health care and for them to motivate an increased participation on the part of the client in her own health care.

Laboratory tests that help to establish base line data about the client's state of general health include the following:

1. Complete blood count (CBC) and differential indicate that the numbers of cellular components of blood and hemoglobin are within normal limits (see Appendix G).
2. Blood tests are negative for VDRL (Veneral Disease Research Laboratories) test for treponema antibodies (nonspecific test for syphilis) and sickle cell (in susceptible populations).
3. Urinalysis is negative for infection and for protein, acetone, and sugar.
4. Cervical and vaginal smears are negative for gonorrhea, *Chlamydia trachomatis*, herpes, or other infections and for cellular dysplasia (Papanicolaou smear).

Fig. 11.1
Cervical changes during menstrual cycle.

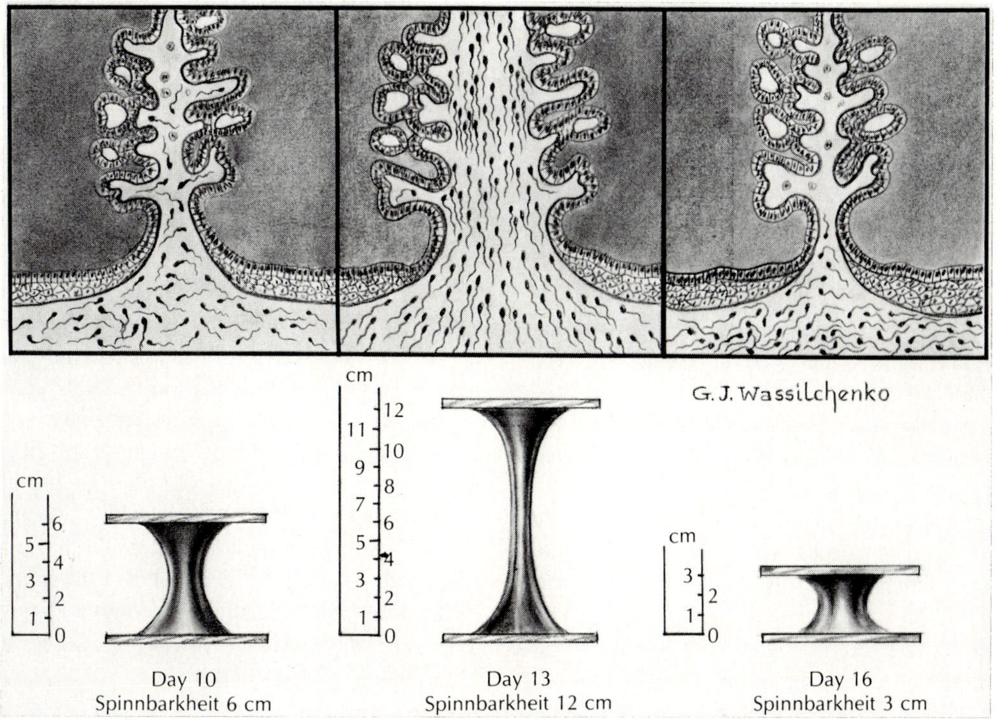

Profile of a Fertile Man: Assessment Data

Physical examination of a sexually mature man with a normally functioning reproductive system reveals the following data:

1. His developmental history does *not* include conditions that *may* affect fertility, for example, cryptorchidism (undescended testes), hypospadias, or orchitis (due to infection such as mumps). Prompt surgical intervention, if surgery were needed, for undescended testes or hypospadias may have prevented the development of a potential problem that would interfere with fertility.
2. His developmental history reveals normal development of secondary sexual characteristics, for example, growth spurts, appearance and pattern of facial hair, and voice change.
3. His history does not include exposure to toxic agents (e.g., x rays, lead, chemicals), antihypertensive medications; or accidents that involve the pelvic area.
4. Physical findings are within normal limits: hair patterns, normotensive readings, genital structures (p. 76), and neurologic signs, including vision.

Other Factors Contributing to Fertility

Age. The age for maximal fertility for both the female and the male is 25 years.

Length of exposure. For two thirds of couples who are at the maximal age for fertility, conception occurs within 5 to 6 months of regular intercourse if no contraceptive methods have been used; within 12 months, all but four to seven couples out of 100 will conceive.

Intercourse. Frequency of intercourse and timing of intercourse with ovulation (coital exposure) are important to fertility.

Health promotion. Fertility cannot be ensured for everyone. However, some guidelines (given below) are available for nurses who provide anticipatory guidance for clients and their families.

The incidence of *vaginal infection* may be avoided or decreased by observing the following cautions. Maintain normal vaginal pH by avoiding diets high in refined sugar and avoiding douching. Watch for vaginal infections when the woman is taking antibiotics or if the woman has diabetes mellitus or other debilitating disease. Antibiotic therapy and certain disease conditions change the vaginal pH and therefore change the body's natural defenses against infection. Choose sexual partners carefully; for example, avoid direct contact with infected lesions. In addition to the possibility of acquiring an infection that may progress to pelvic inflammatory disease (PID) that is directly implicated in infertility (p. 178), herpetic infection also primes the woman to cervical carcinoma under certain conditions (see Chapter 36).

Damage from infections of the reproductive tract can be minimized if the infection is recognized and treated early.

If the young man does not acquire mumps, he should be immunized against parotitis before puberty to avoid *mumps orchitis* which can result in infertility or sterility.

Before using a *contraceptive method,* each method is considered carefully in light of future fertility. Women need to wait until menstrual cycles are well established before starting hormonal suppression of ovulation (birth control pills). Women need to watch for early signs of PID and obtain prompt treatment, especially when wearing an intrauterine device (IUD) (p. 179).

If the *intrauterine cavity* is to be entered for any reason (e.g., endometrial biopsy, currettage, completion of a spontaneous abortion), women need to know the following information. Laminaria* atraumatically dilate the cervix that is firm and has a tight os. Traumatic dilation is avoided to prevent injury to the internal os. Such injuries may result in an incompetent cervix later (p. 781). Postprocedure infections require early diagnosis and treatment. Poor nutrition before or following a procedure predisposes the women to infection.

Good hygiene and the wearing of loose-fitting clothing reduce the incidence of vulvar-vaginal infections. Clothing that prevents air circulation in the vulvar area (tight jeans, pantyhose without cotton crotches) keeps the area dark and moist—good conditions for the development of microorganisms. Good hand washing before and following touching the vulvar area prevents self-reinnoculation with infectious material but also prevents spread to other people. Nurses may need to remind some women that perineal pads or tampons need to be changed frequently. Perineal pads should be changed every time a woman voids or defecates; tampons need to be changed about every 2 to 3 hours. Occasionally, women need to be reminded to wipe "front to back" once with each tissue and to avoid wiping back over the vulvar area after touching the area around the anus.

Abstention from coitus until age 18 and avoidance of multiple sexual partners decrease the incidence of infection and cervical dysplasia (p. 829). Such conditions may result in the need for cervical surgery (see discussion of incompetent cervix, Chapter 35).

Severe or prolonged *emotional stress* decreases the body's defense against infection. Knowledge that stress affects the body adversely alerts the individual of the need to employ stress reduction methods.

There is a *peak time* during reproductive life when the potential for fertility is greatest; fertility decreases after age 35 in the woman and after age 40 in the man.

Education for fertility begins with adequate knowledge of hygiene, mental health practices, and nutrition. Sex education in the schools and in the home can help individuals to have fertile reproductive lives.

*For a description of laminaria, see Chapter 41.

References and Readings

Anthony, C.P., and Thibodeau, G.A.: Textbook of anatomy and physiology, ed. 11, St. Louis, 1983, The C.V. Mosby Co.

Beacham, D.W., and Beacham, W.D.: Synopsis of gynecology, ed. 10, St. Louis, 1982, The C.V. Mosby Co.

Benson, R.C., editor: Current obstetric and gynecologic diagnosis and treatment, ed. 4, Los Altos, Calif., 1982, Lange Medical Publications.

Eschenback, D.A.: A guide to diagnosis and treatment of vaginal infection, Contemp. Obstet. Gynecol. **20**(3):203, 1982.

Fogel, C.I., and Woods, N.F.: Health care of women: a nursing perspective, St. Louis, 1981, The C.V. Mosby Co.

Guyton, A.C.: Textbook of medical physiology, ed. 5, Philadelphia, 1976, W.B. Saunders Co.

Lowrey, G.H.: Growth and development of children, ed. 7, Chicago, 1978, Year Book Medical Publishers, Inc.

Malasanos, L., et al.: Health assessment, ed. 2, St. Louis, 1981, The C.V. Mosby Co.

Moore, K.L.: The developing human, ed. 2, Philadelphia, 1977, W.B. Saunders Co.

Moore, K.L.: Before we are born: Basic embryology and birth defects (revised reprint), Philadelphia, 1977, W.B. Saunders Co.

Shangold, M.M: Advising patients about tampons and other sanitary products, Contemp. Obstet. Gynecol. **20**:73 (special issue), Oct. 1983.

Urban, D.J., et al.: Nurse specialization in reproductive endocrinology, J.O.G.N. Nurs. **11**(3):167, 1982.

Williams, S.R.: Nutrition and diet therapy, ed. 4, St. Louis, 1981, The C.V. Mosby Co.

12
Infertility

- Investigation of Infertility
  - Religious factors leading to infertility problems
  - Use of marijuana (a cannabinoid)
  - General nursing care
- Investigation of Female Infertility
  - Factors implicated in female infertility
  - Identification of infertility factors
  - Fertility tests and examinations
  - Therapy for female infertility
    - Congenital or developmental factors
    - Ovulation
    - Tubal (peritoneal) factors
    - Endometriosis
    - Uterine factors
    - Vaginal-cervical factors
    - In vitro fertilization
- Investigation of Male Infertility
  - Factors implicated in male infertility
  - Identification of infertility factors
  - Therapy for male infertility
    - Artificial insemination
- The Emotional Crisis of Infertility: Implications for Nursing Action
- Summary of Nursing Actions

The inability to conceive and bear a child comes as a tragedy to a surprising number of otherwise healthy adults. Persons requesting assistance for problems of infertility have already decided that they want a child. The experiences of pregnancy and birth, parenthood, and the expression of love through the care and nurturing of another human being represent to them evidence of normal growth of adult sexuality. The idea that fertility is a necessary component of mature and fulfilled sexuality is common throughout the world. Pressures from family or peers may be subtle or obvious. Messages that it is natural to want babies or that only selfishness could be the motivating factor in childlessness can bring much unhappiness to couples. Many people appear anxious and tense as they relate their difficulty in achieving pregnancy and are sensitive to real or imagined criticisms of their sexual ability or, conversely, of their need for a child in this overpopulated world. They look for readily expressed acceptance from the nurse and physician of their need for a child as well as of their infertility problems.

Investigation of Infertility

Infertility is the inability to conceive after at least 1 year of adequate exposure when no contraceptive measures were used or the inability to deliver a live infant after three consecutive conceptions. Generally two thirds of couples who have sexual intercourse without the use of contraceptives achieve pregnancy within 6 months, and 90% within 1 year. For the anxious couple or the older couple (woman over 30 years and man over 40 years, or both), a 6-month effort is sufficient before fertility studies are begun.

Infertility is *primary* if the woman has never been pregnant (or the man has never impregnated a woman); infertility is *secondary* if the woman has been pregnant at least once but has not been able to conceive again or to sustain a pregnancy. Infertility, whether primary or secondary, occurs in one couple in five. For 85% of these couples, the underlying cause can be diagnosed; 50% to 70% can be treated successfully. The incidence of infertility seems to be increasing, probably because of (1) the trend to delay pregnancy until later in life when fertility decreases naturally and (2) the increase in pelvic inflammatory disease.

Investigation of infertility requires the accumulation of extensive data related to factors essential for or contributing to fertility. A theoretic base is necessary to direct the investigator's assessments, to analyze findings, and to plan, implement, and evaluate the management of and therapy for infertility.

Some of the data needed is of a sensitive, personal nature, and obtaining this data may be viewed as an invasion of privacy. The tests and examinations are occasionally painful and intrusive and can take the romance out of lovemaking. A high level of motivation is needed to endure the investigation. The attitude, sensitivity, and caring nature of those who are involved in the assessment of infertility lay the foundation for the client's ability to cope with the subsequent therapy and management.

Members of the health team must respect the clients' rights to privacy and confidentiality of records.

RELIGIOUS FACTORS LEADING TO INFERTILITY PROBLEMS

The Orthodox Jewish husband and wife may face infertility management problems because of religious laws that govern marital relations. According to Jewish law, the couple may not engage in marital relations during menstruation and through the following 7 "preparatory days." The wife then is immersed in a ritual bath (Mikvah) before relations can resume. The 5 menstrual days and 7 preparatory days collectively are called the "nida state." Any vaginal bleeding of physiologic origin marks the beginning of the nida state. Fertility problems can arise when the woman has a short cycle (i.e., a cycle of 24 days or less, when ovulation would occur on day 10 or earlier). Small doses of estrogen may delay ovulation to allow for the time needed to complete the nida state. Other procedures that induce bleeding may delay intercourse for another 12 days to allow for the nida state. Thus Orthodox Jewish clients as well as observant Catholics may at times question proposed diagnostic and therapeutic procedures because of religious proscriptions. These clients are encouraged to consult their rabbi or priest for a ruling.

USE OF MARIJUANA (A CANNABINOID)

Among marijuana smokers there have been observed decreases in sperm number and sperm motility and small decreases in the percentage of spermatozoa in the ejaculate with a normal oval configuration. Therefore marijuana smoking has been shown to have a direct suppressive effect on spermatogenesis. There has been no evidence that marijuana affects the production of testosterone, however. Counseling the infertile couple when the male smokes several marijuanna cigarettes every day includes avoidance of marijuana and frequent semen analyses for at least a minimum of 6 months if pregnancy is desired.

GENERAL NURSING CARE

Nursing actions vary with the nurse's level of education, position held, and policies of the agency. Basic to all nursing actions is knowledge of those factors that are essential to or contribute to fertility, of assessment strategies (history, examinations, and tests), and of management and therapy for infertility. The nurse helps to assess the client's readiness to learn and her or his level of understanding of infertility. Although primary responsibility for teaching the client or clients rests with the physician, the nurse assists in the identification of the client's gaps in knowledge, clarifies information, and reinforces the physician's explanations and instructions. Occasionally the nurse acts as the client's advocate by assisting the client to state a concern or question or to request further explanation from the physician or technician.

The nurse's nonverbal behavior before or during the procedure can reassure and support the client. Often the client is feeling inadequate due to the necessity for testing and the intimidating nature of the tests.

Written and verbal instructions for specific preparation for tests will increase the client's feeling of adequacy and prepare the client for sensations usually experienced during and after the procedure. Therapeutic nursing actions include providing privacy while giving instructions for obtaining specimens and changing clothes, draping, creating a comfortable physical environment, padding the stirrups of the examination table, efficiency in use of equipment, warming the speculum, and coaching for relaxation.

Women often experience anxiety when undergoing a pelvic examination. This anxiety stems from many sources, such as fear of what will be discovered, fear of pain, and fear of embarrassment. Some women tend to relax when they are involved in the examination by viewing themselves with a mirror while the physician or nurse-practitioner examines them. Relaxation of the perineum decreases the amount of perceived discomfort. To assist the client to relax the perineum, ask her to keep her eyes and hands open and to breathe in through her nose and out through her mouth while her relaxed lips form the letter *o*. Clutching onto a grip on the table or to the nurse's hand and pressing one's lips together cause tightening of all of the perineal musculature. The insertion of the speculum is less traumatic if it is done while the woman performs Valsalva's maneuver (taking a deep breath and bearing down toward the vagina).

Following a procedure, after the client is fully dressed and comfortably seated (at the same level as the nurse and physician), she or he benefits from an opportunity to talk about the experience in an unhurried manner. Not only do these behaviors help the client relax, but also they indicate that the recipient of such care is worthy and thus helps build self-esteem. The goal of nursing-medical *care* is to encourage the client to become an active partner in care as well as to establish rapport to ensure that therapy and eventual counseling is facilitated.

The nurse needs to know the correct method for obtaining, labeling, and transporting specimens to the laboratory. A mishandled specimen may lead to misdiagnosis or the need to obtain another specimen. These errors create added expense to the client as well as significant time delays before theapy can be instituted.

In this emotionally charged area, the problem-oriented record with progress notes and flow sheets is one useful method to facilitate consistency of information given to the woman (or couple). Regardless of the method of record keeping, accurate and detailed notes are essential.

Investigation of Female Infertility

FACTORS IMPLICATED IN FEMALE INFERTILITY

Investigation of fertility and identification of the conditions that may be responsible for the infertile state constitute a long and tedious process. Infertility may occur when a single fertility factor is absent. At other times a combination of factors, female and male, is necessary to cause infertility. In Table 12.1 each factor

Table 12.1
Factors Associated With Fertility and Infertility

Factors Required for Fertility	Conditions Associated with Infertility
Development of reproductive tract is normal.	Congenital or developmental factors Abnormal external genitalia (e.g., enlarged clitoris or fused labia) which may suggest masculinization Gynetresia (e.g., absence of vagina or shallow vagina) Vaginal anomalies (e.g., double vagina with single or double cervix and single or double uterus or with one vaginal canal ending blindly, the other vaginal canal ending at entrance to a uterus) Unusual uterus (e.g., congenital small, or "infantile," uterus) Uterine and tubal defects from exposure to DES as embryo/fetus Abnormalities of ovary (see ovulation)
Ovulation: Hypothalamus-pituitary-gonadal axis is normal. An ovum is released from a mature ovarian follicle.	Absence of ovulation Malfunctioning of axis with menstrual irregularities (see p. 177) Abnormal ovaries as seen in Turner's syndrome (see p. 149) or Stein-Leventhal syndrome Hormonal suppression of hypothalamus-pituitary-gonadal axis with birth control medication Emotional problems (e.g., severe psychoneurosis or psychosis or anorexia nervosa, which may be responsible for anovulatory cycles, frequently associated with amenorrhea or oligomenorrhea) Menstrual irregularities from vigorous exercise (jogging, sports), especially in thin women
Tubal: ovum enters fallopian tube promptly after ovulation. Spermatozoa migrate into fallopian tube where fertilization takes place. Fertilized ovum finds its way down tube into endometrial cavity to implant into hormone-prepared endometrium 7 to 10 days after ovulation.	Fallopian tube is blocked or its function is altered. Blockage of tube by scar tissue formation following infection (pelvic inflammatory disease, ruptured appendix followed by peritonitis), or pelvic surgery Blockage of tube by compression or kinking by abnormal growth such as endometriosis and neoplasms Alteration in tubal motility by birth control medication or from emotional stress
Uterine: uterine endometrium is adequately prepared to receive fertilized ovum.	Uterus is malformed or endometrium is unreceptive to fertilized ovum (malfunction of hypothalamus-pituitary-gonadal axis; presence of endometrial infection; presence of intrauterine device [IUD])
Vaginal-cervical: cervical mucus is receptive and supportive to spermatozoa. Cervix is competent.	Absence of mucous characteristics receptive and supportive to spermatozoa (see p. 159) Altered vaginal pH from feminine hygiene preparations or douches, infections, antibiotic chemotherapy, disease states (e.g., diabetes mellitus), poor hygiene, or emotional stress Altered vaginal pH by lubricants used during coitus Presence of spermicidal foams or other preparations used for contraception Development of antibodies (an immunologic response) against a specific male's spermatozoa (see discussion of sperm, pp. 172 and 180
Spermatozoa are normal, adequate in number, and ejaculated into female reproductive tract.	Spermatozoal factors discussed later in this chapter
Conceptus develops normally, reaches viability, and is delivered in good condition.	

essential to fertility is presented, along with a listing of conditions associated with infertility.

IDENTIFICATION OF INFERTILITY FACTORS

The diagnosis of female infertility requires a careful history taken with special reference to growth, development, and general health, as well as to specific illnesses that may compromise fertility (e.g., gonorrhea or tuberculosis) (see p. 178). A careful evaluation of the menstrual history, the occurrence of pregnancy in the past, and the outcome is helpful. Consideration of the woman's emotional makeup, life-style, and habits, as well as her general hygiene, is important. Previous abdominal or vaginal surgery is recorded and may have significance. If contraception has been practiced, the type, duration of use, and any problems arising from the contraceptive method, in addition to the frequency of coitus, are recorded. The family history may be revealing, particularly when genetic or congenital abnormalities, infertility, and loss of early pregnancies are reported.

A thorough physical examination may disclose medical disorders such as goiter or other endocrine problems that can cause infertility. Examination for gynecologic abnormalities must be meticulous.

In addition to routine blood and urine analyses, any or all of the tests or examinations given in Table 12.2 may be necessary for accurate diagnosis and management of various fertility factors.

Table 12.2
Tests and Examinations for Fertility

Fertility Factor	Test or Examination
Ovulation	Basal body temperature (BBT)
	Cervical mucus changes
	Timed endometrial biopsy
	Plasma progesterone level
Tubal	Rubin's test
	Hysterosalpingography or hysterography
	Laparoscopic examination
Uterine	Physical examination
	Hysterosalpingography or hysterography
	Laparoscopic examination
Cervical	Physical examination
	Assessment of cervical mucus changes
	Postcoital test, or Sims-Huhner test
	Sperm immobilization antigen-antibody reaction

FERTILITY TESTS AND EXAMINATIONS

There are several examinations and tests for female infertility. Each method of assessment is discussed under the following headings: which partner is involved in testing or in collection of the specimen, why the test is done, when the test is scheduled, how and where the test is accomplished, the risks involved, the information that is sought, and specific medical and nursing actions pertinent to the situation.

Self-assessment of BBT and cervical mucus involves touching oneself and one's discharges. Therefore self-assessment can be emotionally uncomfortable for some women. The nurse may also be uneasy teaching self-assessment techniques to others.

To assess her BBT, the woman must lubricate and insert a rectal thermometer (see procedure, p. 167), leave it in place for at least 3 minutes, and then remove and wipe it clean. After reading the thermometer, she must enter the finding on a graph and wash the thermometer with soap and tepid water. After teaching the technique, the nurse needs to ask the woman to repeat the directions and demonstrate her ability to read a thermometer and enter the temperature on the graph. (Some women prefer to use oral thermometers.)

Assessment of cervical mucus does not necessarily require internal examination or the use of instruments. The woman (couple) is asked to observe for changes in the physical characteristics of the mucus. The woman is asked to describe whatever characteristics and sensations she has already noticed whether or not she has previously known their significance. Her descriptions give the nurse clues to the words the woman uses and direct the nurse's anticipatory guidance to fit the client's level of understanding. The nurse then reviews mucous findings associated with menstrual cycle phases.

From the last day of the menstrual flow, the woman makes daily observations and recordings of changes in her cervical mucus—its quantity, consistency, color, and sensation.

1. Quantity (e.g., none, copious, sparse).
2. Consistency (e.g., thick, pasty, sticky, tacky, creamy, milky, stretchable [spinnbarkeit], slippery, like raw egg white).
3. Color (e.g., whitish or cloudy, yellowish, clear, blood tinged).
4. Sensation in the vulvar area (e.g., dry, wet, lubricative).

Mucus should be observed several times each day, perhaps before each time the woman empties her bladder. She can obtain the mucus at the vaginal introitus. There is no need to reach into the vagina to the cervix for mucus.

A simulation experience that may facilitate the client's use of this diagnostic aid can be provided by the nurse: using raw egg albumen (in a bowl) that the

Text continued on p. 171.

Basal ("Resting") Body Temperature

Who: Woman

Why: To obtain presumptive evidence of ovulation and an adequate luteal (progesterone) phase

How: Obtain and maintain a record of daily rectal temperatures taken each morning after awakening and before *any* physical activity; any physical activity increases the body's metabolic rate; the increased metabolic rate is reflected in a thermal increase, which then may be mistaken for the thermal rise that accompanies ovulation and the secretory phase of the cycle; one suggestion that may help the woman remain at her basal metabolic rate is to ask her to buy a snooze alarm; the first time the snooze alarm goes off, she inserts her thermometer and snoozes; then when the alarm goes off the second time 5 to 10 minutes later, she can take out the thermometer and set it aside to read later when she is awake and can focus

When: Daily throughout several menstrual cycles

Where: At home in privacy of own bedroom

Risk:
1. Low
2. Requires high level of motivation by woman (and cooperation of sexual partner).
3. May be inconvenient to take temperature before any activity (e.g., shaking down the thermometer, going to the bathroom, engaging in lovemaking)
4. Misinterpretation because other factors, when present, elevate the BBT (e.g., tension, infection, headaches, fever, any activity such as coitus before taking BBT, staying up late the previous night, imbibing in alcoholic beverages the evening before)
5. Misinterpretation because of inability to use and read the thermometer

Procedure

- Woman obtains a BBT thermometer that is calibrated in tenths (Fig. 12.1).
- Woman takes and records her temperature daily (Fig. 12.2) before any activity.
- Woman maintains a record of other events (e.g., fever, tension, cervical mucus characteristics).
- Woman shakes down the thermometer, washes it in tepid water with a mild soap, and replaces it within easy reach by the bedside. Woman resets the snooze alarm for the next morning.

Information Sought

Factors favorable to fertility:
1. The menstrual cycle is biphasic.
2. The elevated temperature persists for 12 to 14 days before menses.
3. At the time of the slight temperature drop that is followed by a persistent elevation, midcycle bleeding or mittleschmerz may occur; or just prior to menses, premenstrual syndrome may occur.*

*NOTE: 20% of ovulating women do *not* show a biphasic temperature curve.

Fig. 12.1
Special thermometer for recording BBT, marked in tenths to enable person to read more easily.

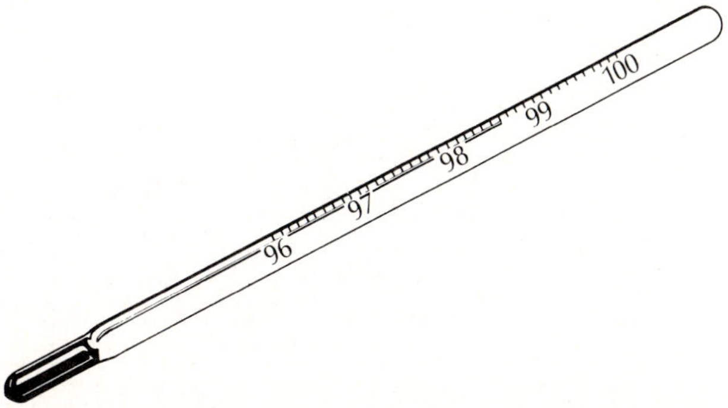

Fig. 12.2

A, Basal temperature record shows drop and sharp rise at time of ovulation. Biphasic curve is indicative of ovulatory cycle. **B,** Monophasic (flat) curve is indicative of anovulatory cycle. **C,** Persistent elevation and amenorrhea are suggestive of pregnancy.

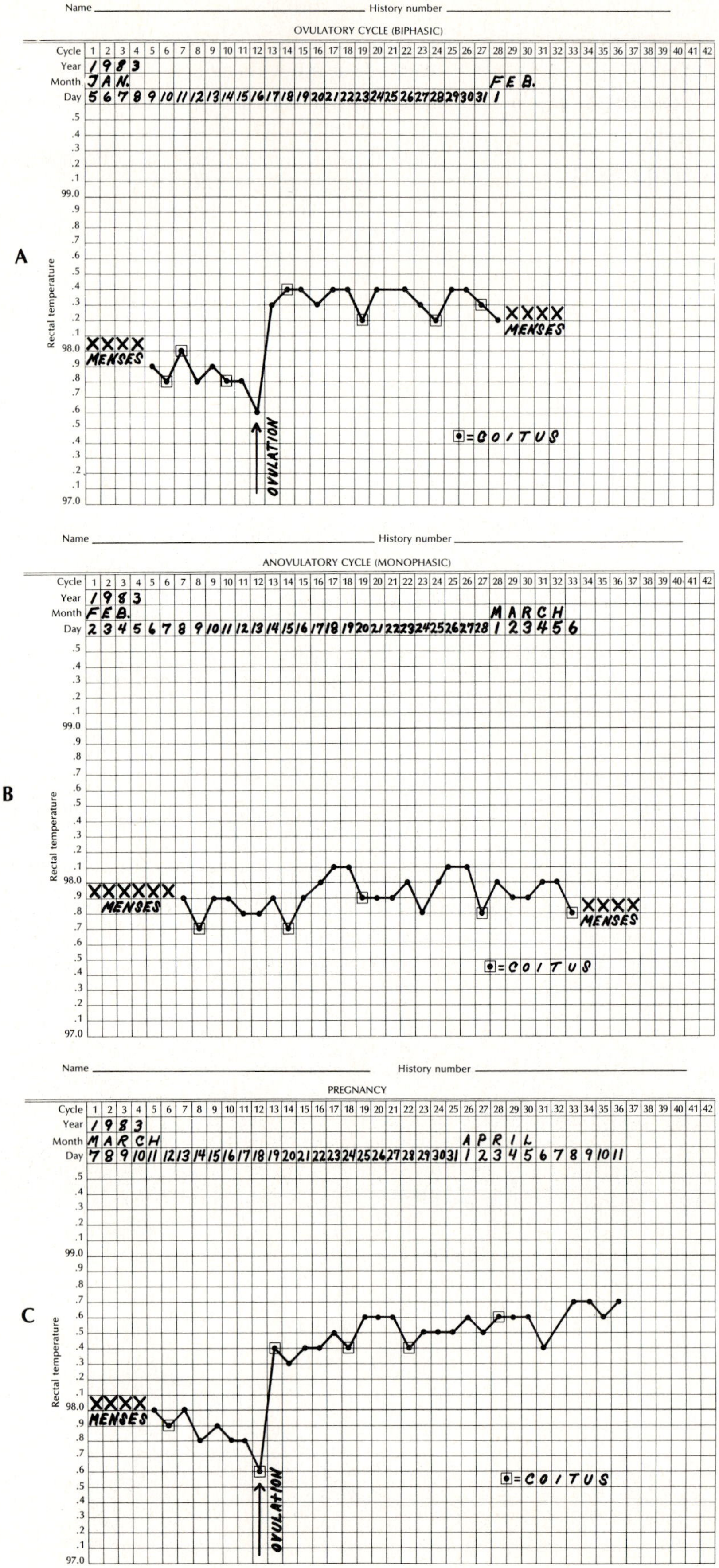

Cervical Mucus Characteristics

Who: Woman (and man)

Why: To obtain presumptive evidence of ovulation and adequacy of estrogen and progesterone phases

How: Obtain and evaluate cervical mucus characteristics through several menstrual cycles (see Fig. 11.1)

When: Daily throughout several menstrual cycles

Where: At home in privacy of own bedroom

Risk:
1. Low
2. Requires high level of motivation by couple
3. Evaluation may be difficult in the presence of vaginal discharge from infection, vaginal menstrual bleeding, contraceptive foams, lubricants, etc.

Procedure

- After carefully washing her hands, woman (or her mate) obtains some cervical mucus and assesses its characteristics.
- Woman records findings on the same record on which her BBT is entered.
- Woman records any other events or feelings.

Information Sought

For findings favorable to fertility see the box on p. 170 and Figs. 12.3 to 12.5.

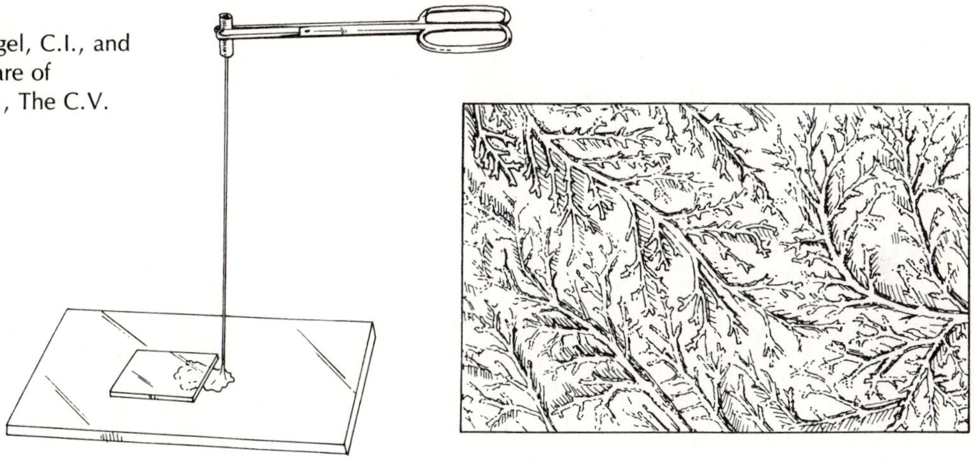

Fig. 12.3
Fern patterns. (From Fogel, C.I., and Woods, N.F.: Health care of women, St. Louis, 1981, The C.V. Mosby Co.)

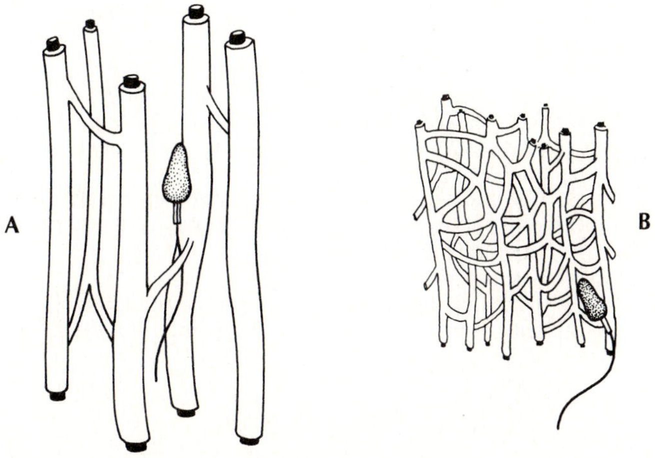

Fig. 12.4
Sperm passage through cervical mucus. **A,** Receptive mucus under estrogen influence. **B,** Nonreceptive mucus under progesterone influence. (From Fogel, C.I., and Woods, N.F.: Health care of women, St. Louis, 1981, The C.V. Mosby Co.)

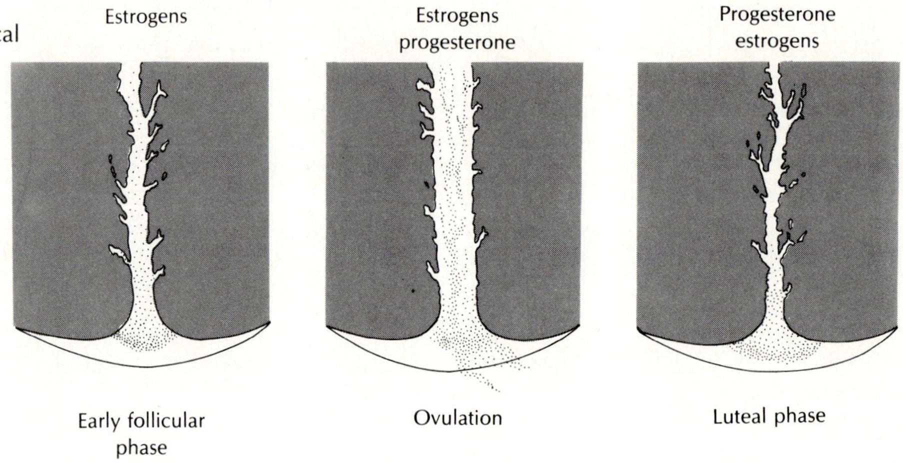

Fig. 12.5
Sperm migration through cervical canal. (From Fogel, C.I., and Woods, N.F.: Health care of women, St. Louis, 1981, The C.V. Mosby Co.)

Summary of Fertility Test Findings Favorable to Fertility

1. Follicular development, ovulation, and luteal development are supportive to pregnancy:
   a. BBT (presumptive evidence of ovulatory cycles)
      (1) Is biphasic
      (2) Reveals temperature elevation that persists for 12 to 14 days just before menstruation
   b. Cervical mucus characteristics change appropriately during phases of the menstrual cycle
   c. Findings from endometrial biopsies taken at different times during menstrual cycle are consistent with day of cycle
   d. Laparoscopic visualization of pelvic organs verifies follicular and luteal development
2. The luteal phase is supportive to pregnancy:
   a. Levels of plasma progesterone are adequate
   b. Endometrial biopsy findings indicate a secretory endometrium
3. Cervical factors are receptive to spermatozoa during expected time of ovulation:
   a. Cervical os is open
   b. Cervical mucus is clear, watery, abundant, and slippery and demonstrates good spinnbarkeit and arborization (fern pattern)
   c. Cervical examination is negative for lesions and infections
   d. Postcoital test findings are satisfactory (adequate number of live, motile, normal spermatozoa present in the cervical mucus)
   e. No immunity to spermatozoa can be demonstrated
4. The uterus and fallopian tubes are supportive to pregnancy:
   a. Uterine and tubal patency is documented by
      (1) Passage of carbon dioxide into peritoneal cavity
      (2) Spillage of dye into peritoneal cavity
      (3) Outlines of uterine and tubal cavities are of adequate size and shape with no abnormalities
   b. Laparoscopic examination verifies normal development of internal genitalia, and absence of adhesions, infections, endometriosis, and other lesions
5. Semen is supportive to pregnancy:
   a. Spermatozoa are adequate in number per milliliter
   b. Majority of spermatozoa show normal morphology
   c. Spermatozoa are motile
   d. No autoimmunity exists
   e. Seminal fluid is normal

nurse and client can feel, the client will be better prepared for the sight and texture of the slippery cervical mucus.

In a menstrual cycle of average length, menses lasts about 5 days. For several days after the cessation of menses, the woman senses no obvious wetness in or near the vagina; these are the "dry" days (Table 11.1). The sensation of dryness disappears as the amount of mucus increases and becomes noticeable outside the vagina. Close to ovulation, the mucus becomes watery, clear, and slippery. At this time the woman notices that the mucus on her panties is like raw egg white and clings and stretches as she takes them off. This type of mucus gives a lubricative sensation. Some women prefer to assess mucus that they remove from near the cervical os, usually with their fingers. If the woman takes the mucus between her thumb and forefinger and separates her fingers, the mucus can be stretched several centimeters. *Spinnbarkeit* (to spin a thread) is the term given to describe the stretchiness of the mucus. The "peak" mucus sign appears just before ovulation (e.g., abundant, watery, clear, cloudy or yellowish, spinnbar keit to 5+ cm [Fig. 11.1], lubricative) and indicates the period of maximal fertility. Sperm deposited in this type of mucus can survive until ovulation occurs. The peak mucus sign may be accompanied by a feeling of

Plasma Progesterone Level

Who: Woman
Why: To assess function of corpus luteum
How: A blood sample is drawn
When: Late in menstrual cycle, just before menstruation
Where: Clinic, physician's office, or hospital laboratory
Risk:
1. Low
2. Discomfort from venipuncture

Procedure	Information Sought
■ Woman has blood drawn at the appropriate time.	Findings favorable to fertility: adequate levels of progesterone are found. Progesterone levels correlate well with BBT and cervical mucus characteristics.

Hormone Analysis

Who: Woman
Why: To assess endocrine function
How: Blood and urine specimens are obtained
When: At varying times during menstrual cycle
Where: Clinic, physician's office, or hospital laboratory
Risk:
1. Low
2. Discomfort from venipuncture
3. Inconvenience of collecting urine and taking to laboratory (when urine specimens are used)

Procedure	Information Sought
	Findings favorable to fertility:
■ Blood sample is drawn.	1. Levels of progesterone, estrogen, FSH, and LH are all appropriate.
■ Urine specimen is obtained.	2. Levels of 17-ketosteroids and 17-hydroxycorticosteroids are within normal limits.

fullness around the vagina, mittelschmerz, and increased physical energy, sense of well-being, and libido. Menstruation should follow in 12 to 16 days.

Assessment of mucus characteristics is best learned with mucus that has not been mixed with semen or discharge from infection. The couple is asked to refrain from ejaculation of semen into or near the vagina for at least one full, infection-free cycle. When intercourse is resumed in the following cycle, the difference between cervical mucus and semen will be apparent.

Good hand washing is imperative to begin and end all self-assessment activities.

Keeping daily records for a long period of time can become annoying. The woman or couple needs to be given an opportunity to ventilate negative feelings, to be complimented on charts that are well done, and to be encouraged in whatever other ways are appropriate.

Sperm immobilization antigen-antibody reaction is another check for infertility. Three principal immune processes are responsible for occasional instances of infertility unexplained in other ways:

1. In men, autoimmunization occurs. Autoimmune antibodies (produced by the man against his own sperm) agglutinate or immobilize spermatozoa in less than 5% of men with infertility.
2. In women, tissue antibodies are formed against spermatozoa.
3. In women, circulatory antibodies (beta-globulin agglutinating antibodies probably attached to a steroid hormone) are formed against spermatozoa.

About 20% of infertile women have sperm antibodies. Spermatozoa may be immobilized within the cervical mucus, or they become incapable of migration into the uterus. A greater incidence of sperm agglutination occurs in women with otherwise unexplained infertility. However, the true significance and reliability of tests for sperm immobilization or agglutination are uncertain.

Laparoscopy* is a diagnostic and surgical endoscopy technique that can be done on an outpatient basis with local or general anesthesia (Fig. 12.8). Marked

*Adapted from the film *Laparoscopy: The View Within,* text by John Marlow, M.D., July 1975, Merrell-National Laboratories. With permission from Merrell-National Laboratories, Division of Richardson-Merrell Inc.

Endometrial Biopsy

Who: Woman; and her driver to take her home

Why: To assess function of corpus luteum and receptivity of endometrium for implantation; and to check for tuberculosis*

How: Sample of endometrium is removed for histologic study

When: Late in menstrual cycle; 3 to 4 days before expected menses

Where: Clinic or hospital surgical suite

Risk:
1. Analgesia/anesthesia may be needed
2. Discomfort from uterine cramping

Procedure

- Couple is cautioned to abstain from intercourse during preceding "fertile" period to avoid dislodging a possible pregnancy during procedure.
- Cervix is dilated with laminaria† 4 to 24 hours before procedure (requires no analgesia).
- Woman assumes lithotomy position, is draped, and has a speculum inserted.
- Laminaria are removed.
- If not previously dilated with laminaria, cervix is dilated now with metal rod dilators. Analgesia/anesthesia is often necessary.
- Small specimen of endometrium is removed from side wall in fundus to avoid an embryo should conception have occurred.‡

Information Sought

Findings favorable to fertility:
1. Endometrium is negative for tuberculosis, polyps, or inflammatory conditions.
2. Endometrium reflects secretory changes normally seen in presence of adequate luteal (progesterone) phase.

*The incidence of tuberculosis is high partly because large numbers of recent refugees have come to the United States with the disease.
†Laminaria are small, thin inserts of packed seaweed, which, when inserted into the cervix, absorb moisture and thus dilate the cervix.
‡When implantation occurs, it is usually high in the fundus, either in the anterior or in the posterior portion.

obesity and previous abdominal surgery may make the procedure more difficult but are not absolute contraindications.

Laparoscopy may be used in the *investigation of infertility* secondary to adnexal disease (disease of the ovaries, tubes, or broad ligaments), unexplained abdominal or pelvic pain, primary or secondary amenorrhea associated with developmental anomalies, suspected endometriosis or ectopic pregnancy, evaluation of masses, assessment of chronic pelvic inflammatory disease, and ovum recovery for in vitro fertilization (test-tube babies).

A number of *surgical procedures* can be accomplished through laparoscopy, for example, tubal insufflation, lysis of adhesions, biopsies of ovary, aspiration cytology, peritoneal biopsies, coagulation of endometriosis, and removal of an intra-abdominal intrauterine device (IUD). (For sterilization procedures, see Table 41.3.)

Laparoscopy permits a wide variety of examinations and surgical procedures. The woman can resume her usual activities in a few days. The woman's outpatient status results in a saving of hospital utilization and the surgeon's time and is cost effective.

Postcoital Test

Who: Both the woman and the man

Why: To test for adequacy of coital technique, cervical mucus, spermatozoa, and degree of sperm penetration

How: Assessment of specimen of cervical mucus following ejaculation of semen into vagina

When: 8 to 24 hours following sexual intercourse that is synchronized with expected time of ovulation (as determined from evaluation of BBT, cervical mucus changes, and usual length of menstrual cycle); performed only in the absence of vaginal infection

Where: Clinic or office

Risk:
1. Low; physically safe; no anesthesia is needed because having this test feels about the same as having a Papanicolaou smear
2. May be difficult to have intercourse with ejaculaton "on schedule"; sex "on demand" may strain the couple's interpersonal relationship
3. Expected day of ovulation may occur when facilities or physician is unavailable

Procedure

- Couple is asked to abstain for 48 hours before test commences.
- Then intercourse with ejaculaton into vaginal vault should occur within the 8 hours before the test.
- Woman may shower but not bathe between time of intercourse and test.
- Within 24 hours after intercourse, but preferably 8 hours, in the office or clinic:
  1. Woman is positioned in lithotomy position and draped; speculum is inserted without lubrication (no lubrication is needed at this time because mucus is abundant and the lubricant may alter the viscosity of the cervical mucus and invalidate the results); cervix is cleansed.
  2. Mucus is removed with a nasal polyp forceps or dressing forceps from the internal and the external cervical os and examined for macroscopic and microscopic characteristics.

Information Sought

Findings favorable to fertility:
1. Coital technique is adequate if sperm are found.
2. Mucus is supportive if many sperm are motile.
3. If more than 20 motile sperm are found, male most likely produces at least 20 mil/ml.*
4. Mucus is clear and abundant, with good spinnbarkeit.
5. A drop of each specimen is used for the fern test (p. 169); with high estrogen at ovulation, fern pattern (arborization) is seen (Fig. 12.3, *B*).

*Postcoital test is *not* a substitute for semen analysis.

Hysterosalpingography

Who: Woman; and her driver to take her home

Why: To assess tubal patency and endometrial cavity to a lesser degree; to assess uterine mobility

How: Fluoroscopic visualization (image intensification fluoroscopy) or spread of radiopaque dye (Fig. 12-6)

When: 2 to 6 days after menstruation to avoid flushing a fertilized ovum out through a tube into the peritoneal cavity; if the woman has pelvic inflammatory disease (PID), she is treated with antibiotics first and the test is rescheduled in 2 to 3 months

Where: Radiology department

Risk:
1. Allergy to radiopaque dye
2. May need premedication
3. Exposure to radiation
4. Discomfort: uterine cramping during procedure; referred shoulder pain after procedure
5. Needs someone to drive her home if medicated or in pain

Procedure

- Woman may be premedicated.
- Woman assumes lithotomy position and is draped.
- Vaginal speculum is inserted.
- Dye is instilled into uterus with a special cannula inserted into the cervical canal. Dye (Ethiodol*) is injected under controlled pressure.
- Usually three films are taken:
  1. Before dye instillation.
  2. As dye spills out from one or both tubes.
  3. After dye has spread throughout cavity.
- The shoulder pain:
  1. Subsides with position change.
  2. Disappears usually within 12 to 24 hours.
  3. Is controlled by mild analgesics.
- Perineal pad is applied to protect clothing from dye.

Information Sought

Findings favorable to fertility:
1. Spilling of dye into peritoneum within 10 to 15 minutes.
2. Spread of dye throughout peritoneal cavity.
3. Shoulder pain. Shoulder pain is indicative of subphrenic irritation from the chemical if the chemical spilled into peritoneal cavity.

Possible therapeutic effects of test:
1. Passage of dye may clear tubes of mucous plugs, straighten kinked tubes, or break up adhesions.
2. Cilia may be stimulated in the lining of the tubes.
3. It may aid healing as a result of the bacteriostatic effect of dye (iodine).

*Ethiodol, a liquid, oil-based dye, produces a better picture, has a lower incidence of injection pain, and results in better posthysterosalpingography pregnancy rates than water-soluble sodium acetrizoate (Salpix). Embolization and possible death are extremely rare but have occurred after hysterosalpingography with either Ethiodol or Salpix. Therefore informed consent should state this fact.

Rubin's Test

Who: Woman; and her driver to take her home

Why: To assess patency of fallopian tube or tubes

How: Tubal insufflation with carbon dioxide gas (Fig. 12-7)

When: 2 to 6 days following menses to avoid forcing possible fertilized ovum through tube into peritoneal cavity; in the absence of infection to avoid forcing infectious material through tubes into abdomen

Where: Clinic or physician's office.

Risk:
1. Low; no exposure to radiation
2. Discomfort: uterine cramping during procedure; referred shoulder pain following procedure
3. False positive readings

Procedure

- Woman assumes lithotomy position and is draped.
- Analgesia may be required.
- Vaginal speculum is inserted; cannula is inserted into cervical os; carbon dioxide gas is passed through cervix to uterus and tubes with the rate and pressure under careful control.

Information Sought

Findings favorable to fertility:
1. Woman experiences referred shoulder pain.
2. Auscultation of abdomen reveals passage of air through tubes.
3. Carbon dioxide pressure is below 150 mm Hg.

False results (tube is patent but gas flow is obstructed) may result from poor technique or spasms of the tubes.

Possible therapeutic effects of test: passage of carbon dioxide may clear out tubes or straighten out kinked tubes.

Fig. 12.6

Hysterosalpingogram showing liquid contrast medium filling uterus (fundus is angulated on cervix), with small gas bubble or polyp in region of lower uterine segment. Normal upper uterine cavity and normal filling of both delicate fallopian tubes, with spillage of medium out of the distal ostii. Note narrow diameter of proximal tubes.
IMPRESSION: Normal patent fallopian tubes.

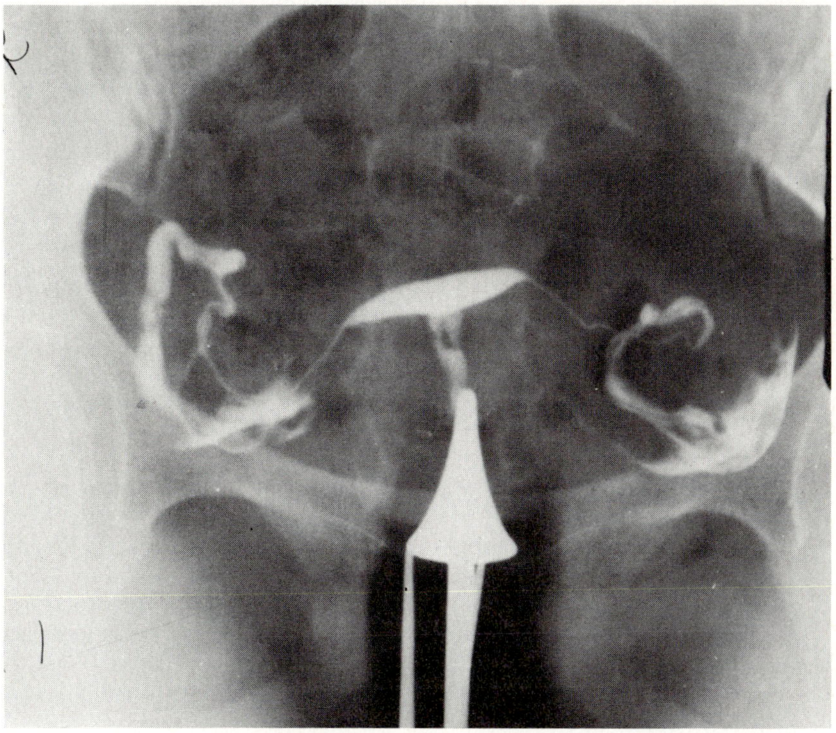

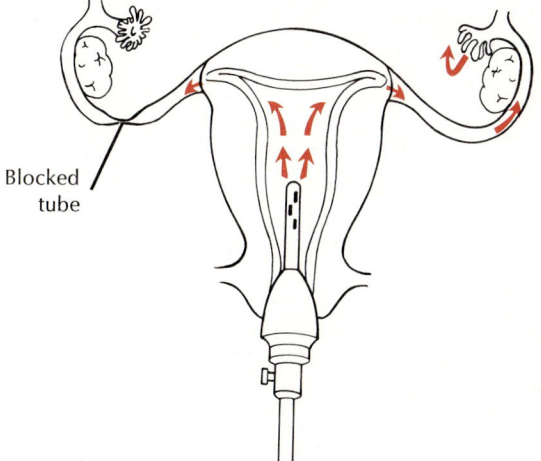

Fig. 12.7

Rubin's test. Carbon dioxide escapes into abdominal cavity through patent left fallopian tube.

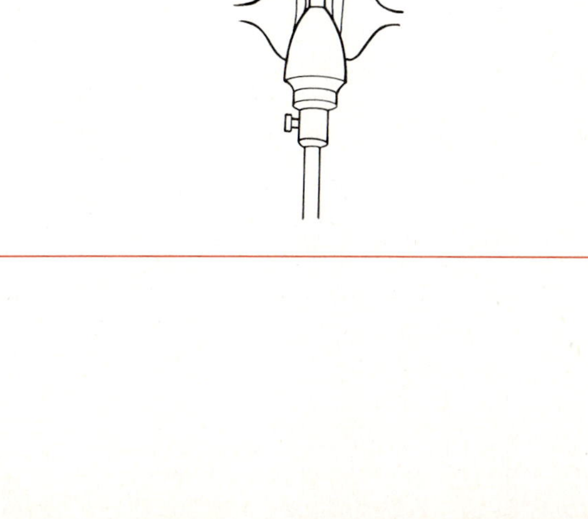

Laparoscopic Examination

Who: Woman; and her driver to take her home

Why: To assess visually the organs in the interior of the abdomen; and to perform minor surgical procedures

How: A small telescope is inserted through a small incision in the anterior abdominal wall using cold fiberoptical light sources that allow for superior visualization of the internal pelvis (Fig. 12-8)

When: Laparoscopy is timed depending on the purpose: if tubal patency is to be assessed, then it is done 2 to 6 days following cessation of menses; if sites of endometriosis are to be treated, any day of the cycle is appropriate

Where: In a surgical suite with an anesthesiologist present (may be done on an outpatient basis)

Risk:
1. Usually general anesthesia is used
2. A pneumoperitoneum is established by insufflation of carbon dioxide gas via a needle inserted through the abdominal wall.
3. Complications are rare (about 1 in 500): infection; electric burns of intraabdominal tissue
4. Postoperative shoulder (referred pain) or subcostal discomfort may occur for a short time

Procedure

- Woman signs informed consent and is prepared verbally for the examination.
- Woman is usually admitted a few hours before surgery having taken nothing by mouth for 8 hours.
- Woman voids just before surgery.
- Her pubic area is shaved only if examination is likely to be followed by laparotomy.
- Anesthesia is given; general anesthesia with intubation; occasionally, local.
- Woman is placed in a modified lithotomy position, with the legs at 45 degrees.
- The vagina, perineum, and abdomen are prepared and draped, and the area from the umbilicus to the vagina is exposed.
- An intrauterine probe is inserted except in cases where intrauterine pregnancy may be present.
- A needle is inserted and a pneumoperitoneum with carbon dioxide gas is established to elevate the abdominal wall from the organs. The needle may be inserted at lower border of umbilicus.
- Examination or procedure is performed.
- After surgery, deflation of most of gas is done by direct expression. Trocar (and needle) sites are closed with a single subcuticular absorbable suture or a skin clip, and an adhesive bandage is applied.
- Postoperative recovery requires taking of vital signs, assessing level of consciousness, preventing aspiration, monitoring IV fluids, and reassurance regarding shoulder discomfort. Discharge from hospital usually occurs in 4 to 6 hours.
- Shoulder or subcostal discomfort (from pneumoperitoneum) usually lasts only 24 hours and is relieved with a mild analgesic.
- Caution the woman against heavy lifting or strenuous activity for 4 to 7 days, at which time she is usually asymptomatic.

Information Sought

Findings favorable to fertility:
1. No developmental abnormalities of pelvic structures.
2. No lesions, infections, or adhesions.
3. No complications occur as a result of the examination or procedure.
4. If tubal insufflation is done, the tubes are found to be patent.
5. If there is a reparable problem (e.g., adhesions that are kinking the fallopian tubes), the problem is repaired through the laparoscope.

Fig. 12.8
Laparoscopy, in which carbon dioxide lifts abdominal wall off intra-abdominal contents, creating an empty space that permits visualization and exploration with laparoscope. Rubin's cannula is used for injections of methylene blue dye to assess for tubal patency.

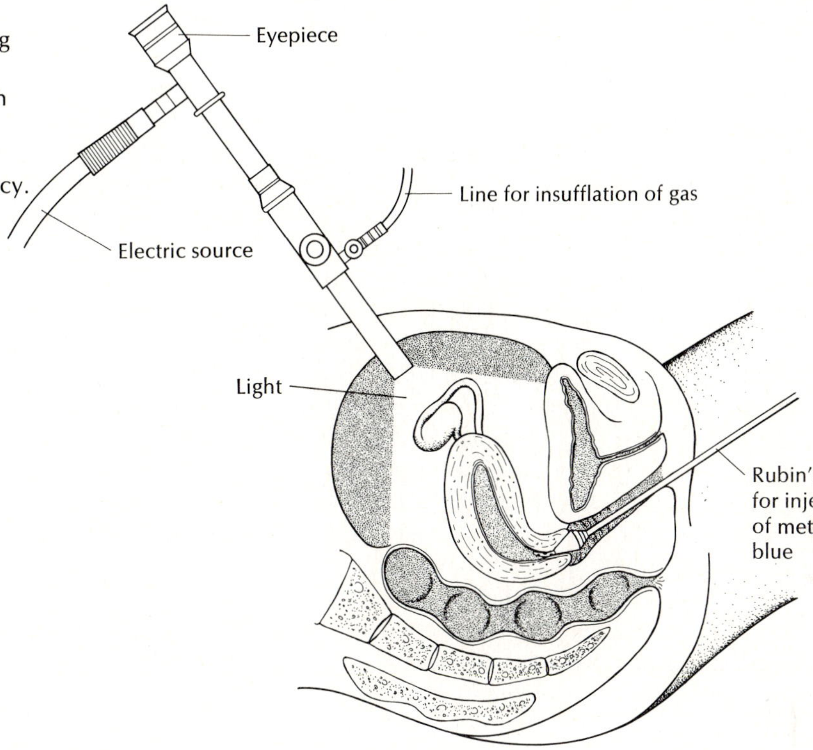

THERAPY FOR FEMALE INFERTILITY

It is estimated that at least 50% of all infertility problems can be diagnosed and treated by medical or surgical means. Diagnosis and treatment require considerable physical, emotional, and financial investment over several months or years.

Congenital or developmental factors. If the woman has abnormal external genitalia, surgical reconstruction of abnormal tissue and construction of a functional vagina may permit normal intercourse. If internal reproductive tract structures are absent, there is no hope for fertility. Surgical intervention depends entirely on the anatomic development, the surgical feasibility, and the individual's actual gender role.

Vaginal and uterine anomalies and their surgical repair vary from individual to individual. If a functional uterus can be reconstructed, pregnancy may be possible. Following surgical repair of the uterus, cesarean delivery is necessary to prevent uterine rupture during labor. Women with ovarian agenesis or dysgenesis are sterile, and no treatment will improve their fertility.

Ovulation. Anovulation may be primary (caused by a pituitary or hypothalamic hormone disorder) or secondary (caused by ovarian disease). In amenorrheic states and instances of anovulatory cycles, hormone studies usually reveal the problem. In some instances endocrine therapy with so-called fertility drugs such as oral clomiphene citrate (Clomid) or with intramuscular human menopausal gonadotropin (HMG) (Pergonal) may induce ovulation in anovulatory women.

Ovarian tumors must be excised; whenever possible, functional ovarian tissue is left intact. Chronic infections, which may cover much or all of the ovary, usually necessitate surgery to free and expose the ovary so that ovulation (release of ova) can occur.

An increasing number of young women are experiencing secondary amenorrhea. Their history reveals a serious interest in jogging and other sports and a considerable weight loss that has been followed by menstrual irregularities. The dietary history may reveal meals that consist of lean red meat and calorie-free soda drinks. Examination results frequently reveal amenorrhea or menstrual irregularities and osteoporosis (from loss of calcium). The woman who engages in vigorous exercise with normal menstrual cycles need have no concern for osteoporosis because she may have actually increased her calcium levels in bones and thereby increased their healthy density. Any woman who has missed two or three periods, however, is urged to consult an endocrinologist or an obstetrician/gynecologist.

In the presence of severe emotional problems, the woman is referred to a mental health therapist. Her condition may require the teamwork of the mental health therapist, the endocrinologist, and an obstetrician/gynecologist.

Tubal (peritoneal) factors

Review of tubal function. The fingerlike processes of the fimbriated end of the fallopian tube and the tube itself need to be free to approach the ovary to "catch" the ovum. The tube must be open, sufficiently long, and capable of ciliary action and peristalsis to carry the ovum into and down the tube. In most cases fertilization occurs in the ampulla of the fallopian tube. Supplied by the ampulla of the tube, some unknown factor, possibly an enzyme, seems to be required for the physiologic change or "conditioning" of the sperm called capacitation (see Chapter 14). Capacitation allows the escape of the enzyme hyaluronidase from the head of the sperm. Hyaluronidase digests a path for the sperm through the covering layers of cells surrounding the ovum and attaches to the surface of the ovum in preparation for penetration and fertilization (see Chapter 14).

Tubal factors leading to infertility are identified through several examinations: hysterosalpingography, Rubin's test, laparoscopy, or laparotomy.

Impairment of tubal function. The motility of the tube and its fimbriated end may be reduced or impossible as a result of infections, adhesions, or tumors. In rare instances there may be congenital absence of one tube, or one tube is relatively short; the latter is often found with an abnormally developed uterus.

Inflammation within the tube or involving the exterior of the tube or the fimbriated ends represents a major cause of infertility. Three types of bacterial tubal infection are recognized: gonococcal infection, postabortal sepsis, and tubercular infection. In addition, tubal adhesions resulting from pelvic infections (e.g., ruptured appendix) may cause infertility. Infection with purulent discharge eventually heals by scar formation. In the process the tube may be blocked anywhere along its length; it can be closed off at the fimbriated end, or it can be distorted and kinked by adhesions. If the tube remains patent after tubercular infection, the tubal lumen may become thickened and rigid with its function severely impaired. Adhesions may permit the tiny sperm to pass through the tube but may prevent a fertilized egg from completing the journey into the intrauterine cavity, resulting in an ectopic pregnancy that may completely destroy the tube (see discussion of ectopic pregnancy, Chapter 35).

In other cases, adhesions of the tubes to the ovary or bowel may follow endometriosis, which commonly involves the tubes and ovaries. In endometriosis, periodic monthly bleeding from endometrial implants causes dense adhesions, making pregnancy difficult or impossible.

For a discussion of tubal sterilization procedures, see Chapter 41.

Treatment for tubal factors. Treatment must include prevention and early adequate management of infection with appropriate antibiotics. Surgery may be necessary when drainage of a serious focus of infection is required. Hysterosalpingography is useful for the identification of tubal obstruction and also for the release of blockage (see p. 174). During laparoscopy, delicate adhesions may be divided and removed and endometrial implants may be destroyed by electrocoagulation. Laparotomy and even microsurgery may be required to do extensive repair of the damaged tube. After any surgery, new adhesions may form. Protection against new adhesion formation may require the insertion of a plastic splint (stent) into the tube or the temporary application of a plastic hood. Unfortunately a second operation is necessary for the removal of the plastic hood. However, a polyethylene splint often can be withdrawn if it is coiled in the uterus for withdrawal through the cervix about 6 weeks after surgery, when tubal healing is complete.

Prognosis. Tubal surgery to correct obstruction or closure after salpingitis may result in a patent mobile tube. Pregnancy is uncommon, however, because the original inflammatory process often prevents capacitation of spermatozoa, that is, the addition of a substance or substances by the tubal epithelium that make fertilization of the ovum possible. Prognosis for reanastomosis of the tubes after tubal sterilization is discussed in Chapter 41.

Endometriosis. Endometriosis is a disease in which endometrial tissue is found outside the uterine cavity. The etiology of this disease, which occurs in about 25% of women aged 20 years through menopause, is unknown although there is a familial tendency. Two basic theories are held: (1) that bits of endometrium pass into the abdominal cavity through the fallopian tubes during menstruation (retrograde menstruation) and subsequently implant and (2) that remnants of fetal tissue later differentiate into endometrial-like tissue. Endometrial cells from these extrauterine implants can spread (metastasize) through the lymphatic or venous systems to any part of the body (e.g., lungs or brain).

The ectopic endometrial tissue responds to hormonal stimulation just like normal endometrium within the uterus. However, its monthly discharge is absorbed by surrounding tissues causing inflammation and constricting scar tissue. Symptoms are related to the site of endometriosis, not to its extent. Classic symptoms include:

1. Pain: dysmenorrhea (painful menstruation), dyspareunia (painful intercourse), sacral backache, and pain noted with bowel movements
2. Infertility
3. Menstrual abnormalities

Endometriosis may become extensive and engulf pelvic organs (e.g., uterus, tubes, or ovaries), bowel, or kidneys, resulting in severe and disabling disease, or it may be so small that it is asymptomatic.

Diagnosis is made by history, pelvic examination, and direct visualization by laparoscopy, laparotomy, or culdotomy.

Treatment varies from mild analgesia for dysmenorrhea to removal of endometrial implants through electrocoagulation or surgical resection. *Danazol,* an antigonadotropin, is being used with good results. Danazol suppresses the pituitary-ovarian axis (depresses output of both FSH and LH), thereby altering the normal and ectopic endometrial tissue so that it becomes inactive and atrophic. Anovulation results because of suppression of ovarian function. Generally the pituitary-suppressive action is reversible; ovulation and menstrual bleeding usually return within 60 to 90 days after treatment ends. Danazol is expensive but has few side effects (e.g., weight gain, edema, break-through bleeding).

Nursing care of women who have surgery for endometriosis (which may involve hysterectomy) includes attention to general postoperative measures and to the emotional significance the client (and her family) may place on her disease and its reproductive implications.

Uterine factors

Review of uterine function. The uterus must be of sufficient size and shape to permit maintenance of a pregnancy to term. The endometrium must be prepared by estrogen and progesterone and must be healthy for implantation to occur.

Uterine factors are identified through several tests or examinations: hysterosalpingography, laparoscopy, endometrial biopsy, and plasma progesterone levels.

Impairment of uterine function. Congenital abnormalities of the uterus are far more common than might be expected. Hysterosalpingography may reveal a double uterus or other anomalous congenital variations that include a T-shaped uterus and a boxlike uterus, which have been described in daughters of women who took diethylstilbestrol (DES) during the early months of pregnancy. Occasionally uterine adhesion or scar tissue from too vigorous curettage (scraping) following an abortion (elective or spontaneous) may partially or totally obliterate the uterine cavity. In addition, endometrial and myometrial tumors (e.g., polyps or myomas) may also be revealed by x-ray studies of infertile women.

Endometritis (inflammation of the endometrium) may result from any of the causes of infection of the fallopian tubes. Women who use an intrauterine device (IUD) are more susceptible to endometrial infection than nonusers.

Treatment and prognosis for uterine factors. A woman with a relatively small uterus may become pregnant, but the uterus may be incapable of accommodating the enlarging fetus, and a spontaneous abortion may result. In such cases repeated or habitual (three or more) spontaneous abortions often occur. No medical therapy has been effective for the enlargement of an abnormally small uterus. Observation suggests that women who do become pregnant but who miscarry often abort at a later time with each successive pregnancy. Finally, after two or three pregnancy losses, they may deliver a viable infant. Apparently actual ''growth'' of the uterus occurs with each pregnancy.

Infertility may result from infections such as endometrial tuberculosis (from an acid-fast bacillus) or schistosomiasis (from a fluke parasite), which are significant health problems in many parts of the world, including the Near East, Puerto Rico, and South America. Although these disorders often involve the tubes and ovaries also, medical cure of the infection may permit pregnancy despite some scarring of the endometrium.

Other disorders of the endometrium are dysfunctional, secondary to abnormalities of the ovarian cycle. The endometrium becomes damaged by cystic glandular hyperplasia that results from anovulation and persistent estrogen stimulation without the ''ripening effect'' of progesterone.

Surgical removal of tumors involving the endometrium or uterus often improves the woman's chance of conceiving and maintaining the pregnancy to viability. Surgical treatment of uterine tumors or maldevelopment that results in successful pregnancy requires delivery by cesarean surgery near term because of potential weakness and subsequent rupture of the area of healing.

Vaginal-cervical factors

Review of vaginal-cervical function. Vaginal fluid is acid (pH of 4 or less), whereas cervical mucus is normally alkaline (pH of 7 or more). Ejaculation should place the sperm at or near the cervical os. The alkalinity of cervical mucus helps support spermatozoa and permits the ascending transportation of sperm at the time of ovulation.

In addition, endocervical mucus normally obstructs or plugs the cervix, acting as a barrier against infection. The latter is important because, in the woman, ascending infection to the peritoneum is virtually unimpeded with a normally patent genital tract. Alkaline mucus in the cervix not only controls procreation but also is a specific protection to life and health. The amount of cervical mucus and its characteristics are influenced by the hormones estrogen and progesterone (see p. 169).

Impairment of vaginal-cervical function. Vaginal-cervical infections (e.g., *Trichomonas* vaginitis) increase the acidity of the vaginal fluid and reduce the alkalinity of the cervical mucus. Thus vaginal infection often destroys or drastically reduces the number of viable, motile spermatozoa before they enter into the cervical canal. The amount of mucus and its physical changes are influenced by the presence of blood, pathogenic bacteria, and such irritants as an IUD or a tumor. Severe emotional stress, antibiotic therapy, and diseases such as diabetes mellitus also increase the acidity of mucus.

Abnormalities of the cervix itself may exist (e.g., an unusually small os, a cervix positioned high and anterior in the vaginal vault, or a cervix that is lacerated extensively and therefore gaping).

Some women have immunologic reactions to spermatozoa. The serum of these women shows elevated antisperm antibody titers and agglutination-immobilization of sperm.

Treatment and prognosis for vaginal-cervical factors. Therapy for lower genital infection requires the elimination of vaginitis or cervicitis, often with appropriate antibiotic or chemotherapeutic drugs. In addition to antibiotics, radial chemocautery (destruction of tissue with chemicals) or thermocautery (destruction of tissue with heat, usually electrical) of the cervix, cryosurgery (destruction of tissue by application of extreme cold, usually liquid nitrogen), or conization (excision of a cone-shaped piece of tissue from the endocervix) is effective in eliminating chronic infection. When the cervix has been deeply cauterized or frozen or when extensive conization has been performed, extreme limitation of mucous production by the cervix may result. Therefore sperm migration may be difficult or impossible because of the absence of a mucous "bridge" from the vagina to the uterus. Artificial insemination may be necessary to carry the sperm directly to the *internal os* of the cervix.

If the cervical os is unusually small, it is often called a pinhole os. In such cases, gentle dilation of the cervix or several shallow radial incisions followed by dilation are often sufficient to open the lower cervix. In contrast, if the cervix is grossly lacerated following delivery and widely gaping, suturing the cervix (trachelorrhaphy) or cryosurgery may be required to reduce the size of the external os for prevention of recurrent infection and the maintenance of a column of mucus.

Good general hygiene must be practiced in order to minimize vaginal infections. The woman benefits from good hand washing before and following elimination of urine and stool. She must wipe from front to back once with each tissue and never wipe back and forth over the perineal area. Feminine deodorants, soaps that are heavily colored and perfumed, bubble-bath salts, and tight clothing are avoided. Good nutrition is practiced with the avoidance of large amounts of unrefined sugars. To maintain a healthy vaginal-cervical pH during antibiotic therapy, the woman once or twice daily may insert one to two applicators full of cultured yogurt (not the pasteurized type of yogurt found in supermarkets, but the cultured yogurt that the woman herself can make at home quite inexpensively). As a general rule, douching is avoided unless by prescription from a physician.

Good mental health helps to prevent some forms of vaginitis that could become secondarily infected. Stress from anxiety, worry, and emotional discomfort changes the vaginal pH so that vaginal infections are more apt to take hold.

Concurrent medical conditions such as diabetes mellitus must be controlled to maintain vaginal-cervical pH within normal range.

Treatment is available for women who have immunologic reactions to sperm. Exposure to semen via the orogenital and anal modes is avoided. The use of condoms during genital intercourse for 6 to 12 months will reduce female antibody production* in the majority of women who have elevated antisperm antibody titers. After the serum reaction subsides, condoms are used at all times except at the expected time of ovulation. Approximately one third of couples with this problem conceive by following this course of action.

• • •

The prognosis for the infertile woman is generally good provided a serious genital or inflammatory disorder is not identified. Most women present numerous so-called minor problems that, although compounded, may be relatively easy to correct (e.g., chronic cervicitis, hypothyroidism). If successful treatment has not been achieved after a year, for example, other alternatives may be considered (e.g., adoption, childlessness, artificial insemination or in vitro fertilization).

In vitro fertilization. The first successful term delivery of an infant conceived by in vitro fertilization (test-tube pregnancy) in 1978 was the culmination of years of study and experimentation by Drs. Robert Edwards and Patrick Steptoe in England. Since then several other "laboratory-conceived" and normal-appearing neonates have been delivered, including a sibling for the first laboratory-conceived child.

*The production of antibodies by one member of a species against something that is commonly found within that species is termed *isoimmunization*.

Many women whose fallopian tubes either are obstructed or have been removed are now potential candidates for similar treatment. Certainly an explanation is due these eager, frustrated, but deserving women. However, because of the complexity of the procedure, the likelihood is that this approach to infertility must remain severely limited for the near future. The following steps, ultrasimplified, are necessary for in vitro fertilization:

1. Ovulation is induced by gonadotropin therapy.
2. Mature follicles are identified by laparoscopy, and needle aspiration of ova is carried out.
3. Ova are transferred to tissue culture media, and the sperm are added.
4. After fertilization, a second tissue culture transfer allows division to approximately a 12-cell blastocyst (3 to 6 days).
5. Progesterone therapy in the interval induces a late secretory type of endometrium, whereupon the blastocyst is transferred to the uterus, where the implantation (nidation) of the zygote occurs and embryonic development proceeds.

Within an 18-month period, overall success rates for in vitro fertilization worldwide have risen from 1% to 8% to almost 20%. This vast improvement is attributable to increased precision in predicting ovulation and in retrieving the ovum. The conventional methods of predicting ovulation—calendar, BBT, cervical mucus, fertility awareness, and laboratory tests such as vaginal cytology and serum hormone determination—can only approximate the moment of ovulation. The more precise methods are beyond the scope of this text but are mentioned here for interest. These methods are (1) stimulating ovulation with clomiphene citrate (Clomid) or human menopausal gonadotropin (HMG) (Pergonal) given at a precise time during the cycle, and (2) monitoring ovulatory function with real-time ultrasound, and (3) performing rapid radioimmunoassay for estrogen level. Through a laparoscope the ovum is retrieved by inserting an aspiration needle into the ripened follicle and removing the ovum. The husband's semen is collected and treated before its use for fertilization of the ovum. The complete procedure is described by Marrs (1982).

Human experimentation and manipulation of this type have been sanctioned by the United States Department of Health and Human Services. The Roman Catholic Church is strongly opposed to in vitro fertilization. Legal aspects of in vitro fertilization are discussed on p. 42.

Investigation of Male Infertility

FACTORS IMPLICATED IN MALE INFERTILITY

Male reproductive failure may be caused by many of the difficulties that also affect women, such as nutritional, endocrine, and psychologic disorders. In addition, male infertility may be caused by one or more of the following specific causes:

1. Timing and frequency of coitus in relation to ovulation.
2. Coital difficulties. Chordee (downward deflection of the penis due to a congenital anomaly [hypospadias] or to infection) or marked obesity may make penile entrance into the vagina difficult or impossible; or sperm may be deposited at the introitus instead of near the cervix.
3. Sperm antibodies; autoimmunization.* Autoantibodies in men may be responsible for interference with normal spermatogenesis or may directly affect the spermatozoa, preventing pregnancy. Trauma, infection, or surgical blockage of the vas deferens (vasectomy) may induce autoimmunity that can result in oligospermia (decreased numbers) or azoospermia (absence of sperm).
4. Abnormalities of sperm or semen. These abnormalities include a very small ejaculatory volume (less than 2 ml), a low sperm count (arbitrarily set at 20 mil/ml or less), increased viscosity, poor initial or reduced sustained motility of the sperm, more than 40% abnormal sperm forms, and low levels of PGs.
5. Testicular abnormalities. These abnormalities include agenesis or dysgenesis of the testes; cryptorchidism; inadequate maturation of the spermatozoa because of endocrine disorder (dysfunction of the hypothalamus, pituitary, thyroid, or adrenal glands) or genetic disorder such as Klinefelter's syndrome (XXY sex chromosomes); previous orchitis after mumps, gonorrhea, or tuberculosis; and physical injury perhaps caused by direct trauma, irradiation, or increased temperature for prolonged periods.
6. Abnormalities of the penis or urethra, including hypospadias or urethral stricture.
7. Abnormalities of the epididymis and vas deferens. These passageways act as reservoirs and means of transport for the sperm specimen. Inflammation or closure may reduce the quantity or viability of the sperm.

---

*The production of antibodies by a person against her or his own tissues.

8. Varicocele (a cystic accumulation of blood in the spermatic cord). Varices within the spermatic cord, resulting in scrotal swelling, reduce fertility probably because of increased temperature of the blood accumulation in the distended vein or veins.
9. Prostate and seminal vesicle abnormalities. Chronic prostatitis or seminal vesiculitis may reduce the number or quality of sperm or may alter the spermatozoa-containing fluid.
10. Severe nutritional deficiencies.
11. Social habits involving nicotine, drug, and alcohol abuse.
12. Psychologic disorders.

IDENTIFICATION OF INFERTILITY FACTORS

A careful *history is taken,* and a complete physical examination is carried out. Special attention is given to physical growth and development, recent excessive weight gain or loss, infection (e.g., mumps orchitis) or illness, injuries, exposure to diethylstilbestrol (DES) in utero or to chemicals or irradiation, type of clothing worn, occupation (e.g., truck driving, which keeps the man away from home for long periods), and operations on or near the genitourinary tract. A sperm analysis is done at least twice to determine whether oligospermia or other abnormalities are likely.

Semen is analyzed early in the diagnostic process. Before collecting a specimen, the man avoids ejaculation for 2 to 3 days. Then he collects a masturbated specimen in a clean glass jar and takes the sealed jar to the laboratory within 2 hours after emission, without warming or chilling it. The Roman Catholic man may prefer to remove ejaculated sperm from the woman's vagina with a Doyle (vaginal) spoon. A condom should not be used for collection of the semen (unless a special sheath manufactured by the Milex Corporation is used), since any residual rubber solvents and sulfur present would alter the specimen. The semen is examined for gross appearance, volume, and pH; sperm are analyzed for number or density, for percentage of motile forms, and for abnormal morphology (see Fig. 6.28).

Endocrinologic study for pituitary, thyroid, adrenal, or testicular problems is warranted in the presence of aspermia or oligospermia.

With maldeveloped or anomalous genitalia, a buccal smear and a chromosomal study should be carried out to *identify genetic disorders* such as Klinefelter's syndrome.

In some cases a biopsy of the testes may be necessary to differentiate between ductal obstruction and a failure to produce sperm (aspermatogenesis).

THERAPY FOR MALE INFERTILITY

Medical therapy for male infertility has been disappointing, especially when pituitary or testicular diseases are discovered. Occasionally it is possible to suppress the production of sperm with injections of testosterone and in that way cause a reduction in the number of autoimmune antibodies present in the man. Following the reduction in sperm autoantibodies, sperm quality improves, and a pregnancy sometimes occurs.

If the difficulty may be caused by timing and frequency of intercourse, the couple is taught about the menstrual cycle, the peak cervical mucus symptom, and appropriate timing of intercourse.

Penile intromission is often difficult because of chordee and obesity. In these situations the couple is advised to alter the positions used for intercourse. Heavy use of alcohol makes penile erection difficult to achieve and maintain until ejaculation so that the man is advised to avoid imbibing alcohol during the time of the woman's ovulation.

Infections (e.g., T mycoplasma) are identified and treated promptly. Poor nutritional state is corrected if it exists. Problems with the thyroid or adrenal glands are corrected.

Surgical reanastomosis following vasectomy is discussed with male surgical sterilization, Chapter 41.

Surgical repair of varicocele* has been relatively successful. A varicocele on the left side is found in a substantial number of subfertile men. Ligation of the varicocele does lead to improvement of the sperm quality and frequently to pregnancy.

Simple changes in life-style may be effective in the treatment of subfertile men. High temperatures in the groin area reduce the number of sperm produced. High temperatures may be caused by the wearing of brief shorts and tight jeans that keep the scrotal sac pressed against the body regardless of environmental temperature changes. The testes are kept at temperatures that are too high for efficient spermatogenesis. Frequent and prolonged hot tubbing has also been implicated in relative infertility. It must be remembered that these conditions only lead to relative infertility and should not be employed as a means of contraception.

Artificial insemination. The term *homologous insemination* (artificial insemination by husband, or AIH) denotes the use of the husband's semen, and the term *heterologous insemination* (artifical insemination by donor, or AID) denotes the use of the semen of a donor other than the husband.

When the husband's sperm has poor quality or motil-

*Varicocele refers to varicose veins of the spermatic vein in the groin. The swollen, distended veins press on the testes and impair their function.

ity, several semen samples are collected from him. The samples consist of split ejaculates, that is, the spermatozoa-rich *first portion* only is collected for freezing and later pooling for AIH. Rapid freezing with liquid nitrogen and subsequent thawing do not cause genetic damage even after 10 years' storage using glycerol. Pooling should increase the sperm count and improve the placement of a portion of the total semen specimen at the cervical os to spare the sluggish spermatozoa a part of their journey. In spite of advanced techniques, few pregnancies have resulted even after repeated attempts, perhaps because poor motility and a low sperm count reflect only a part of the sperm deficiency.

Assuming normal female fertility, AID at or about the time of ovulation has resulted in pregnancy in as many as 70% of cases. Numerous inseminations may be necessary to ensure proper timing at ovulation, usually determined by the basal body temperature (BBT) and cervical mucus record. Approximately 50% of pregnancies with AID will occur within 2 months; almost 90% occur within 6 months.

Insemination directly into the uterine cavity should be avoided because of severe cramping (prostaglandin effect) and possible infection. The recommended procedure is the instillation of about 0.5 ml of the specimen into the cervical canal, with the remainder deposited in a cervical cap or a cleanly washed contraceptive diaphragm to be worn by the woman for about an hour.

Insemination with the husband's semen presents no legal problems, but heterologous insemination (insemination with a combination of husband and donor sperm) involves many legal, ethical, and emotional aspects. The couple must know that there is no guarantee of pregnancy and that in either instance, the spontaneous abortion rate is approximately the same as in a control population. There is no increase in maternal or perinatal complications; that is, the same frequency of anomalies (about 5%) and obstetric complications (between 5% and 10%) that accompanies normal insemination applies also to AID.

The decision for artificial insemination with donor sperm should be made only after thorough consideration and discussion. The implications for the long-term welfare of the child as well as the parents must be considered (see p. 43).

The Emotional Crisis of Infertility: Implications for Nursing Action

Feelings connected to infertility are many and complex.* The origin of some of these feelings are myths, superstitions, misinformation, or "magical" thinking about the cause of infertility. Other feelings arise from the need to undergo many tests and examinations and from being "different" from others.

The woman or couple facing infertility exhibits behaviors that resemble the grieving process that is associated with loss. The loss of one's genetic continuity with the generations to come leads to loss of self-esteem, of a sense of adequacy as a woman (or man), of control over one's destiny, and of a sense of self. The investigative process leads to a loss of spontaneity and control over the couple's marital relationship and sometimes over one's progress toward career and life goals. All people do not experience every one of the reactions described below nor can the length of time be predicted that any one reaction will last for an individual.

The nurse may feel at a loss in knowing how to assist. Table 12.3 presents characteristic behaviors of people experiencing the psychologic impact of infertility along with some suggestions for nursing (or other health professionals') actions.

The support systems of the infertile couple need to be explored. This exploration should include persons available to assist, their relationship to the couple, their ages, their availability, and the cultural or religious support that is available. This type of assessment is suitable for a health team conference where representatives of several disciplines can share ideas and work cooperatively in developing a plan for management.

If the couple conceives, the nurse needs to be aware that the concerns and problems of the previously infertile couple may not be over. Many couples are overjoyed with the pregnancy. However, some are not. Some couples rearrange their lives, sense of self, and personal goals within their acceptance of their infertile state. The couple may feel that those who worked with them to identify and treat infertility expect them to be happy with the pregnancy. The couple may be shocked to find that they themselves feel resentment because the pregnancy, once a cherished dream, now necessitates another change in goals, aspirations, and identities. The couple may choose to abort the pregnancy at this time (see Chapter 41). If the couple wishes to continue with the pregnancy, they will need the care pregnant couples need (see Unit 3). The couple may need extra preparation for the realities of pregnancy, labor, and parenthood, because they have developed fantasies about childbearing when they thought it was beyond their reach. A history of infertility is considered to be a risk factor for pregnancy. The couple who has a history of infertility before this pregnancy faces another label, that of being at high risk for this pregnancy (see Chapter 33).

The couple too may desire information about contra-

*See Chapter 8 for cross-cultural aspects.

Table 12.3
Behavior Associated with Infertility

Behavioral Characteristic	Nursing Actions
Surprise: each person assumes she or he is fertile and that pregnancy is an option.	Point out resemblance to grieving process—a normal, expected reaction to loss. Refer to support group.* Prepare them for length of time it may take to grieve, types of feelings (psychologic, somatic) to expect. Encourage and allow time to talk of past and present feelings of sexuality, self-image, and self-esteem.
Denial: "It can't happen to me!"	Allow time for denial because it gives the body and mind time to adjust a little at a time. Do not feed into the client's denial; instead say, "It must be hard to believe such a devastating report."
Anger: toward others (perhaps even at the nurse) or themselves.	Explain that the reaction to loss of control and to a feeling of helplessness is often anger, which can easily be projected onto another person. Without release, anger can lead to chronic depression. Anger is a natural feeling. Allow time to express anger at losing their sense of control over their bodies and destinies; identify and direct energy directly at the problem. Airing one's own anger often eases the intensity of the emotion. A helpful approach may be, "It's OK to be angry . . . at those who are pregnant, at people who want abortions, at self, at mate, at care givers, and so forth."
Bargaining: "If I get pregnant, I'll dedicate the child to God."	
Depression:	
Isolation: personal	Allow time for both woman and man to talk about how it feels whenever a sight, event, or word serves as a reminder of own infertile state. Develop role playing situations to practice interactions with others under various circumstances to increase the couple's ability to cope and to problem solve (increases their self-confidence). The nurse may say, "You must feel so terribly alone sometimes."
Guilt/unworthiness	Allow time to identify feelings that may be based on earlier behaviors (e.g., abortion, premarital sex, contact with sexually transmitted disease [STD]). Goal: couple or person comes to the realization that "unworthiness" and infertility are unrelated.
Acceptance (resolution)	Clients need to know that grief feelings are never laid away forever; they may be activated by special reminders (e.g., anniversaries).

*RESOLVE, Inc., P.O. Box 474, Boston, Mass. 02178.

ception following the birth of this baby. If the previously infertile couple desires additional children, the couple is advised about those contraceptive methods that are least likely to cause damage and infertility.

If the couple does not conceive, they are assessed regarding their desire to be referred for help with adoption, artificial insemination, or with choosing childlessness. The couple would find a list of such agencies within their particular community helpful. Examples of community agencies, besides RESOLVE, are OURS* (an adoptive organization); ARENA* (an adoptive organization); and National Organization for NonParents* (for those who choose to remain childless).

*Lists of such groups throughout the United States can be obtained from OURS, Inc., 20140 Pine Ridge Dr., Anoaka, MN 55303.

Summary of Nursing Actions

Based on knowledge of infertility, the nurse is equipped to assist with the management of a plan of care for the infertile couple. The nursing actions are planned in collaboration with the physician in light of the nurse's level of expertise, and with other members of the health team and the couple to achieve certain mutually determined goals. These same goals, outcomes, or evaluative criteria are reference points for evaluating effectiveness of nursing actions and redirecting the nurse to alter actions as necessary. For the nursing student the evaluative criteria in the box below serve as a guide for the review of content relevant to infertility.

Evaluative (Outcome) Criteria

1. Couple is educated in the anatomy and physiology of the reproductive system.
2. Any abnormalities identified through various tests and examinations are treated (e.g., infections, blocked fallopian tubes, sperm allergy, varicocele).
3. Couple receives an estimate of their chances to conceive.
4. Couple resolves guilt feelings and does not need to focus blame.
5. Couple conceives or, failing to conceive, decides on an alternative that is acceptable to both of them (e.g., childlessness, adoption, or artificial insemination).
6. Couple finds acceptable methods for handling pressures they may feel from peers and relatives regarding their childless state.

References and Readings

Alexander, N.J.: Cover story—symposium: when you suspect infertility is immunologic, Contemp. Obstet. Gynecol. **14**(5):92, 1979.

Archer, D.F.: Treating endometriosis with lose-dose danazol, Contemp. Obstet. Gynecol. **19**(6):47, 1982.

Bachmann, G.A., and Kemmann, E.: Prevalence of oligomenorrhea and amenorrhea in a college population, Am. J. Obstet. Gynecol. **144**(1):98, 1982.

Beacham, D.W., and Beacham, W.D.: Synopsis of gynecology, ed. 10, St. Louis, 1982, The C.V. Mosby Co.

Benson, R.C., editor: Current obstetric and gynecologic diagnosis and treatment, ed. 4, Los Altos, Calif., 1982, Lange Medical Publications.

Bernhard, L.A.: Endometriosis, J.O.G.N. Nurs. **11**(5):300, 1982.

Bernstein, J., and Mattox, J.H.: An overview of infertility, J.O.G.N. Nurs. **11**(5):309, 1982.

Donnez, J., et al.: Luteal function after tubal sterilization, Obstet. Gynecol. **57**(1):65, 1981.

Edgar, H.S.: The legal implications (in vitro fertilization): are restraints likely? Contemp. Obstet. Gynecol. **20**(5):233, 1982.

Gaines, F.L.: Secondary amenorrhea. Part 2, The Nurse Practitioner **6**(5):14, 1981.

Garcia, C., et al.: Current therapy of infertility, 1982-1983, St. Louis, 1983, The C.V. Mosby Co.

In vitro fertilization: the work continues, Contemp. Obstet. Gynecol. **19**(5):40, 1982.

Jansen, R.P.: Spontaneous abortion incidence in the treatment of infertility, Am. J. Obstet. Gynecol. **143**(4):451, 1982.

Luciano, A.A.: A guide to managing endometriosis, Contemp. Obstet. Gynecol. **19**(5):211, 1982.

Machol, L.: Update on in vitro fertilization technology, Contemp. Obstet. Gynecol. **20:**63 (special issue), 1982.

MacVicar, M.G., et al.: What do we know about the effects of sports training on the menstrual cycle? M.C.N. **7**(1):55, 1982.

Marrs, R.P.: In vitro fertilization's future looks bright, Contemp. Obstet. Gynecol. **20**(3):135, 1982.

McCormick, R.A.: Ethical questions (in vitro fertilization): a look at the issues, Contemp. Obset. Gynecol. **20**(5):227, 1982.

McCormick, T.M.: Out of control: one aspect of infertility, J.O.G.N. Nurs. **9**(4):205, 1980.

McCusker, M.P.: The subfertile couple, J.O.G.N. Nurs. **11**(3):157, 1982.

Menning, B.E.: The psychosocial impact of infertility, Nurs. Clin. North Am. **17**(1):155, 1982.

Mishell, D.R.: State of the art (in vitro fertilization)—what can we offer patients? Contemp. Obstet. Gynecol. **20**(5):219, 1982.

Moghissi, K.S.: What causes habitual abortion? Contemp. Obstet. Gynecol. **20**(5):45, 1982.

Nurses' Association of the American College of Obstetrics and Gynecology: Infertility: an overview, O.G.N. Nursing Practice Resource, no. 7, Nov. 1982.

Petrie, R.H.: Taking a fresh look at in vitro fertilization, Contemp. Obstet. Gynecol. **20**(5):194, 1982.

Problem-patient conference. New methods of diagnosing and treating Asherman syndrome (a condition caused by intrauterine adhesions), Contemp. Obstet. Gynecol. **14**(5):117, 1979.

Rehns, M.: Genes and miscarriage, Am. Baby Childbirth Educator **1**(2):14, Winter 1981-82.

Sanborn, C.F., et al.: Is athletic amenorrhea specific to runners? Am. J. Obstet. Gynecol. **143**(8):859, 1982.

Sawatzky, M.: Tasks of infertile couples, J.O.G.N. Nurs. **10**(2):132, 1981.

Shane, J.M., et al.: The infertile couple: evaluation and treatment, Clin. Symp. **28**(5):1, 1976.

Shane, J.M.: What can the family physician do for infertility? The Female Patient, p. 94, 1979.

Shangold, M.M., and Levine, H.S.: The effect of marathon training upon menstrual function, Am. J. Obstet. Gynecol. **143**(8):862, 1982.

13 Control of Fertility

- Methods of Control of Fertility
  - Natural family planning (biologic periodic abstinence)
    - Rhythm or calendar method
    - Basal body temperature
    - Cervical mucus method
    - Sympto-thermal method
    - Fertility awareness method
  - Oral hormonal therapy
    - Mode of action
    - Combined oral hormone therapy
  - Injectable medication
  - Intrauterine device
    - Procedure for insertion of the IUD: client preparation
  - Diaphragm with spermicide
    - Procedure for insertion and follow-up
  - Cervical cap
  - The 48-hr contraceptive
  - Vaginal spermicides
  - Male contraception
    - Condom
    - Other methods of male contraception
- Nursing Actions
  - Evaluative criteria
  - Assessment
  - Planning and implementation
  - Evaluation

The fertile period in humans is relatively short. It is limited to the 24 to 36 hours following ovulation. If 100 normal couples have frequent intercourse, 25% of the couples will conceive the first month, 19% the second, 14% the third, and over the remainder of the year all but four to seven couples will conceive. Therefore, if conception is not desired, it is recommended that some method be used to prevent pregnancy.

Contraception is the voluntary prevention of pregnancy; it has both individual and social implications. It has been established that more than 90% of couples in the United States have used or intend to use some method of birth control (contraception). Family planning is accepted in principle by all religions, but the Roman Catholic Church insists that it be achieved by periodic abstinence alone. The availability of reliable and safe techniques for controlling fertility has meant that parenthood, with its tasks and responsibilities as well as its pleasures, can be willingly assumed by adults who wish to do so. Recent advances in the physiologic safety of prenatal, perinatal, and postnatal existence can now be combined with the psychologic safety of being a wanted child.

Spacing of children is important for promotion of the health not only of the mother but also of her children. Quality of the offspring rather than quantity is now emphasized. Moreover, to control excessive world population, voluntary limitation of family size has become important.

Before studying techniques for control of fertility, a brief overview of the risks of pregnancy are compared to those of contraception. Pregnancy in emerging countries (where contraception is not used) involves a maternal death rate of 300/100,000 births, which is contrasted to 15/100,000 births in developed countries. Mortality from any method of pregnancy prevention (or termination of pregnancy under controlled conditions) should be less than the deaths from pregnancy. Statistics from developing countries indicate that there is a mortality rate of 10/100,000 births from oral contraceptive use; for those who use the intrauterine device (IUD) the rate is 15/100,000 births. In developed countries the rates have been dramatically reduced: for those

Table 13.1
Estimated Annual Deaths Associated with Fertility Control and No Control per 100,000 Fertile Women

	Age (yr)					
Method	**15-19**	**20-24**	**25-29**	**30-34**	**35-39**	**40-44**
No method	5.5	5.2	7.1	14.0	19.3	22
Abortion only (legal)	2.3	2.5	2.5	5.2	9.8	6.6
Oral contraceptive only (nonsmoker)	1.3	1.4	1.4	2.2	4.5	3.1
Oral contraceptive only (smoker)	1.5	1.6	1.6	10.8	13.4	59
IUD only	1.1	1.2	1.2	1.4	1.6	1.4
Traditional contraception* only	1.1	1.4	1.9	3.7	4.7	4.0
Traditional contraception with abortion	0.3	0.4	0.4	0.8	1.4	0.8

*Family planning methods, spermicides, and/or condoms.

Table 13.2
Risk Factors and Degree of Associated Risk by Age for Users of Oral Contraceptives

	Age (yr)		
Risk	**≤29**	**30-39**	**≥40**
Heavy smokers (≥15 cigarettes)	2*	3	4
Light smokers (≤14 cigarettes	1	2	3
Nonsmokers with no added risk conditions	1	1,2	2
Nonsmokers with added risk conditions	2	2,3	3,4

*1 = Use associated with low risk; 2 = use associated with moderate risk; 3 = use associated with high risk; 4 = use associated with very high risk.

Table 13.3
Contraceptive Methods and Pregnancies per 100 Women

Method of Contraception	**Contraceptive Failures (no. of pregnancies)**
No method	60-80
Calendar only	14-47
Periodic abstinence	1-47
Jellies/creams	4-36
Condom	3-36
Aerosol foams	2-29
Mucous method	1-25
Diaphragm with spermicide	2-20
BBT only	1-20
BBT with intercourse during postovulatory time	1-7
IUD	1-6

using oral contraceptives or the IUD, there is less than one death (mortality) per 100,000 births.

Methods of Control of Fertility

There are various contraceptive techniques used in North America. The ideal contraceptive should be safe, easily available, economical, acceptable, simple to use, and promptly reversible. Although no means or method may ever achieve all these objectives, impressive progress has been made recently. Before choosing the "right" contraceptive method, several topics need to be discussed: frequency of coitus (once every so often or several times per week); one sexual partner or several; what level of involvement does each partner wish to assume; does the woman or couple object to any method. The woman or couple must be fully informed of the risks (Tables 13.1 and 13.2), effectiveness, reversibility, and the alternatives (Table 13.3) (see the discussion of informed consent, p. 41).

Contraception employs one or more of the following methods* (Fig. 13.1):

1. Methods that require periodic medical examination and prescription†
   a. Hormonal therapy: estrogen or progestogen preparations or a combination of these compounds
   b. Mechanical barrier: cervical uterine occlusion by caps or diaphragms
   c. Intrauterine contraceptive devices
2. Methods available to people without prescription
   a. Natural family planning: biologic periodic abstinence

*Surgical interruption of fertility (sterilization procedures) will be discussed in Chapter 41.
†Certified nurse-midwives and some certified nurse-practitioners may be educated to provide this service too.

Fig. 13.1
Medications and appliances in control of fertility

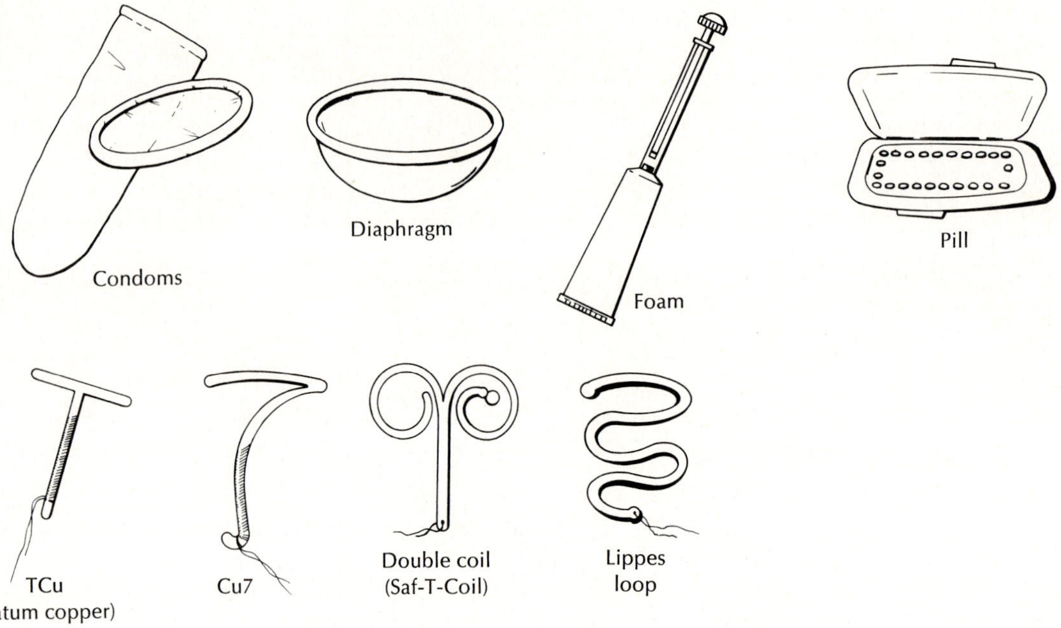

b. Chemical barriers: spermicidal creams, gels, or vaginal suppositories
c. Mechanical barrier: condoms or sheaths

NATURAL FAMILY PLANNING (BIOLOGIC PERIODIC ABSTINENCE)

Natural family planning methods employ a combination of the following:

1. Rhythm or calendar method
2. Basal body temperature (BBT) method
3. Cervical mucus (Billings, ovulation) method
4. Sympto-thermal method
5. Fertility awareness method

The five methods of natural family planning necessitate periodic abstinence from sexual intercourse. Each depends on the continuous observation and recording of events of the menstrual cycle. The woman or couple must be able to assess hormone-induced signs and symptoms that indicate whether she is in the fertile or infertile part of the menstrual cycle. While teaching a woman about fertility awareness, the nurse uses this opportunity for helping the woman or couple learn a great deal about their bodies.

The *mode of action* for these methods of contraception is abstention from intercourse during the fertile period. The sperm remain motile in the woman's reproductive tract for about 24 (up to 72) hours; the ovum within the fallopian tube is fertilizable for 12 (up to 24) hours. Therefore fertilization is *most likely* during a 36-hour period. However, the exact moment of ovulation is unpredictable and the exact life spans for the sperm and egg are not known; extra precaution must be taken to prevent pregnancy. Because the life span of the sperm within the female reproductive tract may exceed 24 hours, the couple must abstain from coitus at least 2 days *before* anticipated ovulation. Because the life span of the egg may exceed 12 hours, the couple must abstain from coitus for at least 1 day *after* ovulation. This brings the total number of days of abstinence to 3; for added insurance, an extra day of abstinence before and after the fertile period (for a total of 5 days) is considered good practice.

It is possible for sperm deposited on the vulva or within the reproductive tract of the female 2 to 3 days before ovulation to fertilize the ovum. If fertilization does occur under these circumstances, the fetus would most likely be female because the X-carrying sperm live longer than the Y-carrying sperm.

Each of the five methods of natural family planning utilizes various means of determining the day of ovulation so that coitus can be avoided during the woman's fertile period.

Rhythm or calendar method. For this discussion the rhythm method and the calendar method are combined in one method. The calendar method is based on a formula that takes into consideration the fact that ovulation occurs about 14 days before the next men-

Fig. 13.2
M = menstrual flow. x = absolute abstention from sexual intercourse or use of diaphragm, condom, or spermicide; o = abstention from sexual intercourse for added "safety" or use of diaphragm, condom, or spermicide. Ovulation occurs 14 days *before* the onset of menstruation. If within an 8- to 12-mo period, the woman's cycles vary from 24 to 30 days, the date of ovulation varies accordingly. Using the calendar method only, the woman has no way of predicting the length of the current cycle. During each cycle, the couple must abstain or use a second form of contraception during the fertile (unsafe) days, for example, in a 24-day cycle, the fertile days are 6 to 13; in a 26-day cycle, 8 to 15; and in a 30-day cycle, days 12 to 19. Therefore this couple must abstain from day 6 to day 19 (14 days).

	Cycle length (days)	1	2	3	4	5	6	7	8	9	10	11	12	13	14	15	16	17	18	19	20	21	22	23	24	25	26	27	28	29	30	31	32
A.	Cycle variations in past 12 mo.	M	M	M	M	M					Ovulation															M	M	M	M	M			
	Shortest cycle						o	o	x	x	x	x	x	o	o																		
B.		M	M	M	M	M							Ovulation															M	M	M	M	M	
									o	o	x	x	x	x	x	o	o																
C.	Longest cycle	M	M	M	M	M											Ovulation															M	M
													o	o	x	x	x	x	x	o	o												
D.	Current cycle	M	M	M	M	M	Abstain from sexual intercourse																			?M		?M				?M	

strual period, the life span of the ovum, and the life span of the sperm. In this method, extra days are added before and after the probable day of ovulation so that the total number of days of abstinence is about 8 days.

Each month the woman calculates her probable fertile period based on the menstrual pattern of the previous 8 to 12 months. A formula has been developed that takes into consideration the length of both the life span of the sperm and the life span of the ovum, as well as adding a padding of 2 days before ovulation and 1 day following ovulation for added safety. From the longest cycle, subtract 11; from the shortest, subtract 18. The formula is applied to the cycles in Fig. 13.2.

Shortest cycle	**Longest cycle**
24	30
−18	−11
6th day	19th day

If the woman's cycles over the last 8 to 12 months varied from 24 to 30 days, this month the couple would have to abstain from day 6 to day 19 (14 days).

If the woman has very regular cycles of 28 days each, the formula indicates the fertile days to be:

Shortest cycle	**Longest cycle**
28	28
−18	−11
10th day	17th day

To avoid pregnancy, the couple abstains from day 10 to day 17, as ovulation occurs on day 14 (13 to 15).

Basal body temperature. Since the occurrence of ovulation often can be identified by the basal (resting) body temperature (BBT) (see p. 167 for a discussion of fertility and p. 83 for a discussion of the menstrual cycle), the postovulatory period may in fact be "safe," or infertile. The BBT during the menses and for approximately 5 to 7 days thereafter usually varies from 36.2° to 36.3° C (97.2° to 97.4° F). If ovulation fails to occur, this pattern of lower body temperature continues throughout the cycle. However, as stated previously, infection, fatigue, less than 3 hours of sleep per night, awakening late, and anxiety may cause temperature fluctuations, altering the expected pattern. If a new BBT thermometer is purchased, this fact is noted on the chart because the readings may vary slightly. Jet lag, alcohol taken the evening before, or sleeping in a heated water bed must also be noted on the chart because each will affect the BBT.

About 24 to 36 hours *before* ovulation, the temperature may drop 0.2° to 0.3° F and then rise 0.7° to 0.8° F within 24 to 48 hours *after* ovulation. The temperature remains on an elevated plateau until the day before menstruation, when it drops to the low levels recorded during the previous cycle.

The drop and subsequent rise in temperature are referred to as the *thermal shift*. When the entire month's temperatures are recorded on a graph, the pattern described above is more apparent; however, it is more difficult to perceive day-to-day variations. To determine if a rise in temperature is indeed the thermal shift, the woman must be aware of other signs of approaching ovulation while she continues to assess the BBT. She needs to do the following:

1. Assess the cervical mucus characteristics.
2. Assess for opening of cervical os and rise of cervix in vagina.*
3. Note other symptoms (e.g., increased libido).
4. Compare the rise in temperature to the highest BBT of the previous 6 days:
   a. If the rise is at least 0.3° F over the previous highest recorded temperature, and if the temperature remains elevated for at least 3 days, then the thermal shift has occurred, and the woman is in the infertile phase of this cycle.
   b. If the BBT drops after the first or second day, no thermal shift has occurred and the woman must assume that unprotected intercourse at this time could lead to pregnancy.

Because of sperm and ovum life spans and duration of receptive cervical mucus, the fertile period extends from 48 hours before ovulation to 48 (up to 72) hours after the onset of elevated temperature. Assuming regularity (unlikely for many women), the preovulatory and postovulatory safe periods can be estimated more accurately by using the BBT and the calendar methods together.

Cervical mucus method. The cervical mucus method, also called the *Billings method* or the *ovulation method,* depends on the characteristic changes in the amount and consistency of cervical mucus at the time of ovulation (see Table 11.1 and Figs. 12.3 and 12.4). These changes are easily learned by most couples. The first task is to learn to distinguish changes in the cervical mucus. To ensure accurate assessment of changes, the cervical mucus should be free of semen, contraceptive gels or foams, and blood or discharge from vaginal infections for at least one full cycle. Other factors that create difficulty in identifying mucous changes include douches and vaginal deodorants, being in the sexually aroused state, and medications such as antihistamines, which dry up the mucus.

The days of menstrual flow are noted on a chart. For the first few days (3 to 4 or none) after the end of flow, the vagina usually feels dry. Dryness is followed by the appearance of sticky (i.e., sticks to finger but does not stretch), cloudy mucus. As the production of estrogen increases, the mucus increases in quantity and becomes more like raw egg white—clear, stringy, slippery (lubricative), and stretchable (spinnbarkeit). Quantity alone is not a good indicator; extra mucus is produced when a woman has a cold. The woman looks for a sensation of wetness. The onset of the peak mucus sign (slipperiness and a sensation of wetness) signals that ovulation is imminent and that to avoid the possibility of conception, the couple must practice sexual abstinence until the fourth day after the peak mucus sign (the first day of the peak mucus, plus 3 more days).

After ovulation, cervical mucus is under progesterone influence. It becomes sticky, thick, and cloudy and diminishes in amount. Each of these changes is entered on the continuous record.

If it is difficult to evaluate the mucus because of the presence of semen or discharge from vaginal infection, the woman double checks for fertility by assessing her BBT record and other symptoms of fertility. (NOTE: Each woman has her own unique pattern of mucous changes.)

Whether or not the individual wants to use this method for contraception, it is to the woman's benefit to learn to recognize mucous characteristics at ovulation. Assessing changes in cervical mucus can be useful diagnostically for any of the following purposes:

1. To alert the couple to the reestablishment of ovulation while breast feeding and after discontinuation of oral contraception
2. To note anovulatory cycles at any time and at the commencement of menopause
3. To assist couples in planning a pregnancy

Sympto-thermal method. The sympto-thermal method combines the BBT and cervical mucus methods with awareness of secondary, cycle phase-related symptoms. Both partners take responsibility for assessments, recordings, and evaluation of their findings. Together they determine the days for abstinence.

*Check with a family planning clinic or with a women's health center for technique for self-assessment of vagina using a speculum, mirrors, and light source.

The couple gains in fertility awareness as they learn the woman's individual psychologic and physiologic symptoms that mark the relatively infertile (menstrual) period, fertile (secretory phase) period, and infertile (proliferative phase) period. Secondary symptoms (see Table 11.1) include increased libido, midcycle spotting, mittelschmerz, pelvic fullness or tenderness, and vulvar fullness. The couple, perhaps using a speculum, looks at the cervix to assess for changes indicating ovulation; that is, the os dilates slightly, the cervix softens and rises in the vagina, and cervical mucus is copious and slippery. To complete their records, the couple notes days on which coitus, changes in routine, illness, and so on have occurred (Fig. 13.3).

Fig. 13.3

Example of completed sympto-thermal method chart. (From Fogel, C., and Woods, N.F.: Health care of women, St. Louis, 1981, The C.V. Mosby Co.)

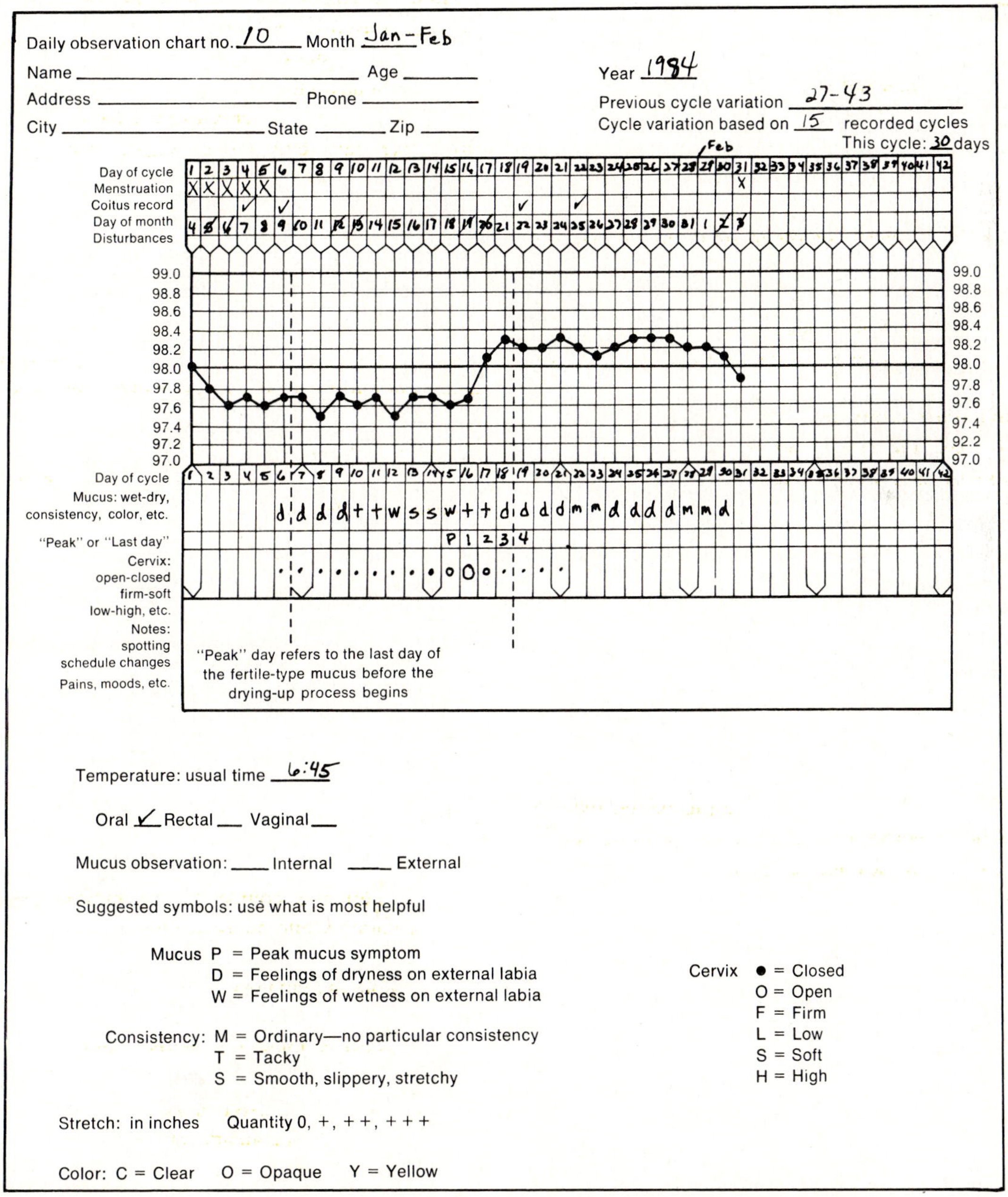

Couples who use the sympto-thermal method frequently report an improvement in their sexual relationship.

Effectiveness of the sympto-thermal method with abstinence during the fertile period ranges between 85% and 97%. For couples who *do not* want a pregnancy, effectiveness may reach 99% during the first year and about 98% during the second year. For couples who only wish to *delay* pregnancy, effectiveness usually approaches 86% during the first year of use and then drops to 73% during the second year.

Fertility awareness method. The fertility awareness method is a combination of the sympto-thermal method and barrier contraception. During the fertile period the couple has the choice of abstinence from genital-genital contact or the use of barrier contraception. After ovulation the couple may enjoy freedom from contraception for the remaining, nonfertile days of the menstrual cycle.

ORAL HORMONAL THERAPY

Mode of action. Progesterone and estrogen compounds (steroid sex hormones) prevent pregnancy by inhibiting the hypothalamus and anterior pituitary so that ovulation does not occur. In addition, hormonal therapy inhibits fertility by doing the following:

1. Altering the secretion of mucin and the motility of the fallopian tubes
2. Inadequately developing the endometrium, thereby making it unsuitable for implantation
3. Keeping cervical mucus unreceptive and unsupportive of sperm

Combined oral hormone therapy. The "pill," originally a combination of a synthetic estrogen (mestranol) and a synthetic progestogen (norethynodrel) (Enovid), is still a popular and successful product. Many subsequent combinations, some of considerably lower dosage (e.g., Loestrin 1/20), now are available. A dosage program common to all these products requires the administration of one tablet daily, beginning on the fifth day of the cycle and continuing for 20 to 21 days. Generally *withdrawal bleeding* begins 1 to 4 days after the last tablet is taken. Withdrawal bleeding is bleeding brought about by abrupt withdrawal of the steroid sex hormones that have been maintaining the endometrium; it is not true menstrual flow. The next container of pills is begun on the fifth day of the cycle.

Some pharmaceutical companies have added seven blanks (lactose or ferrous sulfate tablets) to follow the last combination hormone tablet so that the woman can take one pill every day. This pattern is easier to remember and is more likely to ensure regular menses. To benefit from the ferrous sulfate tablets, the woman is instructed to take this iron supplement with a source of vitamin C, for example, orange juice.

Advantages and benefits. Taken exactly as directed, oral contraceptives prevent ovulation and pregnancy cannot occur; the overall effectiveness rate is almost 100%. Almost all failures (i.e., pregnancy occurs) are caused by omission of one or more pills during the regimen.

There are several advantages to women receiving combined oral hormone therapy. For motivated women it is easy to take an oral contraceptive (OC) at about the same time each day. Taking the pill does not relate directly to the sexual act; this fact increases its acceptability to some women. Frequently, there is an improvement in sexual response once the possibility of pregnancy is not an issue. For some, it is convenient to know when to expect the next "menstrual" flow. The regular cyclic stimulation of the endometrium may help regulate menstrual cycles and make it possible for conception to occur at a later time. Occasionally, using oral hormone therapy for a period of time may decrease or eliminate premenstrual tension and dysmenorrhea (menstrual cramps).

Women who use OCs have less risk for endometrial carcinoma. The risk rate for endometrial carcinoma is decreased by 50% probably because of the regular cyclic stimulation and shedding of the endometrium. In addition, the use of OCs decreases the woman's risk of ovarian cancer, a rare but often fatal carcinoma of older women. There is growing evidence that women using OCs may have a decreased incidence of pelvic inflammatory disease (PID). These new findings need additional study.

Occurrence of ectopic pregnancy is decreased among OC users. Ectopic pregnancy is now the second most common cause of pregnancy-related mortality in the United States. OC use decreases the need for surgical removal of ovarian cysts, the fifth most common surgical procedure for women.

The amount of bleeding is often less than with non-OC–regulated menstrual cycles so that women lose less blood and therefore less iron with each cycle.

And finally, the risk of death from thromboembolism associated with the pill is less than the risk of death from thromboembolism during pregnancy (excluding deaths from illegal abortion) in the United States and the United Kingdom. This last comment is only true for women who did not have a history of thromboembolism before use of OCs or pregnancy.

Contraindications. Before starting oral contraception and again every 6 to 12 months during therapy, it is imperative that each woman have a complete health assessment including history, physical examination including Papanicolaou smear, and laboratory studies. Prevention of pregnancy through hormonal therapy is contraindicated when any one of the following exists:

1. Family history of vascular accident (stroke), diabetes mellitus, or breast cancer
2. History of hepatitis or hepatic insufficiency, jaundice, thromboembolic disease, sickle cell disease, moderate or severe hypertension, smoking more than 15 cigarettes per day, or psychic depression
3. History of conditions that can be aggravated by fluid retention, for example, migraine headache, convulsive disorders, asthma, or cardiac or renal insufficiency
4. Physical examination: age 30 years or older, presence of hormone-dependent tumors, breast nodules, fibrocystic disease, abnormal mammogram, or varicose veins

Disadvantages and precautions. Before OCs are prescribed and periodically throughout hormone therapy, the woman is alerted to stop taking the pill and to report any of the following symptoms to the physician immediately. The word *aches* helps in retention of this list:

A—Abdominal pain: may indicate a problem with the liver or gallbladder

C—Chest pain or shortness of breath: possible clot problem with lungs or heart

H—Headaches (sudden or persistent): may be caused by cardiovascular accident or hypertension

E—Eye problems: may indicate vascular accident or hypertension

S—Severe leg pain: may indicate a thromboembolic process

Several side effects have been attributed to the use of oral hormonal contraceptives:

1. Thromboembolic disorders and other vascular problems including cerebrovascular disorders and myocardial infarction
2. Estrogen excess or deficiency and progestin excess or deficiency
3. Alterations in metabolism, especially of carbohydrates and B vitamins
4. Fetal effects after discontinuing OCs
5. Amenorrhea after discontinuing OCs
6. Neoplastic disease
7. Hypertension
8. Adverse drug interactions

Thromboembolic disorders and other vascular problems. Thromboembolic disease, which is life threatening, must always be considered because estrogen is one factor implicated in the process. Women are started on the product with the lowest amount of estrogen, 0.05 mg or less, that is acceptable to her to minimize this problem. However, about 1 in 2000 women who use OCs will be hospitalized each year for vascular thrombosis and embolism.

A study, conducted in the United Kingdom, regarding the mortality rate per 100,000 women per year from diseases of the circulatory system for users and nonusers of OCs according to age, smoking habits, and duration of use found that the overall death rate annually from circulatory diseases for OC users was estimated at 20/100,000; by age categories, the death rate was cited as follows:

15- to 34-year-old group	5/100,000
35-•to 44-year-old group	33/100,000
45- to 49-year-old group	140/100,000

The risk is highest in older women, in those with long duration* of use, and in cigarette smokers. In older women, risk for adverse effects from OCs is further increased by other underlying risk factors that may be age related, for example, hypertension, obesity, and diabetes mellitus.

NOTE: As a precaution against postsurgical thrombophlebitis, it is advisable to discontinue oral contraception for 4 to 8 weeks before anticipated surgery.

NOTE: To lessen the risk of thromboembolic disease after miscarriage or elective abortion and to initiate contraception before ovulation, the following schedule is often used:

Gestation Length	Start of Oral Contraception
12 weeks or less	Immediately
13 to 28 weeks	After 1 week
28 weeks or more	After 2 weeks, if not lactating

The risk for myocardial infarction is greater among (1) users of OCs, especially for women past 35 years of age, (2) those suffering from other conditions such as hypertension, obesity, or diabetes, and (3) those who smoke. Thromboembolic disorders, including coronary thrombosis, are greater when higher dosages of estrogen are used in oral contraceptives. However, the quantity of estrogen may not be the sole factor involved.

Estrogen excess/deficiency and progestin excess/deficiency. Certain side effects of anovulatory drugs are attributable to estrogen or progestin or both. Side effects of *estrogen excess* include nausea and vomiting, dizziness, edema, leg cramps, increase in breast size, chloasma (mask of pregnancy), visual changes, hypertension, and vascular headache. Side effects of *estrogen deficiency* include early spotting (days 1 to 14), hypomenorrhea, nervousness, atrophic vaginitis leading to painful intercourse (dyspareunia). Side effects of *pro-*

*"Long duration" has not been defined.

gestin excess include increased appetite, tiredness, depression, breast tenderness, vaginal yeast infection, oily skin and scalp, hirsutism, and postpill amenorrhea. Side effects of *progestin deficiency* include late spotting and break-through bleeding (days 15 to 21), heavy flow with clots, and decreased breast size.

In the presence of side effects, especially those that are bothersome to the woman, a different product, a different drug content, or another method of contraception may be required. The "right" product for a woman contains the lowest dose of sex steroid hormones that prevents ovulation and that has the fewest and least harmful side effects. There is no way to predict the "right" dose* for any particular woman; trial and error is the main method for prescribing OCs, starting with the lowest possible estrogen dose.

Alteration in metabolism. The *changes in glucose tolerance* that occur in some women taking OCs are similar to those changes that occur during pregnancy. OCs challenge the islets of Langerhans to produce more insulin. If the individual is prediabetic, the use of oral contraception can induce the frank expression of diabetes mellitus.

The OC also affects the woman's *general nutritional needs,* especially for B vitamins. There is considerable evidence that OCs are implicated in deficiencies of vitamin B_6 (pyridoxine) and folic acid in about 20% to 30% of users. Among some OC users, symptoms such as headaches, nausea and vomiting, and emotional disturbances and depression have been alleviated by dietary supplementation of vitamin B_6.

Symptoms of folic acid deficiency are rare, since folate is plentiful in the North American diet. However, if a pregnancy occurs soon after the pill is discontinued, folic acid deficiency is to be expected. Clinical symptoms of folic acid deficiency are those of megaloblastic anemia: increasing fatigue, pallor, moderate depapillation of the tongue, and changes in peripheral blood and bone marrow. Symptoms are rapidly reversed with supplementation of folic acid or if the OC is discontinued.

Although not yet proven, there may be some deficiency of vitamin C and vitamin B_{12} (cobalamin). Vitamins whose metabolism is suspected of being altered by OCs are vitamin A, vitamin B_2, and niacin.

Some women complain of edema, which is associated with administration of estrogens; however, if the dose of estrogen is sufficiently low, fluid retention is not likely to occur or can be compensated for by decreasing the oral intake of sodium compounds.

The clinical significance of altered metabolism of the nutrients listed above and other nutrients and of reduced (rather than deficient) levels of the nutrients discussed above is unknown at this time.

*Fetal effects after discontinuing the pill.** Women who discontinue oral contraception for a planned pregnancy frequently ask whether they should wait before attempting to conceive. Although data are controversial, there does seem to be some evidence of increased incidence of chromosomal changes in abortuses when pregnancy occurs during the first few (usually one or two) cycles after discontinuation of oral contraception.

Postpill amenorrhea. After discontinuing oral contraception there is usually a delay before ovulation and menstrual cycles recur. However, amenorrhea exceeding 6 months should be investigated.

Neoplastic disease. Some neoplasms of the breast, benign or malignant, may be stimulated by estrogens. If another hormone-dependent tumor is suspected (e.g., of the endometrium), oral contraception is contraindicated.

There is an association between long-term use of contraceptive pills by women over 30 years of age and the occurrence of a liver tumor known as hepatocellular adenoma (HCA). The risk of developing HCA is higher with increasing use of OCs. The annual incidence of HCA is approximately 3 or 4 per 100,000 long-term users of OCs. In comparison the annual occurrence rate is approximately 1 to 1.3 per 1 million in women aged 16 to 30 years and in women aged 31 to 34 who have never used OCs or have used them for 24 months or less. Of the women who develop HCA, 88% are long-term users of OCs. The development of HCA can be minimized when the lowest possible dose that provides protection against pregnancy is used. Hepatic adenomas are also associated with the use of OCs. Because hepatic adenomas may rupture and cause death through hemorrhage, they should be considered in women with abdominal pain and tenderness, an abdominal mass, or shock.

Hypertension. Infrequently hypertension is first noted after the woman begins oral contraception, especially if she is 30 years of age or older. In some women, higher blood levels of angiotensinogen and plasma renin have been found. It is thought that these factors play a part in the hypertension experienced by some women. After discontinuing oral contraception, hypertension subsides.

Miscellaneous side effects and precautions. Some *laboratory values* may be altered in women taking OCs. These changes are listed, not for memorization, but only for interest and to alert the nurse to the need to ask about contraceptive use when taking a health history. The following laboratory values may be increased:

*Warn women, young and old, that using another woman's OCs may not prevent ovulation, if the dose is not correct for them.

*For a discussion of effects of the pill on the fetus when the woman continues with oral contraception after conception, see Appendix H.

bromsulphalein (BSP), serum glutamic oxaloacetic transaminase (SGOT), serum glutamic pyruvic transaminase (SGPT), alkaline phosphatase, and thyronine-binding protein (a thyroid hormone).

Some conditions are aggravated by fluid retention. Women who are susceptible to *migraine headaches* may notice an increase in headaches when taking the pill. Since headache is also a symptom of cerebral thrombosis, there may be confusion with correct diagnosis. Therefore women who experience migraine headaches are counseled to use other forms of contraception. Although many women with *epilepsy* tolerate OCs well, others tend to have an increase in the incidence of seizures.

Some women who wear *contact lenses* experience a change in the curvature of the cornea. Although the reason for this change is unknown, the woman is advised to discontinue use of the contact lenses.

More serious *neuroocular lesions* are associated with use of OCs. Optic neuritis or retinal thrombosis, although rare, has been reported. Symptoms such as sudden or gradual and partial or complete loss of vision and double vision require immediate diagnosis and treatment. **Women must stop taking OCs at the first sign of visual disorders.**

There is an increased risk of *gallbladder disease* after 2 years of use of OCs. The risk doubles after 4 to 5 years of pill use.

Oral contraceptives and drug interactions. The effectiveness of OCs is decreased along with an increased possibility of break-through bleeding if the woman is receiving any of the following drugs:

- Rifampin (for tuberculosis)
- Barbiturates (for sedation)
- Phenylbutazone (for arthritis or bursitis; treatment for superficial thrombophlebitis)
- Phenytoin sodium (for seizure disorders)
- Ampicillin (for infections)
- Tetracycline (for infections)

Long-term use of OCs slows diazepam (Valium) clearance by the liver; therefore higher blood levels of the drug increase the risk of an overdose of diazepam. Planned Parenthood facilities keep current information about newly identified drug interactions as it becomes available.

Procedure for taking the pill: client counseling. If used according to prescription, this method of contraception is very efficient (99.7%). The woman needs to take the pill at the same time each day to maintain constant blood levels of estrogen and progesterone for 21 days. If one pill is missed, she takes that pill as soon as she remembers it; she takes the next pill at the regularly scheduled time. If she misses two pills, she takes both as soon as she remembers to do so. A second form of contraceptive (e.g., diaphragm with spermicide) for the rest of that cycle is advised. If three pills are missed, the remainder of the pills in that packet are discarded and use of a back-up type of contraceptive is advised. A new packet of pills is begun on the fifth day of the next cycle. (Bleeding should begin within 2 to 3 days after she misses the pills; day 1 of the new cycle is the first day of bleeding.)

• • •

The *minipill* is a progesterone-only pill containing norethindrone, 0.35 mg, and is taken daily. *Ovulation may occur;* however, daily progesterone ingestion blocks conception by altering the endometrium and rendering the cervical mucus nonreceptive to sperm. The minipill is useful to those who must avoid estrogens and reduces the side effects experienced with the other oral preparations. However, women who use the minipill may complain of menstrual irregularity, uterine cramping, and lumps in the breast. The minipill is slightly less effective than the combination pill but can reach 98% reliability if taken exactly as prescribed.

The *morning-after pill* is an estrogen compound, diethylstilbestrol (DES), 25 mg, and is used primarily by rape victims. DES must be started within 72 hours after intercourse. One tablet is taken two times daily for 5 consecutive days (10 doses = 250 mg). The estrogen suppresses the hypothalamic-pituitary axis to prevent ovulation and alters the endometrium to discourge implantation. Menstruation (called withdrawal bleeding) occurs within 5 days after the last dose is taken. Nausea and vomiting are the chief complaints during therapy.

The greatest disadvantage to the morning-after pill is that *ovulation may occur*. If pregnancy does occur, the embryo may be damaged by the DES. DES predisposes the female child to delayed reproductive tract disorders, including cancer (e.g., clear cell adenoma), which may occur in adolescence and early adulthood. There may also be a relationship between male infertility and increased incidence of testicular cancer in male embryos exposed to DES.

The woman who is being considered for therapy with the morning-after pill is advised that should pregnancy occur anyway, elective abortion by cervical dilation and currettage (D and C) is indicated. The effectiveness of the morning-after pill reaches 100% if hormone therapy is followed by D and C.

INJECTABLE MEDICATION

Medroxyprogesterone acetate (Depo-Provera), 150 mg, is administered by intramuscular injection every 90 days. This compound suppresses the function of the hypothalamic-pituitary axis, primarily by inhibiting production of luteinizing hormone (LH), which in turn inhibits development of the graafian follicle and endometrium. Due to lack of stimulation, the endometrium atrophies and uterine bleeding is either irregular or absent. The greatest disadvantage is that the reestablishment of regular ovulation and true menstrual flow may be delayed longer than 1 year after discontinuing the medication.

INTRAUTERINE DEVICE

The intrauterine device (IUD) is an object made of plastic or nonreactive metal (nickel-chromium alloy) that fits inside the uterine cavity and is manufactured in several shapes (e.g., loop, coil, and spiral). *Effectiveness* has been cited as 97% to 99%.

An IUD is *indicated* when the woman is unable to, or prefers not to, use oral hormones for fertility control or when she (or the couple) cannot learn or lacks the motivation to use other contraceptive methods.

The *mode of action* of the IUD is thought to be that it causes a chronic inflammatory response in the endometrium, which discourages implantation of a fertilized ovum. Ovulation continues to occur; conception can and does occur. If implantation occurs, early spontaneous abortion usually follows.

Note the following:

1. Women for whom abortion is not acceptable should *not* use an IUD for contraception.
2. Chronic inflammation of the endometrium (endometritis) predisposes the wearer to intrauterine and intratubal infection and pelvic inflammatory disease (PID) with possible consequent infertility/sterility.

Advantages of the IUD include low production costs, increased spontaneity of intercourse, increased convenience (no schedule or pills), no interference with hormonal regulation of the woman's menstrual cycles, and the possibility of retention for prolonged periods of time.

There are several *disadvantages* to use of the IUD. IUDs are *contraindicated* if there is any inflammatory condition or infection of the reproductive tract structures or PID, abnormalities of the uterus, or severe dysmenorrhea or uterine bleeding of unknown etiology or if pregnancy is suspected. Some IUDs are not suitable for women who have not carried a pregnancy to viability (the nulliparous woman) because of the small size of the uterine cavity. *Complications from and adverse reactions* to the use of the IUD have been identified. For some women, manipulation of the cervix, such as dilation and insertion of an IUD, or stretching of the intrauterine cavity stimulates a vagal nerve response recognized by diaphoresis, faintness and syncope (fainting), pallor, and tachycardia. Some women perceive the procedure as painful.

The increased risk of PID is a significant disadvantage. Since infections heal by scar formation, there is potential for the following to occur:

1. *Sterility* by enclosing the ovary and preventing ovulation, by direct blockage of the lumen of the tube, or indirectly by kinking or distorting the fallopian tube.
2. *Infertility* from the same mechanisms that result in sterility. The tube may be blocked partially so that fertilization can occur but the ovum's passage into the uterine cavity is prevented. Ectopic pregnancy followed by surgical removal of the tube (salpingectomy) is more common in IUD wearers than in other women.
3. *Medical-surgical intervention* for complications such as twisted ovary, bowel obstruction, unilateral tuboovarian abscess.

Because of the possibility of infection and scar tissue–related complications, the IUD may not be a suitable method for the woman who desires children in the future. The women at greatest risk to develop PID are nulliparas 25 years or younger, women with a history of PID, and women who have more than one sex partner or who change partners frequently.

Other complications include perforation of the uterus during insertion or later, at a rate of 1/1500 women users. The IUD may be expelled, especially during the first months of use. Expulsion occurs at a rate of 1 to 20 per 100 women users. IUD-caused uterine cramping and vaginal bleeding (and consequent anemia) are the most common causes for removal. These conditions are related to the size of the IUD and the size of the uterine cavity. If pregnancy does occur, the physician will determine the feasibility of removal of the IUD. The rate of spontaneous abortion with an IUD in place is 25% to 50% with a greater possibility of sepsis (infection). If the IUD cannot be removed, and pregnancy continues, the fetus usually suffers no ill effects (unless the IUD is copper coated) because the IUD is outside the sac enclosing the pregnancy. Part of the contraceptive effect of a copper IUD is the cytotoxic property of copper on sperm; it is thought that the slow release of copper that occurs continuously may harm the developing conceptus.

One out of twenty pregnancies that occur while an IUD is in place is ectopic. The reason for the ectopic location of the pregnancy is not always known.

The following list summarizes possible IUD-related complications and adverse reactions:

1. Uterine perforation
2. Expulsion

3. Dysmenorrhea
4. Increased blood loss (anemia)
5. PID
6. Ectopic pregnancy
7. Spontaneous abortion
8. Surgical intervention
9. Infertility/sterility

A number of different *types of IUDs* are currently on the market:

1. *Nonmedicated:* These IUDs do not require periodic removal and replacement.
   a. *Lippes loop* is available in four sizes (A [small] to D [large]). This IUD is used more frequently than other devices and can be fitted to the size of the uterus. The woman who has never borne children is usually fitted with size A.
   b. *Saf-T-Coil* is available in two sizes, small and large. This type is easy to insert and fills the intrauterine cavity.
2. *Medicated:* Medications enhance the contraceptive action of the IUD. These medicated IUDs do require periodic removal and replacement.
   a. *Copper-7 (Cu 200)* is available in one size only. This type needs to be replaced every 3 years because the available copper, released at the rate of 10 to 50 μg/24 hr, is depleted by then. Copper has a direct spermicidal effect. Insertion is easier because of the small size of this device. There is less pain during and after insertion and less postinsertion bleeding (50 to 60 ml of blood vs. 70 to 80 ml of blood with the loop type of IUD). The rare sensitivity to copper, manifested principally by a skin rash or unusual allergic reaction, necessitates removal of the IUD.
   b. *Copper-T (T-Cu 200)* (tatum copper–bearing IUD) retains its contraceptive effectiveness for 3 years. Fertility is restored promptly after removal of either of the copper-bearing IUDs in the majority of women.
   c. *Progestasert-T* is available in one size only. Progesterone, 65 μg, is released each day for 1 year. The Progestasert has been discontinued in the United Kingdom because of decreased effectiveness when compared to other devices.

Procedure for insertion of the IUD: client preparation

1. A thorough health assessment is essential and includes the following:
   a. A health history that includes description of mental status, life-style, desire for future pregnancies, and menstrual characterisitics
   b. Physical examination that includes assessment for uterine anomalies or disorders and size of intrauterine cavity
   c. Laboratory testing for anemia and vaginal infections; Papanicolaou smear for cytology
2. A full explanation of the IUD is given: advantages, contraindications, use-effectiveness, and mode of action; description of the IUD; directions for its insertion, use, and removal/replacement; complications and adverse reactions and warnings; cautions regarding pregnancy; and alternative methods for fertility control. The woman is instructed about her responsibilities for self-examination and reporting adverse reactions. After the individual understands the explanation given, she is legally prepared to sign an informed consent. She should then be given an informed consent to sign.
3. Insertion (or removal) of an IUD ideally is timed during menstruation for three reasons: insertion is technically easier through a slightly dilated cervical os, women are less concerned about bleeding at this time, and the presence of an early pregnancy is less likely. Aseptic insertion is accomplished following antiseptic preparation of the cervix and vagina. A tenaculum is applied to the anterior lip of the cervix to straighten the uterus, which decreases the risk of uterine perforation during insertion. Application of the tenaculum is usually felt as a pinch; the paucity of nerve endings in the cervix decreases physical pain experienced by many women. However, insertion may be accomplished under paracervical block (see Chapter 25).
4. During the first month after insertion of an IUD, the woman should use an additional form of contraception (e.g., foam). If a woman is changing from oral contraception to an IUD, she continues on the pills for 1 month.
5. The attached string suture is trimmed to 2.5 cm (about 1 in) below the external cervical os. The woman is instructed to check for the presence of the IUD suture (tail)* before intercourse and after each menstrual cycle to identify early expulsion of the device, which occurs unnoticed in 1 to 20 out of 100 users. At body temperature the suture is usually not noticed by the sexual partner. Sutures that feel "too long" may indicate beginning expulsion.
6. The woman receives instruction about possible

*The IUD suture tail may act as a wick for the passage of microorganisms from the vagina into the intrauterine cavity. In the future this tail may no longer be a part of IUDs.

adverse reactions that should be reported immediately. This list includes the following signs:
   a. Perforation—abdominal and low back pain
   b. Pelvic or vaginal infection—chills/fever; unusual vaginal discharge
   c. Expulsion—inability to locate strings or tail
   d. Pregnancy
   e. Uterine irritation—dysmenorrhea, increased menstrual flow (menorrhagia), bleeding between periods (metrorrhagia)
7. The woman is provided with a wallet-sized card indicating the type of IUD inserted, insertion date, date for replacement (if appropriate), and emergency phone numbers.

An IUD can be placed immediately after first-trimester abortion, at 2 weeks after second-trimester abortion, and at 6 weeks after delivery. Insertion is delayed after delivery to decrease the risks of uterine perforation and expulsion during involution (for discussion of involution, see p. 687). There is an expulsion rate of approximately 30% of IUDs inserted during the puerperium.

DIAPHRAGM WITH SPERMICIDE

The vaginal diaphragm is a shallow, dome-shaped rubber device with a flexible wire rim that covers the cervix. The upper edge of the diaphragm fits snugly under the symphysis pubis, the dome covers the cervix, and the lower edge rests in the posterior vaginal vault. The diaphragm should feel comfortable. The use of a contraceptive gel or cream with the diaphragm offers both mechanical and chemical barriers to pregnancy. The *effectiveness* of this combined method is approximately 83% to 90%. Highly motivated women may achieve rates of 99%.

The *mode of action* of mechanical barriers is to prevent the union of sperm and ovum. The diaphragm holds the spermicide in place against the cervix for the 4 to 6 hours it takes to destroy the sperm.

There are several *advantages* to this method. Except for occasional allergic response to the diaphragm or spermicide, there are no side effects from a well-fitted device. Ill-fitting devices may cause severe rubbing and ulcer formation in the vaginal mucosa, especially in the area behind the symphysis pubis. The diaphragm can be inserted several hours before intercourse. Some women object to the presence of a foreign body inside their uterine cavity (the IUD), or they are unable or unwilling to take medications to prevent ovulation (OCs). In some instances the woman who engages in intercourse infrequently may choose this barrier method. The spermicide does offer additional lubrication if it is needed. A decreased incidence of vaginitis and cystitis is noted among women who use contraceptive creams, foams, and gels with the diaphragm.

For the woman with relaxation of her pelvic support expressed as uterine prolapse or a large cystocele or for the woman who is uninformed, this method is *contraindicated*. *Disadvantages* include the reluctance of some women to insert and remove the diaphragm. A cold diaphragm and a cold gel temporarily reduce vaginal response to sexual stimulation if insertion of the diaphragm occurs immediately before intercourse. Some women or couples object to the "messiness" of the spermicide. These annoyances of diaphragm usage, along with failure to insert the device once foreplay has begun, are the most common reasons for failures of this method.

There are three main *types* of diaphragms. The oval-shaped device is useful for women with small cystoceles. The type with a coil spring is the most common. It ranges in size from 6 to 10 cm (2½ to 4 in). The diaphragm with an arc spring has two hinges and is indicated with a retroverted uterus and cervix that is anterior in the vaginal vault.

Procedure for insertion and follow-up. After a general health assessment that includes a health history, physical examination, and laboratory tests, the woman is measured for the diaphragm. The depth of the vagina is estimated and the largest diaphragm that will fit comfortably is chosen. A diaphragm that is too small may be dislodged during intercourse. The physician or nurse-practitioner demonstrates the proper application of spermicide and insertion following careful hand washing. The physician assists the woman to feel her cervix to determine that the diaphragm is properly placed. Approximately 1 teaspoonful of spermicide is placed inside the diaphragm and a small amount is spread around the rim. To remove the diaphragm, the woman reaches behind her symphysis pubis and lifts the diaphragm out by the rim. The physician or nurse demonstrates proper care (washing of the diaphragm in warm water with mild, unperfumed soap, followed by light dusting with cornstarch to maintain the condition of the rubber), teaches the woman to check the device for defects, and cautions her to store it in a cool, dry place away from a source of heat. With proper care, the diaphragm may last 3 to 5 years.

The device may be inserted several hours before intercourse; however, it is recommended that intercourse occur within 1 hour following insertion. If intercourse occurs more than 6 hours after insertion, or if repeated intercourse occurs, an additional application of the spermicide is necessary. Under no circumstances must the diaphragm be removed until at least 6 hours after the last intercourse to allow for full spermicidal activity.

The woman is informed that she needs an annual gynecologic examination and that the device must be refitted after the loss or gain of 4.5 kg (10 lb) or more or if she gives birth.

CERVICAL CAP

Cervical caps come in two types: one is presized in small, medium, and large, and one is custom fitted. The custom cervical cap is a plasticlike cap about 2.5 cm (1 in) in diameter and is fitted to conform to the individual woman's cervix. This cap has several advantages: (1) It can be made in the physician's office in approximately 20 minutes. A mold of the cervix is made with a nontoxic substance used to make contact lenses. A plaster cast is made of the mold, and then the cap is fitted onto the cast. (2) Its design allows menstrual flow out through the cervix and self-cleaning with natural mucous flow, while preventing sperm from entering the cervix. (3) No foreign-matter reaction has been noted in users of this device. (4) It can be left in place indefinitely.

The presized cervical cap, however, cannot be left in place indefinitely. The custom cervical cap and the presized cervical cap are not yet approved for sale in the United States. They are only available in those clinics involved in studies of this method of contraception.

THE 48-HR CONTRACEPTIVE

The 2-day contraceptive is a soft, 5 cm (2 in) plastic sponge impregnated with spermicide. It is inserted into the vagina, soaks up semen, and blocks sperm from entering the cervix. There is no need to add additional spermicide. There is an estimated failure rate of 10%. (Testing of 2000 women began in 1977 in the United States; it has been in use in Great Britain since the summer of 1982.) An added note: The FDA's Fertility and Maternal Health Advisory Committee states that a link between the sponge and the bacteria thought to cause toxic shock syndrome is "very unlikely." The sponge will be sold over the counter without a prescription.

VAGINAL SPERMICIDES

Spermicides are available as creams, jellies, gels, suppositories, foam, and tablets. All except the tablets are effective immediately. The tablets require up to 10 minutes to dissolve. *Effectiveness* ranges between 20 and 45 pregnancies per 100 women users of spermicides without diaphragm or condom. The *mode of action* of spermicides is to (1) destroy sperm, decrease their motility, or incapacitate them before they reach the ovum; and (2) block passage of sperm. *Advantages* to the use of spermicides include ready availability, the need for very little instruction for their use, and ease of application. Also they increase effectiveness of mechanical barriers, add to lubrication, do not require previous medical examination or prescription, and may offer some protection against some sexually transmitted diseases through bacteriostatic action.

The only *contraindication* for use is possible allergy to the preparation. There are no medical *complications* except chemical vaginitis. Some couples describe spermicides as "messy." Messiness is compounded by the necessity of reapplication of spermicide each time intercourse is to be repeated. Tactile sensation may be dulled for some users.

MALE CONTRACEPTION

The development of effective contraception for males has long been neglected. Two barrier methods—the condom that prevents the deposition of sperm in or near the vagina and spermicides that destroy or incapacitate sperm after being deposited in the vagina—are the only approved safe methods available today.*

Condom. The condom is a thin, stretchable rubber sheath worn over the penis by the man during intercourse. The *effectiveness* of this method varies but is about the same as for the diaphragm if a spermicide is also used. There may be a failure rate (pregnancy rate) of from 7% to 28% without the spermicide. Effectiveness is increased significantly if a spermicide is used and if the sheath is held in place while the still slightly erect penis is withdrawn, thus preventing spillage of sperm in or near the vagina. The *mode of action* of this method is to prevent the entry of sperm into the vagina (if the sheath does not tear).

The chief *advantage* of this method is its safety—there are no side effects. The sheath does provide some protection against the spread of sexually transmitted infections. The basic type of condom is relatively inexpensive. There are no medical *complications* attributed to the use of the condom. *Disadvantages* have been noted by some couples; that is, interruption of foreplay is one disadvantage. It does take time to apply the sheath over the slightly erect penis. If some pre-ejaculatory fluid escapes before the application of the condom, pregnancy from the few sperm that are found in these drops may occur even if the fluid only reaches the vulvar area. The sheaths now are lubricated and allow the man to retain or enhance his perception of sensation. Condoms are available in most drugstores and can be purchased without prescription or prior health assessment by a physician. Contact dermatitis has been reported.

Condoms are used by 10% to 15% of couples in the United States and are very popular in Japan, Sweden,

*Coitus interruptus, a method practiced for centuries, is mentioned here only to caution couples against this type of unreliable method. This method requires the man to withdraw before ejaculation. Extreme self-discipline is needed, and the sexual relationship may be strained. The danger of pregnancy from sperm in the pre-ejaculatory drops is ever present. No advantages are given for this method, which has a low rate of effectiveness.

and the United Kingdom. In the United States use of the condom is increasing as more women are opting not to use the IUD or hormonal or chemical contraceptives. The shelf life (length of safe storage time before deterioration) of the latex condom is 2 years.

Procedure for application. The man is directed to follow the instructions on the box for proper use of the condom: (1) apply over entire erect penis before vaginal penetration; (2) leave a reservoir at the tip to retain semen; (3) use an adequate water-soluble lubricant such as spermicidal foam (never use petrolatum, since this erodes the sheath and can cause tearing); and (4) withdraw the penis after ejaculation, simultaneously holding the condom against the base of the penis before the penis becomes flaccid, to avoid spilling the semen into or near the vagina.

Other methods of male contraception. Efforts to suppress spermatogenesis or to inhibit maturation of sperm have been relatively unsuccessful. Steroid hormones can suppress spermatogenesis, but unacceptable side effects have prevented their use. Some adverse reactions were (1) unpredictability in time needed to establish infertility or delay or absence in reversing the infertility effect, (2) erectile problems (impotence), and (3) Antabuse symptoms.* Some nonhormonal preparations tested had serious toxicity with resultant destruction of testicular interstitial cells.

Trials of *5-thio-D-glucose* inhibition of spermatogenesis indicate reversibility after discontinuance of therapy. The product is nontoxic and does not alter libido or ability to achieve an erection (potentia). Studies are continuing.

Gossypol, a male contraceptive pill first developed in China, is being evaluated in the United States. This phenol extract is made inexpensively from cottonseed. It has proved to be 99.8% effective in 4000 Chinese men and 99.1% effective in approximately 8806 men in

*Antabuse produces a sensitivity to alcohol that results in a highly unpleasant reaction even if only small amounts of alcohol are ingested.

Table 13.4
Contraceptives in Common Use, Their Modes of Action, and Female/Male Involvement

Contraceptive	Woman	Man	Mode of Action	Involvement Time: Periodic	Involvement Time: Daily
Natural family planning					
Rhythm/calendar	X		Couple cooperation: abstinence during fertile periods	Mathematical formula calculated once every month	
BBT	X		Couple cooperation: abstinence during fertile periods	Ovulation determined from daily record of BBT	X
Cervical mucus	X		Couple cooperation: abstinence during fertile periods	Ovulation determined from daily record of cervical mucus characteristics	X
Sympto-thermal	X	Assists	Couple cooperation: abstinence during fertile periods	Combination of BBT, cervical mucus observation, and record of secondary symptoms by couple	X
Oral contraceptives	X		Suppress ovulation by inhibiting hypothalamus and pituitary	Ingestion of OC at same time each day; physical examination by physician every 6 mo.	X
IUDs (unmedicated)	X		Prevent implantation within uterus	Inserted into uterus by trained person; placement checked often; IUD changed every 2-3 yr, prn	
Mechanical barriers					
Diaphragms	X		Prevent sperm migration into uterus	Inserted into vagina over cervix before intercourse	
Condoms		X	Prevent sperm migration into uterus	Applied to penis before intercourse	
Chemical barriers: foams, gels, suppositories*	X	X	Destroy sperm or make them immobile within vaginal vault	Inserted into vagina before each intercourse; applied with diaphragm or condom	
Fertility awareness	X	X	Family planning method combined with a barrier method of contraception		

*Chemicals may be combined with other forms of contraception to enhance their effectiveness (e.g., Cu-7 IUD; spermicide with diaphragm or condom).

the United States. In 99.1% of those tested, sperm counts have been reduced to below 4 million/ml of ejaculate. The antifertility effect is present within 2 to 3 months after initiating this oral contraceptive and persists for a few weeks after therapy is discontinued. Initially, to establish the antifertility effect, gossypol is taken daily for 3 months; thereafter the antifertility effect is maintained with two doses per week. Gossypol is effective in inhibiting spermatogenesis. It does not damage the interstitial cells that are responsible for gametogenesis, levels of LH and testosterone are unchanged, and libido and potentia (ability to achieve and maintain an erection) are unaffected. The drug is considered safe and effective. The study results from China did not mention delay or absence of reversibility of the antifertility effect. Of the men studied in the United States, reversibility was incomplete in 25% of the 2000 subjects who were observed. Reported side effects consisted of fatigue (12%), gastrointestinal symptoms (7%), decreased libido (6%), and decrease in potassium levels (hypokalemia). Research is still needed to investigate the mechanism of action of gossypol and the reversibility of this drug before it can be made available to the public.

Because of the lag in the development of male contraception, the use of the condom and submitting to vasectomy (see p. 999), unsatisfactory though either may be, are the only reliable male contraceptive methods to date.

In Table 13.4, contraceptives in common use, their modes of action, and female/male involvement are compared and contrasted. In Table 13.5, fertility factors and the contraceptive techniques or appliances that block those factors are summarized.

Table 13.5
Contraceptive Techniques or Appliances to Block Fertility, in Common use

Fertility Factor	Contraceptive Method
Female	
Ovulatory	Hormonal therapy: OCs and injectable (primary site of activity at anterior pituitary to prevent ovulation)
	Abstention during fertile period
Tubal	Hormonal therapy alters motility and therefore rate of egg's passage
	Temporary blockage with hood or clip (surgical procedure required) (see Chapter 41)
Uterine	Hormonal therapy alters preparation of endometrium
	IUDs (nonmedicated) alter endometrium
Vaginal-cervical	Hormonal therapy (progesterone) keeps mucus unreceptive to sperm
	Barriers: mechanical (diaphragm) and chemical (spermicides) prevent sperm from reaching ovum
	Abstention during fertile period
Male	
Sperm	Abstention during fertile period
	Barriers: mechanical (condom) and chemical (spermicides) prevent sperm from reaching ovum

Nursing Actions

Nursing actions in the area of contraceptive counseling will vary with the nurse's preparation in the field, the type of role specified in the job description of the nurse, the clients with whom the nurse comes in contact, and the policies of the agency in which the nurse functions. Because of this wide range of involvement and responsibility the nurse may have, the nursing actions presented are broad in scope.

EVALUATIVE CRITERIA

In the area of contraceptive counseling, there are evaluative criteria that direct the type of care the client should be able to expect. The evaluative criteria serve as a guide for the health care *team* and are not the sole responsibility of the nurse. The nurse can best function when all members of the team have an adequate theoretical base. The recipients of health care related to contraception should be able to expect that the woman or couple is or will become:

1. Aware of the biologic and psychologic components of sexuality and possible outcomes of sexual activity
2. Able to plan for a desired (wanted) pregnancy or prevent an unwanted one
3. Knowledgeable concerning the advantages and disadvantages of the contraceptive method selected
4. Skilled in the use of chemical, hormonal, or mechanical techniques or knowledgeable about the technical processes involved in surgical contraception
5. Aware of community resources for assistance with sexuality problems
6. Aware of legal rights and responsibilities concerning adult sexual activity
7. Provided with continuity of care based on records established and maintained by the health care team

ASSESSMENT

The nurse may assess for, or contribute to the health history, information about the following:

1. The woman's (couple's) knowledge of the
   a. Biologic and psychologic components of human sexuality
   b. Various methods to prevent conception
   c. Physical and emotional responses of the woman to the phases of the menstrual cycle
2. The willingness (motivation) of the woman or couple to assess her body and keep records of findings on a daily basis
3. The willingness (motivation) of the woman or couple not to be "spontaneous" all the time in their sexual relationship, but to consider abstinence or participate in some contraceptive activities
4. The need for fertility control in the following situations:
   a. Woman or couple is sexually active now or plans to be
   b. Woman has a disease process incompatible with pregnancy (e.g., nephritis) and therefore must use some form of contraception
   c. Woman has just experienced a pregnancy
5. Determination of whether method selected for the woman meets the following criteria:
   a. It is safe for her use (e.g., the pill is contraindicated under certain conditions, for instance, during lactation)
   b. It is suitable to her life-style (e.g., she wants to become pregnant in the future or does not want any children)
   c. It is compatible with her religious or moral convictions
   d. She can afford the protective technique chosen
   e. She or they are able to learn the protective technique chosen

PLANNING AND IMPLEMENTATION

1. Refute myths and misconceptions with factual information. In some instances the nurse may be the one who identifies the client's information needs, but the physician may prefer to do the teaching about the following:
   a. Biology of sexuality
   b. Consequences of sexual activity (e.g., woman may become pregnant as early as the third postnatal week—before menstruation resumes; may become pregnant on first exposure to intercourse; may become pregnant after deposit of semen on labia minora without vaginal penetration by penis; may become pregnant after menses have become irregular with approach of menopause)
   c. Contraceptive methods: assemble reading material (pamphlets) in language understood by the client; assemble various samples of contraceptives for client to observe and handle; set aside time for client to ask questions; explain the mode of action, advantages, possible side effects, effectiveness, and proper technique for implementation; demonstrate use, application, and removal of contraceptives, using plastic models as necessary; demonstrate taking, reading, and recording of BBT
2. Provide safe, open, accepting environment to enable woman or couple to come to a decision regarding the choice of method to be used
3. Provide supportive, nonjudgmental care for woman in clinic or hospital settings, including careful explanation of procedures, relief of discomfort, use of gentle touch and tone of voice and closeness in space to convey interest, privacy, and presence of family or friend or both, if woman desires this
4. Establish with woman a future plan of care, such as the need for an annual physical examination while taking OCs or the need to have a diaphragm refitted if weight is gained or lost.

EVALUATION

The effectiveness of the goals, the plan of care, and the care delivered is determined during the evaluation phase of the nursing process. The nurse may use a number of different methods to evaluate the effectiveness of the care given to the client. Suggestions for evaluating the client's knowledge vary with the situation and may include any of the following:

1. Encourage feedback from the client:
   a. Rhythm or calendar method: ask client to calculate fertile times for a variety of cycle lengths.
   b. BBT: ask woman to take her temperature, read the thermometer, and record it on a graph.
   c. Cervical mucus method: present client with mucous characteristics and have her identify the proper phase of the cycle.
   d. Diaphragm: physician, nurse-midwife, or nurse-practitioner asks the woman to demonstrate application of spermicide on diaphragm, folding the device, inserting it, and checking herself for correct placement behind the symphysis pubis and over the cervix. The woman then assumes the lithotomy position while the physician or nurse examines the woman's

placement of the diaphragm. The woman is then asked to remove the diaphragm and demonstrate proper care of the appliance. She is asked to wear the diaphragm for about 8 hours per day for a few days and return to be rechecked to confirm proper fit.

e. Condom: ask woman (couple) to demonstrate condom application and removal from a plastic pelvic model, or ask woman to repeat verbally, directions for application and removal.
f. OC: ask woman to describe action she would take if she misses one, two, or three OCs.

2. During return visits, the nurse evaluates the client's experiences with the chosen contraception; the nurse knows that the woman has learned to use the protective technique well and that the method is acceptable and effective, if
   a. Records show daily entries, correctly noted for the BBT, cervical mucus changes, and sympto-thermal markers for ovulation.
   b. Negative experiences or side effects are absent.
   c. No pregnancy occurs.
   d. The woman confers with the physician immediately if unexpected symptomatology occurs.

References and Readings

Beacham, D.W., and Beacham, W.D.: Synopsis of gynecology, ed. 10, St. Louis, 1982, The C.V. Mosby Co.

Benson, R.C., editor: Current obstetric and gynecologic diagnosis and treatment, ed. 4, Los Altos, Calif., 1982, Lange Medical Publications.

Britt, S.S.: Fertility awareness: four methods of natural family planning, J.O.G.N. Nurs. **6**(2):9, 1977.

Canavan, P.A.,and Lewis, C.A.: The cervical cap: an alternative contraceptive, J.O.G.N. Nurs. **10**(4):271, 1981.

Cates, W.: Sex and spermicides; preventing unintended pregnancy and infection (editorial), J.A.M.A. **248**(13):1636, 1982.

Darney, P.D.: Evaluating the pill's long-term effects, Contemp. Obstet. Gynecol. **20**(3):57, 1982.

Editorial Board: Postcoital contraception for unprotected intercourse, Contemp. Obstet. Gynecol. **20**(6):79, 1982.

Garcia, C., et al.: Current therapy of infertility, 1982-1983, St. Louis, 1983, The C.V. Mosby Co.

Hastings-Tolsma, M.T. The cervical cap: a barrier contraceptive, M.C.N. **7**(6):382, 1982.

Keith, L.G., et al.: Effective use of vaginal contraception, a method for the 1980's, Contemp. Obstet. Gynecol. **19**(6):64, 1982.

Keith, L.G., et al.: Perspective on vaginal contraception: a method for the 1980's, Contemp. Obstet. Gynecol. **19**(5):63, 1982.

Kelaghan, J., et al.: Barrier method contraceptives and pelvic inflammatory disease, J.A.M.A. **248**(2):184, 1982.

Mishell, D.R.: Noncontraceptive health benefits of oral steroidal contraceptives, Am. J Obstet. Gynecol. **248:**184, 1982.

Oral contraceptives can benefit women, Health Education Bulletin, no. 29, July, 1982, National Clearinghouse for Family Planning Information.

Rosenthal, T.: Voluntary childlessness and the nurse's role, M.C.N. **5**(6):398, 1980.

Roy, S., et al.: Comparison of metabolic and clinical effects of four oral contraceptive formulations and a contraceptive vaginal ring, Am. J. Obstet. Gynecol. **136**(7):920, 1980.

Prenatal Period

14 From Conception to Birth
15 Anatomic and Physiologic Adaptations to Pregnancy
16 Family Responses to Pregnancy
17 Nursing Care During the Prenatal Period
18 Maternal and Fetal Nutrition
19 Preparation for Parenting

UNIT THREE

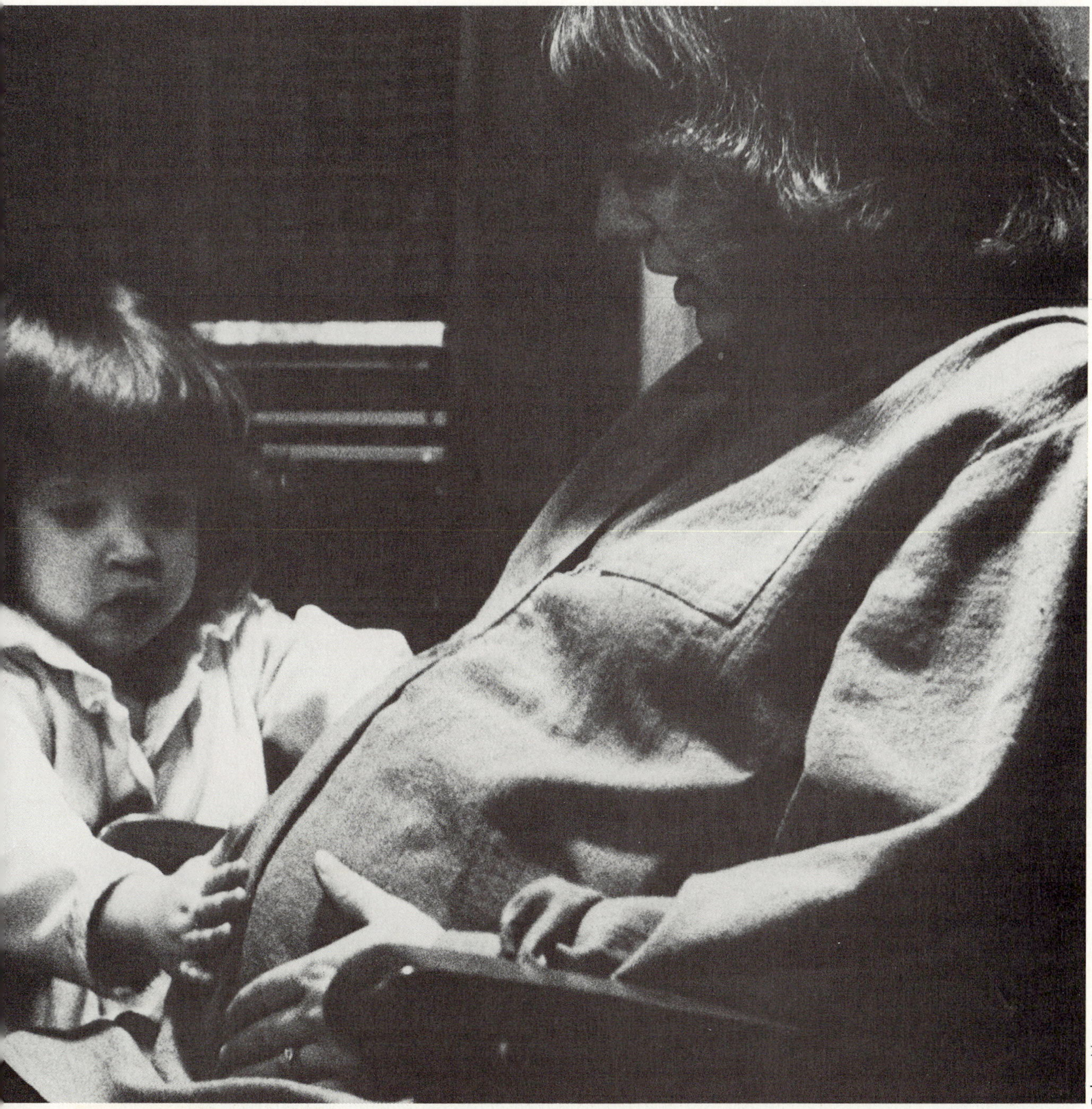

Robert Maust

14

From Conception to Birth

- Conception
  - Developmental stages
    - Ovum
    - Embryo
    - Fetus
  - Gestational time units
  - Implantation (nidation)
  - The decidua
  - Placentation
  - Fetal membranes
  - Umbilical cord
  - Placenta
    - Placental physiology
    - Placental transfer
    - Placental variations
  - Amniotic fluid
- Embryonic Development and Fetal Maturation
  - Cardiovascular system
  - Hematopoietic system
  - Respiratory system
  - Renal system
  - Neurologic system
    - Fetal neuromuscular behavior
  - Gastrointestinal system
    - Metabolism
    - Meconium
  - Hepatic system
  - Endocrine system
  - Reproductive system
    - Female genital development and function
    - Male genital development and function
  - Immune system
- Viability

Each human life begins with the union of two single cells, an ovum and a sperm, which form a single cell called the zygote (Fig. 14.1). Once united, this cell begins to divide, differentiate, and grow into a person, a replica of humanity's continuing generations and yet a unique individual. The growth that takes place from conception to birth is more rapid than at any other time in a person's life; the microscopic union of sperm and ovum increases in size more than 200 billion times during this period.

Before conception can occur, a process called *gametogenesis* occurs. Gametogenesis is the production of specialized sex cells, or *gametes*. As these cells mature, the number of chromosomes that they contain is reduced by half (meiosis) to the haploid number of 23. In the male, continuous spermatogenesis in the testes produces small, highly motile sperm. In the female, cyclic oogenesis in the ovaries produces large, nonmotile ova (see Chapter 10 for more details).

Conception

During sexual intercourse 2 to 5 ml of semen, usually containing more than 300 million sperm, is ejaculated into the female vagina. By flagellar movement, the sperm make their way through the fluids of the cervical mucus (if the mucus is receptive) (see Chapter 11 for further dicussion), across the endometrium, and into the fallopian tube to meet the descending ovum in the ampulla of the fallopian tube.

Before fertilization the sperm undergo a physiologic change called *capacitation* and a structural change called *acrosome reaction*. Capacitation refers to the removal of a protective coating from the sperm. Enzymes produced by the lining of the fallopian tubes assist in capacitation of the sperm. The acrosome reaction refers to the small perforations that form in the anterior head of the sperm. Enzymes (e.g., hyaluronidase) escape through these perforations and digest a path for the sperm through the corona radiata and zona pellucida of the ovum. Only one sperm is required for actual fertil-

Fig. 14.1
Sperm and ovum.

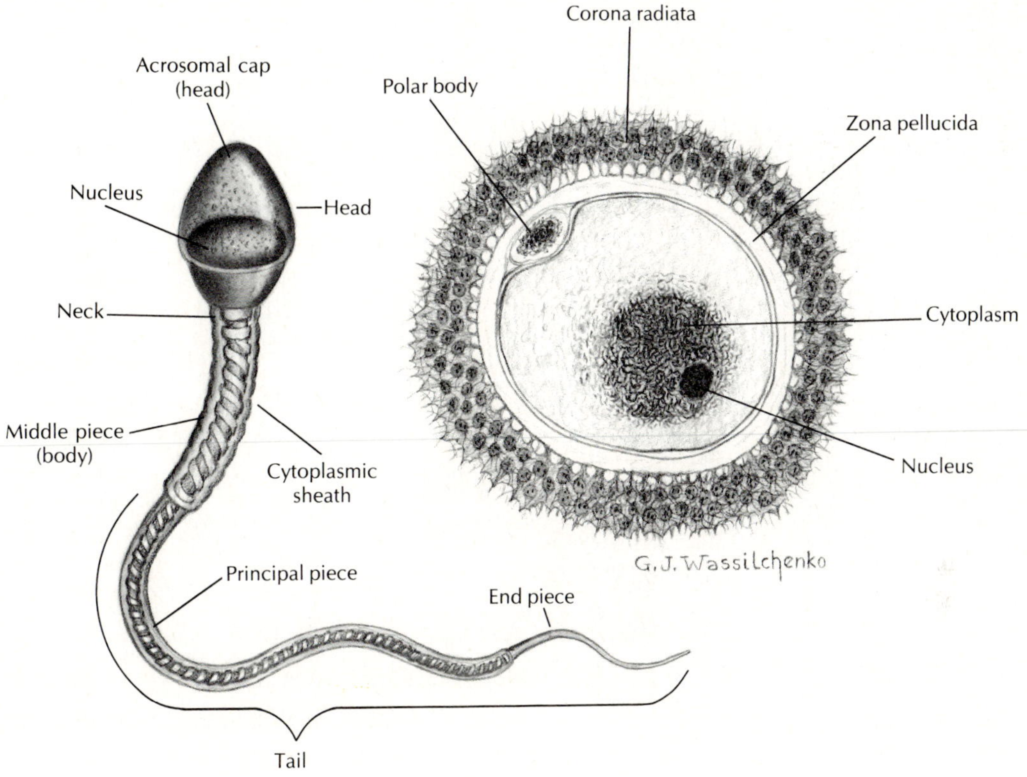

ization, but the presence of many increases the chances for one to penetrate.

Each normal sperm carries a haploid number of chromosomes, either 22 autosomes and an X chromosome or 22 autosomes and a Y chromosome.* Each normal ovum contains 22 autosomes and an X chromosome. When the sperm and the ovum meet and their nuclei fuse to form a *zygote* (fertilized ovum), the diploid number of chromosomes (44 autosomes and 2 sex chromosomes) is restored, the sex of the new human is determined, and the blueprints for the growth, development, and maturation of a new individual are laid down. An ovum fertilized by a sperm bearing a Y chromosome results in a male zygote, whereas an ovum fertilized by an X-bearing sperm results in a female zygote.

DEVELOPMENTAL STAGES

The fusion of the nuclei of the two gametes, called conception, fertilization, fecundation, or impregnation, initiates the first of the three stages of human prenatal development: ovum, embryo, and fetus.

Ovum. The organism is called an ovum during the period from conception until primary villi appear, approximately 12 to 14 days (4 weeks since the last menstrual period [LMP]). By the end of this period, implantation (nidation) is complete; that is, the conceptus is totally within the endometrium and is covered by the surface epithelium.

Embryo. The organism is called an *embryo* during the period from the end of the ovum stage until it measures approximately 3 cm from crown to rump, normally 54 to 56 days (10 weeks since LMP). This period is characterized by rapid cell division and is the most critical time in the development of an individual (Fig. 14.2). All the principal organ systems are being established and are highly vulnerable to environmental agents (e.g., teratogens such as viruses, drugs, radiation, or infection). Developmental interference during this time can result in major congenital (existing before birth) abnormalities. By the end of this period the beginnings of all the main systems have been established. The embryo attains characteristics that establish it as unquestionably human and is then referred to as a *fetus*, a Latin word meaning *offspring*.

*NOTE: It is the male who supplies the genetic material (an X or a Y sex chromosome) that determines the sex of the child.

Fig. 14.2
Sensitive, or critical, periods in human development. Solid red denotes highly sensitive periods; stippled red indicates stages that are less sensitive to teratogens. (From Moore, K.L.: The developing human: clinically oriented embryology, ed. 2, Philadelphia, 1977, W.B. Saunders Co.)

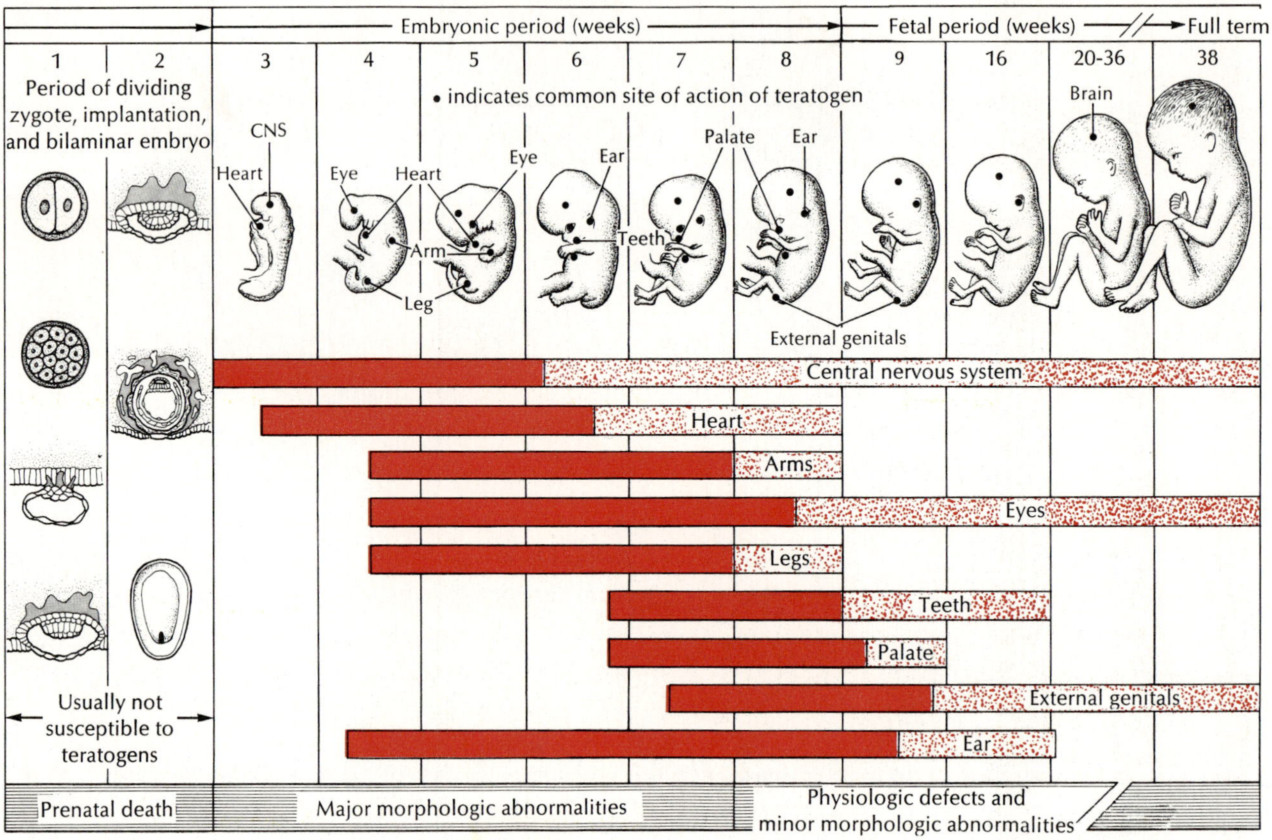

Fetus. The embryo is called a fetus during the period from the end of the embryo stage until the pregnancy is terminated. Changes occurring during the fetal period, although important, are not as dramatic as those in the preceding period. During this period the fetus is less vulnerable to the teratogenic effects of drugs, viruses, or radiation—*malformations*. However, these noxious agents may interrupt normal *functional development* of organs, especially the brain.

GESTATIONAL TIME UNITS

The chronology of pregnancy may be referred to in several ways, for example, 10 lunar months (of 4 weeks each), 40 weeks of gestation, or 9 calendar months (3 trimesters of 3 months each). (*In this chapter, age in weeks refers to the time since fertilization.* In clinical practice however, the term *gestational age* [or *menstrual age*] refers to the time since the first day of the LMP. see Table 14.1 for a comparison of these two time limits.) A summary of the development of the embryo and fetus during the 38 weeks of gestation is shown in Fig. 14.3.

Table 14.1
Comparison of Gestational Time Units

	Reference Point	
	Fertilization*	**Last Menstrual Period**
Days	266	280
Weeks	38	40
Calendar months	8¾	9
Lunar months	9½	10

From Moore, K.L.: Before we are born: basic embryology and birth defects, Philadelphia, 1974, W.B. Saunders Co.

*The date of birth is calculated as about 266 days after fertilization, or 280 days after the onset of the last normal menstrual period. From fertilization to the end of the embryonic period, age is best expressed in days; thereafter age is commonly given in weeks. Because ovulation and fertilization are usually separated by not more than 12 hours, these events are more or less interchangeable in expressing prenatal age.

Fig. 14.3

Timetable of human prenatal development (weeks 1 to 38). **A,** Maturation of a follicle containing a developing ovum (egg), ovulation, and menstrual cycle. *Development begins at fertilization,* about 14 days after onset of last menstruation in a 28-day cycle. Cleavage of zygote in uterine tube, implantation of blastocyst, and early development of embryo are also shown.

TIMETABLE OF HUMAN PRENATAL DEVELOPMENT
1 to 6 weeks

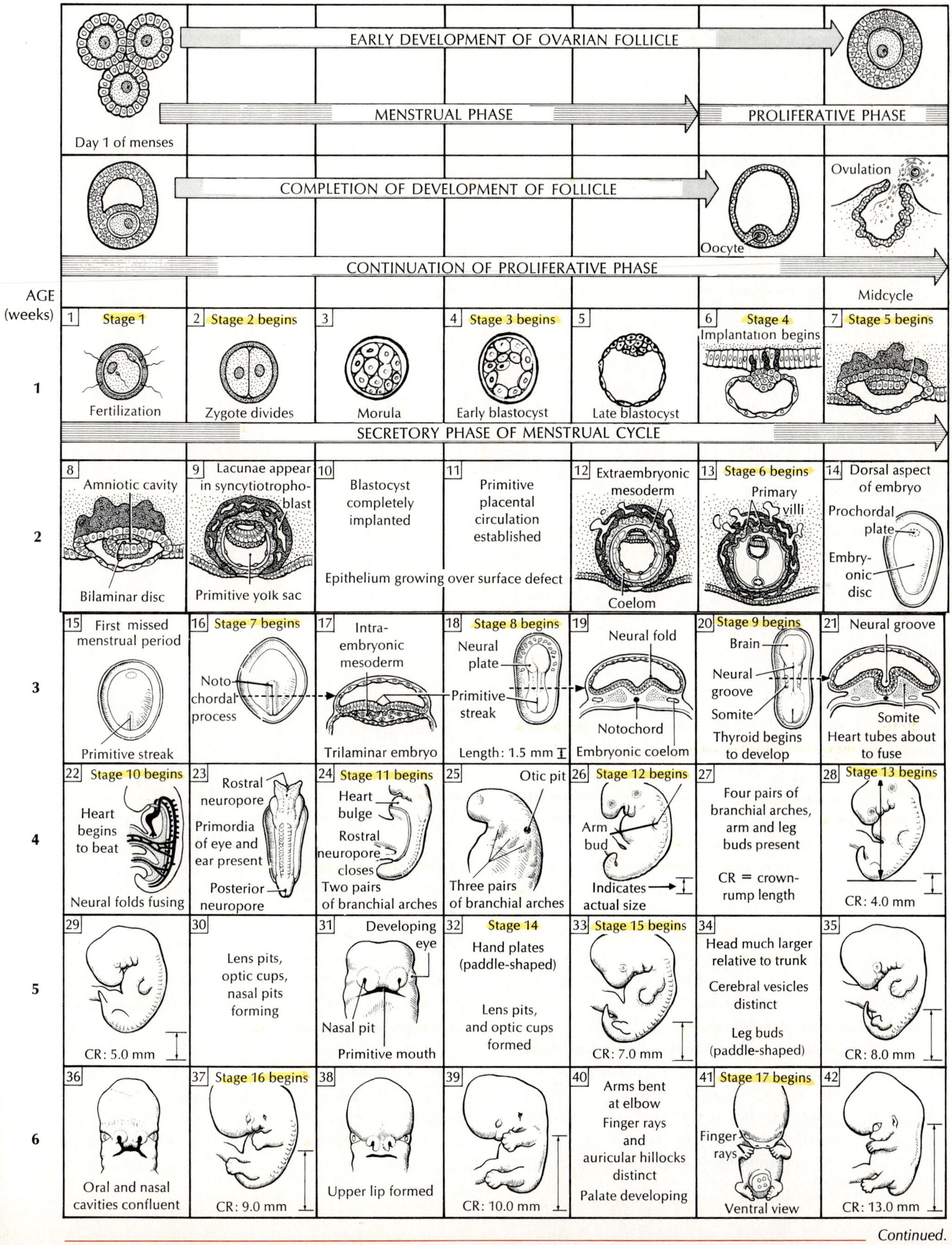

A

Continued.

Fig. 14.3, cont'd
For legend see p. 209.

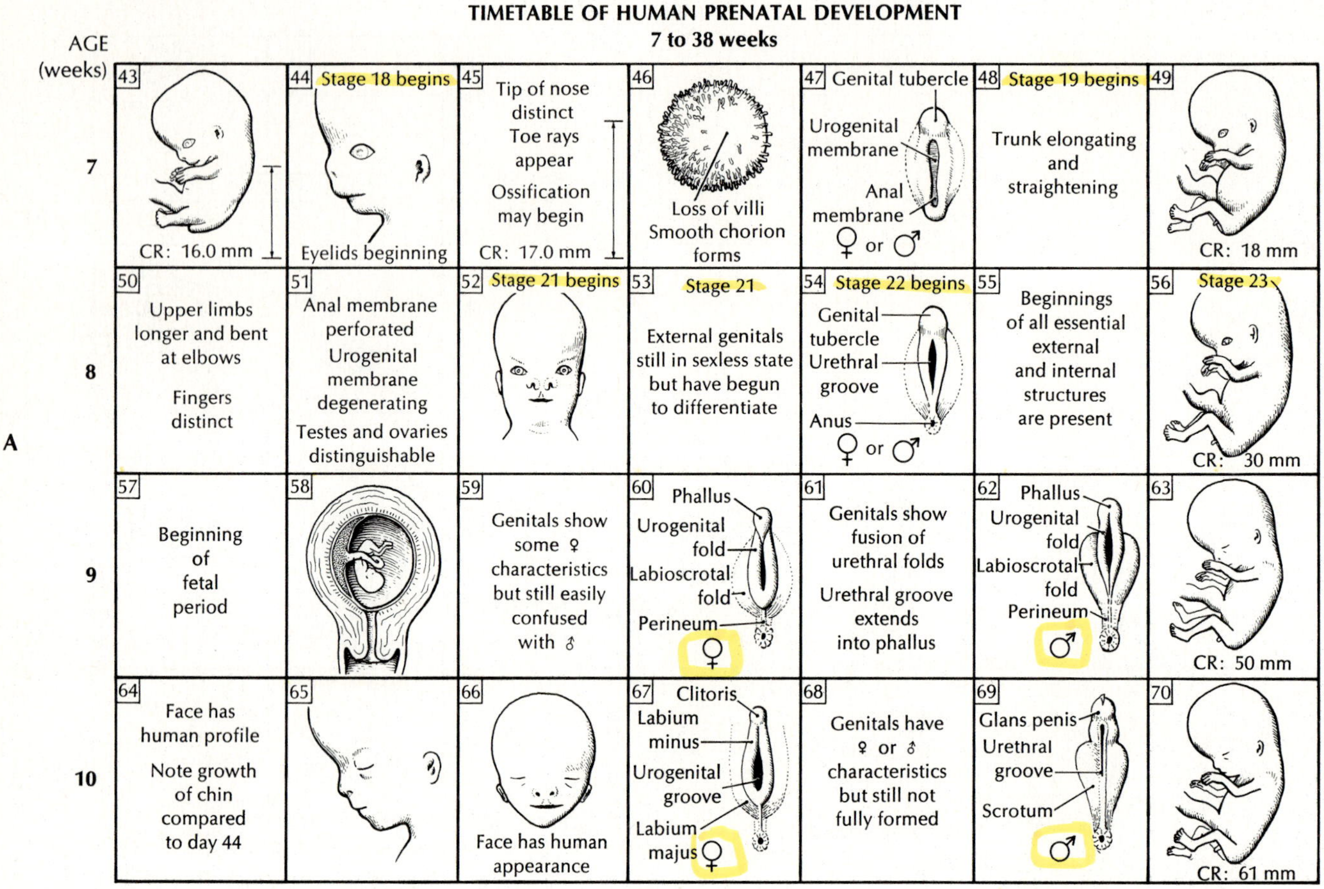

IMPLANTATION (NIDATION)

After conception, the zygote, propelled by ciliary action and irregular peristaltic contractions, starts to move through the fallopian tube into the uterine cavity. During the 3- to 4-day period it takes to travel down the fallopian tube, the zygote begins a process of rapid cell division called *mitosis*, or *cleavage*. The initial division of the zygote results in two *blastomeres*, which subsequently divide into progressively smaller blastomeres. At the end of 3 to 4 days, the developing individual comprises about 16 blastomeres arranged in a ball-like structure called a *morula*. After the morula enters the uterus, a cavity forms within the dividing cells, changing the morula into a *blastocyst*. The blastocyst remains free in the uterus for 1 or 2 days, and then the exposed cells of the *trophoblast* (cellular wall of the blastocyst) implant, generally in the endometrium of the anterior or posterior fundal region. About 7 to 10 days elapse between conception and the completion of implantation (days 21 to 24 after LMP).

Occasionally implantation will occur in the lower uterine segment, and varying degrees of placenta previa can result (see Chapter 35).

Cells of the attaching portion of the trophoblast secrete proteolytic (causing breakdown of proteins) and cytolytic (causing breakdown of cells) enzymes to help them burrow their way into the compact layer of the endometrium. This burrowing into the endometrium is called *nidation, or implantation,* and may cause slight bleeding, called *implantation bleeding,* which the woman may notice as small spots of blood on her panties. In almost all cases, trophoblastic burrowing stops before it reaches the myometrium. The blastocyst usually implants itself at a point high in the uterus on either the front or back wall and is fully embedded by the fourteenth day after ovulation (4 weeks or 28 days since LMP).

During the first few weeks after nidation, trophoblasts (primary villi) appear over the entire blastodermic vesicle. Trophoblasts are vascular processes that have the power of cytolysis and are able to tap maternal blood vessels as sources of nourishment and oxygen for

Fig. 14.3, cont'd

B, An embryo becomes a fetus at end of eighth week; by this time, beginnings of all essential structures are present. Fetal period, extending from ninth week until birth, is characterized by growth and elaboration of structures. Sex is clearly distinguishable at about 12 weeks. The 11- to 38-wk fetuses are about half their actual size. NOTE: This timetable is calculated from the time of fertilization. For *gestational* age, as the term is used clinically, see Table 14.1. (From Moore, K.L.: The developing human: clinically oriented embryology, ed. 2, Philadelphia, 1977, W.B. Saunders Co.)

B

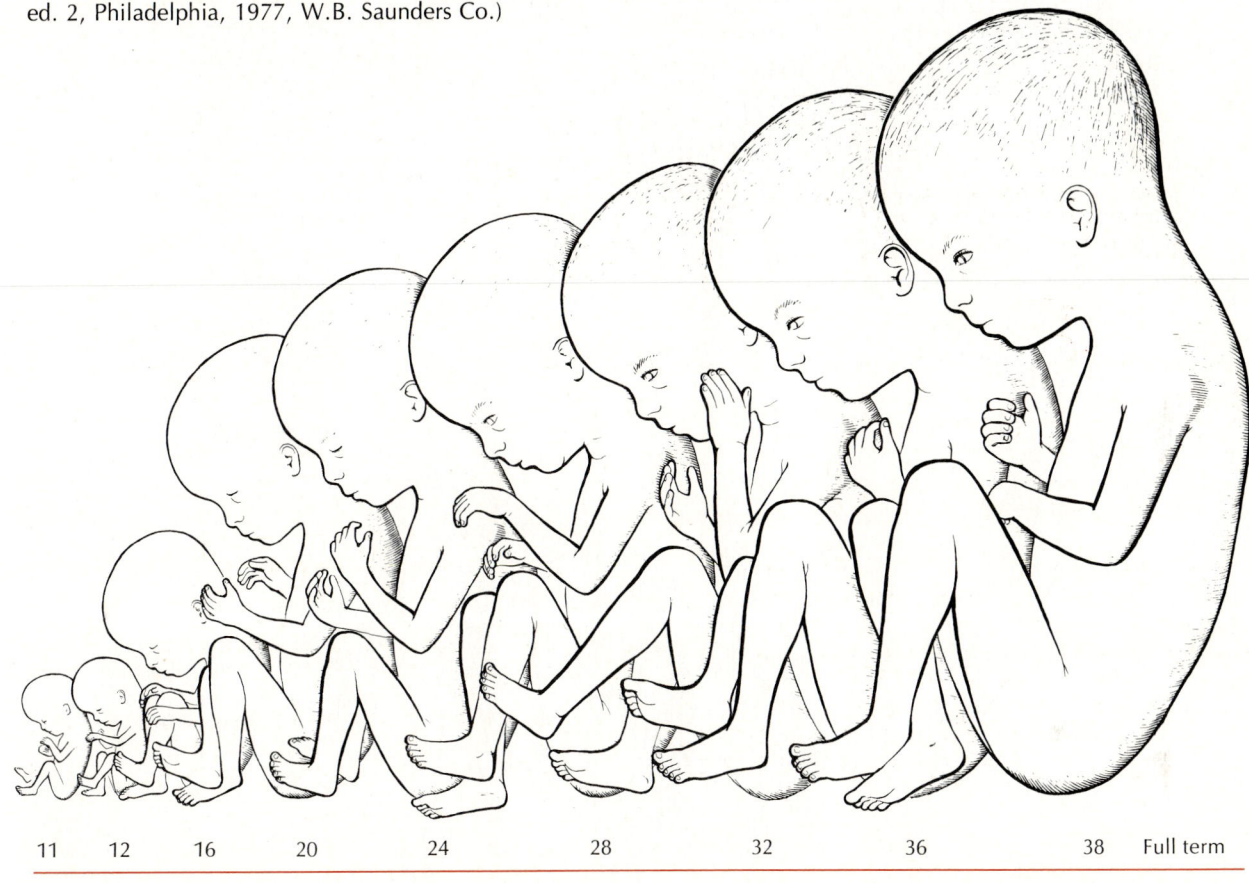

the embryo. These villi are the first stage of the developing *chorionic villi* (fingerlike projections) that secrete the chorionic gonadotropic hormone (HCG) and synthesize proteins and glucose for approximately 12 weeks; by then, the fetal liver can supply its own glucose (and insulin). HCG stimulates continued secretion of progesterone and estrogen by the corpus luteum, thus preventing ovulation and menstruation during pregnancy.

THE DECIDUA

As part of the morphologic changes in the endometrium during the secretory phase (phase of the corpus luteum) of the cycle, the blood vessels enlarge and the entire lining becomes more succulent and richer in glycogen. After conception the vascularity of the uterine wall increases greatly under the influence of the ovarian hormones, principally progesterone.

After implantation the endometrium is called the *decidua,* which means "to cast off," or "to discard," since this is actually what happens after the infant is born: the prepared lining of the endometrium *is* cast off in a vaginal discharge called lochia (see Chapter 31).

This decidua is divided into three areas (Fig. 14.4):

1. *Decidua vera (parietalis)* is the uterine lining exclusive of the area engrossed by the embryo, or that part of the endometrium not directly associated with the development of the embryo.
2. *Decidua basalis* is the portion of the decidua vera where nidation takes place; that is, the area where chorionic villi (frondosum) invade the maternal blood vessels and develop into the placenta.
3. *Decidua capsularis* is the portion of the decidua vera that covers the blastocyst after nidation occurs, isolating it from the other portions of the uterus. It appears to fuse with the chorion, a fetal membrane, as pregnancy advances.

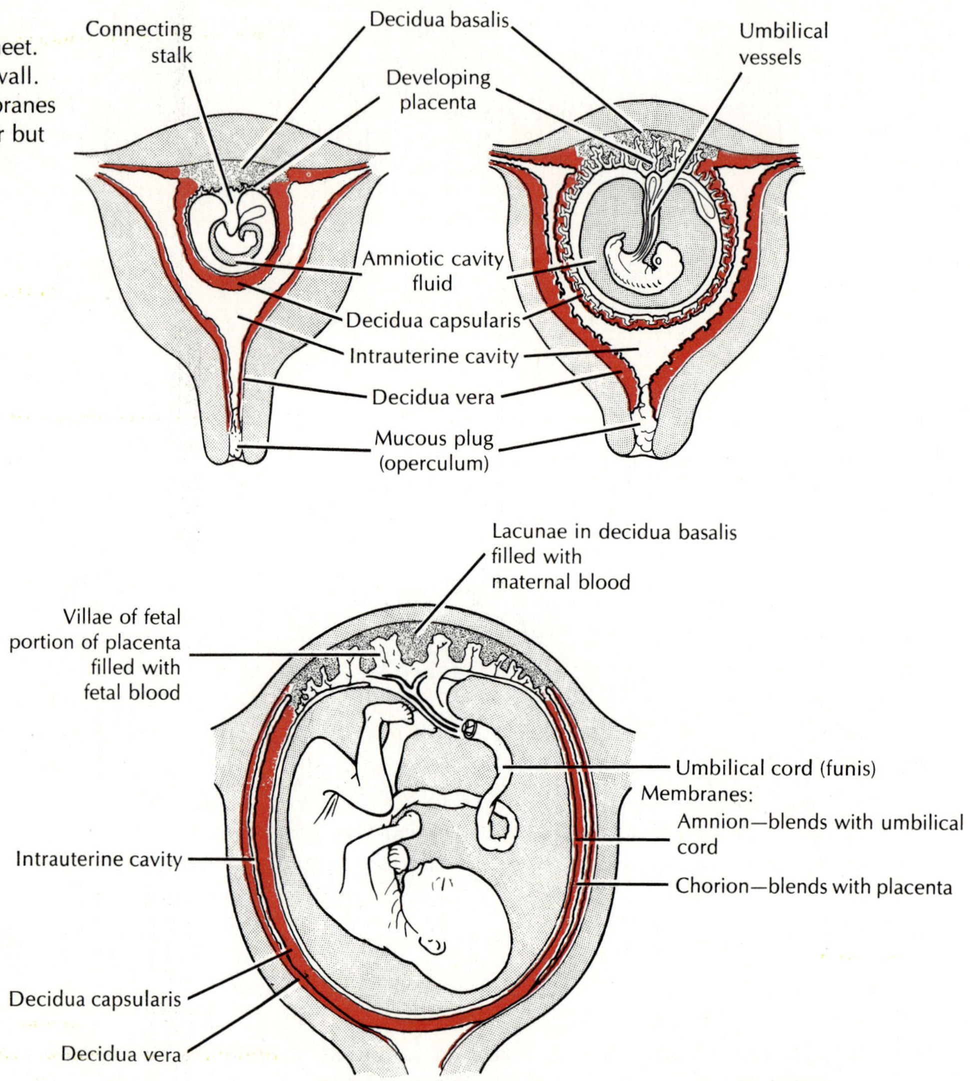

Fig. 14.4
Development of fetal membranes. Note gradual obliteration of intrauterine cavity as decidua capsularis and decidua vera meet. Also note thinning of uterine wall. Chorionic and amniotic membranes are in apposition to each other but may be peeled apart.

PLACENTATION

The chorionic villi invade the endometrium by enzyme action that occasionally opens a maternal vein and artery causing the formation of lacunae (small blood lakes) in the decidua basalis. This rich blood supply causes the adjacent villi to multiply rapidly. These villi become the *chorion frondosum,* or fetal portion, of the future placenta.

FETAL MEMBRANES

Two closely applied but separate membranes surround the developing embryo-fetus (Fig. 14.4). Both membranes, the *amnion* (inner membrane) and the *chorion* (outer membrane), arise from the zygote. As the chorion develops, it blends with the fetal portion of the placenta; the amnion blends with the fetal umbilical cord, or *funis*. These deceptively strong, translucent membranes contain not only the fetus but also the amniotic fluid, and they are continuous with the margins of the placenta.

UMBILICAL CORD

The umbilical cord (funis) is the lifeline that links the embryo and the placenta. It extends from the um-

Fig. 14.5
Cross section of umbilical cord. Note collapsed appearance of thin-walled umbilical vein and contour of thicker, muscular-walled arteries.

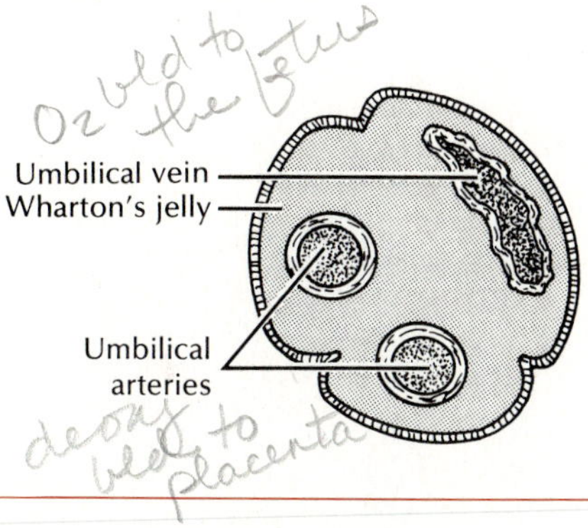

bilicus to the fetal portion of the placenta and is attached either centrally or eccentrically. At term this light gray, smooth, vascular attachment is 50 to 55 cm long, slightly longer than the fetus, and is approximately 2 cm in diameter.

The surface of the cord is composed of thin squamous epithelium and is an extension of the skin of the fetus; however, *it contains no pain receptors*. The cord normally contains two umbilical arteries and one umbilical vein (Fig. 14.5). The vein carries oxygenated blood to the fetus, and the arteries return deoxygenated blood to the placenta. Frequently these vessels are longer than the cord and consequently become coiled on themselves, giving the cord a lumpy appearance. They are supported by a loose connective tissue containing a cushioning mucoid material called *Wharton's jelly*. This jelly prevents kinking of the cord in utero and interference with circulation to the fetus.

Approximately 400 ml of blood flows through the cord every minute. The pressure exerted by this rapid flow makes the cord relatively stiff and not flexible as it is after birth. If fetal movements cause the cord to loop, its stiffness prevents the loops from kinking and from knotting tightly. The high water content of Wharton's jelly causes the cord to shrink quickly after birth. In addition, several naturally occurring prostaglandins in Wharton's jelly have a vasoconstrictive effect that inhibits bleeding from the umbilical cord stump when it is cut after birth.

It is always important for the physician or nurse to note the number of vessels in the cord, because in at least 1% of neonates a two-vesseled cord (one umbilical vein and one umbilical artery) will be noted. Various anomalies (defects or malformations) are present in at least 10% of these neonates and are more common in multiple births (i.e., twins, triplets).

PLACENTA

The maturing placenta (Greek: flat cake) develops into 15 or 20 subdivisions called *cotyledons*. Each of these is partially separated from other cotyledons by fenestrated septa (windowed partitions); thus in essence each cotyledon is a functioning unit.

Growth of the thickness of the placenta continues until 16 to 20 weeks' gestation. However, the placental circumference continues growing until later pregnancy. The fully developed placenta (afterbirth) is a reddish, discoid organ 15 to 20 cm (6 to 10 in) in diameter and 2.5 to 3 cm (about 1 in) thick (Fig. 14.6). The weight of a term placenta is 400 to 600 g (1 lb to 1 lb, 5 oz) or approximately one sixth the weight of the newborn. About four fifths of the placenta by weight is of fetal origin; the remainder is maternal.

The maternal surface of the placenta, the area originally adherent to the decidua basalis of the uterus, is rough and beefy red. The cotyledons stand out as segments with shallow clefts between. The fetal surface of the placenta is shiny and slightly grayish. The umbilical vessels that enter the cord can be seen as a branching system just beneath the membranes (Fig. 14.6). The fetal membranes cover the fetal surface of the placenta and extend from the placental margins to envelop the fetus and its amniotic fluid.

In multiple pregnancy, one or more placentas will be present. The number depends on the number of fertilized ova and the manner of ovum segmentation (see discussion of twinning, Chapter 37).

Placental physiology. The placenta functions as a transport mechanism between embryo and mother. Maternal nutrients pass through the placenta to the embryo, and waste materials move from the embryo to the mother by way of the placenta.

In addition to its anabolic (metabolism that builds up substances) and catabolic (metabolism that breaks down substances) functions, the placenta serves as an effective lung, kidney, stomach, and intestine, as well as an endocrine gland, for the fetus. It also serves as a protective barrier against the harmful effects of certain drugs and microorganisms.

The placenta's life span is measured by its oxygen consumption, which reflects intense metabolic activity until term is approached, whereupon function progressively decreases until delivery.

Placental function depends almost entirely on maternal circulation. Maternal circulation depends on the woman's blood pressure, condition of her blood vessels, maternal position, and uterine contractions. *Optimal circulation to the placenta and fetus is possible when the woman is lying on her left side* (see p. 236). When she is supine, the third-trimester uterus compresses the vena cava and the venous return from the

Fig. 14.6

Photographs of full-term placentas, *about one-third actual size.* **A,** Maternal (or uterine) surface, showing cotyledons and grooves. **B,** Fetal (or amniotic) surface, showing blood vessels running under amnion and converging to form umbilical vessels at attachment of umbilical cord. **C,** Amnion and smooth chorion are arranged to show that they are (1) fused and (2) continuous with margins of placenta. **D,** Placenta with a marginal attachment of the cord, often called a battledore placenta because of its resemblance to bat used in medieval game of battledore and shuttlecock. (From Moore, K.L.: The developing human: clinically oriented embryology, ed. 2, Philadelphia, 1977, W.B. Saunders Co.)

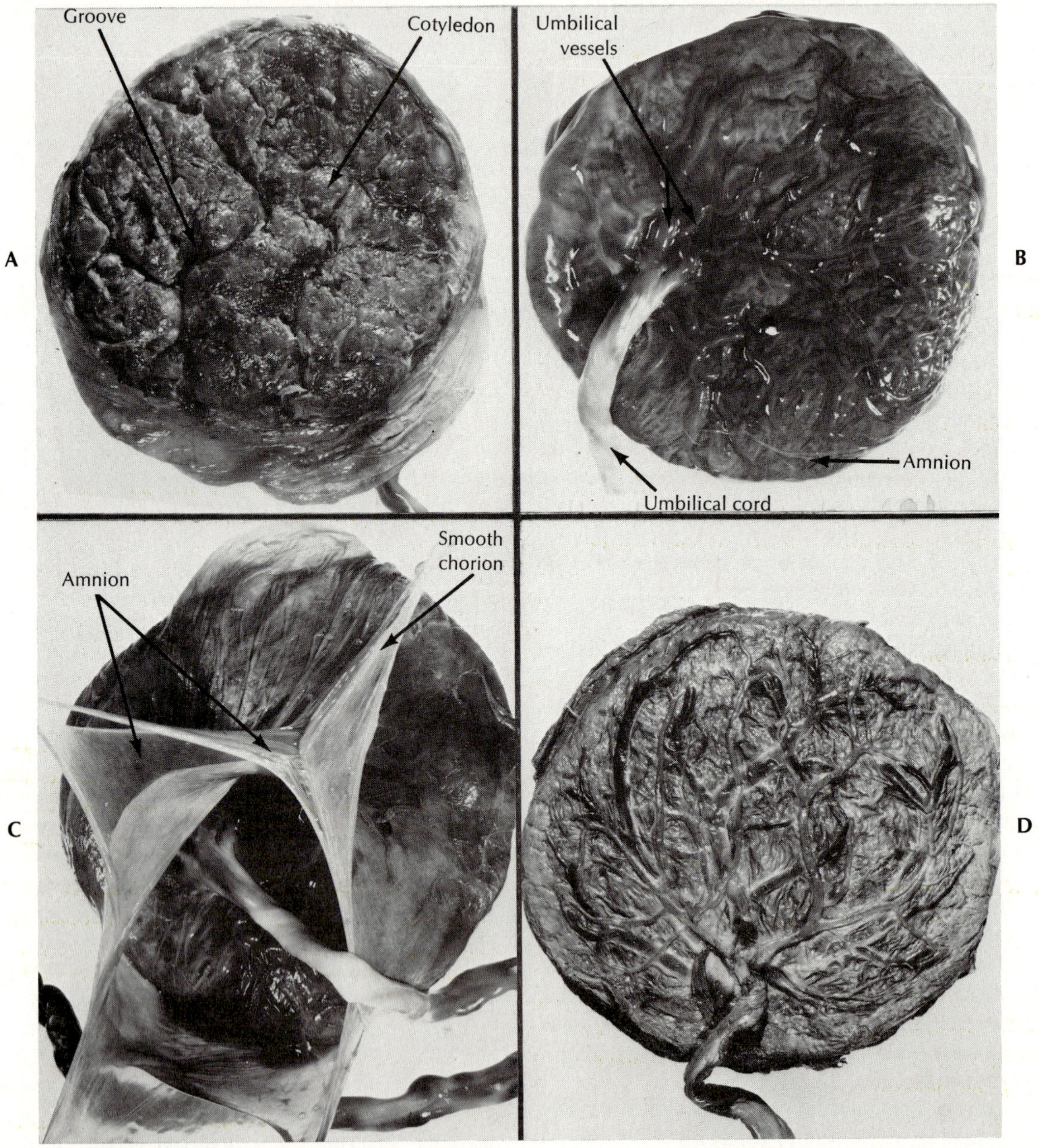

uterus and lower extremities is significantly impeded, producing vena cava syndrome (see Fig. 21.11). The aorta and internal iliac arteries may be compressed as well when the uterus becomes very heavy.

Contrary to popular assumption, before labor the placental lakes *fill during uterine contractions* (Braxton Hicks), not during relaxation. This is accomplished by closure of the maternal venous apertures beneath the placenta. In contrast, the heavier arteries to the placental site remain open during uterine contractions; hence blood flows in. With uterine relaxation, blood drains out of the placental sinusoids into the maternal circulation.

This process by which blood fills and drains the placental lakes suggests a sluggish circulation. However, the placental capacity is large, and a considerable volume of maternal blood (approximately 500 ml/min) at term clears the placenta. In contrast, only about 400 ml/min of fetal blood passes through the placenta, which is obviously advantageous to the fetus.

The placenta is an endocrine organ that produces all of the hormones or their precursors except for ACTH. These hormones are discussed in several sections of the book (see index) and in Chapter 15.

Placental transfer. Only two layers of cells separate maternal and fetal circulation for the first 12 weeks of gestation. During the second and third trimesters, only one cell layer separates the two bloodstreams. This so-called *placental barrier* is a partial (semipermeable) barrier; it can afford only very limited protection to the fetus.

Passage of materials to and from the fetus is effected by four principal mechanisms:

1. *Diffusion,* such as across a membrane, allows passage of oxygen, carbon dioxide, anesthetic gases, water, electrolytes, and other substances of low molecular weight.
2. *Active,* or *facilitated, transfer,* often by enzyme action, results in the passage of glucose, amino acids, calcium, iron, and other substances of higher molecular weight.
3. *Pinocytosis* is a mechanism by which minute particles, including fats, may be engulfed and carried across the cell.
4. *Leakage* as a result of small defects in the trophoblastic surface *allows slight mixing of maternal and fetal blood cells and plasma.*

Nutrients. The transfer of vitamins to the fetus is only partially understood, but vitamins A, B complex, C, E, and K are transmitted to the fetus. It is not known whether vitamin D is produced by the fetus or supplied by the mother (see discussion of maternal nutrition, Chapter 18).

Microorganisms. Because of their small size, some viruses traverse the placenta with ease; the larger bacteria rarely involve the fetus except when inflammation of the placenta develops. Placentitis is generally the result of an intranatal infection from an ascending invasion of bacteria from vagina and cervix associated with ruptured membranes and prolonged labor but may occur even if membranes are intact. Maternal and fetal and neonatal infections are discussed in Chapter 36.

Drugs. Many drugs cross the placenta readily (e.g., caffeine, alcohol, nicotine, carbon monoxide, and the over 1000 other toxic substances and gases* inhaled from cigarette smoke, antibiotics, antihistamines, sedatives, analgesics, narcotics, anesthetics, etc.). Most drugs promptly cross the placenta, and many are deleterious to the human fetus. Harmful drugs may be grouped into categories as follows:

1. Established teratogenic drugs
2. Possible teratogenic drugs
3. Fetotoxic drugs

Examples of these drugs, to which may be added vaccines and excessive amounts of certain vitamins, are given in Appendix H. Because medications may contain elements harmful to the fetus, all but essential medications should be avoided, particularly during the first trimester of pregnancy.

Oxygen. For a discussion of oxygen transfer, see the discussion of fetal hemoglobin, p. 217.

Placental variations. Rarely, the placenta may be divided into two or more separate lobes. Each lobe has a distinct circulation; the vessels collect at the periphery, and the main trunks unite eventually to form the vessels of the cord. Blood vessels joining the lobes may be supported only by the fetal membranes and are therefore in danger of tearing during labor or during the birth of the baby or of the placenta. During delivery of the placenta, one or more of the separate lobes may remain attached to the decidua basalis, preventing the uterus from contracting. Bleeding and infection are possible consequences. Therefore the margins of the placenta are always examined for torn vessels, and if the latter are found, the retained lobes are manually removed.

AMNIOTIC FLUID

The full-term fetus is immersed in about 1000 ml (range of 800 to 1200 ml) of clear, slightly yellowish liquid that has a faint characteristic (not foul) odor. The specific gravity of amniotic fluid is 1.007 to 1.025, and the pH is neutral to slightly alkaline (7.0 to 7.25). It contains albumin, urea, uric acid, creatinine, lecithin, sphingomyelin, bilirubin, fat, fructose, inorganic salts, epithelial cells, a few leukocytes, various enzymes, and lanugo hairs. Amniotic fluid, replaced every 3 hours, is thought to have multiple origins and a composition that changes during pregnancy. Early in pregnancy it probably originates from maternal serum, but as pregnancy proceeds a greater proportion of it is derived from fetal urine. It accomplishes numerous functions for the fetus, including the following:

1. Protects from direct trauma by distributing and equalizing any impact the mother may receive

*Hydrogen cyanide is also present in cigarette smoke. This is the same gas used to execute prisoners in gas chambers.

2. Separates the fetus from the fetal membranes
3. Allows freedom of fetal movement and permits musculoskeletal development
4. Facilitates symmetric growth and development of the fetus
5. Protects from loss of heat and maintains a relatively constant fetal body temperature
6. Is a source of oral fluid for the fetus
7. Acts as an excretion-collection system

There is still much to be learned about amniotic fluid. However, study of its components has provided a great deal of knowledge concerning the sex, state of health, and maturity of the fetus. Amniocentesis (see p. 152) has made it possible to detect diseases and abnormalities that may suggest the options of therapeutic abortion or intrauterine treatment.

During pregnancy the amniotic fluid volume increases at an average rate of 25 ml/wk from 1 to 15 weeks' gestation, and 50 ml/wk from 15 to 28 weeks' gestation. There is great variation within the normal volume; however, more than 2 L (hydramnios) or less than 300 ml (oligohydramnios) is usually associated with fetal disease or abnormality (see Chapter 40).

Embryonic Development and Fetal Maturation

Fetal maturation takes place in an orderly and predictable pattern (Fig. 14.3 and Table 15.5). There is a steady increase in overall growth, and organ systems develop from the three primary germ layers: the ectoderm (ecto = outside), the entoderm (ento = inner), and the mesoderm (meso = middle). The *ectodermal* germ layer gives rise to such tissues as the skin and nails, the nervous system, and tooth enamel. The *entodermal* germ layer develops into such tissues as epithelial inner linings of the gastrointestinal and respiratory tracts, endocrine glands, and auditory canal. The *mesodermal* germ layer forms tissues such as the connective tissue, teeth (except for the enamel), muscles, and blood and vascular systems.

CARDIOVASCULAR SYSTEM

The first system to function in the developing human is the cardiovascular system (Fig. 27.2). Blood vessel formation begins early in the third week; it follows the first missed menstrual period of the mother. The cardiovascular system must form early to bring nourishment and oxygen from the mother to the embryo. The cardiovascular system is functional (heart is beating) before the mother's menstrual period is 1 week late. At this time (3 weeks since conception), circulation of blood begins the fetomaternal exchange of oxygen, nutrients, and waste products. This exchange is necessary because the fetal lungs and digestive system are not functional until after birth.

The single umbilical vein carries oxygen-enriched blood from the placenta. Upon entering the liver, the vein gives off a number of branches and then enters the ductus venosus. About half the oxygenated blood bypasses the liver through the ductus venosus into the inferior vena cava. There it mixes with deoxygenated blood from the fetal lower extremities, abdomen, and pelvis. Most of this blood then enters the right atrium and is pumped through the foramen ovale into the left atrium, where it mixes with a small amount of deoxygenated blood returning from the lungs through the pulmonary veins. The blood then flows into the left ventricle and exits through the ascending aorta. *As a result, the vessels leading to the heart, head, neck, and upper limbs receive well-oxygenated blood.* This circulatory pattern is the reason for the embryo's cephalocaudal (head-to-tail) development, which persists in subsequent motor development, making it possible for the infant to manipulate his hands long before being able to walk.

A small quantity of oxygenated blood from the inferior vena cava remains in the right atrium and mixes with deoxygenated blood from the superior vena cava and coronary sinus. It then flows into the right ventricle and pulmonary artery, passing through the ductus arteriosus into the aorta; a small amount is diverted to the nonfunctional lungs.

The paired umbilical arteries return most of the mixed blood from the descending aorta to the placenta. There the fetal blood simultaneously gives up carbon dioxide and waste materials and takes up oxygen and nutrients from the maternal blood. The remaining blood circulates through the lower part of the fetal body and ultimately enters the inferior vena cava.

The pattern of blood flow* is as follows:

1. Placenta
   ↓
   Umbilical vein ↗ Liver, sinusoids, hepatic veins ↘ Inferior vena cava
   Umbilical vein ↘ Ductus venosus ↗ Inferior vena cava
2. Inferior vena cava→Right atrium→*Foramen ovale*→Left atrium→Left ventricle→Aorta
3. Inferior vena cava→Right atrium→Right ventricle→Pulmonary artery→Small amount to nonfunctional lungs but most of it through the *ductus arteriosus*→Aorta→Hypogastric arteries→*Umbilical arteries*→Placenta

Following are a number of compensatory circulatory

*The four structures that differentiate fetal circulation from extrauterine circulation are shown in italic type. The foramen ovale and ductus arteriosus allow fetal blood to bypass the fetal lungs.

factors that benefit the fetus (these values are those of the fetus near term):

1. The fetal heart rate (FHR) is 120 to 160 beats/min, and the fetal cardiac output is approximately 350 to 400 ml/kg/min, or about that of the adult at rest.
2. The hemoglobin of the fetus is primarily fetal hemoglobin (HgF), a type synthesized before birth. HgF is capable of maintaining a high oxygen saturation at a lower pressure (Po_2). It has been estimated that HgF can carry as much as 20% to 30% more oxygen than can maternal hemoglobin.
3. The hemoglobin concentration of the fetus is about 50% higher than that of the mother.

As a result of these compensatory circulatory factors, greater amounts of oxygen can be transported to the fetal tissues.

HEMATOPOIETIC SYSTEM

Hematopoiesis (formation and development of blood cells) begins in the liver about the sixth week of gestation, when vascular channels have been formed. Later, blood formation occurs in the spleen, bone marrow, and lymph nodes.

Platelets are present in the circulation by the eleventh week of gestation. The isoagglutinogens (e.g., the Rh factor) that determine blood grouping are present in the red blood cells soon after the sixth week. Because of the early appearance of red blood cells, the Rh-negative woman needs to be protected against isoimmunization after each pregnancy that lasts longer than 6 weeks as well as after the birth of each child who is Rh positive (for extensive discussion, see Chapter 40).

RESPIRATORY SYSTEM

As previously mentioned the fetal lungs do not function until after delivery. Simple diffusion (passing from higher to lower concentration across a semipermeable membrane) across the placenta explains the exchange of oxygen and carbon dioxide in the fetus.

Development of human lungs occurs in four overlapping phases:

1. *Pseudoglandular period* (5 to 17 weeks' gestation): formation of bronchi and terminal bronchi
2. *Canalicular period* (13 to 25 weeks' gestation): enlargement of lumens of bronchi and terminal bronchioles, development of respiratory bronchioles and alveolar ducts, increased vascularity of lung tissue
3. *Terminal sac period* (24 weeks' gestation to birth): growth of primitive alveoli (terminal air sacs) from alveolar ducts; fetuses younger than 24 weeks are not likely to survive if born before the terminal sac period begins
4. *Alveolar period* (late fetal period to approximately 8 years of age): formation of characteristic pulmonary alveoli as the lining of the terminal air sacs thins, with the number of alveoli increasing six to eight times between birth and age 8 years

During the terminal sac period, *pulmonary surfactants** (phospholipid substances) are produced in increasing amounts by the alveolar cells. These substances cover the internal surface of the alveoli before birth. Pulmonary surfactant comes up from the lung fluid and mixes with amniotic fluid in the upper respiratory tract. Pulmonary surfactants reduce the alveolar surface tension during extrauterine respiration, facilitating expansion of the lungs at birth and preventing collapse at end-expiration. If insufficient surfactants are present, the lungs cannot be properly inflated, and respiratory distress syndrome (RDS)† may develop.

Lecithin, a major component of surfactant, builds up in the amniotic fluid from about the twenty-fourth week, and sphingomyelin, another pulmonary phospholipid, remains unchanged. Hence, by determining the amount of lecithin present, or the *lecithin-sphingomyelin (L/S) ratio,* an appraisal of fetal lung maturity is possible. RDS is unlikely when the L/S ratio is greater than 2:1.‡

Periodic fetal hiccough can be seen and palpated, and rhythmic fetal respiratory movements can be demonstrated by ultrasonography in advanced pregnancy. Fetal cellular wastes (squamae) and lanugo fragments are commonly found in the fetal respiratory passages. Hence respirations at birth appear to be an extension of intrauterine respiratory activity.

A reduction in the rate and depth of maternal respiration may be reflected in fetal oxygenation. Excessive amounts of barbiturate, narcotic analgesia, or maternal hypoxia during anesthesia may reduce the fetal Po_2. Moreover, heavy maternal sedation by those drugs that readily cross the placenta may depress the fetal CNS respiratory center to further jeopardize the baby at birth. Breathing of pure oxygen (10 to 12 L/min) by the mother before delivery and again before cessation of pulsation in the cord after delivery may aid the infant.

RENAL SYSTEM

The placenta is the major fetal excretory organ and effectively eliminates waste products from fetal blood. The placenta, in collaboration with maternal lungs and kidneys, maintains fetal water, electrolyte, and acid-

---

*Testing for pulmonary surfactants is one of the tests for fetal lung maturity.

†Also known as hyaline membrane disease (HMD).

‡This may not hold true if the mother is diabetic.

base balance. Kidneys are *not* necessary for fetal growth and development. In fact, an infant may be born without kidneys. However, renal excretory and regulatory functions must begin immediately after delivery to maintain life and health.

In preparation for extrauterine existence, the fetal kidneys develop rapidly. The kidneys appear in the fifth week and begin to function during the eighth week. Urine is excreted into and mixes with the amniotic fluid that the fetus swallows.

NEUROLOGIC SYSTEM

The *neural plate* (a thickened area of embryonic ectoderm), from which the infant's nervous system develops, appears during the third week of gestation. The *neural tube** and *neural crest* evolve from this structure, the first differentiating into the CNS (the brain and cord) and the second into the peripheral nervous system.

The brain, which is formed at the cranial end of the neural tube, consists of the forebrain, midbrain, and hindbrain. The cerebrum develops from the forebrain; the adult midbrain develops; and the pons, cerebellum, and medulla oblongata evolve from the hindbrain. The longest part of the neural tube ultimately becomes the spinal cord.

The human brain is only partially developed and functional at birth. It grows in three stages: first, prenatally by hyperplasia (an increase in cell number); second, during the first 6 months of life by a combination of hyperplasia and hypertrophy (an increase in size of existing cells); and third, thereafter until puberty by hypertrophy. An adequate supply of protein and calories is required for this process, particularly during the first and second stages. Prenatal maternal anemia and malnutrition compromise fetal brain development: if the fetus does not receive adequate nutrition early in development, there is a smaller number of cells developed; if the fetus continues to receive inadequate nutrition, the existing cells are smaller in size.

The brain needs adequate nutrition after birth because it doubles its weight during the first year and triples its weight by the sixth year. The growth rate then slows, and the adult level is reached about the time of puberty.

The late fetal and early neonatal phases of maturation are especially critical to later achievement. Disease, trauma, or unfavorable environmental factors may irreparably alter the development of the CNS.

Hypoxia attributable to maternal causes (e.g., premature separation of the placenta), fetal causes (e.g., cord entanglement), or iatrogenic causes (e.g., maternal hypotension after being given spinal anesthesia) may be critical to the infant. Many of the survivors of severe asphyxia develop cerebral palsy, mental retardation, or other neurologic deficits. Newborns of 36 weeks' gestational age or younger are less sensitive to hypoxia but are more sensitive to birth trauma than mature newborns. Fortunately, however, the infant has remarkable powers of recuperation, and many depressed babies appear to recover satisfactorily. See Chapter 27 for more information on newborn neurologic function.

Fetal neuromuscular behavior. Fundamental to the successive development of behavior patterns is the development of neuromuscular structure and functioning.

Behavior advances through five stages: (1) myogenic (originating in the muscle) response, (2) neuromotor (muscle movement stimulated by nerves) response, (3) reflex response, (4) integration of simple reflexes, and (5) integration and control from higher centers. Fetal development of the nervous system parallels fetal behavior.

By approximately 8½ weeks of age, the fetus responds to tactile stimulation; the fetus will flex the trunk and extend the head because by this time the necessary neural components of the reflex arc are present.

By 14 weeks the fetus shows specific rather than generalized reflex responses; for example, in response to pain stimuli he will move his limb away from the source of pain (avoidance). By the twentieth week the sucking reflex is present and respiratory movements are recognizable. From 28 weeks to term the fetus shows steady progression in patterns of behavior, as evidenced by the premature or full-term neonate (see Chapters 27, 28, and 37).

GASTROINTESTINAL SYSTEM

The digestive system forms during the fourth week. The middle portion of the intestine projects out into the umbilical cord during the fifth week of development because there is not enough room in the abdomen (the liver and kidneys are taking up considerable space at this time). The intestines return to the abdomen during the tenth week. Failure of the intestines to return to the abdomen results in a condition known as omphalocele.

Intrauterine nutrition and elimination occur through the placenta, making it unnecessary for the slowly developing gastrointestinal system to function before birth. During the second trimester the fetus begins to swallow and subsequently to excrete amniotic fluid by way of the kidneys; however, this system is still physiologically immature at birth.

Metabolism. While in utero the fetus exists in a non-

*The nurse may need to explain to parents about neural tube defects, one of several malformations that can be identified in utero through amniocentesis (see test for alpha-fetoprotein, p. 288).

demanding physical environment. Constant ambient temperature, minimal physical activity, depressed muscle tone, and effective insulation against heat loss all contribute to a relatively low metabolic rate. The fetus maintains a temperature about 0.4° C (32° F) above maternal temperature. Oxygen consumption is about one third that of the neonate. Most of the caloric intake, which consists primarily of glucose from the mother, is used to accomplish growth and development.

The fetus receives its glucose, its main source of energy, from the mother. Maternal insulin does not pass to the fetus; the fetus secretes insulin. The fetus synthesizes glycogen and anabolizes (forms) his own fat rather than receiving these nutrients in these forms from the mother.

Meconium. As term approaches, increasing amounts of meconium (the end product of fetal metabolism) are found in the fetal intestinal tract. Normal meconium is a sterile, dark, greenish brown, semisolid residue of bile and embryonic secretions, plus cellular waste (squamous epithelial cells) and hair swallowed in utero. The presence of meconium in amniotic fluid before delivery usually indicates fetal hypoxia (see Chapter 21).

HEPATIC SYSTEM

Liver function begins at about the fourth week of gestation. Hematopoiesis starts at about the sixth week of intrauterine life; this activity is primarily responsible for the rapid growth and relatively large size of the liver during the second month.

The fetal liver at term is proportionately much larger than the liver of the 1-year-old infant. It is a metabolic and glycogen storage organ that also secretes bile and acts as a depot for iron. Full liver function is not achieved until well after delivery, however. For example, coagulation factors contributed to or produced by the liver and fibrinogen are low at the time of delivery but adjust in early infancy.

The production of fetal liver enzymes is limited, especially in the fetus of less than 36 weeks' gestational age. Therefore the conjugation and excretion of bilirubin are impaired in the premature infant (see Chapter 37). Poor metabolism of drugs by the immature fetal liver also may pose problems for the infant. The congenital absence of certain liver enzymes causes *inborn errors of metabolism* (e.g., phenylketonuria and Tay-Sachs disease).

ENDOCRINE SYSTEM

The fetal *adrenal cortex,* or outer part of the gland, produces cortisol. Increasing amounts of cortisol may be important in the initiation of labor.

The *thyroid* gland is the first endocrine gland to develop in the fetus. By the fourth week the thyroid can synthesize thyroxine. When the mother's thyroid function is depressed, the fetal thyroid will support the inadequate maternal thyroid function. However, this increased fetal thyroid function increases the gland's size. If the fetal thyroid is excessive in size it could compromise fetal respirations at birth by compressing the trachea. Because maternal thyroxine stimulates fetal growth and development, however, antithyroid drugs crossing the placenta may adversely affect the fetus.

By the twelfth week insulin may be extracted from the beta cells of the fetal *pancreas*. The fetus must supply whatever is needed for its metabolism of glucose. Insulin is the primary hormone regulating the rate of fetal growth. If the mother is diabetic, the response of the beta cells of the fetal pancreas to repeated stimuli of hyperglycemia (caused by high levels of maternal glucose) will be hyperplasia (increased amount of tissue) of all body structures except the brain. This is thought to account for the large size of the infants of diabetic mothers and the hyperinsulinism found in these neonates immediately after birth.

REPRODUCTIVE SYSTEM

Until the end of the ninth week, male and female external genitalia appear somewhat similar (see Fig. 6.1). It is not until the twelfth week that external genitalia are well enough developed so as to be easily distinguishable.

Female genital development and function. The fetal ovary (see Fig. 6.16) has many primordial (primitive) follicles and produces small but increasing amounts of estrogen. It is the high level of maternal estrogen that stimulates the fetal endometrium; the rapid drop in maternal estrogens in fetal circulation following birth is followed by withdrawal bleeding. Withdrawal bleeding accounts for the brief mucoid vaginal discharge and even slight bloody spotting that may be noted in female neonates.

During childhood a small but continuing secretion of estrogen occurs. Before puberty a much greater production of estrogen accounts for the development of female secondary sex characteristics (see Table 6.8).

Male genital development and function. Early in embryonic development, the gonads of the genetically male fetus (fetus with a Y chromosome) play a critical role in the formation of the genital tract. As the gonads evolve in the testicular pattern, presumably under the influence of maternal HCG, LH, and fetal adrenal hormones, the testes produce androgenic hormones that result in growth and differentiation of male genitalia.

After delivery a slow increase in the production of

androgen and traces of estrogen continue until just before puberty, when much larger amounts of testosterone, in particular, are secreted. This increase causes development of the male secondary sex characteristics (see Table 6.10).

IMMUNE SYSTEM

See Chapter 27 for a discussion of the immune system.

Viability

The capability of a fetus to survive outside the uterus at the earliest gestational age is termed viability. Until recently it was believed that viability was reached when the fetus weighed more than 1000 g and had reached at least 28 weeks' gestational age. Improvement in maternal and neonatal care now suggests that a new standard of viability must be established. On the basis of current published literature, the criteria for viability are now believed to be a weight of at least 601 g and a gestational age of at least 24 weeks. There is a problem with a lack of accuracy in estimating gestational age so that it is difficult to establish definite criteria.

Survival outside the uterus is dependent on (1) the maturity of the fetal CNS to direct rhythmic respirations and to control body temperature and (2) the maturity of the lungs.

References and Readings

Athey, P.A., and Hadlock, F.P.: Ultrasound in obstetrics and gynecology, St. Louis, 1981, The C.V. Mosby Co.

Kremkau, F.W.: How safe is obstetric ultrasound? Contemp. Obstet. Gynecol. **20**(6):182, 1982.

Lowrey, G.H.: Growth and development of children, ed. 7, Chicago, 1978, Year Book Medical Publishers, Inc.

Moore, K.L.: Before we are born: basic embryology and birth defects, Philadelphia, 1977 (revised), W.B. Saunders Co.

Moore, K.L.: The developing human, ed. 2, Philadelphia, 1977, W.B. Saunders Co.

Page, E.W., et al.: Human reproduction: essentials of reproductive and perinatal medicine, ed. 3, Philadelphia, 1981, W.B. Saunders Co.

Plauche, W.C., et al.: Phosphatidylglycerol and lung maturity, Am. J. Obstet. Gynecol. **144**(2):167, 1982.

Williams, S.R.: Nutrition and diet therapy, ed. 4, St. Louis, 1981, The C.V. Mosby Co.

Wohlgemuth, D.J., and Blake, E.M.: Changes in egg and sperm before and during fertilization, Contemp. Obstet. Gynecol. **20**(5):196, 1982.

15

Anatomic and Physiologic Adaptations to Pregnancy

- Female Reproductive System: External Structures
- Female Reproductive System: Internal Genitalia
  - Ovaries and fallopian tubes
  - Uterus
    - Enlargement
    - Arrangement of muscle fibers
    - Shape and consistency
    - Position
    - Contractility
    - Auscultation of intrauterine sounds
    - Uterine blood flow
    - Isthmus
    - Posture
    - Implications for nursing actions
  - Cervix
  - Vagina and vulva
    - Implications for nursing actions
  - Breasts
    - Implications for nursing actions
- Cardiovascular System
  - Anatomic changes: cardiac size and position
  - Auscultatory changes
  - Changes in hemodynamics
  - Hematologic changes: changes in blood constituents
  - Vascular headache
  - Implications for nursing actions
- Respiratory System
  - Anatomic changes
  - Pulmonary function
  - Basal metabolism rate
  - Acid-base balance
  - Implications for nursing actions
- Kidneys and Renal Function: an Overview
- Urinary System
  - Anatomic changes
    - Renal pelves and ureters
  - Implications for nursing actions
  - Bladder and urethra
  - Renal function changes
    - Renal plasma flow
    - Glomerular filtration rate
    - Fluid and electrolyte balance
    - Implications for nursing actions
    - Nutrient, including glucose, excretion
    - Proteinuria
- Skin Changes
  - Pigmentation
  - Striae gravidarum
  - Vascular abnormalities: spider angiomas, palmar erythema, and epulis
  - Oily skin and acne
  - Hirsutism
  - Fingernail changes
  - Implications for nursing actions
- Changes in the Musculoskeletal System
  - Implications for nursing actions
- Neurologic Changes
  - Implications for nursing actions
- Gastrointestinal Changes
  - Mouth
  - Teeth
  - Appetite
  - Esophagus and stomach
  - Small intestine
  - Colon
  - Gallbladder
  - Liver
  - Abdominal pain
  - Implications for nursing actions

■ **Endocrine Changes**
Pituitary gland
Fetoplacental hormone production
Ovary
Thyroid gland
Parathyroid glands
Adrenal glands
Pancreas

The difference between normal maternal physiologic adaptations and pathologic changes during pregnancy may only be a matter of degree. Although pregnancy is a normal phenomenon, problems can occur. The nurse needs an adequate foundation in normal maternal physiology to accomplish the following:

1. Assist the mother to understand the anatomic and physiologic changes during pregnancy
2. Allay the mother's (and family's) anxiety that may result from lack of knowledge
3. Teach the mother (and family) signs and symptoms that must be reported to the physician
4. Identify potential or actual deviation from normal adaptation

Among the expected adjustments to pregnancy are changes that are found in some disease states, for example, low hemoglobin levels, high erythrocyte sedimentation rate, dyspnea at rest, and alterations in cardiac function and endocrine balance. These changes reflect the body's effort to protect the mother and the fetus. An understanding of these changes is necessary for anyone who participates in the care of the mother and the fetus. Some of the changes are recognized as signs and symptoms of pregnancy.

Female Reproductive System: External Structures

External structures of the *perineum* are enlarged during pregnancy because of an increase in vasculature, hypertrophy of the perineal body, and deposition of fat (Fig. 15.1).

The labia majora of the nullipara approximate and obscure the vaginal introitus; those of the parous

Fig. 15.1
A, Pelvic floor in nonpregnant woman. **B,** Pelvic floor at end of pregnancy. Note marked projection (growth of tissue) below line joining tip of coccyx and inferior margin of symphysis. Urethra is elongated, and fat deposits are increased.

A

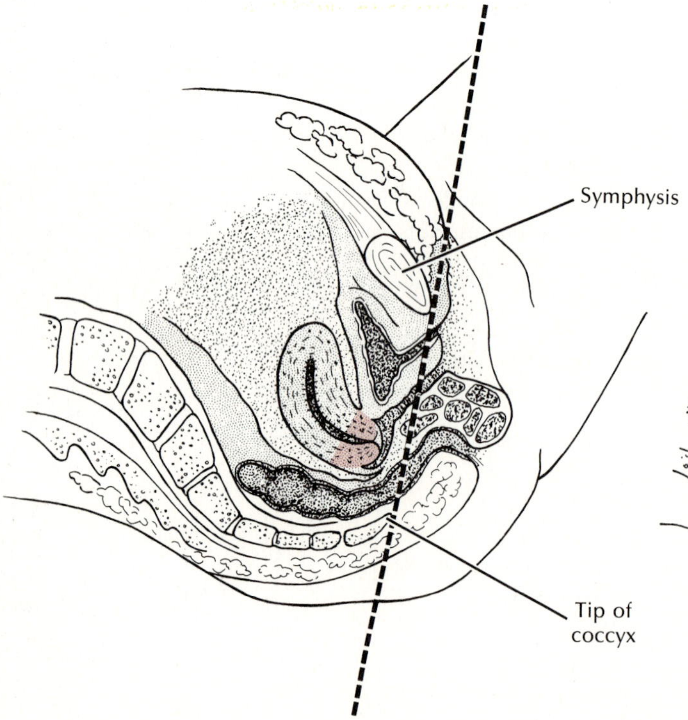

B

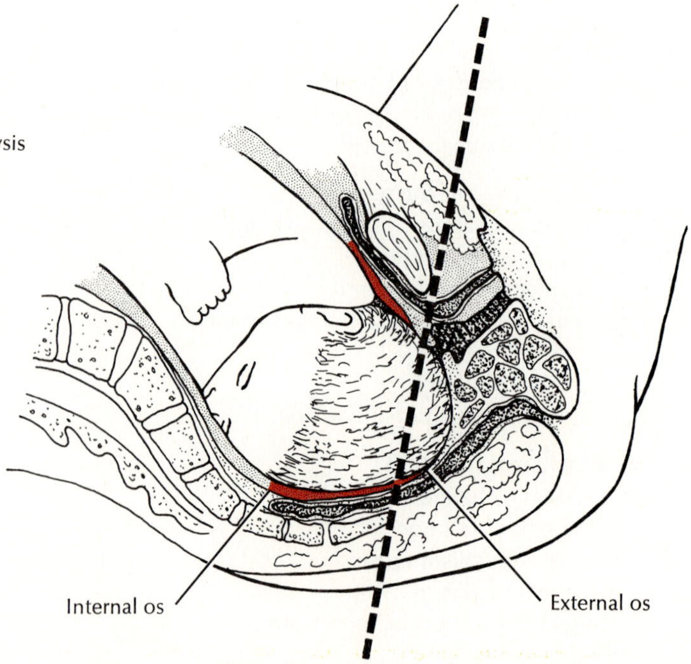

woman separate and gape after childbirth and perineal or vaginal injury.

Torn residual tags of the hymen remain after the use of tampons, coitus, and vaginal delivery.

Increased pelvic congestion, relaxation of smooth muscle of veins, constipation, bearing down during birth, multiparity, and obesity cause or aggravate anal and vulvar varices.

Female Reproductive System: Internal Genitalia

OVARIES AND FALLOPIAN TUBES

Ovulation does not occur during pregnancy. Anovulation is the result of the suppression of follicle-stimulating hormone (FSH) and luteinizing hormone (LH) by the elevated levels of estrogen and progesterone. Estrogen and progesterone are secreted during the first 8 to 10 weeks of pregnancy by the corpus luteum, after which the placenta takes over this function. The corpus luteum remains active following conception because of stimulation from HCG (see p. 246). Its function is crucial for maintaining the pregnancy for the first 8 to 12 weeks. During this time, it is typical for the corpus luteum to enlarge to a diameter of 2 to 3 cm (1 in), reaching its largest size about 7 weeks after the last menstrual period and then gradually decreasing in size and function. The growing placenta must be able to take over the production of estrogen and progesterone as corpus luteal function decreases, if pregnancy is to continue.

The fallopian tubes show very little change during pregnancy. They do elongate, however, and together with the ovaries, appear suspended from the sides of the greatly enlarged uterus.

The veins draining the ovaries and fallopian tubes are dilated to approximately three times their nonpregnant state, evidence of the generalized increase in vascularity seen during pregnancy.

UTERUS

Enlargement. Uterine enlargement to accommodate the growing fetus is the most distinctive characteristic of pregnancy. Its growth is phenomenal (Table 15.1), and it causes significant changes in the physiology of adjacent structures. The uterus develops from a small, almost solid organ into a thin-walled, muscular sac that can contain a fetus, placenta, and an average of 800 ml of amniotic fluid at term (40 weeks).

The endocrine system and mechanical factors are responsible for the enlargement of the uterus. Estrogen and progesterone provide the hormonal stimulus for (1) increased vascularity and dilation of blood vessels, (2) hyperplasia (production of new muscle fibers and fibroelastic tissue) and hypertrophy (enlargement of preexistent muscle fibers and fibroelastic tissue), and (3) development of the decidua. The growing products of conception increase the uterine size by mechanical stretching and dilation as they increase in volume. However, the most significant single factor responsible for uterine growth is the enlargement of preexistent muscle fibers—from seven to eleven times longer and two to seven times wider than those in the nonpregnant uterus (Fig. 15.2). As these bands of muscles enlarge, the new fibroelastic tissue forms a network between them, adding considerable strength to the uterine wall.

Hyperplasia of uterine muscle fibers is most prominent for the first 6 weeks of pregnancy; after the first trimester, hypertrophy of uterine muscle fibers and dilation of blood vessels are responsible for most of the subsequent increase in size.

The uterine wall develops from a thickness of 1 cm at conception to almost 2 cm at the end of the first few months of pregnancy and then thins to 0.5 cm or less at term. At term the thin and soft uterine wall permits effective palpation of the fetus by the examiner.

As the uterus increases in size, it also changes

Table 15.1
Comparison of Uterine Measurements for Nonpregnant and Pregnant at 40 Wk*

Measurement	Nonpregnant	Pregnant (40 wk)
Length	6.5 cm (2½ in)	32 cm (12½ in)
Width	4.0 cm (1½ in)	24 cm (9½ in)
Depth	2.5 cm (1 in)	22 cm (8½ in)
Weight	60-70 g (2½ oz)	1100-1200 g (2½ lb)
Volume	1-2 ml	5000 ml

*Note that references vary as to the exact values but all references agree on the magnitude of the growth the uterus undergoes during pregnancy.

Fig. 15.2
Growth of smooth muscle cells of uterus. **A,** Before pregnancy. **B,** During pregnancy. **C,** In puerperium.

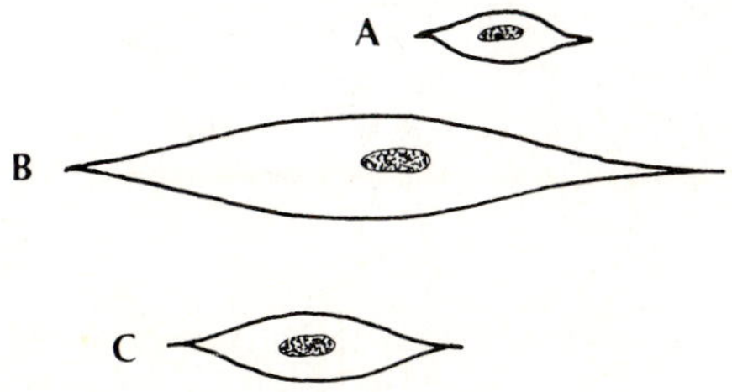

in weight, shape, and position. For information on changes in the intrauterine lining, see p. 211.

Arrangement of muscle fibers. The musculature of the uterus is unique since it not only provides for support and delivery of its contents but is also a natural physiologic defense against postdelivery hemorrhage. A brief review of the muscles of the uterus (see p. 63) will emphasize the importance of that arrangement to the mechanism of parturition (labor).

There are three muscle layers in the uterine wall (see Fig. 6.11). The outer layer consists of longitudinal fibers, which extend up and over the fundus and down its posterior aspect. These longitudinal fibers are arranged and distributed so that when they contract, they act to shorten the uterus, to efface the cervix by pulling it up, and to push the fetus outward. The middle layer consists of fibers entwined in a figure-eight formation around the large blood vessels. The fibers of this middle stratum supply much of the force of the uterine contractions. During contractions they constrict the blood vessels; between contractions they allow the blood to flow freely through the venous channels. After the placenta is separated, these interlacing fibers (the living ligature) contract and exert pressure on the blood vessels to prevent hemorrhaging. The inner layer consists of circular fibers that encompass the corpus and lower uterine segment (see p. 63).

Shape and consistency. As the size of the uterus increases, it also changes in weight, shape, and position. At conception the uterus is shaped like an upside-down pear. During the second trimester it is spheric or globular. Later, as the fetus lengthens, the contour of the uterus becomes more ovoid. The ovoid shape further increases the effectiveness of uterine contractions during labor by exerting maximal force from the fundus downward.

During the early weeks of pregnancy the uterus becomes perceptibly and progressively softer. It is believed by some that the nonsteroid ovarian hormone, relaxin, may act synergistically along with progesterone, contributing to a relaxing effect not only in the uterus but throughout various parts of the body (e.g., walls of blood vessels, joints). Relaxin appears in the blood early in pregnancy and increases in volume gradually to term. The hormone then disappears within 24 hours of delivery.

NOTE: In the nonpregnant woman, cervical or uterine anomalies, tumors, chronic passive congestion (with a retroflexed uterus), or "pelvic congestion syndrome" may mimic the previously discussed signs. A misinterpretation of findings in the obese or tense woman may lead to a false diagnosis of pregnancy.

Position. As the uterus grows it is elevated out of the pelvic area and may be palpated above the symphysis pubis sometime between the twelfth and sixteenth weeks of pregnancy (Figs. 15.3 and 15.4). It rises gradually to the level of the umbilicus at about 22 to 24 weeks and nearly reaches the xiphoid process at term.

Generally the uterus is rotated to the right as it elevates, probably because of the presence of the rectosigmoid colon on the left side. However, the extensive hypertrophy (enlargement) of the round ligaments keeps the uterus in line. Eventually the growing uterus touches the anterior abdominal wall and displaces the intestines to either side of the abdomen.

In primigravidas the uterus gradually sinks downward and forward about 2 weeks before term when the fetus's presenting part (usually the fetal head) descends into the true pelvis. This settling is called *lightening* or "dropping" and usually happens gradually; after it occurs, women feel less congested and breathe more easily. However, there is usually more bladder pressure as a result of this shift and, consequently, a return of urinary

Fig. 15.3
Height of fundus by weeks of gestation. These measurements refer to the normally growing, single conceptus within the uterus. It must be remembered that fundal height measurements are offset by numerous factors, for example, molar pregnancy, multiple pregnancy, growth retarded fetus (small for gestational age [SGA]), or abnormally large fetus (large for gestational age [LGA]).

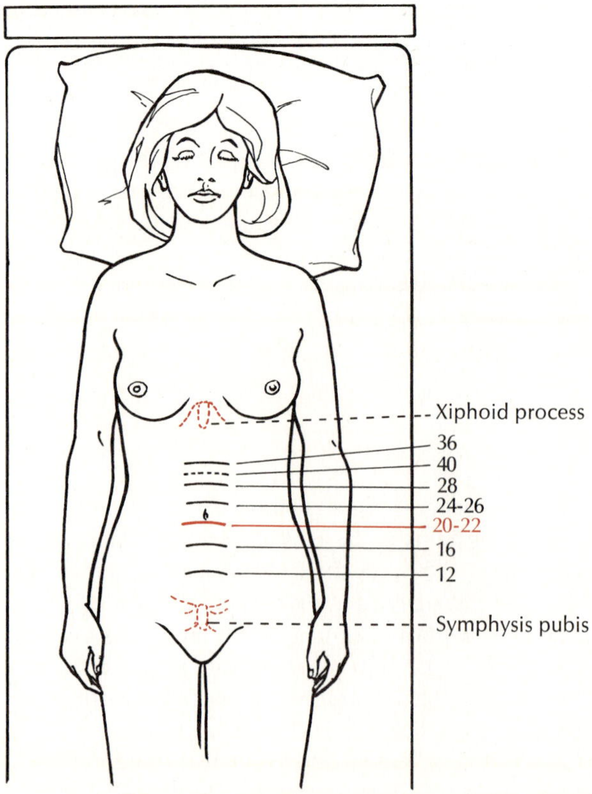

frequency. In multigravidas, lightening may not take place until after uterine contractions are established and true labor is in progress. The height of the fundus and the time when lightening occurs provide rough estimates of the duration of pregnancy (see p. 224).

Contractility. Braxton Hicks contractions are discussed in Chapter 17, p. 275. Monitoring of uterine activity by manual palpation of the uterine fundus and by intrauterine catheter and tocotransducer are discussed in Chapter 24, p. 471. For a discussion of uterine activity during labor, see Chapter 20; for uterine changes following delivery, see Chapter 31.

The contractions can be felt through the abdominal wall soon after the fourth month and are called Braxton Hicks contractions. Braxton Hicks contractions are merely a continuation of the irregular, painless contractions that occur intermittently throughout each menstrual cycle. Braxton Hicks contractions are felt as uterine firmness through the abdominal wall or are evident because the contractions raise the uterus and push it forward. They are caused by the upper uterine segment's stretching the longitudinal muscle fibers of the lower uterine segment and the cervix. The purpose of these contractions is to facilitate the return of venous blood to the placenta and so to aid in the oxygenation of fetal blood. Although Braxton Hicks contractions are not ordinarily painful some women do complain that they are annoying. They may become strong enough during the last few weeks to be confused with the beginning of labor. In that case they are called "false labor" (see p. 396).

Fig. 15.4
Lightening: descent of presenting part into true pelvis. Pressure on diaphragm is relieved, and breathing is easier; pressure on bladder increases, as does urinary frequency and varices.

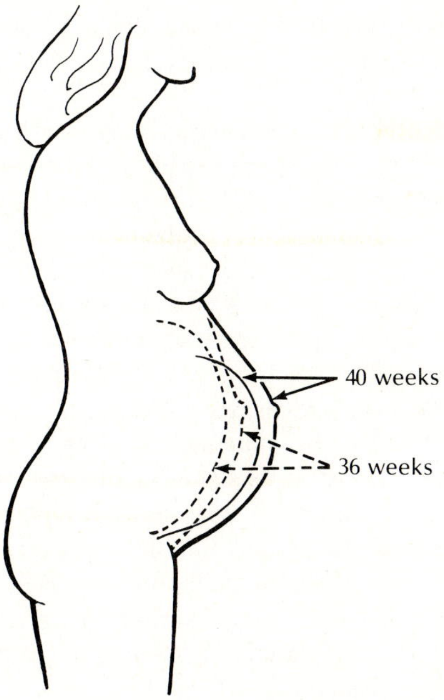

Auscultation of intrauterine sounds. Using an ultrasound device or a fetal stethoscope, the physician or nurse may hear (1) the *uterine souffle* or bruit, a rushing sound of maternal blood going to the placenta that is synchronous with the maternal pulse, (2) the *funic souffle* caused by fetal blood coursing through the umbilical cord and is synchronous with the fetal heart rate, and (3) the *fetal heart rate* (FHR). For further discussion, see Chapter 17.

Uterine blood flow. In a normal term pregnancy, one sixth of the total maternal blood volume is within the uterine vascular system, the rate of blood flow through the uterus averages 500 ml/min, and oxygen consumption of the gravid uterus averages 25 ml/min. Maternal arterial pressure, contractions of the uterus, and maternal position are three factors known to influence blood flow to this organ throughout pregnancy. Maternal malnutrition and hemorrhaging affect the blood flow to the uterus and the conceptus; the former problem results in chronic problems such as small-for-gestational age (SGA) babies and metabolic disease of late pregnancy, and the latter one results in acute problems such as fetal distress and asphyxiation.

Isthmus. The isthmus is located between the body of the uterus and the cervix. It differs from the body of the uterus in that is does not contain any mucus-secreting glands. As the uterus enlarges during gestation, the isthmus increases in length to about 2.5 cm and becomes quite soft. The isthmus is gradually incorporated into the uterine cavity, and as it expands during labor, it forms part of the lower uterine segment. Noted at about the eighth week, isthmic softening (Hegar's sign) appears (Fig. 15.5). Hegar's sign is a presumptive, objective sign of pregnancy.

Posture. When a pregnant woman stands, the major part of her uterus rests against the anterior abdominal wall and alters her center of gravity. To compensate for the increased pressure on her abdomen, the woman walks with her head and shoulders thrust backward and with her chest protruding. This gives her a characteristic stride called the *pride of pregnancy*. However, this posture (dorsolumbar lordosis) places increased strain on muscles and ligaments of the thighs and back and thus contributes to the musculoskeletal aches and cramps so characteristic of pregnancy (see Chapter 17).

Implications for nursing actions. The nurse's descriptions of anticipated uterine changes are often reassuring to the woman who is unaware of the uterus's capacity to adapt to the pregnancy and especially to the labor process. By learning from a nurse various self-

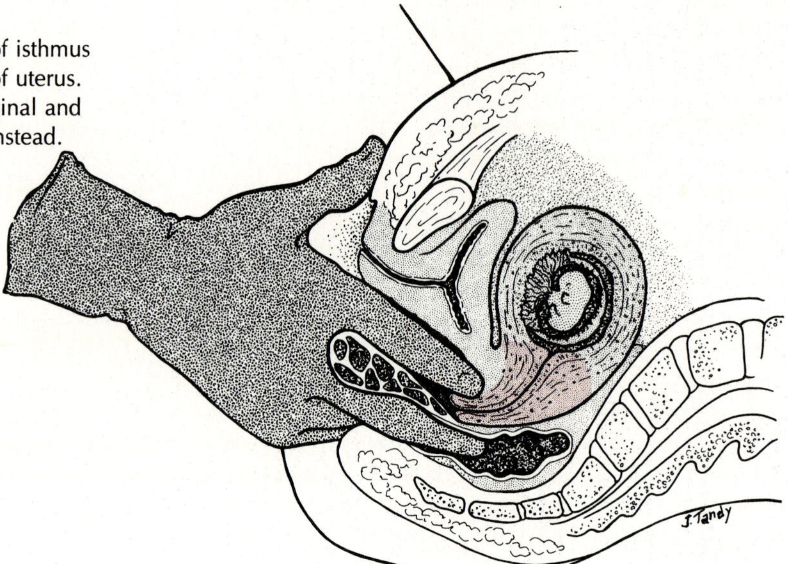

Fig. 15.5
Hegar's sign. Rectovaginal examination for softening of isthmus between cervix and body of uterus. Bimanual examination (vaginal and suprapubic) may be used instead.

help techniques to increase her comfort during the pregnancy, the woman builds up her pool of knowledge, self-confidence, and self-esteem for meeting the demands of labor, postdelivery recovery, and parenthood. Nursing actions relevant to the discomforts of back and leg aches, Braxton Hicks contractions, and round ligament pain are discussed in Table 17.10.

CERVIX

The softening of the cervix during pregnancy is brought about by increased vascularity, slight hypertrophy, and hyperplasia of the muscle and connective tissue. The connective tissue becomes loose, edematous, highly elastic, and increased in volume. The changes in the cervix (as well as those of the vagina) help to prepare the birth canal for the fetus's passage through it. Cervical softening (Goodell's sign) occurs at about 6 weeks since the last menstrual cycle; a violet-bluish hue (Chadwick's sign) from the enhanced blood supply is seen at about 8 weeks. Friability is increased (e.g., the cervix bleeds easily when scraped or touched); thus a few drops of blood after coitus with deep penetration or vaginal examination are usually within normal limits.

The changing consistency of the cervix may be likened to the feel of the following: prepregnant—the tip of the nose; pregnant (early and at midterm)—the earlobe; and pregnant (term)—the lips. At term the spongelike cervix thins (effaces) and the os widens (dilates) to allow the insertion of 1 cm (a fingertip) in primigravidas and even of 2 cm or more (several fingertips) in multigravidas.

The cervix of the nullipara is a rounded, almost conical, rather firm body with an external diameter of approximately 2 to 2.5 cm (about 1 in). The length of the cervix is about the same as its width. The cervix protrudes into the vaginal vault, and it should feel smooth. Lacerations of the cervix almost always occur during the birth process. With or without lacerations, the cervix becomes more oval in the horizontal plane, and the external os appears as a transverse slit following childbirth (Fig. 6.12).

The endocervix (inside the cervix, the cervical canal), which is composed of a vast number of crevices, clefts, and tunnels (but no tubular or branching glands), is covered by columnar mucus-producing cells that are supported by light, musculofibrous tissue. During pregnancy, under the influence of estrogen and progesterone, hypertrophy and hyperplasia of all elements occur, and edema of the connective tissue becomes notable (Fig. 15.6). The tissues soon lose their rigidity; the folds thin and become more delicate. Considerable mucus is produced, and because of the progesterone effect, *ferning* (see Chapter 13) does *not* occur in the dried cervical smear. The mucus fills the endocervical canal resulting in the formation of the mucous plug (operculum), which acts as a barrier against bacterial invasion during pregnancy. Normal leukorrhea of pregnancy is described in Chapter 17.

Fig. 15.6
A, Cervix in nonpregnant woman.
B, Changes in cervix during pregnancy.

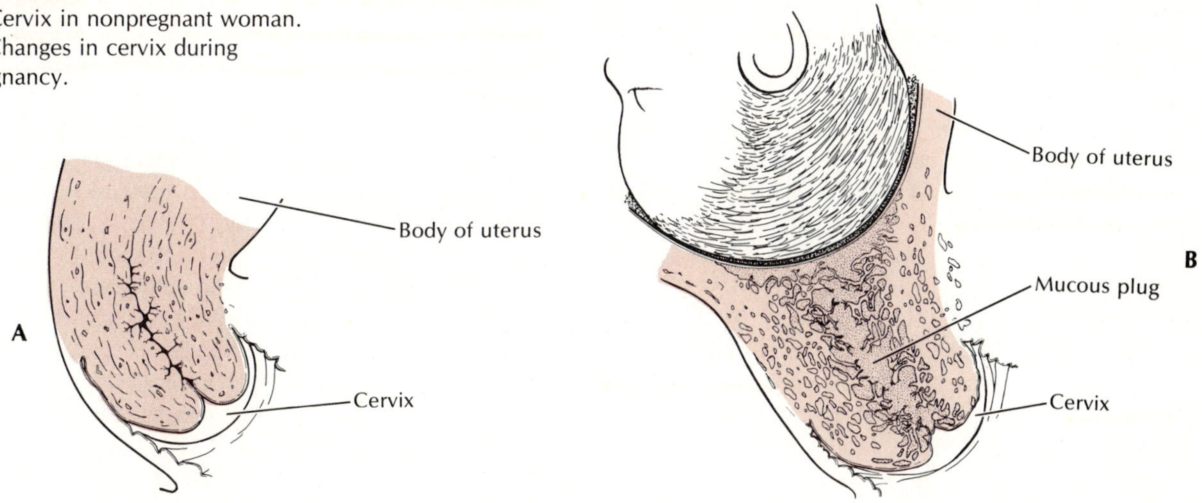

VAGINA AND VULVA

Striking changes are seen in the vulva, but especially in the vaginal walls in preparation for distention during labor. The vaginal squamous epithelium and elastic tissues undergo progressive hypertrophy and hyperplasia throughout pregnancy. The result is a thickened vaginal mucosa, loosened connective tissue, hypertrophied smooth muscle, and an increase in the length of the vaginal vault.

At about the eighth week of pregnancy the vaginal mucosa changes color because of the increase in vascularity and takes on a violet hue. The physician may observe this change during a pelvic examination and may use it as an early clinical diagnostic sign (Chadwick's sign). Chadwick's sign is a presumptive, objective sign of pregnancy.

This estrogen-induced activity causes heavy desquamation (or exfoliation) of the vaginal, glycogen-rich cells. The cells that are shed contribute to a thick whitish vaginal discharge, *leukorrhea,* which can be profuse and annoying, and which is a common complaint of pregnant women and their spouses. In the mucoid vaginal fluid, leukocytes (WBCs) are numerous, red blood cells (RBCs) are absent, and a mixed bacterial flora, perhaps with lactobacilli predominating, is typical.

The acid medium of normal adult vaginal secretions (pH of 4 to 5) allows Doderlein's bacilli to flourish; these bacilli help to keep pathogenic organisms that grow only in alkaline media from invading the vaginal canal. However, during pregnancy, the pH varies from 3.5 to 6. As the pH becomes less acid (pH between 5.5 to 6.5) it favors the growth of monilial (yeastlike) organisms (i.e., *Candida albicans*) and increases the possibility that the woman will contract a monilial infection (see Chapter 36).

The increased vascularity of the vagina and other pelvic viscera results in a marked increase in sensitivity and may lead to a high degree of sexual interest and arousal, especially during the second trimester of pregnancy. As pregnancy progresses there is more venous engorgement of the entire vaginal canal, causing the orgasmic platform to become almost completely obtruded. During orgasm the rhythmic contractions of the orgasmic platform are felt but are not observable. Because of the increased congestion and a resolution period that is less complete, some women become multiorgasmic for the first time. The increased congestion plus the relaxed walls of blood vessels and the heavy uterus may result in edema and varicosities of the vulva that will resolve during the postpartal period.

Implications for nursing actions. Many women will ask if they can douche because of the leukorrhea. They need to know that douching poses some danger during pregnancy.* In addition, douching will not lessen the vaginal discharge or the odor. In expectant fathers' groups, men will often voice their dislike (or outright revulsion) of vaginal discharge. Ventilation of these

*NOTE: Pressure-type (hand-held) douche ensembles are contraindicated during pregnancy because the mucous plug may be dislodged. If fluid is forced into the cervix, there is danger of douche fluid or air embolism that could lead to maternal death.

negative feelings and finding support from other men in the same situation often help them cope with their feelings (see p. 259). Frequent bathing with warm water and mild soap, wearing cotton panties, and perhaps wearing "light day" perineal pads will increase the woman's comfort. The woman is reminded that eating large quantities of sugars (soda, cookies, and candy) can make the vaginal environment even more suitable for a yeast infection.

BREASTS

Vascularity to the breasts increases early in pregnancy and is responsible for the presumptive (subjective) signs. Fullness, heightened sensitivity, tingling, and heaviness of the breasts are progressive after the missed period. About the same time a secondary pinkish areola may be apparent. Nipples and areolae become more pigmented, and nipples more erectile. Hypertrophy of the sebaceous glands embedded in the primary areola, called *Montgomery's tubercles,* may be seen around the nipples. These sebaceous glands may have a protective role by keeping the nipples lubricated. The richer blood supply dilates the vessels beneath the skin. Previously barely noticeable, now the blood vessels become visible, often appearing in an intertwining pattern. Venous congestion in the breasts is more obvious in primigravidas. Striae may appear at the outer aspects of the breasts.

During the second and third trimesters, growth of the mammary glands accounts for the progressive increase in breast size. The high estrogen-progesterone levels in pregnancy promote proliferation of the ducts and lobule-alveolar tissue, so that the breasts may feel nodular.

Although development of the mammary glands is functionally complete by midpregnancy, lactation is inhibited until a drop in estrogen level occurs after delivery of the fetus and placenta. A thin precolostrum secretion, however, may be expressed from the nipples by the end of the sixteenth week.* This secretion thickens as term approaches and is then known as colostrum. Colostrum, the creamy, white to yellowish premilk fluid, may be expressed from the nipples during the third trimester. Near term, protection may be needed if colostrum leaks from the breast, soiling the clothing.

Initiation of lactation is dependent on a complex interaction of estrogens, progesterones, human chorionic somatomammotropin (HCS) (also known as human placental lactogen [HPL]), and prolactin (PRL). For the discussion of lactation, see Chapter 30.

*References differ as to the gestational week during which precolostrum can be expressed. Some references cite week 16 as the earliest time at which fluid may be expressed from the breasts.

Implications for nursing actions. Anticipatory guidance early in pregnancy includes reassurance about the breast symptoms the woman is experiencing and prepares her for changes expected as pregnancy progresses. She is advised to wear a supportive maternity brassiere to add to her comfort and to prevent overstretching of fibrous suspensory ligaments supporting the breasts. A cotton brassiere is preferred with wide adjustable straps that cross over her back. The crossed straps pull the weight to the opposite shoulder and prevent deep ruts forming over her shoulders. The cups should be large enough to allow for growth of the breasts and the size adequate for the increase in her anteroposterior chest diameter. After the fourth month (sixteenth week) she may want to insert cotton pads, cut pieces from perineal menstrual pads, or clean, folded handkerchiefs in the cups to absorb any leakage from the breasts. Caution the woman against using a nonabsorptive pad (e.g., plastic) because the moisture retained against the skin may macerate the nipples and open a portal of entry for infection.

The breasts should be cleansed with warm water alone to avoid washing off the protective oils. If the woman insists on using soap, advise her to use a mild soap without added coloring or perfume.

The woman and her mate benefit from counseling about sexual activity. The increased tenderness of the breasts during the first trimester may necessitate their changing their position for sexual activity to avoid pressure on her breasts.

The *pinch test* identifies whether the woman's nipples will invert (draw in) or evert (protrude). To do the pinch test, pressure is applied with the thumb and forefinger to the outside of the areola where the newborn's gums would be during feeding. If the woman's nipples invert, the baby will have difficulty latching on. Therefore, to try to bring the nipples out more, the woman may benefit from wearing a Swedish milk cup during the last trimester of pregnancy (see p. 300 and Fig. 17.16).

Cardiovascular System

Maternal adjustments to pregnancy involve extensive changes in the cardiovascular system, both anatomic and physiologic. Cardiovascular adaptations serve to protect the woman's normal physiologic functioning, to meet the metabolic demands pregnancy imposes on her body, and to provide for fetal developmental and growth needs. The cardiovascular adaptations are thought to be caused by the hormones of pregnancy.

ANATOMIC CHANGES: CARDIAC SIZE AND POSITION

Slight cardiac enlargement is noted. Slight cardiac hypertrophy (enlargement) or dilation is probably secondary to increased blood volume and cardiac output. As the diaphragm is displaced upward, the heart is elevated upward and to the left (Fig. 15.7). The apical impulse (PMI) is shifted upward and laterally about 1 to 1.5 cm (½ in). The degree of shift depends on the duration of pregnancy and the size and position of the uterus.

AUSCULTATORY CHANGES

Auscultatory changes accompany the changes in heart size and position. Increases in blood volume and cardiac output also contribute to auscultatory changes common in pregnancy. A summary of heart sounds follows:

1. First heart sound: exaggerated splitting with increased loudness of the mitral and tricuspid components
2. Second heart sound: the normal slight splitting during inspiration is more obvious during pregnancy
3. Third heart sound: loud, easily heard; usually heard after 20 weeks

The third heart sound results from ventricular wall vibrations caused by rapid ventricular filling. These vibrations are best heard with the bell of the stethoscope over the apex of the heart. The sound is commonly heard in normal children, young adults, and pregnant

Fig. 15.7
Changes in position of heart, lungs, and thoracic cage in pregnancy. *Broken line,* Nonpregnant. *Solid line,* Change that occurs in pregnancy.

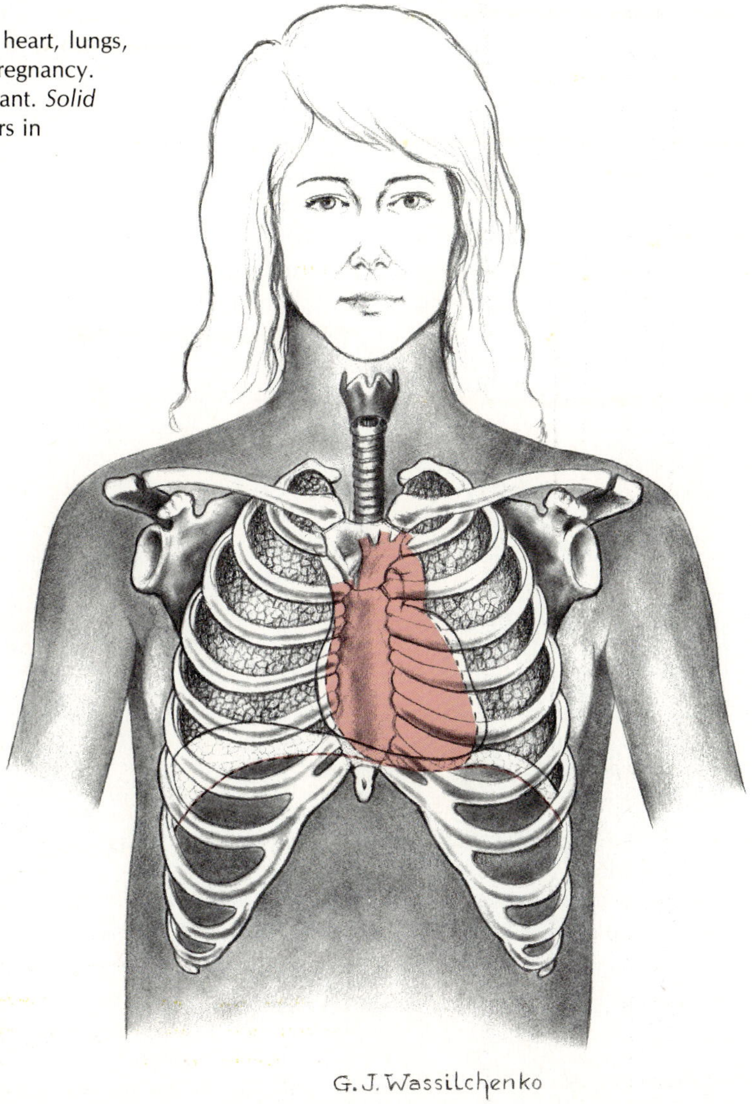

women. In these instances, the sound is known as "physiologic S_3." It is heard shortly after S_2 when the atrioventricular (AV) valves (the mitral and tricuspid valves) are open.

Low-grade (grade II) systolic (but not diastolic) ejection murmurs may be heard over the pulmonary valve (second intercostal space, left sternal border) and at the apex of the heart. These murmurs are secondary to increased blood flow.

CHANGES IN HEMODYNAMICS

The increased level of progesterone causes a generalized relaxation of smooth muscle and arteriolar dilation, which result in vasodilation. This increased capacity of the vascular bed accommodates the increase in blood volume, while maintaining a normal blood pressure.

During pregnancy, *blood volume* increases by 47%, by approximately 1500 ml* (normal value: 8.5% to 9% of body weight). The increase is made up of 1000 ml plasma plus 450 ml red blood cells (RBCs). The increase begins by the first trimester and peaks by 30 to 40 weeks. Peripheral vasodilation maintains normal blood pressure. The increased volume is a protective mechanism. It is essential for (1) the hypertrophied vascular system of the enlarged uterus, (2) adequate hydration of fetal and maternal tissues when the woman assumes an erect or supine position, and (3) fluid reserve for blood loss during the delivery and puerperium (Table 15.2). During labor, hemoconcentration varies with degree of muscular activity and dehydration. During delivery and in the immediate postpartal period, approximately one third of volume surplus is lost (500 ml for a vaginal delivery of a single fetus; 1000 ml for a vaginal delivery of twins or for cesarean birth). Following delivery, the loss of placental hormones decreases vasodilation and the loss of uteroplacental circulation reduces maternal vascular system by 10% to 15%. During the puerperium, by the end of the first week, another one third of the volume surplus is lost through diaphoresis and urine; by the end of the third week, the prepregnant level returns unless the woman is breast feeding.

The cardiac output increases about 30% during the first and second trimester (Fig. 15.8). The cardiac output remains elevated until term (40 weeks) largely as a result of increased stroke volume and in response to increased tissue demands for oxygen (normal value is 5 to 5.5 L/min). The cardiac output decreases with the woman in the supine position (see discussion of supine hypotension, p. 236). Cardiac output increases with any exertion (labor and delivery). During the first week after delivery, the cardiac output remains slightly elevated at about 13% above prepregnant levels and then returns to prepregnant levels.

The normal heart of a healthy woman can make the necessary adjustments and take on the added work load. The woman with heart disease is especially at risk for cardiac decompensation (1) during pregnancy, between weeks 28 and 35 when blood volume and cardiac load reach their peak, and (2) during labor and immediately after delivery when rapid hemodynamic changes occur (For a discussion of cardiac complications, see Chapter 36.)

*Expansion of blood volume: primigravidas, 1250 ml; multigravidas, 1500 ml; twin pregnancies, 2000 ml.

Table 15.2
Regional Increases in Blood Flow During Pregnancy*

Structure	Maternal Adaptation
Uterus	Major target for increased blood flow; flow increases throughout pregnancy and at term reaches 20 to 40 times non-pregnant value, or approximately 500ml/min *Purpose:* local maternal growth needs and fetal needs
Skin	Increased warmth generally, and hands may feel clammy; perfusion rate of 500 ml/min achieved early in pregnancy Increased fingernail growth; hair gets thicker and is less apt to break or fall out Mucosal congestion *Purpose:* eliminate heat generated by fetus and increased maternal metabolism
Kidneys	Increased blood flow begins early in pregnancy, to about 400 ml/min (or 25-50% increase) above prepregnant level by start of second trimester *Purpose:* Enhance elimination
Breasts	Evidence of increased blood flow appears early in pregnancy and includes sudden enlargement, and engorgement, feeling of tingling and warmth, dilated skin veins *Purpose:* Growth to prepare breasts for lactation
Gastro-intestinal tract	No direct evidence of increased blood flow; indirect evidence includes more efficient digestion and absorption

*See also Fig. 15.8.

Fig. 15.8
Distribution of increased cardiac output in pregnancy.

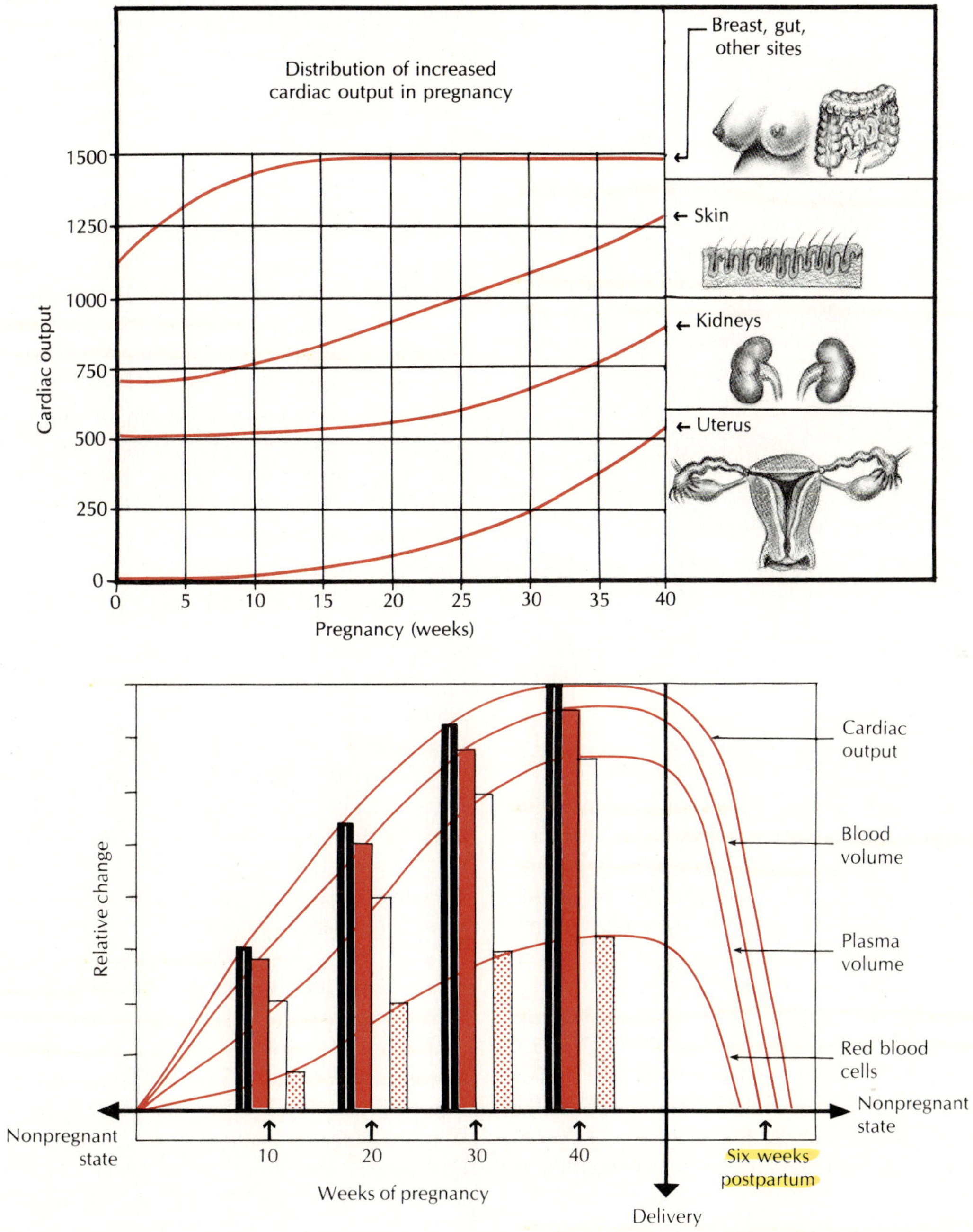

As a result of the cardiovascular changes during pregnancy, the *heart rate* increases by 15 to 20 beats/min. The maximal increase is noted in the last trimester. Occasionally the woman complains of palpitation or a ''racing'' heart beat.

Arterial blood pressure (brachial artery) varies with age. Average findings of systolic/diastolic pressure in women (in mm Hg) are as follows:

10 years of age: 103/70
20 years of age: 120/80
30 years of age: 123/82
40 years of age: 126/84
50 years of age: 130/86

Blood pressure findings vary with the position of the woman: it is highest when she is sitting, lowest when she is lying in the left lateral recumbent position, and intermediate when she is supine. During the first half of pregnancy, there is a decrease in both systolic and diastolic pressure of 5 to 10 mm Hg. The decrease in blood pressure is probably the result of peripheral vasodilation from hormonal changes during pregnancy. During the third trimester, maternal blood pressure should return to the values obtained during the first trimester. Therefore third-trimester blood pressure readings are not compared to midtrimester readings but instead to first-trimester recordings (under the same circumstances [e.g., sitting up, left arm]) to determine if a current reading is normal or is instead indicative of hypertensive disease of late pregnancy.

HEMATOLOGIC CHANGES: CHANGES IN BLOOD CONSTITUENTS

During pregnancy there is an accelerated production of *RBCs* (normal is 4 to 5.5 million/mm^3). The percentage of increase depends on the amount of iron available. The RBC mass increases by 30% by term if an iron supplement is taken, but it increases by only 17% if no supplement is taken. For the discussion of iron therapy see nutrition, p. 321.

Normal *hemoglobin* values (12 to 16 g/dl blood) and *hematocrit* values (37% to 47%) decrease. The decrease is more noticeable during the second trimester, when rapid expansion of blood volume takes place. If the hemaglobin value drops to 10 g/dl or less, or if the hematocrit drops to 35% or less, the woman is considered anemic.

To facilitate oxygen transfer to the fetus, red cell 2,3-diphosphoglycerate (DPG) rises during pregnancy.

The total *white cell count* increases during the second trimester and peaks during the third trimester. This increase is primarily in the leukocytes; the lymphocyte count stays about the same throughout pregnancy. At the onset of labor, the white cell count is as high as 25,000/mm^3 (normal is 5000 to 10,000/mm^3).

There is a greater *tendency to coagulation* during pregnancy because of increases in various clotting factors. Fibrinolytic activity (the splitting up or the dissolving of a clot) is depressed during pregnancy; activity returns within 15 minutes of delivery; then it is depressed again during the postpartum period. The result is that the chance of thromboembolism during the postpartum period is three times greater than during pregnancy; the chance of thromboembolism is greater during pregnancy than during the nonpregnant state.

VASCULAR HEADACHE

In rare instances, vascular headaches may occur during pregnancy. This type of headache is benign, although the symptoms are severe. The vascular headache is characteristically throbbing and is associated with blurred vision and transient neurologic signs such as dizziness, slurred and garbled speech, and perhaps numbness in an extremity. It is important for physicians to consider benign vascular headache before proceeding with a complete invasive neurologic workup, which could have a serious deleterious effect on both the mother and her fetus.

IMPLICATIONS FOR NURSING ACTIONS

The gravida and her family benefit from understanding the importance of a good diet even before the woman gets pregnant. The woman who has a good store of iron and who is not anemic when she becomes pregnant is in a better state to provide oxygen to her fetus and to maintain her own stores of this vital nutrient. If the woman needs information about foods that provide iron (see p. 324) and help her build RBCs, the nurse helps her choose foods that provide the most nutrients and that fit within her food preferences and budget. When iron supplementation* is ordered, the woman is advised to take the medication with water or fruit juice (vitamin C helps with iron absorption and utilization) 20 minutes after a meal, to decrease gastrointestinal irritation. She needs to know that taking iron medication will darken the color of her stools and that it can cause diarrhea or constipation. Some iron medications contain stool softeners; the nurse must therefore thoroughly research all the ingredients in a medication and inform the woman of their effects.

There is a greater risk of thromboembolism during pregnancy. Because of this increased risk, the woman

*The World Health Organization (WHO) recommends supplemental iron during pregnancy.

Table 15.3
Cardiovascular System: Maternal Adaptations and Implications for Nursing

Function	Maternal Adaptation	Implications for Nursing Actions
Heart rate	Between 14 and 20 wk, pulse increases slowly up to 10-15 beats/min, which then persists to term; palpitations may occur; bradycardia may occur after delivery and persist for 1 wk	1. Inform woman of expected changes. Maintain accurate record. 2. Establish base-line rate of BP before twentieth wk if possible.
Blood pressure Arterial	No significant change in systolic pressure; Diastolic pressure drops slightly at midpregnancy	3. Record position of woman when her BP is assessed.
Venous	Arms: no change Legs: continued gradual increase after eighth wk, especially when woman is supine, sitting, or standing	4. Ass for varicosities in legs, vulva, and rectum (hemorrhoids). Counsel her about support hose, avoiding constrictive clothing, and resting with hips and legs elevated.
Cardiac output	Increases between 30-50% by thirty-second wk of pregnancy; declines to about a 20% increase at 40 wk	5. Advise woman that lying in the left lateral recumbent position facilitates blood flow.
Total body water	Increases between tenth and fortieth wk of pregnancy	6. Counsel woman about maintaining adequate hydration.
Plasma and blood volume	Increase starts about twelfth wk, peaks at about 25-40% at thirty-second wk, then decreases slightly to fortieth wk	7. Counsel woman about adequate dietary intake.
RBC mass	Increases by 10-15% (450 ml) between eighth and fortieth wk; total RBC volume increases average of 33%	
Circulation time	Decreases slightly (13-11 sec) by wk 32, then returns to normal near term	

needs to learn about signs and symptoms that may occur (e.g., pain in the calf of her leg). She is taught not to massage or use heat over the painful area but to dorsiflex the foot while keeping her knee extended (she is to point her heel). (See leg cramps, Table 17.10, and Chapter 31, p. 692.) If the pain increases (a positive Homan's sign), she is to call the physician immediately and stay seated in a chair or in bed until someone takes her into the emergency room or the physician's office. If the pain is relieved by pointing her heel, then she has no need to call her physician, for the problem is then related to muscular cramping, which is associated with a calcium deficiency or a phosphorus excess.

A summary of cardiovascular changes during pregnancy is presented in Table 15.3.

Respiratory System

Respiratory adaptations occur during pregnancy to provide for both maternal and fetal needs. Maternal oxygen requirements increase in response to the acceleration in metabolic rate and the need to add to the tissue mass in the uterus and breasts. The conceptus (embryo or fetus) requires oxygen and a way to eliminate carbon dioxide.

ANATOMIC CHANGES

Increased vascularization in response to elevated levels of estrogen also occurs in the respiratory tract. As the capillaries become engorged, edema and hyperemia develop within the nose, pharynx, larynx, trachea, and bronchi. This congestion within the tissues of the respiratory tract gives rise to several conditions commonly seen during pregnancy: nasal and sinus stuffiness, epistaxis (nosebleed), changes in one's voice, and marked inflammatory response to even a mild upper respiratory infection. Increased vascularity swells tympanic membranes and eustachian tubes, giving rise to symptoms of impaired hearing, earaches, or a sense of fullness in the ears. Women need to be cautioned against taking cold or allergy medication for pregnancy-induced nasal stuffiness or eustachian tube blockage to avoid possible damage to the conceptus (see Appendix H).

Before the uterus is large enough to affect intraabdominal pressure, the length of the lungs decreases. Broadening of the thorax in the anteroposterior and transverse diameters compensates for the shortening in the length of the lungs. The lower part of the rib cage flares out as pregnancy progresses so that the substernal angle increases from the usual 68 degrees (first trimester) to slightly over 100 degrees toward the end of the third trimester. The resulting 5 to 7 cm increase in thoracic circumference plus the increase in breast size necessitates supportive brassieres specially made for pregnant women. Hormone-induced softening of the ligaments of the rib cage allows for the increase in thoracic diameters. After delivery, the joints of the rib cage do not always return to the prepregnant state.

The level of the diaphragm rises by as much as 4 cm during pregnancy. Mechanical pressure upward from the enlarging uterus only partially accounts for this upward displacement. With advancing pregnancy, thoracic breathing replaces abdominal breathing and descent of the diaphragm with inspiration becomes less possible.

PULMONARY FUNCTION

Three pulmonary functions undergo little if any change during normal pregnancy: *respiratory rate* increases by about two breaths per minute; *vital capacity*, the volume of air that can be expelled from the lungs by the most forcible expiration following deepest inspiration; and *maximal breathing capacity* (MBC), the greatest amount of air that can be breathed voluntarily during a 10- to 30-sec period.

Some components of lung function are modified as the woman adapts to pregnancy. The pregnant woman breathes deeper (increases *tidal volume*, the amount of gases exchanged with each breath) but increases her respiratory rate only slightly.

Functional residual capacity and *residual volume* of air are decreased because of elevation of the diaphragm. The increase in tidal volume and decrease in residual volume result in more efficient exchange of lung gases in the alveoli and an increase in *minute oxygen uptake*. The oxygen-carrying capacity of the blood is increased accordingly.

The increase in tidal volume, without a great increase in respiratory rate, increases the amount of air expired per minute *(minute ventilation or volume)* by 40% to 50% above normal between the sixteenth and fortieth week of pregnancy. *Alveolar ventilation* is increased by 65% to 70%. This lowers alveolar PCO_2, resulting in lowered plasma PCO_2 and development of mild respiratory alkalosis. The respiratory alkalosis is compensated for by kidney function, with one notable exception: the rapid and shallow respirations (hyperventilation) lower arterial PCO_2 and increase pH values to harmful levels. Hyperventilation in the pregnant woman may be noted as a response to stress such as the discomfort of a labor contraction. Hyperventilation, its signs and symptoms and treatment, is discussed in Chapter 19, p. 349. The lowered alveolar PCO_2 seen during pregnancy is also found during the luteal phase of each menstrual cycle.

During pregnancy, changes in the respiratory center result in a lowered threshold carbon dioxide. Progesterone and estrogen are presumed to be responsible for the increased sensitivity of the respiratory center. In addition, pregnant women experience increased awareness of the need to breathe; some may complain of dyspnea at rest.

BASAL METABOLISM RATE

Basal metabolism rate (BMR) gradually increases by 15% to 25% because of increased oxygen consumption as a result of metabolic activity of fetal and maternal tissues.

ACID-BASE BALANCE

By about the tenth week of pregnancy, there is a decrease of about 5 mm Hg in PCO_2. Progesterone may be responsible for increasing the sensitivity of the respiratory center receptors so that tidal volume is increased and PCO_2 falls. As PCO_2 falls, the base excess (HCO_3, or bicarbonate) falls, and pH rises (becomes more basic). These alterations in acid-base balance indicate that pregnancy is a state of respiratory alkalosis compensated by mild metabolic acidosis. Episodes of hyperventilation potentially can be harmful to the mother and fetus because of existing acid-base imbalance. When the woman is in labor, these alterations are accentuated.

Metabolic changes during pregnancy are discussed in Chapter 18.

IMPLICATIONS FOR NURSING ACTIONS

The pregnant woman welcomes hearing that some of the sensations she is experiencing are expected (e.g., dyspnea at rest, sighing, increased feeling of warmth). The woman is alerted to the fact that dyspnea can occur with slight exertion or even while at rest and that she may find that she is sighing more and taking deep breaths, starting from the first trimester through delivery. The nurse suggests good posture, sitting upright, and breathing in and out slowly until the feeling passes. Because some of the changes during pregnancy mimic pulmonary and cardiac pathologic conditions, the woman is encouraged to inform her physician of the symptoms she is experiencing.

If the gravida feels warm and is complaining of heat intolerance, as her basal metabolic rate (BMR) rises, the nurse suggests the use of cooler clothing and bathing to relieve the distress.

Anticipatory guidance also includes enlisting the woman's help in early diagnosis of potential problems related to respiratory tract function. The woman is advised to report respiratory tract infections to the physician. Although overall pulmonary function is not impaired during pregnancy, with respiratory tract diseases, increased oxygen requirements by the fetus and the mother are jeopardized. *The woman is cautioned against taking unprescribed medications.* Questionable respiratory tract signs and symptoms need to be referred to the physician so that complications such as severe anemia, pulmonary edema, severe acidosis, or excessive pressure on the diaphragm, as that which occurs with hydramnios, can be diagnosed or ruled out. For discussion of complications, see Chapter 41.

The nurse needs to be aware that the rapid exchange in gases in the maternal lungs not only increase the rate at which induction of inhalation anesthesia occurs (the anesthesiologist's problem) but also that her recovery from inhalation anesthesia is more rapid than in the nonpregnant woman (the concern of the nurse who is attending a woman during recovery from anesthesia).

Kidneys and Renal Function: an Overview

The kidneys are vital excretory organs. Their purpose is to maintain the body's internal environment in the relatively constant homeostatic state necessary for the efficient functioning of the body at the cellular level. The kidneys are responsible for maintenance of electrolyte and acid-base balance, regulation of extracellular fluid volume, excretion of waste products, and the conservation of essential nutrients.

Urinary System

Changes in renal structure result from hormonal activity (estrogen and progesterone), pressure from an enlarging uterus, and an increase in blood volume.

ANATOMIC CHANGES

Renal pelves and ureters. As early as the tenth week of pregnancy, the renal pelves and the ureters dilate. Dilation of the ureters is more pronounced above the pelvic brim, occurring most frequently on the right side due to the lie of the uterus. In most women the ureters below the pelvic brim are of normal size. The smooth muscle walls of the ureters undergo hyperplasia (increase in cell number) and hypertrophy (increase in cell size) and relaxed muscle tone. The ureters elongate, become tortuous, and kink. In the latter part of pregnancy, the right renal pelvis and ureter dilate more than on the left, due to displacement of the heavy uterus to the right by the sigmoid colon.

Because of these changes, a larger volume of urine is held in the pelves and ureters and urine flow rate is slowed. Urinary stasis or stagnation has several consequences:

1. There is a lag between the time urine is formed and when it reaches the bladder. Therefore clearance test results may reflect substances contained in glomerular filtrate several hours before.
2. Stagnated urine is an excellent medium for the growth of microorganisms. In addition, the urine of pregnant women contains greater amounts of nutrients, including glucose. Therefore, during pregnancy, women are more susceptible to urinary tract infection.

IMPLICATIONS FOR NURSING ACTIONS

1. Modify collection of urine specimens to increase accuracy of renal function tests.
   a. Encourage the pregnant woman to increase her water intake before the start of the test to increase rate of urine flow.
   b. Ask woman to lie on her left side (left lateral recumbent position) when renal function tests are being performed.
2. Instruct woman regarding her susceptibility to infection and how she can help herself.
   a. Maintain cleanliness; wipe once with each tissue from front to back after defecating or urinating.
   b. Report symptoms that may indicate infection (see Chapter 41).

BLADDER AND URETHRA

There is a decrease in bladder tone, which permits distention of the bladder to approximately 1500 ml. At the same time the bladder is compressed by the enlarging uterus, resulting in the urge to void even if the bladder contains only a small amount of urine.

Urinary frequency results from increased bladder sensitivity and later from compression of the bladder. In the second trimester, the bladder is pulled up out of the true pelvis into the abdomen. The urethra lengthens to 7.5 cm (3 in) as the bladder is displaced upward. The pelvic congestion of pregnancy is reflected in hyperemia of the bladder and urethra. This increased vascularity causes the bladder mucosa to be traumatized and bleed easily.

The causes of dilation of the urine collection and transport system are not fully understood. It had been thought that dilation occurred mainly in response to the high levels of progesterone during pregnancy. There is some evidence that dilation is in response to mechanical pressure as well. Early in pregnancy pressure results from dilated blood vessels, and later, from the enlarging uterus compressing ureters as they pass over the pelvic brim. Generally, the right renal pelvis and ureter are more markedly dilated than the left. The pregnant uterus is dextrorotated (displaced toward the woman's right side) because of the fullness of the sigmoid colon.

RENAL FUNCTION CHANGES

In normal pregnancy, renal function is altered considerably. The woman's kidneys must manage the increased metabolic and circulatory demands of the maternal body and also excretion of fetal waste products. Changes in renal function are caused by pregnancy hormones, an increase in blood volume, the woman's posture, physical activity, and nutritional intake. The malnourished, protein-deficient mother-to-be has a decrease in oncotic pressure, which results in a reduced renal plasma flow, producing the secondary symptoms of kidney malfunction: albuminuria, release of renin and angiotensin, and, eventually, oliguria.

Renal plasma flow. The renal plasma flow (RPF) increases approximately 25% by the second trimester, decreases to nonpregnant levels in the third trimester, and remains below nonpregnant levels until the eighth week after delivery. Normal value is 490 to 700 ml/min.

Glomerular filtration rate. The glomerular filtration rate (GFR) increases approximately 50% and returns to nonpregnant levels in the early puerperium. Normal value is 105 to 132 ml volume.

Renal function is most efficient when the woman lies in the left lateral recumbent position and least efficient when the woman assumes a supine position. Positional differences are noted in the gravida's GFR and RPF from the twentieth week of pregnancy until term. When the woman is upright or supine, the GFR and renal blood flow drop by about 50%. Therefore there is a drop in the excretion of water, sodium, and chloride. When the pregnant woman is lying supine, the heavy uterus compresses the vena cava and the aorta and cardiac output decreases. The result is a drop in maternal blood pressure and fetal heart rate (vena cava or hypotensive syndrome) and a drop in the volume of blood to the kidneys. When cardiac output drops, blood flow to vital organs (brain and heart) is continued at the expense of other organs, including the kidneys. Arterial blood flow to these other organs is reduced because of a reflex vasoconstriction.

When the pregnant woman is standing (or sitting upright), the heavy uterus compresses the common iliac veins and, aided by gravity, fluid pools in the woman's legs. Venous return is reduced, circulating blood volume and cardiac output are decreased, blood pressure drops, and renal vasoconstriction occurs. Decreased blood flow to the kidneys is one cause of proteinuria (see p. 237).

Fluid and electrolyte balance

Sodium balance. Selective renal tubular reabsorption maintains sodium and water balance regardless of changes in dietary intake and losses through sweat, vomitus, or diarrhea. The maintenance of a sodium-water balance is a complex process under ordinary circumstances. During pregnancy, factors that cause sodium retention or loss change.

From 500 to 900 mEq of sodium is normally retained during pregnancy to meet fetal needs. The need for increased maternal intravascular and extracellular fluid volume requires additional sodium to expand fluid volume and to maintain an isotonic state. The resulting tendency to sodium *depletion* can present major problems if the condition is made worse by severe dietary restriction of sodium or by use of diuretics.

Several factors promote renal excretion of sodium; two of these factors are an increase in GFR and high levels of progesterone. The GFR rises to about 50% higher than in the nonpregnant state. The high level of progesterone overcomes aldosterone's sodium retention effect and promotes sodium excretion. To prevent excessive sodium depletion, the maternal kidneys undergo a significant adaptation by increasing tubular reabsorption.

Several other factors enhance sodium reabsorption, two of which are the renin-angiotensin-aldosterone system and the high level of some pregnancy hormones. Renin, secreted into the blood by the kidneys, stimulates the production of angiotensin. Angiotensin is the main regulator of aldosterone secretion by the adrenal cortex. During pregnancy there is a marked increase in both renin activity and aldosterone, a compensatory response, to ensure adequate sodium for fetal needs and increased maternal extracellular fluid volume. As efficient as the renin-angiotensin-aldosterone system is, it can be overstressed by excessive dietary sodium intake or restriction or by use of diuretics. *Severe hypovolemia and reduced placental perfusion are two consequences.*

Estrogen favors sodium retention. Increased levels of placental human chorionic somatomammotropin (HCS), otherwise known as human placental lactogen (HPL), prolactin, and plasma cortisol help to conserve sodium as well.

Water balance. The capacity of the kidneys to excrete water during the early weeks of pregnancy is more efficient than later in pregnancy. Occasionally in early pregnancy, the extent of water loss may cause some women to feel thirsty. The pooling of fluid in the legs in the latter part of pregnancy decreases renal blood flow and GFR. The diuretic response to the water load is triggered when the woman lies down, preferrably on her left side, and the pooled fluid reenters general circulation. This pooling of blood in the lower legs is sometimes referred to as *physiologic edema,* which requires no treatment.

Other factors that may account for the kidney's decreased ability to excrete water in late pregnancy may be the lower osmolar level (quantity of solutes per volume of fluid) or the increased secretion of oxytocin. Oxytocin has some antidiuretic effect.

The total weight gain in pregnancy (average of 12.5 kg [27½ lb]) includes the weight gain from fluid retention (total of 3.68 kg [8.5 lb]). Until the thirtieth week, weight gain is almost entirely due to deposition of fat. After that time, interstitial fluid volume increases by 1 to 2 L, accounting for a greater part of the weight gained during that time. Weight loss during labor and delivery amounts to 5.5 kg (12 lb) as a result of blood loss, insensible water loss, and loss of the fetus, placenta, and amniotic fluid. Weight loss during the puerperium (4 kg [9 lb]) reflects excretion of fluids and electrolytes accumulated during pregnancy. During the puerperium extracellular fluid is lost at a rate of 2 L during the first week and 0.68 kg (1.5 lb) over the next 5 weeks.

Implications for nursing actions. The many urinary tract changes during pregnancy concern many women and their friends and families. Women need to know that physiologic edema is normal and becomes apparent in the lower legs, especially by evening (if she is up all day). Edema is reduced by resting in the left lateral recumbent position. This position improves circulation to the kidneys (and the heart) so that more urine is formed. Therefore the woman can expect to get up to void several times at night (nocturia) and to be free of edema in the morning. Women are cautioned against taking "water pills" (diuretics) because this could cause an electrolyte and fluid imbalance. Gravidas do need sodium in their diets, but the nurse needs to assess each woman's diet for adequate protein intake and excessive sodium intake.

The gravida can be reassured that the extra fluid she is carrying is a protective mechanism—it is there to transport goods to and from the fetus and to meet her fluid needs in case of hemorrhage.

The woman needs to realize that poor posture and restrictive clothing can impede the blood return to the heart and increase edema formation. If the woman's work requires that she stand for long periods of time, the blood flow to her kidneys could be impaired. If the woman must continue to work, she may benefit from knowing what kind of clothes to wear and knowing to avoid garters, to wear support hose, to take rest periods, and to take short walks during the day.

If the edema is generalized so that the woman wakes up with puffy eyes that are "hard to open" and if she can no longer wear any of her rings because her fingers have become "too fat," she needs to be assessed by the physician for pregnancy-induced hypertension (preeclampsia) (see Chapter 35).

Nutrient, including glucose, excretion. Under normal circumstances, the kidney reabsorbs almost all of the glucose and other nutrients from the plasma filtrate. In pregnant women tubular reabsorption of glucose is not as efficient as that of sodium, so that glucosuria does occur at varying times and to varying degrees. Normal values are zero to 20 mg/dl. That is, during any one day, the urine is positive and sometimes it is negative. When it is positive, the amount of glucose varies from 1+ to 4+.

In pregnant women, blood glucose levels must be at 160 to 180 mg/dl before glucose is "spilled" into the urine (not reabsorbed). During pregnancy, glucosuria occurs when maternal glucose levels are lower than 160 mg/dl. Why glucose, as well as other nutrients such as amino acids, are wasted during pregnancy is not understood nor has the exact mechanism been discovered. Although glucosuria may be found in normal pregnancies (indeed, 1+ levels may be seen with increased anxiety states), the possibility of diabetes mellitus must be kept in mind (see Chapter 36).

Implications for nursing actions. At each visit to the physician, the woman's urine is tested for sugar. The nurse follows the directions on the bottle of reagent sticks (Clinitest, Testape, Dextrostix) for checking urine carefully. If glucose is present, ask the woman if she has just eaten and what she had. Occasionally, women will have just finished a candy bar and soda. Both the test results and the woman's answer to questions about the food she has eaten are referred to the physician.

Proteinuria. Albumin and globulin are proteins that are not normal constituents of urine at any time. Small (trace) amounts of protein may occasionally be found in very concentrated urine or in first-voided urine following sleep. However, a measurable amount (over 150 mg in 24 hours) of protein in the urine is a significant sign of renal disease at any time and of pregnancy-induced hypertension (preeclampsia).

Implications for nursing actions. Freshly voided urine is assessed for protein at each prenatal visit using the reagent end of a dipstick. It is important to test a clean-catch midstream specimen (see p. 285) to decrease the possibility of its contamination with vaginal discharge. If the test is positive, the physician is alerted. The nurse reminds the woman to avoid sleeping on her back at any time, but especially during pregnancy, to enhance uterine renal blood flow (Fig. 21.11).

Skin Changes

Alterations in hormonal balance and mechanical stretching are responsible for several changes in the integumentary system during pregnancy. The following outline summarizes integumentary system changes associated with pregnancy:

1. General changes including the following:
   a. The skin thickens, and subdermal fat is increased.
   b. Hyperpigmentation develops.
   c. Increased hair and nail growth is notable in many women.
   d. Sweat and sebaceous gland activity is accelerated.
   e. There is greater fragility of cutaneous elastic tissues, resulting in striae gravidarum, or stretch marks.
   f. Increased circulation and vasomotor activity, as well as dermatographia, are evident.
   g. Cutaneous allergic responses are enhanced.
   h. Vascular permeability is increased.
2. Dermatologic disorders induced by pregnancy include herpes gestationis, noninflammatory pruritus of pregnancy, vascular spiders, palmar erythema, and pregnancy granulomas (including epulides).
3. Skin problems generally aggravated by pregnancy are acne vulgaris (in first trimester), erythema multiforme, herpetiform dermatitis, granuloma inguinale, condyloma acuminatum, neurofibromatosis, and pemphigus.
4. Dermatologic disorders usually improved by pregnancy include acne vulgaris (in third trimester), seborrheic dermatitis, and psoriasis.
5. An unpredictable course during pregnancy may be expected in atopic dermatitis, lupus erythematosus, and herpes simplex.

Several skin changes serve as presumptive signs of pregnancy and add objective data that assist in the diagnosis of pregnancy (see discussion of prenatal period, Chapter 17). These changes are selected for discussion here.

PIGMENTATION

Pigmentation is caused by the anterior pituitary hormone melanotropin, which is increased during pregnancy. Facial *melasma,* also called *chloasma* or *mask of pregnancy,* is a blotchy, brownish hyperpigmentation of the skin over the malar prominences and the forehead, especially in dark-complexioned expectant women. Chloasma appears in 50% to 70% of pregnant women, beginning after the sixteenth week and increasing gradually to delivery. The sun intensifies this pigmentation in susceptible women. Chloasma caused by normal pregnancy usually fades after delivery. Darkening of the nipples, areolae, axillae, and vulva occurs at about the same time.

The *linea nigra* is a pigmented line extending from the symphysis pubis to the top of the fundus in the midline; this line is known as the linea alba before hormone-induced pigmentation (see p. 69). In primigravidas the extension of the linea nigra, beginning in the third month, keeps pace with the rising height of the fundus; in multigravidas, the entire line often appears earlier than the third month.

STRIAE GRAVIDARUM

Striae gravidarum, or stretch marks, which appear in 90% of gravidas during the second half of pregnancy, may be due to action of adrenocorticosteroids. Striae reflect separation within the underlying connective (collagen) tissue of the skin. These marks tend to occur over areas of maximal stretch, (i.e., abdomen, thighs, and breasts). Tendency to the development of striae may be familial. After delivery they usually fade although they never disappear completely.

VASCULAR ABNORMALITIES: SPIDER ANGIOMAS, PALMAR ERYTHEMA, AND EPULIS

The underlying cause of these changes is thought to be high levels of circulating estrogens.

1. *Telangiectasias*. Commonly referred to as vascular spiders, telangiectasias are tiny, stellate or branched, slightly raised and pulsating end-arterioles. The spiders are usually found on the neck, thorax, face, and arms. They are also described as focal networks of dilated arterioles radiating about a central core. Vascular spiders appear during the second to the fifth month of pregnancy in 65% of white women and 10% of black women. The spiders usually disappear after delivery.

2. *Palmar erythema*. Pinkish red, diffuse mottling or well-defined blotches are seen over the palmar surfaces of the hands in about 60% of white women and 35% of black women during pregnancy.

3. *Epulis and bleeding gums*. Epulis (gingival granuloma gravidarum) is a red, raised nodule on the gums that bleeds easily. This lesion may develop around the

third month and usually continues to enlarge as pregnancy progresses. Treatment by excision is initiated only if it becomes excessive in size, causes pain, or bleeds excessively.

OILY SKIN AND ACNE

Oily skin and acne may occur during pregnancy. For other women the skin clears and looks radiant.

HIRSUTISM

An increase in fine hair growth may occur but then tends to disappear after pregnancy; however, coarse or bristly hair growth usually remains. Some women comment that their hair is thickest and most abundant during pregnancy.

FINGERNAIL CHANGES

By the sixth week some women notice thinning and softening of the nails.

IMPLICATIONS FOR NURSING ACTIONS

The woman and her family need to be informed that these changes are to be expected during pregnancy. However, if they have any questions, or if any of the changes occur, the physician is consulted. The woman and her family are encouraged to verbalize their reactions to her skin changes. To prevent deepening of the hyperpigmentation that occurs naturally, the woman is advised to avoid exposure to the sun by covering up or by using sun screen lotions. If the stretching causes a sensation that resembles itching, the woman may use an oil preparation* for relief.

There is an interesting old wives' tale associated with the striae, which, if implemented, results in potential harm to mother and fetus. It is the erroneous belief that the ingestion of laundry starch (e.g., Argo starch) will result in a smooth, unbroken, unstriated skin in pregnancy. Women who then consume this starch (pica) may fulfill caloric requirements (since the Argo starch is a carbohydrate) of pregnancy, but these would be empty calories. The woman would be malnourished, her fetus an SGA infant, and she would be at risk for metabolic disease of late pregnancy. This old wives' tale must therefore be debunked.

Good dental hygiene with mild toothpaste and mouth wash, use of a soft brush, and dental check-ups is necessary during pregnancy. Gingival granulomas may develop as a result of dental calculus that builds up when dental hygiene is poor, or an infection is possible. If fingernail changes occur, nail polish and polish remover may need to be discontinued and the nails kept short to prevent breakage.

*A cooking oil works just as well as more expensive skin preparations and is considerably less costly and more readily available.

Changes in the Musculoskeletal System

The gradually changing body and increasing weight of the pregnant woman cause marked alterations in posture and walking. The great abdominal distention, decreased abdominal muscle tone, and increased weight bearing in late pregnancy require a realignment of the spinal curvatures. An increase in the normal lumbosacral curve develops, and a compensatory curvature in the cervicodorsal region (exaggerated anterior flexion of the head) is required to maintain balance. Large breasts and a stoop-shouldered stance will further accentuate the lumbar and dorsal curves. Locomotion is more difficult, and the waddling gait of the gravid woman, termed "the proud walk of pregnancy" by Shakespeare, is well known. The ligamentous and muscular structures of the mid and lower spine may be severely stressed. These and related changes often cause musculoskeletal discomfort.

The young, well-muscled woman may tolerate these changes without complaint. However, older women or those with a back disorder or a faulty sense of balance may have a considerable amount of back pain during and just after pregnancy.

Slight relaxation and increased mobility of the pelvic joints are normal during pregnancy. This is secondary to exaggerated elasticity of connective and collagen tissue, the result of increased circulating steroid sex hormones and the hormone relaxin. The degree of relaxation varies, but considerable separation of the symphysis pubis and the instability of the sacroiliac joints may cause pain and difficulty in walking. Obesity and multiple pregnancy tend to increase the pelvic disability.

IMPLICATIONS FOR NURSING ACTIONS

The gravida and her family benefit from knowing that pregnancy causes some changes in the musculoskeletal system, which may lead to discomfort. The degree of discomfort experienced could be decreased by the following: rest periods; good posture at all times; good body mechanics while bending, lifting, and getting up; avoidance of heavy lifting; wearing low-heeled, sturdy supportive shoes; wearing a comfortable well-fitted brassiere; moderate exercise (dancing or swimming) designed for pregnant women; the "pelvic rock." For some women, maternity girdles may bring relief. Women who have occupations in which a degree of coordination and balance is required may have to take maternity leave from work. For additional discussion see Table 17.10.

Neurologic Changes

Little is known regarding specific alterations in function of the neurologic system during pregnancy, aside from hypothalamic-pituitary neurohormonal changes. Certainly no characteristic gestational electroencephalography (EEG) variations have been described, although pregnancy-induced hypertension (eclampsia) may grossly distort the normal brain-wave pattern. Specific physiologic alterations caused by pregnancy may cause the following neurologic or neuromuscular symptomatology:

1. Compression of pelvic nerves or vascular stasis caused by enlargement of the uterus may result in sensory changes in the legs, for example, meralgia paresthetica, a condition characterized by objective loss of sensation over the anterolateral aspect of the thigh because of pressure on the lateral cutaneous nerve (L2-3).

2. Dorsolumbar lordosis may cause pain because of traction on nerves or compression of nerve roots; for example, spondylolisthesis (anterior slippage of the sacrum fom the last lumbar vertebral body) may cause severe backache and posterior leg pain. Herniation of an intervertebral disk and sciatic pain may be aggravated by back curvature during pregnancy.

3. Edema involving the peripheral nerves may result in carpal tunnel syndrome, which is characterized by paresthesia (abnormal sensation such as burning or tingling because of a disorder of the sensory nervous system) and pain in the hand, radiating to the elbow, and is caused by edema and compression of the median nerve beneath the carpal ligament of the wrist. Acroesthesia, or numbness and tingling of the hands, is caused by the stoop-shouldered stance during pregnancy and is assciated with traction on segments of the brachial plexus.

4. Hypocalcemia may cause neuromuscular problems such as muscle cramps or tetany.

Tension headache is common when anxiety or uncertainty complicates gestation. Vision problems such as refractive errors, sinusitis, or migraine may also be responsible for headaches. Gravidas with constant throbbing or "splitting" headache in the frontal, sincipital, or occipital area bilaterally, associated with generalized edema, hypertension, or proteinuria, may have preeclampsia (pregnancy-induced hypertension) (see Chapter 35).

"Lightheadedness," faintness, and even syncope (fainting) are common during early pregnancy. Vasomotor instability, postural hypotension, or hypoglycemia may be responsible.

In addition to the problems mentioned, numerous neurologic disorders (e.g., multiple sclerosis and myasthenia gravis) may or may not be altered by pregnancy.

IMPLICATIONS FOR NURSING ACTIONS

See Table 17-10 for nursing actions regarding neurologic changes during pregnancy.

Gastrointestinal Changes

The functioning of the gastrointestinal tract during pregnancy presents a curiously interesting picture: the appetite increases, nausea and vomiting may occur, motility is diminished, intestinal secretion is reduced, liver function is altered, and absorption of nutrients is enhanced.

MOUTH

The gums are hyperemic, spongy, and swollen, and they tend to bleed easily because the rising level of estrogen causes selective increased vascularity and connective tissue proliferation (a nonspecific gingivitis). There is no increase in secretion of saliva. Women do complain of excessive salivation (ptyalism); however, this is just an apparent increase. This perceived increase is thought to be due to a decrease in unconscious swallowing by the woman when nauseated. Epulis and bleeding gums are discussed under Skin Changes.

TEETH

The pregnant woman requires about 1.2 g of calcium and approximately the same amount of phosphorus every day during pregnancy. This is an increase of about 0.4 g of each of these elements over nonpregnant needs. With a well-balanced diet (see Chapter 18), these requirements are satisfied. Serious dietary deficiency, however, may deplete the mother's osseous stores of these elements but does not draw on calcium in her teeth. Demineralization of teeth does not occur during pregnancy. Hence the old adage "for every child a tooth" is untrue. Poor dental hygiene during pregnancy or anytime and gingivitis may contribute to dental caries, which could result in the loss of a tooth.

APPETITE

In early pregnancy the woman may experience an *increase in appetite*. *Nausea and vomiting* that usually begin between the first and second missed periods (weeks 6 to 8) generally suppress the appetite. High levels of HCG and possibly cultural expectation, emotional factors, or hypoglycemia may contribute to this "morning sickness," which can occur at any time during the day. The increased basal metabolism associated with pregnancy secondary to the 24 hour a day (continuous) fetal and maternal body functions predisposes to a state of hypoglycemia, especially after a period of fasting (as between the evening meal and breakfast). This type of morning nausea tends to disappear if the woman eats a high-protein snack at bedtime. Nausea that is secondary to lengthy intervals between meals or to inferior quality of diets (i.e., high carbohydrates, low protein) can be corrected with frequently spaced, small meals of high-quality (protein) foods.

The woman's *taste sense* may be blunted or altered. She may show a preference for fruits, salty foods, or spicy foods, or she may think that "everything smells or tastes like celery." She may develop a dislike for certain foods such as coffee or sweets.

Strange aversions to food or curious food cravings may develop during gestation. The type of substance eaten seems to be based in local tradition and availability. The most common substances ingested in the United States are red clay and starch (Argo laundry starch is most commonly preferred), but cravings for coal, dirt, or plaster have been noted. *Pica* is defined as a craving for unusual substances or a bizarre appetite. The danger of pica lies in substituting nutritionally empty foods for the needed well-balanced diet (see Chapter 18).

ESOPHAGUS AND STOMACH

Although nausea and vomiting may be emotional in origin or occur in response to the presence of HCG or increased levels of progesterone, it may also result from ingestion of iron, hepatitis, dehydration, hypoglycemia, or certain odors. If vomiting persists beyond the first trimester or is excessive at any time, it is termed *hyperemesis gravidarum* (see Chapter 36).

Herniation of the upper portion of the stomach *(hiatal hernia)* occurs after the seventh or eighth month of pregnancy in about 15% to 20% of gravidas. This condition results from upward displacement of the stomach, which causes a widening of the hiatus of the diaphragm. It occurs more often in multiparas and older or obese women.

Increased estrogen production causes decreased secretion of hydrochloric acid. Therefore peptic ulcer formation or flare-up of existing peptic ulcers is uncommon during pregnancy.

Increased progesterone production causes decreased tone and motility of smooth muscles, so that there is esophageal regurgitation, decreased emptying time of the stomach, and reverse peristalsis. As a result the woman may experience "acid indigestion" or *heartburn* (pyrosis).

SMALL INTESTINE

In response to increased needs during pregnancy, iron is absorbed more readily. In general, if the individual is deficient in iron, iron absorption is increased.

COLON

Increased progesterone (causing loss of muscle tone and decreased peristalsis) results in an increase in water absorption from the colon. *Constipation* may result. In addition, constipation is secondary to hypoperistalsis (sluggishness of the bowel), unusual food choice, lack of fluids, abdominal distention by the pregnant uterus, and displacement of intestines with some compression. *Hemorrhoids* (varicose veins of the rectum and anus) may be everted or may bleed during straining at stool. Bowel habits and a characteristic type of stool are established early in life. Variations will be noted with concern and may be perceived as a disease process. A mild ileus (sluggishness, lack of movement) that follows delivery, as well as postdelivery fluid loss and perineal discomfort, contributes to continuing constipation.

GALLBLADDER

Decreased emptying time of the gallbladder is typical. This feature, together with slight hypercholesterolemia from increased progesterone levels, may account for the frequent development of *gallstones* during pregnancy.

LIVER

Hepatic function is difficult to appraise during gestation. However, only minor changes in liver function develop during pregnancy. Occasionally, intrahepatic cholestasis (retention and accumulation of bile in the liver, due to factors within the liver) in response to placental steroids, occurs late in pregnancy and may result in *pruritus gravidarum* (severe itching) with or without jaundice. Oatmeal baths and lotions help ease the itching. These distressing symptoms subside promptly after delivery.

ABDOMINAL PAIN

Intraabdominal alterations that can cause discomfort include pelvic heaviness or pressure, round ligament tension, flatulence, distention and bowel cramping, and uterine contractions. In addition to displacement of intestines, pressure from the expanding uterus increases venous pressure in the pelvic organs. Although most abdominal discomfort is a consequence of normal maternal alterations, the physician is constantly alert to the possibility of disorders such as bowel obstruction or an inflammatory process.

Appendicitis (see p. 989) may be difficult to diagnose. The *appendix* is displaced upward and laterally, high and to the right, away from McBurney's point.

IMPLICATIONS FOR NURSING ACTIONS

Nursing actions for pregnancy-induced gastrointestinal tract discomforts are also presented in Table 17.10.

Endocrine Changes

Profound endocrine changes occur that are essential for pregnancy maintenance, normal fetal growth, and postpartal recovery (Table 15.4).

PITUITARY GLAND

Although slight enlargement of the anterior lobe of the pituitary occurs during pregnancy, prolactin (PRL) is the only hormone that is produced in greater amounts. During pregnancy the anterior pituitary continues to produce all the hormones exhibited in the nonpregnant state, but the amounts noted may be slightly different. This relative inactivity of the anterior pituitary is seemingly due to suppression, principally by HCG. Further support for this opinion is the observation that the levels of follicle-stimulating hormone (FSH) fall to clinically undetectable levels by the tenth day after ovulation and remain there during the entire pregnancy. Secretion of the gonadotropins FSH, LH, and growth hormone (GH) may actually decrease. This inhibition of gonadotropin synthesis and release may be caused by elevated levels of the estrogen and progesterone produced by the fetoplacental unit. FSH remains

Table 15.4
Hormonal Factors in Pregnancy

Hormone and Source	Principal Effects	Clinical Significance
Fetoplacental unit		
Estrogen: produced by ovary and adrenal cortex as in prepregnant state; however, principal source is placenta. Synthesized from precursors from fetal liver and adrenals. Increase in level of E_3 (estriol) by end of fourth wk; by end of pregnancy, 300 × normal. However, low potency of E_3 means estrogenic activity only 30 × normal	Level of circulating estriol rises in pregnancy and so increases in urine and amniotic fluid	Urinary excretion of 30-40 mg/24 hr of estriol by end of pregnancy—an indication of fetal well-being (must be repeated, i.e., serial): Significant decrease indicates fetus in jeopardy (or fetal death) Excessive increase may indicate multiple pregnancy, erythroblastosis fetalis
	Enlargement of uterus: Hypertrophy of musculature Proliferation of endometrium Increase in blood supply	Probable sign of pregnancy Continued growth indicates pregnancy advancing
	Enlargement of breast	Breast tenderness
	Growth of glandular tissue ducts, alveoli, nipples	
	Deposition of fat	
	Enlargement of genitalia	Growth of vagina permits passage of infant
	Nutrient metabolism altered: Increases elastic properties of connective tissue (relaxation of pubic joints and pelvic ligaments; cervix enlarges, softens, is stretchable [theory])	Softening of connective tissue: Backache, tenderness over pubic area, flank pain Cervical dilation
	Decreased secretion of HCl, pepsin	Digestive upsets, nausea, decreased absorption of fat

Table 15.4—cont'd
Hormonal Factors in Pregnancy

Hormone and Source	Principal Effects	Clinical Significance
	Affects thyroid function: thyroxine production increases, but so does production of thyroxine-binding globulin	No major increase in free thyroxine (BMR rises primarily as result of increased O_2 consumption with growth of uterus, fetus, placenta)
	Interferes with folic acid metabolism	
	Increase in total body proteins	Positive nitrogen balance: protein available for fetal growth
	Sodium and water retention by kidney tubules	Increased plasma volume and interstitial fluid volume→edema, fluid reserve
	Hematologic changes:	Safety mechanism vs. hemorrhage
	Hypercoagulability of blood	Tendency for thrombosis to occur (legs)
	Decrease in fibrinolytic activity	Affects use in clinical diagnosis using SR tests (no diagnostic value)
	Increase in sedimentation rate (SR)	
	Vascular changes:	No clinical significance; changes usually disappear after pregnancy
	Telangiectases (spider nevi)	
	Palmar erythema	
	Stimulation of production of melanin-stimulating hormone	Hyperpigmentation (chloasma, linea nigra, areolar tissue, genitalia)
Progesterone: produced by corpus luteum for 2 mo and by placental trophoblastic cells) from about 8-10 days after conception; rises steadily through pregnancy	Promotes development of decidual (secretory) cells in endometrium	Glycogen deposits support nutrition of embryo
	Decreases contractility of gravid uterus	Prevents uterine contractions from causing spontaneous abortion
	Promotes development of secretory portions of lobular-alveolar system	Prepares breasts for lactation
	Nutrient effects:	Nutritional significance:
	Favors maternal fat deposition	Energy available for maternal and fetal needs
	Reduced gastric motility, sphincters relaxed	Regurgitation (heartburn); small, frequent feedings tolerated
	Increases sodium excretion	Hyponatremia may develop
	Increases sensitivity of respiratory center to CO_2	Respiratory rate increases; decreased alveolar and arterial P_{CO_2} (feeling of breathlessness)
	Reduces tone of smooth muscle	Colonic activity diminishes (constipation)
		Reduced tone of bladder and ureters (distention, urinary stasis, urinary tract infections)
		Vascular tone decreases (venous dilation; stasis in lower limbs with edema, varicosities)
		Decreased tone in gallbladder: reduced motility; incidence of gallbladder disease increases
	Raises body temperature 0.5° C	Feelings of warmth, perspiration increases
Human chorionic gonadotropin (HCG): produced by syncytiotrophoblast. Peak level by day 60-70 of gestation; levels fall after fourth mo, disappear 2 wk after pregnancy ends	Maintenance of corpus luteum in early pregnancy	Corpus luteum not necessary after first few weeks—placenta produces sufficient hormones
	Exerts interstitial-cell–stimulating effect on testes of male fetus	Testosterone levels in male fetus rise
	May have immunologic properties	May inhibit lymphocyte response to foreign protein, the fetal portion of placenta
	May cause allergic response	May be cause of hyperemesis gravidarum
		Diagnostic value:
		Persistence of HCG after spontaneous abortion symptomatic of hydatidiform mole or choriocarcinoma
		Basis for hormone test for pregnancy
		Decreased level in threatened abortion
		Increased level with multiple pregnancies

Continued.

Table 15.4—cont'd
Hormonal Factors in Pregnancy

Hormone and Source	Principal Effects	Clinical Significance
Human chorionic somatomammotropic hormone (HCS) (also called human placental lactogen [HPL] or chorionic growth hormone [CGH]): produced by syncytiotrophoblast; detectable by wk 5 or 6; rises steadily, disappears 2 wk after delivery	Similar action to pituitary growth hormone:	
	Glucose metabolism:	Glucose metabolism changes result in:
	Decreases use of glucose for energy by maternal organism by increasing lipolysis to make fatty acids available for energy (carbohydrate sparer)	Glucose available for fetal energy needs (only energy source for fetus)
	Glycogen deposition increased, cells saturated (inhibits glyconeogenesis), causing blood glucose levels to rise	Diabetogenic effect in mother (increased blood glucose levels stimulate β cells of islets of Langerhans to produce more insulin)—may "burn out," producing diabetes mellitus
	Carbohydrates and insulin required for hormone activity	Fetal pancreas produces insulin by wk 12; maternal insulin does not cross placenta. Fetal pancreas may overproduce if continuous hyperglycemic stimulus is present. At birth infant becomes hypoglycemic and brain growth is endangered
	Protein metabolism:	Protein metabolism:
	Increases protein synthesis Decreases breakdown and utilization of protein for energy (mobilizes free fatty acids; if excessive, may cause ketosis)	Protein available for fetal and maternal growth needs
	Acts synergistically with hydrocortisone and insulin in development of alveoli of breast (lactogenic effect)	Preparation of breasts for lactation
	Amount secreted depends on size of placenta	Research to determine whether level of circulating HCS (HPL, CGH) an indicator of normal pregnancy
Origin: multiple organs		
Prostaglandins: widely distributed in human body, including seminal fluid, brain, nerves, most endocrine organs, endometrium, decidua, and amniotic fluid	Reproductive system: play a role in erection, ejaculation, ovulation, formation of corpus luteum, uterine motility, parturition, and milk ejection	Prostaglandins are used to induce labor in second-trimester abortions; may be used (research in progress) for induction of labor at term
	Cardiovascular system: play a role in platelet aggregation, blood pressure increase	
Ovary		
Relaxin	Present in many mammalian species and is thought to: Prevent premature labor Promote relaxation of pelvic joints and cervical softening Stimulate growth of breasts	Same as principal effects
Pituitary		
Pituitary growth hormone: produced by anterior pituitary	Decreases markedly during pregnancy and rises slowly to prepregnancy level 6-8 wk after delivery	May be reason why insulin requirements decrease after delivery (HCS ↓ with delivery of placenta)

Table 15.4—cont'd
Hormonal Factors in Pregnancy

Hormone and Source	Principal Effects	Clinical Significance
Follicle-stimulating hormone (FSH): produced by anterior pituitary	Decreases markedly during pregnancy; remains low for 10-12 days after delivery	Ovulation ceases during pregnancy
	Increases then to follicular-phase concentrations during third week after delivery	Ovulation recurs 6 wk after delivery in 10-15%, 12 wk in 30% of nonlactating women (first menses usually follows anovulatory cycle)
Prolactin (PRL): produced by anterior pituitary	Lactation: stimulates production of fat, lactose, and casein by mammary glandular cells after placenta is delivered May play role in regulation of fluid exchange across fetal membranes, lung maturation, and pregnancy maintenance	Milk not produced prenatally despite high levels because high levels of estrogen have a local inhibitory effect on mammary gland
Oxytocin: produced by *posterior* pituitary	Causes uterus to contract Action suppressed by action of progesterone until production of oxytocin exceeds that of progesterone Stimulates myoepithelial cells in mammary glands to eject milk	May be used to induce or augment labor Spurt of oxytocin during expulsive phase of labor to ensure efficient muscle contraction during and immediately after birth Sensory receptors in nipple stimulate release of oxytocin via reflex arc

low for 10 to 12 days after delivery; it increases to normal concentrations during the third week after delivery. Ovulation recurs 6 weeks after delivery in 10% to 15% of nonlactating women and at 12 weeks in 30% of nonlactating women.

PRL is produced by the *anterior pituitary* of the mother and the fetus. Its level rises with the rising levels of estrogen. Its primary effect, initiation of lactation, does not occur during pregnancy because estrogen has a local inhibiting effect on mammary gland milk production. With the delivery of the placenta, estrogen levels fall rapidly, and prolactin is now free to initiate the production of fat, lactose, and casein by mammary glandular cells. Continued lactation depends on the suckling of the infant (see Chapter 30).

Melanotropic hormone is increased, causing the added pigmentation of skin that is characteristic of pregnancy.

Oxytocin is produced by the *posterior pituitary* in increasing amounts as the fetus matures. There is a spurt of oxytocin during the expulsive phase of labor to ensure efficient muscle contraction during and immediately after delivery. When stimulated by the suckling infant, sensory receptors in the nipple cause the release of oxytocin via a neural reflex arc. During lactation oxytocin stimulates myoepithelial cells in the mammary gland to eject milk.

FETOPLACENTAL HORMONE PRODUCTION

After fertilization the woman's hormonal pattern differs greatly from that observed during the menstrual cycle. The steroid sex hormone effects are clearly reflected in the endometrium after implantation (nidation), as shown in Fig. 15.9.

Estrogens continue to rise after implantation. Placental production of estrogens is evidenced by ovarian inactivity during pregnancy. In contrast, progesterone production begins to rise rapidly at ovulation and continues to rise until the third or fourth week of pregnancy. Then the level decreases until the sixth to eighth week of pregnancy, when responsibility for progesterone production is transferred from the corpus luteum to the placenta. Thereafter the titer rises rapidly again as pregnancy progresses and the placenta increases in size. Progesterone levels may fall just before the onset of labor.

The placenta synthesizes steroid hormones, but to accomplish this, it must receive some essential steroid precursors from other sources. Some of these essential materials, such as estriol, are produced by the fetus; others, such as cholesterol, are produced by the mother.

Of the primary estrogens produced by the fetoplacental unit (i.e., estradiol, estrone, and estriol), estriol probably is the most important estrogen during preg-

Fig. 15.9
Changes in endometrium and corpus luteum if pregnancy occurs (in days).

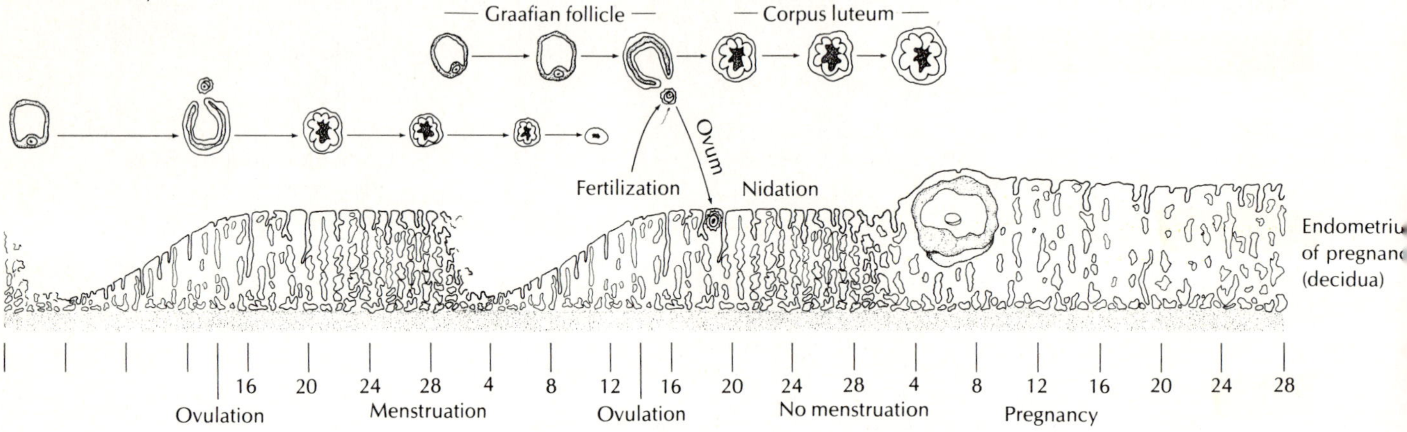

nancy. Fetal and maternal estriol is significant in fetoplacental metabolism. In the presence of an adequately functioning fetoplacental unit and maternal liver and kidneys, maternal urinary estriol values continue to rise from conception to term (40 weeks' gestation).* Because the fetal contribution to estriol production is so considerable (90%), the measurement of the excreted urinary estriol is one *index of fetal well-being*.

HCG, a placental hormone, as measured in the peripheral plasma, rises sharply about 10 days after ovulation to an initial peak at about the sixteenth day after ovulation (a total of 40 days since the first day of the last menstrual cycle). The titer then sinks to a slightly lower level by the twelfth week where it remains for the duration of pregnancy. Although HCG appears to support the corpus luteum early in pregnancy, the function of this hormone later in gestation is unknown. The presence of HCG in maternal serum and urine is the basis for pregnancy tests (see p. 275). Exceedingly high levels of HCG indicate a multiple gestation (twins or triplets) or a serious complication such as hydatidiform mole or choriocarcinoma (see Chapter 35).

In addition to HCG, chorionic somatomammotropin (HCS) (also known as human placental lactogen [HPL]) is the other hormone of strictly placental origin. HCS has an anabolic effect similar to growth hormone and is measured in gradually increasing amounts during pregnancy. Like HCG, HCS slowly dissipates after delivery.

*That is, if there is some disorder that impairs placental function (e.g., hypertension) or if the mother's liver or kidney function is impaired, estriol levels cannot be used as an index of fetal status.

OVARY

The hormone relaxin is produced during pregnancy. Relaxin is thought to prevent premature labor and promote relaxation of pelvic joints and softening of cervix.

THYROID GLAND

Pregnancy induces slight hyperplasia of the thyroid, which results in an increase in iodine metabolism. This is apparent in increased radioactive iodine uptake by the thyroid in experimental animals. Slight but recognizable thyroid gland enlargement occurs by the third month, usually without progression. Iodine is bound to thyroxine in blood. Return to normal size and function can be expected by the sixth postnatal week.

The pregnant woman's basal metabolic rate (BMR) rises by the fourth month and increases almost 25% by term. The elevated BMR actually reflects the demands of the uterus and its contents and the greater oxygen consumption from increased maternal cardiac work. Within a week following delivery, the BMR returns to the nonpregnant level. Elevation of BMR is an objective sign that is one of the presumptive manifestations of pregnancy (see p. 269).

PARATHYROID GLANDS

Pregnancy induces a slight secondary hyperparathyroidism, a reflection of increased requirements for calcium and vitamin D. When the needs for growth of the fetal skeleton are greatest (during the last half of pregnancy), plasma parathormone levels are elevated; that is, the peak level occurs between 15 and 35 weeks' gestation.

ADRENAL GLANDS

The adrenal cortex thickens slightly, and a "pregnancy zone" has been described. Little change in adrenal function occurs during pregnancy, however.

PANCREAS

The fetus requires significant amounts of glucose for its growth and development. To meet its need for fuel, the fetus not only depletes the store of maternal glucose but also decreases the mother's ability to synthesize glucose by siphoning off her amino acids. Maternal blood glucose levels fall. Maternal insulin does *not* cross the placenta to the fetus. As a result, in early pregnancy, the pancreas decreases its production of insulin.

However, as pregnancy continues, the placenta grows and produces progressively larger amounts of hormones (i.e., HCS [HPL], estrogen, and progesterone). Cortisol production by the adrenals also increases. HCS, estrogen, progesterone, and cortisol collectively decrease the mother's ability to utilize insulin. Cortisol stimulates increased production of insulin but also increases the mother's peripheral resistance to insulin (i.e., the tissues cannot use the insulin). Insulinase is an enzyme produced by the placenta to deactivate maternal insulin. Decreasing the mother's ability to utilize her own insulin is a protective mechanism that ensures an ample supply of glucose for the needs of the fetoplacental unit.

The result is an added demand for insulin by the gravida. The normal beta cells of the islets of Langerhans in the pancreas can meet the demand for insulin that continues to increase at a steady rate until term (for a discussion of gestational diabetes mellitus, see Chapter 36).

• • •

In Table 15.5, content from Chapter 14 ("From Conception to Birth") and this chapter is summarized in chronologic order. Events in embryologic/fetal development appear alongside maternal adaptations to pregnancy. (See also Chapter 17, "Nursing Care during the Prenatal Period.")

References and Readings

Benson, R.C., editor: Current obstetric and gynecologic diagnosis and treatment, ed. 4, Los Altos, Calif., 1982, Lange Medical Publications.

Danforth, D.N., editor: Obstetrics and gynecology, ed. 4, Philadelphia, 1982, Harper & Row, Publishers.

Guyton, A.C.: Textbook of medical physiology, ed. 5, Philadelphia, 1976, W.B. Saunders Co.

Malasanos, L., et al.: Health assessment, ed. 2, St. Louis, 1981, The C.V. Mosby Co.

Table 15.5
Summary: Fetoplacental Growth and Development by Calendar Months, and Maternal Response

Menstrual Age	Embryonic and Fetal Development	Uterine Changes	Possible Maternal Signs and Physiologic Changes in Pregnancy
Month: first			
			Menstruation
Week 1		Weight: 60 g (2 oz) Length: 6.5 cm ($2\frac{1}{2}$ in) Capacity: 1-2 ml	
Week 2		Menstrual phase: estrogenic, proliferative, follicular, or preovulatory	Cervical mucus becoming clear, slippery (like raw egg white) with a lubricative sensation; dried mucus shows fern arborization at midcycle
			Ovulation and fertilization
Week 3	Unfertilized ovum to fertilized egg—zygote—to free blastocysts to implanting blastocyst	Menstrual phase: progestational, secretory, luteal, or postovulatory	Basal body temperature remains elevated
			Implantation (nidation)
Week 4	Digestive system forming; primitive blood cells present	Mucosa invaded by trophoblasts; endometrium becomes decidua	Nausea; fatigue; breasts tense and tingling

Table 15.5—cont'd
Summary: Fetoplacental Growth and Development by Calendar Months, and Maternal Response

Menstrual Age	Embryonic and Fetal Development	Uterine Changes	Possible Maternal Signs and Physiologic Changes in Pregnancy
Month: second			*Amenorrhea*
Week 5	Embryonic stages begin 3 wk after ovulation: brain, nervous system, heart forming and beginning to function; reproductive system forming; susceptible to teratogenic effect Length: 3 mm (1/8 in)	Human chorionic gonadotropin (HCG) secreted in quantity by chorionic villi; HCG supports corpus luteum	Some painless uterine bleeding (spotting) experienced by 25% of women—cause unknown; basal body temperature elevated and constant; blood glucose low; endocrine test for human chorionic gonadotropin (HCG) positive
Week 6 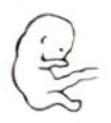	Facial features forming; circulation starts; susceptible to teratogenic effect Length: 4-5 min (3/16 in); weight: 0.4 g	Cervix soft: Goodell's sign	Pressure on bladder from enlarging uterus; turgescence of bladder and urethral walls cause urinary frequency and urgency; breasts heavy
Week 7	Arm and leg buds present (susceptible to teratogenic effect, e.g., thalidomide-produced phocomelia) Length: 14 mm (1/2 in)	Mucous plug forming in cervical canal Uterus—size of a large hen's egg	Profuse vaginal secretions (leukorrhea)—thick, acidic; nausea subsiding; epulis may appear
Week 8	Hands, feet, fingers, and toes forming (susceptible to teratogenic effect); becoming a fetus—ossification of skeleton begins Length: 22-24 mm (about 1 in); weight: about 1 g	Lower uterine segment soft: Hegar's sign Cervix blue: Chadwick's sign	Salivation (ptyalism); breasts larger and nodular; tubercles of Montgomery appear
Month: third			
Week 9	Eyelids forming; genital ridge visible but sexless in character as yet Length: 3 cm (1 1/4 in)	Placenta now secreting progesterone; corpus luteum decreasing in function	
Week 10	Human appearance; respiratory activity evident; becomes a fetus—subsequent development is primarily growth and maturation of existing tissues and structures Length: 4 cm (1 1/2 in); weight: 2 g	Placenta covers one third of uterine wall Uterus: about size of an orange	Vulvar varicosities appear
Week 11	Eyelids fused; sex distinguishable; tooth buds forming; kidney begins secretion; bile present in intestines	Fetal heart tones (FHTs) may be heard by Doppler method in some women by 10-12 wk	
Week 12	External genitalia now show definite signs of male or female sex; fingernails and toenails forming Length: 9 cm (3 1/2 in); weight: 15 g (1/2 oz)	Uterus is size of a grapefruit; fundus is at level of symphysis pubis (SP)	Nausea and vomiting rare now
Week 13 (end of first trimester) 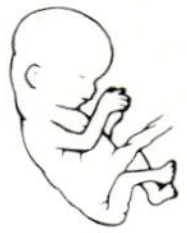	Muscles contract occasionally, weakly; period of organogenesis (organ differentiation and hyperplasia) ends—fetus less susceptible to teratogenic effect from now on; growth continues primarily by hypertrophy (increase in cell size)	Uterus rising from pelvic cavity, becoming an abdominal organ that can be felt above SP	Bladder pressure lessens; blood glucose elevated

Month: fourth			
Week 14	Sex easily distinguishable; thyroid and liver functional; blood forming in bone marrow Length: 10-11.5 cm (4 in); weight: 19 g	Uterus is now an abdominal organ Internal ballottement present (Fig. 17.4)	Blood volume starts to increase; cardiac output increases
Week 15	Lanugo appearing; head hair forming	Uterine contractions occur but are not externally palpable as yet	Physiologic anemia; free hydrochloric acid in gastric juice declines
Week 16	Muscles contracting more vigorously; skin transparent; blood vessels visible Length: 16 cm (6½ in)*; weight: about 100 g (4 oz)	Fundal height: midway between SP and umbilicus (U), or 3-4 fingerbreadths (fb) above SP	Gravida may feel fetal movement, or "quickening" Thin watery fluid may be expressed from nipples (precolostrum)
Week 17	Skeleton visible on anteroposterior x-ray film—a positive sign of pregnancy	Uterine souffle (bruit) heard	Pigmentation changes may occur after sixteenth week: chloasma, nipples, areolae
Month: fifth			
Week 18	Vernix caseosa forming on skin; meconium collecting; fetal heart tones (FHTs) may be heard with a fetoscope; fetal movements (quickening) felt by many women now Length: 19 cm (7 in)	Uterine wall thin; fetal movements generally palpable to examiner now	Decisive increase in blood volume starting; nitrogen storage increasing
Week 19	Onset of rapid growth; iron starts to be stored; enamel and dentine deposited	External ballottement may be elicited by examiner at 4-5 mo	
Week 20	FHTs may be heard more easily with a stethoscope—a positive sign of pregnancy; downy lanugo covers almost entire body; some scalp hair Length: 25 cm (10 in); weight: 300 g (10 oz)	Fundal height: 3-4 fb below U Braxton Hicks contractions usually palpable; examiner may be able to palpate fetal movements	Secondary areolae appear Gravida does feel life now
Week 21	Eyebrows and eyelashes visible; scalp hair forming		U flush with skin; relaxation of smooth muscle, of vein walls, of bladder, etc.
Month: sixth			
Weeks 22 to 23	Skin less transparent and wrinkled; vernix caseosa accumulating		Ureteral dilation marked; linea nigra; chloasma (facial melasma, or mask of pregnancy) may appear
Week 24	Skin wrinkled; if born, infant will attempt to breathe; may be viable Length: 30 cm (12 in); weight: 600 g (1¼ lb)	Fundal height: at the U (21 cm above SP)† External ballottement can be elicited now	Period of greatest weight gain starts—1.8-2.3 kg (4-5 lb)/mo
Week 25	Skin red, shiny, thin; face wrinkled ("old man" appearance)		Striae gravidarum may appear
Week 26 (end of second trimester)	Fetal outline may be felt abdominally—a positive sign of pregnancy		Period of lowest hemoglobin level starts; iron therapy is begun now if not started earlier

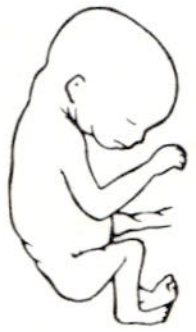

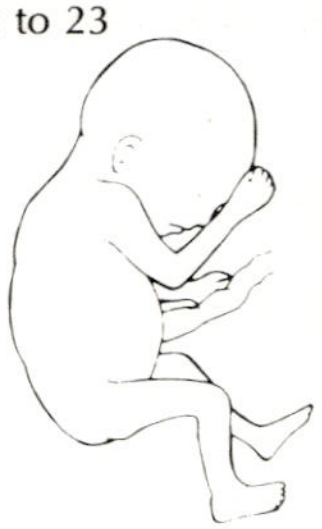

*Haase's rule: for first 5 months, square of lunar month = length in centimeters; for last 5 months, lunar month × 5 = length in centimeters (e.g., fourth lunar month: 4 × 4 = 16 cm; sixth lunar month: 6 × 5 = 30 cm).

†McDonald's rule: Height of fundus in centimeters × 8/7 = duration of pregnancy in weeks (e.g., at 24 wk, fundal height is 21 cm above SP in the average woman/pregnancy).

Continued.

Table 15.5—cont'd
Summary: Fetoplacental Growth and Development by Calendar Months, and Maternal Response

Menstrual Age	Embryonic and Fetal Development	Uterine Changes	Possible Maternal Signs and Physiologic Changes in Pregnancy
Month: seventh			
Week 27	Much iron stored; storage of subcutaneous fat begins; testes begin to descend in male	Uterine wall soft and yielding; start of placental senility	Weight gain continues—1.8 kg (4 lb)/mo
Week 28	Thick, red skin covered with vernix caseosa; eyelids open, fingerprints set; if born, infant can move energetically and cry weakly; viable with appropriate environmental support Length: 35-37 cm (14 in); weight: 1000 g (2½ lb)	Fundal height: 3 fb above U McDonald: 25 cm above SP Spiegelberg: 26.7 cm above SP	Period of lowest hemoglobin level continues
Weeks 29 to 30	Weak cry; more rapid growth starts; start of considerable calcium deposit and storage	Braxton Hicks contractions palpable	Marked protein storage; blood volume highest
Month: eighth			
Week 31	Twice as much calcium deposited as retained by mother; considerable nitrogen stored		Large amount of calcium lost to fetus
Week 32	Presentation: usually vertex—3% breech; testes may descend into scrotal sac Length: 40-42 cm (16 in); weight: 1700-1800 g (4 lb)	Fundal height: 3 fb below xiphoid McDonald: 28 cm above SP Spiegelberg: 30 cm above SP	1.4-1.8 kg (3-4 lb) weight gain this month; striae gravidarum more evident; pelvic joints more relaxed
Weeks 33 to 35	Storage of considerable iron, nitrogen, calcium, and other nutrients; subcutaneous fat storage continues; vernix covers body	Braxton Hicks contractions stronger	Large amount of iron lost to fetus; stomach flaccid, on top of uterus; heartburn common
Month: ninth			
Week 36	Skin thicker and less wrinkled as subcutaneous fat stores accumulate; if born, infant has excellent chance for survival Length: 45-47 cm (18 in); weight: 2000-2500 g (5 lb)	Fundal height: 1-2 fb below xiphoid McDonald: 32 cm Spiegelberg: 32 cm	U protrudes; shortness of breath; hemoglobin level starts to rise

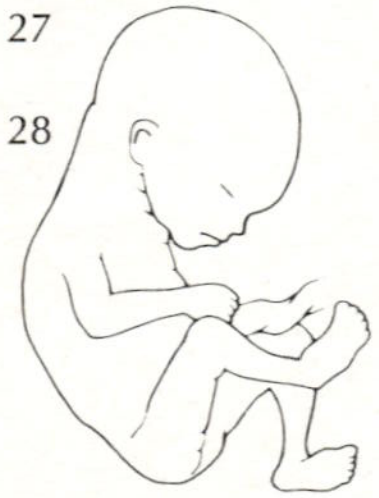

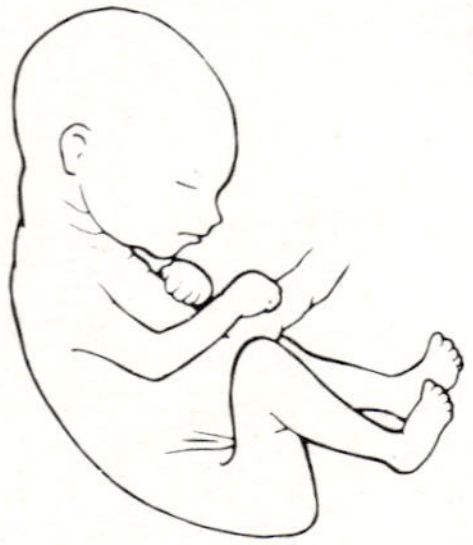

Weeks 37 to 38 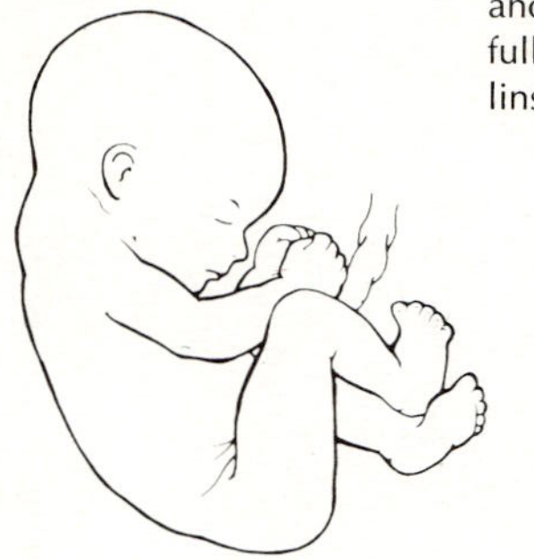	High hemoglobin level, low P_{O_2} tension (cyanotic); body well formed—now considered full term; storage of maternal immunoglobulins to diseases she has had	Fundus at eighth-month level (after engagement in nullipara)	Lightening (nullipara); breathing easier; varicosities more pronounced; ankle edema; urinary frequency
Weeks 39 to 40 (end of third trimester) 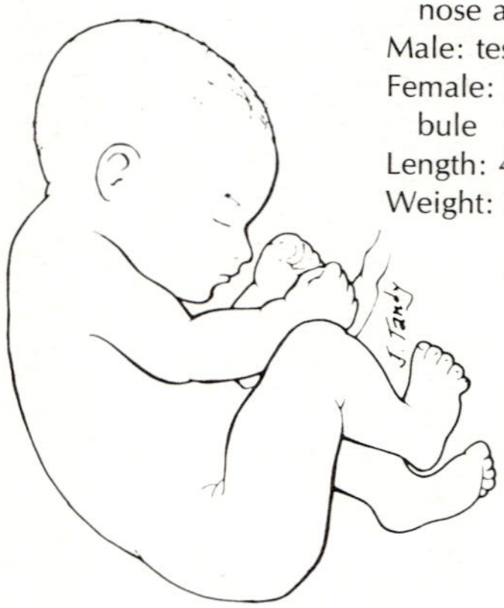	Lanugo shed, except for shoulders, generally; body contours plump; decreased amount of vernix; scalp hair 2-3 cm long; cartilage in nose and ears is well developed Male: testes within well-wrinkled scrotum Female: labia well developed and cover vestibule Length: 45-55 cm (18-22 in) Weight: 3400 g (7½ lb)	Fundal height McDonald: 35 cm Spiegelberg: 37.7 cm Length: 32 cm (12½ in); weight: 1100 g-1200 g (2½ lb) Capacity: 5000 ml Amniotic fluid volume: 500-800 ml to 1200 ml	Lightening with start of labor in parous woman; cervix generally soft, slightly patulous, and partially (nullipara) or totally (para) effaced
Postterm: over 42 weeks	Vernix, lanugo absent; breast tissue: 7 mm; skin dry, thick, desquamating with superficial or deep cracks—parchmentlike Length: bone growth continues; weight may decrease because fetus may need to mobilize own subcutaneous fat to meet metabolic needs	Placental degeneration continues; metabolic exchange diminishing	Impatient for delivery; concern heightened by physician's request for tests to determine fetal well-being; cesarean delivery may be indicated

16
Family Responses to Pregnancy

- Mother-to-be
  - Maternal tasks
    - First trimester
    - Second trimester
    - Third trimester
  - Body image
  - Ambivalence about pregnancy
  - Stress and anxiety
    - Behavior
    - Dependence vs. independence
    - Sexual concerns
    - Adult responsibilities
    - Birth process
    - The child
- Father-to-be
  - Couvade
  - Paternal tasks
    - First trimester
    - Second trimester
    - Third trimester
- Siblings
- Grandparents
- Summary

Pregnancy involves not only the mother-to-be but also the father-to-be, prior offspring, parents, and other family members. All the persons involved react to the event and interpret its meaning in light of their own needs as well as the needs of the others affected. As Colman and Colman (1971) stated, ''Pregnancy is more than simply a biologic event; it is a time of crisis for those involved, a time when identities are changing and new roles are being explored.'' The perceptions of those involved, the coping mechanisms they have evolved, and the situational support systems to which they turn are components in the crisis of pregnancy. To the extent that these three components act to stabilize and reinforce one another, the persons will respond to the crisis event in a positive sense and both they and society will benefit. See Chapter 8 for cultural aspects.

Mother-to-be

Every woman brings to a pregnancy a personalized version of the role of the pregnant woman and the eventual mother. This unique perception has evolved from past experience and will continue to evolve throughout her lifetime. Certain events, such as her own pregnancy, accelerate, intensify, and bring this lifelong process into conscious awareness.

The role of the mother in our culture is undergoing change as women move out of the home and actively participate in the political, economic, and social aspects of the community. However, if a person were asked to select adjectives that would best describe a mother, a career woman, and a lover, the various adjectives used would demonstrate how differently these three roles are conceived. Women today play all three roles and must balance the tasks and responsibilities of each. Regardless of how women now view the relative importance of each role, in actuality they tend to use a classic model of motherhood as a measuring rod for their own endeavors. Although nurses may have accepted the idea of a woman's having a career, they may also view their clients' behavior against what they feel is "right and natural."

The classic model of a mother's role in our culture has been idealized and stereotyped. It may be described as follows: Motherhood and pregnancy are states that are wanted and needed by women to fulfill the natural life cycle. Therefore acceptance of a pregnancy, wanted or not, comes eventually, along with a desire to provide loving and competent care to the child to be born. Mothers-to-be are adults and as such will assume responsibility for their health and their child's health.

It is further expected that the woman will seek, accept, and act on medical advice and care and that she will take participant action in preparing for childbirth and parenthood. That is, she will obtain prenatal care, arrange for a suitable birthing area, preferably in a hospital setting, and attend parent-craft classes.

According to the ideal stereotype, pregnancy is a shared event for the family. As such it is perceived as generally strengthening the family as a unit and permitting the acceptance of atypical maternal behaviors such as increased dependency needs, bizarre desires for food, and rapid mood changes. The time of birth will be shared by a supportive partner, and after the child is born, intuition will assist the mother in being all-wise, all-loving, and all-accepting.

The model is, of course, adapted by each woman in light of her own experiences. Certain experiences seem crucial to this process of adaptation. They include the following:

1. Memories of mothering experienced as a child and the subsequent nature, supportive or nonsupportive, of the mother-daughter relationship
2. The emphasis placed on the primary expression of the feminine role (e.g., dependence vs. independence; motherhood vs. career)
3. The experiences that bolster her self-esteem or that act to lower her feelings of self-worth
4. Stepping-stone roles that have been played (e.g., playing with dolls, taking care of siblings, babysitting)
5. Individuals from the peer group or an older group who acted as negative or positive models and their behaviors that were noted and either emulated or discarded
6. Options open for planning to have children and the here-and-now implications of this pregnancy
7. The use of sexual activity and consequent pregnancy as mechanisms to satisfy needs not necessarily related to the creation of a child and parenthood
8. Economic or social conditions so adverse that the care of another person represents a great burden
9. Social isolation with no family or friends to act as supports

The mother-to-be's perception of her role may be congruent with the model acceptable to her cultural subgroup, or it may be at variance with her subgroup's model. This perception will color her expectations of persons deemed supportive and important to her. However, those who are expected to provide support and care have their own versions of the role of the mother also, and the congruence between these versions and that of the expectant mother will help determine the effectiveness of the support offered and accepted.

MATERNAL TASKS

The prenatal period is a period of preparation for assuming a new role. This period of transition from the nonparent to the parent state (or from the parent of one to the parent of two, etc.) has for many years been divided into three trimesters. These trimesters may be thought of as progressive steps in the emotional development of a new parent, with each step emphasizing a major developmental task. Just as in other developmental sequences, the completion of one task readies the individual for the next. Moreover, there is not an abrupt ending of one task and a beginning of the next, but rather a gradual emergence of the task to follow. Completion of the tasks of the prenatal period means that the woman is ready to move on to the reality phase of the parenthood role.

First trimester

TASK: *To accept the biologic fact of pregnancy. The woman needs to be able to state, "I am pregnant."*

Before the woman can accept the fact that she is indeed pregnant, she must seek an answer to the question, "Am I pregnant?" The hope or fear of being pregnant arises for all sexually active women at some time.

The possibility of pregnancy may come as a result of first intercourse for a teenager: "We, you know, made out last night, and now I'm afraid I'm pregnant"; or "I couldn't be pregnant if it's my first time."

The possibility of being pregnant may follow repeated attempts to become pregnant: "We had been trying to get pregnant for such a long time, and then in the middle of the night I realized I hadn't menstruated. I got so excited thinking that finally it had happened I couldn't sleep the rest of the night."

Once the idea of being pregnant arises, the early symptoms of pregnancy can be used to confirm the idea or dismiss it if denial seems necessary.

For those women prepared to accept a pregnancy, early symptoms prompt them to seek medical validation of pregnancy. Those women who have strong feelings of "not me," "not now," and "not sure" may postpone seeking supervision and care (Rubin, 1970). Many women delay for three missed menstrual periods (fetal age of 10 weeks) before seeking confirmation. This means that a critical period of embryonic-fetal development has passed, and some daily activities, such as the inadvertent taking of drugs, may have had deleterious effects on the developing fetus. For those who will decide to abort the fetus, the time of the least physical effect from the abortion on the woman is limited (Chapter 41).

A positive diagnosis of a suspected pregnancy may be the time when the first overt reactions to its biologic reality are manifested. A woman's emotional response to the confirmation of her suspicions may range from great delight to shock, disbelief, and despair, as seen in the following statements:

> I was just delighted when I heard I was really pregnant. I was so excited I could hardly wait to tell Ron—we talked and talked. I'm still way up there.

> I thought, it can't be; I'm too old! What will he say—we have just finished with the other kids—now to start all over. I can't face it—those 2 AM feedings, diapers, and those terrible 2-year-olds into everything. I feel guilty, but I hate the whole idea.

> I have a terrible time when I'm pregnant; my legs are so swollen and painful and I feel so lumpy and unattractive, but when I am most down I think of the baby and how much she will mean to us, and I get through another day.

Rubin (1970) describes the reaction of many women to confirmation of their pregnancy as the ''someday but not now'' response:

> There is a real pleasure in finding oneself functionally capable of becoming pregnant. There is pleasure in learning that others are pleased with the promise of having, and being given, a child. But these feelings exist independently of the question of time. Personally and privately she is not ready, not now.

Caplan (1959) also reported that the majority of his clients were initially dismayed at finding themselves pregnant. However, dismay gave way to an eventual acceptance of the pregnancy that paralleled the growing acceptance of the reality of the child. He cautioned, however, against assuming that the nonacceptance of the pregnant state can be equated with the rejection of the child, because he believed that women can separate the state of physical pregnancy from the idea of being a parent. Thus a woman may dislike being pregnant but feel love for the child to be born.

In the first trimester, concern centers around the mother's self. There is little appreciation of the child. The pregnancy is experienced as ''something happening to *me*.''

There is often an attempt to conceal the pregnancy from persons other than the father. Society has a stock response to the pregnant woman, ''Oh, how wonderful to be going to have a baby.'' This is not where she is; she would prefer a comment, ''How wonderful *you* are, to be having a baby.''

The pregnant woman's egocentric state needs to be recognized when planning for her care; for example, nutrition counseling should focus on her needs. Emphasis should be placed on her concerns and her discomforts. She needs this ego support while she confronts the idea of her body being a shelter for another. One should not insist on care for the child's good until she has reconciled the nonpregnant and pregnant concepts of herself. She is the one who experiences the symptoms of pregnancy. It is a case of ''I am pregnant.''

Second trimester

TASK: *To accept the growing fetus as distinct from the self. The woman can now state, ''I am going to have a baby.''*

The beginning of future *mother-child relationships* has not been identified through research but by the fifth month most women have accomplished the task of identifying the fetus as a separate being, although still very much a part of themselves. With this acceptance of the reality of the child (hearing the heartbeat and feeling the child move) and with a subsidence of early symptoms, the woman enters a quiet or latent period. At this time she becomes more introspective, and the *fantasy child* takes shape. She appears to withdraw from other relationships and to concentrate her interest on the unborn child. Husbands and children seem to sense this withdrawal. Sometimes husbands will comment on feeling ''left out,'' and children become more demanding in their efforts to redirect the mother's attention to themselves.

If one observes unobtrusively, pregnant women can be seen to hold their abdomens and gently rock them as though they were rocking the child. Many parents talk to the fetus. Conversation reveals the intensity of this intimate woman-baby relationship as women talk freely about the child and their hopes and aspirations for his future. Pet names may be given: ''I called all my babies 'Herman' before they were born.'' Sexual preferences surface: ''I just knew I was going to have a boy this time.'' Some women even begin to plan the child's career: ''I saw her as a ballet dancer.''

The child becomes precious to the woman, and the feeling that ''I am going to have a baby'' supersedes all else.

Third trimester

TASK: *To prepare realistically for the coming of the child and prepare to relinquish it. The woman expresses the thought that ''I am going to be a parent.''*

In the last part of pregnancy, the quiet period is su-

Fig. 16.1
A happy, healthy mother-to-be eagerly awaiting delivery.

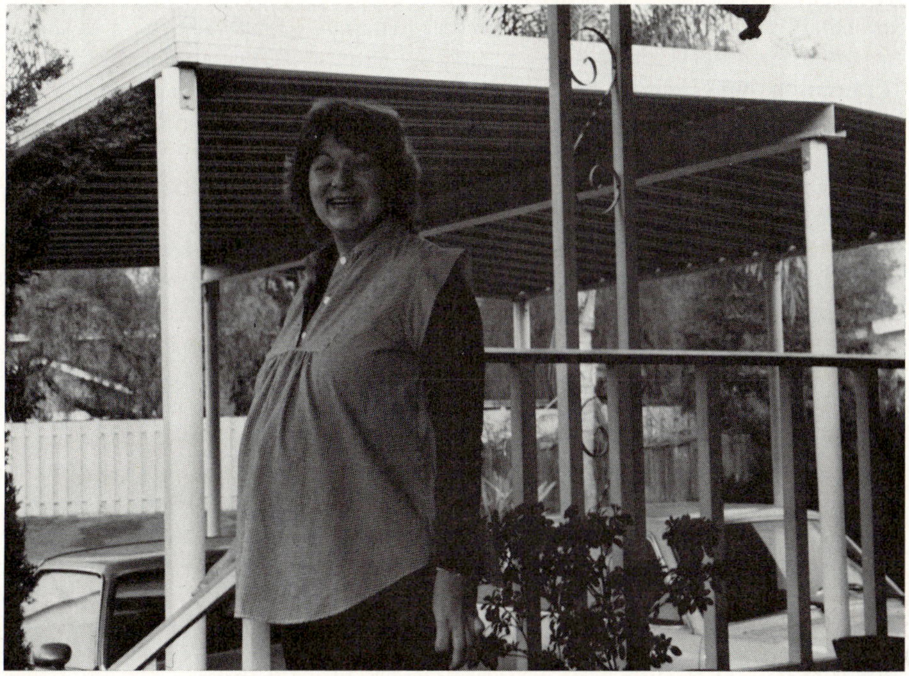

perseded by a more active period that is more oriented to reality on the part of the mother-to-be toward her coming role and toward her child. A recurrence of symptoms brings the physical nature of pregnancy back into the woman's focus of attention. Breathing is difficult, and movements of the fetus become vigorous enough to disturb the mother's sleep. Backaches, frequency and urgency of urination, constipation, and varicose veins become troublesome. The bulkiness and consequent awkwardness of her body impede her ability to care for other children, do routine housekeeping duties, and assume a comfortable position for sleep and rest.

There is a flurry of activity in preparing for the birth. Parents-to-be may enroll in community classes for birth and parenthood. Layettes may be prepared; rooms and cribs are readied for the new arrival. Arrangements are made for the other children's care.

Whether birth is anticipated with joy, dread, or a mixture of both, about the ninth lunar month the majority of women become impatient for labor to begin. There is a strong desire to have the state of pregnancy end, "to be over and done with it." Women at this stage are ready to move on to the next phase: childbirth and assuming their new role as mother (Fig. 16.1).

In addition to accomplishing the developmental tasks of pregnancy certain responses can be identified in pregnant women. These responses relate to changes in body image, ambivalent feelings about the pregnancy, and stress and anxieties relating to herself, her responsibilities, and her child.

BODY IMAGE

The concept we have of our body evolves from the perceptions, feelings, and attitudes we have developed over our life span. This mental picture evolved from our earliest experiences. Children incorporate the perceptions and attitudes of parents; adolescents incorporate those of peer groups; and adults incorporate those of intimates.

A girl who described herself as very tall noted, "Whenever we had visitors my mother would say, 'Stand up and let them see how tall you are.' Now whenever I feel self-conscious I feel tall, tall like the Tower of Pisa."

A young adult who is now thin remarked, "I see myself as very fat. I wonder if I can get through the doorway. When I was a teenager, I was called fatso; that image never leaves me."

The body image may be said to encompass two independent dimensions, one relating to an emotional response to the body and another to its physical appearance as it exists in space.

The physiologic changes of pregnancy result in rapid and profound changes in body contour. The woman's and family's responses to this change become more noticeable as pregnancy advances.

During the first trimester body shape changes little, but by the second trimester obvious bulging of the abdomen, thickening of the waist, and enlargement of the breasts proclaim the state of pregnancy. The woman develops a feeling of an overall increase in the size of her body and of occupying more space. This feeling intensifies as pregnancy advances (Jessner et al., 1970). There is a gradual loss of definite body boundaries that serve to separate the self from the nonself and to provide a feeling of safety from the environment: "I looked in the mirror and wondered if it were really me. I had a sudden feeling that I was ballooning outward, there was no end, and I did not know how to bring it together and be myself again."

These negative feelings may be countered by a "mother earth" feeling, a feeling of being a protective shield for the fetus (Colman, 1969; Deutch, 1945; Rubin, 1970). For most women the feeling of liking or not liking their pregnant bodies is a temporary one and does not cause significant changes in their perceptions of themselves.

AMBIVALENCE ABOUT PREGNANCY

Acceptance of the reality of pregnancy does not seem to be a constant state. Even for those women who are pleased with and accepting of their pregnancies, feelings of hostility toward, and a wishing away of, the unborn child come and go.

Any number of daily events can trigger such feelings, for example, a husband's chance remark about the attractiveness of a slim, nonpregnant woman or hearing about a colleague's promotion when the decision to have a child means relinquishing a job. Even body sensations that come into conscious awareness for the first time can prove unsettling. The concept of pregnancy becomes a set of symptoms—tingling breasts, increased vaginal discharge, frequency and urgency of urination, nausea, vomiting, bizarre food desires, and shortness of breath—all of which under other circumstances would be interpreted as abnormal and in need of treatment. To those who have little knowledge of physiologic responses of the maternal organism to the growing fetus, such symptoms can be alarming as well as uncomfortable. They can give rise to concern about personal safety, wishing for the end of the pregnancy, or regret about having become pregnant.

If birth of a healthy child ensues, memories of these ambivalent feelings are dismissed. If a child with a defect is born, some women remember the times of not wanting the child and feel intensely guilty. Even the most enlightened individuals tend to give credence in times of stress to the "magical powers of thought." Thus a normal and natural response experienced by all persons preparing for a new role is perceived as instrumental in causing the defect of the child.

STRESS AND ANXIETY

Feelings of anxiety are common to all of us. Pregnancy intensifies feelings of anxiety that may be expressed in a number of ways.

Behavior

Mood changes. Disconcerting to the mother-to-be and those around her are the rapid mood changes occasioned by an increased sensitivity to actions and words of those significant to her. Increased irritability, explosions of tears and anger, or feelings of great joy and cheerfulness alternate apparently with little or no provocation. According to one father-to-be:

> I sometimes think she is crazy—we're going somewhere she wants to go—out to dinner or a concert. She goes upstairs happy as a lark and in 2 minutes is down again in a regular temper, won't go, and shouts at me. I really feel bewildered by it all.

Many reasons, such as sexual concerns or fear of pain during delivery, have been postulated to explain this seemingly erratic behavior. It may be that the profound hormonal changes that are part of the maternal response to pregnancy are also responsible for mood changes, much as they are before menstruation or during the menopausal period.

Openness. As pregnancy progresses, another trait becomes noticeable. This is the mother-to-be's openness about her feelings toward herself and others (Caplan, 1959). The layer of reserve that society has hitherto imposed is lifted, and the mother-to-be exhibits a willingness to talk about matters previously not discussed or discussed only within the family confines. She seems to believe that expression of her thoughts and ideas or description of her symptoms will be of interest to and welcomed by the listener. She appears ready to enter into a trusting relationship with the outsider she deems protective. This openness, coupled with a learning readiness, makes working with pregnant women a delight and increases the likelihood of supportive care being therapeutically effective.

Dependence vs. independence. For some women recognition of increasing dependency needs when independence has been attained may give rise to conflict. Pregnancy "shatters the illusion of our separateness and reminds us of our interconnectedness with others" (Colman and Colman, 1974). The woman who is pregnant is never alone, her baby is always with her. She is no longer independent, for she needs both economic and emotional support from her partner. For the woman who equates maturity with "being on her own" and with knowing "who she is," the dependency of pregnancy may seem like regression to a more immature stage of her life. "She may become confused about who she is and what is happening" (Colman and Colman, 1974).

Sexual concerns. Sexual expression during pregnancy is affected by physical, emotional, and interactional factors. The couple's relationship is influenced by myths about sex during pregnancy, sexual dysfunction problems, and physical changes of the woman.

Myths about how the body functions and fantasies about the influence of the fetus as a third party in lovemaking are frequently expressed. Anomalies and mental retardation, as well as other injuries to the mother and fetus, are often attributed to sexual relations at varying points during pregnancy. Many couples have fears that the woman's genitalia will be drastically changed by the birth process. Magical thinking, embarrassment, and hesitancy because of not wanting to appear foolish often prevent couples from expressing these concerns to the health professional.

Dyspareunia (painful intercourse), differing sexual drives, and impotence are the three major dysfunctional problems experienced by pregnant couples. Dyspareunia may be caused by pressure on the pregnant abdomen or deep penile thrusting. In addition to pain during coitus, postcoital cramping and backache may occur. Severe breast tenderness has also been reported by multiparous women during the first trimester.

In addition to dyspareunia, differing sexual drives can create problems for expectant parents. The father-to-be may become frustrated by his partner's sporadic lack of interest in sex. The mother-to-be may have difficulty when her partner becomes confused by her libidinal fluctuations. Changes in the man's level of sexual interest may disturb the woman.

As pregnancy progresses, changes in body shape, body image, and levels of discomfort influence the man's and woman's desire for sexual expression. Whether the pregnant body is perceived as beautiful or repulsive has an impact on the couple's comfort and desire for sexual intimacy. During the first trimester, the woman is frequently plagued by nausea, fatigue, and sleepiness. However, as she progresses into the second trimester, her combined sense of well-being and increased pelvic congestion profoundly increase her desire for sexual release. In the third trimester, fatigue, fetal demands, and physical bulkiness increase her physical discomfort and lower her libidinal interests.

The woman's expanding abdomen may become an object of ridicule and shame or a source of pride for the couple. Some women, who resent losing their shape and wearing waistless maternity clothes, make derogatory comments about their abdomen. Men respond in a variety of ways to their partners' changing shapes. Some say their partners are most beauitful when pregnant, whereas others make derisive comments about the pregnant contours and are repulsed by them.

Communication between the couple is important at this time. Since pregnancy is a developmental crisis, it is a time of emotional upheaval for both the man and the woman. Partners who do not understand the seemingly rapid physiologic and emotional changes of pregnancy can become confused by the woman's erratic behavior. Talking to each other about the changes they are experiencing is of primary importance. When discussed and dealt with constructively, these changes can strengthen the relationship. Unfortunately expectant fathers have received little attention in studies of sex and sexuality during pregnancy. The health professional, however, cannot neglect the problems and concerns expressed by the father.

Adult responsibilities. Realization that pregnancy signals the end of girlhood and the beginning of womanhood and that it is accompanied by new tasks and responsibilities can be shocking and become a source of stress to many young women. Pregnancy, more than any other happening, functions as a rite of passage to maturity in a society that has few other obvious rituals. In many states the pregnant woman is legally an adult regardless of age. She may give personal consent for any type of care for herself or for her newborn. She is entitled to financial and other aid from a government source if needed and, if unwed, is considered the sole legal guardian of her child. As such she retains the right to care for the child herself, place the child in a foster home, or give the child up for adoption.

Birth process. Anxiety can also arise from concern for personal safety during the birth process, or as Rubin (1975) expresses the concern: "seeking a safe passage." This may not be expressed overtly, but cues are given as the nurse listens to the plans most women make for the care of the new baby and other children in case "anything should happen." These feelings persist in spite of the known statistical evidence regarding the safe outcome of pregnancy for the mother. Many women express fear of the pain of delivery. They may fear mutilation because of their ignorance of their body structure and the birth process: "I was afraid I would just split. You know split from front to back—how else would the baby get out—no big baby could come through that small space."

Often women express concern over what behaviors are appropriate during the birth process and how persons caring for them will accept them and their actions. Anxiety about reaching the hospital in time for the birth, practical concerns for the care of children at home, and the uncertainty of being able to plan specific dates for outside help or the partner's vacation combine to make the last few weeks a time of tension. The tension is compounded by a lack of adequate rest.

The child. Parental concern for the health of the child appears to vary over the course of pregnancy (Leifer, 1977). The first concern appears in the first trimester and relates to abortion. One woman related her feelings as follows: "I spotted (blood) off and on. The doctor said, 'If you are going to hold it you will, if you abort it, it is probably just as well.' How could he say 'it'—he was talking about my baby."

As the child becomes more of a reality with movement and an audible heartbeat, parental anxiety is focused on possible defects in either the mental or physical abilities of the child. Parents talk openly about these anxieties and press for confirmation that the child will be all right. Less identifiable in the later stages of pregnancy is the fear about the death of the child; this possibility is evidently a remote one to parents. Death of the infant comes as a great shock; little or no anticipatory grieving has been done.

Father-to-be

The father of her child is probably the most important of those persons who form the pregnant woman's significant others. His thoughts and feelings during pregnancy may in many respects parallel her own. His beliefs about the ideal mother and father and his cultural expectations of appropriate behavior during pregnancy will affect his response to her need for him.

To one individual the pregnant state of his partner may mean freedom to engage in nurturing behavior. To another, it represents a time of loneliness and alienation as the woman becomes physically and emotionally engrossed in her unborn child. He may find himself going outside the home for comfort and understanding, becoming interested in a new hobby, or getting involved with his work. This is often the time of the husband's first extramarital affair. Some men view pregnancy as a proof of their masculinity and as an outcome of their dominant role. To others, pregnancy as a result of intercourse with a woman has no meaning in terms of responsibility to either mother or child. For most women and men, however, pregnancy functions as a time of preparation for the parental role, of fantasy, of great pleasure, and of intense learning.

In parent education classes, in labor units, at the nursery windows, wherever there is an expectant or new father, the complexity and urgency of his needs are dramatically evident. Nursing education and nursing literature once emphasized the mother, her needs, and her relationship to her child. Cartoons, greeting cards, and popular literature perpetuate the image of the expectant father as a comic strip character, anxious and incompetent. He is a figure in the background whose task, aside from that of breadwinner, is to be patient with his wife's moods and bring her flowers. Gradually his existence and strategic position are being recognized; the importance of his role is emerging.

In this chapter, *father* is defined as follows: the male who shares the pregnancy with the female in the psychosocial as well as the biologic sense. The relationship need not be legally sanctioned. Father is used interchangeably with husband, expectant father, or father of a newborn infant. This chapter will not deal with the man who shares the childbearing experience with a woman he knows is pregnant by another man or who was artificially inseminated. No studies have been done to provide data for comparing and contrasting the feelings and needs of these "social" fathers and those of "biologic" fathers.

COUVADE

Couvade (French, "to hatch") is a practice among some primitive peoples in which the man subjects himself to various behaviors and observes taboos associated with pregnancy and giving birth. By enacting the couvade through definite patterns of socially prescribed behaviors, the man's new status is recognized and endorsed. In addition, his responses are channeled into acceptable modes of expression. His behavior acknowledges his psychosocial as well as biologic relationship to the mother and child.

Without a formally recognized and accepted couvade in our society, how do expectant fathers respond to their new status? How do expectant fathers make the transition to their new role with its demands and expectations?

PATERNAL TASKS

The responses of the father-to-be to becoming a father change over the course of pregnancy as do those of the mother-to-be. The behaviors can be grouped into the time periods approximating the three trimesters of pregnancy. The groupings are not mutually exclusive. Threads of each reaction, concern, and informational need span the entire experience but seem to be most obvious in one trimester over another.

First trimester

TASK: *To accept the biologic fact of pregnancy. The man needs to be able to state, "She is pregnant and I am the father."*

The expectant father: I am to become. In essence, the expectant father, like the expectant mother, has been preparing for parenthood for his entire life. Subconsciously he has given some thought to having a wife and children. During courtship and early marriage, the couple's discussion of future plans may even include the number, spacing, and names of their children-to-be. Yet pregnancy and the child remain in the realm of fantasy—illusions that can be savored, elaborated on, toyed with, or cast off at will. The first suspicion of pregnancy actualizes the need for facing role transition *now*. The presumptive signs of pregnancy initiate the first phase of transition from a childless married state to fatherhood.

"I couldn't believe it." "I felt inadequate and apprehensive." "I felt reassured, encouraged, and somewhat relieved that we could get pregnant." These spontaneous remarks, a sampling of men's responses to news of confirmation of pregnancy, voice an inner concern about one's capacity to procreate, a basic human drive, and one's virility. They also reflect an anxiety and uncertainty that accompany role transition. The initial glow (or concern) accompanying confirmation of virility is rapidly followed by a tremendous burst of energy, which finds outlets in diverse activities.

Changing self-concept: provider role identity. The heightened concern for economic security is real. Many young married women are employed outside the home. Although pregnant women and "new" mothers may be employed in a work setting, many childbearing and child-rearing women have a phase of unemployment, the length of which is determined by a combination of factors such as the couple's economic status, the policies of the employer, or the couple's value system. For example, the wife may give up her employment at her husband's insistence: "I can't see a wife of mine working beyond 3 months. For a while I wondered who was going to play the masculine role around here. I'll bring in the bread from now on." Some men attempt to compensate for anticipated needs by keeping their present jobs even though they had planned a change, by putting more effort into earning rapid promotions, by working overtime, or by taking on an extra job.

The concern for providing financially extends beyond the immediate future. Some men take out new or additional insurance at this time.

Even when budgets are inflexible, husbands may arrange for diaper service as early as the sixth month of pregnancy to "help her out." Regardless of budgetary restrictions, husbands often provide for some sort of present for the expectant wife.

Many expectant fathers take an active role in arranging for the wife's medical care. Some search for free clinics. One husband visited the clinic and evaluated the care given before making an appointment for his wife. Those men who wish to participate actively in the event take special care to find physicians who are supportive of the couple's goals. On the other hand, some men think that choosing a physician is women's work and that they need be responsible only for the bills.

Expectant fathers feel more confident during the second trimester. This confidence is overtly expressed in decreased concern about money matters. The initial flurry of activity ends.

Mitleiden: "suffering along." *Mitleiden,* or psychosomatic symptoms of expectant fathers, has long been recognized as a phenomenon of expectant fatherhood. In 1627 Bacon observed, "That loving and kinde Husbands, have a Sense of their Wives Breeding Childe, by some Accident in their owne Body." And in the 1600s, another author commented, "It often falls out, that when the woman is in good health, the husband is sick, yea sometimes being many miles off" (Hunter and Macalpine, 1963).

During discomforts such as nausea, lassitude, aches, and pains the husband sympathizes or identifies with his pregnant wife. Frequently he alone experiences these symptoms. These behaviors can be a positive force bringing the couple closer together and assisting the father to become more responsive to his wife's and child's needs for love and care.

Inquiring about symptoms validates their normalcy and conveys the nurse's understanding of and interest in the couple. Recognizing that the father may be experiencing "pains" brings his needs into focus so they can be dealt with openly. This recognition tends to decrease his tensions and in turn modifies his need to overtly express that tension in actions such as nagging his wife, negating her discomforts, and engaging in potentially dangerous exploits. Before realizing these needs, the nurse may feel annoyed when fathers interrupt their wives to exhibit new wounds (burns, cuts, bruises), to talk of their gas pains and constipation, or to insist that they have bigger and better "potbellies." Fathers were not actually belittling their wives but were trying to convey their feelings in the only way open to them. Acknowledgement of the father's needs by encouraging discussion of feelings results in increased acceptance of each other's responses. This acceptance may facilitate increased openness in other areas of communication between spouses.

The astute nurse can cope with these problems of expectant fathers. Crisis intervention in most cases consists of discussing the problems and anticipations that surround the expectation of a new baby. Only in severe cases is psychiatric referral required.

Second trimester

TASK: *To accept the mother's changing body and the reality of the fetus. The man needs to be able to state, "We are going to have a baby and we are changing."*

Sexuality. Evidence of increased abdominal size and palpable fetal movements heralds a new crisis situation. The man may struggle with feelings about his wife's changing body.*

Discussions on the pros and cons of husbands attending their wives during delivery uncover other areas of concern. Mental pictures of the woman's position during delivery can be upsetting. After seeing a film on delivery, men described their uneasiness when listening to the sounds made by women during the last stage of labor.

In psychoanalytic literature many aspects of the father's behavior are identified as indicators of rivalry. One example is a man's increased frustration and dissatisfaction with his present job—becoming bored with the work or irritated with what is perceived as internal politics and competition among the staff. When the husband is expressing these feelings, the tensions he feels seem to electrify the room. The woman is often amazed and unnerved that her husband is having this type of reaction when he had previously been comfortable and secure in his job. The couple can be forewarned to expect these feelings and discuss them openly when they occur.

Rivalry between the expectant father and his pregnant wife is not new. In Greek legend, Zeus, angered by his wife's superior wisdom after she conceived, swallowed her and later gave birth to Athena, who emerged full grown from his forehead. In the same instant he both punished and replaced his wife.

Direct rivalry with the fetus may be evident, especially during sexual activity. Husbands may protest that fetal movements prevent sexual gratification, making comments such as "we can't have sex with 'that' kicking around in there."

The wife's increased introspection may be a source of anxiety to her husband. He may experience a sense of uneasiness as she becomes preoccupied with thoughts of her mother and sister, with her growing attachment to her male physician, and with her reevaluation of their relationship.

The nurse can prepare the couple for these possible reactions to sexuality and sexual expression during pregnancy and assist the couple in keeping the lines of communication open. When appropriate, the nurse can involve the man in the pregnancy. It has been found that when the husband takes an active role during the pregnancy, the wife is less likely to develop a strong attachment to her male physician.

Father-child relationship. Many fathers are actively and meaningfully involved in the pregnancy, but most find it difficult to relate to the coming child. The woman feels the fetal movements intimately and continuously; the man cannot share this intimacy in the same way. In addition, there is a gap between the time the mother becomes aware of fetal movement and the time when the father can feel the fetus move. The father, however, does have the option to step away physically, intellectually, or emotionally.

Frequently during the second trimester there are attempts to ward off the inevitable with statements such as, "it'll be a while yet" or "the baby isn't really a baby yet." Short excursions or second honeymoons occur during this period. Many wives confide concern about what they perceive to be their husbands' thwarted hopes and dreams. Many men fantasize openly, "If I were single now, I would be going to Australia . . . traveling around the world . . . living in the open with only a knapsack and bedroll . . . taking a chance with a new, exciting job."

In spite of remarks such as those above, many fathers become involved with the coming newborn by means of activities such as picking the child's name, anticipating the child's sex, and discussing the method of feeding the child.

What's in a name? As early as the first month, the name of the child may be selected. Family tradition, religious mandate, and continuation of one's own name or names of relatives and friends are important in the selection process. The names chosen are tried on for fit; for example, the father might emphatically state, "I just cannot picture myself as being a father to a boy named John." Some strive for originality in the name because "a common name just won't do." Armed with several names, one husband said he would decide on his final choice only after he saw the baby, pointing out that "to be named Eric, he *must* be blue eyed and blond."

Concerns in this area center on disagreements between the couple and also between one of the expectant parents and one or both sets of grandparents-to-be. Taking exception to the grandparents-to-be can bring the expectant couple together as a solid front or incite conflict between them. Asking the expectant couple how they arrived at a name can provide data for the nurse's decision to intervene.

Boy or girl? Cultural conditioning colors the couple's

---

*The student is referred to psychoanalytic literature regarding revival of oedipal conflicts, incestuous fantasies, and homosexual/heterosexual drives in the man during pregnancy.

preference for the sex of the firstborn and subsequent children. Women frequently defer to their husband's stated preference. Cultural patterning alone cannot account for all the statements couching personal preference. Men more obviously than women work at finding an internal fit between the anticipated sex of the child and their own comfort with the imagined future relationship with that child.

Most men opt for a son. Some refuse to voice a preference, fearing that verbalization will prevent its coming true. Some refuse to even consider girls' names and will not listen to their wives' prompting to be prepared for a child of either sex.

At the time of birth most parents are able to accept the sex of the child born to them. Although disappointment is evident and often voiced, verbal acceptance is expressed to each other soon after the birth. Frequently personnel assist parents in voicing their disappointment and then point out the positive attributes of the child as soon as it is appropriate. Normally there is a grief reaction and sense of loss at birth as the parents release the fantasized child and begin to accept the real child.

Occasionally the father (or mother) has a marked negative reaction to the "wrong" sex of the child. Disappointment at the birth of a girl prompted one husband to curse the nurses, the physician, his wife, and the wife's relatives. He refused to speak to his wife or even to see her or the child after delivery. There might have been clues to this problem area during the prenatal period that could have prompted intervention and modified this unfortunate outcome.

Breast or bottle? Deciding on the infant's feeding method is of concern when the partners' preferences differ or when one partner has intense reactions. Recognized benefits and disadvantages of one method over another appear to be irrelevant. Some expectant mothers are startled by the husband's strong insistence on one method or the other. Some men insist that the wife breast feed; others are adamantly set against breast feeding. Reasons given for this strong and sometimes vehement antinursing stance include its "animal-like" nature, competition for the wife's breasts, concern that the breasts will sag later on, fear of effects on the baby (e.g., "It makes a sissy of a baby boy"), fear of being tied down, and inability to know (and perhaps control) how much milk the child receives.

When the husband refuses to voice an opinion one way or the other, the wife experiences uneasiness. Inwardly she accuses him of disinterest or feels uncertain about choosing the right way. The wife seems to ask for his support for whatever choice is made. Many couples find it difficult to vent honest feelings without a supportive other, such as the nurse, to open up the subject or mediate the discussion.

Changing self-concept. During the second trimester men seem to become more introspective. There are many discussions about one's relationships with different family members and friends and about one's own philosophy of life, religion, and childbearing and childrearing practices. This parallels the withdrawal response of the mother-to-be discussed earlier.

Rehearsing for fatherhood. Daydreaming is a form of role playing. This form of anticipatory psychologic preparation for the infant is most frequent in the last weeks before delivery. Rarely do men confide their daydreams unless they are reassured that daydreams are normal and fairly prevalent. Questions such as the following assist the nurse and the parent in identifying concerns and informational needs and allow for reality testing: What do you expect the child to look and act like? What do you think it will be like to be a father? Have you thought about the baby's crying? Changing diapers? Burping the baby? Being awakened at night? Sharing your wife with the baby? Occasionally just asking the questions suffices. The father may not wish to share his answers with the nurse at the moment but may need time to think them through or discuss them with his spouse.

If an expectant father can imagine only an older child and has difficulty visualizing or talking about the infant, this area needs to be explored. Frequently he only requires information. He may never have seen a newborn. He may need to talk about the baby or may benefit from early introduction to holding the child. After delivery he should have the opportunity to physically inspect his child and to be reassured that his child's appearance and behavior are normal.

Third trimester

TASK: *To negotiate with his partner the role he is to play in labor and to prepare for the reality of parenthood. The man needs to be able to state, "I know my role during the birth process and I am going to be a parent."*

Changing self-concept. Noticeable changes and reactions occur in the father. During the last trimester it is not unusual to find the clean-shaven expectant father growing a beard or mustache. Meanwhile, his bearded counterpart suddenly decides to shave his face clean. Time, energy, and money are spent fixing up long-existent physical problems. Glasses are replaced with contact lenses. Weight reduction diets are usually successful if attempted. The expectant father may replace his old wardrobe with a new one to show himself and others that he is indeed a new person. Wife, family, and friends are bewildered at this unexplained concentration on self at this crucial time and often react with teasing or open hostility. A wife may believe her husband is withdrawing his attention from her. Anticipatory guidance for this eventuality can reassure and support the couple.

Creative activites. The creative drive is evident in every person. For the woman a direct biologic mode of creative expression is available. Other modes are possible for the man. Whether or not the pregnancy was planned, many men express a profound feeling of awe or pride in being a part of the creation of a human being.

During the last 2 months of pregnancy, expectant fathers experience a surge of energy to create and to achieve in the home and on the job. These behaviors could be interpreted as tangible evidence of sharing the wife's creative experience while channeling the anxiety (or other feelings) of the final weeks before birth. Furthermore, these behaviors earn recognition and compliments from friends, relatives, and wives, and some may even coincide with wives' nesting activities. Dissatisfaction increases with present living space. The need to alter the environment is acted on wherever possible. When a move into a new home or apartment is not possible, other changes are made to accommodate the new self-concept: furniture is rearranged; new furniture or appliances or both are added; pets may be ousted; and acquisition of a new car may be considered.

Coping and defense activities. The days and weeks immediately preceding the expected day of delivery are characterized by anticipation and anxiety. Many husbands (and couples) describe the dimension of time as heavy, slowing down, and distorted. Boredom and restlessness are common. Expectant fathers and their wives focus on the birth process.

The father will spend his heightened energies in diverse ways: conversing with others regarding their experiences; justifying fears of being with his wife in labor by basing these fears on past experiences with blood or needles; teasing and ridiculing his wife's ungainly appearance and movements; projecting hostilities toward homosexuals, landlords, fellow workers, and those of other races, religions, and nationalities; denial may be expressed by refusal to think about the coming event or by planning other activities during his wife's labor; or sleeping and resting to the exclusion of all else.

The expectant mother's reactions to the observed behaviors in her mate vary. One prevailing reaction is concern about the possibility of being deserted physically or emotionally when she is feeling most vulnerable.

A primary concern of the father is his ability to get the mother to a medical facility in time for the birth. It is a convenient and acceptable focus for his fear and anxiety. Initially some fathers fantasize several ridiculously humorous situations and then move on to plan what they will do. Many rehearse the routes to the hospital, timing each route at different times of the day. Suitcase, car, and essential telephone numbers are kept in readiness.

In addition, many fathers want to be able to recognize labor and to determine when it is appropriate to leave for the hospital or call the physician or midwife. The concern here is twofold: getting to the hospital in time and not appearing "stupid."

Many fathers have questions about the labor suite's physical environment and staffing—furniture, nursing staff, location, and availability of physician and anesthesiologist. Other fathers' interests lie in knowing what is expected of them when their wives are in labor.

Fathers have imagined the delivery room as containing "10,000 lights" with "instruments everywhere and a delivery table like a slab." During delivery, men anticipate "lots of blood" and commotion and rushing about, with "people everywhere, moving fast."

The father has fears of mutilation and death for his wife and child. While he harbors these fears within, he cannot listen or help his mate with her unspoken or overt apprehensions. Words such as "dropped," "rupture of bag of waters," "bloody show," "tears and stitches," and "labor pains" have violent overtones.

With the exception of parent education classes, there are few opportunities for a father to learn to be an involved, active, and needed partner in this rite of passage into parenthood. The unprepared, unsupported father may add to the mother's fears. Tensions and apprehensions are readily transmitted and may increase the mother's difficulties. His own self-doubt and fear of inadequacy may be realized if he is not supported. Self-confidence comes from achieving realistic self-goals and earning the approval of others.

Most men whose wives are approaching labor may have their anxieties decreased through intervention before the event. Fantasies can be replaced by knowledge gained through activities such as the following:

1. A hospital tour to accomplish the following: visualize the labor room and waiting areas (This will allow him to envision methods of using the environment when he arrives and to familiarize himself with the delivery room and determine where he will sit and what his role will be.)
2. A demonstration of helping and supportive measures to comfort his wife during labor
3. A brief review of what to expect from his wife during the labor process if she has medication or anesthesia or if she delivers without medication or anesthesia (e.g., irritability, breathing, grunting)
4. A description of what to expect of the staff during his wife's labor

A realistic discussion of all known factors helps the

father more rationally problem solve and plan for the event. Such discussions are ego strengthening, since they focus one's energies toward more appropriate coping strategies and help alleviate anxieties about the unknown. Today many men elect to participate actively during labor and the delivery of their child. However, some men through personal or cultural concepts of the father role neither wish to nor intend to participate. They prefer the *observer role* (May, 1982a). The important concept is that the partners agree on the other's roles. For nurses to advocate any changes in these roles may cause confusion or feelings of guilt.

Father-child relationship. As the birth day approaches, questions regarding fetal and newborn behaviors increase: "What do they do in there (in utero)?" "Is he hiccupping?" "Does he suck his thumb?" "How is he breathing?" "What does a newborn baby look like?" Some fathers express shock or amazement about the small size of clothes and furniture received as gifts for the baby. Other fathers protest, "He'll only be real to me when I can hold him in my arms."

All these activities speak to the father's involvement and concerns in becoming a father to his own child. Throughout the pregnancy but to a heightened degree now, his memories emerge of being fathered as a child. These memories merge with his expectations of himself in the father role that is soon to be *his* role.

Siblings

The response of siblings to pregnancy varies with age and dependence needs. The 1-year-old infant seems largely unaware of the process. However, the 2-year-old child notices the change in his mother's appearance and may comment, "Mummy's fat." The 2-year-old child's need for sameness in his environment makes him very aware of any change. By the third or fourth year of age children like to be told the story of their own beginning and accept its being compared to the present pregnancy. They like to listen to heartbeats and sometimes worry about how the baby is being fed and what it wears. Interference with established routines can cause anger. One 4-year-old boy resented not being able to fit on his mother's lap anymore and was not above punching at his mother's abdomen; his father resolved the issue by making the child a small ski that he could slide down his mother's bosom and over her abdomen ("over the jump"). He could still sit close by, touch her, and accept her abdomen as part of his life.

School-aged children take a more clinical interest in their mother's pregnancy. They may want to know in more detail "how the baby got in there" and "how it will get out." Children in this age group notice pregnant women in stores, in church, and in school and sometimes seem shy if they need to approach the

Fig. 16.2
Mother-to-be and her 5-year-old son look at his baby pictures.

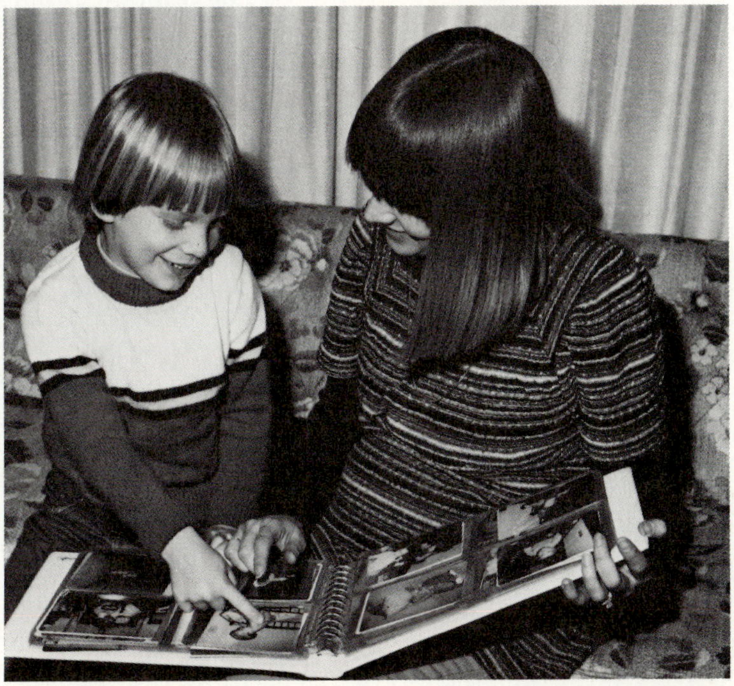

Fig. 16.3
A 5-year-old helps mom get the new baby's clothes ready.

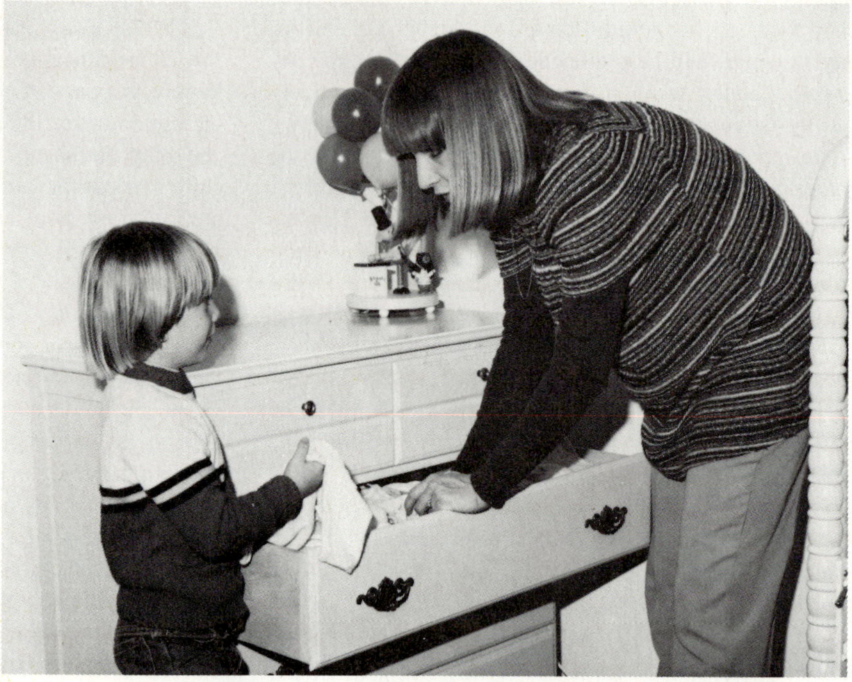

Fig. 16.4
A sibling-to-be checks to see if the crib will be suitable for the new arrival.

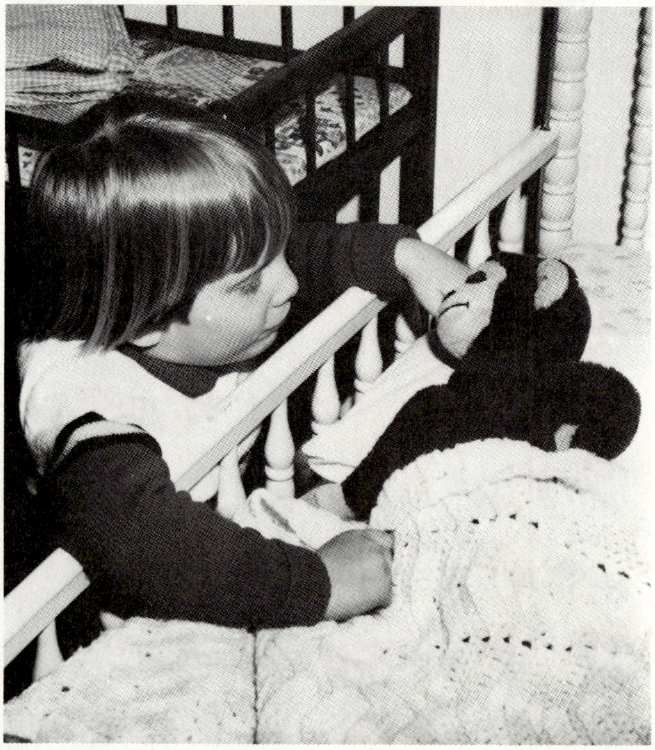

woman directly. On the whole they look forward to the new baby, see themselves as "mothers" or "fathers," and enjoy being included in the preparations, buying baby supplies, and readying a place for the baby. Because they still think very concretely and base judgment on the here and now, they respond positively to their mother's present good health and do not seem to be anxious about a future injury to her or to the unborn child. They need help to cope with any adverse change in the physical or mental status of the parent or newborn, since they do not anticipate such a change.

For early and middle adolescents preoccupied with the establishment of their own sexual identity, the overwhelming evidence of the sexual activity of their parents may prove very difficult to accept. They reason that if they are "too young" for such activity, certainly their parents are "too old." All the uncertainties about the status of their parents and the appearance of their mothers are compounded by the pregnancy. They seem to take on a critical parental role and may ask, "What will people think?" or "How can you let yourself get so fat?" Many pregnant women with teenaged children will confess that their teenagers were the hardest part of the present pregnancy.

On the positive side, just as the parents will someday catch a glimpse of the fine person their adolescent will become, so are parents-to-be suddenly confronted by a warm, sensitive person who is able to restore the mother's self-esteem, as illustrated by the following example:

> I came home one day feeling very pregnant, tired, and heavy and dreading the idea of making dinner and being helpful—you know—the mother bit! Mary (aged 15 years) was cooking some hamburger, had the table set for dinner, and even had a flower centerpiece. For some reason I just started to cry. She came to me and hugged me and said, "I think you're doing the loveliest thing in the world, having a baby." I'll always remember that—she was really *my* mother for the moment.

The late adolescent does not appear to be unduly disturbed. There is a feeling that he or she will be gone from the home. Parents usually report that offspring in this group are very comforting and act more as other adults than as children. One mother delivering her tenth baby remarked, "The only complaint my oldest daughter made was, 'Mother, I'm getting married in August, so don't you dare be too pregnant to come to the wedding.' "

Grandparents

Many women report that their pregnancies bridged the final gap between them and their own mothers. The estrangement that began in adolescence disappeared as the now-pregnant daughter experienced joys, concern, and anxieties similar to those her mother had felt before her.

Some grandparents-to-be do not welcome the new role for their daughters or sons. It may be seen as notice of their aging process or as the victory of the exchild in obtaining an equal role with the parent. Some grandparents-to-be are not only nonsupportive but also use subtle means to decrease the self-esteem of the young parents-to-be. Mothers may talk about their terrible pregnancies; fathers may discuss the endless cost of rearing children; and mothers-in-law may describe the neglect of their son as the concern of others is directed toward the pregnant daughter-in-law.

Most grandparents, however, are delighted with the prospect of a new baby in the family. It reawakens their feelings of their own youth, the excitement of giving birth, and their delight in the behavior of the parents-to-be when they were infants. They set up a memory store of first smiles, first words, and first steps, which can be used later for "claiming" the newborn as a member of the family. Satisfaction comes with the realization that continuity between past and present is guaranteed.

Summary

Pregnancy represents one of the developmental crises of an individual's and a family's life. The concept of crisis implies events that necessitate change in outlook, role responsibilities, and everyday living. The ability to respond to changes with new behaviors and new self-concepts is fostered not only by intrinsic strengths but by extrinsic strengths, such as the love and support of outsiders. Nurses can act as one source of extrinsic strength. The knowledge they possess of the responses of all family members to a pregnancy enables them to use these responses as the cornerstones of nursing care plans. The long-term contact nurses have with clients and their families provides unique opportunities for informed supportive nursing that may have a long-term effect on family life.

References and Readings

Anderson, S.V.: Siblings at birth: a survey and study, Birth Fam. J. **6**(2):9, 1979.

Antle, K.: Psychologic involvement in pregnancy by expectant fathers, J.O.G.N. Nurs. **4**:40, July-Aug. 1975.

Bibring, G.: Some consideration of the psychological processes in pregnancy, Psychoanal. Study Child **14**:113, 1959.

Bibring, G., Dwyer, T.F., and Huntington, D.S.: A study of the psychological processes in pregnancy and of the earliest mother-child relationship. II. Methodological considerations, Psychoanal. Study Child **16**:9, 1961.

Bowen, S., and Miller, B.: Paternal attachment as related to presence at delivery and attendance at preparenthood classes: a pilot study, Nurs. Res. **23**:210, 1974.

Bowlby, J.: Attachment. In Attachment and loss, vol. 1, New York, 1969, Basic Books, Publishers.

Bradley, R.A.: Husband-coached childbirth, New York, 1974, Harper & Row, Publishers.

Bucove, A.: Postpartum psychoses in the male, N.Y. Acad. Med. **40**:961, 1964.

Caplan, G.: Concepts of mental health and consultation, Washington, D.C., 1959, U.S. Department of Health, Education, and Welfare.

Colman, A.D.: Psychological state during the first pregnancy, Am. J. Orthopsychiatry **39**:788, 1969.

Colman, A.D., and Colman, L.L.: Pregnancy: the psychological experience, New York, 1971, Herder & Herder.

Colman, A.D., and Colman, L.L.: Pregnancy as an altered state of consciousness, Birth Fam. J. **1**:7, 1974.

Cowan, C., et al.: Becoming a family: the impact of a first child's birth on the couple's relationship. In Newman, L., and Miller, W., editors: The first child and family formation, Chapel Hill, N.C., 1978, University of North Carolina (Carolina Population Center).

Deutch, H.: The psychology of women, vol. 2, New York, 1945, Bantam Books.

Edwards, M.: Communications: dimensions in childbirth education, Pacific Grove, Calif., 1973, M. Edwards.

Greenberg, M., and Morris, N.: Engrossment: the newborn's impact upon the father, Am. J. Orthopsychiatry **44**:520, 1974.

Griffin, S.: Childbearing and the concept of culture, J.O.G.N. Nurs. **11**:181, 1982.

Halper, M.M., et al.: Life events and acceptance of pregnancy, J. Psychosom. Res. **12**:183, 1968.

Highley, B.L., and Mercer, R.T.: Safeguarding the laboring woman's sense of control, Am. J. Matern. Child Nurs. **3**(1):39, 1978.

Hoffman, L.W.: Changes in family roles, socialization and sex differences, Am. J. Psychol. **32**:644, 1977.

Hunter, R., and Macalpine, I., editors: Three hundred years of psychiatry, 1535–1860, London, 1963, Oxford University Press.

Interprofessional Task Force on Health Care of Women and Children: Joint position statement on the development of family-centered maternity/newborn care in hospitals, Chicago, June 1978.

Jessner, L., Weigert, E., and Foy, J.L.: The development of parental attitudes during pregnancy. In Anthony, E.J., and Benedek, T., editors: Parenthood, Edinburgh, 1970, Churchill-Livingstone.

Josselyn, I.M.: Psychology of fatherliness, Smith Coll. Stud. Soc. Work **26**:1, Feb. 1956.

Lamb, M.E.: Father-infant and mother-infant interaction in the first year of life, Child Dev. **48**:167, 1977.

Leifer, M.: Psychological changes accompanying pregnancy and motherhood, Genet. Psychol. Monographs **95**:57, 1977.

LeMasters, E.: Parenthood as crisis, Marriage and Family Living, Nov. 1957.

Liebenberg, B.: Expectant fathers. Paper presented at Conference of Prenatal Counseling Project, Group Health Association, Inc., Oregon, March 1967.

May, K.A.: A typology of detachment and involvement styles adopted during pregnancy by first-time expectant fathers, West J. Nurs. Res. **2**:445, 1980.

May, K.A.: The father as observer, M.C.N. **7**:319, Sept/Oct. 1982.

May, K.A.: Father participation in birth: fact and fiction, J. Calif. Perinatal Assoc. **2**(2):41, Fall 1982.

Parke, R.D., et al.: Mother-father-newborn interaction: effects of maternal medication, labor and sex of infant, Proc. Am. Psychol. Assoc., pp. 85-86, 1972.

Parke, R.D., et al.: The father's role in the family system, Semin. Perinatol. **3**:25, Jan. 1979.

Phillips, C.R., and Anzalone, J.T.: Fathering: participation in labor and birth, ed. 2, St. Louis, 1981, The C.V. Mosby Co.

Rubin, R.: Body image and self-esteem, Nurs. Outlook **16**:20, June 1968.

Rubin, R: Cognitive style in pregnancy, Am. J. Nurs. **70**:502, 1970.

Rubin, R.: Maternal tasks in pregnancy, Mat. Child Nurs. J. **4**:143, Fall 1975.

Satir, V.: Conjoint family therapy, Palo Alto, Calif., 1967, Science & Behavior Books.

Standley, K., Soule, B., and Copans, S.A.: Dimensions of prenatal anxiety and their influence on pregnancy outcome, Am. J. Obstet. Gynecol. **135**(22):22, 1979.

Sumner, P.: Six years' experience of prepared childbirth in a homelike labor delivery room, Birth Fam. J. **3**:79, Summer 1976.

Willmuth, L.R.: Prepared childbirth and the concept of control, J.O.G.N. Nurs. **4**(5):38, 1975.

Yogman, M.J., et al.: The goals and structure of face-to-face-interaction between infants and fathers. Presentation at the Biennial Meeting, Society for Research in Child Development, New Orleans, 1977.

17

Nursing Care During the Prenatal Period

- **Definitions**
- **Assessment**
  - Diagnosis of pregnancy
    - Presumptive signs and symptoms
    - Probable signs and symptoms
    - Positive signs
    - Laboratory tests
    - Duration of pregnancy and estimated date of confinement
  - Fetal gestational age and health status
    - Ultrasonography
    - Amniocentesis
    - Maternal urinary or plasma estriol level
    - Fetal heart rate
    - Fetal movement
    - Radiography
    - Amnioscopy
  - Maternal and family need for psychosocial care
    - Nursing role
    - Assessment: gravidas
    - Assessment: family
  - Prenatal examination procedures
    - Clean-catch urine specimen
    - Pelvic examination
    - Papanicolaou smear
    - Gonorrheal culture
    - Herpes simplex, types 1 and 2, culture
    - Vaginal discharges
    - Maternal urinary estriol determinations
    - Amniocentesis
- **Nursing Diagnoses in the Prenatal Period**
- **Planning**
  - Initial contact with woman and family
    - Protocol for care
    - Collection of specimens
  - First prenatal visit
    - Protocol for care: comprehensive examination
  - Subsequent visits
- **Implementation**
  - Goals
  - Nursing actions
    - Instruction regarding danger signals
    - Childbirth and parenthood education
    - Nutritional counseling
    - Frequent questions
    - Discomforts of pregnancy
    - Sexual counseling during pregnancy
    - Symptomatology of impending labor
- **Evaluation**

The prenatal period is a preparatory one physically in terms of fetal growth and maternal adjustments and psychologically in terms of anticipation of parenthood. It is one of the maturational crises of our lives and as such can represent a time of growth in responsibility and concern for others. It is a time of intense learning for the woman and man and for those close to them, a time for family unity and development.

The best method for ensuring the health of the expectant mother and her infant is prenatal care. During a woman's life, pregnancy is unique because only then does she seek ongoing health care. Regular prenatal visits, ideally beginning soon after the first missed period, offer opportunities to supervise the course of normal pregnancy, to reassure the woman and her family, and to teach parenting skills. Prenatal health supervision permits diagnosis and treatment of maternal disorders that may have been preexistent or may develop during the pregnancy and is designed to follow the growth and development of the fetus and to identify abnormalities such as pelvic tumors or imminent labor.

The professionals who have contact with the gravida and her family will include a cross section of health workers, for example, nurse, physician, nutritionist, and social worker. It is essential that these individuals work as a team to provide holistic care for their clients.

The first phase of prenatal management consists of verifying the pregnancy, establishing a diagnosis of either a normal or abnormal physical or emotional response, and accepting the decision of the woman to continue or terminate the pregnancy.

The second phase of management consists of establishing a data base for subsequent care, setting up a schedule for ongoing assessment of maternal and fetal health, providing therapeutic and educational care, and initiating remedial care as needed.

The initial visit of the woman to either the physician's office or obstetric clinic is important in setting the tone for her care. The woman needs to feel welcomed and important. The initial visit may include both the diagnosis or verification of pregnancy and the establishment of the data base depending on the duration of gestation.

If pregnancy is too early and cannot be verified, her next appointment is scheduled in 2 weeks. Misdiagnosis may lead to serious emotional and legal consequences; therefore caution is warranted.

Her desire regarding this pregnancy is evaluated; if she is pregnant and does not wish to continue the pregnancy, she is referred for abortion counseling (see Chapter 41). If she is not pregnant but desires to be pregnant, she may be a candidate for fertility diagnostic studies (see Chapter 12). If she is not pregnant and does not wish to be, refer her for family planning, if appropriate (see Chapter 13).

If the woman is pregnant and plans to carry the pregnancy to term (and depending on existing office procedures), the examiner (1) proceeds to the protocol for the first prenatal visit or schedules her for her first prenatal visit in 1 to 2 weeks and (2) begins expectant parent education regarding good health practices (e.g., diet; exercise; rest; avoidance of harmful drugs, infectious diseases, and the taking of x-ray films; self-awareness—physical signs, symptoms, and feelings).

Regardless of the outcome of the history and examination, the examiner responds to the woman's or couple's specific questions and concerns. No opportunity for health teaching is overlooked!

The nursing actions represent the changing care given the pregnant woman as she progresses through pregnancy from her first contact with health professionals to the last prenatal visit that confirms the beginning of labor.

Definitions

The following definitions refer to the pregnant woman. The pregnant woman is termed a **gravida;** when she is in labor, she is a **parturient.** The process of labor and delivery may be termed **parturition** or **confinement. EDC** refers to the expected date of confinement.

Parity refers to the number of *pregnancies* in which the fetus or fetuses reach viability, not the number of fetuses delivered. Whether the fetus is born alive or is stillborn after viability is reached does not affect parity.

nulligravida A woman who has never been pregnant.
primigravida A woman who is pregnant for the first time.
multigravida A woman who has had two or more pregnancies.
nullipara A woman who has *not* completed a pregnancy with a fetus or fetuses that have reached the stage of fetal viability (legal definition: 24 to 28 weeks of gestational age).
primipara A woman who has completed one pregnancy with a fetus or fetuses that have reached the stage of fetal viability.
multipara A woman who has completed two or more pregnancies to the stage of fetal viability.

This information is abbreviated as parity/gravidity. For example, 0/1 means a woman has not carried a pregnancy to viability (nullipara) and is pregnant for the first time (primigravida).

One obstetric abbreviation commonly employed in maternity centers is even more complete. It consists of five digits with dashes for separation. The first digit represents the total number of pregnancies, including the present one; the second digit represents the total number of deliveries; the third indicates the number of premature babies; the fourth identifies the number of abortions; and the fifth is the number of children living at this time. If a woman pregnant only once with twins delivers at the thirty-fifth week and the babies survive, she is "1-1-2-0-2." During her next pregnancy, she is "2-1-2-0-2." Additional examples are given in Table 17.1.

The following terms refer to the periods of pregnancy:

prenatal Prebirth.
perinatal period Period extending from the twentieth or twenty-eight week of gestation through the end of the twenty-eight day after birth.
postnatal After birth.
prepartum Before delivery.
intrapartum Labor and delivery (in reality delivery of fetus and placenta is part of labor).
postpartum After delivery.

The content material pertaining to the care of the maternity client and her family during the prenatal period is extensive. All the previous chapters presented some aspect pertinent to the care. Although presented sepa-

Table 17.1
Parity and Gravidity Using Five-Digit and Two-Digit Systems

	Five-Digit System					Two-Digit System
Condition	**A***	**B**	**C**	**D**	**E**	**F**
Judith is pregnant for the first time.	1	0	0	0	0	0/i
She carries the pregnancy to term and the neonate survives.	1	1	0	0	1	i/i
She is pregnant again.	2	1	0	0	1	i/ii
Her second pregnancy ends in abortion.	2	1	0	1	1	i/ii
During her third pregnancy, she delivers viable twins.	3	2	0	1	3	ii/iii

*A = times uterus has been pregnant; B = no. of deliveries; C = no. of premature deliveries; D = no. of abortions (spontaneous or therapeutic); E = no. of living children; F = parity/gravidity.

rately in this chapter, assessment, planning, implementation, and evaluation are interdependent and interrelated throughout pregnancy.

Assessment

DIAGNOSIS OF PREGNANCY

The clinical diagnosis of pregnancy before the second missed period may be difficult in at least 25% to 30% of women. Physical variability, lack of relaxation, obesity, or tumors, for example, may confound even the experienced obstetrician. Accuracy is most important, however, because social, medical, or legal consequences of an inaccurate diagnosis, either positive or negative, may be extremely serious. Unfortunately even laboratory tests are not invariably correct. A correct last menstrual period (LMP), date of intercourse, or basal body temperature (BBT) record may be of great value in the accurate diagnosis of pregnancy. Reexamination in 2 to 4 weeks may be required for certainty of diagnosis.

Great variability must be admitted in the subjective and objective symptomatology of pregnancy. Hence the diagnosis of pregnancy is classified as follows: presumptive, probable, and positive (Table 17.2). The student is referred to Chapter 15 for an in-depth discussion of the symptomatology caused by maternal adaptations to pregnancy. Many of the signs and symptoms of pregnancy are clinically useful in the diagnosis of pregnancy. Table 17.3 presents the signs and symptoms of pregnancy in order of appearance.

Presumptive signs and symptoms. The following signs and symptoms may make the physician or woman suspicious of pregnancy but are not proof of pregnancy.

Because all the presumptive signs and symptoms of pregnancy can be caused by conditions other than gestation, no one of the following manifestations can be relied on for a final impression, nor are combinations of several manifestations diagnostic (Table 17.4).

Symptoms: subjective data

Amenorrhea. The majority of women have no periodic bleeding (menstruation ceases) after the onset of pregnancy. However, at least 20% have some slight painless spotting during early gestation for unexplained reasons. A great majority of these continue to term and have normal infants.

Secondary amenorrhea may also accompany emotional tension, any serious endocrine disorder, CNS abnormality, ovarian insufficiency or neoplasia, uterine disease, cervical obstruction, or excessive jogging (Table 17.4).

Women who are not menstruating during lactation or who have just had dilatation and curettage (D and C) can also become pregnant.

Nausea and vomiting. Although the colloquialism ''morning'' sickness is widely accepted as descriptive of nausea and vomiting during pregnancy, numerous expectant mothers have nausea later in the day or all day. Regardless of its origin, the nausea and vomiting usually last up to 8 weeks but rarely beyond 12 weeks, only to recur close to term in some pregnancies.

Severe protracted vomiting, or hyperemesis gravidarum (see Chapter 36), necessitates hospitalization.

Nausea and vomiting frequently are associated with conditions other than pregnancy, such as allergies, infection, obstruction, CNS disorders, or viremia.

Breast sensitivity. The sensation varies from mild tingling to frank pain (mastodynia). The sensation may arise as a result of hormone therapy, and mastalgia may be caused by estrogen excess associated with anovulatory menstrual cycles or ovarian tumors.

Urinary frequency and urgency. Bladder irritability, nocturia, and urinary frequency and urgency (without dysuria) frequently may be reported early in pregnancy. Near term a return of bladder symptoms is noted by the woman.

Urinary tract infection is indicated by similar symptoms and dysuria.

Lassitude and fatigability. Listlessness and fatigue after only slight exertion are described by many women in early pregnancy and may persist, along with an increased need for sleep.

Ennui and fatigue may be psychologic or pathologic.

Table 17.2
Summary of Signs and Symptoms of Pregnancy*

Presumptive	Probable	Positive
Subjective symptoms		
Amenorrhea Nausea, vomiting Breast sensitivity Urinary symptoms Lassitude/fatigue Constipation Weight gain Fingernail changes Quickening	Same as presumptive symptoms; when combined with probable signs, strong suspicion of pregnancy	No symptoms positively diagnostic of pregnancy
Objective signs		

Elevation of BBT
Integumentary changes
  Pigmentation
  Chloasma
  Nipples, areola
  Linea nigra
  Striae gravidarum
  Telangiectasis (or "spiders")
  Acne
  Hirsutism
  Epulis
Breast changes
  Enlargement
  Secondary areolae
  Montgomery's tubercles
  Colostrum
Abdominal enlargement
Pelvic changes
  Vagina (Chadwick's sign; leukorrhea)
  Cervix (softening; Goodell's sign; dried mucus in granular pattern)
  Uterus (softening: Ladin's sign, Hegar's sign, McDonald's sign, von Fernwald's sign; enlargement)
  Relaxation of bony pelvic joints and ligaments
	Uterine enlargement
	Uterine contractions (Braxton Hicks' sign)
	Ballottement
	Uterine souffle
	Laboratory tests (except radioimmunoassay of beta subunit of HCG)
		FHT
		  Electronic device (8-11 wk)
		  Electrocardiogram (12 wk)
		  Auscultation (17-24 wk)
		Palpation of fetal outline and movement
		Roentgenographic evidence of fetal skeleton
		Ultrasonographic (echographic) evidence of pregnancy
		Laboratory tests
		  Biologic (before 1960s) (Aschheim-Zondek; Friedman's)
		  Immunologic (6 wk)
		  Radioimmunoassay (beta-subunit of HCG can diagnose pregnancy before missed period)
		  Home pregnancy test (9 days after end of missed period)
		  Clinical test
		  Progesterone withdrawal

*Clinical diagnosis of pregnancy depends on the ability to interpret presumptive, probable, and positive physical signs and symptoms.

One should also consider emotional disorders, anemia, infection, or malignant disease.

Constipation. Constipation appears early and may persist throughout pregnancy.

Weight gain. Rapid weight gain is not associated with early pregnancy; some women experience weight loss. Women who eat to ease emotional tension or boredome may gain excessive weight.

Fingernail changes. By the sixth week some women notice thinning and softening of the nails.

Quickening. The first recognition of fetal movements or "feeling life" by the multiparous woman may occur as early as the fourteenth to sixteenth week, but primigravidas may not notice these sensations until the eighteenth week or later. Quickening is frequently described as a flutter and is difficult to distinguish from peristalsis. Noting the week in which quickening occurs provides a tentative clue in dating the duration of gestation.

Signs: objective data. Although signs are more specific than symptoms, they are not diagnostic. In the presence of hormones common to pregnancy, organs and systems respond to give the following signs.

Table 17.3
Symptoms and Signs of Pregnancy in Order of Appearance

Symptoms and Signs	Approximate Wk of Gestation	Symptoms and Signs	Approximate Wk of Gestation
Amenorrhea	4	Palpable uterine enlargement—size of an orange	10
"Morning" sickness	4	Palpable uterine enlargement—size of an grapefruit; uterus becomes an abdominal organ	12
Bladder symptoms	6	Internal ballottement	14-18
Cervical softening	6	Breast: clear fluid (precolostrum) can be expressed	16
Breasts: increased vascularity and sensation of heaviness	6	Quickening ("feeling life")	16-20
Palpable uterine enlargement—size of a large hen's egg	7	Palpable uterine contractions (Braxton Hicks' sign)	20
Darkening of vaginal mucous membrane and cervix (Chadwick's sign)	8	Palpable fetal movements	20
Softening of lower uterine segment	8	External ballottement	24
Breast: primary areolae become more pigmented and Montgomery's tubercles also more prominent	8	Auscultation of fetal heart (fetal stethoscope)	17-24
Ultrasound detection of fetal heart tones	10-12	Palpable fetal parts (felt by examiner)	26
Vulval varicosities appear	10		

Table 17.4
Differential Assessment of Signs and Symptoms of Pregnancy

Symptoms	Possible Causes of Diagnostic Error
Amenorrhea	Emotional factors: severe emotional shock, tension, fear of (or strong desire for) pregnancy
	Endocrine factors: adrenal or ovarian neoplasms, thyroid or pituitary disorders, lactation, menopause
	Metabolic factors: anemia, malnutrition, diabetes mellitus, degenerative disorders
	Systemic disease: acute or chronic infection (tuberculosis, brucellosis) or malignancy
Nausea or vomiting	Emotional factors: anxiety, pseudocyesis (false pregnancy), anorexia nervosa
	Gastrointestinal disorders: hiatal hernia, ulcers, enteritis, appendicitis
	Systemic disease: acute infection—influenza, encephalitis
Breast sensitivity (mastalgia; mastodynia)	Infectious processes: mastitis, cystic mastitis, premenstrual tension
	Pseudocyesis
Urinary frequency and urgency	Emotional factors: tension
	Metabolic factors: diabetes mellitus
	Pelvic organ disorders: urinary tract infection (UTI), cystocele, tumors
Quickening	Peristalsis; "gas"
Leukorrhea	Infections: vaginal, cervical
	Tumors
Vaginal, cervical color changes	Exogenous progesterone, pelvic tumors, infection
	Pelvic congestion syndrome
Cervical and uterine changes in shape, size, consistency	Tumors, adenomyosis, cervical stenosis with hematometra or pyometra, tuboovarian cysts
Abdominal enlargement	Obesity, abdominal muscle relaxation, tumors, ascites, ventral abdominal hernia
Nipple discharge (milklike)	Drug ingestion: oral contraceptives, psychotropic drugs
	Tumors
	Syndromes (also associated with amenorrhea): hypothalamic or anterior pituitary disorders
Epulis	Infection, dental calculus, vitamin C deficiency
Psuedocyesis	Emotional factors
	Pituitary tumor
Clinical and laboratory findings	
Elevation of BBT	Poor thermometer, faulty use of thermometer, inaccurate recording
	Corpus luteum cyst
	Drug ingestion: progesterone
Pregnancy tests	False results, incorrect interpretation of results
	Elevation of HCG levels for a few days after spontaneous abortion
	Elevation of HCG: hydatidiform mole, choriocarcinoma

Elevation of basal body temperature. If a woman has been recording her basal body temperature (BBT) throughout several menstrual cycles and has noted a persistent temperature elevation spanning 3 weeks since ovulation, pregnancy is a possibility.

Skin changes. Pigmentation is caused by the anterior pituitary hormone melanotropin, which increases during pregnancy. Facial *melasma (chloasma* or *mask of pregnancy)* occurs after the sixteenth week. Darkening of the nipples, areolae, and vulva occurs at about the same time.

In primigravidas the extension of the *linea nigra,* beginning in the third month, keeps pace with the rising height of the fundus; in multigravidas, the entire line often appears earlier than the third month.

Hyperpigmentation of the skin in the nonpregnant woman may result from local causes (e.g., excessive sunlight, tanning creams) or from systemic problems, such as Addison's disease. Chloasma is commonly seen in women taking oral contraceptives because of the pregnancy-like hormones and may not fade after the contraceptive is discontinued.

Fig. 17.1
Softening of uterus. **A,** Ladin's sign. **B,** Hegar's sign. **C,** McDonald's sign. **D,** Tip of cervix. **E,** Braun von Fernwald's sign.

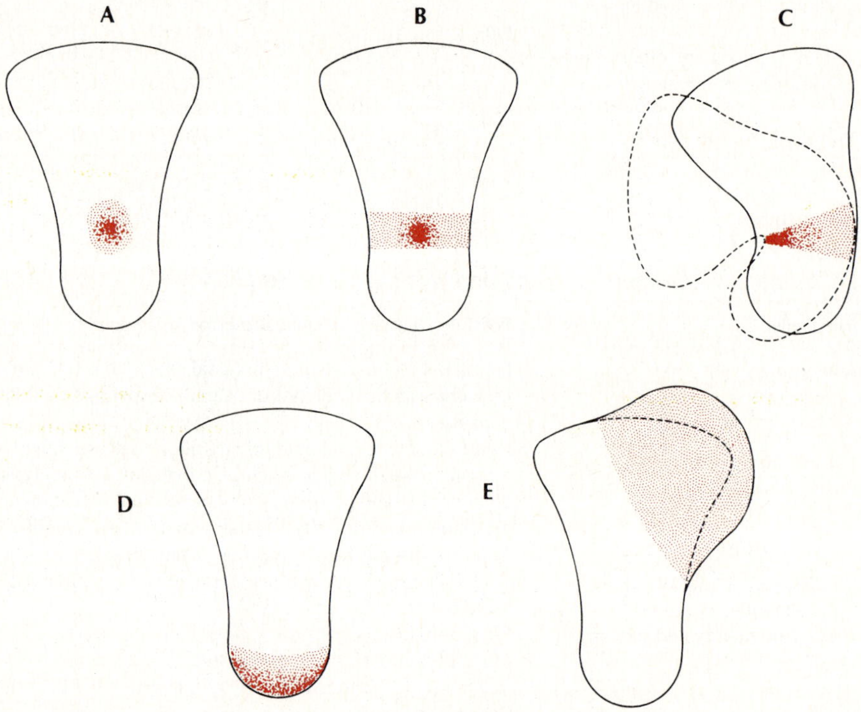

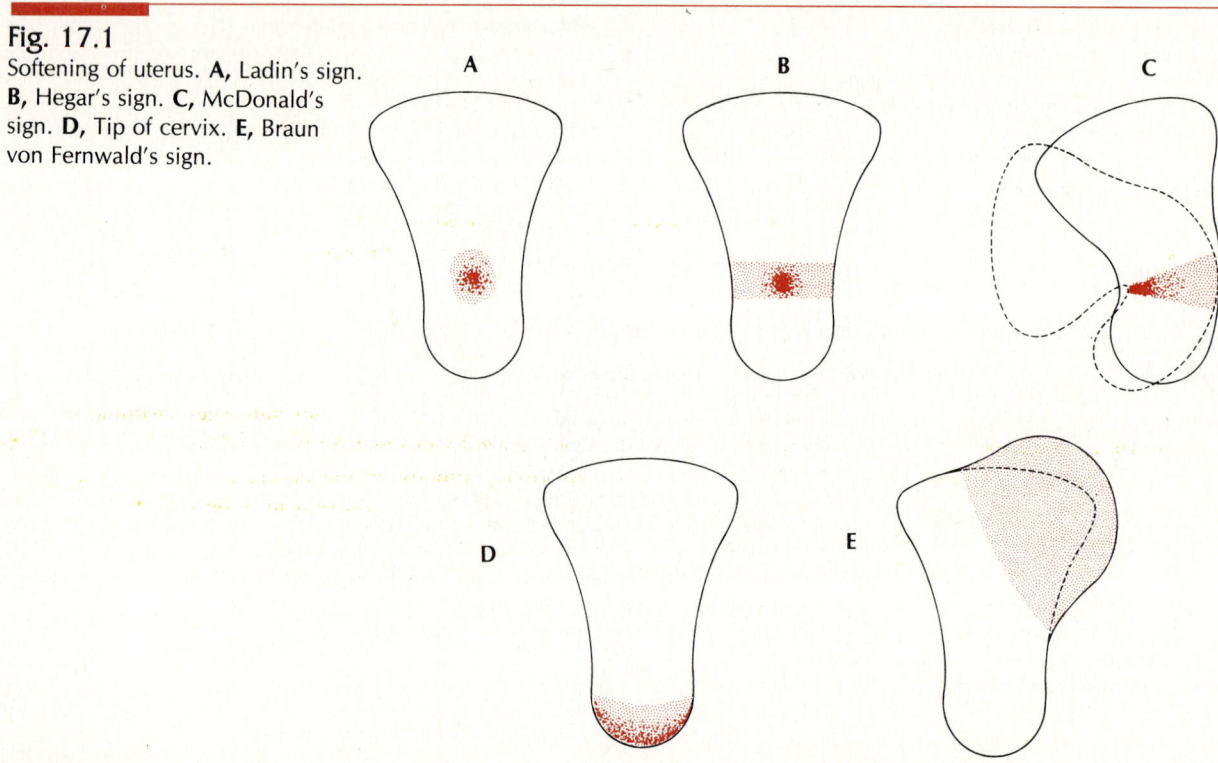

Fig. 17.2
External cervical os as seen through speculum. **A,** Nonparous cervix. **B,** Parous cervix.

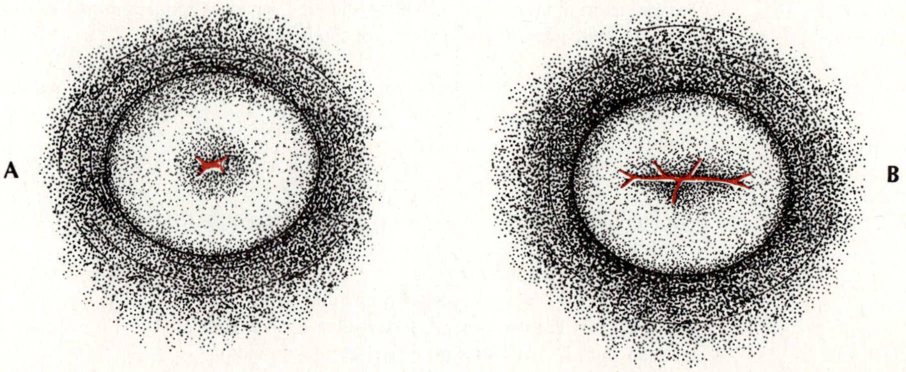

Striae gravidarum, or stretch marks, occur in the second half of pregnancy particularly over the abdomen and breasts.

Commonly referred to as "spiders," *telangiectasias* occur between the second and fifth months of pregnancy.

Oily skin and *acne* may occur during pregnancy.

An increase in fine *hair growth* tends to disappear after pregnancy, but coarse or bristly hair growth usually remains.

Epulis and bleeding gums. Hypertrophy of the gingival papillae may develop during the second and third trimesters of pregnancy.

Gingival granulomas may develop as a result of dental calculus or infection in nongravid women.

Breast changes. Early pregnancy breast changes include enlargement, prominence of veins, and a secondary pinkish areola with prominence of the small sebaceous glands about the nipple (Montgomery's tubercles). These changes can begin as early as the sixth week of gestation. Colostrum, a yellowish premilk secretion, may be expressed manually during the third trimester.

Nipple discharge may be the result of nonpregnancy problems, including breast stimulation, mammary neoplasia, or CNS disease.

Abdominal enlargement. The pregnancy may "show" after the fourteenth week, although this depends to some degree on the woman's height and weight.

Abdominal enlargement may be an expression of obesity, a sign of intraabdominal neoplasm, or evidence of a hernia of the abdominal wall.

Changes in internal genitalia and pelvis. The following are typical changes in the internal genitalia.

Cyanosis, or bluish discoloration of the vagina (Chadwick's or Jacquemier's sign), may be noted as early as the sixth week of pregnancy.

Leukorrhea is a white or slightly gray mucoid discharge with a faint musty odor. Increased estrogen and progesterone stimulation of the cervix produces copious mucoid fluid that is whitish because of the presence of many exfoliated vaginal epithelial cells secondary to normal pregnancy hyperplasia. This vaginal discharge is never pruritic or blood stained.

Cervicitis or vaginitis may be responsible for leukorrhea in nonpregnant women (see Chapter 36). Irritation and discoloration finally will develop in most of these cases.

In the *uterus* softening of the cervical tip may be observed about the fifth week in a normal unscarred cervix. Softening of the cervical-uterine junction (Ladin's sign) may be recorded about the fifth or sixth week (Fig. 17.1). The appearance of the cervix depends on the woman's parity (Fig. 17.2), as well as the hormones of pregnancy. About the seventh week, isthmic softening (Hegar's sign) may be noted (Fig. 17.3). Easy flexion of the fundus on the cervix (McDonald's sign) is usually seen by the seventh to eighth week. Softening

Fig. 17.3
Hegar's sign. Rectovaginal examination for softening of isthmus between cervix and body of uterus. Bimanual examination (vaginal and suprapubic) may be used instead.

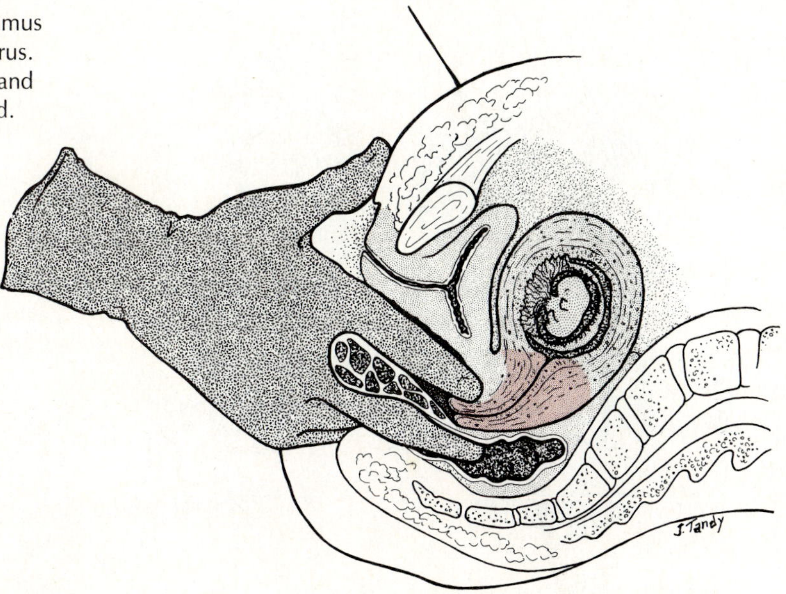

and slight fullness of the fundus near the area of implantation (Braun von Fernwald's sign) or a soft lateral bulge with cornual implantation (Piskacek's sign) may be noted by the eighth week. After the eighth week general enlargement and softening of the uterine corpus are likely. By 10 weeks the uterus generally enlarges to twice its nonpregnant size and is more globular.

In the nonpregnant woman cervical or uterine anomalies, tumors, chronic passive congestion (with a retroflexed uterus), or the pelvic congestion syndrome may mimic the previous signs. A misinterpretation of findings in the obese or tense woman may lead to a false diagnosis of pregnancy.

The *joints and ligaments of the bony pelvis* relax during pregnancy. Relaxation of the symphysis pubis and sacroiliac joint is considerable, resulting in hypermobility of these articulations. Relaxation of the articulation between the sacrum and coccyx permits the movement of the coccyx posteriorly to increase the pelvic outlet. These adaptations permit enlargement of pelvic dimensions.

Probable signs and symptoms

Symptoms: subjective data. Symptoms of pregnancy include all the symptoms considered previously under the presumptive symptomatology of pregnancy.

Signs: objective data

Uterine enlargement. A reasonably accurate correlation of uterine enlargement and the duration of amenorrhea in weeks from the sixth week to term is possible in most normal pregnant women. Variations in the positions of the fundus or the fetus, variations in the amount of amniotic fluid present, or the presence of more than one fetus reduces the accuracy of this estimation of the duration of pregnancy.

Abdominal enlargement may be less apparent in the primigravida with good abdominal muscle tone. Posture also influences the type and degree of abdominal enlargement.

Uterine enlargement may be due to neoplasms, or the normal-sized uterus may be displaced by a pelvic tumor (usually a fibroid tumor or a myoma) of even larger size.

Uterine souffle or bruit. A swishing sound heard just above the symphysis pubis and timed precisely with the mother's pulse is caused by augmented blood flow in the uterine arteries.

A souffle may be heard over a vascular tumor or aneurysm in the nonpregnant woman or may simply be abdominal aortic pulsation, particularly in a thin woman.

Ballottement. Passive movements of the unengaged fetus (ballottement) generally can be identified at about the eighteenth week. Ballottement is a technique of palpating a floating structure by bouncing it gently and feeling it rebound. Internal ballottement of a fetus within a uterus is a probable objective sign of pregnancy: The examiner's finger within the vagina taps gently upward and remains against the cervix; the fetus floats upward; then the fetus sinks and a gentle tap is felt on the finger (Fig. 17.4). This is done by gently palpating the fetus, which moves away and rebounds after a tap by the palpating fingers. This sign is not diagnostic, because it can be elicited in the presence of uterine leiomyomas, ascites, or ovarian cysts.

Fig. 17.4
Internal ballottement (18 weeks).

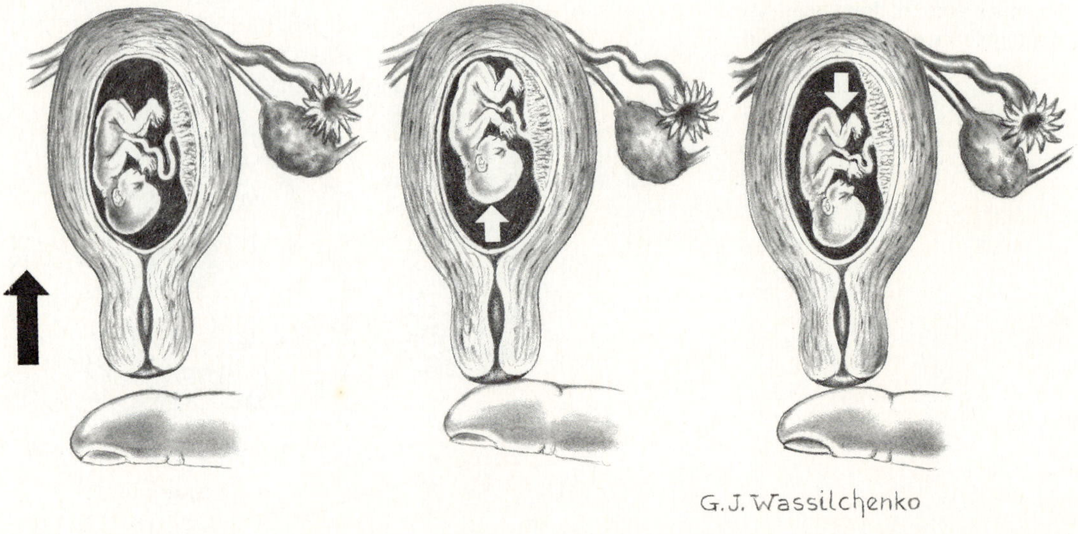

Uterine contractions (Braxton Hick's sign). Occasionally, intermittent uterine contractions may be felt by the woman or observer almost any time after well-established pregnancy. After the twenty-eighth week, contractions become much more definite, especially in slender women. Generally these contractions cease with walking or exercise. Rarely they may be perceived as painful (see also Table 21.1).

Misinterpretations of contractions of muscles of the abdominal wall, intestinal peristalsis, and transmission of the abdominal pulse may be mistaken for the Braxton Hick's sign.

Laboratory tests for pregnancy. Positive laboratory tests for pregnancy are usually catalogued under probable signs. However, the recently developed radioimmunoassay test of the beta subunit of human chorionic gonadotropin (HCG) is so accurate it is regarded as diagnostic (see p. 277). Most currently available laboratory tests for pregnancy, particularly those that test for the presence of HCG in serum or urine, are fairly accurate, simple, and inexpensive; they are available in kit form, so that little practice is needed to perform them.

Improper collection of the specimen, hormone-producing tumors, drugs, or laboratory errors may be responsible for false reports of pregnancy (see box).

Positive signs. Medical and legal proof of pregnancy is based on any one of the following *signs* (objective data). There are no particular symptoms (subjective data) that irrefutably indicate pregnancy.

Fetal heartbeat. Auscultatory or electronic verification of fetal heart activity requires the counting of the fetal heart rate (FHR) or impulse for 1 minute and a comparison with the mother's pulse rate for the same period of time. Electronic devices employing the Doppler principle or fetal electrocardiography may pick up the fetal cardiac impulses (Table 17.2 and Fig. 17.5). Auscultation with a clinical stethoscope may not be successful until the seventeenth or eighteenth week under ideal circumstances.

Doppler ultrasound is *continuous* ultrasound that picks up differing frequencies from the beating fetal

Pregnancy Tests

Indirect tests

Types: Pregnosticon (Organon); Placentex and Pregnosis (Roche); UCG (Wampole); Gest-State (Lederle)
Pregnant: positive test–*no* agglutination (*no* ring formation in bottom of test tube)
Not pregnant: negative test—agglutination

Tube test (2 hours)

Pregnosticon Accuspheres and Pregnosticon tube
Placentex*
UCG-Lyphotest tube
UCG test

False negative readings

Reading error
Excessive amount of antiserum
Gestation too early or too late
Urine too dilute (HCG $<$ 750 IU/L)
Urine left unrefrigerated too long
Disorders of pregnancy: threatened or missed abortion, ectopic implantation

Direct tests

Types: DAP-Test Macro (Wampole)
Pregnant: positive test—agglutination (ring formation or mat evident in bottom of test tube)
Not pregnant: negative test—*no* agglutination

Rapid-slide tests (2 minutes)

Pregnosticon Dri-Dot slide
Pregnosis slide
UCG slide†
DAP-Test Macro†‡
Gest-State†
Gravindex†

False positive readings

Reading error
Proteinuria
Hematuria
Premature or perimenopausal period
Neoplasms: epithelioma, undifferentiated lung cancer, ovarian teratoma
Cysts of corpus luteum
Abscess of tubes and/or ovaries
Drug ingestion: methyldopa (Aldomet), aspirin, marijuana, methadone, phenothiazine, anticonvulsants, antidepressants, L-dopa
Detergent residue from dishes, glasses, or flatware

*One-hr test.
†Less expensive.
‡One-min test.

Fig. 17.5
Detecting fetal heartbeat.
A, Fetoscope. **B,** Stethoscope with rubber band. **C,** Doppler principle.

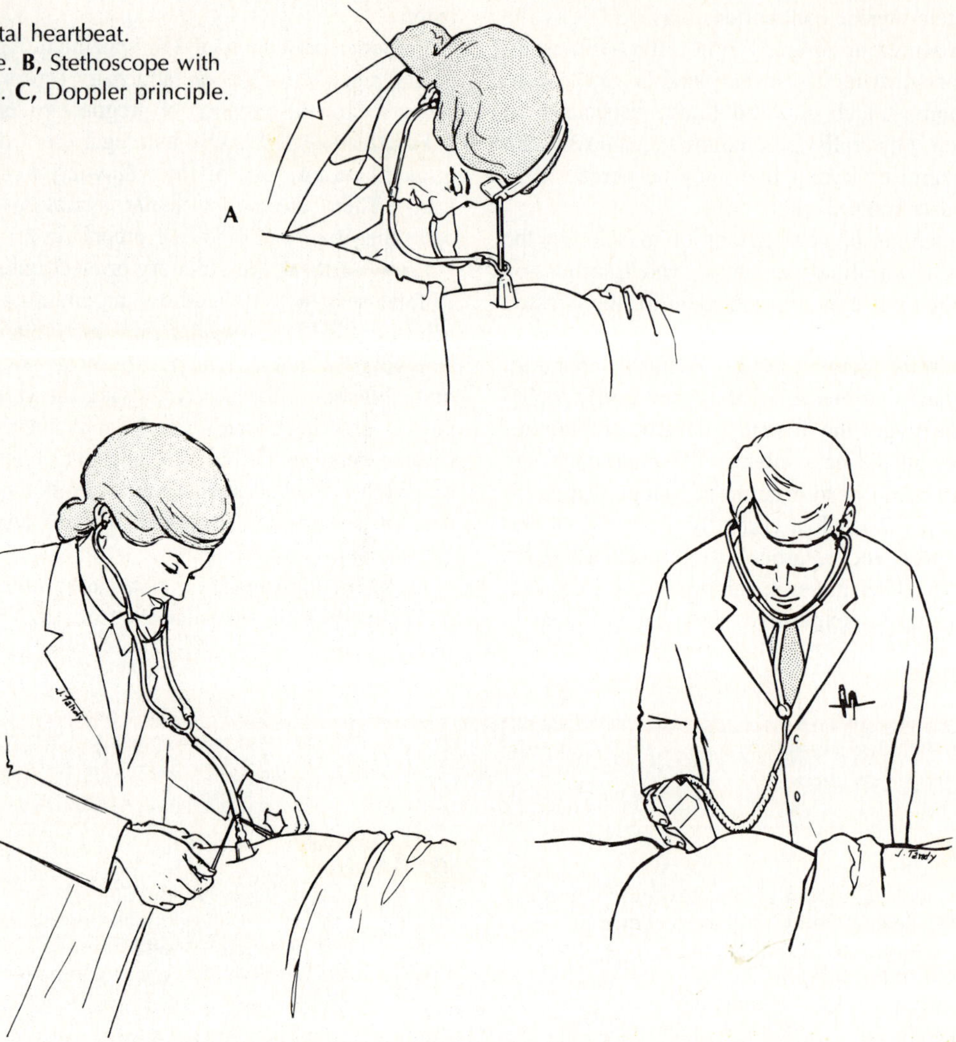

heart. Some evidence (in rats, dogs, and nonhuman primates) suggests that ultrasound at very high intensities may affect fetal development; for example, it may cause anomalies, a delayed neuromotor reflex response, or altered emotional behavior. In 1978 the Food and Drug Administration (FDA) recommended that maximal output for continuous ultrasound be 20 mW/cm^{-2}.

Electrocardiography involves only the picking up of sound; that is, it does not involve sending any type of impulse to the fetus.

Palpation of fetal outline. Palpation of the entire fetus, that is, head, back, and upper and lower small parts, may be outlined in most women, other than the obese woman, particularly after the twenty-fourth week.

Palpation of fetal movements. Active movements of the fetus by an observer other than the mother may be identified after the eighteenth week in some women but are easier to elicit after week 24. Sometimes fetal activity can only be felt on vaginal examination.

Ultrasonographic demonstration of fetus. Ultrasonography has successfully identified an embryo as early as the fourth week; after the third month, this approach is most accurate. Ultrasonography (echography) is a valuable diagnostic aid that uses *pulsed* sound waves traveling through tissues of varying density to obtain a two-dimensional "gray scale" picture of the area under examination. In 1978 the FDA recommended ultrasound maximal outputs for pulse-echo devices to be 10 mW/cm^{-2}.

Radiographic demonstration of fetus. The fetal skeleton can be revealed by x-ray film as early as the twelfth week. In utero the fetus receives total body radiation that may lead to genetic or gonadal alterations, with implications for future generations. Therefore, roentgenography as a diagnostic tool must be used with caution during the woman's childbearing years.

Laboratory tests

Immunologic assays for human chorionic gonadotropin (HCG) have replaced biologic assays because they are convenient, inexpensive, and accurate. Most pharmaceutical companies claim that HCG secreted from the time of implantation (or nidation) can be accurately detected in *urine* 42 days after the LMP. HCG levels peak between days 50 to 90 after the LMP.

The 2-hr tube tests with urine are more reliable, especially if performed on the first-voided morning specimen. Two-minute rapid-slide tests are less expensive but also less sensitive and reliable. Test materials can be stored in a refrigerator for about 1 year. See manufacturers' directions for use. If the woman is to bring a urine specimen for a pregnancy test, she is given the following written directions:

1. Do not eat or drink anything after the evening meal.
2. Collect first urine voided in the morning (concentrated specimen).
3. Refrigerate urine until bringing the specimen to the office.

The *radioimmunoassay (RIA) test for the beta subunit of HCG* is so sensitive that pregnancy can be diagnosed *before* the first missed period. This test is expensive and not readily available.

RIA for HCG, if performed correctly, is virtually 100% accurate by the fifth week. The possibility that this test can cross react with luteinizing hormone (LH) renders it less accurate than the assay for the beta subunit of HCG.

RIA is the most sensitive test but is not always available. It requires about 24 hours to complete. Diagnosis of pregnancy is possible from the second day after implantation, the twenty-third day after the LMP, or about 5 days *before* the first missed period.

The positive tests for pregnancy may be done at the initial visit (e.g. urine tests) or postponed until the appropriate time during pregnancy (e.g., palpation of fetal movements).

Duration of pregnancy and estimated date of confinement

Term pregnancy. A term pregnancy is a gestation of 38 to 42 weeks (see box on p. 278 for correlation of data regarding gestational age). Occasionally women will be certain of the LMP, date of coitus on or just before ovulation, or both. Hence the duration of pregnancy can be assessed with certainty. More often, however, women will have none of these essential data, and estimates of the length of gestation by the physician will be necessary.

In pregnancy, numerous ways of determining the duration of pregnancy may be employed. No one of these is infallible, but a combination of the results of two or three of the following methods is accurate.

Because the precise date of conception generally must remain conjectural, many formulas or rules of thumb have been suggested to calculate the estimated date of confinement (EDC). None of these is accurate, but the approximations below are helpful.

Naegele's rule. Naegele's rule is as follows: add 7 days to the first day of the LMP, subtract 3 months, and add 1 year, or EDC = [(LMP + 7 days) − 3 months] + 1 year; for example, if the first day of the LMP was July 10, 1983, the EDC is April 17, 1984. (In simple terms, add 7 days to the LMP and count forward 9 months.)

Naegele's rule assumes that the woman has a 28-day cycle and that the pregnancy occurred on the fourteenth day. An adjustment is in order if the cycle is longer or shorter that 28 days.

Using Naegele's rule, only about 4% to 10% of gravidas will deliver spontaneously on the EDC. The majority of women will deliver during the period extending from 7 days before to 7 days after the EDC.

Fundal height. During the first and second trimesters of pregnancy, the fundal height, as measured on the anterior abdominal wall, affords a gross estimate of the duration of pregnancy. Measurement of fundal height may aid in identification of such high-risk factors as intrauterine growth retardation (IUGR), multiple gestation, and polyhydramnios.

Among the factors that affect the accuracy of measurement are obesity (subtract 1 cm from the measurement if the gravida weighs 90 kg [200 lb] or more), the amount of amniotic fluid, multiple gestation, the fetal size and attitude, the tilt of the uterus, and the width of the examiner's finger if fingerbreadths(fb) are used.

To measure fundal height a tape measure or a pelvimeter may be used. With a flexible (not stretch) tape measure, measure the height of the fundus from the notch of the symphysis pubis over the top of the fundus without tipping the corpus back. A metal pelvimeter may be used in place of a pliable tape.

To increase measurement reliability and facilitate management, the same person examines the gravida at each of her prenatal visits, and one protocol is established for use by all examiners providing care to a group of gravidas.

The protocol must include the gravida's position on the table and the measuring device and method used. The gravida's position is supine with the knees slightly bent and the head and shoulders slightly elevated. If a pliable measuring tape is used, it should be specified whether the measurement is taken with the tape following the exact contour of the uterus to the fundus (Fig.

Correlation of Data in Determining Fetal Gestational Age

Menstrual history

LNMP*: Date ____________ Duration ____________ Amt ____________
LMP†: Date ____________ Duration ____________ Amt ____________
PMP‡: Date ____________ Duration ____________ Amt ____________
Menarche ____________ Interval ____________ Duration ____________
Hx of menstrual irregularity ____________

Contraceptive history

Type of contraceptive ____________
When stopped ____________

Pregnancy test

Date ____________ Type ____________ Result ____________

Clinical evaluation

First uterine size estimate: Date ____________ Size ____________
FHT first heard: Date ____________ Dopptone ____________ Fetoscope ____________
Date of quickening ____________
Current fundal height ____________ EFW§ ____________
Current weeks' gestation ____________
Ultrasound: Date ____________ Weeks' gestation ____________ BPD|| ____________
Reliability of dates ____________

Impression

EDC ____________ Estimated gestational age ____________
Estimation based on ____________
Comments ____________
Signature ____________ Date ____________

*Last normal menstrual period.
†Last menstrual period.
‡Previous menstrual period (prior to LMP).
§Estimated fetal weight.
||Biparietal diameter.

17.6) or if the measurement is read with the palm of the hand at the fundus and the tape elevated between the forefinger and middle finger (Fig. 17.7).

Authorities disagree on the exact measurement of fundal height appropriate for each week of gestation. There is no identified protocol for the measuring techniques used to obtain the values in Table 17.5.

McDonald's rule adds precision to the measurement of fundal height during the second and third trimesters. Calculate as follows:

$$\text{Height of fundus (cm)} \times 2/7 \text{ (or } + 3.5) = \text{Duration of pregnancy in lunar months}$$

$$\text{Height of fundus (cm)} \times 8/7 = \text{Duration of pregnancy in weeks}$$

Sandberg (1978) states that during the second trimester the height of the uterine fundus in centimeters above the symphysis pubis generally approximates the menstrual age of the gestation in weeks.

Gestational age. The gestational age of the fetus may be used to indicate the duration of pregnancy and the EDC. See p. 281 for details of the methods used in estimating gestational age.

Prolonged pregnancy. Prolonged or postdate pregnancy, by definition, begins 294 days after the LMP, that is, 14 days after the conventionally accepted normal duration of pregnancy (280 days). Prolonged pregnancy occurs in 10% to 12% of all gestations. Perinatal mortality in prolonged pregnancy, as compared with term pregnancy, is increased three times at 43 weeks and five times at 44 weeks. Infants of primigravidas with prolonged pregnancy are at greater risk than those of multiparas.

Although some of the neonates of prolonged pregnancies are well developed and more mature than those born at term, others are postmature—actually dysmature. The latter have dry, cracked, wrinkled, parchmentlike skin with absent vernix caseosa and long, thin arms and legs. These neonates have a higher incidence of fetal distress and perinatal death. The normal-appearing infants do well if fetopelvic disproportion (FPD) does not develop because of their increased size. A

Fig. 17.6
Student practicing taking the measurement of fundal height (McDonald's method).

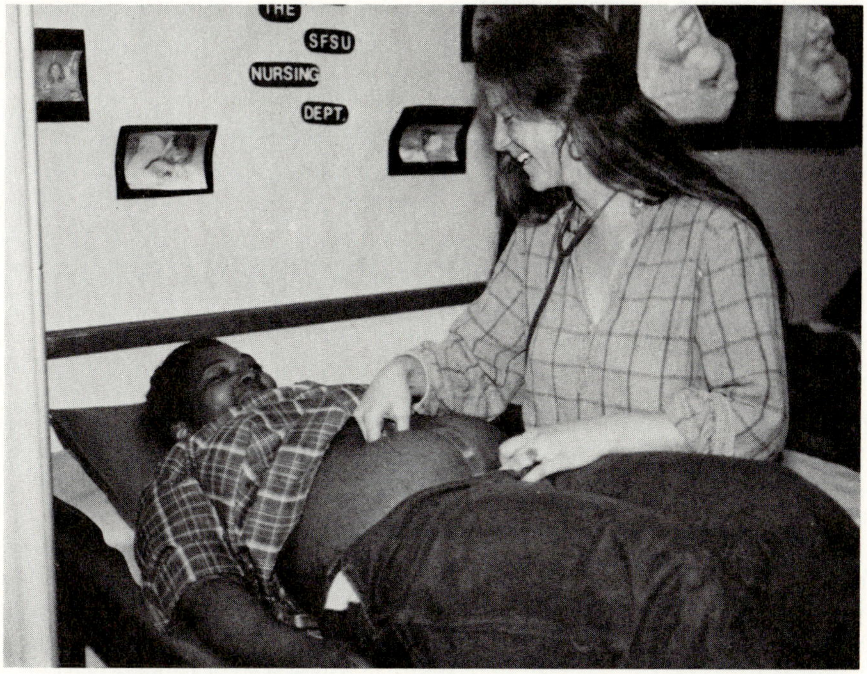

Fig. 17.7
Measurement of fundal height from symphysis.

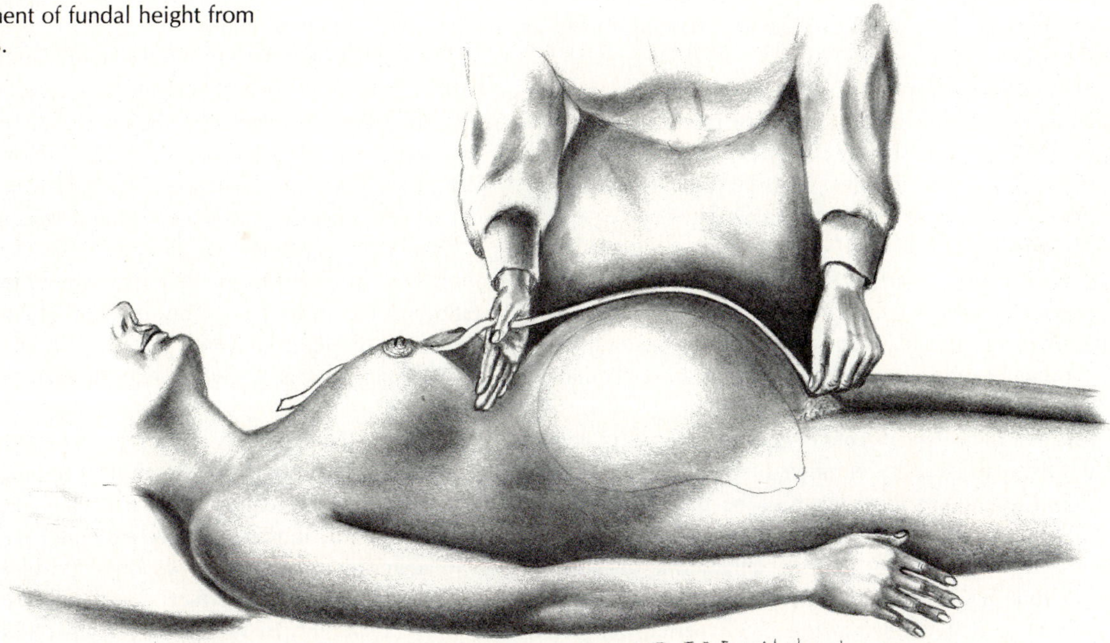

Table 17.5
Comparison of Fundal Heights

	Height in Fingerbreadths (fb) in Relation to Anatomic Landmarks	Height in Centimeters above Symphysis Pubis		
Week	**McLennan and Sandberg**	**Spielberg**	**McDonald**	**Sandberg**
16	3-4 fb above symphysis pubis			
20	2-3 fb below umbilicus		18	20
24	At umbilicus		21	24
28	3 fb above umbilicus	26.7	24.5	28
32	3 fb below xiphoid	29.5-30	28	32
36	2 fb below xiphoid	32	31.5	36
40	2 fb below xiphoid	37.7	35	40

breakdown of perinatal deaths associated with prolonged pregnancy reveals that about one third occurred during the prenatal period; approximately one half occurred during the intranatal period; and about one sixth occurred during the postdelivery period.

When a gravida is 2 weeks overdue, one of the following possibilities and its implications apply:

1. The pregnancy is not prolonged, and therefore there is no threat to the fetus.
2. The pregnancy is prolonged, but the placenta continues to function efficiently and there is no threat to the fetus.
3. The pregnancy is prolonged, and there is acute placental failure with threat to the fetus.
4. The pregnancy is prolonged, there has been chronic placental insufficiency, and the threat to the fetus continues.

For safe delivery of the offspring, it becomes important to determine whether prolonged pregnancy actually has developed and if there is any evidence of fetal jeopardy. Data for determining fetal gestational age is obtained from several sources and correlated.

Verification of the LMP or rejection of this as inaccurate is most important to the diagnosis of prolonged pregnancy. A correlation of the LMP with the estimated duration of pregnancy at two of the earliest obstetric examinations may lead to substantiation or recalculation of the EDC.

If the dates are accurate but the uterus is larger than expected for the duration of pregnancy, hydramnios or multiple pregnancy may be the cause. If the dates seem correct but the size of the fetus is disparate, fetal compromise, such as intrauterine growth retardation (IUGR), may be the problem, particularly in association with pregnancy-induced hypertension (PIH).

The woman's medical status should be reappraised. Diabetic or gestational diabetic mothers have large babies, and this may confuse the estimate of gestational age. Amniocentesis to ascertain the true gestational age is also advised. Preterm delivery of large babies should be avoided.

When the initial diagnosis of pregnancy was made at 20 weeks or less by physical examination, one or more of the *following observations* provide clinical confirmation of prolonged pregnancy:

1. Thirty-six weeks have elapsed since the recorded positive pregnancy test.
2. Thirty-two weeks have elapsed since the recorded FHT by Doppler instrument.
3. Twenty-four weeks have elapsed since recorded fetal movement.
4. Twenty-two weeks have elapsed since recorded FHT by auscultation.

Two serial *ultrasound examinations* and measurement of the *fetal biparietal diameter* should be accomplished 2 weeks apart after the twentieth week. This may confirm or reestablish the EDC. However, the EDC cannot be calculated when the initial biparietal diameter measures 9.5 cm or more (term size).

Other investigations may support the diagnosis of prolonged pregnancy, for example, amniotic fluid L/S ratio and creatinine and x-ray evidence of ossification centers in the fetal skeleton (p. 283).

The management of overly long pregnancy is as follows:

1. When the diagnosis of prolonged pregnancy is uncertain, additional information for or against the diagnosis is required and expectant management with fetal monitoring, for example, fetal activity determination (FAD), weekly cervical assessment for dilatation and effacement, weekly estimate of fetal weight (EFW), nonstress test (NST), and serial estriol determinations, should be carried out.
2. When the diagnosis of prolonged pregnancy is es-

tablished and there is a threat to the fetus, the woman should deliver. If induction (under constant fetal monitoring) is unsuccessful, if labor is unsatisfactory, or if fetal distress develops, cesarean delivery should be done.

FETAL GESTATIONAL AGE AND HEALTH STATUS

During the past decade, a variety of techniques have been developed for appraising the gestational age and health of the fetus. These include (1) ultrasonography, (2) measurements of certain hormones in maternal plasma or urine, (3) amniocentesis, (4) FHR, (5) fetal movement, and (6) other identifiable events.

Ultrasonography. A static-image (beta scanner) or a dynamic (moving) image (real-time scanner) may be used. In obstetrics the real-time scanner is used more frequently since fetal motion and cardiac motion can be visualized. This technology is regarded as accepted practice for the following indications:

1. Establish fetal gestation (head size measurement)
2. Determine placental location (choosing site for amniocentesis)
3. Assess the possibility of multiple pregnancy
4. Exclude fetal death
5. Evaluate possible complicating uterine abnormalities

No adverse biologic effects have yet to be measured using diagnostic ultrasonic intensities. Consequently, the use of *diagnostic* ultrasound is considered to be innocuous (Athey and Hadlock, 1981). However, since the long-term effects are not yet definitively established, this technique is not used routinely for pregnant women by all physicians. If the technique is used, it is performed at 20 weeks and repeated at 32 weeks. The nurse can assure the woman that the procedure is painless and make sure the technician describes the process to the woman. The woman is instructed *not* to empty her bladder before coming for the test. Early in pregnancy the full bladder acts to support the uterus. However, it may obscure certain diagnoses, e.g., placenta previa. It takes only a few minutes to empty the bladder, but the examination may require an additional hour if bladder filling is needed and the woman has not been instructed to report with a full bladder.

If ultrasonography is done, beta-scan fetal biparietal diameter at 36 weeks should be approximately 8.7 cm. Term pregnancy and fetal maturity can be diagnosed with considerable confidence if the biparietal cephalometry by ultrasonography is greater than 9.8 cm (Figs. 17.8 and 17.9 and Table 17.9).

Amniocentesis. Greater accuracy in estimating fetal maturity is now possible through utilization of amniotic fluid or its exfoliated cellular content (for procedure see

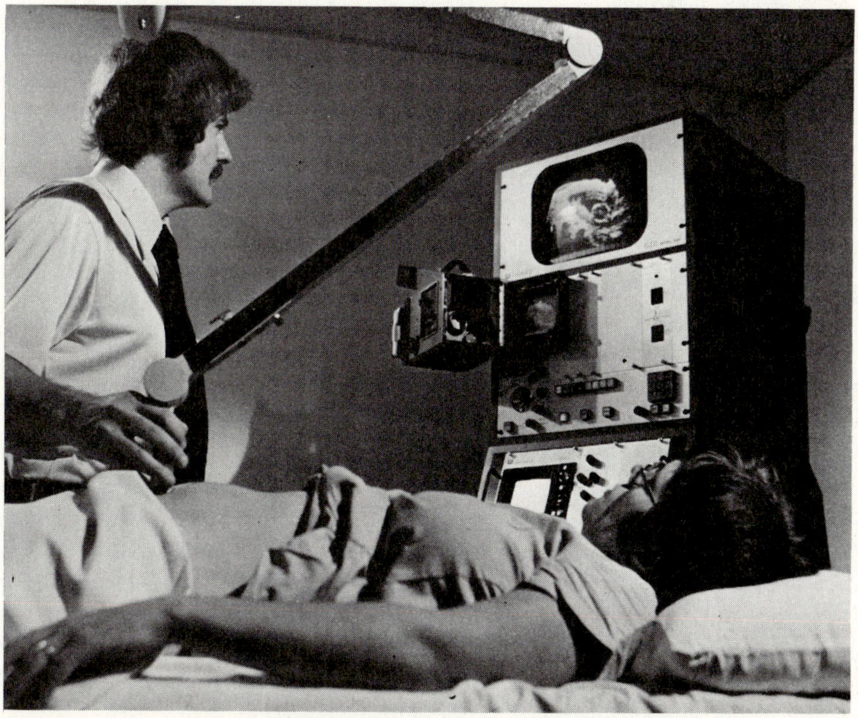

Fig. 17.8
Ultrasonography is noninvasive, painless method of scanning mother's abdomen with high-frequency sound waves to determine fetal growth and development. (Courtesy March of Dimes.)

Fig. 17.9
Biparietal cephalometry by ultrasound.

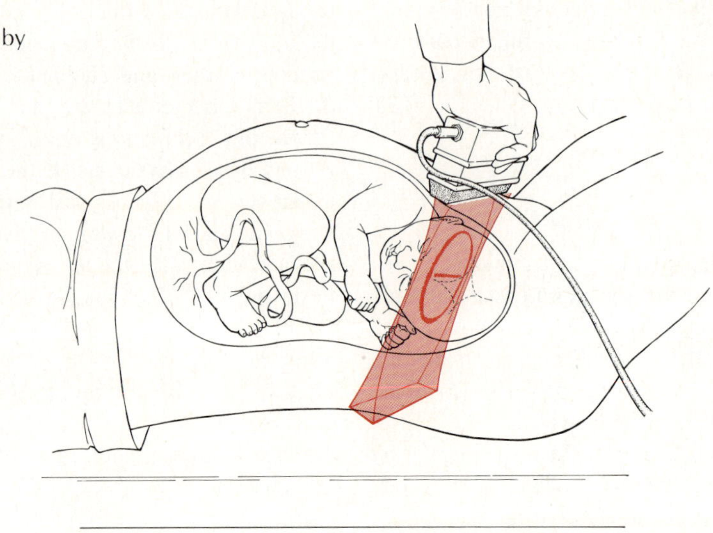

p. 152). Technically, term pregnancy and fetal maturity have been reached if more than one of the following are properly demonstrated by laboratory studies:

1. An *L/S ratio* that is greater than two indicates adequate lung maturity for extrauterine life (see p. 217). This will be achieved if the fetus is older than 36 weeks' gestational age. A practical variation of the L/S ratio is the rapid surfactant test, also known as the shake test or bubble test. Equal parts of fresh amniotic fluid and normal saline solution are added to two parts 95% ethyl alcohol. The mixture is shaken vigorously for 30 seconds. If bubbles are still present at the meniscus 15 minutes after shaking, the fetal lung is judged to be mature.
2. When the optical density of *bilirubinoid pigments* is 450 nm <0.01, this indicates a gestational age of greater than 38 weeks. Bilirubin disappears after 36 weeks. (For further discussion of delta optical density [ΔOD] see Fig. 40.2.)
3. When the *creatinine* (estimate of renal maturity) value is greater then 1.8 mg/dl, the gestational age is greater than 36 weeks in the absence of maternal renal disease, dehydration, or fetal anomaly.
4. After *fetal lipid-containing exfoliated cells* are stained with Nile blue sulfate, a finding of more than 20% orange-staining cells indicates a gestational age of greater than 35 weeks; the fetus probably weighs 2500 g. (For information regarding the use of amniocentesis in estimating fetal health, see Table 17.6.)

Maternal urinary or plasma estriol level. Maternal estriol level in maternal urine (24 hr specimen) is an indicator of the normalcy of the fetoplacental unit. Estriol levels are elevated in multiple pregnancy, but they are extremely low in the presence of a failing pregnancy, anencephaly, or fetal death. Estriol levels fall in dysmaturity, preeclampsia-eclampsia (PIH), complicated diabetes mellitus, and partial separation of the placenta. Serial estriol determinations (never a single estimate) are essential to establish a trend to justify delivery of the fetus (for procedure, see p. 287).

Correct estimates of EDC based on estriol levels in maternal urine are unlikely with obesity, multiple pregnancy, or pelvic tumors, because the EDC will often be an early estimate. Growth retardation of the fetus, oligohydramnios, or fetal death may suggest a false later EDC.

Fetal heart rate. The fetal heart rate (FHR), rapid in early pregnancy, slows to about 120 to 140 beats/min at term. The rate is not a reliable index of the length of gestation. The FHR can be heard relatively early in pregnancy:

1. FHR heard by the Doppler method between weeks 10 and 12
2. FHR heard with a fetoscope at 17 to 19 weeks
3. FHR heard with a stethoscope by eighteenth to twenty-fourth week

Nonstress test. The FHR accelerates in response to fetal movement. This reaction is indicative of fetal health (see Chapter 24 for details of assessment near term).

Oxytocin stress or challenge test (OCT). Cautious uter-

Table 17.6
Summary of Biochemical Monitoring Techniques

Test	Results	Significance of Findings
Maternal urine estriols	High and rising levels	General fetal well-being
	Low and falling levels	Possible fetal jeopardy
Maternal blood		
Human placental lactogen	High levels	Large fetus; multiple gestation
	Low levels	Threatened abortion; IUGR; postmaturity
Unconjugated and plasma estriol	High and rising levels	General fetal well-being
	Low and falling levels	Possible fetal jeopardy
Heat-stable alkaline phosphatase	Normally elevated during pregnancy	Poor correlation with fetal outcome
Oxytocinase	200-400 U at term	General fetal well-being
	Low levels	Associated with fetal death; postmaturity; IUGR
Coombs' test	Titer of 1:8 and rising	Significant Rh sensitization
Amniocentesis		
Color	Meconium	Possible hypoxia/asphyxia
Lung profile		Fetal lung maturity
L/S ratio	>2.0	
PGL*	Present	
Creatinine	>2.0/dl	Gestational age > 36 wk
Bilirubin (ΔOD† 450)	<0015	Gestational age > 36 wk; normal pregnancy
	High levels	Fetal hemolytic disease in isoimmunized pregnancies
Lipid cells	> 10%	Gestational age > 35 wk
Alpha-fetoprotein	High levels after 15 wk gestation	Open neural tube defect
Osmolality	Decline after 20 wk gestation	Advancing nonspecific gestational age
Genetic disorders	Dependent on cultured cells for karyotype and enzymatic activity	
Sex-linked		
Chromosomal		
Metabolic		

From Tucker, S.M.: Fetal monitoring and fetal assessment in high-risk pregnancy, St. Louis, 1978, The C.V. Mosby Co. In an effort to summarize these studies in tabular form, generalization must be made. The reader is referred to the text (Tucker) for a complete description.

*Phosphatidylglycerol.

†Delta optical density.

ine stimulation with careful external FHR electronic monitoring is a simulated test of the fetoplacental functional reserve (see Chapter 24).

Fetal movement. The mother first experiences fetal movement between weeks 17 and 19. She is advised to report cessation or diminution of movement so that the physician may reassess fetal health.

Radiography. The presence of distal femoral ossification centers indicates a fetal age of 36 weeks. If the proximal tibial centers are present, the fetus is 40 weeks' gestational age. X-ray visualization of the distal femoral and proximal tibial epiphyseal centers also indicates term pregnancy. This is used with great caution because of the danger of fetal and maternal gonadal damage.

Amnioscopy. Fetal hypoxia is known to result in meconium passage by the mature fetus. Transcervical visualization of greenish amniotic fluid through the intact membranes indicates fetal asphyxia. Unfortunately the cervix must be more than 1 cm dilated, and special equipment (amnioscope with tungsten lamp) is needed so this technique is used rarely.

MATERNAL AND FAMILY NEED FOR PSYCHOSOCIAL CARE

Nursing role. The nurse functions in a collaborative manner with other members of the health team in providing emotional support for the pregnant woman and her family. In the process of providing such support, the nurse assumes many roles: consultant, counselor, teacher, and advocate.

The extent of the nurse's involvement with the mother-to-be, the family, or both varies with the needs of the individuals concerned. With some persons the nurse's action may consist of noting the presence of adequate situational supports developed by the family and the use of successful methods of coping with stress, commending the individuals for their foresight and planning, and serving as a resource person for information about services available either locally or nationally or in the public or private sector that may be useful for the mother-to-be and her family. With other persons stressful periods may necessitate either intermittent or sustained nursing care. For those women who have symptoms indicating a deep and traumatic rejection of the pregnancy or of parenthood, the nurse may be instrumental in securing the intervention of other health workers—psychiatrist, psychologist, psychiatric nurse specialist, or psychiatric social worker. If the woman is unable to resolve her deep feelings of anger and despair, there may be a carry-over of these attitudes to the postdelivery period, with deleterious effects on the child and other family members. Decisions about the extent of therapy required are of necessity constantly recurring stratagems in the nursing process.

Assessment: gravidas. In providing adequate prebirth support to pregnant women, a major problem is the difficulty in determining those whose emotional status will prove vulnerable to the stress of pregnancy and parenthood. Larsen and associates (1967) found that the woman holding negative attitudes stemming from the areas of interpersonal relationships (with husband, mother-in-law, or mother) and self-esteem (concerning her own body) was more prone to develop severe personality problems.

Gordon and Gordon (1960) theorized that adverse reactions to childbearing stem from the cumulative effect of social stresses. They categorized these stresses as belonging to three groups

1. *Sensitizers*—stresses happening early in life that act to reduce and render inadequate an individual's defense mechanisms (e.g., loss of one's mother before 21 years of age)
2. *Pressurizers*—stresses arising from an individual's everyday environment whether in the home or marketplace (e.g., inadequate income for basic needs)
3. *Precipitators*—unexpected stresses that overwhelm the individual's emotional defenses (e.g., moving to a new community with no relatives or friends to help)

Gordon and Gordon's subsequent research indicated that women who experience 10 or more of the 50 identified social stresses are in need of support to prevent emotional breakdown in the postdelivery period. Those particularly prone to stress were identified as presenting two key patterns, one centering around the amount of personal insecurity and the other around the amount of maternal role conflict present.

Steele and Pollock (1968) used a questionnaire to assist in detection of parent-to-be possessing traits in common with those parents known to have distorted parent-child relationships. Undue anxiety about the crying of infants, the necessity to assume sole responsibility for a child, negative reactions to supervision of child care, and rigid expectations of a child's behavior can be used as indicators for providing additional emotional support.

As a result of their research, Gray and associates (1979) described signs during the prenatal period that may indicate a potential for disorders in parenting:

1. Mother seems overly concerned with baby's sex or performance.
2. Mother exhibits denial of pregnancy (not willing to gain weight, no plans for baby, refusal to talk about situation).
3. This child could be "one too many."
4. Mother is extremely depressed over pregnancy.
5. Mother is very frightened and alone, especially in anticipation of delivery. Careful explanations do not seem to dissipate fears.
6. There is lack of support from husband and family.
7. Mother or father or both formerly wanted an abortion or seriously considered relinquishment and have changed their minds.
8. Parents come from an abusive or neglectful background.
9. Parents' living situation is overcrowded, isolated, unstable, or intolerable to them.
10. They do not have a telephone.
11. There are no supportive relatives or friends.*

Although research is continuing to develop more precise methods of assessing individuals' capabilities in relation to successful coping with the tasks of pregnancy and parenthood (see Chapter 16), much still must be done. Unfortunately for many nulliparas, fantasy about pregnancy and parenthood precludes a real understanding of future commitments. Assessment will therefore need to continue throughout the prenatal, natal, and postdelivery periods if those for whom we have sufficient knowledge to help are actually to receive that help.

The form developed by Funke-Farber is a useful tool for assessing maternal response prenatally to parenthood (see p. 294). It provides questions as guides for the nurse's use while interviewing clients.

Assessment: family. The family also needs to be assessed as a support system for the woman and her child. The family assessment (see p. 293) provides information about family identification, activities, and dynamics.

---

*Reproduced by permission from Gray, J.D., et al.: Prediction and prevention of child abuse, Semin. Perinatol. **3**:86, Jan. 1979.

PRENATAL EXAMINATION PROCEDURES

The examination procedures used during the prenatal period are relatively few in number, and some are common to many clinical areas.

Clean-catch urine specimen

Purpose. A specimen of urine* is needed for examination at the initial visit for routine urinalysis and at subsequent visits for evaluation for glucose and protein.

Procedure. Ideally, the specimen is obtained immediately after rising in the morning. A clean container must be used. The woman should be instructed as follows:

1. Wash hands.
2. Spread labia and wipe from front to back, using moistened toilet paper.
3. Begin voiding and then obtain specimen during midstream in a clean container; 30 to 60 ml (1 to 2 oz) of urine is sufficient.
4. Wash hands.
5. Bring the specimen for analysis (it does not have to be kept cool).

Pelvic examination

Purpose. A pelvic examination (see p. 384) permits visual and digital examination of the external and internal genitalia and pelvic contours.

Preparation. Many women find the pelvic examination to be embarrassing and somewhat frightening. The emotional and psychologic components of the pelvic examination need to be stressed. The examination may be utilized to increase the woman's knowledge of her anatomy and physiology and, if so used, is an important educational tool. Before beginning the examination the nurse or practitioner discusses the procedure and what to expect. The woman can be shown the speculum and how it is to be used. During the examination the woman can be reminded that she will be touched to avoid her suddenly tensing up and experiencing discomfort.

Procedure

1. Have woman void.
2. Select and prepare equipment for use. (Fig. 17.10). The speculum is warmed before inserting.
3. Assist the woman into lithotomy position. Drape her and explain the procedures to follow.
4. Help her to relax by having her pant-breathe, keep her eyes open, keep her fingers relaxed (clenching the fist increases tension in all muscles). *Do not* allow her to squeeze your hand because this also increases tension in all muscles.
5. Involve her in the examination with explanations of what is being touched and why, by maintaining eye contact, and by offering to show her (with the use of a mirror) what is being viewed.
6. During the examination, if the woman becomes pale and breathless and her skin becomes clammy, turn her onto her left side to relieve *supine hypotension syndrome. (Occasionally the same reactions are seen when the cervix is touched. It is thought to be the result of stimulation of the vagal nerve.)*
7. When the examination is complete, assist the woman into a sitting position and then a standing position. Provide wipes for removal of lubricant.

Papanicolaou smear

Purpose. The Papanicolaou (Pap) smear is taken to detect abnormalities of cell growth by examining secretions and cells from the squamocolumnar junction, the cervix, and the vagina.

Preparation. The woman is told the purpose of the test, what sensations she will feel as the specimen is obtained (i.e., pressure but not pain), and that the test should be repeated routinely.*

Procedure. Smears should be obtained at the first opportunity, although bleeding or douching within 12 hours of taking smears may result in a higher percentage of unsatisfactory or negative specimens. Women should be advised routinely that repeat smears may be necessary so that they will not be unduly anxious if asked to return.

The examiner will require a vaginal speculum sized according to the woman's dimensions, a spatula for removal of the specimen, clean glass slides, and cytology fixative such as Spray-Cyte or its equivalent, hair spray (Aqua-Net) (Fig. 17.10). No digital examination should be employed before obtaining the cytologic specimens, because the findings may be distorted. The speculum must be introduced with *no* lubricant (Fig. 17.11). Warm tap water or vaginal fluid may be used to moisten the speculum and assist its introduction.

The cervix should not be wiped, nor should endocervical bacteriologic specimens be taken with cotton swabs before the spatula scraping of the cervix. The mucus may contain the best carcinoma cells. If gross exudate or mucus is present, the excess is gently pushed away from the os with the end of the spatula. The specimen is taken by placing the S-shaped end of the cervical spatula just *within the cervical canal at the external os.* The blade is rotated 360 degrees, so that the

---

*If the urine is to be used for a pregnancy test or estriol determination test, see also p. 275 and p. 287.

*Instead of urging that all women obtain annual Pap tests for cervical cancer, the American Cancer Society now advises that women over the age of 20, and those under 20 who are sexually active, have the test at least every 3 years, *but only after they have had two negative Pap tests a year apart.* A pelvic examination is recommended every 3 years from age 20 to 40 and annually thereafter.

Fig. 17.10
Equipment used for pelvic examination during prenatal care. **A,** Petri dish with media for cultures. **B,** Vaginal speculum. **C,** Swab for cultures. **D,** Vaginal pipette with rubber bulb. **E,** Slides. **F,** Spatula for Papanicolaou smear and cytology. **G,** Preservative. **H,** Slide for hanging drop preparation. **I,** Cotton pledgets. **J,** Forceps. **K,** Uterine sound. **L,** Sterile lubricant; may be antiseptic. **M,** Sterile glove for vaginal examination (clean for rectal examination).

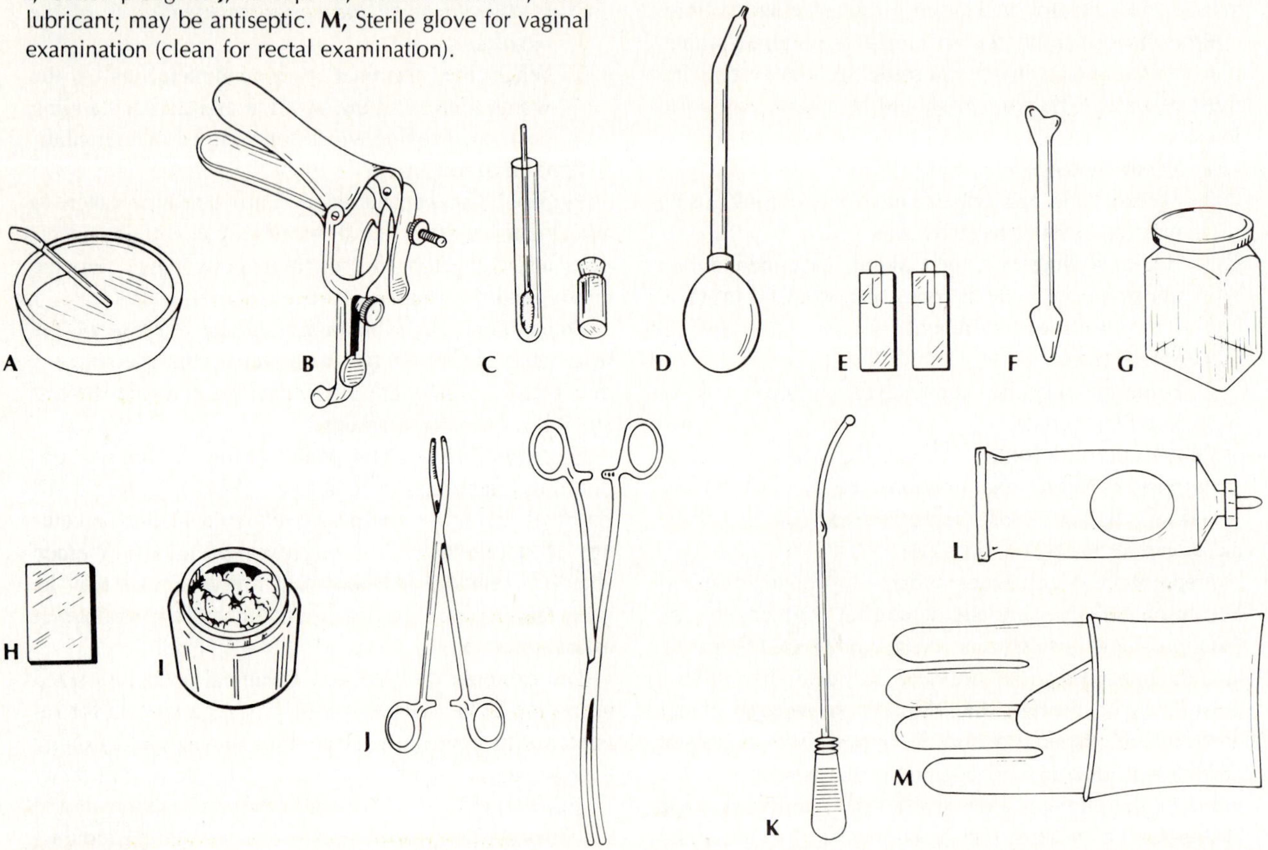

Fig. 17.11
Bivalve speculum examination. Cervix mucosa and vaginal mucosa are exposed by opening blades.

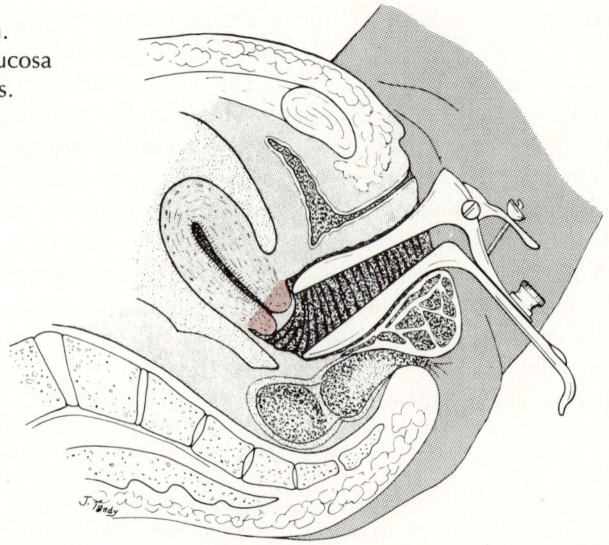

surface at the squamocolumnar junction is firmly scraped. The mucus is spread on a slide without drying or rubbing, sprayed lightly with fixative, and then allowed to dry.

Some mucus is obtained from the *posterior fornix* (vaginal pool) with the rounded end of the spatula, spread on another slide, sprayed, and dried.

The first slide will contain mainly cells from the endocervix and ectocervix in the area where cervical cancer is most often found. The second slide may reveal cells from the endometrium, endocervix, ectocervix, and vagina. Generally the slides are identified not by sites but by the woman's name.

The woman's name, age, parity, and chief complaint or reason for taking the cytologic specimens must be recorded on a form to accompany the slides. They should be sent to the pathology laboratory promptly for staining, evaluation, and a written report, with special reference to abnormal elements, including cancer cells.

Gonorrheal culture

Purpose. The gonorrheal culture screens a woman for gonorrheal infections for protection of the woman, her fetus, and her partner.

Preparation. The woman is told the reason for the test (e.g., test for vaginal infection) and that the test is done routinely at the first prenatal visit and repeated toward the end of pregnancy (thirty-sixth week).

Procedure. The specimen is obtained at the same time as the Papanicolaou smear, and the same precautions regarding use of digital examinations and lubricant are followed. A specimen is obtained from the endocervical canal using a sterile cotton-tipped applicator. The applicator is rolled on a culture plate with a special medium (Thayer-Martin). The plate is then incubated.

Herpes simplex, types 1 and 2, culture. If the Papanicolaou smear is positive, the result may be caused by the presence of herpes simplex, type 2. Open lesions may also be present. A viral culture is obtained and repeated at intervals.

Vaginal discharges. For assessing vaginal discharges other than blood, see p. 273.

Maternal urinary estriol determinations. The steroid precursor produced by the fetal adrenals is synthesized into estriols in the placenta and is excreted by the mother's healthy kidneys.

Purpose. The woman is told the purpose of the urine tests, that is, "to assess the health of your developing baby."

Preparation. The woman is provided with written directions for obtaining the specimens.

Procedure

1. Printed instructions are given to the woman: to void and discard the first morning urine, to collect all urine for the next 24 hours, storing it in the refrigerator, and then to bring it to the laboratory.
2. The following equipment is needed: two collection bottles, one sieve, and one boric acid cup.

Timing of serial determinations

1. Determinations are possible by 20 weeks.
2. A more reliable base line is possible after 28 weeks.
3. Best results are obtained after 32 weeks.

Factors altering results

1. Closely spaced serial evaluations are required to get the slope of increase or decrease. One reading at one point is useless.
2. The same technician should do all the tests for a particular woman to increase reliability of the results.
3. A false reading is likely if the woman is taking any of the following medications: corticosteroids, ampicillin, methenamine mandelate (e.g., Mandelamine) for urinary tract infection.
4. The methods of specimen collection and preservation are also factors.

Results *(see Table 17.6)*

1. High estriol levels with a rising slope are associated with a good prognosis for the fetus.
2. Low estriol levels may be associated with a compromised fetus.
3. Serum assays may be required if the woman's kidney clearance ability is questioned.

Amniocentesis. Amniocentesis is possible after the fourteenth week, when the uterus becomes an abdominal organ and when there is sufficient amniotic fluid for this procedure (Table 17.7).

Indications

1. Prenatal diagnosis of genetic problems (see p. 152).
   a. Karyotype from a cell culture indicating chromosomal aberrations, which appear in fetuses of 1% to 2% of women between 35 to 38 years of age, 2% of women between 39 and 40 years of age, and 10% of women over 45 years of age.

Table 17.7
Typical Amniotic Fluid Increase During Pregnancy

Weeks' Gestation	Amniotic Fluid Volume (ml)
12	50
14	100
16	175
18	250
20	325

From Queenan, J.T.: Contemp. Obstet. Gynecol **15:**61, Feb. 1980.

b. Sex chromatin in fetal cells (no culturing needed) if a sex-linked disorder (especially in the male fetus) is suspected.
c. Biochemical analysis of enzymes produced from a cell culture to detect inborn errors of metabolism (over 60 types are possible now).
d. Determination of alpha-fetoprotein (AFP) levels in supernatant fluid to detect neural tube defects, such as spina bifida and anencephaly. It may also be elevated with severe fetohemolytic disease, esophageal atresia, congenital nephrosis, omphalocele, fetal demise, and fetal hemorrhage into amniotic fluid. The amount of AFP should decrease to 18.5 μg/ml at 15 weeks and to 0.26 μg/ml at term. The recurrence rate of neural tube defects is 5%.

2. Gestational age (see Table 17.6 and Fetal Maturity, p. 281).
3. Identification and follow-up of isoimmune disease (Chapter 40).
   a. First determination is postponed until 24 to 25 weeks, since intrauterine transfusion of packed, Rh-negative, type O red blood cells is not possible before that time.
   b. Transfusion is usually indicated if Coombs' titer is above 1:8 to 1:16.
4. Amniography and fetography (following injection of radio contrast material): These procedures, to detect fetal death or anomaly, are ordered with caution because of concern regarding carcinogenic, teratogenic, and mutagenic effects on future generations.
5. Second-trimester elective abortion (see Chapter 41).
6. Hydramnios: Treat by aspiration of amniotic fluid.

Preparation. An amniocentesis is performed when there is indication of problems with the pregnancy or the fetus (Fig. 17.12). The mother and family are informed of the need for the surgical procedure and appraised of the risks. As with any surgical procedure the client and family will be tense and anxious as to the outcomes. The nurse acts as a support person during the procedure. Before beginning, the nurse reviews the following information:

1. Why such a long needle is used: The needle passes through layers of fat and muscle before reaching the uterus. Actually only a small portion of the needle enters the uterus.
2. Why no local anesthesia is used: The physician will not use a local anesthetic for two reasons: (a) the local anesthetic ''stings'' and (b) it would mean two needles. Once the skin is pierced there is a sensation of pressure but not pain.

Procedure

1. An informed consent statement and a surgical permit are signed by the woman.
2. Ultrasonography is performed to locate the placenta (Figs. 17.13 and 17.14).

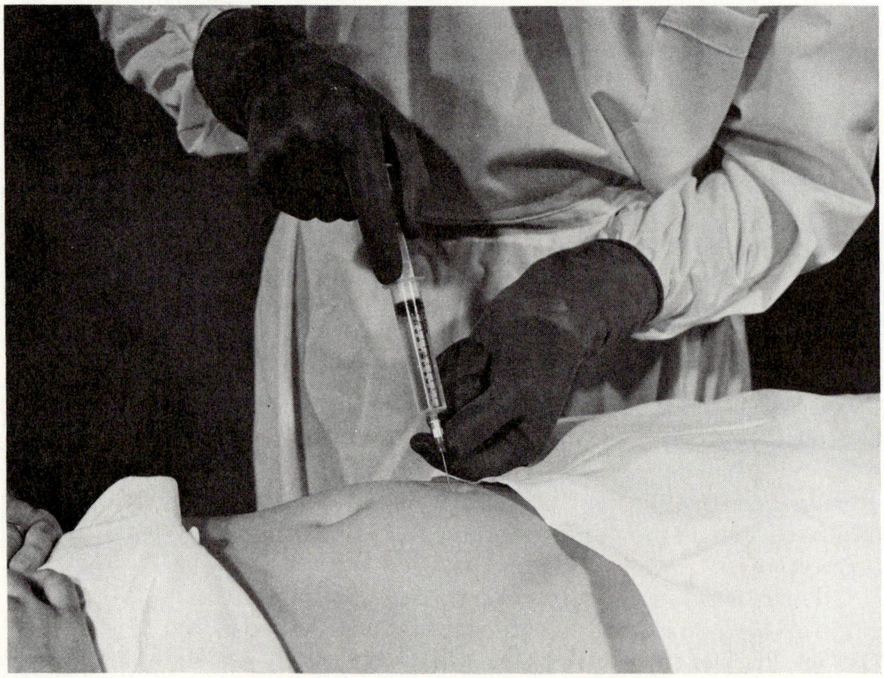

Fig. 17.12
Transabdominal amniocentesis. (Courtesy March of Dimes.)

Fig. 17.13

A, Real-time ultrasound image demonstrates appropriate site *(arrow)* for amniocentesis; this will avoid injury to fetal abdomen *(a)*. **B,** Static-image ultrasound examination demonstrates site for amniocentesis *(arrow)* that will avoid injury to fetal thorax *(t)*. (From Athey, P.A., and Hadlock, F.P.: Ultrasound in obstetrics and gynecology, St. Louis, 1981, The C.V. Mosby Co.)

A

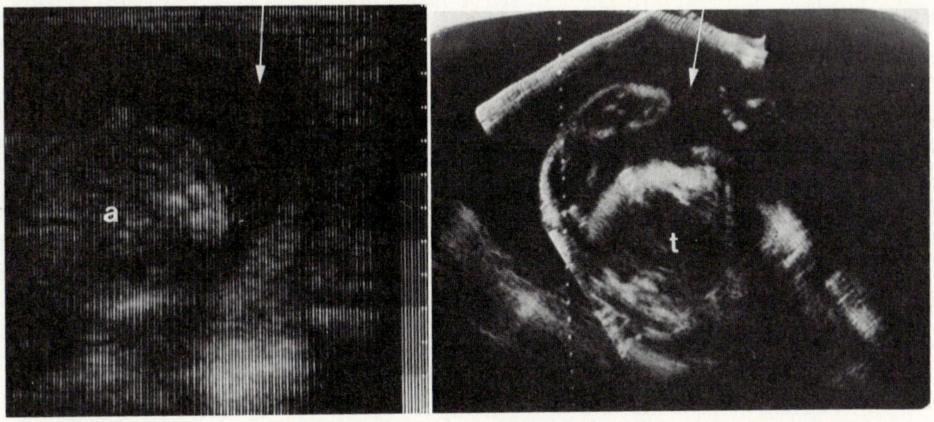

B

Fig. 17.14

A, Amniocentesis and laboratory utilization of amniotic fluid aspirant. **B,** 1a, 2a, 3, 4, 5, and 6 are front views with arrows indicating appropriate sites for amniocentesis varying with placental position. 1b and 2b are side views. (From Whaley, L.F.: Understanding inherited disorders, St. Louis, 1974, The C.V. Mosby Co.)

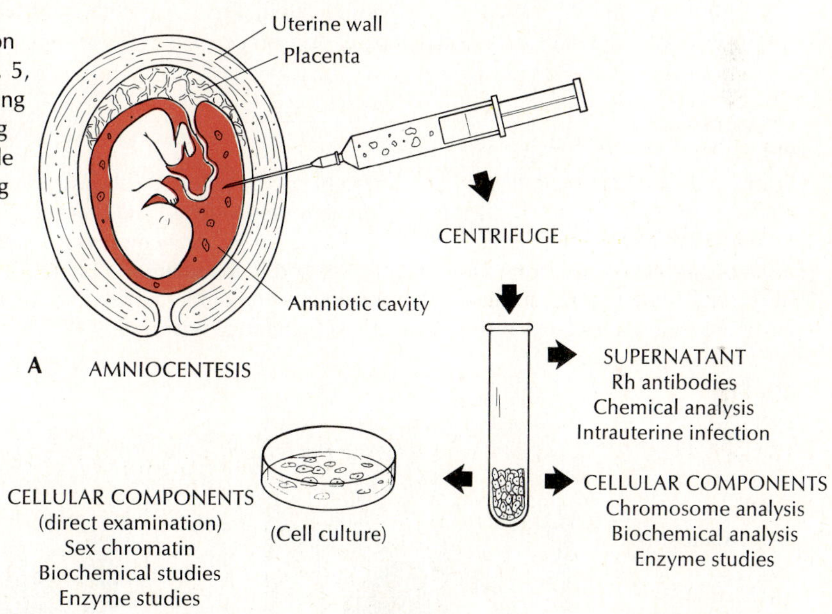

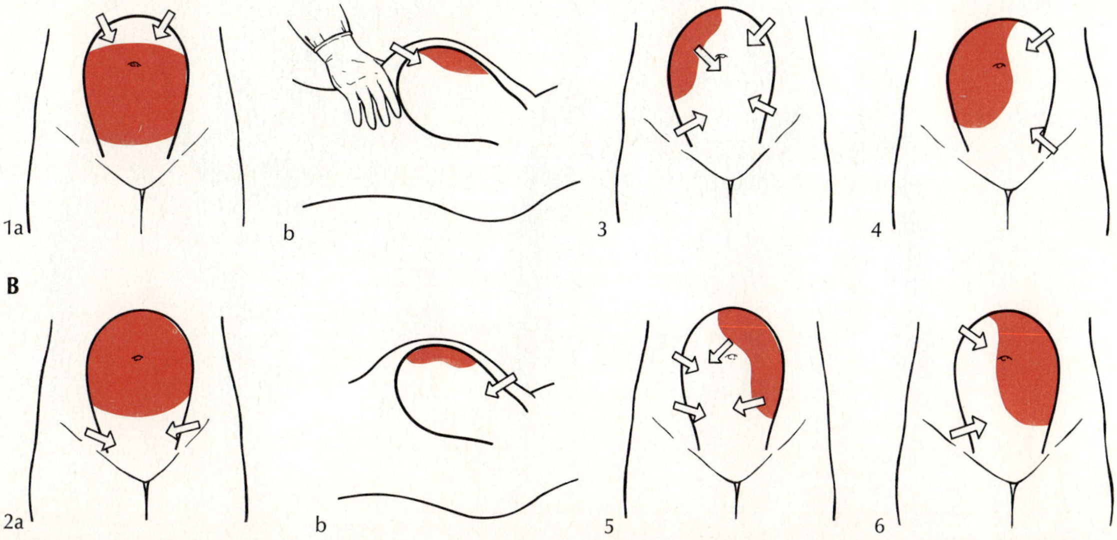

3. Equipment is readied, including an amniocentesis tray, fetal monitor, flashlight, and aluminum foil, or amber-colored test tubes (if a bilirubin determination is to be done), razor, bandage, antibacterial cleanser (pHisoHex), sterile gowns, masks, and gloves.
4. The woman is prepared.
   a. If the pregnancy is less than 20 weeks, a full bladder helps to brace the uterus (see bladder preparation under Ultrasonography, p. 281).
   b. Take base-line vital signs and the FHR; premedicate (if ordered) and place the woman in a supine position with her hands under her head, prepare the abdomen with a shave and scrub (Betadine); draw a blood sample (to compare with a postprocedure blood sample for assessing probable fetomaternal hemorrhage).
5. The nurse assists the physician, monitors and supports the mother, assesses FHR as indicated, assists with the specimens, and records the procedure (Fig. 17.15).
   a. Label three sterile tubes.
   b. If a bilirubin determination is needed, darken the room, use a flashlight, and immediately cover the filled alumnium-wrapped tube—light alters bilirubin so a true reading is not obtained.
   c. After withdrawing fluid, wash all povidone-iodine (Betadine) off the abdomen to prevent skin burn and apply a bandage.
   d. Assist with or draw a blood sample for assessing the presence of fetomaternal hemorrhage.
   e. Continue monitoring the FHR for 30 minutes.

Risks

1. Overall complications are less than 1% for both mother and fetus.
2. Maternal: hemorrhage, fetomaternal hemorrhage with possible maternal Rh isoimmunization, infection, labor, abruptio placentae, inadvertent damage to the intestines or bladder, amniotic fluid embolism.
3. Fetal: death, hemorrhage, infection (amnionitis,

Fig. 17.15
Example of data-recording system for amniocentesis procedures. Following data should be recorded: (1) diagram—abdomen, uterus, fetus, and placenta; (2) placental location; (3) amniotic fluid—volume, clarity, and color; (4) blood aspiration—initial aspiration, during procedure, and at termination; (5) fetal heart rates—before procedure and after procedure; (6) number of needle insertions; and (7) Rh factor, amniotic fluid (AF), and fetal heart rate (FHR).

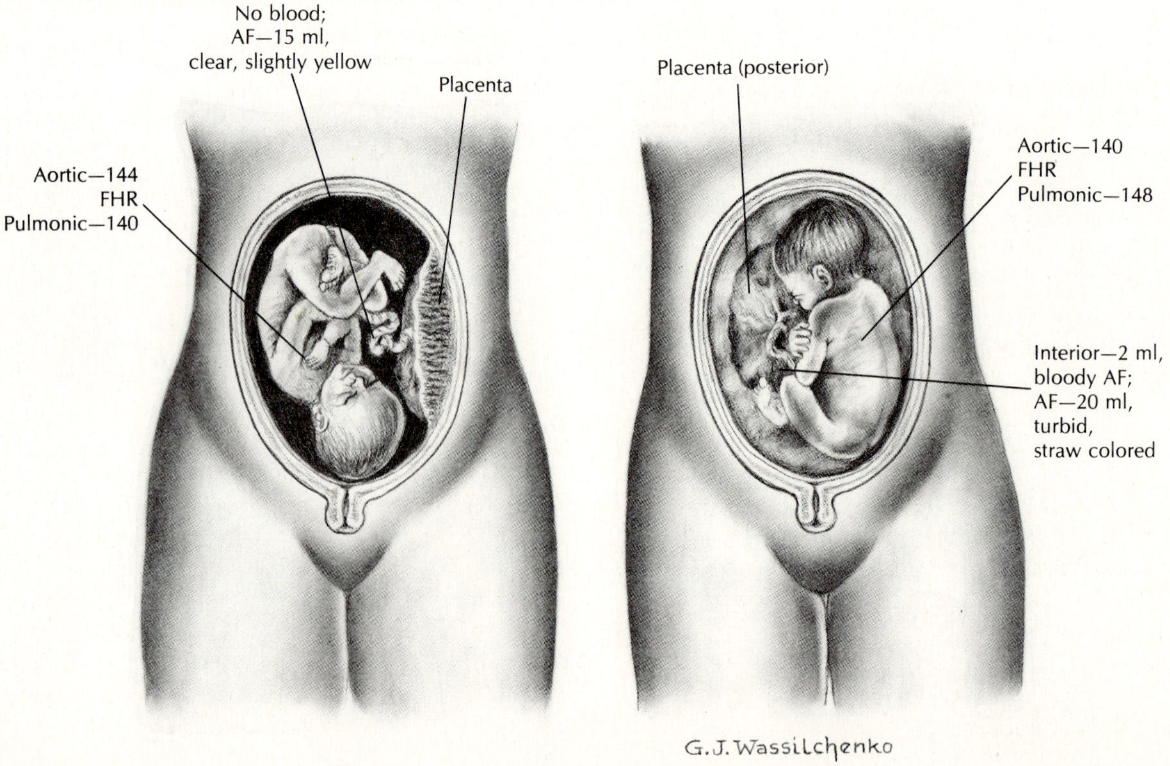

direct injury from the needle, abortion or premature labor, leakage of amniotic fluid.

Nursing Diagnoses in the Prenatal Period

Each client and family will present the nurse with a unique set of responses to pregnancy. In attending to these responses the nurse begins by formulating appropriate nursing diagnoses. The following are examples of nursing diagnoses arising during the course of the prenatal period:

1. Fear of pain during vaginal examination
2. Knowledge deficit regarding normal physical responses to pregnancy
3. Social isolation from lack of understanding of language and cultural expectations of childbirth
4. Alterations in family dynamics because of pregnancy of wife/mother

The nursing diagnosis acts as the stimulus for planning, implementing, and evaluating individualized care for clients. The information that follows is based on the generalized needs of clients and presents an overall picture. Clients will not exhibit all symptoms or needs.

Planning

INITIAL CONTACT WITH WOMAN AND FAMILY

The initial contact with the woman and her family marks the beginning of the nurse-client relationships and the maternity nursing process. The woman initiates the contact because she suspects she is pregnant. The care begun during the first visit is directed toward (1) the diagnosis (confirmation) of the pregnancy and (2) the beginning of the collection of data that acts as a basis for maternity care.

Protocol for care

Interview. The nurse obtains as much information as possible concerning the subjective symptoms of pregnancy and the woman's general health. The information is obtained through interview techniques and questionnaires.

1. Probability of pregnancy and any symptoms noted (e.g., amenorrhea)
2. Menstrual history: date of menarche; duration, amount of flow
   a. Last menstrual period (LMP)
   b. Previous menstrual period (PMP)
   c. Last normal menstrual period (LNMP)
3. Times and frequency of coitus
4. Contraceptive history: type, when used, any problems, when discontinued and reasons
5. Any current health problems
6. Any previous major illnesses, including those in previous pregnancies
7. Outcomes of previous pregnancies
8. All medications being used (the woman is asked to bring these with her at the next visit)
9. Reactions to pregnancy; if pregnant, does she desire it to continue
10. Concerns and questions

Physical examination. The next step in the diagnosis is a careful physical examination by observation, palpation, and auscultation and collection of specimens for laboratory testing.

1. Temperature, pulse, respirations, and blood pressure
2. Height and weight
3. Breast examination for changes: enlargement and vascular engorgement (sixth to eighth week), secondary areola, and colostrum (expressed after sixteenth week)
4. Abdominal examination
   a. Contour of uterus: measurement of fundal height if appropriate
   b. FHR if appropriate
5. Vaginal, bimanual, and rectovaginal examination
   a. Increased vascularity and deepening color of the vestibule and vaginal wall: Chadwick's sign (appears at about 6 weeks)
   b. Increased softening
      (1) Hegar's sign: softening of the lower uterine segment, resulting in its compressibility at about sixth week
      (2) Goodell's sign: cervical softening occurring about fourth to fifth week; infection or fibrosis may mask this presumptive sign
   c. Enlargement of uterus
   d. Leukorrhea

Collection of specimens

1. Clean-catch urine: glucose, protein, and culture to identify significant bacteria, and pregnancy testing
2. Blood: hemoglobin, hematocrit, red cell indexes, serologic tests for syphilis, identification of blood types and abnormal antibodies, and rubella antibody titer
3. Papanicolaou smear for cervical cancer
4. Smears for vaginal infections (e.g., gonorrhea, trichomomas)
5. Viral culture of the cervix for herpes simplex, type 2, if either the Papanicolaou smear or history suggests a herpes infection

FIRST PRENATAL VISIT

The first prenatal visit includes a comprehensive general health evaluation of the woman for the purpose of (1) defining the health status of mother, (2) determining the gestational age of the fetus, and (3) initiating a plan for continuing maternity care.

Protocol for care: comprehensive examination

I. Physical history
  A. Family history
    1. Health status of woman's parents and her siblings (if deceased, note cause of death)
    2. History of tuberculosis, cancer, diabetes mellitus, vascular disease, neuromuscular disease, allergies, other serious illnesses, or complications with pregnancies
  B. Medical history
    1. Age
    2. Racial origin (e.g., sickle cell anemia in blacks)
    3. Ethnic background (e.g., Tay-Sachs disease in Ashkenazic Jews)
    4. Childhood diseases
    5. Other diseases (e.g. sexually transmitted diseases)
    6. Surgery (e.g., abortion may predispose woman to incompetent cervix; uterine surgery or extensive repair of pelvic floor may necessitate cesarean birth; appendectomy rules out appendicitis as cause of right lower quadrant pain; spinal surgery may contraindicate spinal or epidural anesthesia)
    7. Injuries, particularly involving pelvis
    8. Allergies or sensitivities (drugs, foods, previous transfusions)
    9. Immunizations, including rubella
    10. Problems related to body systems; eyes, ears, nose, and throat; cardiovascular; gastrointestinal; urinary
    11. Menstrual history: menarche and present interval, amount of flow, pain; any other accompanying symptoms
    12. Sexual history
      a. Attitudes concerning range of acceptable sexual behavior as defined by such factors as culture, religion, family, and peer group
      b. Sexual self-concept: how one sees oneself sexually influences how one relates to others
      c. Level of knowledge, including knowledge of how body works and of sexual anatomy and physiology in addition to myths and misinformation
      d. Sexual behavior: marital or alternative relationship
      e. Physical status (one's state of health affects both sexual interest and ability to perform sexually)
      f. Contraceptive history (see Chapter 13)
  C. Obstetric history
    1. Gravidity, parity, abortions, stillbirths, living children
    2. If woman is multigravida, description of previous pregnancies: length of gestations; birth weight; fetal outcome; length of labor; presentation and type of delivery; prenatal, natal, and postdelivery complications
    3. Whether woman breast fed or bottle fed a previous infant
    4. If woman is Rh negative, whether she received Rho (D) immune globulin (RhoGAM)
  D. Present pregnancy
    1. See section on diagnosis of pregnancy
    2. Any abnormal symptoms noted
    3. Medications taken, prescription or nonprescription (e.g., aspirin), including alcohol, tobacco, and caffeine
    4. X-ray examinations, if any

II. Social and emotional history (woman's or couple's profile)
  A. Identification: birthplace, marital status or history, education, occupation, employment history
  B. Support systems: family composition and availability of friends, living arrangements, sources of income, health of family members, ages of other children, how family receives this pregnancy and how family supports or frustrates woman, health care concepts (particularly for pregnancy)
  C. Perception of this pregnancy: wanted or not, planned or not, pleased or displeased, accepting or nonaccepting; problems engendered by pregnancy—financial, career, and living accommodations; ideas about childbearing; expectations of infant's behavior; outlook on life and female role; what is expected of physician-woman (couple)-nurse relationship; perceptions related to age, race, or ethnic background
  D. Coping mechanisms: knowledge of preg-

nancy, maternal changes, fetal growth, care of self, and care of newborn (including feeding); attitudes toward natural or medicated childbirth; knowledge of parentcraft classes available; decision-making ability; use of significant others and of community affiliations (church, clubs) as supports; living habits (e.g., exercise, sleep, diet, diversional interests, personal hygiene, clothing)

E. Indicators for parenting potential (see box p. 294).

III. Review of woman's physical systems (or each symptom presented, obtain the following additional data: aggravating or alleviating factors, and associated manifestations [onset, character, course]).

A. General appearance: body type and weight, energy level, grooming, posture

B. Skin, hair, and nails: condition, color, consistency, lesions

C. Head: injury to, aches, dizziness, syncope

D. Eyes: vision, prescription glasses or contact lenses, pain, infections, discharges, swelling

E. Nose and sinuses: pain, bleeding, obstruction, discharge, frequency of colds or sinusitis, sneezing

F. Oral cavity: hoarseness, toothache, dentures, last visit to a dentist, frequency of dental care, state of lips and gums, problems with chewing or swallowing

G. Neck: pain, restriction of movement, swellings

H. Nodes: tenderness, enlargement, discharge

I. Breasts and nipples: pain, lumps, discharge, pigmentation, size, whether woman does breast self-examination

J. Respiratory system: pain or shortness of

Family Assessment Tool

Goal

To determine the support systems available: Who can be supportive to this woman and her unborn baby at this time? What kinds of support are available? What changes might be attempted to produce the needed support now or in the future? What preparation is now being made for the care of the infant?

Item	Findings
1. Family identification a. Who are the family members? Ages? Kinship? b. Where do they live? c. What family boundaries have been established? What family-community interchange exists? Who is permitted to be a family member? d. What relatives or friends are available? 2. Family activities a. What are the family's goals? Plans for the future? b. Who assumes responsibility for resources such as food, clothing, and housing? c. How are decisions made? What criteria are used? d. Who does what family work? Is there men's work, women's work, child's work, or anybody's work? E. How will the new baby be cared for? 3. Family dynamics a. What communication patterns are used? b. What are the attitudes toward health care and particularly, care during childbearing? c. What relationships exist between mother, father, siblings, and in-laws? Is the pregnancy "hers" or "theirs"? Who acts as the mother's primary support? d. What does the new baby mean to the family?	

Assessment of Maternal Psychologic Adaptation to Pregnancy and Parenting at 34 to 36 Weeks' Gestation

1. When did you first see a doctor about your pregnancy? Can you tell me why you chose to go at this particular time?

   Score

   _____ Saw doctor after third missed menstruation; didn't realize was pregnant; thought lack of menstruation may be due to something else; went to see doctor to have this investigated (1 point)
   _____ Saw doctor after second or third missed menstruation; went to see doctor because husband observed wife's irritability; went to have IUD checked (2 points)
   _____ Vague about when visit to doctor was made; thinks she missed two menstruations; unplanned pregnancy; wanted to validate (3 points)
   _____ Saw doctor about 1 week after second missed menstruation; knew she was already pregnant; planned; wanted to validate (4 points)
   _____ Saw doctor about 1 week after first missed menstruation; wanted to have planned pregnancy validated (5 points)

2. As a child, was there someone in your immediate family that you saw as a loving kind of person? Who was the most loving person in your family? Your mother? Your father? What were your parents like?

   Score

   _____ Did not have anyone in family that she saw as a loving person; expresses dislike and negative feelings about early childhood; may have been in numerous foster homes; parents very strict or very lenient (1 point)
   _____ Defines problems in childhood: separations from parents; definite family problems (e.g., alcoholism); parents inconsistent (2 points)
   _____ Vague about family; unable to give definite ideas re "a loving person"; ambivalent feelings expressed; unable to define characteristics (3 points)
   _____ Describes relationship with a parent as being satisfactory, with warmth, but wants relationship with own child to be stronger (4 points)
   _____ Mother or father seen as very positive, very warm person; expresses positive feelings (5 points)

3. What thoughts and ideas have you and your partner had on the changing of life-styles, working hours, or other adjustments pertaining to this pregnancy and new baby?

   Score

   _____ Have thought about it but believe no changes or adjustments are necessary; state that they believe this is important, not to change things for a baby (1 point)
   _____ Haven't thought about adjustments and changes; wonder if there will be a need to change; questioning possibility (2 points)
   _____ Have had some thoughts about changes; think they want to wait to see what it will be like once baby arrives; think that it is easier to do after baby comes (3 points)
   _____ Have already made a few changes; think that there will be a need for further changes; have spent time talking about it; have tentative plans (4 points)
   _____ Have made changes to suit wife's needs for increased rest; have spent time thinking about the changes; have plans for help—baby-sitter, relatives visiting, etc. (5 points)

4. Do you think you will need help when you get home from the hospital? Have you made any plans for help? If so, what are they?

   Score

   _____ No, doesn't want anyone interfering (2 points)
   _____ No, believes can manage well by self (4 points)
   _____ Ambivalent, doesn't know (6 points)
   _____ No help available: has made definite plans on how to try to manage, or plan involves calling someone in case of emergency (8 points)
   _____ Yes, has specific plans for husband or other person to be there for help (10 points)

Adapted from Funke-Furber, J.: Reliability and validity testing of maternal adaptive behavior, Edmonton, Alta., 1978, University of Alberta, Faculty of Nursing.

Assessment of Maternal Psychologic Adaptation to Pregnancy and Parenting at 34 to 36 Weeks' Gestation—cont'd

5. Have you had any thoughts, ideas, or hunches about your baby's appearance and behavior after you bring him home from the hospital?

Score

_____ Describes very unrealistic behaviors, such as regular sleeping or sleeping through the night; or describes three of four negative aspects (3 points)
_____ Describes one or two negative aspects along with two or three fears re not knowing what to do; or has no idea, gives it no thought (6 points)
_____ Unable to describe; can describe only in vague terms; describes fears relating to baby's crying (9 points)
_____ Can describe a few aspects (one or two) of baby's behavior (12 points)
_____ Describes realistically baby's sleeping, feeding, and crying behavior; has a few questions to have clarified (15 points)

Key
8-20: very high risk, intervention needed
21-30: questionable, "at risk," further follow-up needed
31-33: low risk
34-40: no risk

Scoring
Add points from each question:
1. _____
2. _____
3. _____
4. _____
5. _____
TOTAL _____

breath; frequency and types of infection (bronchitis, pneumonitis, pleurisy); cough, sputum, or wheezing, number of pillows (to elevate head) needed to sleep comfortably; number of cigarettes smoked per day and for how many years

K. Cardiovascular system: history of congenital heart disease, rheumatic fever, hypertension, hypotension, or anemia; pain; dyspnea; palpitations
L. Gastrointestinal system: changes in stools, bowel habits, or appetite—including food intolerance; history of disease of gallbladder, liver, or appendix; pain; jaundice; parasites; nausea; vomiting; or diarrhea; drugs taken
M. Genitourinary system; frequency, pain, or discharge; sexual history (see p. 302) and contraception history (see Chapter 13); history of sexually transmitted diseases and treatment
N. Extremities: muscle tone and cramping, vascularity, joint shape, joint pain or stiffness—gout, bone fragility, flat feet
O. Back: pain, stiffness, movement, sciatica or disk problems, curvature
P. Central nervous system: general, mentation, speech, motor, sensory
Q. Hematopoietic system: blood type, Rh, bleeding or coagulation disorders, transfusions, exposure to radiation
R. Endocrine system: history of growth and nutrition, tolerance for heat and cold
S. Immunizations

IV. Physical examination techniques and findings (see I, above)
   A. Head: face, scalp, hair, and hair pattern distribution, eyes, ears, nose, mouth, breath, teeth, gums, tonsils, salivary glands, lymph nodes
   B. Neck: skin, movement, lymph nodes, pulses (jugular, carotid), trachea, thyroid
   C. Thorax
      1. Anterior: heart, lungs, breasts, lymph nodes (include axillary), skin
      2. Posterior: heart, lungs, spine, skin
   D. Abdomen
   E. Extremities: size, contour, muscle mass and tone, vascularity, skin, joint movement, reflexes, nails and nail beds, edema, lymph nodes, pulses, varicosities
   F. Pelvic examination
V. Laboratory tests (Table 17.8)
   A. Tine or PPD (purified protein derivative [of tuberculin]) for exposure to tuberculosis
   B. Cervical and vaginal smears for cytology (Papanicolaou) and for chlamydia, gonorrhea, and herpes simplex, types 1 and 2

Table 17.8
Summary of Laboratory Tests in Prenatal Period

Laboratory Test	Purpose
Hemoglobin/hematocrit	To detect anemia
Hemoglobin electrophoresis	To identify women with hemoglobinopathies (e.g., sickle cell anemia)
Blood type, Rh, and irregular antibody	To identify those fetuses at risk for developing erythroblastosis fetalis or hyperbilirubinemia in neonatal period
Rubella titer	To determine immunity to rubella
VDRL/FTA	To identify women with untreated syphilis
Urinalysis, including microscopic examination of urinary sediment	To identify women with unsuspected diabetes mellitus, renal disease, hypertensive disease of pregnancy
Urine culture	To identify women with asymptomatic bacteriuria
Papanicolaou smear	To screen for cervical intraepithelial neoplasia and herpes simplex, type 2
Gonorrhea culture	To screen high-risk population for asymptomatic infection
Tuberculin skin testing	To screen high-risk population
Renal function tests: BUN, creatinine, electrolytes, creatinine clearance, total protein excretion	To evaluate level of possible renal compromise in patients with a history of diabetes, hypertension, or renal disease
Cardiac evaluation: ECG, chest x-ray film, and echocardiogram	To evaluate cardiac funtion in patients with a history of hypertension or cardiac disease

C. Blood (repeat at 32 weeks as necessary): VDRL test for syphilis, complete blood count (CBC) with hematocrit, hemoglobin, and differential values; blood type and Rh; antibody screen (Kell, Duffy, rubella, toxoplasmosis, anti-Rh); sickle cell; level of folacin when indicated; packed cell volume (PCV)—may be done at each visit in some offices

D. Urine: tests for glucose, protein, and acetone; culture and sensitivity as necessary

SUBSEQUENT VISITS

The gravida should be seen once each month until the thirty-second week, every 2 weeks until the thirty-sixth week, and each week thereafter until delivery. More frequent visits may be required if there are complications.

At subsequent visits the following information should be obtained and recorded in the gravida's record:

1. General well-being, complaints, or problems.
2. Weight and determination of whether gain (or loss) is compatible with overall plan for weight gain (see Fig. 18.4).
3. Gross urinalysis on first-voided morning urine specimen. Note degree (1+ to 4+) of protein and glucose.
4. Blood pressure (right arm, woman sitting).
5. Abdominal palpation.
   a. Height of fundus above symphysis pubis (measured with tape). Identify unusual tenderness, masses, herniation, and other important details.
   b. Determination of fetal presentation (after twenty-fourth week). Auscultate and count FHR. (FHR may be heard from eleventh week using Doppler method.)
   c. Beginning at thirty-second week, identification (with aid of Leopold's maneuvers [see p. 383]) of fetal presentation, position, and station (engagement) and assessment of uterine measurements and size (weight) of fetus as compared with supposed duration of pregnancy. Although some clinicians can estimate fetal weight with unbelievable accuracy, estimations are generally inconsistent and unreliable. Accuracy in estimating fetal weight improves with ultrasound determination of biparietal diameter (Table 17.9). Thus possible growth retardation of the fetus, multiple pregnancy, or inaccuracy of the EDC may be disclosed.
6. Vaginal or rectal examination at any time (unless gravida is bleeding) to investigate leukorrhea, confirm presenting part, corroborate station, and determine cervical dilatation and effacement. This may be especially important if labor is impending or induction is anticipated.
7. Specimen of venous blood for repeat hematocrit

Table 17.9
Correlation of Fetal Weight and Biparietal Diameter

Biparietal Diameter (cm)	Estimated Fetal Weight
8.2	2290 g (5 lb, 1 oz)
8.5	2500 g (5 lb, 8 oz)
8.8	2730 g (6 lb, 0 oz)
9.4	3180 g (7 lb, 0 oz)
10.0	3630 g (8 lb, 0 oz)
10.6	4070 g (9 lb, 0 oz)

or hemoglobin determination to diagnose and treat possible anemia. Repeat anti-Rh titer also if there is a reasonable chance that isoimmunization (Chapter 40) may have developed.

Table 17.10 presents a summary of the discomforts of pregnancy. Instruction and treatment regarding these are part of the care given during the subsequent visits.

Table 17.11 presents the assessments that are made at each prenatal visit and the expected findings as the woman progresses through pregnancy. Any significant deviations prompt further assessment and a revision of the care plan.

Recording complete and concise records during the prenatal period is essential for the documentation of maternal and fetal progress. Many standard printed record forms are available. The best records incorporate medical, laboratory, nursing, and dietary data assessments and plans in an easily readable arrangement from the first through subsequent office or clinic visits.

Implementation

GOALS

The goals of maternity nursing that relate to the client and her family during the prenatal period include goals directed toward both physiologic and psychologic support.

Expectations of success in providing physiologic support include individualized goals such as the following:

1. To detect deviations from the normal progress (see Table 17.11) of pregnancy and to initiate prompt remedial therapy.
2. To provide clients with pertinent knowledge of the adaptation of the maternal body to a developing fetus as a basis for understanding the rationale and necessity for certain modalities of care.

Goals that are more directed to the maternity population as a whole include the following:

1. To develop health services that are available to all pregnant women and their fetuses/neonates and families (see Appendixes A and B).
2. To develop nursing strategies with sound scientific bases.

Expectations of success in the area of emotional supportive care must of necessity be flexible. It is not within the province of any outsider to assure another person of a rewarding, satisfying experience. The mother and those significant to her are crucial elements in that process, and many of their problems are beyond the scope or capabilities of any professional worker. In describing her work with young and poor persons, Edwards (1973) noted: "They did not usually change their living situation and I was not instrumental in modifying home or drug problems." However, this did not deter her from encouraging them to use the decision-making process as a means of coping with problems rather than merely complaining about injustice.

At other times a successful outcome can be readily documented. A woman who early in her pregnancy had predicted a severe depressive state in the postdelivery period was elated when such a state did not materialize. She remarked to the nurse who had provided support during the pregnancy and birth, "You are the best nerve medicine I have ever had!"

In counseling it must be remembered that both the nurse and the client are contributing to the relationship. The nurse has to accept her own responses as a factor in trying to be of help. An example of one nurse-client relationship follows:

> Mrs. ________ had been very forthright in saying that this pregnancy was unplanned but countered this statement with comments such as "all things happen for the best," "we always wanted the boys to have a family to turn to," and "children bring their own love." Over a period of time as our relationship developed to one of *mutual* trust, she complained increasingly of her fear of pain, her hating to wear maternity clothes, and her having to give up helping the family. Finally I ventured to say, "Sometimes when a pregnancy is unplanned, women resent it very much and are angry about it." Her relief was evident. She said, "Oh, you don't know how angry I've been." As a result, the whole tenor of support being offered changed, and the plan was adjusted to meet her real needs.

The nurse must also accept the fact that the woman must be a willing partner in a relationship that is a purely voluntary one. As such, the relationship can be refused or terminated at any time by the pregnant woman or her family.

Supportive care involves developing, augmenting, or changing the mechanisms used by women and families in coping with stress. An effort is made to promote active participation by the individuals in the process of solving their own problems by gathering pertinent information, exploring alternative actions, making decisions as to choice of action, and assuming responsibility for the outcomes. These outcomes may be any or all of the following:

1. Living with a problem as it is
2. Mitigating effects of a problem so it can be accepted more readily
3. Eliminating problem through effecting change

NURSING ACTIONS

The actions the nurse chooses to use in providing support will depend in part on ability to convey interest and a desire to be of help. The nurse may use such strategies for support as development of behavior acquisition or modification, promotion of decision making as crucial in solving problems, and providing pertinent information or teaching care-taking activities.

The initiation of the nurse-client relationship is crucial in setting the tone for further interactions (see also Chapter 4). The techniques of listening with an attentive expression, touching, and use of eye contact have their place, as does recognition of the client's feelings and her right to express them. The intervention may occur in varied settings, formal or informal. For certain individuals involvement in goal-directed health groups is not feasible or acceptable. Encounters in hallways or clinic examining rooms, home visits, or telephone conversations may provide the only opportunities for contact and can be used effectively. One nurse described her intervention with a gravid woman as follows:

> I tried to teach her about relaxation and breathing techniques during childbirth but she was not interested. When she phoned to tell me she was at the hospital in labor she said, ''What was all that stuff you were saying about breathing?'' In between the next few contractions I repeated the salient points.

At other times women may seek information about a particular problem repeatedly, not so much for the advice given but to direct the nurse's attention to themselves. Edwards (1973) discourages such mechanisms by making it a rule to give advice three times and then if it is not acted on, to ask for a client-generated solution and a report of its effectiveness. The need for additional attention is recognized and provided in other ways.

Counseling for emotional tension is related to the problem involved; for example:

1. Sexual relationships with partner: Normalcy of changes in sexuality must be emphasized. Give information about safe and unsafe sexual practices and provide the woman or couple with pertinent reference materials. Discussion of these problems openly is encouraged.
2. Changes in self-image: As body contours change, doubts as to attractiveness may occur. Listening to these doubts, complimenting the woman on her appearance, and providing instruction in prenatal exercises aimed at figure control, diet, and weight gain can be tried for effectiveness; the woman's concern over her ability to be a ''good mother'' may begin in the second trimester. Discuss her concepts regarding mothering. Note her expectations and how realistic they are.
3. Complaints of ''nervousness'': Assess what the woman means by this term. Emphasize the naturalness of anxiety and stress response in all life situations; determine how she previously has coped with her nervousness.

Emotional support techniques such as acceptance of the individual's feelings as normal, continued interest, and the provision of opportunities for ventilation of feelings serve to help people explore methods of coping with pressures with a view of retaining successful methods, rejecting unsuitable ones, and eventually discovering new techniques.

Instruction regarding danger signals. One of the first responsibilities of those involved in the care of pregnant women is to alert them to those signs or symptoms that indicate a potential complication of pregnancy and how to report them (see boxed material). When one is stressed by a disturbing symptom, it is difficult to remember specifics. Because of this, the gravida and her family are more comfortable and alert if they receive a printed form listing the signs and symptoms that warrant an investigation and phone numbers to call in an emergency.

Danger Signals

1. Visual disturbances—blurring, double vision, or spots
2. Swelling of face or fingers
3. Severe, frequent, or continuous headaches
4. Muscular irritability or convulsions
5. Epigastric pain
6. Persistent vomiting beyond first trimester or severe vomiting at any time
7. Fluid discharge from vagina—bleeding or amniotic fluid (anything other than leukorrhea)
8. Signs of infections: chills, fever, burning on urination
9. Burning on urination
10. Severe or unusual pain in abdomen
11. Absence of fetal movements after quickening (some physicians want woman to report any unusual change in pattern or amount of fetal movements)

Childbirth and parenthood education. Formal classes in childbirth and parenthood education have proved successful for some women and couples. The various methods (e.g., Lamaze, Bradley) have certain premises in common:

1. The partners wish to share the birth of their child as part of their concept of family unity.
2. The mother gains the support of a partner who is trained to provide it.
3. There is opportunity to develop mechanisms for coping with pain or discomfort during labor and delivery (relaxation, diversion, disassociation) and thereby maintain self-controlling behaviors and control of one's environment.
4. Parent-craft activities are discussed and practiced.

For a complete discussion of childbirth and parenthood education see Chapter 19.

Nutritional counseling. Nutritional intake is an important factor in the maintenance of maternal health during pregnancy and in its provision of adequate nutrients for fetal development. Assessing nutritional status and providing nutritional information are part of the nurse's responsibilities in prenatal care. For detailed information concerning maternal and fetal nutritional needs see Chapter 18.

Frequent questions. Women and their families have many questions concerning the pregnancy and the physical and emotional changes they experience in themselves, as well as those that they perceive in others. Questions about activities of daily living are common. If the woman or couple does not ask about prenatal classes in preparation for childbirth, the nurse should provide her with information and encouragement to participate. See Chapter 19 for details concerning childbirth education.

Bathing and swimming. Tub bathing is permitted even late in pregnancy, because water does not enter the vagina unless under pressure. Swimming is also permitted during normal pregnancy, although diving is discouraged because of possible traumatic injury. Baths can be therapeutic because they relax tense, tired muscles, help counter insomnia, and make the pregnant woman feel fresh and sweet smelling. Physical maneuverability presents a problem (increased chance of falling) late in pregnancy. Tub bathing is contraindicated after rupture of the membranes.

Clothing. Comfortable, loose clothing is best. Washable fabrics (e.g., absorbent cottons) are often preferred. Since maternity clothes are expensive and rarely wear out, hand-me-downs or used clothes from garage sales can suffice. Tight brassieres and belts, stretch pants, garters, tight-top knee socks, panty girdles, and other constrictive clothing should be avoided. Tightness is uncomfortable, generally. Tight clothing over the perineum encourages vaginitis and miliaria (heat rash). Impaired circulation in the lower extremities favors varices.

A well-fitted maternity girdle,* frequently readjusted, may be welcomed for backache by obese women or those with a multiple pregnancy. An old, even very large, girdle meant for the nonpregnant woman is unsuitable during pregnancy because it pushes the abdomen (uterus) inward. A nonmaternity girdle may also aggravate backache and leg ache.

Maternity brassieres are constructed to accommodate the increased breast weight, chest circumference, and size of breast tail tissue (under the arm); they have drop flaps over the nipples to facilitate preparation of nipples for nursing or for actual nursing. A good brassiere can help prevent neck ache and backache.

Elastic hose or leotards may give considerable comfort to women with large varicose veins or swelling of the legs.

Comfortable shoes that provide firm support and promote good posture and balance are advisable. Very high heels and platform shoes are not recommended because of the woman's changed center of gravity, loosened pelvic girdle, tendency to lose her balance, and, with her pelvis tilted forward, backaches, leg aches, and leg cramps.

Employment. Many women continue to work during pregnancy. Whether the expectant mother can or should work and for how long depends on the physical activity involved, industrial hazards, fetotoxic environment (e.g., chemical dust particles, gases such as inhalation anesthesia†), medical or obstetric complications, and employment regulations of the company. Activities dependent on a good sense of balance should be discouraged, especially during the last half of pregnancy. Frequently, excessive fatigue is the deciding factor in the termination of employment.

Women in sedentary jobs need to walk around at intervals and should neither sit nor stand in one position for long periods. Activity is necessary to counter the usual sluggish dependent circulation that potentiates development of varices and thrombophlebitis. The pregnant woman's chair should provide adequate back support. A footstool can prevent pressure on veins, relieve strain on varices, and minimize swelling of feet. Work breaks are best spent resting in the left lateral side-lying position (employers are required to have an area where women can lie down).

Some women may lose interest in work as they become more introverted. This response may be difficult for the woman who has always been "on top of it" and

---

*Caution gravida to begin fastening girdle from symphysis pubis upward to support uterus from below.

†Operating room personnel who are pregnant should be aware of the dangers of their working environment to the fetus.

independent before pregnancy. Women who plan to return to work after giving birth may appreciate information about day-care centers, breast feeding and working, and the like.

Physical activity. Moderate exercise is encouraged. However, activities continued to the point of exhaustion or fatigue compromise uterine perfusion and fetoplacental oxygenation. Furthermore as gestation advances, the woman's center of gravity changes, her bony pelvic support loosens, her coordination usually decreases, and she notices a sensation of ungainliness.

Travel. Travel is a cause neither of abortion nor of premature labor. In high-altitude regions, lowered oxygen levels may cause fetal hypoxia. Women who travel widely expose themselves to the risk of serious accidents and may find themselves far removed from good maternity care. Use of a seat belt is recommended when traveling by car.

In addition, fatigue or tension, as well as altered regular personal habits and diet during arduous travel, may be detrimental. If long-distance travel is necessary, the trip should be made by air. Perhaps fortuitously, flight regulations do not permit pregnant women aboard during the last month of pregnancy without a statement from an obstetrician.

Many women experience a sense of uneasiness when traveling by any vehicle. They describe feelings of fear for the safety of their unborn.

Body image and pregnancy. Many women actually appear more beautiful during pregnancy. It is true that the altered silhouette and posture differ from those of the nonpregnant woman, but this is temporary and a gradual return to normal after the puerperium is likely. Concern for personal appearance, proper nutrition for the pregnant woman's individual needs, proper breast support, and regular exercise will do much to maintain her figure. Personal neglect, not pregnancy, generally is the cause of a poor figure.

Sexuality and sexual response. For a discussion of sexuality and sexual response during the childbearing cycle, see p. 302.

Feeding the newborn. Pregnant women are usually eager to discuss their plans for feeding the newborn. Breast milk is the food of choice, and breast feeding is associated with a decreased incidence in perinatal morbidity and mortality. However, immaturity of the infant, deep-seated aversion to nursing by mother or father, and certain medical complications, such as pulmonary tuberculosis, are contraindications to nursing. The woman and her partner are better equipped to decide which method of feeding is suitable for them after they have been given information about the advantages and disadvantages of bottle and breast feeding.

The choice of feeding method belongs to the mother or the couple. The woman who breast feeds because it is the "in" thing to do but inwardly is repulsed by the act will communicate this message to her infant, even if she is able to produce sufficient milk.

Fig. 17.16
Breast cup for inverted or retracted nipple. (From Riordan, J.: A practical guide to breastfeeding, St. Louis, 1983, The C.V. Mosby Co.)

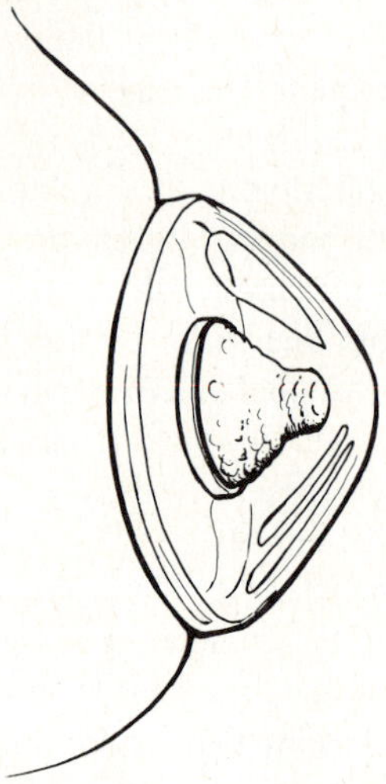

Women desiring to breast feed may determine nipple formation (retracted, flat, or normal) by the pinch test. Place the thumb and forefinger on the areola and squeeze. This causes the nipple to stand erect or flatten (i.e., retract or invert). If retraction occurs, nipple preparation can be started during the last two trimesters of pregnancy. After bathing, nipples are dried with a rough towel and gently rolled between the fingers.

> Special plastic doughnut-shaped cups are available for correcting inversions or retractions (Fig. 17.16). By a continuous, gentle pressure exerted around the areola, the nipple is pushed through a central opening in the inner shield. These cups should be worn during the last 2 trimesters of pregnancy, starting with an hour or two each day and gradually increasing the length of wearing time. Various trade names of these cups are Woolwich, Netsy, La Leche League Cups, Nurse-Dri, Free and Dry, and Hobbit Shields. They can also be worn after childbirth, but the mother should be cautioned against using milk that collects in the cup. Since body warmth can foster rapid bacterial growth and contamination, this milk should be discarded and not fed to the infant. (Riordan, 1983)

The possibility of contaminants in breast milk concerns many women. Many questions are being raised by consumers and professionals about the safety of breast milk. However, there are many beneficial qualities of breast milk such as the following. Breast milk does display immunologic activity resulting in a statistically significant difference in the expected incidence of infection between breast-fed and formula-fed infants. Breast milk also contains the same amount of vitamin D as fortified milk. In addition, breast-fed babies absorb iron and calcium to a greater extent than formula-fed babies. Breast milk contains the least amount of lead (gasoline and paint component) of any milk.

However, breast feeding can be potentially hazardous as well. The mother harboring *Salmonella kottbus* transmits this organism through her milk. The mother who adheres to a strict vegetarian diet deprives her infant of sufficient vitamin B_{12}, with potentially serious consequences. The mother whose milk contains anti-cow's-milk antibodies passes her sensitivity to cow's milk to the infant.

Environmental pollutants tend to concentrate in humans. Dairy farms in Michigan in 1973 and 1974 were accidentally contaminated with polybrominated biphenyl (PBB). Subsequently, high levels of PBB were found in human breast milk. This and other related compounds, polychlorinated biphenyls (PCBs), are environmental pollutants. The long-term effects of contamination with PCBs is as yet unknown. Medications that pass through the mother's milk are listed in Appendix J.

Dental problems. Nausea during pregnancy may lead to poor oral hygiene, and dental caries may develop. Dental care during pregnancy is especially important. Calcium and phosphorus in the teeth are fixed in enamel. No physiologic alteration during gestation can cause dental caries. The old adage "for every child a tooth" need not be true therefore.

There is no scientific evidence that filling teeth or even dental extraction using local or nitrous oxide–oxygen anesthesia causes abortion or premature labor. Antibacterial therapy should be considered for sepsis, however, especially in gravidas who have had rheumatic heart disease or nephritis. Extensive dental surgery is postponed until after delivery for the women's comfort, if possible.

Immunization. Immunization against poliomyelitis (Salk vaccine, not Sabin vaccine) and killed-virus immunizations, such as influenza, are advisable during gestation because of the mother's increased susceptibility to these infections. In contrast, attenuated live virus immunizations such as rubella (German measles), rubeola (measles), and epidemic parotitis (mumps) are contraindicated during pregnancy because of the teratogenicity of the viruses. If antibody screen for rubella is 1:8 or less, the woman requires immunization during the early puerperium. The woman is cautioned against getting pregnant for at least 3 months following immunization (see Chapter 31).

Smallpox vaccination is no longer required, because there has been no case reported (except as a result of laboratory accident) for a number of years.

Drugs (medications). Although much has been learned in recent years about fetal drug toxicity (see Appendix H), the possible teratogenicity of many drugs is still unknown. This is especially true for new medications and combinations of drugs. Moreover, certain subclinical errors or deficiencies in intermediate metabolism in the fetus may convert an otherwise harmless drug into a hazardous one. The greatest danger of causing developmental defects in the fetus from drugs exists from fertilization through the first trimester (i.e., the period of organogenesis). Self-treatment must be discouraged. All drugs, including aspirin, should be limited, and a careful record of therapeutic agents used should be kept.

Alcohol. Occasional alcoholic beverages are not considered harmful to the mother of her infant. Excesses must be avoided; regular drinkers or those who drink heavily during pregnancy have infants who demonstrate fetal alcohol syndrome (see Chapter 39 and Appendix H). Alcohol should be avoided by those on weight control diets because of the nutritionally empty calories in the alcohol.

Smoking. Heavy cigarette smoking (more than six cigarettes per day) or continued exposure to a smoke-filled environment (even if the mother does not smoke) is associated with fetal growth retardation and an increase in perinatal and infant mortality. Laboratory studies indicate a lowered Po_2 level and an elevated Pco_2 level in both mother and fetus when exposed to cigarette smoke. Smoking is deleterious to women with asthma, chronic respiratory infections, and allergy to pollen, dust, or dander. Smoking does not deter the success of lactation, but harmful substances may be transferred to the fetus in the milk.

Radiation. For a discussion of radiation see p. 276 and Appendix H.

Discomforts of pregnancy. The discomforts of pregnancy are a result of physiologic and anatomic adaptations of the woman to pregnancy. Although the discomforts do not reflect a hazard to the woman's health, they are of considerable importance to the woman. Women pregnant for the first time are confronted with symptoms, for example, urinary frequency or shortness of breath, that would, in the nonpregnant state, be considered abnormal. Women experiencing later pregnancies may experience an aggravation of varicose veins or severe backache from postural changes associated with a pendulous abdomen. Such symptoms are frightening and uncomfortable. Much of prenatal care requested by women relates to explanations of the causes of the discomforts and what measures can be taken to relieve them. The discomforts are fairly specific to each trimester of pregnancy (see box). The nurse can anticipate their appearance and provide anticipatory guidance for the woman. Table 17.10 contains information about the physiology, prevention, and treatment of the discomforts.

Sexual counseling during pregnancy. Nurses have many opportunities to counsel pregnant couples. Nurses offer expectant parent classes, work as nurse-practitioners in clinics and physicians' offices, and make home visits as community health nurses. In addition, nurses provide around-the-clock care on hospital maternity units.

Counseling pregnant couples demands self-assessment by the nurse, plus a knowledge of the physical, social, and emotional responses to sex during pregnancy. Pregnant women or couples continue to be sexual beings. The expectant woman or couple needs information about sexual activities and possible changes that may be encountered in feelings and behaviors. Not all maternity nurses are comfortable dealing with the sexual concerns of their clients. The nurse who is aware of her personal strengths and limitations in healing with sexual content is in a better position to make referrals when necessary.

The role of the maternity nurse in sex counseling is defined by the origin and severity of the sexual problem encountered. There are a significant number of clients who merely need *permission* to be sexual during pregnancy. Many other clients need *information* about the physiologic changes that occur during pregnancy and an opportunity to debunk myths associated with sex during pregnancy. Giving permission and providing information are within the purview of the maternity nurse and should be an integral component of providing health care.

A smaller number of couples must be referred for either *sex therapy* or *family therapy*. Couples with sexual dysfunction problems of long standing that may be intensified by pregnancy should be referred for sex therapy. When a couple's sexual problem is a symptom of a more serious interactional problem, they would benefit from family therapy.

Sex counseling during pregnancy is the same process described in Chapter 3.

Assessment: history taking. Following are the areas to be covered, as well as examples of questions to be asked, when taking a client's history:

1. Attitudes
   a. What has your family (partner, friends) told you about sex during pregnancy?
   b. What are your feelings about sex during pregnancy?
   c. Is it all right for married people to masturbate?
   d. How do your ideas and feelings about sex differ from those of your partner?

Discomforts of Pregnancy

First trimester

Pain and tingling in the breasts
Urgency and frequency of urination
Languor and malaise
Nausea and vomiting

Second trimester

Constipation
Heartburn
Increased pigmentation
Leg cramps
Pica

Third trimester

Hemorrhoids
Varicosities
Leg cramps
Hypermobility of joints
Backache
Urinary frequency

2. Sexual selfconcept
   a. How do you feel about the changes in your appearance?
   b. How does your partner feel about your body now?
   c. Do maternity clothes make pregnant women attractive?
3. Marital relationships
   a. What will it be like to have a baby in the home?
   b. How is your life and that of your partner going to change by having a baby?
   c. What plans do having a baby interrupt?
4. Physical status
   a. How is your overall health?
   b. What is your energy level?
   c. When do you feel most alive?

History taking is an ongoing process. Receptivity to changes in attitudes, body image, marital relationships, and physical status has relevance throughout pregnancy. When changes occur, problems may develop that require unexpected interventions.

Nursing actions. The history provides a base line for indentifying the client's knowledge level of female anatomy and physiology, attitudes about sex during pregnancy, as well as perceptions of the pregnancy, the health status of the couple, and the quality of their marital relationship. Identification of the couple's subjective experience provides the direction and focus of sexual counseling. Sexual counseling includes countering misinformation, providing reassurance of normalcy,

Text continued on p. 308.

Table 17.10
Discomforts Related to Maternal Adaptations to Pregnancy

Discomfort	Physiology	Prevention	Treatment
Gastrointestinal tract			
"Morning" sickness—occurs in 50-75% of pregnant women; starts between first and second missed periods and lasts until about fourth missed period; may occur any time during day; if mother does not have symptoms, expectant father may; may be accompanied by "bad taste" in mouth	Cause unknown (may result from hormonal changes, possible HCG; may be partly emotional reflecting pride in, ambivalence about, or rejection of pregnant state)	Avoid empty or overloaded stomach, offending odors, or foods hard to digest; maintain good posture—give stomach plenty of room; stop or decrease smoking	Eat dry carbohydrate upon awakening; remain in bed until feeling subsides, *or* alternate dry carbohydrate one hour with fluids such as hot tea, milk, or clear coffee the next hour until feeling subsides; eat 5-6 small meals per day; avoid fried, odorous, spicy, greasy, or gas-forming foods; consult physician if intractable vomiting (hyperemesis gravidarum, food poisoning, infectious disease); reassurance
Food cravings	Cause unknown; cravings determined by culture or geographic area	Not preventable	Satisfy craving unless it interferes with well-balanced diet; report unusual cravings, (e.g., pica: laundry starch, clay, dirt) to physician
Ptyalism (excessive salivation)—may occur starting 2-3 wk after first missed period	Elevated estrogen levels (?)	Not preventable	Astringent mouth wash; chewing gum
Gingivitis and epulis (hyperemia, hypertrophy, bleeding, tenderness)	Increased vascularity and proliferation of connective tissue from estrogen stimulation	Well-balanced diet with adequate protein and fresh fruits and vegetables; avoid trauma; good dental hygiene	Gentle brushing and good dental hygiene; avoid infection; reassurance that condition will disappear spontaneously 1-2 mo after delivery
Heartburn, pyrosis, or acid indigestion: burning sensation in lower chest or upper abdomen, occasionally with burping and raising of a little sour-tasting fluid	Progesterone slows gastrointestinal motility and digestion, reverses peristalsis, relaxes cardiac sphincter, and delays emptying time of stomach, resulting in reflux of food into esophagus; stomach displaced upward and compressed from enlarging uterus; may be associated with tension, nausea, and vomiting in early pregnancy	Limit or avoid gas-producing or fatty foods and large meals; maintain good posture to give GI tract lots of space; keep torso upright to reach below the waist (bend down at knees)	Sips of milk for temporary relief; hot tea, chewing gum; physician may prescribe antacid (aluminum hydroxide, magnesium trisilicate, or magnesium hydroxide [Amphojel, Gelusil, Maalox, milk of magnesia]) between meals (NOTE: *Do not* use baking soda or Alka-Seltzer [both have high salt content] or patent medicines); flying exercise; refer to physician for persistent symptoms to rule out hiatal hernia or peptic ulcer
Constipation	Gastrointestinal tract motility slowed because of progesterone, resulting in increased resorption of water and drying of stool; intestines compressed by enlarging uterus; predisposition to constipation (some women respond with diarrhea) because of oral iron supplementation	Six glasses of water per day; roughage in diet: bran, coarse ground cereals, fresh fruits and vegetables; moderate exercise; sit on toilet seat with feet supported on footstool and maintain regular schedule for bowel movements; use relaxation techniques and deep breathing	Treatment same as prevention; *do not* take stool softener, laxatives, other drugs, or enemas without first consulting physician; *never* ingest mineral oil as this inhibits absorption of fat-soluble vitamins

Continued.

Table 17.10—cont'd
Discomforts Related to Maternal Adaptations to Pregnancy

Discomfort	Physiology	Prevention	Treatment
Gastrointestinal tract—cont'd			
Hemorrhoids—see Cardiovascular system; flatulence with bloating and belching	Reduced gastrointestinal motility because of hormones, allowing time for bacterial action that produces gas; swallowing air	Chew solid foods slowly and thoroughly; avoid gas-producing foods, fatty foods, large meals	Treatment same as prevention; exercise; regular bowel habits
Cardiovascular system			
Faintness and, rarely, syncope (orthostatic hypotension)	Vasomotor lability or postural hypotension from hormones; in late pregnancy may be caused by venous stasis in lower extremities	Moderate exercise, deep breathing, vigorous leg movement; avoid sudden changes in position* and warm crowded areas; move slowly and deliberately; keep evnrionment cool; avoid hypoglycemia by eating 5-6 small meals per day	Treatment same as prevention; elastic hose; sit down as necessary; if symptoms are serious, refer to physician for possible neurologic disorder or hypoglycemia
Supine hypotension (vena cava syndrome)	Posture induced by pressure of gravid uterus on ascending vena cava when woman is supine; also reduces uterine-placental and renal perfusion	Side-lying position or semisitting posture, with knees slightly flexed	Treatment same as prevention
Palpitations	Unknown; should not be accompanied by persistent cardiac irregularity	Not preventable	Reassurance; refer to physician if accompanied by symptomatology of cardiac decompensation
Ankle edema (nonpitting) to lower extremities	Posture aggravated by prolonged standing, sitting, or hot weather	Good posture; avoidance of prolonged standing or sitting; moderate exercise; avoidance of constrictive clothing (e.g., *garters*); ample fluid intake for "natural" diuretic effect	Treatment same as prevention; put on support stockings before arising; rest periodically with legs and hips elevated; refer to physician if she develops generalized edema even if other symptoms of preeclampsia are not found; diuretics *contraindicated*
Varicose veins (large distended, tortuous, superficial veins)—may be associated with aching legs and tenderness; may be present in legs, vulva, and perianal area (hemorrhoids, piles)	Hereditary predisposition; relaxation of smooth muscle walls of veins because of hormones, causing pelvic vasocongestion; condition aggravated by enlarging uterus, gravity, and bearing down for bowel movements or during second stage of labor; thrombi from leg varices rare but may be produced by hemorrhoids	Avoidance of obesity, lengthy standing or sitting, constrictive clothing, and constipation and bearing down with bowel movements; moderate exercises	Treatment same as prevention; rest with legs and hips elevated; support stockings applied before rising—may need assistance with this as abdominal size increases; thrombosed hemorrhoid may be evacuated; outlet forceps delivery may prevent enlargement of hemorrhoids; relieve swelling and pain with hot sitz baths, local application of astringent compresses (witch hazel)
Spider nevi (telangiectasia)—appear during trimesters 2 or 3 over neck, thorax, face, and arms (in that order) in two thirds of women	Focal networks of dilated arterioles (end-arteries) from increased concentration of estrogens	Not preventable	Reassurance that they fade slowly during late puerperium; rarely disappear completely

*Caution woman to rise slowly and sit on edge of bed or to assume hands-and-knees posture before rising, and to get up slowly after sitting or squatting.

Table 17.10—cont'd
Discomforts Related to Maternal Adaptations to Pregnancy

Discomfort	Physiology	Prevention	Treatment
Cardiovascular system—cont'd			
Palmar erythema occurs in 50% of pregnant women; may accompany spider nevi	Diffuse reddish mottling over palms and suffused skin over thenar eminences and fingertips may be caused by genetic predisposition or hyperestrogenism	Not preventable	Reassurance that condition will fade within 1 wk after giving birth
Respiratory system			
Shortness of breath and dyspnea—occur in 60% of pregnant women	Expansion of diaphragm limited by enlarging uterus (compensated for in part by other maternal adaptations); may be caused by increased sensitivity to or compensation for slight acidosis ("breathing for two")	Not preventable; avoid anemia	Good posture; flying exercise; sleep with extra pillows; avoid overloading stomach; stop or decrease smoking; refer to physician if symptoms worsen to rule out anemia, emphysema, and asthma
Nasal stuffiness	Increased vascularization because of hormones	Not preventable	Reassurance that condition will return to normal during puerperium
Musculoskeletal system			
Leg cramps (gastrocnemius spasm)—especially when reclining	Compression of nerves supplying lower extremities because of enlarging uterus; reduced level of diffusible serum calcium or elevation of serum phosphorus; aggravating factors: fatigue, poor peripheral circulation	Avoid pointing toes when stretching legs and lead with heel of foot when walking; avoid drinking more than 1 L (1 qt) of milk per day (may need to limit to 0.5 L [1 pt]); avoid fatigue and cold legs; diet with adequate calcium	Rule out blood clot by checking for Homans' sign; if Homans' sign negative, use massage and heat over affected muscle; stretch affected muscle by standing up and leaning forward on affected leg or by having another person extend knee and dorsiflex foot of affected leg until spasm relaxes; stand on cold surface; treatment same as prevention; oral supplementation with calcium carbonate or calcium lactate tablets, 0.6 g, three times a day before meals; aluminum hydroxide gel, 1 oz, with each meal removes phosphorus by absorbing it
Joint pain, backache, and pelvic pressure; hypermobility of joints	Relaxation of symphyseal and sacroiliac joints because of hormones, resulting in unstable pelvis; exaggerated lumbar and cervicothoracic curves caused by change in center of gravity from enlarging abdomen	Maternity girdle; good posture and body mechanics; tuck pelvis under baby; bend at knees; avoid fatigue; wear shoes with 5 cm (2 in) heels; conscious relaxation; exercises to strengthen back muscles; firm mattress	Treatment same as prevention; local heat and back rubs; pelvic rock exercise; rest; reassure that condition will go away 6-8 wk after delivery
Renal system			
Urinary frequency and urgency	Vascular engorgement and altered bladder function caused by hormones; bladder capacity reduced by enlarging uterus and fetal presenting part	Not preventable; Kegel exercises to strengthen pubococcygeal muscle (see p. 309); limit fluid intake before bedtime to ensure rest	Treatment same as prevention; reassurance; wear perineal pad; refer to physician for pain or burning sensation

Continued.

Table 17.10—cont'd
Discomforts Related to Maternal Adaptations to Pregnancy

Discomfort	Physiology	Prevention	Treatment
Integumentary system			
Spider nevi—see Cardiovascular system			
Pruritus (noninflammatory)	Unknown cause; various types as follows:	Fingernails short and clean	Refer to physician for diagnosis of cause
	Nonpapular	Not preventable	Symptomatic: Keri baths; mild sedation
	Closely aggregated pruritic papules	Not preventable	As for nonpapular type
	Increased excretory function of skin and stretching of skin possible factors	Distraction; tepid (not hot) baths with sodium bicarbonate or oatmeal added to water	Treatment same as prevention; lotions and oils; change of soaps or reduction in use of soap; loose clothing
Deepened pigmentation (striae gravidarum, chloasma, linea nigra, fingernails, hair) acne, oily skin	See p. 238	See p. 238	Usually resolved during puerperium; reassurance given to women and their families about these manifestations of pregnant stage
Rashes	Various causes; infection, reaction to drugs, allergies	Dependent on underlying condition	Refer to physician for diagnosis: drug reactions; allergies; herpes gestationis
Breast changes, new sensations	Hypertrophy of mammary glandular tissue and increased vascularization, pigmentation, and size and prominence of nipples and areolae caused by hormone stimulation	Not preventable; supportive maternity brassiere with pads to absorb discharge may be worn at night; wash with warm water and keep dry	Treatment same as prevention; see Maternal physiology and sex counseling
Neurologic system			
Feelings during pregnancy (see Chapter 16): mood swings, mixed feelings	Hormonal and metabolic adaptations; plus feelings about female role, sexuality, timing of pregnancy, and resultant changes in one's life and life-style	Not preventable; reassurance and support; supportive significant other who can reassure woman re her attractiveness, etc.; improved communication with her partner, family and others	Treatment same as prevention; both partners need support; refer to social worker, if needed, or supportive services (financial assistance, food stamps)
Faintness and syncope—see Cardiovascular system			
Headaches	Emotional tension (more common than vascular migraine headache); eye strain (refractory errors); vascular engorgement and congestion of sinuses from hormone stimulation	Emotional support; prenatal teaching timed to need (see prenatal teaching guide and p. 342); conscious relaxation	Treatment same as prevention; refer to physician for constant "splitting" headache, either frontal, sincipital, occipital, or bilateral after assessing for PIH (see Chapter 35)
Carpal tunnel syndrome (involves thumb, second and third fingers, lateral side of little finger) (Fig. 17.17)	Compression of median nerve from changes in surrounding tissues: pain, numbness, tingling, burning; loss of skilled movements (typing); dropping of objects	Not preventable	Elevation of affected arms; splinting of affected hand may help; surgery is curative
Periodic numbness, tingling of fingers (acrodysesthesia)—occurs in 5% of pregnant women	Brachial plexus traction syndrome from drooping of shoulders during pregnancy (occurs especially at night and early morning)	Maintain good posture; wear good supportive maternity brassiere	Treatment same as prevention; reassurance that condition will disappear if lifting and carrying baby does not aggravate it

Fig. 17.17
Nurse assessing for carpal tunnel syndrome, a common discomfort during pregnancy.

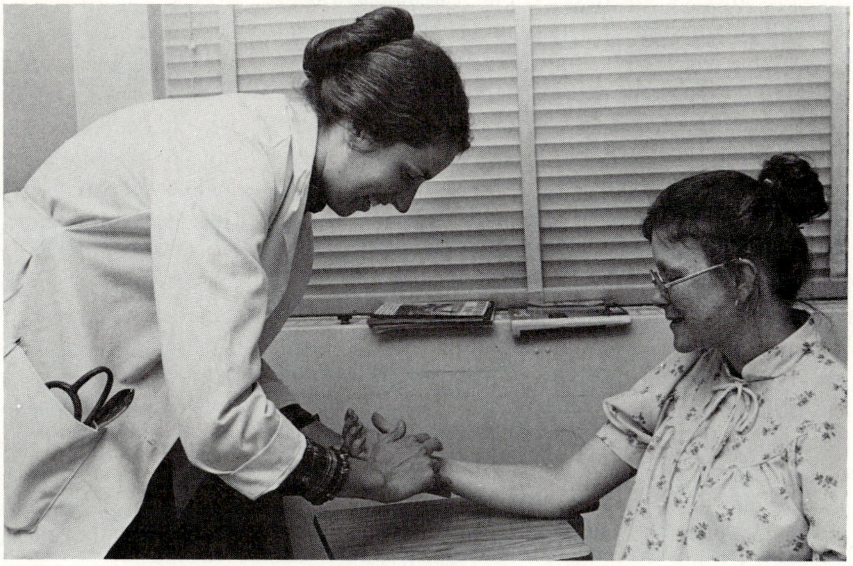

Table 17.10—cont'd
Discomforts Related to Maternal Adaptations to Pregnancy

Discomfort	Physiology	Prevention	Treatment
Miscellaneous conditions			
Fatigue (early pregnancy, usually)	Unexplained; may be due to increasing levels of estrogen, progesterone, and HCG or to elevated BBT	Not preventable; avoid anemia	Reassurance; rest prn; well-balanced diet to prevent anemia
Insomnia (later weeks of pregnancy)	Fetal movements, muscular cramping, urinary frequency, shortness of breath, or other discomforts	Not preventable; conscious relaxation	Reassurance; conscious relaxation; back massage; support of body parts with pillows; warm milk or warm shower before retiring
Abdominal discomfort			
Pressure	Pressure from enlarging uterus, especially when standing or walking; multiple gestation	Not preventable	Rest, conscious relaxation, and good posture; maternity girdle; refer to physician for assessment and treatment if pain is present (appendicitis, urinary tract infection, abruptio placentae, gallbladder disease, torsion of adnexa); if near term, rule out labor
Braxton Hicks' contractions	Intensification of uterine contractions in preparation for work of labor	Necessary uterine function	Reassurance; rest; change of position; practice breathing techniques when contractions are bothersome
Round ligament pain (tenderness)	Stretching of ligament caused by enlarging uterus	Not preventable; avoid further stretching (e.g., to get out of bed, roll on side first, then push self to sitting position with hands)	Reassurance, rest, good body mechanics to avoid overstretching ligament; relieve cramping by squatting or bringing knees to chest
Gastrointestinal discomforts—see Gastrointestinal tract			
Leukorrhea	Hormonally stimulated cervix becomes hypertrophic and hyperactive, producing abundant amount of mucus	Not preventable; do not douche	Hygiene; perineal pads; reassurance; refer to physician if accompanied by pruritis, foul odor, or change in character or color

and suggesting alternative behaviors. The uniqueness of each couple is considered within a biopsychosocial framework.

Countering misinformation. Many myths and much of the misinformation related to sex and pregnancy are masked behind seemingly unrelated issues. For example, a question about the baby's ability to hear and see in utero may be related to the baby's role as a third person in lovemaking. The counselor must be extremely sensitive to questions behind the question when counseling in this highly charged emotional area.

Fetal heart rate decreases during orgasm; however, fetal distress has not been noted. Although it has been suggested that premature delivery may be induced by the effect of oxytocin released during maternal response, by orgasmic contractions, or by prostaglandins in the male ejaculate, researchers have not validated these hypotheses.

When possible the couple is counseled together. Expectant parent education classes can also be an effective way to explore these kinds of concerns because of the support and sharing offered by the group.

Providing reassurance of normalcy. Couples are relieved to learn that their fears and concerns do not make them "weird" or "crazy." A breast-feeding mother may welcome the knowledge that her erotic response to suckling is normal. At the same time the father may be relieved to know that many fathers are jealous of their suckling infants.

It is important for the counselor to view sexuality in its broadest sense. Kissing, hugging, massage, petting, and increased gentleness and sensitivity are valid forms of sexual expression and signs of affection. Each of these behaviors is pleasurable in itself and is not always a secondary behavior leading to intercourse. When a couple cannot or chooses not to have penile-vaginal intercourse, they can express their needs for closeness and intimacy in many other ways.

Suggesting alternative behaviors. The following discussion focuses on some suggested alternatives for sexual practice during pregnancy.

Coitus or orgasm is not contraindicated at any time during pregnancy for the obstetrically and medically healthy woman. However, a history of more than one spontaneous abortion, a threatened abortion in the first trimester, impending miscarriage in the second trimester, or premature rupture of membranes, bleeding, *or* abdominal pain during the third trimester warrants precaution against coitus and orgasm. The woman or couple should also be cautioned against masturbatory activities when orgasmic contractions are contraindicated. Studies have shown that orgasm is often more intense when induced by masturbation. After being cautioned against orgasm, some women require reassurance if they experience erotic dreams.

The United States Collaborative Perinatal Project* analyzed data from almost 27,000 pregnancies between 1959 and 1966, a period when perinatal mortality was higher than today. In the discussion of data, the researcher presented the following facts: amniotic fluid infection occurred at a rate of 156 per 1000 births when mothers reported coitus more than once per week during the month before giving birth and at a rate of 117 per 1000 births to mothers who reported abstinence; 11% of infected infants died if there was coitus, but only 2.4% died when there was no coitus; when mothers reported coitus, the frequencies doubled for infants with low Apgar scores, neonatal respiratory distress, and hyperbilirubinemia. Perinatal rates are lower today, and deaths from "coitus-associated" infections may be less frequent. Naeye (1979) suggests that improved genital hygiene and perhaps other actions may reduce the risk of intrauterine infection and that until we have more data "a reasonable policy might be to recommend the avoidance of intercourse and orgasm in the third trimester in women with a poor reproductive history or in those who, on pelvic examination, have premature ripening of the cervix." In an interview Naeye commented further that he "was not prepared to recommend prolonged abstinence during pregnancy, since this can cause serious marital discord."

Solitary and mutual masturbation and oral-genital and anal intercourse may be *alternatives to penile-vaginal intercourse.* Men who enjoy cunnilingus may feel "turned off" by the normal increase in amount and odor of vaginal discharges during pregnancy. Couples who practice cunnilingus should be cautioned concerning the blowing of air into the vagina, particularly during the last few weeks of pregnancy. There have been cases reported of maternal death from air emboli caused by forceful blowing of air into the vagina. If the cervix is slightly open (as it may be near term), there is the possibility of the air being forced between the membranes and the uterine wall. Some air may enter the maternal placental lakes, thus gaining entrance into the maternal vascular bed.

Pictures of possible variations of *coital position* are often helpful. The female superior, side-by-side, and rear-entry positions are possible alternative positions to the traditional male superior position. The woman astride (superior position) allows her to control the an-

*Authors' comment: The report of the methodology of this study leaves some questions open. The subjects in this retrospective study were not randomized, and there was inadequate control over the data collection. The chi-square statistical formula is not designed to make inferences; the researcher can only say that there *may be* a relationship. Instead, a multiple regression formula would have accounted for the amount of variance among variables as causes of amniotic fluid infections. A prospective study in contemporary populations is necessary.

gle and depth of penile penetration as well as to protect her abdomen. The side-by-side position is the position of choice, especially during the third trimester, because it requires reduced energy and pressure on the pregnant abdomen. For other positions, refer to Bing and Colman (1977) and McCary (1983).

Multiparous women have reported severe *breast tenderness* in the first trimester. A coital position that avoids direct pressure on the woman's breasts and decreased breast fondling during love play can be recommended. The woman should also be reassured that this condition is normal and temporary.

Lactating mothers lose milk in uncontrolled spurts in response to sexual stimulation. The couple who are forewarned can be prepared for this eventuality.

Some women complain of lower abdominal cramping and backache after *orgasm* during the first and third trimesters. A back rub can often relieve some of this discomfort, as well as provide a pleasant experience.

A tonic contraction, often lasting up to a minute, replaces the rhythmic contractions of orgasm during the third trimester. Changes in fetal heart rates without fetal distress have been reported.

Postdelivery intercourse. For a discussion of postdelivery intercourse, see Chapter 31.

Kegel exercises. Kegel exercises (perineal tightening) can be taught at the time the woman is having a vaginal examination. The woman holds a mirror between her legs while the examiner points out external and internal anatomy. The woman is asked to tighten the (pubococcygeus) muscles around the examiner's fingers and to feel and watch the muscle movement. If the woman cannot contract the right muscles now, she is asked to practice by stopping and restarting her flow during urination.

The exercise consists of the woman's tightening the anal sphincter, then the introitus, and then the meatal sphincter, holding for a count of 10, and then relaxing. It may be repeated many times per day (some suggest up to 100 times per day)..

Although there is no definitive proof that they are beneficial, Kegel exercises are thought to be beneficial in the following ways:

1. They increase awareness of genital feelings and body function.
2. They improve pubococcygeal muscle tone—before and after delivery.
3. They enhance the mother's ability to respond to coaching to relax her perineum and to push during delivery.
4. They stimulate blood circulation to the area to maintain health and to aid healing.
5. They increase sexual pleasure, especially when used during coitus.
6. An additional benefit is improved control of the urinary meatus. This exercise is used to treat urinary incontinence.

The well-informed nurse who is comfortable with her own sexuality and the sex counseling needs of pregnant couples can offer counseling in a valuable but often neglected area.

Symptomatology of impending labor. During the third trimester instructions are given concerning preparation for delivery. The symptoms of impending labor and what information to report are reviewed:

1. Uterine contractions: The woman is told to report the frequency, duration, and intensity of uterine contractions. Nulliparas are usually counseled to remain at home until contractions are regular and 5 minutes apart. Parous women are counseled to remain at home until contractions are regular and 10 minutes apart. If the woman lives more than 20 minutes from the hospital or has a history of rapid labors, these instructions are modified accordingly.
2. Rupture of the membranes: See Chapter 21, p. 401.
3. Bloody "show": The "show," or a mucous plug, is noted early in labor. The "show" is scant, pink in color, and sticky (contains mucus).

If the woman or couple is not attending classes in preparation for parenthood, the clinic or office nurse assumes responsibility for instruction in the process of labor and what care to expect; in methods to control pain (e.g., analgesia and anesthesia, and breathing-relaxing techniques); in responsibilities of the spouse, family member, or friend who will be accompanying the woman through labor and delivery; and in the care of the newborn (i.e., clothing, feeding, daily hygienic care).

If a hospital delivery is planned, the woman is required to register at the hospital of choice. Most hospitals now provide pamphlets containing information such as where to report when labor begins and policies pertaining to visitors and visiting hours; many also conduct tours of the facilities to be used.

Counseling is provided to relieve emotional tensions. These tensions often relate directly to the childbirth experience (e.g., anxiety about pain or possible delivery of the child before reaching the hospital). Nursing strategies include providing an opportunity for discussing the woman's specific fears or anxieties, helping her make definite plans concerning what she will do when labor starts, repeating instructions willingly, and having "sharing sessions" with recently delivered mothers. If possible, involve significant others in preparation for the birth and arrange to have them participate in a supportive way during labor and delivery; this may be effective in allaying or defusing anxiety.

Other tensions relate to responsibilities of the soon-to-be assumed role of parent. The nurse promotes discussions with other mothers, helps the woman have a reasonable and attainable expectation of her role, involves other family members as prospective child-care aides, and gives anticipatory guidance regarding possible conflicts of the new mother to minimize problems in the postdelivery period. Tensions may also relate to the husband-wife relationship. In a normal, uncomplicated pregnancy, sexual intercourse with penile penetration is medically sanctioned until the membranes rupture.

Evaluation

Evaluation is a continuous process. To be effective, evaluation needs to be based on measurable criteria. The goal for normal pregnancy is maintenance of maternal and fetal health; therefore the criteria need to reflect the parameters used to measure this goal. Table 17.11 is a summary of the maternal and fetal areas consistently assessed as indicators of maternal and fetal health and the clinical findings that represent normal response.

Table 17.11
Assessment During Pregnancy with Evaluative Criteria

	First and Second Trimesters (wk 1 through 24)	Third Trimester (wk 25 through 38-40[term])
Schedule of care	After initial contact and preliminary assessments, return visit scheduled for 2 wk, thereafter every 4 wk	Medical and nursing care has been increased to permit detection of any abnormal response, maternal or fetal: woman is examined every 2 wk between 32 and 36 wk and every wk between 36 and 40 wk; if indicated, plan of care is modified
Maternal adaptations		
Physical		
Temperature	Normal range established	Normal range
Pulse	Normal range established	Gradual rise of +8 to +10 by thirty-fifth wk
Respirations	18-20/min	18-20/min; occasional shortness of breath and sighing breaths may be troublesome at times
Blood pressure	Normal range of less than +30 systolic and +15 diastolic may decrease slightly in midpregnancy	Systolic no greater than +30 and diastolic no greater than +15 over base line, which is normally higher (+6-+10) as term approaches
Urinalysis	Negative for protein and acetone; no greater than 1+ for glucose; negative for bacteria	Negative for protein and acetone, no greater than 1+ for glucose; lactose is present as hormone prolactin increases
Blood tests		
RBC	At sea level for wk 1-12: Hg, 11 g/dl; hematocrit, 37% Wk 12-24: Hg, 10.5 g/dl; hematocrit 35%	At sea level for wk 24 to term: Hg, 10 g/dl; hematocrit, 33% RBC repeated at 32-34 wk
STS (VDRL)	Negative	Negative
Weight gain	Weeks 1-12: about 3-4 lb (1.4-1.8 kg) Weeks 12-24: 12-14 lb (5.6-6.3 kg) Approximately 0.5 lb (0.23 kg)/wk	Wk 24 to term: no more than 1 lb (0.45 kg)/wk Approximately 24± 4 lb (11 kg) gain over prepregnancy weight (less than 20 lb puts fetus at risk)
Edema	Dependent edema not yet apparent	Dependent edema of lower legs, ankles, and feet
Vagina	Bluish-red hyperemia characteristic of pregnancy, little increase in size No anomalies, including cystocele, rectocele, or relaxed perineum	Highly distensible
Cervix	Long, firm but some softening by midpregnancy Moderate white mucoid discharge	Readiness for labor Cervix becomes more softened as term approaches In parous women, external os of cervix may be about 3 cm dilated by wk 35 Discharge persists
Breasts	Early weeks, breasts tender with tingling sensations By wk 8 breasts increase in size, become nodular; veins become visible beneath skin Nipples become larger, more pigmented, and more erectile No secretions from breasts Topic of infant feeding introduced	Striations may appear if increase in size of breasts extensive Areola becomes larger and more deeply pigmented and glands of Montgomery appear Lactogenesis begins with secretion of colostrum; may be expressed by gentle massage Preparation of breasts for breast feeding begins

Table 17.11—cont'd
Assessment During Pregnancy with Evaluative Criteria

	First and Second Trimesters (wk 1 through 24)	Third Trimester (wk 25 through 38-40[term])
Maternal adaptations—cont'd		
Abdomen	Gradual enlargement: see height of fundus	Enlargement continues: see height of fundus Toward end of pregnancy striae gravidarum may occur; in multipara glistening silvery lines of striae from earlier pregnancies may be seen Linea nigra at midline of abdomen
Uterus	Progressive enlargement to accommodate growing products of conception Fundal height at 12-13 wk: felt just above symphysis pubis; 16 wk: 3-4 cm above symphysis pubis; 20 wk: 2-3 cm below umbilicus; 24 wk: at umbilicus	Continued progressive enlargement of uterus Fundal height at 36 wk: almost to xiphoid process; 40 wk: 2 cm below due to "lightening" Readiness for labor: Braxton Hick's contractions may be felt by wk 34
Pelvis	Pelvic measurements within normal range (examined at second visit, not repeated) Diagonal conjugate 11.5 cm or more Transverse diameter of outlet 8 cm or more Ischial spines not prominent, concavity of sacrum ample, side walls of pelvis do not converge	Pelvic measurements adequate in relation to size of fetus (examined near term)
Skin	Changes not noticeable	May develop chloasma (mask of pregnancy), vascular spiders, palmar erythema (red palms) Varicose veins may appear in lower legs and vulva
Common problems	Woman or couple verbalizes understanding of physiologic basis and treatment of nausea and vomiting up to wk 12; increased skin pigmentation (e.g., linea nigra); heartburn; constipation; leg cramps; pica	Woman or couple verbalizes understanding of physiologic basis and treatment of hemorrhoids, varicosities, leg cramps, hypermobility of joints, backache
Abnormal symptoms	Woman or couple verbalizes understanding of physiologic basis, need for immediate treatment, and how to obtain necessary care Vaginal bleeding Burning or pain on urination Gastroenteritis Exposure to communicable disease (e.g., rubella) Nausea and vomiting beyond wk 12 Abdominal pain	Woman or couple verbalizes understanding of physiologic basis; need for immediate treatment and how to obtain necessary care Vaginal bleeding; at term rule out brownish spotting occurring 8 hr after vaginal examination and/or "show" of pinkish mucus Symptoms of preeclampsia-eclampsia: weight gain over 1 lb/wk, generalized edema, persistent headache, dimness or blurring of vision Cessation, noticeable diminution, or acceleration in amount of fetal movement Rupture of membranes Burning or pain on urination Chills or elevated temperature Abdominal pain Persistent nausea and vomiting
Psychosocial adaptations	Reactions indicative of positive psychologic response to pregnancy, including birth process and parenthood During first trimester, woman may be selfcentered and concerned with her own adjustment to idea of pregnancy During second trimester, woman usually is reasonably free of symptoms; she is more tranquil and at ease; reality of child is now recognized, and most women come to accept their pregnant state; however, feelings of ambivalence come and go During first and second trimesters family members (spouse, others) adjust in a positive manner to the pregnancy although they may express feelings of being "left out" by mother	Responses typical of normal findings in pregnancy Interest centered around preparing for parenthood Anxiety may be expressed over pain of labor, behavior during labor, care of other children Ambivalent feelings persist

Continued.

Table 17.11—cont'd
Assessment During Pregnancy with Evaluative Criteria

	First and Second Trimesters (wk 1 through 24)	Third Trimester (wk 25 through 38-40[term])
Psychosocial adaptations—cont'd	Verbalizes understanding of sexual responses and relates that sexual relationships are mutually accepted and serve as a means of communication	Verbalizes understanding of various modes of sexual expression (which are safe, which to avoid) and of medical acceptance of sexual intercourse with penile penetration until rupture of membranes; feelings of frustration and resentment over abstinence expressed early in third trimester and acceptance expressed in end of third trimester
	Negative feelings about self-image are recognized as temporary; expresses pride or pleasure about being pregnant	Expresses eagerness to be done with pregnancy; complaints about awkwardness, annoyance about symptoms (shortness of breath and backache) expressed; questions asked about how soon appearance will be back to "normal"
Active participation in care	Verbalizes understanding of plan of care; schedule, need for continuity of care, physical examination to be done, reporting of abnormal symptoms	Verbalizes understanding of preparation for delivery; symptoms of impending labor (i.e., uterine contractions, rupture of membranes, bloody "show"), what to report, and where to go for delivery Verbalizes understanding of delivery process; methods to control pain (e.g., analgesia, anesthesia, and breathing-relaxing techniques); responsibilities of spouse, family member, or friend who will be accompanying woman through labor and delivery; and care of newborn (i.e., clothing, feeding, daily hygienic care)
	Complies with care Keeps appointments, reports abnormal symptoms promptly, follows diet plan, takes only prescribed medications, refrains from smoking and drinking alcoholic beverages, exercises Appearance is healthy, grooming adequate, energy level normal Discusses techniques of infant feeding Discusses prenatal education classes	Complies with care As stated earlier Demonstrates relaxation, breathing techniques, etc. to be used in labor as taught in prenatal education classes or by prenatal nurse Demonstrates preparation of nipples for breast feeding Discusses plans for care of newborn, help at home, preparation of siblings
Fetal well-being	FHR heard by dopptone at wk 12, by fetoscope by wk 24	FHR and rhythm are normal (120-160 beats/min) and regular; will be less if fetus is asleep and greater with fetal movement
	Fetal movements felt at 17-19 wk (quickening)	Fetal movements increase with maternal movements, may lessen during fetal sleep; same pattern of movements every 24 hr Height of fundus, abdominal growth, and estimation of weight within normal limits for the estimated gestational age; presentation size of infant and maternal pelvic configuration permit vaginal delivery Engagement occurs about 2 wk before term in nullipara; may not occur until labor is well established in parous woman

References and Readings

Afaf Ibraheim Melias, L.: Arab American women and their birth experiences, M.C.N. **6:**171, May-June 1981.

Affonso, D., and Harris, T.: Postterm pregnancy: implications for mother and infant, challenge for the nurse, J.O.G.N. Nurs. **9**(3):139, 1980.

American Academy of Husband-Coached Childbirth: The Bradley method, Sherman Oaks, Calif., 1974, The Academy.

Arms, S.: Immaculate deception, Boston, 1975, Houghton Mifflin Co.

Athey, P., and Hadlock, F.: Ultrasound in obstetrics and gynecology, St. Louis, 1981, The C.V. Mosby Co.

Bash, D.: Jewish religious practices related to childbearing, J. Nurs. Midwife. **25**(5):39, 1980.

Benedict, T.: Parenthood as a development phase: a contribution to the libido, J. Am. Psychoanal. Assoc. **7:**389, 1959.

Benson, R.C., editor: Current obstetric and gynecologic diagnosis and treatment, ed. 3, Los Altos, Calif., 1980, Lange Medical Publications.

Bentz, J.M.: Missed meanings in nurse/patient communication, M.C.N. **5**:55, Jan./Feb. 1980.

Bing, E., and Colman, L.: Making love during pregnancy, New York, 1977, Bantam Books.

Brown, W.: Psychological care during pregnancy and the postpartum period, New York, 1979, Raven Press.

Caplan, G.: Concepts of mental health and consultation, Washington, D.C., 1959, U.S. Department of Health, Education, and Welfare.

Carter-Jessop, L.: Promoting maternal attachment through prenatal intervention, M.C.N.**6**:107, March/April 1981.

Chung, H.J.: Understanding the Oriental maternity patient, Nurs. Clin. North Am. **12**:67, March 1977.

Colman, A.D., and Colman, L.L.: Pregnancy as an altered state of consciousness, Birth Fam. J. **1**:7, 1974.

Dameron, G.W.: Helping couples cope with sexual changes pregnancy brings, Contemp. Obstet. Gynecol. **21**:23, Feb. 1983.

Debrovner, C.H., and Stubin-Stein, R.: Psychological aspects of vaginal examination, Med. Aspects Hum. Sex **9**:163, March 1975.

Donaldson, J.O.: Neurology of pregnancy. In Major problems in neurology, vol. 7, Philadelphia, 1978, W.B. Saunders Co.

Dossey, B., and Guzzetta, C.: Nursing diagnosis, Part II, Nurs. '81 **11**(6):34, 1981.

Doucette, J.S.: Is breast-feeding still safe for babies? M.C.N. **3**:345, 1978.

Druzin, M.L., et al.: Current status of the contraction stress test, J. Reprod. Med. **23**:222, Nov. 1979.

Edwards, M.: Communications: dimensions in childbirth education, Pacific Grove, Calif., 1973, M. Edwards.

Fogel, C.I., and Woods, N.F.: Health care of women: a nursing perspective, St. Louis, 1981, The C.V. Mosby Co.

Gordon, R., and Gordon, L.: Social factors in prevention of postpartum emotional problems, Obstet. Gynecol. **15**:453, 1960.

Gray, J.D., et al.: Prediction and prevention of child abuse, Semin. Perinatol. **3**:86, Jan. 1979.

Grosso, C., et al.: The Vietnamese American family . . . and Grandma makes three, M.C.N. **6**:177, May-June 1981.

Hogan, L.R.: Pregnant again—41, M.C.N. **4**:174, May-June 1979.

Holt, J.R.: Best laid plans: pre- and postpartum comparison of self and spouse in primiparous Lamaze couples who share delivery and those who do not, Nurs. Res. **29**:20, Jan.-Feb. 1980.

Larsen, V.L., Evans, T., and Martin, L.: Differences between new mothers: psychiatric admissions vs. normals, J. Am. Med. Wom. Assoc. **22**:995, 1967.

Liston, J., and Liston, E.H.: The mirror pelvic examination: assessment in a clinic setting, J.O.G.N. Nurs. **7**:47, March-April 1978.

Luke, B.: Does caffeine influence reproduction? M.C.N. **7**:240, July-Aug. 1982.

Lytle, N.A., editor: Nursing of women in the age of liberation, Dubuque, Iowa, 1977, William C. Brown Co., Publishers.

Magee, J.: The pelvic examination—view from the other end of the table, Minn. Med. **59**:99, 1976.

Malasanos, L., et al.: Health assessment, St. Louis, 1977, The C.V. Mosby Co.

McCary, J.L.: Human sexuality, ed. 2, New York, 1973, Van Nostrand Reinhold Co.

McKay, S.: Smoking during the childbearing year, M.C.N. **5**:46, Jan./Feb. 1980.

Mercer, R.T.: "She's a multip . . . she knows the ropes," M.C.N. **4**:301, Sept.-Oct. 1979.

Mill, J., Harlap, S. and Harley, E.: Should coitus late in pregnancy be discouraged? Lancet **1**:136, 1981.

Miller, G.D.: The gynecological examination as a learning experience, J. Am. Coll. Health Assoc. **23**:162, 1974.

Mocarski, V.: Asymptomatic bacteriuria—a "silent" problem of pregnant women, M.C.N. **5**:238, July/Aug. 1980.

Moore, D.: A comparison of methods for collecting clean catch urine specimens in a clinic population of obstetric patients, Am. J. Obstet. Gynecol. **122**(1), 1975.

Moore, D.: Effect of prepodyne as a perineal cleaning agent for clean catch specimens, Nurs. Res. **25**(4), July-Aug. 1976.

Naeye, R.L.: Coitus and associated amniotic-fluid infections, N. Engl. J. Med. **301**:1198, 1979.

Naeye, R.L.: Coitus and antepartum hemorrhage, Br. J. Obstet. Gynecol. **88**:765, 1981.

Perkins, R.P.: Sexual behavior and response in relation to complications of pregnancy, Am. J. Obstet. Gynecol. **134**:498, 1979.

Popkess, S.: Diagnosing your patient's strengths, Nurs. '81 **11**(7):34, 1981.

Price, M.: Making a concept come alive. Am. J. Nurs. **80**:688, April 1980.

Queenan, J.T.: When and how to do amniocentesis, Contemp. Obstet. Gynecol. **15**:61, Feb. 1980.

Rayburn, W., and Wilson, E.: Am. J. Obstet. Gynecol. **137**:972, 1980.

Riordan, J.: A practical guide to breastfeeding, St. Louis, 1983, The C.V. Mosby Co.

Rubin, R.: Cognitive style in pregnancy, Am. J. Nurs. **70**:502, 1970.

Sandberg, E.C.: Synopsis of obstetrics, ed. 10, St. Louis, 1978, The C.V. Mosby Co.

Satir, V.: Conjoint family therapy, Palo Alto, Calif., 1967, Science & Behavior Books.

Sloane, E.: Biology of women, New York, 1980, John Wiley & Sons.

Snyder, C., et al.: New findings about mothers' antenatal expectations and their relationship to infant development, M.C.N. **4**:354, Nov.-Dec. 1979.

Solola, A., et al.: Gonorrhea during the intrapartum period, Am. J. Obstet. Gynecol. **144**(3):351, 1982.

Steele, B., and Pollock, C.: A psychiatric study of parents who abuse infants and small children. In Helfer, R., and Kempe, H., editors: The battered child, Chicago, 1968, The University of Chicago Press.

Vontner, L.A., et al.: Recurrent genital herpes simplex virus infection in pregnancy: infant outcome and frequency of asymptomatic response. Am. J. Obstet. Gynecol. **143**(1):75, 1982.

Wheeler, L.A.: Sexuality during pregnancy and the puerperium, Perinatal Press **3**:131, Oct. 1979.

Whitely, N.: A comparison of prepared childbirth couples and conventional prenatal class couples, J.O.G.N. Nurs. **8**:109, March-April 1979.

Wiggins, J.D.: Childbearing: physiology, experiences, needs, St. Louis, 1979, The C.V. Mosby Co.

Zalar, M.K.: Human sexuality: a component of total patient care, Nurs. Dig. **3**:40, Nov.-Dec. 1975.

Zalar, M.K.: Sexual counseling for pregnant couples, M.C.N. **1**:176, May-June 1976.

18

Maternal and Fetal Nutrition

- **Physiologic Adjustments and the Basis for Nutrition Needs in Pregnancy**
  - Tissue growth
    - The placenta
    - Blood volume and constituents
  - Functional alterations
    - Alimentary canal
    - Respiratory system
    - Renal function
    - Hormonal effects
  - Weight gain during pregnancy
    - Deviations in weight and weight gain
- **Nutrient Needs**
  - Energy
    - Tissue deposition
    - Metabolic needs
    - Activity
  - Protein
  - Major minerals
    - Iron
    - Calcium
    - Sodium
  - Fat-soluble vitamins
    - Vitamin A
    - Vitamin D
    - Vitamin E
  - Water-soluble vitamins
    - Folic acid
    - Pyridoxine (vitamin B_6)
    - Thiamin (vitamin B_1)
    - Riboflavin (vitamin B_2)
    - Cobalamin (vitamin B_{12})
    - Ascorbic acid (vitamin C)
  - Trace minerals
    - Zinc
    - Fluorine
  - Nutritional supplements: their role in pregnancy
- **Nutrition Risk Factors in Pregnancy**
  - Risk factors at the onset of pregnancy
    - Adolescence
    - Frequent pregnancies
    - Poor reproductive history
    - Economic deprivation
    - Bizarre food patterns
    - Vegetarian diets
    - Smoking, drug addiction, and alcoholism
    - Chronic systemic diseases
    - Prepregnant weight
  - Risk factors in pregnancy
    - Anemia of pregnancy
    - Pregnancy-induced hypertension
    - Inadequate weight gain
    - Excessive weight gain
    - Demands of lactation
- **Guidelines for Management**
  - Nutrition assessment
    - History
    - Physical examination
    - Biochemical tests
    - Dietary assessment
  - Nutrition counseling
  - Referral for additional services
- **Summary of Nursing Care: Maternal and Fetal Nutrition**
  - Goals for care
  - Assessment and analysis
  - Examples of nursing diagnoses
  - Plan and implementation
  - Evaluation

Many factors interact to determine the progress and outcome of human pregnancy (Fig. 18.1). The woman can contribute toward a successful pregnancy and healthy neonate; she can, for example, reproduce at an optimal age and manipulate her environment to avoid harmful agents. Considerable information about nutrition is available such that a woman can select foods and dietary patterns that are associated with a healthy experience of pregnancy and a healthy outcome.

To promote successful reproduction, the dissemination of nutrition information must be directed to persons in all stages of the life cycle, not only to expectant parents, whose motivation to change may temporarily be great. Nutrition education can be effective throughout the life cycle.

The Policy Statement on Nutrition and Pregnancy issued by the American College of Obstetricians and Gynecologists (ACOG) contains the following statements:

> a woman's nutritional status before, during and after pregnancy contributes to a significant degree to the well-being of both herself and her infant. Therefore, what a woman consumes before she conceives and while she carries the fetus is of vital importance to the health of succeeding generations.

Physiologic Adjustments and the Basis for Nutrition Needs in Pregnancy

Many physiologic, biochemical, and hormonal changes occuring during pregnancy influence the need for nutrients and the efficiency with which the body uses them. Several of these changes are apparent early in the first trimester, an indication that they are an integral part of the maternal-fetal system, which creates the most favorable environment possible for the developing child. The changes are necessary to regulate maternal metabolism, promote fetal growth, and prepare the mother for labor, childbirth, and lactation.

TISSUE GROWTH

The placenta. Placentas of poorly nourished mothers often contain fewer and smaller cells that have a reduced ability to synthesize substances needed by the fetus, to facilitate flow of needed nutrients, and to inhibit passage of potentially harmful substances. Therefore it is understandable that the infant of a poorly nourished mother would likewise be poorly nourished and would be small for gestational age (SGA) (see Chapter 37).

Blood volume and constituents. Total blood volume is known to increase about 47% above normal levels, and plasma volume increases 50% in primiparas and higher in multiparas. These increases are needed in part because the blood carries nutrients to the fetus and metabolic waste products away from the fetus.

Red cell production is stimulated during pregnancy, and their numbers gradually rise, but the increase is not as large as the expansion of plasma volume (see p. 230). It is evident that there is a "physiologic [pseudo] anemia of pregnancy," largely reflecting the relatively greater increase in plasma volume than in red blood cell mass. At the same time, a deficiency of iron or of folic acid or both may contribute to the development of anemia.

Fig. 18.1
Examples of factors known to affect course or outcome of pregnancy.

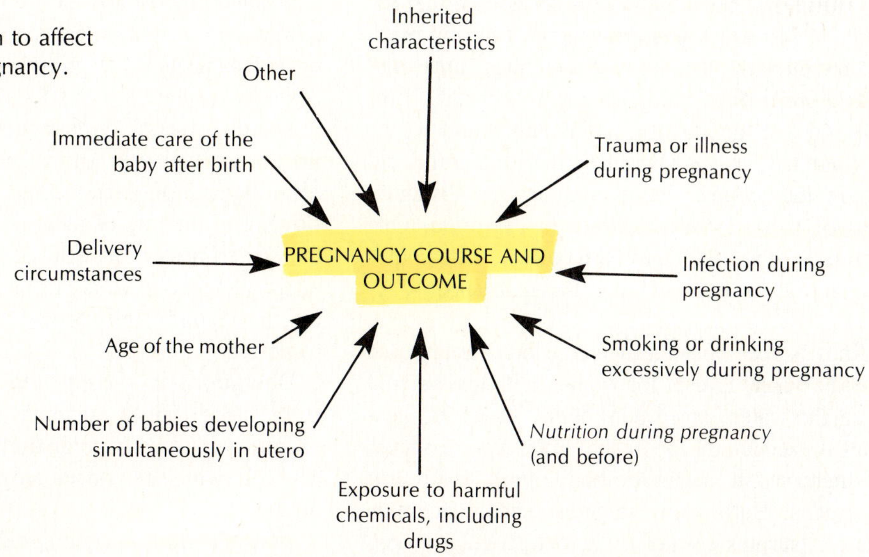

Total protein concentration decreases during pregnancy, largely because albumin falls from about 4 g/dl to between 2.5 and 3 g/dl. Women with pregnancy-induced hypertension (PIH) sustain a much larger drop in albumin as a result of the glomerular membrane leak of protein into the urine.

Most plasma lipid fractions rise during pregnancy. For example, cholesterol increases from under 200 mg/dl to between 250 and 300 mg/dl.

FUNCTIONAL ALTERATIONS

Alimentary canal. A decrease in gastric motility and intestinal tonus, common in pregnancy, has the advantage of slowing the passage of food through the gastrointestinal tract and possibly enhancing absorption of nutrients. On the other hand, it may be a factor in nausea of pregnancy and may lead to considerable discomfort when it results in constipation.

Respiratory system. In addition to serving as a lifeline for nutrients, the placenta also functions in the exchange of respiratory gases and waste products between the mother and fetus. The delivery of oxygen to the fetus is just as important to proper metabolism as an adequate supply of nutrients. Maternal nutrition can influence oxygen exchange through the production of hemoglobin. In the presence of normal concentrations of hemoglobin, the blood can deliver up to 16 ml/dl of oxygen. If maternal hemoglobin levels are depressed, the quantity of oxygen per deciliter (dl) of blood is reduced. Since the fetus can tolerate little variation in the rate at which oxygen is supplied, the mother must compensate by increasing her cardiac output, which increases her basal metabolic rate (BMR) and her need for protein foods.

Renal function. Renal blood flow and glomerular filtration rate (GFR) are increased somewhat during pregnancy to facilitate the clearance of creatinine, urea, and other waste products of fetal and maternal metabolism. Normally most of the glucose, amino acids, and water-soluble vitamins that are filtered by the glomerulus are resorbed in the tubules, but in pregnancy substantial quantities of these nutrients appear in the urine. One explanation is that the high GFR offers the tubules greater quantities of nutrients than they can feasibly resorb.

Pregnancy is accompanied by a considerable increase in total body water. Except for women with generalized edema, all the water gained until about 30 weeks' gestation can be accounted for in the products of conception and increases in maternal blood volume and reproductive organs. Before this stage is reached there is evidence of ''surplus'' water in the extracellular space, but at term there is a surplus of about 1 or 2 L. All or most of the gains are lost through perspiration and urine within 6 to 8 weeks after delivery. These calculations have important implications for monitoring and interpreting body weight gained during pregnancy.

Hormonal effects. During pregnancy the placenta assumes a major role in the production of hormones, becoming the primary source of estrogen and progesterone. Progesterone causes the deposit of fat in subcutaneous tissues over the abdomen, back, and upper thighs. The fat serves as a caloric reserve for both pregnancy and lactation.

Increases in several hormones affect nutrition, including increased secretion of the following:

1. Aldosterone (salt-conserving hormone) by the adrenal gland
2. Thyroxin, which regulates metabolism, by the thyroid gland
3. Parathyroid hormone, which controls calcium and magnesium metabolism, by the parathyroid gland
4. Human chorionic somatomammotropin by the placenta, which also acts as a growth hormone

WEIGHT GAIN DURING PREGNANCY

The weight gained in a normal pregnancy will vary among individual women. The acceptable weight gain for most healthy women of normal weight for height carrying a single fetus is 12 kg (27 lb) (Naeye, 1979) with a range of 10 to 14.5 kg (22 to 32 lb).

Along with growth of the developing fetus itself, a concurrent increase in supporting maternal tissue occurs. The components of maternal weight gain shown in Figs. 18.2 and 18.3 indicate that a normal pregnancy calls for considerable weight gain over and above that represented by the size of the fetus. Thus if the net gain in maternal weight is less than about 10 kg (22 lb), one must assume that the growth of the fetus has caused a depletion of the mother's tissue reserves.

There is general agreement that the normal curve of weight gain should show little gain during the first trimester, a rapid increase during the second, and some slowing in the rate of increase during the third. During the first trimester, growth takes place almost entirely in maternal tissue; gain is primarily in maternal tissue during the second trimester and in fetal tissue in the third trimester.

Deviations in weight and weight gain. Deviations from usual values for either prepregnant weight or weight gain during pregnancy are relatively common. The following are considered to be deviations from the norm:

1. Underweight: prepregnant weight less than 85%

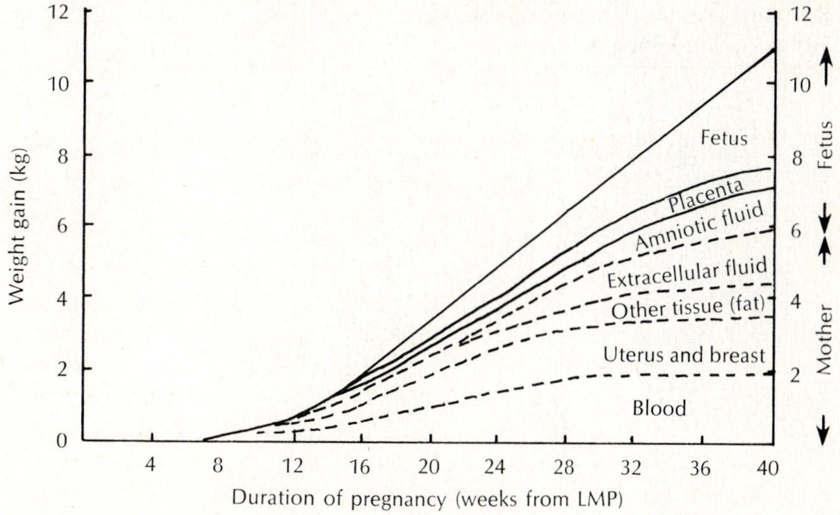

Fig. 18.2
Pattern and components of weight gain throughout course of pregnancy. (From Schneider, H.A., et al.: Nutritional support of medical practice, New York, 1977, Harper & Row, Publishers.)

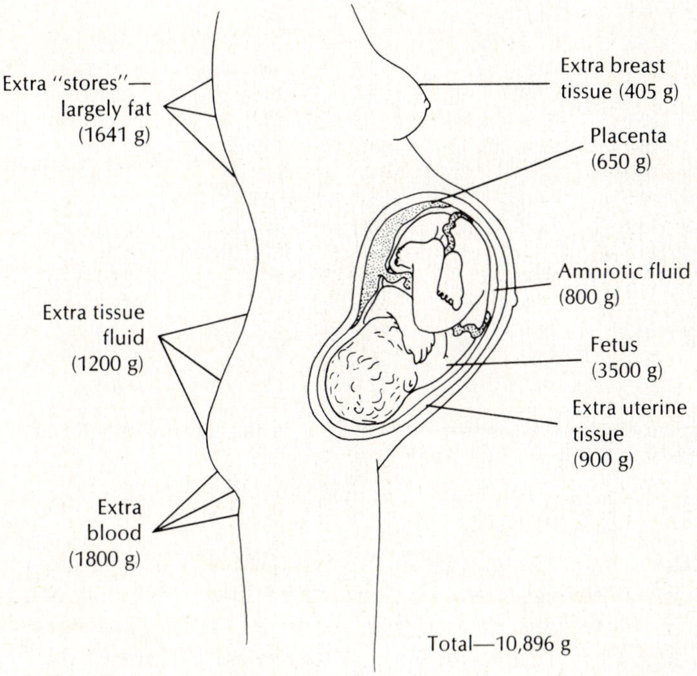

Fig. 18.3
Distribution of extra maternal weight at the end of a normal 40-week pregnancy. (From Worthington-Roberts, B.: Contemporary developments in nutrition, St. Louis, 1981, The C.V. Mosby Co.

of standard weight for age and height* (Table 18.1).

2. Overweight: prepregnant weight more than 120% of standard weight for age and height (Table 18.1).
3. Inadequate gain: gain of 1 kg (2.2 lb) or less per month in the second or third trimester. Weight loss or failure to gain during pregnancy is a sign of nutrition difficulties.
4. Excessive gain: gain of 3 kg (6.6 lb) or more per month is likely to have been caused by tissue fluid retention rather than by excessive caloric intake.

*The female suffering from anorexia nervosa, the ultimate in malnourishment, is usually amenorrheic and therefore would not be capable of conceiving.

Table 18.1
Standard and Deviations from Standard Weight (< 85% and > 120%) for 17- to 24-Year-Old Nonpregnant Women

Height		Underweight (<85%)		Standard Weight		Overweight (>120%)	
cm	in	kg	lb	kg	lb	kg	lb
140	52.2	38.0	84	45	99	53.8	118
142	56.0	39.0	86	46	101	55.0	121
144	56.7	40.0	88	47	103	56.4	124
146	57.5	40.7	90	48	105	57.6	127
148	58.3	41.8	92	49	108	59.0	130
150	59.1	42.8	94	50	110	60.4	133
152	60.0	43.8	96	51	112	61.8	136
154	60.7	44.6	98	52	115	63.0	139
156	61.5	45.6	100	53	117	64.4	142
158	62.2	46.6	103	55	121	65.8	145
160	63.0	47.7	105	56	123	67.4	148
162	63.8	49.0	108	57	126	69.1	152
164	64.6	50.0	110	58	129	70.6	155
166	65.4	51.0	112	59	131	72.1	159
168	66.2	52.0	114	61	134	73.6	162
170	66.9	53.4	118	63	138	75.4	166
172	67.7	54.6	120	64	141	77.2	170
174	68.5	56.0	124	66	145	79.1	174
176	69.3	57.5	127	68	149	81.2	179
178	70.1	59.1	130	69	152	83.4	184
180	70.9	60.6	134	71	157	85.6	189
182	71.7	61.9	137	73	161	87.4	193
184	72.4	63.2	139	74	163	89.3	197
186	73.2	64.5	142	76	167	91.1	201
188	74.0	65.7	145	78	171	92.8	205
190	74.8	66.7	147	79	173	94.2	208
192	75.6	67.7	149	80	175	95.6	211
194	76.4	68.7	152	81	179	97.0	214
196	77.2	69.5	153	82	180	98.2	217
198	78.0	70.4	155	83	182	99.4	219
200	78.7	71.2	157	84	185	100.6	222
202	79.5	72.0	159	85	187	101.6	224

Adapted from Task Force on Nutrition: Assessment of maternal nutrition, Chicago, 1978, The American College of Obstetricians and Gynecologists and the American Dietetic Association.

A total weight gain of over 14.5 kg (32 lb) is associated with higher rates of perinatal mortality.

A pattern of desirable prenatal gain in weight is shown in Fig. 18.4. To monitor the desirable weight gain as compared to deviations in weight gain, the grid should be used for plotting the pregnant woman's weight throughout pregnancy.

There are potential hazards for both mother and infant from restricting weight gain during pregnancy. The mother's weight gain and prepregnancy weight are the two strongest influences (except gestational age) on birth weight. Infant birth weights, in turn, have been studied intensively with respect to infant mortality and morbidity, brain development, and learning disabilities in later life, and as practical indicators of the health and nutrition of a population (Fig. 18.5).

The obese woman entering pregnancy faces an increased risk of severe complications, notably hypertensive disorders and diabetes mellitus, which have adverse effects on pregnancy outcome. Obesity should not be equated with overall good nutrition; excessive caloric ingestion may mask other nutritional problems (e.g., anemia, inadequate protein intake). Some persons have advocated restriction of weight gain in such women so that they conclude pregnancy with a net loss. However, the advisability of such a course seems questionable on several grounds. First, dietary restrictions to limit calories may also result in displacement of other nutrients

Fig. 18.4
Prenatal weight gain grid. (From Committee on Maternal Nutrition, Food and Nutrition Board–National Research Council, National Academy of Sciences: Maternal nutrition and the course of pregnancy, Washington, D.C., 1970, The Committee.)

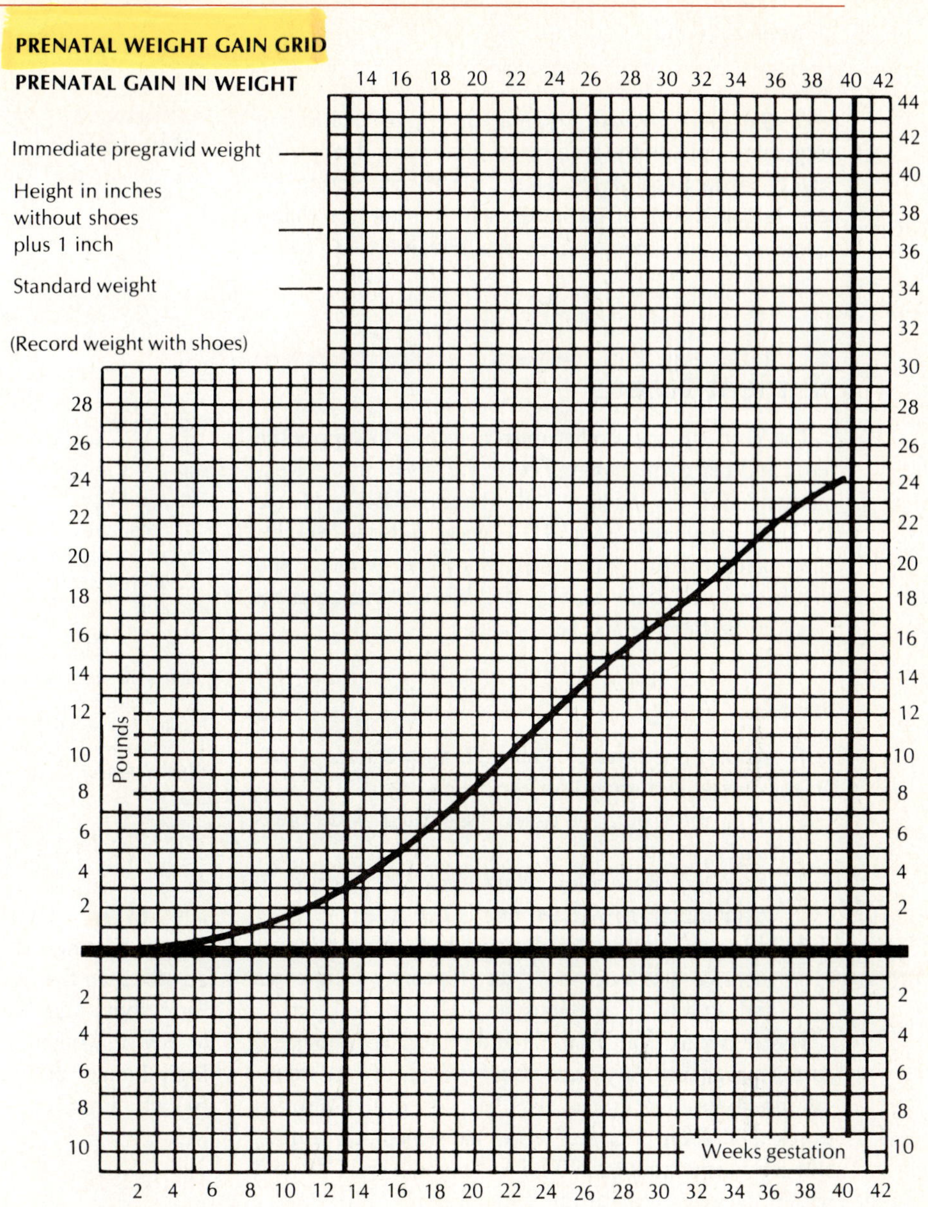

Fig. 18.5
Condition of infants at birth in relation to prenatal diet of mother. (From Mitchell, H.S., et al.: Nutrition in health and disease, ed. 16, Philadelphia, 1976, J.B. Lippincott Co.)

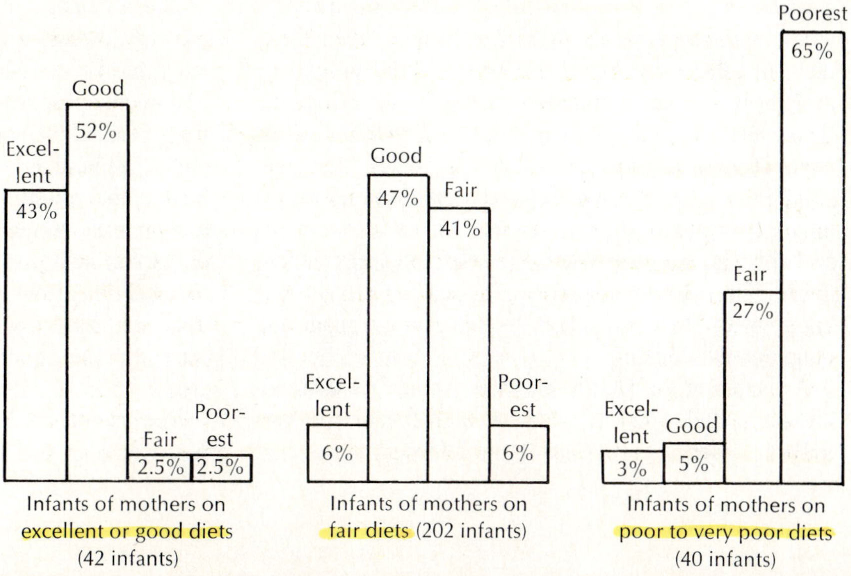

from the diet. Second, optimal protein utilization in pregnancy apparently requires a minimum of approximately 30 kcal/kg/24 hr. Third, dietary restriction results in catabolism of fat stores, which in turn produces ketonemia, which jeopardizes fetal development.

Nutrient Needs

The nutrients the mother must consume to supply the fetus and her own changing body are given in the Recommended Daily Dietary Allowances (RDAs) (Table 18.2) for pregnancy. The RDAs vary with the weight, age, health status, and activity of the woman and should be used only as a guide. Weight management needs to be flexible and personalized.

ENERGY

To support good energy status during pregnancy, sufficient energy is required for the following:

1. Deposition of new tissue associated with pregnancy
2. Increased metabolic expenditure of energy to maintain the new tissue that is deposited
3. Increased activity level associated with the movement of a heavier body as pregnancy progresses and with other activities such as work and play

Tissue deposition. Both fat and protein are deposited during pregnancy. By term about 3.8 kg of fat, representing about 36,000 kcal, has been deposited. Protein stores total about 925 g at term, and deposition of protein represents about 5200 kcal. Thus the total fat and protein deposits require about 41,000 kal.

Metabolic needs. Basal metabolic rates (BMR), when expressed as kilocalories per minute, are about 20% higher in pregnant women than in nonpregnant women, or about 0.9 to about 1.1 kcal/min. This increase includes the energy cost for tissue synthesis. The increased basal energy need over the entire pregnancy period plus the energy needed for new tissue brings the total energy cost for pregnancy to about 80,000 kcal, or about 300 kcal/24 hr.

Activity. Energy required for activity essential for ordinary living as well as for planned physical exercise is probably the most variable contributor to energy expenditure. The additional energy required for activity per kilogram of body weight is the same in pregnant and nonpregnant women.

As stated in the RDAs, pregnant women need an additional 300 kcal/24 hr. This recommendation covers only the energy cost of synthesis and maintenance of new tissue. If the woman participates regularly in weight-bearing activities, her energy needs will be greater than that recommended. Since the energy needs for activity vary from one woman to another, it is best to advise women to eat enough to satisfy their physiologic hunger and to support a gain of about 0.4 kg (4 oz)/wk during the final three fourths of pregnancy.

Table 18.2
Recommended Daily Dietary Allowances of Some Selected

Nutrients	Nonpregnant Girl 12-14 yr, 47 kg (103 lb)	Nonpregnant Girl 14-18 yr, 55 kg (120 lb)	Nonpregnant Woman, 25 yr, 58 kg (128 lb)
Calories	2200	2100	2000
Protein (g)	46	46	44
Calcium (g)	1.2	1.2	0.8
Iron (mg)	18	18	18
Vitamin A (RE)*	800	800	800
Thiamin (mg)	1.1	1.1	1.0
Riboflavin (mg)	1.3	1.3	1.2
Niacin equivalent and tryptophan (mg)	15	14	13
Ascorbic acid (mg)	50	60	60
Vitamin D (μg)‡	10	10	5

National Research Council, 1980 revision.
From Williams, S.R.: Nutrition and diet therapy, ed. 4, St. Louis, 1981.
*Retinol equivalents.
†Required iron supplement, 30-60 mg.
‡Cholecalciferol; 10 μg equals 400 IU vitamin D.

PROTEIN

Requirements for protein during pregnancy are based on the needs of the nonpregnant woman plus the extra amount needed for growth.

The efficiency of protein utilization depends on the protein's digestibility and amino acid composition. Proteins that do not contain all eight essential amino acids in amounts proportional to human requirements are utilized less efficiently, but the utilization of even high-quality protein is only about 70%. Utilization from a mixed diet or from one in which protein is supplied totally from vegetable sources is less efficient. Protein utilization also depends on caloric intake. This means that calories from nonprotein sources (i.e., carbohydrate, fat) have a sparing effect on protein. If these calories are inadequate, protein requirements would increase.

Because of these considerations, the Food and Nutrition Board of the National Academy of Sciences–Na-

Nutrients for Pregnancy and Lactation

Pregnancy				Lactation (850 ml daily)			
Added Need	Girl 12-14 yr	Girl 14-18 yr	Woman, 25 yr	Added Need	Girl 12-14 yr	Girl 14-18 yr	Woman, 25 yr
300	2500	2400	2300	500	2700	2600	2500
30	76	76	74	20	66	66	64
0.4	1.6	1.6	1.2	0.4	1.6	1.6	1.2
+	18+	18+	18+	†	18+	18+	18+
200	1000	1000	1000	400	1200	1200	1200
0.4	1.5	1.5	1.4	0.5	1.6	1.6	1.5
0.3	1.6	1.6	1.5	0.5	1.8	1.8	1.7
2	17	16	15	5	20	19	18
20	70	80	80	40	90	100	100
5	15	15	10	5	15	15	10

The C.V. Mosby Co.

tional Research Council recommends an additional 30 g protein per day from the second month of pregnancy to the end of gestation (Table 18.2). This allowance will provide for maternal protein storage as well as fetal weight gain and will cover the individual variability in protein requirements. To adjust protein intake to the body size of individuals, the following guidelines are suggested:

1. Mature women: 1.3 g protein per kilogram of pregnant weight
2. Adolescent girls (15 to 18 years of age): 1.5 g protein per kilogram of pregnant weight
3. Younger girls: 1.7 g protein per kilogram of pregnant weight

A greater amount is recommended for adolescents and younger girls to support possible continued maturation. If a multiple birth (e.g., twins) is expected, there is then a concomitant need for increases in protein and other nutrients in the mother's diet.

MAJOR MINERALS

Iron. The changes in maternal blood volume accompanying pregnancy represent a fundamental physiologic adjustment. The total elemental iron requirements of pregnancy amount to 600 to 800 mg. Since full-term average-for-gestational-age (AGA) infants are born with high hemoglobin levels of 18 to 22 g/dl and with a supply of iron stored in the liver to last 3 to 6 months, the maternal organism transfers about 300 mg of iron to the fetus during gestation. In addition to this need for fetal growth, maternal needs are 70 mg for the placenta, 500 mg for the formation of hemoglobin (the result of the increase in maternal blood volume), and 280 mg to replace basal losses in skin, hair, and sweat.

If dietary iron is not available to meet these needs, iron stores will be depleted and there will be a reduction in expansion of the maternal red cell mass rather than impairment of fetal iron reserves. If the mother has no iron reserves, which occurs frequently in young women, especially teenagers, maternal hemoglobin levels will drop more than usual and iron deficiency anemia may be superimposed on the physiologic anemia of pregnancy.

The Food and Nutrition Board recommended that dietary allowances of 18 mg suggested for the nonpregnant woman be supplemented with 30 to 60 mg of elemental iron (150 to 300 mg of ferrous sulfate). Iron preparations are taken with a source of vitamin C (orange juice) to aid absorption and utilization of iron. Iron supplementation is usually started during the second trimester to maintain maternal reserves and to meet fetal requirements during pregnancy.

Calcium. Almost all the additional calcium required during pregnancy is utilized by the fetus. The current RDA for calcium in pregnancy is 1200 mg, an increase of 400 mg over the allowance for the nonpregnant adult woman. This would seem to provide adequate amounts, particularly considering the body's adaptive ability to increase absorption and decrease excretion at times of need, such as during pregnancy. Because it is virtually impossible to meet these requirements with foods other than dairy products, milk is considered by many to be particularly essential during pregnancy, 1200 mg of calcium is precisely the amount contained in 1 L of milk. Individuals who do not consume milk or milk products—for example, persons with lactose intolerance—will require calcium supplementation.

Since calcium and phosphorus are found in the same foods, if calcium needs are met, adequate phosphorus will be assured.

Sodium. During pregnancy, there is a slight increase in the need for most nutrients, including sodium. Diets low in calories and sodium place the normal mother and her fetus at risk, especially for PIH. When sodium is restricted, the maternal organism undergoes a series of hormonal and biochemical changes in an effort to conserve sodium.

To restrict sodium, important foods, such as cheeses, meats, fish, and milk, would need to be avoided. Products devoid of nutritive value and excessively high in sodium (e.g., pretzels, potato chips, soft drinks, bouillon cubes) are discouraged. Fresh fruits, vegetables, and meats are preferred over canned and processed foods that tend to have excess amounts of sodium.

The use of diuretics during pregnancy should be discouraged because their use leads not only to a loss of sodium but also to electrolyte imbalance. Diuretics are of no benefit in preventing PIH (see Chapter 35).

FAT-SOLUBLE VITAMINS

Vitamin A. The RDA for vitamin A during pregnancy is 1000 RE (retinol equivalents) (5000 IU) daily, an increase of 25% over the allowance for the nonpregnant adult woman. The added allowance for pregnancy relates to fetal storage of the vitamin. An intake of this magnitude can readily be provided by dietary sources, and there appears to be no need for routine supplementation. Certain food faddists advocate massive amounts of vitamin A, but pregnant women should be cautioned against this practice. Since urinary excretion is at a minimal level, toxicity (hypervitaminosis A) represents a potential danger to both the pregnant woman (liver damage) and to her unborn child (congenital malformations).

Vitamin D. Vitamin D plays an important role in promoting positive calcium balance in pregnancy. It is present naturally in only a few animal foods, such as fatty fish, eggs, butter, and liver. It is also produced in the skin by the action of ultraviolet light on dehydrocholesterol. The RDA for vitamin D in adults is 5 to 10 μg (200 to 400 IU) daily; during pregnancy it is 10 to 15 μg (400 to 600 IU). Excessive amounts (hypervitaminosis D) may result in hypercalcemia in infants. Since most milk in the United States is fortified with vitamin D at a level of 10 μg per quart, the consumption of a quart of milk daily will provide the full allowance of vitamin D as well as that of calcium for most gravidas.

Vitamin E. Vitamin E (tocopherol) levels in the serum gradually rise throughout pregnancy, reaching a level by term nearly double that of the nonpregnant state. The RDA for vitamin E is 8 mg daily in the nonpregnant adult female and 10 mg daily during pregnancy, the difference intended to provide for fetal deposition.

WATER-SOLUBLE VITAMINS

The water-soluble vitamins, in contrast to those soluble in fat, are readily excreted in urine. Thus storage is less, accounting for a diminished reserve against deprivation as well as lessened likelihood of toxicity with overdosage. Furthermore, in contrast to fat-soluble vitamins, maternal serum concentrations of many water-soluble vitamins decrease during the course of pregnancy.

Folic acid. The augmented maternal erythropoiesis of pregnancy requires substantially increased amounts of folic acid. Moreover, because folic acid, or folacin, is intimately involved in DNA synthesis, requirements are particularly high in rapidly growing cells such as fetal and placental tissues. The current RDA for folic acid in pregnancy is 800 μg. In view of the evidence indicating increased folic acid needs during pregnancy and dietary survey data suggesting that the usual American diet is marginal in folic acid content, some authorities have advised routine folic acid supplementation for pregnant women. If folic acid supplements are given, daily doses of 200 to 400 μg appear appropriate.

Pyridoxine (vitamin B_6). Vitamin B_6 is another important nutrient concerned with amino acid metabolism and protein synthesis. Urinary excretion of vitamin B_6 metabolites during pregnancy is 10 to 15 times higher than in nonpregnant women, whereas blood values are typically reduced. For some time there have been efforts to link B_6 to PIH because urinary excretion is even higher in women who develop PIH than in normal pregnant women. It is likely that the observed values are the results of PIH rather than a cause of it. A dietary allowance of 2.5 mg/24 hr of vitamin B_6 is recommended in pregnancy. However, since no clinically significant conditions that are commonly observed can be attributed to inadequate levels of vitamin B_6, the Food and Nutrition Board does not believe that oral supplements are justified.

Thiamin (vitamin B_1). Thiamin requirements in general are related to energy (calorie) intake. The current RDA for thiamin in the nonpregnant adult female is 1 mg daily, to which an addition of 0.3 mg daily is recommended for pregnancy.

Riboflavin (vitamin B_2). Riboflavin requirements are thought to be increased during pregnancy. Traditionally the allowance for riboflavin has been set on the basis of energy (calorie) intake. The current RDA for females is 1.4 mg daily at 15 to 22 years of age and 1.2 mg daily at 23 years of age and older, to which an allowance of 0.3 mg daily is added during pregnancy. Allowances of this magnitude can readily be provided by the diet.

Cobalamin (vitamin B_{12}). Serum vitamin B_{12} levels decline progressively throughout gestation, and approximately one third of women at term have low values judged by standards for nonpregnant women. These changes are probably related to an increase in urinary excretion. It has been confirmed that fetal blood levels of B_{12} are higher than maternal blood levels even when maternal levels are depleted. Low maternal levels are associated with prematurity and occur more often in smokers than in nonsmokers. The capacity to absorb vitamin B_{12} is increased in pregnancy, but a large amount is transferred to the fetus. The recommended daily intake of vitamin B_{12} to maintain constant serum levels is 4 μg. If these amounts are not supplied, the serum vitamin B_{12} levels drop but return to normal without supplementation after pregnancy.

Ascorbic acid (vitamin C). The current RDA for ascorbic acid for nonpregnant women is 60 mg daily, and the recommended amount is increased by 20 mg daily during pregnancy. The entire requirement may be readily provided by the diet.

The possibility of beneficial effects of extremely large ascorbic acid supplements (up to 5 g daily) for prevention of the common cold has created considerable interest. Aside from the controversial aspect of this type of pharmacologic treatment, its use in pregnancy is open to serious question. Although no specific complications of fetal hypervitaminosis C are known, the possibility exists that fetal metabolism could be adversely affected by high levels of an oxidizing agent such as ascorbic acid. Therefore, at least for the present, pregnant women should be cautioned against use of excessive supplementation.

TRACE MINERALS

Zinc. The metal zinc is a constituent of numerous enzymes involved in major metabolic pathways. During pregnancy, total body zinc increases parallel to increased body protein. At the same time zinc levels in maternal plasma and hair decrease during pregnancy. The significance of these changes, specifically whether they reflect physiologic adjustments or deficiency, is unclear. It is perhaps noteworthy that maternal zinc deficiency is highly teratogenic in rats, and the incidence of malformations of the CNS in humans appears to be increased in geographic areas where zinc deficiency is prevalent. The current RDA for zinc in pregnancy is 20 mg daily, an increase of 5 mg daily over the allowance for the nonpregnant woman.

Flourine. Flourine in small amounts (1 part per million in drinking water) is associated with dental health. Excessive flourine acts on teeth in their budding stage of formation so that by the time they erupt, the enamel is mottled, pitted, and discolored.

NUTRITIONAL SUPPLEMENTS: THEIR ROLE IN PREGNANCY

Nutrition counselors (nurses, nutritionists) must assess whether the woman has appropriate knowledge and motivation and enough income to follow the nutrition guidance given. If needs can be met through diet, vitamin and mineral supplementation may not be necessary. However, in some instances a careful selection of vitamin and mineral supplements is of some value if problems are anticipated in a particular person. It must be noted that supplementation cannot compensate for poor food habits, and in some instances the prescriptions of supplements may give both the woman and the health care professional a false sense of security.

NOTE: One additional basis for caution in the use of high-level nutritional supplementation during pregnancy has been brought to light: the infant may become conditioned to a high intake during fetal life if the intake of the maternal organism is high. This may be reflected in the neonate's increased need in the postdelivery period.

A summary of nutrient needs of pregnancy, reasons for increased nutrient need in pregnancy, and food sources is presented in Table 18.3.

Table 18.3
Nutrient Needs of Pregnancy

Nutrient	Amount (NRC) Nonpregnant Adult Need (19-22 yr)	Amount (NRC) Pregnancy Need	Reasons for Increased Nutrient Need in Pregnancy	Food Sources
Protein	44 g	74-100 g	Rapid fetal tissue growth Amniotic fluid Placental growth and development Maternal tissue growth: uterus, breasts Increased maternal circulating blood volume: Hemoglobin increase Plasma protein increase Maternal storage reserves for labor, delivery, and lactation	Milk Cheese Egg Meat Grains Legumes Nuts
Calories	2100	2400	Increased BMR, energy needs Protein sparing	Carbohydrates Fats Proteins
Minerals				
Calcium	800 mg	1200 mg	Fetal skeleton formation Fetal tooth bud formation Increased maternal calcium metabolism	Milk Cheese Whole grains Leafy vegetables Egg yolk
Phosphorus	800 mg	1200 mg	Fetal skeletal formation Fetal tooth bud formation Increased maternal phosphorus metabolism	Milk Cheese Lean meats
Iron	18 mg	18+ mg (+30-60 mg supplement)	Increased maternal circulating blood volume, increased hemoglobin Fetal liver iron storage (primarily in third trimester) High iron cost of pregnancy	Liver Meats Egg Whole or enriched grain Leafy vegetables Nuts Legumes Dried fruits
Iodine	100 μg	125 μg	Increased BMR—increased thyroxine production	Iodized salt
Magnesium	300 mg	450 mg	Coenzyme in energy and protein metabolism Enzyme activator Tissue growth, cell metabolism Muscle action	Nuts Soybeans Cocoa Seafood Whole grains Dried beans and peas
Vitamins				
A	800 RE* (4000 IU)	1000 RE* (5000 IU)	Essential for cell development, hence tissue growth Tooth bud formation (development of enamel-forming cells in gum tissue) Bone growth	Butter Cream Fortified margarine Green and yellow vegetables
D	5-10 μg† (200-400 IU)	10-15 μg† (400-600 IU)	Absorption of calcium and phosphorus, mineralization of bone tissue, tooth buds	Fortified milk Fortified margarine
E	8 mg alpha-TE‡	10 mg alpha-TE‡	Tissue growth, cell wall integrity Red blood cell integrity	Vegetable oils Leafy vegetables Cereals Meat Egg Milk

From Williams, S.: Handbook of maternal and infant nutrition, Berkeley, Calif., 1976, SRW Productions, Inc.
*Retinol equivalents (RE) replace international units (IU).
†400 IU (international units) = 10 μg of pure crystalline vitamin D_3 (cholecalciferol).
‡Total vitamin E activity, estimated to be 80% as alpha-tocopherol and 20% as other tocopherols.

Table 18.3—cont'd
Nutrient Needs of Pregnancy

Nutrient	Amount (NRC) Nonpregnant Adult Need (19-22 yr)	Amount (NRC) Pregnancy Need	Reasons for Increased Nutrient Need in Pregnancy	Food Sources
C	60 mg	80 mg	Tissue formation and integrity Cement substance in connective and vascular tissues Increases iron absorption	Citrus fruits Berries Melons Tomatoes Chili peppers Green peppers Green leafy vegetables Broccoli Potatoes
Folic acid	400 μg	800 μg (+200-400 μg supplement)	Increased metabolic demand in pregnancy Prevention of megaloblastic anemia in high-risk women Increased heme production for hemoglobin Production of cell nucleus material	Meat Peanuts Beans and peas Enriched grains
Riboflavin	1.2 mg	1.5 mg	Coenzyme in energy metabolism Coenzyme in protein metabolism Coenzyme in energy metabolism and protein metabolism	Milk Liver Enriched grains
Thiamin	1.1 mg	1.5 mg	Coenzyme for energy metabolism	Pork, beef Liver Whole or enriched grains Legumes
B_6 (pyridoxine)	2.0 mg	2.6 mg	Coenzyme in protein metabolism Increased fetal growth requirement	Wheat, corn Liver Meat
B_{12}	3.0 μg	4.0 μg	Coenzyme in protein metabolism, especially vital cell proteins such as nucleic acid Formation of red blood cells	Milk Egg Meat Liver Cheese

Nutrition Risk Factors in Pregnancy

To assess effectively the nutritional status of the pregnant or lactating woman, the counselor (nurse, nutritionist) needs to understand the major risk factors and their implications for nutrition. Nutrition risk factors include those present at the onset of pregnancy and those that may occur during the course of pregnancy.

RISK FACTORS AT THE ONSET OF PREGNANCY

Adolescence. See Chapter 38 for a discussion of the nutrition risk factors for pregnant adolescents.

Frequent pregnancies. The woman who has had three or more pregnancies within 2 years, as well as the multiparous woman who has progressed from one pregnancy directly to another, is considered to be at increased risk and is prone to depleted nutrient stores. This situation can potentially compromise maternal and fetal health and well-being.

Poor reproductive history. Special attention should be paid to the woman's obstetric history. Poor weight gain in pregnancy, PIH, a previous stillbirth or delivery of a low–birth weight infant, premature delivery, and perinatal infection are all more common in women who are or have been poorly nourished in the past. As a result, the woman with a poor reproductive history may need more than the usual nutrition guidance.

Economic deprivation. For economically deprived women there are several programs that help with the purchase of food or that offer supplements, for example, the federal food stamp program and the supplemental food program for women, infants, and children, sometimes known as the WIC program.

Bizarre food patterns. A woman may enter pregnancy either having been or continuing to be on a faddish or otherwise nutritionally inadequate diet. The woman who practices pica may not consume adequate levels of nutrients. Pica is defined as regular and excessive ingestion of nonfood items (Argo starch or red clay) or of foods with limited nutritional value. The practice often relates to cultural or geographic factors or both (pp. 118 and 241).

Recently megavitamin supplementation and various types of vegetarian diets have become popular. Persons on a megavitamin regimen ingest massive amounts of vitamins far above the RDA levels. Although there is no documentation that these large amounts of vitamins are beneficial, there is evidence that consumption of large numbers of fat-soluble vitamins (e.g., vitamin A), which are stored in the body, may lead to toxicity.

Vegetarian diets. There are various types of vegetarian diets (see p. 335). The lactoovovegetarian eats no meat, fish, or poultry but will use either eggs (ovo) or dairy products (lacto) or both. Of particular concern is the strict vegetarian (vegan), who eliminates all products of animal origin, including meat, poultry, fish, cheese, eggs, and milk. The pregnant woman who practices strict vegetarianism may not receive ample quantities of complementary and complete proteins and may not obtain enough vitamin B_{12}. Particularly intense nutrition counseling will be required to work out a diet pattern for a strict vegetarian during the prenatal period.

Smoking, drug addiction, and alcoholism. The person who is a heavy smoker (more than 6 cigarettes per day), drug addict, or alcoholic (chronically using more than 150 ml [5 oz] of whiskey per day or its equivalent of beer or wine) is likely to have major physiologic problems. The effects of smoking during pregnancy include reduction in gestation length (with onset of premature labor) and infants who are small for gestational age (SGA). In addition, there is always the possibility that women who indulge excessively in the use of cigarettes, drugs, or alcohol may not consume sufficient quantities of nutritious food. (For detailed discussion, see Chapter 39 and Appendix H.)

Chronic systemic diseases. Medical problems such as anemia, thyroid dysfunction, and chronic medical or surgical gastrointestinal disorders may be associated with interference with the ingestion, absorption, or utilization of nutrients. Drugs utilized in treatment of these conditions may also affect nutrition by similar interference. Nutrition counseling should combine general nutrition guidelines for prenatal care *and* diet therapy recommended for a particular woman's medical condition.

Prepregnant weight. If a woman begins pregnancy at a weight below 85% of the standard weight for height (e.g., less than 46 kg [100 lb] in weight for a height of 152 cm [60 in]), she is considered to be at increased risk to enter pregnancy. The woman is also at risk if she is obese, or weighs more than 120% of the standard weight (Fig. 18.5).

RISK FACTORS IN PREGNANCY

Anemia of pregnancy. The iron needs during pregnancy are obtained from maternal iron stores, diet, and supplementation. True anemia occurring during pregnancy is most often caused by iron deficiency. Many healthy American women do not have iron stores large enough to meet the demands of pregnancy. Iron supplementation will aid greatly in maintaining the hemoglobin at normal levels.

Pregnancy-induced hypertension. The cause of pregnancy-induced hypertension (PIH) is not known. It is characterized by an elevation in blood pressure, proteinuria, and rapid weight gain caused by edema. There is considerable controversy over the influence of nutrition on the development of PIH. This disorder occurs more frequently in pregnant women with poor diets and particularly in those with low protein intake than in those receiving good diets.

In the past few years a question has arisen about the relation of sodium to PIH. The Committee on Maternal Nutrition of the Food and Nutrition Board (1975) discourages the routine use of salt restriction and diuretics during pregnancy.

Inadequate weight gain. Normal pregnancy is a time of progressive maternal weight gain. The following are presumptive signs of maternal and fetal malnutrition: (1) failure to gain weight (less than 0.9 kg [2 lb]/mo during the second and third trimesters), (2) actual weight loss, (3) significant nausea and vomiting during early pregnancy, and (4) poor or delayed uterine-fetal growth.

Inadequate maternal weight gain, less than 0.9 kg (2 lb)/mo in the second and third trimesters, has been associated with lowered birth weight and evidence of intrauterine growth retardation (IUGR). It is therefore important to document the pattern of weight gain in pregnancy as well as the total amount gained.

Excessive weight gain. Total maternal weight gain during the 40 weeks of pregnancy averages 11.5 kg (25 lb). This amounts to about 1.4 to 1.8 kg (3 to 4 lb)/mo. Rapid accumulation of weight in a singleton pregnancy—that is, 0.9 to 2.3 kg (2 to 5 lb)/wk—results only from tissue fluid retention and may be associated with PIH. The woman must be carefully assessed for development of this condition.

Excessive weight gain associated with accumulation

of fat is less dramatic and is best assessed by evaluating the woman's eating habits and by measuring subcutaneous fat stores by means of skinfold calipers. Sources of calorically rich but nutritionally poor food should be sought and eliminated. Weight reduction in pregnancy or lactation by dietary manipulation or drug administration or both is contraindicated because of the potentially adverse and possibly toxic effects on fetal nutrition, growth, and development.

Demands of lactation. Increased nutritional demands of lactation can also be a risk factor. Storage of 2 or 3 kg of fat during pregnancy provides the gravida with a reservoir of some 14,000 to 24,000 kcal for lactation needs. Ordinarily, fat stores will be gradually utilized for the first 4 to 6 months of lactation. Without these stores the nursing mother faces the difficult task of increasing food consumption 50% to be able to provide the 1000 kcal required for production of 800 to 900 ml of milk.

Without the demands of nursing, fat stores may remain a permanent addition to the maternal frame and increase the potential for obesity with advancing age and parity. A modest reduction in caloric intake after delivery is appropriate for the woman who does not nurse her infant. This is particularly true if she uses an oral contraceptive agent. For discussion of nutrition and the contraceptive pill, refer to p. 194.

Guidelines for Management

The basic nutrition guidelines for normal pregnancy are based on recommendations of the Committee on Maternal Nutrition of the National Academy of Sciences–National Research Council and the Committee on Nutrition of the American College of Obstetricians and Gynecologists, as adapted by the California Department of Health Services.

To obtain the woman's compliance with the guidelines, the following elements required to deliver quality prenatal nutrition care must be considered:

1. Nutrition assessment evaluation
2. Intervention
3. Monitoring and evaluation

NUTRITION ASSESSMENT

An individual assessment of nutritional status must be made at the beginning of prenatal care and supported by continuing evaluation throughout the pregnancy. The following methods of assessment provide the data necessary to determine need:

1. Clinical observation, including history and physical examination
2. Biochemical tests of serum
3. Dietary assessment

History. Data from the pregnant woman's history are among the most important elements in nutrition assessment. These data must include basic information carefully taken from the medical, obstetric, nutrition, family and social portions of the history, all of which have a bearing on nutritional status.

Physical examination. Two problems bear on the validity of the physical examination. First, the lack of standard definitions and the nonspecificity of most clinical manifestations of malnutrition result in considerable variation in interpretation of physical signs. Second, pregnancy may complicate specific interpretation of physical signs. Despite these shortcomings the physical assessment of nutritional status can be useful if it is utilized in conjunction with the biochemical analyses and dietary assessment (Table 18.4).

General screening for dental health status provides helpful information on nutritional status. The most common clinical nutrition-related disorders that are likely to be encountered during the reproductive years are caries and periodontitis. These conditions cause mechanical and mastication difficulties that interfere with the ingestion of certain types of food.

Biochemical tests. Laboratory data provide vital base-line information for nutrition assessment at the beginning of pregnancy as well as a means of monitoring nutritional status throughout gestation. In general, laboratory tests provide a more objective and precise determination of nutritional status than do other assessment indexes.

Blood-forming nutrients. Measures of the blood-forming nutrients—iron, folacin, and vitamins B_6 and B_{12}—are important guides for use in preventing and treating anemias often associated with pregnancy (see Chapter 36). The following can be measured in routine tests:

1. Hemoglobin levels
2. Hematocrit levels
3. Mean corpuscular volume (MCV)
4. Mean corpuscular hemoglobin concentration (MCHC)
5. Serum iron levels and percentage of concentration in saturation
6. Transferrin levels

Other tests include those for folic acid deficiency:

1. MCV
2. Hypersegmented polymorphonuclear leukocytes
3. Serum folic acid
4. RBC folic acid
5. Serum protein

Some of these tests are expensive. Care must be taken to order those that benefit the client most, at the least expense.

Table 18.4
Physical Assessment of Nutritional Status

Body Area	Signs of Good Nutrition	Signs of Poor Nutrition
General appearance	Alert, responsive	Listless, apathetic, cachectic
Weight	Normal for height, age, body build	Overweight or underweight (special concern for underweight)
Posture	Erect, arms and legs straight	Sagging shoulders, sunken chest, humped back
Muscles	Well developed, firm, good tone, some fat under skin	Flaccid, poor tone, undeveloped, tender, "wasted" appearance, cannot walk properly
Nervous control	Good attention span, not irritable or restless, normal reflexes, psychologic stability	Inattentive, irritable, confused, burning and tingling of hands and feet (parasthesia), loss of position and vibratory sense, weakness and tenderness of muscles (may result in inability to walk), decrease or loss of ankle and knee reflexes
Gastrointestinal function	Good appetite and digestion, normal regular elimination, no palpable organs or masses	Anorexia, indigestion, constipation or diarrhea, liver or spleen enlargement
Cardiovascular function	Normal heart rate and rhythm, no murmurs, normal blood pressure for age	Rapid heart rate (above 100 beats/min: tachycardia), enlarged heart, abnormal rhythm, elevated blood pressure
General vitality	Endurance, energetic, sleeps well, vigorous	Easily fatigued, no energy, falls asleep easily, looks tired, apathetic
Hair	Shiny, lustrous, firm, not easily plucked, healthy scalp	Stringy, dull, brittle, dry, thin and sparse, depigmented, can be easily plucked
Skin (general)	Smooth, slightly moist, good color	Rough, dry, scaly, pale, pigmented, irritated, easily bruised, petechiae
Face and neck	Skin color uniform, smooth, pink, healthy appearance, not swollen	Greasy, discolored, scaly, swollen, skin dark over cheeks and under eyes, lumpiness or flakiness of skin around nose and mouth
Lips	Smooth, good color, moist, not chapped or swollen	Dry, scaly, swollen, redness, angular lesions at corners of mouth, fissured, scarred (cheilosis, stomatitis)
Mouth, oral membranes	Reddish pink mucous membranes in oral cavity	Swollen, boggy oral mucous membranes
Gums	Reddish pink, healthy, no swelling or bleeding	Spongy, bleed easily, marginal redness, inflamed, gums receding
Tongue	Healthy pink or deep reddish in appearance, not swollen or smooth, surface papillae present, no lesions	Swollen, scarlet and raw, magenta color, beefy (glossitis), hyperemic and hypertrophic papillae, atrophic papillae
Teeth	No cavities, no pain, bright, straight, no crowding, well-shaped jaw, clean, no discoloration	Unfilled caries, absent teeth, worn surfaces, mottled (fluorosis), malpositioned
Eyes	Bright, clear, shiny, no sores at corners of eyelids, membranes moist and healthy pink color, no prominent blood vessels or mound of tissue on sclera, no fatigue circles beneath	Eye membranes pale (pale conjunctiva), redness of membrane (conjunctival injection), dryness, signs of infection, Bitot's spots, redness and fissuring of eyelid corners (angular palpebritis), dryness of eye membrane (conjunctival xerosis), dull appearance of cornea (corneal xerosis), soft cornea (keratomalacia)
Neck (glands)	No enlargement	Thyroid enlarged
Nails	Firm, pink	Spoon shaped (koilonychia), brittle, ridged
Legs, feet	No tenderness, weakness, or swelling; good color	Edema, tender calf, tingling, weakness
Skeleton	No malformations	Bowlegs, knock-knees, chest deformity at diaphragm, beaded ribs, prominent scapulas

From Williams, S.R.: Nurtitional guidance in prenatal care. In Worthington, B.S., Vermeersch, J., and Williams, S.R.: Nutrition in pregnancy and lactation, St. Louis, 1977, The C.V. Mosby Co.

Serum albumin. An adequate level of serum albumin is important during pregnancy because of its function in helping to maintain normal flow of tissue fluids from the circulating blood through the tissue for nourishment of cells and back into circulation by means of capillary fluid shift mechanisms. A protein deficit would contribute to a lowered plasma albumin level and in turn to an imbalance in the fluid shift mechanism, resulting in edema. An acceptable level of serum albumin during pregnancy is 3.5 g/dl or above.

Other minerals and vitamins. Depending on individual situations, tests for other vitamin and mineral levels may be performed, including determinations of the water-soluble vitamins (thiamin, riboflavin, niacin, and vitamin C), the fat-soluble vitamins (A, D, E, and K), and trace minerals.

Blood lipids, glucose, and enzymes. Routine testing for urine sugar and ketone bodies will screen for latent diabetes mellitus or gestational glycosuria. Other tests may be performed if there is a complicating chronic disease, particularly heart disease or renal disease.

Dietary assessment. Since pregnancy is a time in the life cycle when nutrition is of special importance, it is essential to learn who the mother is, where she is, what her needs are, and how these needs can best be met. Only in this context can realistic guidance be provided. Dietary assessment in pregnancy involves three basic areas: background data, diet history, and diet analysis.

Background data. Food habits and attitudes cannot be viewed in isolation: life situations and values as well as physical and emotional factors must also be considered. Thus, if nutrition counseling is to be valid, it must be based on an individual plan of care.

A woman's living situation will have an influence on her eating behavior. Therefore the data on the home setting, housing, life-style, family members, occupation, general socioeconomic status, food assistance needs, and family roles and attitudes concerning foods are important. Cultural-ethnic food practices should be explored, including types of food, ethnic dishes, methods of cooking, and taboos associated with pregnancy (Table 18.5). It is important to determine special diet practices such as faddist or unusual patterns. Strict vegetarian diets or various forms of pica may be nutritionally unsound. Food allergies and milk or lactose intolerance* need to be explored. The use of *all* medications and supplements should be discussed with the woman.

A *nutrition questionnaire* covering the background information is a useful tool in dietary assessment. the California Department of Health Services developed an excellent instrument to be used specifically by the physician, nurse, dietitian, or nutritionist with the pregnant woman. The nutrition questionnaire given in the box below groups questions into 11 sections that identify factors that may influence prenatal nutrition.

*Lactose intolerance is a problem of certain ethnic groups and individuals. The nurse should help the family plan for protein and calcium intake from sources other than milk and alert the family to watch for this condition in the newborn. One food, tofu (soybean cake), contains considerable calcium but no lactose. Of the cheeses, Swiss cheese contains the least lactose.

Table 18.5
Characteristics of Some Cultural Food Patterns

Ethnic Group	Milk Group	Meat Group	Fruits and Vegetables	Breads and Cereals	Possible Dietary Problems
American Indian (many tribal variations; many "Americanized")	Fresh milk Evaporated milk for cooking Ice cream Cream pies	Pork, beef, lamb, rabbit Fowl, fish, eggs Legumes Sunflower seeds Nuts: walnut, acorn, pine, peanut butter Game meat	Green peas, beans Beets, turnips Leafy green and other vegetables Grapes, bananas, peaches, other fresh fruits Roots	Refined bread Whole wheat Cornmeal Rice Dry cereals "Fry" bread Tortillas	In California, major problems: obesity, diabetes, alcoholism, nutritional deficiencies expressed in dental problems and iron deficiency anemia Inadequate amounts of all nutrients Excessive use of sugar
Middle Eastern (Armenian, Greek, Syrian, Turkish)	Yogurt Little butter	Lamb Nuts Dried peas, beans, lentils	Peppers Tomatoes Cabbage Grape leaves Cucumbers Squash Dried apricots, raisins	Cracked wheat and dark bread	Fry many meats and vegetables Lack of fresh fruits Insufficient foods from milk group (use olive oil* in place of butter) Like sweetenings, lamb fat, and olive oil

*Olive oil is all fat, with no other nutrient value.

Continued.

Table 18.5—cont'd
Characteristics of Some Cultural Food Patterns

Ethnic Group	Milk Group	Meat Group	Fruits and Vegetables	Breads and Cereals	Possible Dietary Problems
Black	Milk Ice cream Puddings Cheese: longhorn, American	Pork: all cuts, plus organs, chitterlings Beef, lamb Chicken, giblets Eggs Nuts Legumes Fish, game	Leafy vegetables Green and yellow vegetables Potato: white, sweet Stewed fruit Bananas and other fresh fruit	Cornmeal and hominy grits Rice Biscuits, pancakes, white breads Puddings: bread, rice Molasses†	Extensive use of frying, "smothering," or simmering Fats: salt pork, bacon drippings, lard, and gravies Like sweets Insufficient citrus and enriched breads Vegetables often boiled for long periods Limited amounts from milk group
Chinese (Cantonese most prevalent)	Cheese Milk: water buffalo	Pork sausage‡ Eggs and pigeon eggs Fish Lamb, beef, goat Fowl: chicken, duck Nuts Legumes	Many vegetables Radish leaves Bean, bamboo sprouts Soybean curd (tofu)§	Rice/rice flour products Cereals, noodles Wheat, corn, millet seed	Tendency of northern China (Mandarin), coastal China (Shanghai), and inland China (Szechwan) immigrants to use more grease in cooking Limited use of milk and milk products Often low in protein, calories, or both May wash rice before cooking Soy sauce, ginger
Filipino (Spanish-Chinese influence)	Flavored milk Milk in coffee Cheese: gouda, cheddar	Pork, beef, goat, deer, rabbit Chicken Fish Eggs Nuts Legumes	Many vegetables and fruits	Rice, cooked cereals Noodles: rice, wheat	Limited use of milk and milk products Tend to prewash rice May have only small portions of protein foods
Italian	Cheese Some ice cream	Meat Eggs Dried beans	Leafy vegetables Potatoes Eggplant Spinach Fruits	Macaroni White breads, some whole wheat Farina Cereals	Prefer expensive imported cheeses; reluctant to substitute less expensive domestic varieties Tendency to overcook vegetables Limited use of whole grains Enjoy sweets Extensive use of olive oil Insufficient servings from milk group
Japancese (Isei, more Japanese influence; Nisei, more westernized)	Increasing amounts being used by younger generations	Pork, beef, chicken Fish Eggs Legumes: soya, red, lima beans Nuts	Many vegetables and fruits Seaweed Tofu	Rice, rice cakes Wheat noodles Refined bread, noodles	Excessive salt: pickles, salty crisp seaweed Insufficient servings from milk group May use refined or prewashed rice

†Light molasses (first extraction): 1 tbsp = 50 calories, 33 mg of calcium, 0.9 mg of iron, 0.01 mg each of vitamins B_1 and B_2; dark molasses (third extraction): 1 tbsp = 45 calories, 137 mg of calcium, 3.2 mg of iron, 0.02 mg of vitamin B_1, 0.04 mg of vitamin B_2, 0.4 mg of niacin.
‡Lower in fat content than Western sausage.
§Good source of protein.

Table 18.5—cont'd
Characteristics of Some Cultural Food Patterns

Ethnic Group	Milk Group	Meat Group	Fruits and Vegetables	Breads and Cereals	Possible Dietary Problems
Mexican-Spanish	Milk Cheese Flan Ice cream	Beef, pork, lamb, chicken, tripe, hot sausage, beef intestines Fish Eggs Nuts Dry beans: pinto, chick-peas (often eaten more than once daily)	Spinach, wild greens, tomatoes, chilies, corn, cactus leaves, cabbage, avocado Pumpkin, zapote, peaches, guava, papaya, citrus	Rice, oats, cornmeal Sweet bread Tortilla: corn, flour Biscuits Vermicelli *(fideo)*	Limited meats primarily due to economics Limited use of milk and milk products Some tendency toward increasing use of flour tortillas over more nutritious corn tortillas Large amounts of lard *(manteca)* Abundant use of sugar Tendency to boil vegetables for long periods
Polish	Milk Sour cream Cheese Butter	Pork (preferred) Chicken	Vegetables Cabbage Roots Fruits	Dark rye	Like sweets Tendency to overcook vegetables Limited fruits (especially citrus), raw vegetables, and meats
Puerto Rican	Limited use of milk products Coffee with milk *(café con leche)*	Pork Poultry Eggs (Fridays) Dried codfish Beans (habichuelas)	Avocado, okra Eggplant Sweet yams Starchy vegetables and fruits *(viandas)*	Rice Cornmeal	Use small amounts of pork and poultry Use fat, lard, salt pork, and olive oil extensively Lack of butter and other milk products
Scandinavian: Danish, Finnish, Norwegian, Swedish	Cream Butter	Wild game Reindeer Fish Eggs	Fruit berries Dried fruit Vegetables: cole slaw, roots, avocado	Whole wheat, rye, barley, sweets (molasses for flavoring)	Insufficient fresh fruits and vegetables Like sweets, pickled salted meats, and fish

Diet history and analysis. There are several methods to determine food intake and provide an overview of the woman's dietary pattern. The two most commonly used are (1) recalling foods consumed during the previous 24 hours and (2) describing consumption of food in terms of frequency over a period of time.

NUTRITION COUNSELING

The nurse or nutritionist must give consideration to understanding the client's problems and concerns, recognizing that other persons—such as family members, peers, colleagues, and other members of the health team who interact with the pregnant woman—may have considerable influence on the client's eating habits as well.

The screening and assessment results are the first tools to be used in determining a care plan for nutrition counseling. Counseling may be carried out to obtain more information about the woman and her family, to teach new information, to review and strengthen acquired knowledge and desirable habits, or to help the woman set her own goals and make her own decisions.

There are several tools that are useful in providing nutrition information to the pregnant woman. The tools include a daily food guide and a list of food groups, a sample meal pattern and sample menus, and information on ethnic preferences and vegetarian diets.

Daily food guide and list of food groups. A diet consisting of a variety of foods can supply needed nutrients. The increased quantities of essential nutrients needed during pregnancy may be met by skillful planning around a daily food guide based on the RDAs.

The California Department of Health Services has developed an excellent food guide that uses an exchange list system to provide flexibility in the selection of a nutritious diet (Table 18.6 and boxed material, pp. 333 and 334). The list of food groups presents six categories according to the nutrients they contribute. Comparable amounts of specific nutrients are provided in each group, although portion sizes differ for various foods. Because of the comparable amounts of specific nu-

Nutrition Questionnaire

Name: ______________________ **Date:** __________

Please answer the following by checking the appropriate box or filling in the blank. Answer only those questions that apply to you. All information is confidential.

1. a. Before this pregnancy, what was your usual weight? ______ kg (____________ lb)
   ☐ Don't know
   b. During your last pregnancy, how much weight did you gain? ______ kg (____________ lb)
   ☐ Don't know
   c. How much weight do you expect to gain during this pregnancy? ______ kg (____________ lb)
   ☐ Don't know
   d. Have you ever had any problems with your weight?
   ☐ Yes ☐ No If yes, what? ☐ Underweight ☐ Overweight ☐ Other ______
2. a. How would you describe your appetite?
   ☐ Hearty ☐ Moderate ☐ Poor
   b. With this pregnancy, have you experienced either of the following? ☐ Nausea ☐ Vomiting
3. How would you describe your regular eating habits?
   ☐ Regular ☐ Irregular
4. a. Indicate the person who does the following in your household?
   Plans the meals ____________
   Buys the food ____________
   Prepares the food ____________
   b. How much is spent on food each week for your household? ______ ☐ Don't know
   How many people does this feed? ______
   c. Indicate the type of kitchen equipment you have in your home:
   ☐ Refrigerator ☐ Hot plate ☐ Stove
5. a. Are you *now* taking any vitamin or mineral supplement? ☐ Yes ☐ No
   b. Do you take any pills to control your weight?
   ☐ Yes ☐ No
   c. Do you take diuretic (water) pills? ☐ Yes ☐ No
6. a. Are you now on a diet to lose weight?
   ☐ Yes ☐ No
   b. Are you *now* on a special diet (low salt, diabetic, gallbladder, etc.)? ☐ Yes ☐ No
   If yes, what kind of diet? ____________
   c. If you have been on a special diet in the past, indicate what kind and when. ____________
   ____
   ____
7. a. Is there any food you *cannot* eat? ☐ Yes ☐ No
   If yes, what food(s)? ____________
   ____
   What happens when you eat this food? ______
   ____
   b. Do you have any cravings for things such as:
   ☐ Cornstarch ☐ Plaster ☐ Dirt or clay
   ☐ Other ____________
8. Do you have either of the following problems?
   ☐ Constipation ☐ Diarrhea
9. a. Do you smoke? ☐ Yes ☐ No
   b. Do you drink any alcoholic beverages (liquor, wine, beer)? ☐ Yes ☐ No
10. Are you receiving either of the following?
   ☐ Food stamps ☐ WIC vouchers
11. How do you want to feed your baby? ☐ Breast milk ☐ Evaporated milk formula ☐ Commercial formula ☐ Undecided

Adapted from Nutrition during pregnancy and lactation, Sacramento, Calif., 1975, Maternal and Child Health Branch, California Department of Health Services.

Table 18.6
Daily Food Plan for Pregnancy and Lactation

Food	Nonpregnant Woman	Pregnant Woman	Lactating Woman
Milk, cheese, ice cream, skimmed milk or buttermilk (food made with milk can supply part of requirement)	2 C	3-4 C	4-5 C
Meat (lean meat, fish, poultry, cheese, occasional dried beans or peas)	1 serving (3-4 oz)	2 servings (6-8 oz); include liver frequently	2½ servings (8 oz)
Eggs	1	1-2	1-2
Vegetable* (dark green or deep yellow)	1 serving	1 serving	1-2 servings
Vitamin C–rich food* Good source—citrus fruit, berries, cantaloupe Fair source—tomatoes, cabbage, greens, potatoes in skin	1 good source or 2 fair sources	1 good source and 1 fair source or 2 good sources	1 good source and 1 fair source or 2 good sources
Other vegetables and fruits	1 serving	2 servings	2 servings
Bread† and cereals (enriched or whole grain)	3 servings	4-5 servings	5 servings
Butter or fortified margarine	As desired or needed for calories	As desired or needed for calories	As desired or needed for calories

From Williams, S.R.: Nutrition and diet therapy, ed. 4, St. Louis, 1981, The C.V. Mosby Co.
*Use some raw daily.
†One slice of bread equals 1 serving.

Food Groups

Protein foods include both animal and vegetable foods. Animal protein foods supply protein, iron, riboflavin, niacin, vitamins B_6 and B_{12}, phosphorus, zinc, and iodine. Vegetable protein foods supply protein, iron, thiamin, folacin, vitamins B_6 and E, phosphorus, magnesium, and zinc.

Animal protein foods*

A serving is a 60-90 g (2-3 oz) cooked (boneless) of the following unless otherwise noted.

- Bacon, 6 slices
- Beef: ground, cube, roast, chop
- Canned tuna, salmon, crab, etc., ½ C
- Cheese (see milk list)
- Chitterlings (tripe)
- Clams, 4 large or 9 small
- Crab
- Duck
- Eggs, 2
- Fish: fillet, steak
- Fish sticks, breaded, 4
- Frankfurters, 2
- Hog maws
- Lamb: ground, cube roast, chop
- Lobster
- Luncheon meat, 3 slices
- Organ meats: liver, kidney, sweetbreads, heart, tongue
- Oysters, 10-15 medium
- Pigs' feet, ears, snouts
- Pork, ham: ground, roast, chop
- Poultry: ground, roast
- Rabbit
- Sausage links, 4
- Shrimp, scallops, 5-6 large
- Spareribs, 6 medium ribs
- Veal: ground, cube, roast, chop

Vegetable protein foods

A serving is 1 C cooked unless otherwise stated.

- Canned garbanzo, lima, kidney beans
- Canned pork and beans
- Dried beans and peas
- Lentils
- Nut butters, ¼ C
- Nuts, ½ C
- Sunflower seeds, ½ C
- Tofu (soybean curd)

Milk and milk products constitute an exchange group of foods containing calcium, phosphorus, vitamin D, and riboflavin. In addition, these foods supply protein, vitamins A, E, B_6, and B_{12}, magnesium, and zinc. For some people, milk and milk products serve as primary sources of protein in the diet.

A serving is 240 ml (8 oz, or 1 C) unless otherwise noted.

- Cheese: hard and semisoft (except blue, Camembert, and cream), 42 g (1½ oz)
- Cheese spread, 56 g (2 oz)
- Cottage cheese, creamed, 1⅓ C
- Cow's milk: whole, nonfat, low fat, nonfat dry reconstituted, buttermilk, chocolate milk, cocoa made with milk
- Cream soups made with milk, 360 ml (12 oz)
- Evaporated milk, 90 ml (3 oz)
- Goat's milk (low B_{12} content)
- Ice cream, 1½ C
- Ice milk
- Instant breakfast made with milk, 120 ml (4 oz)
- Liquid diet beverage, 150 ml (5 oz)
- Milkshake, commercial, 240 ml (8 oz)
- Puddings, custard (flan)
- Soybean milk (low B_{12} content)
- Yogurt

NOTE: Tofu is also a source of calcium; 1 C tofu may be exchanged for one serving of the above foods.

Grain products supply thiamin, niacin, riboflavin, iron, phosphorus, and zinc. This exchange group is divided into two parts: whole grain items and enriched products. The enriched breads, cereals, and pastas provide significantly lower amounts of magnesium and zinc. For this reason, people should be urged to choose whole grain products.

Whole grain items

- Brown rice, ½ C
- Cereals, hot: oatmeal (rolled oats), rolled wheat, cracked wheat, wheat with malted barley, ½ C cooked
- Cereals, ready-to-eat: puffed oats, shredded wheat, wheat flakes, granola, ¾ C
- Cracked and whole wheat bread, 1 slice
- Wheat germ, 1 tbsp

Enriched breads, cereals, and pastas

NOTE: California law requires that bread and bakery products be made with enriched flours. The following should comply with this requirement.

- Bread, 1 slice (all other forms)
- Cereals, hot: cream of wheat, cream of rice, farina, cornmeal, grits, ½ C
- Cereals, ready-to-eat, ¾ C
- Cornbread, 1 piece (5 cm [2 in] square)
- Crackers, 4 (all kinds)
- Macaroni, noodles, spaghetti, cooked, ½ C
- Muffin, biscuit, dumpling, 1
- Pancake, 1 medium
- Rice, cooked, ½ C
- Roll, bagel, 1
- Tortilla, corn, 2

Adapted for Nutrition during pregnancy and lactation, Sacramento, Calif., 1975, Maternal and Child Health Branch. California Department of Health Services.

*An alternate protein food is a combination of animal (70%) and vegetable (30%) protein foods. Most commonly used is a mixture of meat and textured vegetable protein (TVP). Such foods have the advantage of being more economical than 100% animal protein foods.

Continued.

Food Groups—cont'd

Tortilla, flour, 1 large
Waffle, 1 large

Vitamin C–rich fruits and vegetables supply ascorbic acid. Fresh, frozen, or canned forms may be used, although vitamin C content of canned products is lower.

Juices
- Orange, grapefruit, 120 ml (4 oz)
- Tomato, pineapple, 360 ml (12 oz)
- Fruit juices and drinks enriched with vitamin C, 180 ml (6 oz)

Fruits
- Cantaloupe, ½
- Grapefruit, ½
- Guava, ¼ medium
- Mango, 1 medium
- Orange, 1 medium
- Papaya, ⅓ medium
- Strawberries, ¾ C
- Tangerine, 2 small

Vegetables
- Bok choy, ¾ C
- Broccoli, 1 stalk
- Brussels sprouts, 3-4
- Cabbage, cooked, 1⅓ C
- Cabbage, raw, ¾ C
- Cauliflower, raw or cooked, 1 C
- Greens: collard, kale, mustard, Swiss chard, turnip greens, ¾ C
- Peppers, chili, ¾ C
- Peppers: green, red, ½ medium
- Tomatoes, 2 medium
- Watercress, ¾ C

Leafy green vegetables are an exchange group containing folacin. In addition, these foods supply vitamins A, E, and B_6, riboflavin, iron, and magnesium.

A serving is 1 C raw, or ¾ C cooked.
- Asparagus
- Bok choy
- Broccoli
- Brussel sprouts
- Cabbage
- Dark, leafy lettuce: chicory, endive, escarole, red leaf, romaine
- Greens: beet, collard kale, mustard spinach, Swiss chard, turnip
- Scallions
- Watercress

Other fruits and vegetables include yellow fruits and vegetables that supply significant amounts of vitamin A. Vitamin A is also found in outstanding amounts in the leafy green vegetable group. Other fruits and vegetables also contribute varying amounts of B-complex vitamins, vitamin E, magnesium, zinc, and phosphorus.

A serving is ½ C (fresh, frozen, or canned) unless otherwise indicated.

Vegetables
- Artichoke
- Bamboo shoots
- Bean sprouts: alfalfa, mung
- Beet
- Burdock root
- Carrot
- Cauliflower
- Celery
- Corn
- Cucumber
- Eggplant
- Beans: green, wax
- Hominy
- Lettuce: head, Boston, bib
- Mushrooms
- Nori seaweed
- Onion
- Parsnip
- Peas
- Pea pods
- Potato
- Radishes
- Summer squash
- Sweet potato
- Winter squash
- Yam
- Zucchini

Fruits
- Apricot, fresh, 1 large
- Nectarine, 2 medium
- Peach, fresh, 1 medium
- Persimmon, 1 small
- Prunes, 4 (also significant iron source)
- Pumpkin, ¼ C
- Apple, 1 medium
- Banana, 1 small
- Berries
- Cherries
- Dates, 5
- Figs, 2 large
- Fruit cocktail
- Grapes
- Kumquats, 3
- Pear, 1 medium
- Pineapple
- Plums, 2 medium
- Raisins (also significant iron source)
- Watermelon

trients, it is possible to substitute, or "exchange," foods within each group. The six food groups are described in some detail, and the list includes nutrients found in significant amounts and foods that can be exchanged.

Sample meal pattern and sample menus. It is necessary to show the woman how the daily food guide and list of food groups can be used. Table 18.7 provides a sample daily meal pattern and sample menus.

The use of the daily food guide and the list of food groups will ensure an average intake of essential nutrients that will meet the metabolic needs of pregnant women. However, the RDAs for folacin and iron cannot be met by diet alone. Therefore daily supplementation of 400 to 800 μg folacin and 30 to 60 mg iron is recommended. For adequate calories the woman should be counseled to include additional foods in her diet by increasing servings of the food groups and by using combinations of foods in casseroles.

The food guide contains more protein than indicated in the RDA. Unless a higher level of protein is provided, nutrients such as B_6, iron, and zinc will not be adequate.

Ethnic influences on dietary practices. Consideration of a woman's cultural food preferences enhances the communication between her and her counselor, thus providing a greater opportunity to obtain compliance with a prescribed diet. However, within one cultural group there may occur several variations. Thus careful exploration of individual preferences is needed (Table 18.5).

Vegetarian diets. Vegetarianism has gained popularity in recent years. Foods basic to almost all vegetarian diets are vegetables, fruits, legumes, nuts, and grains. Vegetarian diets may not satisfy all nutrient requirements for the pregnant and lactating woman. The use of eggs and of milk and milk products varies.

There are four basic types of vegetarians:

1. *Lactoovovegetarian.* The vegetable diet is supplemented with milk, eggs, and cheese. There is no problem in securing adequate protein with this diet.

Table 18.7
Sample Menus

	Nonpregnant Woman	Pregnant Woman	Lactating Woman
Breakfast	120 ml (4 oz) orange juce ½ C oatmeal 240 ml (8 oz) milk Coffee or tea*	120 ml (4 oz) orange juice ½ C oatmeal 240 ml (8 oz) milk Coffee or tea*	120 ml (4 oz) orange juice ½ C oatmeal 240 ml (8 oz) milk Coffee or tea*
Morning snack		Fruit and/or cheese†	Fruit and/or cheese†
Lunch	1 tuna fish sandwich made with: 2 slices whole wheat bread ½ C tuna fish Diced celery and onion to taste. mayonnaise,* lettuce* 1 medium apple 240 ml (8 oz) milk	1 tuna fish sandwich made with: 2 slices whole wheat bread ½ C tuna fish, 1 hard-boiled egg Diced celery and onion to taste,* mayonnaise,* lettuce* 1 medium apple 240 ml (8 oz) milk	1 tuna fish sandwich made with: 2 slices whole wheat bread ½ C tuna fish, 1 hard-boiled egg Diced celery and onion to taste,* mayonnaise,* lettuce* 1 medium apple 240 ml (8 oz) milk
Afternoon snack		½ C salted peanuts 120 ml (4 oz) milk	½ C salted peanuts 240 ml (8 oz) milk
Dinner	84 g (3 oz) roast beef ½ C egg noodles* with sautéed poppy seeds* ¾ C cut asparagus Salad made with: 1 C torn spinach Sliced mushrooms and radishes to taste* Oil and vinegar* Coffee or tea†	168 g (6 oz) roast beef ½ C egg noodles* with sautéed poppy seeds,* 1 pat butter ¾ C cut asparagus Salad made with: 1 C torn spinach Sliced mushrooms and radishes to taste,* tomato Oil and vinegar* 240 ml (8 oz) milk Coffee or tea	168 g (6-9 oz) roast beef ½ C egg noodles* with sautéed poppy seeds,* 1 pat butter ¾ C cut asparagus Salad made with: 1 C torn spinach Sliced mushrooms and radishes to taste,* tomato Oil and vinegar* 240 ml (8 oz) milk Coffee or tea*
Evening snack		1-2 oatmeal raisin cookies* 120 ml (4 oz) milk	2 oatmeal raisin cookies* 240 ml (8 oz) milk

Adapted from Nutrition during prgnancy and lactation, Sacramento, 1975, Maternal and Child Health Branch, California Department of Health Services.
*This food is optional and is added to the basic diet.
†Serving size determined by caloric or dietary need.

2. *Lactovegetarian.* The vegetable diet is supplemented with milk and cheese. Milk products add complete protein to this diet.
3. *Pure vegetarian, or vegan.* The all-vegetable diet includes vegetables, fruits, legumes, nuts, and grains but is not supplemented with any animal foods, dairy products, or eggs. More careful planning is required to achieve combinations providing the necessary amounts of the essential amino acids. Vitamin B_{12} deficiency is a potential problem.
4. *Fruitarian.* The fruitarian diet consists of raw or dried fruits, nuts, honey, and olive oil. Potential inadequacy is greater in this diet than in other diets.

In general, protein is not a problem for the vegetarian when caloric intake is adequate and a wide variety of plant proteins are selected. It is necessary to eat certain combinations of plant foods to obtain complete proteins. These complete proteins contain the eight essential amino acids in amounts necessary for growth and maintenance. Unlike animal foods, most plant foods do not contain all the essential amino acids in these appropriate amounts. If one essential amino acid is missing, the protein is incomplete and cannot be utilized to build body tissues. The appropriate combination of two or more plant foods eaten at the same meal can make a ''complete'' protein. Tables 18.8 and 18.9 illustrate combinations of plant foods that are complementary, that is, constitute complete proteins.

A problem of sufficient income to purchase foods may cause an individual to have a nutritionally inadequate diet. Nutrients such as protein and iron are among those more likely to be deficient in diets of low-income groups. To help improve the nutritional quality of the diet, the person with limited income should be encouraged to participate in federal food programs such as the supplemental feeding program for women, infants, and children (WIC) and the food stamp program. Nutrition education and counseling are important to ensure the benefits of such programs.

REFERRAL FOR ADDITIONAL SERVICES

The referral system has two functions. First, a comprehensive network of services can offer solutions to problems that a particular program may not have the resources to solve. Second, the referral system informs women about a program by making them aware of their needs for benefits from that service. Food assistance programs such as the WIC program are a particularly good example of resources that can be tapped for pregnant women.

Table 18.8
Modified Food Guide for Vegetarian Diets

	Recommended No. of Servings			
	Lactovegetarian		Lactoovovegetarian	
Food group	Adult	Pregnant Adult	Adult	Pregnant Adult
Milk	4	5	4	5
Protein				
Eggs (2 = 1 serving)	0	0	½	1
Legumes	2	3	2	3
Nuts	1	1	1	1
Fruits and vegetables				
Vitamin C	3	3	3	3
Vitamin A	1½	2	1½	2
Other	3	4	3	3
Whole grain products	6	7	5	6
Others	0	1	0	1

Summary of Nursing Care: Maternal and Fetal Nutrition

GOALS FOR CARE

By the end of the second prenatal visit

1. The gravida is assessed for nutritional status.
2. Nutrition risk factors are identified.
3. A nutrition care plan is developed and initiated (e.g., education, mineral/vitamin supplementation).

Throughout pregnancy

4. Gravida's pattern of weight gain is within normal limits (Fig. 18.4); gravida gains approximately 454 g (1 lb) per month during the first trimester, and 425 g (15 oz) per week during the last two trimesters.
5. Gravida's hematocrit remains at or above 33% and her hemoglobin at or above 12 g/dl.
6. Intrauterine fetal growth remains appropriate for gestational age.
7. Gravida's urine remains negative for glucose and for ketones.
8. Referrals are made to community agencies as necessary for assistance with acquisition of necessary foods, food preparation, and food storage.
9. Gravida's dietary intake is maintained at appropriate levels for calories and all needed nutrients (Table 18.2).

By end of pregnancy

10. Gravida has attained appropriate weight gain.

Table 18.9
Vegetarian Food Guide*

General guidelines†

1. Follow nutrition guide for regular food plan during pregnancy.
2. Eat a wide variety of foods, including milk and milk products and eggs.
3. If no milk is allowed, use a supplement of 4 μg of vitamin B_{12} daily. If goat and soy milk are used, partial supplementation may be needed.
4. If no milk is taken, also use supplements of 12 mg of calcium and 400 IU of vitamin D daily. Partial supplementation will be necessary if less than 4 servings of milk and milk products are consumed.
5. Select a variety of plant foods (especially grains, legumes, nuts, and seeds) to obtain "complete" proteins by complementary combinations, as indicated in the list below.
6. Use iodized salt.
7. Increase intake of legumes, dried seeds, and nuts for protein and iron.
8. Increase intake of dairy foods for calcium, protein, and vitamin B_{12}.
9. Cut "empty" calories (sugars, concentrated sweets, and visible fats) at least by half.
10. Increase intake of whole grain breads and cereals for B vitamins, protein, and iron.
11. Increase intake of fruits and vegetables for vitamins A and C and for minerals.

Complementary plant protein combinations‡

Careful planning is necessary to complement incomplete plant proteins with each other and with dairy foods.

Food	Amino acids deficient	Complementary protein food combinations
Grains	Isoleucine Lysine	Rice + legumes Corn + legumes Wheat + legumes Wheat + peanut + milk Wheat + sesame + soybean Rice + brewer's yeast
Legumes	Tryptophan Methionine	Legumes + rice Beans + wheat Beans + corn Soybeans + rice + wheat Soybeans + corn + milk Soybeans + wheat + sesame Soybeans + peanuts + sesame Soybeans + peanuts + wheat + rice Soyeans + sesame + wheat
Nuts and seeds	Isoleucine Lysine	Peanuts + sesame + soybeans Sesame + beans Sesame + soybeans + wheat Peanuts + sunflower seeds
Vegetables	Isoleucine Methionine	Lima beans, Green beans, Brussels sprouts, Cauliflower, Broccoli } + Sesame seeds or Brazil nuts or mushrooms Greens = millet or rice

*Adapted from Williams, S.R.: Nutritional guidance in prenatal care, In Worthington, B.S., Vermeersch, J., and Williams, S.R.: Nutrition in pregnancy and lactation, St. Louis, 1977, The C.V. Mosby Co.

†Nutritional considerations when meat, poultry, and fish are omitted from the diet.

‡Adapted from Lappe, F.M.: Diet for a small planet, New York, 1971, Friends of the Earth/Ballantine.

11. Gravida is knowledgeable regarding nutrition: calories, needed nutrients, food preparation, and so on.
12. Gravida is knowledgeable regarding effects of drugs, alcohol, and tobacco on nutrition; pica; weight below and above normal limits; special needs for the adolescent (if appropriate); nutrition-related conditions (PKU, and diabetes mellitus where appropriate).
13. Gravida has had the opportunity to explore the choices for feeding the neonate (breast, bottle).

Pregnancy outcome

14. Pregnancy reaches term.
15. Mother suffers no adverse sequelae.

16. Neonate's weight and condition are within normal limits.

ASSESSMENT AND ANALYSIS

1. Maternal physiologic status is assessed for following:
    a. Age
    b. Prepregnancy weight
    c. Previous obstetric history (e.g., pregnancy intervals)
    d. Present physical examination and laboratory tests
    e. Concurrent medical problems with nutritional base (e.g., diabetes, cystic fibrosis, PKU, anemia: hematologic values), lactose intolerance
    f. Activity level (housewife, office worker, farm laborer)
2. Sociocultural assessment pertinent to nutrition
    a. What is individual's life-style?
    b. If gravida is not responsible for buying, selection, and preparation of food, who is responsible?
    c. How does religion, culture, or ethnic group influence usual dietary patterns? During pregnancy?
    d. Does gravida (and other in immediate environment) depend on welfare or food stamps? What is allotment?
    e. Are there other "special" circumstances (e.g., is she a model or dancer)?
    f. How many people eat together for each meal? How many meals?
3. Dietary assessment
    a. How many meals are served per day and how are they spaced?
    b. Typical daily menu: foods, quantities, preferences, dislikes?
    c. How are foods selected and cooked?
    d. Any special diet woman may be following is reviewed (e.g., diabetes mellitus).
4. Identify nutrition-related folklore and myths
5. Does she smoke, drink alcohol, or take drugs? Amount? Type of drugs?
6. Is she influenced by food fads?
7. Identify her level of understanding of good nutrition

EXAMPLES OF NURSING DIAGNOSES

1. Poor weight gain because of lack of knowledge of the relationship between good nutrition and normal weight gain in pregnancy
2. Poor compliance with good nutritional practice because of lack of understanding that an adequate supply of nutrients promotes normal development of the infant and normal weight gain
3. Inability to implement good nutritional practice because of lack of money (refrigeration, cooking facilities, transportation to grocery store, etc.)

PLAN AND IMPLEMENTATION

Involve the woman as a participant in her own care.

1. Refer woman to physician and nutritionist* for special dietary and pharmaceutic prescriptions for unique circumstances (e.g., PKU, cystic fibrosis, diabetes, anemia). Confer with physician and nutritionist or refer to flow sheet regarding these therapies to ensure team approach to care.
2. Act as resource person for following:
    a. Dietary suggestions and alternatives (Table 18.10 describes one protocol that can be used for nutrition counseling for pregnancy.)
    b. Channeling woman (and family) to appropriate community agencies for additional assistance as needed (school, welfare, public health nurse)
3. Acknowledge effort woman makes in altering or maintaining diet. Praise when appropriate.
4. Monitor weight gain throughout pregnancy. Weighing in should be ego building and psychologically unthreatening. (Many women "quiver in their shoes" while waiting to hear disgust and condemnation for "gaining too much." Some starve evening before visit or take diuretics to avoid such unpleasant encounters; both alternatives are detrimental to health.)
5. Check to see how she is managing her iron, vitamin, and mineral supplements.
6. Share with woman laboratory results, weight, and blood pressure. Discuss how these reflect her nutritional status. Point out areas where her laboratory values reflect her efforts to improve her nutrition.
7. Discuss nutrition-related folklore and myths with woman (e.g., "eating for two," "a tooth for every pregnancy," "if you eat green peppers, your baby will be hairy").
    a. Utilizing openings gained from identifying myths, explore realities in myths and clarify or correct misconceptions without talking down to her.

*In some rural and other areas, nutritionists may not be readily available. It then becomes the nurse's and physician's responsibility to be thoroughly informed as to particular food habits in that community, that is, nutritive values, usual means of preparation, and other characteristics.

Table 18.10
Pregnancy Protocol for Nutrition Counseling

Knowledge Needs	Behavioral Objectives	Suggested Learning Activity	Examples of Assessment
Why are nutrient needs increased during pregnancy?	Woman will know reason for increased nutrient and energy needs during pregnancy.	Explain that pregnancy is like building a house (the baby). You need materials (nutrients) and labor (energy). If you do not have enough materials or labor, the house will not be big or strong. This is also true for the baby.	Woman will explain why she needs more nutrients and energy while she is pregnant.
What are extra nutrients needed during pregnancy? How can they be obtained?	Woman will know additional nutrients needed during pregnancy and how to fulfill this need. Woman will meet her nutrient needs.	Explain that although all nutrient needs are increased during pregnancy, seven nutrients are particularly essential: *calories, protein, calcium, iron supplements, vitamin A, vitamin C,* and *folic acid.* Use 24-hr recall to point out areas of concern. Discuss daily food guide (see Table 18.6).	Woman will identify which nutrients should be increased, including calories, protein, calcium, iron, vitamin A, vitamin C, and folic acid. Woman will suggest how she might fulfill these needs.
What is normal pattern of weight gain during pregnancy? What are components of normal weight gain in pregnancy?	Woman will know normal weight gain pattern and components of total weight gain during pregnancy.	Explain that normal weight gain pattern is about 1.4 kg (3 lb) in first trimester, 4.5 kg (10 lb) in second, and 4.5 kg (10 lb) in third. Discuss components of total weight gain as follows: 27%, fetus 12%, placenta and fluid in uterus 50%, increased maternal organs 10%, increased blood volume	Woman will explain what normal weight gain pattern is and will list following components that make up total weight gain: 27%, fetus 12%, placenta and fluid in uterus 50%, increase in maternal organs (uterus, fat, breasts) 10%, increased blood volume
What is relationship between good nutrition and normal weight gain in pregnancy?	Woman will know that good nutrition leads to normal weight gain in pregnancy.	Explain that monitoring weight is a way to measure whether fetus is receiving adequate supply of nutrients.	Woman will state that adequate supply of nutrients promotes normal development of infant and normal weight gain.
What is my weight gain?	Woman will achieve normal weight gain.	Explain that normal weight gain indicates that fetus is receiving adequate nutrients.	Woman will state how much she has gained.
How does it compare to average weight gain?	Woman will know how her weight gain compares to average weight gain.	Using pregnancy gain-in-weight grid, record weight gain at each visit. Discuss weight gain pattern.	Complete each time throughout second and third trimesters. Woman will state how her weight gain compares to average.
What are dangers of poor nutrition during pregnancy?	Woman will know that poor nutrition can lead to anemia, preeclampsia-eclampsia, obesity, or prematurity.	Explain that poor nutrition during pregnancy may lead to several problem conditions. Poor supply of iron, folic acid, protein, or vitamin C may lead to *anemia.* Generally poor nutrition may lead to *prematurity.* Poor selection of food may lead to *obesity.*	Woman will identify following problems that may result from poor nutrition in pregnancy: anemia, preeclampsia-eclampsia, obesity, and prematurity.

Adapted from Pregnancy protocol for nutrition counseling, Phoenix, 1978, Nutrition Services, Arizona Department of Health; and Detroit, 1979, Nutrition Division, City of Detroit Department of Health.

b. If some beliefs are firmly held (e.g., ''green peppers . . .'' myth), discuss foods of same nutritive value to substitute.
c. Some physiologic demands on nutrition and body stores may be discussed in same context.

8. Based on analysis of woman's understanding of nutrition and food preparation briefly discuss physiologic demands (maternal and fetal) on body stores and daily intake.
9. The woman and her family's preferences, pocketbook, and other resources (cooking equipment,

refrigeration, space) form context in which to review following:

a. Review her present weight.
b. Divide current diet into basic four groups. Compliment her on all nutritionally sound aspects of diet.
c. Confer with her about types of food she would and could add to or subract from that diet. Discuss any possible problems she may encounter with other family members, purchasing, or preparing.
d. Decide on alternatives to c. Set appointment at next visit to review successes or failures experienced in interim.

10. Discuss discomforts of pregnancy that can be managed by means of foods and fluids (e.g., nausea and vomiting, constipation, leg cramps, fatigue).
11. Make suggestions regarding best time and method to take iron pills if prescribed. Forewarn her regarding black color of stools and possible constipation (or diarrhea) while on iron therapy.

EVALUATION

The nurse can be assured that care was effective if the goals of care have been met. Also, if the behavioral objectives in column 2 of Table 18.11 are met, the nurse is justified in evaluating her care as being effective.

References and Readings

Brennan, R.E., Caldwell, M., Rickard, K.A.: Assessment of maternal nutrition, J. Am. Diet. Assoc. **75:**152, Aug. 1979.

Brewer, G.S., and Brewer, T.: What every pregnant woman should know, New York, 1977, Random House.

Committee on Nutrition: Nutrition in maternal health care, Chicago, 1974, The American College of Obstetricians and Gynecologists.

Edwards, L.E., et al.: Pregnancy in the massively obese: course, outcome and obesity prognosis of the infant, Am. J. Obstet. Gynecol. **131:**479, 1978.

Edwards, L.E., et al.: Pregnancy in the underweight woman: course, outcome and growth patterns of the infant, Am. J. Obstet. Gynecol. **135:**297, 1979.

Food and Nutrition Board: Recommended dietary allowances, rev. ed., Washington, D.C., 1979, National Academy of Sciences–National Research Council.

Frank, D.A., et al.: Nutrition in adolescent pregnancy, J. Calif. Perinatal Assoc. **3**(1):21, 1983.

Guthrie, H.A.: Introductory nutrition, ed. 4, St Louis, 1979, The C.V. Mosby Co.

Haworth, J.C., et al.: Fetal growth retardation in cigarette-smoking mothers is not due to decreased maternal food intake, Am. J Obstet. Gynecol. **137:**719, 1980.

Hurley, L.S.: Developmental nutrition, Englewood Cliffs, N.J., 1980, Prentice-Hall, Inc.

Jensen, M.D., and Bobak, I.M.: Handbook of maternity care: a guide for nursing practice, St. Louis, 1980, The C.V. Mosby Co.

Laboratory indices of nutritional status in pregnancy, pub. no. F-427, Washington, D.C., Sept. 1977, National Academy of Sciences–National Research Council.

Naeye, R.L.: Weight gain and the outcome of pregnancy, Am. J. Obstet. Gynecol. **135:**3, 1979.

Naeye, R.L.: Teenaged and pre-teenaged pregnancies: consequences of the fetal-maternal competition for nutrients, Pediatrics **67:**146, 1981.

Nutrition during pregnancy and lactation, Sacramento, Calif., 1975, Maternal and Child Health Branch, California Department of Health Services.

Williams, S.R.: Nutrition and diet therapy, ed. 4, St. Louis, 1981, The C.V. Mosby Co.

Worthington, B.S., Vermeersch, J., and Williams, S.R. Nutrition in pregnancy and lactation, St. Louis, 1977, The C.V. Mosby Co.

Zuspan, F.P., and Quilligan, E.J., editors: Practical manual of obstetrical care: a pocket reference for those who treat the pregnant patient, St. Louis, 1982, The C.V. Mosby Co.

19

Preparation for Parenting

- **Parent Education**
  - Early pregnancy classes
  - Midpregnancy classes
  - Late pregnancy classes
  - After-birth classes
- **Childbirth Preparation**
  - Historical overview
  - Effectiveness of methods
    - Psychophysical components
    - Psychologic components
    - Intellectual components
  - Methods of childbirth preparation
    - Dick-Read method: childbirth without fear
    - Lamaze (PPM) method
    - Bradley method
  - Breathing techniques
    - Cervical dilatation to 3 cm
    - Cervical dilatation of 4 to 7 cm
    - Cervical dilatation of 8 to 10 cm
    - Expulsion breathing
  - Childbirth exercises
    - Exercises for the pelvic floor (Kegel exercise)
- **Pain in Childbirth**
  - Causes of pain in labor
  - Reactions to pain
- **Nursing Actions**
- **Preparation for Becoming a Grandparent**
  - Assessment and planning
  - Intervention
  - Evaluation
  - Conclusion
- **Organizations Involved in Parent Education**

Parent Education

In its publication *Guidelines for Childbirth Education* (1981) the Nurses' Association of the American College of Obstetricians and Gynecologists (NAACOG) defines childbirth education as follows:

> . . .The process designed to assist parents in making the transition from the role of expectant parents to the role and responsibilities of parents of a new baby which includes the period from the time of conception to approximately three months after birth.

This last statement implies that childbirth education is more than *preparation for a labor and birth experience*. It is also *preparation for parenting*.

In order to meet the numerous and varied learning needs of expectant and new parents, comprehensive parent education programs are needed. Classes in preparation for the birth itself are only one part of preparation-for-parenthood programs. Such programs recognize that pregnancy is not a disease state but is a state of wellness, during which people move from the role of expectant parents to the role and responsibilities of parents of a new baby, as a new family. Pregnancy can be a meaningful growth experience and can increase the family's self-confidence with the help of education for parenting.

A typical preparation-for-parenthood program recognizes that childbearing people have different interests and information needs as the pregnancy progresses; and consequently, the program is designed to meet the concerns of the people at the three major stages of pregnancy, and after birth.

EARLY PREGNANCY CLASSES

Early pregnancy (''early bird'') classes provide fundamental information about early development, physiologic and emotional changes of pregnancy, human sexuality, and the nutritional needs of the mother and fetus.

MIDPREGNANCY CLASSES

Midpregnancy classes provide information on preparation for breast and bottle feeding, basic hygiene, health maintenance (rest, exercise, nutrition), and infant health.

LATE PREGNANCY CLASSES

Late pregnancy classes include preparation for childbirth classes, teenage classes, cesarean birth classes, refresher classes, and parenting discussion groups.

Throughout the series of classes there is discussion of support systems persons can use during pregnancy and after delivery, so that they can function independently and effectively by developing their own health awareness and health maintenance behavior. During all the classes the open expression of feelings and concerns about any aspect of pregnancy, birth, and parenting is welcomed.

AFTER-BIRTH CLASSES

After-birth classes (''What do we do now?'') include coping mechanisms for the reality of parenting, support systems, infant care and growth and development, birth control methods, human sexuality, and adapting to new roles (wife-lover ⇆ mother and husband-lover ⇆ father).

Many innovative programs also include grandparents' classes and sibling classes. When the families are preparing for birth in alternative birth centers (in-hospital or freestanding) or birthing rooms, there are mandatory preparation classes for birth in those particular settings.

Preparation-for-parenthood programs are multiplying throughout the country as more and more satisfied new parents tell friends and neighbors and families about their prepared births. It is very exciting to watch well-informed, interested persons become active, intelligent consumers of health care. The box below presents an excellent prenatal teaching guide.

Fig. 19.1 presents an example of childbirth education classes in a private obstetric practice.

Prenatal Teaching Guide

Weeks 1-12

Woman more concerned with herself, physical changes with pregnancy, and her feelings about the pregnancy.

- Changes that are normal for pregnancy
  - Breast fullness
  - Urinary frequency
  - Nausea and vomiting
  - Fatigue
- EDC—Calculate and explain
  - Compare with uterine size
- Expectation for care
  - Initial visit
  - Subsequent visits
  - Clinic appointments
- Need for iron and vitamins
- Resources available
  - Education
  - Dental evaluation
  - Medical service
  - Social service
  - Emergency room
- Danger signs
  - Drugs, self-medication
  - Spotting, bleeding
  - Cramping, pain

Weeks 12-24

Woman has usually resolved the issue of the pregnancy and becomes more aware of the fetus as a person.

- Growth of fetus
  - Movement
  - FHR
- Personal hygiene
  - Comfortable clothing
  - Breast care and supportive bra
  - Recreation, travel
  - Vaginal discharge
- Employment or school plans
- Method of feeding baby
  - Breast or bottle
  - Give literature re. methods
- Avoidance or alleviation of the following:
  - Backache
  - Constipation
  - Hemorrhoids
  - Leg ache, varicosities, edema, cramping
  - Round ligament pain
- Nutritional guidance
- Weight gain
- Balanced diet
- Special nutritional needs

Adapted from Roberts, J.: Priorities in prenatal education, J.O.G.N. Nurs., pp. 18-19, May-June 1976.

Prenatal Teaching Guide—cont'd

Weeks 24-32

Woman becomes more interested in baby's needs as a corollary to her own needs now and after birth.

- Fetal growth and status
  - Presentation and position
  - Well-being—FHR
- Personal hygiene
  - Comfortable clothing
  - Body mechanics and posture
  - Positions of comfort
- Physical and emotional changes
- Sexual needs/changes; intercourse
- Alleviation of the following:
  - Backache
  - Discomfort from Braxton Hicks' contractions
  - Dyspnea
  - Round ligament pain
  - Leg ache or edema
- Confirm infant feeding plans
  - Prepare for breast or bottle feeding
  - Nipple preparation
  - Massage and expression of breast
- Preparation for baby
  - Supplies
  - Household assistance
- Danger signs
  - Preeclampsia
  - Headache, excessive swelling, blurred vision
- Tubal ligation (papers prepared ahead)

Weeks 32-36

Woman anticipates approaching labor and caring for baby after birth.

- Fetal growth and status
- Personal hygiene
  - Positions of comfort
  - Rest and activity
  - Vaginal discharge
- Alleviation of discomfort
  - Backache
  - Round ligament pain
  - Constipation or hemorrhoids
  - Leg ache or edema
  - Dyspnea
  - Recognition of "false labor"—Braxton Hicks' contractions
  - How to cope and "practice" with these
- Nature of "true labor"—signs; difference between "bloody show" and vaginal bleeding
- What happens during labor
  - Labor contractions and progress
  - What she will experience
- Relaxation techniques
- Breathing techniques
  - Abdominal
  - Accelerated pattern
  - Panting and pushing
- Involvement of husband or significant other
- Provision for needs of other children
  - Anticipation of baby
  - Care for children at home while mother is in hospital

Week 36 to term

Woman should feel "ready" for labor and for the assumption of care-taking responsibilities for baby, even though she may feel anxious about both of these as well.

- Review signs of labor (or teach)
- Review or continue instruction re. relaxation and breathing techniques
- Finalize home preparations
- Anticipation of hospitalization
  - Admission (ER and labor admitting room)
  - Examination, IV, possible shave, possible enema
  - Care in labor
  - Medication and anesthesia available
  - Postnatal care
  - Supplies needed: bra, personal items, money
  - May have two visitors
  - Tour of maternity unit
- Confirm plans to get to hospital (when to go and where); care of other children
- Consider family planning needs
- Emergency arrangements
  - Precipitate delivery
  - Premature rupture of membranes with or without contractions
  - Care away from home
  - Vaginal bleeding
  - Danger signals (see box, p. 298)

Fig. 19.1
Information on the Harbor Medical Group childbirth education classes. (From Phillips, C.R., and Anzalone, J.T.: Fathering: participation in labor and birth, ed. 2, St. Louis, 1982, The C.V. Mosby Co.)

Harbor medical group
childbirth education classes

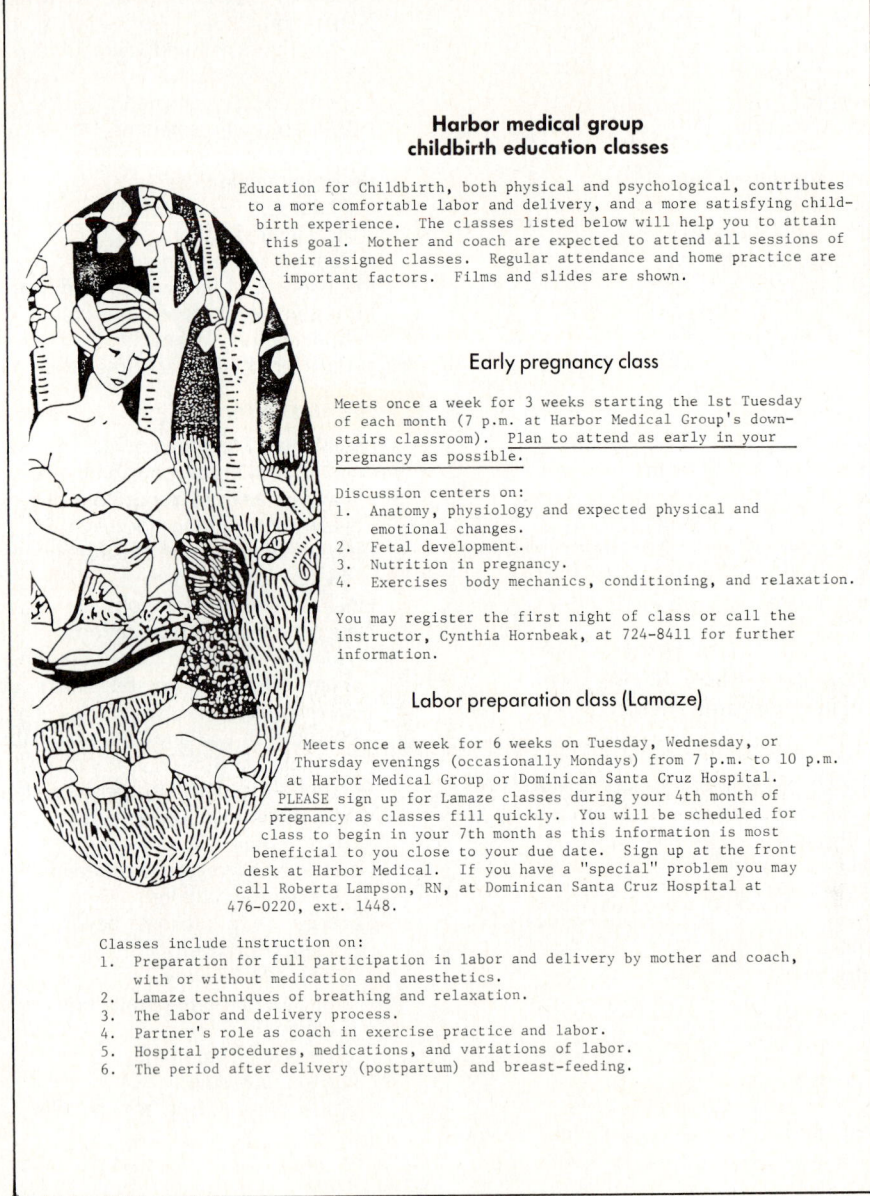

Education for Childbirth, both physical and psychological, contributes to a more comfortable labor and delivery, and a more satisfying childbirth experience. The classes listed below will help you to attain this goal. Mother and coach are expected to attend all sessions of their assigned classes. Regular attendance and home practice are important factors. Films and slides are shown.

Early pregnancy class

Meets once a week for 3 weeks starting the 1st Tuesday of each month (7 p.m. at Harbor Medical Group's downstairs classroom). Plan to attend as early in your pregnancy as possible.

Discussion centers on:
1. Anatomy, physiology and expected physical and emotional changes.
2. Fetal development.
3. Nutrition in pregnancy.
4. Exercises body mechanics, conditioning, and relaxation.

You may register the first night of class or call the instructor, Cynthia Hornbeak, at 724-8411 for further information.

Labor preparation class (Lamaze)

Meets once a week for 6 weeks on Tuesday, Wednesday, or Thursday evenings (occasionally Mondays) from 7 p.m. to 10 p.m. at Harbor Medical Group or Dominican Santa Cruz Hospital. PLEASE sign up for Lamaze classes during your 4th month of pregnancy as classes fill quickly. You will be scheduled for class to begin in your 7th month as this information is most beneficial to you close to your due date. Sign up at the front desk at Harbor Medical. If you have a "special" problem you may call Roberta Lampson, RN, at Dominican Santa Cruz Hospital at 476-0220, ext. 1448.

Classes include instruction on:
1. Preparation for full participation in labor and delivery by mother and coach, with or without medication and anesthetics.
2. Lamaze techniques of breathing and relaxation.
3. The labor and delivery process.
4. Partner's role as coach in exercise practice and labor.
5. Hospital procedures, medications, and variations of labor.
6. The period after delivery (postpartum) and breast-feeding.

Childbirth Preparation

HISTORICAL OVERVIEW

Since colonial times in America, women shared their information on childbirth with other women. Births occurred in the families' homes with midwives in attendance. However, in the nineteenth century, male physicians gradually came to be recognized as experts to whom women went for information about birth. By 1900 physicians had usurped women's age-old skills concerning childbirth and became, for many, the sole authorities.

In the United States the first formal classes in childbirth education were offered nationally in 1913 by the American Red Cross. The Maternity Center Association

Fig. 19.1 cont'd

For legend see opposite page.

Exercise classes

In addition to birth classes, Harbor Medical Group offers to its patients, prenatal and postpartum exercise classes.

The classes stress general body fitness, good muscle tone, relaxation, and stamina in preparation for birth. Special emphasis is placed on the woman's body as it is directly involved in pregnancy and birthing. No registration is required. The classes are ongoing at Harbor Medical Group's downstairs classroom. For more information call instructors Cynthia Hornbeak at 724-8411 or Patty Smith at 429-6412.

TUESDAY		THURSDAY	
9:00 10:00 a.m.	Prenatal exercise class, older children welcome.	9:00 10:00 a.m.	Prenatal exercise class, older children welcome.
10:00 11:00 a.m.	Postpartum babies only.	10:00 11:00 a.m.	Postpartum babies only.
11:00 12:00 a.m.		11:00 12:00 a.m.	
5:30 6:30 p.m.	Prenatal exercise class.		

Infant care class
Additional class (offered through Dominican Hospital)

The class fee is $10.00. The class is offered every other month. It meets once a week for 3 weeks with instruction on:

1. Planning for the new baby, including layette and equipment.
2. Bathing, feeding, and dressing demonstrations and practice.
3. Keeping baby well and healthy.
4. Growth and development.

For more information and registration call Roberta Lampson, RN, at 476-1220, ext. 1448.

NOTES:

in New York City followed with classes for expectant parents as early as 1919. Literature on these early attempts at childbirth education revealed that the first classes for childbirth were developed out of a public health need to teach mothers basic hygiene.

An English physician, Dr. Grantly Dick-Read, published two books in which he theorized that pain in childbirth is socially conditioned and is caused by a fear-tension-pain syndrome. His first book, *Natural Childbirth,* was publised in 1933. Dr. Dick-Read's second bood, *Childbirth Without Fear,* was published in the United States in 1944. Dr. Dick-Read's work became the foundation for the first organized programs of preparation for childbirth and teacher training. The first of such groups to organize was the International Childbirth Education Association (ICEA) founded in 1960.

At about the same time, the Lamaze method, also known as the psychoprophylactic method (PPM), was gaining popularity in the United States. PPM opened new perspectives into preparation for childbirth by emphasizing mind control. Marjorie Karmel introduced PPM to the United States in her book, *Thank You, Dr. Lamaze,* which was published in the United States in 1959. Others have written extensively on PPM. This system grew out of Pavlov's work on the higher nervous activity of humans and animals in which he proposed that every vital activity of an organism is a complex reflex process capable of conditioning.

In 1960 the American Society for Psychoprophylaxis in Obstetrics (ASPO) was formed in New York as a national organization to promote use of the Lamaze method and prepare teachers of the method. The National Association of Childbirth Education, Inc. (NACE) (formerly the Childbirth Without Pain Education League, Inc. [CWPL]), was formed in 1970 to teach the Lamaze method and prepare teachers. The Council of Childbirth Education Specialists, Inc. (CCES) was founded in New York City in 1971 and offered teacher training seminars throughout the United States.

A Denver obstetrician, Dr. Robert Bradley, published *Husband-Coached Childbirth* in 1965. In this book he advocates what he proposes is the true natural childbirth, without any form of anesthesia or analgesia and with a husband-coach and breathing techniques for labor. The American Academy of Husband-Coached Childbirth (AAHCC) was founded to make the Bradley method available and to prepare teachers.

Of the other techniques developed, the most widely known include the work of Kitzinger and Wright, developed in England. Wright's work is based on PPM and is described as "levels of breathing." Kitzinger's work is designed around a psychosexual approach, which proposes that birth is a sexual experience. As such, birth is perceived as a normal physiologic process in which the woman works in harmony with her body.

Hypnosis as a method of relieving pain in childbirth has been used since the 1800s. Through hypnosis the woman reaches a trancelike state, remaining awake but responsive to the hypnotist. The use of hypnosis requires an extensive time commitment of the hypnotist. It is impractical for use with large numbers of women.

EFFECTIVENESS OF METHODS

Chertok (1967) summarized and evaluated the effectiveness of preparation for birth and suggested that all preparation techniques had three components: (1) psychophysical, (2) psychologic, and (3) intellectual.

Psychophysical components. Various studies have been undertaken to determine the physiologic effectiveness of prepared childbirth methods in terms of the amount of pain experienced during labor and birth, maternal and fetal complications, and the length of labor. Chertok (1967) and Velvovsky and co-workers (1960) reviewed many studies in which investigators demonstrated the effectiveness of preparation-for-birth approaches to pain relief during childbirth. Huttel and coworkers (1972) reported observations of less "complaint" and "tension" behaviors among women who were prepared for birth compared with women who did not attend preparation classes. Huttel suggested that preparation for birth enables the mother to experience a shorter labor.

Psychologic components. Although the physiologic benefits of prepared childbirth are important, additional benefits have been claimed. A review of the literature by Buxton in 1962 concluded by emphasizing the critical importance of the psychologic benefits of preparation for birth. Unlike some of the contradictory material found on physiologic effects, research on psychologic effects continues to be overwhelmingly in agreement. Tanzer (1967) found that prepared women had a more positive subjective experience during delivery. It is particularly notable in this research how many of the women stressed the importance of having either their husband or another support person present during labor. Tanzer's results indicate that women experience a positive and highly desirable effect when their mates are present during birth. Other studies report that support and participation in labor and birth by the infant's father contribute to positive perceptions of the birth experience.

Intellectual components. The intellectual components of preparation for childbirth are closely tied to the psychologic components, since research has indicated that the more knowledge a woman gains concerning pregnancy, labor, and birth as a result of childbirth preparation classes, the more favorable will be her resultant attitude toward the pregnancy and labor and delivery experience. A woman's perception of maintaining control is closely associated with satisfaction, according to studies by Willmuth (1975) and Felton (1978). Although the mechanisms by which preparation-for-childbirth classes affect the birth experience are not yet fully understood, it is clear that these classes affect the subjective experience in a positive manner.

METHODS OF CHILDBIRTH PREPARATION

Major methods taught in the United States are (1) the Dick-Read method, (2) the Lamaze method (PPM), and (3) the Bradley method.

Dick-Read method: childbirth without fear

Psychophysical component. Dick-Read basically recommended three techniques: deep breathing both in abdominal respirations and thoracic respirations; shallow breathing; and breath holding for the second stage of labor. The Dick-Read method also incorporates physical exercise to prepare the body for labor.

For most of labor the pattern of breathing is basically abdominal breathing. The women is taught to force her abdominal muscles to rise during a contraction. In this way she lifts the abdominal muscles off the uterus as it rises forward during a contraction. Teachers of the Dick-Read method contend that the weight of the abdominal musculature on the contracting uterus increases pain.

Relaxation is also an important part of the Dick-Read method. Women are taught to use passive relaxation methods that involve progressive relaxation of the muscle groups in the entire body. Consequently, during labor, the woman is able to relax completely between contractions. Using passive relaxation techniques, some women are actually able to sleep between contractions (Fig. 19.2).

Psychologic component. According to Dick-Read (1959):

> . . . Fear, tension, and pain are three veils opposed to the natural design which have been concerned with preparation for and attendance at childbirth. If fear, tension, and pain go hand in hand, then it must be necessary to relieve tension and to overcome fear in order to eliminate pain. The implementation of my theory demonstrates the methods by which fear can be overcome, tension may be eliminated and replaced by physical and mental relaxation.

Intellectual component. Dick-Read's program educated women in order to exchange understanding and confidence for fear of the unknown. Adequate prenatal education included information on nutrition and basic hygiene as well as information concerning labor and birth.

In the Dick-Read method, provision of support for the woman in labor was *originally* to be provided by nursing and medical labor attendants. However, in the adaptations of the Dick-Read method in use today, labor support is provided by the father or a support person chosen by the mother.

Lamaze (PPM) method. The terms *psychoprophylaxis* (or *mind prevention*) and *Lamaze* are used interchangeably.

Psychophysical component. Controlled muscular relaxation and breathing techniques are combined in the Lamaze method. Active relaxation is an integral part of the Lamaze method. The woman is taught to relax uninvolved muscle groups (neuromuscular control) while she contracts a specific muscle group. By this process the woman can relax the uninvolved muscles in her body while her uterine musculature contracts.

The breathing techniques use the chest muscles. Lamaze teachers feel that chest breathing lifts the diaphragm off the contracting uterus, thus giving it more room to expand. These chest breathing patterns vary according to the intensity of the contractions and the progress of labor.

Psychologic component. According to the Lamaze method, pain in labor is a conditioned response and women can be conditioned not to experience pain in

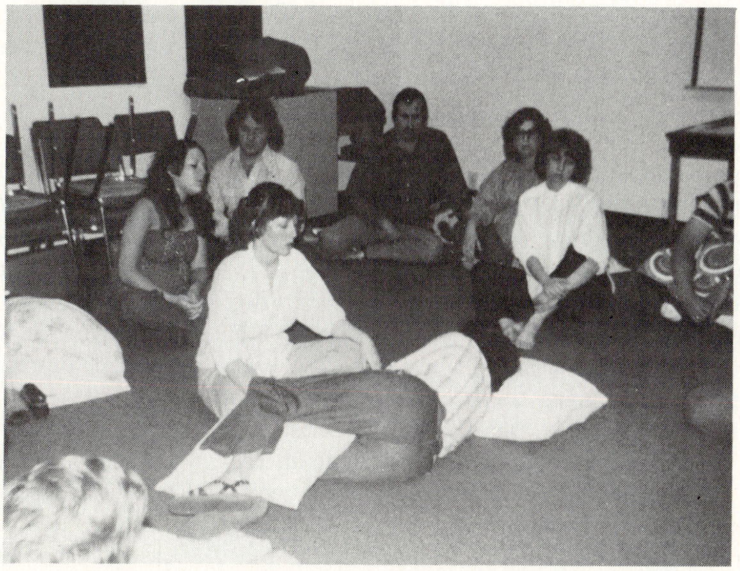

Fig. 19.2
Teaching relaxation. (From Phillips, C.R.: Family-centered maternity/newborn care, St. Louis, 1980, The C.V. Mosby Co.)

labor. Instead of crying out and losing control during uterine contractions, women are taught to respond with conditioned relaxation and breathing patterns.

Intellectual component. The Lamaze method emphasizes understanding the body and how it works. It offers a flexible but structured program to remove fear by education, thus eliminating distressing associations. This method finds its rationale in the neurophysiology of pain.

In the Lamaze method, provision of support for the woman in labor is provided by her husband or other support person. Specially trained labor attendants termed *monitrices* sometimes provide support for the Lamaze laboring mother.

Bradley method

Psychophysical component. Breath control, abdominal breathing, and general body relaxation are utilized in the Bradley method. Working in harmony with the body is emphasized. Dr. Bradley based his method on observations of animal behavior during birth. His technique focuses on environmental variables such as darkness, solitude, and quiet to make childbirth a more natural experience. Women using the Bradley method often appear to be sleeping during labor. However, they are not asleep but simply in a state of deep mental relaxation.

Psychologic component. The importance of the husband's support is foremost in this method. In fact, the method is also referred to as "husband-coached childbirth."

Intellectual component. Preparation-for-birth teaching concentrates on minimizing the need for analgesics or anesthetics for birth. There is also an emphasis on nutrition, omitting foods containing preservatives and added salt and sugar.

• • •

Each of the three methods just discussed emphasizes intellectual and physical components. However, the Dick-Read and Bradley methods emphasize the naturalness of childbirth, while Lamaze emphasizes active mental and physical conditioning. These methods have mutually influenced each other so that it is unusual to find classes in a pure "method" anymore. Also, different teachers find their own methods, which may change with each group of pregnant couples. Education in preparation for birth is continually evolving. The teachers themselves are being taught by the experiences of each childbearing couple. Books, journal articles, magazine articles, and audiovisual aids on childbirth education are proliferating. A list of some of the organizations involved in parent education can be found at the end of this chapter.

BREATHING TECHNIQUES

As the summary of methods of childbirth preparation indicated, there are varying techniques for using breathing as a tool to help women cope with labor. In the first stage, breathing techniques can promote relaxation of abdominal muscles and thereby increase the size of the abdominal cavity and lessen friction and discomfort between the uterus and the abdominal wall. Since the muscles of the genital area also become more relaxed, they do not interfere with descent. In the second stage, breathing is used to increase abdominal pressure and thereby assist in expelling the fetus. It is also used to relax the pudendal muscles to prevent precipitate expulsion of the head.

For those couples who have prepared for labor by practicing such techniques, occasional reminders to the couple may be all that is necessary (Fig. 19.3). For those who have had no preparation, instruction in simple breathing and relaxation can be given early in labor and is often surprisingly successful. Motivation is high, and learning readiness is enhanced by the reality of labor.

Cervical dilatation to 3 cm. As the woman feels the onset of a contraction, she takes a deep, cleansing breath in through the nose and out through pursed lips. Then she is encouraged to concentrate on slow, rhythmic chest breathing (6 to 9 breaths/min) through the contraction (Fig. 19.4). When the contraction is over, she takes a final deep breath in and out and then "blows the contraction away." She may focus on a chosen fixed point or simply close her eyes.

Cervical dilatation of 4 to 7 cm. Breathing during this phase is similar to that advocated in the early phase. When cervical dilatation reaches 5 cm, some women begin to concentrate seriously on the strength of the contractions and the discomfort accompanying them. At this time a change to shallower, lighter breathing can be suggested (no more than 16 breaths/min to prevent hyperventilation). Other women can be helped by changing to slow abdominal breathing. Another technique that is often successful is to have the woman slowly raise her abdomen as she breathes in, following the support person's hand "up the ceiling" or "out to the side of the bed." This focusing mechanism results in the lifting of the abdominal wall away from the contracting uterus.

Cervical dilatation of 8 to 10 cm. The most difficult time to maintain control during contractions comes when cervical dilatation reaches 8 to 10 cm (transition). Even for the woman who has prepared for labor, concentration on breathing techniques is difficult to maintain. The type used may be the 4:1 pattern: breath, breath, breath, breath, puff (as though blowing out a candle). This ratio may increase to 6:1 or 8:1. These

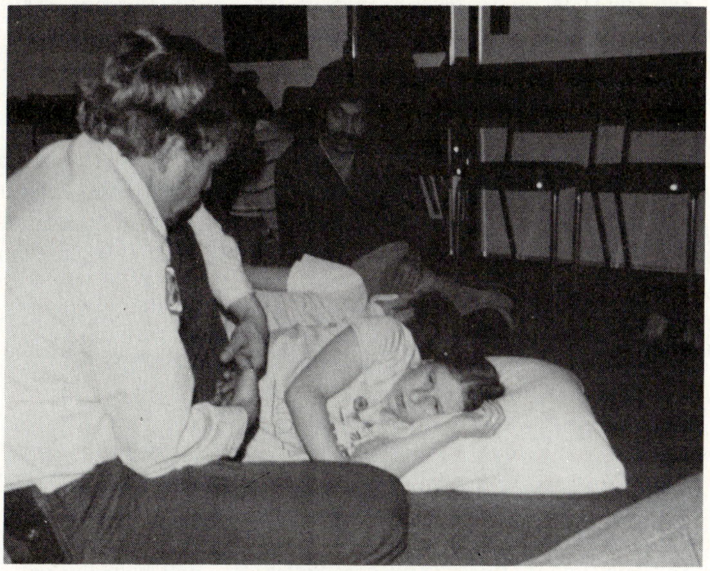

Fig. 19.3
Preparing for labor. (From Phillips, C.R.: Family-centered maternity/newborn care, St. Louis, 1980, The C.V. Mosby Co.)

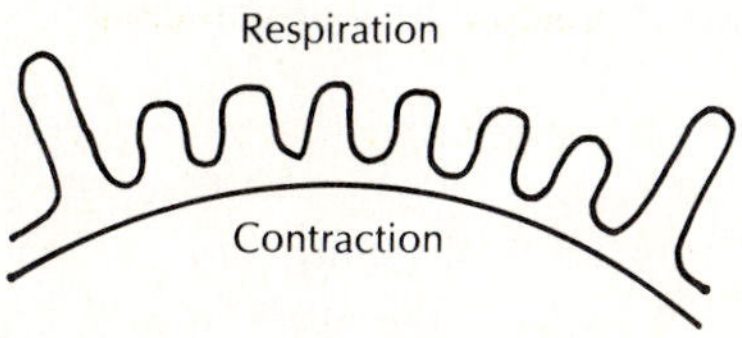

Fig. 19.4
Slow chest breathing. (From Phillips, C.R.: Family-centered maternity/newborn care, St. Louis, 1980, The C.V. Mosby Co.)

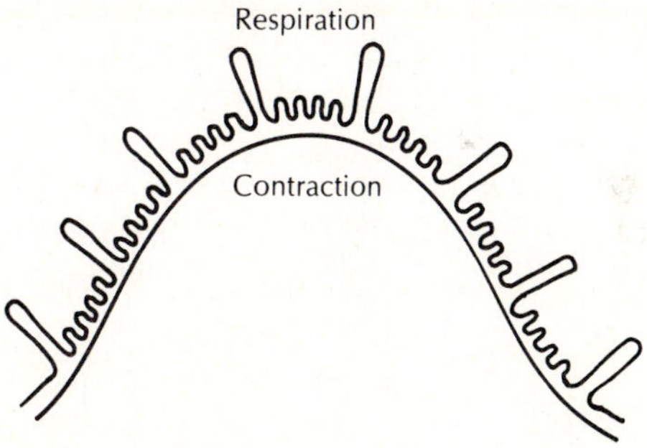

Fig. 19.5
Expulsion breathing. (From Phillips, C.R.: Family-centered maternity/newborn care, St. Louis, 1980, The C.V. Mosby Co.)

patterns begin with the routine cleansing breath and end with a deep breath that "blows the contraction away." An undesirable side effect of this type of breathing may be **hyperventilation.** The woman must be aware of the accompanying symptoms of the resultant respiratory alkalosis: lightheadedness, dizziness, tingling of fingers, or circumoral numbness. Alkalosis may be overcome by having the woman breathe into a paper bag that is tightly held around the mouth and nose, enabling her to rebreathe carbon dioxide and replace the bicarbonate ion.

As the fetal head reaches the pelvic floor, the woman will experience the urge to push and will automatically begin to exert downward pressure by contracting her abdominal muscles. Descent cannot continue until the cervix is fully dilated and the presenting part is free to move down the birth canal. Pushing before full dilatation is reached compresses the cervix between the fetal head and the pubic bone, resulting in fetal distress or trauma or in cervical edema. It may even slow the dilatation process. The woman can control the urge to push by taking panting breaths or by slowly exhaling through pursed lips. This is good practice for the type of breathing to be used as the fetal head is slowly delivered.

Expulsion breathing. Sometimes you will hear coaches helping women push by saying, "Push as though you were going to have a bowel movement." One must remember that this woman is pushing a baby out through the vagina and needs to relax the vagina and pelvic floor to do this. Talking to her about having a bowel movement may only serve to confuse her pushing efforts. Therefore, coach her to "push the baby out of the vagina (or birth canal)."

Also, sometimes you will hear helping persons ask a woman to ''hold her breath'' and push as long as she can before coming up for air. Dr. Caldeyro-Barcia reported at the International Childbirth Education Association Biennial Conference in Kansas City in June, 1978, that when a woman holds her breath for more than 6 or 7 seconds as she pushes, there is greatly reduced exchange of gases across the placenta to the fetus. This reduction in perfusion could be dangerous to the fetus by causing a reduced oxygen supply. When coaching women to push, the nurse encourages them to push as *they* feel like pushing, without holding their breath more than 5 seconds at a time, if at all possible (Fig. 19.5).

CHILDBIRTH EXERCISES

Numerous exercises are taught to prepare women for childbirth and to keep them physically fit.

Exercises for the pelvic floor (Kegel exercise). Many women are not aware of the muscles of the pelvic floor until it is pointed out that these are the muscles used when urinating and during sexual intercourse and are therefore consciously controlled. Since pelvic floor muscles ring the outlet through which the baby must pass, it is important that they be exercised, because an exercised muscle can stretch and contract readily at the time of birth. In order to locate these muscles, a woman can practice stopping the flow and starting it again while urinating.

Once the muscles are located, they should be contracted repeatedly every day for the rest of the woman's life. This exercise needs to be practiced many times a day to be effective. A good time to practice is during trips to the bathroom, but additional practice at other times is even more beneficial. Since it is not obvious when a woman is practicing she might practice anytime and anywhere.

The procedure is to tighten the pelvic floor muscles as in holding back urine, hold for 10 seconds, and then release or to think of the vagina as an elevator and practice ascending and descending slowly. This exercise can be done ten times in a row, five to ten times or more a day. Although some people recommend doing this exercise as many as 100 times in a row, this only fatigues the pelvic floor muscles. After delivery, this exercise will help the pelvic floor muscles to return to normal functioning. Kegel exercises should be started immediately after delivery.

• • •

Figs. 19.6 to 19.9 illustrate postures and exercises usually taught in preparation-for-childbirth classes.

Fig. 19.6

A, Relaxed position. Some women prefer upper leg to be supported by pillow also. **B,** Squatting helps to relax pelvic floor and is preferred to bending over at waist. (Bending over at waist causes or aggravates heartburn from reflux of gastric contents into esophagus.) **C,** Rising in this manner aids in maintaining balance.

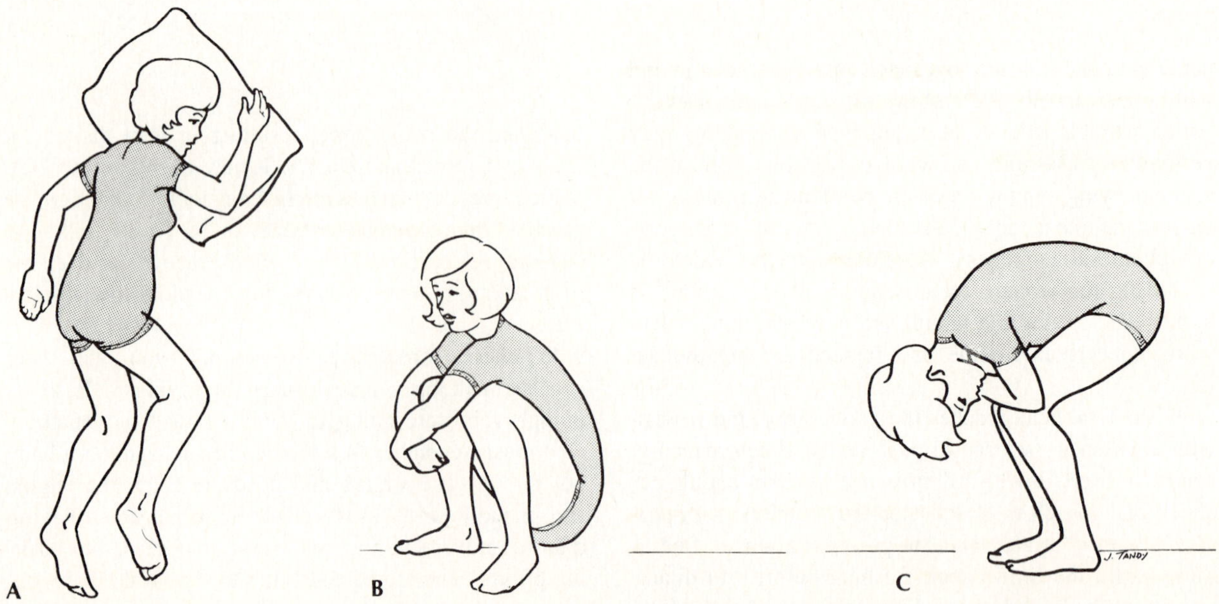

Fig. 19.7

Pelvic rocking to relieve low backache (excellent for relief of menstrual cramps as well). **A,** Hands-and-knees position. **B,** Standing position. **C,** Supine position.

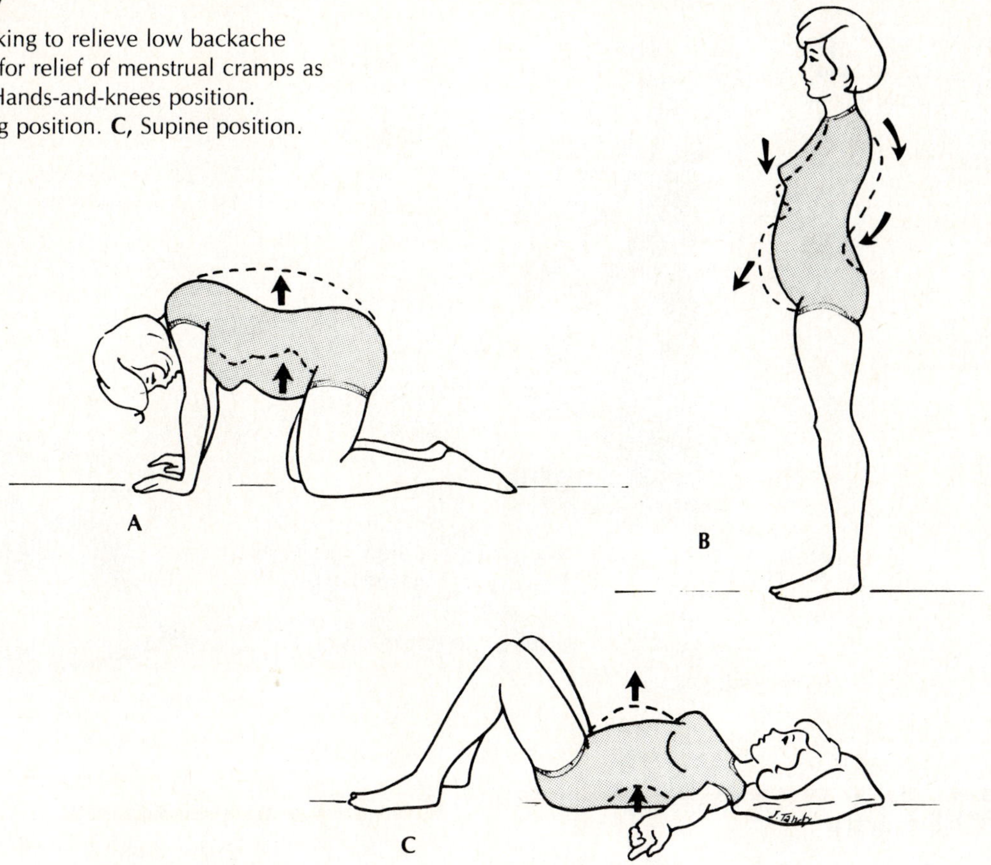

Fig. 19.8

Positions for rest and relaxation. These postures and exercises are usually taught in preparation-for-childbirth classes. **A,** Abdominal breathing aids relaxation and lifts abdominal wall off uterus. **B,** Tailor sitting position aids in relaxing muscles of pelvic floor. **C,** Position for pushing.

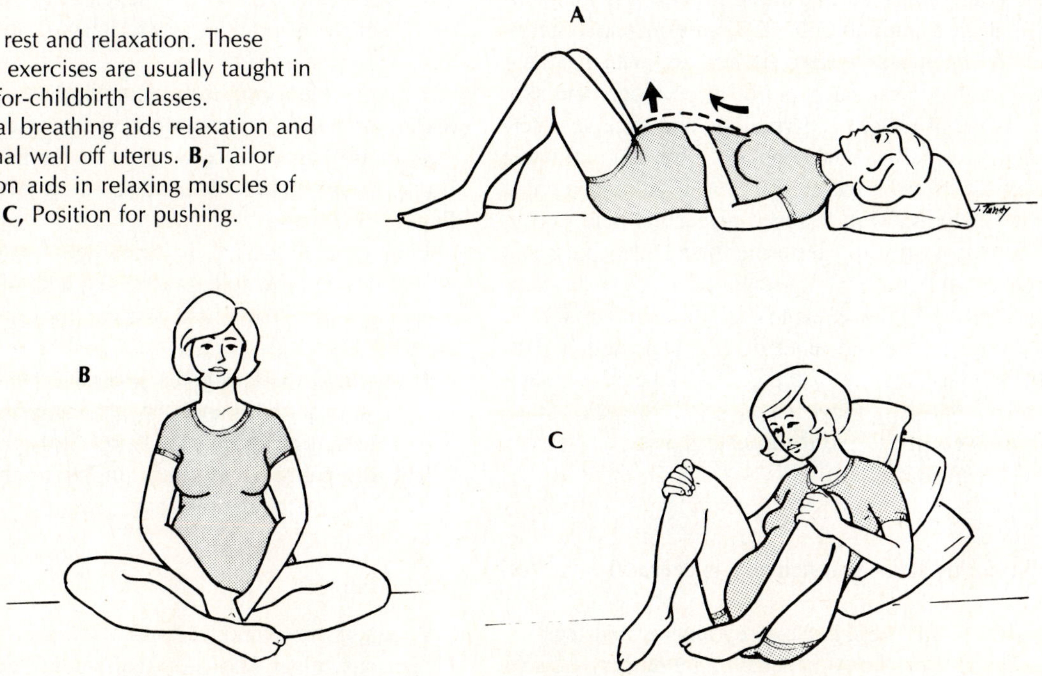

Fig. 19.9
Position in which to rest legs and reduce swelling, edema, and varicosities. Encourage woman with vulvar varicosities to add pillow under her hips.

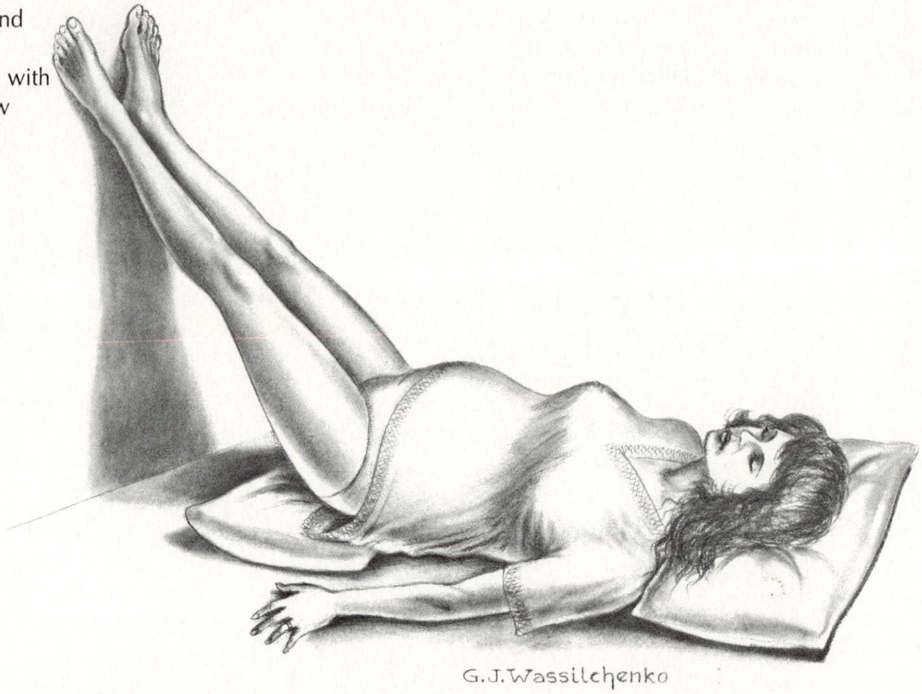

Pain in Childbirth

Pain results in both reflex physical and psychic reactions. The quality of physical pain has been described as pricking, burning, aching, throbbing, sharp, nauseating, or cramping. Pain in childbirth gives rise to symptoms that are identifiable. It may cause increased activity of the sympathetic nervous system, with resultant changes in blood pressure, pulse, respirations, and skin color. Bouts of nausea and vomiting and excessive perspiration are also commonplace. Certain affective expressions of suffering are familiar to all and include increasing anxiety with lessened perceptual field, writhing, crying, groaning, gesturing (hand clenching and wringing), and excessive muscular excitability throughout the body. Childbirth pain is of a limited duration (at most 2 to 3 days), and relief of this pain must be balanced by consideration of the goal of a healthy mother and baby. It is important not to jeopardize the baby's safety in order to relieve the mother's pain.

CAUSES OF PAIN IN LABOR

Pain during labor and delivery is caused by the following:

1. *Emotional tension* caused by anxiety and fear
2. *Traction* on the peritoneum and uterocervical supports during contractions or expulsive efforts
3. *Pressure* by the presenting part on the bladder, bowel, or other sensitive pelvic structures
4. *Hypoxia* caused by circulatory stasis in the myometrium and adjacent tissues, during and immediately after strong uterine contractions; may cause a local oxygen deficit (the pain has been compared to angina pectoris associated with myocardial hypoxia)

Pain may be *local,* with cramplike uterine pain and a tearing or bursting sensation because of distention and laceration of the cervix, vagina, or perineal tissues; or it may be *referred,* with the discomfort felt in the back, flanks, or thighs.

Pain impulses during the first stage of labor are transmitted through the spinal nerve segment of T11-12 and accessory lower thoracic and upper lumbar sympathetic nerves.

Pain impulses during the second stage of labor are carried through S1-4 and the parasympathetic system. Pain experienced during the third stage, as well as so-called afterpains, is uterine, similar to that described early in the first stage of labor.

REACTIONS TO PAIN

Although the pain threshold is remarkably similar in all persons, regardless of sexual, social, ethnic, or cultural differences, these factors play a definite role in the individual's perception of the pain experience. The reasons for the effects of such factors as culture, use of counterstimuli, or distraction in coping with pain are not fully understood. The meaning of pain and the verbal and nonverbal expressions given to pain are apparently learned from interactions within the primary social group and are personalized for each individual. As pain is experienced, people develop various coping mechanisms to deal with it. Pain or the possibility of pain that has unknown qualities can induce fear in which anxiety borders on panic. At times, pain stimuli that are particularly noxious can be ignored. It has been postulated that certain nerve cell groupings within the spinal cord, brain stem, and cerebral cortex have the ability to modulate the pain impulse through a blocking mechanism. This *gate control theory,* as it is known, is helpful in understanding the approaches used in education-for-childbirth programs or the use of hypnosis in labor. According to this theory, local physical stimulation such as massage or stroking of the woman in labor can balance the pain stimuli by closing down a hypothetical "gate" in the spinal cord that blocks pain signals from reaching the brain. Also, when the laboring woman performs neuromuscular and motor skills, activity within the spinal cord itself further modifies the transmission of pain. In addition, cognitive activities of concentrating on breathing and relaxation skills require selective and directed cortical activity, which activates and closes the gating mechanism as well.

This gate control theory emphasizes the need for a supportive setting for birth. In such an environment, the laboring woman can relax and allow the various higher mental activities to be implemented.

Nursing Actions

Even if the laboring woman and her partner (or family or support persons) are well prepared, the nurse remains still an important member of the childbirth team. Labor is a crisis time and all people, no matter how well prepared, enter labor with some level of anxiety. The following are some helpful actions that the nurse as a support person may use in order to offer both verbal and "hands on" support during labor:

1. Remember that labor is stress even if the couple is prepared. Continually encourage relaxation. They need you. Do not leave them totally alone. Provide support when they need it—and privacy when they need it.
2. Minimize adverse environmental stimuli. Control glaring lights. Decrease traffic flow and noise in the birth setting.
3. Provide privacy and a space with adequate room temperature and ventilation.
4. Talk of contractions, not pains. Remember, the woman is having "contractions"!
5. Relax and get as near to the woman's level as possible. Sit by the bedside. Do not tower over her. Touch!
6. Adjust the labor bed to provide a comfortable position (usually elevating the top of the bed to 45 degrees). She should never be flat on her back because the weight of the uterine contents puts too much pressure on major blood vessels, thus reducing the blood flow back to the brain. Use pillows to support all dependent body parts.
7. Use comfort measures such as cold cloths, backrubs, and ice chips. Showers or bed baths may be taken depending on the progress of labor. Allowing warm water to strike the lower part of the back may be very relaxing.
8. Try effleurage (a light rhythmic stroking over the woman's abdomen in rhythm with breathing during contractions). Effleurage is best done by the woman herself, although it may be done for her.
9. Carry on a conversation only between contractions if necessary.
10. Talk with the father or other support person. Give reassurance and remember that the father has needs for nourishment, rest, and elimination as well as the mother. Let him know where the bathroom is and where he may purchase food. Also, reassure him that you will stay with the laboring woman if he needs to leave for a while in order to tend to his own needs.
11. Do not ask irrelevant questions. Keep talk to a minimum. It utilizes energy needed to cope. Be aware of attitudinal changes as labor progresses.
12. Keep your voice well modulated at all times.
13. Remind the mother to urinate frequently. A full bladder can slow down the descent of the baby.
14. Encourage rest between contractions.
15. Keep the couple informed of what is happening: how many centimeters dilated, station, effacement, and fetal position.
16. Assure the mother she is doing well, offer encouragement, agree with her is she says it hurts but offer positive comments too.
17. Do not distract her during contractions. Wait until a contraction is over to do a nursing procedure.
18. Remember that transition (8 to 10 cm) may be the most intense time during labor. Because the woman may fall asleep between contractions, they may get ahead of her. She may become very irritable.

Table 19.1
Summary of Support Measures

	Woman	Support Person
Dilatation of cervix 0-3 cm		
Contractions 10-30 sec long, 5-30 min apart, mild to moderate Mood: alert, happy, excited, mild anxiety	Settles into labor room; selects focal point Rests or sleeps if possible Uses breathing technique Begin contraction with deep breath in through nose and out through pursed lips Slow chest breathing, 6-9/min through contraction End contraction with deep breath in and out Uses effleurage (gentle stroking of abdomen, using both hands, begin at pubes and stroke upward and outward); focusing and relaxation techniques	Provides encouragement, feedback for relaxation, companionship Assists with contractions Alerts woman to the following: Beginning of contraction Time called out at 15 sec, 30 sec, etc. Ending of contraction Uses focusing techniques Concentration on fixed point in room "Listen to me and follow my breathing" "Watch my face" Concentration on breathing technique Uses comfort measures Position most comfortable for woman Keeps aware of progress, explains procedures and routines Gives praise Offers ataractics as ordered (Chapter 25)
Dilatation of cervix 4-7 cm		
Contractions 30-40 sec long, 3-5-min apart, moderate to strong Mood: seriously labor oriented, concentration and energy needed for contractions, alert, more demanding	Continues relaxation, focusing techniques Uses breathing techniques Begin contraction with deep breath in and out, then slow chest breathing until contraction intensifies, then shallow, effortless breathing, moderate pace, high in chest through peaking of contraction; slow chest breathing as contraction subsides *or* Use abdominal breathing to raise abdominal wall away from uterus; end contraction with deep breathing in and out	Acts as buffer, limits assessment techniques to between contractions Assists with contractions May need to encourage woman to help her to maintain breathing techniques Uses same instructions Uses same focusing devices as in early phase Uses comfort meaures Positions woman on side to minimize pressure of uterus on vena cava and aorta Encourages voluntary relaxation of muscles of back, buttocks, thighs, and perineum; effleurage Uses counterpressure to sacrococcygeal area Encourages and praises Keeps aware of progress Offers analgesics and anesthetics as ordered Checks bladder, encourages to void Gives mouth care, ice chips
Dilatation of cervix 8-10 cm		
Contractions 45-60-90 sec long, 2-3 min apart, strong Mood: irritable, intense concentration, symptoms of transition	Continues relaxation, needs greater concentration to do this Breathing techniques Uses 4:1 pattern if possible Uses panting to overcome response to urge to push	Stays with woman, provides constant support Assists with contractions Probably will need to remind, reassure, and encourage to reestablish breathing pattern and concentration If sedated or drowsy, woman needs warning to begin breathing pattern before contraction becomes too intense If woman begins to push, institutes panting respirations Uses comfort measures Accepts woman's inability to comply with instructions Accepts irritable response to helping, such as counterpressure Supports woman who has nausea and vomiting, gives mouth care as needed, gives reassurance regarding symptomatology of end point of first stage Uses countertension techniques (effleurage and voluntary relaxation) Keeps aware of progress, tells woman when time to push

19. During the actual birth stage, trust her and work with her body. This is not an athletic contest; the goal is pelvic floor release and relaxation. Encourage a series of quick breaths, holding one for 5 seconds while pushing and then taking another breath. Give verbal support such as, "Beautiful! Go with it! Let it flow! Open up below! Soft and loose! Open the door!" You might even give the woman a mirror so that she can watch her own progress as she pushes the baby out.
20. Give the father or other support person the clothes to wear in the delivery room well in advance so that there is no last-minute rush.
21. As you encourage relaxation, encourage *release* toward your touching hand on her body. This will help the woman to increase her body awareness.
22. Always encourage the breathing that *feels* right for each woman. She may have practiced one type of breathing before labor only to find that it is not helpful during a certain part of labor. If this happens, be flexible. Encourage her to find what is working for her and stick with it.
23. There is no failure! Some people who have prepared faithfully for a "natural" childbirth will not be able to achieve that goal because of circumstances beyond their control. They may need analgesia, anesthesia, or a cesarean birth. If they are disappointed, encourage them to talk about their disappointment and then help them to work through it by emphasizing that there is no failure. When they have achieved a meaningful and *safe* birth experience, they have achieved their goal.
24. Throughout the entire labor process be constantly and consistently aware of the needs of the fetus. When the couple has prepared diligently for labor and are extremely intent on what they are doing, it is often easy for the support person to get caught up in that intensity and feel reluctant to do any procedure that might "spoil" their experience. Continually think of yourself as a fetal advocate and use your knowledge and skills to make sound judgments that will lead to a meaningful and safe birth experience for all family members.
25. Share in the couple's joy (or in their grief).

The helpful actions for labor support given in this unit are very useful for all laboring people. However, if there is no family or friend to support the laboring woman, then the nurse's role becomes even more crucial. A woman should never have to labor alone! If the realities of staffing shortages prevent your constant attendance to women laboring alone, you could seek labor support persons from community volunteer groups. A few days spent in teaching and preparation of these volunteers could provide countless hours of labor support for women alone at this crisis time in their lives. Until labor support groups can be formed, you can communicate openly and honestly with women laboring alone. Inform them of the constraints on your time and let them know where you will be when you leave their side, how they can communicate with you, and when you will be coming back.

Women alone or couples who have not attended preparation-for-birth classes can learn relaxation and slow chest breathing techniques with your help during labor. Inform them that there are ways to cope with labor and that you can help them to learn these techniques right then and there. A motivated learner is the best learner, and most laboring women are highly motivated for relief of discomfort.

There are times when no matter how much support you offer and no matter what you do, the woman or couple will choose not to cope with labor and request analgesia or anesthesia (total or partial). Each person has a right to labor and give birth in whatever way she chooses, provided the way is safe for both mother and baby.

Preparation for Becoming a Grandparent

Margaret Mead (1970) defines cultures as being postfigurative, in which children learn primarily from their forebearers (parents and grandparents), cofigurative, in which both children and adults learn from their peers, and prefigurative, in which adults learn also from their children. She states that the latter is a reflection of the period in which we currently live. Certainly, this is exemplified today by the predominance of nuclear families in which the childbearing generation lives apart from the grandparent generation.

Most expectant families rely heavily on information gained from mass media, books, magazines, friends, and childbirth educators to teach them how to experience pregnancy, birth, and early parenting. Grandparents may recall their own birth and early parenting experiences quite differently from how their children do today. Very few modern grandfathers coached their wives in labor or witnessed the births of their own babies. Grandmothers remember little, if any, preparation for labor; they experienced longer hospitalizations and rigid feeding schedules. They may hear and learn from their children that their experiences are outdated. Consequently, their advice may be ignored. Other grandparents may realistically feel unprepared to offer advice and assistance at the time a new baby arrives, even when asked. Actress Virginia Graham recently stated that to be a grandmother in today's society is to be "a prophet without a portfolio." Goode (1976) expresses it this way: "For me and for every woman I know, no matter what we have expected. . . , becoming a grandmother has been a totally new and wonderful, but also somewhat strange experience for which nothing seems to prepare us in advance."

If grandparents are outdated and generally unprepared to assume a meaningful role in the lives of their expectant or new-parent children, is there a need for grandparents at all?

Mead (1970) states that "with the removal of grandparents physically from the world in which the child is reared, the child's experiences of his future are shortened by a generation and his links to the past are weakened." More specifically, it is now recognized that the transition to parenthood creates profound physical and emotional stressors for new parents.

In the United States, new parents who deliver their infants in an alternative birth center or experience high-risk delivery most often can expect medical and/or nursing follow-up care in the early weeks at home with their infant. However, there is still a large gap in professional support for most families between the day of discharge from the hospital and the 4- to 6-wk postpartum checkup.

Grandparents, then, outdated and old fashioned as they may first appear, are most assuredly needed and may be in the best position to provide continuing emotional support, advice, and nurturing to young families during this sensitive and vulnerable time.

How can nurses best assist expectant parents and grandparents to achieve homeostasis within the family unit during the predictable crisis of the fourth trimester?

There is little available literature that focuses on the role of the expectant or new grandparent. Nursing research is needed to identify specific problems modern grandparents face in their own transition to a new life role and to explore appropriate coping mechanisms in a complex and fast-changing world.

A prenatal workshop called the Grandparent Class that deals with the transition to parenthood and focuses specifically on the grandparent has been developed at Hoag Memorial Presbyterian Hospital, Newport Beach, California. Designed to meet the needs of its participants, it is now included as an option for expectant families in two Orange County, California, hospitals where comprehensive prenatal education programs are offered. The class, taught by registered nurse-educators, is offered monthly and is announced through local newspapers and at ongoing prepared-childbirth classes. General topics include the myths of traditional grandparenting, the realities and styles of modern grandparenting, the modern birth experience, common fourth-trimester stressors for parents and siblings, appropriate coping mechanisms and health-promoting behaviors for grandparents, essential infant care skills, and local community resources for families.

The basic concept of the class (Spradley, 1981) is derived from principles of community health nursing where the overall goal is the promotion of high-level wellness or health and the prevention of disease for communities and groups as well as for families and individuals. The promotion of client participation and self-responsibility toward the attainment of this goal is a major characteristic of community health nursing and is stressed in this program. Teaching modalities were developed utilizing adult learning theories and the nursing process.

ASSESSMENT AND PLANNING

Expectant parents and grandparents are encouraged to preregister for the grandparent class by telephone and are, at that time, asked to identify with the nurse-educator specific concerns and needs. Objectives are then mutually defined according to the family's individual needs. After 2 years of monthly classes, nurse-educators have found the most common grandparent-identified needs are family role clarification (who will do what?) and lack of knowledge about prepared childbirth and the birth experience, community resources, and early infant care skills.

INTERVENTION

Class sessions encourage group discussion, role playing, and anticipatory problem solving through games and simulations. Short lecture sessions, a birth film, tour of the maternity unit, and infant care demonstrations are teaching modalities utilized. One problem-solving tool requires that each family (expectant parents and grandparents) discuss among themselves and decide who will do such things as the following:

1. Drive Mom to the hospital
2. Coach her during labor and delivery
3. Contact other friends and relatives following the birth
4. Visit: when and for how long
5. Feed baby
6. Assume most of infant care
7. Help with infant care when Mom and Dad are resting
8. Plan, cook, and clean up meals for 3 weeks

9. Do laundry
10. Be the "go for" (groceries, sanitary pads, etc.)
11. Offer encouragement to Mom and Dad when they are tired and overwhelmed
12. Take 2-year-old brother to park each afternoon
13. Take pictures
14. Dust, vacuum, etc.

Families can identify for themselves potential areas of problems or misunderstanding and can develop coping mechanisms before the fact.

EVALUATION

At the conclusion of each class session, all families are asked to complete a written posttest that is designed to measure behavioral objective outcomes. Families are invited to discuss questions with the nurse-educators and then keep their own posttest for further family discussion at home. Additionally, participants complete a class evaluation tool measuring teacher effectiveness, overall usefulness/applicability of class, demonstration/audiovisual materials, and physical environment of the class setting.

CONCLUSION

In today's fast-changing society the role of grandparenting is no longer bound by the traditional mores of the past. Yet during maturational crisis, such as the transition to parenthood, grandparents, when available and willing to help, are often the best providers of continuing close support and reassurance for new parents. Nurses can encourage the mobilization of existing support systems, provide families with opportunities to increase intergeneration communication, explore alternative styles of grandparenting, anticipate fourth-trimester stressors, and plan appropriate coping mechanisms to maintain equilibrium within the family unit. The grandparent class is but one example of an innovative approach that can fill the gap in the continuity of care for childbearing families.

Organizations Involved in Parent Education

The following organizations can provide information on parent education:

American Academy of Husband-Coached Childbirth (AAHCC)
P.O. Box 5224
Sherman Oaks, CA 91413

American Society for Psychoprophylaxis in Obstetrics (ASPO)
1411 K Street N.W., Suite 200
Washington, DC 20005

Council of Childbirth Education Specialists, Inc. (CCES)
168 West 86th Street
New York, NY 10024

International Childbirth Education Association (ICEA)
P.O. Box 20048
Minneapolis, MN 55420

National Association of Childbirth Education, Inc. (NACE)
3940 11th Street
Riverside, CA 92501

Nurses Association of the American College of Obstetricians and Gynecologists (NAACOG)
600 Maryland Avenue, S.W. #300
Washington, DC 20024

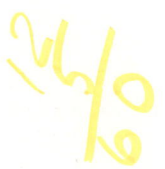

References and Readings

American Academy of Husband-Coached Childbirth: The Bradley method, Sherman Oaks, Calif., 1974, The Academy.

American Society for Psychoprophylaxis in Obstetrics: You want to be a certified childbirth educator? Washington, D.C., 1979, The Society.

Andersen, J.: A clarification of the Lamaze method, J.O.G.N. Nurs. **7**(2):53, 1977.

Arms, S.: Immaculate deception, Boston, 1975, Houghton Mifflin Co.

Barker-Benfield, G.L.: The horrors of the half-known life, New York, 1977, Doubleday Co.

Beals, P., editor: ICEA teacher's guide, ed. 2, Milwaukee, 1975, International Childbirth Education Association.

Benedict, T.: Parenthood as a development phase: a contribution to the libido, J. Am. Psychoanal. Assoc. **7**:389, 1959.

Benson, R.C., editor: Current obstetric and gynecologic diagnosis and treatment, ed. 3, Los Altos, Calif., 1980, Lange Medical Publications.

Bing, E.: Six practical lessons for an easier childbirth, New York, 1969, Bantam Books.

Bing, E., and Colman, L.: Making love during pregnancy, New York, 1977, Bantam Books.

Bobak, I.M.: Self-image: a universal concern of women becoming mothers, C.N.A. Bull. **9**:7, April 1969.

Bradley, R.: Husband-coached childbirth, New York, 1965, Harper & Row, Publishers, Inc.

Buxton, C.L.: A study of psychological methods for relief of pain in childbirth, Philadelphia, 1962, W.B. Saunders Co.

Chabon, I.: Awake and aware, New York, 1966, Dell Publishing Co., Inc.

Chertok, L.: Psychosomatic methods of preparation for birth, Am. J. Obstet. Gynecol. **98**(5):698, 1967.

Childbirth Without Pain League: Bylaws of the Childbirth Without Pain League, Riverside, Calif., 1979, The League.

Colman, A.D., and Colman, L.L.: Pregnancy as an altered state of consciousness, Birth Fam. J. **1**:7, 1974.

Cronenwett, L., and Newmark, L.: Father's responses to childbirth, Nurs. Res. **23**(3):210, 1974.

Deutsch, R.M.: The key to feminine response in marriage, New York, 1968, Random House, Inc.

Dick-Read, G.: Childbirth without fear, ed. 2, New York, 1959, harper & Row, Publishers, Inc.

Donaldson, J.O.: Neurology of pregnancy. In Major problems in neurology, vol. 7, Philadelphia, 1978, W.B. Saunders Co.

Edwards, M.: Communication: dimensions in childbirth education, Pacific Grove, Calif., 1973, M. Edwards.

Ehrenreich, B., and English, D.: For her own good: 150 years of the experts' advice to women, New York, 1978, Harper & Row, Publishers, Inc.

Ewy, D., and Ewy, R.: Preparation for childbirth, New York, 1972, New American Library.

Felton, G.S., and Segelman, F.B.: Lamaze childbirth training and changes in belief about personal control, Birth Fam. J. **5**:141, Fall 1978.

Goode, R.: A book for grandmothers, New York, 1976, Macmillan Publishing Co., Inc.

Hassis, P.: Textbook for childbirth educators, New York, 1978, Harper & Row, Publishers, Inc.

Hathaway, T., and Hathaway, M., editors: The Bradley method, Sherman Oaks, Calif., 1974, American Association of Husband Coached Childbirth.

Holt, J.R.: Best laid plans: pre- and postpartum comparison of self and spouse in primiparous Lamaze couples who share delivery and those who do not, Nurs. Res. **29**:20, Jan.-Feb. 1980.

Hommel, F.: Painless? childbirth, J. Am. Soc. Psychoproph. Obstet. **2**:4, 1969.

Huprich, P.A.: Assisting the couple through a Lamaze labor and delivery, M.C.N. **2**(4):245, July-Aug. 1977.

Huttel, F.A., et al.: A quantitative evaluation of psychoprophylaxis in childbirth, J. Psychosom. Res. **16:**81, 1972.

Keuscher, M.B., and Oliver, M.: An overview of childbirth education, J. Calif. Perinatal Assoc. **2**(1):79, 1982.

Kitzinger, S.: The experience of childbirth, Middlesex, England, 1970, Pelican Publishing Co., Inc.

Klopher, F., Cogan, R., and Henneborn, W.: Second stage medical intervention and pain during childbirth, J. Psychosom. Res. **19:**289, 1975.

Lamaze, F.: Painless childbirth: the Lamaze method, Chicago, 1970, Henry Regnery Co.

Mead, M.: Culture and commitment: a study of the generation gap, Garden City, N.Y., 1970, Natural History Press/Doubleday & Co., Inc.

Mercer, R.T.: "She's a multip . . . she knows the ropes," M.C.N. **4:**301, Sept.-Oct. 1979.

Naeye, R.L.: Coitus and associated amniotic-fluid infections, N. Engl. J. Med. **301:**1198, Nov. 29, 1979.

Nurses' Association of the American College of Obstetricians and Gynecologists: Guidelines for childbirth education, Washington, D.C., 1981, The Association.

Nurses' Association of the American College of Obstetricians and Gynecologists: Preparation for parenthood. NAACOG technical bulletin no. 3, Washington, D.C., 1978, The Association.

Oehrtman, S.: Assessment and crisis intervention: a model for the family. In Hall, J., and Weaver, B., editors: Nursing of families in crisis, Philadelphia, 1974, J.B. Lippincott Co.

Olson, M.L.: Fitting grandparents into new families, M.C.N. **6**(6):419, Nov.-Dec. 1981.

Osipow, S., and Walsh, W.: Strategies in counseling for behavioral change, New York, 1970, Appleton-Century-Crofts.

Otto, S., editor: ICEA 1978 biennial report, Milwaukee, 1978, International Childbirth Education Association.

Parfitt, R.R.: The birth primer: a source book of traditional and alternative methods in labor and delivery, Philadelphia, 1977, Running Press.

Rubin, R.: Cognitive style in pregnancy, Am. J. Nurs. **70:**502, 1970.

Sasmor, J.L.: Childbirth education: a nursing perspective, New York, 1979, John Wiley & Sons, Inc.

Smith, B.A., Priore, R.M., and Sterm, M.K.: The transition phase of labor, Am. J. Nurs. **73:**448, March 1973.

Spradley, B.W.: Community health nursing: concepts and practice, Boston, 1981, Little, Brown & Co.

Stevens, R.J.: Psychological strategies for management of pain in prepared childbirth. I. A review of the research, Birth Fam. J. **3:**4, 1977.

Stevens, R.J.: Pyschological strategies for management of pain in prepared childbirth. II. A study of psychoanalgesia in prepared childbirth, Birth Fam. J. **4:**1, 1977.

Sweet, P.T.: Prenatal classes especially for children, M.C.N. **4:**82, March-April 1979.

Tanzer, D.: Why natural childbirth? New York, 1972, Doubleday & Co., Inc.

Tanzer, S.: The psychology of pregnancy and childbirth. An investigation of natural childbirth, unpublished doctoral dissertation, Waltham, Mass., 1967, Brandeis University.

Vellay, P.: Psychoprophylaxis and its evolution, Birth Fam. J. **2:**19, 1975.

Velvovsky, I., et al.: Painless childbirth through psychoprophylaxis, Moscow, 1960, Foreign Languages Publishing House.

Wertz, R.W., and Wertz, D.C.: Lying in: a history of childbirth in America, New York, 1977, The Free Press.

Wiggins, J.D.: Childbearing: physiology, experiences, needs, St. Louis, 1979, The C.V. Mosby Co.

Willmuth, L.R.: Prepared childbirth and the concept of control, J.O.G.N. Nurs. **4**(5):38, 1975.

Wright, E.: The new childbirth, New York, 1966, Hart Publishing Co., Inc.

The Birth Period

20 Essential Factors of Labor

21 First Stage of Labor

22 Second Stage of Labor

23 Third and Fourth Stages of Labor

24 Fetal Monitoring

25 Pharmacologic Control of Discomfort During the Birth Period

26 Alternative Settings for Childbirth

UNIT FOUR

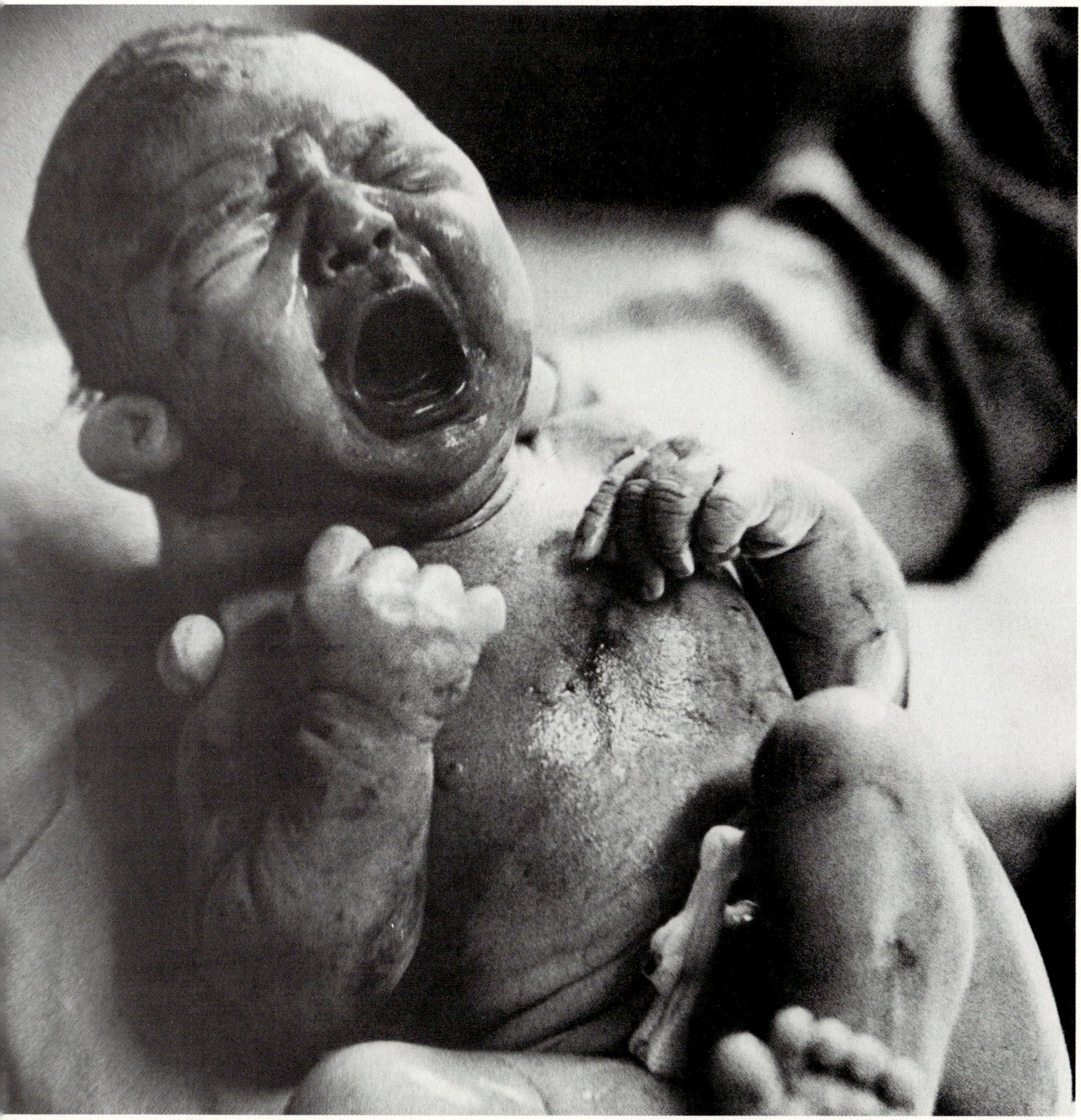

Robert Maust

20
Essential Factors of Labor

- Essential Factors in Labor: Basis for Assessment
  - The passenger
    - Fetal head
    - Shoulders and pelvic girdle
    - Fetal lie
    - Presentation
    - Attitude
    - Position
  - The passageway
    - Pelvis
    - Soft tissues
  - The powers
    - Uterine contractions
    - Voluntary bearing-down efforts
    - Implications for nursing care
  - The placenta
  - Psychologic response
- Techniques for Assessment
  - Abdominal palpation
  - Auscultation
  - Vaginal examination
    - Effacement of the cervix
    - Dilatation of the cervix
    - Station
  - Conventional x-ray films
  - Computed tomography
  - Ultrasonography
- Process of Labor
  - Changes preliminary to onset of labor (prodromal labor)
  - Onset of labor
  - Mechanism of labor
    - Phases of the mechanism of labor in vertex presentation
    - Persistent occiput posterior or occiput transverse position
  - Duration of labor
    - First stage of labor
    - Second stage of labor
    - Third stage of labor
    - Fourth stage of labor

The time to be born signals the end of the preparatory fantasy phase for parenthood and the beginning of the reality phase of parenthood. It is a time of physical and emotional crisis that requires collaborative care between the obstetric team and the pregnant woman or couple. This chapter and those that follow first present labor as a process, providing a theoretical base and then discuss the application of the nursing process with women and their families during the stages of labor and with the neonate immediately following birth.

Labor (parturition, childbirth, birthing) is the process by which the fetus and placenta are expelled from the uterus and the vagina into the external environment. For the infant the repetitive stress of labor culminates in delivery and the necessity for sucessful transition from a dependent to an independent biologic state. For the mother, labor is an essentially normal process but one that carries a potential risk of disability for herself and the child she bears. For the mother and father childbirth marks the time when each assumes the role of parent with its personal and social connotations.

The goals of the health team are the safe delivery of mother and child and the promotion of emotional fulfillment for the parents.

Essential Factors in Labor: Basis for Assessment

Parturition is the birth process. A *parturient* is a woman in labor. *Labor* is a coordinated sequence of involuntary uterine contractions that result in effacement and dilatation of the cervix and voluntary bearing-down efforts that result in delivery, the actual expulsion of the products of conception, the fetus and placenta. *Toko-* and *toco-* (Greek) are combining forms meaning childbirth or labor: *eu*tocia is normal labor; *dys*tocia is abnormal or difficult labor.

Health care professionals involved in maternity care recognize that few factors will shorten labor but many will prolong the process. In every labor five essential factors affect the process. These are more easily remembered as the five P's*:

1. *Passenger:* size, presentation, and position of the passenger or fetus
2. *Passageway:*
   a. Configuration and diameters of the maternal pelvis
   b. Distensibility of the lower uterine segment, cervical dilatation, and capacity for distention of vaginal canal and introitus
3. *Powers:* strength, duration, and frequency of uterine contractions (so-called primary powers of labor)
4. *Placenta:* site of insertion of the placenta
5. *Psychology:* psychologic state of the woman

THE PASSENGER

The passage of the fetus through the birth canal is influenced by the size of the fetal head and shoulder, the dimensions of the pelvic girdle, and the fetal presentation and position.

Fetal head. Because of its size and relative rigidity, the fetal head has a major effect on the birth process. The bony skull is made up of the larger and more compressible cranial vault and the smaller, incompressible face and base of the skull.

The external cranial vault is composed of two parietal bones, two temporal bones, the frontal bone, and the occipital bone. These bones are united by membranous *sutures:* the sagittal, lambdoidal, and coronal. At the points of intersection, these sutures become enlarged to form the *fontanels* (''soft spots'') (Figs. 20.1 and 20.2). The two most important fontanels are the anterior and posterior fontanels. The anterior fontanel is found at the intersection of the sutures of the two parietal and the frontal bones. The larger of the two, it is diamond shaped and closes at about 18 months of age. The posterior fontanel is at the junction of the sutures of the two parietal bones and one occipital bone and is therefore triangular in shape. It is smaller than the anterior fontanel and closes by about the twelfth week of life.

The bones of the cranial vault are not firmly united, and slight overlapping of the bones, or *molding* of the shape of the head, occurs during labor (Figs. 20.3 and 20.4). This capacity of the bones to slide over one another permits adaptation to the various diameters of the pelvis. Molding can be extensive, but with most neonates the head assumes its normal shape within about 3 days after birth.

The fetal head can move on the neck about 45 degrees in flexion or extension and approximately 180 degrees during rotation. This movement permits smaller diameters of the fetal head to present during descent through the birth canal.

Principal measurements of the fetal skull are as follows (in centimeters):

1. Anteroposterior diameters (Fig. 20.5)
   a. Occipitomental (OM): 13.5

*A sixth *P* is emerging in the literature. It refers to *position* of the mother during labor: walking, Fowler's, or flat in bed.

Fig. 20.1
Neonate's head at term.

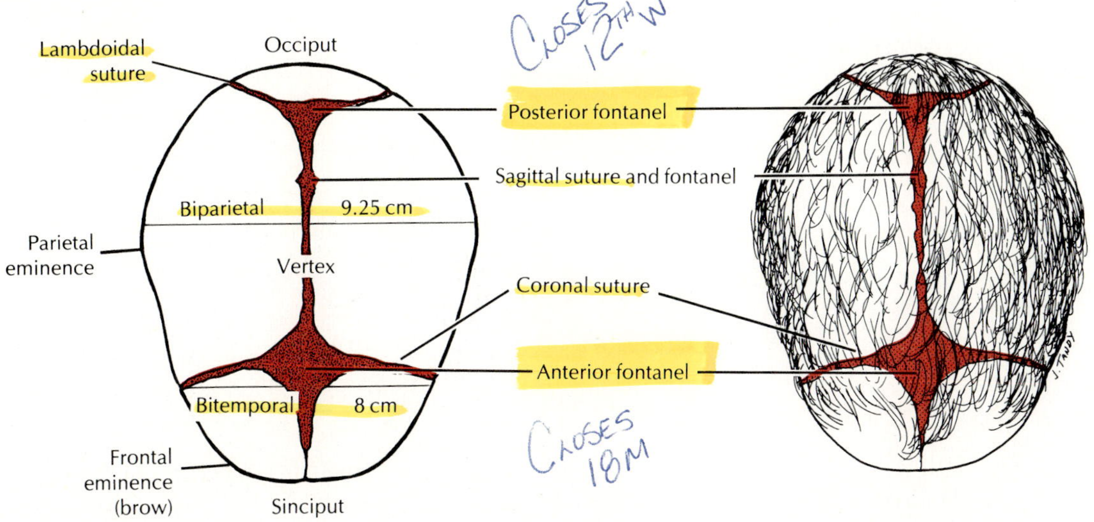

Fig. 20.2
Head at term showing fontanels and sutures.

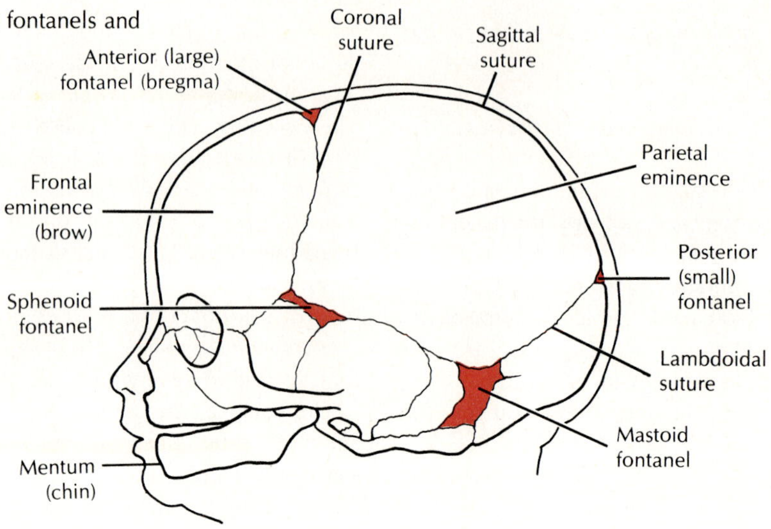

Fig. 20.3
Molding during birth process. Shaded area indicates stationary, noncompressible portions of skull: face and base of skull. **A,** Overlapping (molding) of cranial bones during labor. **B,** Realignment of cranial bones by third day of life to normal position.

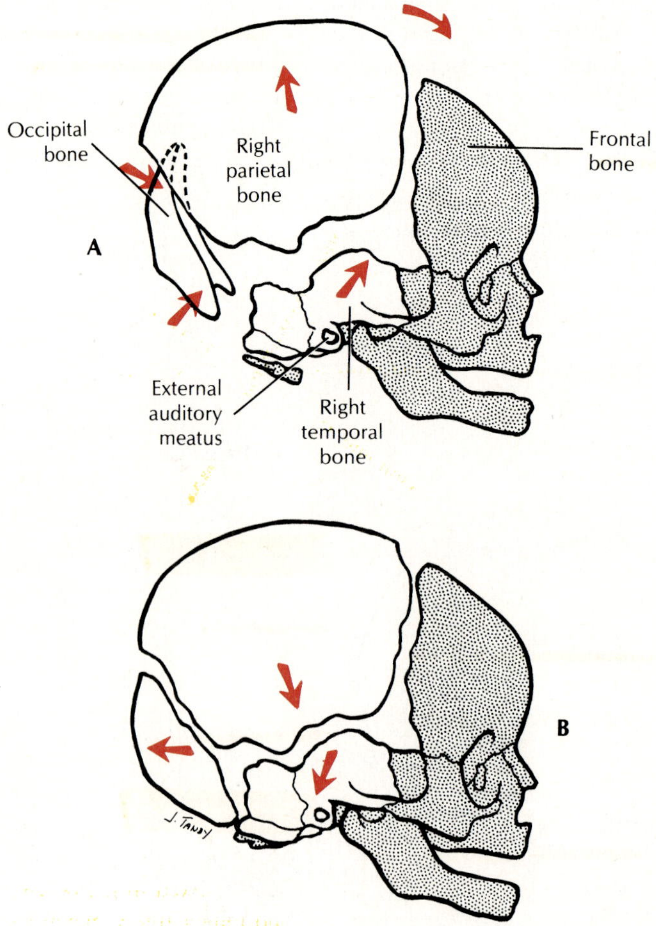

Fig. 20.4
Molding of head *(red)* in cephalic presentations. **A,** Occipitoanterior. **B,** Occipitoposterior. **C,** Brow. **D,** Face. In face presentations, soft tissues of face become edematous and ecchymotic.

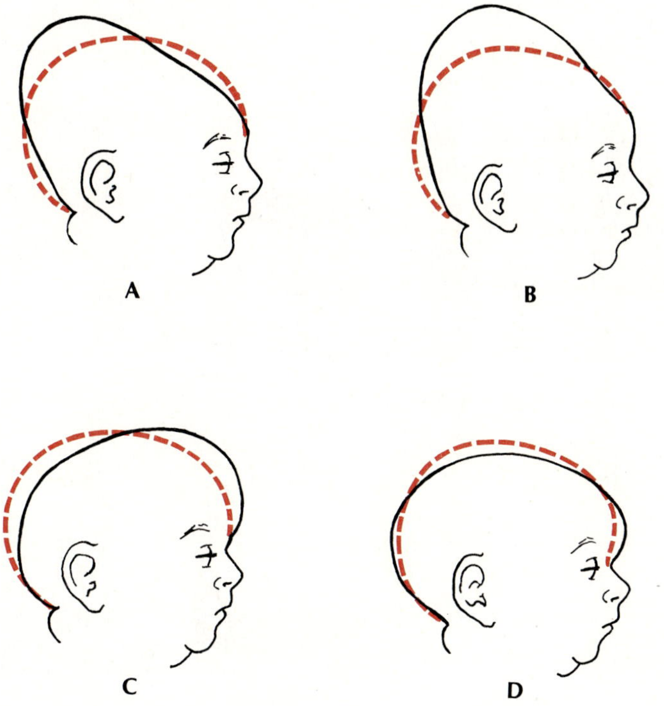

Fig. 20.5
Head at term showing diameters.

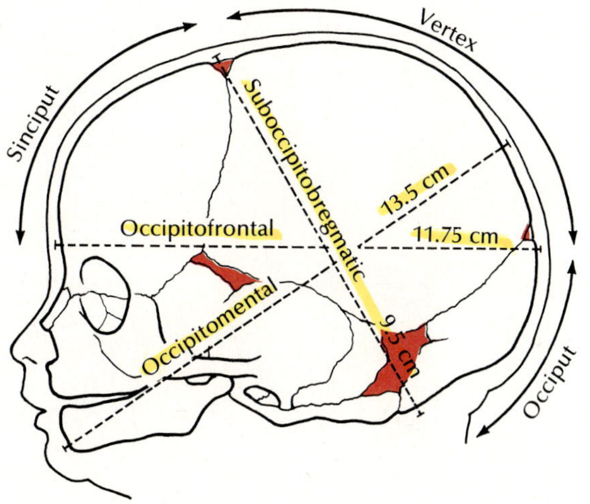

b. Occipitofrontal (OF): 11.75
c. Suboccipitobregmatic (SOB): 9.5

2. Transverse diameters (Fig. 20.1)
    a. Biparietal (Bip): 9.25
    b. Bitemporal (Bit): 8.0

The biparietal diameter is the largest of the transverse diameters. When the biparietal diameter has descended past the inlet (brim, or superior strait), the head becomes fixed in the pelvis, is said to be *engaged,* and is no longer freely movable.*

*Most medical texts on obstetrics use this definition for engagement.

Fig. 20.6

Head entering pelvis.
A, Suboccipitobregmatic diameter: complete flexion of head on chest so that smallest diameter enters. **B,** Occipitofrontal diameter: moderate extension (military attitude) so that large diameter enters. **C,** Occipitomental diameter: marked extension (deflection) so that largest diameter, which is too large to permit head to enter pelvis, is presenting.

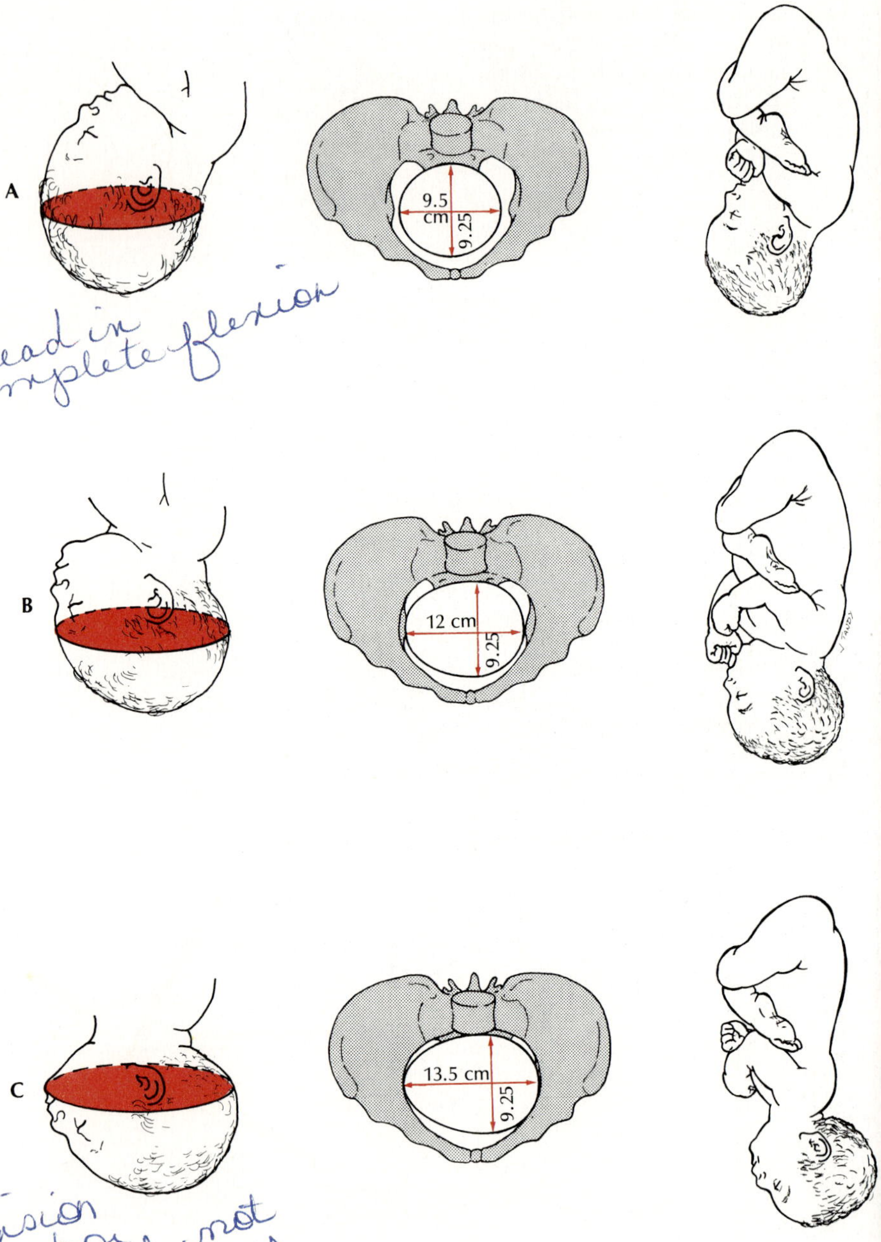

Of the anteroposterior diameters shown in Figs. 20.6 and 20.8, it can be seen that the attitudes of flexion or extension allow diameters of different sizes to enter the pelvis. The smallest diameter (suboccipitobregmatic) to present is with the head in complete flexion and thus able to enter easily, whereas the largest diameter, with the head in hyperextension, is too large for the head to enter the average pelvis, and therefore the birth process will not progress.

Shoulders and pelvic girdle. Because of their mobility, the position of the shoulder (the shoulder girdle) can be altered during labor, so that one shoulder may occupy a lower level than the other. This permits a small shoulder diameter to negotiate the passage. The circumference of the hips, or pelvic girdle, is usually small enough not to create problems.

Fetal lie. Lie is the relationship of the long axis (spine) of the fetus to the long axis (spine) of the mother. There are two lies: *longitudinal,* in which the long axis of the fetus is parallel with the long axis of

Fig. 20.7
A, Cephalic landmarks.

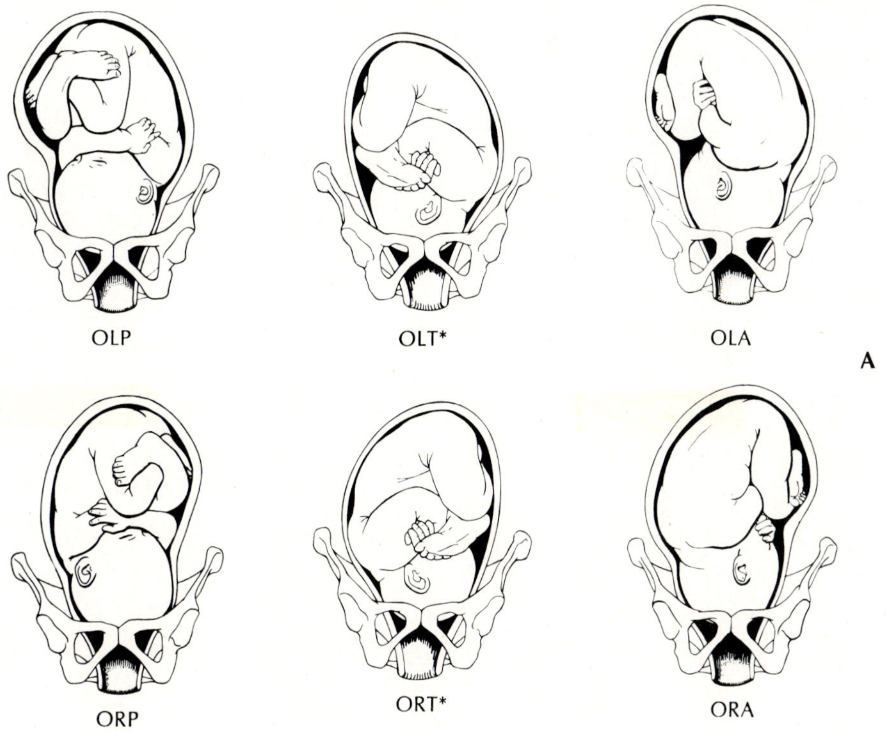

Lie: vertical
Presentation: vertex
Reference point: occiput
Attitude: complete flexion

Fetal reference point	Maternal pelvis: Side	Maternal pelvis: Quadrant
O—Occiput	L—Left	A—Anterior
M—Mentum	R—Right	T—Transverse
S—Sacrum		P—Posterior
Sc—Scapula		

*Illustration adapted from Hellman, L.M., and Pritchard, J.A.: Williams' obstetrics, ed. 14, New York, 1971, Appleton-Century-Crofts, p. 322.

Obstetric presentations and positions will be designated by indicating fetal presentation first, followed by maternal side and quadrant (e.g., OLA = occiput left anterior). In these vertex presentations, the occiput (O) is the reference point. (Courtesy Ross Laboratories, Columbus, Ohio.)

Continued.

the mother, and ***transverse,*** in which the long axis of the fetus is at right angles to that of the mother (Fig. 20.7: compare *A* and *B* to *C*).

Longitudinal lies are either cephalic (head) or pelvic (breech) presentations, depending on the fetal structure that first enters the mother's pelvis.

Presentation. Presentation refers to that portion of the fetus that enters the pelvis first and covers the internal os of the cervix, such as cephalic (vertex, head), breech, or shoulder (Fig. 20.7). Presentation may also be more precisely described as a presenting part; for example, in cephalic presentation, the presenting part varies with the attitude of the fetus; in breech presentation either the sacrum (frank breech) or a foot (footling breech) may present.

Attitude. Attitude is the relationship of the fetal body parts to each other. The fetus assumes a characteristic posture (attitude) in utero partly because of the mode of fetal growth and partly because of accommodation to the shape of the uterine cavity. The shape is roughly

Fig. 20.7, cont'd
B, Pelvic landmarks. **C,** Shoulder presentation.

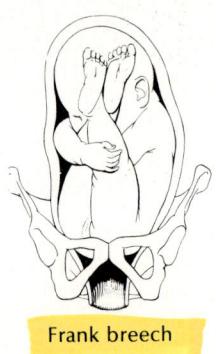

Frank breech

Lie: vertical
Presentation: breech (incomplete)
Reference point: sacrum
Attitude: flexion, except for legs at knees

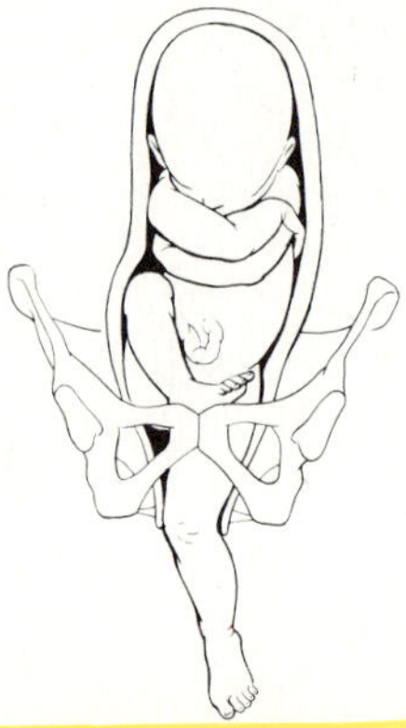

Single footling breech

Lie: vertical
Presentation: breech (incomplete)
Reference point: sacrum
Attitude: flexion, except for one leg extended at hip and knee

B

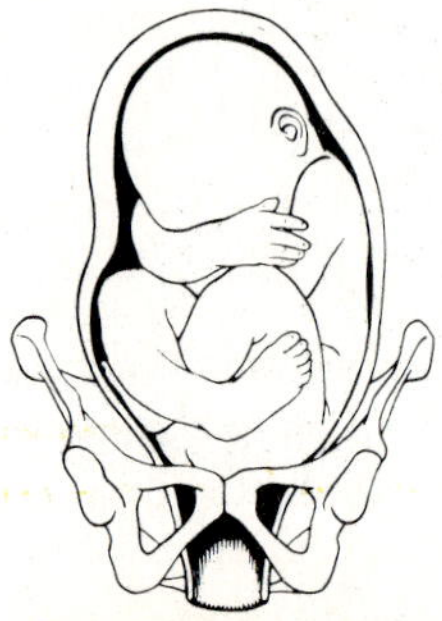

Complete breech

Lie: vertical
Presentation: breech (sacrum and feet presenting)
Reference point: sacrum (with feet)
Attitude: general flexion

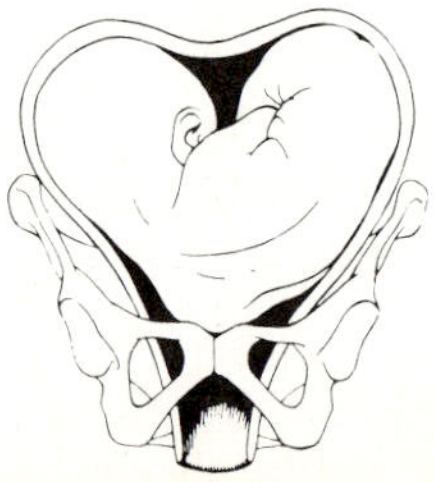

C

Shoulder presentation.

Lie: horizontal or transverse
Presentation: shoulder
Reference point: scapula (Sc)
Attitude: flexion

ovoid, the back is markedly flexed, the head is flexed on the chest, the thighs are flexed on the abdomen, the knees are flexed at the knee joints, and the arches of the feet rest on the anterior surface of the legs; this is the attitude of "general flexion." The arms are crossed over the thorax, and the umbilical cord lies between them and the legs. In cephalic presentations the degree of flexion of the head on the chest determines the presenting part:

1. If the head is fully flexed on the chest, the occiput (vertex) presents first and *the posterior fontanel is palpable on vaginal examination;* this is termed an *occipital,* or *vertex, presentation* (Fig. 20.8, *A*).
2. If the head is partially flexed or not flexed (moderate flexion), the anterior fontanel presents and is palpable on vaginal examination; this is termed a *sinciput presentation* or a *military attitude* (Fig. 20.8, *B*).

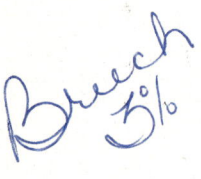

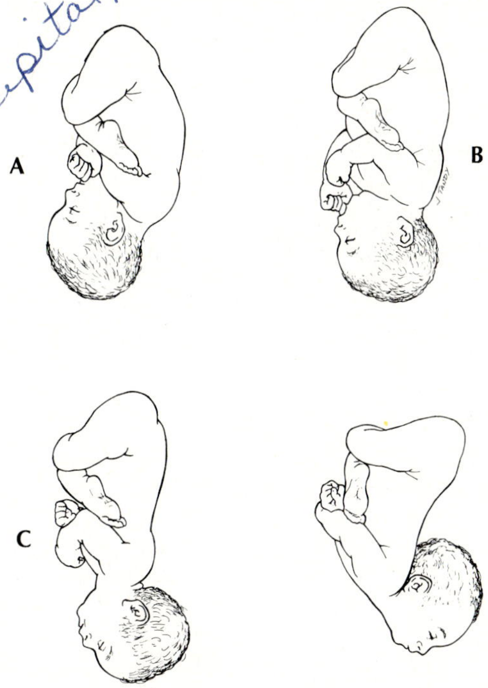

Fig. 20.8
Differences in attitude of fetal head cause different presentations. **A,** Complete flexion: *vertex* presentation. **B,** Moderate flexion (military attitude): *sinciput* presentation. **C,** Marked extension (deflection): *brow* presentation. **D,** Excessive extension (deflection): *face* presentation.

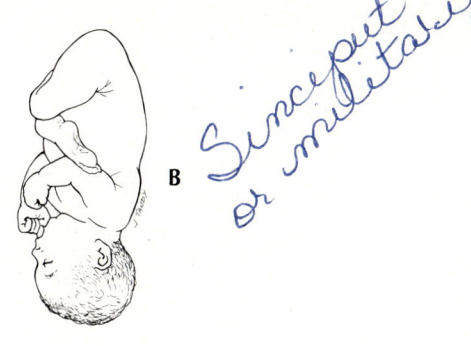

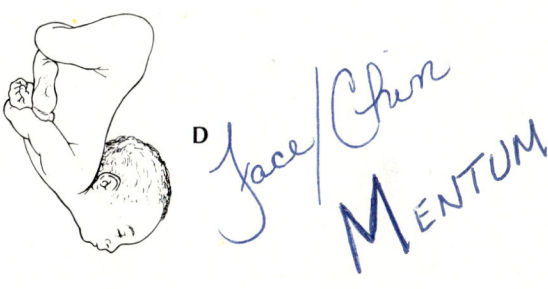

3. If the head is markedly extended, the brow is the presenting part; this is termed a *brow presentation* (Fig. 20.8, *C*).
4. If the head is hyperextended, the chin (mentum) is the presenting part; this is termed a *face* or *chin presentation* (Fig. 20.8, *D*).

In pelvic (breech) presentation the thighs may be flexed on the abdomen and the legs extended (frank breech presentation), the legs may be flexed on the thighs so that buttocks and feet present (complete breech), or one or both feet may extend downward (single or double footling breech) (Fig. 20.7, *B*).

Transverse lies are referred to as *shoulder presentations* (Fig. 20.7, *C*). Unless the fetus rotates or is rotated to a longitudinal presentation, birth is possible only by cesarean delivery.

The most common presentations are vertex (96%) and breech (3%). The others are rarely encountered, but they act to slow or prevent the birth process.

Position. Position is the relationship of the fetal reference point (e.g., occiput, brow, chin or mentum, or sacrum) to one of the four quadrants of the mother's pelvis; that is, the most prominent and dependent portion of the presenting part is related to one of the four quadrants of the mother's pelvis. These quadrants, formed by drawing an imaginary line from the mother's sacral promontory to the upper edge of the symphysis pubis and bisecting it transversely with a line from one side to the other, are termed the *right posterior* and *anterior quadrants* and the *left posterior* and *anterior quadrants* (Fig. 20.9). In a vertex presentation, if the occiput (fetal reference point) is the most prominent portion of the presenting part and is located in the right anterior quadrant, the position is noted as right occiput anterior (ROA*). A summary of lies and positions and additional examples are given in Table 20.1

THE PASSAGEWAY

The passageway, or birth canal, is composed of the rigid bony pelvis and the soft tissues of the cervix, vagina, and introitus.

Numerous constrictions and changing contours characterize the birth canal. Therefore the passage is not like a smooth, bent tube; instead it resembles a curved pipe with baffles (deflectors). The baffles direct the presenting part, and the narrower portions require the head, for example, to turn, seeking the easiest way

*In this traditional method expressing fetal position, the first and last initials refer to the maternal pelvis, and the middle initial refers to the fetal reference point. See legend for Fig. 20.7 for further clarification.

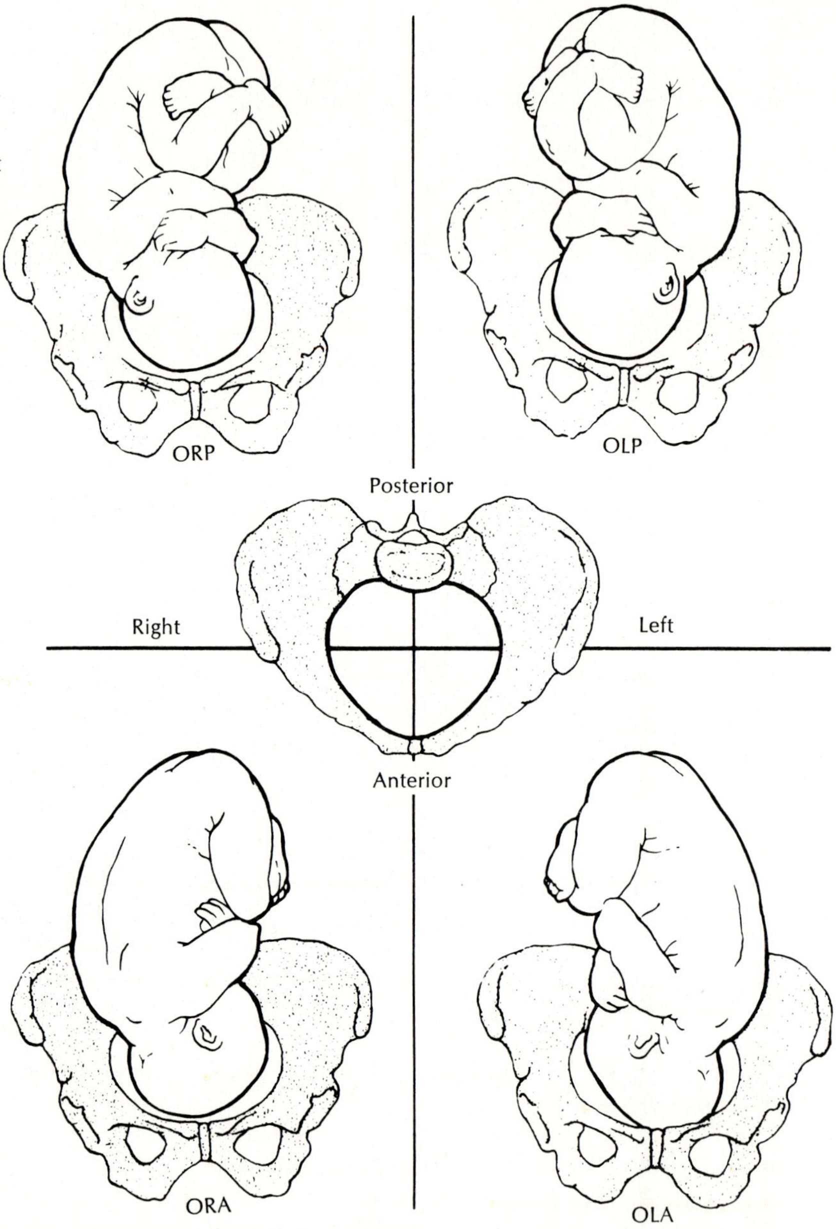

Fig. 20.9
Examples of fetal vertex (occiput) presentations in relation to quadrant of maternal pelvis. **A,** If occiput is in either right or left posterior quadrant, examiner feels lumpy fetal arms and legs more easily. **B,** If occiput is in either right or left anterior quadrant, examiner feels smoother fetal back more easily. (Adapted from Iorio, J.: Childbirth: family-centered nursing, ed. 3, St. Louis, 1973, The C.V. Mosby Co.)

through. Both bony and soft parts serve to restrict or deflect the presenting part, but the fetus, always a passive participant, is propelled by the forces of labor (i.e., analogous to maneuvering a big piano through a narrow door).

Pelvis. In Chapter 6 the anatomy of the pelvis was reviewed. A further discussion of the significance of pelvic configurations in labor is necessary at this point.

Assessment of the bony pelvis. The purpose of the examination of the bony pelvis is to determine if the pelvic cavity is of adequate size to allow for the passage of a full-term infant. This examination may be performed during the first prenatal evaluation and need not be repeated if the pelvis is of adequate size. However, if findings indicate that the pelvis is of borderline adequacy or if the examination could not be done because the woman was tense, the examination is repeated between 32 and 36 weeks' gestation. In the third trimester of pregnancy, the examination may be more thorough and results more accurate because there is a relaxation

Fig. 20.10
Female pelvis from above pelvic brim (inlet, linea terminalis, or ileopectineal line).

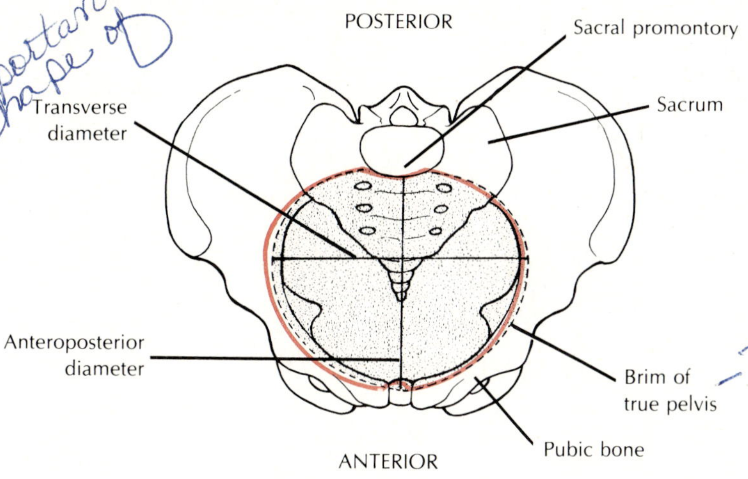

Table 20.1
Fetal Lie and Position

	Presenting part	Example of position
Longitudinal lie		
Cephalic		
Vertex	Occiput	*Left occiput posterior* (LOP)
Face (chin) (rare)	Mentum	*Right mentum posterior* (RMP)
Brow	Brow	*Left brow anterior* (LBA)
Pelvic		
Breech	Sacrum	*Right sacrum anterior* (RSA)
Transverse lie		
Shoulder	Scapula	*Right scapula anterior* (RScA)

of pelvic joints and ligaments, and the woman may be more accustomed to examination.

Pelvic joints. The four pelvic joints are the symphysis pubis, the right and left sacroiliac joints, and the sacrococcygeal joint (see Fig. 6.17). The joints of the pelvic bones are synchondroses (joints in which the surfaces are connected by plates of cartilage) that allow little movement in the nonpregnant state; the hormones of pregnancy, especially the ovarian hormone progesterone, cause considerable mobility to develop. Widening of the symphyseal joint and instability may cause pain in any or all of the joints.

Because the examiner does not have direct access to the bony structures and because the bones are covered with variable amounts of soft tissue, estimates are approximate. Precise bony pelvis measurements can be determined using computed tomography and ultrasound, or x-ray films. However, x-ray examination is not indicated for the vast majority of gravidas (see techniques of assessment, p. 373).

The bony pelvis is separated by the brim or inlet into two parts: the *false pelvis* and the *true pelvis* (see Fig. 6.18). The false pelvis is that part above the brim and is of no obstetric interest.

The *true pelvis* is divided into three planes: the inlet or brim, the midpelvis or cavity, and the outlet:

1. The *pelvic inlet,* or brim of the pelvis, is formed anteriorly by the upper margins of the pubic bone, laterally by the iliopectineal lines along the innominate bones, and posteriorly by the anterior, upper margin of the sacrum, the sacral promontory (Fig. 20.10).

2. The *pelvic cavity,* or midpelvis, is a curved passage having a short anterior wall and a much deeper concave posterior wall. It is bounded by the posterior aspect of the symphysis pubis, the ischium, a portion of the ilium, and the sacrum and coccyx (see Fig. 6.19).

3. The *pelvic outlet* when viewed from below is ovoid, somewhat diamond shaped, bounded by the pubic arch anteriorly, the ischial tuberosities laterally, and the tip of the coccyx posteriorly (Fig. 20.11). In the latter part of pregnancy, the coccyx is movable (unless it had been broken in a fall while skiing, skating, etc. and had fused to the sacrum during healing).

The pelvic canal varies in size and shape at various levels. The diameters at the plane of the pelvic inlet,

Fig. 20.11
Female pelvic outlet (from below).

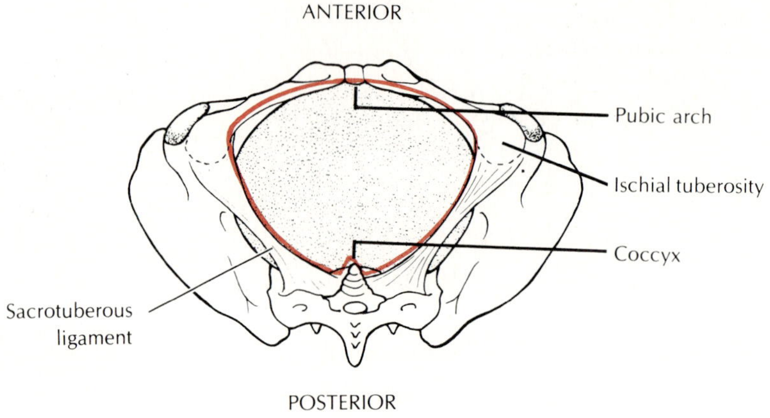

Fig. 20.12
Planes of true pelvis. **A,** Sagittal section. **B,** Coronal section. Outlet plane not shown.

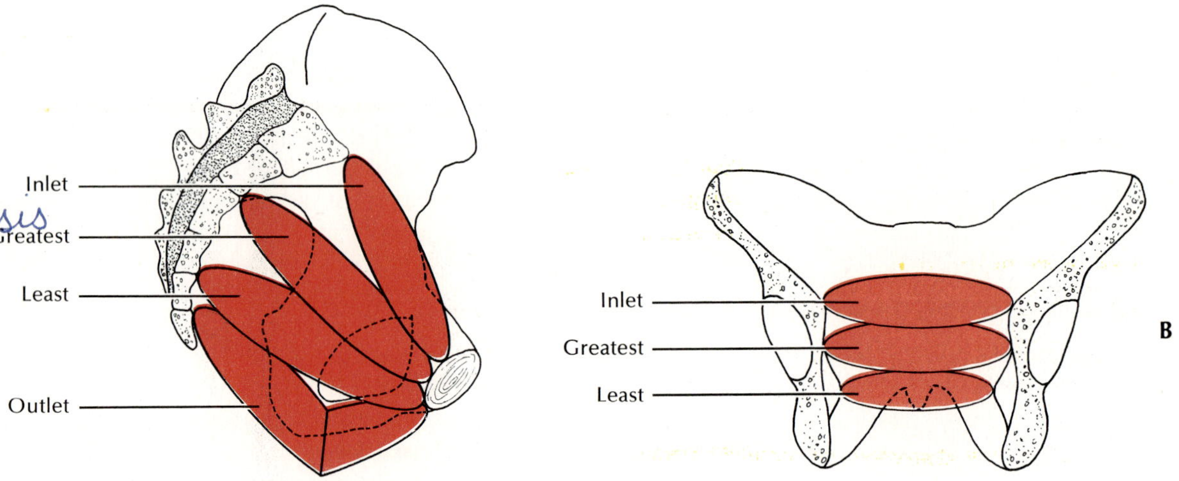

midpelvis, and outlet (Fig. 20.12) and the axis of the birth canal (Fig. 20.15) determine whether vaginal delivery is possible and the manner by which the fetus may pass down the birth canal (mechanism of labor).

External measurement yields little worthwhile information regarding the size and shape of the true, or internal, pelvis, except in cases of gross deformity.

Pelvic type and woman's body build. The pelvic type occasionally may be suspected from the woman's body build. Small women of slight stature generally have small, rounded, generally contracted gynecoid (female) pelves (see Fig. 6.20). Fortunately most of these women will have small babies, despite the fact that their husbands may be appreciably larger.

In contrast, the short, fat, or heavyset woman with broad shoulders may have difficulty in labor. Her pelvis may be predominantly android, and she may experience dystocia. However, hirsutism (excessive growth of hair), male physique, or other characteristics generally do not indicate an android pelvis.

By and large, the tall, slender woman, perhaps with wide shoulders, often has a favorable, long, oval (anthropoid) pelvis. She does well in labor and usually delivers without difficulty. No general body index exists that will accurately predict the type of pelvis and suggest the obstetric prognosis.

Problems can be expected in women with rickets, osteomalacia, or paralysis of one or both extremities or

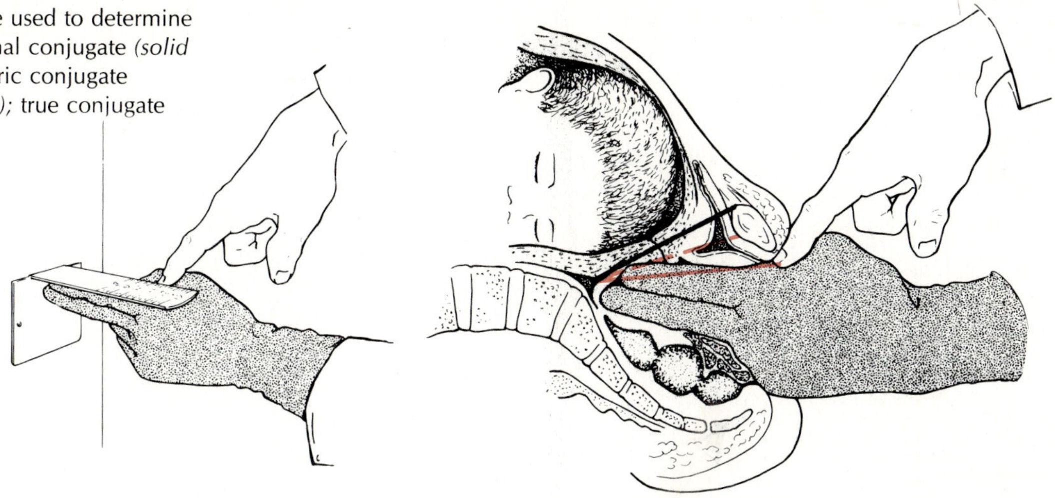

Fig. 20. 13
Metal wall scale used to determine length of diagonal conjugate *(solid red line)*; obstetric conjugate *(broken red line)*; true conjugate *(black line)*.

following a motor vehicle accident in which the woman experienced a crushed pelvis. The pelvis may be grossly deformed and the pelvic canal so distorted as to preclude vaginal delivery of a full-term fetus.

Great importance now centers on internal pelvimetry for pelvic dimensions and capacity, cephalometry for size and shape of fetal head, and the internal configuration of the birth canal. See techniques of assessment that follow.

Obstetric measurements

Plane of inlet (superior strait). The principal pelvic diameters of the plane of the inlet are as follows:

1. Anteroposterior diameters (Fig. 20.13):
   a. The *true conjugate*, or conjugata vera (11 cm or more), is the distance from the upper margin of the symphysis to the sacral promontory. This dimension usually is a radiographic or ultrasonic measurement.
   b. The *diagonal conjugate* (12.5 to 13 cm) is the distance from the lower border of the symphysis pubis to the promontory of the sacrum. The diagonal conjugate is the only dimension of the superior strait (inlet) that can be obtained by vaginal examination. Its length is used to estimate the obstetric conjugate; it is 1.5 to 2 cm greater than the obstetric conjugate.
   c. The *obstetric conjugate* is the distance between the inner surface of the symphysis pubis slightly below its upper border and the sacral promontory. The obstetric conjugate determines whether the presenting part can enter the true pelvis because it is the smallest diameter. Therefore this diameter is the most important measurement of the inlet. Unfortunately, it can be obtained only by radiographic measurement or ultrasonography. The obstetric conjugate is estimated by subtracting 1.5 to 2 cm from the diagonal conjugate depending on the length and inclination of the symphysis pubis (Fig. 20.14).

Fig. 20.14
Estimation of length and inclination of symphysis pubis. (From Malasanos, L., et al.: Health assessment, ed. 2, St. Louis, 1981, The C.V. Mosby Co.)

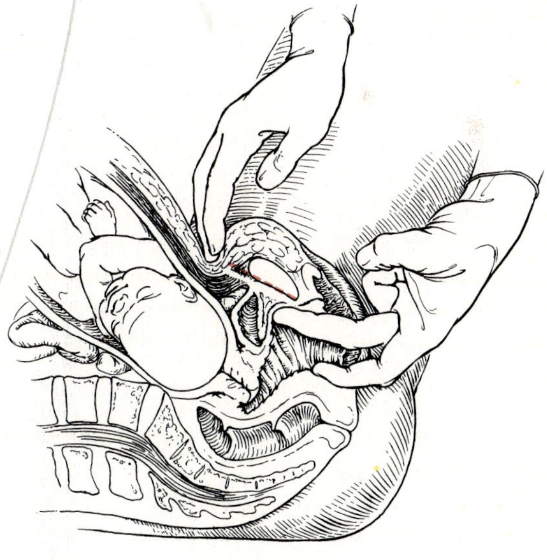

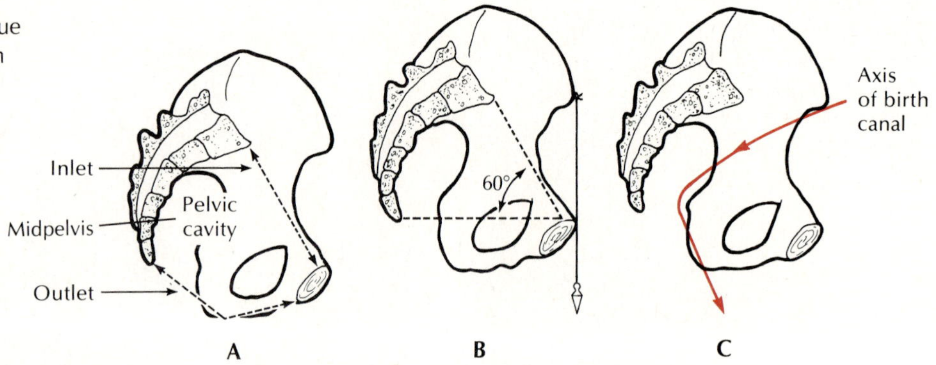

Fig. 20.15
Pelvic cavity. **A,** Cavity of true pelvis. Note curve of sacrum and tilt of pelvis posteriorly. **B,** Pelvic inclination with woman standing. **C,** Axis of birth canal.

2. The transverse diameter of the inlet (13.5 cm or more) is an important determinant in assessing the shape of the inlet (Fig. 20.10).
3. The oblique diameter (12.75 cm or larger) is directed from the sacroiliac joint on one side to the opposite iliopectineal prominence. The fetal head often enters the pelvis in the oblique diameter because the colon fills part of the left pelvis and the sacral promontory protrudes into the area of the transverse diameter.

The plane or inclination of the pelvic inlet (brim) normally describes an angle of approximately 60 degrees with the horizontal when the woman is standing (Fig. 20.15). The pelvic inclination, or tilt of the pelvis, measured by ultrasonograpy or computed tomography, is altered with exaggerated posture. Straightening the lumbar curve reduces the inclination, and increasing the curve increases pelvic inclination. Therefore good posture while standing or in the squatting position straightens out this curve somewhat. This inclination may greatly influence the progress of labor (see maternal position during labor, p. 411).

Midplane of the pelvis. The midplane of the pelvis normally contains the planes of greatest and shortest pelvic dimensions (Fig. 20.12):

1. Anteroposteriorly the greatest dimension is from midsymphysis to the sacrum at the fused second and third sacral vertebras. This measurement should be 12.75 cm or more.
2. Extending from the middle of the posterior borders of the ischial bones are the ischial spines. The distance between these spines (10.5 cm) represents the shortest transverse diameter of the true pelvic cavity. The ischial spines are the bony attachments for the pelvic floor muscles and are at the same level as the vaginal vault. They can be reached during vaginal examination (Fig. 20.16).

Fig. 20.16
Measurement of interspinous diameter. (From Malasanos, L., et al.: Health assessment, ed. 2, St. Louis, 1981, The C.V. Mosby Co.)

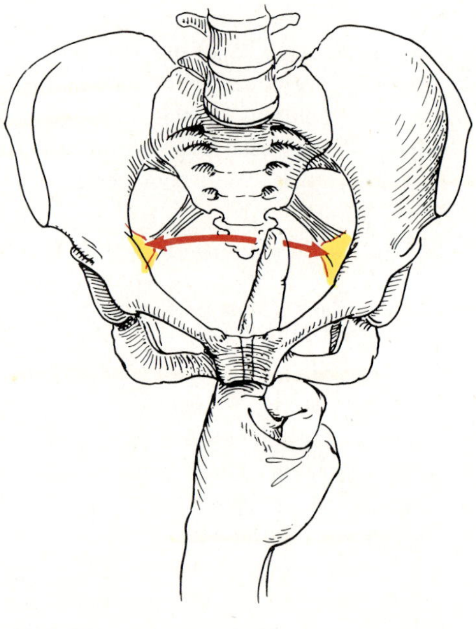

The ischial spines also serve as landmarks in determining station, or the level to which the presenting part of the fetus has descended into the pelvic cavity (see p. 386).

Although the midplane is comparatively large, critical shortening of any of these measurements of the midplane may cause pelvic dystocia.

Plane of pelvic outlet. The outlet presents the smallest plane of the pelvic canal (Figs. 20.11 and 20.12)

Fig. 20.17
Measurement of intertuberous diameter. **A,** Use of fist to estimate intertuberous diameter. Examiner knows the span of her or his own fist and estimates diameter accordingly. **B,** Use of Thom's pelvimeter to measure intertuberous diameter. (From Malasanos, L., et al.: Health assessment, ed. 2, St. Louis, 1981, The C.V. Mosby Co.)

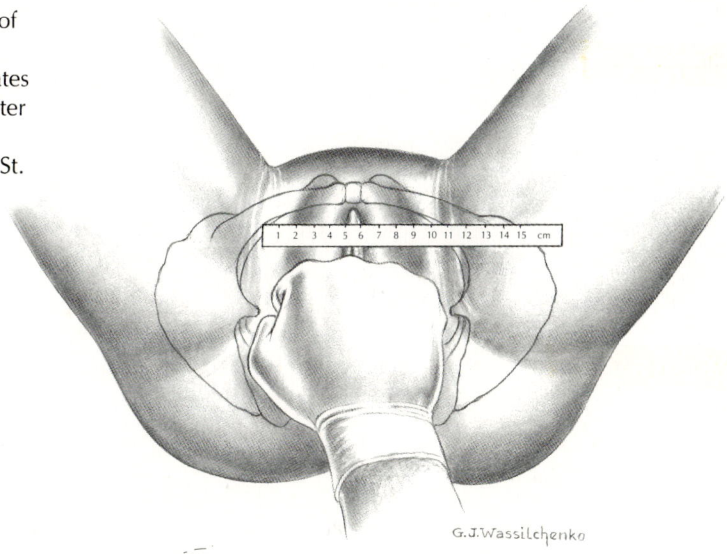

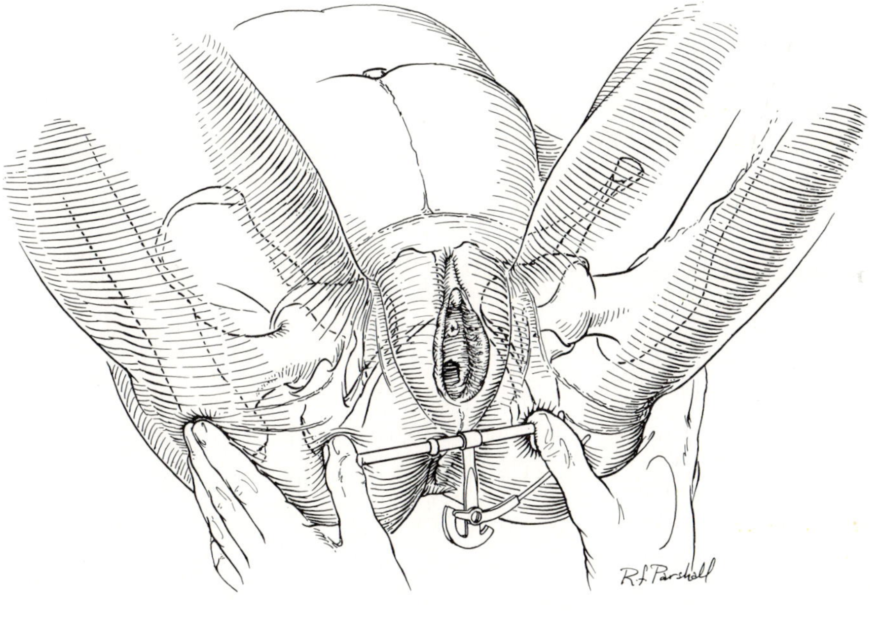

and is the easiest structure to evaluate. The significant diameters are as follows:

1. The *anteroposterior diameter* (about 11.9 cm) extends from the lower margin of the symphysis to the sacrococcygeal joint rather than the tip of the coccyx. The mobility of the never-damaged coccyx, because of the relaxation of the sacrococcygeal joint, permits its backward displacement during labor.
2. The *transverse* or *intertuberous diameter* of the outlet is measured from the inner border of one ischial tuberosity to the other (about 10 to 11 cm) (Fig. 20.17).
3. The *posterior sagittal diameter* (about 9 cm) of the outlet is projected from the tip of the sacrum to a point in space where the intertuberous diameter transects the anteroposterior projection.

A summary of obstetric measurements is given in Table 20.2.

The *subpubic angle,* which indicates the type of pubic arch, together with the length of the pubic rami and the intertuberous diameter, is of great importance. Because the presenting part must pass beneath the pubic arch, a narrow subpubic angle will be less favorable than a rounded, wide arch. Measurement of the subpubic arch is shown in Fig. 20.18. If the subpubic angle

Table 20.2
Obstetric Measurements

Plane of inlet (superior strait). The principal pelvic diameters of the plane of the inlet are as follows:		
Conjugates		
Diagonal	12.5-13.0 cm	From *inferior border* of SP* to sacral promontory
Obstetric: measurement that determines whether presenting part can engage or enter superior strait	1.5-2.0 cm greater than diagonal (radiographic)	From *posterior surface* of SP to sacral promontory
True (vera) (anteroposterior)	≥11.0 cm (12.5) (radiographic)	From *upper margin* of SP to sacral promontory
Transverse diameter	≥13.0 cm	Usually colon obscures this by filling left pelvis
Oblique diameter (R or L)	≥12.75 cm	From sacroiliac joint on one side to opposite iliopectineal prominence
Midplane of pelvis. The midplane of the pelvis normally is its largest plane and the one of greatest diameter.		
Anteroposterior	≥11.5 cm	From midsymphysis to sacrum (at fused second and third sacral vertebras)
Transverse (interspinous)	10.5 cm	Narrowest transverse diameter in normal pelvis
Posterior sagittal diameter	4.5 cm	Segment of anteroposterior diameter dorsal to line between ischial spines; although midplane is comparatively large, critical shortening of interspinous or posterior sagittal diameter of midplane may cause pelvic dystocia
Plane of pelvic outlet. The outlet presents the smallest plane of the pelvic canal. It encompasses an area including the lower portion of the symphysis pubis, the ischial tuberosities, and the tip of the sacrum. The significant diameters are as follows:		
Anteroposterior diameter	11.9 cm	From lower border of SP to tip of sacrum; coccyx may be displaced posteriorly during labor and is not considered to be a fixed bone
Transverse diameter	≥8.0 cm	From inner border of one ischial tuberosity to other
Posterior sagittal diameter	9.0 cm	Projected from tip of sacrum to a point in space where intertuberous diameter transects anteroposterior projection

*Symphysis pubis.

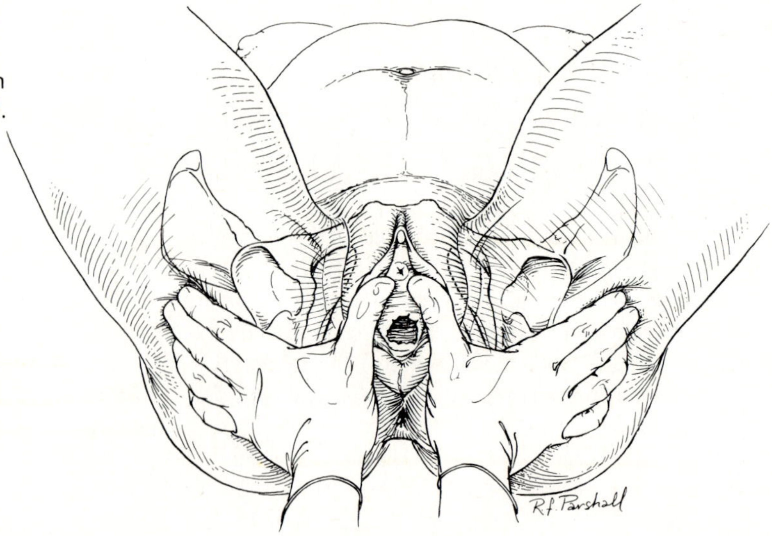

Fig. 20.18
Estimation of angle of subpubic arch. Using both thumbs, examiner externally traces descending rami down to tuberosities. (From Malasanos, L., et al.: Health assessment, ed. 2, St. Louis, 1981, The C.V. Mosby Co.)

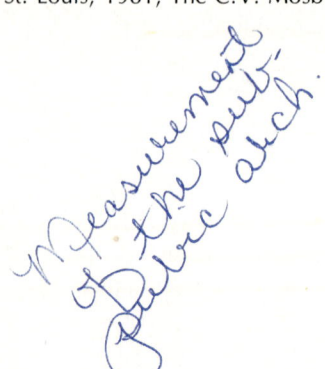

Fig. 20.19
X-ray pelvimetry chart. (Courtesy Picker Corporation, Cleveland.)

◄— Anteroposterior Diameters*

X-RAY PELVIMETRY CHART

(Colcher-Sussman Technique)

Transverse Diameters* —►

*Centimeter rule markings from the films are transferred to the sides of the chart. The sides of the chart then become actual ruler.

(Date)________________ 19____

Name:________________________________

Age________

Referring Physician:________________________________

Due Date:________

Para. 0. 1. 2. 3. ____

INTERSECTING DIAMETERS

Three levels embody all salient bony landmarks of the true pelvis.

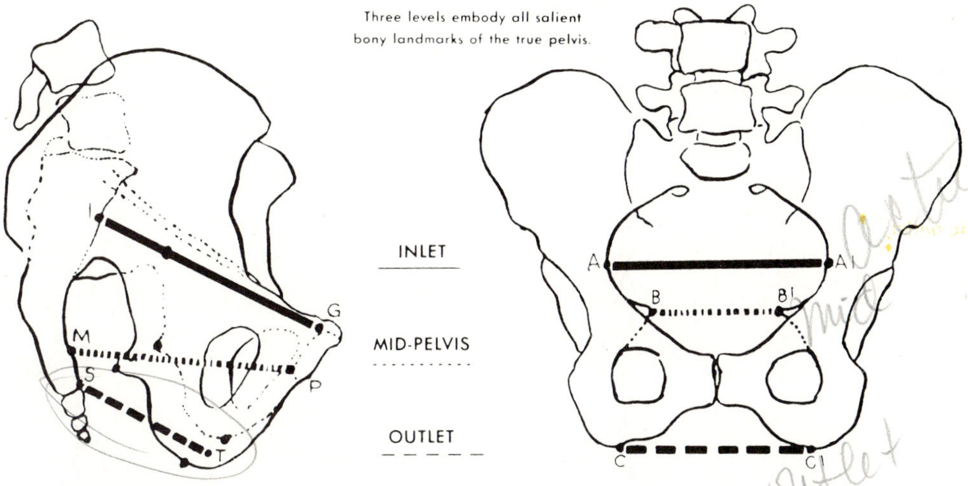

DIAMETERS				TOTAL	AVERAGE NORMAL	AVERAGE TOTAL	LOW NORMAL
ACTUAL INLET	Anteroposterior	I to G			12.5	25.5	22.0
	Transverse	A to A¹			13.0		
MID-PELVIS	Anteroposterior	M to P			11.5	22.0	20.0
	Transverse (Bispinous)	B to B¹			10.5		
OUTLET	Anteroposterior (Post. Sagittal)	S to T			7.5	18.0	16.0
	Transverse (Bituberal)	C to C¹			10.5		

FETAL HEAD — Anteroposterior View: Longest Diameter________ Shortest Diameter________ Average (10cm)________
Lateral View: Longest Diameter________ Shortest Diameter________

Position of Fetal Head:
Position of Fetal Spine:
Location of Vertex:
Moulding of Fetal Head:

Separation of Symphysis:
Coccyx:
Sacrum:
Sub-Pubic Angle: (75°)

SHAPE OF INLET

○ ROUND ⬭ FLAT
0 OVAL ♡ HEART

Remarks:

____
Roentgenologist

PICKER CORPORATION CLEVELAND, OHIO

Printed in U.S.A.

is narrow, the fetal head, for example, is forced backward toward the coccyx, and the extension of the head may be difficult. The result is known as *outlet dystocia* (difficult labor at the pelvic outlet). Forceps delivery frequently is required, and fetal injury or deep maternal lacerations may result.

Descent of the fetus through the birth canal follows an orderly process (see p. 388). Generally the fetal head (usually presenting first) enters the inlet to the true pelvis in transverse fashion. Descent continues in a slightly backward and downward direction to the ischial spines.

An almost right-angled anterior turn occurs in the birth canal at the ischial spines. When the head turns to pass between the ischial spines, it contacts the forward-sloping pelvic floor musculature and sacrum and is generally directed forward and downward (Fig. 20.5). The fetal head thus is guided into the direction of the pelvic outlet and the vagina.

The obstetric measurements are organized into a pelvimetry chart that can be utilized for a rapid evaluation of the maternal pelvis (Fig. 20.19).

Classification of pelves. The four basic types of pelves are as follows (see also Fig. 6.20):

1. Gynecoid (the classic female type)
2. Anthropoid (resembling the pelvis of anthropoid apes)
3. Platypelloid (the flat pelvis)
4. Android (resembling the male pelvis)

Major gynecoid pelvic features can be expected in about half of all pregnant women; significant anthropoid features will be present in slightly less than one fourth of gravidas; android configuration will affect almost one fifth of pregnant women; and the small remainder of gravidas will have a platypelloid pelvis. Examples of pelvic variations or mixed types are given in Fig. 20.20.

The *gynecoid pelvis* is the most favorable for normal

Fig. 20.20
Female pelves; pure and mixed types. Note differences in shape of inlets.

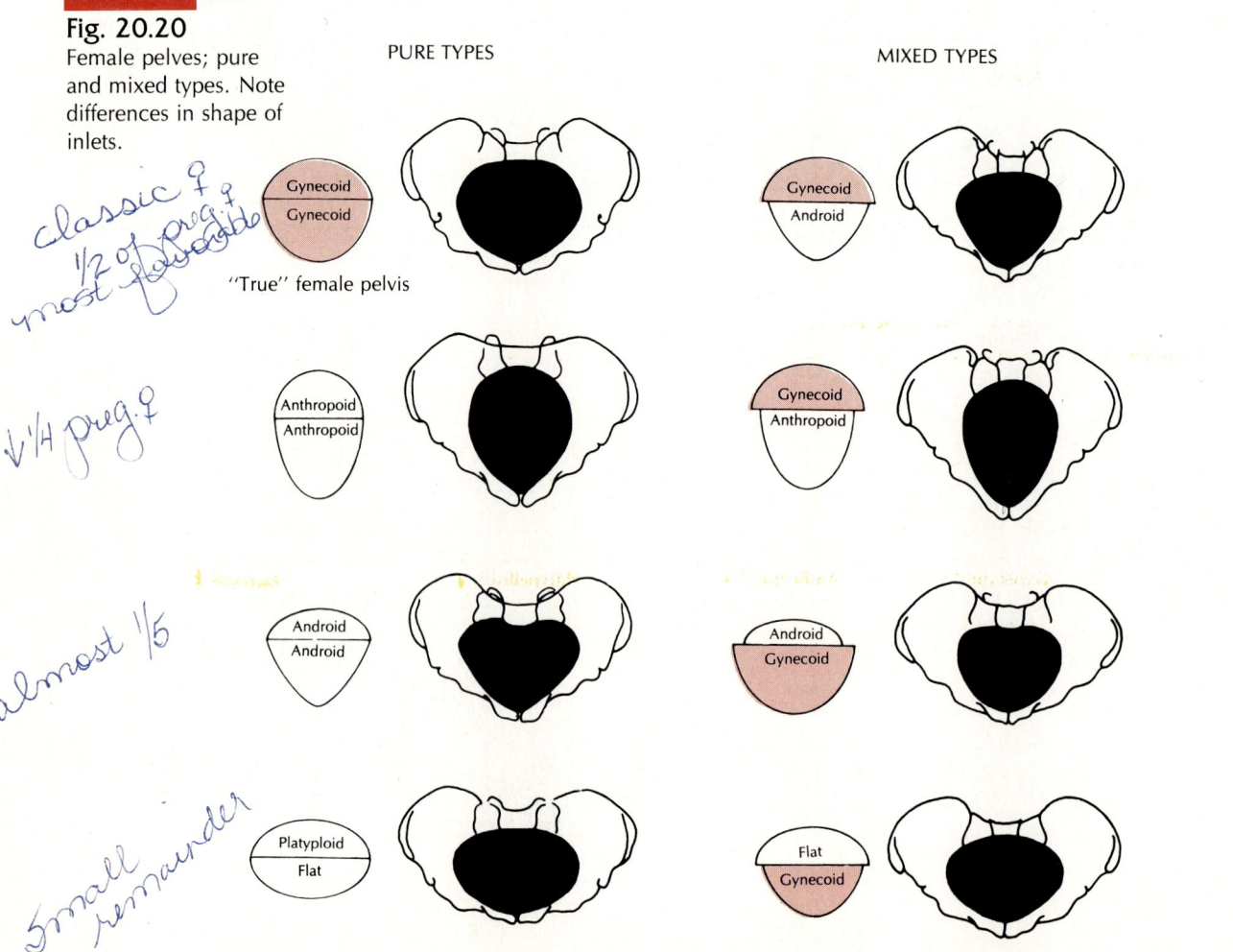

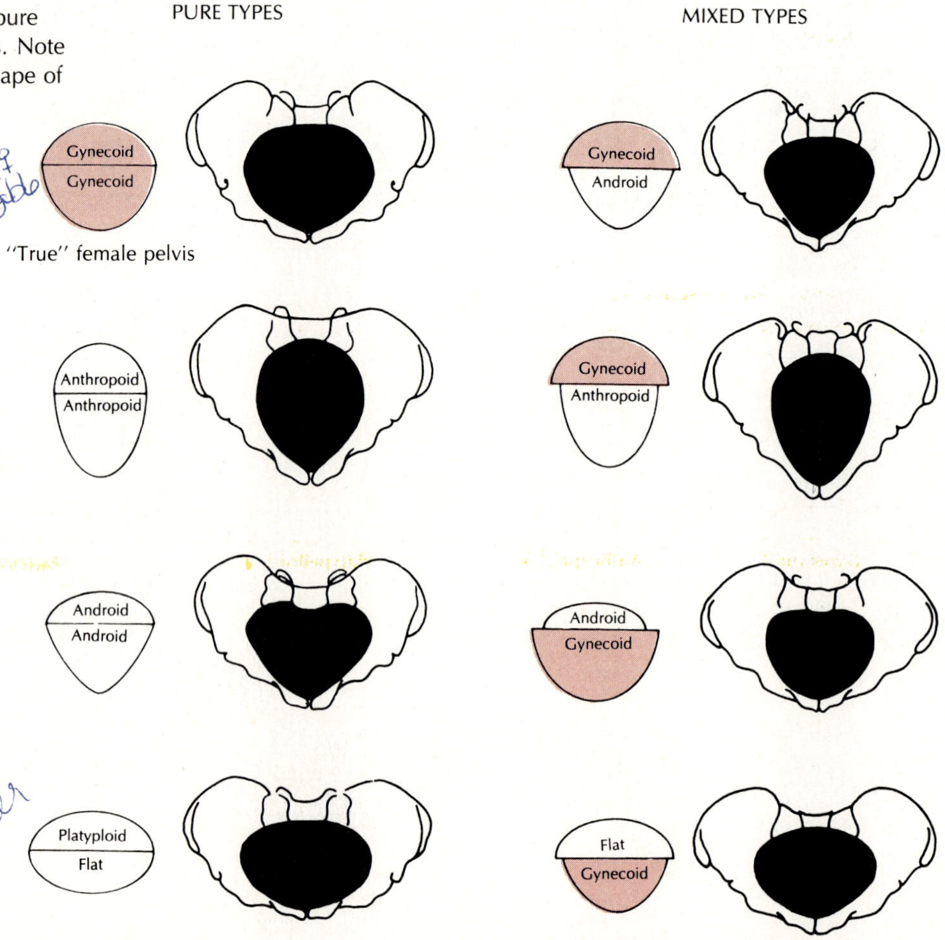

delivery. Engagement usually is in the transverse or oblique diameter, descent is rapid, rotation occurs in the midpelvis, and delivery of the vertex in an occiput anterior position (OA) often occurs spontaneously. The "female" gynecoid pelvis is compared to other pelvic types as to characteristics and usual type of delivery each necessitates (Table 20.3).

Implications for nursing care. The examination of the bony pelvis can be uncomfortable for the gravida (see procedure, p. 373). It should be done after the internal examination of the soft pelvic organs. The preparation of the woman includes an explanation of the procedure, a request for her to empty her bladder, coaching her for relaxation, and maintaining eye contact with her whenever possible.

Whenever the woman is in a supine position for a procedure, place a pillow under her head and ask her to flex her knees. Drape her as necessary. Offer her the option of a mirror to view her perineum and vaginal vault during the examination while explaining to her what is occurring.

If she shows signs of supine hypotension or the vagal nerve reflex (see p. 411) (e.g., she becomes pale, breathless, and faint, and her skin becomes clammy), turn her onto her left side to relieve the signs and symptoms.

Soft tissues. The soft tissues of the passage include the distensible lower uterine segment, cervix, and vaginal canal.

Before labor begins, the uterus is composed of the uterine body (corpus) and cervix. After labor has begun, the uterine contractions cause the uterine body to differentiate into a thick and muscular upper segment and a thin-walled passive muscular tube, the lower segment. A physiologic retraction ring separates the two (Fig. 20.21). The lower uterine segment gradually distends to accommodate the intrauterine contents as the walls of the upper segment become thicker and its content is reduced.

The downward pressure caused by contraction of the fundus is transmitted to the cervix, and it effaces and dilates sufficiently to allow descent of the presenting part into the vagina. Actually, the cervix is drawn upward and over the presenting part as the vertex or breech descends.

The vagina in turn distends to permit passage of the fetus into the external world. As noted earlier, the soft tissues of the vagina develop throughout pregnancy until at term the vagina can dilate to accommodate the fetus.

Implications for nursing care. Women who do not realize the extent of this distensibility may be fearful of the fetus's "tearing them" to emerge. It may relieve the woman's apprehension to remind her that the vagina has expanded considerably since the initial examination from a size that only accommodated the speculum to one that will accommodate the examiner's entire hand. The rugae of the vagina become smooth, and the surface enlarges, similar to the spreading out of a piece of corrugated paper.

THE POWERS

The forces acting to expel the fetus and placenta are derived from three sources:

1. Involuntary uterine contractions
2. Voluntary bearing-down efforts
3. Contraction of the levator ani muscles

Table 20.3
Comparison of Pelvic Types

	Gynecoid	Anthropoid	Platypelloid	Android
Brim	Slightly ovoid or transversely rounded	Oval, wider anteroposteriorly	Flattened anteroposteriorly, wide transversely	Heart shaped, angulated
Depth	Moderate	Deep	Shallow	Deep
Side walls	Straight	Straight	Straight	Convergent
Ischial spines	Blunt, somewhat widely separated	Prominent, often with narrow interspinous diameter	Blunted, widely separated	Prominent, narrow interspinous diameter
Sacrum	Deep, curved	Slightly curved	Slightly curved	Slightly curved, terminal portion often beaked
Subpubic arch	Wide	Narrow	Wide	Narrow
Usual mode of delivery	Vaginal Spontaneous OA position	Vaginal Forceps/spontaneous OP or OA position	Vaginal Spontaneous	Cesarean Difficult vaginal, with forceps

Fig. 20.21
Progressive development of segments and rings of uterus at term. Note comparison between nonpregnant uterus, **A,** uterus at term, **B,** and uterus in normal labor in early first stage, **C,** and second stage, **D.** Passive segment is derived from lower uterine segment (isthmus) and cervix, and physiologic retraction ring is derived from anatomic internal os. **E,** Uterus in abnormal labor in second-stage dystocia. Pathologic retraction (Bandl's) ring that forms under abnormal conditions develops from physiologic ring. (Adapted from Willson, J.R., and Carrington, E.R.: Obstetrics and gynecology, ed. 6, St. Louis, 1979, The C.V. Mosby Co.)

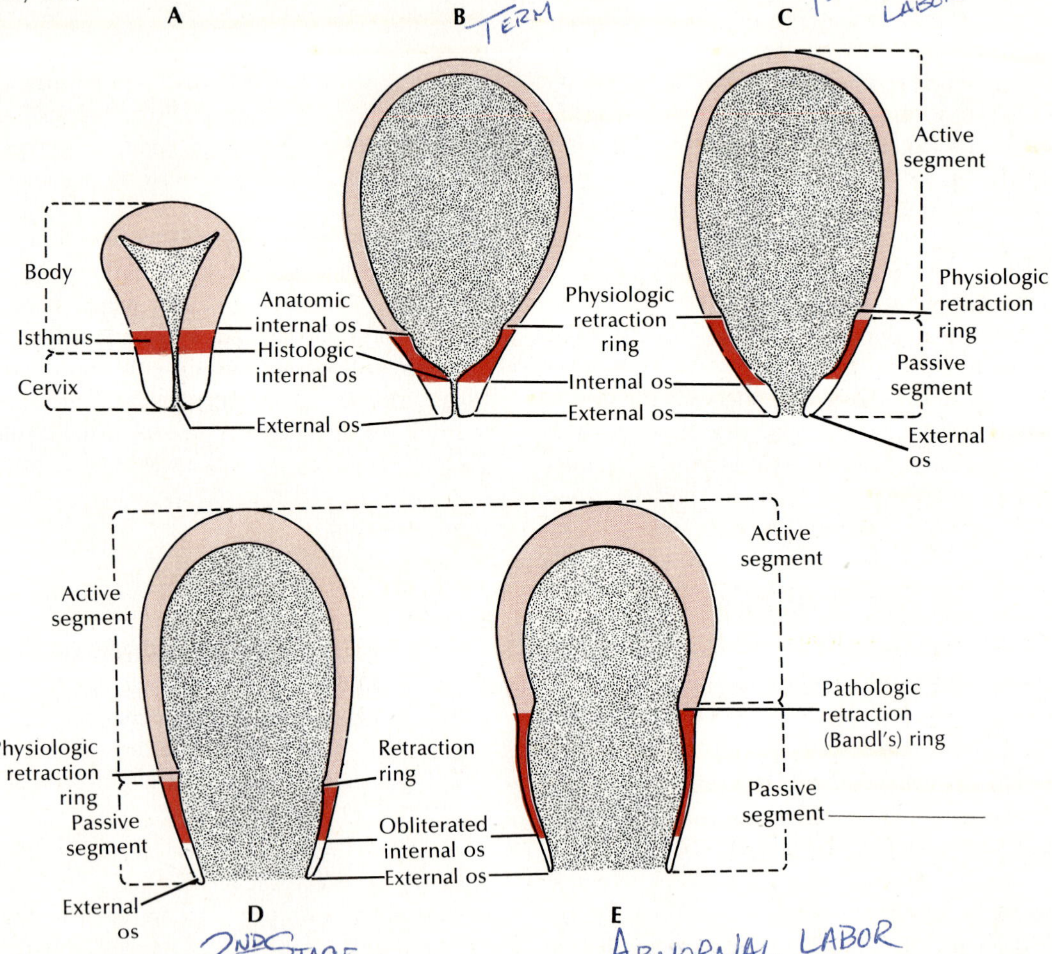

Uterine contractions. Uterine contractions (primary powers) are involuntary. This is attested to by the observations that paraplegics can deliver vaginally and that uterine action is not stopped by use of spinal anesthesia. However, certain events act to inhibit uterine contractions. For example, women in active labor find that once they are admitted to the hospital, the labor may cease for a short time because of the emotional impact of coming to the hospital or that active labor can be interrupted briefly after analgesia or anesthesia is administered.

Description of uterine contractions. In describing a uterine contraction (Fig. 20.22), reference is made to the following characteristics:

1. *Frequency.* Contractions occur intermittently throughout labor. They begin at about 20 to 30 minutes apart and become closer together until, at the height of the expulsive efforts, they are as frequent as every 2 to 3 minutes.
2. *Regularity.* Contractions occur more and more regularly as labor becomes well established.
3. *Duration.* The length of time a contraction lasts increases from 30 seconds to between 60 and 90 seconds near full dilatation of the cervix. Then the duration becomes about 60 seconds until delivery of the fetus is accomplished.
4. *Intensity.* The strength of the contraction also increases as labor progresses, from weak contrac-

Fig. 20.22
A, Changes in abdominal contour before and during uterine contraction. **B,** Assessing contractions: frequency in minutes—interval from beginning of one contraction to beginning of next; duration in seconds—how long contraction lasts (e.g., 45 seconds); regularity—whether intervals are same length or uneven lengths (e.g., every 4 minutes [regular] or every 4 to 7 minutes [irregular]); intensity—how strong contraction is (e.g., strong, moderate, weak). Length of relaxation period is rarely recorded. *Red line,* Some practitioners assess interval between contractions from acme of one contraction to acme of the next.

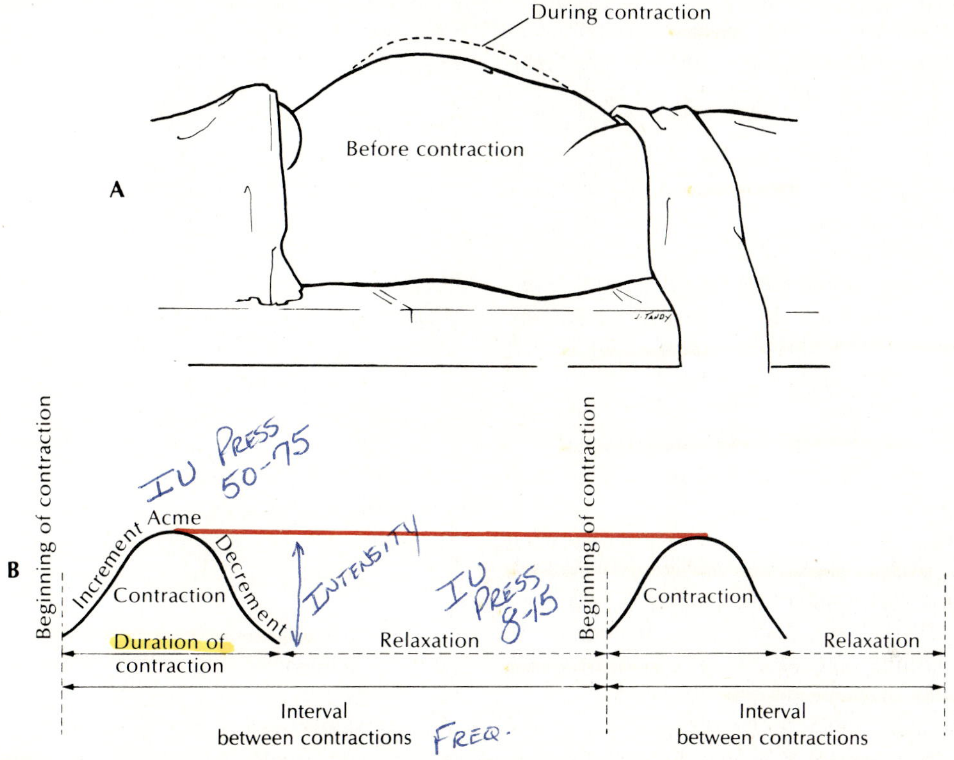

tions noted early in labor to strong expulsive contractions (intrauterine pressure measured at 50 to 75 mm Hg) evidenced near the time of delivery.*

Each contraction exhibits a wavelike pattern; it begins with a slower increment, gradually reaches an acme, and then diminishes rather rapidly (decrement). Next there is an interval of rest (intrauterine pressure is 8 to 15 mm Hg), which is broken when the next contraction begins. Contractions that have been augmented by administration of oxytocin tend to increase more rapidly. Women describe them as sharper, harder, and more uncomfortable contractions.

*Uterine contractions are measured in Montevideo units in some parts of the United States; the intensity of the contractions is measured in total mm Hg per 10 minutes. Until the thirtieth week of pregnancy, contractions are fewer than 20 Montevideo units. Contractions increase thereafter from 30 to 80 Montevideo units as pregnancy approaches term. During early labor, uterine activity averages 80 to 120 Montevideo units. Near the end of labor (five contractions per 10 minutes) the average of 250 Montevideo units is reached.

Assessment of uterine contractions. There are three methods of assessing contractions. The first is the subjective description given by the woman; the second, palpation and timing by a nurse or physician; and the third, use of electronic monitoring devices.

When the woman reports that contractions have begun, she is asked, ''When did they start? How often are they coming? Are they coming regularly? Would you say they are weak or strong?'' Depending on the woman's knowledge, her answers can be definite or vague, but they serve as a basis for deciding whether she should be admitted to the hospital.

The second method is used routinely throughout labor by the attending nurse. Palpations are done by using the fingertips, not the palmar surface, and the fingers must be kept moving. The uterus begins to contract in the fundal portion, and as the contraction proceeds, the uterus is less easily indented; at the height of the contraction, the uterus feels very firm or even hard. Then as the contraction diminishes, the fingers can again indent the uterine surface. The woman is not aware of the sensation of the uterus's contracting until the contraction is fairly well established. Frequently, her description of the end of the contraction is related to the end of the pain sensation (felt in the lower portion of the uterus, not the fundus), and this can remain after the contraction is completed. Therefore her description may not be as accurate as that obtained by the nurse.

External monitoring devices measure the frequency and duration of the contractions. Internal monitors measure these factors and also the strength of contractions. The findings are automatically recorded by the machine (see Chapter 24).

Voluntary bearing-down efforts. As soon as the presenting part reaches the pelvic floor, the woman experiences an urge to push, a voluntary bearing-down effort (secondary power). The bearing-down effort is similar to that used in the process of defecation. However, a different set of muscles is used; the parturient contracts her diaphragm and abdominal muscles and pushes out the contents of the birth canal (see Chapters 19 and 22 for instructions for the woman). Bearing-down results in increased intraabdominal pressure. The pressure compresses the uterus on all sides and adds to the power of the expulsive forces.

Implications for nursing care. This bearing-down reflex must be held in check until full cervical dilatation (10 cm). If this is disregarded, the cervix can be bruised and traumatized as it is forced against the symphysis pubis during pushing. The result may be cervical edema due to chronic passive congestion. The edema can act to delay cervical dilatation and predisposes the cervix to laceration. However, the woman can control the urge to push by taking panting breaths similar to blowing out candles. These expulsive reflexes are diminished or lost with anesthesia (Chapter 25), but the woman can be told when to push with a contraction so that delivery is not impeded (see Chapters 19 and 22).

THE PLACENTA

Since the ovum usually implants in the fundal portion of the uterus, the developed placenta rarely acts as an impediment to labor. When implantation takes place in the lower uterine segment, the placenta may cover part of all of the internal cervical os to act as a barrier to birth of the fetus. This condition, known as *placenta previa,* and other placental problems necessitate medical intervention (see Chapter 35).

PSYCHOLOGIC RESPONSE

Women who are relaxed, knowledgeable, and capable of actively participating in the control of the birth process usually experience shorter, less intense labors. Preparation-for-childbirth classes are based on such premises (see Chapter 19).

Techniques for Assessment

Provisional determination of fetal presentation, position, and descent may be made by the following techniques:

1. External palpation after the sixth month of pregnancy
2. Identification of the location of the maximal intensity of the fetal heart rate (FHR) through auscultation
3. Vaginal examination

Certain confirmation of fetal presentation or position and the maternal pelvis is possible with the following:

1. Conventional x-ray films (radiographic pelvimetry), which are not recommended because of danger to the fetus, fetal gonads, and maternal gonads
2. Computed tomography
3. Ultrasonography

ABDOMINAL PALPATION

Use of the four maneuvers of Leopold provides a systematic examination (Fig. 20.23). Proficiency in determining presentation and position by abdominal palpation requires considerable practice, and thus every learning opportunity must be utilized. Gross maternal obesity, excessive amniotic fluid (hydramnios), or tumors may make it hard to feel the fetal contours.

Abdominal palpation is done as follows: The woman empties her bladder before the examination is begun and lies on her back with one pillow under her head and her knees slightly flexed. The examiner stands facing the woman on her right if she or he is right-handed (and vice versa if left-handed). The examiner keeps the following assessment in mind while carrying out the procedure:

1. Is there one fetus or more than one?
2. What is the presentation (lie)?
3. What is the position?
4. Is the presenting part engaged?
5. Is there fetal movement?
6. Do the uterine size and fundal height correspond with the due date (expected date of confinement [EDC]) according to MacDonald's rule (see p. 277)?
7. Is there any indication of uterine, pelvic, or fetal abnormality?

Fig. 20.23

Leopold's maneuvers. Palpation as in left occiput anterior position. For **A** to **C,** examiner faces woman's head. For **D,** examiner faces woman's feet. **A,** Palpation of superior pole. **B,** Palpation of fetal back and small parts. **C,** Assessment of presenting part: cephalic prominence, flexion, and engagement. **D,** Palpation of cephalic prominence to determine attitude.

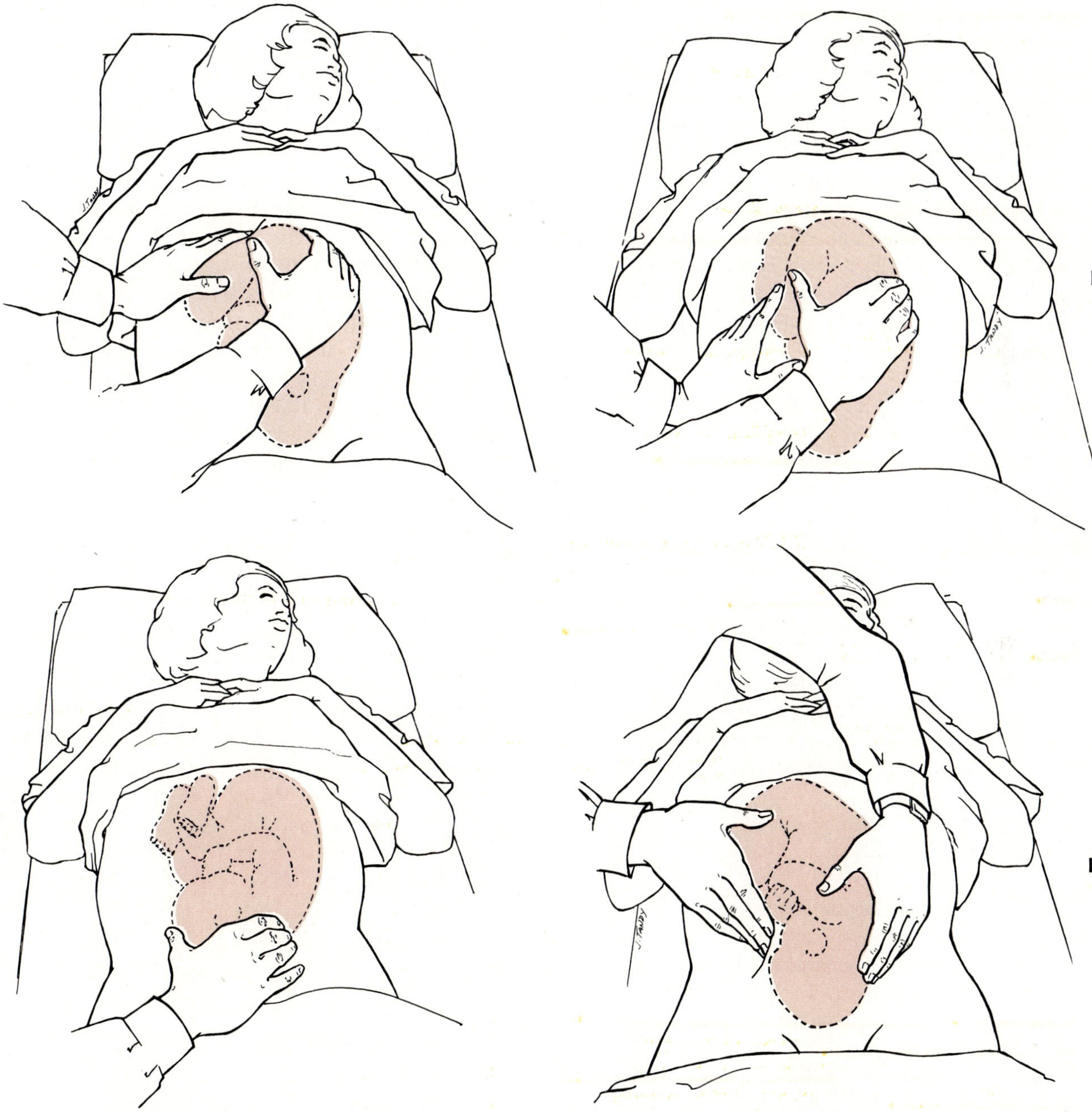

Leopold's maneuvers are as follows:

1. The fetal part that occupies the fundus of the uterus is identified first. The head feels round, firm, freely movable, and palpable by ballottement; the breech feels less regular and softer (Fig. 20.23, *A*).

2. The back is then identified by using the palmar surface of the hand to note a smooth convex contour anteriorly or to one side. The fetal ventral (front) surface is concave and soft, and the small parts (feet, hands, elbows) are irregularities felt on the side opposite the back (Fig. 20.23, *B*).

3. The examiner should next determine with the right

hand which fetal part is presenting over the inlet to the true pelvis. This is done by gently grasping the lower pole of the uterus between the thumb and fingers and pressing in slightly. If the fetus is at term, the rounded head presents, and if it is not engaged, it may be rocked gently from side to side (Fig. 20.23, *C*).

If the presenting part is not engaged, the next step is to determine the attitude of the head. If the cephalic prominence is found on the same side as the small parts, the head must be flexed; this is a vertex presentation. If the cephalic prominence is on the same side as the back, the presenting head is extended.

If the presenting part has entered the pelvis, the maneuver also determines whether or not the presenting part is fixed in the pelvis (engaged).

4. Finally, the degree of descent is estimated. To do this, the examiner faces the woman's feet and uses both hands (Fig. 20.23, *D*). When the presenting part has descended deeply, only a small portion of it may be outlined.

2. AUSCULTATION

The area of maximal intensity of the FHR (i.e., the location of the maternal abdomen where the FHR sounds the loudest) is an aid in determining the fetal position (Fig. 20.24). For example, in vertex and breech presentations, FHRs are best heard through the back of the fetus. In face presentations, however, FHRs generally are loudest when transmitted through the fetal chest.

In vertex presentations FHRs commonly are heard below the mother's umbilicus in a lower quadrant of the abdomen (Fig. 20.24, *B*), but in breech presentation they are heard above the level of the umbilicus (Fig. 20.24, *A*).

3. VAGINAL EXAMINATION

The vaginal examination has virtually replaced the rectal examination because clinical studies have indicated that there is not a significant increase in infection with vaginal examinations. The vaginal examination is more accurate in determining the condition, effacement, and dilatation of the cervix. It is less painful and requires less manipulation. Prolapse of the cord and compound presentations (e.g., the hand presenting alongside the fetal head) can be detected more readily.

The examination must be done carefully, gently, and under aseptic conditions. Sterile gloves are used, as well as an antiseptic solution.* For the first examination in labor, sterile water can be used as a solution to lubricate the fingers, because lubricants can alter the response of the phenaphthazine (Nitrazine Paper) (see page 397) used to diagnose rupture of membranes.

Vaginal examinations must never by performed by a nurse if bleeding (as distinguished from bloody show) is present because the examination could exacerbate the bleeding (puncturing the placenta), thereby endangering both mother and fetus. If bleeding is copious, the physician may do the vaginal examination in the operating room so that a cesarean delivery can be performed immediately if necessary (see discussion of double set-up, p. 793).

The woman lies in a supine position. If the supine position is contraindicated, a small rolled towel under her right hip will keep the uterus off the inferior vena cava and aorta and not affect the examination. A pillow is placed under her head, her knees are slightly flexed and separated (the lithotomy position), and she is suitably draped. While the woman is being positioned, she is told that she is to be examined internally to assess her progress and that although the procedure may be uncomfortable, it should not be painful.

The examining hand is then gloved, and the other hand may be placed on the abdomen to steady the fetus

Fig. 20.24
Areas of maximal intensity of FHR for differing positions: *RSA,* right sacrum anterior; *ROP,* right occiput posterior; *RMA,* right mentum anterior; *ROA,* right occiput anterior; *LSA,* left sacrum anterior; *LOP,* left occiput posterior; *LMA,* left mentum anterior; and *LOA,* left occiput anterior. **A,** Presentation is *breech* if FHR is heard *above* umbilicus. **B,** Presentation is *vertex* if FHR is heard *below* umbilicus.

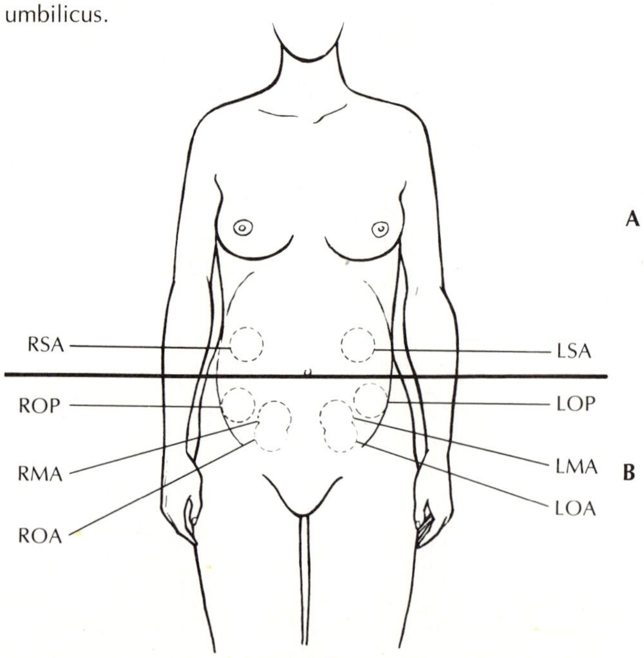

*The nurse assesses for known allergy to iodine because Betadine is usually used.

and to exert a gentle downward pressure, which applies the presenting part more closely to the cervix. The index and middle fingers are introduced into the vagina. Discomfort is less if the examining fingers are directed with the palmar surface downward so that the initial pressure is directed toward the less sensitive posterior vaginal wall. Then the fingers may be rotated. Assessment consists of answering the following questions:

1. Is the cervix soft or firm? What is the degree of effacement and dilatation of the cervical os?
2. Are the membranes intact? If so, are they bulging through the cervical os?
3. What is the presentation: vertex, breech, or other (e.g., hand, face)?
4. What is the position? If the vertex presents, the sagittal suture is located and traced to the posterior fontanel (triangle shaped) if the head is well flexed (Fig. 20.25) or to the anterior fontanel (diamond shaped) if the head is extended. Once the fontanel is located, its position must be determined in relation to the quadrants of the mother's pelvis. The most common position is the left occiput anterior (LOA) (i.e., the fetal occiput [O] is located on the mother's left [L] and anterior [A] or front part of her pelvis. In this position the fetus is facing toward the mother's right and back).
5. What is the station?
6. How well is the presenting part applied against the cervix?

To accomplish the foregoing assessment, the nurse must understand the following terms in addition to those related to presentation and position.

Effacement of the cervix. Effacement of the cervix means the shortening and thinning of the cervix during the first stage of labor. The cervix, normally 2 to 3 cm in length and about 1 cm thick, is obliterated or "taken up" by a shortening of the uterine muscle bundles during the thinning of the lower uterine segment in advancing labor. Eventually only a thin edge of the cervix can be palpated when effacement is complete. Effacement generally is advanced in primigravidas at term before more than slight dilatation occurs. In multiparas, effacement and dilatation of the cervix tend to progress together. Degree of effacement is expressed in percentages (e.g., a cervix that is 50% effaced) (Fig. 20.26).

Dilatation of the cervix. Dilatation of the cervix is the enlagement or widening of the cervical os and the cervical canal during the first stage of labor. The diameter increases from perhaps less than 1 cm to approximately 10 cm to allow delivery of a term fetus. When the cervix is fully dilated (and completely retracted), it can no longer be palpated (Figs. 20.26 and 20.27).

Dilatation of the cervix is involuntary and occurs by the drawing upward of the musculofibrous components of the cervix with strong uterine contractions. Pressure exerted by the amniotic fluid while the membranes are intact or force applied by the presenting part also encourages cervical dilatation. Scarring of the cervix as a result of infection or surgery may retard cervical dilatation.

Voluntary bearing-down efforts by the woman are counterproductive to cervical dilatation. Straining will exhaust the woman and cause cervical trauma (p. 382).

Fig. 20.25
Vaginal palpation of sagittal suture line. Note position of hand: two fingers are introduced into vagina and thumb rests on symphysis pubic externally. The other fingers are kept curled and away from the anus.

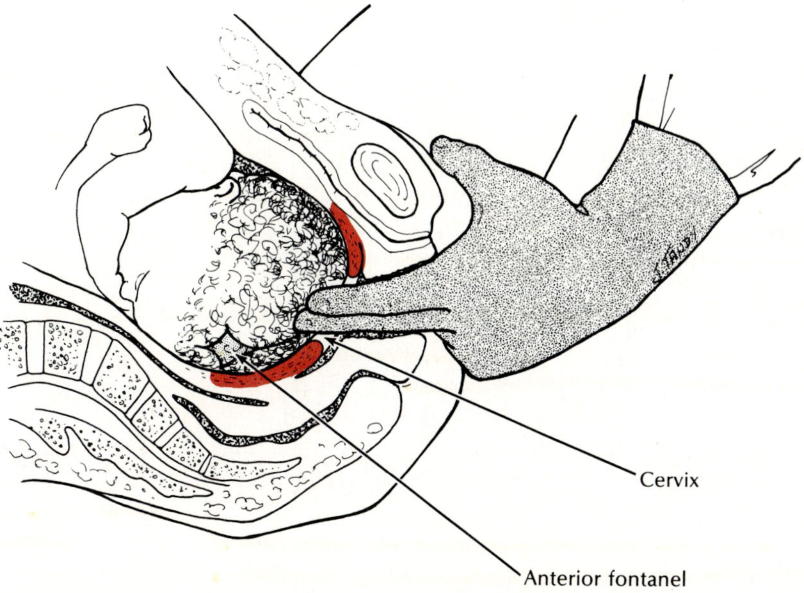

Fig. 20.26
Cervical effacement and dilatation. Note how cervix is drawn up around presenting part (internal os). Membranes are intact, and head is not well applied to cervix. **A,** Before labor. **B,** Early effacement. **C,** Complete effacement (100%). **D,** Complete dilatation (10 cm). NOTE: Membranes are intact, and head is *not* well applied to the cervix.

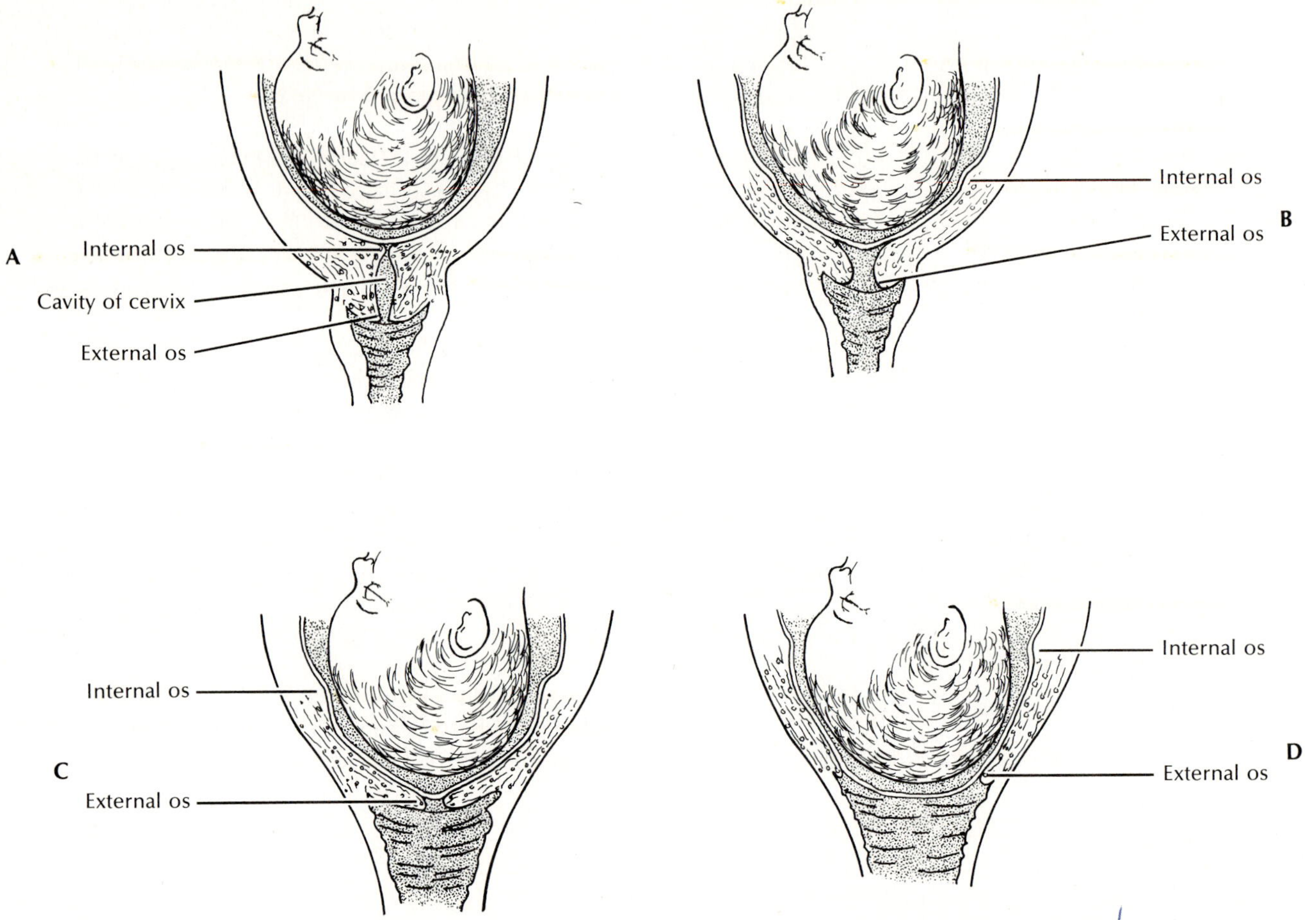

Station. Progress in the descent of the presenting part is determined by vaginal examination until the presenting part can be seen at the introitus. The level of the ischial spines is considered to be station 0, and the position of the head (the bony prominence, not the edematous scalp or caput), or the fetal sacrum with a breech presentation, is described in centimeters minus (above the spines) or plus (below the spines) (Fig. 20.28). In a vertex position the presenting part is definitely engaged when the biparietal diameter of the fetal skull has passed the inlet. At this time the palpable portion of the presenting part is below the level of the spines.

The speed of descent increases in the second stage of labor. In nulliparas this descent is slow but steady; in multiparas the descent may be very rapid.

CONVENTIONAL X-RAY FILMS

Conventional x-ray films expose the fetus to radiation in an amount that has been implicated in a small but significant risk of childhood cancer. Therefore this method of internal assessment is used with great caution. (See also Chapter 17.)

COMPUTED TOMOGRAPHY

Computed tomography (CT) is relatively new to obstetrics. It can determine whether a woman's pelvis is wide enough to permit vaginal delivery more accurately and with 97% less radiation to the fetus and the mother's ovaries than conventional film pelvimetry. CT pelvimetry uses digital radiographs, which means that the

Fig. 20.27
Aid for visualization of cervical dilatation. Cervical dilatation of 1 cm usually admits one finger; 3 cm dilatation usually admits 2 fingers.

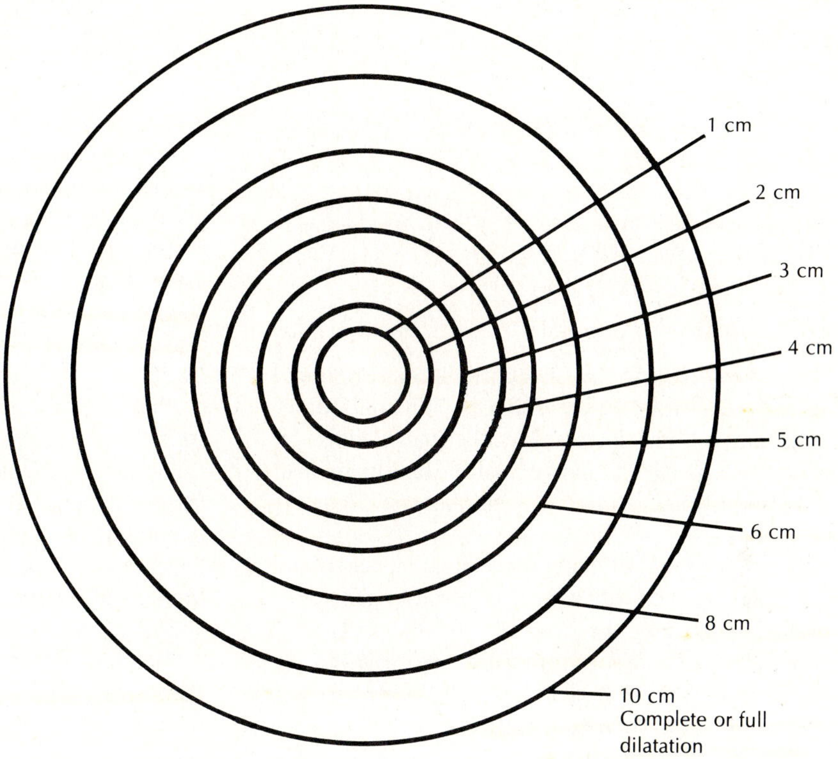

Fig. 20.28
Location of presenting part in relation to level of ischial spines is designated *station* and indicates degree of descent of presenting part through pelvis. Head is *engaged* when biparietal diameter is at inlet. When head is engaged, palpable portion of fetal head may be below station 0, approximately at station +2, depending on degree of molding.

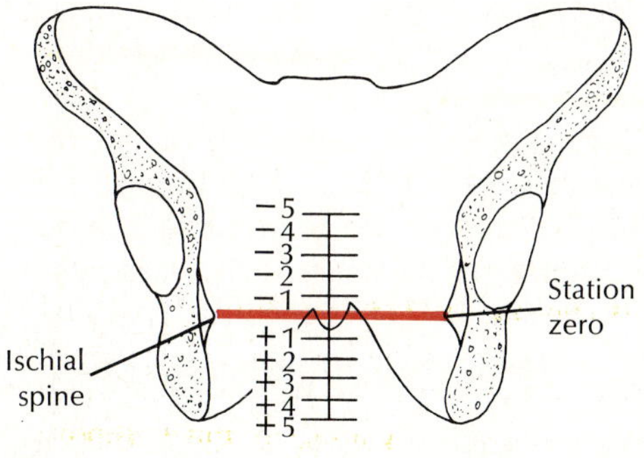

image is not printed out on film but is stored in numerical form in a computer.

ULTRASONOGRAPHY

Ultrasonography is discussed on pp. 152 and 281.

Process of Labor

CHANGES PRELIMINARY TO ONSET OF LABOR (PRODROMAL LABOR)

The head descends into the pelvis in most primigravidas 2 to 3 weeks before delivery. With this descent (lightening), some increased pelvic and bladder pressure is noted, but the mother can breathe more easily. In multigravidas, descent and the onset of labor often coincide.

Before the onset of labor, the vaginal mucus becomes more profuse, and a brownish or blood-tinged cervical mucous plug may be passed. Streaks of blood or brownish secretion (bloody show) may be noted. Frequently this type of discharge is noted within 48 hours after a vaginal examination or coitus.

Persistent low backache may be described, and occasionally strong, frequent, but irregular uterine contractions may be identified by the woman.

The cervix becomes soft, partially effaced, or dilated. The membranes may rupture spontaneously.

ONSET OF LABOR

The onset of labor cannot be ascribed to a single cause; multiple factors, including changes in the maternal uterus, cervix, and pituitary, are involved. Hormones produced by the normal fetal hypothalamus, pituitary, and adrenal cortex probably contribute to the initiation of labor. Progressive uterine distention, increasing intrauterine pressure, and aging of the placenta resulting in changing concentrations of estrogen, progesterone, and prostaglandins seem to be associated with increasing myometrial irritability. In actuality, many factors may be responsible for initiating labor and the mutually coordinated effects of these factors result in strong, regular, rhythmic uterine contractions, which normally terminate in the birth of the fetus and the delivery of the placenta. How certain alterations trigger others and how proper checks and balances are maintained are still not completely understood.

Afferent and efferent nerve impulses to and from the uterus alter its contractility. Although nerve impulses to the uterus will stimulate contractions, the denervated uterus still contracts well during labor because oxytocin in the circulating blood is the regulator of labor. Therefore some women who are paralyzed can still deliver vaginally (p. 66).

MECHANISM OF LABOR

The female pelvis has varied contours and diameters at different levels, and the presenting part of the passenger is large in proportion to the passageway. For delivery to occur, therefore, the fetus must adapt to the birth canal during its descent. The turns and other adjustments that are necessary in the human birth process are termed the *mechanism of labor* (Figs. 20.29 and 20.30).

Phases of the mechanism of labor in vertex presentation. The phases of the mechanisms of labor are called (1) engagement, (2) descent, (3) flexion, (4) internal rotation, (5) extension, and (6) external rotation (restitution is a phase of external rotation). Although these phases will be discussed separately, a combination of movements is going on simultaneously. For example, engagement involves both descent and flexion.

Engagement. When the biparietal diameter of the head passes the pelvic inlet, the head is said to be engaged, or fixed, in the pelvis. In most nulliparous women this occurs 2 weeks before the onset of active labor because the firmer abdominal muscles direct the presenting part into the pelvis, whereas in multiparous women with more relaxed musculature the head often remains freely movable above the pelvic brim (e.g., ''floating'') until labor is established. In the majority of cases, the head of a normal-sized infant enters the pelvis with the sagittal suture in the transverse diameter.

Descent. Descent refers to the progress of the presenting part through the pelvis. As labor curves (Figs. 21.1 and 21.2) indicate, there is little progress in descent during the latent phase of the first stage of labor. Descent becomes more rapid in the latter part of the active phase, when the cervix has become dilated to 5 to 7 cm and especially when the membranes have ruptured.

Descent depends on four forces: (1) pressure of the amniotic fluid, (2) direct pressure of the contracting fundus on the buttocks of the fetus, (3) contraction of the maternal diaphragm and abdominal muscles in the second stage, and (4) the gradual straightening of the fetus and close approximation of the extremities to the body as a result of the uterine contractions. The effects of these forces are modified by the size and shape of the maternal pelvic planes and the size and malleability (capacity to mold) of the fetal head.

If the fetal head enters the pelvis with the plane of the biparietal diameter parallel to the plane of the inlet and the sagittal suture midway between the pubis and

Fig. 20.29
Mechanism of labor in left occiput anterior (LOA) presentation. **A,** Onset. **B,** Flexion. **C,** Internal rotation to OA. **D,** Extension. **E,** Restitution. **F,** External rotation. (Courtesy Ross Laboratories, Columbus, Ohio.)

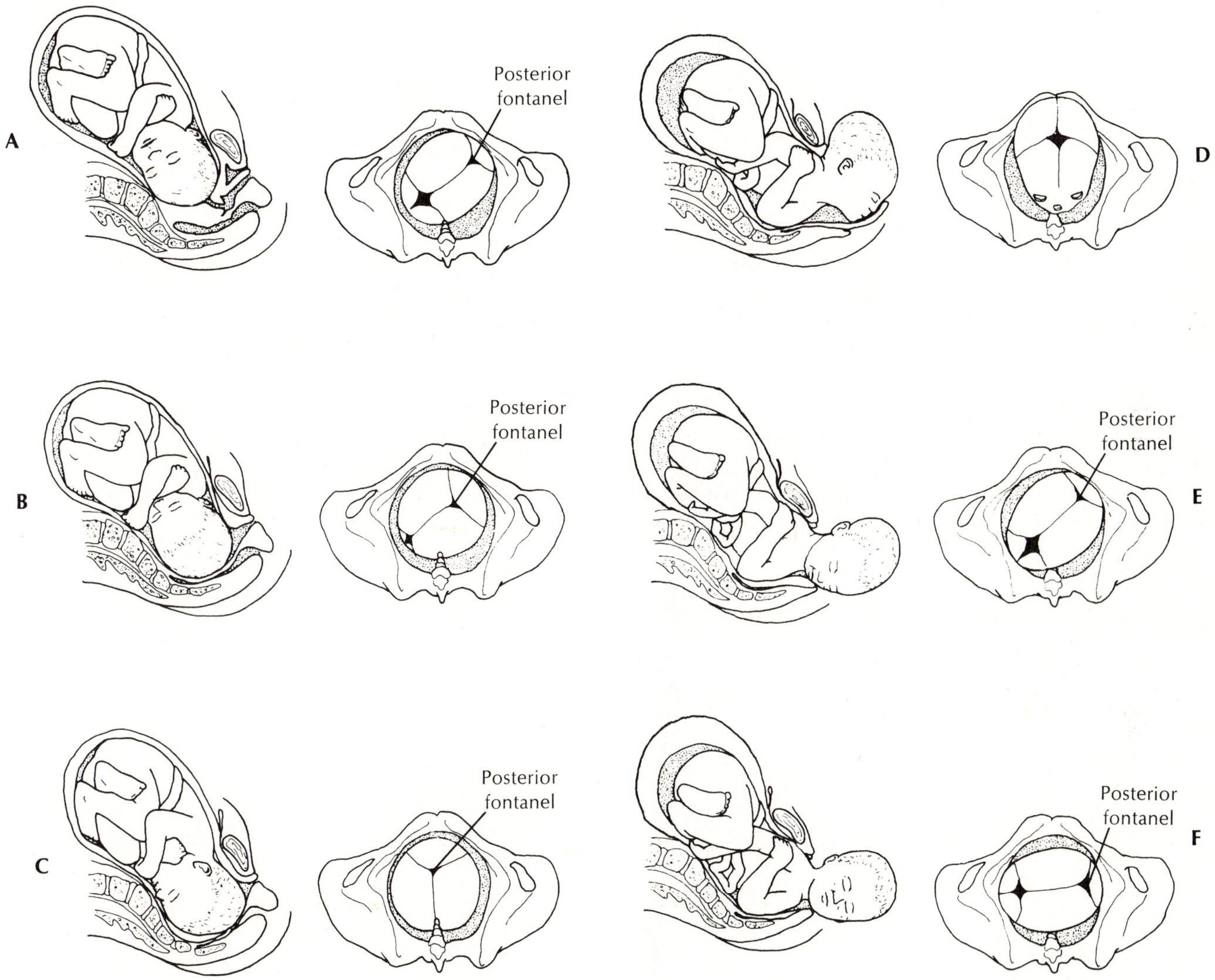

the sacrum, the relationship is termed *synclitism* (Fig. 20.31, *A*). Slight lateral flexion of the head, when the sagittal suture is closer to either the symphysis pubis or sacrum, is termed *asynclitism* (Fig. 20.31, *B*). Moderate degrees of asynclitism are found in most normal labors. As the head moves either toward the symphysis pubis (anterior) or toward the sacrum (posterior), descent is facilitated because the presenting part takes advantage of the largest diameter of the pelvic cavity. (For estimating amount of descent [station], see Fig. 20.28.)

Flexion. As soon as the descending head meets resistance from the cervix, pelvic wall, or pelvic floor, flexion normally occurs and the chin is brought into more intimate contact with the fetal chest (Fig. 20.32). The fetal skull may be thought of as a lever with unequal arms; the longer arm is made up of the anterior portion of the head, and the shorter arm is made up of the posterior portion. The fixed point of articulation of the two arms is called the fulcrum. When the descending head meets resistance as noted above, the force exerted on each of the arms is equal. Its effect, however, is great-

Fig. 20.30
Steps in normal mechanism of labor (head passing through birth canal): **A,** increased flexion; **B,** descent and engagement; **C,** internal rotation; **D,** internal rotation and beginning of extension; and **E,** extension (external rotation not shown). **F,** Summary of steps in normal mechanism of labor with the fetus presenting as LOA. (Courtesy Ross Laboratories, Columbus, Ohio.)

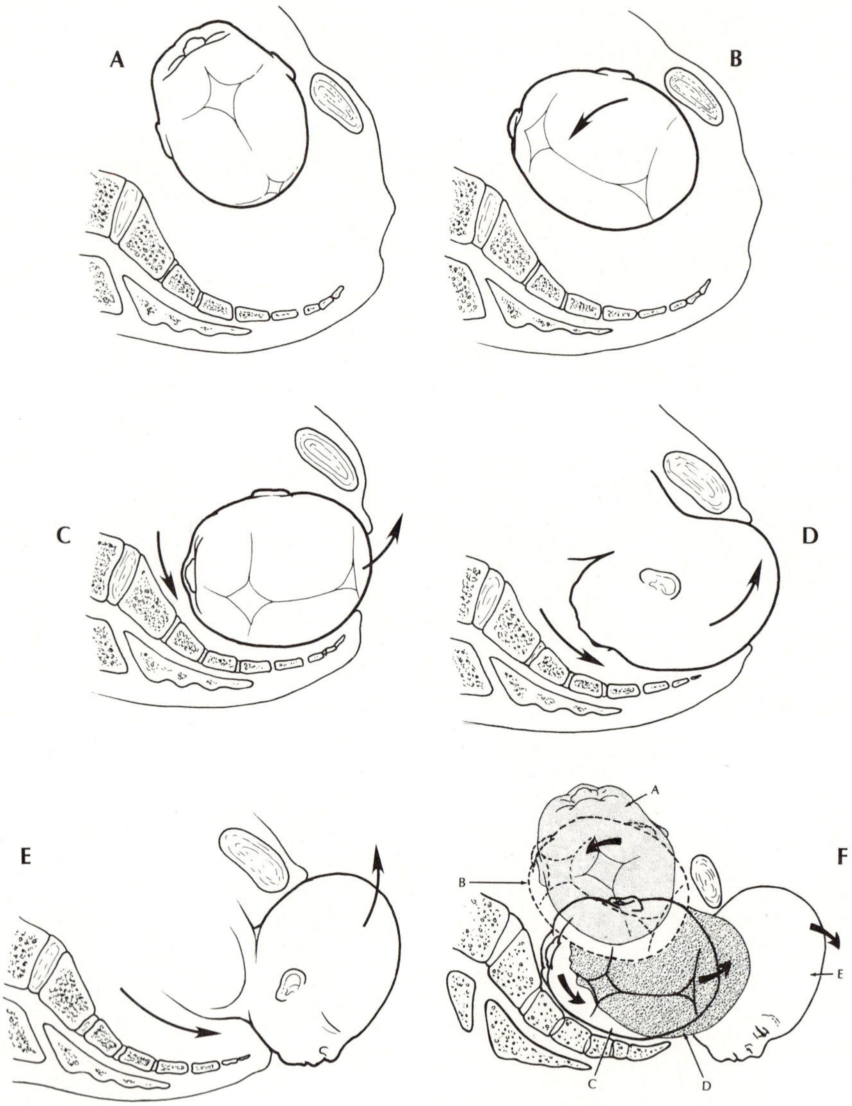

est on the longer lever arm, and as a result the shorter arm (the occiput) advances more rapidly and flexion is increased. This permits the shorter suboccipitobregmatic diameter (9.5 cm) rather than the larger occipitofrontal diameter (11.75 cm) to present to the outlet.

Internal rotation. Internal rotation permits the long axis of the fetal skull to change from the transverse diameter in which it passed the pelvic inlet and descended to the midpelvis (level of the spines) to an anteroposterior diameter at the outlet. The bispinous diameter is too small to permit passage of a normal-sized head; therefore the head is rotated obliquely by simple pressure from the protuberant spines that occurs with each contraction. By these maneuvers, the head passes the midpelvis. Rotation to the final anteroposterior diameter is accomplished by pressure from the bony pelvis and levator ani muscles with each uterine contraction. The head is almost always rotated by the time it reaches the pelvic floor.

Extension. When the fetal head reaches the perineum

Fig. 20.31

A, Synclitism. Head entering pelvis with plane of biparietal diameter parallel (or synclitic) to place of inlet. Dotted lines indicate changes in position as head advances.
B, Asynclitism. Before engagement, head is laterally flexed, and attitude is referred to as anterior synclitism or posterior parietal bone presentation. Subsequent changes in attitude, noted by dotted lines, are caused by both adaptation of head to pelvis and effect of lower uterine segment and cervix.

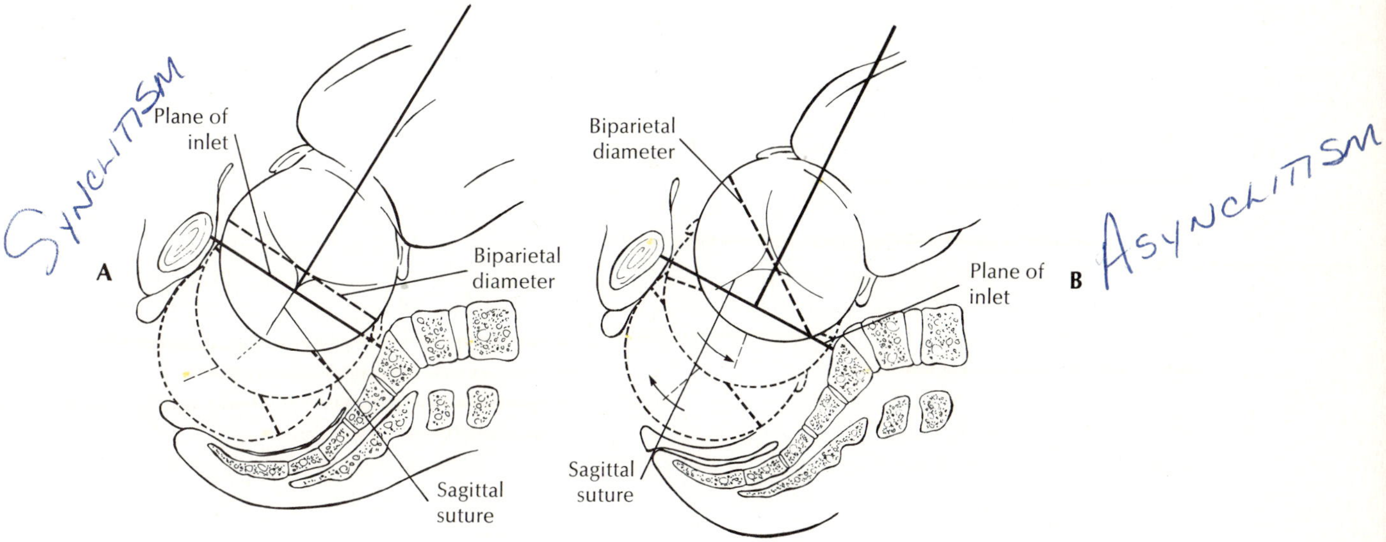

Fig. 20.32

A, Relation of head to spinal column before flexion. **B,** Relation of head to spinal column after flexion has occurred. Effect of force is greater on long arm of lever, so shorter arm (occiput) descends first and smaller diameter presents.

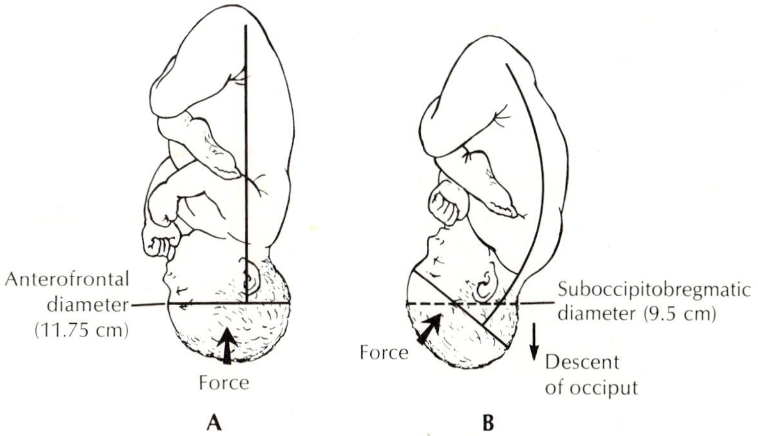

to be born, it is deflected anteriorly by the perineum. The occiput acts as the fulcrum as it passes under the lower border of the symphysis pubis. As a result the head is born by extension: first the occiput, then the face, and finally the chin.

External rotation. After delivery of the head, it rotates briefly to the position that it occupied when it was engaged in the inlet (restitution). This 45-degree movement realigns the infant's head with its back and shoulders. The head can then be seen to rotate further. This rotation occurs as the shoulders (with which the head is aligned) engage and descend in maneuvers similar to those of the head. As noted earlier the anterior shoulder presents first and, when it reaches the outlet, remains impinged beneath the pubic arch, and the posterior shoulder is forced up over the perineum until it is free of the introitus. The head then falls toward the maternal anus and the anterior shoulder is delivered. Subsequently the body of the infant is delivered without any particular mechanism. When the *entire infant* has

Table 20.4
Stages of Labor and Comparison of Mean Durations for Nulliparas and Multiparas

	Stages of Labor			
	First (stage of the cervix)	Second (stage of the baby)	Third (stage of the placenta)	Fourth (stage of recovery)
Nulliparas	13 hr	60 min	3-4 min	2 hr
Multiparas	8 hr	20 min	4-5 min	2 hr

emerged from the mother, birth is said to be complete. *This is the time noted on the records.*

Persistent occiput posterior or occiput transverse position. Prolongation of the first or second stage of labor may be caused by a persistent occiput posterior or occiput transverse position. During the normal mechanism of labor, the occiput may be directed posteriorly, particularly in an android pelvis. In any event, dilatation of the cervix may be delayed because the head does not fit the pelvis well or because it does not press with equal firmness around the internal os. As a consequence, labor may be slowed (for discussion of dystocia, see Chapter 37).

DURATION OF LABOR

Normal labor (eutocia) is recorded when the woman is at or near term, without complications, when a single fetus presents by vertex, and when labor is completed within 24 hours.

The course of normal labor is remarkably constant and consists of three concomitant subprocesses: (1) regular progression of uterine contractions, (2) effacement and progressive dilatation of the cervix, and (3) progress in descent of the presenting part. Four stages of labor are recognized; the mean duration of the first three stages is approximately 13 hours for primigravidas and about 8 hours for multigravidas.

A description of the labor experience of a significant number of parturients is given in Figs. 21.1 and 21.2. Friedman and Sachtleben (1965) utilized the information to predict the duration of normal labor for the first and second stages.

First stage of labor. The first stage of labor is considered to last from the onset of regular contractions to full dilatation of the cervix. Frequently the onset of labor is difficult to establish; the woman may be admitted to the labor floor just before delivery so that the beginning of labor may be only an estimate. The first stage is much longer than the second and third combined, averaging about 12 hours for nulliparas and approximately 6 hours for multiparas. Great variability is the rule, however, depending on the essential factors discussed earlier. Some multiparas may become fully dilated in less than an hour, or, infrequently, a nullipara may not be completely dilated in 24 hours.

The first stage of labor has been divided into two phases: a *latent phase* and an *active phase*.* During the latent phase there is more progress in effacement of the cervix and little increase in descent. During the active phase there is more rapid dilatation of the cervix and descent of the presenting part. If the degree of dilatation and descent is plotted in a graph, it forms an S curve. This curve can be used as a basis for assessment of progress in labor (Figs. 21.1 to 21.4).

Second stage of labor. The second stage of labor lasts from full dilatation of the cervix to delivery of the fetus. The mean duration of the second stage of labor is 20 minutes for multiparas and 1 hour for nulliparas. Labor of up to 2 hours is considered within the normal range for the second stage.

Third stage of labor. The third stage of labor lasts from delivery of the fetus to delivery of the placenta. The placenta normally separates with the third or fourth strong uterine contraction after the infant has been delivered. Then it should be delivered with the next uterine contraction after placental separation. Unusual adherence of the placenta (Chapter 35) or mismanagement of the third stage of labor may result in placental retention (see Chapter 23). The actual duration of the third stage of labor depends on how this stage is managed by the physician. Manual removal or expression of the placenta may be necessary.

Placental separation usually begins with the contraction that delivers the baby's trunk and is usually completed with the first contraction after the birth of the baby: within 3 or 4 minutes for the primipara and 4 or 5 minutes for the multipara. However, delivery of the placenta within 45 to 60 minutes is within normal limits usually.

Fourth stage of labor. The fourth stage of labor ar-

*Transition is a part of the active phase of the first stage of labor (see Chapters 19 and 21).

bitrarily lasts about 2 hours after delivery of the placenta. It is the period of immediate recovery, when homeostasis is reestablished, and is an important period of observation for complications, such as abnormal bleeding.

See Table 20.4 for a comparison of mean durations of nulliparas and multiparas for the four stages of labor.

References and Readings

Friedman, E.A., and Sachtleben, M.R.: Station of the fetal presenting part, Am. J. Obstet. Gynecol. **93:**522, 1965.

Hickman, M.A.: An introdution to midwifery, London, 1978, Blackwell Scientific Publications, Inc.

Howe, C.L.: Physiologic and psychosocial assessment in labor, Nurs. Clin. North Am. **17**(1):49, 1982.

Jensen, M.D., Benson, R.C., and Bobak, I.M.: Maternity care: the nurse and the family, ed. 2, St. Louis, 1981, The C.V. Mosby Co.

Liggins, G.C.: New concepts of what triggers labor, Contemp. Obstet. Gynecol. **19**(5):131, 1982.

Malinowski, J.S., et al.: Nursing care of the labor patient, ed. 2, Philadelphia, 1983, F.A. Davis Co.

Varney, H.: Nurse-midwifery, London, 1980, Blackwell Scientific Publications, Inc.

Wiggins, J.D.: Childbearing: physiology, experiences, needs, St. Louis, 1979, The C.V. Mosby Co.

21
First Stage of Labor

- Assessment: Review of Client's History
- Initial Assessment
  - Is she in labor?
  - How far has she progressed?
  - Have the membranes ruptured?
  - Are there complications that may require treatment?
  - What is her psychologic response to the beginning of labor?
- Progress in Labor
  - Cervical dilatation and descent
  - Uterine contractions
    - Characteristics
    - Assessing uterine contractions
  - Rupture of membranes and amniotic fluid
    - Tests for rupture of membranes
    - Assessment of amniotic fluid
    - Complications
- Stress in Labor
  - Fetal stress
    - Monitoring techniques
  - Maternal stress
  - Paternal stress
- Nursing Diagnoses
- Planning
- Implementation
  - Procedures
  - Preparation of the vulva: the "mini-prep"
  - Enema
  - Intravenous therapy
  - Assisting the physician with vaginal examinations
  - Emergency procedures
    - Prolapsed cord
    - Fetal distress or abnormal FHR pattern
    - Uterine contractions
  - Motherhood with dignity
    - Admission to the labor unit
    - Intake and output
    - Maternal position during labor
    - Comfort measures
    - General hygiene
    - Atmosphere of the labor and delivery area
    - Touch
    - Pain and its relief
  - Fatherhood with dignity
    - Birth process as seen through father's eyes
    - Father in labor suite
    - Supporting the father during labor
  - Preparation for delivery
- Evaluation

The first stage of labor begins with the onset of regular contractions and is complete when the cervix is fully dilated. The symptoms the expectant mother has been prepared to recognize herald the beginning of labor. The waiting period of pregnancy is at an end. The time has come for the child to be born. The mother or couple are about to undergo one of the most stressful yet meaningful events of their lives. Only with adequate preparation for childbirth will most couples make this an easier experience.*

During the first stage the forces that efface and dilate the cervix and cause descent of the fetus are limited to the uterine contractions, the primary powers. The woman who is relaxed and able to work with these forces tends to hasten the process. However, effort on her part directed toward voluntary bearing-down or pushing has negative effects, that is, exhaustion of the mother and possible trauma to the fetus or cervix.

The goals for care during this stage are to confirm labor, identify any abnormalities that would interfere with normal progress and fetal and maternal health, and support the woman's and her family's desire to partici-

*The psychosocial components of childbirth are of such magnitude that several chapters have been devoted to the discussion of this aspect of the event, that is, Chapters 7, 8, 9, 16, 19, 26, and 32.

pate as fully as they desire in this momentous event in their lives.

Care of the woman in labor begins with the woman's report of the following:

1. Onset of progressive, strong, frequent, sustained uterine contractions
2. Rupture of the membranes
3. Bloody vaginal discharge (bloody show)

If a hospital delivery has been elected, the woman is admitted to the labor unit, and if a home or birthing center delivery has been planned, the family follows the instructions previously agreed upon. (See Chapter 26 for a discussion of alternative settings for childbirth.)

Assessment: Review of Client's History

Before the nurse's first meeting with the woman who is in labor, a review of her prenatal record is made and significant items are noted:

1. Obstetric history
   a. Age and estimated date of confinement (EDC)
   b. Parity, or gravidity, and previous obstetric history (problems, type of labor, abortions, stillbirths)
   c. Maternal vital signs, blood pressure
   d. Fetal heart rate (FHR); rate, rhythm, and area of maximal intensity
   e. Results of laboratory tests: urinalysis (protein, acetone, glucose) and blood tests (hemoglobin, hematocrit, Rh factor, blood group, sickle cell trait, antibody titer, serum albumin and serum total protein, BUN, and creatinine). The serum albumin and total protein are drawn to determine malnourishment and therefore predisposition to metabolic disease of late pregnancy and BUN and creatinine are drawn to determine the quality of kidney function secondary to hypovolemia and metabolic disease of late pregnancy.*
   f. Type of analgesia and/or anesthesia requested
   g. Any problems listed and their past or current management
2. Client profile: preparation for childbirth; problems (e.g., no supportive persons available, negative ethnic or cultural influences, anxieties about pain, fear of injections or needles); plans for newborn care (method of feeding; pediatrician)
3. General history: any pertinent notations

*The controversy about pregnancy-induced hypertension (PIH) continues. Some authorities use "metabolic disease of late pregnancy" to refer to PIH or one of its components, preeclampsia-eclampsia (see Chapter 35).

Should the woman not have had any prenatal care, the above information must be obtained on admission so that her data base report may be completed before active labor begins.

Initial Assessment

The initial examination serves to confirm the advent of true labor and to provide assessment of the woman's current clinical condition. The questions to be answered are as follows:

1. Is she in labor?
2. How far has she progressed?
3. Have the membranes ruptured?
4. Are there complications that may require treatment?
5. What is her psychologic response to the beginning of labor?

IS SHE IN LABOR?

False labor may be experienced from the thirty-eighth week onward. It is frustrating for the woman to find that the contractions she was experiencing were not true labor and that she must return home until more definitive symptoms are present. For those who experience false labor two or three times, the onset of true labor comes as an anticlimax, and only attentive care eradicate the feelings of disappointment and even anger. (For a comparison of false and true labor, see Table 21.1.)

HOW FAR HAS SHE PROGRESSED?

The nullipara, because of eagerness to complete labor, may come to the hospital very early in the first stage. If she lives near the hospital, she may be asked to return home to wait for further progress either in frequency and strength of contractions or in amount of show. She is encouraged to walk about but is asked to restrict ingestion to clear fluids. Clear fluids are those fluids one can see through, for example, tea with honey and lemon, homemade broth (not salt-loaded bouillon), and apple juice. If she lives a considerable distance from the hospital, she may be admitted, and the same care will be given. (For progression of labor, see Table 21.2.)

The degree of progress is established as follows:

1. Assess the character of the contractions.
   a. Have the woman describe when the contractions began and what they are like now.

Table 21.1
Comparison of Labors

True Labor	False Labor	Complicated Labor (examples)
Show: usually present; pinkish mucus; may be mucous plug from cervix	Show: usually none or brownish-stained mucus (inquire whether she had vaginal examination within last 48 hr)	Hemorrhage: woman reports blood trickling down legs as she stands or has soaked perineal pad with bright red blood
Contractions: occur regularly; interval between has shortened; intensity has gradually increased; located in lower back (may feel like gastrointestinal upset with some diarrhea); intensified by walking	Contractions: occur irregularly; intervals remain long; intensity unchanged; located in abdomen; relief with walking or no effect (Braxton Hicks contractions)	Contractions: suddenly intensify, then cease; abdomen becomes rigid and boardlike; woman feels very ill, nervous, shocked
Cervix: becomes effaced and dilates progressively	Cervix: no change	Cervix: excessive vaginal bleeding precludes vaginal examination
Fetal movement: no significant change	Fetal movement: intensifies (for a short period) or remains the same	Fetal movement: intensifies but then ceases altogether

Table 21.2
Maternal Progress in First Stage of Labor within Normal Limits

Cervix			
Dilatation*	0-3 cm	4-7 cm	8-10 cm
Effacement†			
Duration	About 8-10 hr	About 3 hr	About 1-2 hr
Contractions			
Magnitude (strength)	Mild	Moderate	Strong to expulsive
Rhythm	Irregular	More regular	Regular
Frequency	5-30 min apart	3-5 min apart	2-3 min apart
Duration	10-30 sec	30-45 sec	45-60 sec (few to 90 sec)
Descent			
Station of presenting part	Nulliparous: 0 Multiparous: 0 to −2 cm	About +1 to +2 cm About +1 to +2 cm	+2 to +3 cm +2 to +3 cm
Show			
Color	Brownish discharge, mucous plug or pale, pink mucus	Pink to bloody mucus	Bloody mucus
Amount	Scant	Scant to moderate	Copious
Behavior and appearance	Excited; thoughts center on self, labor, and baby; may be talkative or mute, calm or tense; some apprehension; pain controlled fairly well; alert, follows directions readily; open to instructions	Becoming more serious, doubtful of control of pain, more apprehensive; desires companionship and encouragement; attention more inner directed; fatigue evidenced; malar flush; has some difficulty following directions	Pain described as severe; backache common; feelings of frustration, fear of loss of control, and irritability surface; vague in communications; amnesia between contractions; writhing with contractions; nausea and vomiting, especially if hyperventilating; hyperesthesia; circumoral pallor, perspiration on forehead and upper lips; shaking tremor of thighs; feeling of need to defecate, pressure on anus

*The pace of progress in cervical dilatation (according to Friedman and Sachtleben, 1965) varies as follows: from 0 to 2 cm (latent phase), progress is slow; from 2 to 4 cm (phase of acceleration), pace quickens; from 4 to 9 cm (phase of maximal acceleration), pace is most rapid; and from 9 to 10 cm (phase of deceleration), pace slows again (Figs 21.1 and 21.2).

†In the nullipara, effacement is often complete before dilatation begins; in the multipara, it occurs simultaneously with dilatation.

b. Assess their duration, intensity (in some parts of the United States, the terms *strength* or *magnitude* are used instead), frequency, and regularity (see discussion that follows).

2. Assess the nature of the vaginal discharge and its amount, color, and character. Bloody show must be distinguished from bleeding. Show is pink in color and feels sticky from the mucus it contains. It is scant to begin with and increases with effacement and dilatation of the cervix. A woman may report a scant brownish discharge. This may be attributable to trauma to the cervix as a result of vaginal examination or coitus within the last 48 hours.
3. Complete a vaginal examination or assist physician (p. 384) to assess the following:
   a. Effacement and dilatation of the cervix
   b. Presentation and position of the fetus
   c. Station of the presenting part
   d. Degree of molding of the fetal head
   e. Presence and amount of stool in the rectum

HAVE THE MEMBRANES RUPTURED?

Labor is initiated by spontaneous rupture of the membranes (SRM) in almost 25% of gravidas. The lag period, rarely exceeding 24 hours, precedes the onset of labor. The length of uterine inactivity is directly related to the duration of pregnancy. If the woman is only 32 weeks pregnant, for example, several days may pass before labor begins. If she is at term, labor usually ensues within 12 hours of rupture of the membranes. After a delay of 24 hours, the woman is said to have premature or prolonged rupture of the membranes (PROM). If they are ruptured, note the color and character of the amniotic fluid, ask for the time of rupture, and check the vaginal discharge with phenaphthazine (Nitrazine Paper) for pH (positive = dark blue) because pH is weakly basic at 7.2. Rupture of membranes is discussed in the section on preliminary care that follows and in Chapter 22.

ARE THERE COMPLICATIONS THAT MAY REQUIRE TREATMENT?

Although some complications of labor are anticipated, others appear only in the clinical course of labor (see Unit Seven). Knowledge of the pregnancy, careful initial assessment, and follow-up of progress are necessary during normal labor as well as during an abnormal labor:

1. Check the vital signs and blood pressure (if the latter is elevated, repeat procedure 30 minutes later to obtain a true reading after the woman has relaxed).
2. Check for edema of the legs, face, hands, or sacrum.
3. Obtain a specimen of urine for routine analysis and the presence of protein, glucose, or acetone.
4. Inquire regarding symptoms of infection (e.g., diarrhea, cold, cough, sore throat).
5. Recheck for allergies: mention names of drugs routinely used, such as meperidine hydrochloride (Demerol) or mepivacaine hydrochloride (Carbocaine).
6. Check the woman's dietary intake for the last 4 hours. Gastric motility is inhibited with uterine contractions, and the possibility of vomiting involves danger of aspiration of vomitus and consequent respiratory complications.
7. Perform Leopold's maneuvers to determine fetal presentation, lie, position, and engagement (see p. 382).
8. Assess FHR for rate and regularity; mark the area of maximal intensity.

WHAT IS HER PSYCHOLOGIC RESPONSE TO THE BEGINNING OF LABOR?

The woman's general appearance and behavior (and that of her partner) provide valuable clues as to the type of supportive care she will need. The nurse notes the following:

1. *Verbal interaction*. Is she talkative or mute? Does she talk to staff members freely or only in response to questions? How does she talk to her support person? Does that person do all the talking?

2. *Body posture and set*. Is she relaxed or tense? What is her anxiety level? Does she lie rigidly on her back or sit up tailor fashion? Where does her partner sit?

3. *Perceptual acuity*. Does she have any helpful or harmful background knowledge? Does her anxiety level require repeated explanations? Does she understand what the nurse says? Can she repeat what has been said or demonstrate that she understands (e.g., use the call bell correctly)?

4. *Energy level*. Does she look tired? How much rest has she had in the previous few days? Does excitement mask a depleted energy reserve?

5. *Discomfort or pain*. How much does the woman relate what she is experiencing? How does she react to a contraction?

6. *Cultural background*.

Progress in Labor

The symptomatology of progress in labor is well defined, and careful assessment provides the cues for selection and implementation of nursing actions, both therapeutic and educational. *The nurse assumes much of the responsibility for making the assessment of progress and for keeping the physician informed as to progress and any deviations from normal.*

In normal labor (eutocia), progress of effacement and dilatation of the cervix and descent of the presenting part occur in a predictable fashion (Figs. 21.1 and 21.2). The character of the woman's uterine contractions and her behavior and appearance correlate with the phase of labor she is experiencing.

The woman's response to labor may also be reflected in vital signs and blood pressure. Hemorrhage, pregnancy-induced hypertension, infection, and panic states can cause alterations in the base-line findings in these areas. Frank hemorrhage also alters the appearance and character of the bloody show; it becomes more blood-like and less like mucus (sticky).

Continued fetal well-being is monitored through assessment of the FHR and of the character of the amniotic fluid discharge. Tables 21.1 and 21.2 summarize the symptomatology of progress.

The routine for assessment of progress and of the continued well-being of the mother and fetus is usually set on a minimal level by hospital policy (Table 21.3). Any untoward findings would prompt an increase in the timing of assessment procedures.

CERVICAL DILATATION AND DESCENT

Thanks to the clinical research of Friedman and Sachtleben (1965), the early recognition of normal and abnormal labor patterns has been facilitated. The graphic recording of cervical dilatation and descent of the presenting part provides a concise guide for instituting remedial care in dystocia of either fetal or maternal origin.

The normal pattern of cervical dilatation presents an S-shaped curve and may be divided into two phases:

1. The *latent phase* begins with the onset of true labor (regular contractions and an average cervical dilatation of 1 cm in the nullipara and 3 cm in the parous woman).
2. In the *active phase* the rate of cervical dilatation increases rapidly. It is divided into the acceleration phase (rate of dilatation begins to increase), the phase of maximal slope (cervical dilatation is almost complete), and the deceleration phase (rate slows; may not be noticeable).

The normal pattern of cervical dilatation and descent in a nulliparous labor is shown in Fig. 21.1, and the pattern in a parous labor is shown in Fig. 21.2.

Each time an assessment is made, the findings are plotted on the graphic chart and a pattern emerges (Fig. 21.3).

1. Cervical dilatation patterns
   a. Normal (Figs. 21.1 and 21.2)
   b. Abnormal (Fig. 21.4): report to physician
      (1) Prolonged latent phase: 20 hours or longer in the nullipara and 14 hours or longer in the parous woman
      (2) Protracted active phase: cervical dilatation of less than 1.2 cm/hr in the nullipara and less than 1.5 cm/hr in the parous woman
      (3) Arrest of the active phase: no progress in the active phase for more than 2 to 4 hours
      (4) Precipitate labor: labor of less than 3 hours
2. Descent patterns
   a. Normal (Figs. 21.1 and 21.2)
   b. Abnormal (Fig. 21.4): report to physician
      (1) Protracted descent pattern in the active phase: rate of descent less than 1 cm/hr in the nullipara and less than 2 cm/hr in the parous woman
      (2) Arrest of descent in the active phase: no progress for 1 hour or more in the nullipara and 30 minutes in the parous woman

UTERINE CONTRACTIONS

Characteristics. For a detailed discussion see Chapter 20 (p. 380 and Fig. 20.22).

Assessing uterine contractions. There are three methods of assessing contractions. The first is the subjective description given by the woman; the second, palpation and timing by a nurse or physician; and the third, use of electronic monitoring devices.

When the woman reports that contractions have begun, she is asked, "When did they start?" "How often are they coming?" "Are they coming regularly?" "Would you say they are weak or strong?"

For some women, contractions may never get closer than 20 to 30 minutes apart; I assisted a woman to give birth the moment she stepped through the delivery room door. The woman kept waiting for her contractions to get closer than every 20 to 30 minutes before coming in! Occasionally, there are women who never feel their contractions; they have so-called "silent" labors. These women often present themselves in the emergency room just before, or indeed, just after the baby is born.

The intensity or magnitude of the contractions has been described in the following manner:

Fig. 21.1
Relationship between cervical dilatation and descent of presenting part in nulliparous labor. *L,* Latent phase; *A,* acceleration phase; *M,* phase of maximal slope; *D,* deceleration phase; *2,* second stage.

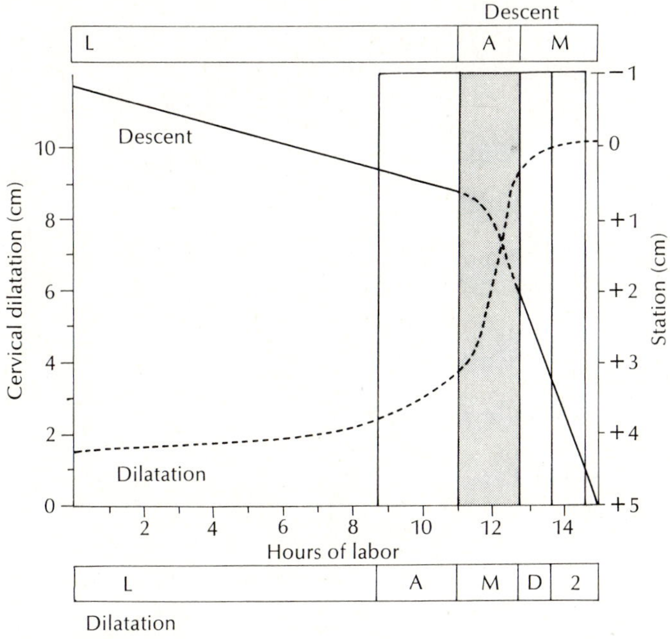

Fig. 21.2
Relationship between cervical dilatation and descent of presenting part in parous labor. *L,* Latent phase; *A,* acceleration phase; *M,* phase of maximal slope; *D,* deceleration phase; *2,* second stage. (Adapted from Friedman, E.A., and Sachtleben, M.R.: Am J. Obstet. Gynecol. **93:**522, 1965.)

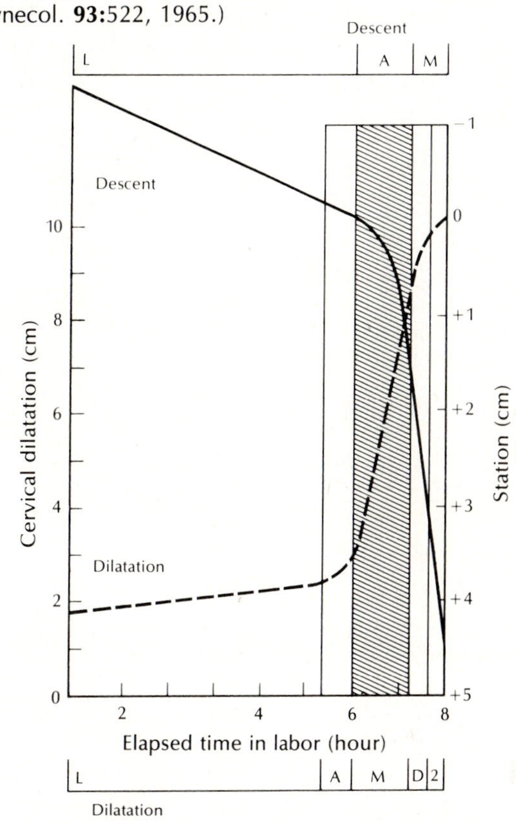

Table 21.3
Minimal Reassessment of Progress of First Stage of Labor

	Cervical Dilatation		
	0-5 cm	**6-7 cm**	**8-10 cm**
Vital signs*	Every 4 hr	Every 4 hr	Every 4 hr
Blood pressure	Every 60 min	Every 60 min	Every 60 min
Contractions	Every 30 min to 1 hr	Every 15 min	Every 5-10 min
FHR	Every 15 min†	Every 15 min†	Every 5 min†
Show	Every 60 min	Every 30 min	Every 10-15 min
Behavior, appearance, energy level	Every 30 min	Every 15 min	Every 5 min
Vaginal examination‡	To be done only for following reasons: 1. To confirm diagnosis when symptoms indicate change (e.g., strength, duration, or frequency of contractions; increase in amount of bloody show; membranes rupture; or woman feels pressure on her rectum) 2. To determine whether dilatation and descent are sufficient for administration of anesthetic 3. To reassess progress if labor takes longer than expected 4. To determine station of presenting part		

*If membranes have ruptured, check temperature every 2 hr.
†For a period of 30 sec immediately after a uterine contraction (Zuspan et al., 1979).
‡In presence of vaginal bleeding, physician performs vaginal examination, usually under double setup.

Fig. 21.3
Assessment sheet for cervical dilatation and descent of presenting part. Individual woman's labor patterns *(red)* superimposed on prepared graph *(black)*. **A,** Nulliparous labor. **B,** Parous labor.

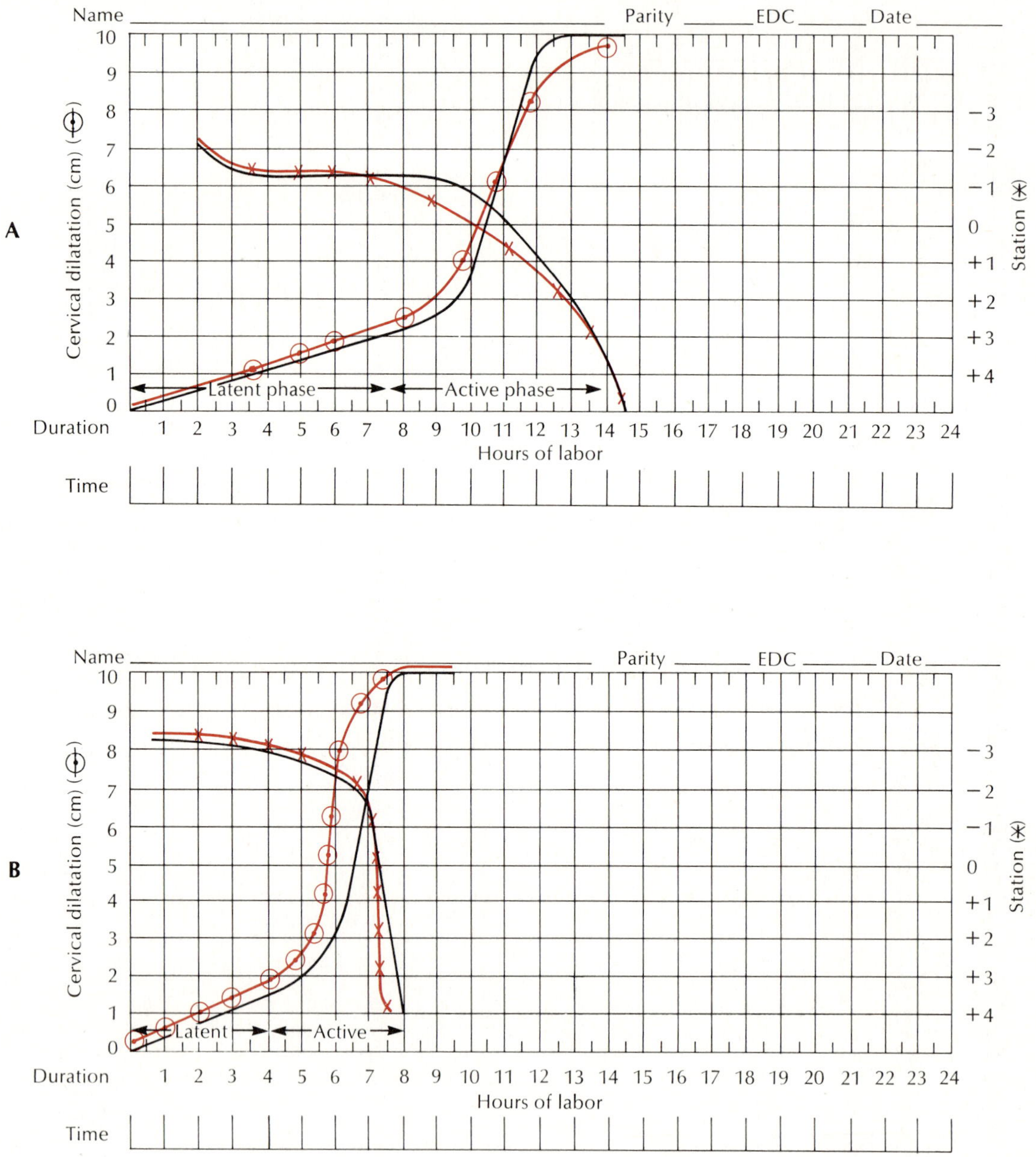

Mild—Slightly tense fundus that is easy to indent with fingertips
Moderate—Firm fundus that is difficult to indent with fingertips
Strong—Rigid boardlike fundus that is almost impossible to indent

The woman is not aware of the sensation of the uterus's contracting until the contraction is fairly well established. Frequently, her description of the end of the contraction is related to the end of the pain sensation (felt in the lower portion of the uterus, not the fundus), and this can remain after the contraction is completed.

Fig. 21.4
Major types of deviation from normal progress of labor may be detected by noting dilatation of cervix at various intervals after labor begins. If a woman exhibits an abnormal labor pattern as depicted by broken lines, physician should be notified immediately.

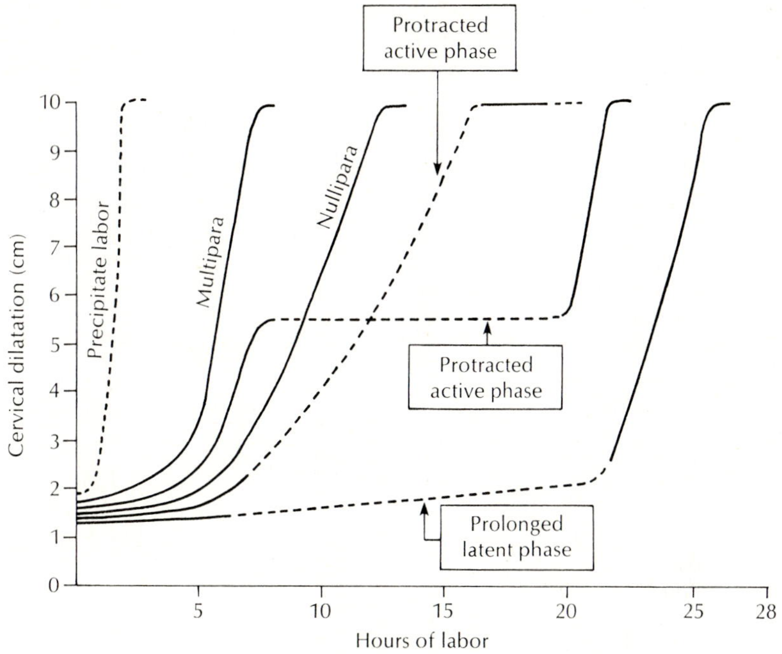

Therefore her description may not be as accurate as that obtained by the nurse.

RUPTURE OF MEMBRANES AND AMNIOTIC FLUID

Rupture of the membranes must be noted if it has not already occurred. When the membranes do rupture, the routine for assessment is as follows.

Tests for rupture of membranes. Drainage of amniotic fluid may be an obvious prelude to labor. Questionable leakage of amniotic fluid usually is not an indication for the induction of labor. If obvious loss of fluid does not persist, one probably should await the onset of uterine contractions in pregnancies of doubtful viability (gestations of 28 weeks or less). Loss of urine by the incontinent woman or leukorrhea in the woman with vaginitis must be differentiated from amniotic fluid for proper maternity management.

The following simple procedures are useful in the diagnosis of ruptured membranes:

1. Spread a drop of the fluid on a clean side. Allow the fluid to dry. Dried amniotic fluid (in the absence of blood or gross infection) will show a frondlike crystalline pattern when viewed under a microscope. This result is known as a *positive fern test*. It should not be confused with the cervical mucus test, which also shows a fernlike formation. Urine, vaginal discharge, or blood will not show a crystalline pattern.

2. Determine the pH of the vaginal fluid. Amniotic fluid is slightly alkaline; urine or pus is acidic. Place sterile glove on examining hand*; place piece of pH paper at cervical os to test for amniotic fluid. Phenaphthazine (Nitrazine Paper) moistened with amniotic fluid will turn dark blue in the alkaline range.

3. Fetal lanugo hairs or fetal squamous cells may be noted under the microscope if amniotic fluid is the test material. Moreover, some of the squamous cells, presumably derived from sebaceous glands, contain lipids that stain yellow after the addition of aqueous Nile blue stain; other squamous cells and hairs stain blue.

Assessment of amniotic fluid

Color. Amniotic fluid is normally pale straw colored. If it is greenish brown, the fetus has probably undergone a hypoxic episode resulting in relaxation of the anal sphincter and passage of meconium from the bowel.

Yellow-stained fluid may indicate (1) fetal hypoxia that occurred 36 hours or more before rupture of the membranes or (2) fetal hemolytic disease (Rh or ABO incompatibility, intrauterine infection).

Meconium-stained amniotic fluid is a normal finding in breech presentation. Frank meconium may often be seen exuding into the birth canal (see p. 877). However, even in the case of a breech presentation, the pas-

*Sterile water is the preferred lubricant. It does not interfere with the test results.

sage of meconium may indicate fetal distress and not just pressure on the fetal rectum.

If an iodine preparation is used as a vaginal disinfectant during vaginal examinations, it may be difficult to differentiate iodine staining from meconium staining.

Although meconium-stained fluid may be noted with fetal asphyxia, its presence is not always diagnostic of prospective fetal distress. However, it should be promptly reported and recorded and the FHR monitored very closely. Port wine–colored amniotic fluid is one indicator of premature separation of the placenta (abruptio placentae) (see Chapter 35).

Character. Thick consistency and unpleasant odor are associated with infection.

Amount. *Polyhydramnios,* an excessive amount of amniotic fluid (more than 2000 ml), is frequently associated with congenital anomalies in the neonate (see Chapter 40).

*Oligohydramnios,** an abnormally small amount or virtual absence of amniotic fluid (less than 500 ml), may be accompanied by such abnormalities as agenesis or malformation of the ears. In the presence of oligohydramnios, also observe for genitourinary tract anomalies, particularly renal agenesis (see Chapter 40).

Complications. Complications associated with ruptured membranes may include infection and prolapsed cord.

Infection. Once the membranes have ruptured, the "clock of infection" begins to tick. The frequency of chorioamnionitis follows a progressive linear course after a period of about 4 hours. Fulminating, clinically evident sepsis often is notable after 72 hours. Therefore, if it can be assumed that the fetus is definitely viable (weight of 2000 g and gestational age of 34 weeks or more), the physician may stimulate labor with dilute oxytocin solution administered intravenously when 6 to 8 hours have passed without the onset of spontaneous labor. If the survival of the fetus is doubtful because of immaturity, watchful expectancy is the better policy. Once clinical amnionitis does occur, induction of labor is indicated (see Chapter 37). If induction is unsuccessful, cesarean birth may be required.

Prophylactic antibiotic therapy rarely will protect against chorioamnionitis. In most cases such treatment often results in the development of antibiotic-resistant strains of many pathogenic organisms.

In the presence of intact membranes and herpetic vaginal lesions (herpes simplex virus type I or type II), cesarean birth is indicated to protect against direct transmission of the virus as the neonate passes through the birth canal. If rupture of the membranes occurred as long as 4 hours previously, the fetus is considered infected already; vaginal birth may thus be permitted (for further discussion of herpetic infections and childbirth, see pp. 827 and 839).

Prolapsed cord. See discussion of emergencies, p. 407.

*The nurse should not be too quick to diagnose oligohydramnios or polyhydramnios on the basis of the amount that trickles or gushes out when the membranes rupture or are ruptured artificially.

Stress in Labor

FETAL STRESS

Since labor represents a period of stress for the fetus, continuous monitoring of fetal health is instituted as part of the nursing care during labor.

Fetal well-being during labor is measured by the response of the FHR to uterine contractions and by fetal blood gas studies. In general, normal, active labor is characterized by (1) an FHR between 120 and 160 beats/min with normal variability and no ominous periodic changes and (2) uterine contractions with a frequency of about every 3 to 5 minutes, a duration of 30 to 60 seconds, an intensity resulting in a rise in intrauterine pressure to 50 to 75 mm Hg at the peak of a contraction, and an average resting intrauterine pressure (tonus) of between 8 and 15 mm Hg.

Monitoring techniques. Following are methods of determining the degree of fetal distress throughout labor:

1. Assessment of the rate and rhythm of the fetal heart
2. Fetal blood sampling (pH and concentration of oxygen and carbon dioxide [Po_2 and Pco_2]) (see p. 491)
3. Nonstress test (NST) or oxytocin challenge (stress) test (OCT) (see p. 496)
4. Assessment for presence of meconium-stained amniotic fluid (see p. 401)
5. Fetal activity or movements (see p. 496)

Fetoscope monitoring. *Periodic auscultation of the fetal heart* may reveal tachycardia (compensation), bradycardia (decompensation), or arrhythmia that may occur during the brief examinations. In the low-risk woman, auscultation of the FHR may be done every 15 minutes in the first stage and every 5 minutes during the second stage, in both instances throughout a contraction and for a period of 30 seconds immediately after a uterine contraction. However, serious or even critical jeopardy interspersed with or not recurring during the periods of auscultation may pass unrecognized by the examiner. Therefore only marked degrees of fetal distress can be identified by listening to the FHR periodically.

An improved method that is more likely to aid in diagnosing fetal compromise in the high-risk pregnancy is the counting of FHR during sequential contractions and for a full 3 minutes thereafter. Persistent, postcontraction bradycardia (e.g., FHR of 100 beats/min or a persistent drop of 30 beat/min or more below base line) or gross irregularity indicates fetal distress and chronic decompensation.

Naturally the woman becomes anxious if the examiner cannot count the FHR. For the inexperienced listener it often takes time to locate the heartbeat and find the area of maximal intensity (see p. 384). For a vertex presentation, it is suggested that the student use a fetoscope (see Fig 17.4) and start at the umbilicus and move in a widening half circle below the umbilicus until the beat can be heard. The mother can be told that the nurse is ''finding the spot where the sounds are loudest.'' If it has taken considerable time to locate them, offer the mother (and father) an opportunity to hear them too, to reassure her (them).

Electronic fetal monitoring. Electronic fetal monitoring (EFM) probably is not necessary for monitoring the fetus during a normal labor.* However, if either the mother or the fetus is considered to be at high risk, the more precise measurement of fetal response in indicated. For an extensive discussion of fetal monitoring, FHR patterns, and the implementation of related nursing actions, see Chapter 24.

MATERNAL STRESS

Although women and their families approach labor with a feeling of satisfaction that the preparatory phase of pregnancy is now at an end and that within a relatively short time their child will be born, most women have two major concerns. First, a woman may ask, ''Will my child be all right?'' Second, she may ask, ''Will my labor be as I expected? How will I act? Will I be okay?''

Further assessment of the woman's first question by asking her why she is so worried is probably not appropriate at this time.

Her second question needs to be assessed further now. Her (or the couple's) goals for this labor may be noted in her prenatal record. For example, she or they may have indicated preferences for the following:

1. Medicated or unmedicated labor
2. Support person she wants with her—husband, mother, coach, other
3. Electronic monitor or not
4. Episiotomy or not

*The National Institute of Health (NIH) does not recommend EFM for normal labor, only for high-risk labors.

Some women and couples want an active role in decision making; others want to leave it all in the hands of the physicians and nurses. Each individual has her or his own self-expectations and expectations of others. Regardless of the actual labor and delivery experience, the woman's or couple's *perception* of the birth experience is most positive if she or they evaluate the events and performance as meeting expectations.

Women from various cultures are taught from childhood the ''right'' way to behave during labor. They are taught that they should moan, scream, remain silent, or be totally anesthetized, depending on the culture. If a woman can follow through with the social expectations of her culture, she perceives herself as having mastery, as having had control over her labor. Her self-esteem receives a boost.

The woman's level of anxiety may rise when she does not understand what is being said. Observe the facial expression and body language of the woman who has just been examined vaginally when the physician, within the parturient's hearing, tells the nurse, ''She's a primigravida, EDC 2 weeks from now. She's 50% effaced but I can barely get a fingertip in there. She has bloody show but she'll have to drop the head some yet. If her membranes don't break by themselves, I'll pop them myself. The contractions are weak now; they'll have to get a lot harder to get the job done.'' To the nurse, the physician may say, ''Do a mini-prep on her.'' Understandably, the woman who is unfamiliar with these terms could panic. Many of the terms—bloody show, drop the head, membranes break—sound violent and could conjure up thoughts of injury or pain. If she had thought that her ''weak'' contractions were uncomfortable, she may become tense anticipating the more intense uterine contractions that are needed ''to get the job done.''

The woman's or couple's body language, facial expressions, and verbal cues (e.g., ''Huh?'' ''What's wrong?'') are all noted by the observant nurse. Symptoms and signs of discomfort are described and discussed in Chapter 19.

PATERNAL STRESS

The father's behavior is also assessed. Is he hesitant to go into the labor room? Does he appear confident? Does he appear aggressive or hostile as he strides into the labor room? (He may be asserting his felt need to be with his wife or just covering up his anxieties.) Is he hungry? (He could faint from low blood sugar.) Is he sleepy, red eyed, or glassy eyed from fatigue? Does he look worried? Does he pull back and say that he is ''just an onlooker'' (observer)?

The nurse assesses the father's and mother's perception and preference as to the type and amount of participation he is to have. Is he prepared through classes? Which kind? How does the couple interpret information given them in classes (e.g., does natural childbirth mean the woman is not to receive medication?) Does he want to provide comfort measures? Which comfort measures does he need to learn? Is he considering accompanying her at the birth?

Has the father been on a hospital tour? Does he want a tour? Is he oriented to the unit? To this hospital? What questions does he have regarding the mother's room, delivery area, nursery, and postdelivery care?

Nursing Diagnoses

Nursing diagnoses lend direction to types of nursing actions needed to implement a plan of care. Before establishing nursing diagnoses, the nurse analyzes the significance of findings collected during assessment:

1. Prenatal record
   a. Obstetric history
   b. Client profile
   c. General history
2. Initial examination
3. Progress in labor
   a. Cervical dilatation and descent
   b. Uterine contractions
   c. Rupture of membranes and amniotic fluid
4. Stress in labor
   a. Fetal
   b. Maternal
   c. Paternal

Analysis of findings results in the identification of nursing diagnoses. The following is a list of 10 examples of possible nursing diagnoses. This list is not exhaustive.

1. Potential alteration in parenting of child at home because labor began before expected due date (EDC)
2. Ineffective individual coping because of lack of familiarity with labor unit, staff, and hospital policies
3. Potential fluid volume deficit because of fluid restrictions during labor
4. Fear because of unfamiliar sensations during the labor process
5. Impaired gas exchange because of hyperventilation
6. Alteration in nutrition of the parturient (and her family) because of long labor and involvement in the labor process
7. Ineffective individual coping because of exhaustion from long labor (or sleep deficit or unexpected happenings, etc.)
8. Alteration in mobility because of station of fetal presenting part and status of fetal membranes
9. Alteration in mobility because of fetal monitoring
10. Alteration in urinary elimination because of bed rest during labor, analgesia or anesthesia, or other reason

Nursing diagnoses developed for the parturient become the bases for planning individualization of nursing actions.

Planning

Planning for nursing actions that assist in meeting the goals for care identified in the introduction to this chapter is essential if goals are to be met. Planning is essential for the implementation of the following:

1. Continuous, comprehensive assessment of physical and emotional response to labor
2. Coordination of the efforts of the health care team
3. Rapid identification of and intervention in medical-surgical and obstetric emergencies
4. Support of the family's chosen level of involvement and control
5. Formulation of nursing diagnoses individualized to specific parturients and their families

Implementation

PROCEDURES

Before starting any procedures, recheck the physician's order and the labels on any solutions, ointments, or other material used in the procedure; if hospital sterilized packs are used, check for sterility by noting appropriate sign of sterility (e.g., disks or crystals that change color or diagonal black stripes over the tape) and the date; check the woman's identification band and hospital number. Even with prepackaged supplies, such as intraveneous fluid bags and bottles, check for defects (cracks in bottle) and possible contamination (floating particles).

A calm manner, gentleness in carrying out necessary procedures with a thorough explanation of what is being done, and acceptance of the woman's definition of discomfort or pain serve as nursing support (caring) measures. The nurse must be willing to repeat instructions and modify the time taken to carry out procedures. The responsibility for initiating and maintaining such a therapeutic relationship rests with the nurse.

PREPARATION OF THE VULVA: THE "MINI-PREP"

The "mini-prep" (or *no* prep) has taken the place of shaving the parturient's pubic hair and vulva. Shaving is undesirable because even in expert hands, the razor leaves nicks and scrapes that serve as portals of entry for infection; there may be small warts or moles that could be cut inadvertently; the procedure is uncomfortable especially if the woman is trying to work with her contractions; and regrowth of the hair is accompanied by severe itching. A mini-prep—depending on the hospital—is either a clipping of vulvar hair with scissors or a shaving of a very small area between the vagina and the anus, the site for episiotomies. The vulvar area is cleansed with a soap solution or nonirritating detergent preparation on admission and repeated after elimination, vaginal examinations, or vaginal discharge.

ENEMA

Historically, in North American hospitals, enemas were given to women in early labor to add to the space available for stretching of the birth canal by emptying the bowel and to prevent bowel movements later in labor. However, if the onset of labor was preceded by diarrhea, a common occurrence, there is no need for the enema. Enemas do add to the discomfort (and unpleasantness) of labor, but there are times when an enema is necessary: when the rectum is full and could impede the progress of the fetus through the vaginal canal, and to stimulate reflex uterine contractions.

When an enema is necessary, a physiologic solution (several prepared formulas in individual dose bottles are available commercially), *never* a soapsuds enema*, is given according to directions on the label. The fluid is inserted slowly *between* contractions.

Because enemas stimulate uterine contractions, they are not given in the presence of vaginal bleeding. The bleeding may be caused by a placenta previa (see Chapter 35) and the contractions could result in cervical dilatation, separation of the placenta, and life-threatening (to the fetus) complications especially hemorrhage. Uterine contractions for the woman whose premature labor is being suppressed (Chapter 37) could stimulate the onset of labor. If the presenting part is not yet engaged, uterine contractions could cause rupture of membranes and possible prolapsed cord (see p. 407).

*Soapsuds enemas have been implicated in soapsuds emboli and damage to intestinal mucosa (Mitchell, 1981).

Times Not to Give an Enema

1. Vaginal bleeding
2. Premature labor
3. Presenting part not engaged or abnormal (e.g., breech, transverse lie)

INTRAVENOUS THERAPY

Intravenous (IV) procedures have become routine in many hospitals. If the parturient has an intravenous line in place, the nurse follows the hospital's protocols for its care. These protocols may include the following:

1. Solution: Recheck physician's order with label on solution container; monitor flow rate accurately and record level of solution every hour; check for possible contamination of solution (cloudy or discolored fluid).
2. Check patency of all tubing.
3. Check venipuncture site for pain, warmth, redness, swelling, leakage of fluid or oozing of blood, position of extremity, and security and comfort of tape. The tape at the venipuncture site should have written on it the type of needle that is in place and the date and time it was started.
4. Assess woman for circulatory overload: headache, tachycardia, neck vein distention, elevated blood pressure, respiratory distress, shortness of breath, shock, and pulmonary edema.
5. Be alert for the following symptoms if the intravenous therapy has continued for more than 24 hours: pyrogenic reaction (inflammation or infection) signaled by elevated temperature, tachycardia, and hypotension.
6. The woman is informed of the purpose and importance of intravenous fluid therapy and is cautioned not to touch the tubing or lie on it.

Intravenous therapy has several advantages: it provides a ready "lifeline" if complications occur and the woman requires fluids for the treatment of hypovolemic shock or if she needs medications. It provides fluids and calories when she may be unable to take anything by mouth for a period of time. It prevents dehydration that can result in fatigue, increased temperature, and generalized discomfort.

Intravenous fluids are not necessary for every woman in labor. The woman whose labor is progressing normally, who is able to take oral clear fluids with sugar, and who is planning to receive no analgesics or anesthetics is not usually in need of intravenous fluid. Each woman should be evaluated as an individual.

Fig. 21.5
Vaginal examination.

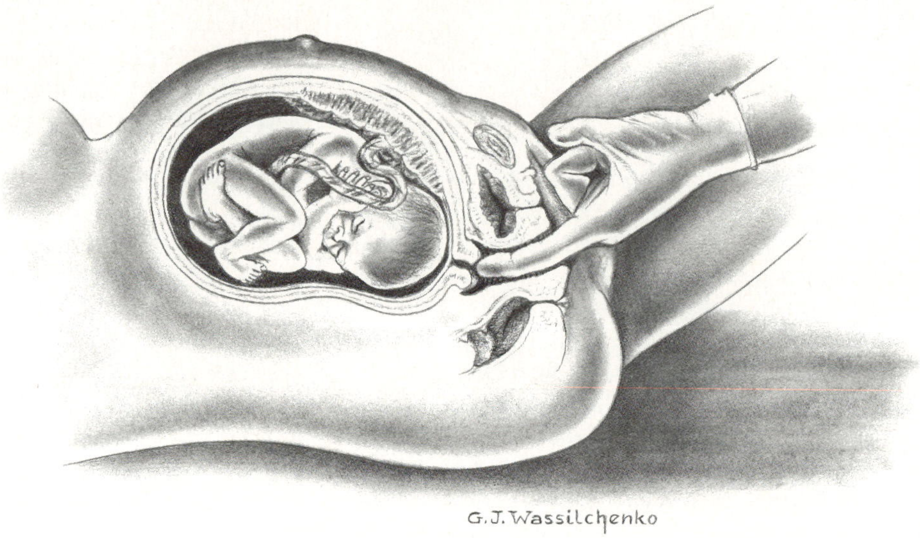

Fig. 21.6
Prolapse of umbilical cord. Note pressure of presenting part on umbilical cord, which endangers fetal circulation. **A,** Occult (hidden) prolapse of cord. **B,** Complete prolapse of cord. **C,** Cord presenting in front of fetal head and may be seen within vagina. **D,** Breech presentation with prolapsed cord.

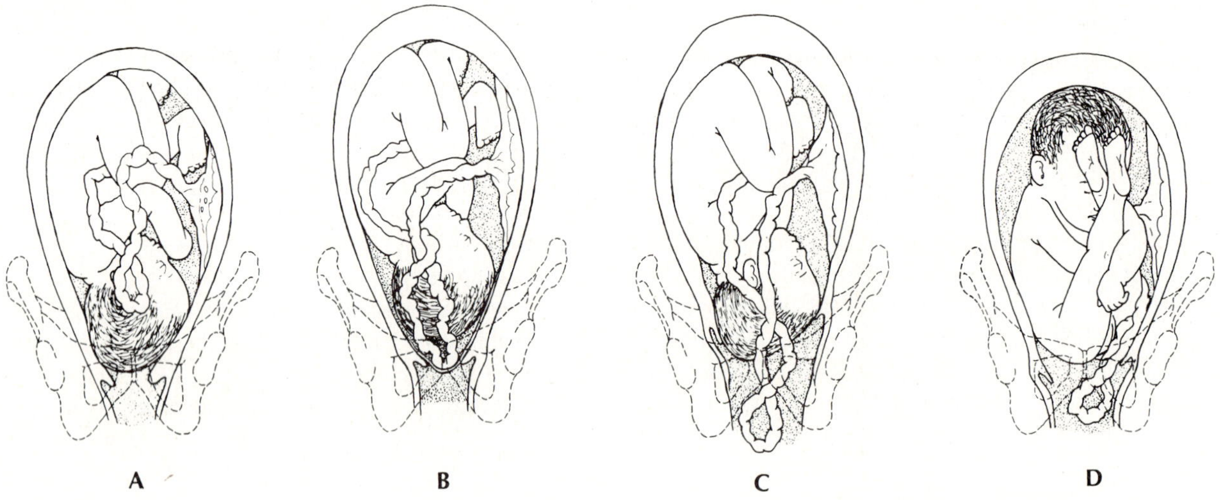

ASSISTING THE PHYSICIAN WITH VAGINAL EXAMINATIONS

The nurse fan-folds the parturient's covers to the foot of the bed, helps her assume the lithotomy position, drapes her suitably, and positions the light, (if needed) for better viewing of her vulva. The nurse offers the physician, midwife, or other nurse gloves and lubricant or antiseptic solution for the internal examination (Fig. 21.5). During the examination, the nurse coaches the woman with breathing or focusing. Remember, the woman is more capable of relaxing her pelvic floor if she does not squeeze her eyes closed, if she does not squeeze the nurse's hands or bed rail, and if she can keep her mouth relaxed.

After the examination, clean the parturient's vulva if necessary, place a clean pad on the bed under her, and reposition her bed covers according to her preference. If she has questions about what the physician told her about the findings of the examination, repeat the explanations and clarify any misunderstandings.

The physician or examiner records findings on the appropriate record immediately following the examination. *Each* entry onto the labor record is noted with the time and ended with the examiner's signature or initials.

• • •

For *coaching, breathing, and focusing techniques,* see Chapter 19.

For a discussion of *fetal monitoring,* see Chapter 24.

EMERGENCY PROCEDURES

Prolapsed cord. Prolapse of the umbilical cord is displacement of the cord downward, often below the presenting part (Fig. 21.6). Occasionally, the cord may even slip through the cervix into the vagina or beyond. A long, loose cord and an unengaged presenting part or breech presentation, frequently associated with rupture of membranes, may allow prolapse of the cord because the cord may be carried downward with a sudden gush of fluid. The gravida may feel the cord slither into the vagina when the membranes rupture. More often, vaginal examination by an alert nurse or physician immediately after a sudden gush of fluid may lead to the diagnosis of prolapsed cord. Prompt recognition of prolapse of the cord, which occurs in 1 of every 400 late pregnancies and more often in immature gestations (under 37 weeks), is important because the cord may be compressed between the presenting part and the bony pelvis. Fetal hypoxia from prolonged cord compression (i.e., more than 5 minutes) usually causes central nervous system (CNS) damage or death of the fetus.

Both the woman's knee-chest or Trendelenburg's position and the vaginal support of the presenting part to keep the presenting part away from the prolapsed cord are continuously maintained until delivery is accomplished (see p. 408). Immediate cesarean birth is indicated unless cervix is fully dilated, in which case rapid forceps delivery of a vertex or extraction of a breech presentation may be feasible. Prompt delivery in the manner least harmful to mother and infant is imperative.

Fetal Distress or Abnormal FHR Patterns

1. Change maternal position:
   a. For late deceleration, place mother in the left lateral position.
   b. For prolapsed cord, place mother in knee-chest position or any other position that corrects the problem.
2. Correct maternal hypotension:
   a. Elevate her legs.
   b. Increase rate of maintenance IV.
3. Stop stimulation of uterine contractions by discontinuing oxytocin infusion.
4. Administer oxygen by face mask at 10 to 12 L/min.

Inadequate Uterine Relaxation*

1. Change maternal position.
2. Stop stimulation of uterine contractions by discontinuing oxytocin infusion.
3. Notify physician.
4. Administer oxygen by tight face mask at 10 to 12 L/min until physician arrives and permits oxygen to be discontinued.

*Contractions lasting longer than 90 seconds; relaxation between contractions inadequate or less than 30 seconds.

Fetal distress or abnormal FHR pattern. Fetal distress may occur in the absence of prolapsed cord. If distress is noted, the nurse implements the measures given in the box above.

The physician should be notified immediately of the fetal distress or abnormal FHR pattern, the nursing actions implemented, and the fetal response to the interventions recorded. For further discussion, see Chapter 24.

Uterine contractions. Uterine contractions can be stressful to the fetus. To prevent possible damage to the fetus, the nurse continuously assesses uterine contractions to identify those that can lead to fetal jeopardy.

Rupture of Membranes and Prolapse of the Cord

1. Auscultate FHR immediately after rupture of the membranes and perform a vaginal examination. If no prolapse is evident at that time, reassess FHR within 10 minutes; strong uterine contractions stimulated by rupturing of membranes can force the cord down to beside or in front of the presenting part.
2. If prolapse is suspected, immediately:
   a. If possible, glove the examining hand rapidly and insert two fingers into the vagina to the cervix. With one finger to one side of the cord—do not compress the cord with the fingers—exert upward pressure against the presenting part to relieve the compression of the cord (Fig. 21.7), or
   b. Assist or direct others to assist the woman into the knee-chest position or extreme Trendelenburg's position so that gravity pulls the presenting part down and thus relieves the compression of the cord (Fig. 21.8).
3. If the cord is protruding from the vagina, direct others to wrap it loosely in a sterile towel wet with sterile normal saline.
4. Direct others to apply a face mask for oxygen. Give oxygen at 10 to 12 L/min until delivery is accomplished.

Fig. 21.7
The arrow indicates direction of pressure of examiner's fingers against presenting part to relieve compression of prolapsed umbilical cord in vertex presentation, **A,** and in breech position, **B.**

A

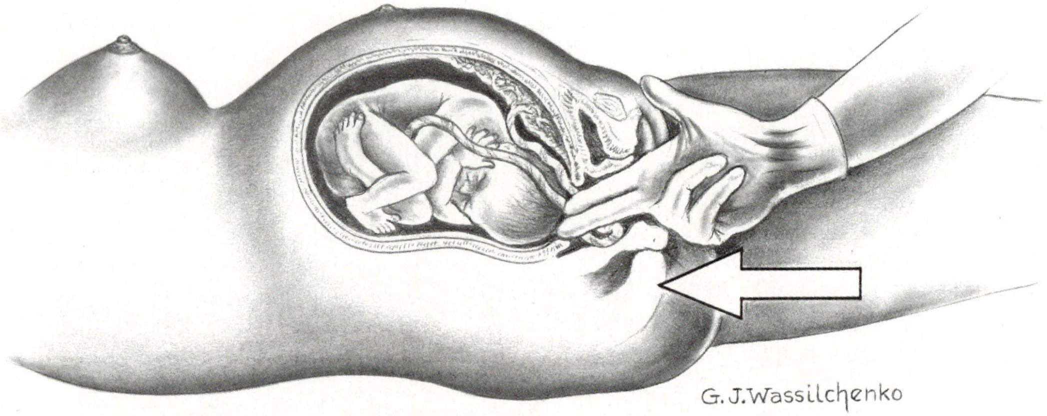

B

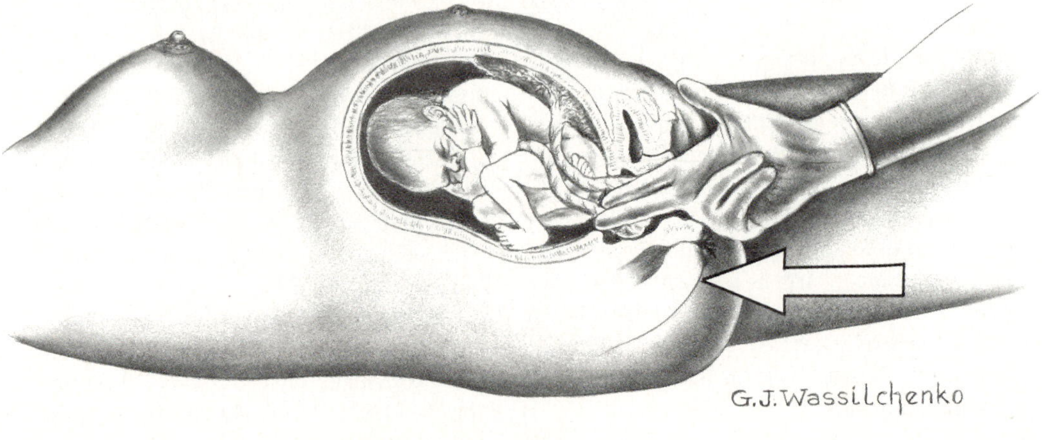

Fig. 21.8
Changes in maternal position that assist in relief of pressure of presenting part on prolapsed umbilical cord. **A,** Knee-chest position. **B,** Modified Sims position. Note: hips are elevated as high as possible with pillows.

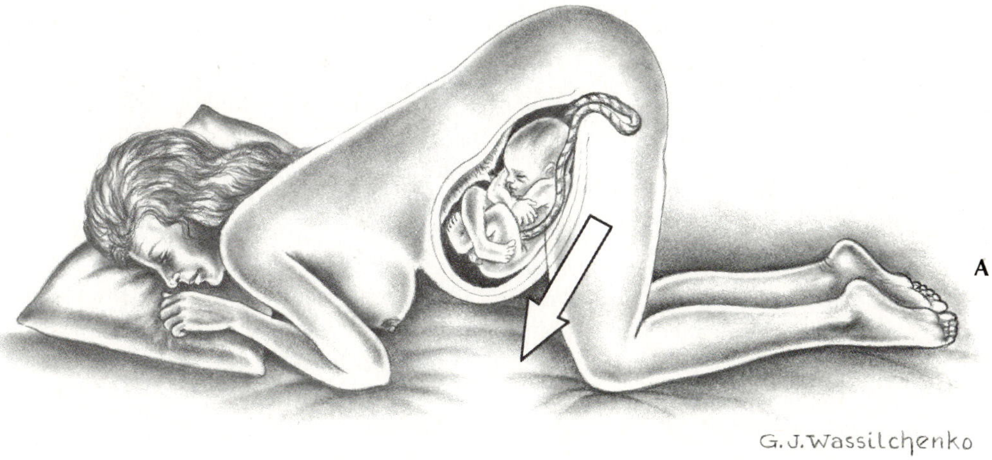

A

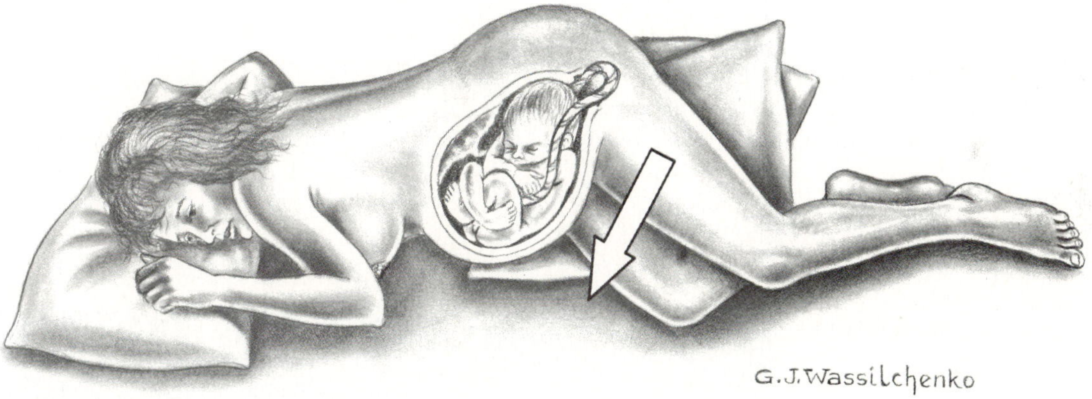

B

MOTHERHOOD WITH DIGNITY

Admission to the labor unit. First impressions are vivid. The woman and her partner or family need to feel welcome. The nurse addresses them by name and introduces herself. The nurse then determines whether the woman wishes her partner or family member to stay throughout the examination. If not, the partner may be directed to the waiting area. Then the woman is asked to undress and get into bed, and her personal belongings are put away safely. For legal reasons, most hospitals have a check list or other method of recording her belongings that becomes part of her permanent record. If the woman prefers to wear some items of her own (e.g., knee socks), these are noted on her chart.

Her understanding of the use of the call bell (or light) is checked, and she is told the reasons that bathroom privileges are permitted or not (if the membranes have ruptured, have her remain in bed until assessment for potential prolapse of the umbilical cord is completed). The routine of care is reviewed, that is, which techniques will be used to assess progress, the reasons for using them, and how the woman or couple may assist in reporting her progress.

She then signs the necessary papers giving permission for care for herself and her newborn, and her identification bracelet is secured. Legally, a permit for care must be signed before the woman receives any medication for discomfort.

If parking is a problem at that facility, the nurse inquires if she came by car and where the car is parked. The nurse may need to advise a family member to repark the car, or, as in a recent case where the woman drove in herself and therefore could not repark the car, the nurse must inform the hospital's security forces.

Some women, especially those who arrive in labor unexpectedly (e.g., directly from the physician's office), welcome the offer of a telephone to notify their families. In some instances the nurse may have to make the calls to the family.

Do not increase the woman's anxiety by quizzing her about her understanding of terms commonly used during labor. As the nurse reviews the woman's prenatal record, the nurse can add short definitions or explanations for technical terms and abbreviations. The woman's interest and response serve to guide the nurse in chosing the depth and breadth of the explanations. The nurse's openness and willingness to explain can be reassurance in itself—it indicates to the woman and her family that there need be no ''secrets.''

For the minimal schedule for reassessment of progress during the first stage of labor, see Table 21.3.

Intake and output. Dietary intake (if the woman is not NPO) must be limited to clear fluids as ordered by the physician (Fig. 21.9). Some women bring lollipops to suck, or ice chips can be offered (if ordered). Frequent cleansing of the mouth with a toothbrush or washing the teeth with an ice-cold wet washcloth helps to counteract the dry, thirsty feeling, a complaint of many women. An infusion of 1000 ml of 5% dextrose in Ringer's lactated solution at a slow drip rate may be ordered. Small amounts of antacids may be given to prevent possible tracheal irritation in case of vomiting.

The woman is encouraged to void at least every 2 hours. If the presenting part is engaged or the membranes are not ruptured and the woman is not medicated, the physician usually orders bathroom privileges; otherwise, she uses a bedpan.* Side rails are then used, since labor beds are usually narrow and women can fall off the bedpan used in the bed.

Techniques for stimulating voiding are often helpful (e.g., turning on the tap, pouring warm water over the vulva, ensuring privacy). If the woman is unable to void, she should be catheterized to prevent overdistention of the bladder. Overdistention may cause bladder atony and injury and difficulty in voiding postnatally. A full bladder may also impede descent of the presenting part. Danger of infection is increased because the urethra has usually been traumatized by the pressure of the presenting part. The catheter is inserted between contractions to avoid going counter to the force of the descending head; it is inserted far enough to account for

*Only a registered nurse should give and remove bedpans for women in labor. Women often misinterpret rectal pressure from the presenting part as the need to defecate; the nurse assesses the situation each time.

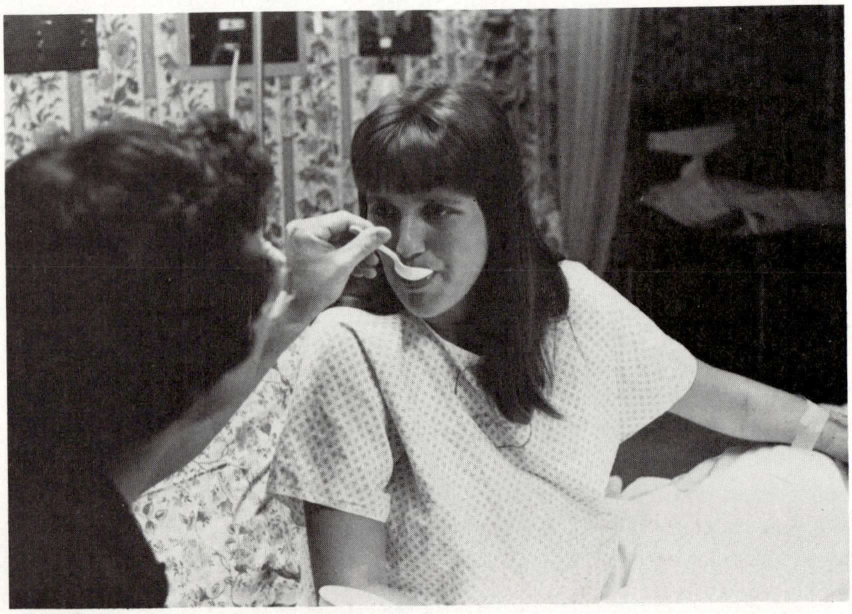

Fig. 21.9
Father providing comfort during labor by offering ice chips. (Photograph by M. Pyle.)

the slight elongation of the urethra during pregnancy.

Maternal position during labor. The position women assume during labor and birth has not been dictated as much by physiology as by culturally patterned behavior. Women may ambulate, stand, squat, sit, or kneel (Fig. 21.10). There is apparently no "right" position; each has a positive and a negative effect. For example, the squatting position in the second stage of labor enlarges the pelvic outlet and makes use of the forces of gravity; however, if assumed before engagement, it impedes descent. Research has shown that women in the upright position during labor and birth have stronger and more efficient contractions, shorter labor duration, and increased comfort.

The dorsal recumbent or semirecumbent position came into use in the nineteenth century with the advent of the obstetric forceps. It is still advocated in most developed countries because it is more convenient for auscultation of the fetal heart, administration of anesthetics, application of forceps, and management of postdelivery hemorrhage. However, this position* results in the development of supine hypotension (Fig. 21.11). The weight of the gravid uterus compresses the ascending vena cava, impeding blood return to the right atrium with a resultant drop in cardiac output and maternal hypotension. To maintain placental perfusion the systolic pressure (brachial artery) must remain above 100 mm Hg. To minimize this danger, any woman who desires or is required to remain in bed during labor should assume a left lateral position or, if supine, have a wedge placed under the right hip to maintain a tilt to the left. She is encouraged to assume a sitting position (45-degree angle) as much as possible.

Many authorities are now suggesting that women in labor ambulate and assume any position that feels comfortable. Delivery occurs with the woman supported in a semisitting or semireclining position, her feet resting on the bed and her legs supported with pillows. Beds and chairs are now designed to function both for labor and for birth (see Chapter 22). The traditional delivery table is still widely used, however.

Much research is presently being directed toward a better understanding of the physiologic and psychic effects of maternal position in labor. It is important to appreciate that clinical entities such as fetal presentations or mechanisms of labor may be helped or hindered by maternal posture. No fixed approach seems to have contributed to progress in labor and the physical well-being of the mother and the child.

Comfort measures. Important components of the nursing care of the woman in labor relate to (1) helping the parturient participate to the extent she wishes in the delivery of her infant, (2) meeting her goals for herself, (3) assisting her to conserve her energy, and (4) helping her in the control of her discomfort.

*For other factors that impede circulation to the maternal-fetal-placental unit, see discussion of fetal monitoring, Chapter 24.

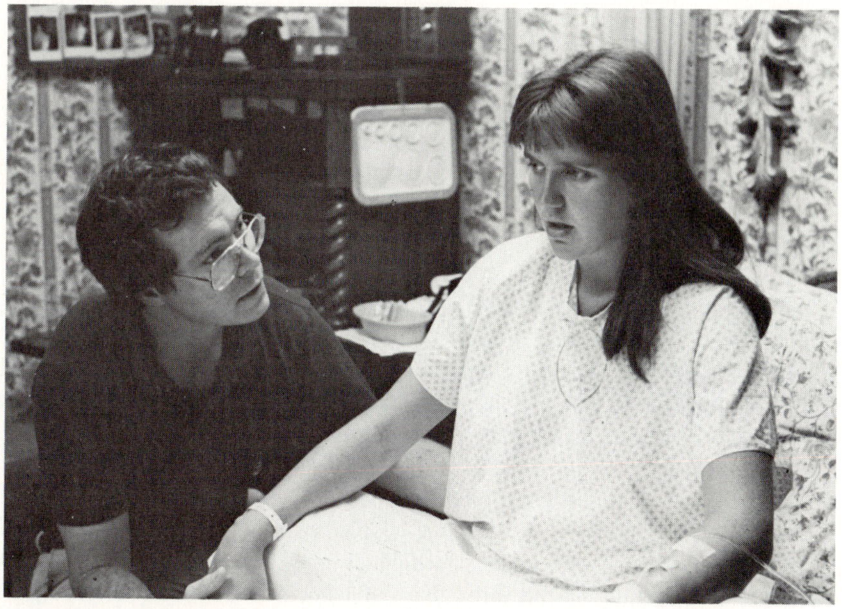

Fig. 21.10
Father coaching mother during first stage of labor. Note intense concentration of couple during contraction. Mother is sitting tailor fashion; fluid, electrolyte, and caloric needs are being met with intravenous infusion (Photograph by M. Pyle.)

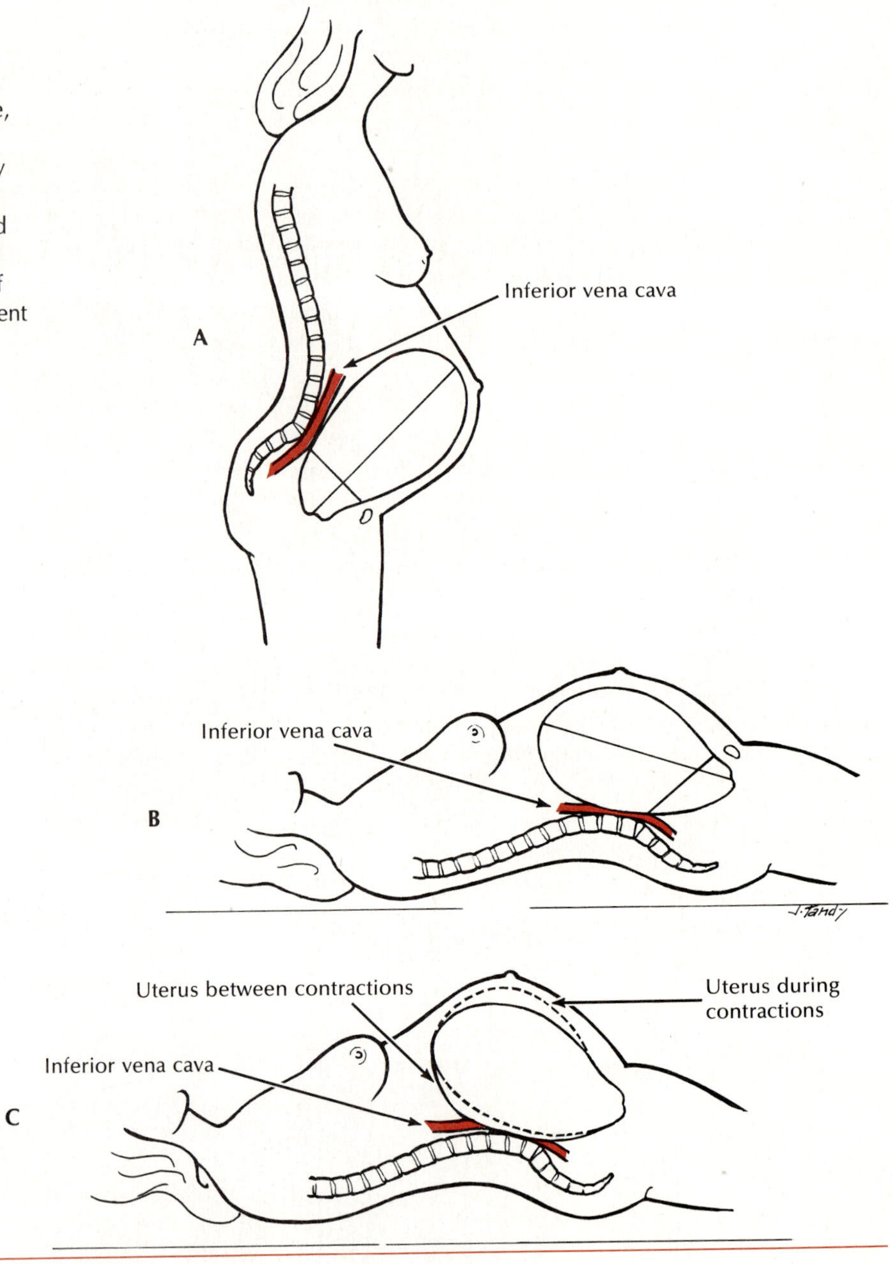

Fig. 21.11
Vena cava syndrome. Note relationship of gravid uterus to ascending vena cava in standing posture, **A,** and in supine posture, **B.** Note how enlarged uterus compresses vena cava, especially during contraction, **C,** reducing return of blood to heart. Reduced cardiac output causes maternal hypotension and reduced flow of blood to placenta, with consequent fetal distress.

An understanding, competent nurse acts as an advocate for the woman and her family. Couples who have attended childbirth education programs using the psychoprophylactic approach will have knowledge of the labor process, coaching techniques, and comfort measures (see Chapter 19 and Fig. 21.12). However, the staff's role is to continue to be supportive and to keep them informed of progress. Even if the couple has not attended such classes, the various techniques may be taught to a degree during the early phase of labor; the nurse will be expected to do more of the coaching and give supportive care. If the woman is alone, the nursing staff acts as the substitute family, coaching and supporting her, and helping her to use her energy constructively in relaxing and in working with the contractions.

Comfort measures vary with the situation (Fig. 21.13). Some have been discussed in Chapter 19. The nurse can draw on the couple's repertoire of comfort measures learned during the pregnancy. The comfort measures to be discussed below include general hygiene, including mouth care; maintaining a comfortable, supportive atmosphere in the labor and delivery

Fig. 21.12
Father providing comfort, **A,** by supplying warmth with an extra blanket, and, **B,** with a cool cloth to forehead. (Photograph by M. Pyle.)

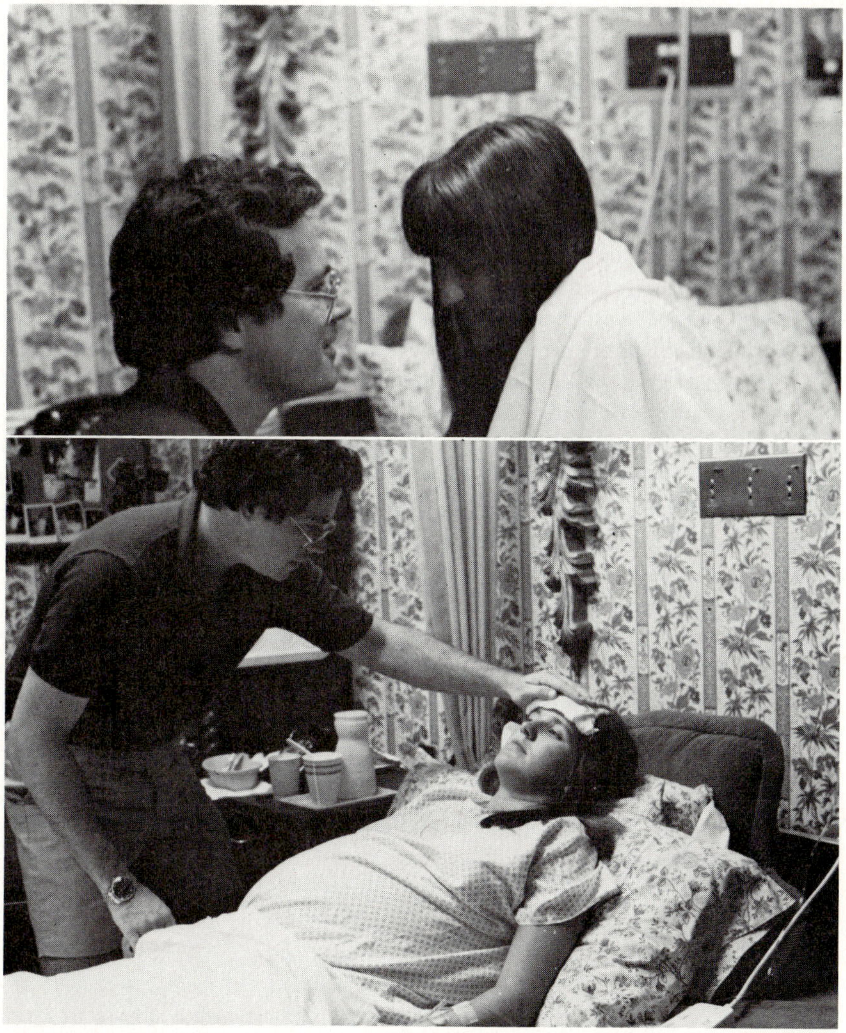

Fig. 21.13
Parents-to-be supporting each other during labor. (Photograph by M. Pyle.)

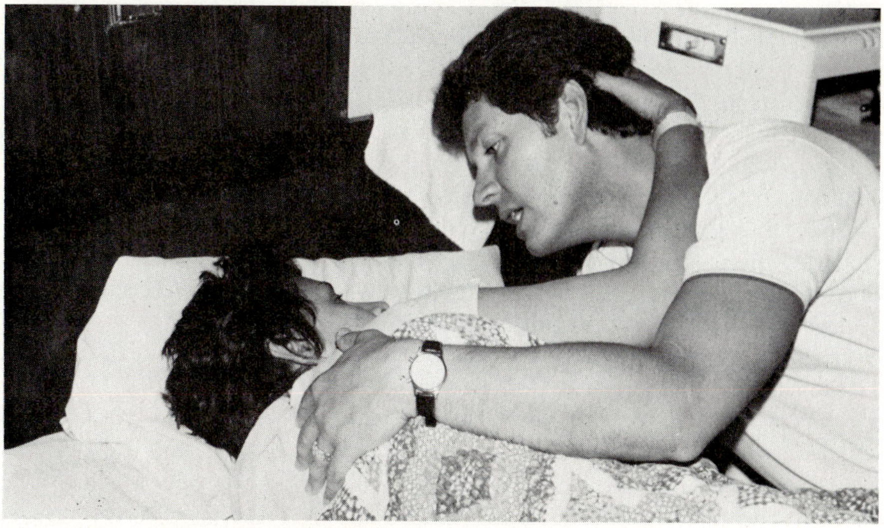

area; using touch therapeutically; and administering analgesics when necessary; but, most of all, just *being there*.

General hygiene. Showers or bed baths may be taken depending on the progress of labor. Allowing warm water to strike the lower part of the back may be very relaxing; care is taken to avoid chilling. The vulva is cleansed with soap and water on admission and cleansed before and after vaginal examinations, defecating, and voiding or when soiled by vaginal secretions. Oral hygiene may need to be done every hour or more often. Mouth washes of the woman's choice can be used. Good mouth hygiene helps relieve the feeling of dryness that occurs at this time. If the woman does not want or cannot use the mouth wash or brush her teeth during the labor, a cold washcloth wiped over her teeth gives her a feeling of cleanliness and helps decrease thirst. The parturient's gowns and linens are changed, even if not soiled but only wrinkled and used for a period of time. Clean linen and a fluffed-up pillow do wonders for the woman's morale.

Atmosphere of the labor and delivery area. Labor rooms need to be light and airy. However, the bright overhead lights are turned off when not needed. The area should be large enough to accommodate the woman's partner in a comfortable chair, as well as the monitoring equipment and hospital personnel. In some hospitals, couples are urged to bring extra pillows to help make the hospital surrounding more homelike. Labor areas *should be constructed with windows* that can be hung with colorful curtains. When people stay in any area for a period of time and do not have access to a view of the outside world, it is easy to become disoriented to time and to focus unnaturally on whatever is happening to them.

The room temperature is kept at a comfortable level—between 20° and 22.2° C (68° and 72° F). Although most women feel very warm during labor, a number complain of feeling cold. A warm blanket placed over the woman and one wrapped around her feet are comforting. Many women wish to wear socks. For those who feel too warm, a cool moist cloth placed on the forehead can be soothing, as can ice chips given for sucking (where permissible).

Touch. Most women respond positively to touch in labor. They appreciate gentle handling by the staff. Effleurage may be effective in helping them relax between contractions. Counterpressure against the sacrum during a contraction results in relief from discomfort. Back rubs, including over the sacral area and the buttocks (especially for women who have been in labor a long time), every hour or two and as necessary between contractions help to ease tension. If possible, warm foot baths followed by foot massage can result in general body relaxation. The woman's awareness of the soothing qualities of touch changes as labor progresses. Many women develop hyperesthesia (increased sensitivity, especially in the skin) as labor progresses. They may tell their coach to "leave me alone," or they may say, "Don't touch me." The partner who is unprepared for this normal response may feel rejected and may react by withdrawing active support. The nurse can point out that this response on the part of the woman is a positive indication that the first stage is ending and that the transitional stage is approaching. The woman's aggressive behavior is accepted; negative comments are unwarranted and inappropriate.

Sound is the touching of sound waves against the tympanic membrane of the ear. The nurse can use soft tones in speaking to the woman. Even firm commands to breathe a certain way or to pant-breathe to avoid pushing at the wrong time can be done without resorting to harsh, vibrant speech.

We believe that the manner in which a woman is touched during her labor is immediately reflected in the manner in which she touches (including her voice) her infant after birth; she must get before she can give.

Pain and its relief. The alleviation of pain is important. Frequently it is not the amount of pain the woman experiences, but *whether or not she meets her goals for herself in coping with the pain* that influences her perception of the birth experience as "good" or "bad." The observant nurse looks for cues to identify the woman's desired level of control in the management of pain and its relief.

The pain associated with parturition was accepted as a necessary part of childbirth until the discovery of the first anesthetics, nitrous oxide and ethyl ether. Since that time much research has gone into the development of methods of pain control that can bring effective relief for the mother without harm to the child. The perfect solution is yet to be found; therefore at times the safety of the child must take precedence over the comfort of the mother.

Nonmedicated methods of relief of discomfort are taught in many different types of prenatal preparation classes and are available in various books and magazines (see Chapter 19).

The nursing process and pharmacologic methods in the control of discomfort are discussed in Chapter 25.

FATHERHOOD WITH DIGNITY

Miller (1966) remarked, "There is joy in having a baby, and joy is an experience worth sharing." Conception is a psychologic as well as a physiologic experience of a man and woman creating a new life; birth can be no less. Conception is the experience of two persons; birth, the experience of three (or more) persons.

Involving the father in the birth of his child dispels feelings of alienation, isolation, impotence, helpless inaction, and insignificance. *Ethnic definition and role expectations govern the type and degree of the individual's involvement.*

Individual preference for the kind of involvement spans a full spectrum of possibilities. One family, recent arrivals from Italy, is a case in point. The father absented himself to the waiting room while the female relatives took turns attending his wife and reporting her progress to him at intervals. After delivery wife and son were wheeled back to the labor area. The father entered proudly as the female relatives stepped aside. He made what sounded like endearing comments to wife and son and kissed them both; then all the relatives left. The new mother beamed. The students present expressed negative reactions about this father, whose participation in this event was perceived as tangential and unsupportive. One student was assigned to this mother's postdelivery care and to make a home visit. Her report and discussion of her experience with the group clarified the situation as "right" for this family.

Other men seek a different type of involvement. What are their hopes and expectations for this experience for themselves and their wives? What is the nurse's role in relation to their decisions? These questions will be discussed in the following sections.

Birth process as seen through father's eyes. The nurse should recall her feelings the first time she witnessed a woman in active labor. The father's experience can be no less intense. In addition, the woman in labor is not a client to him; she is birthing their baby.

During the delivery he may see the following:

1. Her facial and physical expression of pain; grimace and effort written on her face while pushing
2. Blood, mucus, and watery drainage from her vagina
3. Fecal discharge
4. Bulging perineum just before birth
5. Episiotomy, if done, and repair
6. Delivery by forceps, if used
7. Her postures for vaginal examinations, for observations of the perineum, and for delivery
8. Dry heaves or vomiting

He may hear the following:

1. Her moans and grunts (especially while pushing)
2. Dry heaves or efforts at vomiting
3. Hospital noises (e.g., call lights, page systems, clanging, sterilizer buzzers, fetal monitoring devices)
4. Protests about fathers who "belong in a waiting room" and who "should leave this to us"
5. Extraneous, irrelevant social or business chatter among staff

He may smell the following:

1. Vaginal drainage
2. Fecal drainage
3. Vomitus (occasionally)
4. Cleaning solutions or anesthetics

With the emergence of the infant, the father will see and hear the following:

1. Small patch of scalp and hair at the introitus
2. Prolonged (usually) emergence of the molded fetal head (e.g., one father commented, "and then when all that kept coming out was head and more head and no eyes or ears, I wondered when they would come")
3. Blue-purple coloration of the fetal scalp and body along with blood, amniotic fluid, vernix, and occasionally meconium
4. Cord being loosened around the child's neck and or being eased over his head or shoulders
5. Mucus draining from nose and mouth and the physician or nurse suctioning the infant
6. Sounds of suctioning
7. Cutting the cord
8. Verbal communications between physician and nurse regarding position, cord, placement of episiotomy, and similar medical matters in terms often unfamiliar to him.

Father in labor suite. "He'll just be underfoot." "He'll add confusion and increase the chance of infections and the number of lawsuits." These typical statements for years kept the father apart from his wife and child. These fears proved largely unfounded when fathers were reunited with their laboring wives. Fathers proved helpful, comforting, and reassuring to their wives. There was no change in the incidence of infection or lawsuits. Furthermore, it was found that it was easier for the physician and parents to cope with the birth of a child with a defect when both parents were active participants on an adult-to-adult level with the physician.

The father may be an adjunct to the nurse-physician team in several ways. For example, he may assist with comfort measures such as pillows, ice chips, washcloths to forehead, and back rubs. He may provide almost constant companionship to offset the aloneness of labor and the anxiety it can foster. Should something occur when the nurse or physician is out of the room, the father can call for help. In addition, he is usually better equipped to interpret the mother's wishes and needs to the staff.

Participation in the birth is ego building. The father *can* be of assistance; his presence *is* important. It is frequently observed that a caring person can be worth his (her) weight in Demerol (meperidine). Recently a 16-year-old unwed mother in labor with her first child thrashed about, moaning and screaming with each contraction. A nurse remained at her bedside, coaching and comforting to no avail. The unwed adolescent father arrived and was immediately escorted into her room. The young woman continued her labor calmly and unmedicated through delivery.

When the father is active and supportive, the mother turns to him; the physician remains the medical-surgical expert, without his taking on the father-or husband-surrogate role as well. The couple's future relationship and their relationship to their child may be positively influenced. Mutuality is fostered when the mother can turn to the father and say, "I could never have done it without you. You were my pillar of strength."

Supporting the father during labor. Supporting the father* as well as the mother in labor elevates the nurse's role. It is another step forward from merely providing custodial care to enacting a therapeutic role.

Supporting the father reflects the nurse's orientation and commitment to the person, the family, and the community. Therapeutic nursing actions convey to the father several important concepts.

First, he is of value as a person. He is not a comic strip character, inept and bungling or idle, nervous, and inconsequential. Second, he can learn to be a partner in the mother's care. Finally, childbearing is a partnership.

Even if the father enters the labor unit without any parent education classes, he can be taught "on the job," and his choices can be supported. The nurse can support the father in the following ways:

1. Regardless of the degree of involvement desired, orient him to the maternity unit, including wife's labor room and what he can do there (sleep, telephone, smoke or not), restroom, cafeteria, Dads' Room, nursery, visiting hours, and names and functions of personnel present.
2. Respect his or their decisions as to his degree of involvement whether the decision is active participation in the delivery room or just being kept informed. When appropriate, provide data on which he or they can base decisions; offer freedom of choice as opposed to coercion one way or another. This is *their* experience and *their* baby.
3. Indicate to him when his presence has been helpful.
4. Offer to teach him comfort measures to the degree he wants to know them. Reassure him that he is not assuming the responsibility for observation and management of his wife's labor. Supportive behavior can be classified into three categories:
   a. Physical care
   b. Nonverbal care (e.g., holding her hand, smiling, kissing)
   c. Verbal care (e.g., coaching breathing and relaxation techniques, complimenting)
5. Communicate with him frequently regarding her progress and his needs. Keep father or couple informed of procedures to be done, what to expect from procedures, and what is expected of him.
6. Prepare him for changes in her behavior and physical appearance.
7. Remind him to eat; offer snacks and fluids if possible.
8. Relieve him as necessary; offer blankets if he is to sleep in chair by bedside. Acknowledge the stress of the situation on each partner and identify normal responses. The nonjudgmental attitude of staff helps the father and mother accept their own and the other parent's behavior.
9. Attempt to modify or eliminate unsettling stimuli (e.g., extra noise, extra light, chatter); keep the woman clean and dry.

A well-informed father can make a significant contribution to the health and well-being of the mother and child, their family interrelationship, and his self-esteem. It has been found that a significantly lower percentage of women suffered postdelivery emotional upsets when their partners received support and assistance from prenatal classes, physicians, and nurses throughout the childbearing cycle and from community health nurses in the home.

PREPARATION FOR DELIVERY

The delivery room attendant is responsible for seeing that the facility is properly prepared and that all supplies and equipment are in working order at all times. The role of the woman's partner is reviewed and suitable operating room clothing provided. It is essential that the woman's record* be up to date, because her condition can change quickly.

The following are suggestions for preparation for delivery. These items may vary among different facilities so that the protocols from each facility's procedure manual should be consulted.

*These measures recognize parents' need for the nurse to be psychologically as well as physically present. They may be accomplished by the physician or nurse as the situation warrants.

*NOTE: All nursing care and the woman's or couple's responses must be recorded to (1) ensure continuity of care, (2) ensure appropriate assessment of the woman's progress; and (3) document the nursing and other care given. Courts of law insist that the nursing and medical care that is not documented on the client's record has *not* been given.

1. Scrubbing facilities, scrub brushes, cuticle sticks, cleaning agent, and masks are available.
2. The following have been done:
   a. Sterile gowns and gloves for physician or nurse-midwife, sterile drapes and towels for draping the woman, and sterile instruments and other supplies (e.g., sutures, anesthetic solutions) are arranged for convenience in use on sterile table.
   b. Sterile basin and water for hand washing during delivery process are readied for use.
   c. Supplies for cleansing vulva are available (e.g., sterile basin, sterile water, and cleansing solution).
   d. Delivery area is warmed and free from drafts.
   e. Infant receiving blankets and heated crib are readied. Material for prophylactic care of infant's eyes is available (see p. 442).
3. Equipment is in working order: delivery table (bed or chair), overhead lights, and mirror.
4. Emergency equipment, anesthesia, cardioscope, and supplies are available and in working order if needed for emergency situations such as control of maternal hemorrhage or fetal respiratory distress.
5. Additional supplies (anesthetics, oxytocics for injection, obstetric forceps) are available.
6. Woman's record is up-to-date and ready for use in delivery area. In areas such as labor unit, recordings are made concomitantly as symptoms are noted, assessments are made, and care is given. Since woman's condition can change quickly, it is imperative to have recordings complete at all times.

Evaluation

See the summary of the goals for the first, second, third, and fourth stages of labor in Table 23.2.

References and Readings

Friedman, E.A., and Sachtleben, M.R.: Station of the presenting part, Am. J. Obstet. Gynecol. **93:**522, 1965.

Hickman, M.A.: An introduction to midwifery, London, 1978, Blackwell Scientific Publications, Ltd.

Howe, C.L.: Physiologic and psychosocial assessment in labor, Nurs. Clin. North Am. **17**(1):49, 1982.

Jensen, M.D., Benson, R.C., and Bobak, I.M.: Maternity care: the nurse and the family, ed. 2., St. Louis, 1981, The C.V. Mosby Co.

Kitzinger, S.: The experience of childbirth, Baltimore, 1972, Pelican Books.

Lang, R.: The birth book, Ben Lomond, Calif., 1972, Genesis Press.

Liggins, G.C.: New concepts of what triggers labor, Contemp. Obstet. Gynecol. **19**(5):131, 1982.

Malinowski, J.S., et al.: Nursing care of the labor patient, ed. 2, Philadelphia, 1983, F.A. Davis Co.

Miller, J.S.: Return the joy of home delivery with fathers in the delivery room, Hosp. Top. **44:**105, Jan. 1966.

Mitchell, P.H.: Concepts basic to nursing, New York, 1981, McGraw-Hill Book Co.

Phillips, C.R., and Anzalone, J.T.: Fathering: participation in labor and birth, ed. 2, St. Louis, 1982, The C.V. Mosby Co.

Stark, J.L.: BUN/creatinine: your keys to kidney function, Nurs. '80 **10**(5):33, 1980.

Varney, H.: Nurse-midwifery, London, 1980, Blackwell Scientific Publications. Ltd.

Wiggins. J.D.: Childbearing: physiology, experiences, needs, St. Louis, 1979, The C.V. Mosby Co.

Zuspan, F.P., et al.: Predictors of intrapartum fetal distress: the role of electronic fetal monitoring. Report of the National Institute of Child Health and Human Development Consensus Development Task Force, Am. J. Obstet. Gynecol. **135:**287, Oct. 1979.

22

Second Stage of Labor

- **Mechanism of Delivery**
  - Delivery of head
  - Delivery of shoulders
  - Delivery of body and extremities
- **Nursing Care of Mother and Fetus**
  - Goals
  - Assessment
    - Examples of nursing diagnoses
  - Plan
  - Implementation
    - Maternal position
    - Bearing-down efforts
    - Amnesia
    - Fetal heart rate
    - Coach
    - Care for delivery
- **Nursing Care of the Newborn**
  - Goals
  - Assessment
    - Examples of nursing diagnoses
  - Plan and implementation
- **Parent-Child Relationships**
- **Emergency Child Birth: When the Nurse Assists the Mother To Give Birth**
  - Emergency birth of fetus in vertex presentation
  - Unusual occurrences during and after birth
    - Lateral Sims' position for delivery
    - Shoulder dystocia
    - Prebirth passage of meconium with fetus in vertex presentation
    - Tight nuchal cord
    - Maternal postdelivery hemorrhage
  - Emergency birth of fetus in breech presentation
  - Birth and management of preterm infant

When the cervix is fully dilated, the second stage of labor begins, and it ends with the delivery of the baby. As noted earlier, the transition period between the first and second stages is marked by more frequent contractions and sometimes increased discomfort.

The *forces* at work in this stage are uterine contractions, which occur every 2 to 3 minutes and last 50 to 60 seconds, and in addition the contractions of the diaphragm, abdominal musculature, and pelvic floor musculature, which exert a downward pressure on the fetus and decrease the size of the abdominal cavity. These latter forces can be voluntarily controlled, and efficient use of them expedites descent, crowning, and delivery of the head. The combined forces overcome the resistance of the soft tissues of the vagina and introitus, and the baby is born.

The *emotional responses* to entering the second stage of labor are usually excitement at the prospect of the imminent birth of the baby and eagerness to participate actively in the expulsion of the child. Even if parents have not attended childbirth classes, they are most amenable to suggestions as to how they can cooperate and share in this important event in their lives.

The *duration* of the second stage for a multipara is about 20 minutes, and for a nullipara it is approximately 50 minutes. Once the head reaches the pelvic floor (the outlet), fewer than 10 contractions probably will be required for delivery if the woman previously has given birth to a full-term infant. For a first delivery about 20 contractions will be necessary. Many labors are considerably shorter, however; hence one must be ready for the delivery when the head reaches the introitus. Care of the mother is based on a knowledge of the forces at work and an understanding of the mechanism of delivery.

The second stage of labor brings added stress to the infant. The mother may experience discomfort and fatigue, but the stress of labor can be harmful to the fetus. Therefore, continuous assessment of the fetus is mandatory. The second stage of labor includes the delivery of the infant. Thus the immediate care of the newborn and beginning parent-child relationships will be discussed in this chapter.

Mechanism of Delivery

There are three phases to a spontaneous, noninstrument delivery of the fetus in a vertex presentation*:

1. Delivery of the head
2. Delivery of the shoulders
3. Delivery of the body and extremities

The presenting part, in this instance the vertex, advances with each contraction and recedes slightly as the contraction wanes; descent is constant, and late in the second stage the head reaches the pelvic floor. The occiput generally rotates anteriorly, and with voluntary bearing-down efforts, the head distends the introitus. Although more and more caput may be seen with each push, the head "crowns" when its widest part (the biparietal diameter) distends the vulva just before birth (Fig. 22.1). Immediately before delivery, the perineal musculature becomes greatly distended. If an episiotomy is necessary, it is done at this time to minimize soft tissue damage.

*Review Figs 20.29 and 20.30.

DELIVERY OF HEAD

The vertex first appears, followed by the forehead, face, chin, and neck (Fig. 22.2). The speed of delivery of the head must be controlled, or sudden birth of the head may cause severe lacerations through the anal sphincter or even into the rectum. The physician or nurse-midwife controls the birth of the head by (1) applying pressure against the rectum, drawing it down-

Fig. 22.1
Changes in shape of introitus as dilatation of introitus occurs. **A,** Slitlike. **B,** Oval. **C,** Round. **D,** Crowning of head.

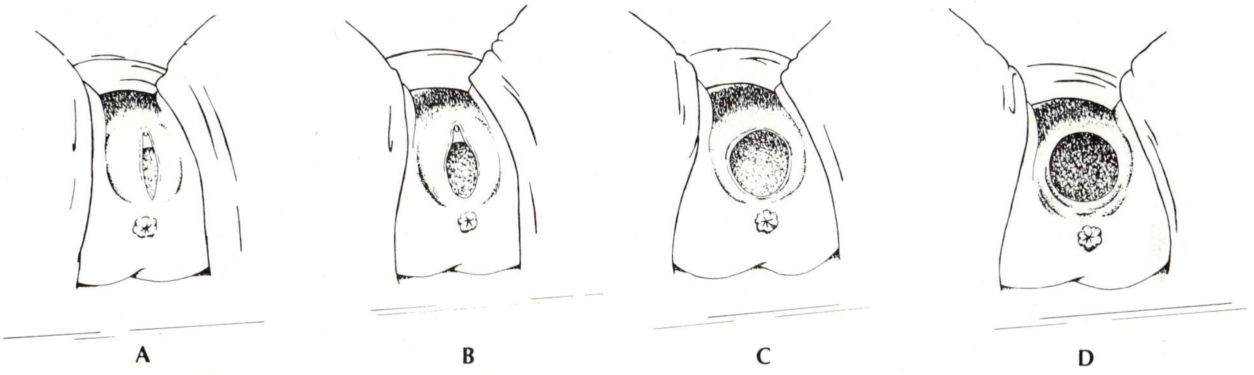

Fig. 22.2
Delivery of head (compare with Fig. 20.31). **A,** Extension. **B,** Delivery. **C,** Restitution. **D,** External rotation.

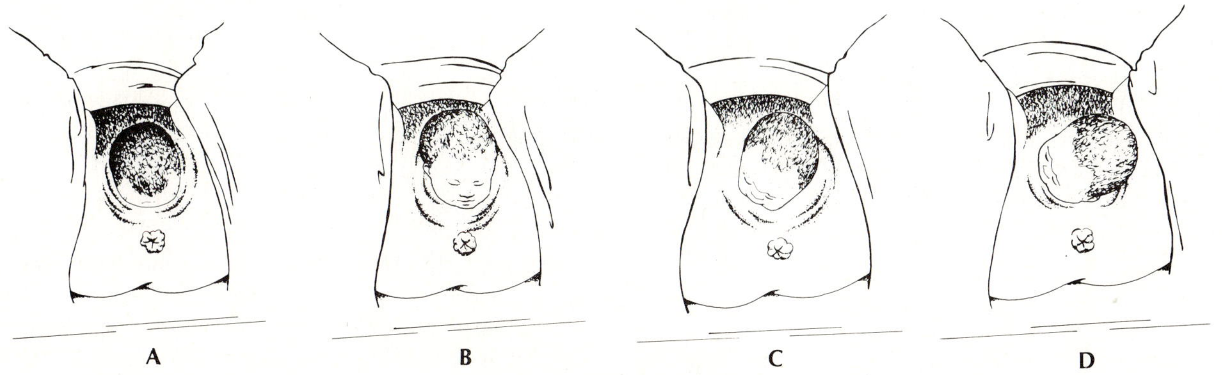

Fig. 22.3
Delivery of head by modified Ritgen maneuver. Note control to prevent rapid delivery of head.

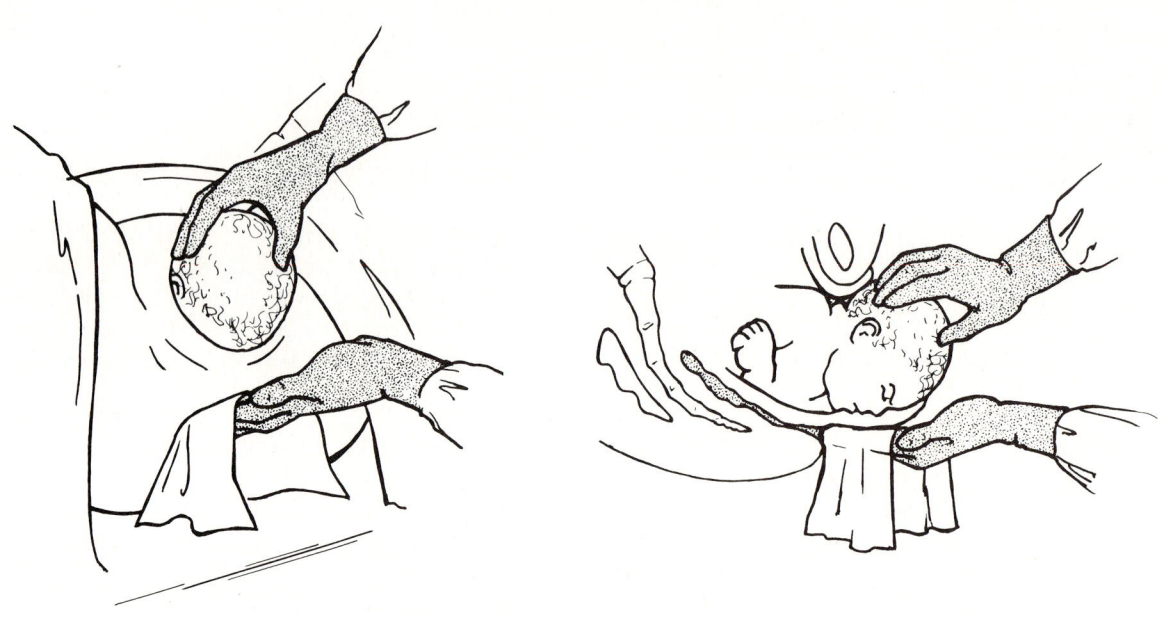

ward to aid in flexing the head as the back of the neck catches under the symphysis pubis; (2) then applying upward pressure from the coccygeal region (modified Ritgen maneuver) to extend the head during the actual delivery, thereby protecting the musculature of the perineum (Fig. 22.3); and (3) assisting the mother with voluntary control of the bearing-down efforts by coaching her to pant. Gradual delivery is imperative to prevent fetal intracranial injury.

The cord often encircles the neck but rarely so tightly as to cause critical hypoxia. The cord should be slipped gently over the head. If there is a tight or second loop, the cord is clamped twice, severed between the clamps, and unwound from around the neck, and then the delivery is continued. Mucus, blood, or meconium in the nasal or oral passages may prevent the newborn from breathing. Moist gauze sponges are used to wipe the nose and mouth. A bulb syringe is inserted into the mouth and throat (oral pharynx) to aspirate contents. The nares are cleared similarly while the head is being supported (see discussion of suctioning the neonate in Chapter 29).

DELIVERY OF SHOULDERS

Before the shoulders can be delivered, they must engage in the pelvic inlet. For this to occur the head is drawn back slightly toward the perineum, and external rotation of the head must occur. Then the shoulders pass through the pelvic inlet.

Now the head is drawn downward and backward to aid the anterior shoulder to impinge against the symphysis pubis and slide beneath the arch of the symphysis. If the head is then lifted upward, the posterior shoulder may be seen to distend the perineum. Several fingers gently inserted into the vagina allow delivery of the posterior arm. Slight downward traction is applied to the head to deliver the anterior shoulder and arm. On occasion, it may be easier to deliver the anterior shoulder first; however, if spontaneous rotation does not occur, the shoulders are rotated slowly to the anteroposterior diameter of the outlet.

Occasionally a hand may present with or after the head. If this occurs, the hand and arm are swept out gently before delivery of the shoulder. Traction and pressure must be limited to avoid damage to the brachial plexus or the neck vessels (see Chapter 37).

DELIVERY OF BODY AND EXTREMITIES

Easy, gradual traction should now deliver the baby. Slight rotation to the right or left may facilitate the birth. The ''time to be born'' has come. The infant, with all his potential, is now part of this world.*

*See Unit 5.

Nursing Care of Mother and Fetus

GOALS

The nurse provides continuous care during the second stage to accomplish the following:

1. Check for progress in descent of the presenting part
2. Monitor the quality and rate of contractions and the rate and regularity of fetal heart rate (FHR)
3. Assist the woman in controlling the voluntary bearing-down efforts

The nurse assumes responsibility for maintaining accurate records. Recording must be done concurrently with care because the course of labor and the maternal and fetal-neonatal response may change without warning.

ASSESSMENT

One indication of the beginning of the second state is lessening of discomfort, and contractions may become further apart. Other symptoms are an increase in bloody show and a feeling of pressure on the rectum, accompanied by a desire to defecate and an urge to bear down with each contraction. A vaginal examination confirms full dilatation (10 cm) of the cervix and station of the presenting part.

During the second stage *each* contraction is monitored for frequency, strength, duration, intensity, and fetal response (see evaluation criteria). If the FHR is monitored intermittently with a fetoscope, the FHR is checked after every contraction or every 5 minutes. If continuous FHR monitoring is used (Chapter 24), the nurse checks the tracings on the monitor with each contraction. Descent of the presenting part (usually the head or vertex) is confirmed by vaginal examination until the presenting part can be seen at the introitus (Fig. 22.1). Show is checked for evidence of excessive bleeding. The amniotic fluid is checked for meconium staining and amount. The vital signs, including BP, are checked (must be taken between contractions). The presence of amnesia between contractions is noted. The partner's or father's response is assessed.

Examples of nursing diagnoses. To establish nursing diagnoses the nurse correlates the events of the second stage, maternal (paternal) responses, and ethnic or cultural identity. The following are examples of nursing diagnoses:

1. Inability to follow coaching because of exhaustion, panic (loss of control), or amnesia
2. Alteration in self-concept caused by feeling that "pushing" efforts are inadequate (i.e., head recedes slightly as contraction wanes)
3. Potential injury because of inappropriate positioning of mother's legs in stirrups
4. Alteration in self-concept of mother because of inability to carry out plan for unmedicated childbirth
5. Alteration in self-concept of father because of inability to support mother during final stage of labor

PLAN

The nurse plans to monitor constantly (1) the events of the second stage and mechanism of delivery, (2) maternal physiologic and emotional responses to the second stage, (3) paternal response to the second stage, and (4) fetal response to the stress of the second stage.

The nurse plans to continue to provide comfort measures for the mother such as positioning, mouth care, maintaining clean, dry bedding, and avoiding extraneous noise, conversation, or other distractions (e.g., laughing, talking of attending personnel in or outside the labor area).

If the woman is to be transferred to another area for delivery, the nurse plans to make the transfer early enough to avoid rushing the client. The delivery area is readied for the birth (see Chapter 21).

IMPLEMENTATION

Maternal position. The woman may want to assume positions such as squatting. For this position a firm surface (not the mattress on a bed) is required, and the woman will need side support. Another position is the side-lying position with the upper leg held by the nurse or coach or placed on a pillow. Some women prefer Fowler's position (can be attained with the support of a wedged pillow or the father can support the woman). Others prefer the hands-knees position when bearing down.

Bearing-down efforts. The natural urge to push is coupled with positioning, breathing, and relaxation techniques to make effective use of the woman's expulsive efforts. The woman uses breathing to increase intraabdominal pressure. As the fetal head reaches the pelvic floor, most women experience the urge to push. Automatically the woman will begin to exert downward pressure by contracting her abdominal muscles while relaxing her pelvic floor. When helping women to push, the nurse encourages them to push as *they* feel like pushing. The nurse monitors the woman's breathing so that the woman does not hold her breath more than 5 seconds at a time. Holding one's breath for more than 5 seconds diminishes the perfusion of oxygen across the placenta and results in fetal hypoxia. The nurse reminds the woman to take deep breaths to refill her lungs.

To ensure slow delivery of the fetal head, the nurse encourages the woman to control the urge to push. The

Fig. 22.4

Delivery room. **A,** Starting at left top of picture and proceeding to right and bottom: door to warmer; roller; x-ray viewing box; fetal heart monitor; Apgar scoring chart; suction; socket for stirrup. Nurse is responsible for seeing that room is kept clean and ready for use at a moment's notice. **B,** Behind delivery table on left is seen anesthesia machine, intravenous pole with fluid, table of supplies and emergency cart, second clock and regular clock with second hand, and, on extreme right, doors to warmer.

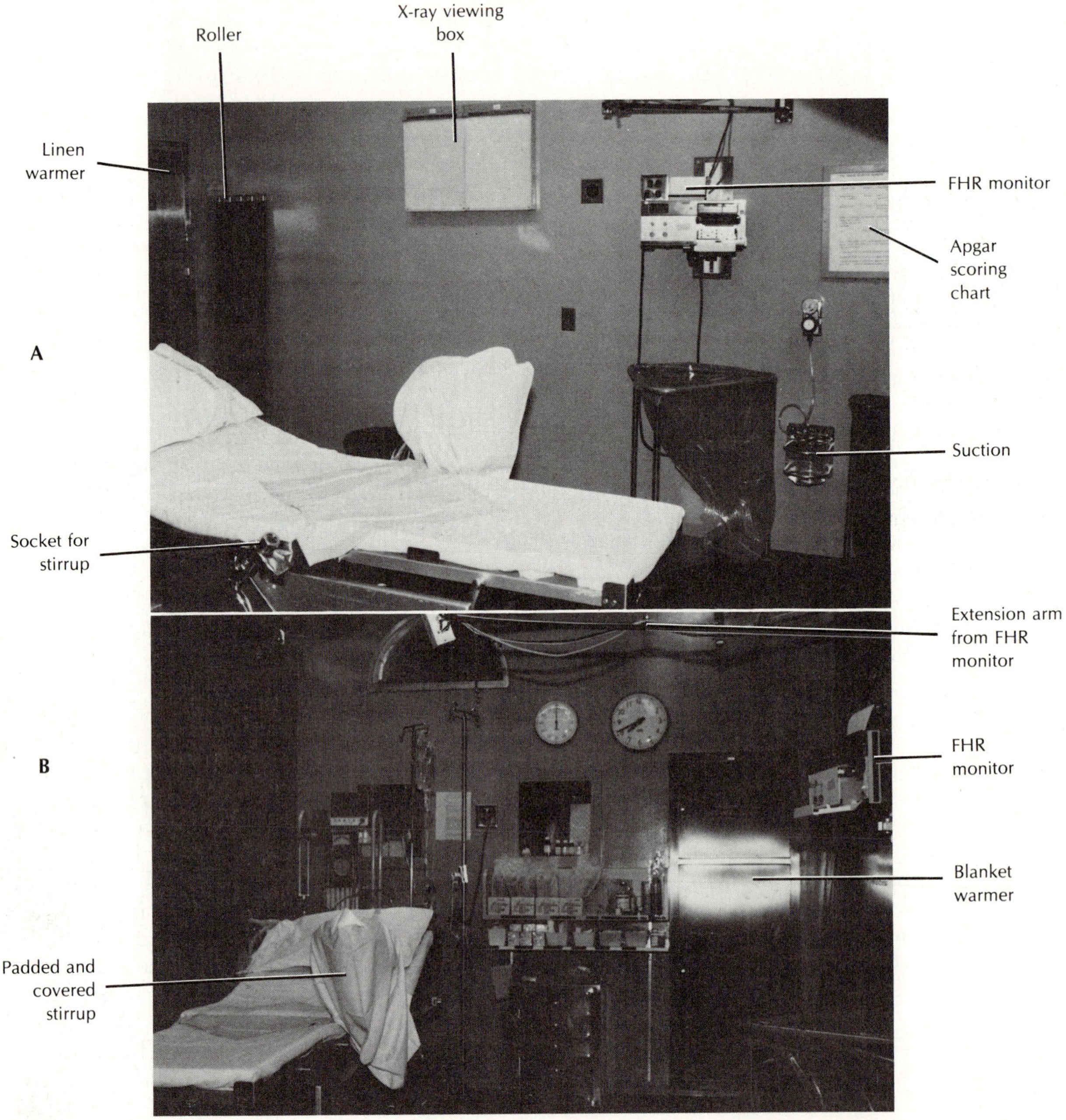

Fig. 22.4, cont'd

C, Fetal heart monitor with its extension arm that swings over mother is out of the way. Suction bottle is seen under monitor. Overhead light has a small adjustable mirror on its support. Cupboards contain forceps, gowns, packs, and other sterile supplies. **D,** Head of delivery table. Note wedge pillow under head; foot pedal to raise and lower entire table; crank to raise or lower head or foot; lever to loosen or tighten stirrup; and hand grip for woman to use as she wishes. Nurse needs to know how to operate this table. One foot pedal is not shown—the pedal that stabilizes (brakes) the table.

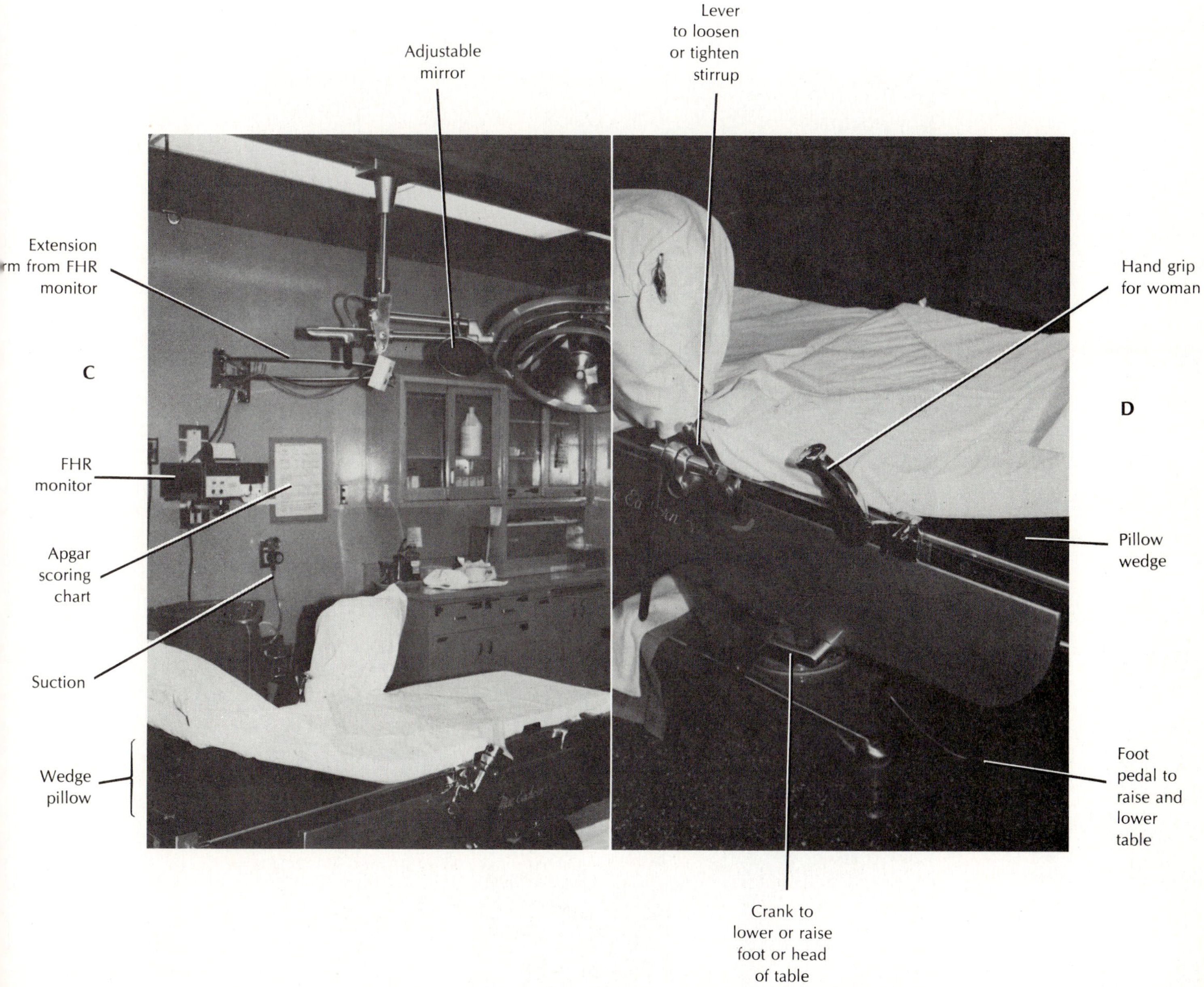

Continued.

Fig. 22.4, cont'd

E, Sterile delivery pack with a strip of nonsterilized heat-sensitive tape to illustrate difference between a pack that has been sterilized and one that has not. Lower pack illustrates proper labeling and dating of packs. Nurse is responsible for ensuring that all supplies used are sterile. **F,** View of delivery instrument and supply table and infant resuscitation equipment from head of delivery table. (Courtesy Stanford University Medical Center, Stanford Calif.)

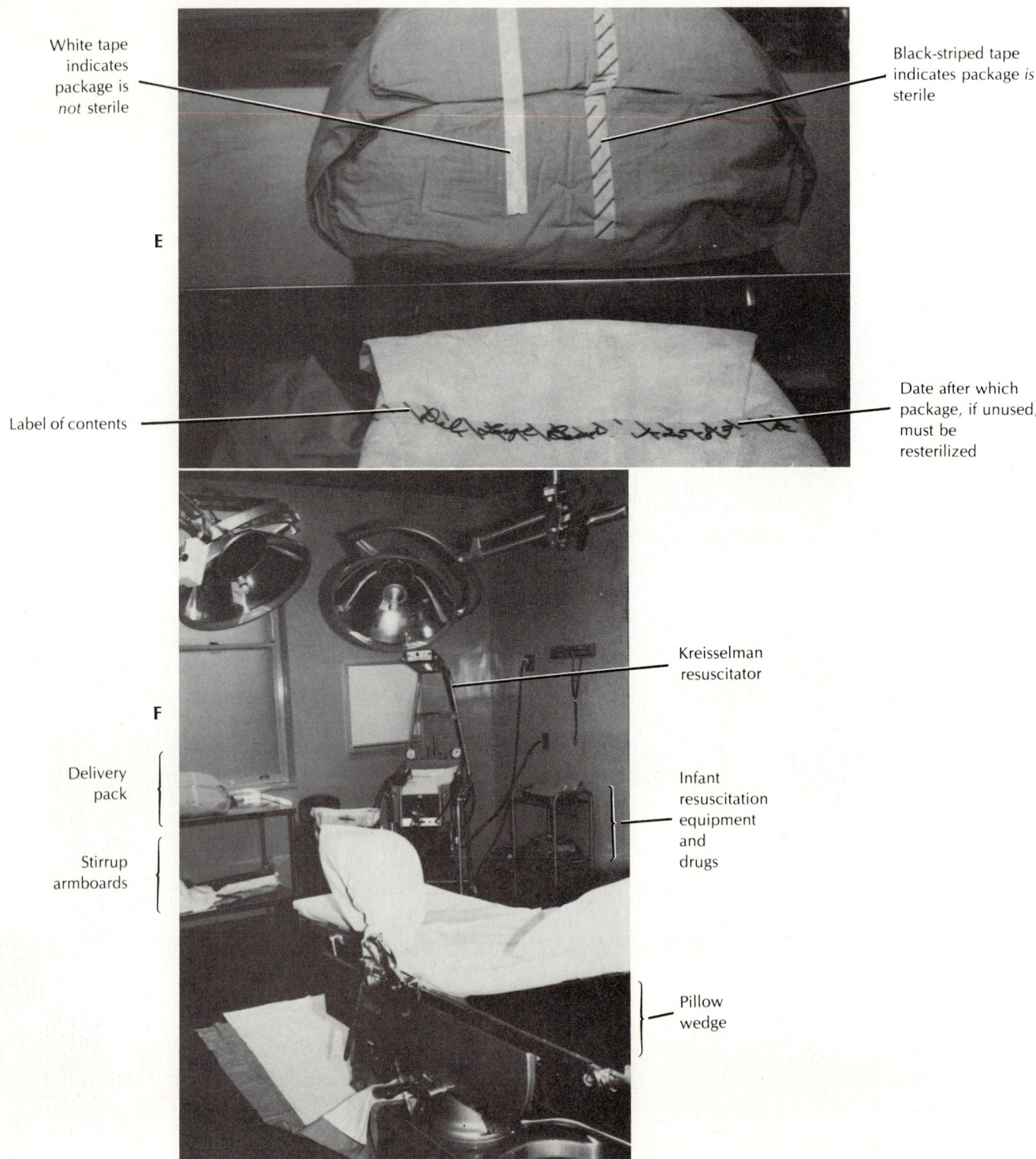

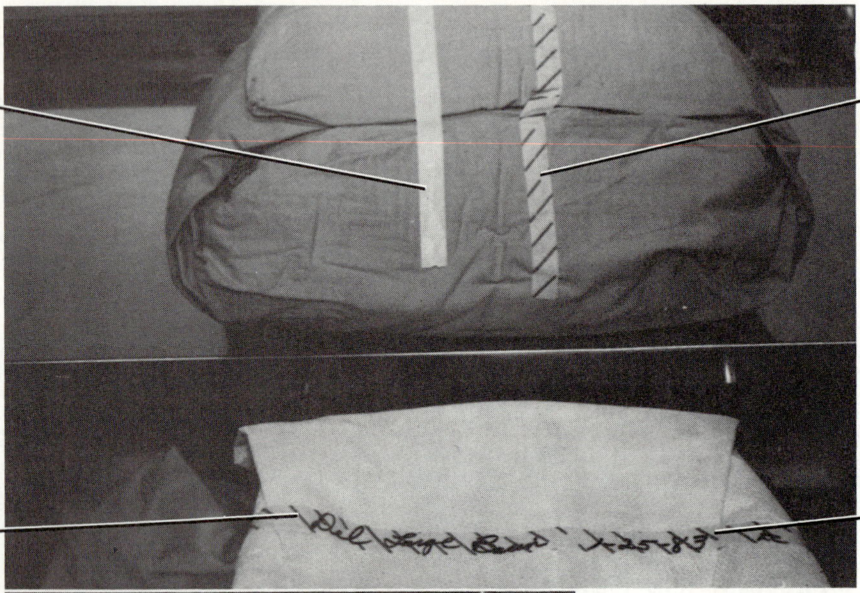

E

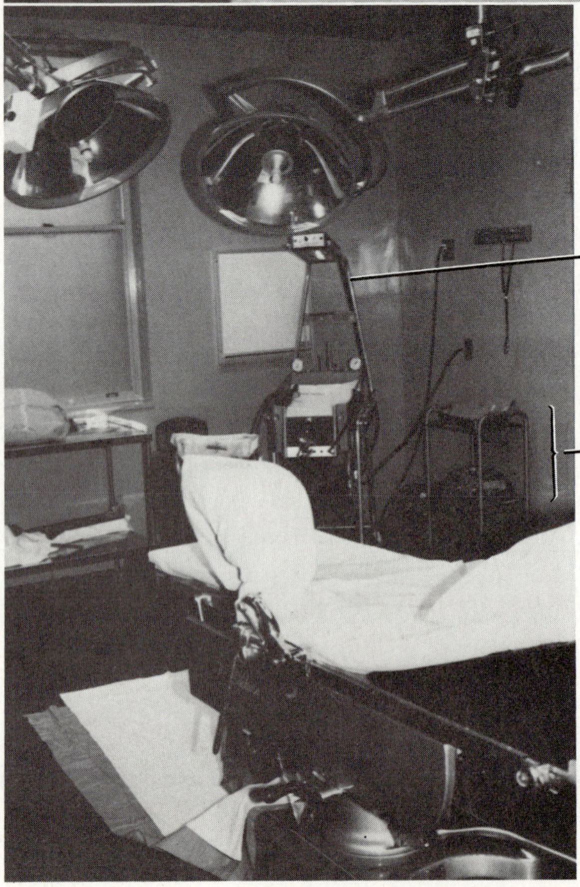

F

urge to push is controlled by coaching the woman to take panting breaths or to exhale slowly through pursed lips as the baby's head crowns. The woman needs simple clear directions from *one* coach (see also Chapter 19).

Amnesia. Amnesia between contractions is pronounced in the second stage, and the woman may have to be roused to cooperate in the bearing-down process. Parents who have attended childbirth classes devise a set of verbal cues for the parturient to follow. It is helpful if they print these on a card that may be attached to the head of the bed so that the nurse can better substitute as coach if the partner has to leave.

Fetal heart rate. Fetal heart rate (FHR) must be checked as noted above. If the rate begins to drop, the woman can be turned on her side to reduce the pressure of the uterus against the ascending vena cava and descending aorta, and oxygen can be administered by mask at 10 to 12 L/min. This is often all that is required to restore the normal rate. If it does not, report this immediately; medical intervention to hasten the birth may be indicated.

Coach. During the second stage the woman needs continuous support and coaching. The coaching process can be physically and emotionally tiring for the father. The nurse can offer him nourishment, fluids, and short breaks. If the father is to attend the delivery, he is given instructions as to donning cover gown, mask, hat, and shoes and he is advised as to areas in which he has freedom to move and what support he can give his wife (some husbands are prepared to do coaching for pushing and panting).

Care for delivery. If the woman is to be transferred to a delivery area for completion of the birth process, the nurse uses the following guidelines:

1. Multipara: toward end of first stage if presenting part is +1 or +2
2. Nullipara: when vertex can be seen at introitus with each contraction

Both will need assistance to move from the labor bed to the delivery table. If this is done between contractions, the mother can help, but because of her awkwardness, she cannot be rushed.

Delivery rooms are specifically designed to facilitate care during delivery (Fig. 22.4). The delivery table is designed with many features: the entire table can be raised or lowered, and the head or foot may be raised or lowered. A wedge pillow or bolster can be inserted under the top of the mattress to raise it slightly, or the head of the table can be raised to prevent hypotension and to facilitate pushing. The table is equipped with stirrups for supporting the legs and handle grips to aid in bearing down. If stirrups are used, the bed can be "broken"; that is, the lower half of the bed can be lowered and rolled back to fit under the top half.

Sterile techniques. The nurse is responsible for ensuring asepsis by implementing the sterile techniques shown in Fig. 22.5:

1. Lifting sterile instruments (Fig. 22.5, *A*)
2. Opening sterile packages (Fig. 22.5, *B*)
3. Adding sterile supplies to the instrument table (Fig. 22.5, *C*)
4. Pouring sterile water into sterile basin.
5. Gloving (Fig. 22.5, *D*)
6. Unwrapping and handing sterile forceps to physician or midwife (Fig. 22.5, *E*)

• • •

Text continued on p. 430.

Fig. 22.5

A, Lifting sterile instruments using ring forceps (uterine forceps or sponge sticks). For beginners this is a good grip. Curved Kelly forcep is balanced and is far from surface of table. Note sharp hooked instruments used for clipping drapes together in lower right corner of photograph.

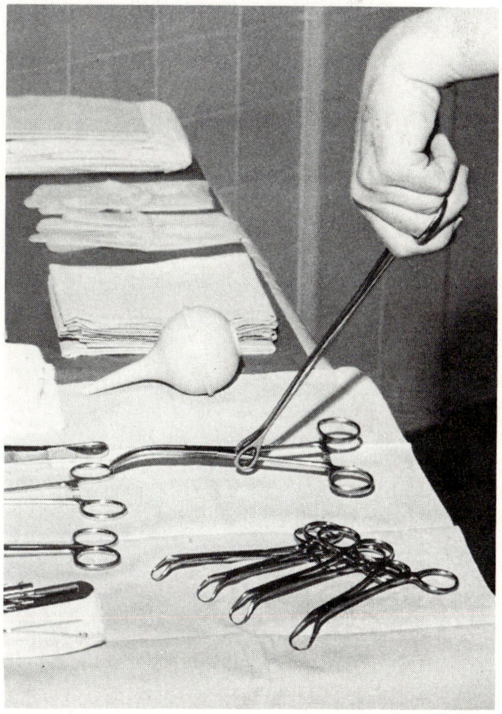

A

Continued.

Fig. 22.5, cont'd
For legend see opposite page.

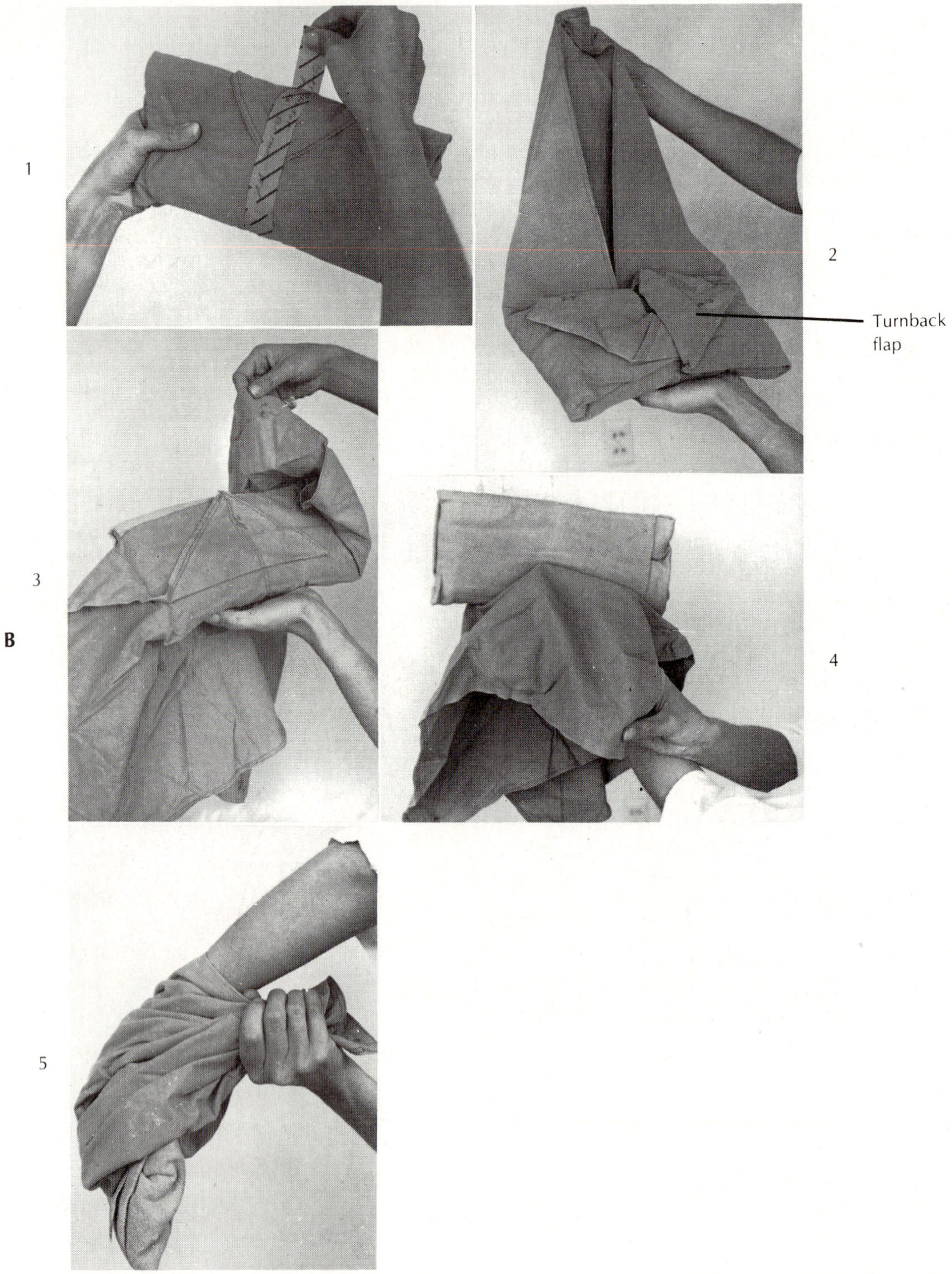

Fig. 22.5, cont'd

B, Opening sterile packages. *1,* Remove heat-sensitive tape closing package and check tape for color change indicating sterility. Start unwrapping package with point of wrapper facing you. In this way the part of the package next to you will remain covered and protected for the longest period possible. *2,* Pull back point and let it drop down after assuring that outside of dangling wrapper will not contaminate any nearby sterile surface. *3,* Pull back two side folds by little turnback flaps. Uncover end on side, supporting under hand first, then side next to active hand. If you are preparing inner package for a drop onto a sterile surface, stabilizing pack by bringing your thumb over top of wrapper before completely exposing inner pack is sometimes helpful. *4,* Pull back last fold covering inner wrap to expose sterile surface. Inner pack can now be picked up by a gloved associate or it can be "scooted" onto a sterile table while ends of outer wrapper are held back to prevent contamination. *5,* If hand thumb grip is used, pack can be dropped in manner pictured. Care must be taken not to get too close to a sterile table or field while adding supplies. **C,** *1,* Extracting a sterile catheter with ring forceps from a commercially prepared peel-back package. *2,* Dropping sterile suture from a commercially prepared peel-back package.

1

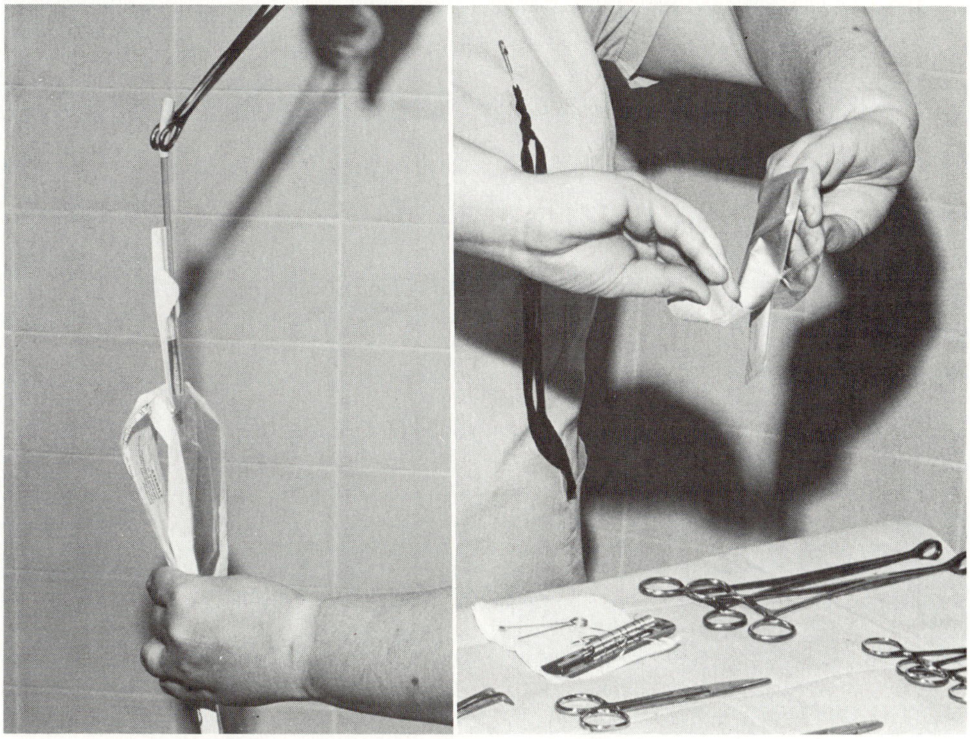

2 **C**

Continued.

Fig. 22.5, cont'd

D, Gloving procedure. *1,* Sterile gloves usually lie side by side with thumbs on top at outside edges, left glove on left and right glove on right. Pick up glove by pinching cuff folded down over palm of glove. If right-handed, slide on right-hand glove first. Your bare fingers may touch any area of the glove that represents the inside of the glove. *2,* Slide your hand in with a rotating motion while pulling on turned-down cuff. *3,* Pick up second glove with your gloved hand by sliding your sterile fingers *under* turned-down cuff. *4,* Place your other hand into glove, sliding and rotating your hand as you pull out and up against inside of cuff with your gloved fingers. Keep your thumb back out of the way. Remember, your arm and top of cuff are contaminated and must not be touched with your fingers. When only gloves are worn, it is permissible to retain narrow cuffs at tops of gloves, but they, of course, are not sterile and should not be treated as such. *5,* After you are gloved, you may adjust the fingers. Learning to glove takes time, patience, and usually more than one pair of gloves.

1

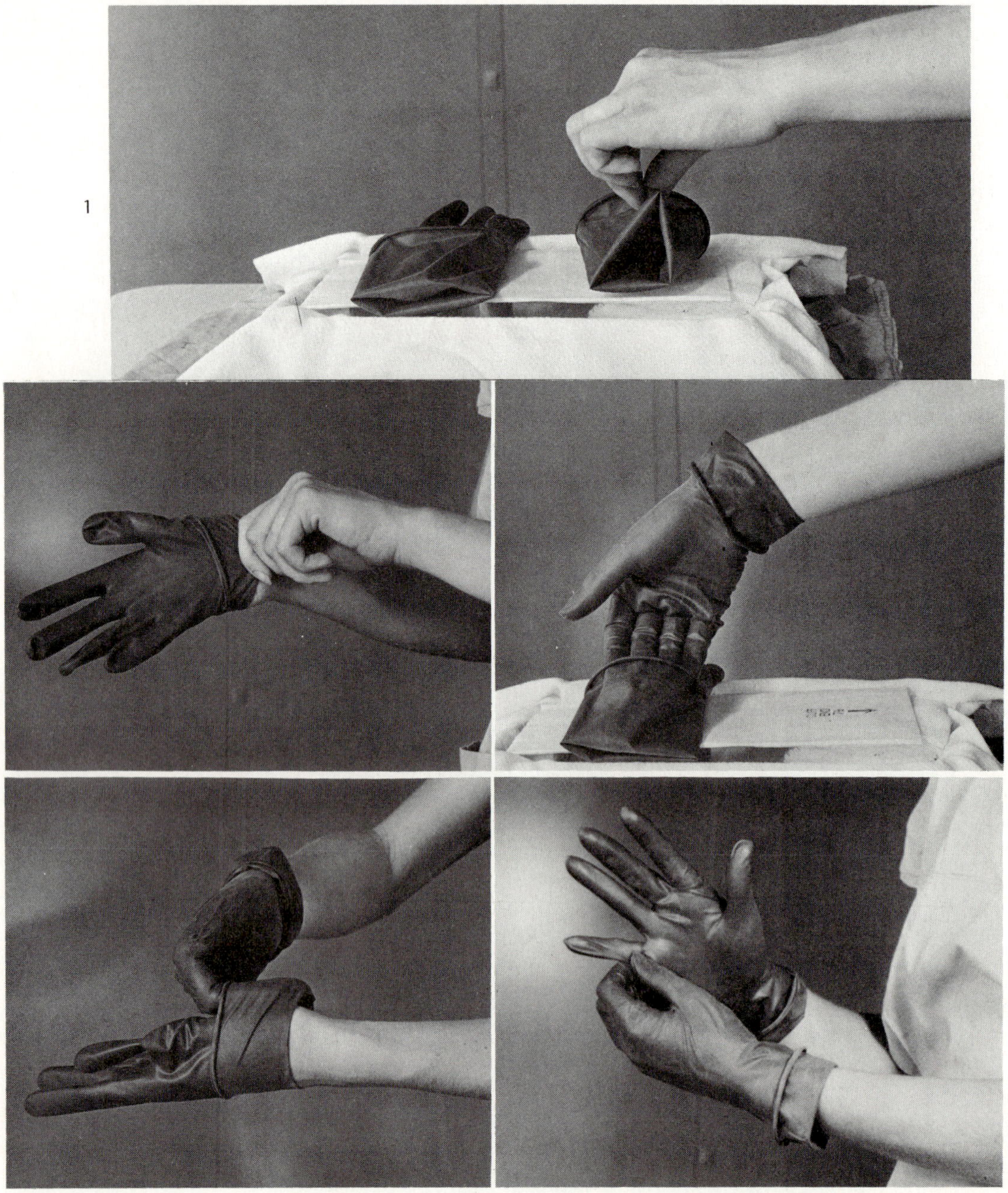

D 2

3

4

5

Fig. 22.5, cont'd

E, Steps in unwrapping sterile forceps to hand to physician. *1,* Grasp one end of package, remove outer tape, and unwind outer wrapper. *2,* Pull back inner turnback at top of package and continue to uncover inner wrap (rather like peeling a banana!). *3,* Grasp carefully all dangling ends of outer wrap and pull them out of the way toward your wrist. Do not touch inner wrap! (From Ingalls, A.J., and Salerno, M.C.: Maternal and child health nursing, ed 5, St. Louis, 1983, The C.V. Mosby Co.)

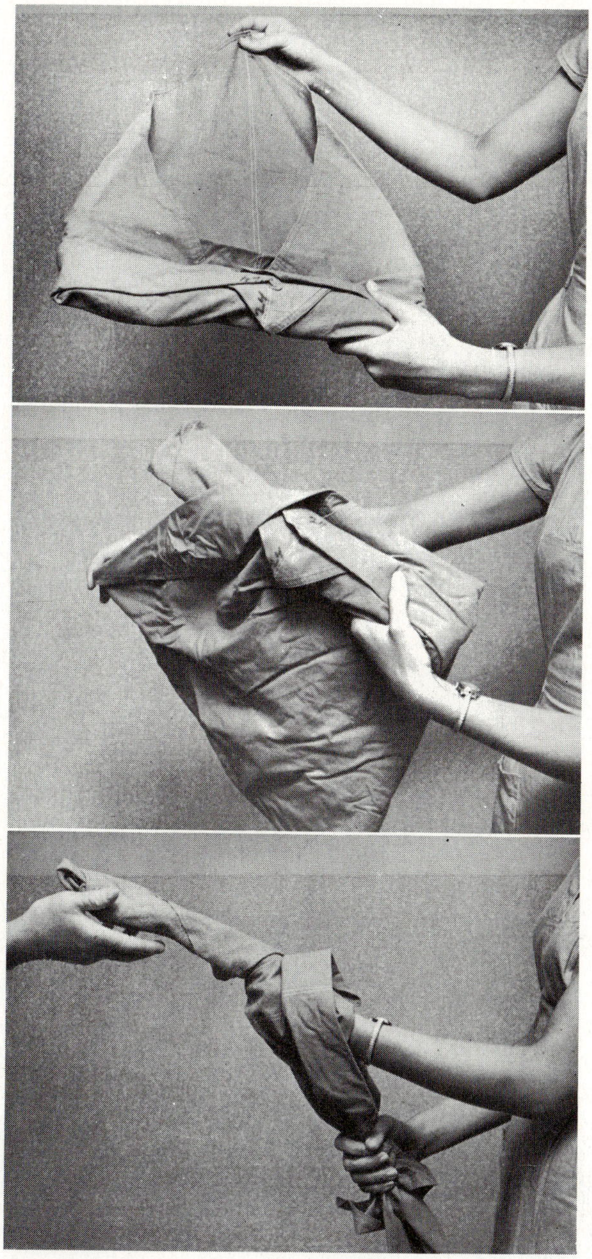

1

2

3

E

The position assumed for delivery may be (1) modified Sims' position (if this is the case, the attendant will need to support the upper leg), (2) a dorsal position, or (3) a lithotomy position.

The following is a description of the lithotomy position for delivery. The lithotomy position is used most often in hospitals because it is more convenient for the physician to deal with any complications that arise. For this position the buttocks are brought to the edge of the table, and the legs are placed in stirrups. Care must be

Fig. 22.6
Steps in perineal cleansing. Use cotton swabs or gauze squares well moistened with disinfectant solution. Discard swab after each step. Finish cleansing with wash of sterile water.

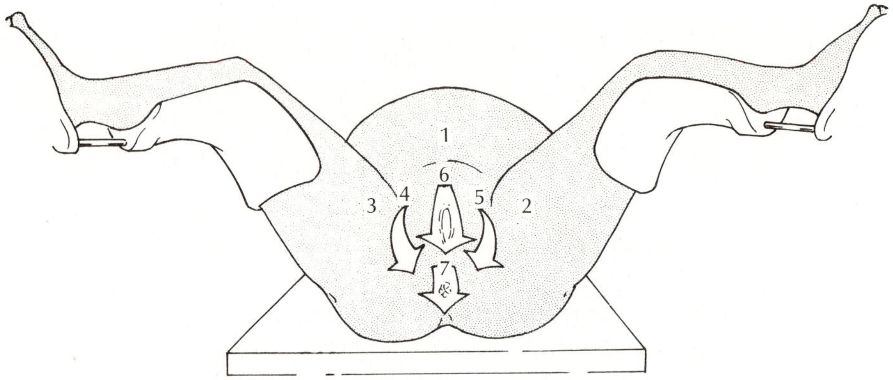

Fig. 22.7
Instrument table (all equipment sterile). *Top, left to right:* receiving blanket, perineal pad, vaginal roll, medicine glasses (for anesthetic agent), hand cover for spotlight, urine specimen bottle, towels, and placenta bowl and paper towel for covering scales. *Bottom, left to right:* syringe (anesthetic) needle guard, episiotomy scissors, bulb syringe (covered with gauze for aspirating newborn), two artery forceps, scissors, cord clamp, ring forceps, needle holder, thumb forceps (for repair of episiotomy), extra instruments (ring forceps, small artery forceps, toothed forceps, Allis clamps, and sharp hook forceps for holding drapes in place) and kidney basin.

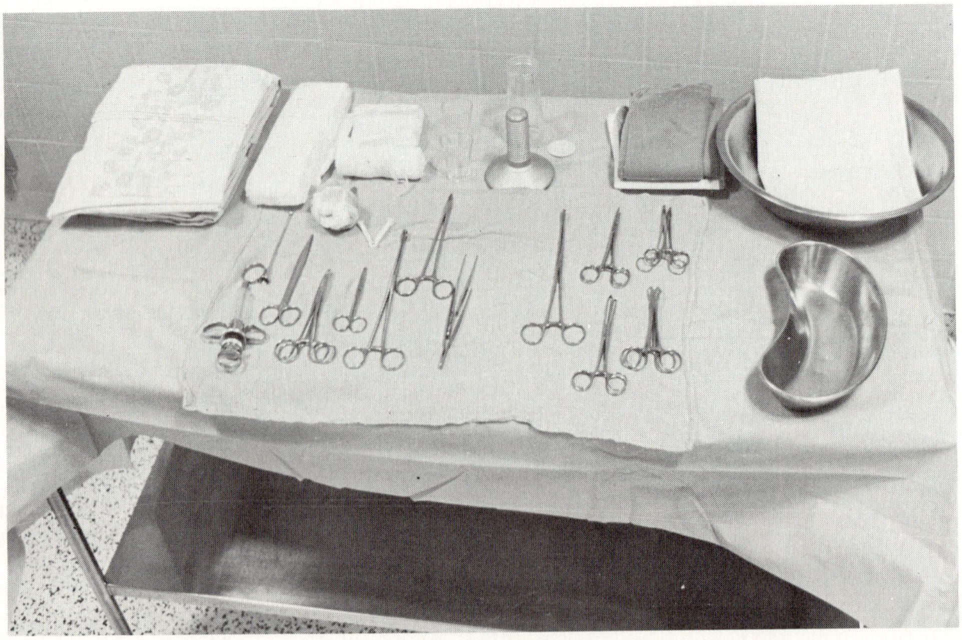

taken to pad the stirrups, raise and place both legs simultaneously, and adjust the shank of the stirrups so that the calf of the leg is supported and there is no pressure on the popliteal space. If the stirrups are uneven in height, the woman can develop strained ligaments in her back as she bears down. This strain causes considerable discomfort in the postdelivery period.

The lower portion of the table may be dropped down and rolled back under the top.

Once the woman is positioned for delivery, the vulva is washed thoroughly with soap and water or a surgical disinfectant (Fig 22.6). The physician or midwife dons cap and mask, scrubs hands, and puts on the sterile gown and gloves. The woman may then be draped with sterile towels and sheets. The husband or coach helps the mother to remember not to touch the sterile drapes.

The delivery table is prepared. Fig. 22.7 illustrates one way to arrange the table.

The circulating nurse will continue to coach and encourage the parturient. Once the woman's legs are in the stirrups, the handle grips can be used to pull against, keeping the elbows bent as before. The nurse will check FHR after every contraction and notify the physician as to the rate and regularity. The equipment for taking the blood pressure should be readied for instant use if signs of shock develop. However, the readings are distorted (increased) by the increase in thoracic and abdominal pressures as the woman pushes. A reading will be taken after delivery before transferring the woman to the recovery room. The oxytocic medication such as Syntocinon may be prepared for administration after delivery, supplies for the infant organized, and observations and procedures recorded on the chart.

Fathers are encouraged to be present at the birth of their infants if this is in keeping with their cultural expectations. The psychologic closeness of the family unit is maintained, and the father can continue the supportive care given in labor. The father needs as much opportunity as does the mother to initiate the attachment process with the baby. Studies indicate, however, that it is the continuous long-term contact between father and child that acts to cement the bonds.

The father is usually gowned in a clean scrub outfit and wears a cap and a mask. These supplies need to be provided in ample time for him to don them before the delivery. If the couple has decided that the father is not to be present, this position should be respected.

Contact with parents is maintained by touch and verbal comforting instructions as to reasons for care, assistance with coaching during contractions, and sharing in parents' joy at birth of their child. Crib and equipment are readied for the infant. The nurse notes and records the time of birth (i.e., when infant is born completely).

In some hospitals, parents have the option to labor and give birth in one room, without changing rooms or beds. Figs. 22.8 to 22.19 record the experience of one couple's birth experience.

Text continued on p. 436.

Fig. 22.8
Side-lying position for second stage. Mother is sleeping between contractions. (Photograph by Jacqueline Capra, Santa Cruz, Calif.)

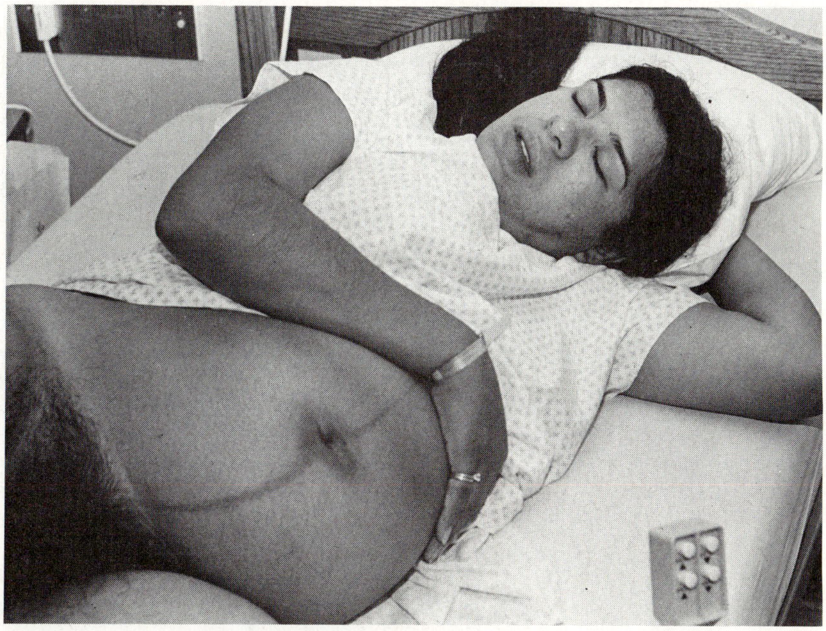

Fig. 22.9
Side-lying position for pushing during second stage. (Photograph by Jacqueline Capra, Santa Cruz, Calif.)

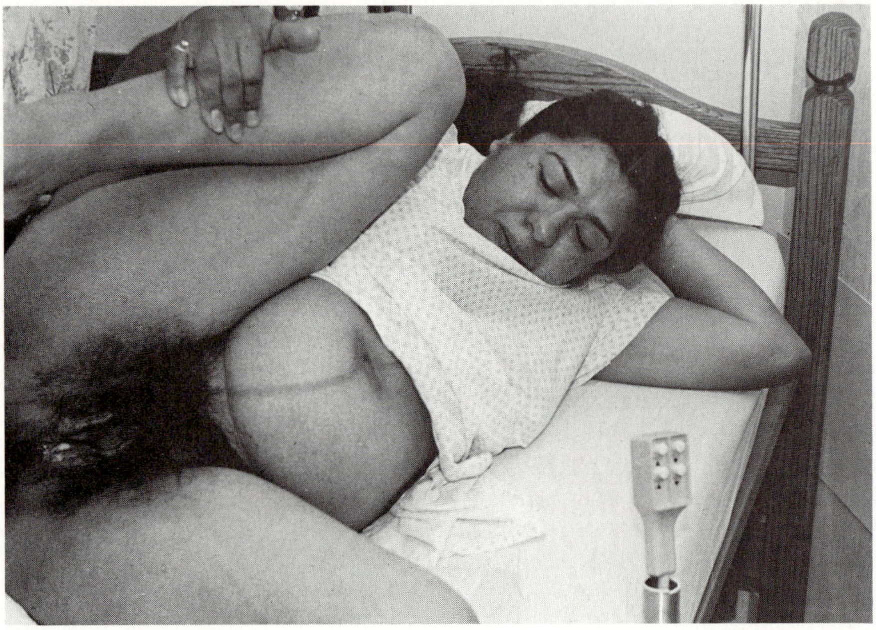

Fig. 22.10
Caput visible at introitus. NOTE: No perineal shave had been done. (Photograph by Jacqueline Capra, Santa Cruz, Calif.)

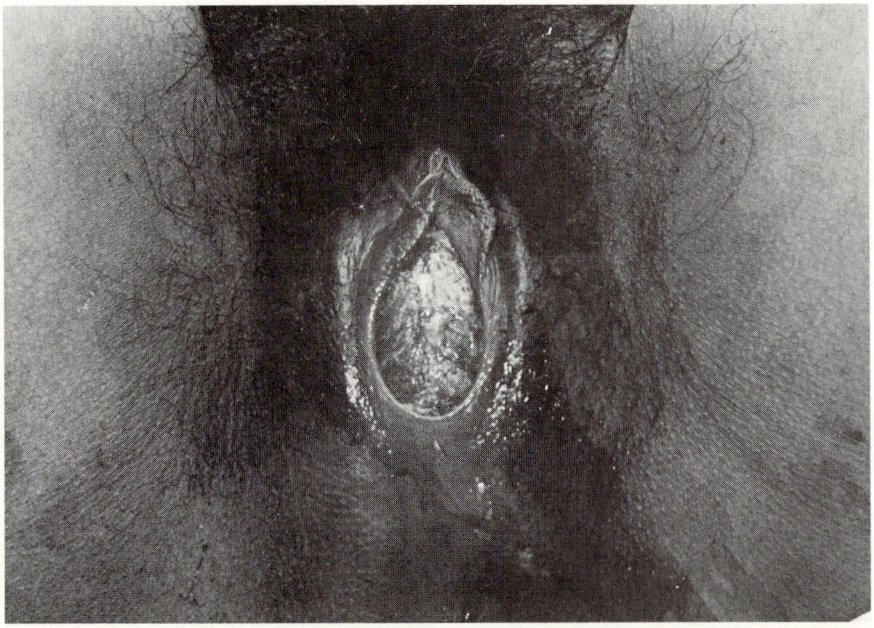

Fig. 22.11
Controlled birth of head with no episiotomy. (Photograph by Jacqueline Capra, Santa Cruz, Calif.)

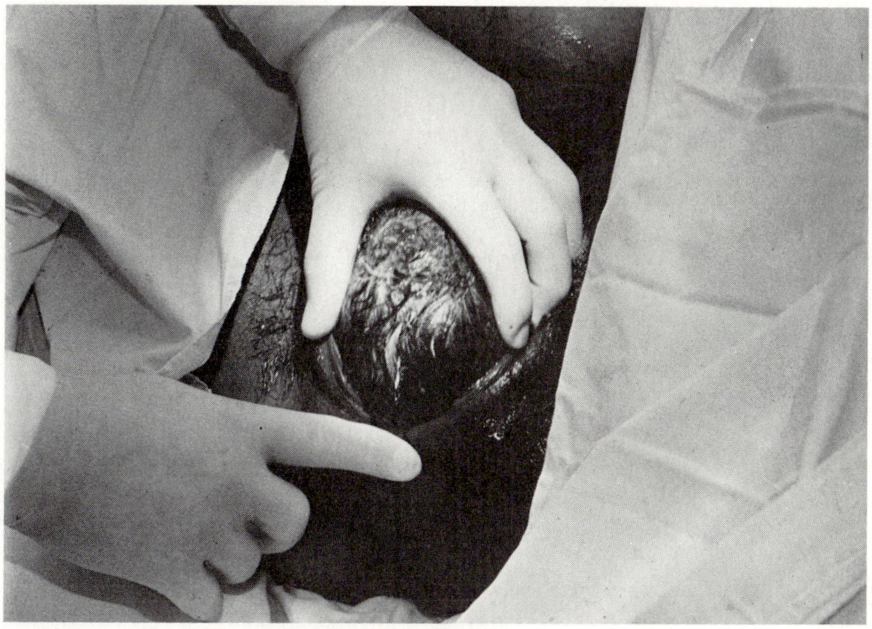

Fig. 22.12
Infant's head is born; note molding and caput succedaneum. (Photograph by Jacqueline Capra, Santa Cruz, Calif.)

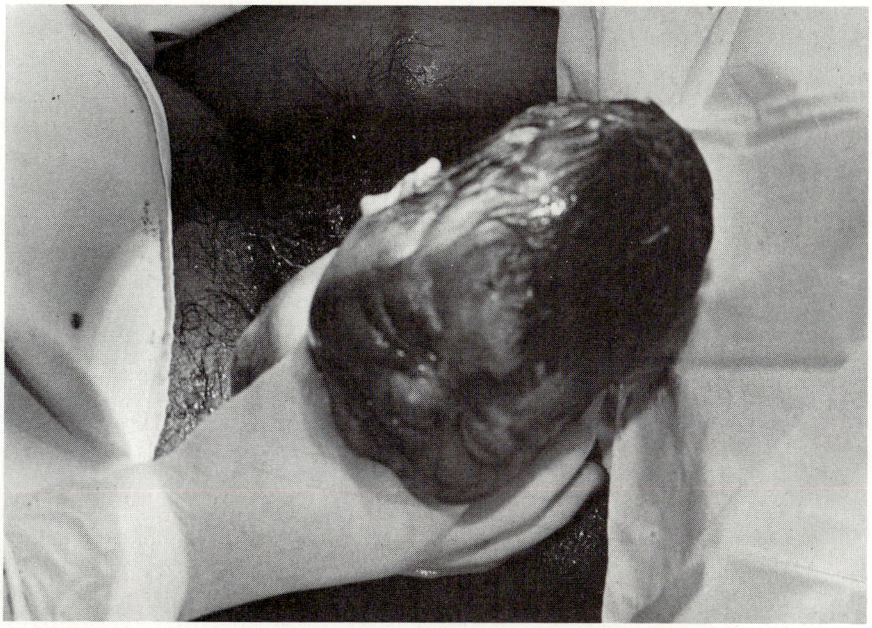

Fig. 22.13
Birth of shoulders, body, and upper extremities. (Photograph by Jacqueline Capra, Santa Cruz, Calif.)

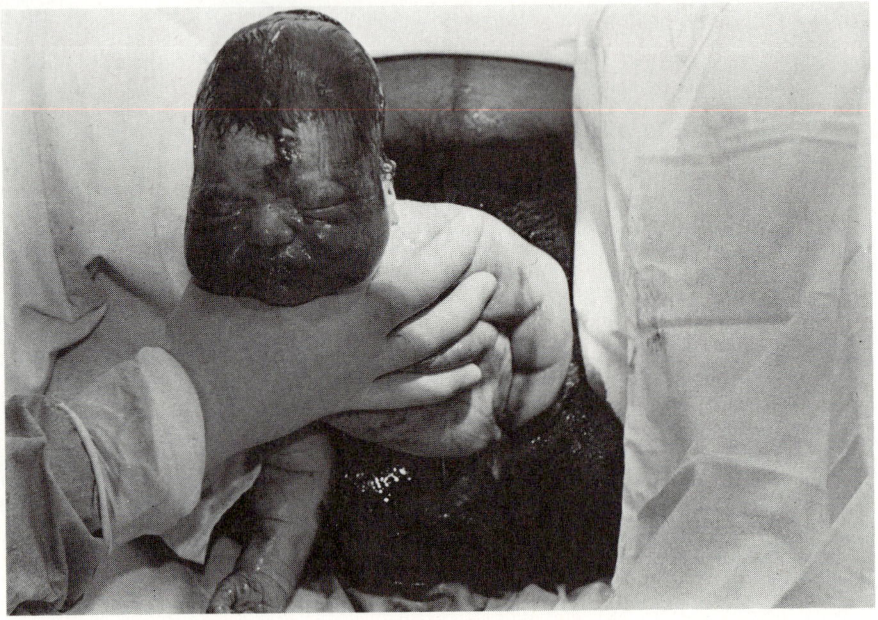

Fig. 22.14
Mother glances toward husband with joy as baby rests on her abdomen. Nurse holds bulb syringe ready to aspirate mucus from baby's mouth and nose if necessary. (Photograph by Jacqueline Capra, Santa Cruz, Calif.)

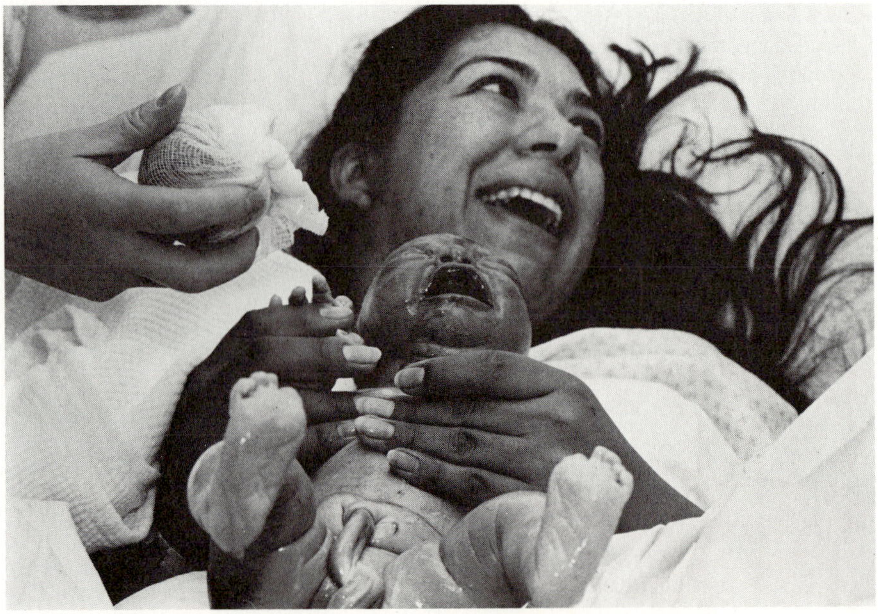

Fig. 22.15
Father admires his newly born child. (Photograph by Jacqueline Capra, Santa Cruz, Calif.)

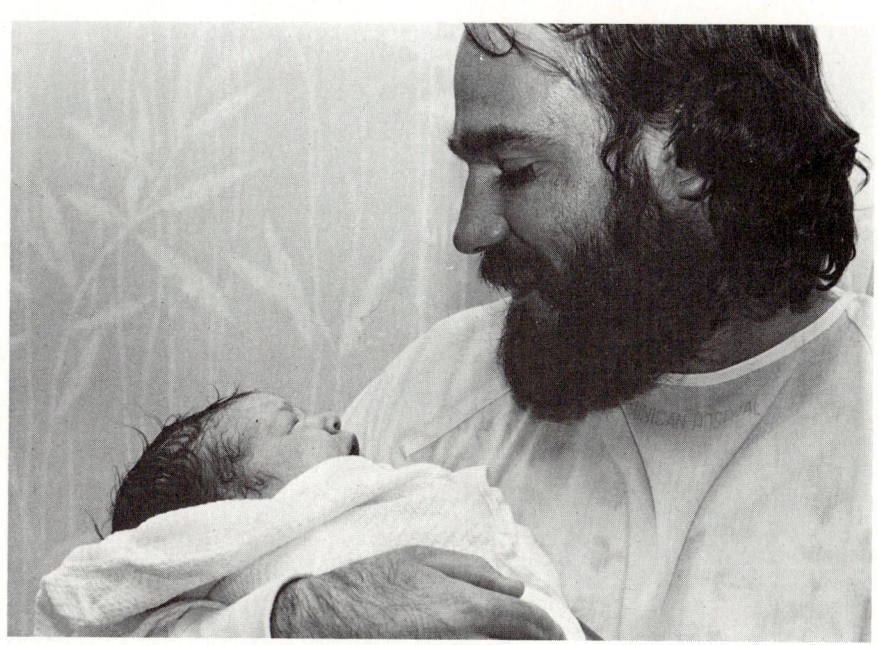

Fig. 22.16
Mother is crying with joy as she cuddles baby to her body. (Photograph by Jacqueline Capra, Santa Cruz, Calif.)

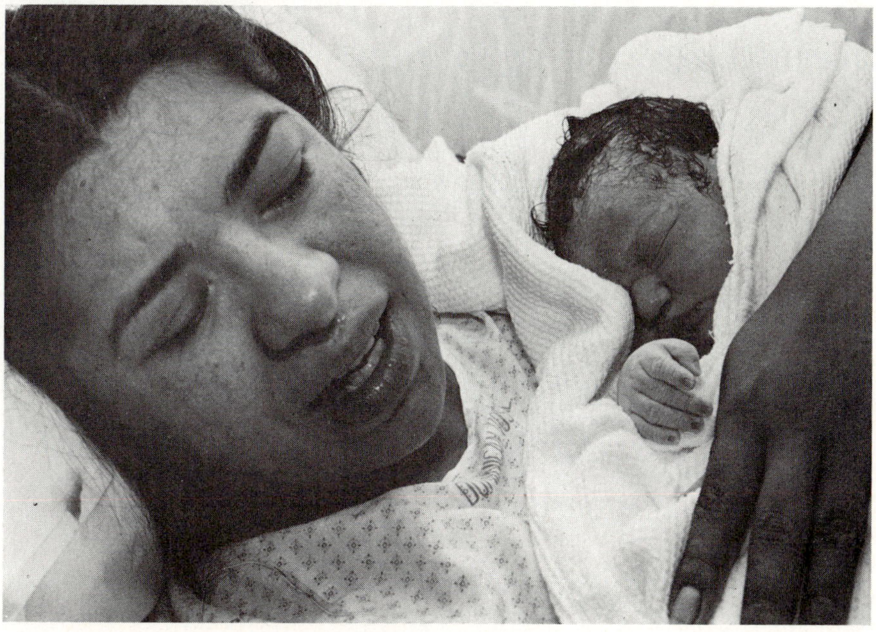

Fig 22.17
In her first reactive state baby nurses well shortly after birth. Baby knows how to suckle at birth because of extensive practice in utero. (Photograph by Jacqueline Capra, Santa Cruz, Calif.)

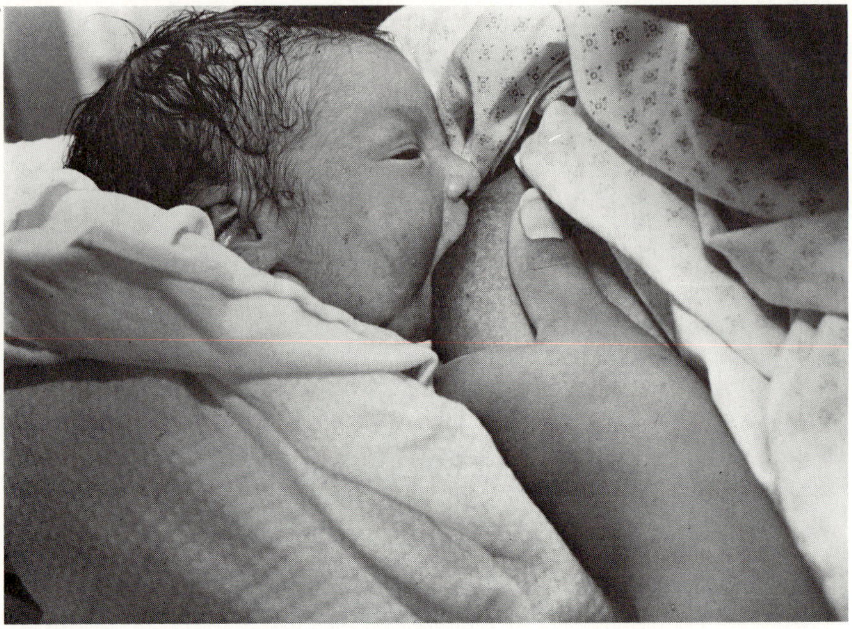

Fig. 22.18
Initiating parent-child relationship Note how carefully newborn is wrapped to prevent heat loss. (Photograph by Jacqueline Capra, Santa Cruz, Calif.)

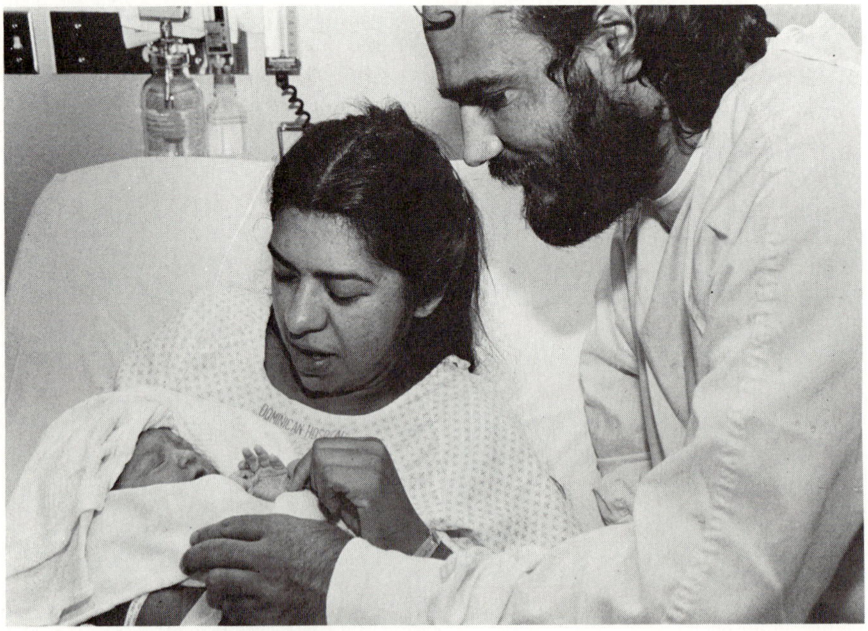

There is no single ideal position for childbirth. Labor is a dynamic, interactive process between the mother's uterus, pelvis, and voluntary muscles. Angles between the baby and the mother's pelvis constantly change as the infant turns and flexes down the birth canal. If able to, a mother will constantly change position in labor. The Borning Bed (Figs. 22.20 and 22.21) changes shape according to her needs. The mother can squat, kneel, recline, or sit, whatever is most comfortable. At the same time, there is excellent exposure for exami-

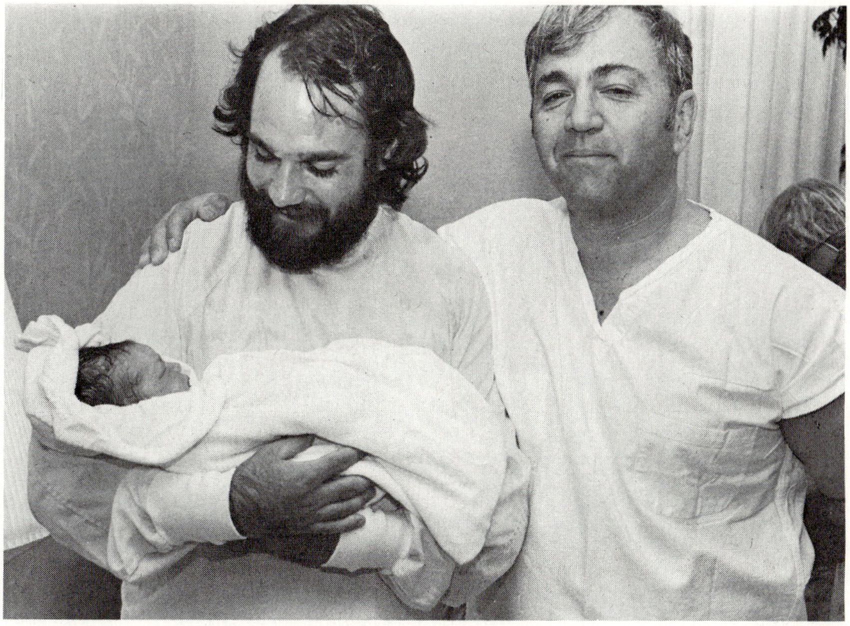

Fig. 22.19
Physician shares parents' joy at birth of their baby. (Photograph by Jacqueline Capra, Santa Cruz, Calif.)

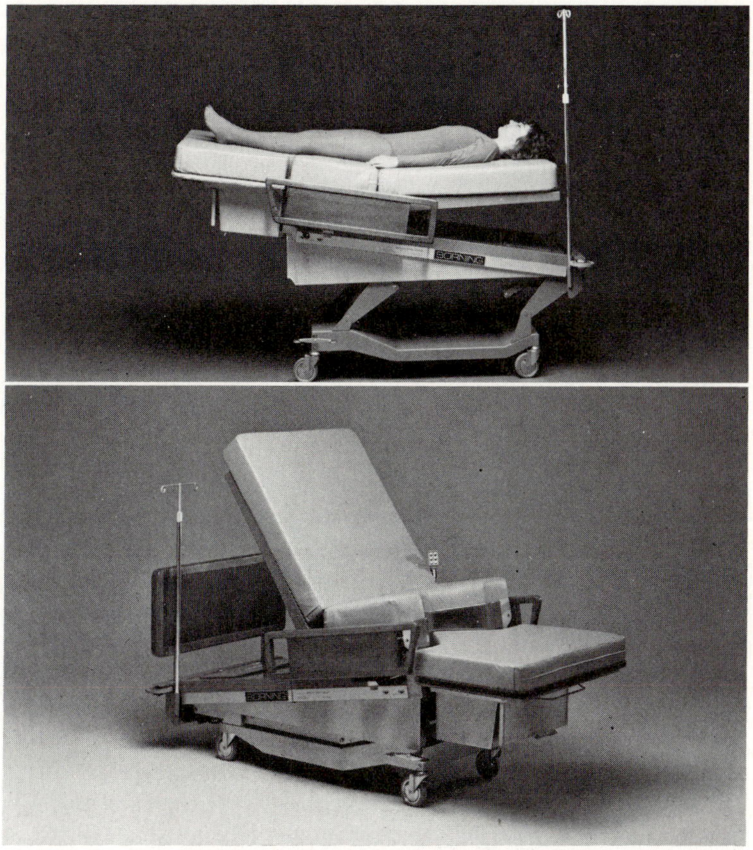

Fig. 22.20
The Borning 800 birth chair/childbearing bed. (Courtesy The Borning Corporation, Spokane, Wash.)

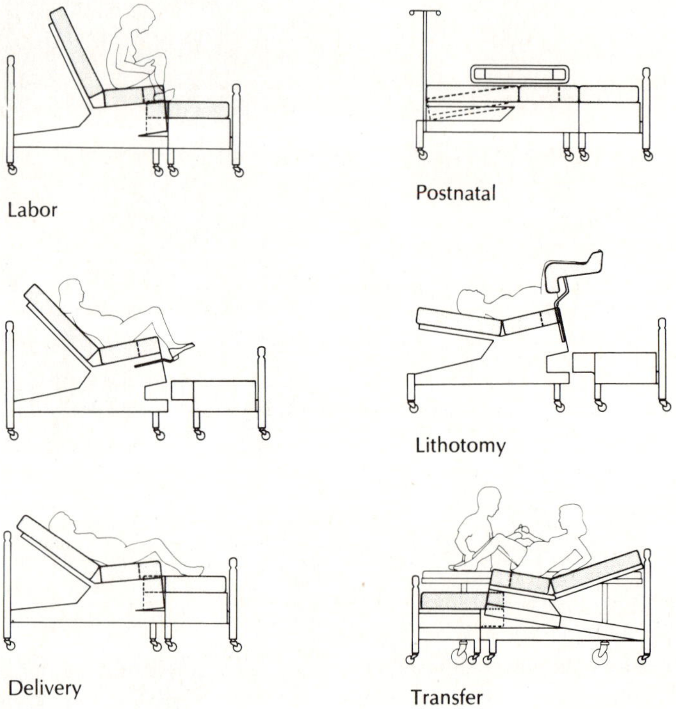

Fig. 22.21
The Borning 800 birth chair/childbearing bed positioned for labor, delivery, postnatal recovery, lithotomy, and transfer to another unit. (Courtesy The Borning Corporation, Spokane, Wash.)

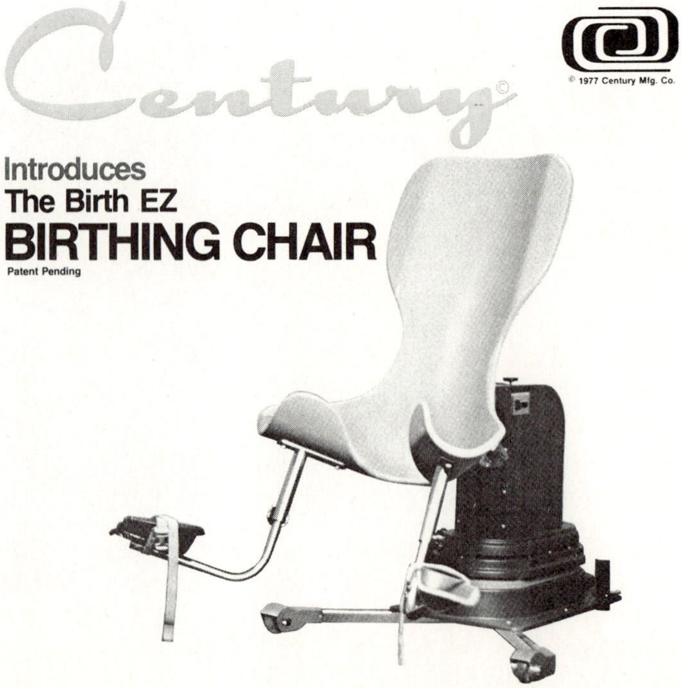

Fig. 22.22
The Birth EZ Birthing Chair. (Courtesy Century Manufacturing Co., Aurora, Neb.)

nation, electrode placement, fetal scalp sampling, and delivery. The mother has full control of both seat and back functions, so she can adjust her position for maximal comfort. The mother and father can maintain close personal contact and a new degree of involvement in the birth if they desire. The bed can be positioned for administering anesthesia, the V-shaped perineal cut-out is adaptable to both forceps and spontaneous birth, and the bed can be used for transport to surgery in the event of a cesarean birth.

The birth chair (Fig. 22.22) provides the woman with a better physiologic position during childbirth. In this position the duration of labor may be shortened, women often experience less pain, episiotomies are required less frequently, the force of gravity assists the labor and delivery process, the maternal pelvic measure enlarges by 0.5 to 1.5 cm in the sitting position, pressure on abdominal blood vessels is avoided, and circulation to the lower extremities is not restricted. There are psychologic advantages as well: the woman is able to participate more fully because her view is not obstructed and the sitting position is more natural than the horizontal position associated with illness. The chair is designed so that, in the event of emergency, it can be adjusted to the horizontal or Trendelenburg's position.

Nursing Care of the Newborn

GOALS

The nurse provides continuous care during the neonate's initial adjustment to extrauterine life by doing the following:

1. Maintaining a clear airway to facilitate respirations
2. Preventing heat loss (cold stress) to conserve neonate's energy
3. Providing a safe environment (e.g., to prevent infection)
4. Identifying any potential or actual problem that may require immediate medical intervention.

The nurse assumes responsibility to facilitate the parents' attachment to or acquaintance with the neonate.

The nurse assumes the responsibility to maintain accurate records.

ASSESSMENT

Before birth, the nurse evaluates the maternal history, including labor, to identify potential problems for the neonate. Although an extensive examination will be performed later, a minimal examination of the neonate is completed immediately following birth. The physician or nurse performs the following:

1. Assesses respirations and neonate's ability to keep airway clear
2. Estimates infant's health status using Apgar rating at 1 and 5 minutes of age
3. Examines the cord for anomalies and verifies the presence of two arteries and one vein
4. Collects cord blood for analysis (Rh factor, blood grouping, and hematocrit)
5. Assesses weight, length, and gestational age
6. Notes passage of meconium or urine
7. Performs minimal physical examination and assessment of neonate such as the following:
   a. *External:* notes skin color, staining, peeling, or wasting (dysmaturity); considers length of nails and development of creases on soles of feet; checks for presence or absence of breast tissue; assesses nasal patency by closing one nostril at a time while observing infant's respirations and color; notes meconium staining of cord, skin, fingernails, or amniotic fluid (may indicate fetal hypoxia; offensive odor may indicate intrauterine infection)
   b. *Chest:* palpates for site of maximal cardiac impulse and auscultates for rate and quality of heart tones; compares and notes character of respirations and presence of rales or rhonchi by holding stethoscope in each axilla
   c. *Abdomen:* palpates and percusses liver for consistency and enlargement (3 cm or more below costal margin; causes of hepatomegaly: infection, pneumothorax with depression of diaphragm, erythroblastosis fetalis, etc.)
   d. *Neurologic:* checks muscle tone and reflex reaction and appraises Moro's reflex (at 1 and 5 minutes); palpates large fontanel for fullness or bulge; notes by palpation the presence and sizes of the sutures and fontanels
   e. *Other observations:* notes gross structural malformations obvious at birth (described in general terms and recorded on delivery record)
8. Assesses parent's response to newborn and to each other

Examples of nursing diagnoses. Before establishing nursing diagnoses, the nurse correlates any pertinent information from the prenatal record, labor, and delivery. Examples of nursing diagnoses include the following:

1. Ineffective airway clearance because of mucus in neonate's mouth
2. Loss of body heat because of parents' uncovering baby for too long a period while examining their neonate
3. Alterations in parenting caused by mother's energy deficits following long labor
4. Potential disturbance in parenting caused by parental disappointment in child's appearance or sex

PLAN AND IMPLEMENTATION

After delivery of the infant, the following measures must be effected immediately:

1. Ensure a clear airway. The newborn baby is held with the head lowered (10 to 15 degrees) to expedite drainage and prevent aspiration of amniotic fluid, mucus, and blood. The oral pharynx is suctioned with a small bulb syringe as soon as the head is delivered; next the nares are aspirated. It should be noted that if the sequence is reversed, the infant may aspirate amniotic fluid, mucus, or blood because aspiration of the nares stimulates the neonate to take a breath.

Do not use deep suction on the nasal passages with a catheter, since bradycardia and laryngospasm may occur; *do not* suspend infant by ankles—hyperextension of the baby whose entire development occurred in the flexed position is detrimental to the spine, ankles, and brain and is painful.

2. When breathing is unimpeded, the neonate is held at about the same level as the uterus, until pulsations of the cord cease. If the infant is held higher, for example, on the mother's abdomen, fetal blood may drain to the placenta; if he is held lower, excessive blood may flow to the neonate before cord pulsations stop. Cord pulsations usually cease within seconds after respiration is initiated.

3. The cord is clamped or tied close to the umbilicus approximately 30 seconds after delivery when cord pulsations cease, if the neonate appears normal and mature (Figs. 22.23 to 22.25). However, if the need for transfusion is likely, such as in erythroblastosis, an 8 to 10 cm proximal length of cord is left. The cord is examined for two arteries and one vein (normal), and any cord abnormalities are noted (see p. 972).

Fig. 22.23
Hesseltine cord clamp.

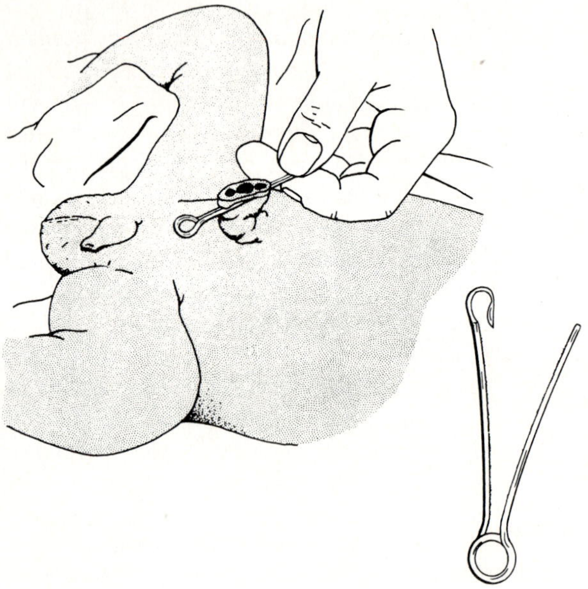

Fig. 22.24
Hollister cord clamp. **A,** Position clamp close to umbilicus. **B,** Secure cord. **C,** Cut cord. **D,** Remove clamp, using scissors, after cord dries (about 24 hours).

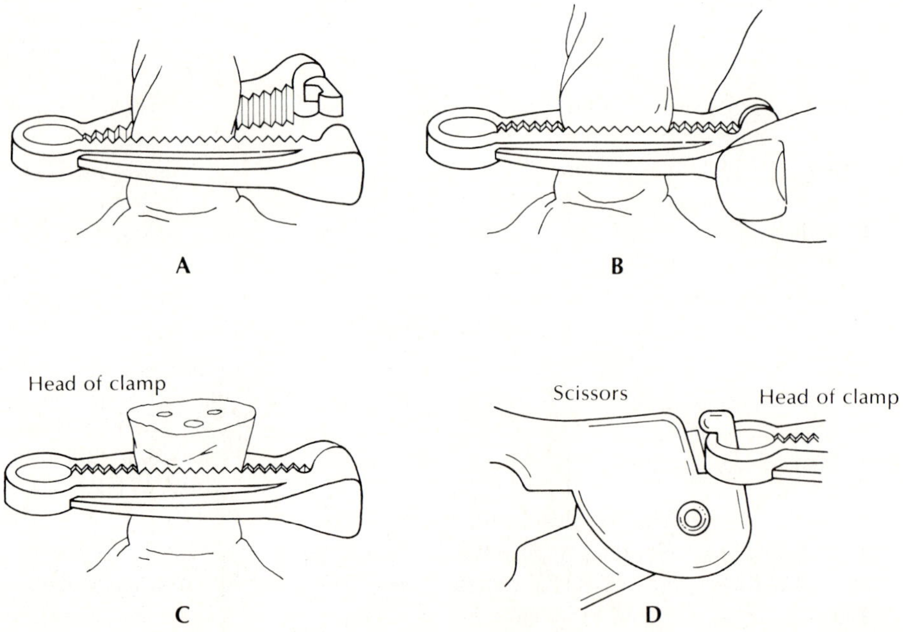

Some parents want the baby to receive an extra supply of blood and advocate "stripping" (milking) the cord toward the baby. Ordinarily it is unwise to strip the cord before clamping and cutting because postdelivery red blood cell destruction, which normally occurs neonatally, will be increased and hyperbilirubinemia (see p. 807) may ensue. In addition, polycythemia (increased number of red blood cells) increases blood viscosity, leading to cardiopulmonary problems in the neonate.

4. If the neonate is full term, of adequate weight for gestational age, and in good condition, he can be placed on a warmed blanket on the mother's abdomen; the parents are assisted to dry the infant immediately. The mother's body provides the neonate with sufficient warmth to prevent cold stress. The nurse must ensure the neonate's warmth by providing warmed blankets and taking care to cover the head.

5. The condition of the neonate is appraised at 1 minute and again at 5 minutes. The scoring method of Apgar is the simplest and most practical method clinically available. The Apgar score permits a rapid and semiquantitative assessment based on five signs indicative of the physiologic state of the neonate (Fig. 22.26): heartbeat (auscultatory); respiration, based on observed movement of the chest wall; color (pallid, cyanotic, or

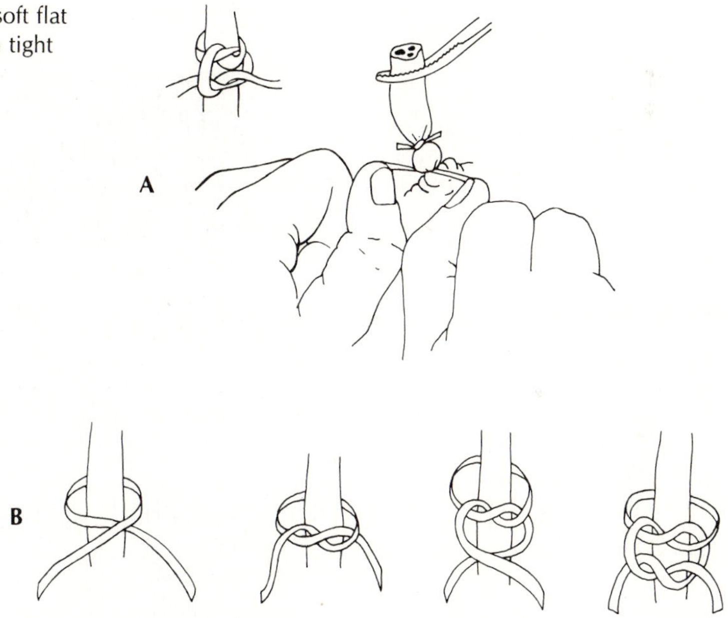

Fig. 22.25
Technique of tying off umbilical cord using, **A,** soft flat tie to prevent cutting through cord as it is drawn tight and, **B,** square knot to prevent slippage.

Fig. 22.26
Apgar scoring chart.

Sign	0	1	2
Heart rate	Absent	Slow (below 100)	Over 100
Respiratory effort	Absent	Slow, irregular	Good, crying
Muscle tone	Flaccid	Some flexion of extremities	Active motion
Reflex irritability	No response	Grimace	Cry
Color	Blue, pale	Body pink, extremities blue	Completely pink

Abnormal Neonatal Breathing

If the infant fails to breathe normally after delivery, immediate resuscitative measures (e.g., aspiration of the trachea through an infant laryngoscope, administration of oxygen by mask) are initiated (Fig 22.27). Obtain immediate pediatric assistance if needed. Transfer the critical or seriously compromised infant to the pediatric neonatal intensive care unit as soon as possible. Parents should be informed that additional care in an intensive care nursery is required.

pink); muscle tone, based on movement of the extremities; and reflexes, based on gentle slaps on the soles of the feet. The 5-minute score correlates with neonatal mortality and morbidity.

6. It is a legal requirement for all newborns to have treatment to prevent gonococcal or pneumcoccal or chlamydial infection in the conjunctiva. Such infections or ophthalmia neonatorum can lead to blindness (Figs. 22.28 to 22.30). The recommendations of the National Society to Prevent Blindness, NSPB Committee on Ophthalmia Neonatorum (June 15, 1981), are given in the box on p. 445. Clients who refuse eye prophylaxis for their neonate are requested to sign an informed con-

Fig. 22.27
A, Infant Kreisselmann resuscitator with overhead heat panel. Emergency equipment and supplies and drug tray are positioned next to the resuscitator under infant-sized stethoscope. Nurse is responsible for seeing that resuscitator is plugged in and functional at all times in event of an emergency.

A

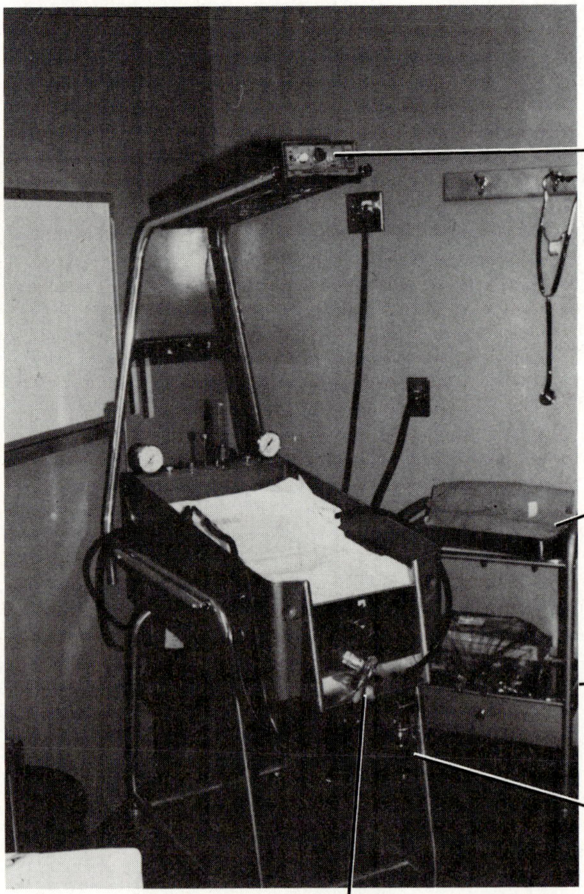

sent. A note to this effect must be entered in the neonate's record.

7. The baby is weighed and measured. (This may be delayed until the newborn is admitted to the nursery.)

8. Although rare, an occasional mix-up in the identity of newborns occurs, causing much anxiety and legal complications. As a precaution, newborns are identified by one of a number of techniques *before leaving the delivery area*. One technique uses Identibands, one to be attached to the mother's wrist and two others to the infant's wrist and ankle. Some hospitals take handprints and footprints of the baby. Others make up bead necklaces spelling out the infant's name. Most hospitals have policies that require the mother to acknowledge the identity of her baby before discharge from the delivery room.

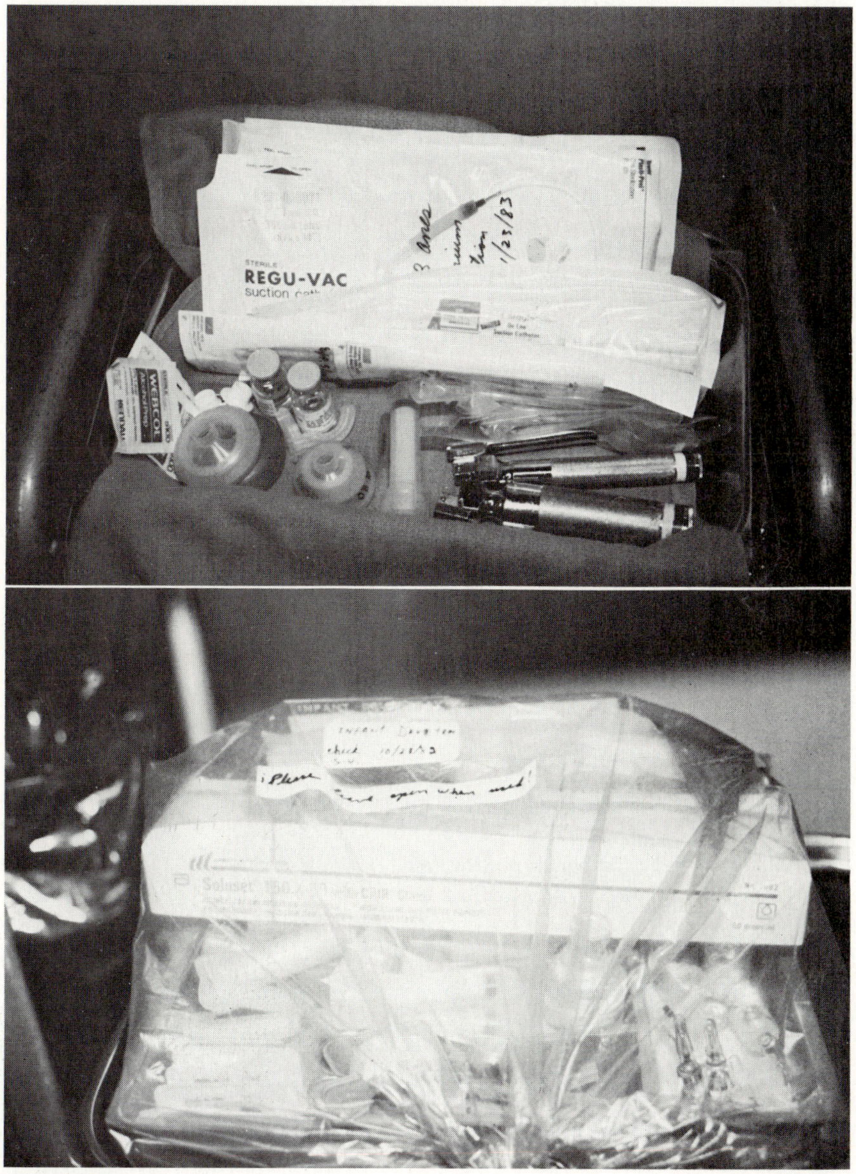

B

C

Fig. 22-27, cont'd
B, Equipment and supplies for emergency resuscitation of depressed neonate are always kept in readiness for all births. Nurse is responsible to see that this tray is always stocked and that batteries and light bulbs for laryngoscopes are functional. **C,** Infant drug tray. Nurse is responsible for seeing that tray is replaced when its expiration date is reached. (Courtesy Stanford University Medical Center, Stanford, Calif.)

Fig. 22.28

Silver nitrate for prophylactic eye care of newborn. **A,** Silver nitrate, 1%, in wax containers. **B,** Puncture wax containers with needle. **C,** Squeeze to release drops. Administer by placing 1 or 2 drops in lower conjunctival sac of lower lid and close eye to spread medication. **D,** New-style sterile container with twist-off top for silver nitrate in a see-through package.

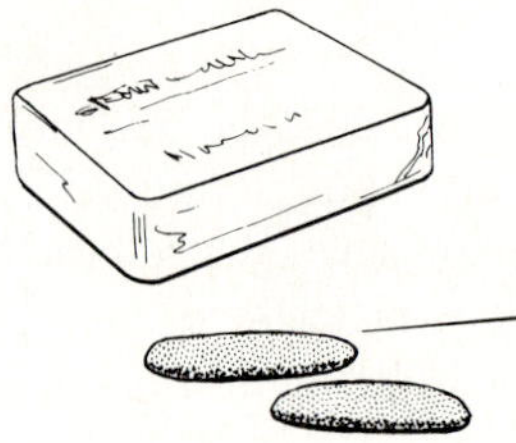

A

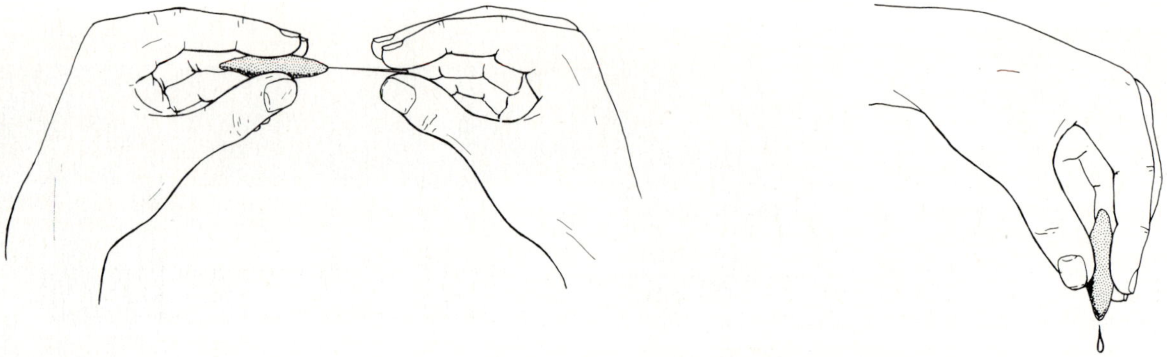

B

C

D

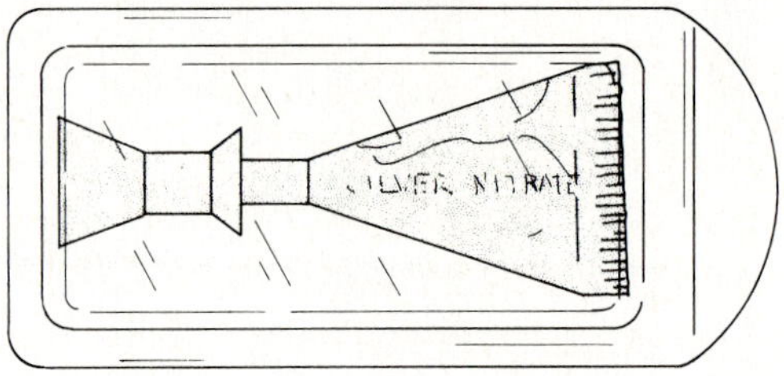

Fig. 22.29

Silver nitrate for prophylactic eye care of newborn. (From Ingalls, A.J., and Salerno, M.C.: Maternal and child health nursing, ed. 5, St. Louis, 1983, The C.V. Mosby Co.)

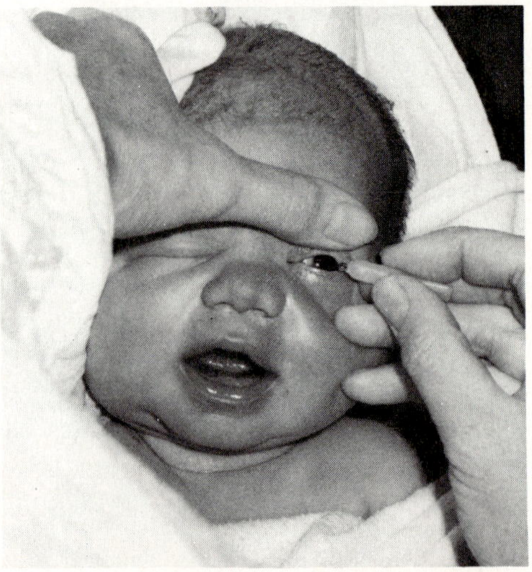

Fig. 22.30
Instillation of ophthalmic erythromycin drops using a needleless syringe. Drops are instilled into conjunctival sac. (Courtesy Stanford University Medical Center, Stanford, Calif.)

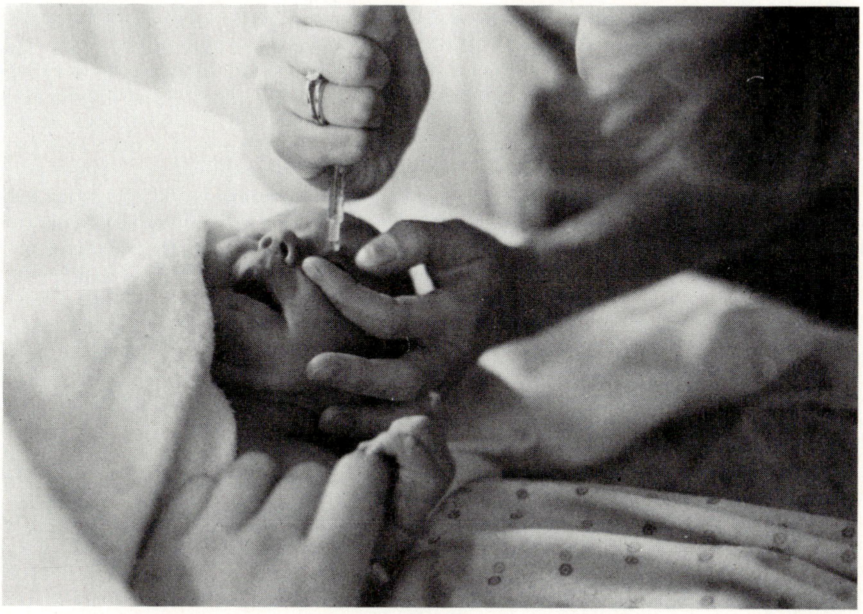

Recommendations for Neonatal Treatment of Conjunctiva

1. Instillation of a prophylaxis agent in the eyes of all newborn infants.
2. Acceptable prophylactic agents that prevent gonococcal ophthalmia neonatorum include the following:
   a. Silver nitrate solution (1%) in single-dose ampules
   b. Erythromycin (0.5%) ophthalmic ointment or drops in single-use tubes or ampules
   c. Tetracycline (1%) ophthalmic ointment or drops in single-use tubes or ampules
3. Acceptable prophylactic agents that prevent chlamydial ophthalmia neonatorum include the following:
   a. Erythromycin (0.5%) ophthalmic ointment or drops in single-use tubes or ampules
   b. Tetracycline (1%) ophthalmic ointment or drops in single-use tubes or ampules
   Silver nitrate does not prevent chlamydial infections.
4. Prophylaxis agents should be given shortly after birth. A delay of up to 1 hour* is probably acceptable and may facilitate initial maternal-infant bonding.
5. The importance of performing the instillation so the agent reaches all parts of the conjunctival surface is stressed. This can be accomplished by careful manipulation of the lids with fingers to ensure spreading of the agent. If medication strikes only the eyelids and lid margins but fails to reach the cornea, the instillation should be repeated. Prophylaxis should be applied as follows:
   a. Silver nitrate
      (1) Carefully clean eyelids and surrounding skin with sterile cotton, which may be moistened with sterile water.
      (2) Gently open baby's eyelids and instill two drops of silver nitrate on the conjunctival sac. Allow the silver nitrate to run across the whole conjunctival sac. Carefully manipulate lids to ensure spread of the drops. Repeat in the other eye. Use two ampules, one for each eye.
      (3) After 1 minute, gently wipe excess silver nitrate from eyelids and surrounding skin with sterile water. *Do not irrigate eyes.*
   b. Opthalmic ointment (erythromycin or tetracycline)
      (1) Carefully clean eyelids and surrounding skin with sterile cotton, which may be moistened with sterile water.
      (2) Gently open baby's eyelids and place a thin line of ointment, at least 1 to 2 cm (½ in), along the junction of the bulbar and palpebral conjunctiva of the lower lid. Try to cover the whole lower conjunctival area. Carefully manipulate lids to ensure spread of the ointment. *Be careful not to touch the eyelid or eyeball with the tip of the tube.* Repeat in other eye. Use one tube per baby.

From National Society to Prevent Blindness, NSPB Committee on Ophthalmia Neonatorum (June 15, 1981).
*Center for Disease Control, Atlanta, specifies up to 2 hours' delay is safe.

Continued.

Recommendations for Neonatal Treatment of Conjunctiva—cont'd

(3) After 1 minute, gently wipe excess ointment from eyelids and surrounding skin with sterile water. *Do not irrigate eyes.*

c. Ophthalmic drops (erythromycin or tetracycline)

(1) Apply as for silver nitrate.

6. The eye should not be irrigated after instillation of a prophylaxis agent. Irrigation may reduce the efficacy of prophylaxis and probably does not decrease the incidence of chemical conjunctivitis.
7. Infants born to mothers infected with agents that cause ophthalmia neonatorum may require special attention and systemic therapy as well as prophylaxis. A single does of aqueous crystalline penicillin G, 50,000 units/kg body weight for term and 20,000 units for low–birth weight infants should be administered intravenously to infants born to mothers with gonorrhea.
8. The detection and appropriate treatment of infections in pregnant women, which may result in ophthalmia neonatorum, are encouraged.
9. All physicians and hospitals should be required to report cases of ophthalmia neonatorum and etiologic agents to state and local health departments so that incidence data may be obtained to determine the effectiveness of the control measures.

Parent-Child Relationships

The mother's reaction* to the sight of her newborn may range from excited outbursts of laughing, talking, and even crying to apparent apathy. A polite smile and nod may acknowledge the comments of nurses and physicians. Occasionally the reaction is one of anger or indifference; the mother turns away from the baby, concentrates on her own pain, and sometimes makes hostile comments. These varying reactions can arise from pleasure, exhaustion, or deep disappointment. Whatever the reaction and cause may be, the mother needs continuing acceptance and support from all the staff. A written form accompanying the baby's chart should record the parents' reaction at birth. How do parents *look?* What do they *say?* What do they *do?*

Most parents, however, enjoy being able to handle, hold, and examine the baby right after birth (Figs. 22.14 and 22.19). The newborn infant is placed on the mother's abdomen, which has been draped with a warm receiving blanket. Both parents can assist with the thorough drying of the infant.

The mother may cut the cord or the cord may be left long enough so that the father can clamp it and cut off the extra portion. The mother can hold the newborn infant next to her skin to maintain his body heat and provide skin contact; care must be taken to keep the head warm as well. It is the nurse's responsibility to make sure the baby is kept warm and is in no danger of slipping from the parents' grasp (Fig. 23.12).

*See Chapter 32 for further discussion of parent-child relationships.

Warning Signs During Delivery

1. Passive reaction, either verbal or nonverbal (Parents do not touch, hold, or examine baby or talk in affectionate terms or tones about baby.)
2. Hostile reaction, either verbal or nonverbal (Parents make inappropriate verbalization, glances, or disparaging remarks about physical characteristics of child.)
3. Disappointment over sex of baby
4. No eye contact
5. Nonsupportive interaction between parents (If interaction seems dubious, talk to nurse and physician involved with delivery for further information.)

Reproduced by permission from Gray, J.D., Christy, A.C., Dean, G.D., and Kempe, C.H.: Prediction and prevention of child abuse, Semin. Perinatol. **3:**85, Jan. 1979.

Many women wish to begin to breast feed their infants at this time to take advantage of the infant's alert state and to stimulate the production of oxytocin that promotes contraction of the uterus (Fig. 22.17). Others wish to wait until the infant, mother, and father are together in the recovery room.

While the physician carries out the postdelivery vaginal examination and, if necessary, repairs the episiotomy, the mother usually feels discomfort. Therefore, while this process is being completed, the infant can be weighed and measured, wrapped in warm blankets, and given to the father to hold.

Parents are responsive to praise of their newborn.

Many require reassurance that the blue appearance of the baby after delivery is normal until respirations are well established. The reason for the molding of the baby's head must be reviewed with parents. Information about hospital routine as to future parent-child contacts can be repeated. The hospital staff, by their interest and concern, can do much to make this a satisfying experience for both parents.

Emergency Childbirth: When the Nurse Assists the Mother to Give Birth

EMERGENCY BIRTH OF FETUS IN VERTEX PRESENTATION

The following measures are necessary for the emergency birth of a fetus in the vertex position:

1. Position the woman comfortably. She will usually assume the position most suitable for her. If she is in a bed and there is time, elevate the head of the bed about 45 degrees. This position, in addition to facilitating perfusion of the uterus, allows you to maintain eye-to-eye contact with the woman. Occasionally the woman will assume the crawling position, on hands and knees.
2. Reassure her verbally with eye-to-eye contact and a calm, relaxed manner. If there is someone else available (e.g., the father), that person could help support her in position, assist with coaching, and compliment her on her efforts.
3. Wash your hands with soap and water or wash-and-dry pledgets if possible.
4. Place under her buttocks whatever clean material or clean newspapers are available.
5. Avoid touching the vaginal area to decrease the possibility of infection. (If there is time, scrub your hands and fingernails for 5 minutes before touching the parturient.) If hands can be clean or sterile gloves are available, massage or support perineum as needed.
6. The perineum thins and distends. As the head begins to crown, the birth attendant should do the following:
   a. Tear the amniotic membrane (caul) if it is still intact.
   b. Instruct woman to pant or pant-blow, thus avoiding the urge to push.
   c. Place the flat of the hand on the exposed fetal head and apply *gentle* pressure toward the vagina to prevent the head from "popping out." The mother may participate by placing her hand under yours on the emerging head. (NOTE: Rapid delivery of the fetal head must be prevented because (1) it is followed by a rapid change of pressure within the molded fetal skull, which may result in dural or subdural tears, and (2) it may cause vaginal or perineal lacerations.)
7. Instruct the mother to pant or pant-blow as you check for an umbilical cord. If the cord is around the neck, try to slip it up over the baby's head or pull *gently* to get some slack so that it can slip down over the shoulders.
8. Support fetal head as restitution (external rotation) occurs. After restitution, with one hand on each side of the baby's head, exert *gentle* pressure downward so that the anterior shoulder emerges under the symphysis pubis and acts as a fulcrum; then as *gentle* pressure is exerted in the opposite direction, the posterior shoulder, which has passed over the sacrum and coccyx, is delivered.
9. Be alert! Hold the baby securely because the rest of his body may deliver quickly. He will be slippery!
10. Cradle the baby's head and back in one hand and the buttocks in the other, keeping the head down to drain away the mucus. (NOTE: Do not hold the baby upside down by his ankles because to do so (1) hyperextends the spine, which has been flexed since conception, (2) increases intracranial pressure and the danger of capillary rupture, (3) may cause direct tissue trauma to his ankles, and (4) increases the possibility of dropping a wet, slippery baby.)
11. Dry the baby rapidly (to prevent rapid heat loss), keeping him at the same level as the mother's uterus. (NOTE: Keep the baby at the same level to prevent gravity flow of baby's blood to or from the placenta and the resultant hypovolemia or hypervolemia. Also, do not "milk" the cord: hypervolemia can cause respiratory distress initially or hyperbilirubinemia subsequently [Chapters 29 and 30]; and if isoimmunization has occurred, the baby may receive an additional inoculation of harmful antibodies [e.g., anti-Rh positive or anti-A or anti-B antibodies].)
12. As soon as infant is crying, place him on mother's abdomen, cover him (remember to keep his head warm too) with her clothing, and have her cuddle him. Compliment her (them) on a job well done and on the baby if appropriate. (If something appears to be the matter with the baby, do not lie!) She may wish to expose the part of the baby that will be touching her skin for skin-to-skin contact. (NOTE: Soon after the Wharton's jelly in the cord is exposed to cool air and expands and the infant cries, the umbilical vessels stop pulsating, and the

blood flow ceases. The baby's presence on the mother's abdomen stimulates the release of oxytocin from the posterior pituitary and thus stimulates uterine contractions, which aid in placental separation.)

13. *Wait* for the placenta to separate; *do not* tug on the cord. (NOTE: Injudicious traction may tear the cord, separate the placenta, or invert the uterus. Signs of placental separation include (1) a slight gush of dark blood from the introitus, (2) lengthening of the cord, and (3) change in uterine contour from discoid to globular shape.)
14. Instruct the mother to push to deliver the separated placenta. Gently ease out the placental membranes, using an up-and-down motion until membranes are removed. To minimize complications do not cut the cord without proper clamps or ties and a sterile cutting tool and inspect the placenta for intactness. Place the baby on the placenta and wrap the two together for additional warmth. (NOTE: There is no hurry to cut the cord. The infant will not lose blood through the placenta because the cord circulation ceases [clots] within minutes of birth.)
15. Check the firmness of the uterus. Gently massage the uterus and demonstrate to the mother how she can massage her own uterus properly.
16. Clean the area under the mother's buttocks.
17. Prevent or minimize hemorrhage.
    a. Hemorrhage from uterine atony.
        (1) *Gently* massage fundus to stimulate uterine musculature to contract. (NOTE: Overstimulation may fatigue the myometrium and cause atony.)
        (2) Put the baby to the breast as soon as possible. Sucking or nuzzling and licking the breast stimulate the release of oxytocin from the posterior pituitary. (NOTE: If the baby does not nurse, manually stimulate the mother's breasts.)
        (3) If medical assistance is delayed, do not allow the mother's bladder to become distended.
        (4) Expel any clots from her uterus. (NOTE: The fundus should be firm to prevent accidental inversion during this procedure. While holding the bottom of the uterus just above the symphysis pubis, apply gentle pressure on the firm fundus downward toward the vagina.)
    b. Hemorrhage from perineal lacerations.
        (1) Apply a clean pad to the perineum.
        (2) Instruct the mother to press her thighs together.
18. Comfort or reassure the mother and her family or friends. Keep her and the baby warm. Give her fluids if available and tolerated.
19. If this is a multiple birth, identify the infants in order of birth.
20. Make notations on the birth.
    a. Fetal presentation and position
    b. Presence of cord around neck or other parts and number of times cord encircles part
    c. Color, character, and amount of amniotic fluid
    d. Time of delivery
    e. Estimate of Apgar score, resuscitation, and ultimate condition of baby
    f. Sex of baby
    g. Approximate time of placental expulsion, its appearance, and completeness
    h. Maternal condition: affect, amount of bleeding, and status of uterine contractions
    i. Any unusual occurrences during the delivery

Lateral Sims' position for delivery. A lateral Sims' posture may be the position of choice for delivery when (1) the delivery is progressing rapidly and there is insufficient time for slow distention of the perineum; (2) the fetal head seems too large to pass through the introitus without laceration, and episiotomy is not possible; or (3) the apparent size of the fetus* is consistent with possible shoulder dystocia.

In the lateral Sims' position, less stress is placed on the perineum and better visualization of the perineum is possible. In the event of shoulder dystocia, lateral Sims' posture increases the space needed for delivery.

UNUSUAL OCCURRENCES DURING AND AFTER BIRTH

Shoulder dystocia. Shoulder dystocia may occur unexpectedly. It results when the bisacromial diameter exceeds the anteroposterior, or oblique, diameter of the pelvic inlet. The following measures serve to decrease the fetal bisacromial diameter and enlarge the maternal pelvic inlet. (1) Ask the mother to flex her thighs on her abdomen or ask her husband (or other person) to help her achieve and maintain this position. (2) Apply *suprapubic* (not fundal) pressure to collapse the diameter of the shoulders. The assistant places the flat of one hand over that of the other, keeps the arms straight, and applies pressure downward. Fracture of the clavicle while using this technique is rarely seen.

Prebirth passage of meconium with fetus in vertex presentation. Anal sphincter relaxation and release of meconium occur in the fetus stressed by a diminished

*There is no one size of fetus that is "too large," since size is relative to the maternal structures. However, a large head and lack of progress in expulsion raise the possibility of shoulder dystocia.

supply of oxygen. Meconium in the amniotic fluid is expected to enter the fetal air passages as the fetus gasps in response to oxygen lack. Without appropriate suction equipment it is not possible to remove meconium trapped in the lower levels of the respiratory tree.

Tight nuchal cord. The cord may be so tightly coiled around the fetal neck or body that no amount of slack is possible and it cannot be unwound. The birth attendant may have no way to tie (clamp) the cord and no sterile scissors to cut it to permit release of the cord before birth. In that event, deliver the fetus as described above and unwind the cord as soon as possible. Three complications may occur: (1) fetal respiratory hypoxia and depression, (2) tearing of the cord or placenta, thus compromising timely and total placenta removal, and (3) inversion of the uterus. Complications may not occur from a tight nuchal cord, and the newborn may be in good condition.

Maternal postdelivery hemorrhage. Postdelivery hemorrhage is possible from the uterus, cervix, and vagina and from perineal lacerations and may be life threatening. (For control of *uterine* hemorrhage, see the discussion of the delivery process, above.)

A precipitate labor or a large baby may be responsible for *cervical* or *vaginal* tears. Until the services of a medical facility or physician are available, the birth attendant can help the mother control her blood pressure by using the Trendelenburg position and keeping her quiet.

Bleeding from *perineal laceration* is easier to contain. Possible measures to control or stop the bleeding include direct pressure on the wound with your hand, a perineal pad, or a cloth compress (see Chapter 35).

EMERGENCY BIRTH OF FETUS IN BREECH PRESENTATION

Should it become necessary for an individual to deliver a breech infant, one must remember the following points:

1. The infant's body should be elevated during the birth process.
2. Traction and compression should be avoided, thus preventing the arms from being upward above the head and blocking delivery.
3. The body should be brought upward as the head is being born to ensure a patent airway (see Chapter 37).

BIRTH AND MANAGEMENT OF PRETERM INFANT

The actual process of birthing the preterm infant does not vary from that of the term infant. However, the care of the infant after birth requires some modification as follows:

1. Warmth is essential.
2. Minimize handling, maintain a clear airway, and feed and change the infant.
3. Nutrition may be a problem if a medical facility is not available. Although the infant may be unable to nurse at the breast, slow feeding is important, using a medicine dropper, for example.
4. Urge the preterm infant to breathe by stimulating him *gently* when he "forgets."
5. Transport the infant to a medical facility equipped to handle preterm infants as early as possible (see Chapter 37).

References and Readings

Blair, C., and Mahoukis, C.: Comparing notes: the nurse as patient/the nurse as labor coach, M.C.N. **5**(2):102, 1980.

Childbirth sitting up, Newsweek, p. 79, March 2, 1981.

Grad, R.K.: Breaking ground for a birthing room, M.C.N. **4**(4):245, 1979.

Hickman, M.A.: An introduction to midwifery, London, 1978, Blackwell Scientific Publications, Ltd.

ICEA Review: Maternal position during labor and birth, Milwaukee, 1978, International Childbirth Education Association, Inc.

ICEA Review: Second stage labor: labor, Milwaukee, 1978, International Childbirth Education Association, Inc.

Jensen, M.D., Benson, R.C., and Bobak, I.M.: Maternity care: the nurse and the family, ed. 2, St. Louis, 1981, The C.V. Mosby Co.

Malinowski, J.S., et al.: Nursing care of the labor patient, ed. 2, Philadelphia, 1983, F.A. Davis Co.

Maloni, J.: The birthing room: some insights into parents, M.C.N. **5**(5):314, 1980.

Shannon-Babitz, M.: Addressing the needs of fathers during labor and delivery, M.C.N. **4**(6):378, 1979.

Sumner, P.E., and Phillips, C.R.: Birthing rooms: concept and reality, St. Louis, 1981, The C.V. Mosby Co.

Varney, H.: Nurse-midwifery, London, 1980, Blackwell Scientific Publications, Ltd.

Wiggins, J.D.: Childbearing: physiology, experiences, needs, St. Louis, 1979, The C.V. Mosby Co.

Wimberly, D.: Intrapartal care, Am. J. Nurs. **79**(3):451, 1979.

23 Third and Fourth Stages of Labor

- Third Stage
  - Separation and delivery of placenta
    - Assessment for placental separation
  - Immediate care of mother
    - General assessment of mother
    - Assessment of the birth canal
    - Factors associated with uterine atony
    - Pharmacologic stimulation of uterine contractions after delivery of placenta
  - Nursing diagnoses
  - Plan and implementation
- Fourth Stage
  - Maternal recovery
    - Goals of care
    - Assessment
    - Nursing diagnoses
    - Plan and implementation
  - Neonatal adjustment to extrauterine existence
- Evaluative Criteria for Care During Four Stages of Labor

Third Stage

The third stage of labor extends from the birth of the baby until the delivery of the placenta. The goal in the management of the third stage of labor is the prompt separation and expulsion of the placenta, achieved in the easiest, safest manner. Outmoded procedures such as kneading the corpus (Credé's maneuver) and pushing the fundus downward have been abandoned because of the serious hazards of uterine bleeding, retention of the placenta, contamination of the cervix outside the introitus, and possible inversion (turning inside out) of the uterus.

SEPARATION AND DELIVERY OF PLACENTA

The placenta is attached to the myometrium beneath the extremely thin endometrium of the basal plate by numerous, randomized, fibrous anchor villi—much like a postage stamp is attached to a sheet of postage stamps. After the fetus is delivered, in the presence of strong uterine contractions, the placental site is markedly reduced in size. This reduced size causes the anchor villi to break and the placenta separates from its attachments. Normally the first few strong contractions 5 to 7 minutes after the birth of the baby shear the placenta from the myometrium. A placenta will not be easily freed from a flaccid (relaxed) uterus because the placental site is not reduced in size.

NOTE: Although manipulation (such as massaging) of the fundus may cause fundal contractions, the irritation may also cause the cervix to contract. Therefore after being partially separated, the placenta may be trapped within the uterus, and bleeding may be dangerously profuse before the placenta can be extracted.

Assessment for placental separation. Placental separation is indicated by the following, in sequence (Fig. 23.1).

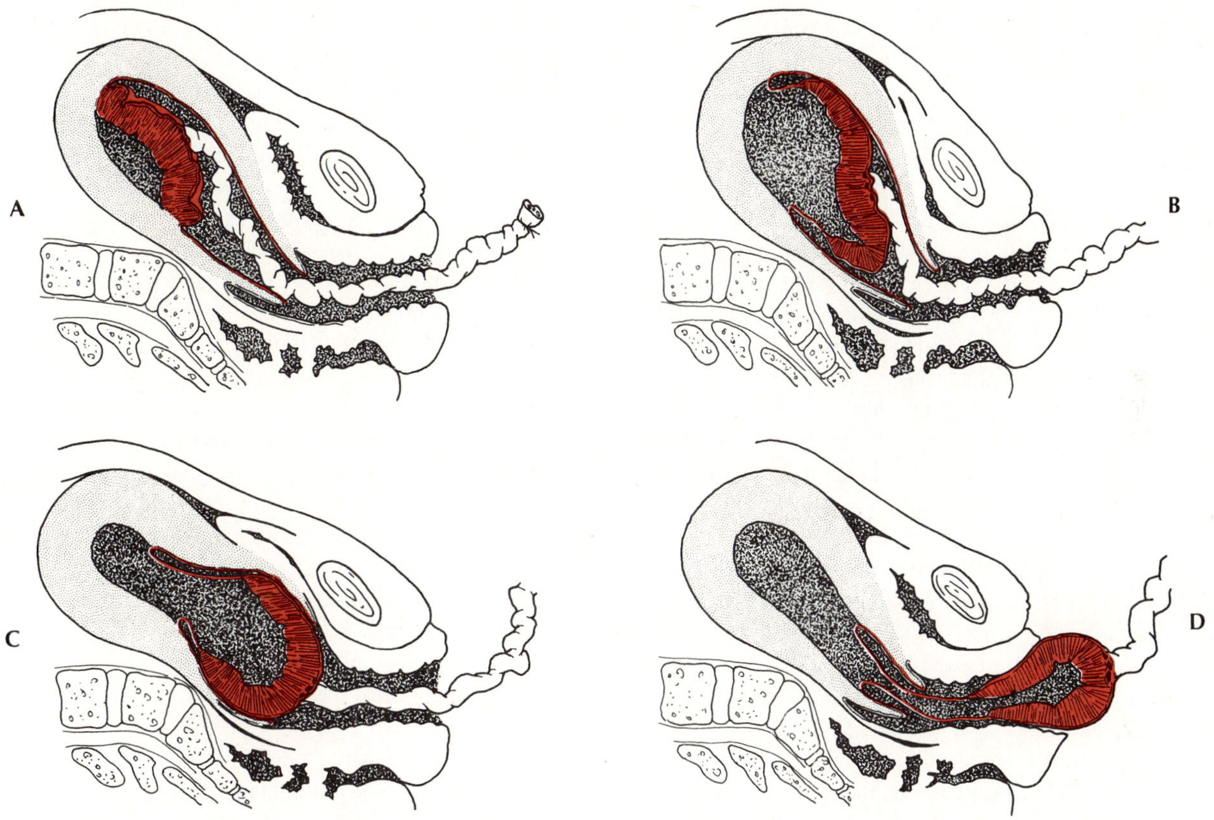

Fig. 23.1
Third stage of labor. **A,** Placenta begins by separating in central portion with retroplacental bleeding. Uterus changes from discoid to globular shape. **B,** Placenta completes separation and enters lower uterine segment. Uterus is globular in shape. **C,** Placenta enters vagina, cord is seen to lengthen, and there may be increase in bleeding. **D,** Expression (birth) of placenta and completion of third stage.

1. A firmly contracting fundus
2. A change in the uterus from a discoid to a globular shape
3. A visible and palpable rounded bulge above the symphysis (the bladder must be empty to avoid confusing a full bladder with a change in the uterus)
4. A sudden gush of dark blood from the introitus
5. Apparent lengthening of the umbilical cord as the placenta gets closer to the introitus
6. A vaginal fullness (the placenta) noted on vaginal or rectal examination, or fetal membranes seen at the introitus

Whether the placenta presents by the shiny fetal surface (Schultze mechanism) or whether it turns to show first its dark roughened maternal surface (Duncan mechanism) is of no clinical importance. At one time it was believed that the Duncan mechanism was associated with a significantly greater blood loss, but this has been disproved. After the placenta is born, it is examined for intactness to be certain that no portion of it remains in the uterine cavity (that is, no retained placental fragments).

IMMEDIATE CARE OF MOTHER

General assessment of mother. Physiologic changes following delivery are profound. The cardiac output is increased rapidly as maternal circulation to the placenta ceases and the pooled blood from the lower extremities is mobilized. The pulse rate slows in response to the change in cardiac output. Pulse rates tend to remain slightly slower than before pregnancy during the first 7 to 10 days after delivery.

The blood pressure usually returns to normal prenatal levels shortly after delivery. Several factors contribute to an elevated blood pressure: the excitement of the second stage, certain medications, and the time of day (blood pressure is highest during the late afternoon). Analgesics and anesthetics may lead to hypotension in the hour following birth.

Even as the physician or nurse-midwife is completing the third stage of labor, the nurse observes the mother for signs of an altered level of consciousness (LOC) or alterations in respirations. Because of the rapid cardiovascular changes (e.g., the increased intracranial pressure during pushing and the rapid increase in cardiac output), this period presents the risk of rupture of a preexisting cerebral aneurysm and of pulmonary emboli. The risk for pulmonary emboli arises from another source as well. As the placenta separates, there is a possibility of amniotic fluid entering the maternal circulation if the uterine musculature does not contract rapidly and well. The incidence of these possible complications is small; however, the alert nurse can contribute to their immediate recognition and the prompt initiation of therapy.

Assessment of the birth canal. Assessment of the birth canal is performed immediately after delivery of the placenta and before the physician or nurse-midwife completes a thorough examination. The gloved hands are rinsed in sterile solution (usually available from a basin in a stand on wheels), and the introitus is swabbed with wet sponges. It is unnecessary to change the drapes. The perineum, vagina, and cervix are inspected for lacerations, extensions of the episiotomy, or hematomas (blood "tumors").

The cupped hand is inserted into the vagina and, if possible, through the cervix. The other hand on the mother's abdomen steadies the uterus and pushes it downward gently. In this way the uterine cavity can be examined manually and the placental site identified. Any *retained placental fragments* may be removed manually and any membrane strands grasped with an appropriate forceps for removal. Retained fragments of placenta or pieces of membrane prevent the uterus from contracting effectively to control bleeding and, if left in place for a few days, from becoming infected. Infection from retained fragments was one of the causes of "child-bed fever" (puerperal sepsis) that caused many maternal deaths until the advent of modern obstetrics.

To examine the vaginal canal, vaginal retractors may be used to hold the canal open, the cervix is grasped with a sponge (also called stick, long, or ring) forceps (Fig. 22.5, *A*), and its entire circumference is systematically inspected. *The nurse assists the physician or nurse-midwife* by supplying the appropriate equipment for the delivery table, repositioning the light if necessary, and by elevating the fundus (under the direction of the physician). Elevation of the fundus is done by dipping the fingers down behind the woman's symphysis pubis and moving the uterine body up away from the symphysis pubis, thus opening and tenting the vaginal fornices. The lateral and posterior fornices can then be examined together with the areas beneath the bladder and over the ischial spines. Pudendal block or, rarely, light inhalation anesthesia is entirely adequate for examination and repair of most lacerations.

In routine postdelivery examinations of the uterus and vaginal canal, unsuspected cervical lacerations 2.5 cm (about 1 in) long may be found in 5% to 7% of women. Retained membranes may be identified in almost 5% of cases, and vaginal lacerations, including an extension of the episiotomy, may be identified in about the same percentage of women. Retained placental tissue may be expected in about 2% to 4% of cases. Uterine anomalies and pelvic tumors are occassionally identified for the first time during this examination.

Factors associated with uterine atony. Excessive blood loss during the third stage of labor or within the first hour thereafter may be caused by uterine atony (inability of the uterus to contract); often associated with one of more of the following:

1. Excessive analgesia or anesthesia
2. Traumatic delivery
3. Multiple pregnancy (twins, triplets)
4. Polyhydramnios (excessive amount of amniotic fluid)
5. Uterine neoplasm
6. Hypertensive cardiovascular renal disease
7. Grand multiparity (more than six pregnancies reached viability)

A poor labor, especially when caused by uterine inertia (poor or absent uterine contractions), may be followed by postdelivery uterine hypotonia (inadequate contractions), faulty placental separation, or hemorrhage (see Chapter 35). A distended bladder forces the uterus up into the abdomen and thus may contribute to uterine relaxation and hemorrhage. Contraction of the uterine myometrium, the "living ligature" (see p. 63), is essential to control blood loss. If an early problem such as uterine atony or hypotonia can be anticipated and properly treated, it may be possible to avoid a later complication such as postdelivery hemorrhage.

Pharmacologic stimulation of uterine contractions after delivery of placenta. Ergot causes firm contraction of the uterus. For this reason, ergot products such as ergonovine maleate, 0.2 mg, or methylergonovine (Methergine), 0.2 mg, are useful after the placenta has separated to prevent or control postabortal or postdelivery bleeding. One parenteral dose or repeated oral doses may be given.

NOTE: Ergot is a vasoconstrictor also; thus hypertension may be a side effect of ergot medications. Therefore these drugs are avoided in women with elevated blood pressure. The nurse must remember to assess the woman's previous blood pressures and take the blood pressure just before administering ergot products.

Synthetic oxytocin (Syntocinon, 10 units, or Pitocin, 10 units) may be administered either intramuscularly or intravenously to accomplish the same purpose. The effect lasts about 30 minutes. If excessive bleeding continues, an intravenous infusion of 1000 ml of Ringer's lactated solution with 10 to 20 units of oxytocin may be ordered.

NURSING DIAGNOSES

Before establishing nursing diagnoses, the nurse correlates the events of the third stage and the mother's physical and emotional responses to the third stage of labor. The following are examples of nursing diagnoses:

1. Ineffective individual coping by mother because of lack of knowledge of sensations to expect during the third stage of labor
2. Abnormal vaginal bleeding caused by inadequate contractions of the uterine myometrium

PLAN AND IMPLEMENTATION

To assist in the delivery of the placenta, the nurse or coach instructs the mother to push as contractions are felt. If an oxytocin medication is ordered, the nurse administers the medication in the dosage and by the route indicated by the physician or nurse-midwife. When the delivery of the placenta is complete and the episiotomy is sutured, the vulva is gently cleansed with sterile water by the physician or nurse-midwife. The circulating nurse (sometimes assisted by the physician) then performs the following:

1. Applies a sterile perineal pad
2. Removes the drapes
3. Repositions the delivery table or bed
4. Lowers the mother's legs simultaneously from the stirrups
5. Assists the woman onto her bed if she is to be transfered from the delivery area to the recovery area (The nurse will need assistance to move the woman from a delivery table onto a bed if the woman has had anesthesia and does not have full use of her lower extremities.)
6. Dresses the woman in a clean gown and covers her with a warmed blanket
7. Raises the side rails of the bed during the transfer (In some hospitals, the mother is given the baby to hold during the transfer; in some hospitals, the father carries the baby; in other hospitals; the nurse carries the baby either to the nursery or to the recovery area for the duration of the mother's recovery period.)

NOTE: The nurse is to observe excellent body mechanics to avoid injury to own back or other body structure. The nurse may use a roller. To use the roller, one nurse covers the roller with a blanket and stands on the right side of the woman's bed; the other nurse rolls the woman over onto her left side away from the bed. The roller is moved under the woman, and the woman is rolled back onto the roller. Care is taken not to entangle the woman's hair, intravenous tubing, or anything else in the roller. Using good body mechanics, the nurse on the right side of the bed pulls the blanket covering the roller while the other nurse assists. Someone else—the physician or another nurse—takes care that the mother's legs move safely onto her bed. The woman is turned onto her side, and the roller is removed. Transferring the woman from the delivery table to her bed without a roller can be accomplished if she can use her legs safely or there are several people to lift her.

If the woman plans to bottle feed and she understands and has signed an informed consent, the nurse may administer an intramuscular injection of antilactogenic hormones soon after the placenta is delivered. See Chapter 30 for further discussion of suppression of lactation.

If the woman labors, gives birth, and recovers in the same bed and room, she is refreshed as described above and the delivery area is cleaned as necessary (see Chapter 22).

Fourth Stage

The fourth stage of labor, the stage of recovery, is a critical period for the mother and neonate. While both the mother and neonate are recovering from the physical process of birth, they are also initiating new relationships.

During the next 2 hours, the maternal organism makes its initial readjustment to the nonpregnant state, and body systems begin to stabilize; therefore the immediate physical response of the mother to the birth process is kept under careful scrutiny. The neonate's anatomy and physiology continue with the transition from intrauterine to extrauterine existence and are also kept under careful scrutiny.

MATERNAL RECOVERY

Goals of care. The goals for nursing actions during the fourth stage are the following:

1. Prevent hemorrhage from uterine atony

2. Identify and report immediately hemorrhage from lacerations or the formation of a hematoma
3. Meet fluid and nutrient needs as ordered
4. Prevent bladder distention
5. Help the mother begin to integrate the birth experience by listening and answering questions she and father may have about the experience
6. Note and report immediately any findings that are not within normal limits (e.g., hypotension or hypertension, tachycardia, dyspnea; remember the blood pressure of a woman who has given birth is normally lower than her previous blood pressure)
7. Facilitate parent-child and acquaintance attachment
8. Maintain mother's physical comfort and facilitate rest

Assessment. To assess the mother during the fourth stage of labor, the nurse does the following:

1. Notes factors on the prenatal and labor record that could predispose the new mother to hemorrhage (e.g., factors associated with uterine atony or hypotonia)
2. Reviews length of labor and progress in labor
3. Initiates routine assessment for this stage of labor (Table 23.1 and Figs. 23.2 and 23.3)
4. Notes the character and location of discomfort (e.g., "afterpains," pain from site of episiotomy, unusual pain from a hematoma)
5. Notes evidence of fatigue or exhaustion, hunger, or thirst and level of recovery from analgesics or anesthesia if used
6. Notes response to birth (e.g., excitement or disappointment, fatigue, drowsiness [urge to sleep may come within the hour])
7. Notes responses of parent or parents to child

Nursing diagnoses. Before establishing nursing diagnoses, the nurse correlates the findings from the assessment. Examples of nursing diagnoses may include the following:

1. Potential uterine relaxation caused by filling urinary bladder
2. Alterations in physical comfort because of pain in the episiotomy area
3. Inability to void because of effects of labor and delivery on urinary tract sensation
4. Potential alteration in self-concept of parent or parents because of poor self-evaluation of behavior during birth experience

Plan and implementation. The period of recovery is a very busy and crucial one for the nurse who is attending the family. The nurse is concerned about the maternal position in bed, the prevention of hemorrhage, the prevention of urinary bladder distention, the maintenance of cleanliness, the maintenance of comfort, the maintenance of fluid balance and nutrition, and the support of parental emotional needs before the transfer of the family to the postdelivery unit.

Maternal position. The nurse settles the woman comfortably in bed. A new mother needs to remain in bed for at least 2 hours even if she had had an unmedicated delivery. The rapid decrease in intraabdominal pressure results in a dilation of blood vessels supplying the intestines (known as splanchnic engorgement). Splanchnic engorgement pools blood in the viscera; therefore when the woman stands up, she may feel faint (orthostatic hypotension). Women and their families need to be forewarned so that she knows to call for assistance, especially the first time or two that she gets out of bed.

The woman who had received analgesics needs to be watched until she is fully recovered from the medications (i.e., vital signs are stable and she is fully awake). Women who have had saddle block anesthesia will need to remain flat in bed (on their sides, abdomens, or backs) with the head raised not more than 15 to 20 cm

Table 23.1
Physical Assessment of the Mother During Fourth Stage

	Minimal Assessment	Findings and Comments
Fundus	Every 15 min	Firm: midline, 2 cm below or at umbilicus Soft: massage until firm and express clots until contracted to midlevel Right of midline: check bladder for distention
Lochia	Every 15 min (in conjunction with assessment of fundus)	Moderate flow: normal; if flow comes in spurts, suspect cervical tear Heavy flow: recheck in 3-5 min and report
Perineum	Check in conjunction with assessment of lochia	Condition of episiotomy and perineum: clean, edematous, discolored, stitches intact
Blood pressure	Every 15 min for 1 hr or until stable, then every 30 min times two	Slightly elevated from excitement and effort of delivery; returns to normal within 1 hr
Pulse	Every 15 min	Normal rate for individual within 1 hr

Fig. 23.2

Nurse prepares to assess for blood pressure, pulse, and respirations. As she interacts with new mother, nurse also assesses for maternal alertness, signs of discomfort, and cues to reaction to her birth experience and newborn. (Courtesy Stanford University Medical Center, Stanford, Calif.)

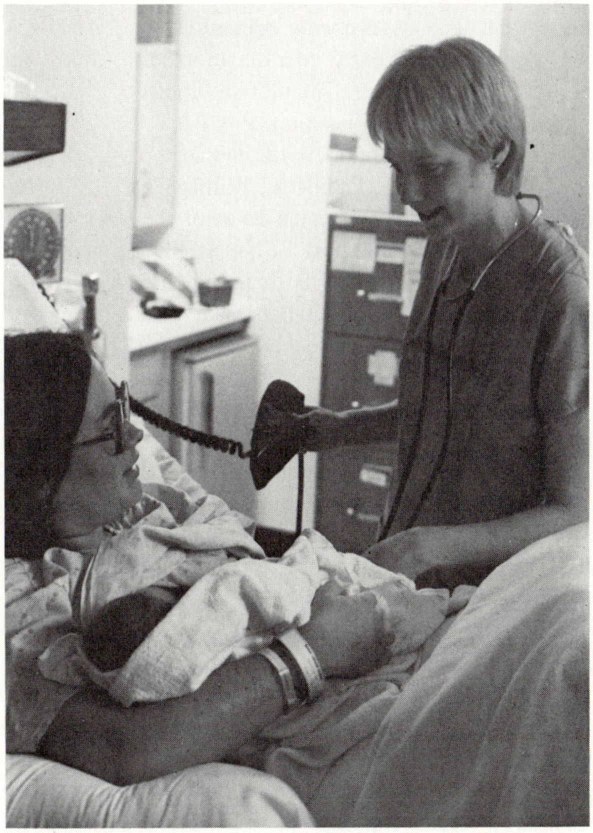

Fig. 23.3

Palpating fundus of uterus during first hour after delivery. Note that upper hand is placed over fundus; lower hand dips in above symphysis pubis and supports uterus while it is massaged gently.

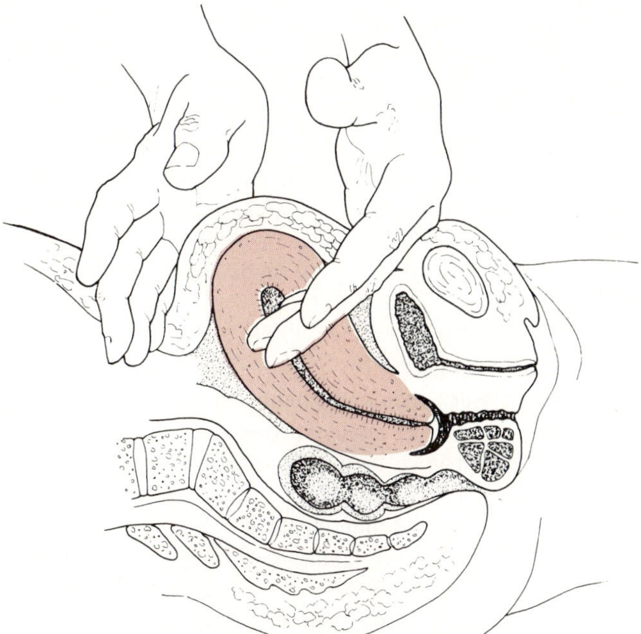

(6 to 8 in) for 8 to 12 hours to prevent development of a ''spinal'' headache (see Chapter 31).

Prevent hemorrhage. The assessments presented in Table 23.1 are designed for early identification of events that may lead to hemorrhage. The uterine fundus is palpated to note consistency and position (Fig. 23.3). Immediately after delivery the fundus is located in the midline about 2 cm below the umbilicus. Within an hour it usually rises to slightly above the level of the umbilicus and remains there for the next 12 hours. Normally the fundus remains firm or may be returned to a state of firmness with intermittent gentle massage. As noted earlier, *atony* of the uterine musculature may occur, and as the relaxed uterus distends with blood and clots, blood vessels in the placental site are not clamped off by the ''living ligature,'' and hemorrhage results. It is necessary to express gently the accumulated blood and clots before the uterus can again contract. If the atony is not controlled by such treatment, medical intervention must be instituted (see Chapter 35).

Palpation to determine the amount of *bladder distention* accompanies the palpation of the fundus. A distended bladder may also contribute to postdelivery hemorrhage. The full bladder forces the uterus upward and to the right of the midline. Such a position interferes with the contractibility of the uterine muscle, and hemorrhage results. The nurse encourages the woman to void, or if necessary, obtains an order for catheterization.

The nurse notes the amount of lochia. Lochia may be described as scant, moderate, or marked (profuse). As the effect of the oxytocic medication administered after delivery wears off, the amount of lochia will increase because the myometrium relaxes somewhat. The nurse always checks under the mother's buttocks as well as on the perineal pad. Bleeding may flow between the buttocks onto the linens under the mother while the amount on the perineal pad is slight. If a perineal pad is soaked through from tail to tail (100 ml) in 15 minutes or blood is found to be pooled under the buttocks, continuous observation of blood loss, vital signs, and maternal color and behavior is indicated.

NOTE: Immediate medical intervention will be necessary if any of the following occur:

1. Marked bleeding persists; that is, the mother soaks a second perineal pad in 15 minutes (whether or not bleeding is accompanied by a change in vital signs or maternal color or behavior).
2. Mother complains of feeling light-headed, ''seeing stars,'' or feeling ''funny and sick to [her] stomach'' (symptoms of shock).
3. Mother begins to act anxious, her color turns ashen or grayish, her skin feels cool and clammy (wet), or she exhibits air hunger (signs of shock).

If the mother exhibits symptoms or signs of shock (also see p. 800), the nurse does the following:

1. Calls for help fast (pushes emergency button and yells, if necessary)
2. Tilts woman onto her side and checks the uterus for firmness (If it is not firm, the nurse massages it gently and when firm, expresses any clots.)
3. Increases the flow rate of intravenous fluids and adds medication, such as oxytocin (Pitocin), if it is ordered
4. Raises woman's legs *high* for fast return of blood to her head
5. Administers oxygen (when available) with a tight face mask at 8 to 10 L/min

If bleeding is in the form of a continuous trickle or is seen to come in spurts, lacerations of the vagina or cervix or the presence of an unligated vessel in the episiotomy is suspected. The woman will most likely be returned to the delivery area to permit visualization of the site and surgical correction.

If blood pressure values begin to fall and pulse rate begins to increase, notify the physician immediately. If symptoms and signs of shock appear, implement steps listed above while awaiting the physician.

Prevent bladder distention. In addition to the possibility of causing uterine relaxation, distention of the urinary bladder can result in atony of the bladder wall. Atony leads to urinary retention; retention provides a favorable environment for infection. The nurse encourages the woman to void naturally employing one or more of the following: the nurse places a bedpan under the mother, gives her water to drink if the physician has ordered oral fluids, turns on the water faucet, ambulates her (if ordered), and provides privacy. If the woman cannot void, most physicians write an order for catheterization. If the woman is catheterized, a urine specimen is saved for laboratory studies as necessary (e.g., culture and sensitivity).

Spirits of peppermint are sometimes used to aid the woman to void naturally. ''Spirits'' are concentrated alcohol solutions of volatile substances; they are also known as essences. Spirits of peppermint give off vapors. These vapors have an external, local relaxing effect on the sphincter muscle of the urinary meatus. Use of *peppermint spirits* may make it unnecessary to catheterize. The nurse places a bedpan under the woman and then pours a few drops of peppermint spirits *into the bedpan*. The vapors rise to flow over the vulvar area, the urinary meatus relaxes, and urine is released. Nothing touches the woman except the vapors; the woman feels no sensation, only notices the aroma of peppermint. We know of no hospital that requires a physician's order for this technique.

Maintain cleanliness. The nurse changes perineal pads

as necessary and cleanses the vulvar area with each pad change. As the nurse demonstrates good hand-washing technique before touching the mother's perineal area, she verbally emphasizes the action. The nurse reminds the woman to cleanse the vulvar area using a separate tissue for one swipe from front to back, applying the pad from front to back and then rewashing the hands. Some hospitals routinely offer a bed bath during this period.

The nurse refreshes the mother, her bed, and the area around the bed as necessary.

Maintain comfort. *Cleanliness* is one measure that increases the mother's comfort.

Uterine contractions may result in discomfort known as *afterpains*. The volume within the uterus is decreased after delivery. The force of the myometrial contractions is considerable; the intrauterine pressure is much greater than that during labor, reaching 150 mm Hg or more.

During the first 12 hours following delivery, uterine contractions are regular and strong, especially in multiparas. The nurse adds to the woman's comfort by the following measures:

1. Explaining the normal physiology of afterpains
2. Helping the mother keep her urinary bladder empty
3. Providing a warmed blanket to the mother's abdomen
4. Administering analgesics ordered by the physician
5. Encouraging relaxation and breathing exercises

A filling bladder pressing up against the uterus causes it to relax. The uterus attempts to stay firm by increasing the force of contractions, thereby increasing the discomfort of afterpains.

Gentle massage of the fundus increases uterine contractions, thereby intensifying afterpains. To help the new mother cope with the discomforts of assessment measures, the nurse explains what is being done and why.

The *episiotomy area* or *hemorrhoids* may contribute to the new mother's discomfort. Ice packs wrapped in gauze or other protective cloth are placed against the area of the episiotomy to numb the area and to minimize the amount of edema that occurs, thus reducing discomfort. The ice pack is most effective in minimizing edema if used for the first hour or two following delivery. The physician may order any one of several antiseptic or anesthetic ointments or sprays to ease discomfort in the perineal area. A side-lying position relieves direct pressure on the area.

If the woman had had a saddle block or other regional anesthetic, the nurse's description of sensations to expect as the anesthetic wears off can be very reassuring (see Chapter 25).

Some women experience intense *tremors* after delivery that resemble the shivering of a chill. This chilling may be related to the sudden release of pressure on pelvic nerves. According to another theory, chilling* may be symptomatic of a fetus-to-mother transfusion that sometimes occurs during placental separation. The nurse can help the woman to relax or to feel comforted by providing her with warmed blankets and an explanation that the tremors are commonly seen after delivery and are not related to infection.

If the nurse administers analgesics (Fig. 23.4), the

*The feeling of a "chill" may be a reaction to adrenalin production during delivery.

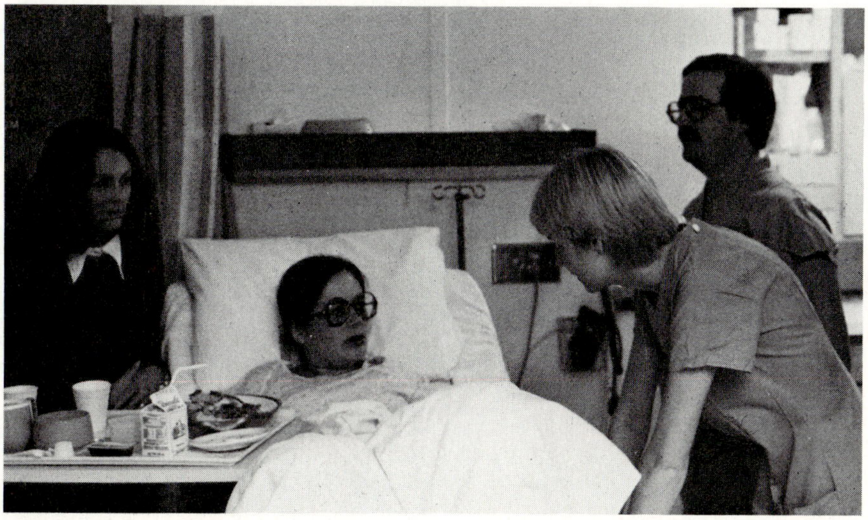

Fig. 23.4
Nurse is validating her suspicions that mother is uncomfortable. Mother indicated that she was uncomfortable. Nurse responded by repositioning her in bed to ease pressure on episiotomy and hemorrhoid sites and administered an analgesic. An ice pack had been in place over episiotomy site and was refilled, recovered, and replaced at this time. Woman's bladder had been assessed as empty. (Courtesy Stanford University Medical Center, Stanford, Calif.)

sedating effect of these analgesics necessitates such protective care as raising side rails, placing call bell within reach, and cautioning about remaining in bed. The woman must be warned about the ''head-spinning'' effect of the medications.

Maintain fluid balance and meet nutritional needs. Because of the restrictions on fluid intake and the loss of fluids (blood, perspiration, or emesis) during labor, many women are thirsty and request fluids soon after giving birth. If fluids are ordered, the nurse may offer any clear fluids in moderate amounts and should instruct the mother to drink slowly (Fig. 23.5). Excessive fluids or drinking too quickly often precipitates bouts of nausea and vomiting. After the first hour, the nurse may offer the mother a light diet. The nurse records the type of fluids and foods taken, the time, the amount, and the mother's tolerance of the fluids or foods ingested. The physician may order continued parenteral fluids at a ''keep open'' rate in the event of hemorrhage or need for intravenous medications.

Support parental emotional needs. It is acceptable for the nurse openly to share in the excitement and joy of birth. The nurse assists the parents by accepting any expressions of disappointment (about the child's sex or

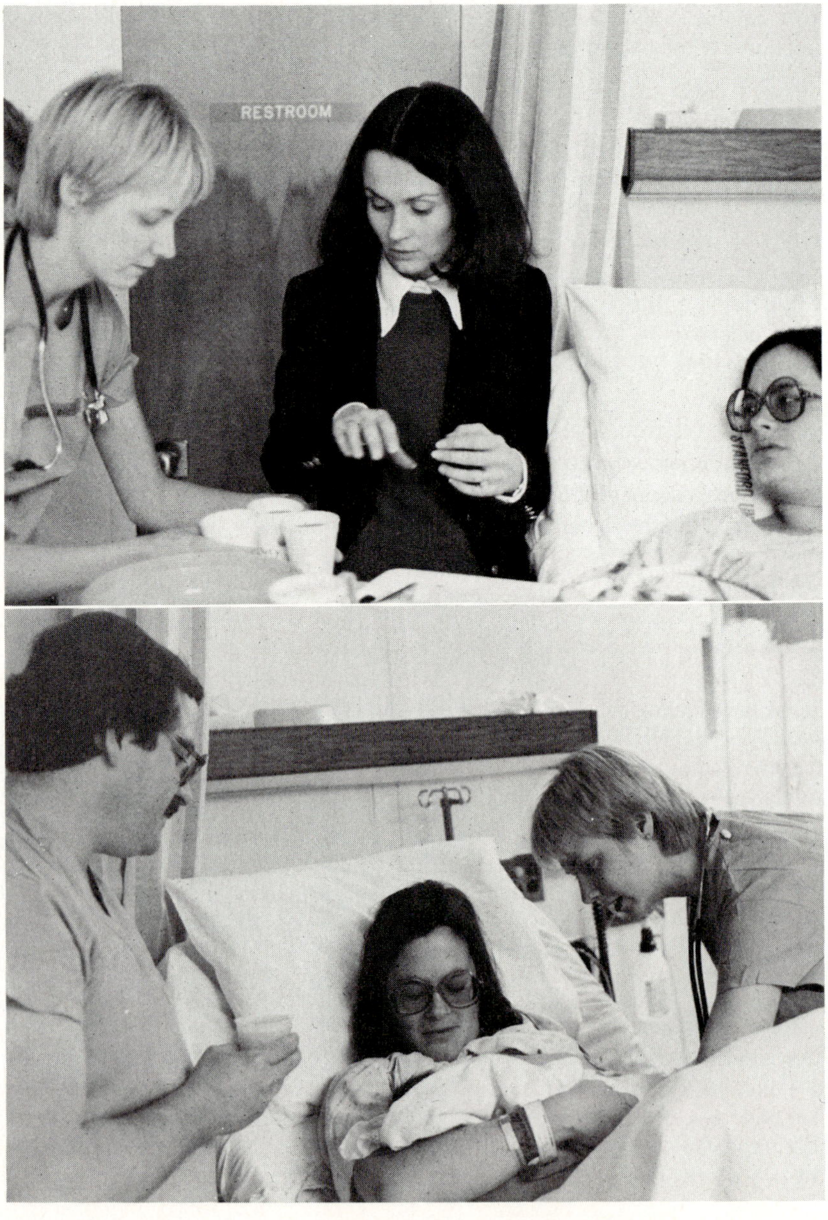

A

B

Fig. 23.5
A, Food and fluid are being offered to mother and fluids are brought to her family. **B,** Husband offered his wife orange juice while she breast fed their baby. Nurse is explaining newborn characteristics and technique of breast feeding. (Courtesy Stanford University Medical Center, Stanford, Calif.)

Fig. 23.6
Support from husband. (Courtesy Stanford University Medical Center, Stanford, Calif.)

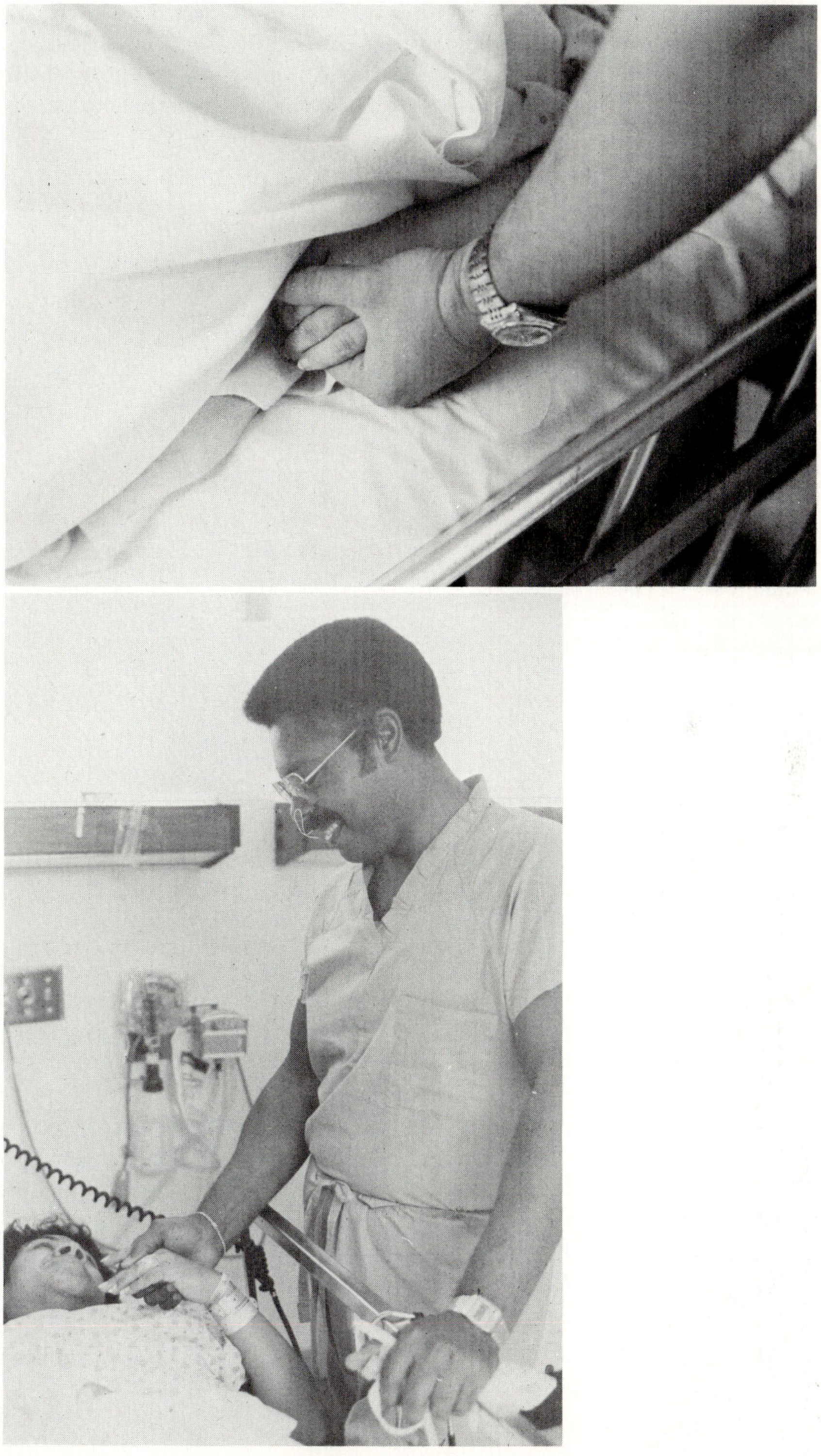

appearance) and reassures them that these feelings are within normal limits. The nurse may reassure the mother that her behavior during labor was acceptable if the mother appears worried about this.

Psychic states of new mothers range from euphoria, a feeling of well-being, to a sleepy state marked by an unawareness of surroundings. As noted earlier, first reactions of new mothers and fathers to their newborns vary widely. These reactions give the obstetric team cues to use in individualizing plans of care. Women who have experienced long, difficult labors or are in pain are frequently too exhausted to extend interest to the child. The nurse can offer to take the baby to the nursery until the mother is rested. After sufficient rest their attitudes can be surprisingly different. The child unwanted for diverse reasons may continue to be rejected or given only mild interest. The attitude of the husband is often reflected in the mother. His pleasure arouses a responsive pleasure (Fig. 23.6), or his disappointment arouses corresponding disappointment.

Fig. 23.7
A, A proud father's pensive moment with his son. **B,** Sharing the news and the joy. (Courtesy Stanford University Medical Center, Stanford, Calif.)

A

B

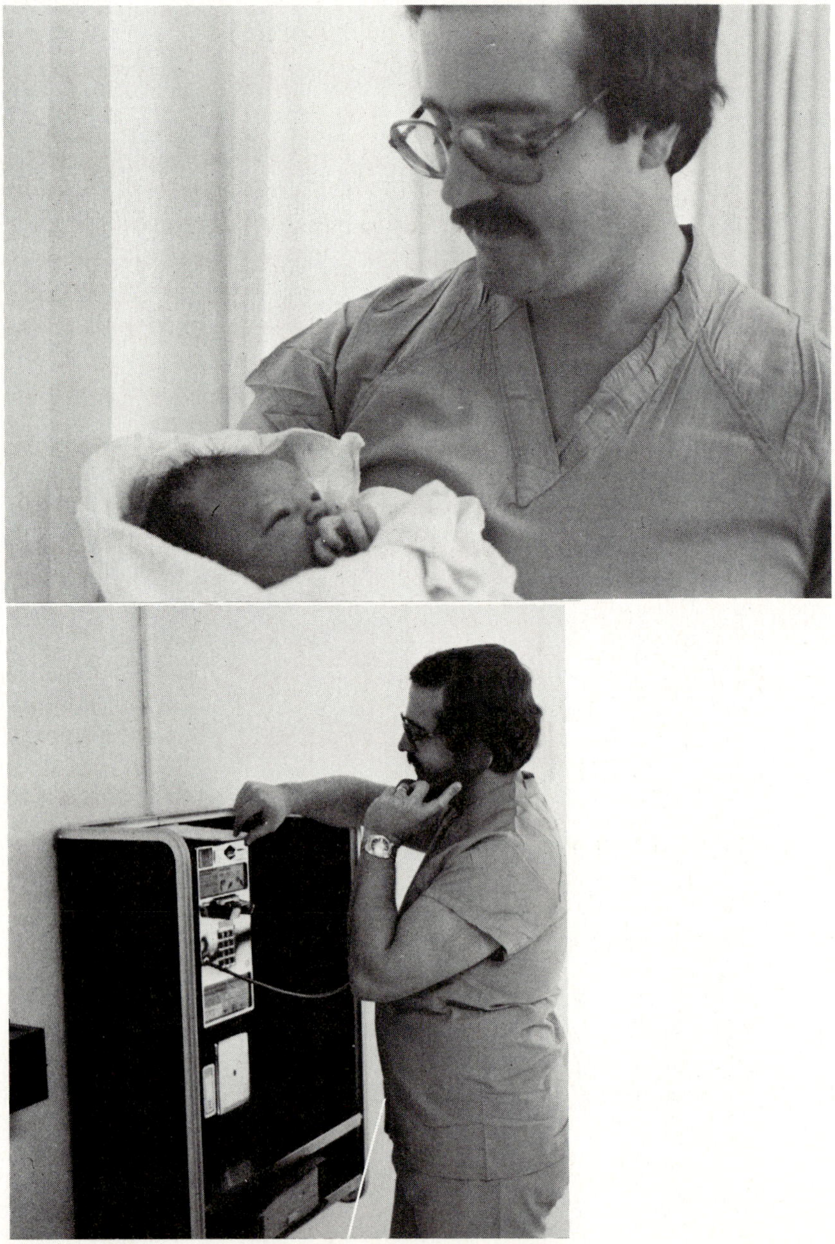

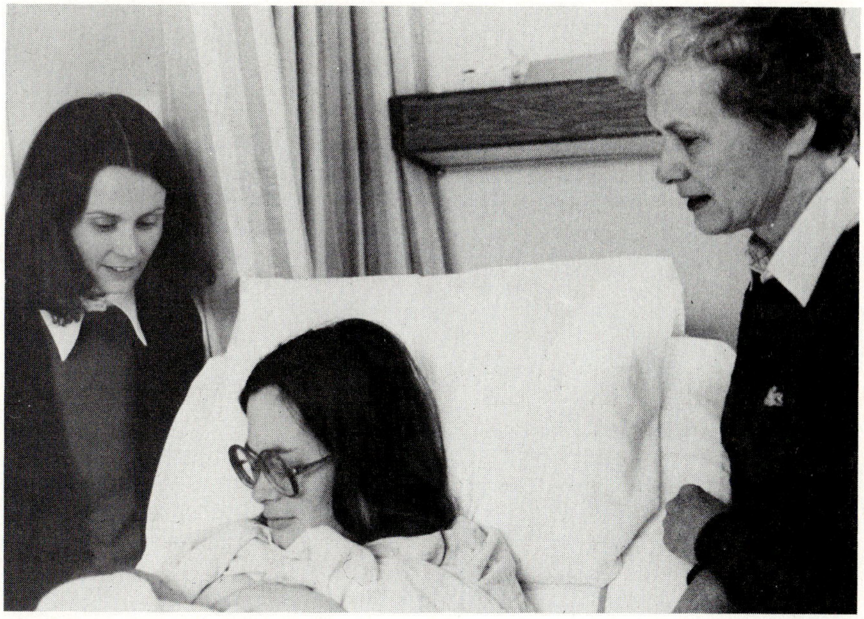

Fig. 23.8
Admiration and support from neonate's aunt and grandmother. Mother looks content as neonate suckles. (Courtesy Stanford University Medical Center, Stanford, Calif.)

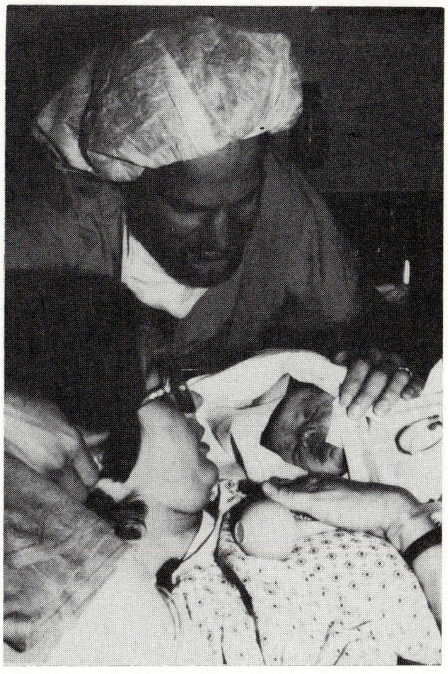

Fig. 23.9
Shared joy. Note neonate's head is well covered to prevent heat loss and bulb syringe is readily available.

Ethnic or cultural origins dictate behaviors that are deemed appropriate for special occasions. Some parents may not be able to express their delight openly; others wish to welcome the newcomer noisily.

The single mother may think that she is not expected to express joy or pleasure in her baby. The nurse can encourage the woman to express her feelings of pleasure. If the single mother does not wish to see or touch the child, the nurse, verbally and nonverbally, can indicate to the mother that her decision is acceptable.

Some mothers, particularly with their firstborn, are surprised and disturbed by the passivity or disinterest they experience on seeing their long-awaited infant. The nurse can reassure the mother of the normalcy of these feelings. The idealized mother love does not necessarily come into being right after delivery. The gradual growth of such love comes to some as they assume the care of and responsibility for their child.

The nurse can facilitate parent-child attachment or acquaintance by providing a warm, quiet, darkened environment (infant opens his eyes more readily when it is somewhat dark) and encouraging parents to hold the infant (Figs. 23.7 to 23.9) so that he is able to bring their faces into focus because he focuses best at about 20.3 cm (8 in). Body odor can be noticed (mothers have remarked that each child smells different), and the infant can be put to breast (Fig. 23.5, *B*).

Transfer of mother and neonate to postdelivery area. At the end of the second hour after delivery, the nurse

Fig. 23.10
Nurse charts assessments and care every 15 minutes. (Courtesy Stanford University Medical Center, Stanford Calif.)

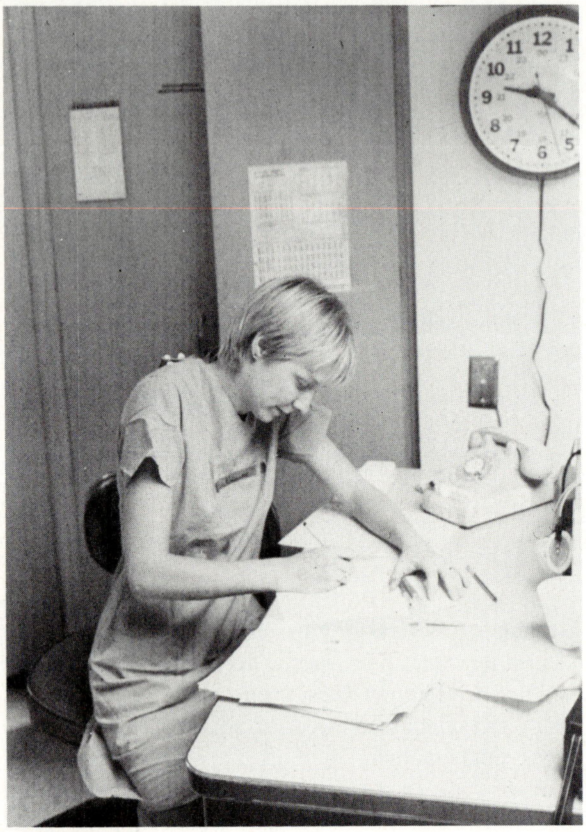

assesses the new mother thoroughly (Fig. 23.10), and if her physical state has stabilized, the mother has completed the fourth stage of labor. The mother is ready for transfer to the postdelivery area. The nurse checks the mother's record for completeness and prepares the record for transfer to the postdelivery area.

In the postpartum area, the delivery nurse assists the mother into bed and introduces her to the nurse on the postpartum unit and to other women who may be sharing her room. The delivery nurse gives a report to the postpartum nurse concerning any problems encountered in the prenatal period; the type of labor and delivery; state of fundus, amount of lochia, vital signs, and blood pressure; whether episiotomy was done; whether medication for pain had been given, what it was, dosage, and time of administration; condition and sex of infant; whether breast or bottle feeding of the infant is desired; whether she has voided; and intravenous fluids and foods that were given.

The neonate is transferred to the nursery (Fig. 23.11).

NEONATAL ADJUSTMENT TO EXTRAUTERINE EXISTENCE

The recovery of the neonate is discussed in detail in Chapter 22 and in Unit Five.

Fig. 23.11
Nurse accompanies father as he carries his son to nursery. Here father is beginning to uncover his son's head in preparation for placing him in covered bassinet. (Courtesy Stanford University Medical Center, Stanford, Calif.)

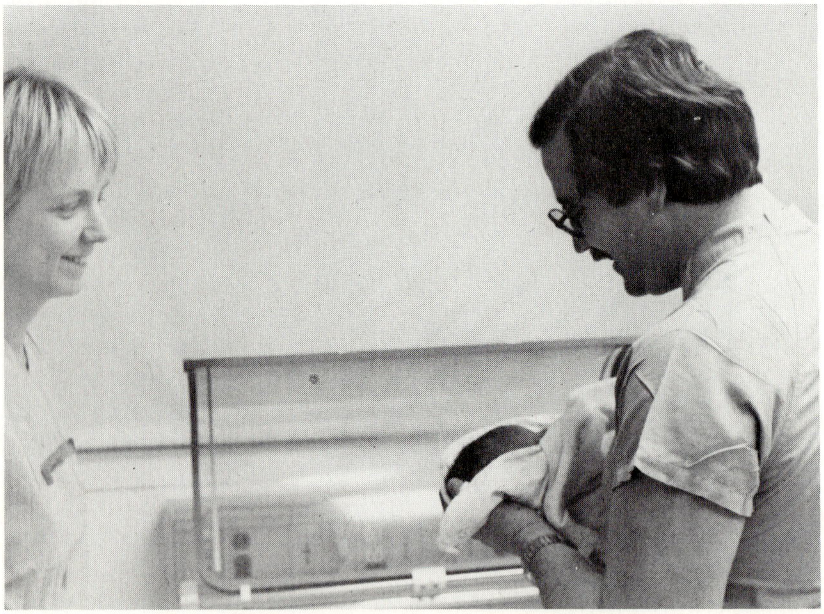

Evaluative Criteria for Care During Four Stages of Labor

The nurse assesses the nursing care given by comparing the clients' responses against a set of criteria. In Table 23.2, evaluation criteria for care during all stages of labor are outlined in detail. The table can also be used for a rapid review of the content presented in Chapters 21, 22, and 23.

• • •

One mother's experience of birth is shown in Fig. 23.12. Every mother has her own reaction to birth—some are bubbly and elated, others are quiet.

Table 23.2
Evaluation Criteria for Care During Labor

First Stage of Labor	Second Stage of Labor	Third and Fourth Stages of Labor
Parturient	**Parturient-mother**	**Mother**
Vital signs and blood pressure: remain within normal limits Temperature: does not increase beyond 37.2° C (99° F) as a result of dehydration and labor Pulse: same as during antepartum period Respirations: change with use of breathing techniques and pain Blood pressure: may be elevated during a contraction or with excitement	Vital signs and blood pressure: remain within normal limits Pulse: not usually assessed Respirations: altered by pushing; hyperventilation prevented Blood pressure: altered by pushing or anesthesia; hypertension or hypotension prevented Temperature: not assessed	Vital signs and blood pressure: remain within her normal range Pulse may be slow
Maternal progress in labor: within normal limits Time (duration): within normal limits for nullipara or multipara Cervix: 0-10 cm dilatation; 0-100% effacement Contractions Magnitude: from mild to moderate to strong to expulsive Rhythm: from irregular to regular Frequency: from 30 min to 2-3 min Duration: from 10-60 sec (few at 90 sec) Descent (station): from floating to +2 or +3 cm Show: from scant, brownish pink mucus to copious bloody mucus Membranes: rupture of membranes may occur at any time; amniotic fluid is pale straw colored; FHR remains stable; cord does not prolapse	Maternal progress through second stage: within normal limits Time (duration): within normal limits for nullipara or multipara Cervix: completely effaced and dilated; lacerations do not occur during birth Contractions: magnitude is expulsively powerful (50-75 mm Hg); frequency, 2-3 min; duration, 60 sec; rhythm, regular Descent: constant For nulliparas, it takes ½-1 hr for descent from station +1 to station +4; from station +4 cm to birth of infant, approximately 20 contractions needed For multiparas, it takes 10-30 min for descent from station 0 cm to station +4 cm; from station +4 cm to birth of infant, approximately 10 contractions needed Show: copious amounts of mixed blood and mucus Birth: no lacerations	Maternal progress through third and fourth stages of labor: within normal limits Placenta: delivered intact with membranes within 30 min (usually 3-5 min) Uterine muscles: contract sufficiently to limit loss of blood from placental site Bleeding from cervical tears: within normal limits or controlled by ligation of torn vessels After delivery, uterus remains firm, positioned in midline At birth: 2 cm below or at the umbilicus Two hr after delivery: at or slightly above umbilicus
Fluids/nutrients: Intravenous fluids may be started with Ringer's lactated solution and 5% dextrose and water; ice chips; in some hospitals, tea with lemon and sugar and hard sour candy suckers are given	Fluids/nutrients: intravenous flow rate maintained; lips may be moistened with cold wet washcloths but oral fluids are usually prohibited	Fluids/nutrients: taken as desired (in most cases); may be ravenously hungry; start with light meal at first (tea, toast)

Continued.

Table 23.2
Evaluation Criteria for Care During Labor—cont'd

First Stage of Labor	Second Stage of Labor	Third and Fourth Stages of Labor
Elimination: woman voids every 2 hr or oftener if bladder is palpable over symphysis pubis; bladder emptied before anesthesia	Elimination: bladder and urethra not traumatized by delivery; bladder catheterized if fullness is seen as interfering with descent or in danger of trauma	Elimination: voids sufficiently to prevent bladder distention
Maternal behavior: from excited (usually) and alert to introspective (concentrating on self and what is happening inside her); to perhaps irritable, vague in communication, amnesic between contractions; to appearance of circumoral pallor, perspiration on forehead and upper lip, shaking, feeling need to defecate	Maternal behavior and appearance: pain sensations decrease in early phases of second stage; urge to push controlled only by panting; woman eager to cooperate and give birth to infant and fretful and irritable if progress is not deemed fast enough; needs coaching to work with contractions and will experience amnesia between contractions; fatigue becomes apparent, especially in nulliparas; woman can follow simple, clear directions; will often comment with surprise at sensation of birth	Maternal behavior and appearance: within normal limits Initial excitement replaced with drowsy satisfaction Desire to rest not curtailed because of discomfort from pain, thirst, or hunger or emotional upset
Fetus	**Fetus**	
Fetal response throughout first stage indicates continued well-being; FHR as follows: Rate: between 120-160 beats/min; auscultated between contractions Normal base-line variability No abnormal variability	Well-being continues FHR: within normal pattern No evidence of meconium staining of amniotic fluid (in vertex presentations)	
	Neonate	**Neonate**
	Neonate in good health Apgar rating of 7-10 (at birth); respirations present; color dusky to pink; muscle tone good; if neonate is crying, crying is strong; reflexes present; no obvious malformations Cord clamped and cut after pulsations cease and respirations are established; no obvious malformations noted Gestational age characteristics are appropriate for EDC	Physical health is satisfactory as measured by following: Apgar score: 7-10 (at 5 min) Respirations: established within 30-60 sec Temperature: 37° C (98.6° F) Data base established through physical examination and assessment for gestational age; by end of 2 hr after birth, baby is weighed, length and suboccipital bregmatic diameter measured, eye prophylaxis completed Infant identified Infant alert with eyes open during first 30-60 min, followed by sleep; during alert period when sucking reflex is vigorous, may be put to breast Bonding process between infant and parents facilitated
	Maternal behavior and appearance	
	Immediate maternal response to infant within normal limits (e.g., open expression of concern for infant's health, joy or disappointment tempered by her physical state and amount of pain or fatigue experienced); reactions vary from euphoria to sleepy exhaustion, with lack of awareness of surroundings	
Family	**Family**	**Family**
Mate or support person participates in supporting relaxation and in providing comfort measures; partner meets self and parturient's expectations	Parent(s) have opportunity to begin attachment to (or acquaintance with) their neonate	Initial mother (father)-child interactions enough to satisfy need to touch, hold, and examine infant; to reassure as to normalcy of infant's appearance and behavior; to provide eye contact with infant (if possible); and to initiate breast feeding of infant (if desired)
Recording	**Recording**	**Recording**
Completed concurrently with care; preparation for delivery completed	Completed concurrently with care given	Completed concurrently with care given

Fig. 23.12

A, Mother in labor room. **B.** Infant handed to mother.

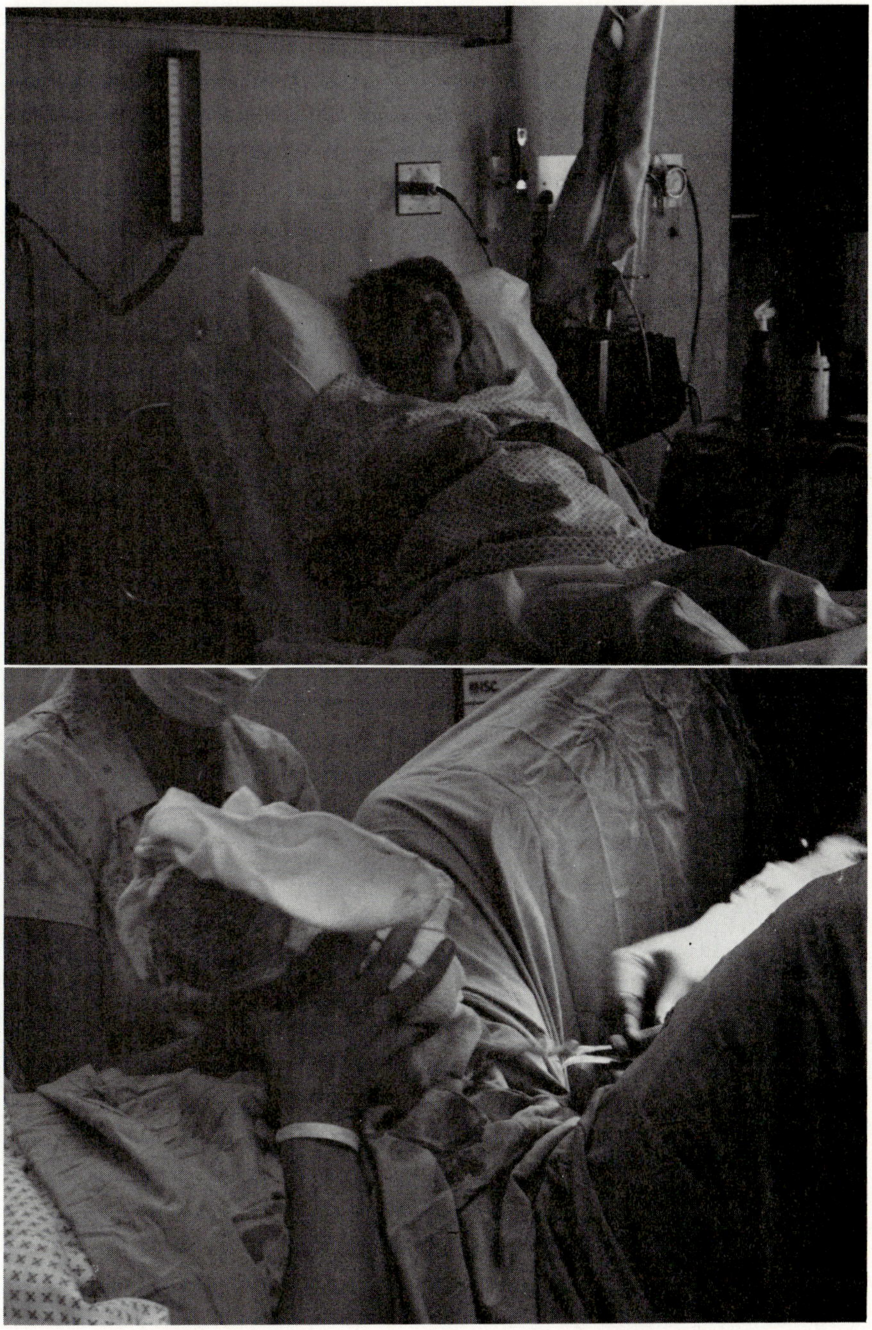

A

B

Continued.

Fig. 23.12, cont'd
C, Mother cutting cord. **D,** Fourth stage: weary—labor completed.

C

D

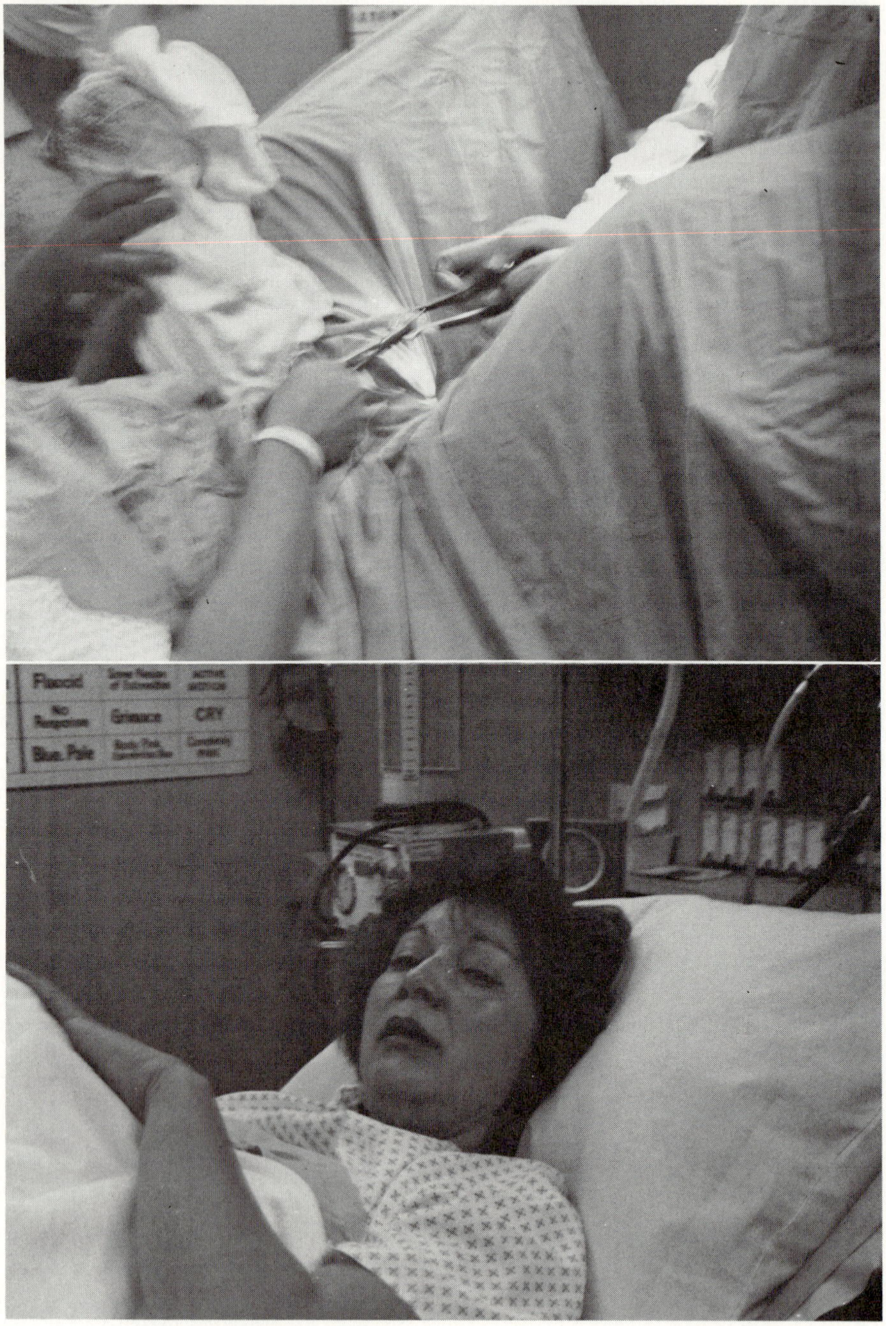

References and Readings

Benson, R.C., editor: Current obstetric and gynecologic diagnosis and treatment, ed. 4, Los Altos, Calif., 1982, Lange Medical Publications.

Caldeyro-Barcia, R.: Report given at ICEA International Convention, Kansas City, Mo., June 1978.

Danforth, D.: Obstetrics and gynecology, ed. 4, Philadelphia, 1982, Harper & Row, Publishers.

International Childbirth Education Association: Focusing on today's issues in perinatal care. Maternal position during labor and birth, ICEA Review **2:**3, Summer 1978.

Natelovitz, M.: Commentary, ICEA Review **2:**3, Summer 1979.

Towler, J., and Butler-Manuel, R.: Modern obstetrics for student midwives, Chicago, 1973, Lloyd-Luke Publication.

Varney, H.: Nurse-midwifery, Boston, 1980, Blackwell Scientific Publications, Inc.

Zuspan, F., and Quilligan, E., editors: Practical manual of obstetric care, St. Louis, 1982, The C.V. Mosby Co.

24
Fetal Monitoring

- History
- Objectives
- Physiologic Basis of Monitoring
  - Uteroplacental and fetal circulation
    - Factors affecting circulation
  - Fetal heart rate regulation
- Instrumentation for Monitoring
  - External mode of monitoring
    - Fetal heart rate
    - Uterine activity: tocotransducer
  - Internal mode of monitoring
    - Fetal heart rate: spiral electrode
    - Uterine activity: intrauterine catheter
- Pattern Recognition
  - Display of fetal heart rate and uterine activity on chart paper
  - Base-line fetal heart rate
    - Tachycardia and bradycardia
    - Variability
  - Periodic changes
    - Prolonged decelerations
  - Uterine activity monitoring
    - Increased uterine activity
  - Fetal distress
    - Fetal blood sampling
- Nursing Care
  - Prepared childbirth
  - Monitor care
  - Charting
  - Legal aspects
- Antepartum Testing
  - Nonstress testing/fetal activity determination
  - Oxytocin challenge test
  - Daily fetal movement count

History

It was not until the seventeenth century that the first fetal heart tones were heard or described. Periodically during the next 200 years, physicians would describe fetal heart tones and uterine souffle in medical journals. Then in 1917, David Hillis, an obstetrician at Chicago Lying-In-Hospital, reported on a head stethoscope or fetoscope as is used today. In 1922, J.B. DeLee, the chief of staff at the same institution, published a report regarding a similar instrument. A controversy developed, as DeLee claimed to have had the idea before Hillis's report. The instrument eventually became known as the DeLee-Hillis stethoscope and has remained essentially unchanged in design and use.

In 1958 Edward Hon of the Yale University School of Medicine published a report on continuous fetal electrocardiographic (ECG) monitoring from the maternal abdomen. Obstetricians Caldeyro-Barcia of Uruguay in 1966 and Hammacher in Germany in 1967 reported their observations of fetal heart rate (FHR) patterns associated with fetal distress. In 1968 Ralph Benson, M.D., and co-workers reported results of the collaborative study that had been commissioned by the National Institute of Neurologic Diseases and Blindness. Some 24,863 deliveries were evaluated, and it was demonstrated that there was no correlation between the FHR as determined with fetoscope and neonatal condition, except in the most extreme circumstances. This was almost always fetal bradycardia auscultated before death. Hon had reported 10 years earlier the unreliability of counting FHR when he asked 15 obstetricians to count several rates from a tape recording of the fetal heart and found a wide divergence in counting.

As investigators throughout the world made similar observations of FHR decelerations and fluctuations from base line, a confusing array of terminology developed. At an international conference on FHR monitoring in December of 1971 in New Jersey and later in March, 1972, in Amsterdam, Hon and Caldeyro-Barcia and their colleagues developed standard nomenclature for FHR monitoring. However, agreement on paper

Fig. 24.1

A, Leffscope. **B,** DeLee-Hillis scope. **C,** Ultrasound fetoscope; amplifies sound to those in immediate area. **D,** Ultrasound stethoscope; amplifies mechanical movement of fetal heart to listener by means of ear pieces. (From Ingalls, A.J., and Salerno, M.C.: Maternal and child health nursing, ed. 5, St. Louis, 1983, The C.V. Mosby Co.)

A

B

C

D

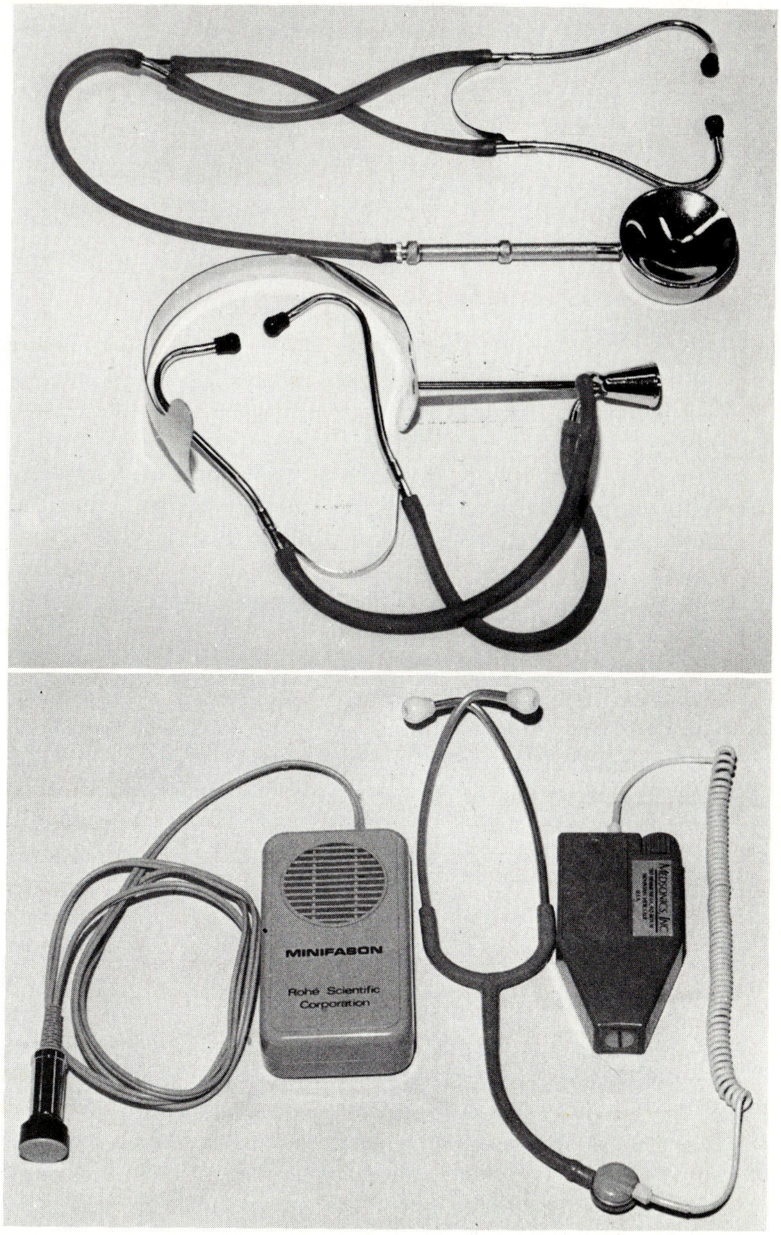

Fig. 24.2

Corometrics fetal monitor. (Courtesy Corometrics Medical Systems, Inc., Wallingford, Conn. From Tucker, S.M.: Fetal monitoring and fetal assessment in high-risk pregnancy, St. Louis, 1978, The C.V. Mosby Co.)

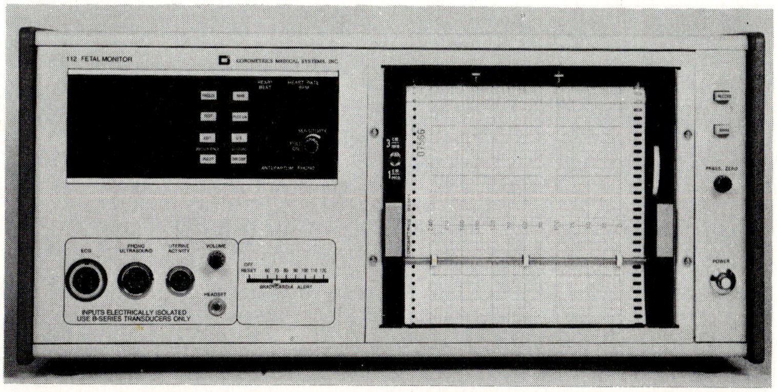

speed and universal scales was not reached and remains somewhat variable.

Since the first generation of commercially available fetal monitors in the late 1960s, technologic advances have improved the quality and accuracy of the tracing. There is currently a proliferation of monitors on the market with variations in capabilities; however, the basic components are the same.

Objectives

Electronic fetal monitoring of high-risk gravidas has become routine. Practice varies with continuous monitoring of low-risk pregnant women. Because early informed judgments can be critical in the assessment of FHR patterns and intervention for fetal distress, the nurse must have a working knowledge of the following factors:

1. Physiologic processes of the maternal-fetal-placental unit
2. Use of the fetal monitor
3. Interpretation of FHR patterns
4. Intervention for fetal distress
5. Clinical implications of antepartum testing
6. Application of the nursing process in caring for the obstetric client
7. Legal aspects related to fetal monitoring

Physiologic Basis of Monitoring

FHR monitoring provides reliable and predictive information about the condition of the fetus as it relates to oxygenation. Characteristic FHR patterns are demonstrated as the result of hypoxic and nonhypoxic stresses to the uterofetoplacental unit. Therefore it is important for the nurse to have a basic understanding of the factors involved in fetal oxygenation including uteroplacental and fetal circulation and physiology of FHR regulation.

UTEROPLACENTAL AND FETAL CIRCULATION

The placenta serves as a liaison between the fetal and maternal circulations. Uterine spinal arterioles must pass through the full thickness of the myometrium to reach the intervillous space. The maternal blood spurts through these arterioles into the intervillous space. Oxygen, nutrients, and inherent warmth are absorbed by the thin-walled fetal capillaries contained within the chorionic villus of the placenta. These are eventually carried to the fetus via the umbilical vein.

Carbon dioxide and fetal waste products circulate back to the placenta through the umbilical arteries and fetal capillaries (contained within the chorionic villi) where they cross back through the intervillous space to the maternal circulation (see p. 213).

Factors affecting circulation. Uterofetoplacental circulation can be affected by many factors, which include maternal position, exercise, uterine contractions, surface area of the placenta, hypertension, and umbilical cord flow.

Maternal position markedly affects circulation to the fetus. In the supine position, the gravid uterus compresses the vena cava thereby decreasing the return of blood to the heart. As maternal cardiac output decreases, hypotension develops, causing a reduction in uterine blood flow. This mechanism is referred to as supine hypotension or vena cava syndrome. An increase in circulation is produced when the mother is at rest in the lateral position.

Maternal exercise may decrease uterine blood flow by diverting blood to the major muscle groups. Diversion of blood in gravidas with normal uteroplacental function probably does not exceed uteroplacental reserve. However, rest may be important in women with decreased uteroplacental respiratory reserve, such as those women with high-risk conditions resulting in uteroplacental insufficiency.

Uterine contractions tend to decrease circulation through the spinal arteries and subsequent perfusion through the intervillous space. This stress seems to be well within the ability of the fetus to compensate for in most gestations. However, a normal fetoplacental unit may have its reserve exceeded by uterine hypertonus or tetanic contractions, as are often produced by oxytocin stimulation and abruptio placentae. In pregnancies in which the margin of fetal reserve is abnormally low, a decrease in perfusion because of contractions can result in fetal distress.

Any reduction in the maternal surface area of the placenta has the potential of producing uteroplacental insufficiency and fetal hypoxemia. Reduced placental area is associated with maternal hypertension, diabetic vascular disease, abruptio placentae, placenta previa, placental infarctions, and fetal growth retardation.

Hypertension affects uteroplacental circulation by decreasing blood flow through the intervillous space. This is caused by vasoconstriction and spasm or by chronic atherosclerotic changes in the uterine arterial blood supply.

Umbilical cord flow can be disrupted by compression as the fetus moves. Uterine contractions can cause intermittent cord occlusion, especially if the cord is trapped between the presenting part and the maternal pelvis or when it is around the fetus's neck (nuchal cord) or other body part. Generally, evidence of umbilical cord occlusion is not observed when there is a sufficient amount of amniotic fluid present.

Several factors then can interfere with optimal uteroplacental and fetal circulation. The nurse's role is to prevent those that are preventable, such as supine hypotension syndrome, and to promote maximal circulation when possible, including positioning the mother in the lateral position.

FETAL HEART RATE REGULATION

The FHR is regulated by several factors, some of which include baroreceptors, chemoreceptors, hormones, blood volume, electrolytes, and the sympathetic and parasympathetic divisions of the autonomic nervous system. Stimulation of the sympathetic division produces an increase in FHR. Conversely, stimulation of the parasympathetic division produces a vagal response and decreases the heart rate. It is the interaction of these divisions of the autonomic nervous system that produces variability of the FHR, which is characterized by uneven intervals between successive heart beats.

The average FHR at term is 140 beats/min with the normal range from 120 to 160 beats/min. Earlier in gestation, the FHR is higher with an average of approximately 160 beats/min at 20 weeks' gestation. The rate progressively decreases as the maturing fetus reaches term.

Instrumentation for Monitoring

There are two modes of electronic monitoring. The external mode employs the use of external transducers placed on the maternal abdomen to assess heart rate and uterine activity. The internal mode uses a spiral electrode applied to the fetal presenting part to assess the fetal electrocardiogram and the intrauterine catheter to assess uterine activity and pressure. A brief description contrasting the external and internal modes of monitoring is provided in Table 24.1. A detailed explanation of application and use follows.

Each of the modes of monitoring in the table is described in detail in terms of application, use, nursing care, and removal of the device. The external mode of monitoring FHR will be described first followed by external assessment of uterine activity as obtained with the tocodynamometer, or tocotransducer. This will be followed by a description of the internal mode of monitoring, which includes the spiral electrode and intrauterine catheter. An outline sequential format is provided to assist the reader in a step-by-step approach.

EXTERNAL MODE OF MONITORING

Fetal heart rate

Ultrasound transducer

1. Explain the procedure to the woman (and her family).
2. Gather necessary equipment: fetal monitor, ultra-

Table 24.1
External and Internal Modes of Monitoring

	External Mode	Internal Mode
Fetal heart rate	Ultrasound transducer: High-frequency sound waves reflect mechanical action of the fetal heart (easiest and most reliable external method to use during the antepartum and intrapartum periods). Phonotransducer: Microphone amplifies sound, reflects excessive noise when woman is in labor. It is used infrequently for antepartum monitoring. Abdominal electrodes: Fetal ECG is obtained when electrodes are properly positioned. It is used infrequently for antepartum monitoring because of ease and reliability of ultrasound transducer.	Spiral electrode: Electrode converts fetal ECG as obtained from the presenting part to FHR via a cardiotachometer. This method can only be used when membranes are ruptured and cervix sufficiently dilated during the intrapartum period. Electrode penetrates fetal presenting part 1.5 mm and must be on securely to ensure a good signal.
Uterine activity	Tocotransducer: This instrument monitors frequency and duration of contractions by means of a pressure-sensing device applied to the maternal abdomen. It can be used during both the antepartum and intrapartum periods.	Intrauterine catheter: This instrument monitors frequency, duration, and *intensity* of contractions. Catheter is filled with sterile water, which is compressed during contractions placing pressure on a strain gauge converting the pressure into mm Hg on the uterine activity panel of the strip chart. It can be used when membranes are ruptured and cervix sufficiently dilated during the intrapartum period.

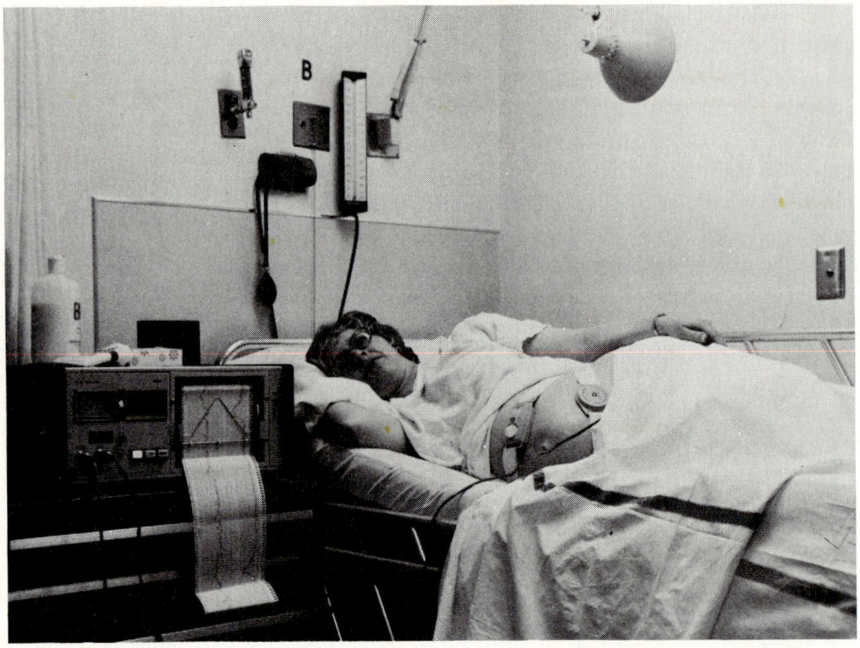

Fig. 24.3
External mode of monitoring with woman in side-lying position. (From Tucker, S.M.: Fetal monitoring and fetal assessment in high-risk pregnancy, St. Louis, 1978, The C.V. Mosby Co.)

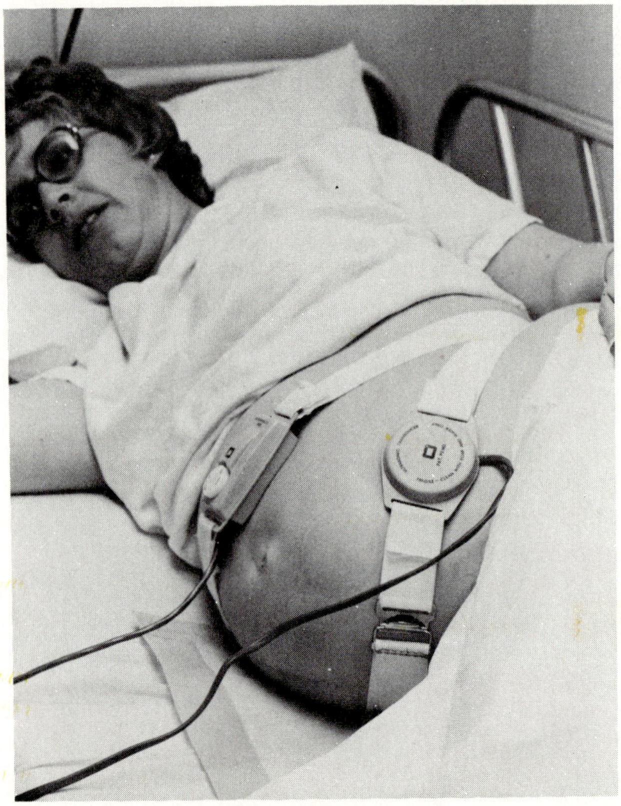

Fig. 24.4
Placement of external transducers. Tocotransducer is above umbilicus with ultrasound transducer below umbilicus. (From Tucker, S.M.: Fetal monitoring and fetal assessment in high-risk pregnancy, St. Louis, 1978, The C.V. Mosby Co.)

Fig. 24.5
Diagrammatic representation of external mode of monitoring with tocotransducer and ultrasound transducer.

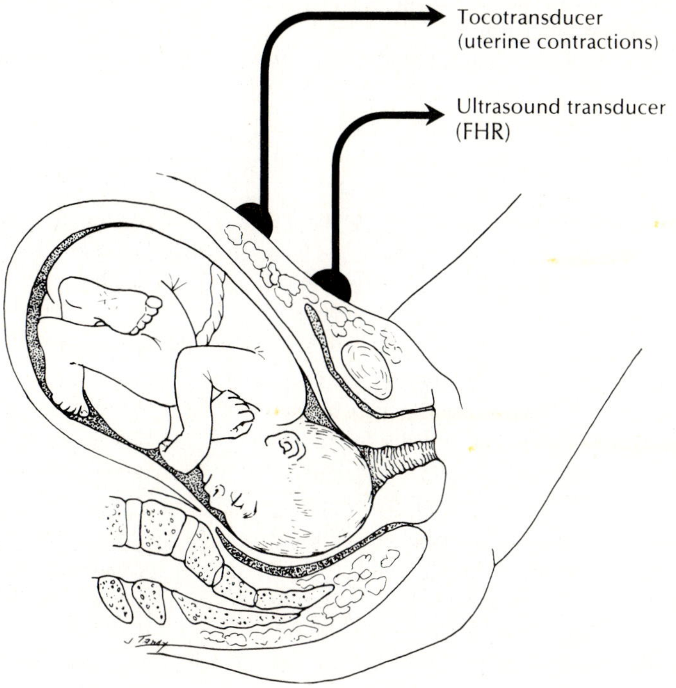

sound transducer, and either tocotransducer or intrauterine catheter apparatuses to assess uterine activity, ultrasonic coupling gel, and abdominal belt.

3. Position the abdominal belt around the woman and place her in a semilateral position of comfort.
4. Insert the ultrasound transducer plug into the appropriate monitor connector labeled "ultrasound" or "cardio."
5. Turn the power on and gently touch the ultrasound diaphragm to elicit an equal audio response.
6. Select the nondirectional Doppler mode initially if the monitor has that option.
7. Apply ultrasound coupling gel to the underside of the transducer to be placed on the maternal abdomen.
8. Place the transducer on the abdomen below the level of the umbilicus in a full-term pregnancy of cephalic presentation or above the level of the umbilicus in a full-term pregnancy of breech presentation (Fig. 20.24).
9. Turn the audio/volume control knob while moving the transducer over the abdomen to obtain the strongest fetal signal.
10. Select the directional Doppler mode if the monitor has that option. The directional Doppler more closely approximates short-term variability and is thus preferred to conventional Doppler. Monitors with autocorrelation are the most accurate in demonstrating both long- and short-term variability.
11. Secure the ultrasound transducer with the abdominal belt.
12. Observe the indicator light, which will flash simultaneously with each fetal signal, and observe the oscilloscope for a consistent wave form, which ensures correct placement of the transducer.
13. If the monitor has both edit and unedit capabilities, select the edit button in order to ensure an interpretable tracing. Some monitors "edit" automatically during external monitoring. Editing reduces artifact and jitter obtained during external monitoring by providing an averaging mechanism, which makes the tracing clearer.
14. Turn the recorder on at 3 cm/min paper speed and observe the FHR on the strip chart. **Obtain the base-line FHR *between* contractions or periodic changes.**
15. Depress the test button for 10 seconds and make a notation of this on the tracing. The monitor will print out a predetermined number, usually

120 or 150 beats/min on the corresponding line of the chart paper according to guidelines in the manufacturer's operating manual.

16. Periodically clean the transducer and maternal abdomen with a damp cloth to remove dried gel. Reapply ultrasonic coupling gel and use talcum powder to dust under the abdominal belt to keep the skin dry and promote the woman's comfort.
17. Reposition the transducer whenever the fetal signal becomes unclear, such as when the mother moves or the fetus descends in the pelvis. It is important to ensure a clear interpretable tracing during fetal monitoring.
18. When removing the ultrasound transducer, exercise caution that it is not dropped or allowed to swing against any equipment in order to protect the ultrasound crystals. Clean the transducer according to the procedure of the facility or follow the directions in the manufacturer's operating manual.
19. Loosely coil the cable and secure this with a rubber band or place loosely coiled in a secure area. This is to prevent damage to the wires, as can occur with tight coiling, resulting in a loss of or inadequate fetal signal.
20. Dispose of disposable abdominal belt, if used. If a reusable belt is used, it should be washed according to the facility's procedure before the next woman's use.

Phonotransducer

1. Explain the procedure to the woman (and her family).
2. Gather necessary equipment: fetal monitor, phonotransducer, tocotransducer to assess uterine activity, and an abdominal belt.
3. Position the abdominal belt around the woman and place her in a semilateral position of comfort.
4. Insert the phonotransducer plug into the appropriate monitor connector labeled "phono" or "cardio."
5. Turn the power on and gently touch the phonotransducer to elicit a good audio response.
6. Place the phonotransducer on the clean and dry maternal abdomen. (Do not apply any type of gel or paste, as this will impede the amplified sounds.) Previous auscultation of the FHR with a fetoscope or stethoscope will help to more quickly identify an optimal location for the phonotransducer.
7. Turn the audio/volume control knob while holding the phonotransducer on the abdomen to ensure that the strongest fetal signal has been obtained.
8. Secure the phonotransducer with the abdominal belt. If there is too much extraneous noise because of movement of the belt, tape the phonotransducer to the maternal abdomen.
9. Avoid amplification of unwanted sounds, such as bed sheets, by positioning these so as not to come in contact with the phono. Request the woman's cooperation to avoid unnecessary movement in order to ensure a clear, interpretable tracing.
10. Observe the indicator light, which will flash simultaneously with each fetal signal and observe the oscilloscope for a consistent wave form, which ensures correct placement of the transducer.
11. If the monitor has both edit and unedit capabilities, select the edit button in order to ensure an interpretable tracing. Some monitors "edit" automatically during external monitoring. Editing reduces the artifact and jitter obtained during external monitoring by providing an averaging mechanism, which is able to make the tracing clearer.
12. Turn the recorder on at the 3 cm/min paper speed and observe the FHR on the strip chart. Obtain the base-line FHR between contractions or periodic changes.
13. Depress the test button for 10 seconds and make a notation of this on the tracing. The monitor will print out a predetermined number, usually 120 or 150 beats/min on the corresponding line of the chart paper according to guidelines in the manufacturer's operating manual.
14. Reposition the transducer whenever the fetal signal becomes unclear. Allow a few seconds for the sound to stabilize before moving the transducer to another area.
15. Periodically massage any reddened skin areas caused by pressure of the belt or transducer. Use talcum powder to dust under the abdominal belt to keep the skin dry and promote the woman's comfort.
16. When removing the phonotransducer, exercise caution that it is not dropped. Clean the transducer according to the procedure of the facility or follow the directions in the manufacturer's operating manual.
17. Loosely coil the cable and secure this with a rubber band or place loosely coiled in a secure area. This is to prevent damage to the wires, as can occur with tight coiling, resulting in a loss of or inadequate amplification of sound.
18. Dispose of disposable abdominal belt, if used. If a reusable belt is used, it should be washed according to the facility's procedure before the next woman's use.

Abdominal ECG

1. Explain the procedure to the woman (and her family).
2. Gather necessary equipment: fetal monitor abdominal electrodes, tocotransducer or intrauterine catheter to assess uterine activity, electrode paste, and cable.
3. Identify the fetal head and buttocks by palpating the maternal abdomen using Leopold's maneuvers (see p. 382).
4. Select the electrode application sites according to the manufacturer's operating manual. Generally, one electrode will be positioned over the fetal head and one over the fetal buttocks. The third electrode is the reference and will be positioned below the umbilicus.
5. Prepare the skin sites with alcohol swabs by using a scrubbing motion. Then allow this to dry.
6. If a built-in cleaner pad is affixed to the electrode protective cover, use it to gently abrade the skin at the selected electrode sites.
7. Apply the two pregelled disposable electrodes: one to the maternal skin site over the fetal head and the other just under the umbilicus.
8. Squeeze a thin bead of electrode paste around the rim of the suction electrode.
9. Apply the suction electrode to the maternal skin site over the fetal buttocks. CAUTION: Do not leave a suction electrode in one location for more than 15 minutes—hematomas may result.
10. Attach the lead wires to the electrodes according to the manufacturer's operating manual. Generally, the lead wire with the white clip should be attached to the electrode over the fetal head. The lead wire with the green clip should be attached to the electrode over the fetal back (just below the maternal umbilicus). The lead wire with the black clip should be attached to the electrode over the fetal buttocks.
11. Insert the electrode cable plug into the appropriate monitor connector labeled "ECG" or "cardio."
12. Turn the power on and depress the edit button.
13. Observe the oscilloscope for a consistent ECG wave form.
14. Turn the recorder on at the 3 cm/min paper speed and observe the FHR on the strip chart.
15. If the recording is clear, replace the suction cup with a disposable electrode. Be sure to clean the electrode paste off the skin site and prepare the skin with alcohol, as described in steps 5 and 6.
16. If a good recording cannot be obtained, a search procedure must be done.
    a. Begin by moving the suction electrode over the fetal buttocks in a circular pattern from the original position to obtain the clearest fetal signal. Replace the suction electrode with a disposable electrode once the best location has been determined.
    b. If the signal continues to be unacceptable, replace the electrode over the fetal head with the suction electrode and move this in a circular pattern from the original position to obtain the clearest fetal signal. Replace the suction electrode with a disposable electrode after preparing the skin site once the best location has been determined.
    c. If the signal is still not acceptable, remove the reference electrode from below the maternal umbilicus and place it with the suction electrode on the gravida's right leg until maximal signal is obtained. If the signal has improved, replace the suction electrode with a disposable electrode after preparing the skin site.
    d. Should the signal continue to be unacceptable following repositioning of the three electrodes, another method of monitoring FHR should be used.
17. If the monitor has both edit and unedit capabilities, select the mode preferred by the physician.
18. If the monitor has the capability of displaying the maternal heart rate on the light-emitting diode (LED) and printing this out on the chart paper, it can be obtained by depressing the maternal heart rate (MHR) button for as long as the maternal heart rate is desired.
19. Observe the indicator light, which will flash simultaneously with each ECG complex and the oscilloscope, which will display both fetal and maternal ECGs to verify a clear signal source.
20. Depress the test button for 10 seconds and make a notation of this on the tracing. The monitor will print out a predetermined number, usually 120 or 150 beats/min, on the corresponding line of the chart paper according to guidelines in the manufacturer's operating manual.

It may be difficult or impossible to obtain an interpretable reading in the following situations: with maternal obesity, at gestational age less than 34 weeks because of a low-voltage fetal signal, and during periods of maternal muscle activity and tension, such as the active phase of labor.

Uterine activity: tocotransducer

1. Explain the procedure to the woman (and her family).
2. Gather the necessary equipment: fetal monitor, tocotransducer (tocodynamometer), and the equipment desired to monitor the FHR.
3. Position the abdominal belt around the woman's

upper abdomen, over the uterine fundus, and place her in a semilateral position of comfort.

4. Insert the tocotransducer plug into the appropriate monitor connector labeled "uterine activity,""toco," or "utero."
5. Place the transducer on the maternal abdomen over the fundus where there is the least amount of maternal tissue between the pressure-sensing button and the uterus.
6. Secure the tocotransducer with the abdominal belt.
7. Turn the power on.
8. Turn the recorder on at the 3 cm/min paper speed and observe the strip chart.
9. Adjust the pen-set knob between contractions to make the stylet print approximately at the 20 mm Hg line on the chart paper. This is done to prevent a grinding noise that occurs when the stylet drops below 0, as occurs with maternal movement and deep inspiration.
10. Test the tocotransducer by applying slight pressure and observe the strip chart for a relative inflection of momentary increase from the "base line."
11. Monitor the frequency and duration of the contractions and document this in the nurse's notes. The tocotransducer *cannot* measure intensity of contractions nor resting tone between contractions, since the depression of the pressure-sensing button varies with the amount of maternal adipose tissue. The information should, therefore, not be relied on to assess need for analgesia in relation to strength (painfulness) of contractions as registered by the machine.
12. When monitoring is in progress, readjust the abdominal strap hourly and massage any reddened skin areas. A small amount of powder can be applied under the belt to promote comfort.
13. Palpate the fundus every 15 to 30 minutes to assess intensity of uterine contractions, as described on p. 381.
14. Reposition the transducer periodically and secure the abdominal belt snugly to promote comfort and ensure a good recording.
15. When removing the tocotransducer, follow the cleaning procedure of the facility or follow the directions in the manufacturer's operating manual.
16. Loosely coil the cable and secure this with a rubber band or place loosely coiled in a secure area. This is to prevent damage to the wires, as can occur with tight coiling.
17. Dispose of disposable abdominal belt, if used. If a reusable belt is used, it should be washed according to the facility's procedure before the next woman's use.

INTERNAL MODE OF MONITORING

Fetal heart rate: spiral electrode. The spiral electrode monitors the fetal electrocardiogram (ECG) from the presenting part. It can only be applied after the

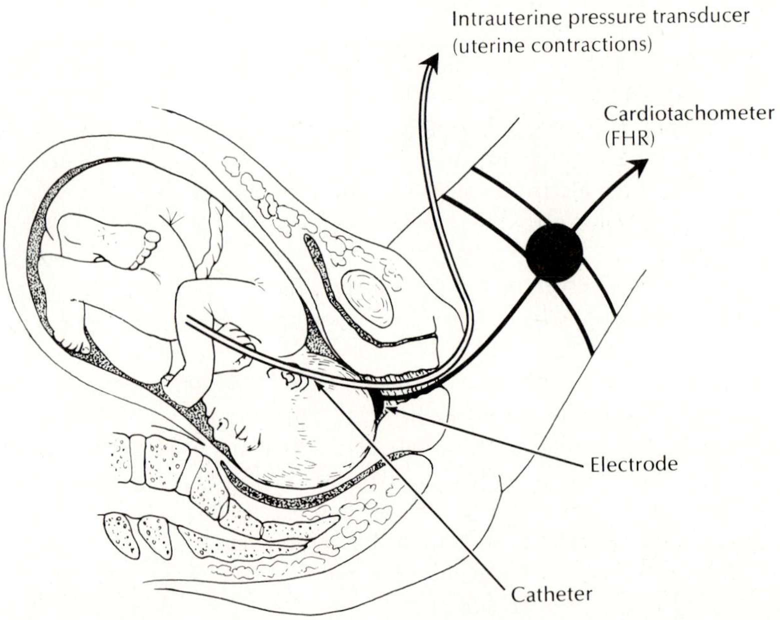

Fig. 24.6
Diagrammatic representation of internal mode of monitoring with intrauterine catheter and spiral electrode in place.

membranes are ruptured, when the cervix is 2 to 3 cm or more dilated, and when the presenting part is accessible and identifiable. Therefore the spiral electrode can be used only during the intrapartum period.

1. Explain the procedure to the woman (and her family).
2. Gather necessary equipment: fetal monitor, disposable spiral electrode, leg plate with cable, leg plate strap, and electrode paste.
3. Position the leg plate strap around the woman's thigh, securing the leg plate to the thigh. Gently lift the leg plate and apply electrode paste to the underside.
4. Insert the cable into the appropriate monitor connector labeled ''ECG'' or ''cardio.''
5. Assist the physician or nurse in performing a sterile vaginal examination in order to apply the spiral electrode. The electrode must be on se-

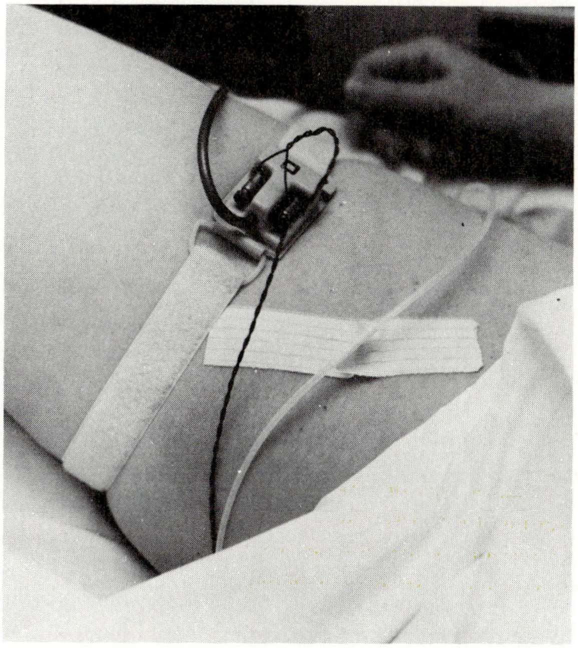

Fig. 24.7
Intrauterine catheter and electrode wires secured to thigh for internal mode of monitoring. (From Tucker, S.M.: Fetal monitoring and fetal assessment in high-risk pregnancy, St. Louis, 1978, The C.V. Mosby Co.)

Fig. 24.8
Spiral electrode. (Courtesy Corometrics Medical Systems, Inc., Wallingford, Conn.)

APPLICATION OF COROMETRICS® SPIRAL ELECTRODE*

WARNING: Because the tip of this electrode is designed to penetrate the fetal epidermis, the possibility of trauma, hemorrhage and infection exists. It should therefore be used only under aseptic conditions. Membranes must be ruptured prior to attachment of spiral electrode.

CONTRAINDICATIONS: The electrode should NOT be applied to the fetal face, fontanels or genitalia, or used when placenta previa is present or when it is not possible to identify the portion of the fetal body where application is contemplated.

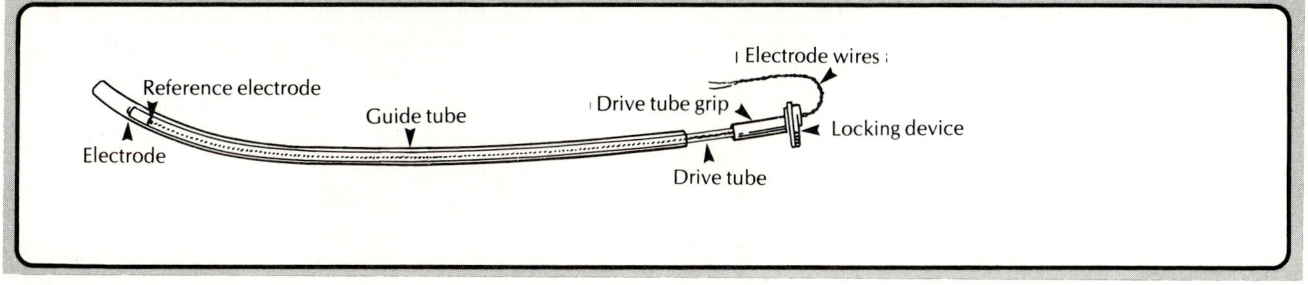

Fig. 24.9
Application of spiral electrode. (Courtesy Corometrics Medical Systems, Inc., Wallingford, Conn.)

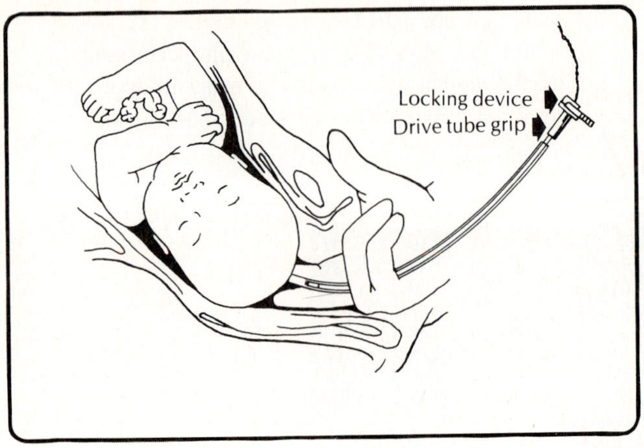

curely to assure a good signal. The fetal face, fontanels, and genitalia are avoided, and the electrode penetrates the skin of the presenting part 1.5 mm.

6. Attach the color-coded wires to the matching colored posts on the leg plate.
7. Turn the power on and observe the oscilloscope for the fetal ECG, allowing at least 15 seconds for the monitor to warm up.
8. Turn the recorder on at the 3 cm/min paper speed and observe the FHR on the strip chart.
9. Depress the test button for 10 seconds and make a notation of this on the strip chart. The monitor will print out a predetermined number, usually 120 or 150 beats/min, on the corresponding line of the chart paper according to the guidelines of the manufacturer's operating manual.
10. During monitoring, the leg plate is checked periodically and electrode paste is reapplied as needed to ensure transmission of the signal.
11. When removing the spiral electrode, turn one and one half turns counterclockwise, or until free from the fetal presenting part. *Do not* pull the electrode from the fetal skin. Disconnect the electrode from the leg plate.
12. Remove the leg strap and dispose of it, if disposable, or wash if reusable.
13. Clean the leg plate according to the procedure of the facility or follow the directions in the manufacturer's operating manual.
14. Loosely coil the cable and secure with a rubber band or place loosely coiled in a secure area. This is to prevent damage to the wires, as can occur with tight coiling, resulting in a loss of or an inadequate fetal signal.
15. Clean the fetal insertion site with a povidone-iodine swab unless otherwise directed by hospital policy or procedure.

Uterine activity: intrauterine catheter. The intrauterine catheter (Fig. 24.10) monitors contraction frequency, duration, intensity, and resting tone. A small fluid-filled plastic catheter is introduced vaginally by the physician or nurse into the uterus after the cervix is dilated 2 to 3 cm and the fetal membranes have been ruptured. The catheter is compressed during uterine contractions, moving the diaphragm of a strain gauge. The pressure is then reflected on the strip chart in the form of millimeters of mercury (mm Hg) pressure.

1. Explain the procedure to the woman (and her family).
2. Gather necessary equipment: fetal monitor, disposable intrauterine kit, strain gauge, injectable sterile distilled water, 18 gauge, 1½-in sterile needle, sterile gloves, and other equipment to perform a sterile vaginal examination.
3. Insert the cable from the strain gauge into the appropriate monitor connector labeled "uterine activity," "toco," or "utero." Adjust the height of the strain gauge until it is level with the middle of the uterus; this is about the same height as the maternal xiphoid process.
4. Assist the physician in performing a sterile vaginal examination in order to insert the intrauterine catheter. Before insertion fill the catheter with 5 ml sterile water, leaving the syringe attached to the catheter. Insertion is complete when the black mark on the catheter reaches the introitus.
5. Slide the catheter guide away from the introitus and remove it, or, after cleaning the guide, tape it securely over the top or across the side of the monitor.
6. Tape the catheter securely to the woman's leg.
7. Remove the syringe, maintaining sterility of the tip and connect the catheter to the male end of the three-way stopcock.
8. Rotate the stopcock lever so that the OFF arrow points *away from* the woman, opposite to the intrauterine catheter.
9. Connect the end of the stopcock opposite the catheter to the angle fitting of the strain gauge (Fig. 24.11).
10. Attach the sterile water-filled syringe to the female fitting of the stopcock perpendicular to the catheter.

Fig. 24.10
Insertion of intrauterine catheter. (Courtesy Corometrics Medical Systems, Inc., Wallingford, Conn.)

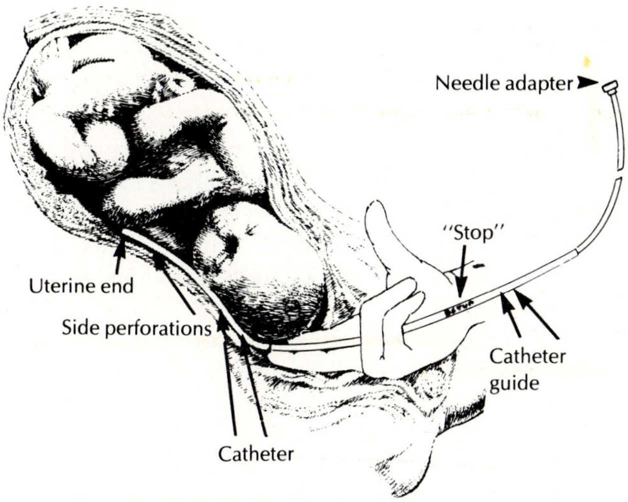

Fig. 24.11
Intrauterine catheter and syringe connected to stopcock and strain gauge in order to monitor intrauterine pressure. (Courtesy Corometrics Medical Systems, Inc. Wallingford, Conn.)

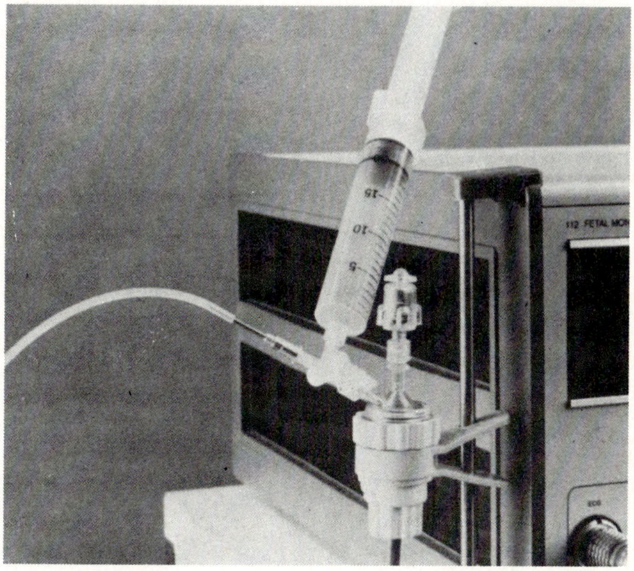

11. Maintaining the stopcock off to the strain gauge, flush the catheter with 5 ml sterile water.
12. Rotate the stopcock lever so that the OFF position points to the catheter.
13. Lift the pressure relief valve on top of the strain gauge dome and inject water from the syringe through the stopcock and dome until all air bubbles are removed.
14. Release the pressure relief valve and then remove the syringe from the stopcock maintaining its sterility. This opens the system to atmospheric pressure.
15. Turn the power on and press the record button.
16. Observe the stylus or pen, which should read on the zero line of the uterine activity section of the chart paper. Turn the pressure knob to ensure that the pen reads just as the zero line of the chart paper. (Do not turn it to go below zero.)
17. Depress the test button for 10 seconds and make a notation of this on the tracing. The monitor will print a predetermined number usually at the 50 mm Hg line of the chart paper, according to the manufacturer's operating manual. If it does not read 50, adjust the pressure knob to ensure that the pen points at the zero line of the chart paper and then test it again.
18. Reattach the syringe to the stopcock.
19. Rotate the stopcock lever so that the OFF position is pointing to the syringe. The uterine pressure system is now ready for monitoring.
20. During monitoring, flush the catheter with sterile water every 2 hours or as necessary.
21. The proper functioning of the catheter can be checked by gently tapping the catheter, asking the woman to cough, or applying fundal pressure and observing a simultaneous inflection on the chart paper.
22. Apply gentle traction when removing the catheter and dispose of it in an appropriate manner.*

Pattern Recognition

Many factors must be evaluated in order to determine if an FHR pattern is reassuring or nonreassuring. This includes an assessment and evaluation of base-line rate, variability, accelerations, and decelerations, as well as consideration of uterine contraction frequency and strength. These factors must be evaluated based on other obstetric information, including parity, maternal and obstetric complications, progress in labor, and an estimate of anticipated delivery time. Intervention and

*Every disposable item should be disposed of, never reused.

interruption of labor are therefore based on medical judgment of a complex, integrated process.

It is the responsibility of the labor and delivery room nurse to assess FHR patterns, perform independent nursing interventions, and report nonreassuring patterns to the physician. In order to assist the nurse with pattern recognition, the following have been discussed in separate sections: base-line FHR, periodic changes, uterine activity, and fetal distress.

DISPLAY OF FETAL HEART RATE AND UTERINE ACTIVITY ON CHART PAPER

The upper section of the chart paper is used to record the FHR by both the external and internal modes of monitoring. The vertical scale relates to FHR, which can be recorded between 30 and 240 beats/min. The horizontal scale is divided into 1-min sections, which are subdivided by six sections representing 10 seconds of time. The lower section is used to record uterine activity. The vertical scale relates to intrauterine pressure, which can be recorded from 0 to 100 mm Hg pressure and which can only be done with the intrauterine catheter/strain gauge. The student should carefully read the legend for Fig. 24.12.

BASE-LINE FETAL HEART RATE

Baseline FHR is that heart rate occurring at the following times:

1. When the woman is not in labor
2. Between uterine contractions
3. During the interval between periodic changes

FHRs are usually between 120 and 160 beats/min in the normal full-term fetus.

Tachycardia and bradycardia. Variations in base-line FHR include tachycardia, bradycardia, and variability (Table 24.2).

Variability. Variability is the normal irregularity of the cardiac rhythm, caused by a continuous balancing interaction of the sympathetic (cardioacceleration) and parasympathetic (cardiodeceleration) divisions of the autonomic nervous sytem. Good variability on the FHR panel is demonstrated by *cyclic fluctuations* and *beat-to-beat changes* of heart rate in the base line. Absence of these fluctuations and irregularities indicates central nervous system depression.

Fig. 24.12
Display of fetal heart rate and uterine activity on chart paper. **A,** External mode with ultrasound and tocotransducer as signal source. **B,** Internal mode with spiral electrode and intrauterine catheter as signal source. (From Tucker, S.M.: Fetal montoring and fetal assessment in high-risk pregnancy, St. Louis, 1978, The C.V. Mosby Co.)

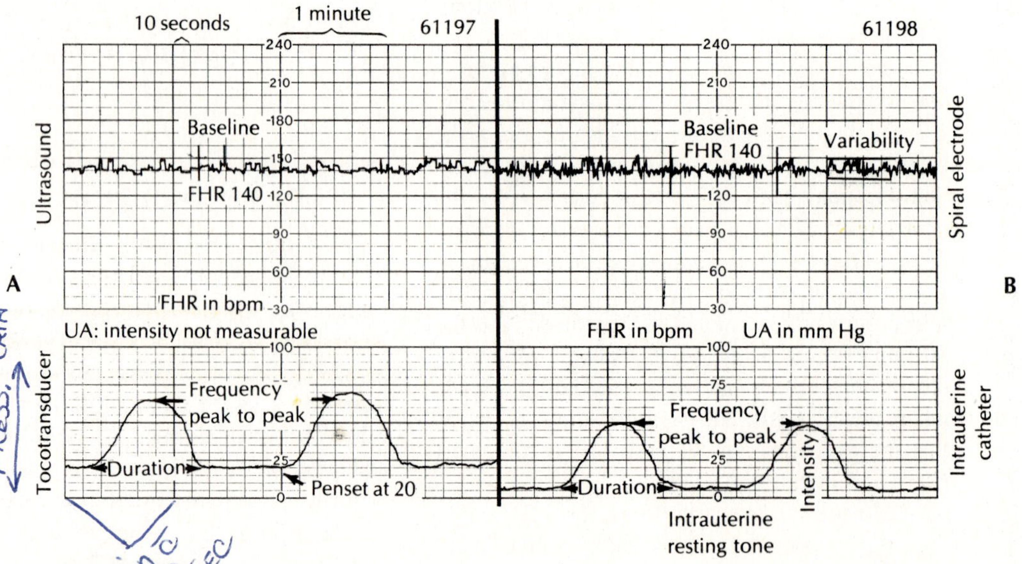

Table 24.2
Tachycardia and Bradycardia

	Tachycardia	Bradycardia
Definition	FHR above 160 beats/min lasting longer than a 10-min period	FHR below 120 beats/min lasting longer than a 10-min period
Description	See Fig. 24.13	See Fig. 24.14
Cause	Early fetal hypoxia Maternal fever Parasympatholytic drug (atropine, hydroxyzine pamoate [Vistaril]) Betasympathomimetic drugs (ritodrine, [isoxsuprine]) Amnionitis Maternal hyperthyroidism Fetal anemia Fetal heart failure Fetal cardiac arrhythmias	Late fetal hypoxia Beta-adrenergic blocking drugs (propanolol; anesthetics for epidural, spinal, caudal, and pudendal blocks) Maternal hypotension Prolonged umbilical cord compression Fetal congenital heart block
Clinical significance	Persistent tachycardia in absence of periodic changes: does not appear serious in terms of neonatal outcome (especially true if tachycardia is associated with maternal fever); tachycardia is an ominous sign when associated with late decelerations, severe variable decelerations, or absence of variability	Bradycardia with good variability and absence of periodic changes: not a sign of fetal distress if FHR remains above 80 beats/min; bradycardia caused by hypoxia is an ominous sign when associated with loss of variability and late decelerations
Nursing intervention	Dependent on cause; reduce maternal fever with antipyretics as ordered and cooling measures; oxygen* at 10-12 L/min may be of some value; carry out physician's orders based on alleviating cause	Dependent on cause; intervention not warranted in fetus with heart block diagnosed by ECG; oxygen at 10-12 L/min may be of some value; carry out physician's orders based on alleviating cause

*Some hospital protocols specify oxygen rates of 7-8 L/min.

Fig. 24.13
Fetal tachycardia with minimal variability. (From Perez, R.H.: Protocols for perinatal nursing practice, St. Louis, 1981, The C.V. Mosby Co.)

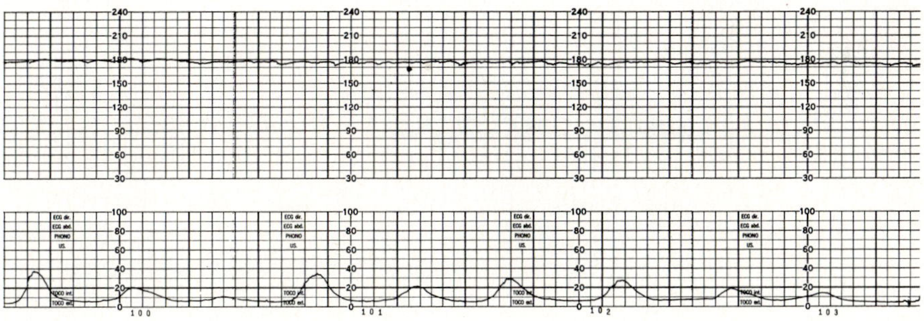

Fig. 24.14
Fetal bradycardia. (From Tucker, S.M.: Fetal monitoring and fetal assessment in high-risk pregnancy, St. Louis, 1978, The C.V. Mosby Co.)

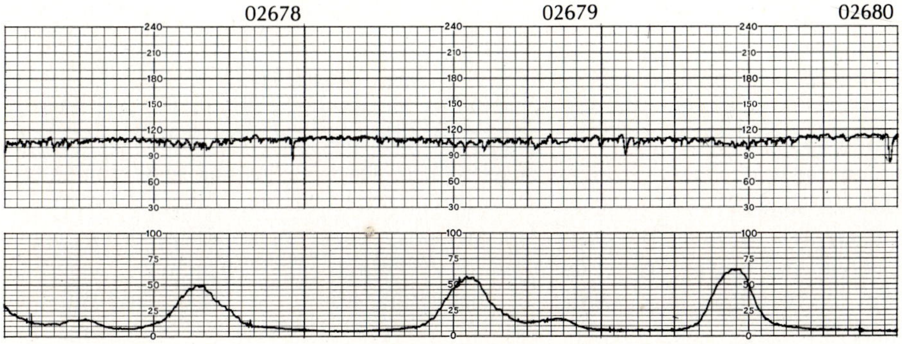

Fig. 24.15
Short-term variability (absence of long-term variability). (From Tucker, S.M.: Fetal monitoring and fetal assessment in high-risk pregnancy, St. Louis, 1978, The C.V. Mosby Co.)

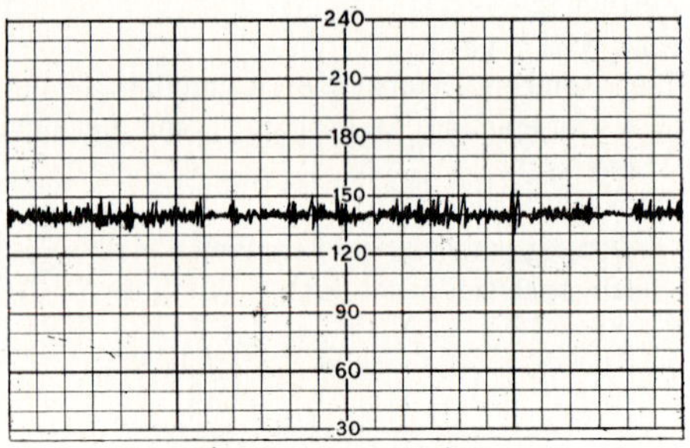

Short-term variability,
absence of long-term variability

Fig. 24.16
Long-term variability (absence of short-term variability). (From Tucker, S.M.: Fetal monitoring and fetal assessment in high-risk pregnancy, St. Louis, 1978, The C.V. Mosby Co.)

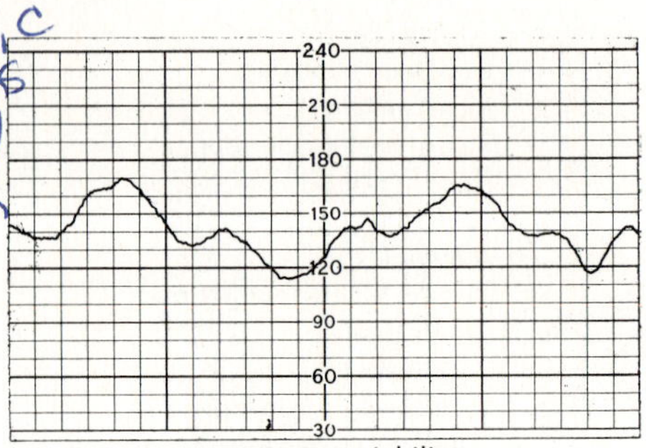

Long-term variability,
absence of short-term variability

Fig. 24.17
Increased variability. (From Tucker, S.M.: Fetal monitoring and fetal assessment in high-risk pregnancy, St. Louis, 1978, The C.V. Mosby Co.)

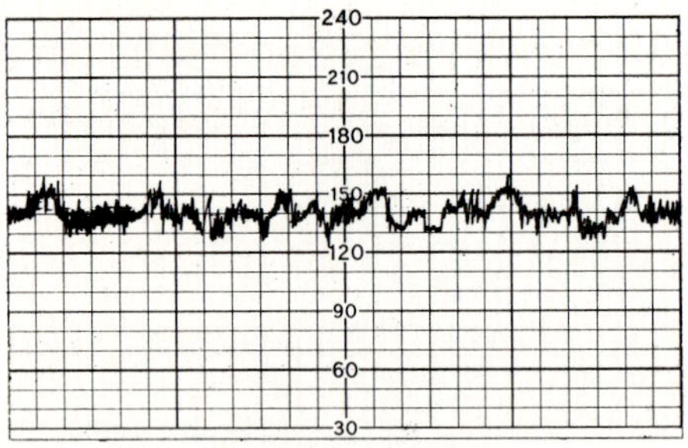

Both short- and
long-term variability

Fig. 24.18
Decreased variability. (From Tucker, S.M.: Fetal monitoring and fetal assessment in high-risk pregnancy, St. Louis, 1978, The C.V. Mosby Co.)

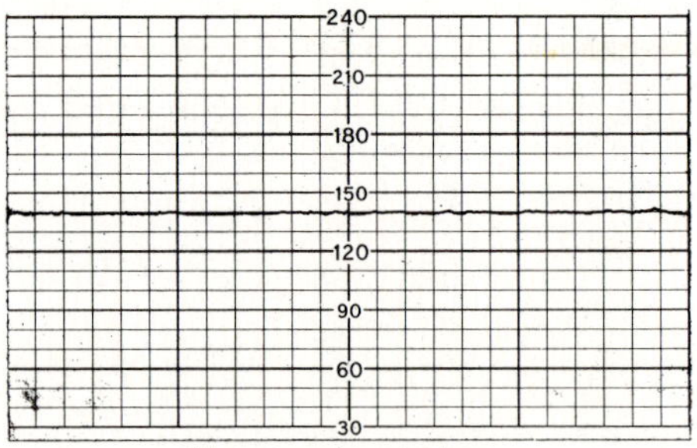

Absence of both short-
and long-term variability

Short-term variability is a change in FHR from one beat to the next. Fig. 24.15 shows an example of short-term variability.

Long-term variability consists of rhythmic fluctuations and waves, generally 3 to 5 cycles/min. Fig. 24.16 shows an example of long-term variability.

The following list gives additional information regarding signal source and short- and long-term variability:

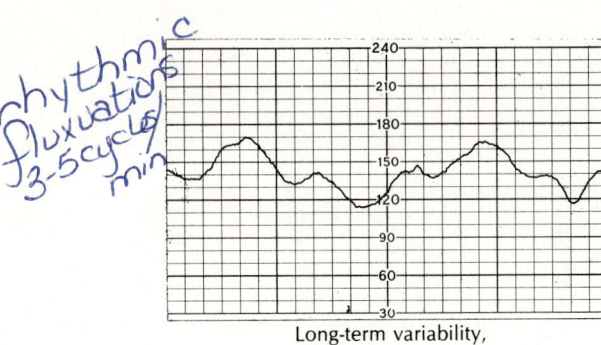

1. Direct FHR monitoring via the spiral electrode provides an accurate display of both long- and short-term variability.
2. Of the external ultrasound methods, external ul-

Table 24.3
Increased and Decreased Variability

	Increased Variability	**Decreased Variability**
Cause	Early mild hypoxia Fetal stimulation by: Uterine palpation Uterine contractions Fetal activity Maternal activity	Hypoxia/acidosis CNS depressants Analgesics/narcotics Meperidine hydrochloride (Demerol) Alphaprodine hydrochloride (Nisentil) Morphine sulfate Pentazocine (Talwin) Barbiturates Secobarbital sodium (Seconal) Pentobarbital sodium (Nembutal) Amobarbital (Amytal) Tranquilizers (Diazepam [Valium]) Ataractics Promethazine hydrochloride (Phenergan) Propiomazine hydrochloride (Largon) Hydroxyzine pamoate (Vistaril) Promazine hydrochloride (Sparine) Parasympatholytics (Atropine) General anesthetics Prematurity Fetal sleep cycles Congenital abnormalities Fetal cardiac arrhythmias
Clinical significance	Significance of marked variability not known; Increased variability from a previous average variability, earliest FHR sign of mild hypoxia	Benign when associated with periodic fetal sleep states, which last 20 to 30 min; if caused by drugs, variability usually increases as drugs are excreted Decreased variability considered ominous if caused by hypoxia/asphyxia; occurring with late decelerations, decreased variability associated with fetal acidosis and low Apgar scores
Nursing intervention	Observe FHR tracing carefully for any sign of fetal distress including decreasing variability and late decelerations; if using external mode of monitoring, consider using internal mode (spiral electrode)	Dependent on cause; intervention not warranted if associated with fetal sleep states or temporarily associated with central nervous system depressants; consider application of internal mode (spiral electrode) with physician; assist physician with fetal blood sampling for pH if ordered; prepare for delivery if so indicated by physician

trasound with autocorrelation most accurately demonstrates both long-and short-term variability.

3. External ultrasound with directional Doppler compares more favorably with both the spiral electrode and ultrasound autocorrelation than with conventional Doppler.
4. External abdominal ECG and phonotransducer can fairly accurately assess long-term variability but inconsistently demonstrate short-term variability because of limitations encountered during monitoring including parturient movement and muscle activity.

Increased variability (Fig. 24.17) and decreased variability (Fig. 24.18) are contrasted in Table 24.3.

The term sinusoidal pattern (Figure 24.19) is used to describe a *sine wave of cyclic long-term variability with minimal to absent short-term variability*. The heart rate cycles in a uniform pattern of about 4 to 8 cycles/min. This pattern is most often associated with severe fetal anemia, as occurs with Rh_o isoimmunization, but it has also been observed with severe fetal hypoxia before fetal death. A pseudosinusoidal pattern has been observed during antepartum testing and is rarely seen in the intrapartum period except as secondary to maternal administration of parenteral alphaprodine (Nisentil). The pseudosinusoidal pattern is self-correcting with maternal metabolism of the narcotic and does not indicate fetal distress.

Fig. 24.19
Sinusoidal pattern.

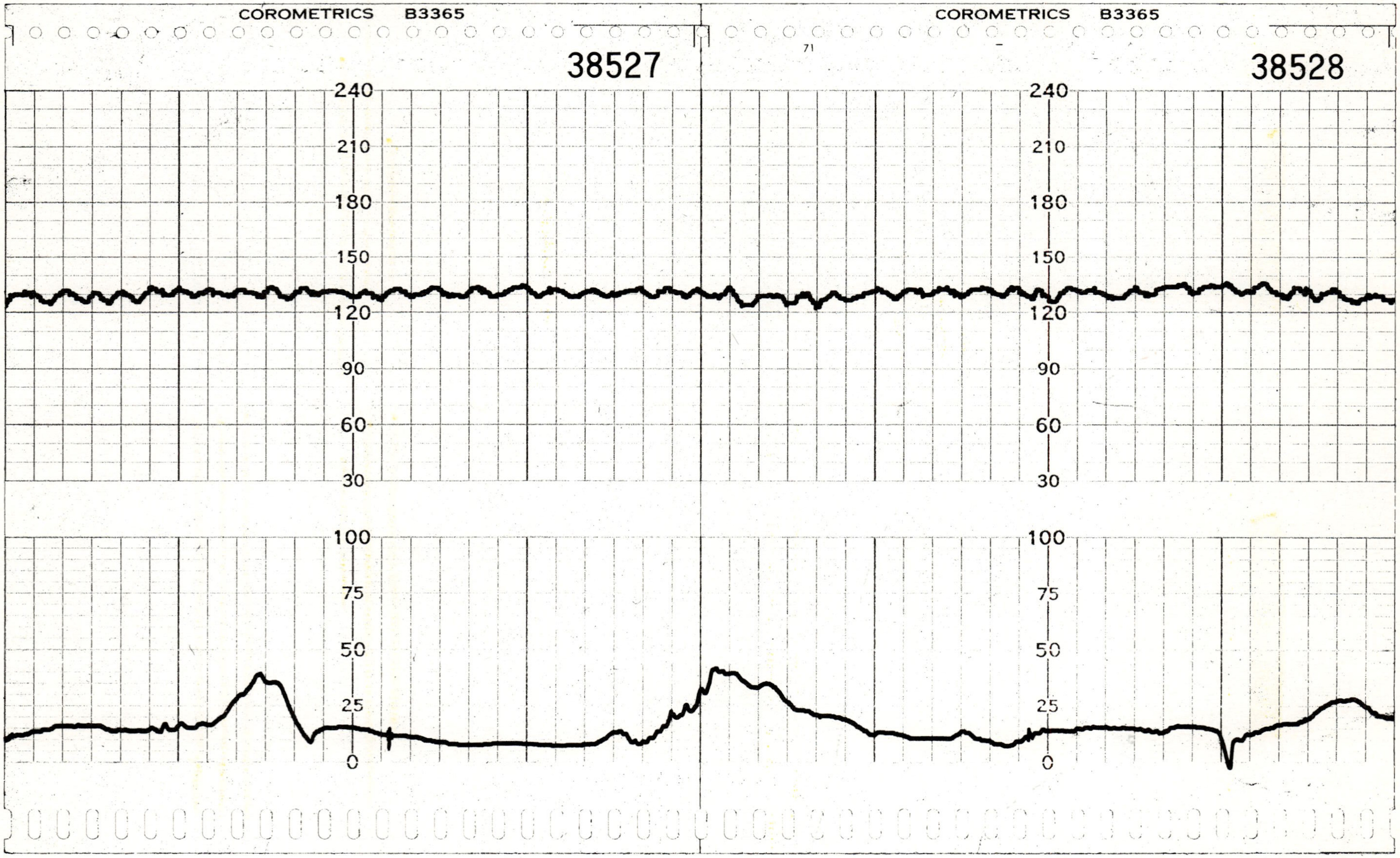

PERIODIC CHANGES

Periodic changes in FHR are *accelerations or decelerations from the base line with the FHR returning to the base line*. They usually occur in response to uterine contractions but also occur with fetal movements. Table 24.4 contrasts accelerations and early decelerations, and Table 24.5 contrasts late decelerations vs. variable deceleration.

Prolonged decelerations. Prolonged decelerations are difficult to classify, as they can occur in many situations.

Generally the benign causes are as follows:

1. Pelvic examination
2. Application of spiral electrode
3. Rapid fetal descent
4. Sustained maternal Valsalva's maneuver

Other prolonged decelerations are caused by progressive severe variable decelerations, sudden umbilical cord prolapse, and hypotension produced by spinal or epidural anesthesia. Paracervical anesthesia, a tetanic contraction, and maternal hypoxia as occurs during a seizure often produce prolonged decelerations. When the duration of the deceleration is longer than 2 to 3 minutes, a loss of variability with rebound tachycardia usually occurs. Occasionally, a period of late decelerations follows this. These responses normally clear spontaneously. However, when a prolonged deceleration is seen late in the course of severe variable decelerations or during a prolonged series of late decelerations, the prolonged deceleration may occur just before fetal death.

The nurse's responsibility is to notify the physician immediately on seeing a prolonged deceleration and initiate treatment of fetal distress.

UTERINE ACTIVITY MONITORING

Manual palpation of the uterine fundus has been the traditional method of monitoring uterine contractions. The intensity of the contractions has been described in the following manner (see also assessment of uterine contractions, p. 381):

Mild—Tense fundus; easy to indent with fingertips
Moderate—Firm fundus; difficult to indent with fingertips
Strong—Rigid boardlike fundus; almost impossible to indent

With the advent of FHR monitoring, additional information regarding uterine activity is obtainable. Table 24.6 lists the uterine activity information and the signal source through which this information can be obtained.

Since the depression of the pressure-sensing button of the tocotransducer is dependent on placement, maternal adipose tissue, and snugness of the abdominal belt,

Text continued on p. 490.

Table 24.4
Acceleration and Early Deceleration

	Acceleration	Early Deceleration
Description	Transitory increase of FHR above base line	Transitory decrease of FHR below base line concurrent with uterine contractions
Shape	May resemble shape of uterine contraction	Uniform shape; mirror image of uterine contraction
Onset	Variable; often precedes or occurs simultaneous with uterine contraction	Early in contraction phase before peak of contraction
Recovery	Variable	By end of contraction as uterine pressure returns to its resting tone
	Amplitude: Usually above 15 beats/min	Usually proportional to amplitude of contraction; rarely decelerates below 100 beats/min
Base line	Usually associated with average base-line variability	Usually associated with average base-line variability
Occurrence	Variable; may be repetitive with each contraction	Repetitious (occurs with each contraction); usually between 4 and 7 cm dilatation and in second stage of labor
Cause	Spontaneous fetal movement Vaginal examination Breech presentation Occiput posterior position Uterine contractions Fundal pressure Abdominal palpation	Head compression resulting from the following: Uterine contractions Vaginal examination Fundal pressure Placement of internal mode of monitoring
Clinical significance	Acceleration with fetal movement signifies fetal well-being representing fetal alertness or arousal states	Reassuring pattern not associated with fetal hypoxia, acidosis, or low Apgar scores
Nursing intervention	None required	None required

Fig. 24.20
Acceleration of fetal heart rate.

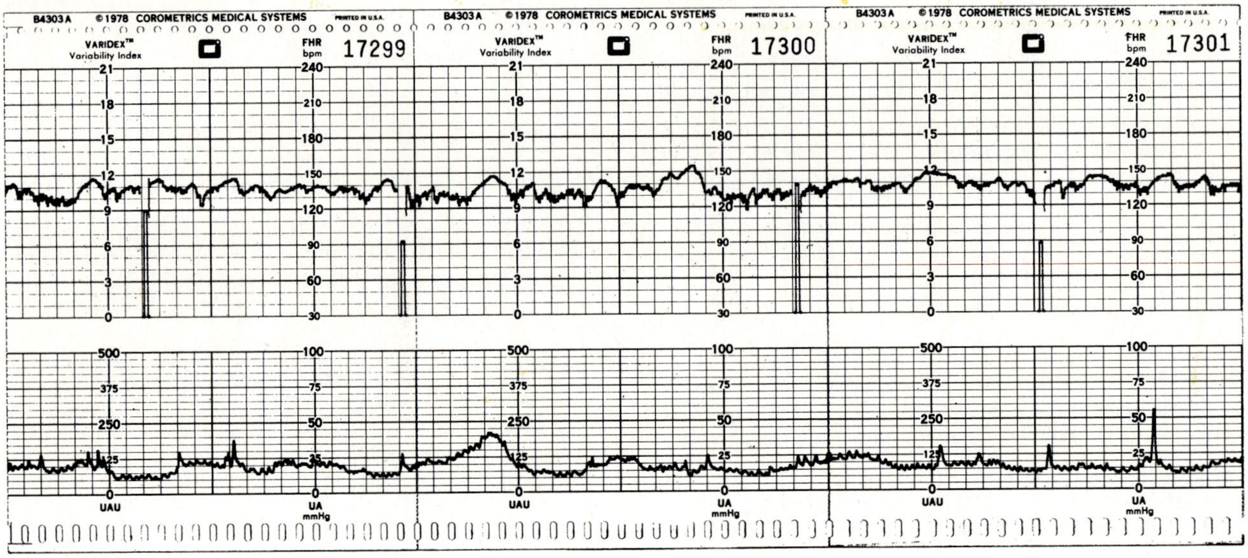

Fig. 24.21
Early decelerations. (From Perez, R.H.: Protocols for perinatal nursing practice, St. Louis, 1981, The C.V. Mosby Co.)

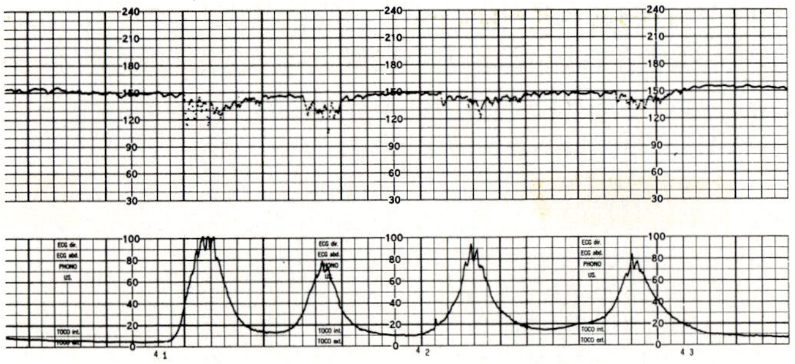

Fig. 24.22
Late decelerations. (From Perez, R.H.: Protocols for perinatal nursing practice, St. Louis, 1981, The C.V. Mosby Co.)

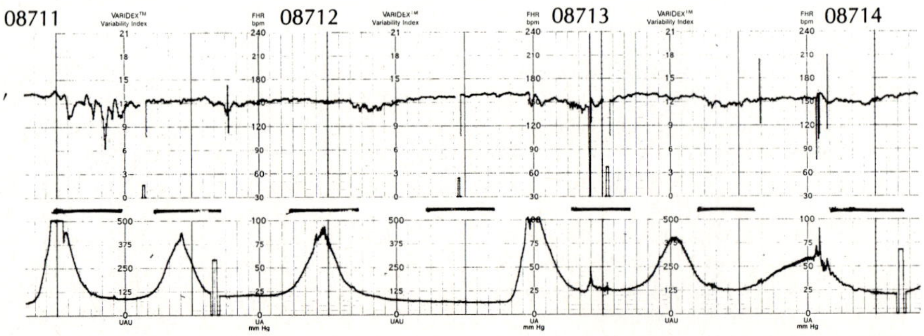

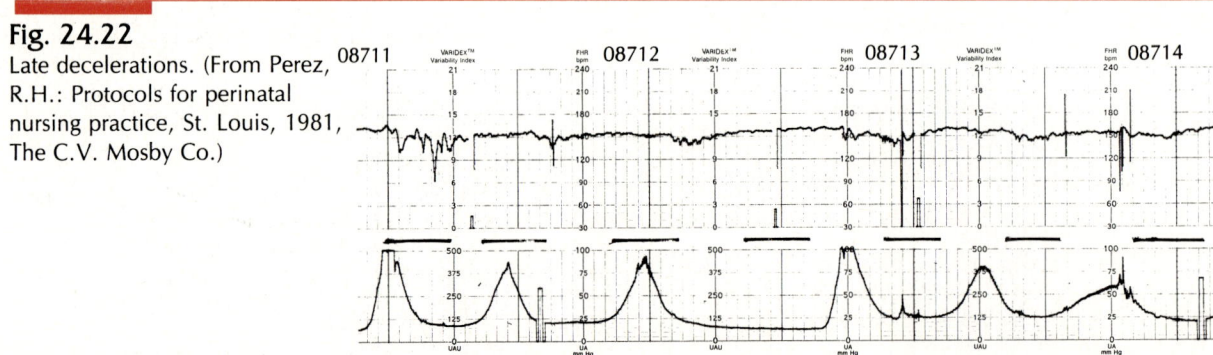

Table 24.5
Late Deceleration vs. Variable Deceleration

	Late Deceleration	**Variable Deceleration**
Description	Transitory decrease in FHR below base-line rate in contracting phase	Abrupt transitory decrease in FHR that is variable in duration, intensity, and timing relative to contractions
Shape	Uniform shape; mirror image of uterine contraction	Variable shape; characterized by sudden drop in FHR in a V or wide U shape
Onset	Late in contraction phase; after peak of the contraction; low point of deceleration occurs well after peak of contraction	Variable times in contracting phase; often preceded by transitory acceleration
Recovery	Well after end of contraction	Return to base line is rapid, sometimes with transitory acceleration (overshoot) or shouldering (acceleration immediately preceding and following deceleration); slow return to base line seen with severe variable decelerations
Deceleration	Usually proportional to amplitude of contraction; rarely decelerates below 100 beats/min	*Mild:* decelerates to any level, less than 30 sec with abrupt return to baseline *Moderate:* decelerates above 80 beats/min, any duration with abrupt return to base line *Severe:* decelerates below 70 beats/min for greater than 30 sec with slow return to base line
Base line	Often associated with loss of variability and increasing base-line rate	Mild variables usually associated with average base-line variability; moderate and severe variables often associated with decreasing variability and increasing base-line rate
Occurrence	Repetitious (occurs with each contraction); proportional to strength and duration of contractions, so may appear minimal to absent with weaker contractions	Variable; frequently observed late in labor with fetal descent and pushing
Cause	Uteroplacental insufficiency caused by the following: Uterine hyperactivity/hypertonus (often from oxytocin augmentation or induction of labor) Maternal supine hypotension Epidural/spinal anesthesia Placenta previa Abruptio placentae Hypertensive disorders Postmaturity Intrauterine growth retardation Diabetes mellitus Amnionitis	Umbilical cord compression caused by the following Maternal position with cord between fetus and maternal pelvis Cord around fetal neck, arm, leg, or other body part Short cord Knot in cord Prolapsed cord
Clinical significance	Nonreassuring, worrisome pattern associated with fetal hypoxia, acidosis, and low Apgar scores; considered ominous if persistent and uncorrected, especially when associated with fetal tachycardia and loss of variability	Variable decelerations occur in about 50% of all labors and are usually transient, correctable phenomena not associated with low Apgar scores; mild variable decelerations reassuring; decelerations progressing from moderate to severe associated with fetal acidosis, hypoxia, and low Apgar scores; severe variable decelerations with good base-line variability just before delivery usually well tolerated
Nuring intervention	Change maternal position Correct maternal hypotension Elevate legs Increase rate of maintenance IV Discontinue oxytocin if infusing Administer oxygen* at 10 to 12 L/min with tight face mask Assist physician with fetal blood sampling if ordered Assist physician with termination of labor if pattern cannot be corrrected	Change maternal position; if decelerations do not yet meet criteria for mild variable deceleration, proceed with measures below. Discontinue oxytocin if infusing Administer oxygen at 10-12 L/min with tight face mask Assist with vaginal or speculum examination If cord is prolapsed, examiner will elevate (push up on) fetal presenting part with cord between gloved fingers until cesarean delivery is accomplished (Figs. 21.7 and 21.8) Assist with fetal blood sampling if ordered Assist with delivery

*Some hospital protocols specify 7-8 L/min.

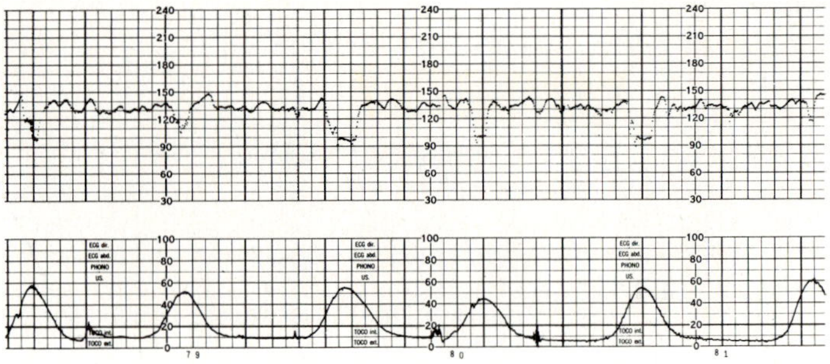

Fig. 24.23
Mild variable decelerations. (From Perez, R.H.: Protocols for perinatal nursing practice, St. Louis, 1981, The C.V. Mosby Co.)

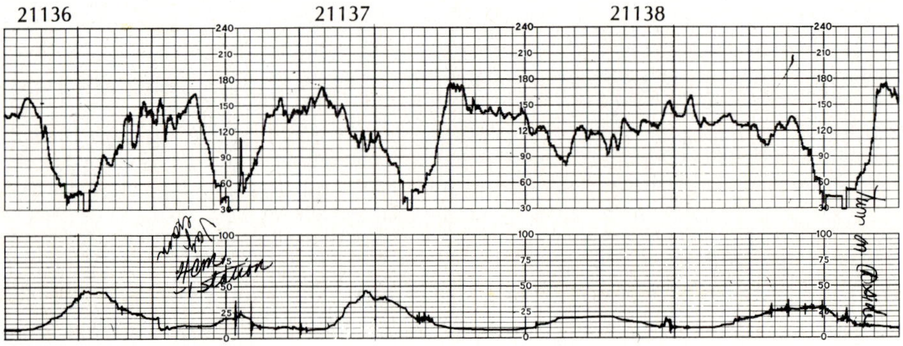

Fig. 24.24
Severe variable decelerations. (From Tucker, S.M.: Fetal monitoring and fetal assessment in high-risk pregnancy, St. Louis, 1978, The C.V. Mosby Co.)

Fig. 24.25
A, Early deceleration caused by head compression.

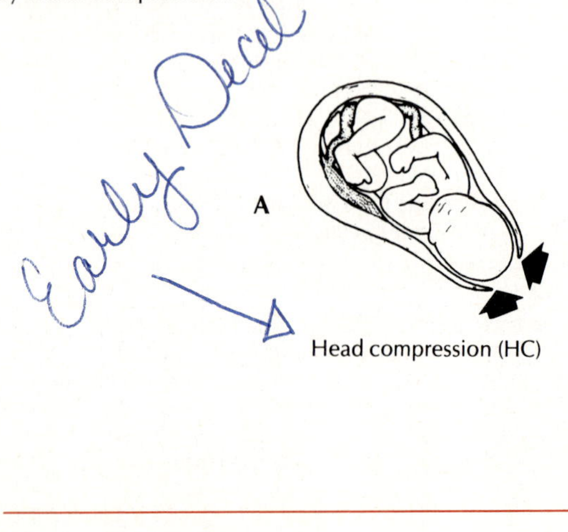

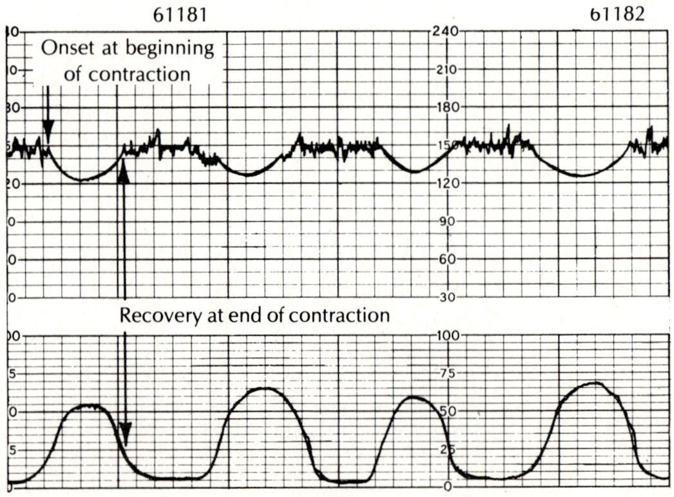

Fig. 24.25, cont'd

B, Late decelerations caused by uteroplacental insufficiency. **C,** Variable deceleration caused by cord compression. (From Tucker, S.M.: Fetal monitoring and fetal assessment in high-risk pregnancy, St. Louis, 1978, The C.V. Mosby Co.)

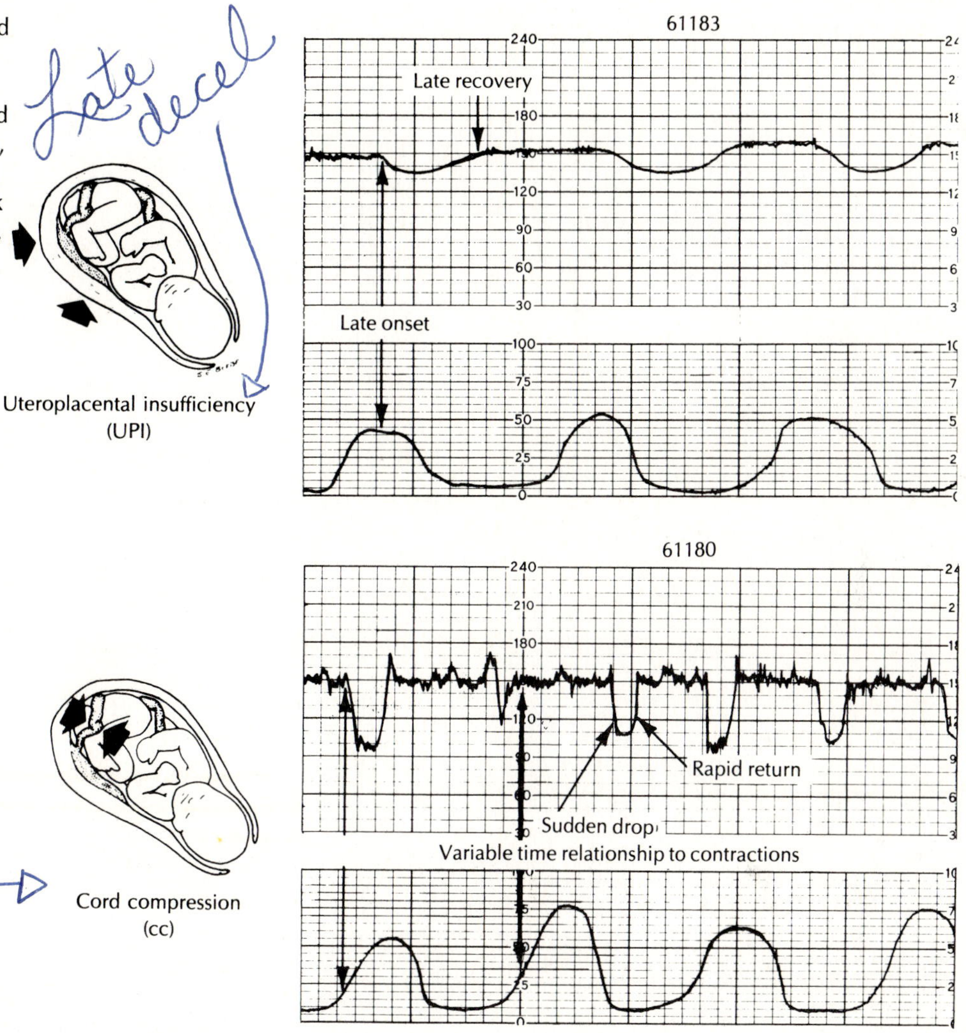

Fig. 24.26

Severe variable decelerations. (From Tucker, S.M.: Fetal monitoring and fetal assessment in high-risk pregnancy, St. Louis, 1978, The C.V. Mosby Co.)

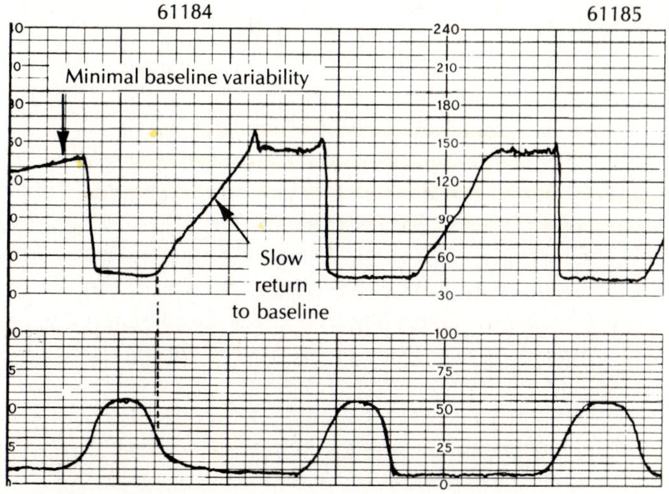

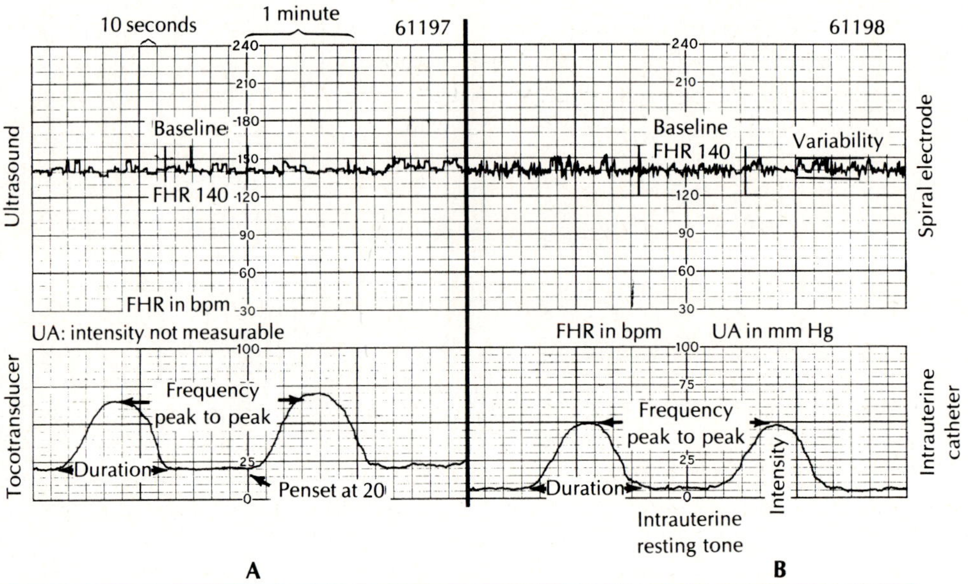

Fig. 24.27
Strip chart with uterine activity displayed both externally via tocotransducer and internally via spiral electrode in order to contrast type of information that can be obtained. (From Tucker, S.M.: Fetal monitoring and fetal assessment in high-risk pregnancy, St. Louis, 1978, The C.V. Mosby Co.)

Table 24.6
Uterine Activity Information and Signal Source

Uterine Activity	Signal Source
Frequency of contractions (measured from peak to peak)	Intrauterine catheter and tocotransducer
Duration of contractions (from beginning to end)	Intrauterine catheter and tocotransducer
Intensity (actual pressure [mm Hg] at peak of contraction)	Intrauterine catheter only
Resting tone (actual pressure [mm Hg] between contractions)	Intrauterine catheter only

the tocotransducer cannot measure intensity nor resting tone of contractions.

During a normal labor, uterine contractions occur about every 3 to 5 minutes with a duration of 30 to 60 seconds, an intensity of 50 to 75 mm Hg and a resting tone between 8 and 12 mm Hg pressure (see p. 381 for Montevideo units). In addition to this information, evidence of fetal movement can be observed on the chart panel as spikes or momentary increases in uterine pressure. The importance of observing fetal activity is described in the antepartum testing section.

During electronic fetal monitoring, the uterine activity and contractions are displayed on the lower section of the strip chart. Each major horizontal division represents 25 mm Hg pressure with the subdivisions representing 5 mm Hg. The vertical scale has been previously described.

Uterine hyperstimulation caused by oxytocin induction or augmentation of labor can be observed on the strip chart as well as the normal laboring pattern. The following section describes factors related to increased uterine activity.

Increased uterine activity

Observations

1. Contractions lasting longer than 90 seconds
2. Relaxation between contractions less than 30 seconds
3. Inadequate relaxation between contractions with intrauterine resting tone above 15 mm Hg
4. Peak intrauterine pressure of contractions above 80 mm Hg

Causes

1. Hyperstimulation of the uterus with oxytocin
2. Abruptio placenta
3. Pregnancy-induced hypertension
4. Drugs
   a. Narcotics (e.g., meperidine hydrochloride [Demerol])
   b. Catecholamines (adrenergics) (e.g., norepinephrine [Noradrenalin, Levarterenol])
   c. Beta-blocking agents (e.g., propranol [Inderal])
   d. Prostaglandins (e.g., prostaglandin F_2 alpha [$PGF_2\alpha$; Dinoprost])
   e. Pituitary hormones (e.g., vasopressin [Pitressin])

Intervention

1. Decrease oxytocin if infusing and increase rate of maintenance intravenous infusion
2. Change maternal position (left lateral preferred)
3. Consider administration of oxygen* at 10 to 12 L/min by tight face mask depending on FHR response

Clinical significance. Hyperstimulation of the uterus or a tetanic contraction can result in fetal distress because of lack of placental perfusion. The most common cause of uterine hyperstimulation is the injudicious use of oxytocin. When an oxytocin infusion is discontinued, uterine relaxation usually occurs within 10 minutes.

Since it has been well documented that uterine contractions are known to decrease the rate of blood flow through the intervillous space and that most fetuses are well able to tolerate this, it is important for the nurse to monitor attentively uterine activity as well as FHR. In pregnancies where the margin of fetal reserve is low, this phenomenon can cause commensurate decreases in FHR, earlier described as late decelerations. The physician should be notified promptly when there is evidence of uterine hyperstimulation with or without an associated heart rate response.

FETAL DISTRESS

Fetal distress is a compromise in fetal well-being. It can be an acute or chronic condition depending on antepartum and intrapartum events with the possibility of an acute insult superimposed on a condition of chronic fetal distress.

The goal of intrapartum FHR monitoring is the early detection of mild fetal hypoxia and the prevention of severe fetal hypoxia. The nurse must be thinking continually in terms of whether FHR pattern is reassuring and whether one can consider that fetal oxygenation is good. A differentiation can be made of reassuring patterns, nonreassuring or warning FHR patterns generally indicative of mild fetal hypoxia, and worrisome or ominous patterns where there is evidence of severe fetal hypoxia. Reassuring FHR patterns are given in the following list:

1. Base-line FHR in the normal range of 120 to 160 beats/min with no periodic changes and average base-line variability
2. Early decelerations
3. Mild variable decelerations
4. Accelerations

Nonreassuring (warning) FHR patterns are given in the following list:

1. Progressive increase or decrease in base-line heart rate
2. Tachycardia of 160 beats/min or above
3. Progressive decrease in base-line variability

Administration of oxygen to the mother may be of some value with the preceding patterns.

Ominous FHR patterns and the appropriate nursing intervention are given on p. 492.

Fetal blood sampling. Assessment of fetal pH is done by fetal blood sampling after rupture of the membranes and some cervical dilatation. A decrease in blood pH becomes a measure of the degree of fetal hypoxia. This information is an important adjunct to the definitive diagnosis of fetal distress.

Fetal blood sampling is indicated when the FHR pattern is suggestive of hypoxia. (Not all hospitals have 24-hr access to microblood gas analysis with a 10- to 15-min turnaround time and this is therefore not done.) Results of fetal pH are most helpful when the FHR pattern is confusing, when the base line is flat without periodic changes, and when uncorrectable late decelerations occur with good variability.

The physician performs the procedure with the woman in lithotomy position. The presenting part is swabbed before the puncture is made with a small blade. The blood is collected in a long capillary tube, which is sealed until the sample is analyzed.

Collection of a maternal venous blood sample for pH may also be requested by the physician. A heparinized syringe is used to withdraw the venous sample preferably without the use of a tourniquet.

The normal range of pH in an adult is 7.35 to 7.45. The average fetal range is 7.30 to 7.35, with values above 7.25 considered acceptable. A value between 7.20 and 7.24 is considered preacidotic, and sampling is usually repeated within 15 minutes. Expeditious delivery by low forceps or cesarean surgery is done when values are below 7.20 (see Chapter 37).

Factors influencing fetal pH include maternal acidosis or alkalosis, caput succedaneum, laboratory error, stage of labor, and time relationship of blood sampling to uterine contractions. Fetal blood sampling complements FHR monitoring and has proved of value in providing additional information about fetal condition. Maternal blood sample should be collected for pH in a heparinized syringe from a vein without a tourniquet.

Nursing Care

Nursing care of the woman who is monitored is the same as that given to the woman who is not monitored. The nurse must exercise caution that the monitor does

*Some hospital protocols specify oxygen rates of 7 to 8 L/min.

Ominous FHR Patterns and Nursing Interventions

Ominous FHR Patterns	Nursing Intervention
Severe variable deceleration; definition: FHR below 70 beats/min lasting longer than 30-60 sec with any of following: Rising base-line FHR Decreasing variability Slow return to base line; may be with "overshoot"	With severe variable deceleration: Change maternal position Perform vaginal or speculum examination or both Discontinue oxytocin if infusing Administer oxygen at 10-12 L/min by tight face mask Termination of labor considered by physician if pattern cannot be corrected to meet criteria of mild variable deceleration
Late decelerations of any magnitude—more serious if associated with decreasing variability or rising base line	Intervene in step-by-step approach proceeding to next step *only* if pattern is uncorrected Place woman on side Correct maternal hypotension; elevate legs, increase rate of maintenance IV infusion Discontinue oxytocin if infusing Administer oxygen at 10-12 L/min by tight face mask Assist physician with fetal pH if done; pH >7.20: repeat pH in 10 to 15 min; pH <7.20: prepare for immediate delivery Expeditious delivery considered by physician if pattern cannot be corrected
Absence of variability	Correct identifiable cause; if uncorrectable, assist physician with termination of labor
Prolonged deceleration	As above
Severe bradycardia	As above

not receive more care than does the woman and her family. However, the woman who is monitored needs additional personal attention based on the mode of monitoring used. When the external mode is used, the ultrasound transducer needs to be cleaned and transmission gel reapplied every 2 hours as needed. The belts and tocotransducer are repositioned every 1 to 2 hours to massage any reddened skin areas. A light dusting of powder under the belts often promotes comfort. Repositioning of the leg plate strap when ECG paste is reapplied to the leg plate can also promote comfort.

In order to allay anxiety, the nurse explains the basic functions of the monitor to the woman and her family. The nurse describes briefly the type of information that is printed on the upper and lower panels of the chart paper and explains that the information regarding fetal status can be assessed continuously, even during contractions. The nurse explains that although the digital display cannot print out every heart beat, it provides a sampling of FHR. Because of the fluctuations and variability in the heart rate, the woman may observe numbers such as 88 and 156 when the base-line rate is actually 120 beats/min. Should the woman express concern about these variations in numbers, she can be told that the main reason for the digital display is not to demonstrate base-line heart rate, but to be used for testing and calibrating the instrument. Acceptance of the monitor by the woman and her family can usually be gained by a thorough explanation of the factors producing anxiety.

In contrast, for some women, the audible beep with each fetal heart beat is often reassuring and encouraging.

PREPARED CHILDBIRTH

Couples who have taken prepared childbirth classes are usually informed about the monitor and adapt accordingly. Effleurage usually performed on the maternal abdomen can be difficult with the external mode of monitoring, but it can be done on the upper thighs to elicit the same effect.

In performing breathing techniques during labor, it is important to identify the onset of the contraction well before the peak. This is sometimes difficult for the woman to do if she dozes between contractions. The labor coach can observe the increase in intrauterine pressure on the uterine activity panel of the strip chart, alerting the woman as to the onset of a contraction in order to start the desired breathing sequence before she senses the contraction. The coach can note the peak of the contraction and relay this information to the woman so that she knows the contraction is half over and that the intensity will diminish.

Couples who are adamantly opposed to the fetal monitor may be required to sign a release form at the hospital, depending on hospital policy. This release is signed only after the physician has provided them with enough information to enable them to give an *informed consent* (see p. 41). Most labors and deliveries are normal processes, but neither the physician nor hospital staff can accurately predetermine who will be at risk during the intrapartum period.

MONITOR CARE

Trouble shooting the monitor is done on a systematic basis. Any time there is an apparent malfunction of equipment, the FHR is auscultated with a stethoscope, fetoscope, or ultrasonic stethoscope. The procedure for application and use of the particular mode of monitoring is reviewed systematically until the source of the problem is identified. The check list for fetal monitoring on p. 494 may be useful for this purpose.

The equipment should be well maintained and in working order. Small care-taking tasks can be important in ensuring the quality of the signal source. These include those described previously with each mode of monitoring as well as careful use of the ultrasound to avoid dropping it and damaging the crystals, and not tightly rolling any of the cords, which can cause damage to the wires resulting in an unsatisfactory signal. A few moments of care are well worth the time when the validity of the signal can be depended on to reflect fetal status.

CHARTING

Charting of pertinent items should appear on the monitor strip.

Preprinted labels may be placed on the chart paper when monitoring is initiated. Whether these are available or not, the nurse should note the following items at the initiation of monitoring:

1. Woman's name
2. Date
3. Hospital record number
4. Part number (i.e., 1 of 3)
5. Physician's name
6. Woman's age
7. Gravida _______ Para _______
8. Expected date of confinement (EDC)
9. Membranes—whether intact, or ruptured with time and color of fluid
10. TPR and BP
11. Number of monitor
12. Time of initiation of monitoring
13. Dilatation and station
14. High-risk factors

During monitoring, the nurse enters frequent notations regarding the following, directly on the chart paper:

1. Vaginal examinations (dilatation)
2. Maternal positioning and repositioning in bed
3. Analgesia or anesthesia
4. Medications
5. BP and TPR
6. Voidings
7. Emesis
8. Pushing
9. Adjustments of signal source
   a. Relocation of transducers
   b. Flushing catheter
   c. Replacement of spiral electrode
   d. Replacement or expulsion of intrauterine catheter
10. Interventions for fetal distress
11. Signature time, date each time strip is evaluated per hospital policy (e.g., every 10 to 15 minutes)

These notations are important for retrospective audit and teaching purposes, but they are of utmost importance in identifying a cause of a specific FHR response to nursing or medical action.

On completion of monitoring and delivery, the nurse should make the following summary notations at the end of the chart paper:

1. Woman's name
2. Delivery date and time
3. Type of delivery
4. Anesthesia
5. Sex of infant
6. Presentation
7. Both 1- and 5-min Apgar scores
8. Complications

The completed strip chart then presents a complete picture of the woman's labor.

The following box summarizes items to be checked and charted during fetal monitoring.

LEGAL ASPECTS

The nurse is held accountable for performing fetal monitoring according to the established standard of care (see p. 40). Documentation of nursing care and the woman's responses are important in providing a clear picture of intrapartum events. Understanding the functions of the monitor is imperative if the nurse is to validate and define the information printed on the strip chart. All equipment is checked and tested periodically to ensure that it is in good working order.

The *legal significance* of complete and accurate charting cannot be overemphasized (see p. 41). Basically, if some aspect of care is not written on the chart, it is considered not to have been done. Because litigation often occurs a few years after the event, nurses cannot rely on memory to recollect specific observations and actions.

Essentially, nurses are held accountable for what they know. If the nurse has become an expert in fetal monitoring and recognizes persistent, uncorrectable late decelerations, the standard of care would dictate that the physician should be notified. A *reasonably prudent nurse* (see p. 40) would note the time and name of the physician notified and the physician's response. In the rare event that the physician was totally unavailable, another resource physician would be sought. It is incumbent on the nurse to follow the appropriate hospital-designated chain of command until the situation is remedied. Mere notification of another person does not absolve the nurse of the responsibility to continue pursuing appropriate medical action on behalf of the fetus.

Checklist for Fetal Monitoring Equipment

Name: ______________________ Evaluator: ______________________

Date: ______________________

Items To Be Checked	Yes	No	Remarks
Preparation of monitor 1. Is the paper inserted correctly? 2. Are transducer cables plugged into appropriate outlet of monitor?			
Ultrasound transducer 1. Has ultrasound transmission gel been applied to the crystals? 2. Was the FHR tested and noted on the chart paper? 3. Does a consistent wave form appear on the oscilloscope? 4. Is the strap secure and snug?			
Tocotransducer 1. Is the tocotransducer firmly strapped where the least maternal tissue is in evidence? 2. Has it been applied without gel or paste? 3. Are there any accumulations of gel around the pressure button? 4. Was the penset adjusted between 20 and 25 mm marks and noted on chart paper? 5. Was this setting done between contractions? 6. Is the strap secure and snug?			
Spiral electrode 1. Are the wires attached firmly to the posts on the leg plate? 2. Is the spiral electrode attached to the presenting part of the fetus? 3. Is the inner surface of the leg plate covered with electrode paste? 4. Is the leg plate properly secured to the woman's thigh?			

From Tucker, S.M.: Fetal monitoring and fetal assessment in high-risk pregnancy, St. Louis, 1978, The C.V. Mosby Co.

Items To Be Checked	Yes	No	Remarks
Internal catheter/strain gauge 1. Is the strain gauge located about half the height of the uterus (approximately at maternal xiphoid)? 2. Is the catheter filled with sterile water? 3. Is the black line on the catheter visible at the introitus? 4. Is it noted on the chart paper that stopcock was opened to room air (reading 0 on paper)? 5. Was the UA tested at 50 for 10 seconds? 6. Was the testing written on the chart paper? 7. Is the stopcock turned off to the syringe during monitoring?			
Charting 1. Are testings of FHR/UA written on chart paper at least every 4 hours? 2. Is the chart paper properly labeled with the following: a. Woman's name b. ID number c. Date d. Time monitor attached and mode e. High-risk conditions (PIH, diabetes, etc.) f. Membranes intact or ruptured g. Gestational age h. Dilatation and station 3. Are the following noted? a. Maternal position and repositioning in bed b. Vaginal examinations c. Paracervical block d. Medication given e. BP and TPR f. Voidings g. O_2 given h. Emesis i. Pushing j. Fetal movement k. Notations of base-line or periodic changes l. Any change in mode of monitoring m. Adjustments of equipment, i.e., (1) Relocation of transducers (2) Flushing catheter (3) Replacement of electrode (4) Replacement of catheter			

Comments:

Antepartum Testing

Evaluation of fetal well-being and maturity is essential in the management of the high-risk pregnancy. The nonstress test (NST), or fetal activity determination (FAD), and the oxytocin challenge test (OCT) have been widely employed for the determination of fetal well-being. In addition, daily fetal movement count (DFMC), as recorded by the expectant mother, has proved to be an additional method of assessing fetal well-being.

The desired goals of antepartum monitoring are to prevent intrauterine fetal death and avoid unnecessary premature intervention.

Indications for both the NST and the OCT are the following:

1. Maternal diabetes mellitus
2. Chronic hypertension
3. Hypertensive disorders in pregnancy
4. Intrauterine growth retardation
5. Sickle cell disease
6. Maternal cyanotic heart disease
7. Suspected postmaturity
8. History of previous stillbirth
9. Rh sensitization (isoimmunization)
10. Meconium-stained amniotic fluid (at amniocentesis)
11. Abnormal estriol excretion pattern
12. Hyperthyroidism
13. Collagen diseases
14. Older gravida (≥ 40 weeks' gestation)
15. Chronic renal disease

There are no contraindications for the NST. Absolute contraindications for the OCT are rupture of membranes and previous classical cesarean delivery. The following are considered relative contraindications for the OCT: multiple pregnancy, previous premature labor, placenta previa, hydramnios, and previous low transverse cesarean delivery.

NONSTRESS TESTING/FETAL ACTIVITY DETERMINATION

The basis for the NST or FAD is that the normal fetus will produce characteristic heart rate patterns. Acceleration of FHR in response to fetal movement is the desired outcome of the NST/FAD. This then allows most high-risk pregnancies to continue, with the test being repeated twice a week. A reactive pattern suggests fetal well-being with an associated good perinatal outcome.

The nurse observes the strip chart for signs of fetal movement and a concurrent acceleration of FHR. If evidence of fetal movement is not apparent on the chart paper, the woman is asked to depress a button on a hand-held event marker that is connected into the appropriate outlet on the monitor when she feels fetal movement. The ''event'' of fetal movement is then noted by a spike or arrow printed by the stylus on the uterine activity panel of the strip chart. The test usually takes 20 to 30 minutes but may take longer if the fetus needs to be moved or awakened because of a sleep state.

A guide for the interpretation of the nonstress test follows:

Result	**Interpretation**
Reactive	Two or more accelerations of FHR of 15 beats/min lasting 15 seconds or more associated with each fetal movement in a 10-min period
Nonreactive	Any tracing with either no FHR accelerations or accelerations less than 15 beats/min or lasting less than 15 seconds throughout any fetal movement during testing period
Unsatisfactory	Quality of FHR recording not adequate for interpretation

The clinical significance of the interpretation of the NST is as follows:

Reactive NST	As long as twice weekly NSTs remain reactive, most high-risk pregnancies are allowed to continue.
Nonreactive NST	Further indirect monitoring may be attempted with abdominal fetal electrocardiography in an effort to clarify FHR pattern and quantitate variability. External monitoring should continue and an OCT be done.
Unsatisfactory	Test is repeated in 24 hours or an OCT is done, depending on the clinical situation.

OXYTOCIN CHALLENGE TEST

The basis for the OCT is that a healthy fetus can withstand a decreased oxygen supply during the physiologic stress of an oxytocin-stimulated contraction, while a compromised fetus will demonstrate late decelerations that are nonreassuring and indicative of uteroplacental insufficiency.

The woman is monitored indirectly, and the nurse observes the strip chart for 10 minutes before the administration of IV-piggybacked oxytocin. Should the woman have three or more spontaneous contractions within a 10-min period, the oxytocin need not be initi-

Fig. 24.28

Nonstress test (NST). **A,** Decreased variability caused by fetal sleep cycle. **B,** Reactive nonstress test 15 minutes later. (From Perez, R.H.: Protocols for perinatal nursing practice, St. Louis, 1981, The C.V. Mosby Co.)

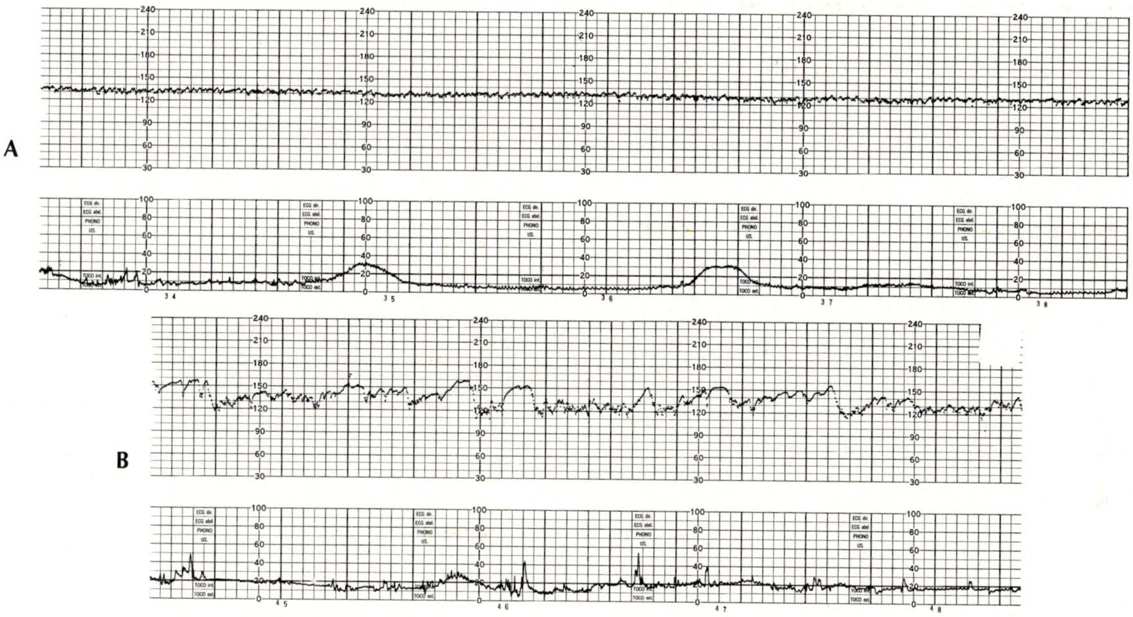

ated. If less than three spontaneous contractions occur within the period and if late decelerations do not occur with intermittent spontaneous contractions, oxytocin can be initiated. The physician orders the dosage, which usually starts at 0.5 mU/min.* The oxytocin, which is always diluted in an IV solution and piggybacked into the tubing of the main IV, is usually delivered via an infusion pump or controller to ensure accurate dosage. The oxytocin infusion is usually increased by 0.5 mU/min at 15- to 20-min intervals until three uterine contractions of good quality are observed within a 10-min period. The FHR pattern is then interpreted. The oxytocin infusion is discontinued, and the maintenance IV solution infused until such time as uterine activity has returned to the preoxytocin infusion level. The IV is then removed, the fetal monitor is discontinued, and the woman can be sent home.

A guide for the interpretation of the OCT follows:

Result	Interpretation
Negative	No late decelerations with a minimum of three uterine contractions lasting 40 to 60 seconds within a 10-min period
Positive	Persistent and consistent late decelerations occurring with more than half the contractions
Suspicious	Late decelerations occurring with less than half the uterine contractions once an adequate contraction pattern has been established
Hyperstimulation	Late decelerations occurring with excessive uterine activity (contractions more often than every 2 minutes or lasting longer than 90 seconds) or a persistent increase in uterine tone
Unsatisfactory	Inadequate uterine contraction pattern or tracing too poor to interpret

The clinical significance of the OCT is as follows:

Negative OCT	Reassurance that the fetus is likely to survive labor, should it occur within 1 week; more frequent testing may be indicated based on the clinical situation.

*See Table 37.2, p. 888, for calculating dosage of Pitocin and drops per minute.

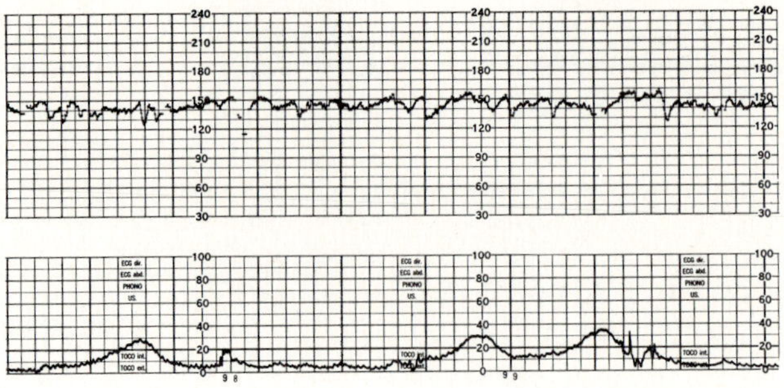

Fig. 24.29
Negative oxytocin challenge test. (From Perez, R.H.: Protocols for perinatal nursing practice, St. Louis, 1981, The C.V. Mosby Co.)

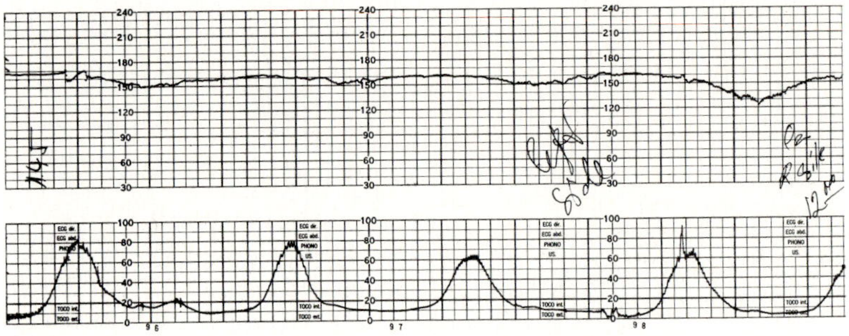

Fig. 24.30
Positive oxytocin challenge test. (From Perez, R.H.: Protocols for perinatal nursing practice, St. Louis, 1981, The C.V. Mosby Co.)

Result	Interpretation
Positive OCT	Management lies between utilization of other tools of fetal assessment and termination of pregnancy. A positive test indicates that the fetus is at increased risk for perinatal morbidity and mortality. The physician may perform an expeditious vaginal delivery following a successful induction or may proceed directly to cesarean delivery.
Suspicious, hyperstimulation, or unsatisfactory	NST and OCT should be repeated within 24 hours. If interpretable data cannot be achieved, other methods of fetal assessment must be used.

DAILY FETAL MOVEMENT COUNT

Frequent movements of the fetus, as perceived by the mother, have been reassuring signs for centuries. Various investigators have recently reported a marked decrease in fetal movement before an episode of fetal distress or fetal death.

Daily fetal movement counts (DFMCs), as reported by the mother, have been compared with movements recorded electronically, revealing that almost 90% of all fetal movements can be identified by the mother. This simple, inexpensive, readily applied ''test'' is continuously available away from the clinical area and relatively easy for the woman to do accurately.

Should a woman complain of decreased fetal movement, she may be asked by the physician to lie down for a period of 1 hour and count all the fetal movements. If she feels three or more during that time, she can be reassured. However, she is cautioned to continue to be aware of fetal movements and report the hourly observations should the problem recur. An immediate NST is usually performed if two or less movements are felt. If the NST is reactive, no further testing is done unless there are some other risk factors. A nonreactive NST would be followed by an OCT, the potential outcomes and significance of which have been previously described.

References and Readings

Bobak, I.M., and Jensen, M.D.: A modular study guide to maternity care, St. Louis, 1983, The C.V. Mosby Co.

Freeman, R.K., and Garite, T.J.: Fetal heart rate monitoring, Baltimore, 1981, Williams & Wilkins.

Jensen, M.D., Benson, R.C., and Bobak, I.M.: Maternity care: the nurse and the family, ed. 2, St. Louis, 1981, The C.V. Mosby Co.

Nursing photobook. Managing I.V. therapy. Nursing '82 books, Springhouse, Pa., Intermed Communications, Inc.

Nursing photobook. Using monitors. Nursing '81 books, Horsham, Pa., Intermed Communications, Inc.

Perez, R.H.: protocols for perinatal nursing practice, St. Louis, 1981, The C.V. Mosby Co.

Pritchard, J.A., and MacDonald, P.C.: Williams' obstetrics, New York, 1980, Appleton-Century-Crofts.

Tucker, S.M.: Fetal monitoring and fetal assessment in high-risk pregnancy, St. Louis, 1978, The C.V. Mosby Co.

25

Pharmacologic Control of Discomfort During the Birth Period

- Introduction
  - Goals of care
  - Informed consent
  - Choices of pharmacologic control of discomfort during birth period
  - Origin of discomfort during labor
  - Definitions
  - Intravenous and intramuscular routes of administration of medications
    - Intravenous route
    - Intramuscular route
- General Nursing Care
- Pharmacologic Analgesia and Anesthesia
- Combination Anesthesia for Cesarean Birth
- Intraspinal Narcotic Method
- Nonpharmacologic, Noninvasive Relief of Discomfort
  - Transcutaneous electrical nerve stimulation (TENS)

Introduction

The use of analgesia and anesthesia was not generally accepted as part of obstetric management until Queen Victoria used chloroform during the birth of her son in 1853. Since that time much study has gone into the development of pharmacologic control of discomfort* during the birth period. The goal of researchers is to develop methods that will provide adequate pain relief to women without adding to maternal or fetal risk.

All the drugs and procedures used to alleviate the discomforts of giving birth have some advantage or desirable characteristic, but none is perfect. In fact, widespread reappraisal of medications and methods used to relieve pain in obstetrics is important because at least 10% of maternal deaths are now due to anesthesia problems, mainly aspiration of vomitus and complications of high spinal anesthesia. Moreover, perinatal morbidity and mortality are greatly dependent on the analgesia and anesthesia employed. However, the specific effects of drugs on the fetus during labor and delivery are not easily interpreted.

GOALS OF CARE

Nursing management of obstetric analgesia and anesthesia combines the nurse's expertise in obstetrics with knowledge and understanding of techniques, drugs, and their potential complications. A general knowledge of analgesia and anesthesia is basic to implementation of the nursing process in relation to use of medications during labor.

The goals for nursing care related to pharmacologic control of discomfort include the following.

*See Chapter 19 for discussion of the nonpharmacologic control of discomfort.

1. To differentiate between the woman's need for pharmacologic or physiologic control of discomfort
2. To select the most effective techniques for each woman
3. To inform parents of their needs and rights in relation to use of analgesia or anesthesia
4. To prepare the medication, select the most advantageous route of administration, and administer it correctly
5. To monitor the effects of pharmacologic control on maternal and fetal well-being and maternal pain relief

INFORMED CONSENT

The anesthesiologist is responsible for informing clients of the alternative methods of pharmacologic pain relief that are available in the hospital setting. The description of the anesthetic techniques is essential to informed consent, even if the woman has received information about analgesia and anesthesia earlier in her pregnancy. This interview should take place just before or early in labor so the woman has time to consider the alternatives. The obstetric nurse plays a part in the informed consent by clarifying or further describing the procedures or by asking the anesthesiologist for further explanations. The explanation of the procedure to be used for anesthesia must include maternal position for administering the anesthetic, skin preparation, degree of discomfort, time requirement, and interval before the anesthetic is effective. The client must be informed that the anesthetic is not always effective and that there are potential side effects for both mother and fetus. Fig. 25.1 provides an example of an informed consent form in English and in Spanish.

CHOICES OF PHARMACOLOGIC CONTROL OF DISCOMFORT DURING BIRTH PERIOD

Today many obstetric clients generally are well informed as to their choices of analgesia and anesthesia. The *limitations* present in each hospital setting must be remembered, that is, whether or not there is an anesthesiologist physically present in the delivery suite, the availability of nursing staff to care for the woman following anesthetic administration, the skill and expertise of the staff, and the adequacy and availability of appropriate equipment.

Usually the woman has received information regarding anesthesia and analgesia in the obstetrician's office or clinic, in childbirth education classes, during hospital tours, or from family or friends. This information can be interpreted in various ways, and a lack of clear understanding can result in concern by the woman, her family, or care providers. The obstetric nurse or physician needs to spend time with the woman to be certain that she has a clear understanding of the information she has received.

Many factors enter into a woman's choice of analgesia or anesthesia, namely, her physical reserve (is she well rested or fatigued), length of labor, and position and size of the baby. The knowledgeable nurse or physician can suggest available alternatives to meet the woman's wishes for her labor and comfort. The choices for women during labor include the following:

1. Some analgesic administered intravenously in small doses
2. Analgesic during early labor followed by a regional block anesthetic
3. Analgesic during early labor followed by a local block anesthetic

Many women benefit from knowing the different techniques of administering anesthetics. Generally, the choices are offered to her within the limitations of the hospital and other contributing factors. There are times when high-risk factors require that the decision be made by the physician and presented to the woman (and her family).

ORIGIN OF DISCOMFORT DURING LABOR

The discomfort during labor has two origins. During the *first* stage of labor, the stage of the cervix, uterine contractions cause (1) the cervix to dilate (stretch) and to efface (thin out) and (2) uterine ischemia from contraction of the arteries to the myometrium.

The discomfort from cervical changes and uterine ischemia is *visceral*. The discomfort is located over the lower abdomen and radiates to the lumbar area of the back and down the thighs. Usually the woman experiences discomfort only during contractions and is free of pain between contractions.

During the *second* stage of labor, the stage of expulsion of the baby, the woman experiences perineal or *somatic* pain. Perineal discomfort results from the stretching of the vagina and perineum.

DEFINITIONS

analgesia The alleviation of pain; the raising of one's threshold for pain perception.

anesthesia The abolition of pain perception by interrupting the nerve impulses going to the brain.

The obstetric client's response to analgesic medications and anesthesia differs from that of the general sur-

Fig. 25.1
Consent form. **A,** English.

STANFORD UNIVERSITY HOSPITAL
STANFORD MEDICAL CENTER

CONSENT TO OPERATION, ADMINISTRATION OF ANESTHETICS, AND FOR DIAGNOSTIC OR THERAPEUTIC PROCEDURES

Date ______________ ______________________________
NAME OF PATIENT

Hour ______________ ______________________________
NAME OF ATTENDING PHYSICIAN

____
NAME OF SURGEON OR PHYSICIAN PERFORMING PROCEDURE

1. Your physician(s) has determined that the operation or procedure listed below may be beneficial in the diagnosis or treatment of your condition. All surgical operations and diagnostic and therapeutic procedures involve risks of complication, injury, or even death, from both known and unknown causes. No warranty or guarantee has been made as to result or cure.

2. OPERATION/PROCEDURE TO BE PERFORMED: ______________________________

____

____

3. Physicians performing professional services, such as anesthesia, radiology, pathology and the like, are not employees of the Hospital. These physicians are either in private practice in the community or faculty members of the Stanford University School of Medicine.

4. Stanford University Hospital and Clinics is an educational institution, and as part of the medical education program residents, interns, medical students, postgraduate fellows, and other health care students may, under the supervision of the attending physician, participate in the care of teaching patients.

5. **As a patient you have a right to receive as much information as you may need in order to give informed consent or to refuse the recommended course of treatment. Except in emergencies, your physician(s) should describe in language you can understand the proposed treatment or procedure, the medically significant risks involved, and the alternate courses of treatment or nontreatment, including the respective risks of each. If you have questions, you should consult your physician(s) prior to giving your written consent to such operation or procedure.**

Having read the above and having received the above information from my physician(s), I hereby authorize the above-named physician(s) and any associates or assistants of my physician(s) to perform the above-named operation or procedure and to provide such additional services as may be deemed medically reasonable and necessary, including, but not limited to, the administration and maintenance of anesthesia and services involving pathology and radiology. I further authorize the pathology service to use its discretion in the disposal of any severed tissue or member, except: ______________________________ .

____
SIGNATURE OF PATIENT, LEGAL GUARDIAN, CONSERVATOR OR LEGAL REPRESENTATIVE

____
SIGNATURE OF WITNESS

(If patient is a minor or unable to sign, complete the following.)

Patient is a minor_____ , or is unable to sign because ______________________________ .

______________________________ ______________________________
SIGNATURE OF FATHER SIGNATURE OF MOTHER

____
LEGAL GUARDIAN, CONSERVATOR, OR LEGAL REPRESENTATIVE

15-01 (Rev. 1/81) (Vea en el reverso la versión española)

Fig. 25.1, cont'd

Consent form. **B,** Spanish. (Courtesy Stanford University Hospital, Palo Alto, Calif.)

HOSPITAL DE LA UNIVERSIDAD DE STANFORD
CENTRO MEDICO DE STANFORD

PERMISO PARA OPERACION, PARA LA APLICACION DE ANESTESICOS Y PARA PROCEDIMIENTOS DIAGNOSTICOS O TERAPEUTICOS

Fecha ____________________ ______________________________________
NOMBRE DEL PACIENTE

Hora ____________________ ______________________________________
NOMBRE DEL MÉDICO DE CABECERA

____
NOMBRE DEL CIRUJANO O MÉDICO A CARGO DEL PROCEDIMIENTO

1. Su Médico (o Médicos) ha determinado que la operación o procedimiento que se consigna más adelante puede ser de beneficio para el diagnóstico o tratamiento de su estado de salud. Todas las operaciones quirúrgicas y procedimientos diagnosticos y terapeuticos inplican riesgos de complicación, lesión o aún muerte, de causas conocidas o desconocidas. Ninguna garantía o seguridad se ha determinado en cuanto al resultado o cura.

2. OPERACION/PROCEDIMIENTO A EJECUTAR: ______________________________________

____

____

3. Los médicos que prestan servicios profesionales tales como anestesia, radiología, patología y servicios semejantes no son empleados del hospital. Estos médicos se dedican a la práctica privada en la comunidad o son miembros de la Facultad de Medicina de la Universidad de Stanford.

4. El Hospital y la Clínica de la Universidad de Stanford constituyen una institución educacional, y como parte del programa de educación médica, los residentes, los internos, los estudiantes de medicina, los becarios graduados y otros estudiantes del cuidado de la salud pueden, bajo la supervisión del Médico en asistencia, participar en el cuidado de los pacientes que están bajo el plan de estudios.

5. **Como paciente, usted tiene derecho a recibir tanta información como usted pueda necesitar a fín de dar el correspondiente permiso, o a rechazar o negar el curso del tratamiento recomendado. Excepto en casos de emergencia su Médico (o Médicos) deben describir, en lenguage que usted pueda entender, el tratamiento o procedimiento propuesto, los significantes riesgos médicos comprendidos y los métodos alternativos de tratamiento o no tratamiento, incluyendo los respectivos riesgos de cada uno. Si usted desea saber algo o tiene preguntas que hacer, usted debe consultar a su Médico (o Médicos) antes de otorgar su permiso por escrito para tal operación o procedimiento a seguir.**

Habiendo leído lo explicado anteriormente y habiendo recibido la información anterior de mi Médico (o Médicos), por la presente autorizo al Médico (o Médicos) mencionado anteriormente y a cualquiera de sus colaboradores o ayudantes de mi Médico (o Médicos) para llevar a cabo la operación que se detalla anteriormente o procedimiento a seguir y a proveer tales servicios adicionales como fueren razonables y necesarios desde el punto de vista médico, incluyendo, pero no limitados, la aplicación y mantenimiento de anestesia y servicios de patologia y de radiologia. También autorizo al servicio patológico para usar su criterio en la disposición de cualquier tejido o miembro removido, excepto: ______________________________________ .

____
FIRMA DEL PACIENTE, TUTOR, ENCARGADO, O REPRESENTATANTE LEGAL

____
FIRMA DEL TESTIGO

(Si el Paciente es menor de edad o no puede firmar, complete lo siguiente.)

El Paciente es menor de edad _____, o no puede firmar porque ______________________________________ .

______________________ ______________________
FIRMA DEL PADRE FIRMA DE LA MADRE

____
FIRMA DEL TUTOR, DEFENSOR O REPRESENTANTE LEGAL

Table 25.1
Comparison of General Surgical Client and Obstetric Client

Factor	Obstetric Client	General Surgical Client
Psychologic status	Many women wish to be active participants in event	Desire for total relief from pain
Persons affected	Mother and fetus	Client only
Physiologic functions		
Sensitivity to anesthetics, analgesics, tranquilizers	Increased	No specific alteration
Upper airway	Edema present in late pregnancy	As above
Oxygen requirement	Increased; greater risk of hypoxia	As above
Pulmonary minute ventilation	Increased; increases speed of induction of inhalation anesthesia	As above
Risk of pulmonary aspiration of stomach contents	Increased; may have eaten within previous few hours; gastric relaxation and delay in emptying increase likelihood of food in stomach; gravid uterus displaces stomach upward and compresses its volume	As above; with few exceptions is NPO for 8 hr before surgery
Cardiovascular system	Heavy, large gravid uterus can compress aorta and vena cava resulting in sudden hypotension and cardiovascular collapse, and fetus may suffer hypoxia and acidosis	Client with a large heavy tumor also may be subject to sudden hypotension and cardiovascular collapse

gical client. These differences are presented in Table 25.1.

INTRAVENOUS AND INTRAMUSCULAR ROUTES OF ADMINISTRATION OF MEDICATIONS

Intravenous route. The preferred route of administration is through intravenous tubing (Fig. 25.2). The medication is given slowly in small doses at the *beginning* of three to five consecutive contractions. During uterine contractions, the blood flow through the intervillous spaces of the placenta is diminished; therefore the amount of drug crossing the placenta to the fetus is minimized. With decreased placental transfer, the mother's degree of pain relief is maximized. The intravenous route has the following results:

1. Pain relief with smaller doses of the drug
2. A predictable onset of pain relief
3. A predictable duration of effect

Intramuscular route. Intramuscular injections of analgesics, although still used, are no longer the preferred route of administration to the laboring woman. Some of the identified disadvantages with the intramuscular route include the following:

1. Onset of pain relief is delayed for several minutes.
2. Higher doses of medication are required.
3. Medication is released from the muscle tissue at an unpredictable rate and is available for transfer across the placenta to the fetus.

Intramuscular injections are given in the upper arm if regional anesthesia is planned later in the labor. The autonomic blockade from the regional anesthesia (e.g., epidural) increases blood flow to the gluteal region and accelerates absorption of the drug. The maternal plasma level of the drug necessary to bring pain relief usually is reached 45 minutes after injection, followed by a decline in plasma levels. The maternal drug levels (after intramuscular injections have been given) are unequal because of uneven distribution (maternal uptake) and metabolism.

The advantage of giving intramuscular injection is quick administration.

General Nursing Care

The implementation of the nursing process during the birth period may be accomplished on several levels:

1. The first day a nursing student arrives on a labor unit, she may feel intimidated and unable to see what nursing care she can provide. Yet, even on the first day, the student comes with several years' experience in communicating with people, expressing concern, providing comfort measures, and seeking assistance when unable to answer questions or to determine the next course of action. The presence of a caring human being during a trying time is valuable in itself.

2. As the student develops a sounder theory base and acquires more experience with the nursing process, she can take an increasingly active role in management of discomfort during the birth period.

Fig. 25.2
Intravenous narcotic analgesia method of administration. Drug is administered at beginning of a contraction so that drug circulates through mother first and reaches baby when intervillous space has a diminished blood flow, thus minimizing amount of drug that reaches fetus.

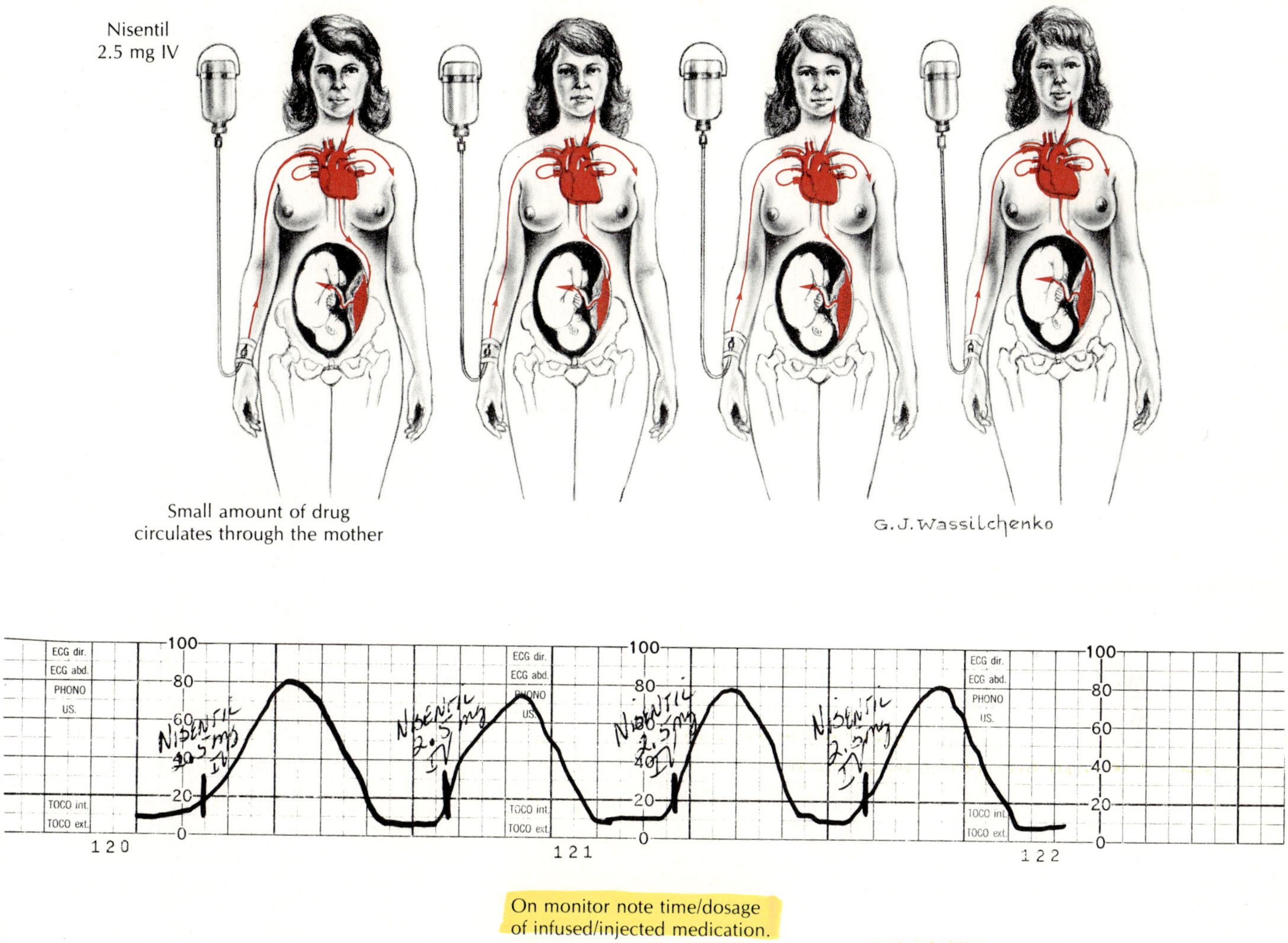

3. For the motivated nurse, it takes about 2 years of full-time nursing on a busy labor unit to develop the high level of competence needed for accurate assessment, analysis, planning, and implementation in regard to pharmacologic control of discomfort during the birth period. The rewards and professional satisfaction are worth the investment of time, energy, and even sweat and tears.

Following are some examples of nursing diagnoses relevant to pharmacologic control of discomfort during the birth period:

1. Inability of the mother to cooperate while being positioned for nerve block analgesia because of lack of knowledge of procedure, expected sensation, and her role
2. Increased anxiety (mother, father, family) because of lack of awareness of options for analgesia and anesthesia
3. Potential dystocia or injury to bladder from bladder distention because of loss of sensation following nerve root block anesthesia
4. Inability to bear down during second stage because of loss of sensation following nerve root block anesthesia

General Nursing Actions

Assessment

1. *On admission* of the woman, the nurse does the following:
   a. Notes history of allergies and liver or renal disease; inquires again whether woman remembers having an unusual reaction to medications, cleansing agents, tape, and so on (Fig. 25.3)
   b. Notes degree of hydration by assessing intake and output, moisture of mucous membranes, and skin turgor
   c. Inquires if woman has a respiratory problem (cold) and the time and type of food taken at her last meal
   d. Notes woman's level of understanding of analgesia and anesthesia
   e. Notes woman's need for pain relief
2. *Throughout the labor* the nurse assesses the woman's need for pain relief (see symptomatology, p. 352).

Implementation	Rationale
1. *During preparation for administering medications* the nurse does the following:	
a. Provides explanation of procedure and what will be asked of woman	The unknown and the unexpected are very ego weakening. Knowledge assists the woman to cooperate or to follow directions (e.g., for maintaining correct position).
b. Asks woman to void	Sensation of bladder filling is diminished or lost. Bladder distention can delay or inhibit baby's passage through birth canal, and the baby's passage can result in trauma to the bladder.
c. Obtains base-line values for pulse, respirations, and blood pressure; notes frequency, duration, and intensity of contractions as well as station	If values differ from earlier values, report to physician stat. Some values do change with medication; changes from base line following the procedure may require medical or nursing intervention. Until the nurse has become experienced in labor management, she should check out all analyses of assessment with experienced personnel.
d. Obtains fetal heart rate (FHR)	If FHR differs from previous values, alert physician stat, before medication is administered. Following procedure, changes from previous FHR may require medical or nursing intervention.
2. *During the procedure* the nurse does the following:	
a. Ensures safety by selecting wrapped supplies that are sterile and are not outdated; prepares mother's skin (nurse [and physician] practices *good handwashing techniques*)	Prevent infection
b. Assists woman into proper position and assists her to maintain appropriate position	Woman's attention span and ability to follow directions may be decreased because of discomfort of labor, fatigue, previous medications, and anxiety. Injury may occur from the needle if woman moves. Needle may be jarred from intended site.
c. Assists physician, as appropriate, if needed; opens sterile trays and packages; adds medications	Prevent infection. Administer correct medication. Read label of drug, then insist the physician read the label aloud.
d. Coaches woman regarding sensations she can expect	Prevent or minimize anxiety caused by unexpected sensations.
e. Raises side rails; places call bell in easy reach; monitors medicated woman closely	Prevent injury from falls.
f. Avoids prolonged pressure on an anesthetized part (e.g., lying on one side with weight on one leg; tight bed clothes on feet) or if stirrups are used, pads stirrups; adjusts stirrups at same level and angle; places both legs into stirrups simultaneously and avoids pressure to popliteal angle; applies restraints without restricting circulation	Prolonged pressure on leg may result in decreased sensation, which may persist for months; pressure on feet may result in footdrop. Prevent injury to nerves (popliteal nerve), to muscles (straining muscles by not placing or removing legs from stirrups simultaneously), or to tissue (tight restraints on feet).

Continued.

Fig. 25.3

Obstetric labor admission record. (Courtesy Stanford University Hospital, Palo Alto, Calif.)

(addressograph stamp)

STANFORD UNIVERSITY HOSPITAL
Stanford University Medical Center
Stanford, California 94305

OBSTETRICAL LABOR
ADMISSION RECORD

Admission Date ________ Time ________ M.D. Notified ________ Time ________
Patient's Age ______ EDC ______ Parity ________ Patient's Blood Type ______ Father's Blood Type ________
☐ In Labor: Began On ______ 19 ______ Time ______ Membranes ________
☐ Not in Labor: Admitted for ☐ Induction ☐ Suspected Labor ☐ Other ________
Anesthesia Preferred ________ Feeding: ☐ Breast ☐ Bottle
Time of Last Meal ______ Type of Food ______ Pediatrician ________
Room Type ________ Rooming In ________

COMPLICATIONS AND MEDICATIONS DURING PREGNANCY

Initial Visit:
☐ 1st trimester
☐ 2nd trimester
☐ 3rd trimester

Diagnostic Studies Done:
☐ None
☐ Estriols
☐ NST & CST
☐ NST only
☐ CST only
☐ Ultrasound
☐ Amniocentesis: ☐ L/S ☐ Shake ☐ Other ________

Cardiovascular:
☐ None
☐ Mild pre-eclampsia
☐ Severe pre-eclampsia
☐ Eclampsia
☐ Chronic hypertension
☐ Heart Disease

Bleeding ($\geqslant$ 20 wks GA):
☐ None
☐ Placenta previa
☐ Abruptio placenta
☐ Vasa previa
☐ Other bleeding

Diabetes:
☐ None
☐ Non-insulin
☐ Insulin dependent
☐ With vascular disease
☐ Suspected macrosomia

Pre-term Labor
($\geqslant$ 20 wks and $<$ 37 wks GA):
☐ None
☐ Spontaneous w/o underlying cause
☐ PROM
☐ Pre-eclampsia
☐ Eclampsia
☐ Bleeding
☐ Multiple births
☐ Hydramnios
☐ Infection
☐ Incompetent cervix
☐ Other uterine anomalies
☐ Other known etiology ________

Other Problems:
☐ None
☐ Anemia
☐ Renal disease
☐ Urinary tract infection
☐ Rh incompatibility
☐ Other ________

Medications Used:
☐ None
☐ Antibiotics
☐ Antihistamines
☐ Aspirin
☐ Barbiturates
☐ Decongestants
☐ Diuretics
☐ Iron/Vitamins
☐ Tranquilizers
☐ Insulin
☐ Tocolytic ________
☐ Steroids ________
☐ Other ________

ADMISSION PREPARATION AND EXAMINATIONS

Admission Preparations: ☐ Half Prep. ☐ Abdominal Prep. ☐ Enema ☐ No Prep.
Temp. ______ R. ______ P. ______ BP. ______ Ht. ______ Wt. ______
Head: ☐ Normal ☐ Other ________ Neck: ☐ Normal ☐ Other ________
Heart: ☐ Normal ☐ Other ________ Lungs: ☐ Normal ☐ Other ________
Abdomen: ☐ Normal ☐ Other ________
Fetal presentation ________ Estimated Fetal Wt. ________
Fetal Heart Rate ________ Uterine Contractions ________
Vagina: Dilation ______ Effacement ________ Consistency ______ Position ________
Fetal Position ________ Station ________
Other Significant Findings: ________

________ M.D. ________ R.N.

☐ Taken to Delivery Room without further examinations.

15-108 Rev. 6/82 WHITE - Mother's Medical Record CANARY - Nursery PINK - Perinatal Outreach

General Nursing Actions—cont'd

Implementation	Rationale
3. *Following the procedure* the nurse does the following: a. Repeats all nursing actions implemented when preparing the woman for the procedure: (1) Answers questions (2) Keeps woman's bladder empty (3) Monitors vital signs, blood pressure, contractions, and FHR	Rationale remains the same.
b. Monitors woman's response to medication: (1) Level of pain relief (2) Return of sensations and perception of pain (3) Allergic or untoward reactions (e.g., hypotension)	Physician needs to be kept informed so that pain relief is maintained without untoward reactions.

Recording

The nurse records the following:

1. Evidence of need for analgesia or anesthesia
2. Request for medication order from physician if necessary; medications may appear on the physician's order sheet as prn orders.
3. Medication—dosage and route of administration
4. Effects on woman, e.g., "discomfort lessened," or effects on fetus, "FHR, 145 bpm"

Table 25.2
Four General Categories of Pharmacologic Analgesia and Anesthesia

Category	Definition	Examples
Systemic medication	Medication that is ingested or injected with a syringe; affects central and peripheral nervous systems, but total unconsciousness does not result	Narcotics Sedatives Tranquilizers Amnesics
Inhalation analgesia	Inhalation of drugs in subanesthesia concentrations; some may be self-administered	Methoxyflurane Nitrous oxide
General anesthesia	Medication administered intravenously or by inhalation resulting in unconsciousness	IV: thiopental sodium (Pentothal) Inhalation: halothane (Fluothane)
Regional (conduction) anesthesia	Local anesthetics injected to block primary sensory (pain) neuropathways that pass from uterus to spinal cord by accompanying sympathetic nerves	Pudendal block Local infiltration Peridural-epidural or caudal Spinal Paracervical block*

*Paracervical block is well suited for gynecologic procedures. Its use during labor has decreased because fetal bradycardia results frequently.

Pharmacologic Analgesia and Anesthesia

Nonpharmacologic techniques for management of discomfort during labor are discussed in Chapter 19.

There are four general categories of analgesia and anesthesia (Table 25.2). A number of these approaches to pain relief are applicable to home as well as hospital delivery.

All the drugs and procedures used to alleviate the discomforts of giving birth have some advantage or desirable characteristic, but none is perfect. In fact, widespread reappraisal of medications and methods used to relieve pain in obstetrics is important because at least 10% of maternal deaths are now caused by anesthesia problems, mainly aspiration of vomitus and complications of high spinal anesthesia. Moreover, perinatal morbidity and mortality are greatly dependent on the analgesia and anesthesia employed. However, the specific effects of drugs on the fetus during labor and delivery are not easily interpreted.

In Table 25.3, three of the four general categories of analgesia and anesthesia are discussed under the following headings: category with examples, routes of administration, and goals; nursing actions: assessment and analysis; and nursing actions: planning and implementation. For the fourth general category, regional or conduction analgesia and anesthesia, additional headings are added, namely, characteristics of each type of technique and a description of each method.

Table 25.4 is a quick reference to assist the nurse in deciding what medication may be best suited for the different phases and stages of labor.

Text continued on p. 524.

Table 25.3
Pharmacologic Control of Discomfort During the Birth Period and the Nursing Process

Category and Goals	Nursing Actions: Assessment and Analysis	Nursing Actions: Planning and Implementation
Systemic medication		
Examples: sedatives Short duration: pentobarbital (Nembutal) Intermediate: amobarbital (Amytal Sodium) Long duration: phenobarbital sodium (Luminal Sodium) Goals: relieve anxiety and induce sleep without depressing maternal respiration or fetus	Before administration of medication: Review chart for allergies, history of liver or kidney damage Stage of labor; progress in labor Degree of apprehension Woman states she is anxious Woman is clenching fists, restless, seems tense Woman is *not* experiencing pain Following administration of medication: Strength and frequency of uterine contractions should not decrease appreciably Little change in maternal vital signs; with decreased anxiety, pulse, respirations, and blood pressure do decrease but should not fall below woman's normal base line in her prenatal record Assess woman's response to medication Assess FHR Assess for pain	Alert physician if chart reveals history of drug allergy, liver or kidney damage Administer if: Woman is apprehensive, tense Woman is in early latent phase of first stage of labor Do not give without an analgesic if woman has pain Continue with comfort measures and general hygiene given to any woman in labor If changes occur in contractions, maternal and/or fetal vital signs, record and notify physician If woman begins to get uncomfortable, confer with physician re. need for analgesic relief
Examples: narcotic analgesics Morphine Meperdine hydrochloride (Demerol) Pentazocine (Talwin) Fentanyl (potent synthetic narcotic with analgesic activity; has 100 times the potency of morphine, with a rapid onset of action and a short duration of activity) Goals: relief of severe, persistent, or recurrent pain, without nausea and vomiting or respiratory depression of mother or fetus	Before administration of medication: Review chart to note history of: Drug allergies Liver and kidney damage Substance (drug) abuse History of asthma Stage of labor; progress in labor: Nullipara: before full dilatation Multipara: before 7 cm dilatation Degree of discomfort: mother states she is having pain; cries out with pain; clenches teeth, fists Maternal and fetal vital signs	Do not administer if birth is expected within 2 hr Explain expected effect
	Following administration of medication: Note time between administration of narcotic and time of baby's birth Maximal effect (IM) in 15 min, duration of 2 hr Drug may slow labor or it may accelerate labor as woman relaxes	If baby is born when drug reaches maximal effect, baby may be depressed and require resuscitation; prepare Narcan (0.05 mg) to be given into baby's umbilical vein

Continued.

Table 25.3—cont'd
Pharmacologic Control of Discomfort During the Birth Period and the Nursing Process

Category and Goals	Nursing Actions: Assessment and Analysis	Nursing Actions: Planning and Implementation
Systemic medication—cont'd		
	Assess for adverse side effects every 15-30 min: Respiratory depression FHR deceleration and loss of short-term variability noted by electronic fetal monitor Nausea, vomiting, dizziness, sweating, dysphoria Bronchospasm in women who suffer from asthma	
Examples: narcotic antagonists Naloxone hydrochloride (Narcan)* Levallorphan tartrate (Lorfan) Nalorphine (Nalline) Goal: Reversal of narcotic depression of mother and/or baby	Note which drug was given, time, amount, route; respiratory depression from any drug other than a narcotic cannot be reversed with these drugs	Do not give Narcan to mother addicted to narcotics because this causes instant withdrawal symptoms; Narcan given to mother reverses pain relief instantly, so that she must be prepared for return of pain or a second form of pain relief is given (e.g., epidural)
Examples: analgesics—potentiating drugs (ataractics, tranquilizers) Promethazine hydrochloride (Phenergan) Propiomazine hydrochloride (Largon) Hydroxyzine pamoate (Vistaril) Promazine hydrochloride (Sparine) Route: IV, IM Goals: increase desirable effect of analgesics without increasing dose of analgesics (i.e., ataractic potentiates effects of analgesic that is given with it and acts as antiemetic	Same as for narcotic analgesics	Same as for narcotic analgesics
Example: amnesics, e.g., scopolamine (belladonna alkaloid) Route: IM Goal: dulls memory and parasympathetic nervous system	After administration, assess for excitation and restlessness caused by hallucinations; assess for fetal tachycardia or bradycardia; monitor maternal heart rate	Generally not recommended; if woman is given this drug, *stay with her constantly* to protect her from injury; nurse must also take precautions against being hurt by woman; restrain if necessary; if drug is given, it is given with narcotic to decrease possibility of excitation and hallucinations If FHR and variability are changed, or if maternal heart rate falls below 70 beats/min, physician may want to order an antagonist (phenothiazine or diazepam)
Inhalation analgesia		
Mother breathes subanesthetic concentrations of inhalation anesthetic; if given properly, woman remains conscious but has profound pain relief Examples: Trichloroethylene (Trilene) Methoxyflurane (Penthrane)	Monitor vital signs closely (be alert for cardiac arrhythmias) every 30 min and FHR every 15 min	Stay with woman; never administer drug for woman because overdose is a risk

*Preferred drug because it does not intensify depressive effects if depression is caused by drugs other than narcotics.

Table 25.3—cont'd
Pharmacologic Control of Discomfort During the Birth Period and the Nursing Process

Category and Goals	Nursing Actions: Assessment and Analysis	Nursing Actions: Planning and Implementation
Inhalation analgesia—cont'd		
Route: self-administered (usually) from a capsule and mask strapped to wrist; physician sets desired concentration; mother inhales drug during contractions Goal: profound analgesia while remaining conscious; some amnesia for painful events	Mother should remain conscious and not become delirious or excited	Alert physician and remove from mother's hand if: Mother has cardiac arrhythmia Mother loses consciousness; FHR abnormalities occur
Example: nitrous oxide (N_2O_2) Route: administered by trained personnel, during contractions, or continuously Goal: analgesia	Monitor maternal-fetal; vital signs every 15 min; assessment carried out by trained personnel	Trained personnel must remain with woman
General anesthesia		
Rarely indicated for uncomplicated vaginal delivery; woman is not awake; danger of aspiration and respiratory depression; safer than regional anesthesia for hypovolemic clients; does not depress neonate unless mother is anesthetized deeply	Anesthetist assesses woman continuously	If general anesthesia is being considered, keep woman NPO and see that an intravenous infusion is established
Examples: Thiopental (Pentothal) sodium (IV)—produces rapid induction of anesthesia; depresses neonate; useful in controlling convulsions Halothane (fluothane) (inhalation)—relaxes uterus quickly, facilitates intrauterine manipulation, version, and extraction	Postanesthesia recovery Assess every 15 min until vital signs are stable and woman is alert and reactive Routine postpartum assessment If woman delivered by cesarean birth, do routine postsurgery assessment—wound assessment, intake and output, etc.	Recovery room care Maintain open airway Maintain cardiopulmonary functions Prevent postpartal hemorrhage
Goals: produces general loss of sensitivity to touch, pain, or other stimulations	Postrecovery period Routine postpartum assessment Assess readiness to see baby Assess her response to anesthesia and event that necessitated general anesthesia delivery (e.g., giving birth by cesarean delivery when vaginal delivery was anticipated)	Postrecovery period Routine postpartum care Facilitate parent-child attachment as soon as possible Answer mother's questions
Regional (conduction) anesthesia		
Local anesthetics injected to block primary neuropathways that result in temporary interruption of conduction of nerve impulses, notably pain; mother remains awake Examples: common agents in 0.5-1.0% solution Procaine hydrochloride (Novocain) Lidocaine (Xylocaine) hydrochloride Bupivacaine (Marcaine) hydrochloride Tetracaine (Pontocaine) hydrochloride Mepivacaine hydrochloride (Carbocaine)		

Continued.

Fig. 25.4
Membranes and spaces of spinal cord.

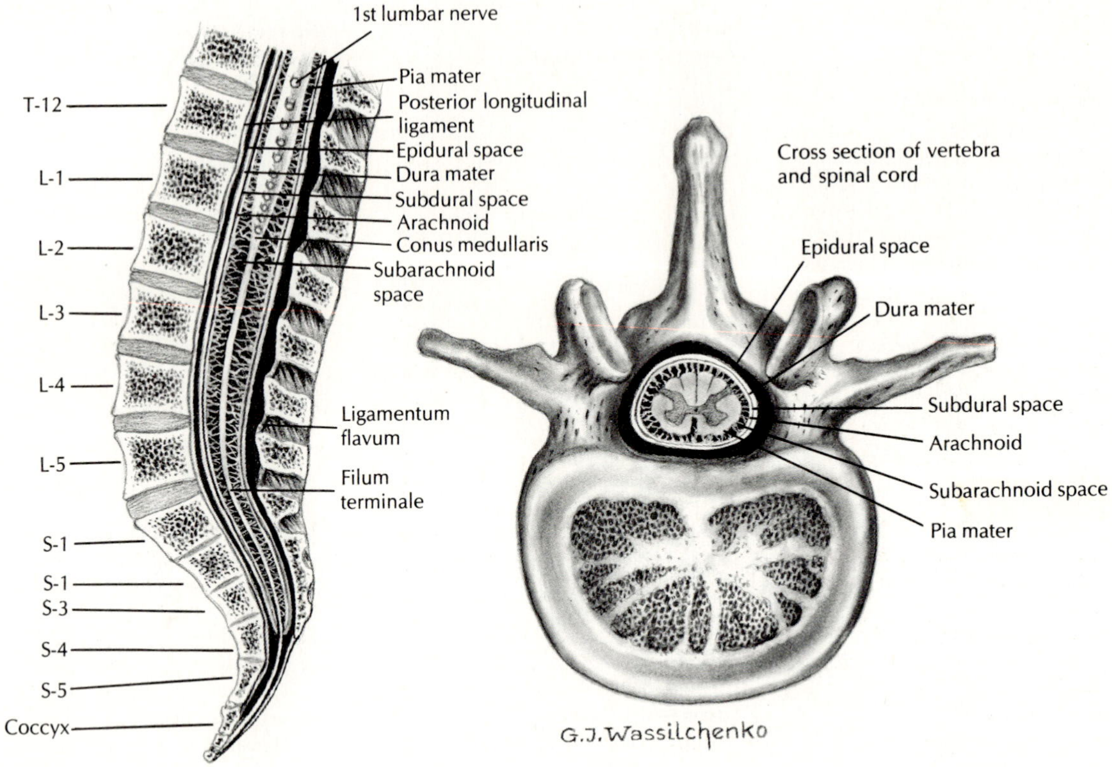

Fig. 25.5
Pain pathways and sites of interruption.

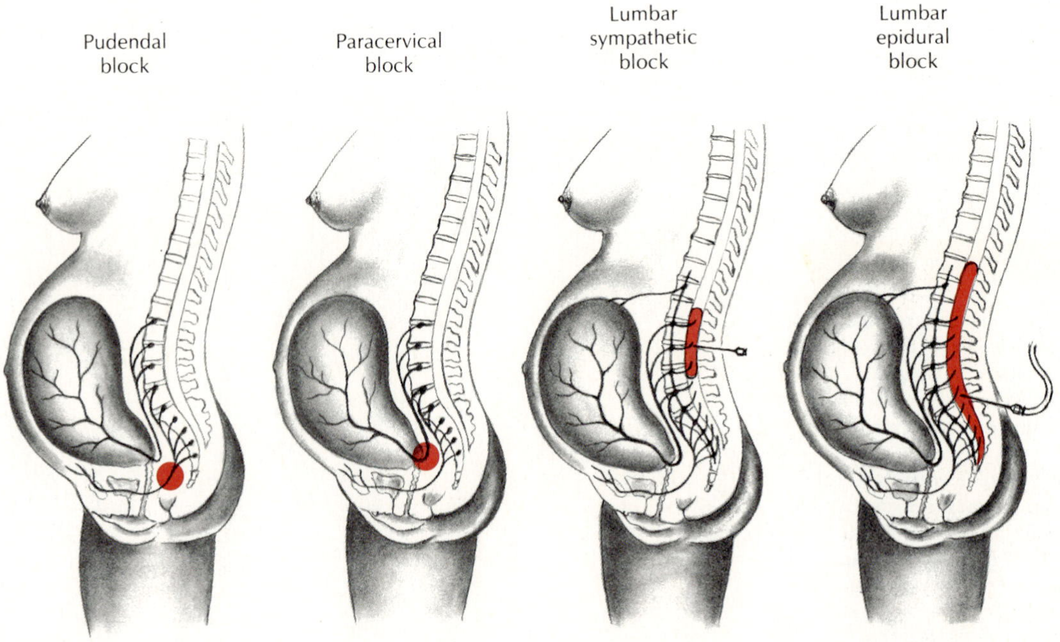

Table 25.3—cont'd
Pharmacologic Control of Discomfort During the Birth Period and the Nursing Process

Category and Goals	Nursing Actions: Assessment and Analysis	Nursing Actions: Planning and Implementation
Regional (conduction) anesthesia—cont'd		
Peripheral nerve block (Fig. 25.4)		
Pudendal (5-10 ml on each side): anesthetizes lower two thirds of vagina and perineum; of short duration (30 min)—given for delivery and repair; local anesthesia, may be done by physician or anesthetist; simple and safe, does not depress neonate; may inhibit bearing-down reflex	Physician or anesthetist is responsible	See general nursing actions
Paracervical block (5-10 ml on each side)*	Physician or anesthetist is responsible	See general nursing actions
Local infiltration: useful for perineal repairs (Fig. 25.5)	Physician or anesthetist is responsible	See general nursing actions
Nerve root block (Fig. 25.6): requires trained anesthesiologist; with proper administration, relieves pain completely, may prolong labor if given too early; hypotension from vasodilation (below anesthesia level) is likely; fetal bradycardia may occur as a result of maternal hypotension; bearing-down reflex partially or completely eliminated, necessitating outlet forceps at delivery: mother remains awake throughout delivery; absence of pain may facilitate maternal-child attachment; postanesthesia headache if medication mixes with cerebrospinal fluid; fosters postnatal uterine and bladder atony; can be used for women with metabolic, lung, and heart diseases	General assessment for all nerve blocks: note degree of hydration, history of allergy, skin infection over back, previous neural or spinal injury or disease, and attitude toward anesthesia Predelivery monitor Maternal vital signs and FHR Assess for return of pain Monitor labor if nerve root block is established during late first stage Rate of IV fluid infusion Perineum to see if delivery is imminent (or monitor progress by vaginal examination)	General nursing actions for all nerve blocks Hydrate by intravenous infusion Explain to woman expected feeling as anesthesia begins (warm toes) and as it wears off (tingling); help position her, offering reassurance and support; it is very frightening to not be able to see the procedure and to deal with only sensations and sounds; do not make promises of complete pain relief; each woman may have a differing perception of pain, or block may not provide complete relief Treatment of hypotension (with resultant fetal bradycardia): turn from supine to lateral position or elevate legs; administer humidified oxygen by mask at 10-12 L/min; increase rate of IV fluids If contractions become less frequent, of less intensity, or of shorter duration, report to physician immediately; physician may need to augment labor; assist as necessary Add forceps to delivery table
	Postdelivery monitor Uterine tone Bladder tone Return of sensation	Provide assistance to move from delivery table to bed; maintain good uterine tone; prevent bladder distention; prevent injury by keeping side rails up and assisting her when she ambulates
Peridural nerve block	These sterile procedures are performed by skilled anesthetists; for each of the nerve blocks:	Assist with positioning woman
Epidural (Figs. 25.7): useful during first and second stages; can be given as "one shot" or over a period of time; given on top of (or over) dura through third, fourth, or fifth lumbar interspace; risk of dural puncture	Injection site is cleansed, wiped dry, and draped; physician makes a skin wheal over site to anesthetize skin and ligaments; short, beveled, 18-gauge needle inserted into interspace; resistance to injection of saline or air disappears as needle enters epidural space; aspira-	For introduction of epidural anesthesia, woman is positioned as for a spinal injection or in a modified Sims' position (Fig. 25.8); for modified lateral Sims' position, woman is placed on her left side, shoulders parallel, legs slightly flexed, and back kept straight (If she

*Rarely used during labor because of its effect on fetus; an effective technique for gynecologic procedures (see Fig. 25.5)

Continued.

Fig. 25.6
A, Use of needle guide ("Iowa trumpet") in pudendal anesthetic block. **B,** Pudendal block technique. Superficial and deep innervations on both sides are injected through only two skin wheals. Dotted lines show paths of needle infiltrating both pudendal and ilioinguinal nerves. (**A** from Benson, R.C.: Handbook of obstetrics and gynecology, ed. 5, Los Altos, Calif., 1974, Lange Medical Publications. **B** from McLennan, C.E., and Sandberg, E.C.: Synopsis of obstetrics, ed. 9, St. Louis, 1974, The C.V. Mosby Co.)

A

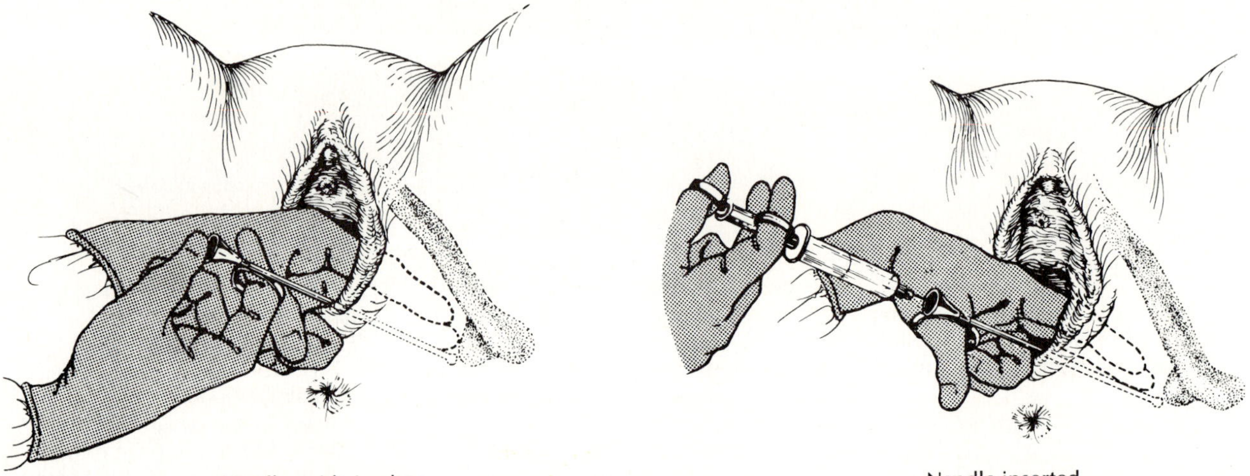

Needle guide in place on ischial spine

Needle inserted through needle guide

PUDENDAL

B

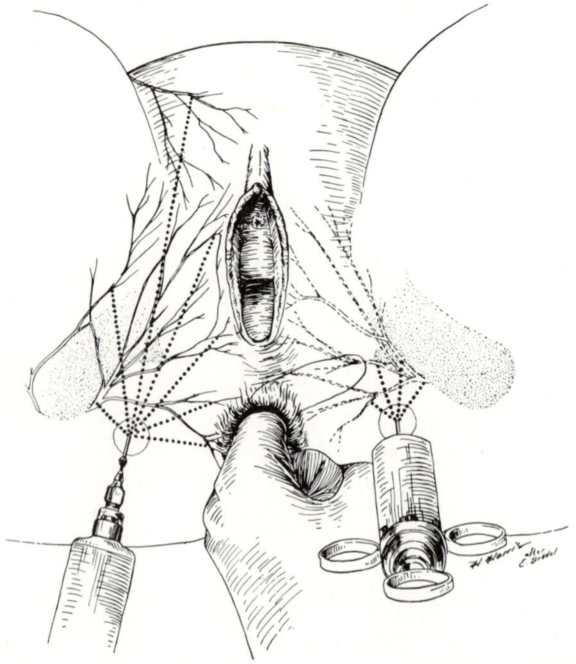

Fig. 25.7
Tray for local infiltration anesthesia. (Courtesy Stanford University Hospital, Stanford, Calif.)

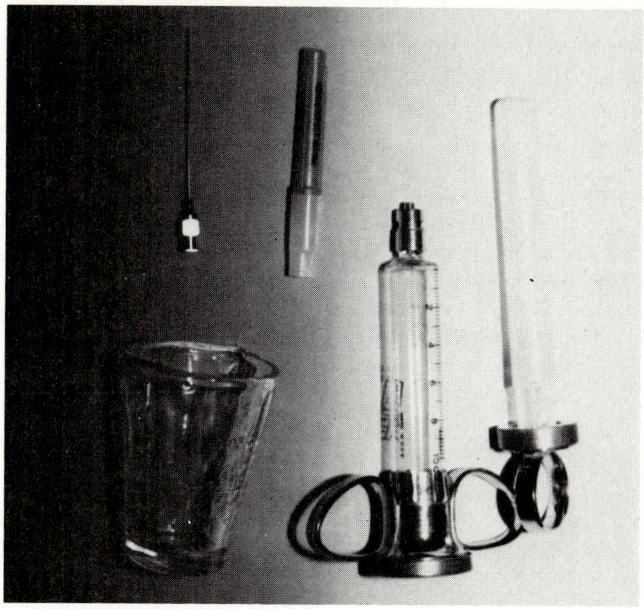

Fig. 25.8
A, Regional anesthesia in obstetrics. **B,** Level of anesthesia necessary for cesarean delivery and for vaginal delivery. (Courtesy Ross Laboratories, Columbus, Ohio.)

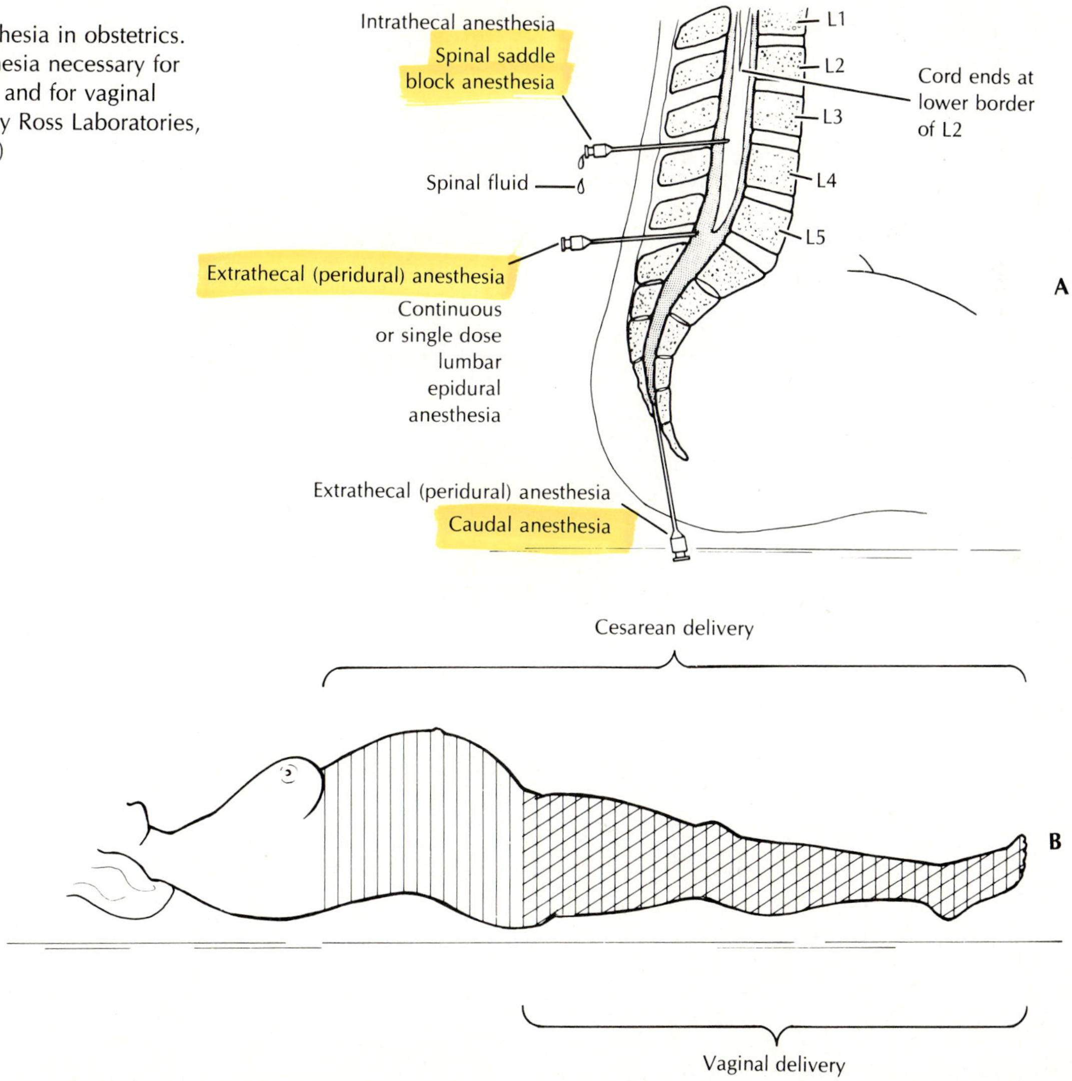

Table 25.3—cont'd
Pharmacologic Control of Discomfort During the Birth Period and the Nursing Process

Category and Goals	Nursing Actions: Assessment and Analysis	Nursing Actions: Planning and Implementation
Regional (conduction) anesthesia—cont'd		
Epidural—cont'd During labor, analgesic doses are given For delivery, anesthetic dose is given	tion rules out entrance into blood vessel or subarachnoid space; test dose of anesthetic is injected, followed in 5 min by anesthetic dose; if medication is to be given over time, catheter is threaded 3-5 cm beyond tip of needle and needle is removed; catheter is taped in place; test dose is given first	were to arch her back, epidural space would be decreased.) If catheter is threaded, woman may feel a momentary twinge down her leg, hip, or back; anesthetist or nurse reassures her it is not a sign of injury
Caudal (through sacral hiatus) (Fig. 25.9): useful during first and second stages; can be given as "one shot" or over a period of time; given in peridural space through sacral hiatus	Once needle and plastic catheter have been inserted into caudal canal, test dose is given; after 5 min anesthesiologist checks anal sphincter for relaxation and temperature of lower extremities (relaxation of anal sphincter and increased warmth of feet indicate proper placement of catheter in caudal canal); remainder of dose is then given; relief is experienced in a few minutes, and repeated doses may be administered as effect wears off; catheter and syringe are taped securely in position so that woman is free to move about in bed	Woman is placed in a modified knee-chest or lateral Sims' position, with upper leg well flexed at hip and knee and lower leg extended
Subarachnoid (low spinal, saddle nerve block [Fig. 25.10]); usually given as "one shot" when fetal head is on perineum; medication is mixed with cerebrospinal fluid in subarachnoid space; injected through third, fourth, or fifth lumbar interspace	Double-needle technique is used; 20- to 21-gauge needle with stylet is placed into epidural space; then 25- to 26-gauge needle is inserted into larger needle and advanced through dura into subarachnoid space; when stylet is removed, a drop of clear (cerebrospinal) fluid can be seen at hub of needle; anesthetic is injected and needle removed	Woman is positioned in a sitting position with her buttocks near edge of delivery table, feet supported on a stool; woman is asked to place her arms between her knees, flex her head, and arch her back "like a rainbow"; after medication is injected, she remains sitting up for 20-30 sec; then she is placed supine with a pillow under her head, and a pelvic wedge to displace uterus to left Postdelivery: encourage oral fluids; lying flat in bed for 8-12 hr; observe for spinal headache (see p. 703) and bladder and uterine atony

Fig. 25.9
A, Epidural tray. Clockwise from top: three gauze sponges; two medicine glasses; ampules of normal saline and 1% xylocaine; sponges for sponge holder; epidural catheters; needles; Tuohy needle with stylet; syringes. **B,** Tuohy needle with curved tip. **C,** Crawford needle with stylet. (Courtesy Stanford University Hospital, Palo Alto, Calif.)

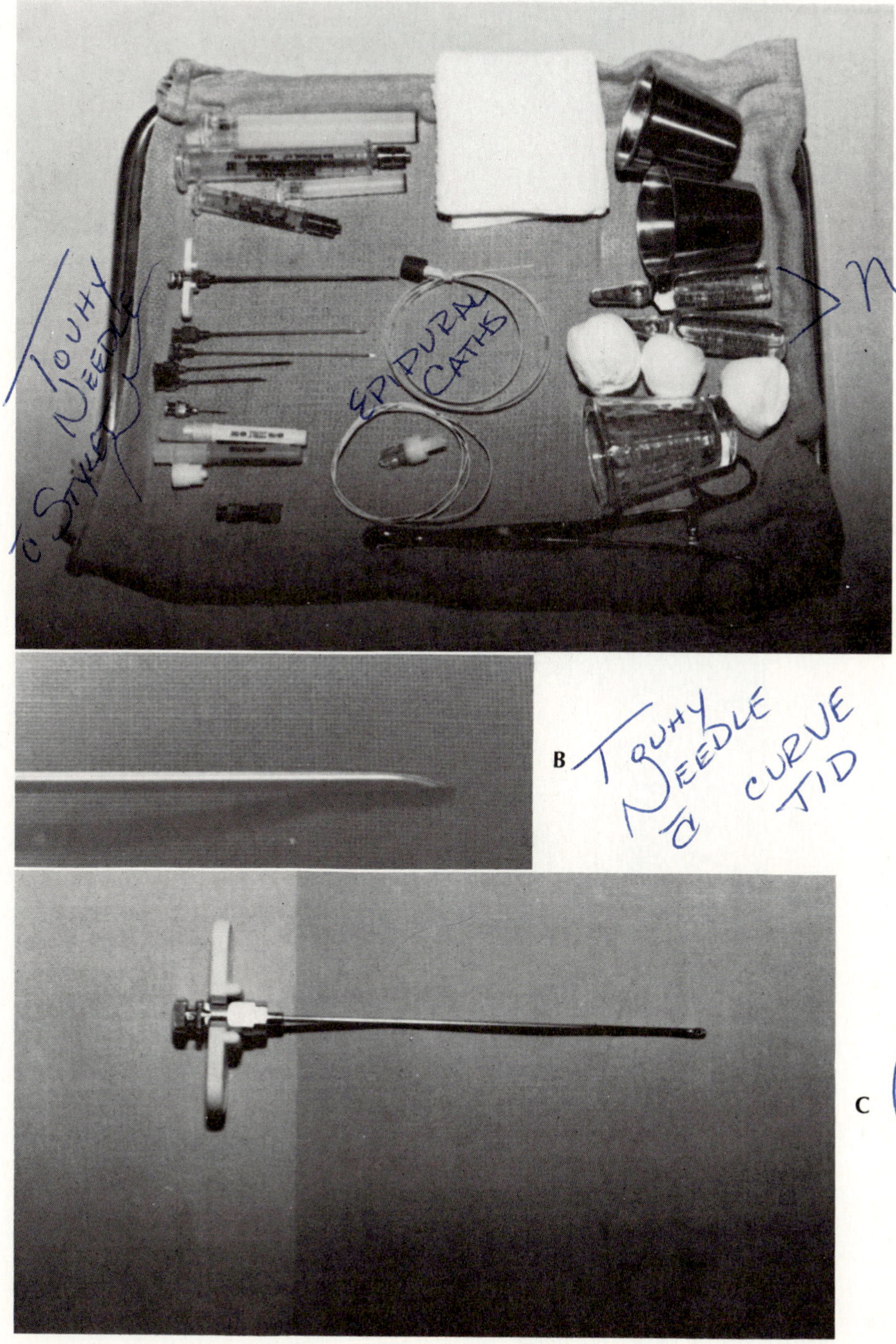

A

B

C

Fig. 25.10
Epidural anesthesia. **A,** Skin is prepared with antiseptic solution (Betadine). Anesthesiologist is explaining the procedure step by step. **B,** Area is draped with sterile towels. Nurse continues to support woman. (Courtesy Stanford University Hospital, Palo Alto, Calif.)

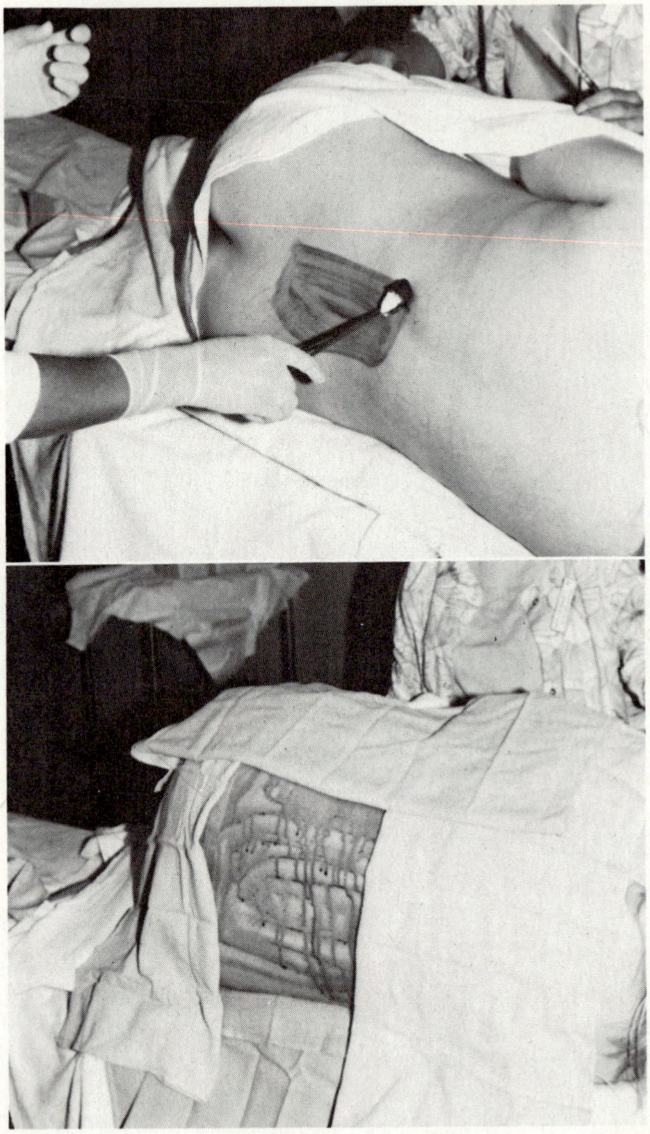

A

B

Fig. 25.10, cont'd

C, Landmarks are palpated; correct area is selected. **D,** "Skin wheal" is made when local anesthetic is injected with a small-gauge, short needle.

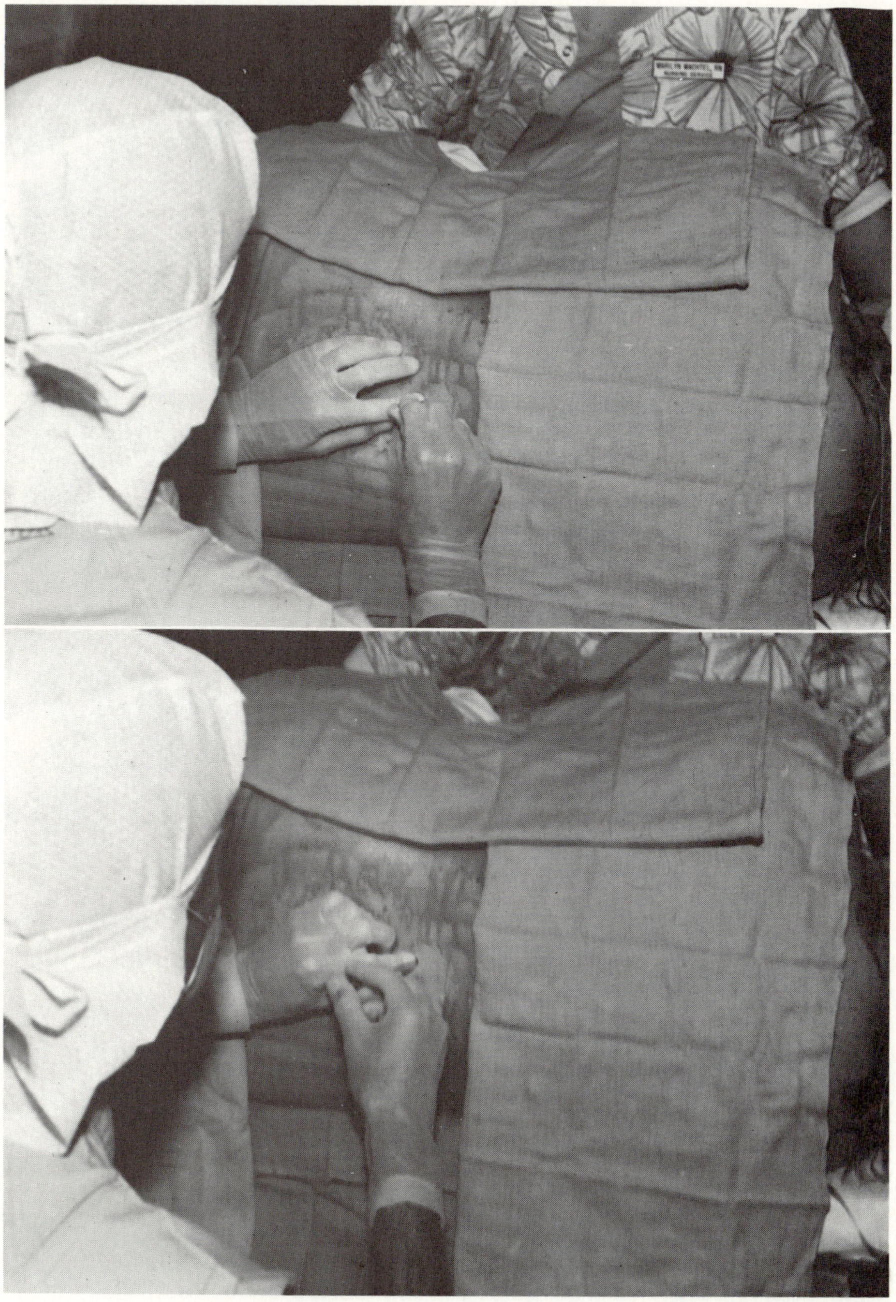

C LANDMARKS PALPATED

D SKIN WHEAL

Continued.

Fig. 25.10, cont'd
E, Local anesthetic is infiltrated with a longer needle. **F,** Tuohy needle with stylet is advanced into epidural space.

Local Anes

E

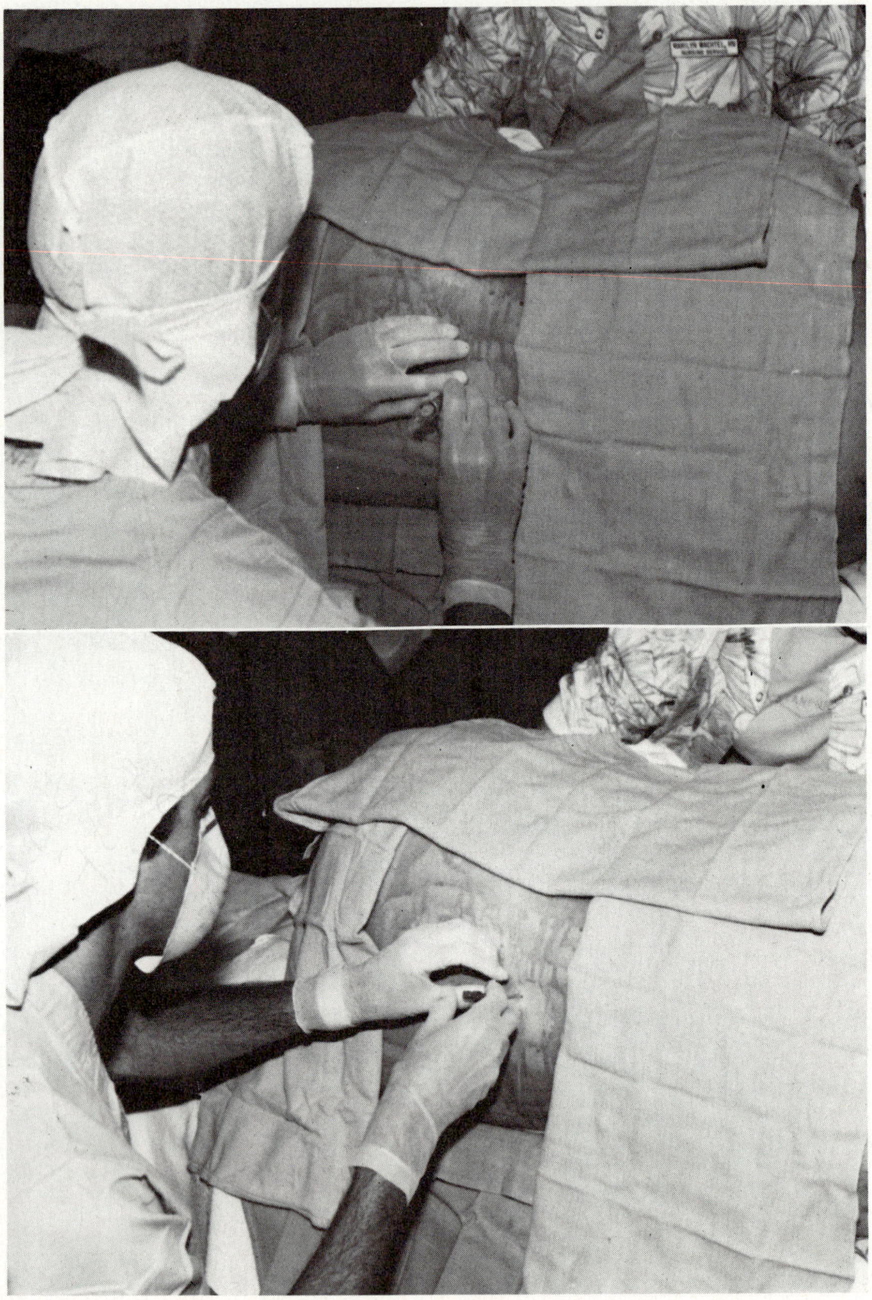

Touhy Needle c̄ Stylet to epidural space

F

Fig. 25.10, cont'd

G, Tuohy needle in place. **H,** Test dose is administered.

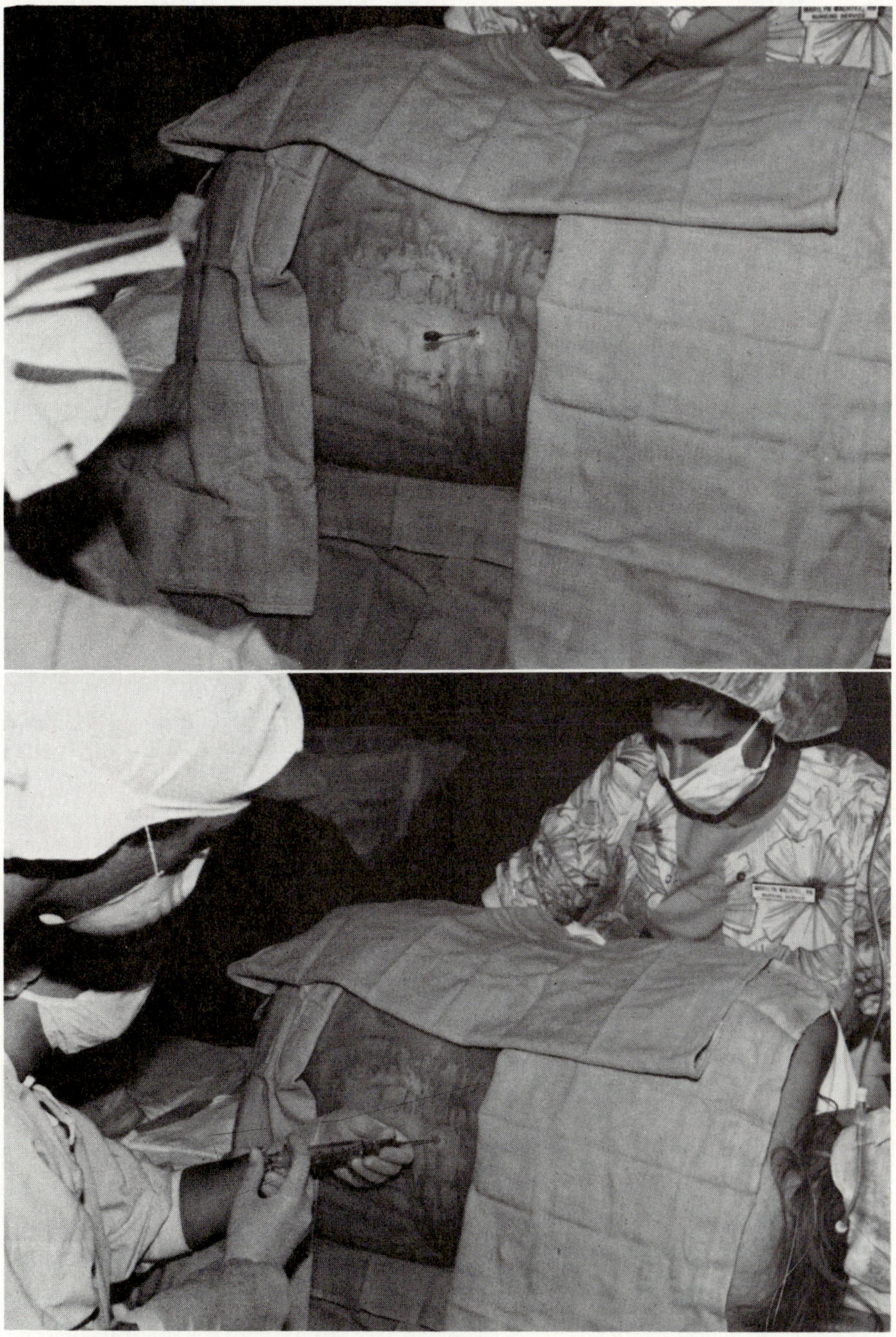

G

TUOHY NEEDLE IN PLACE

H

TEST DOSE ADMIN

Continued.

Fig. 25.10, cont'd

I, Polyethylene catheter is threaded through needle into epidural space. **J,** Local anesthetic is administered into catheter. **K,** Catheter is taped to woman's back; port segment is taped near her shoulder.

CATH THRU NEEDLE

I

LOCAL ANES ADMIN THRU CATH

J

CATH TAPED

K

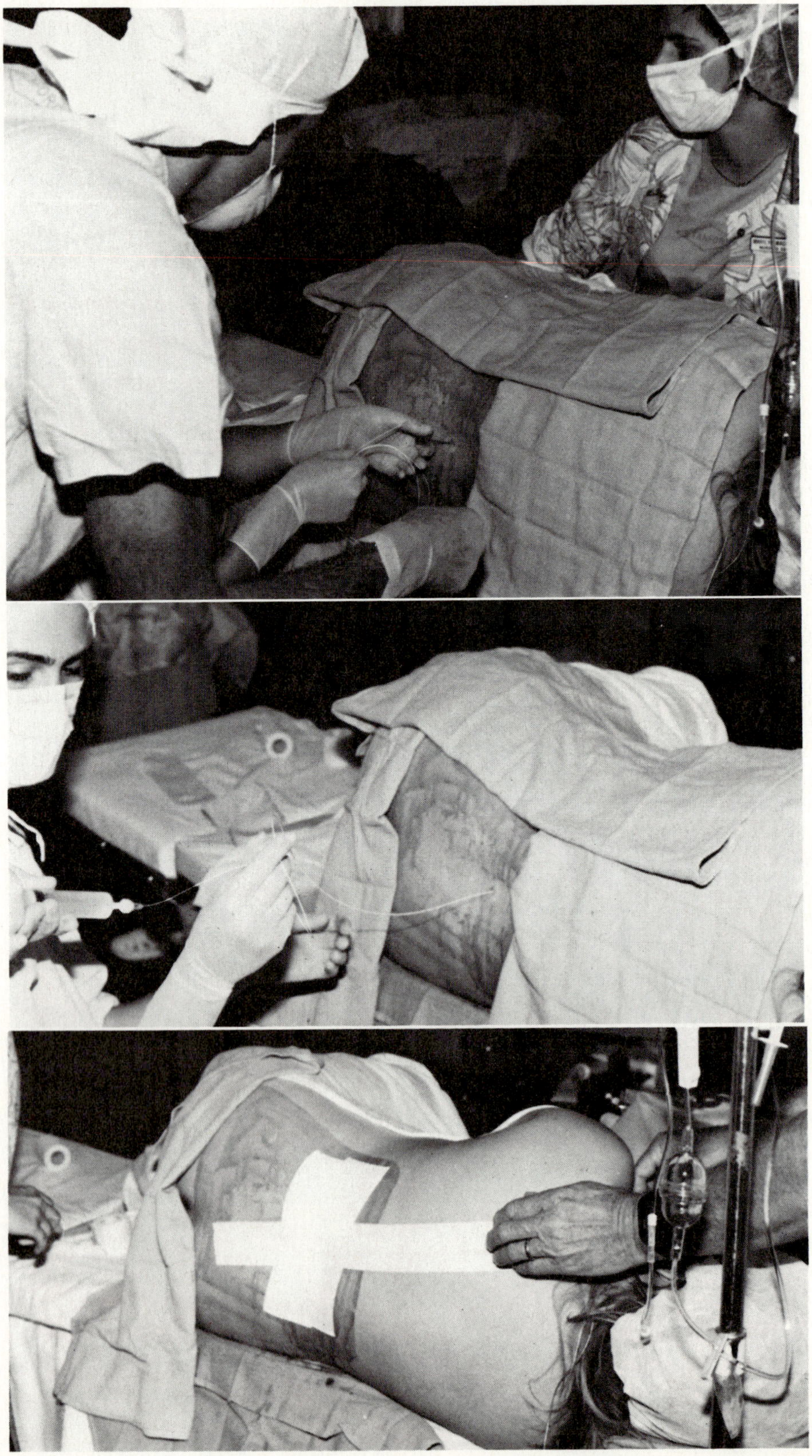

Table 25.4
Comparison of Modalities for Obstetric Analgesia

Therapeutic Modality Drug	Usual Parenteral Dose	Time of Administration	Advantages for Parturient	Disadvantages for Neonate	Nursing Concerns
Psychoprophylaxis		Late pregnancy Labor stages 1-3	No drugs Training in self-reliance	None	Pain controlled but not eliminated
Hypnosis		Late pregnancy Labor stages 1-3	No drugs In rare women, pain free	None	Suggestion reinforcement essential
Medications					
Amnesics					
Scopolamine hydrobromide	0.4 mg IM or IV	Late stage 1	Amnesia profound	Possible injury if woman is disoriented, uncooperative	Delusions, hallucinations, hyperactivity necessitate constant supervision
Alphaprodine (Nisentil)*	40-60 mg subcutaneously or IV	Late stage 1	Amnesia partial plus good analgesia	Slight CNS depression	Routine
Narcotic analgesics					
Morphine	8-15 mg IM or IV	Mid stage I	Analgesia excellent	Moderate to marked CNS depression if delivery <2 hr after administration	Emesis common
Meperidine	50-100 mg IM or IV	Mid stage 1	Analgesia good	Slight CNS depression	Routine
Narcotic antagonists					
Nalorphine (Nalline)	Adult—5 mg IM or IV Neonate—0.5 mg IM or IV	Stage 2 or to neonate	Prompt termination of narcotic effect but ineffective against depression caused by barbiturates or anesthetics	Overdose may be toxic	Physical resuscitation of mother or neonate may be necessary despite narcotic antagonist
Levallorphan tartrate (Lorfan)	Adult—1.0 mg IM or IV Neonate—0.05-0.1 mg IM or IV	Same as above	Same as above	Same as above	Same as above
Naloxone hydrochloride (Narcan)	Adult—0.4 mg IM or IV Neonate—0.01 mg/kg body weight, IV or subcutaneously	Same as above	Same as above	Same as above	Abrupt reversal of narcotic reaction (nausea, vomiting, tachycardia, hypertension, tremors in narcotics addicts)
Sedatives-hypnotics					
Secobarbital sodium (Seconal)	50-100 mg IM	Early or mid stage 1 or postdelivery	Disinhibition or somnolescence (no pain relief in usual doses)	Hypoactive, "sleepy" neonate	Either subdued or excited; may become dehydrated
Pentobarbital sodium (Nembutal)	50-100 mg IM	Same as above	Same as above	Same as above	Same as above
Tranquilizers					
Promethazine (Phenergan)	25-50 mg IM	Early or mid stage 1 or postdelivery	Apprehension, anxiety, depression relieved; narcotic effects potentiated, but antiemetic	Drug enhances narcotic effect (CNS depression)	Closer supervision may be necessary because of mild pseudohypnotic state
Promazine (Sparine)	50 mg IM	Early or mid stage 1 or postdelivery	Apprehension, anxiety, depression relieved; narcotic effects potentiated, but antiemetic	Drug enhances narcotic effect (CNS) depression	Closer supervision may be necessary because of mild pseudohypnotic state
Hydroxyzine pamoate (Vistaril)	25-50 mg IM	Same as above	Same as above	Same as above	Same as above
Diazepam (Valium)	5 mg IM or IV	Same as above	Same as above	Same as above	Same as above

*Alphaprodine hydrochloride (Nisentil) was removed from the market in October 1980 but subsequently was reinstated.

Combination Anesthesia for Cesarean Birth

Light general anesthesia, considered by many to be ideal for cesarean delivery, is achieved with a combination of *thiopental, nitrous oxide–oxygen, and succinylcholine*. An individual experienced in anesthesiology is required, however.

Thiopental, 200 to 300 mg in solution, is administered intravenously for induction just before the skin incision is made. When the parturient is somnolent, nitrous oxide–oxygen, 75%:25%, is given. After about 3 minutes the mixture is reduced to equal volumes. Then a skeletal muscle relaxant (succinylcholine chloride [Anectine]) is administered to the woman to facilitate intubation.

Excellent tolerance of the anesthetic and rapid resuscitation of the mother and even small-for-gestational-age (SGA) or growth-retarded infants are widely reported.

Intraspinal Narcotic Method

Intraspinal narcotic usage in obstetrics is being reported in the literature. There is a high concentration of receptors in the spinal column that are open to the action of the opiates to block pain. These receptors are reached by a catheter placed in the epidural space (see discussion of epidural nerve block).

Some work has been done with labor and delivery clients and for postoperative pain following cesarean delivery (Fig. 25.11). The morphine sulfate used was one without preservative. When used in labor, 1.5 mg morphine sulfate was administered via the epidural catheter. The women felt contractions, but no pain was noted by them or observers. The pushing reflex was not lost, so the mother could cooperate during delivery. Maternal vital signs were normal during labor, and no motor or sympathetic block was noted. All of the women experienced itching of the face, mouth, and eyes. These symptoms were treated with promethazine or metaclopramide.

Fig. 25.11
Caudal anesthesia. **A,** Caudal tray. **B,** Woman assumes modified knee-chest or lateral Sims' position to permit access to sacral hiatus. Once needle and catheter are in place, she may assume any position in bed. Note cervix is approximately 5 cm dilated.
(**A** courtesy Standford University Hospital, Palo Alto, Calif. **B** courtesy Ross Laboratories, Columbus, Ohio.)

A

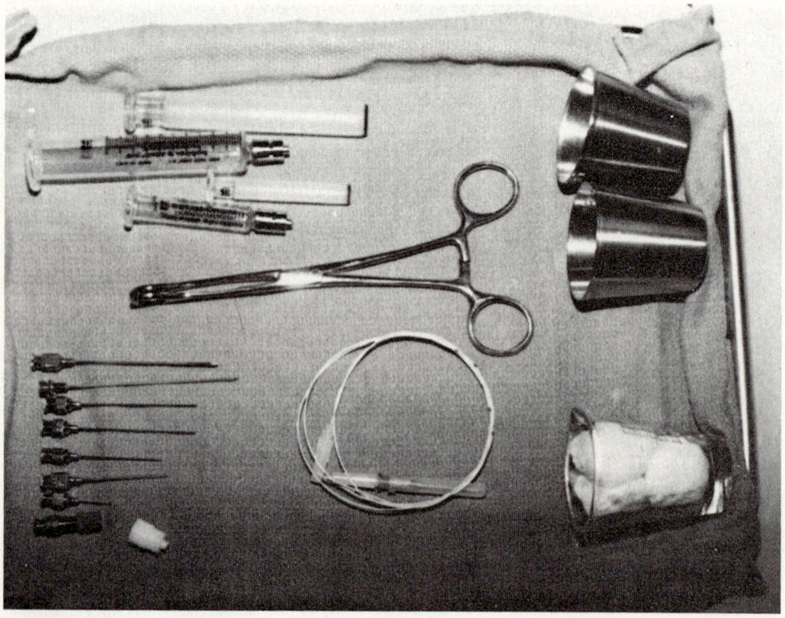

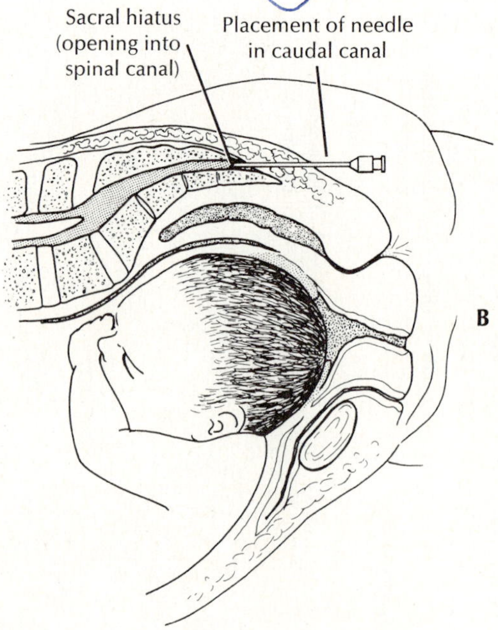

B

The reversal drug for morphine is naloxone, 0.4 mg. Morphine is believed to have no effect on the course of labor. The pain relief continues up to 11 hours after injection.

Women who deliver by the abdominal route are given epidural morphine 1 hour postoperatively through the epidural catheter. The catheter is then removed, and the women are pain free for 24 hours. Ability to be up with ease and to care for the baby are two of the advantages to epidural morphine. The women cannot believe the effects of the morphine on pain. To any woman who had a previous cesarean delivery with the usual postoperative pain, the effects of the epidural morphine seem miraculous.

The side effects of intraspinal morphine are nausea, vomiting, pruritus (itching), urinary retention, or delayed respiratory depression. Antiemetics and antipruritics are used to relieve the nausea, vomiting, and pruritus. Early ambulation and freedom from pain facilitate bladder emptying.

The serious concern is for delayed respiratory depression. The women are observed frequently and are placed on an apnea monitor for 24 hours. Delayed respiratory depression is caused by absorption of morphine from the spinal fluid by the respiratory centers in the brain.

The nurse caring for the woman who has been given epidural morphine generally is amazed at her ease in ambulation and relative freedom from pain.

Fig. 25.12

Spinal tray. (Courtesy Stanford University Hospital, Palo Alto, Calif.)

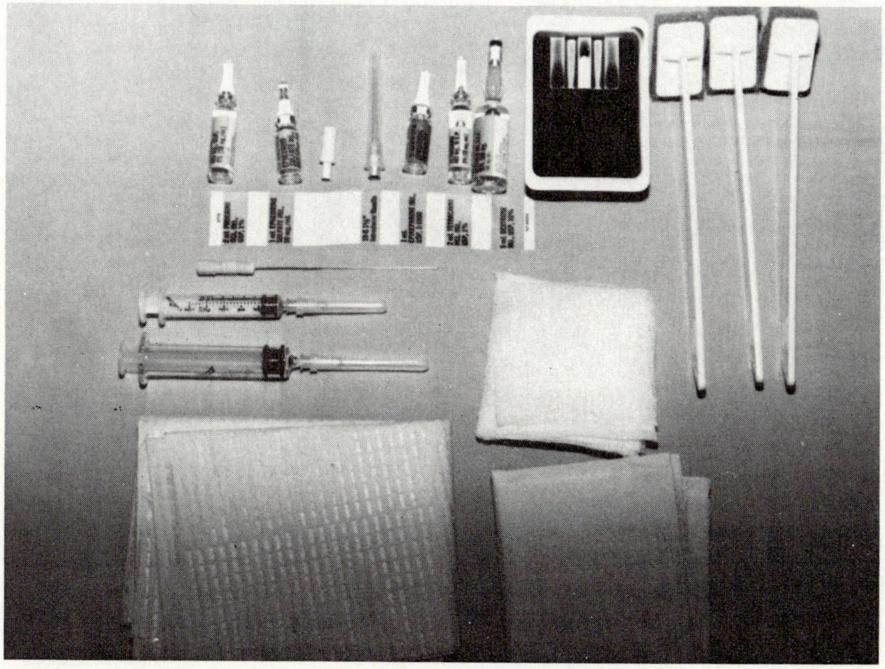

Fig. 25.13

A, Epidural morphine. Following epidural anesthesia for cesarean delivery, dose of morphine is injected into indwelling catheter. Anesthetist is applying apnea monitor on woman. Her respirations will be monitored for 24 hours. **B,** Husband supports wife as nurse begins routine postpartum assessments following cesarean birth.

A

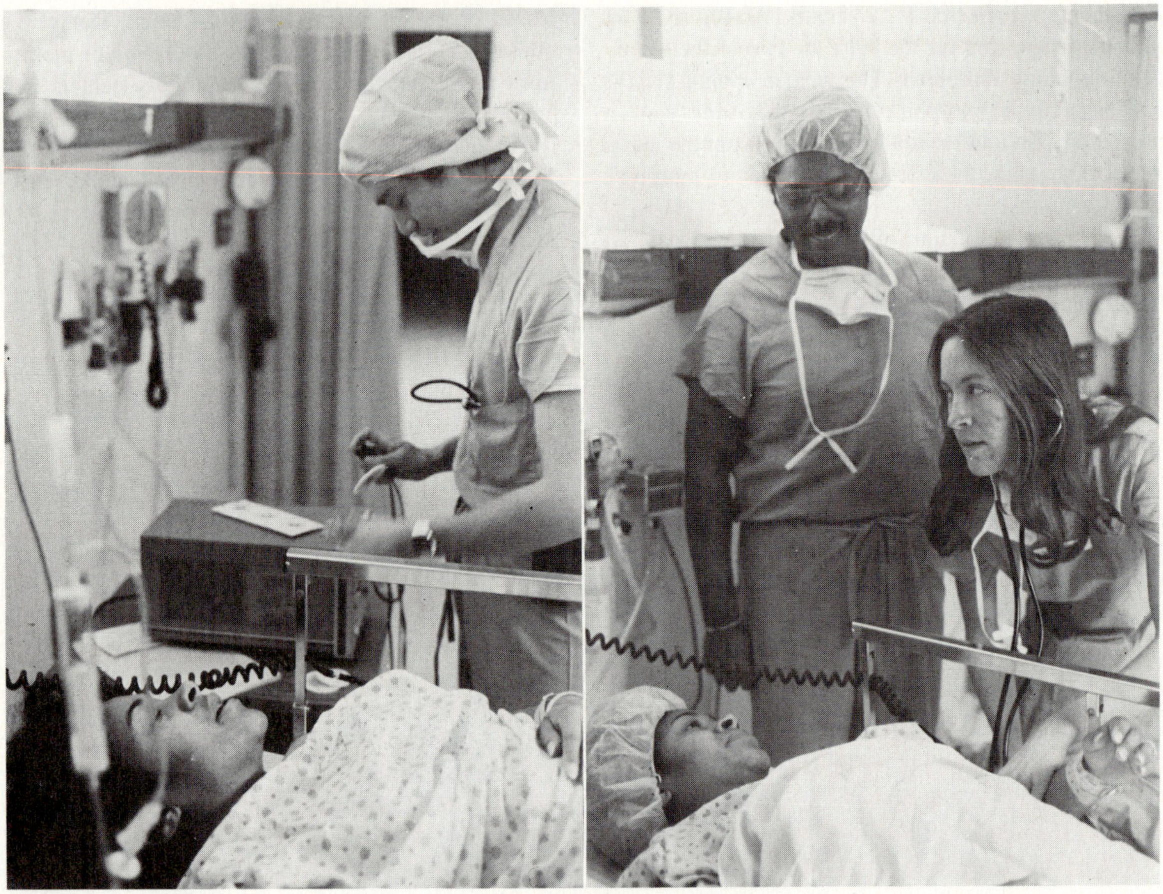

B

Fig. 25.13, cont'd

C, Nurse palpates fundus following cesarean birth. Woman experiences no discomfort during assessment. **D,** Nurse records findings concurrently with assessment. **E,** Neonate born by cesarean delivery. Neonate's Apgar score and neurologic assessment show no adverse reactions to epidural anesthesia. NOTE: Foot is being warmed before heel stick for blood glucose level in this big baby. Also note linea nigra caused by maternal hormones.

C

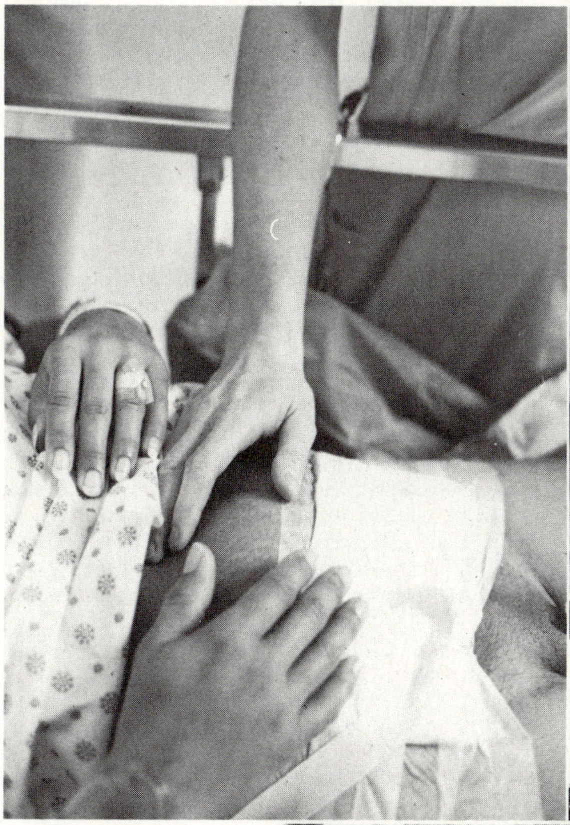

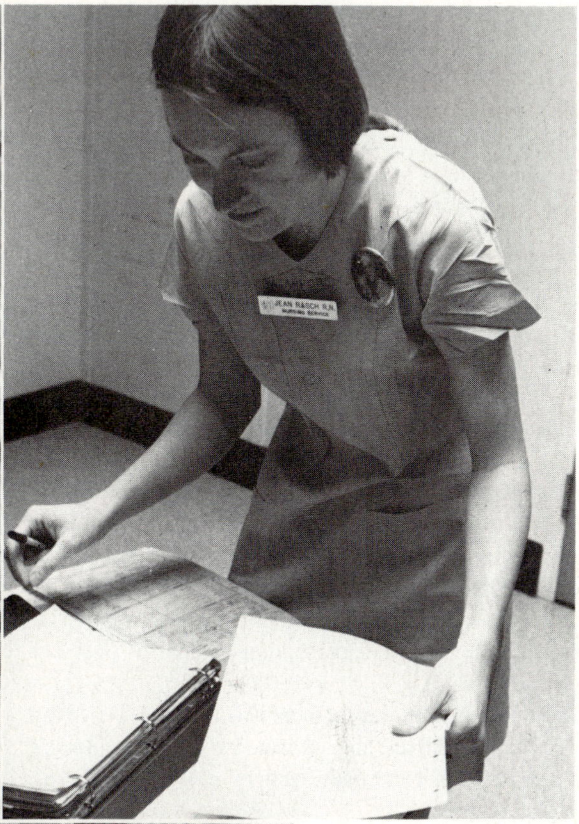

D

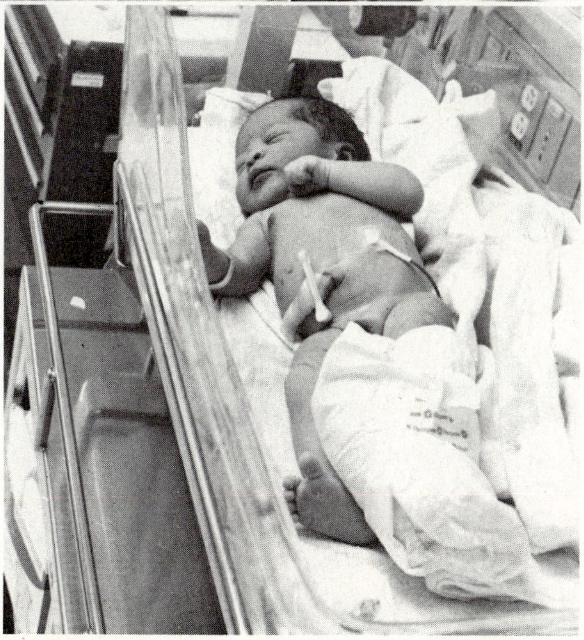

E

Nonpharmacologic, Noninvasive Relief of Discomfort

TRANSCUTANEOUS ELECTRICAL NERVE STIMULATION (TENS)

The application of pressure to or rubbing of a part of the body that is sore is an age-old remedy to relieve discomfort. Effleurage and sacral pressure or massage are two methods that have brought relief to many women during the first stage of labor. The "gate control theory" may supply the reason for the effectiveness of these measures (see p. 353). TENS may operate on the same principle. TENS may also be effective because of the "placebo effect"; i.e., confidence in TENS may stimulate the release of endogenous opiates (enkephalins) in the woman's body and thus alleviate the discomfort.

Two pairs of electrodes are taped on either side of the thoracic and sacral spine. Continuous mild electrical currents are applied from a battery-operated device. During a contraction the woman increases the stimulation by turning control knobs on the device. Women describe the sensation as a tingling or buzzing and pain relief as good or very good. The use of TENS poses no risk to the mother or fetus. TENS is credited with reducing or eliminating the need for analgesia and with increasing the woman's perception of control over her experience.

The nurse assists the mother who is using TENS by explaining the device and its use, by carefully placing and securing the electrodes, and by closely evaluating its effectiveness.

References and Readings

Abonleish, E.: Pain control in obstetrics, Philadelphia, 1977. J.B. Lippincott Co.

Albright, G.A.: Anesthesia in obstetrics, Menlo Park, Calif., 1978, Addison-Wesley Publishing Co.

Bromage, P.R., Camporesi, E., and Chestnut, D.: Epidural narcotics for postoperative analgesia, Anesthes. Analges. **59:**473, 1980.

Cavanaugh, D., Woods, R.E., and O'Connor, T.C.F.: Obstetrical emergencies, ed. 2, Hagerstown, Md., 1978, Harper & Row, Publishers.

Clark, R.B.: Conduction anesthesia, Clin. Obstet. Gynecol. **24**(2):601, 1981.

Datta, S., et al.: Neonatal effect of prolonged anesthetic induction for cesarean section, Am. J. Obstet. Gynecol. **58**(3):331, 1981.

Dilts, P.V.: Selection of analgesia and anesthesia, Clin. Obstet. Gynecol. **24**(2):521, 1981.

Fishburne, J.I.: Systemic analgesia during labor, Clin. Perinatol. **9**(1):29, 1982.

Gibbs, C.P.: Maternal physiology, Clin. Obstet. Gynecol. **24:**2, 1981.

Hughes, S.C.: Intraspinal narcotics in obstetrics, Clin. Perinatol. **9**(1):167, 1982.

Kryc, J.J.: Anesthesia for the high risk obstetrical patient, Clin. Perinatol. **9**(1):113, 1982.

MacLaughlin, S.M., and Taubenheim, A.M.: Epidural anesthesia for obstetric patients, J.O.G.N. Nurs. **10**(1):9, 1981.

Moore, D.E., Blacker, H.M.: How effective is TENS for chronic pain? Am. J. Nurs. **83**(8):1175, 1983

Redick, L.F.: Epidural anesthesia, Clin. Perinatol. **9**(1):63, 1982.

Shnider, S.M.: Choice of anesthesia for labor and delivery, Am. J. Obstet. Gynecol. **58**(5):24, 1981.

Solomon, R.A., et al.: Reduction of postoperative pain and narcotic use of transcutaneous electrical nerve stimulation, Surgery **87**:142, Feb. 1980.

Taylor, A.G., et al.: How effective is TENS for acute pain? Am. J. Nurs. **83**(8):1171, 1983.

Yurth, D.A.: Placental transfer of local anesthetics, Clin. Perinatol. **9**(1):13, 1982.

26

Alternative Settings for Childbirth

- Historical Perspective
- Impetus of Consumerism
- Family-Centered Care
- Birth Choices
- Birthing Rooms
- Alternative Birth Centers
  - High-risk factors excluding admission to the alternative birth center
  - High-risk factors developing after admission requiring transfer to labor and delivery
- Freestanding Birth Centers
- Nurse-Midwifery
- Cesarean Birth
- Home Birth
  - Advantages
  - Disadvantages
  - Contraindications
  - Family's preparation for home birth
- Choice and the Nurse

Historical Perspective

From America's colonial days until the early years of the twentieth century the vast majority of births in America took place at home, attended by midwives. It was not until the mid to late 1800s that the birth process and infant care were viewed as worthy of the physician's attention. Like so many aspects of our society, childbirth also felt the impact of the Industrial Revolution. As is frequently the case in scientific discovery, the technical aspects of childbirth were emphasized and maternity care was developed with the chief intention of reducing perinatal morbidity and mortality.

By the end of the nineteenth century it had become fashionable in America to give birth in a hospital with a male physician in attendance instead of giving birth at home attended by a midwife. Urbanization had separated families so that there were fewer networks of women relatives and friends to help one another. Servants were less common, and the hospital confinement was often viewed as a vacation from the usual chores at home. It seemed easier to remove from the home the physical aspects of birth and the need to clean up afterward. American hospitals actively fostered the idea that they were pleasant, safe, and comfortable places in which to give birth.

At about the time of the First World War, the importation of "twilight sleep" from Europe carried the concept of comfortable birth even further. In this technique, morphine and scopolamine (an amnesic) were given to the mother during labor and ether or chloroform was administered when the baby entered the birth canal. The method did not do away with the pain of childbirth but produced a light sleeplike state in the mother and rendered her passive. As a result, women had no memory of pain in labor or at birth. Many prominent women endorsed twilight sleep publicly, and American women began to request painless deliveries using twilight sleep. The use of twilight sleep coupled with the use of new anesthetic agents changed child-

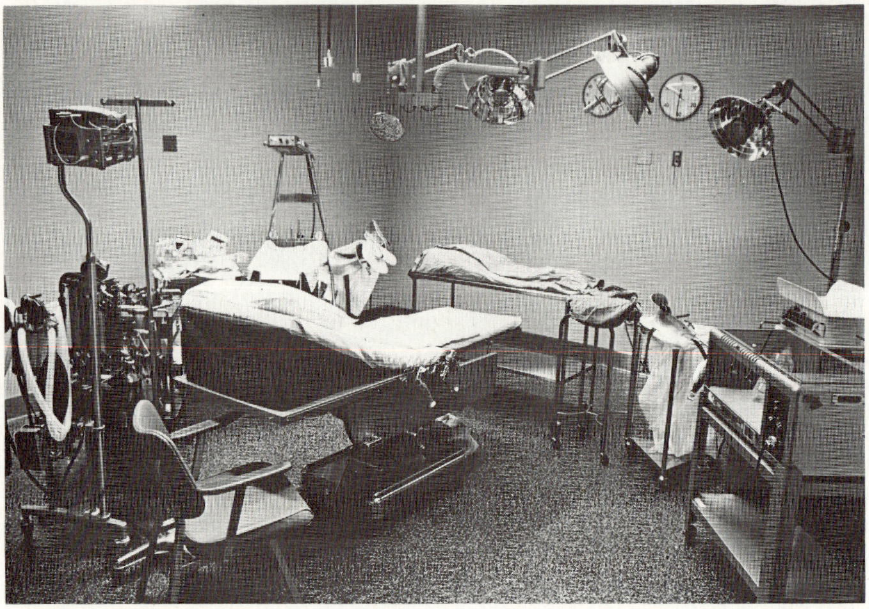

Fig. 26.1
Context of major surgery. (From Phillips, C.R., and Anzalone, J.T.: Fathering: participation in labor and birth, ed. 2, St. Louis, 1982, The C.V. Mosby Co.)

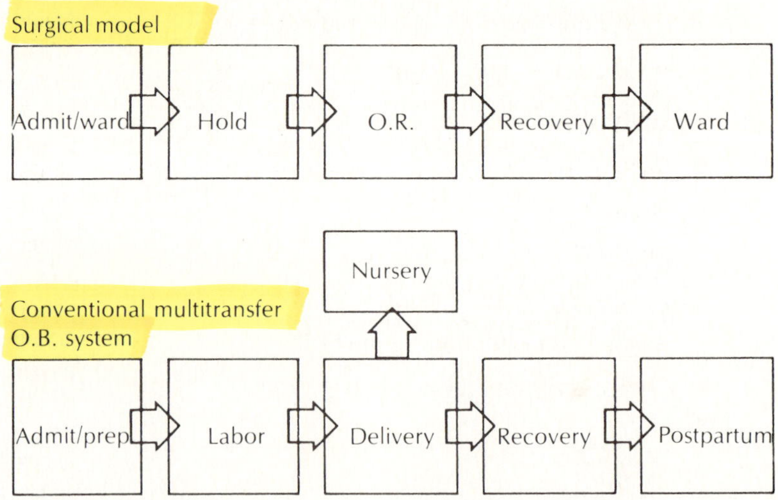

Fig. 26.2
Surgical transfer system. (From Phillips, C.R., and Anzalone, J.T.: Fathering: participation in labor and birth, ed. 2, St. Louis, 1982, The C.V. Mosby Co.)

birth from a physiologic and social event occurring in the familiar environment of home to a medical-surgical event occurring in the context of major surgery, controlled by specialists. Most of the hospital obstetric units in use throughout the United States today were created to provide care for women receiving twilight sleep for labor and anesthesia for birth. Their design is based on the surgical transfer system.

The shift of childbirth from home to hospitals in the United States accelerated rapidly in the 1930s. Although in 1900 less than 5% of all American babies were born in hospitals, by 1940 that percentage increased to 50% and to 99.2% by 1975. Since 1977, however, there has been an interesting change in these statistics showing a small but steady decline in the number of hospital births in the United States. According to Marieskind (1980): "In 1977, for example, 98.5% of all babies were born in hospitals with a physician or midwife in attendance, as were 98.6% of white babies and 98.3% of babies of all other ethnicities."

Estimates for 1982 were that 1.8% of all births in the United States occurred out of hospitals. Along with this recent decline in hospital births is a steady increase in the number of hospitals offering families alternatives to traditional compartmentalized, fragmented, and depersonalized U.S. maternity care. "Innovations" that were commonplace practices before childbirth was institutionalized (e.g., father and sibling presence during labor, midwife attendance) are being reinstated in response to consumer request. The high economic costs of childbearing are prompting both the consumers and the providers of care to explore alternatives to traditional hospital delivery room birth and the 3- or 4-day postpartum hospitalizations for well mothers and babies. Lack of an extended family is creating a need for more supportive care both before and after delivery, since the new mother is often without family help. Changing life-styles and values are allowing men more freedom to be nurturing fathers and participate fully in pregnancy, labor, birth, and child care. At the same time, more families are becoming actively involved in decisions about their births and are making new choices about childbirth.

Impetus of Consumerism

Although the prepared childbirth movement actually began in the 1930s, it gained strength and momentum in the United States in the last 2 decades. The work of Grantly Dick-Read, Lamaze, and Bradley provided women with breathing and relaxation techniques to conquer the fear and pain associated with labor. As women began to experience childbirth awake and aware, they began to feel increased self-esteem and control over their lives. Also, the social significance of the birth experience became very clear to many women and their mates.

Organizations such as the International Childbirth Education Association (ICEA), the American Society for Psychoprophylaxis in Obstetrics (ASPO), and the National Association of Parents and Professionals for Safe Alternatives in Childbirth (NAPSAC) have increased the public's knowledge of prepared childbirth techniques and their impact on birth outcomes. The prepared childbirth movement has fostered an increased acceptance of birth as a normal, rather than a pathologic, event and has encouraged expectant parents to become more knowledgeable about and accountable for their participation. Consumer response has been varied, demonstrating the intensely personal quality of every birth experience and the need for safe, sensible choices in care during this important life event. Some couples wish to exercise maximal control over the birth of their child, with minimal technology and intervention by the health care team. Other couples choose a more traditional approach. The key element in optimal care of the childbearing family is *informed choice* about the place of birth, the plan of care, and the persons present. In fact, the ICEA has always subscribed to the motto, "Freedom of choice based on knowledge of alternatives."

Family-Centered Care

In the 1980s maternal mortality in the United States has become almost nonexistent and neonatal mortality has declined substantially. This allows us to concentrate on the psychologic and social aspects of childbirth. Recent research indicates that the quality of the birth experience can affect parental-infant attachment and couple relationships in both positive and negative ways. Anesthesia and analgesia may limit both the mother's and the newborn's ability to engage in early behaviors important to maternal-infant attachment. Immediate and prolonged separation of parents and their infant may also interfere with the development of parental-infant affectionate bonds. Birth is a life event having a significant impact on human behavior. Childbirth requires sensitive management and attention to the psychosocial health of the family.

In June 1978 the American College of Obstetricians and Gynecologists (ACOG) published a joint statement entitled "The Development of Family-Centered Maternity/Newborn Care in Hospitals." The statement was prepared by the Interprofessional Task Force on Health Care of Women and Children, which included representatives from the American Academy of Pediatrics (AAP), the American College of Nurse-Midwives (ACNM), the American Nurses' Association (ANA), ACOG, and the Nurses' Association of the American College of Obstetricians and Gynecologists (NAACOG). In this statement these five organizations endorsed the concept of family-centered childbirth and supported efforts to develop alternative childbirth centers along the lines described in the statement. The American Hospital Association also added its support. The definition of family-centered care in the joint statement (American College of Obstetricians & Gynecologists, 1978) follows:

> Family-centered maternity/newborn care can be defined as the delivery of safe, quality health care while recognizing, focusing on, and adapting to both the physical and psychological needs of the client-patient, the family, and the newly born. The emphasis is on the provision of maternity/newborn

health care which fosters family unity while maintaining physical safety.

The joint statement recommends significant changes in hospital maternity care, including the following:

1. The option of a homelike birthing room
2. Flexible rooming-in with maximal mother-child contact during the first 24 hours
3. Breast feeding and handling of the baby immediately after delivery
4. Allowing the father or other support person to be present throughout the labor, delivery, and recovery periods
5. Allowing siblings to visit in a special family room
6. Optional early release from the hospital with careful follow-up after discharge
7. Childbirth preparation classes offered by the hospital

The alternative birth movement is the practical application of the family-centered concept of maternity-newborn care. However, family-centered care requires more than just a proper physical environment. The attitude of the health care providers is the most important aspect of family-centered care. Family-centered care recognizes birth as a vital life event and not a surgical procedure. The philosophic approach to family-centered care and alternative childbirth programs is aimed at combating paternalism in the health care system by giving people the right to make informed choices regarding their childbirth experiences.

Birth Choices

In many hospitals rigid rules, procedures, and attitudes are being reevaluated, and, when found to be without a scientific basis, they are being revised and adjusted to fit the concept of family-centered maternity-newborn care. Some institutions have already pioneered family-centered care and have now moved on to even more dynamic and progressive family-care units designated as Alternative Birth Centers (ABCs) or birth rooms in the hospital. Hospital ABCs as well as freestanding birth centers were originally designed to offer families an alternative to home birth, that is, a compromise between hospital and home. Their developers conceived of these units in response to the growing number of parents who chose to boycott the institutions they felt did not meet their childbirth needs and to deliver their babies at home, sometimes with skilled attendants and sometimes without. However, as time has passed, it has become clear that there is a small segment of the birthing population that will choose home birth no matter how many hospital or freestanding ABCs exist. As a result, the hospital's motivation to provide ABCs or birth rooms to the population is usually no longer one of offering an alternative setting to home birth. Instead, the alternative birth movement is becoming a way to offer a humanistic setting for childbirth that is, an alternative to the traditional surgical model accepted since the 1930s.

A survey of ABCs in the United States was undertaken in the spring of 1979 and repeated again 2 years later. Questionnaires were sent to ABCs identified from a published request in the *Newsletter* of the ACOG, a list of ABCs collected by Ross Laboratories, and a list prepared by the ACOG Resource Center. Of the 158 questionnaires mailed in 1979, there were 78 respondents (50%). Of the 242 questionnaires mailed in 1981, there were 151 respondents (62%). It is interesting to note that the great majority of ABCs have opened within the 4-yr period of 1978 to 1982. Comparison of the two surveys suggests that ABC availability is increasing, and that utilization of ABCs is increasing.

In 1976 only one Washington State hospital offered an ABC. In 1981, responses to a mailed questionnaire from 78 of 82 (95%) Washington State hospitals with maternity units disclosed that alternative birth rooms were in existence or planned in 63% of responding hospitals. Acceptance and utilization of ABCs and birth rooms by consumers and professionals are rapidly increasing as they are demonstrated to be a safe alternative to birth in a traditional delivery setting. It is impossible to accurately estimate the numbers of ABCs, birthing rooms, and freestanding birth centers in operation in the United States. As consumer requisites for more humane births increase and competition for the childbearing families occurs, hospitals are responding with alternatives to traditional childbirth routines. Major building and renovation programs are underway in U.S. hospital maternity units. A childbirth revolution has begun in the United States.

Birthing Rooms

In Manchester, Connecticut, an obstetrician, Philip Sumner, and his colleagues have had over 12 years of experience with labor and birth in hospital birthing rooms. Unlike ABCs in hospitals, there is very little admission or risk criteria for the use of these rooms. The program at Manchester Memorial Hospital incorporates labor support by highly trained nurses, or *monitrices*. Prenatal education is stressed, and client feedback is overwhelmingly positive. Women labor, give birth, and spend the first bonding time with their fami-

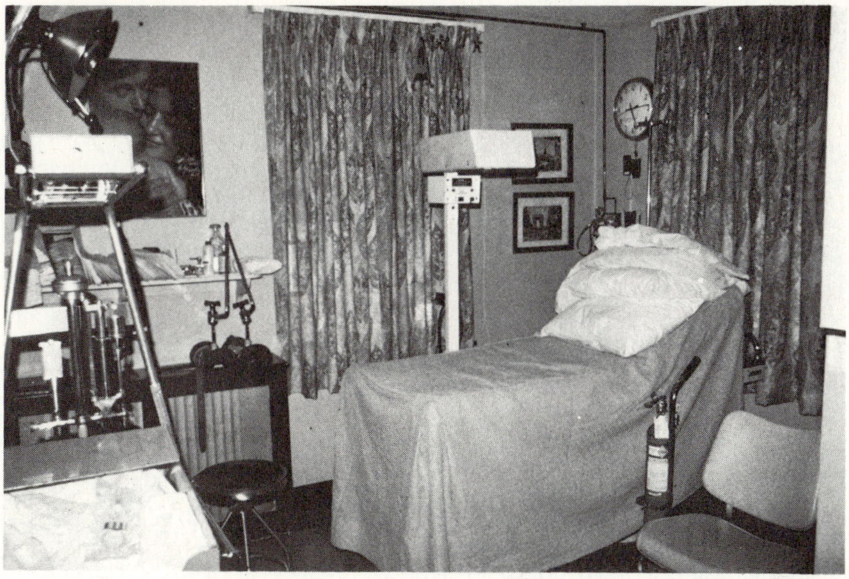

Fig. 26.3
First birth room at Manchester Memorial Hospital, Manchester, Conn. (From Sumner, P.E., and Phillips, C.R.: Birthing rooms: concept and reality, St. Louis, 1981, The C.V. Mosby Co.)

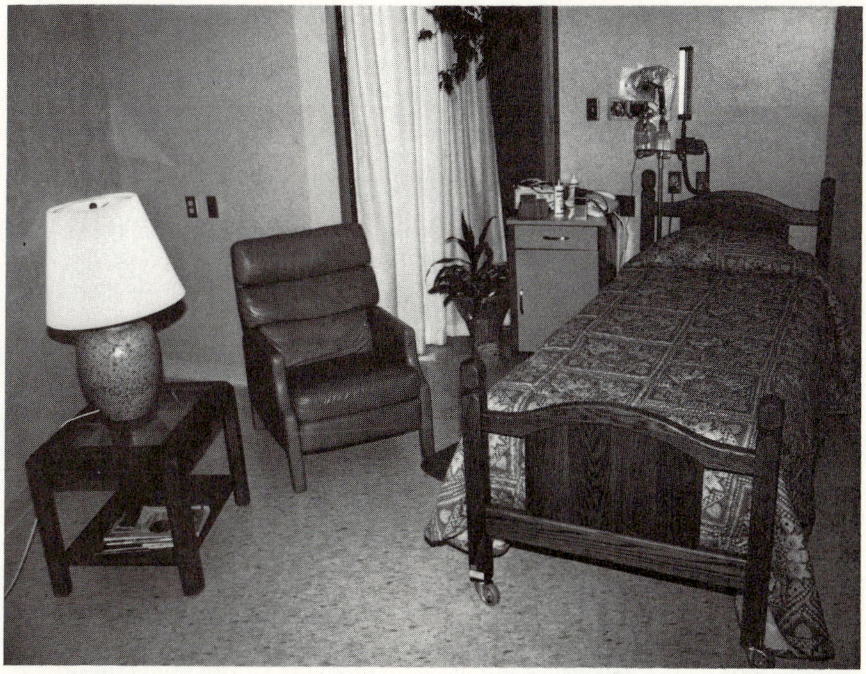

Fig. 26.4
Comfortable private space. (Courtesy Dominican Santa Cruz Hospital, Santa Cruz, Calif.)

lies in birthing rooms. Transfer to a postpartum room is usually the only room change they have to make.

Variations in the birthing room concept are found in many hospitals today. Some of these rooms offer compromises between traditional delivery rooms and ABCs. The birth rooms at Dominican Hospital, Santa Cruz, California, offer families a comfortable private space for childbirth. These rooms are equipped with the *Borning Bed,* which provides safe options for positioning of the mother in the event of labor or birth complications. The borning bed has the ability to ''break,'' so the woman can quickly be put into stirrups. Generally, this

Fig. 26.5
The Borning Bed.

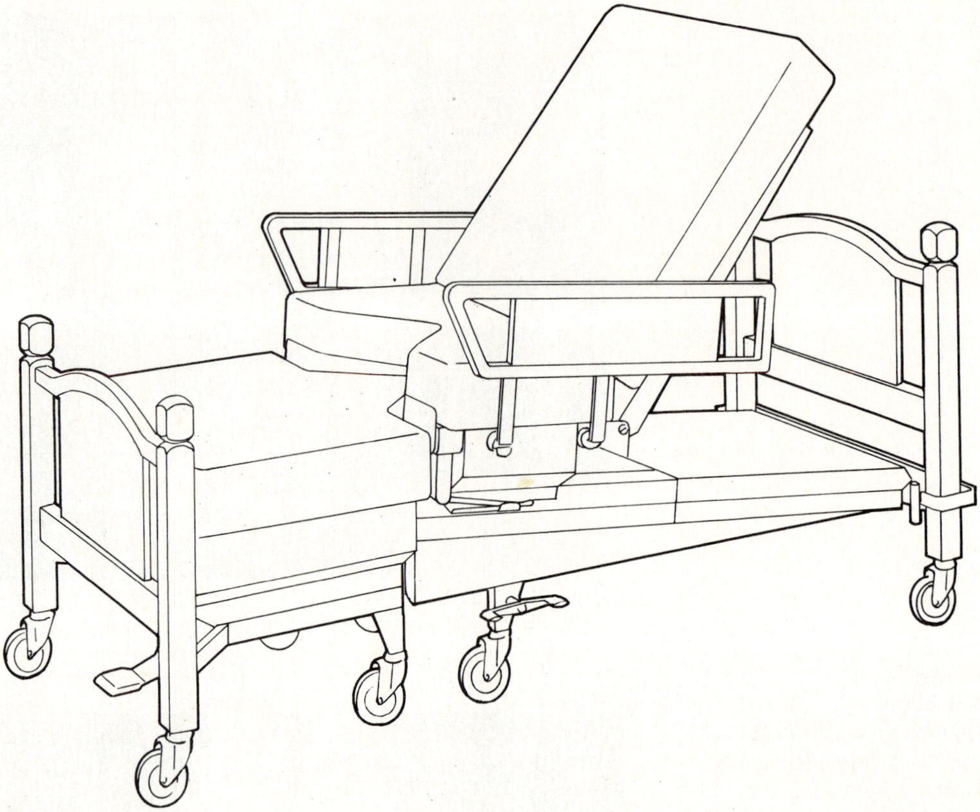

option is not used unless an episiotomy is performed or laceration occurs. Even in the unbroken mode a simple push of a button will cause the upper half of the bed to raise approximately 25 cm (10 in) and allow the easy management of an unsuspected shoulder dystocia.

Giving birth in a birth room rather than moving from a labor room to a delivery room has the advantage of not interfering or disrupting the progress of labor. The woman is able to concentrate on pushing her baby out without expending energy moving to a stretcher and then moving again to the delivery table. Her vital signs may be taken continuously if necessary, and the fetal monitor may remain in place until the baby is born. Also, the father is able to provide continuous support and does not have to be redirected to the new location. If rapid delivery is necessary, the woman's legs may be placed in the leg supports and the baby born quickly without time being wasted in transport to a delivery room. Other advantages of a birth room include the following:

1. The nursing staff no longer has to make decisions on when to move the mother to the delivery room.
2. There is no second room to be set up, so the nurses have ample time to prepare for an in situ delivery.
3. It may be possible to reduce costs, since fewer rooms are used, less laundry and equipment are involved, and there is better utilization of hospital space.

The concept underlying hospital birthing rooms is that of humanizing the birth experience, minimizing intervention, and affording continuity of care. Since these facilities are not a response to the home birth movement, they do not employ rigid screening criteria. Instead, they offer a two-tiered model of care (i.e., low risk and high risk) and emphasize individualizing the birth experience. When deemed necessary by the physician, nurse, or mother, local anesthesia, forceps, fetal monitoring, and so on are used to facilitate a safe but still joyous birth.

Alternative Birth Centers

Alternative Birth Centers (ABCs) usually are in hospital suites away from the traditional obstetric department but close to the delivery and operating rooms and medical or neonatal intensive care facilities for use when serious problems arise.

Fig. 26.6
Alternative birth center. (From Phillips, C.R., and Anzalone, J.T.: Fathering: participation in labor and birth, ed. 2, St. Louis, 1982, The C.V. Mosby Co.)

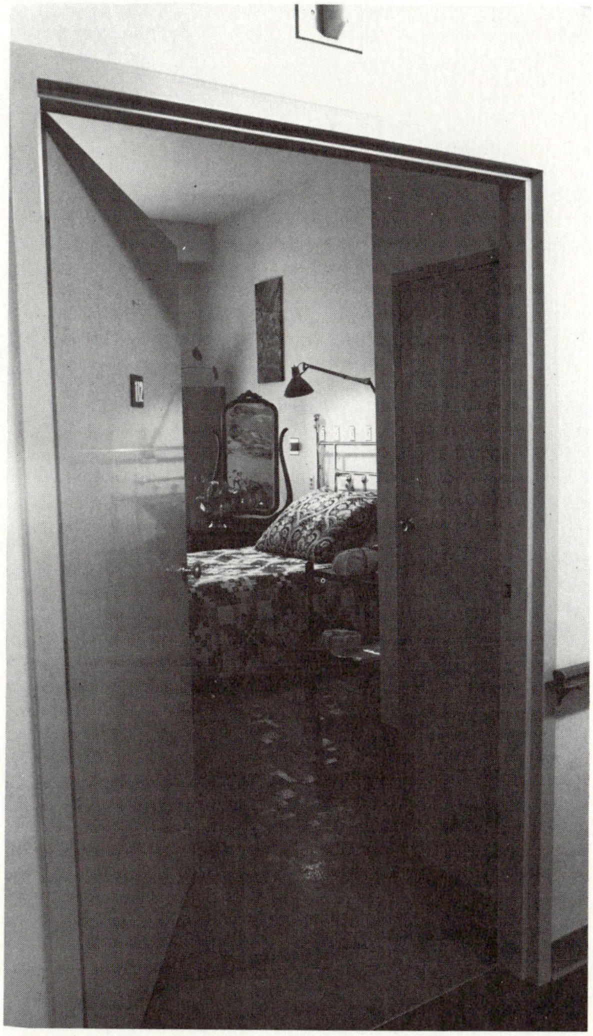

ABCs have homelike accommodations, including a double bed for the couple and a crib for the newborn. Emergency equipment and drugs are discretely stored within cupboards, out of view, but easily accessible. Private bathroom facilities are incorporated into each birth center. Also, there may be an early labor lounge or living room and small kitchen. There is careful screening of each applicant so that the ABC can rule out women with risk factors; that is, only low-risk and prepared women or couples are accepted.

The family is admitted to the ABC, labors there, gives birth there, and may remain there until discharge if the time interval and requirements for room utilization permit. If the family has to remain in the hospital for more than 24 hours postpartum, the demand for use of the ABC by more prospective families may require transfer of the new family to a regular postpartum room.

Ideally, the ABC becomes the private space for one childbearing family throughout their birth experience and until they are ready to go home. It is a warm, private, friendly space within a complex, fully equipped medical constellation. While emphasizing normalcy, natural methods, self-help, and family participation, ABCs are fully supported by the presence of an obstetric nurse or nurse-midwife and by the availability of obstetric and pediatric house staff at all times, with attending staff back-up.

If a situation that could threaten the safety of the mother or baby should arise at any time in labor, the mother would be moved to the regular labor and delivery area. In such a situation the ABC nurse and the father of the baby would also go with her.

Families who choose birth in the ABC may experience a warm, positive, family-centered, highly personalized, highly emotional birth within a structure offering safe and preventive perinatal care. Immediately outside the door of their alternative birth space, this family has available to them the sophistication of technical resources for management of complicated obstetric situations—truly the best of two worlds!

By agreement, medication and instrumentation (forceps, monitoring) are limited. Delivery can be accomplished in the woman's bed with skin-to-skin contact on the mother's abdomen after (usually) spontaneous birth. During labor and delivery, family, including older siblings, and friends of the mother's choosing may remain. Early discharge from the center, often during the day of delivery, must meet medical criteria. Many centers arrange for the mother and infant to be seen within 24 hours of discharge by a nurse-midwife or neonatal nursing specialist.

The fundamental philosophic difference between the ABC concept and a birthing room is screening criteria that divide the birthing population.

Ideally, an ABC should also offer childbearing couples alternative prices, in contrast to the high cost of obstetric care. Since alternative birth requires that the family occupy fewer spaces, less hospital time, and fewer supplies, linen, staff, and so on, it is usually possible to reduce the overall cost of birth to the hospital and consumer.

The establishment of an ABC requires the hospital maternity personnel, childbirth educators, physicians, and parents to come together to develop a common philosophy out of which can be elicited specific goals and

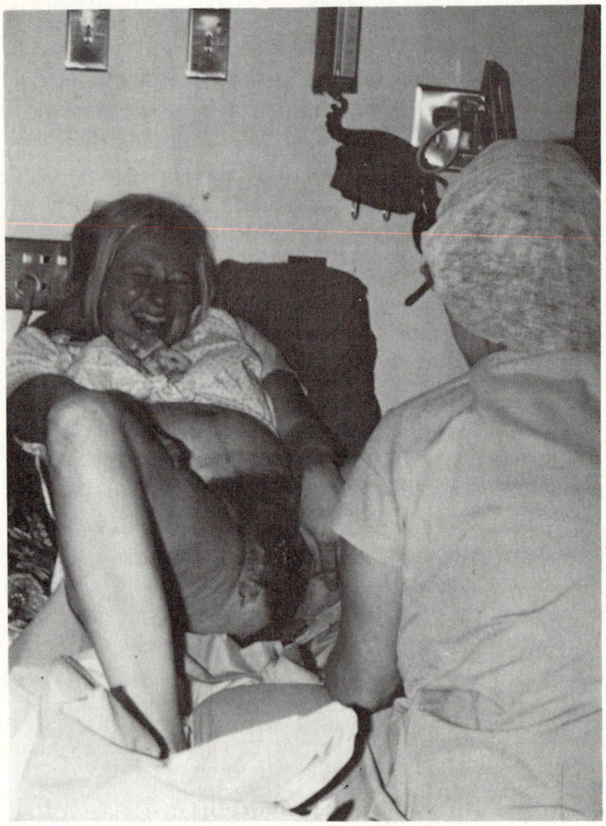

Fig. 26.7
Crowning. (From Sumner, P.E., and Phillips, C.R.: Birthing rooms: concept and reality, St. Louis, 1981, The C.V. Mosby Co.)

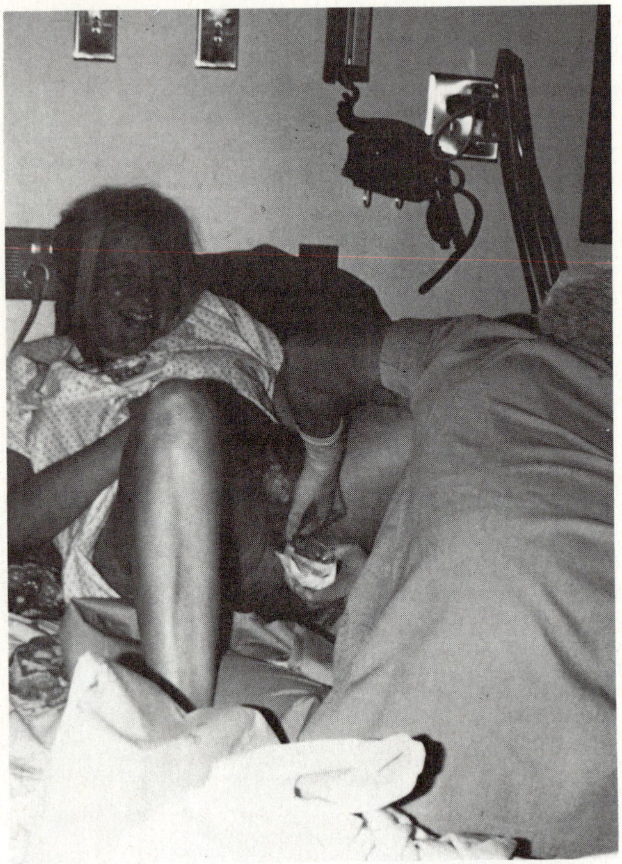

Fig. 26.8
Birth. (From Sumner, P.E., and Phillips, C.R.: Birthing rooms: concept and reality, St. Louis, 1981, The C.V. Mosby Co.)

objectives. The next step is to develop specific policies and procedures to provide uniform standards that will achieve the designated goals. An example of criteria relative to a couple's admission to an ABC follows (Sumner and Phillips, 1981).

HIGH-RISK FACTORS EXCLUDING ADMISSION TO THE ALTERNATIVE BIRTH CENTER

1. Social factors
   a. Less than three prenatal visits
   b. Maternal age*: nullipara greater than 35 years of age; multipara greater than 40 years of age
2. Preexisting maternal disease
   a. Chronic hypertension
   b. Moderate or severe renal disease
   c. Heart disease, classes II to IV
   d. History of PIH with seizures
   e. Diabetes mellitus
   f. Anemia; hemoglobin less than 9.5 g/dl*
   g. Tuberculosis
   h. Chronic or acute pulmonary problem
   i. Psychiatric disease requiring major tranquilizer
3. Previous obstetric history
   a. Previous stillbirth of unknown etiology
   b. Previous cesarean delivery
   c. Rh sensitivity
   d. Multiparity greater than five†

*Relative contraindication—may use center after period of fetal monitoring in the active phase of labor.

*Should the problem resolve, the woman may be transferred back to the ABC or give birth in the labor room.
†May use center with intravenous line during labor.

Fig. 26.9
A happy compromise to home birth. (From Sumner, P.E., and Phillips, C.R.: Birthing rooms: concept and reality, St. Louis, 1981, The C.V. Mosby Co.)

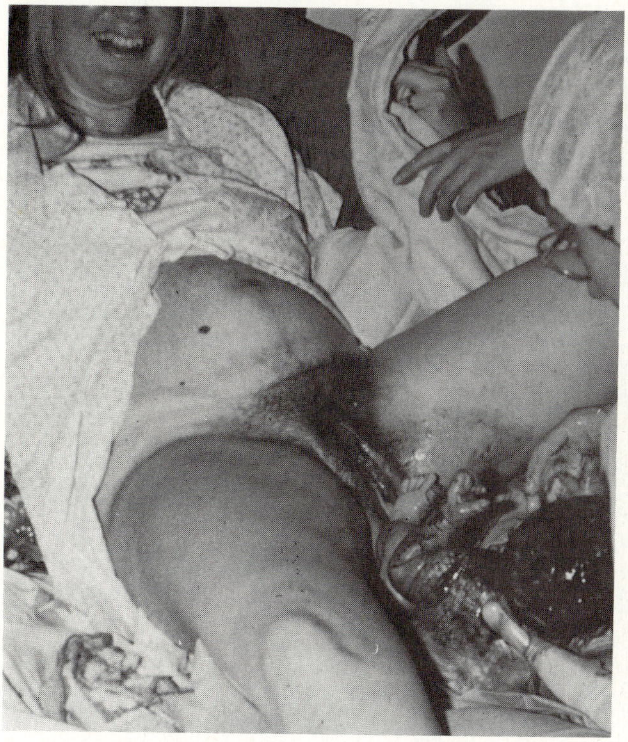

Fig. 26.10
Waiting for the placenta. (From Sumner, P.E., and Phillips, C.R.: Birthing rooms: concept and reality, St. Louis, 1981, The C.V. Mosby Co.)

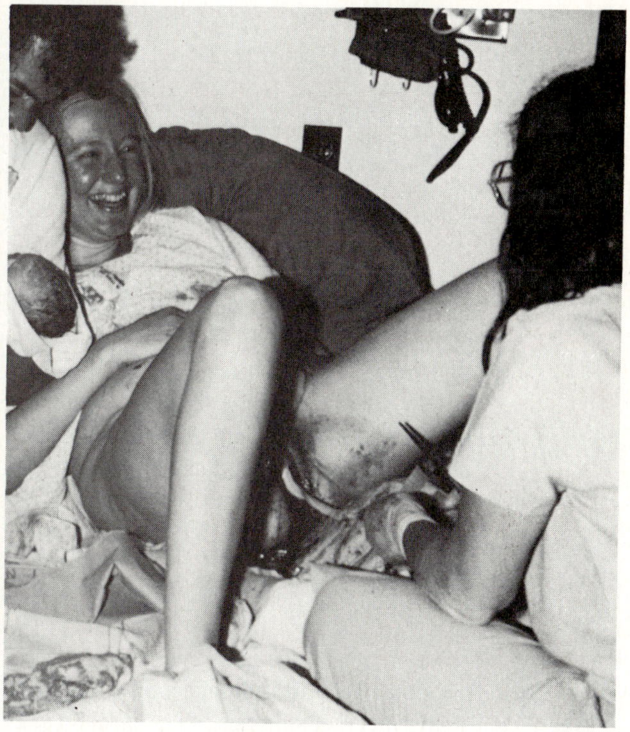

Fig. 26.11
Mother and baby. (From Sumner, P.E., and Phillips, C.R.: Birthing rooms: concept and reality, St. Louis, 1981, The C.V. Mosby Co.)

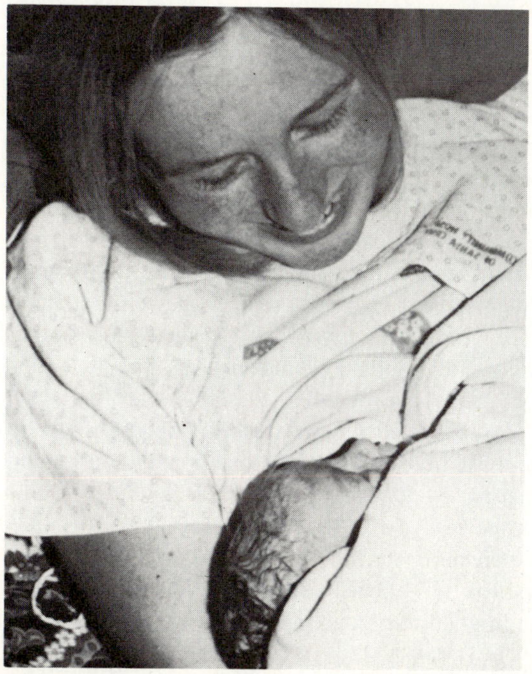

Fig. 26.12
Father and baby. (From Sumner, P.E., and Phillips, C.R.: Birthing rooms: concept and reality, St. Louis, 1981, The C.V. Mosby Co.)

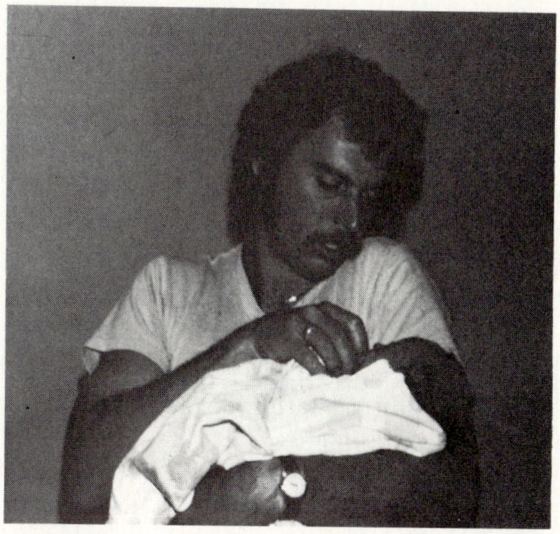

e. Previous infant with respiratory distress syndrome at same gestation

4. Present pregnancy
   a. PIH
   b. Gestational age less than 37 weeks or greater than 42 weeks
   c. Multiple pregnancy
   d. Abnormal presentation (nullipara with a fetus with floating head will need evaluation by her obstetrician)
   e. Third-trimester bleeding or known placenta previa
   f. Prolonged ruptured membranes greater than 24 hours
   g. Evidence of intrauterine growth retardation
   h. Contracted pelvis on any plane
   i. Pelvic diseases (e.g., adnexal masses, uterine malformation, polyhydramnios, pelvic tumors, genital herpes)
   j. Treatment with reserpine, lithium, or magnesium
   k. Induction: intravenous or buccal oxytocin (Pitocin)
   l. Spinal or general anesthesia
   m. Any other acute or chronic medical or psychiatric illness that in opinion of medical staff would increase risk to mother or infant

HIGH-RISK FACTORS DEVELOPING AFTER ADMISSION REQUIRING TRANSFER TO LABOR AND DELIVERY*

1. Hemoglobin: 9.5 g/dl or less†
2. Temperature: 38° C (100.4° F) or higher
3. Significant variation of maternal blood pressure from previously recorded values in office; fall or rise of maternal blood pressure of greater than 30/15 mm Hg
4. Deeply stained meconium in amniotic fluid
5. Abnormal fetal heart rate (FHR) or pattern
6. Prolonged true labor greater than 24 hours
7. Arrest of labor in active phase
8. Second-stage labor: greater than 2 hours for nullipara; greater than 1 hour for multipara
9. Significant vaginal bleeding
10. Development of any factor that requires continuous FHR monitoring
11. Any labor pattern or maternal or fetal complication that attending physician or nurse believes requires more sophisticated diagnosis or treatment than can be done in ABC

*Should the problem resolve, the woman may be transferred back to the ABC or give birth in the labor room.

†Must have intravenous line during labor.

Freestanding Birth Centers

Although most ABCs or birthing rooms are located within existing hospitals, there is a growing number of freestanding birth centers. These units are outside the hospital but are often close to a major hospital so that quick transport to that institution is possible if necessary. Although out-of-hospital birth centers are controversial, they are proliferating rapidly in the United States. However, there is a confusing array of state health regulations for these facilities and even lack of standards and regulations in some states. This confusion has frequently created barriers to adequate insurance reimbursement for families wishing to utilize out-of-hospital birth centers.

A demonstration model for out-of-hospital birth centers has been the Maternity Center Association's Childbearing Center, which opened in 1975 in New York City. Located in a former townhouse, the Childbearing Center has two labor-birth rooms. An early labor lounge and a garden are also available for couples to use when in early labor. Families are accommodated in the center for prenatal care, classes in preparation for childbirth and infant care, labor and delivery, pediatric examination, and postpartum care. The environment is personalized and homelike, emphasizing family involvement and parent responsibility.

The mother and baby are discharged to home within 12 hours of delivery and follow-up care at home is provided by the Visiting Nurses Association of New York. As in hospital birth centers, careful prenatal screening is done and only well mothers without complications are accepted. With thorough record keeping to validate their experiences, the staff of the Child-bearing Center has demonstrated that low-risk pregnancies and deliveries can occur safely in an out-of-hospital center and at a cost substantially below that of birth in a hospital.

Most freestanding birth centers are staffed by physicians who have privileges at the local hospital, and certified nurse-midwives. Both groups are equipped to attend low-risk gravidas through the puerperium. Ambulance service and emergency procedures are readily available. Fees vary with the services provided and the ability of the family to pay (reduced-fee sliding scale). Several insurance companies, as well as Medicaid, recognize and reimburse these clinics.

Services provided by the freestanding birth centers include those necessary for safe management during the childbearing cycle. There are some significant additions, however:

1. Attendance at childbirth and parenting classes is required of all clients. Prenatal supervision of the woman in good nutritional and health status must begin

Fig. 26.13
A, New Beginnings, Inc., freestanding birth center, Warwick, R.I. **B,** Entrance to labor lounge, New Beginnings, Inc.

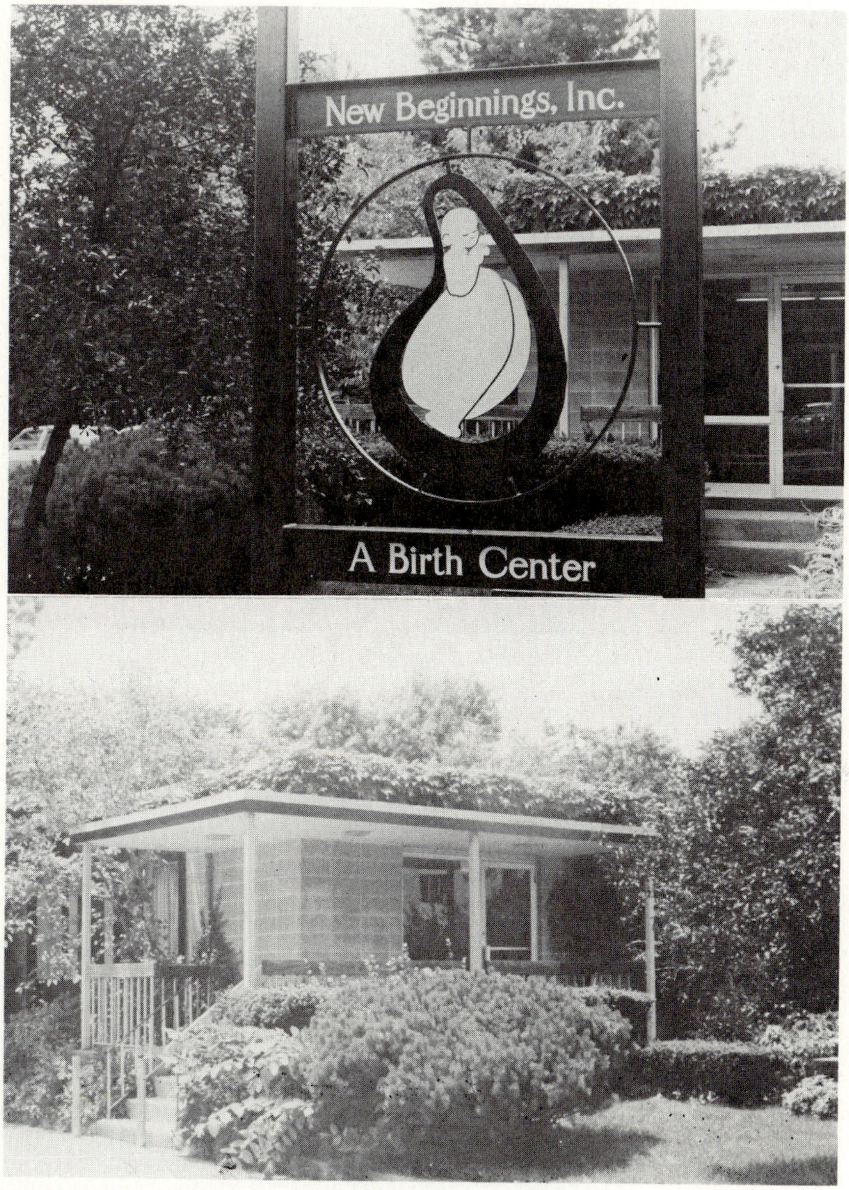

in the first trimester. All clients must be familiar with situations requiring transfer to a hospital.

2. Each expectant family identifies their "birth plan" (Arms, 1978). This is an explanation of practices and procedures they would like to include in or exclude from their childbirth experience. Although the family is given a wide range of choices, they are asked to "assume that there will be no overriding medical or legal necessity for or against any of them in (their) individual case." A sampling of choices follows:

a. *Preparation:* enema, "miniprep," hospital gown instead of own clothing?

b. *Labor:* electronic monitor or fetoscope, freedom to choose positions and activity in labor (walking, squatting), analgesia, presence of siblings, translator?

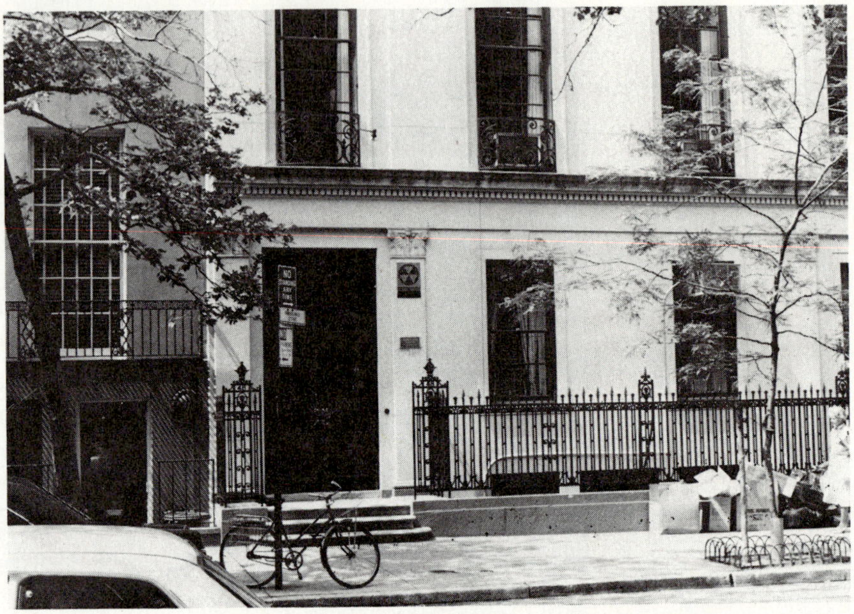

Fig. 26.14
Maternity Center Association, New York.

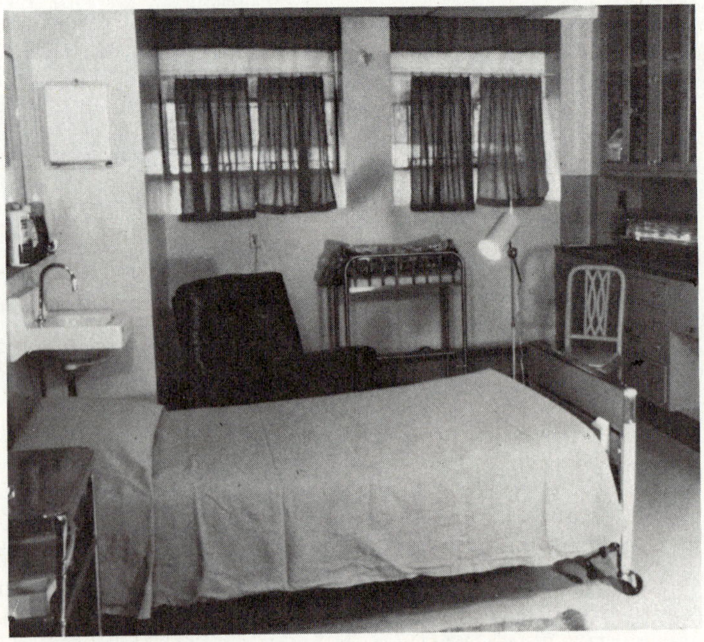

Fig. 26.15
Birth room, Maternity Center Association, New York. (From Sumner, P.E., and Phillips, C.R.: Birthing rooms: concept and reality, St. Louis, 1981, The C.V. Mosby Co.)

c. *Birth:* presence of mate or chosen person, presence of siblings, draping, mirror, dimmed lights, Leboyer bath?

d. *Recovery:* recovery with or without baby or mate or chosen person?

e. *After recovery:* rooming-in, sibling visitation, vitamin K for baby, circumcision, demand feeding—breast or bottle?

Birth centers usually have available a lending library, reference files on related topics, recycled maternity clothes and baby clothes and equipment, supplies and reference materials for childbirth educators, and referral files for community resources that offer services relating to childbirth and early parenting, including support groups (e.g., single parents, postdelivery support group, parents of twins), genetic counseling, women's issues, and consumer action.

A cooperative birth center network has available information on setting up freestanding birth centers.*

Statistics on maternal and infant morbidity and mortality differ from center to center; however, they are consistently comparable with hospital statistics, indicating that birth in a birth center is probably very safe. Studies dealing with questions such as economics, safety, personnel, quality control, and malpractice impact are currently being conducted by numerous hospitals with birth centers as well as by some state health departments.

Nurse-Midwifery

In many hospitals nurse-midwifery services are successful and growing, and in most freestanding birth centers throughout the United States the midwife is the primary care giver. Nurse-midwives are individuals who are educated in both the discipline of nursing and the discipline of nurse-midwifery. A certified nurse-midwife (CNM) is a nurse-midwife who has been certified according to the requirements of the American College of Nurse-Midwives (ACNM). The ACNM defines nurse-midwifery practice as follows:

> . . . the independent management of care of essentially normal newborns and women, antepartally, intrapartally, postpartally, and/or gynecologically, occurring within a health-care system which provides for medical consultation, collaborative management, or referral and is in accord with the *Functions, Standards, and Qualifications for Nurse-Midwifery Practice* as defined by the American College of Nurse-Midwives.

*For information contact CBCN, Box 1, Route 1, Perkiomenville, PA 18074.

At Mount Zion Hospital, San Francisco, certified nurse-midwives have had hospital privileges since 1978. Since 1975, the certified nurse-midwives at San Francisco General Hospital (SFGH) have attended the deliveries of over 1000 low- to high-risk women. At SFGH alternative labor and delivery practices offering more homelike birth settings are available. The SFGH Nurse-Midwifery Service outcome statistics are comparable to those of the obstetrics department in general.

At the Hennepin County Medical Center (HCMC), Minnesota, a Nurse-Midwife Service was initiated in 1973. By January of 1980, the service had had experience with over 2400 births. Maternal and neonatal morbidity has been low, and the service has demonstrated that highly individualized care for normal childbearing women can be provided by nurse-midwives with good results.

Despite an increasing awareness on the part of the consumer and the health professional that nurse-midwives are valuable and often essential members of the health team, the number of lay midwives in this country is growing. A lay midwife may be exceptionally well prepared for practice through self-study, apprenticeship, formal study in the basic sciences, and teaching from sympathetic health professionals. In some states lay midwives may become licensed. Conversely, a lay midwife may have very little preparation or education. Since there is no formal licensing of lay midwifery practice, a wide range of skills can be found among lay midwives. In several states bills have been proposed to combine lay and nurse-midwives and licensed lay midwives and sometimes to develop education programs for nonnurse midwifery. While the controversy about these proposals grows, the number of lay midwives continues to grow. Just as the issue of home birth will eventually have to be addressed, so will the issue of lay midwifery.

Cesarean Birth

Families who are having cesarean births are also in need of the sensitive and supportive care recommended by the Interprofessional Task Force on Health Care of Women and Children. Since 10% to 15% of all births in this country are cesarean births, it is important to acknowledge the needs of these families, too. For couples who want to share the birth of their baby, and who have taken classes to prepare for family-centered birth, an unplanned cesarean delivery can be a cruel blow. In many hospitals today care of parents experiencing a cesarean birth is family centered rather than surgery centered. Education on cesarean birth is being incorporated into prenatal classes, and couples are becoming aware of options available to them if a cesarean delivery is necessary.

Some of the alternatives available to women and their families who experience cesarean birth include the following:

1. Cesarean delivery performed in the labor and delivery area, rather than in the general surgery area
2. The choice of regional instead of general anesthesia, whenever possible
3. The option of having a support person (preferably father) present during the birth
4. The opportunity for skin-to-skin contact with baby and parents immediately after birth
5. Initiation of early rooming-in with help from staff until mother is able to assume responsibility for baby care
6. Encouragement of breast feeding
7. Extended and unlimited visiting privileges for the immediate family members

Cesarean delivery is a birth experience and must be incorporated as such. The goal is a positive birth experience brought about by cooperation between parents, physicians, and hospital personnel.

Home Birth

Home birth has always been popular in certain advanced countries, such as Great Britain, Sweden, and the Netherlands. In developing countries, hospitals or adequate lying-in facilities often are unavailable to most pregnant women, and home birth is a necessity. In the United States and Canada home birth is rapidly gaining popularity.

According to the California Health Department, reported home births in 1975 rose to 3516 from 2038 four years previously. This figure (3516) represents 1.1% of the total births in California in 1975, and these are only those home births that were reported. There are estimates in some communities in California that 10% of the births may occur at home.

According to a study reported by the ACOG, 1.09% of all births in the 47 states studied occurred out of hospitals. Years covered were generally 1975 to 1976 since these were the most recent years in which these data were available. Although in this study only 11 states were able to link mortality in the fetus and newborn with the place of delivery, the data from several states were particularly alarming. For example, in California there were 25 stillbirths per 1000 births for out-of-hospital deliveries as opposed to 9.9 stillbirths per 1000 hospital births in 1975. In Michigan reports on newborn death rates in the first 28 days of life revealed 10.5 per 1000 live births for hospitals and 42.7 per 1000 live births for out-of-hospital births in 1975. Unfortunately, in this study most states had very limited detailed information and only two were able to identify both unplanned precipitate deliveries at home and planned home births. Also, the qualifications of the birth attendants and circumstances of the births were not documented. Until much more detailed statistics on home birth can be compiled, the controversy over the safety of home birth will continue.

National groups supporting home birth are HOME (Home Oriented Maternity Experience) and NAPSAC (National Association of Parents for Safe Alternatives in Childbirth). These groups support changes toward more humane childbearing practices at all levels, integrating the alternatives for childbirth to meet the needs of the total population.

The literature on childbirth contains excellent statistics on medically directed home birth services with skilled nurse-midwives and medical back-up. Two examples of such services are the Chicago Maternity Center with 12,000 home births from 1950 to 1960 without a single maternal death and the home delivery statistics of the Frontier Nursing Service in Appalachia with 23 years without a single maternal death. In the United States today there are reports of very low-risk home delivery populations who have very low levels of difficulty and consequently have excellent statistics. However, there is danger in taking these data on very select populations and applying them to the total population. It must be recognized that even though labor and delivery are normal physiologic events, they do present potential hazards to the mother and fetus both before and after birth. These hazards require provisions for emergency intervention and medical back-up that are available only in hospitals and some birthing homes or in independent birth centers.

Selective home birth in uncomplicated pregnancies is feasible, provided those women at high risk can be identified during the prenatal period and referred for hospital delivery and assuming that a transport system is available for transfer of women with suddenly complicated labors to a nearby adequate medical facility. Another acceptable plan provides for specialist care to be brought to the home by means of a so-called flying squad service, which is utilized in Great Britain, for example.

Collaboration with and supervision of midwives are the obstetrician's duty in many countries. Moreover, obstetric nursing practitioners or nurse-midwives have proved to be invaluable components of the health care team. Thus nurse specialists, general practitioners, and obstetric specialist consultants have become incorporated into home delivery units. A midwife or general practitioner can call on or refer women or infants to numerous essential back-up services for study or specialty care during pregnancy and the early puerperium.

When a woman is to be assisted by a midwife, it is the practice in most areas for the general practitioner to supervise her; meanwhile, both are under the direction of the obstetric specialist.

Although some physicians and nurses are proponents of home births that utilize good medical and emergency back-up systems, most health care professionals regard this practice as exposing the mother and the fetus to unnecessary danger.

ADVANTAGES

One advantage of home birth is that delivery may be more natural or physiologic in familiar surroundings. The mother may be more relaxed and less tense than she might be in the impersonal, sterile environment of a hospital. The family can assist in and be a part of the happy event, and mother-father-infant (and sibling-infant) contact is sustained and immediate. In addition, home birth may be less expensive than a hospital confinement. Serious infection may be less likely, assuming strict aseptic principles are followed. Persons generally are relatively immune to their own home bacteria.

DISADVANTAGES

Because home births are not generally accepted by the medical community, a family may have difficulty finding a qualified health care professional to give prenatal care and to attend the delivery. Also, back-up emergency care by a physician in a hospital may be difficult to arrange in advance. And, emergency transfer to a hospital could be life threatening if the hospital were more than a 10-min distance from the home or if emergency care were not available during the transfer from home to hospital.

Text continued on p. 548.

Fig. 26.16
Out-of-hospital birth. Caput appears at introitus. Perineum is supported using sterile cloth.

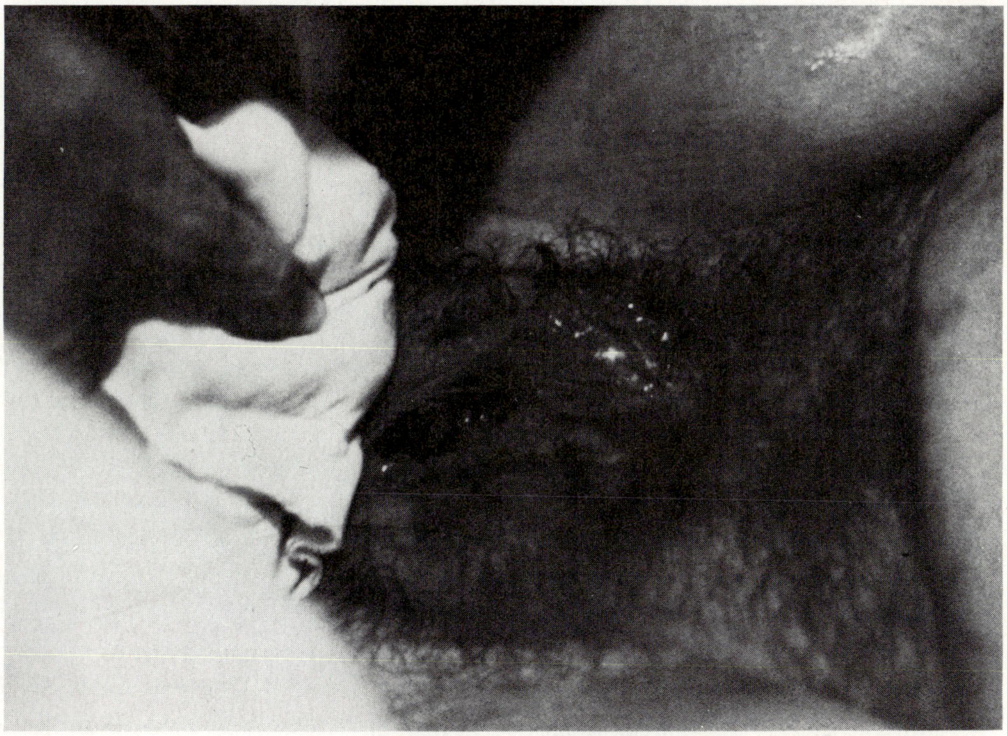

Fig. 26.17
Gentle pressure to back of head is applied with clean hand to control birth of head.

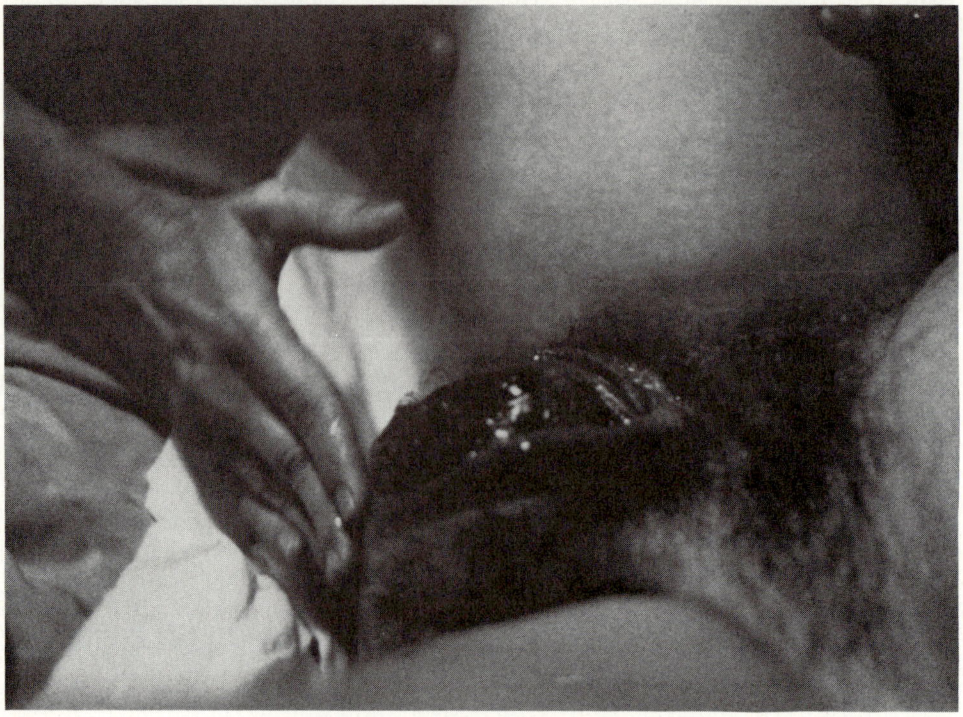

Fig. 26.18
Crowning. Perineum supported using sterile cloth.

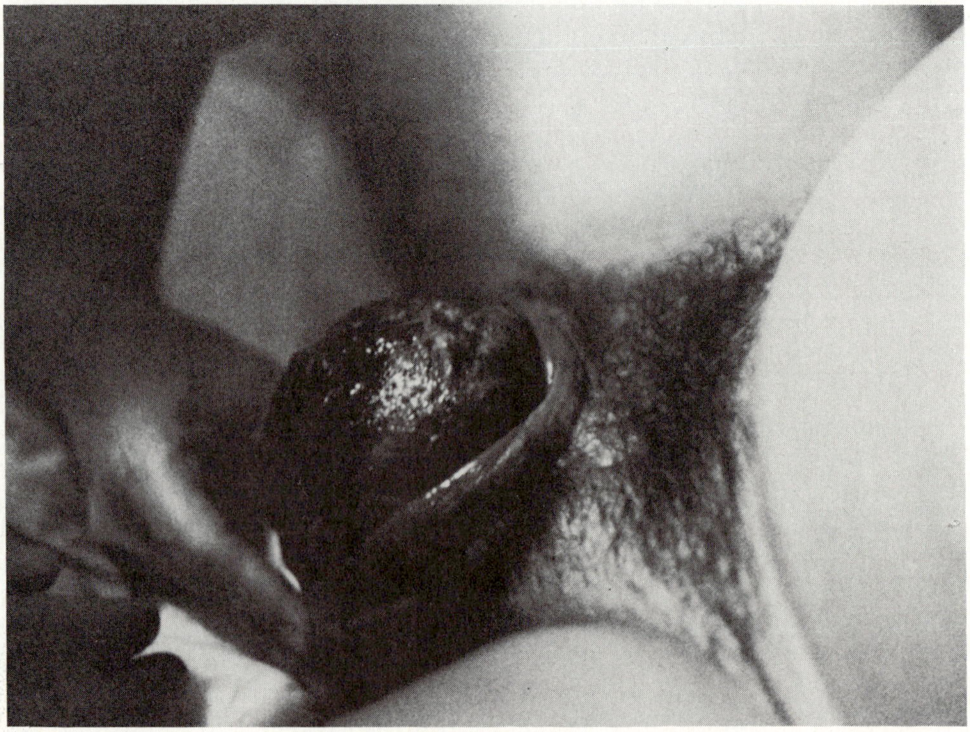

Fig. 26.19
Head is born. Head is supported while restitution occurs.

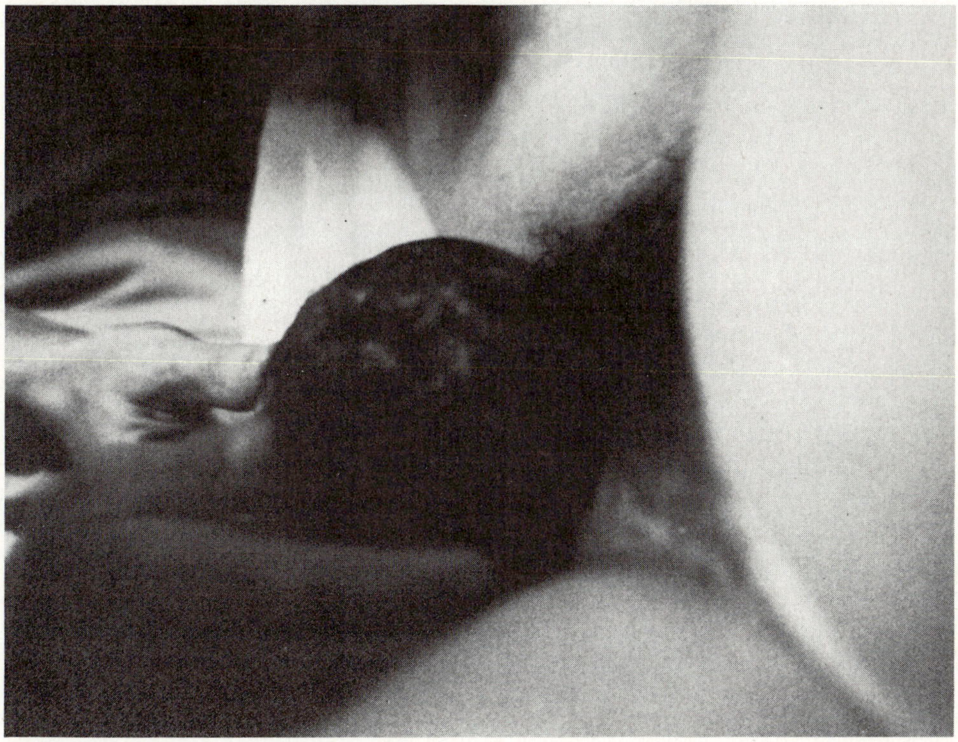

Fig. 26.20
Shoulders are born.

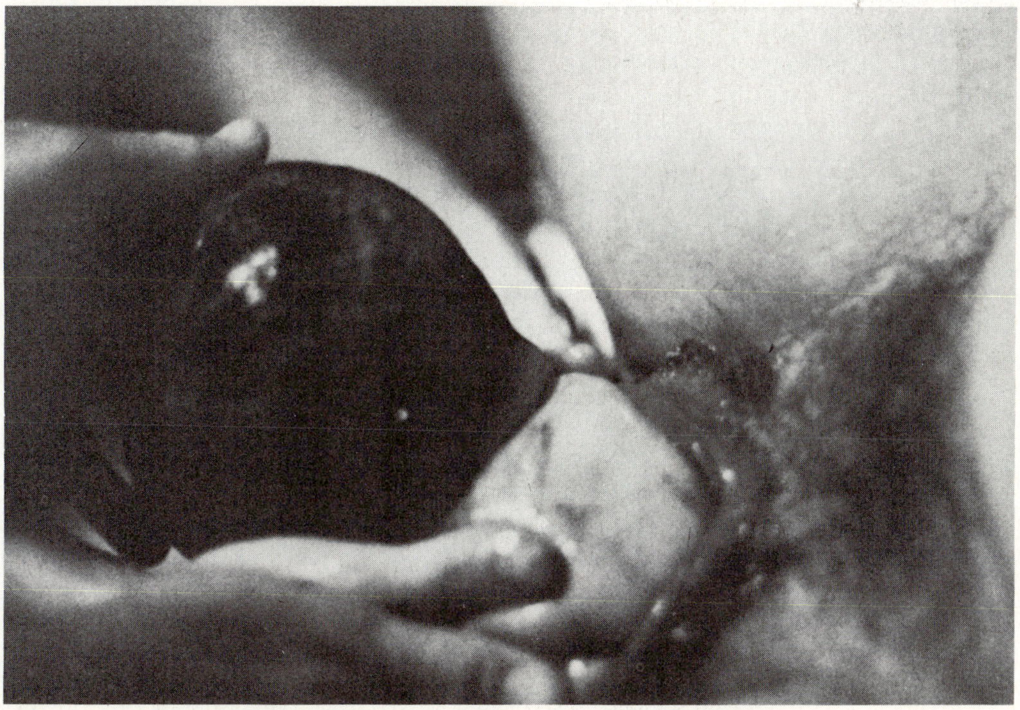

Fig. 26.21
Body emerges rapidly.

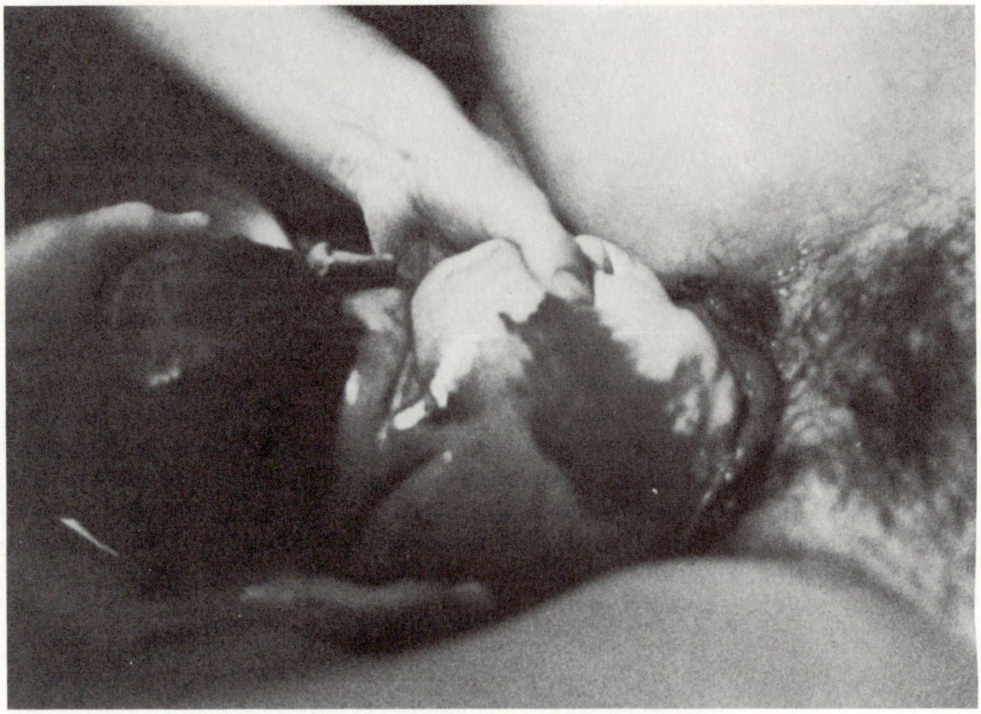

Fig. 26.22
Massaging body while infant is submerged in tub of warm water. Note relaxed, contented expression.

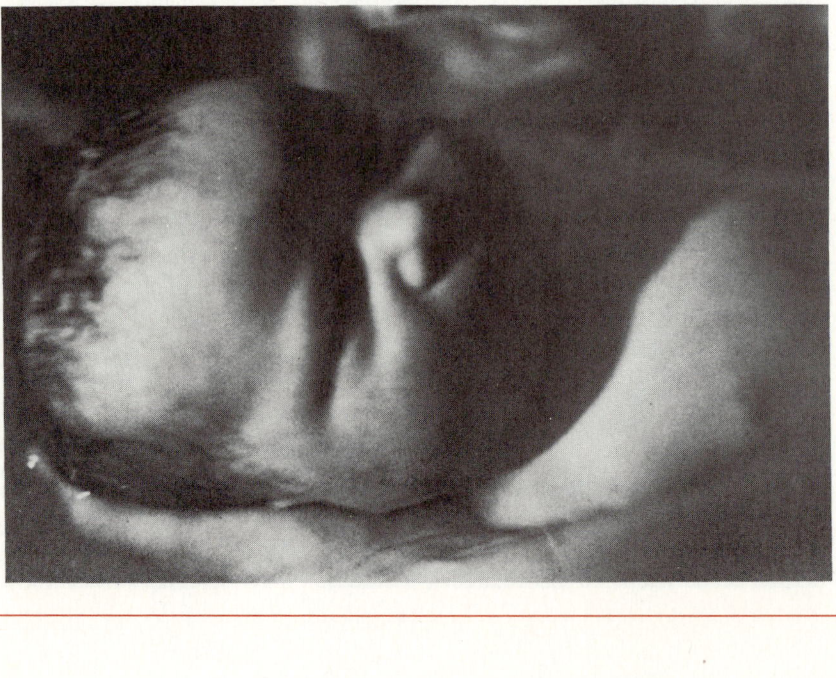

Fig. 26.23
Infant at breast.

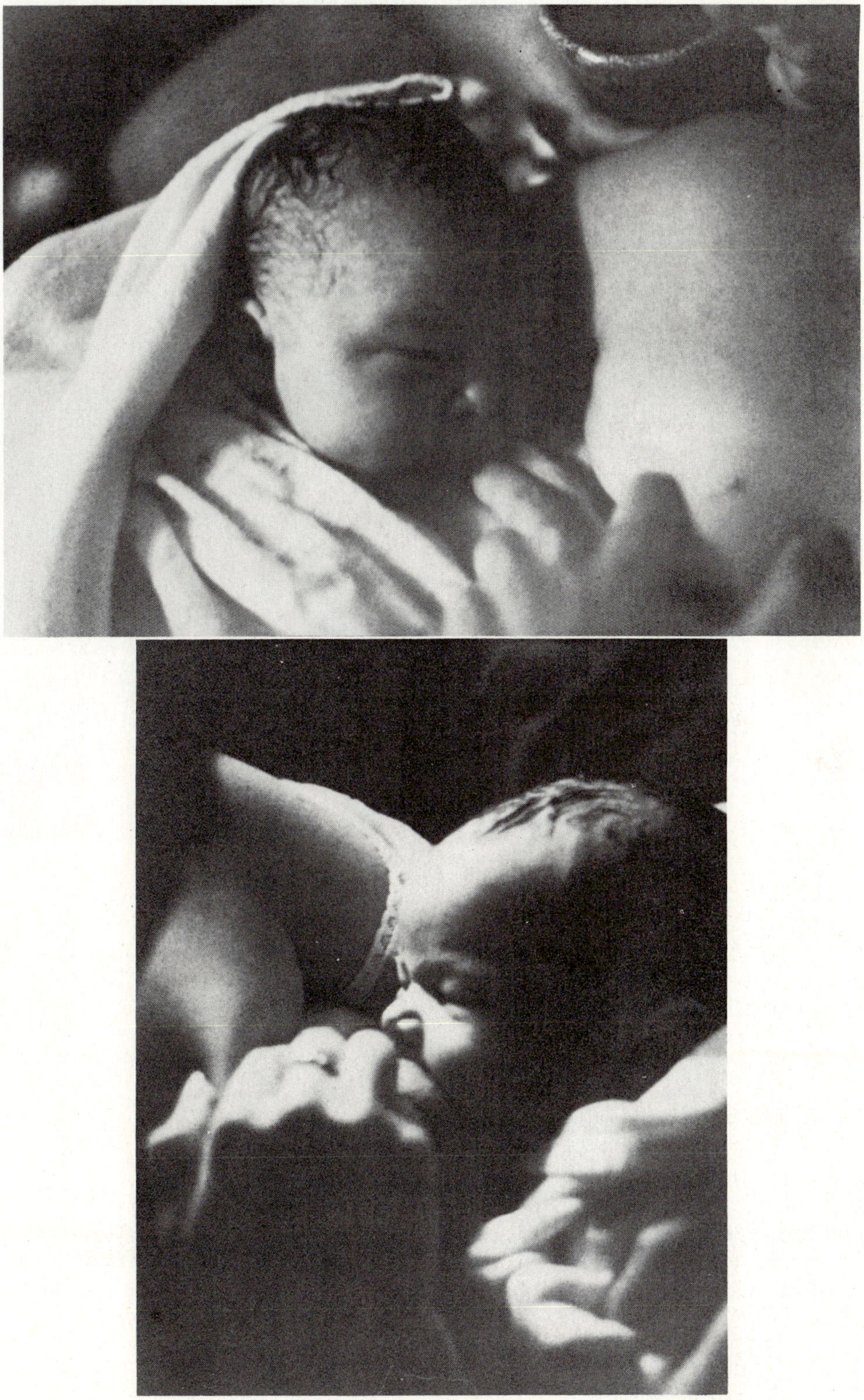

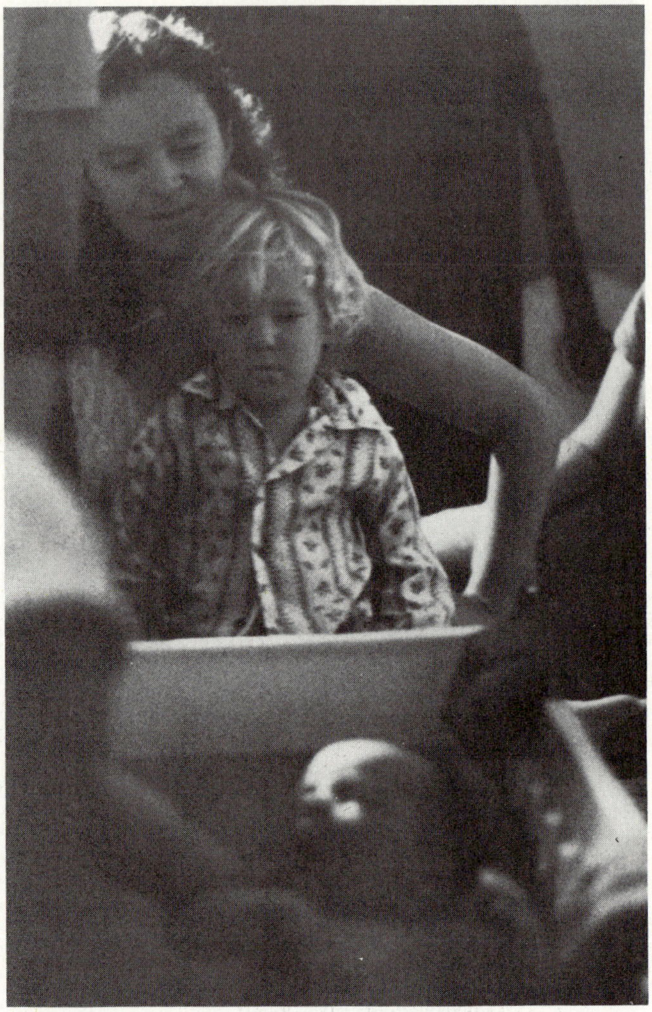

Fig. 26.24
While being held by mother, older child catches first glimpse of baby brother.

CONTRAINDICATIONS

Hospital, not home, birth is indicated for the following:

1. High-risk women (fetal or maternal jeopardy)
2. Women with a history of premature or postdate delivery in their last gestation
3. Women suffering serious medical or surgical complications in this or prior pregnancies
4. Women who cannot be transferred easily to a hospital should the need arise unexpectedly
5. Women who are opposed to home birth
6. Women with inadequate home facilities

FAMILY'S PREPARATION FOR HOME BIRTH

If a home birth is planned, it will usually be possible to obtain and store the necessary articles in advance. In contrast, if birth in the home or elsewhere is an emergency or is determined by circumstances beyond control, considerable improvisation may be necessary.

Facilities and supplies can approximate those available in hospitals. The family will work closely with the physician, nurse, or midwife to complete preparations well in advance of delivery. Attendance by both parents-to-be at childbirth classes (prenatal classes for vaginal and abdominal birth; instructions about the actual delivery of the child if this should occur before the midwife, physician, or other attendant arrives) adds to the competence and also to the pleasure of the parents and other family members. Classes for siblings and grandparents are becoming more available.

Detailed descriptions for preparation are required and may be obtained from either the physician's office or from local health agencies. The agencies may provide some of the equipment and supplies.

A visit to the home by the community health nurse is recommended well before the expected date of birth. At that time the process of birth can be discussed, so that all are aware of the characteristics of normal labor and birth and of the newborn, deviations from normal, and the plan of care for each stage.

Home birth is a selected alternative to hospital birth for some women and couples and a necessity for many. A physically and emotionally safe outcome can be anticipated for most women and couples and their infants, especially if they are prepared and have adequate health care support.

Choice and the Nurse

Since choices for childbirth vary widely from one community to the next, nurses should be aware of all alternatives available in their community. Nurses should evaluate their own values and beliefs about childbearing and attempt to understand why they feel as they do. During their educational and socialization process, nurses have been socialized into a provider culture. The "provider" emphasis in professional socialization tends to view health care from an illness perspective or medical-model viewpoint. This unique preparation of nurses can create values and beliefs that often do not sanction any methods of health care other than those that are "scientifically proved." As a result, there is often incongruity of beliefs and value systems between nurses and consumers. Such incongruity can lead to conflict between the family's choices for childbirth and what the nurse sees as the best choice.

Understanding why families choose alternatives to traditional hospital birth is imperative. Cohen (1982) compared women choosing two different childbirth alternatives (hospital vs. freestanding ABC). He found that women choosing the birth center planned to emphasize autonomy and independence rather than intimacy in their child rearing. Also, their closest relationships were much more supportive and involved in the birth than those women choosing hospital births. Women delivering at the Childbearing Childrearing Center (CCC) at the University of Minnesota, Minneapolis (Rising and Lindell, 1982) reported the three major reasons they chose the center were (1) to have control over their experience, (2) to have family-centered care, and (3) to have no routine procedures administered. Kieffer (1980) compared the attitudes of 109 women before and after experiencing birth using the birthing room concept. The four highest ranking reasons for choice of the birthing room were (1) philosophy, (2) no separation of mother and baby, (3) personal involvement in the birth, and (4) freedom to make choices regarding labor and birth. These studies seem to indicate that attitudes toward issues of choice in the childbirth experience are related to the degree of control that families expect to exert over the birth event.

Most persons who choose home birth are very sincere and concerned about their own safety and the health and safety of their unborn child. In fact, there are probably as many sincere and well-considered reasons for choosing home birth as there are home births. For many individuals experiencing home birth, birth is a very special, intensely personal event to be shared only with family and friends, and not with assorted hospital personnel who are strangers. For many others, birth is an intensely spiritual experience for which a hospital setting is totally inappropriate. Still others do not relish giving up responsibility for their births to hospital personnel; instead, these people want to control their own experience. Most people choosing home birth understand fully the risk involved but also understand that there are also risks in hospital birth.

The concern of nurses is to encourage expectant couples to explore the birth alternatives available to them so that they can make a responsible informed decision. It is also the responsibility of nurses to become actively involved in ensuring that a variety of options for safe childbirth are available in communities.

References & Readings

Alternative Birth Center policies and procedures, San Francisco, April 1976, Mount Zion Hospital and Medical Center, Department of Obstetrics and Pediatrics.

American College of Nurse-Midwives: Statement of qualifications, standards and functions; philosophy and definitions, Washington, D.C., The College.

American College of Obstetricians and Gynecologists, District II: Position paper on out-of-hospital maternity care, ICEA News **15**:2, Spring 1976.

American College of Obstetricians and Gynecologists: The development of family-centered maternity/newborn care in hospitals, Washington, D.C., 1978, The College.

American College of Obstetricians and Gynecologists: Alternative Birth Centers (a questionnaire survey), Washington, D.C., 1981, The College.

Anderson, S., et al.: The choice of home birth in a metropolitan county in Arizona, J.O.G.N. Nurs. **7**:41, March-April, 1978.

Arms, S.: Immaculate deception: a new look at women and childbirth, Boston, 1975, Houghton Mifflin Co.

Arms, S.: Five women, five births, 1978. (Film.)

Averitt, S.S.: Adapting the birthing center concept to a traditional hospital setting, J.O.G.N. Nurs. **9**:103, March-April 1980.

Ballard, R., et al.: An alternative birth center: concepts and operation. In Taylor, P. M., editor: Parent-infant relationships, New York, 1980, Grune & Stratton, Inc.

Barton, J.L., et al.: Alternative birthing center: experience in a teaching obstetric service, Am. J. Obstet. Gynecol. **137**:3, June 1980.

Benton, D.: A study of how women are reflected in nursing textbooks used to teach obstetrics-gynecology, Nurs. Forum **16**(3):268, 1977.

Bodnar, C.: Alternative birthing network under way, Calif. Nurs., p. 7, Dec. 1979.

California: furor over home births, Medical World News, p. 32, April 4, 1977.

Candy, M.M.: Birth of a comprehensive family-centered maternity program, J.O.G.N. Nurs. **8**:80, March-April 1979.

Caplan, G.: Family support systems in a changing world. In Anthony, J., and Chiland, C., editor: The child and his family: children and their parents in a changing world, New York, 1978, John Wiley & Sons, Inc.

Carlson, B., and Sumner, P.E.: Hospital "at home" delivery: a celebration, J.O.G.N. Nurs. **5**:21, Jan.-Feb. 1976.

Chess, S., and Thomas, A.: Infant bonding: mystique and reality, Am. J. Orthopsychiatr. **52**:2, April 1982.

Cohen, R.L.: A comparative study of women choosing two different birth alternatives, Birth **9**:1, Spring 1982.

Dobbs, K.B. and Shy, K.K.: Alternative birth rooms and birth options, Obstet. Gynecol. **58**:5, Nov. 1981.

Edwards, M: Unattended home birth, Am. J. Nurs. **73**:1332, 1973.

Englemann, G.: Birth among primitive peoples: book reviews, Birth Fam. J. **2**:92, 1982; **2**:76, Summer 1975.

Enkin, M.: The family in labour, Birth Fam. J. **2**:133, Fall-Winter 1975-1976.

Estes, M.N.: A home delivery service with expert consultation and back-up, Birth Fam. J. **5**:151, Fall 1978.

Fenwick, L., and Dearing, R.: The Cybele cluster system: single room maternity care for high and low risk families, Spokane, Wash., 1981, The Cybele Society.

Fullerton, J.D.T.: The choice of in-hospital or alternative birth environment as related to the concept of control, J. Nurse-Midwife. **27**:2, March-April 1982.

Gillett, J.: Childbirth in Pithiviers, France, Lancet, P. 894, Oct. 27, 1979.

Hazell, L.D.: A study of 300 elective home births, Birth Fam. J. **2**:11, Fall-Winter 1974-1975.

Hazell, L.D.: Commonsense childbirth, Berkeley, Calif., 1976, Berkeley Windhover Books.

Hewett, M.A., and Hangsleven, K.L.: Nurse-midwives in a hospital birth center, J. Nurse-Midwife. **26:**5, Sept.-Oct. 1981.

Interprofessional task force on health care of women and children: Joint position statement: the development of family-centered maternity/newborn care in hospitals, J.O.G.N. Nurs. **7:**55, Sept.-Oct. 1978.

Kieffer, M.J.: The birthing room concept at Phoenix Memorial Hospital. II. Consumer satisfaction during one year, J.O.G.N. Nursing, p. 158, May-June 1980.

Lang, R.: Birth book, Ben Lomoand, Calif., 1972, Genesis Press.

L'Experance, C.M.: Home birth—a manifestation of aggression? J.O.G.N. Nurs. **8:**227, July-Aug. 1979.

Lubic, R.W.: The impact of technology on health care—the childbearing center: a case for technology's appropriate use, J. Nurse-Midwife. **24:**1, Jan.-Feb. 1979.

Lubic, R.W., and Ernst, E.K.M.: The childbearing center: an alternative to conventional care, Nurs. Outlook **26**(12):754, 1978.

Mann, R.J.: San Francisco General Hospital nurse-midwifery practice: the first thousand births, Am. J. Obstet. Gynecol. **140:**6, July 1981.

Marieskind, H.I.: Women in the health system: patients, providers, and programs, St. Louis, 1980, The C.V. Mosby Co.

Mather, S.: Women's interests in alternative maternity facilities, Nurse-Midwife. **25:**3, May-June 1980.

Mehl, L., et al.: Complications of home birth, Birth Fam. J. **2**(2):123, 1975.

Nielsen, I.: Nurse-midwifery in an alternative birth center, Birth Fam. J. **4:**24, Spring 1977.

Parfitt, R.R.: The birth primer: a source book of traditional and alternative methods in labor and delivery, Philadelphia, 1977, Running Press.

Patterson, K.A., and Peterson, V.L.: The Alternative Birth Center movement in the San Francisco and Bay area, Nurse-Midwife. **25:**2, March-April 1980.

Pearse, W.H.: Home birth (editorial), J.A.M.A. **241:**1039, 1979.

Phillips, C.: The essence of birth without violence, Am. J. Mat. Child Nurs., p. 162, May-June 1976.

Rising, S.S., and Lindell, S.G.: The Childbearing Childrearing Center: a nursing model, Nurs. Clin. North Am. **17:**1, March 1982.

Ritchie, C.A., and Swanson, L.A.: Childbirth outside the hospital—the resurgence of home and clinic deliveries, M.C.N. **1:**372, 1976.

Roberts, J.E.: Maternal positions for childbirth: a historical review of nursing care practices, J.O.G.N. Nurs. **8:**24, Jan.-Feb. 1979.

Rosen, E.L.: The birth room: implementation of an alternative, Can. Nurs., p. 30, March 1980.

Searles, C.: The impetus toward home birth, J. Nurse-Midwife. **26:**3, May-June 1981.

Simkin, P., and Reinke, C., editors: Kaleidoscope of childbearing: preparation, birth and nurturing. Highlights of the Tenth Biennial Convention of the International Childbirth Education Association, Inc., Seattle, 1978, The Pennypress.

Snyder, C., et al.: New findings about mother's antenatal expectations and their relationship to infant development, M.C.N. **4:**345, Nov.-Dec. 1979.

Spector, R.: Cultural diversity in health and illness, New York, 1979 Appleton-Century-Crofts.

Standards of maternal-child nursing practice, Am. Nurse, p. 16, July 1974.

Stewart, David, and Lee: Safe alternatives in childbirth, June 1976, National Association of Parents and Professionals for Safe Alternatives in Childbirth.

Sumner, P., and Phillips, C.: Birthing rooms: concept and reality, St. Louis, 1981, The C.V. Mosby Co.

Nursing Care of the Normal Newborn

27 Biologic and Behavioral Characteristics of the Newborn

28 Nursing Assessment and Diagnosis of the Newborn

29 Planning, Implementing, and Evaluating Care of the Newborn

30 Newborn Nutrition and Feeding

UNIT FIVE

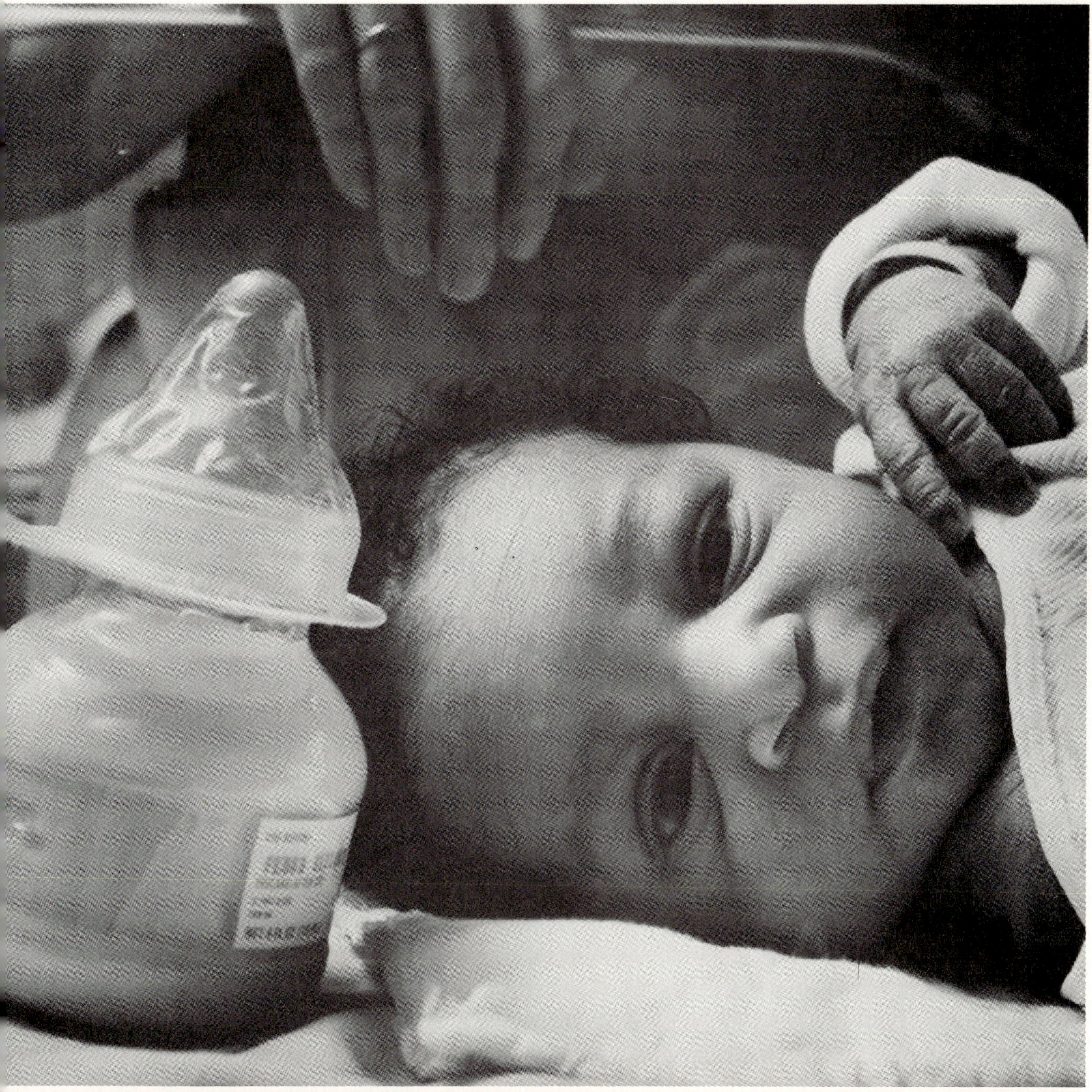

27

Biologic and Behavioral Characteristics of the Newborn

- **Biologic Characteristics**
  - Cardiovascular system
  - Hematopoietic system
  - Respiratory system
  - Renal system and water balance
  - Digestive system
  - Hepatic system
    - Physiologic hyperbilirubinemia
    - Breast milk jaundice
  - Immunity
    - IgG
    - IgM
    - IgA
  - Neurologic system
  - Integumentary system
  - Thermogenesis
    - Heat production
    - Heat loss
    - Temperature regulation
    - Cold stress
  - Reproductive system
- **Behavioral Characteristics**
  - Sensory behaviors
    - Vision
    - Hearing
    - Touch
    - Taste
    - Smell
  - Sleeping and waking behaviors
    - Sleep-wake cycles
  - Social behaviors
  - Feeding behaviors
  - Elimination behaviors

Extrauterine existence imposes a number of developmental tasks on the neonate, which must be accomplished in order to achieve autonomy. By term the infant's various anatomic and physiologic systems have reached a level of development and functioning that permits a physical existence apart from the mother and a readiness for social interaction (Fig. 27.1).

The physiologic tasks involve (1) establishing and maintaining respirations; (2) ingesting, retaining, and digesting nutrients, a transition from maternal parenteral to infant enteral nutrition; (3) elimination of wastes; (4) regulation of temperature; and (5) regulation of weight.

Lewis and Zarin-Ackerman (1977) have described three major interrelated behavioral tasks the neonate must also accomplish:

1. First, he must establish homeostasis, that is, regulated behavioral tempo independent of the mother. This involves self-regulation of arousal, self-monitoring of changes in his state, and patterning of sleep.
2. The second task is cognitive in nature. He must process, store, and organize the multiple stimuli to which he is exposed.
3. The third task is to establish a relationship with a primary caretaker and with his environment (see Chapter 32).

Although in reality the neonate functions as a complex of biologic and social behaviors, for the purpose of clarity a separation of biologic and behavioral characteristics has been made in the following presentation.

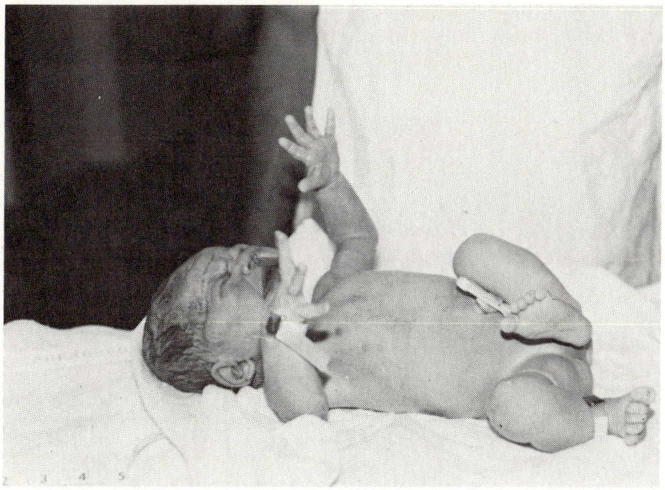

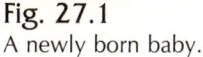

Fig. 27.1
A newly born baby.

Biologic Characteristics

The profound biologic responses that occur at birth make possible the infant's transition from intrauterine to extrauterine life and set the stage for his future growth and development. The neonatal period, from birth through day 28, represents a time of dramatic change for the newborn.

CARDIOVASCULAR SYSTEM

The infant's first breath inflates his lungs, markedly reducing pulmonary vascular resistance to pulmonary blood flow and producing a drop in pulmonary artery pressure. This sequence is the major mechanism by which pressure in the *right atrium declines*. The increased pulmonary blood flow returned to the left side of the heart *increases* the pressure in the *left* atrium.

This change in pressures causes a functional closure of the foramen ovale; anatomic closure, however, may take from several weeks to a year. Because of this nonanatomic closure, an increase in pressure in the right atrium (as from crying) can cause a right-to-left shunt; however, most infants show a left-to-right shunt during the first 24 hours (Fig. 27.2). By 8 days only a few continue to do so (Jegier and co-workers, 1964).

The ductus arteriosus constricts in response to the increased Po_2; however, there is also much controversy over the time of its anatomic closure. It is felt that its continued patency is responsible for the shunting of the blood the first few days after birth. Eventually it occludes and becomes a ligament as do the other fetal vessels, the hypogastric arteries.

With the clamping and severing of the cord, the umbilical vein and ductus venosus close immediately and are eventually converted into ligaments (Table 27.1).

By term the infant's heart lies midway between the crown of the head and the buttocks, and the axis is more transverse than that of the adult (Fig. 28.9). By the third year of life the cardiac shadow is practically the same as the adult cardiac shadow. The size of the heart does not change significantly in the first 4 to 6 weeks. After that period the heart grows steadily, with two major growth periods: from 1 to 9 years and during adolescence. The *heart rate* averages 140 beats/min at birth with variations noted during sleeping and waking states. At 1 week of age the mean heart rate is 128 beats/min asleep and 163 beats/min awake; at 1 month of age, it is 138 beats/min asleep and 167 beats/min awake. Sinus arrhythmia (irregular heart rate) may be considered a physiologic phenomenon in infancy and an indication of good heart function (Lowrey, 1978). By the second to fourth year the rate has decreased to an average of 105 beats/min, and the adult average rate of 80 to 100 beats/min is reached by the end of adolescence. *Heart sounds* during the neonatal period are of higher pitch, shorter duration, and greater intensity than during adult life. The first sound is typically louder and more dull than the second sound, which is sharp in quality.

Most heart murmurs heard during the neonatal period have no pathologic significance, and more than half disappear by 6 months. Blood pressure in infants varies

Fig. 27.2
Fetal circulation. (Courtesy Ross Laboratories, Columbus, Ohio.)

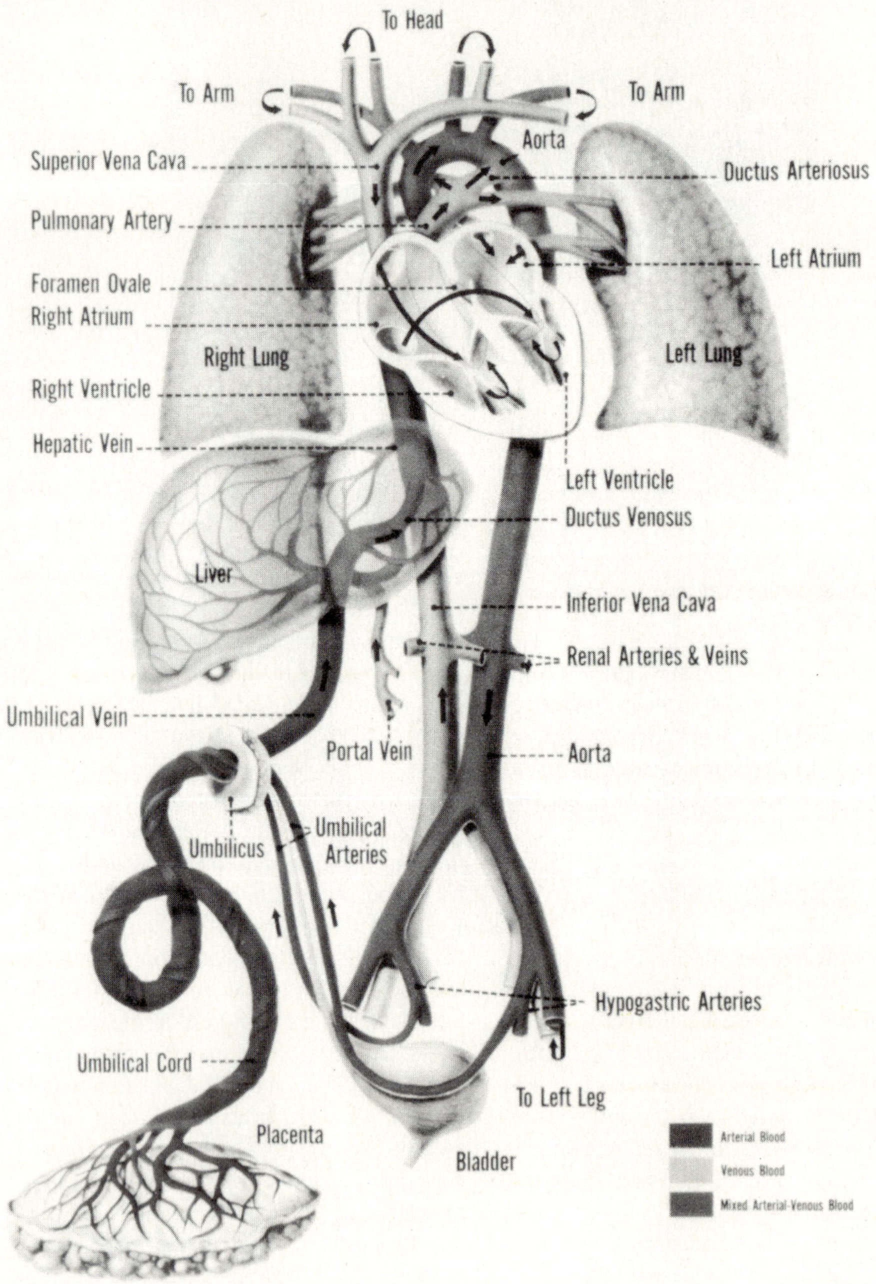

Table 27.1
Cardiovascular Changes at Birth

Prenatal Status	Postdelivery Status	Associated Factors
Primary changes		
Pulmonary circulation: high pulmonary vascular resistance; increased pressure in right ventricle and pulmonary arteries	Low pulmonary vascular resistance; decreased pressure in right atrium, ventricle, and pulmonary arteries	Expansion of collapsed fetal lung with air
Systemic circulation: low pressures in left atrium, ventricle, and aorta	High systemic vascular resistance; increased pressure in left atrium, ventricle, and aorta	Loss of placental blood flow
Secondary changes		
Umbilical arteries: patent; carry blood from hypogastric arteries to the placenta	Functionally closed at birth; obliteration by fibrous proliferation may take 2-3 mo; distal portions become *lateral vesicoumbilical ligaments;* proximal portions remain open as *superior vesical arteries*	Closure precedes that of umbilical vein; probably accomplished by smooth muscle contraction in response to thermal and mechanical stimuli and alteration in oxygen tension; mechanically severed with cord at birth
Umbilical vein: patent; carries blood from placenta to ductus venosus and liver	Closed; after obliteration, it becomes *ligamentum teres hepatis*	Closure shortly after umbilical arteries; hence blood from placenta may enter neonate for short period after birth; mechanically severed with cord at birth
Ductus venosus; patent; connects umbilical vein to inferior vena cava	Closed; after obliteration, it becomes *ligamentum venosus*	Loss of blood flow from umbilical vein
Ductus arteriosus; patent; shunts blood from pulmonary artery to descending aorta	Functionally closed almost immediately after birth; anatomic obliteration of lumen by fibrous proliferation requires 1-3 mo; becomes *ligamentum arteriosum*	High systemic resistance increases aortic pressure; low pulmonary resistance reduces pulmonary arterial pressure Increased oxygen content of blood in ductus arteriosus creates vasospasm of its muscular wall
Foramen ovale: forms a valve opening that allows blood to flow from right to left atrium	Functionally closes at birth; constant apposition gradually leads to fusion and permanent closure within a few months or years in majority of persons	Increased pressures in left atrium together with decreased pressure in right atrium cause closure of valve over foramen

From Whaley, L.F., and Wong, D.L.: Nursing care of infants and children, St. Louis, 1979, The C.V. Mosby Co.

from day to day. A drop in systolic blood pressure (about 15 mm Hg) the first hour after birth is common. Values from several hours after delivery through the neonatal period average a systolic pressure of 78 and a diastolic pressure of 42 (see discussion of Doppler technique, Chapter 24). Crying and moving results in changes in blood pressure, especially systolic.

Total *blood volume* in the newborn ranges from 80 to 110 ml/kg (average total: 200 ml) during the first several days and doubles by the end of the first year. The newborn has approximately 10% greater blood volume and nearly 20% greater red blood cell mass but about 20% less plasma volume when compared by kilogram of body weight with the adult. In further contrast the infant born about the thirty-fifth or thirty-sixth week will have a greater blood volume than the term neonate. This is because of the baby's greater plasma volume, rather than a greater red blood cell mass. The time of clamping of the cord also affects the newborn's circulation:

> Early or late clamping of the cord will cause a number of differences in the circulatory dynamics of the newborn. With so-called placental transfusion from late clamping, there is an expansion of blood volume, increase in heart size, higher systolic blood pressure and an increased respiratory rate, as compared to the controls with no transfusion. These changes persist for about 48 hours. Pulmonary rales and transient cyanosis are encountered more frequently in the group with late clamping. The increase in blood volume by using this technic may average 166 ml, or an increase of close to 60%. The value to the infant, if any, of one method over the other has yet to be determined.*

*Reproduced with permission from Lowrey, G.H.: Growth and development of children, ed. 7. Copyright © 1978 by Year Book Medical Publishers, Inc., Chicago.

HEMATOPOIETIC SYSTEM

At birth the average values of hemoglobin and red blood cells are higher than those values in the adult, but these fall and reach the average levels of 11 to 17 g/dl and 4.2 to 5.2/cu mm, respectively, by the end of the first month. These blood values may be affected by delayed clamping of the cord, which results in a rise in hemoglobin, red blood cells, and hematocrit. The source of the sample is also significant, since capillary blood will give higher values than venous blood. Also, the time after birth when the blood sample was obtained is significant, since the slight rise in red blood cells after birth is followed by a substantial drop. Cord blood contains about 80% fetal hemoglobin, but because of the shorter life span of the cells containing fetal hemoglobin, the percentage falls to 55% by 5 weeks and 5% by 20 weeks. Fortunately iron stores generally are sufficient to sustain normal red blood cell production for 6 months, and thus the slight brief anemia is not serious.

Leukocytosis, with the white blood cell count approximately 18,000/cu mm, is normal at birth. The number, largely polymorphs, increases to about 23,000 to 24,000/cu mm during the first day after birth. A resting level of 11,500/cu mm normally is maintained during the neonatal period. Serious infection is not well tolerated by the newborn, and a marked increase in the white blood cell count is unlikely even in critical sepsis. In most instances sepsis is accompanied by a decline in white cells, and in neutrophils particularly. There is a gradual increase in the strength of the isoagglutinogens determining blood groupings, although the blood group is established early in fetal life.

Platelet count and aggregation are essentially the same in neonates as in adults with the exception of infants of mothers who had taken acetylsalicylic acid (aspirin) or chlorpromazine, which interfere with the release of adenosine diphosphate (ADP). Bleeding tendencies in the neonate are rare, and unless there has been a marked vitamin K deficiency, clotting is sufficient to prevent hemorrhage. The activity of the marrow is accurately reflected by the numbers of circulating cells—both erythrocytes and leukocytes. The early high white blood cell count of the newborn decreases rapidly. A relative leukopenia found in black children and adults is apparent by 1 year of age and is primarily caused by a decreased number of neutrophils. By 6 years of age the peripheral blood picture is approximately the same as that of an adult. (See Appendixes G and I.)

RESPIRATORY SYSTEM

At birth, air must be substituted for fluid that has filled the respiratory tract to the alveoli. During the course of normal vaginal delivery, between 7 and 42 ml of amniotic fluid is squeezed or drained from the neonate's lungs (Aladjem et al., 1979). After delivery the major portion of the fetal lung fluid is absorbed across the alveolar membrane into the blood capillaries. This is largely a result of the pressure gradient from alveoli to interstitial tissue to blood capillary. Reduced vascular resistance also accommodates this flow of lung fluid; however, it is the diminished intravascular pressure that is ultimately responsible.

Initial breathing probably is the result of a reflex triggered in part by pressure changes, chilling, noise, light, and other sensations related to the birth process. In addition, the chemoreceptors in the aorta and carotid bodies initiate neurologic reflexes when the arterial Po_2 falls from 80 to 15 mm Hg, arterial Pco_2 rises from 40 to 70 mm Hg, and arterial pH falls below 7.35 (when these changes are extreme, however, depression ensues). In most cases an exaggerated respiratory reaction follows within 1 minute of birth, and the infant takes his first gasping breath and cries.

With the first breath the infant develops a considerable negative intrathoracic pressure. Air is drawn in, and about half of this remains as residual pulmonary volume. Normally only a few breaths are required to expand the lungs well; subsequently the pressure will be lower than at the onset of respiration.

Once respirations are established, they are shallow and irregular, ranging from 30 to 60 breaths/min, with short periods of apnea (less than 15 seconds). However, any apneic period should be evaluated. Infants are obligatory nose breathers. However, since the normal response to nasal obstruction, that is, opening the mouth to maintain the airway, is not present in most babies for 3 weeks after birth (may occur earlier in certain races [Freedman, 1979]), cyanosis or asphyxia may occur with nasal blockage.

The chest circumference is approximately 30 to 33 cm (12 to 13 in) at birth. The ribs of the infant articulate with the spine at a horizontal rather than a downward slope; consequently the rib cage cannot expand as readily as the adult's with inspiration. Neonatal respiratory function is largely a matter of diaphragmatic contraction. The negative intrathoracic pressure is created by the descent of the diaphragm, much like negative pressure is created in the barrel of a syringe when medication is drawn up by retracting the plunger. The infant's chest and abdomen rise simultaneously with inspiration (Fig. 27.3). Seesaw respirations are not normal (Fig. 27.4).

Auscultation of the chest of an infant reveals loud, clear breath sounds that seem very near, since little chest tissue intervenes. Apnea (less than 15 seconds) and periodic breathing are characteristically present in

Fig. 27.3
Normal respiration. Chest and abdomen rise with inspiration. (Courtesy Mead Johnson & Co., Evansville, Ind.)

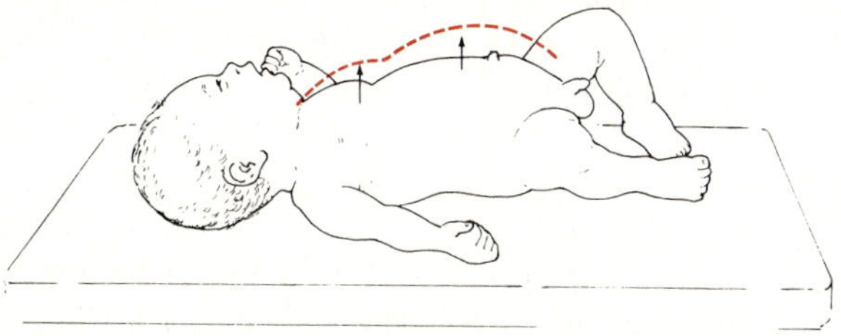

Fig. 27.4
Seesaw respiration. Chest wall retracts and abdomen rises with inspiration. (Courtesy Mead Johnson & Co., Evansville, Ind.)

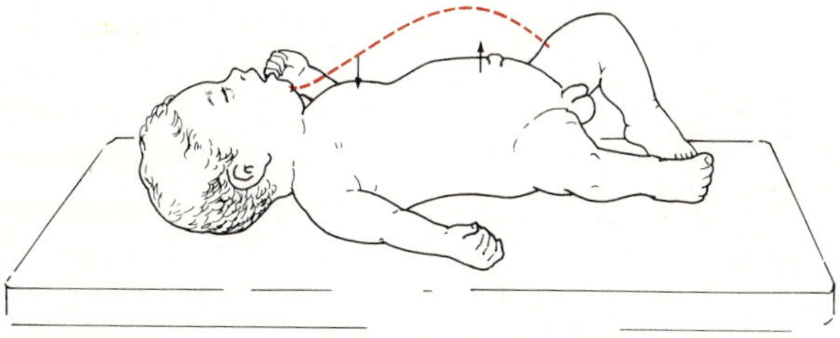

the neonate. They occur most often during the active (rapid eye movement [REM]) sleep cycle and decrease in frequency and duration with age.

Several significant differences exist between the respiratory tract of the infant and that of the adult:

1. Infants are obligate nose breathers.
2. The infant's tongue is relatively large (macroglossia), whereas the glottis and trachea are small.
3. All lumens of the infant are narrower and more easily collapsed.
4. Respiratory tract secretions of the infant are more abundant than the adult's.
5. The mucous membranes of the infant are more delicate and therefore more susceptible to trauma. The ciliated columnar epithelium just below the vocal cords is especially prone to edema.
6. The alveoli of the infant are more sensitive to changes in pressures.
7. The capillary network of the infant is less well developed. Capillaries are more friable and have less well developed vasoconstrictive and dilatative ability.
8. The infant's bony rib cage and respiratory muscles are not as well developed.

RENAL SYSTEM AND WATER BALANCE

At term the kidneys occupy a large portion of the posterior abdominal wall. The bladder lies close to the anterior abdominal wall and is partially an abdominal, as well as a pelvic, organ. In the newborn almost all palpable masses in the abdomen are renal in origin. Maturation of kidney function comparable to the adult is well advanced only after the first year of life. The inability of the kidneys to regulate internal environment, the relatively high hydrogen ion concentration, and the lowered plasma osmotic pressure mean that the neonate has a minimal level of chemical balance and safety. Diarrhea, infection, or improper feeding can lead rapidly to acidosis and fluid imbalances—dehydration or edema. Renal immaturity also limits the neonate's ability to excrete drugs.

Differences from adult physiologic response include the following:

1. Distribution of extracellular and intracellular fluid. About 40% of the body weight of the newborn is extracellular fluid, whereas in the adult it is 20%.
2. Rate of exchange of extracellular fluid. The newborn daily takes in and excretes 600 to 700 ml of water, which is 20% of the total body fluid, or 50% of his extracellular fluid. In contrast, the adult exchanges 2000 ml of water, which is 5% of the total body fluid and 14% of the extracellular fluid.
3. Composition of body fluids. There is a higher concentration of sodium, phosphates, chloride, and organic acids and a lower concentration of bicarbonate ions. These findings mean that the newborn is in a compensated acidotic state and in a state of potential manifest edema.
4. Glomerular filtration rate is about 30% to 50%

that of the adult. This results in a decreased ability to remove nitrogenous and other waste products from the blood. However, the neonate's ingested protein is almost totally metabolized for growth.

5. Decreased ability to excrete excessive sodium results in hypotonic urine compared to plasma.
6. Sodium reabsorption is decreased as a result of a lowered sodium-potassium–activated adenosine triphosphatase (ATPase) activity.
7. The neonate can dilute urine down to 50 milliosmols (mOsm).* Capacity to dilute urine exceeds capacity to concentrate it. There is some limitation in the ability to increase urinary volume.
8. The neonate can concentrate urine—as high as 600 to 700 mOsm compared to the adult's capacity of 1400 mOsm. The inability to concentrate urine is not absolute, but in terms of adult function, it is somewhat limited.
9. A higher renal threshold for glucose.
10. Small amounts of urine are usually present in the bladder at birth; however, the neonate may not void for 12 to 24 hours. Voiding after this period is frequent. Six to ten voidings of pale, straw-colored urine are indicative of adequate fluid intake. The usual urinary output by 10 days is 50 to 300 ml/24 hr.

DIGESTIVE SYSTEM

In the normally hydrated infant, the mucous membrane of the mouth appears moist and pink. Pallor and cyanosis of the mucous membrane normally are not noted. Some drooling of mucus is common in the first few hours after birth; excessive drooling occurs with esophageal atresia. The palate is visualized to rule out clefts. Retention cysts, or small whitish areas, are commonly found on the gum margins and at the juncture of the hard and soft palate. The cheeks appear to be full because of well-developed sucking pads. These, like the labial tubercles (sucking calluses) on the upper lip, disappear when the sucking period is over.

Although limited in function, the intestinal tract of the normal infant is proportionately longer than that of an adult. Its elasticity, musculature, and control mechanisms continue to develop until the child is 2 to 3 years of age, when adult levels of gastrointestinal function are achieved.

Normally bacteria are not present in the newborn's gastrointestinal tract. Soon after birth, oral and anal orifices permit entrance of bacteria and air. Bowel sounds can be heard 1 hour after birth. Generally the highest bacterial concentration is found in the lower portion of the intestine, particularly in the large intestine. The normal intestinal flora help synthesize vitamin K, folic acid, and biotin.

A special mechanism present in normal newborns weighing more than 1500 g coordinates the breathing, sucking, and swallowing necessary for oral feeding. Sucking in the newborn infant takes place in small bursts of three or four sucks at a time. In the term neonate, longer and more efficient sucking attempts occur in only a few hours. The infant is unable to move food from his lips to his pharynx; therefore it is necessary to place the nipple (breast or bottle) well inside the baby's mouth. Peristaltic activity in the esophagus is uncoordinated in the first few days of life but quickly becomes coordinated in normal infants. Persistent uncoordinated motility patterns and swallowing difficulties may indicate brain damage.

The capacity and emptying time for the stomach of the normal newborn are highly variable. Several factors, such as time and volume of feedings, type and temperature of food, and psychic stress, may affect the emptying time (between 1 and 24 hours).

Two principal types of cells make up the stomach: *chief cells,* which synthesize and secrete pepsinogen and aid in protein digestion; and *parietal cells,* which secrete hydrochloric acid. The infant's gastric acidity at birth normally equals the adult level but is reduced within a week and may remain reduced for 2 to 3 months. Gastric acidity and the enzyme pepsin are necessary for preliminary digestion of milk before its entrance into the small intestine.

Further digestion and absorption of nutrients from the stomach occur in the small intestine. This complex process is made possible by pancreatic secretions, secretions from the liver through the common bile duct, and secretions from the duodenal portion of the small intestine.

The infant's ability to digest carbohydrates, fats, and proteins is regulated by the presence of certain enzymes. Most of these are functional at birth. One exception is *amylase,* produced by the salivary glands after about 3 months and by the pancreas at about 6 months of age. This enzyme is necessary to convert starch into maltose. The other exception is *lipase,* also secreted by the pancreas; it is necessary for the digestion of fat. Thus the normal newborn is capable of digesting simple carbohydrates and proteins, but he has a limited ability to digest fats (see Chapter 30).

At birth the lower intestine is filled with meconium. Meconium is greenish black and viscous and contains occult blood. The first meconium passed is sterile, but within hours all meconium that is passed contains bac-

*Osmol is a measure of total number of particles. One gram mol of nondiffusible and nonionizable substance is equal to 1 osmol.

teria. It is passed by 24 hours in 94% of normal infants.

The number of stools varies considerably during the first week, being most numerous between the third and sixth days. Transitional stools (thin, slimy, and brown to green) are passed from the third to sixth day. Thereafter, the stools of breast-fed babies and bottle-fed babies differ. The stools of the breast-fed baby are loose, golden yellow in color, and nonirritating to the infant's skin. The baby may have a bowel movement after each feeding or one every three to four days. Even if the latter is the case, the stools remain loose or unformed. The stools of the bottle-fed baby are formed but soft, are a pale yellow in color, and have a typical stool odor. They tend to be irritating to the infant's skin. The number of stools decreases in the first 2 weeks from five or six each day (after every feeding) to one to two per day.

Distention of the stomach muscles causes a corresponding relaxation and contraction of the muscles of the colon. As a result, infants often have bowel movements during or just after a feeding. (Breast-fed babies are more likely to stool during a feeding than bottle-fed babies.) Stooling at these times has been attributed to the gastrocolic reflex.

HEPATIC SYSTEM

Physiologic immaturity of hepatic function in the neonate has a number of results.

Hyperbilirubinemia occurs when the serum bilirubin levels rise above acceptable norms. The pigment bilirubin is derived from the hemoglobin released with the breakdown of red blood cells (90% to 95%). The remaining pigment is derived from the myoglobin in muscle cells. The hemoglobin is phagocytized by the reticuloendothelial cells, converted to bilirubin, and released in an unconjugated form. This relatively insoluble substance is rapidly bound to circulating albumin. In the liver the unconjugated bilirubin is detached from the plasma protein and is conjugated with glucuronide in the presence of the enzyme glucuronyl transferase. The conjugated form of bilirubin (direct, soluble) is excreted from liver cells. Along with other components of bile, direct bilirubin is thus excreted into the biliary tract system, beginning with the smallest of these ducts (the bile canaliculi) and ultimately ending at the common bile duct, which inserts into the duodenum. There, through the action of the bacterial flora, bilirubin is converted to urobilinogen and stercobilin. Urobilinogen is excreted in urine and feces; stercobilin is excreted in the feces.

The unconjugated (indirect) bilirubin circulates bound to plasma albumin. Where not bound to albumin, bilirubin permeates other extravascular tissues (e.g., the brain, the skin, sclera, oral mucous membranes), and the resultant yellow coloring is termed *jaundice*.

The full-term neonate's liver is usually sufficiently mature and the production of glucuronyl transferase adequate enough to prevent pathologic levels of bilirubin (12 mg/dl or more). In the absence of asphyxia neonatorum, cold stress, hypoglycemia, and maternal ingestion of drugs such as sulfa drugs and aspirin (salicylates), adequate serum albumin–binding sites should also be available. The number and kind of red blood cells necessary to the fetus, but that are superfluous in the neonate, are broken down in the early neonatal period.

Physiologic hyperbilirubinemia. Physiologic hyperbilirubinemia (jaundice) is considered a normal occurrence in the neonatal period. About 50% of full-term and 80% of preterm neonates will demonstrate it *after 24 hours of life*. Fetal red blood cells have a shorter life span than adult red blood cells; therefore the end products of their destruction accumulate more rapidly and bilirubin levels rise. Total serum bilirubin is the sum of conjugated (direct, water-soluble) and unconjugated (indirect) bilirubin.

In the term infant the levels for serum bilirubin (total) increase as follows: up to 24 hours, 2 to 5 mg/dl; up to 48 hours, 9 mg/dl; and up to 3 to 5 days, under 12 mg/dl. Bilirubin concentration in the term infant peaks about the fifth day and does not exceed 12 mg/dl. In the premature infant it peaks on the sixth or seventh day and usually does not exceed 15 mg/dl. Physiologic hyperbilirubinemia is apparent in white infants at 4 to 5 mg/dl of total bilirubin and in black infants at 5 to 6 mg/dl of total bilirubin. Because of the neonate's circulatory pattern (cephalocaudal developmental progression), jaundice is noticeable first in the head and then progresses gradually toward the abdomen and extremities. The appearance of jaundice in the various body locations gives a rough estimate of the circulating levels of unbound bilirubin (see boxed material).

Several nursery practices may influence the appearance and degree of physiologic hyperbilirubinemia. For

Level of Hyperbilirubinemia by Cephalocaudal Distribution

Nose: 3 mg
Face: 5 mg
Chest: 7 mg
Abdomen: 10 mg
Legs: 12 mg
Palms: 20 mg

example, early feeding tends to keep the serum bilirubin level low by stimulating intestinal activity and the passage of meconium and stool. Removal of intestinal contents prevents the reabsorption (and recycling) of bilirubin from the gut, a residual mechanism left over from fetal life.

Chilling of the neonate may result in acidosis, and it also raises the level of free fatty acids. In the presence of acidosis, albumin binding of bilirubin is *weakened* and bilirubin is freed. Bilirubin is *displaced* from its albumin-binding sites by the free fatty acids.

Kernicterus, the most serious *complication* of neonatal hyperbilirubinemia, is caused by the precipitation of bilirubin in neuronal cells, causing their destruction (see Chapter 40). Cerebral palsy, epilepsy, and mental retardation are expected in survivors.

With the increase in numbers of mothers and infants being discharged from the hospital between 12 and 48 hours after birth (early discharge; see Chapter 31) and with the choice of birth at home, the professional attendant may not be available to assess pathologic rises in circulating unbound bilirubin. *Therefore all parents need instruction in how to assess jaundice and to whom to report the findings*.

Breast milk jaundice. Jaundice from ingestion of breast milk occurs in a very small proportion of full-term neonates (the incidence is less than 0.5% [Seligman, 1977]). An enzyme present in the milk of some women inhibits the enzyme glucuronyl transferase, which is necessary for the conjugation of bilirubin. Guthrie (1978) states that although breast milk jaundice is a form of physiologic jaundice, it occurs after the mature milk has come in and persists longer—up to 6 weeks. Unconjugated bilirubin rises beyond physiologic limits (15 to 20 mg/dl) by the seventh day. The levels subside by 5 to 10 mg if nursing is discontinued for 12 to 24 hours, and usually 3 to 5 days pass before the previous level is again reached. Guthrie feels that it is not necessary to completely discontinue breast feeding. It is unfortunate that many breast-feeding women have been made to feel their milk is pathogenic for their offspring because physiologic jaundice normally occurring after 24 hours was labeled ''breast milk jaundice.''

IMMUNITY

Resistance to infection (immunity) includes both specific and nonspecific protective mechanisms. The specific mechanisms, so called because they are directed toward a single organism, involve the antigen-antibody complex. An antigen is any substance that causes special types of cells to produce a protein antibody. The antibody may be attached to a cell or circulate freely (humoral antibodies). The humoral antibodies are known as immunoglobins, and the three major classes of immunoglobins (Ig) are called IgG, IgM, and IgA.

IgG. The IgG class contains antibodies to the majority of bacterial and viral organisms previously encountered by the individual during a lifetime experience with infection. During pregnancy maternal IgG (but not IgM or IgA) crosses the placenta. This transfer constitutes the infant's passive immunity. IgG derived from the mother has been detected in the fetus as early as the third month of gestation and levels increase markedly in the third trimester.* The placental transfer of this class of maternal antibodies results in the newborn having an ample supply of protective antibodies to bacterial and viral agents. This includes gram-positive cocci (pneumococcus, streptococcus), meningococcus, *Haemophilus influenzae,* the viruses, and the toxins of diphtheria and tetanus bacilli. The presence of these antibodies in the newborn may explain, in part, the low incidence of these infections during the neonatal period, since most mothers possess antibodies to them. However, the IgG class does not contain antibodies against the enteric gram-negative rods; thus the infant is not protected against these infections by maternal antibody. The natural destruction of the maternal antibodies (catabolism) after birth results in their depletion by about 3 months of age. During the 3 months following birth the infant begins synthesis of IgG, and the production reaches a level by 3 months that compensates for the loss of maternal antibodies.

IgM. By the twentieth week, the fetus can produce significant amounts of IgM. As noted earlier, maternally derived IgM does not cross the placenta; therefore the fetus must synthesize this (active immunity). Intrauterine infection may result in the fetus producing greater amounts. Detection of increased levels in the newly delivered infant indicates the presence of an infection, but not specifically what the causative organism is. Unlike the adult, IgM production in the fetus and neonate is stimulated by almost all infectious agents.

IgA. In most normal infants IgA is not detectable at birth; it does not cross the placenta. A form of IgA known as *secretory IgA* is present in colostrum and breast milk. Secretory IgA, unlike IgA, IgM, and IgG, is not destroyed by the action of gastric and intestinal enzymes and is specific for microbial agents present in the mother's own gastrointestinal tract. As the neonate is being freshly colonized, *these antibodies limit bacterial growth in the gastrointestinal tract and protect against overgrowth*. This information helps health care professionals to plan for the use of polio vaccine in breast-fed infants. According to Korones (1981):

*NOTE: The prematurely born infant does not benefit from a transfer of antibodies during the latter part of pregnancy.

Oral polio vaccine depends, for its effectiveness, on multiplication in the intestinal tract. The vaccine fails to immunize babies on breast milk from mothers with high antibody titers to poliovirus because vaccine virus is inactivated in the gut by secretory IgA from breast milk.

The *ability* to protect against antigens by formation of antibodies *develops sequentially*. The fetus or infant must be developmentally capable of responding to antigens. This is the reason for planning sequential immunizations in infants.

Much remains to be learned concerning the role of *nonspecific immunity* in the infant. It is apparent that the skin serves as an important barrier. Increasingly frequent generalized infections caused by enteric organisms, usually noninvasive, suggest that the gastrointestinal mucosa may be a portal of entry. Local or generalized circulatory changes may change the intestinal lining, which is normally impermeable to bacteria. During the neonatal period septicemia is far more common than at any other age. Some viral infections, for example, cytomegalic inclusion disease or herpes simplex virus, at this time are serious conditions with high mortality. The protective mechanisms of the neonate are still inadequate, making him highly vulnerable to certain septic processes.

NEUROLOGIC SYSTEM

The neonate's nervous system is extremely immature anatomically and differs from that of the adult in both chemical and physiologic properties. Neurologic functioning is primarily but not exclusively of brain stem and spinal cord level reflex activity, largely uninhibited by cerebral control. This does not preclude, however, a social response on the part of the newborn during the first hours and days of life.

Complete assessment of neurologic functioning (in the presence of an intact musculoskeletal system) includes evaluation of muscle tone, reflex responses, sensory capabilities, and behaviors.

Postdelivery growth of the brain follows a predictable pattern: rapid during infancy and early childhood, more gradual during the remainder of the first decade, and minimal during adolescence. The cerebellum ends its growth spurt, which began at about 30 gestational weeks, by the end of the first year. This is perhaps why it is vulnerable to nutritional or other trauma in early infancy. For example, see discussion of newborn nutrition, Chapter 30, and kernicterus, Chapter 40.

The brain requires glucose as a source of energy and a relatively large supply of oxygen for adequate metabolism. Oxygen requirements range from 5 to 8 ml/100 g. Such requirements signal a need for careful assessment of the infant's ability to maintain an open airway and of respiratory conditions requiring oxygen therapy, as well as an awareness of those neonates who may have hypoglycemic episodes.

Spontaneous motor activity may be evidenced in transient tremors of mouth and chin, especially when crying, and of extremities, notably the arms and hands. Persistent tremors or tremors involving the total body may be indicative of pathologic conditions. Marked tonicity, clonicity, and twitching of facial muscles are signs of convulsions. There is a need to differentiate among normal tremors, tremors of hypoglycemia, and CNS disorders so corrective care can be instituted, if necessary.

Neuromuscular control in the neonate, although still very limited, can be noted, however. For example, if the newborn is placed facedown on a firm surface, he will turn his head to the side to maintain an airway. He attempts to hold his head in line with his body if he is raised by his arms. Various reflexes act to promote his safety and an adequate food intake (see Table 28.2).

INTEGUMENTARY SYSTEM

The epidermis (skin) of the term newborn possesses the characteristic five layers of the adult, that is, strata germinativum, spinosum, granulosum, and corneum and, on the palmar and plantar surfaces, stratum lucidum underneath the stratum corneum. In the neonate the stratum corneum is thin and fused with the vernix caseosa (a reason for not removing the vernix at birth). The stratum corneum later becomes the effective skin barrier.

Caput succedaneum (Fig. 27.5, *A*) is a localized, easily identifiable edematous area of the scalp. The sustained pressure of the presenting vertex against the cervix results in compression of local vessels, thus slowing venous return. The slower venous return causes an increase in tissue fluids within the skin of the scalp, and an edematous swelling develops. This boggy edematous swelling is present at birth, extends across suture lines of the fetal skull, and disappears spontaneously within 3 to 4 days. Excessive pressure to the presenting vertex as it passes over the bony maternal pelvis may cause a cephalhematoma to develop.

Cephalhematoma. Cephalhematoma* is a collection of blood between a skull bone and its periosteum. Therefore a cephalhematoma never crosses a cranial suture line (Fig. 27.5, *B*). Cephalhematoma is caused by pressure during delivery. Bleeding may occur with spontaneous delivery (from pressure against the maternal bony pelvis) or easy forceps delivery, as well as

*NOTE: If there is a soft, fluctuating mass over the occipital bone at the base of the skull, an x-ray evaluation is necessary to rule out a neural tube defect (see Chapter 40).

Fig. 27.5
Differences between caput succedaneum and cephalhematoma. **A,** Caput succedaneum: edema of scalp noted at birth and crosses suture lines. **B,** Cephalhematoma: bleeding between periosteum and skull bone, appears within first 2 days, and does not cross suture lines.

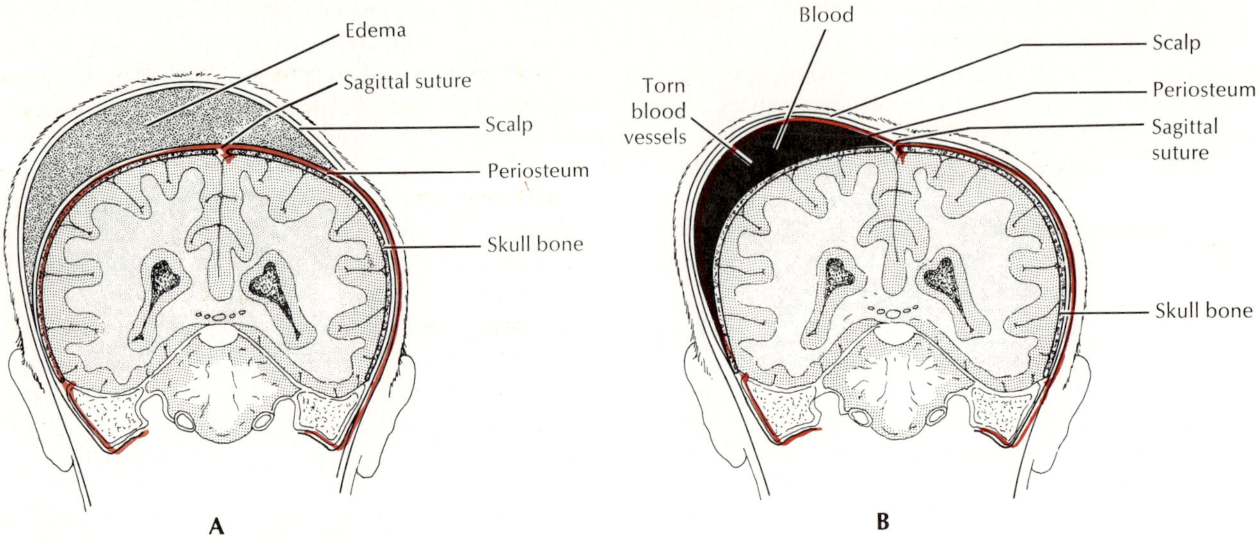

difficult forceps rotation and extraction. This soft, fluctuating, irreducible fullness does not pulsate or bulge when the infant cries. It appears several hours after birth or the day after delivery or becomes apparent following absorption of a caput succedaneum (Fig. 27.5, *A*). It is usually largest on the second or third day, when the bleeding stops. The fullness of cephalhematoma spontaneously resolves in 3 to 6 weeks. It is not aspirated because infection may develop if the skin is punctured.

Nursing care is directed primarily to supporting the parents. The physician's explanations may need to be reaffirmed; that is, the bleeding is not into the brain and no treatment is warranted. The parents may need to talk about their reactions to having a child with a misshapen head, albeit a temporary disfigurement.

Hyperbilirubinemia may occur as the hematoma resolves. Jaundice may not appear until the neonate is home. Therefore the parents are instructed to observe the newborn for jaundice and may be asked to bring the infant in to be rechecked before the usual 4-wk visit.

Sweat glands are present at birth but do not function effectively (i.e., respond to increases in ambient or body temperature), perhaps because the neurogenic stimuli are still immature. There is some fetal *sebaceous gland* hyperplasia and secretion of sebum as a result of the hormonal influences of pregnancy. Vernix caseosa, a cheeselike substance, is a product of the sebaceous glands. Distended sebaceous glands, noticeable in the newborn, particularly on the cheeks and nose, are known as *milia*. Although sebaceous glands are well developed at birth, they are only minimally active during childhood until androgen production increases before puberty.

Desquamation of the skin of the term infant does not occur until a few days after birth. If present at birth it is an indication of postmaturity. *Subcutaneous fat* accumulated during the last trimester acts to insulate the newborn. The preterm infant has difficulty maintaining an even body temperature because of the lack of this fat.

The term infant has an erythematous skin (beefy red) for a few hours after birth, after which it fades to its normal color. It often appears blotchy, especially over the extremities. The hands and feet appear slightly cyanotic. This bluish discoloration, *acrocyanosis,* is caused by vasomotor instability, capillary stasis, and a high hemoglobin level; it is normal, transient in occurrence, and persists over the first 7 to 10 days, especially with exposure to cold.

The healthy term newborn is plump, and the skin may feel slightly tight, suggesting fluid retention. Fine *lanugo hair* may be noted over the face, shoulders, and back. Actual edema of the face and *ecchymosis* (bruising) may be noted as a result of face presentation or forceps delivery. *Mongolian spots,* bluish-black areas of pigmentation, may appear over any part of the extensor surface of the body, including the extremities. They are more commonly noted on the back and buttocks. The occurrence of Mongolian spots is not primarily related to race. Rather its worldwide distribution is more ethnic than racial. Thus these pigmented areas are noted in babies whose origins are from the shores of the Mediterranean, Latin America, Asia, or a number of other areas in the world. They are more common in dark-skinned individuals regardless of race. They fade gradually over a period of months or years.

Telangiectatic nevi, known as "stork bites," are pink and easily blanched (Fig. 27.6). They appear on the upper eyelids, nose, upper lip, lower occiput bone, and nape of the neck. They have no clinical significance and fade between the first and second years. Other birthmarks include nevus vasculosus (strawberry mark) (Fig. 27.7) and nevus flammeus (port-wine stain) (Fig. 27.8).

An evanescent rash, *erythema toxicum* (also called *erythema neonatorum,* or "fleabite" dermatitis), with lesions in different stages (erythematous macules, papules, or small vesicles) may appear suddenly anywhere on the body. The cause is unknown, and although the appearance is alarming, it has no clinical significance and requires no treatment.

The intact skin of the infant acts as an effective barrier to infection; however, the fragility of the skin makes it more vulnerable to disruption of the surface when traumatized by too vigorous handling, rubbing, or excoriation.

Fig. 27.6
Stork bite (telangiectatic nevi). Pale pink or mauve spots seen frequently on eyelids, glabella, and occipital areas of newborn infants are considered by some to be type of nevus flammeus, or true vascular nevus. Certainly they behave differently from nevus flammeus in other skin areas. They are lighter in color, blanch on pressure, and almost invariably fade promptly and disappear completely before end of first year. They are rare in older infants and so common among light-complexioned newborns as to be almost routine finding. (Courtesy Mead Johnson & Co., Evansville, Ind.)

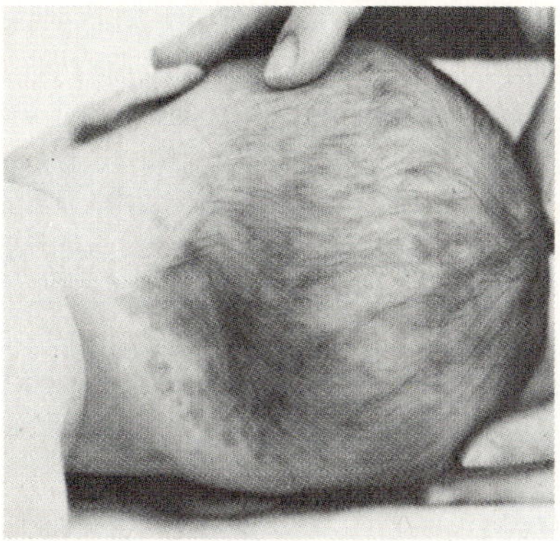

Fig. 27.7
Nevus vasculosus, or strawberry mark, is second most common type of capillary hemangioma and consists of dilated, newly formed capillaries occupying entire dermal and subdermal layers, with associated connective tissue hypertrophy. Typical lesion is raised, sharply demarcated, bright or dark red, and rough-surfaced swelling that resembles an outside slice of ripe strawberry. Lesions are usually single but may be multiple, and 75% occur in head region. (Courtesy Mead Johnson & Co., Evansville, Ind.)

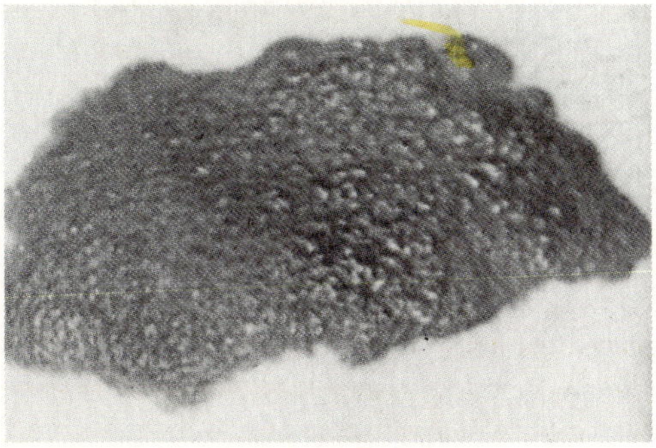

Fig. 27.8
Port-wine stain, or nevus flammeus, is usually observed at birth and is composed of plexus of newly formed capillaries in papillary layer of corium. It is red to purple in color; variable in size, shape, and location; and not elevated. True port-wine stains do not blanch on pressure and do not disappear spontaneously. (Courtesy Mead Johnson & Co., Evansville, Ind.)

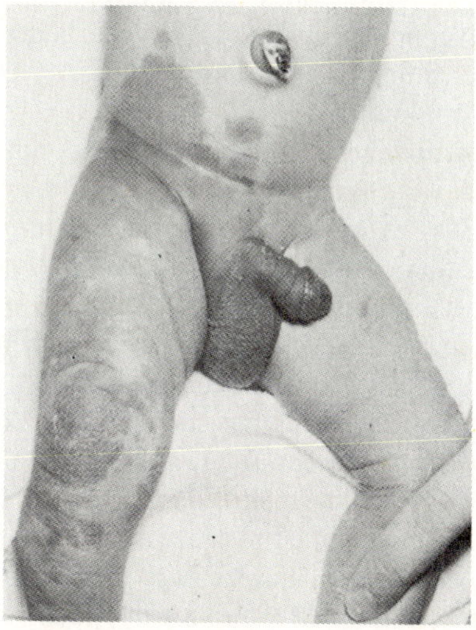

THERMOGENESIS

Effective neonatal care is predicated on the maintenance of an optimal thermal environment. In homoiothermic individuals the narrow limits of normal body temperature are maintained by producing heat in response to its dissipation. Hypothermia from excessive heat loss is a prevalent and dangerous problem in neonates. Although the newborn infant's ability to produce heat often approaches the capacity of the adult, his tendency toward rapid heat loss in a suboptimal thermal environment is increased and is often hazardous to his well-being.

Heat production. The shivering mechanism of heat production is rarely operable in the neonate. Nonshivering thermogenesis is accomplished primarily by brown fat and secondarily by increased metabolic activity in the brain, heart, and liver. Brown fat is unique to the neonate and is located in superficial deposits in the interscapular region and axillas, as well as in deep deposits at the thoracic inlet, along the vertebral column, and around the kidneys. Brown fat has a richer vascular and nerve supply than ordinary fat. Heat produced by intense lipid metabolic activity in brown fat can warm the neonate by increasing heat production as much as 100%. Reserves of brown fat, usually present for several weeks after birth, are rapidly depleted with cold stress. The less mature the infant, the less reserve he has of this essential fat at birth.

Heat loss. Heat loss occurs in four ways:

1. *Convection:* the flow of heat from the body surface to cooler ambient air. For this reason nursery ambient temperatures are kept at 24° C (75° F) and newborns are wrapped to protect them from the cold.
2. *Radiation:* the loss of heat from the body surface to cooler solid surfaces not in direct contact but in relative proximity to each other. Nursery cribs and examining tables are placed away from outside windows.
3. *Evaporation:* the loss of heat that occurs when a liquid is converted to a vapor. In the newborn heat loss by evaporation occurs as a result of vaporization of moisture from the skin. This process is invisible and is known as insensible water loss (IWL). This heat loss can be intensified by not drying the newborn directly after birth or by bathing and drying the infant too slowly.
4. *Conduction:* the loss of heat from the body surface to cooler surfaces in direct contact. The newborn when admitted to the nursery is placed in a warmed cot to minimize heat loss. Loss of heat must be controlled to protect the infant. As noted above, control of such modes of heat loss is the basis for care-taking policies and techniques.

Temperature regulation. Anatomic and physiologic differences among the neonate, child, and adult are notable:

1. The neonate's thermal insulation is less than an adult's. Blood vessels are closer to the surface of the skin. Changes in environmental temperature alter that of blood, thereby influencing temperature-regulating centers in the hypothalamus.
2. The neonate has a larger body surface to body weight (mass) ratio. The flexed position that the newborn assumes is a safeguard against heat loss because it substantially diminishes the amount of body surface exposed to the hostile thermal environment.
3. Vasomotor control is less well developed in the neonate; however, the ability to constrict subcutaneous and skin vessels is approximately as efficient in premature infants as it is in adults.
4. Heat is produced primarily by nonshivering thermogenesis.
5. Although sweat glands are present in the neonate, they have little homoiothermic function until the fourth week or later of extrauterine life.

In response to lower environmental temperature, the normal term infant may try to increase his body temperature by crying or by increased motor activity. Crying increases his work load, and the cost of energy (calories) may be expensive, particularly in the compromised infant.

Cold stress. Cold stress imposes metabolic and physiologic problems on all infants, regardless of gestational age and condition. The respiratory rate is increased as a response to the increased need for oxygen when the oxygen consumption increases significantly in cold stress. Oxygen consumption and energy in the cold-stressed infant are diverted from maintaining normal brain cell and cardiac function and growth to thermogenesis for survival.

If the infant cannot maintain an adequate oxygen tension, vasoconstriction follows and jeopardizes pulmonary perfusion. As a consequence, arterial blood gas levels of Po_2 are decreased and the blood pH drops. These changes aggravate existing respiratory distress syndrome (RDS), also known as hyaline membrane disease (HMD). Moreover, decreased pulmonary perfusion and oxygen tension may maintain or reopen the right-to-left shunt across the patent ductus arteriosus.

The basal metabolic rate will be increased with cold stress, and if cold stress is protracted, anaerobic glycolysis occurs, resulting in increased production of acids. Metabolic acidosis develops, and if there is a defect in respiratory function, respiratory acidosis also develops. Excessive fatty acids displace the bilirubin from the albumin-binding sites. The increased level of circulating unbound bilirubin that results increases the risk of kernicterus even at serum bilirubin levels of 10 mg/dl or less.

REPRODUCTIVE SYSTEM

At birth the ovaries contain thousands of primitive germ cells. These represent the full complement of potential ova, since no oogoniums form after delivery in term infants. The ovarian cortex is made up primarily of primordial follicles and forms a thicker portion of the ovary in the neonate than in the adult. The number of ova decreases from birth to maturity by approximately 90%.

The hyperestrogenism of pregnancy causes a swelling of the breast tissue in infants of both sexes, and in a few a thin discharge (witch's milk) can be seen. The finding has no clinical significance, requires no treatment, and will subside as the maternal hormones are eliminated from the infant's body. The same hyperestrogenism followed by a drop after delivery results in a mucoid vaginal discharge and even some slight blood spotting. The infant's uterus also responds by undergoing involution in the first weeks of life and decreasing in size and weight. Vaginal tags are common findings and have no clinical significance.

The testes have descended into the scrotum in 90% of newborn boys. Although this percentage drops with premature birth, by 1 year of age the incidence of undescended testes in all boys is less than 1%. Spermatogenesis does not occur until puberty (see Chapter 6).

Adhesions of the foreskin (prepuce) are almost universally present in newborn boys. During prenatal development the tissue of the prepuce is continuous with the epidermis that covers the glans. Gradually, the preputial space between the prepuce and the glans forms. The complete separation of the two tissue areas is generally not complete at birth, and for this reason the prepuce of the newborn is usually not retractable. In a study (Gairdner, 1949) of 100 newborn boys, the prepuce was fully retractable in only 4%. The prepuce was nonretractable in 80% of 6-month-old boys, 50% of 12-month-old boys, 20% of 2-year-old boys, and 10% of 3-year-old boys. Gairdner (1949) found that the prepuce was nonretractable among 6% of boys 5 to 13 years of age, generally because of only a few strands of connective tissue. Among the older boys, smegma was present in the preputial area, which was not the case among boys younger than 3 years.

Gairdner suggests that the prepuce functions to protect the glans during the early years, before toilet training is complete, when the glans might be irritated or injured by contact with wet diapers. He points out that meatal ulcers are seen among circumcised male infants or, occasionally, in an uncircumcised boy with a loose prepuce. In cleansing the penis the foreskin is *not* retracted to expose the glans penis. Adherence of the prepuce to the glans contraindicates any attempt at retraction.

STOP

Behavioral Characteristics

Through the first half of this century, the focus of developmental research was on how the infant was affected by the environment. Infants were considered to have been born with neither personality nor ability to interact. However, research now indicates that individual personalities and behavioral characteristics of infants play a major role in the ultimate relationship between infants and their parents.

Brazelton (1973) and others have brought the behavioral states of the neonate into prominence. It is their contention that the behavioral responses of infants are more indicative of their cortical control, responsiveness, and eventual management of the infant environment than is the Apgar rating or the traditional reflex assessment. They emphasize the importance of infant-parent interaction. Through his responses the infant acts to either consolidate relationships or alienate the persons in his immediate environment. By his actions he may encourage or discourage attachment and care-taking activities. The development of parent-child love does not occur without feedback; the absence of feedback because of either separation or incorrectly interpreted feedback can act to impair the growth of parental love.

One of the first tasks parents must accomplish is to become aware of the unique behavioral responses of their child. Brazelton (1969) demonstrated that normal babies are all very different in such things as activity (active, average, quiet), feeding patterns, sleeping patterns, and responsiveness from the moment of birth. He suggests that the parents' reactions and the infants' effect on their environment are determined in part by these differences. Parental knowledge of the significance infant behaviors have on their responses coupled with stimulation of the infant physically (holding, cuddling) and socially (talking to, smiling at) is necessary for the eventual growth and development of the child.

The nurse's knowledge of the behavorial characteristics of the newborn and the parents' responses to them will assist the nurse in planning holistic care.

SENSORY BEHAVIORS

From birth, infants possess sensory capabilities, which indicate a state of readiness for social interaction. The infant is able to use behavioral responses very effectively in establishing his first dialogues. These reponses, coupled with the neonate's "baby appearance" (the face is proportioned so that the forehead and eyes are larger than the lower portion of face) and his smallness and helplessness, rouse a feeling of wanting to hold, protect, and interact with him.

Vision. Because muscle control and coordination are immature, the infant's eyes drift off target. This glancing away actually permits the image being viewed to fall on the fovea more directly. The clearest visual distance is 17 to 20 cm (7 to 8 in), which is about the distance the infant's face is from the mother's face as she breast feeds or cuddles him. Infants are sensitive to light, will frown if a bright light is flashed in their eyes, will turn toward a soft red light, and if the room is darkened, will open their eyes widely and look about. This is noticeable when the delivery area is darkened after birth. By 2 months of age they can detect color, but under 5 days of age they seem more attracted by black-and-white patterns (Frantz, 1966).

Response to movement is noticeable. If a bright object is shown to neonates (even at 15 minutes of age), they will visually follow it, and some will even turn their heads to do so. Because human eyes are bright, shiny objects, newborns will track their parents' eyes. Parents will comment on how exciting this behavior is.

Visual acuity is surprising; even at 2 weeks of age infants can distinguish patterns with stripes 3 mm (⅛ in) apart, and by 6 months their vision is as acute as that of an adult (Frantz and Miranda, 1975). They prefer to look at patterns rather than plain surfaces, even if the latter are brightly colored, and they prefer more complex patterns to simple ones. They prefer novelty (changes in pattern) by 2 months of age. This is significant knowledge, since it means the infant of a few weeks of age is capable of responding actively to an enriched environment.

From birth onward, infants are able to fix their eyes and gaze intently at objects. They gaze at their parents' faces and respond to changes in them with apparent imitative effect. This ability permits parents and children to gaze into each other's eyes, and a subtle communication pattern is thereby set up. Some researchers have indicated that there may be an ethnic component to this pattern. Freedman (1979) reported a study comparing Navaho and Anglo mothers in their efforts to get the attention of the baby. The Anglo mothers became animated, smiled, and used gestures and high-pitched vocal sounds. The Navaho mothers gazed quietly at their babies until their eyes met and the infant gazed quietly back. It is conjectured that such responses may persist over time and influence behavior, as indicated by the following example:

> A 7-month-old Indian infant who was admitted for treatment of an ear infection seemed lonely and depressed. He would stare solemnly at me with his big brown eyes. I tried to cheer him by talking and shaking toys at him, but he would lie stiffly in my arms and gave no indication of noticing me. One evening when giving him his bottle I did not respond to his look by talking (I don't know why) but just looked back at him. After a bit he seemed to give a sigh, I could feel his little body relax against mine, and he reached up and patted the bottle.

Whether such conjectures are true or not, the need to have eye contact is a compelling one. Children of blind parents and parents who have blind children must circumvent this obstacle for the formation of a relation (see Chapter 32).

Hearing. Within 2 minutes of birth, neonates move their eyes in the direction of sound. High-pitched sounds elicit attentive behaviors followed by agitation. Lang (1972) reported that after delivery mothers pitch their voices higher. This acts to alert the child and prompts him to turn to the mother. On the other hand, low-pitched voices have a soothing effect. Parents have noted that their child becomes quiet when the father talks to him, and traditionally mothers have crooned to their babies to comfort them. There are indications that the fetus can hear during the last 3 months of prenatal life. Nurses in intensive care units have commented on how a loud motor in an isolette will disturb a premature infant. One of the authors (M.J.) remembers a mother in the transitional stage of labor who gave a sudden loud scream when a contraction began. The nurse was listening to the fetal heart tones at the time and noted that both she and the fetus jumped with surprise. Neonates accustomed in the uterus to hearing the regular rhythm of the mother's heartbeat respond by relaxing and ceasing to fuss and cry if a regular heartbeat simulator is placed in their cribs.

Touch. Response to pain by crying or withdrawal is considered to be somewhat limited in the first days of life. However, infants are responsive to touch. The newly delivered mother uses touch as one of the first attachment behaviors: fingertip touch, soft stroking of the face, and gentle massage of the back.

Since touch between strangers is avoided in our culture, it would seem that this automatic maternal touching behavior evidences an already intimate relationship. Birth trauma or stress and depressant drugs taken by the mother decrease the infant's sensitivity to touch or painful stimuli.

Taste. Through taste sensations, infants 1 to 3 days of age show evidence of differentiating sweet and sour substances. They have the ability to distinguish between two sweet substances with different sugar concentrations: sucrose and glucose, and if a few drops of lemon juice are put on their tongues, they will grimace.

Smell. By the fifth day of life the infant's sense of

smell is acute enough to help him distinguish his owr mother's breast pads from those of other mothers.

SLEEPING AND WAKING BEHAVIORS

Brazelton (1973) has noted that the infant's *state of consciousness* is the most important element in assessing his reactions to stimulation. This state is affected by a number of variables: hunger, nutrition, dehydration, and the infant's sleep-wake cycle. Description of variations in the infant's state of consciousness by Brazelton (1973) and others indicates that there are two sleep states and four wake states (Table 27.2).

Infant variations in state of consciousness form a continuum with deep sleep, narcosis, or lethargy at one end and extreme irritability at the other end. The various phases (Fig. 27.9) are termed *arousal states*. The optimal state of arousal is defined as "that which allows sustained attention to external stimuli, purposeful hand-eye coordinated movements, and active manipulation of the outside world" (Lewis and Zarin-Ackerman, 1977).

Fig. 27.9
Optimal state of arousal.

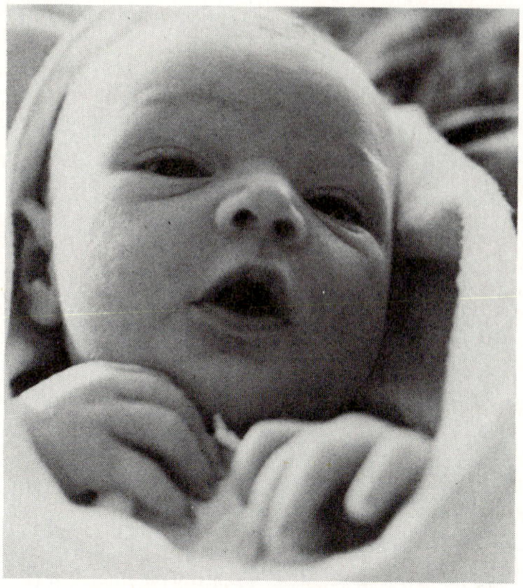

Table 27.2
Sleeping and Waking States

State	Behavior	Duration	Implications for Parenting
Sleep states			
(1) Regular sleep	Closed eyes, no eye movement Regular breathing No movement except for sudden body jerks	4-5 hr/day, 10-20 min/ sleep cycle	External stimuli will not arouse infant. Usual house noises should continue. If sudden loud noise awakens infant and he cries, leave him alone; he will usually fall back to sleep.
(2) Irregular sleep	Closed eyes, rapid eye movements (REM) under closed lids Irregular breathing Slight muscular twitching of body Occasional sucking movements	12-15 hr/day, 20-45 min/ sleep cycle	External stimuli that did not arouse infant during regular sleep may minimally arouse him now. Periodic groaning or crying is usual and should not be interpreted as an indication of pain or discomfort.
Wake states			
(3) Drowsiness	Eyes may be open Irregular breathing Active body movement	Variable	Most stimuli will arouse infant. He should be picked up during this time rather than left in crib.
(4) Alert inactivity	Responds to environment by active body movement and staring at close-range objects	2-3 hr/day	Infant's needs, such as hunger, must be satisfied. He should be placed in that part of home where activity is continuous. He should not be left in crib or playpen with no stimuli close by. Objects should be within 17-20 cm (7-8 in) of viewing. Constant stimulation will initiate and prolong this state.
(5) Waking activity	Eyes open; often begins with whimpering and slight body movement; few spontaneous startles; may or may not be fussy	1-4 hr/day	Behavior provoked by intense internal or external stimuli; such stimuli must be removed for termination of this state.
(6) Crying	Progresses to strong, angry crying and uncoordinated thrashing of extremities		Variable duration. Rocking and swaddling may decrease crying.

Adapted from Whaley, L.F., and Wong, D.L.: Nursing care of infants and children, St. Louis, 1979, The C.V. Mosby Co.

The infant employs purposeful behavior in order to maintain this optimal arousal state. Brazelton and associates (1973) report four behavior modalities for dealing with conditions that interfere with arousal control: (1) active withdrawal by increasing physical distance, (2) a rejecting motion of pushing away with hands and feet, (3) decreasing sensitivity by falling asleep or breaking eye contact by turning the head, or (4) use of signaling behavior, fussing, or crying. Use of such modalities permits the infant to quiet himself and reinstate the base level of readiness to interact again.

Although environment (amount of stimuli, etc.) affects self-regulation or arousal states, the infant himself is also an active contributor to the interaction through his predisposed *temperament*. This temperament has been defined by Chess and Thomas (1977) as a combination of focus and distractibility, intensity of reaction and adaptability, and mood and energy expenditures. It appears to exist at birth and affect the infant's behavioral characteristics by encouraging or discouraging his cognitive development, that is, his ability to organize stimuli. As discussed earlier, the infant's sensory system is capable of processing information (stimuli) from the environment; however, his energy level of distractibility regulates the amount of information processed.

Learning processes have been demonstrated in the neonate. He can learn to make a response in order to cause an event to occur. For example, he is capable of two sucking behaviors to obtain fluid, one by pressing the nipple against the roof of his mouth and the other by creating a vacuum in the oral cavity. If one is not effective, he quickly switches to the other. Also, as noted earlier, infants even as young as 24 hours of age will decrease their attention to a stimuli constantly repeated and eventually will fail to respond. This represents *habituation* and indicates that the infant's nervous system is capable of excluding redundant information. When a new stimulus is presented, the infant shows a recovery of interest, demonstrating that the lack of response was caused by boredom, not fatigue. By 1 month of age the infant has learned to discriminate between the mother's face, voice, and discrepancies and those of a stranger (Lewis and Zarin-Ackerman, 1977).

Sleep-wake cycles. Desmond and associates (1966) noted that infants pass through phases of instability in the first 6 to 8 hours after birth; these phases collec-

Fig. 27.10
Some physiologic changes occurring in neonate in his adjustment to extrauterine life. (From Pierog, S., and Ferrara, A.: Medical care of the sick newborn, ed. 2, St. Louis, 1976, The C.V. Mosby Co.; adapted from Desmond, M.M., Rudolph, A.J., and Phitaksphraiwan, P.: Pediatr. Clin. North Am. **13:**651, 1966.)

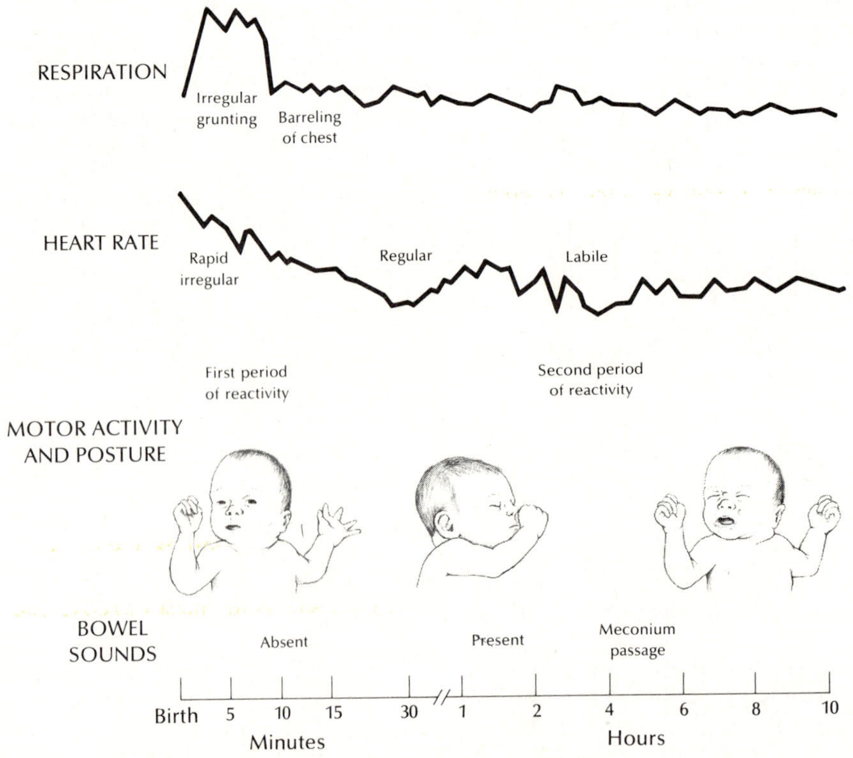

tively are termed the *transitional period* between intrauterine and extrauterine existence (Fig. 27.10). The first phase lasts up to 30 minutes after birth and is called the *first period of reactivity*. The *second period of reactivity* occurs at about the fourth to eighth hour after birth. This sequence occurs in all neonates, regardless of gestational age or type of delivery: vaginal or cesarean. There will be variations, however, in the length of time the periods last, depending on amount and kind of stress experienced by the fetus. Following are the clinical findings in the first period:

1. Infant is awake, alert, and active; his eyes are open, he looks around, and he may appear hungry; he has a good sucking reflex.
2. Respirations are rapid and irregular; there may be some grunting and barreling of chest.
3. Heart rate is rapid (tachycardia) with some irregularity.
4. Body temperature falls.

The infant's activity gradually diminishes, his alertness fades, and sleep comes. Air enters the gastrointestinal tract, and by about the end of the first hour bowel sounds can be heard.

In the second period the infant again wakens and is alert. There is usually a gagging episode with regurgitation of mucus and maternal blood from the birth canal. The meconium stool is usually passed, and the infant again appears hungry and ready to suck.

The first 6 weeks of life involve a steady decrease in the proportion of active REM sleep to total sleep and a steady increase in the proportion of quiet sleep to total sleep time. There is also a 25% increase in wakefulness over the first 3 or 4 weeks. For the first few weeks the wakeful periods seem dictated by hunger, but soon thereafter a need for socializing appears to function as well. The neonate sleeps a total of about 17 hours a day, with the periods of wakefulness gradually increasing. By the fourth week of life, some infants are staying awake from one feeding session to the next. It is not until the child is 4 or 5 years of age that he achieves the adult pattern of sleeping.

SOCIAL BEHAVIORS

Social behavior refers to the following infant behavioral patterns:

1. Crying: Most mothers can describe the difference in their infants' cries as they experience hunger, pain, desire for attention, or fussiness:

> I can tell when she's hungry. Crying starts in a plaintive way and then becomes more and more demanding. When she is hurt, she lets out a startled yell as though she couldn't believe it was happening to her. Sometimes when she is put down to sleep, she starts a kind of talking cry, jerky and demanding; it gets louder, and if nothing happens, fades away in little spurts. The fussy cry is the hardest to take—nothing seems to work—such a complaining sound, it goes on and on.

A report such as this means that this mother and baby are communicating effectively.

2. Smiling, vocalizing, and synchrony: Even during the first day of life, smiling is evident in a surprising number of infants (Wolff, 1969b). They seem to watch their parents' faces carefully and respond to other persons' talking to them. They move their bodies in coordination with the parent's voice and the simultaneous movement of the parent's body (Condon and Sander, 1974). Brazelton (1969) notes that this "dancing in tune" gives feedback to the speaker and encourages more interaction. Infants have been shown to imitate parents' actions by 2 weeks of age (Meltzoff and Moore, 1977). Many begin a type of vocalizing by 2 weeks of age, making cooing, small, throaty noises while feeding.

FEEDING BEHAVIORS

Variations among infants regarding interest in food, symptoms of hunger, and amount ingested at any one time are noticeable from birth. If put to breast, some infants nurse immediately, whereas others require a learning period of up to 48 hours before nursing can be said to be effective. Random hand-to-mouth movement and sucking of fingers have been seen in utero. These actions are well developed at birth and are intensified with hunger. The amount that the infant takes at any one bottle feeding will depend, of course, on the size of the infant, but other factors also seem to play a part:

> The mother reported her 6-day-old infant (2604 g [5 lb, 13 oz]) had taken 90 ml (3 oz) at 11 PM, 45 ml (1.5 oz) at 3 AM, 30 ml (1 oz) at 6 PM, and now at the 10 AM feeding, "was sleepy and seemed to want only 45 ml (1.5 oz)." The nurse suggested she keep track of the total amount taken over 24 hours. The mother interrupted to say, "I know what is wrong—yesterday all the relatives visited and held him. I think he's tired out." The nurse agreed that this could be so.
>
> The next day the mother reported he was eating very well and commented. "I'm glad my instincts were right—it was just too busy a day for him."

Mothers need positive feedback to develop a feeling of confidence in their own ability. Often just listening and praising is the most effective intervention. Feeding is an emotionally charged area of infant care. Culturally, the size and growth of an infant are equated with excellence and evidence of mothering ability. The infant who is a fussy eater can serve to raise parental anxiety levels. The anxious parent appears to compound the problem, and a vicious cycle can develop. If relatives or friends can take over a feeding period or two, this seems to break the cycle so that the mother can view the feeding session in a more relaxed manner, not as a condemnation of her care.

ELIMINATION BEHAVIORS

The infant develops an elimination pattern by the second week of life. It appears to be associated with the frequency and amount of feedings (gastrocolic reflex). The stools of breast-fed and bottle-fed babies differ (see p. 560). The stress in the U.S. cultures for daily bowel movements (regularity) makes most mothers see this process as an indication of health and therefore a judgment concerning the quality of the care they have given. With the addition of solid food, the baby's stool gradually assumes the characteristics of an adult stool, and mothers need to be aware of the change.

Urination increases from about three to four times each day in the first few days to five to six times each day later in the first week; voiding six to ten times each day is a good indicator of adequate fluid intake (hydration) thereafter (see also p. 559).

• • •

The nurse utilizes the knowledge of the biologic and behavioral characteristics of the newborn as a basis for the care of the infant and the teaching and counseling of the parents. Chapter 28 presents the assessment strategies and tools that provide information for devising nursing diagnoses. Chapter 29 presents the plan and implementation of nursing actions for the care of the child and the criteria used to evaluate progress toward the goal of a healthy, happy infant.

References and Readings

Ainsworth, M.D.S.: The development of mother-infant attachment, Rev. Child Dev. Res. **3**:1, 1973.

Aladjem, S.A., Brown, A.K., and Sureau, C.: Clinical perinatology, ed. 2, St. Louis, 1979, The C.V. Mosby Co.

American Academy of Pediatrics: Report of the Committee on Infectious Diseases, ed, 17, Evanston, Ill., 1974, The Academy.

Barnett, C.R., et al.: Neonatal separation: the maternal side of interactional deprivation, Pediatrics **45**:197, Feb. 1970.

Behrman, R.: Neonatal-perinatal medicine: diseases of the fetus and infant, ed. 2, St. Louis, 1977, The C.V. Mosby Co.

Bernal, J.: Crying during the first 10 days of life and maternal responses, Dev. Med. Child Neurol. **14**:362, 1972.

Bowlby, J.: Nature of a child's tie to his mother, Int. J. Psychoanal. **39**:350, 1958.

Bowlby, J.: Attachment and loss, vol. 1, New York, 1960, Basic Books, Publishers.

Brazelton, T.: Infants and mothers, ed. 2, New York, 1983, Dell Publishing Co.

Brazelton, T.: Effect of maternal expectations on early infant behavior, Early Child Dev. Care **2**:259, 1973.

Brazelton, T.B.: Does the neonate shape his environment? Birth Defects **10**:131, 1974.

Brown, M.S.: How to tell if a baby has cerebral palsy, Nurs. '79 **9**:99, 1979.

Chess, S., and Thomas, A.: Temperament and the parent-child interaction, Pediatr. Ann. **6**(9):26, 1977.

Chess, S., Thomas, A., and Birch, H.G.: Your child is a person, New York, 1965, Viking Press.

Clark, A., and Affonso, D.: Childbearing: a nursing perspective, Philadelphia, 1976, F.A. Davis Co.

Clark, D.A.: Times of first void and first stool in 500 newborns, Pediatrics **60**:457, Oct. 1977.

Condon, W.S., and Sander, L.W.: Neonate movement is synchronized with adult speech: interactional participation and language acquisition, Science **183**:99, 1974.

Craig, M.: Normal neonatal behavior patterns the first week of extrauterine life, Child. Fam. **9**:303, 1970.

Desmond, M.M., et al.: The transitional care nursery, Pediatr. Clin. North Am. **13**:651, 1966.

Farmby, D.: Maternal recognition of infant's cry, Dev. Med. Child Neurol. **9**:293, 1967.

Fleming, J.: Common dermatologic conditions in children, M.C.N. **6**:346, Sept.-Oct. 1981.

Foss, B.M., editor: Determinants of human behavior, New York, 1963, John Wiley & Sons.

Frantz, R.L.: Pattern discrimination and selective attention as determinants of perceptual development from birth. In Kidd, A.J., and Rivaire, J.L., editors: Perceptual development in children, New York, 1966, International Universities Press.

Frantz, R.L., and Miranda, S.B.: Newborn infant attention to form and contour, Child Dev. **46**:224, 1975.

Freedman, D.G.: Ethnic differences in babies, Hum. Nature, p. 4., Jan. 1979.

Gairdner, D.: The fate of the foreskin: a study of circumcision, Br. Med. J. **2**:1433, 1949.

Gleiss, J., and Stuttgen, G.: Morphologic and functional development of the skin. In Stave, U., editor: Physiology of the perinatal period, vol. 2, New York, 1970, Appleton-Century-Crofts.

Gordon, T., and Foss, B.M.: The role of stimulation in the delay of onset of crying in the newborn infant, Q. J. Exp. Psychol. **18**:79, 1966.

Goren, C., Sarty, M., and Wu, P.: Visual following and pattern discrimination of face-like stimuli by newborn infants, Pediatrics **56**:544, 1975.

Greenberg, M.M.N.: Engrossment: the newborn impact upon the father, Am. J. Orthopsychiatry **44**:520, 1974.

Guthrie, R.A.: Breast milk and jaundice; keep abreast, J. Hum. Nutr. **3**:47, Jan.-March 1978.

Guyton, A.: Textbook of medical physiology, Philadelphia, 1980, W.B. Saunders Co.

Honig, A.: The role of the nurse in stimulating early learning, J. Nurs. Educ. **9**:11, 1970.

Horoniety, E., et al.: Newborn and four-week retest on a normative population using the Brazelton newborn assessment procedure. Paper presented at the Annual Meeting of the Society for Research in Child Development, Minneapolis, 1971.

International Childbirth Education Association: Focusing on today's issues in perinatal care. Amniotomy, I.C.E.A. Review **3**:2, Summer 1979.

Jegier, W., et al.: The changing circulatory pattern of the newborn infant studied by the indicator dilution technique, Acta Paediatr. Scand. **53**:541, Nov. 1964.

Kohn, C.L., et al.: Gravidas' responses to realtime ultrasound fetal image, J.O.G.N. Nurs. **9:**77, March-April 1980.

Korones, S.B.: High-risk newborn infants: the basis for intensive nursing care, ed. 2, St. Louis, 1981, The C.V. Mosby Co.

Kempe, C.H., Silver, H.K., and O'Brien, D., editors: Current pediatric diagnosis and treatment, Los Altos, Calif., 1976, Lange Medical Publications.

Klaus, M., and Fanaroff, A.: Care of the high-risk neonate, ed. 2, Philadelphia, 1979, W.B. Saunders Co.

Lang, R.: Birth book, Ben Lomond, Calif., 1972, Genesis Press.

Leifer, A.D., et al.: Effects of mother-infant separation on maternal attachment behavior, Child Dev. **43:**1203, Dec. 1972.

Lewis, M., and Zarin-Ackerman, J.: Early infant development. In Behrman, R.E., Driscoll, J.M., Jr., and Seeds, A.E., editors: Neonatal-perinatal medicine: diseases of the fetus and infant, ed. 2, St. Louis, 1977, The C.V. Mosby Co.

Loggie, J., et al.: Renal function and diuretic therapy in infants and children, J. Pediatr. **86:**485, 1975.

Lowrey, G.: Growth and development of children, ed. 7, Chicago, 1978, Year Book Medical Publishers.

McClinton, B., and Meier, B.: Beginnings: psychology of early childhood, St. Louis, 1978, The C.V. Mosby Co.

Meltzoff, A., and Moore, M.: Imitation of facial and manual gestures by human neonates, Science **198:**75, 1977.

Minegeot, R., and Herbert, M.: The functional status of the newborn infant: a study of 5,370 consecutive infants, Am. J. Obstet. Gynecol. **115:**1138, 1973.

Moore, M.L.: Newborn, family and nurse, ed. 2, Philadelphia, 1981, W.B. Saunders Co.

Pierog, S.H., and Ferrara, A.: Medical care of the sick newborn, ed. 2, St. Louis, 1976, The C.V. Mosby Co.

Poole, C.: Neonatal circumcision, J.O.G.N. Nurs. **8**(4):207, 1979.

Prechtl, H.F.R.: Patterns of reflex behavior related to sleep in the human infant. In Clemente, C.D., Purpura, D.P., and Mayer, F.E., editors: Sleep and the maturing nervous system, New York, 1972, Academic Press.

Ringler, N., et al.: Mother-to-child speech at two years—effects of early postnatal contact, J. Pediatr. **86:**141, 1975.

Schachter, J., et al.: Heart rate and blood pressure in black newborns and white newborns, Pediatrics **58:**283, 1976.

Seil, E., and Carrigan, J.: Platelet counts, fibrinogen concentrations and factor V and factor VII levels in healthy infants according to gestational age, J. Pediatr. **82:**1028, 1973.

Seligman, J.W.: Recent and changing concepts of hyperbilirubinemia and its management. In Andrews, B.F., editor: Symposium on the newborn, Pediatr. Clin. North Am. **24:**514, Aug. 1977.

Slumek, M.: Screening infants for hearing loss, Nurs. Outlook **19:**115, 1971.

Vaughan, V.C., and McKay, R.J., editors: Nelson's textbook of pediatrics, ed. 10, Philadelphia, 1975, W.B. Saunders Co.

Whaley, L.F., and Wong, D.L.: Nursing care of infants and children, ed. 2, St. Louis, 1983, The C.V. Mosby Co.

Winick, M.: Malnutrition and brain development, J. Pediatr. **74:**667, 1969.

Wolff, P.H.: The natural history of crying and other vocalizations in early infancy. In Foss, B.M., editor: Determinants of infant behavior, vol. 4, New York, 1969a, Barnes & Noble Books.

Wolff, P.H.: Observations on newborn infants, Psychosom. Med. **21:**110, 1969b.

Wolff, P.H.: Observations on the early development of smiling. In Stone, L.J., Smith, H.T., and Murphy, L.B., editors: The competent infant, research and commentary, New York, 1973, Basic Books, Publishers.

Yu, V.: Body position and gastric emptying, Arch. Dis. Child. **50:**500, 1975.

28

Nursing Assessment and Diagnosis of the Newborn

- Facilities and Personnel
- Assessment
  - Physical assessment
  - Neurologic assessment
  - Behavioral assessment
    - Brazelton Neonatal Behavioral Assessment Scale
    - Factors influencing behavior of the newborn
  - Assessment strategies and tools for normal newborn: first day (2 to 24 hours)
    - Respirations
    - Temperature
    - Cardiovascular system
    - Integumentary system
    - Cord and circumcised penis
    - Defecation
    - Urination
    - Physical assessment
    - Neurologic assessment
    - Behavioral assessment
    - Newborn nutrition
    - Parenthood
  - Summary of assessment strategies and tools for normal newborn: days 2 to 14
  - Summary of assessment strategies and tools for normal newborn: days 15 to 28 (first well-baby visit)
- Nursing Diagnoses
- Planning

Although most infants make the necessary biopsychosocial adjustment to extrauterine existence without undue difficulty, their continued life depends on the care received from others (see Appendix B). Care is dictated by the infant's need for the following:

1. Close observation and monitoring of physiologic response to permit early detection of distress and institution of corrective medical intervention or nursing actions
2. Protection from infection and trauma
3. Provision of warmth, nutrition (see Chapter 30), and body hygiene
4. Parenting

Facilities and Personnel

In the hospital the newborn's environment consists of the personnel who assume responsibility for his care, the facilities provided for his care, and his parents, who may or may not participate in his care. These three components are linked by policies—administrative, medical, and nursing—that reflect the standards of care the agency undertakes to provide for the newborn.

Increased interest on the part of medical and nursing groups in the study of the fetus and care of the neonate during the perinatal period has led to the development of perinatology as a branch of health care. This specialty manages the normal and abnormal infant and the varying environmental influences that increase or detract from the probability of optimal development. Nursing personnel may vary in degree and kind of preparation, but all need to demonstrate ability in detecting abnormal responses in infant or parent and in instituting necessary diagnostic and supportive nursing measures.

The infant is transferred from the delivery unit to the

observational area (transitional nursery). Its location, types of equipment, supplies, and skills of assigned personnel reflect the infant's need for intensive care during the critical transitional period (Fig. 29.13). Once the infant's condition is stabilized, he can be admitted to a mother-infant unit, such as a *rooming-in unit,* where the infant shares accommodations with the mother and full participation of parents in the infant's care is encouraged.* These units provide excellent learning areas for new mothers and serve to foster early and sustained parent-child relationships. In areas where rooming-in units are not feasible or the mother either prefers less direct involvement in infant care or is not physically able to participate, the infant may be lodged in a normal newborn nursery. The implementation of family-centered care is possible under these circumstances through longer mother-child contacts at feeding times and demonstrations and lectures relating to infant care. In some areas early discharge to the home is being introduced. This requires careful preparation of parents, a healthy infant, and regular follow-up services if the infant is not to be placed in jeopardy (see Chapter 31).

For the infant designated as "high-risk," transfer to an intensive care unit is indicated (see Unit Seven).

Construction, maintenance, and operation of nurseries in accredited hospitals are directed by national professional organizations such as the American Academy of Pediatrics and local or state governing bodies. Prescribed standards include areas such as the following:

1. *Environmental factors:* provision of adequate lighting, elimination of potential fire hazards, safety of electric appliances, adequate ventilation, and controlled temperature (warm and free of drafts) and humidity (lower than 50%)
2. *Measures to control infection:* adequate floor space to permit positioning bassinets at least 60 cm (24 in) apart, hand-washing facilities, techniques for safe formula preparation and storage, and cleaning and sterilizing of equipment and supplies

In addition, hospital personnel develop their own policies and procedures directed toward protection of the neonates under their care; for example:

1. Nursery personnel are restricted to those directly involved in the care of mothers or infants. This restriction minimizes the number of persons to whom each infant is exposed, thereby reducing the introduction of pathogenic organisms. In this respect children born at home are at an advantage because other persons who come in contact usually are family members. In hospitals this home environment is somewhat duplicated when the infant and mother "room together" and the mother and father are active in the care, thereby reducing the number of nursing personnel involved. In many hospitals, nurseries are constructed with anterooms, where physicians carry out examinations and procedures such as circumcisions, or where parents may come to feed or hold their infants who must remain in the hospital for care.

2. Personnel assigned to the nursery wear special uniforms or cover gowns, and before beginning the care of infants, they carry out a *hand-washing technique* (Fig. 28.1).

3. Any persons coming from an "outside" area are expected to gown and *wash their hands* before contact with either infants or equipment. Such persons include nurses, physicians, parents, department supervisors, electricians, and housekeepers.

4. Individuals with infectious conditions are excluded from contact with neonates; this includes persons with

Fig. 28.1
Hand washing.

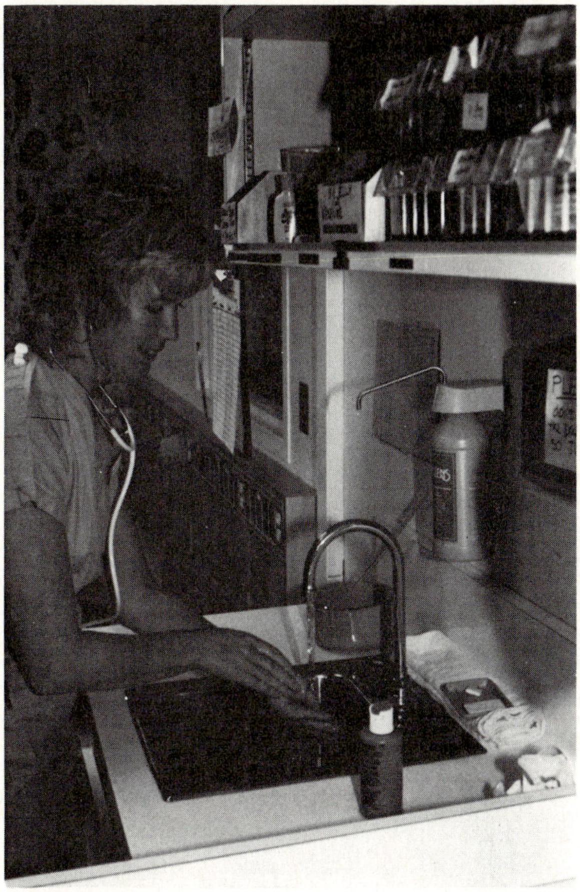

*In some instances healthy newborns are transferred directly to the mother's rooming-in unit.

upper respiratory tract infections, gastrointestinal tract infections, and infectious skin conditions. Most agencies have now coupled this day-to-day screening of personnel with yearly health examinations.

More detailed information concerning standards of care for newborn nurseries may be obtained from a number of sources.*

Assessment

PHYSICAL ASSESSMENT

During the neonatal period the prenatal and postdelivery characteristics of the infant emerge, and only gradually do the former disappear as the infant continues to grow and mature in the extrauterine environment. The first *physical assessment* of the infant is done at birth, using the Apgar scoring technique and a physical assessment (see Chapter 22). The assessment for gestational age, if it is deemed necessary, must be done within the first 2 hours after birth (see p. 919).

A second, more thorough physical examination is done within 24 hours after delivery (Tables 28.1 and 28.2). The *goal* is to provide a complete record of the newborn that will act as a data base for subsequent assessment and care. Having the parents present during the examination permits prompt discussion of parental concerns and actively involves the parents in health care of their child from birth. As the same time, *parental interactions with the child* can be observed, and early diagnosis of problems in parent-child relationships can be facilitated.

The area used for the examination should be well lit, warm, and free of drafts. The child is undressed as needed and placed on a firm, flat surface. The infant may need to be picked up and cuddled at times for reassurance. The examination can be carried out in a systematic manner, beginning with a general evaluation of such characteristics as appearance, maturity, nutritional status, activity, and state of well-being, and then specific observations can be made (Table 28.1).

Text continued on p. 594.

*The American Academy of Pediatrics, 1801 Hinman Ave., Evanston, IL 60202 *(Standards and Recommendations for Hospital Care of the Newborn,* ed. 6, 1977; *Standards of Child Health Care, Council on Pediatric Practice,* ed. 2, 1972); American College of Obstetricians and Gynecologists, 600 Maryland Ave., S.W., Washington, DC 20024 *(Standards for Obstetric-Gynecological Hospital Service,* 1969); American Hospital Association, 840 North Lake Dr., Chicago, IL 60611 *(Infection Control in the Hospital,* 1970); The Nurses' Association of the American College of Obstetricians and Gynecologists, 600 Maryland Ave., S.W., Suite 300, Washington, DC 20024 *(Standards for Obstetric, Gynecologic, and Neonatal Nursing,* ed. 2, 1981).

Table 28.1
Physical Assessment of Newborn*

Evaluation Criteria and Appraisal Procedure	Normal Findings: Average Findings	Normal Findings: Normal Variations	Deviations from Normal Range (Possible Problems)
Posture			
Inspect neonate before disturbing him for assessment Refer to maternal chart for fetal presentation, position, and type of birth (vaginal, surgical), since neonate readily assumes prenatal position	Vertex: arms, legs in moderate flexion; fists are clenched (Fig. 28.2) Neonate resists having extremities extended for examination or measurement and will cry when this is attempted Crying ceases when allowed to reassume curled-up fetal position Normal spontaneous movement is bilaterally asynchronous (legs move in bicycle fashion) but equally extensive in all extremities	Frank breech: more straight and stiff, so that neonate will assume his intrauterine position in repose for a few days Prenatal pressure of limb or shoulder may cause temporary facial asymmetry (Fig. 28.3) or resistance to extension of extremities	Lack of muscle tone, relaxed posture while awake: prematurity or hypoxia in utero Hypertonia: drug dependence, CNS disorder Opisthotonos: CNS disturbance Limitation of motion in any of extremities: see Extremities, below

*See Chapter 37 for assessment of gestational age.

Fig. 28.2
Arms flexed and fists clenched.

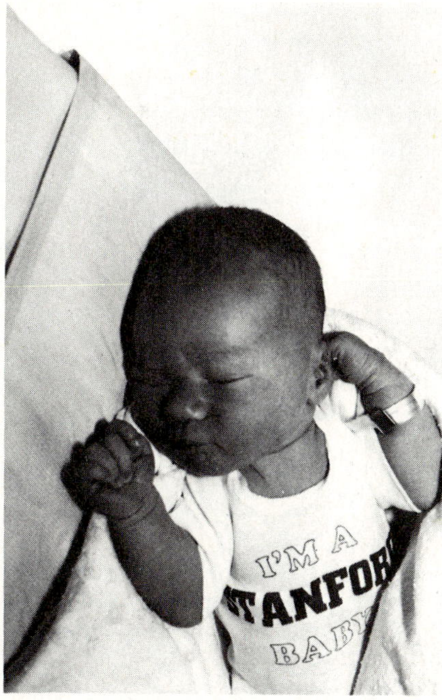

Fig. 28.3
A, Facial asymmetry. Asymmetric appearance is caused by displacement of mandible and presence of more or less pronounced fossa, or excavation, in neck, representing former position of shoulder. Some malocclusion is apparent. Confirmatory evidence may be provided by observing position of comfort that newborn often assumes. **B,** Lopsided appearance disappears spontaneously in few weeks or months, depending on its severity. (Courtesy Mead Johnson & Co., Evansville, Ind.)

A

B

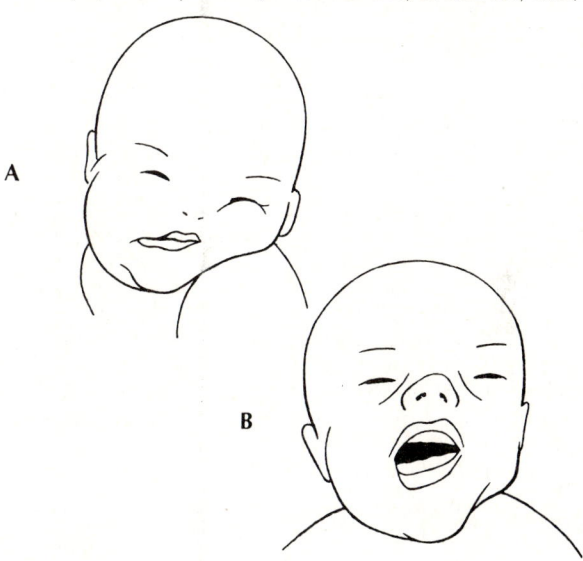

Table 28.1—cont'd
Physical Assessment of Newborn

Evaluation Criteria and Appraisal Procedure	Normal Findings: Average Findings	Normal Findings: Normal Variations	Deviations from Normal Range (Possible Problems)
Measurements			
Weight*			
Adjust scale to 0 and put protective liner cloth or paper in place (Fig. 28.4) Take weight at same time each day Protect neonate from heat loss	3400 g (7 lb 8 oz) Regains birth weight within first 2 wk	2500–4000 g (5 lb 8 oz to 8 lb 13 oz) (Fig. 28.5) Acceptable weight loss: 10% or less (to estimate percent of weight loss, see Chapter 33)	Weight ≤ 2500 g Prematurity Small for gestational age (SGA) Multiple gestation Rubella syndrome Weight ≥ 4000 g Large for gestational age (LGA): maternal diabetes Hereditary: normal for these parents Weight loss over 10%: dehydration?
Length			
Measure recumbent length from top of head to heel; difficult to measure in full-term infant because of presence of molding, incomplete extension of knees (Fig. 28.6)	50 cm (20 in)	45-55 cm (18-22 in)	Chromosomal aberration Heredity: normal for these parents

*NOTE: Weight, length, and head circumference should all be close to same percentile for any child.

Continued.

Fig. 28.4
Weighing infant. Note hand is held over infant as safety measure. Scale is covered to provide warmth and protection against cross infection. Scale is adjusted to zero reading after cover is in place. Note neonate's flexed extremities.

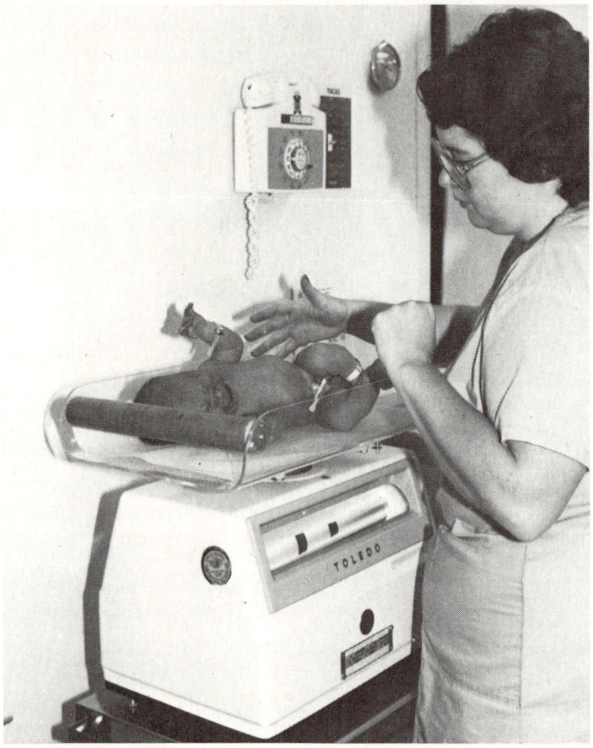

Fig. 28.5
Intrauterine growth status as determined by birth weight at various gestational ages.

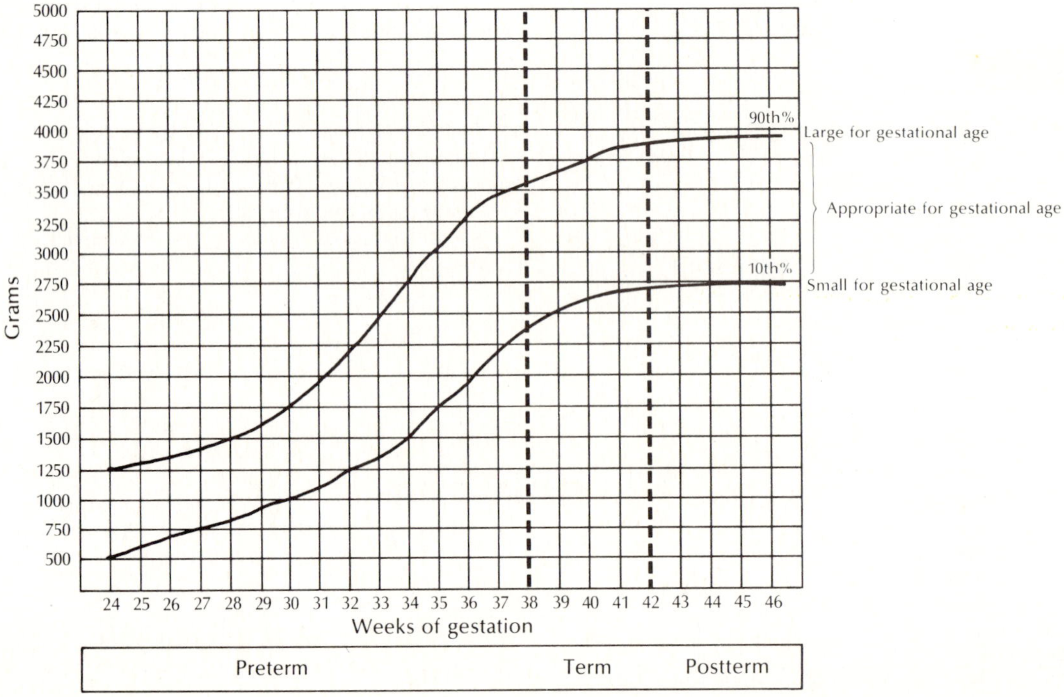

Fig. 28.6
Measuring infant's length, crown to rump. To determine total length, add to length of legs.

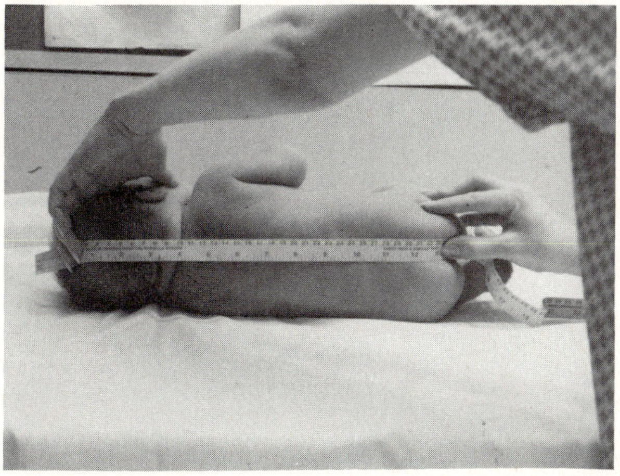

Fig. 28.7
Measuring circumference of head.

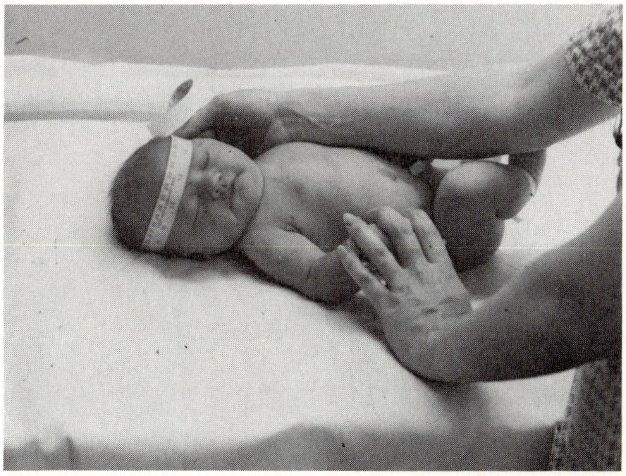

Fig. 28.8
Measuring circumference of chest.

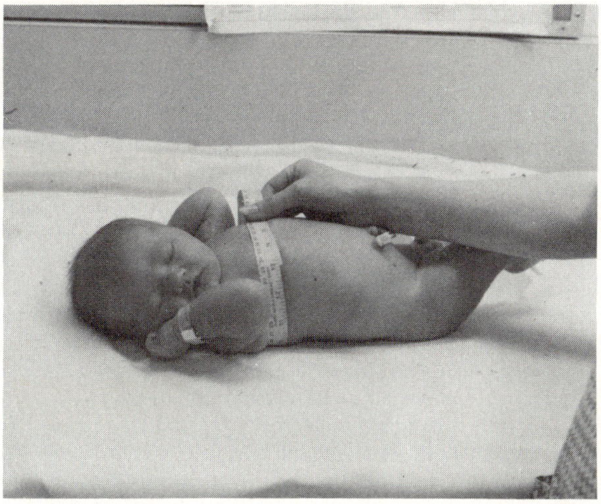

Fig. 28.9
Location of apical pulse in neonate.
A, Apical impulse (PMI) in the neonate is at the fourth intercostal space and to the left of the midclavicular line. The PMI is often visible. **B,** Apical impulse (PMI) in the adult is at the fifth intercostal space at or just medial to (to the right of) the midclavicular line. The PMI is usually displaced upward and to the left by the gravid uterus. (From Whaley, L.F., and Wong, D.L.: Nursing care of infants and children, ed. 2, St. Louis, 1983, the C.V. Mosby Co.)

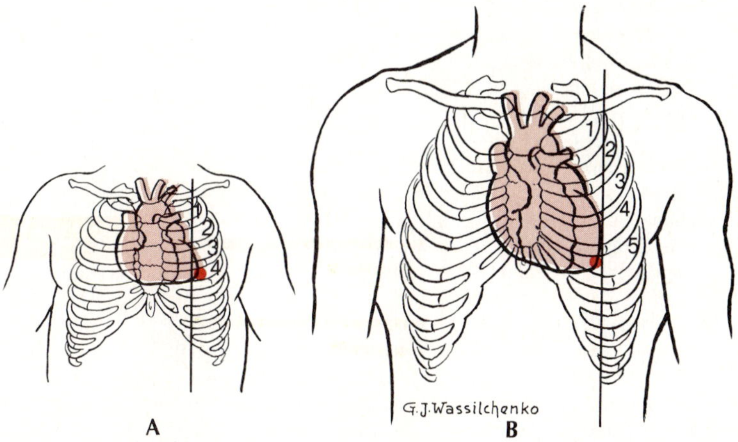

Table 28.1—cont'd
Physical Assessment of Newborn

Evaluation Criteria and Appraisal Procedure	Normal Findings: Average Findings	Normal Findings: Normal Variations	Deviations from Normal Range (Possible Problems)
Measurements—cont'd			
Head circumference			
Measure head at greatest diameter: occipitofrontal circumference (Fig. 28.7) May need to remeasure on second or third day after resolution of molding and caput succedaneum	33-35 cm (13-14 in) Circumferences of head and chest may be about the same for first 1 or 2 days after birth	32.5-37.5 cm (12½-14½ in)	Microcephaly (under 32 cm) Rubella Toxoplasmosis Cytomegalic inclusion disease (CMV) Hydrocephaly (≥ 4 cm more than chest) Increased intracranial pressure Hemorrhage Space-occupying lesion
Chest circumference			
Measure at nipple line (Fig. 28.8)	2 cm (¾ in) less than head circumference; averages between 30-33 cm (12-13 in)		Prematurity: ≤ 30 cm Postmaturity: some SGA and some LGA
Vital signs			
Blood pressure (BP)			
Electronic monitor BP cuff: BP cuff width affects readings; use cuff 2.5 cm (1 in) wide and palpate radial pulse	75/42 (approximately) At birth Systolic: 60-80 mm Hg Diastolic: 40-50 mm Hg At 10 days Systolic: 95-100 mm Hg Diastolic: slight increase	Varies with change in activity level: awake, crying, sleeping	Difference between upper and lower extremity pressures may provide early clue to coarctation of aorta Hypotension Hypertension: coarctation of aorta
Heart rate and pulses			
Thorax Inspection Palpation Auscultation Apex: mitral valve Second interspace, left of sternum: pulmonic valve Second interspace, right of sternum: aortic valve Junction of xiphoid process and sternum: tricuspid valve	Pulsations visible in left midclavicular line; fifth intercostal space Apical pulse; fifth intercostal space 120-140/min (Fig. 28.9) Quality: *first sound* (closure of mitral and tricuspid valves) and *second sound* (closure of aortic and pulmonic valves) should be sharp and clear	100 (sleeping) to 160 (crying); may be irregular for brief periods, especially after crying Murmurs, especially over base or at left sternal border in interspace 3 or 4 (foramen ovale closes at about 1 yr) Average pulses 2 yr: 105 6 yr: 100 8-12 yr*: 85-90 16 yr*: 80 18 yr*: 70	Tachycardia (persistent; ≥ 170): RDS Bradycardia (persistent; ≤ 120): congenital heart block Murmurs: may be functional Arrhythmias: irregular rate Sounds Distant: pneumomediastinum Poor quality Extra Heard on right side of chest: dextrocardia (often accompanied by reversal of intestines)
Femoral pulse palpation: flex thighs on hips; place fingers along inguinal ligament about midway between symphysis pubis and iliac crest; feel bilaterally at same time (Fig. 28.10)	Femoral pulses should be equal and strong		Weak or absent femoral pulses Hip dysplasia Coarctation of aorta Thrombophlebitis
Temperature			
Axillary (Fig. 28.11): method of choice until 6 yr of age Rectal (Fig. 28.12): before passage of meconium, check for patent anus; insert thermometer with great caution, gently; hold in place, keeping legs immobilized	Axillary: 36.5°-37° C (97.6°-98.6° F) Rectal: 35.5°-37.5° C (96°-99.5° F): may be misleading—even in cold stress may remain unchanged until metabolic activity can no longer maintain core temperature	35.7°-37.2° C (96°-99° F) Heat loss: 200 kcal/kg/min from evaporation, conduction, convection, radiation	Subnormal—may reflect the following: Prematurity Infection Low environmental temperature Inadequate clothing Dehydration Increased (pyrexia)—may reflect the following:

*Slightly faster for girls.

Fig. 28.10
Palpating femoral pulse.

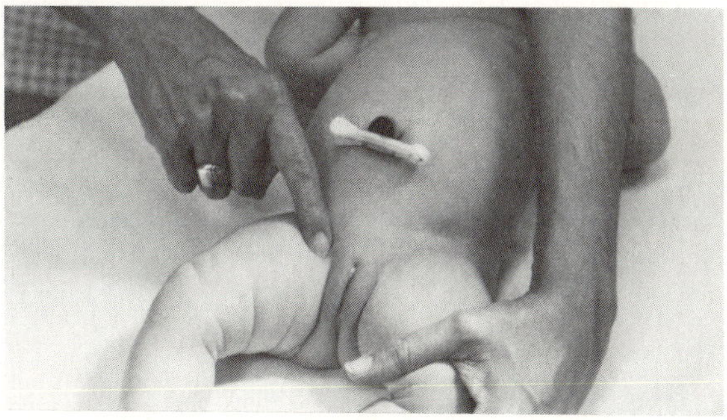

Fig. 28.11
Taking axillary temperature.

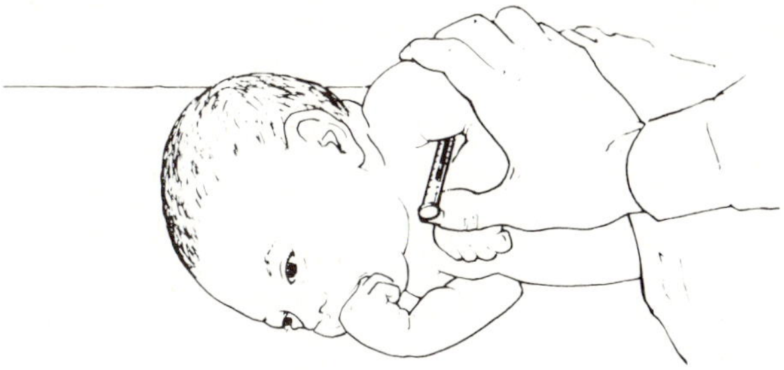

Fig. 28.12
Support of legs for rectal temperature. Attendant maintains support during entire procedure.

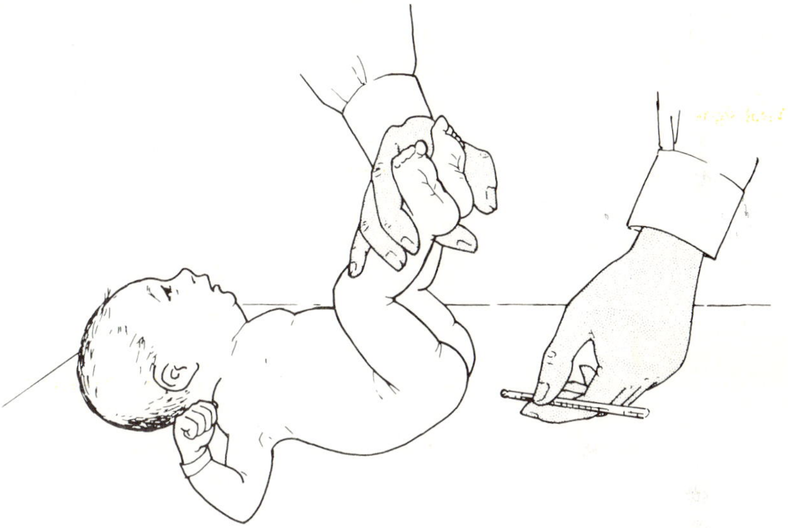

Table 28.1—cont'd
Physical Assessment of Newborn

Evaluation Criteria and Appraisal Procedure	Normal Findings: Average Findings	Normal Findings: Normal Variations	Deviations from Normal Range (Possible Problems)
Vital signs—cont'd			
Electronic: thermistor probe (avoid taping over bony area)	Temperature stabilization by 8-10 hr of age Shivering mechanism undeveloped		Infection High environmental temperature Excessive clothing Proximity to heating unit or in direct sunshine Drug addiction (following increased activity level of infant) Diarrhea and dehydration Temperature not stabilized by 10 hr after birth If mother received magnesium sulfate, neonate is less able to conserve heat by vasoconstriction; maternal analgesics may reduce thermal stability in neonate

Continued.

Table 28.1—cont'd
Physical Assessment of Newborn

Evaluation Criteria and Appraisal Procedure	Normal Findings: Average Findings	Normal Findings: Normal Variations	Deviations from Normal Range (Possible Problems)
Vital signs—cont'd			
Respiratory rate and effort			
Observe respirations when infant is at rest Count respirations for full minute Apnea monitor Listen for sounds audible without stethoscope	40/min Tend to be shallow, and when infant is awake, irregular in rate, rhythm, and depth No sounds should be audible on inspiration or expiration	30-60/min May appear to be Cheyne-Stokes with short periods of apnea and with no evidence of respiratory distress	Apneic episodes: ≥ 15/sec Preterm or premature infant: "periodic breathing" Rapid warming or cooling of infant
Observe respiratory effort	Breath sounds: bronchial; loud, clear, near	First period (reactivity): 50-60/min Second period: 50-70/min Stabilization (1-2 days): 30-40/min	Bradypnea: ≤ 25/min Maternal narcosis from analgesics or anesthetics Birth trauma Tachypnea: ≥ 60/min RDS Aspiration syndrome Diaphragmatic hernia Sounds Rales, rhonchi, wheezes Expiratory grunt Distress Nasal flaring Retractions Chin tug Labored breathing
Integument			
Color			
Inspection and palpation Inspect naked neonate in well-lit, warm area without drafts; natural daylight provides best lighting Inspect neonate when he is quiet and when he is active	Varies with ethnic origin; skin pigmentation begins to deepen right after birth in basal layer of epidermis Generally pink Acrocyanosis, especially if chilled	Mottling (Fig. 28.13) Harlequin sign Plethora Telangiectases ("stork bites" or capillary hemangiomas) Erythema toxicum neonatorum ("newborn rash")	Dark red: prematurity Pallor Cardiovascular problem CNS damage Blood dyscrasia; blood loss; twin transfusion Nosocomial problem (e.g., infection) Cyanosis Hypothermia Infection Hypoglycemia Cardiopulmonary diseases Malformations: cardiac, neurologic, or respiratory
Check for jaundice (see p. 561)			Jaundice (see p. 561) Gray: hypotension, poor perfusion
		Petechiae over presenting part	Petechiae over any other area may be caused by the following: Clotting factor deficiency Infection
		Ecchymoses from forceps in vertex births or over buttocks and legs in breech births	Ecchymoses in any other area: hemorrhagic disease
Birthmarks			
Inspect and palpate for location, size, distribution, characteristics, color	Transient hyperpigmentation Areolae Genitalia Linea nigra	Mongolian spotting Infants of black, Oriental, and American Indian origin: 70% Infants of white origin: 9%	Hemangiomas (vascular tumors) Nevus flammeus (port-wine stain) Strawberry mark Cavernous hemangiomas

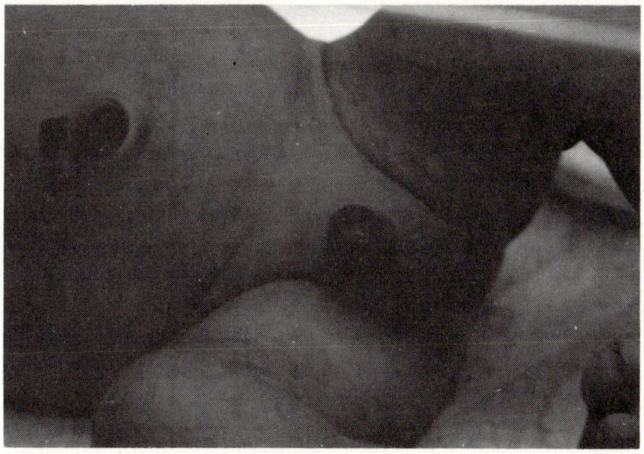

Fig. 28.13
Mottling. Note also dry cord with clamp removed, newly circumcised penis, and wrinkled scrotal sac.

Table 28.1—cont'd
Physical Assessment of Newborn

Evaluation Criteria and Appraisal Procedure	Normal Findings: Average Findings	Normal Findings: Normal Variations	Deviations from Normal Range (Possible Problems)
Integument—cont'd			
Condition			
Inspect and palpate for intactness, smoothness, texture, edema	No skin edema Texture: thick; superficial or deep cracking Opacity: few large blood vessels seen indistinctly over abdomen	Slightly thick; superficial cracking, peeling, especially of hands, feet No blood vessels seen; a few large vessels clearly seen over abdomen Some fingernail scratches	Prematurity Edema on hands, feet; pitting over tibia Texture thin, smooth, or of medium thickness; rash or superficial peeling seen Numerous vessels easily seen over abdomen Postmaturity Texture thick, parchmentlike Skin tags; webbing Papules, pustules, vesicles, ulcers, maceration: impetigo, candidiasis, herpes Diaper rash
Hydration and consistency			
Weigh infant routinely Inspection and palpation Gently pinch skin between thumb and forefinger over abdomen and inner thigh to check for turgor	Dehydration: best indicator of loss of weight After pinch is released, skin returns to original state immediately	Normal weight loss after birth is up to 10% of birth weight May feel puffy	Loose, wrinkled skin Prematurity Postmaturity Dehydration: fold of skin persists after release of pinch Tense, tight, shiny skin: edema, extreme cold, shock, infection
Check subcutaneous fat deposits (adipose pads) over cheeks, buttocks		Amount of subcutaneous fat varies	Lack of subcutaneous fat (e.g., clavicle or ribs prominent): prematurity, malnutrition
Check voiding	Voids 6-10 times per day		
Vernix caseosa			
Observe amount		Amount varies; usually more is found in creases, folds	Absent or minimal: postmaturity Excessive: prematurity

Continued.

Table 28.1—cont'd
Physical Assessment of Newborn

Evaluation Criteria and Appraisal Procedure	Normal Findings: Average Findings	Normal Findings: Normal Variations	Deviations from Normal Range (Possible Problems)
Integument—cont'd			
Observe its color and odor before bath or wiping If not readily apparent over total body, check in folds of axilla and groin	Whitish, cheesy, odorless		Yellow color Possible fetal anoxia 36 hr or more before birth Rh or ABO incompatibility (see Chapter 40) Green color: possible in-utero release of meconium because of fetal anoxia less than 36 hr before birth or presence of bilirubin Odor: possible intrauterine infection (e.g., amnionitis)
Lanugo Inspect for this fine, downy hair: amount, distribution	Over shoulders, pinnas of ears, forehead	Amount varies	Absent: postmaturity Excessive: prematurity, especially if lanugo is abundant and long and thick over back
Body segment			
Head Palpate skin	See Skin, p. 563	Caput succedaneum; may show some ecchymosis	Cephalhematoma (appears after first day)
Palpate, inspect, measure fontanels	Anterior: 5 cm diamond; increases as molding resolves Posterior: triangle; smaller than anterior	Size varies with degree of molding Fontanels may be difficult to feel because of molding	Fontanels Full, bulging: possible intracranial lesion (e.g., tumor, hemorrhage, infection) Large, flat, soft: malnutrition, hydrocephaly, retarded bone age (hypothyroidism) Depressed: dehydration Large mastoid and sphenoid fontanels: hydrocephaly
Palpate sutures	Sutures palpable and not joined	Sutures may overlap with molding	Sutures Widely spaced: hydrocephaly Premature synostosis (closure)
Inspect pattern, distribution, amount of hair; feel texture	Silky, single strands, lies flat; growth pattern is toward face and neck	Amount varies	Fine, wooly: prematurity Unusual swirls, patterns, hairline or coarse, brittle: endocrine or genetic disorder
Inspect shape and size	Makes up one fourth of body length Molding	Slight asymmetry from intrauterine position	Molding (Fig. 28.14) Severe molding may result from birth trauma Lack of molding: prematurity, breech presentation, cesarean birth Circumference ≥ 4 cm larger than chest circumference: hydrocephaly; ≤ 32 cm: prematurity, microcephaly

Continued.

Fig. 28.14
Molding.

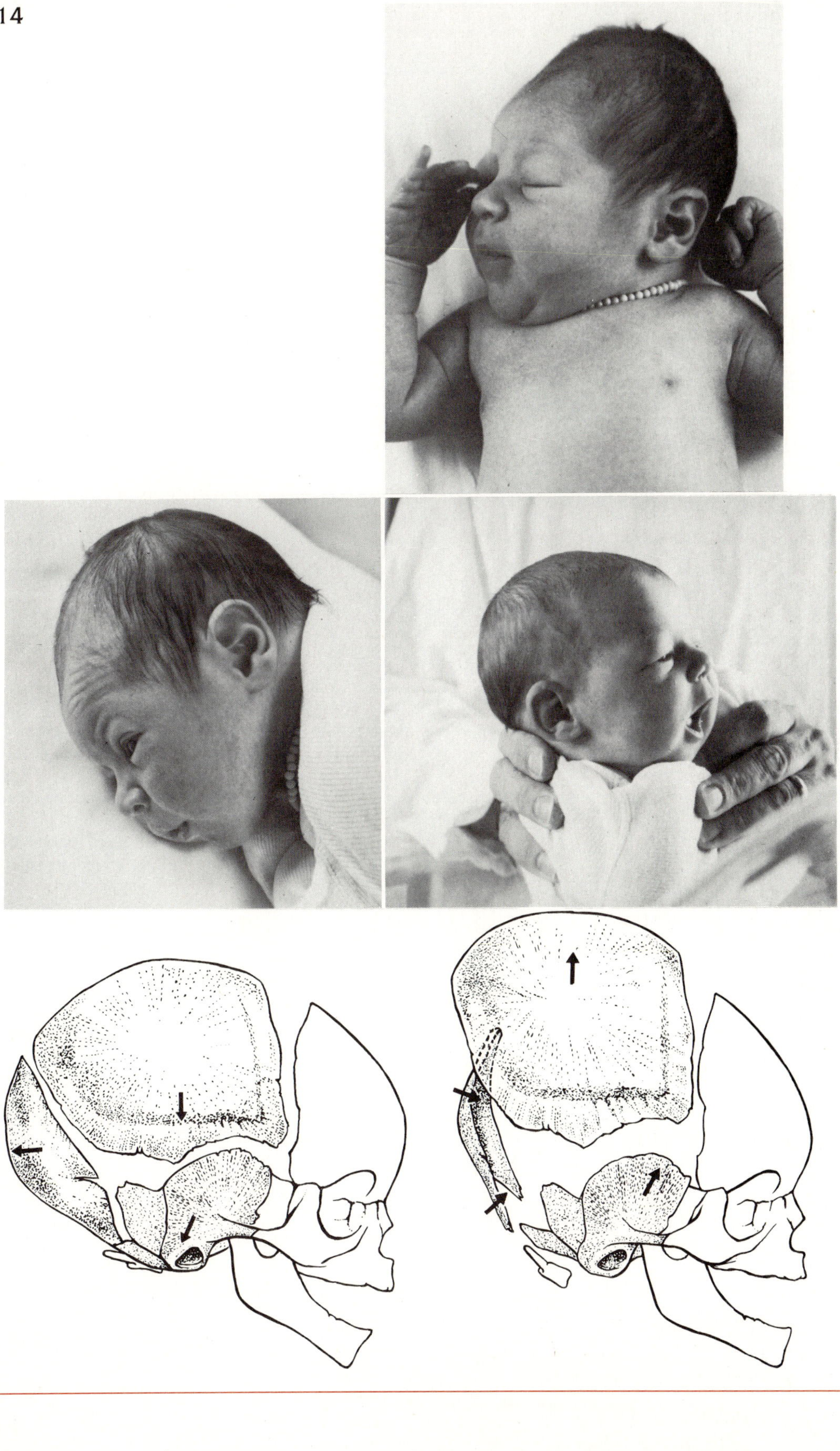

Table 28.1—cont'd
Physical Assessment of Newborn

Evaluation Criteria and Appraisal Procedure	Normal Findings: Average Findings	Normal Findings: Normal Variations	Deviations from Normal Range (Possible Problems)
Body segment—cont'd			
Eyes (Fig. 28.15)			
Placement on face			
Symmetry in size, shape	Symmetric in size, shape		
Eyelids: size, movement, blink	Size and movement symmetric Blink reflex	Edema from instilling silver nitrate	Agenesis or absence of one or both eyeballs Small eyeball size: rubella syndrome Lens opacity or absence of red reflex: congenital cataracts, possibly from rubella Lesions: coloboma (absence of part of iris) Strabismus Epicanthal folds: when present with other signs, may be caused by chromosomal disorders (e.g., Down's syndrome, cri du chat syndrome) Pink color of iris: albinism Jaundiced sclera Discharge: purulent Pupils: unequal, constricted, dilated, fixed
Discharge	None No tears	Some discharge from silver nitrate	
Eyeballs: presence, size, shape	Both present and of equal size; both round, firm	Occasionally has some tears Subconjunctival hemorrhage	
Eyeball movement	Random, jerky, uneven; can focus momentarily, can follow to midline	Transient strabismus or nystagmus until third or fourth month	
Eyebrows: amount, pattern	Distinct		
Nose			
Observe shape, placement, patency, configuration of bridge of nose	Midline Apparent lack of bridge, flat, broad Some mucus but no drainage Obligatory nose breathers Sneezes to clear nose	Slight deformity from passage through birth canal	Copious drainage, with or without regular periods of cyanosis at rest and return of pink color with crying: choanal atresia, congenital syphilis Malformed: congenital syphilis, chromosomal disorder Flaring of nares
Ears			
Observe size, placement on head, amount of cartilage, open auditory canal Hearing	Correct placement: line drawn through inner and outer canthi of eye should come to top notch of ear (at junction with scalp) Well-formed, firm cartilage	Size: small, large, floppy Darwin's tubercle (nodule on posterior helix)	Agenesis Lack of cartilage: possible prematurity Low placement: possible chromosomal disorder, mental retardation, kidney disorder Preauricular tags Size: may have overly prominent or protruding ears
Facies			
Observe overall appearance of face	Infant looks "normal"; features are well placed, proportionate to face	"Positional" deformities (Fig. 28.3)	Infant looks "odd" or "funny" Usually accompanied by other features, such as low-set ears and other structural disorders
Mouth			
Inspection and palpation Placement on face Lips: color, configuration, movement, rooting reflex, sucking	Pink gums Symmetry of lip movement Tongue does not protrude, is freely movable; symmetric in shape, movement	Transient circumoral cyanosis Short frenulum	Gross anomalies Placement, size, shape Cleft lip and/or palate, gums Cyanosis; circumoral pallor

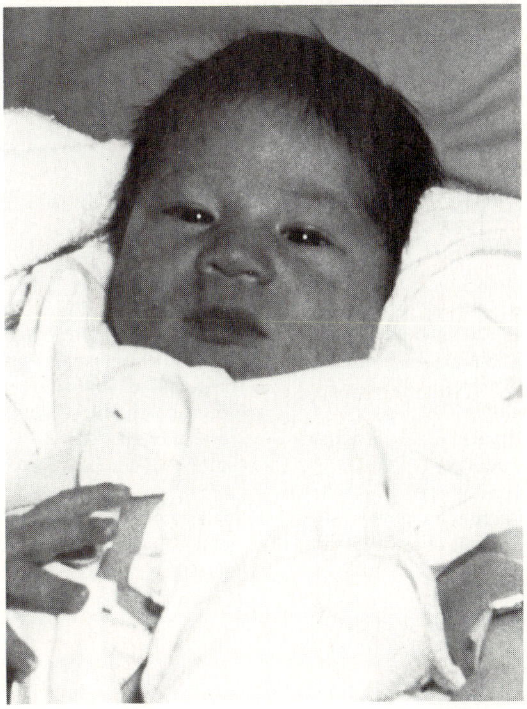

Fig. 28.15
Eyes. Pseudostrabismus. Inner epicanthal folds cause eyes to appear malaligned; however, corneal light reflexes fall perfectly symmetric. Eyes are symmetric in size and shape and well placed. Note that *folds of cheeks* are present and symmetric, indicating an absence of facial palsy. *Hair* on head consists of individual strands and is growing toward face. *Eyebrows* are well shaped and do not converge in midline. *Mouth* is of appropriate size and has a distinct vermilion border.

Table 28.1—cont'd
Physical Assessment of Newborn

Evaluation Criteria and Appraisal Procedure	Normal Findings: Average Findings	Normal Findings: Normal Variations	Deviations from Normal Range (Possible Problems)
Body segment—cont'd Gums Tongue: attachment, mobility, movement, size Cheeks Palate (soft, hard) Arch Uvula Saliva: amount, character Chin Reflexes	Sucking pads inside cheeks Soft and hard palates intact Uvula in midline Reflexes present	Anatomic groove in palate to accommodate nipple; disappears by 3-4 yr of age Epstein's pearls (Bohn's nodules): whitish, hard nodules on gums Reflex response dependent on state of wakefulness and hunger	Asymmetry in movement of lips: seventh cranial nerve paralysis Macroglossia Prematurity Chromosomal disorder Excessive saliva Esophageal atresia Tracheoesophageal fistula Micrognathia: Pierre Robin or other syndrome Teeth: predeciduous or deciduous Thrush: white plaques on cheeks or tongue that bleed if touched
Neck Inspection and palpation Length Movement of head Sternocleidomastoid muscles; position of head Trachea: position; thyroid gland	Short, thick, surrounded by skinfolds; no webbing Head held in midline, i.e., sternocleidomastoid muscles are equal; no masses Freedom of movement from side to side and flexion and extension; cannot move chin past shoulder	Transient positional deformity apparent when neonate is at rest: head can be moved passively	Webbing Restricted movement; head held at angle: possible torticollis (wryneck), opisthotonos Masses: enlarged thyroid Distended veins: cardiopulmonary disorder

Continued.

Table 28.1—cont'd
Physical Assessment of Newborn

Evaluation Criteria and Appraisal Procedure	Normal Findings: Average Findings	Normal Findings: Normal Variations	Deviations from Normal Range (Possible Problems)
Body segment—cont'd			
Reflex response (Table 28.2)	Thyroid not palpable		Skin tags Positive owl's sign: prematurity Absence of head control: prematurity; Down's syndrome
Chest			
Inspection and palpation Shape Clavicles Ribs Nipples: size, placement, number Breast tissue Respiratory movements Amount of cartilage in rib cage Auscultation Heart tones and rate and breath sounds (see Vital signs, above)	Almost circular; barrel shaped Symmetric chest movements; chest and abdominal movements synchronized during respirations Breast nodule: approximately 6 mm Nipples prominent, well formed; symmetrically placed	Occasional retractions, especially when crying Breast nodule: 3-10 mm Secretion of witch's milk	Bulging of chest Pneumothorax Pneumomediastinum Malformation: funnel chest (pectus excavatum) Fracture of clavicle Nipples Supernumerary, along nipple line Malpositioned or widely spaced Lack of breast tissue: possible prematurity Poor development of rib cage and musculature: possible prematurity Sounds: bowel sounds (see Abdomen, below) Retractions with or without respiratory distress signs
Abdomen			
Inspect, palpate, and smell umbilical cord	Two arteries, one vein (AVA) Whitish gray Definite demarcation between cord and skin; no intestinal structures within cord Dry around base; drying Odorless	Reducible umbilical herniation	One artery: internal anomalies Bleeding or oozing around cord: hemorrhagic disease Redness or drainage around cord: infection, possible persistence of urachus Hernia: herniation of abdominal contents into area of cord (e.g., omphalocele); defect covered with thin, friable membrane; may be extensive Gastroschisis: congenital fissure of abdominal cavity Meconium stained: intrauterine distress
Inspect size of abdomen and palpate contour (Fig. 28.16)	Rounded, prominent, dome shaped because abdominal musculature is not fully developed No distention	Some diastasis of abdominal musculature	Distention At birth Ruptured viscus Genitourinary masses or malformations: hydronephrosis; teratomas Abdominal tumors Mild Aerophagia Overfeeding High gastrointestinal tract obstruction

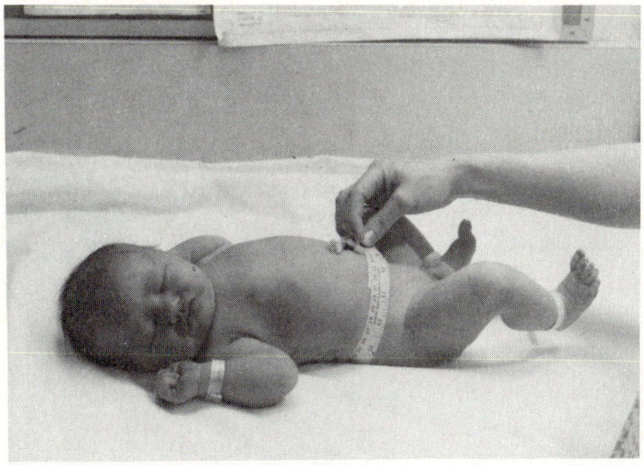

Fig. 28.16
Measuring abdominal circumference.

Table 28.1—cont'd
Physical Assessment of Newborn

Evaluation Criteria and Appraisal Procedure	Normal Findings: Average Findings	Normal Findings: Normal Variations	Deviations from Normal Range (Possible Problems)
Body segment—cont'd			
			Marked Lower gastrointestinal tract obstruction Imperforate anus Intermittent or transient Aerophagia Overfeeding Partial intestinal obstruction from stenosis of bowel Annular pancreas Malrotation of bowel or adhesions Sepsis
Auscultate bowel sounds and note number, amount, and character of stools, and behavior—crying, fussiness—prior to or during elimination	Sounds present within 1-2 hr after birth Meconium stool passed within 24-48 hr after birth		Scaphoid, with bowel sounds in chest and respiratory distress: diaphragmatic hernia
Color		Linea nigra may be apparent; possibly caused by hormone influence during pregnancy	
Movement with respiration	Respirations primarily diaphragmatic; abdominal and chest movements synchronous		Decreased abdominal breathing Intrathoracic disease Diaphragmatic hernia
Genitalia (Fig. 28.17)			
Female			
Inspection and palpation			
General appearance	Female genitalia	Increased pigmentation caused by pregnancy hormones	Ambiguous genitalia—enlarged clitoris with urinary meatus on tip; fused labia: chromosomal disorder; maternal drug ingestion
Clitoris	Usually edematous		
Labia majora	Usually edematous; cover labia minora in term neonates	Edema and ecchymosis following breech birth	

Continued.

Fig. 28.17

A, Genitalia in male term infant. **B,** Genitalia in female term infant. Note also well-formed ear, good muscle tone, domed abdomen, well-formed nipples, deep creases covering entire sole of foot. **C,** Uncircumcised penis. Rugae cover scrotum, indicating term gestation. **D,** Normal term female genitalia. Note mucoid vaginal discharge.

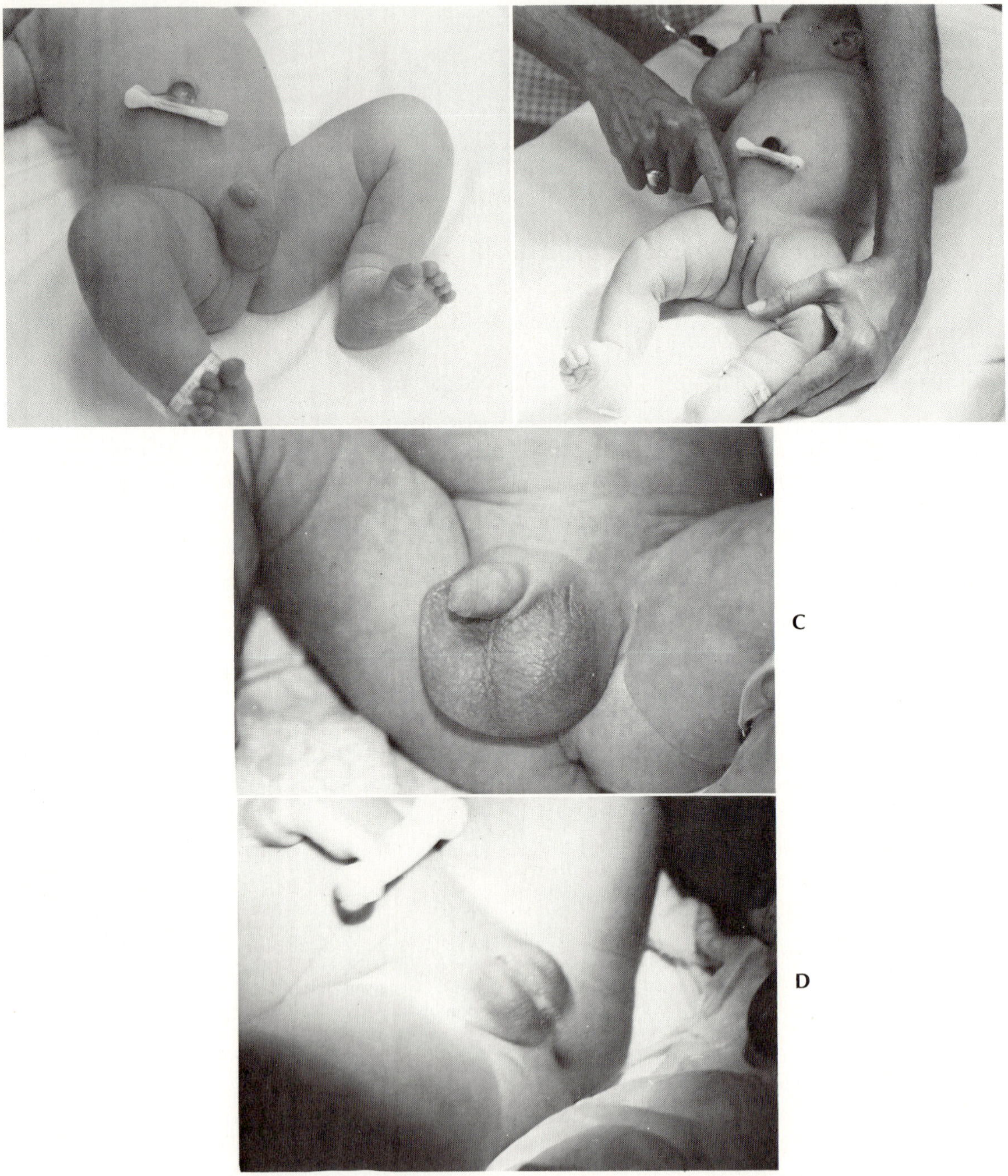

A

B

C

D

Table 28.1—cont'd
Physical Assessment of Newborn

Evaluation Criteria and Appraisal Procedure	Normal Findings: Average Findings	Normal Findings: Normal Variations	Deviations from Normal Range (Possible Problems)
Body segment—cont'd			
Labia minora	May protrude over labia majora	Vaginal tag	Stenosed meatus
Discharge	Smegma	Blood-tinged discharge from pseudomenstruation caused by pregnancy hormones	Labia majora widely separated and labia minora prominent: prematurity
Vagina	Orifice open Mucoid discharge	Rust-stained urine (uric acid crystals)*	Absence of vaginal orifice or imperforate hyman
Urinary meatus	Beneath clitoris; hard to see—watch for voiding	Some vernix caseosa may be between labia	Fecal discharge: fistula
Male			
Inspection and palpation			
General appearance	Male genitalia	Increased size and pigmentation caused by pregnancy hormones	Ambiguous genitalia
Penis Urinary meatus seen as slit Prepuce	Meatus at tip of penis; prepuce (foreskin) covers glans penis and is not easily retractable (for about 6 mo) Voiding before 24-48 hr, stream adequate, amount adequate	Prepuce removed at circumcision Size of genitalia varies widely Edema and ecchymosis if breech birth	Urinary meatus not on tip of glans penis Hypospadias, Epispadias } may be associated with other anomalies Adherent or tight prepuce: phimosis
Scrotum Rugae (wrinkles)	Large, edematous, pendulous; covered with rugae	Hydrocele, small, noncommunicating	Scrotum smooth and testes undescended: prematurity, cryptorchidism
Testes	Palpable on each side	Bulge palpable in inguinal canal	Hydrocele
Reflexes Erection	Erection may occur when genitalia are touched	Rust-stained urine (uric acid crystals)	Inguinal hernia Round meatal opening
Cremasteric	Testes are retracted, especially when neonate is chilled		
Extremities			
General			
Inspection and palpation Degree of flexion Range of motion Symmetry of motion Muscle tone	Assumes position maintained in utero Attitude of general flexion Full range of motion, spontaneous movements	Transient (positional) deformities	Limited motion: malformations Poor muscle tone Positive scarf sign (see Chapter 37)
Arms			
Inspection and palpation Color Intactness Appropriate placement Number of fingers Palpate humerus Joints Shoulder Elbow Wrist Fingers Reflex: grasp (Table 28.2)	Longer than legs in newborn period Contours and movement are symmetric Should be intact Fist often clenched with thumb under fingers Full range of motion; symmetric contour	Slight tremors may be seen at times Some acrocyanosis, especially when chilled	Asymmetry of movement Fracture Brachial nerve trauma Malformations Asymmetry of contour Malformations Fracture Amelia or phocomelia Webbing of fingers: syndactyly Absence or excess of fingers Palmar creases Simian line (commonly seen in Down's syndrome) seen with short, incurved little fingers Strong, rigid flexion; persistent fists; fists held in front of mouth constantly: CNS disorder Increased tonicity, clonicity, prolonged tremors (especially if whole body is involved): CNS disorder

*To determine whether rust color is caused by uric acid or blood, wash under running warm tap water. Uric acid washes out, blood does not.

Continued.

Fig. 28.18
Method of assessing for Ortolani's sign.

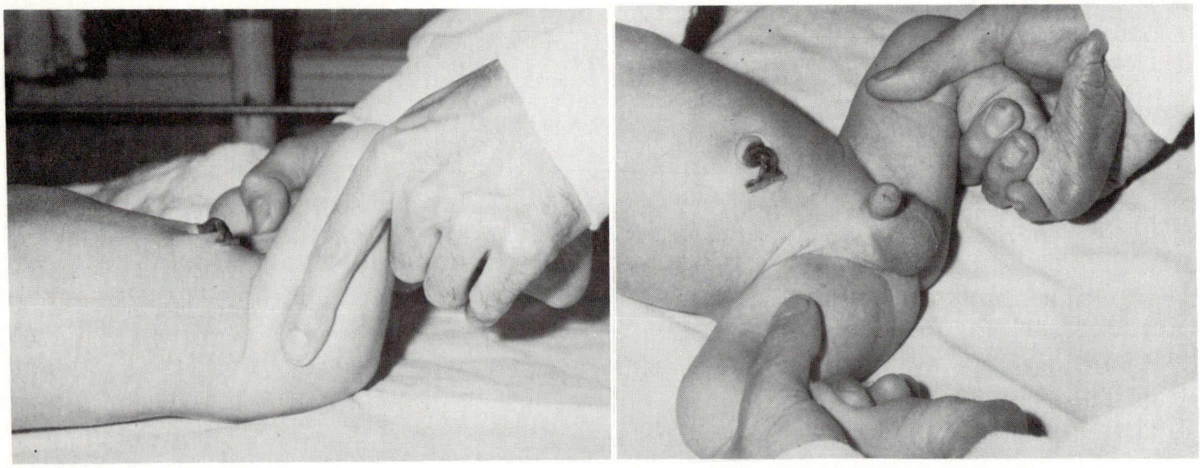

Fig. 28.19
Normal absence of arch in newborn.

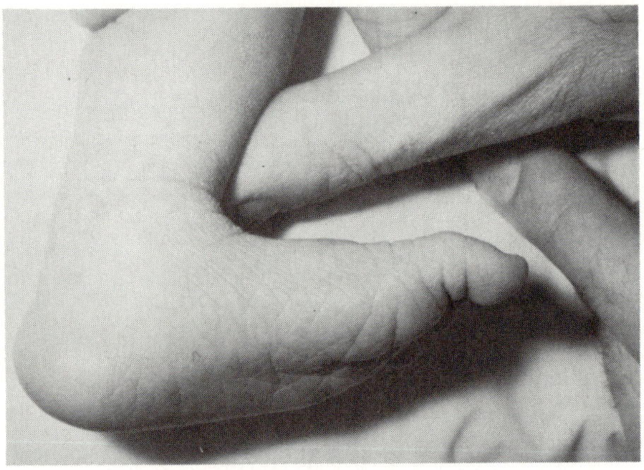

Fig. 28.20
Examining back. Infant's back should be slightly flexed, freely movable, and free of defects. Infant should kick both legs.

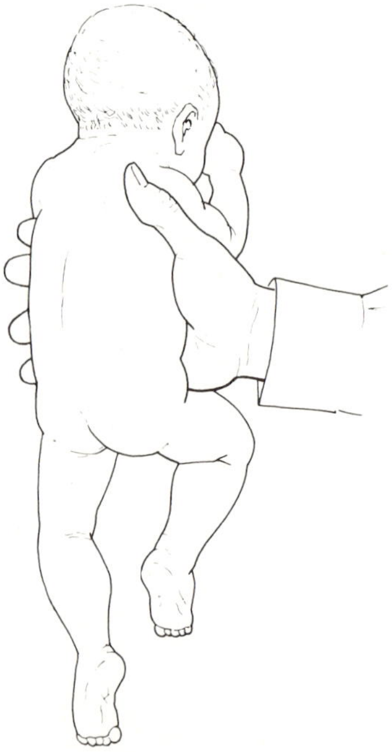

Table 28.1—cont'd
Physical Assessment of Newborn

Evaluation Criteria and Appraisal Procedure	Normal Findings: Average Findings	Normal Findings: Normal Variations	Deviations from Normal Range (Possible Problems)
Body segment—cont'd			
Legs Inspection and palpation Intactness Length—in relation to arms and body and to each other Major gluteal folds Number of toes Femur Head of femur as legs are flexed on hips and adducted; placement in acetabulum; femoral pulses (Fig. 28.18) Color	Appear bowed since lateral muscles more developed than medial muscles Major gluteal folds even Femur should be intact No click should be heard; femoral head should not override acetabulum Feet flat; soles well lined (or wrinkled) over two thirds Plantar fat pad gives flat-footed effect (Fig. 28.19) Inspection and palpation Joints Hip Knee Ankle Toes Reflexes (Table 28.2)	Feet appear to turn in but can be easily rotated externally, also positional defects tend to correct while infant is crying Acrocyanosis	Amelia, phocomelia Chromosomal defect Teratogenic effect Webbing, syndactyly: chromosomal defect Absence or excess of digits Chromosomal defect Familial trait Femoral fracture: after difficult breech delivery Congenital hip dysplasia Absent femoral pulses Soles of feet Poorly lined: prematurity Covered with lines: postmaturity Simian line: Down's syndrome Congenital clubfoot Hypermobility of joints: Down's syndrome Yellowed nail beds Temperature of one leg differs from that of the other
Back Anatomy (Fig. 28.20) Inspection and palpation Spine Shoulders Scapulae Iliac crests Base of spine—pilonidal area	Spine straight and easily flexed Infant can raise and support head momentarily when prone Shoulders, scapulae, and iliac crests should line up in same plane	Temporary minor positional deformities, which can be corrected with passive manipulation	Limitation of movement: fusion of deformity of vertebras Pigmented nevus with tuft of hair when located anywhere along the spine is often associated with spina bifida occulta Spina bifida cystica Meningocele Myelomeningocele
Reflexes (spinal related) Test reflexes (Table 28.2)			
Anus Inspection and palpation Placement Number Patency Test for patency and sphincter response (active "wink" reflex) Observe for following: Abdominal distention Passage of meconium Passage of fecal drainage from surrounding orifices	One anus with good sphincter tone Passage of meconium within 24 hr after birth Good "wink" reflex of anal sphincter	Passage of meconium within 48 hr after birth	Low obstruction: anal membrane (thermometer cannot be inserted) High obstruction: anal or rectal atresia (thermometer may be inserted, but there is no passage of meconium) Drainage of fecal material from vagina in female or urinary meatus in male: possible rectal fistula
Stools	See p. 560		

NEUROLOGIC ASSESSMENT

Assessment of the neonate's early reflexes provides useful information on the normal infant's nervous system and state of neurologic maturation. Many of these reflex behaviors are important for survival, for example, sucking and rooting. Others act as safety mechanisms, for example, gagging, coughing, and sneezing. This assessment needs to be carried out as early as possible because abnormal signs that are present in the early neonatal period may disappear only to reappear months or years later as abnormal functions. Table 28.2 gives the techniques for eliciting significant reflexes and characteristic responses.

Text continued on p. 602.

Table 28.2
Assessment of Newborn's Reflexes

Reflex	Eliciting the Reflex	Characteristic Response	Comments
Sucking and rooting (Figs. 28.21 and 28.22)	Touch infant's lip, cheek, or corner of mouth with nipple	Infant turns head toward stimulus, opens mouth, takes hold, and sucks	Difficult if not impossible to elicit after infant has been fed; if weak or absent, consider prematurity or neurologic defect Parental guidance Avoid trying to turn head toward breast or nipple; allow infant to root Disappears after 3-4 mo but may persist up to 1 yr

Fig. 28.21
Rooting reflex is apparent when corner of newborn infant's mouth is touched. Bottom lip lowers on same side; tongue moves toward stimulus. (Courtesy Joan Edelstein.)

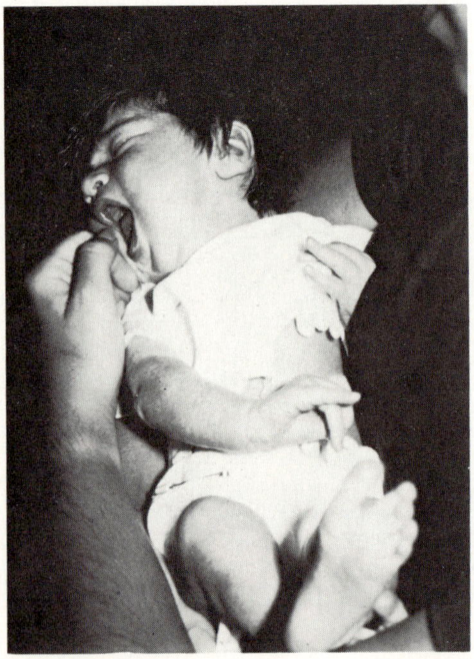

Fig. 28.22
Sucking. Also note hand-to-mouth facility with prolonged sucking. (Courtesy Joan Edelstein.)

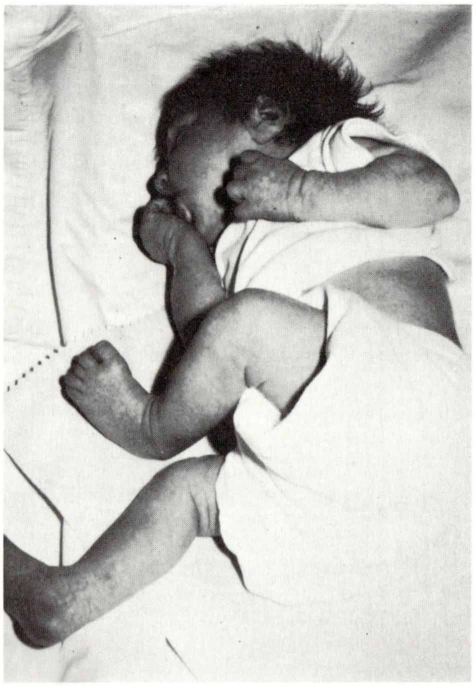

Table 28.2—cont'd
Assessment of Newborn's Reflexes

Reflex	Eliciting the Reflex	Characteristic Response	Comments
Swallowing	Swallowing usually follows sucking and obtaining fluids; suck and swallow are often uncoordinated in early-born infant and may also occur during first few hours of term (normal) infant's life	Swallowing is usually coordinated with sucking and usually occurs without gagging, coughing, or vomiting	If weak or absent, may indicate prematurity or neurologic defect
Extrusion	Touch or depress tongue	Neonate forces tongue outward	Disappears at about fourth mo
Glabellar (Myerson's)	Tap over forehead, bridge of nose, or maxilla of neonate whose eyes are open	Neonate blinks for first 4 or 5 taps	Continued blinking with repeated taps is consistent with extrapyramidal disorder
Tonic neck or "fencing" (Fig. 28.23)	With infant falling asleep or sleeping, turn head quickly to one side	With infant facing his left side, arm and leg on that side extend; opposite arm and leg flex (turn his head to right, and extremities assume opposite postures)	Responses in legs are more consistent Complete response disappears by 3-4 mo; incomplete response may be seen until third or fourth yr After 6 wk, persistent response is possible sign of cerebral palsy

Continued.

Fig. 28.23
A, Classic pose in spontaneous tonic neck reflex finds infant on his back with head turned to one side and arm and leg on same side extended. If baby's head is passively rotated in opposite direction, reversal of position of extremities may occur. **B,** Tonic neck reflex is absent. (**A** courtesy Mead Johnson & Co., Evansville, Ind. **B** courtesy Joan Edelstein.)

A

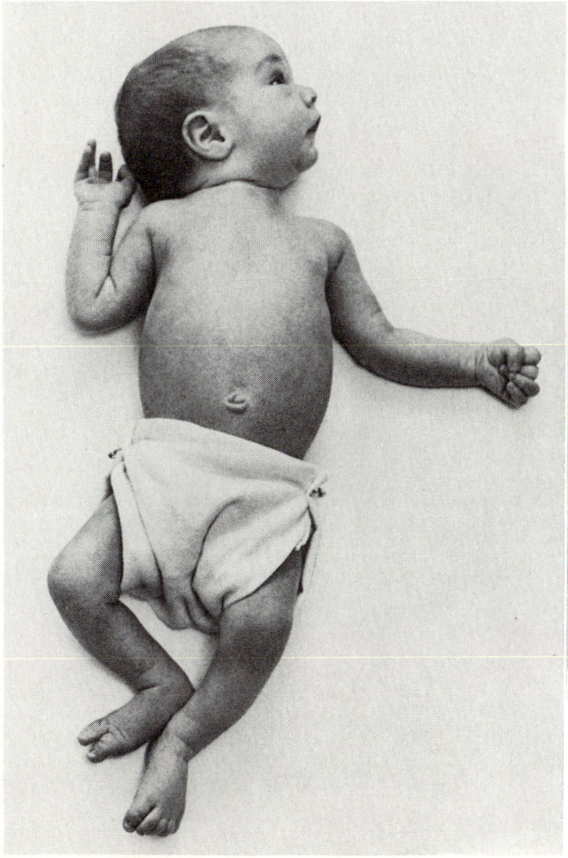

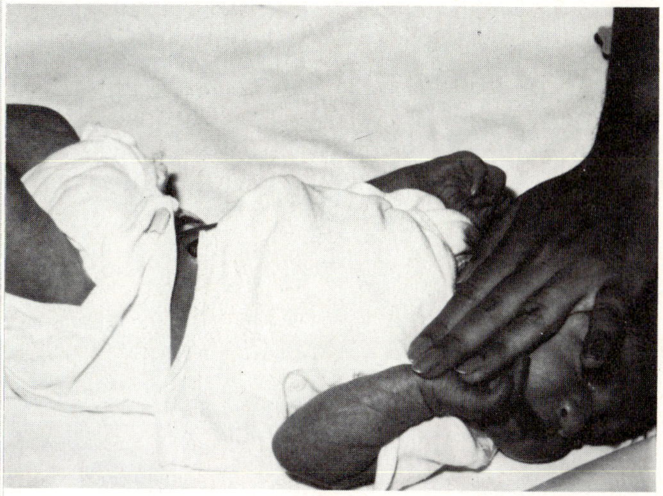

B

Table 28.2—cont'd
Assessment of Newborn's Reflexes

Reflex	Eliciting the Reflex	Characteristic Response	Comments
Grasp (Fig. 28.24) Palmar Plantar	 Place finger in palm of hand Place finger at base of toes	Infant's fingers curl around examiner's fingers; toes curl downward	Palmar response lessens by 3-4 mo; parents enjoy this contact with infant; plantar response lessens by 8 mo
Moro (Fig. 28.25)	Hold infant in semisitting position; allow head and trunk to fall backward to an angle of at least 30 degrees Place infant on flat surface; strike surface to startle infant	Symmetric abduction and extension of arms; fingers fan out and form a C with thumb and forefinger; slight tremor may be noted; arms are adducted in embracing motion and return to relaxed flexion and movement Legs may follow similar pattern of response Premature infant does not complete "embrace"; instead, arms fall backward because of weakness	Present at birth; complete response may be seen until 8 wk* of age; body jerk only, between 8-18 wk; absent by 6 mo if neurologic maturation is not delayed; may be incomplete if infant is deeply asleep; give parental guidance about normal response Asymmetric response: possible injury to brachial plexus, clavicle, or humerus Persistent "embrace": possible mental retardation

*All durations for persistence of reflexes are based on time elapsed since 40 weeks' gestation, that is, if this neonate was born at 36 weeks' gestation, add 1 month to all time limits given.

Fig. 28.24
A, Palmar (hand) grasp. **B,** Plantar grasp. (Courtesy Joan Edelstein.)

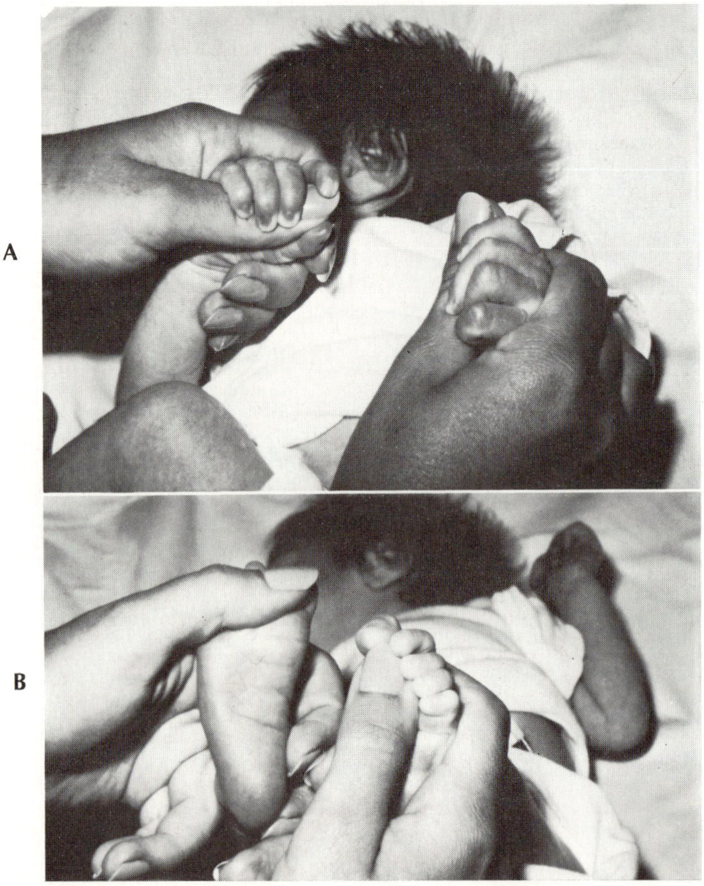

Table 28.2—cont'd
Assessment of Newborn's Reflexes

Reflex	Eliciting the Reflex	Characteristic Response	Comments
Moro—cont'd			Persistent response after 6 mo: possible brain damage
Startle	Loud noise or sharp hand clap elicits response; best elicited if neonate is 24-36 hr old or older	Arms abduct with flexion of elbows; hands stay clenched	Should disappear by 4 mo Elicited more readily in premature newborn (inform parents of this characteristic)
Traction	Pull infant up by wrists from prone position	Head will lag until infant is in upright position; then head will be held in same plane with chest and shoulders momentarily before falling forward; head will right itself spontaneously for a few moments	Depends on general muscle tone and maturity and condition of infant

Continued.

Fig. 28.25
A, Position of rest. **B,** Moro's reflex consists predominantly of abduction and extension of arms. **C,** Interesting subtlety of Moro's response in newborn infants is **C** position of fingers: digits extend, except index finger and thumb, which are often semiflexed, forming shape of C. (Courtesy Mead Johnson and Co., Evansville, Ind.)

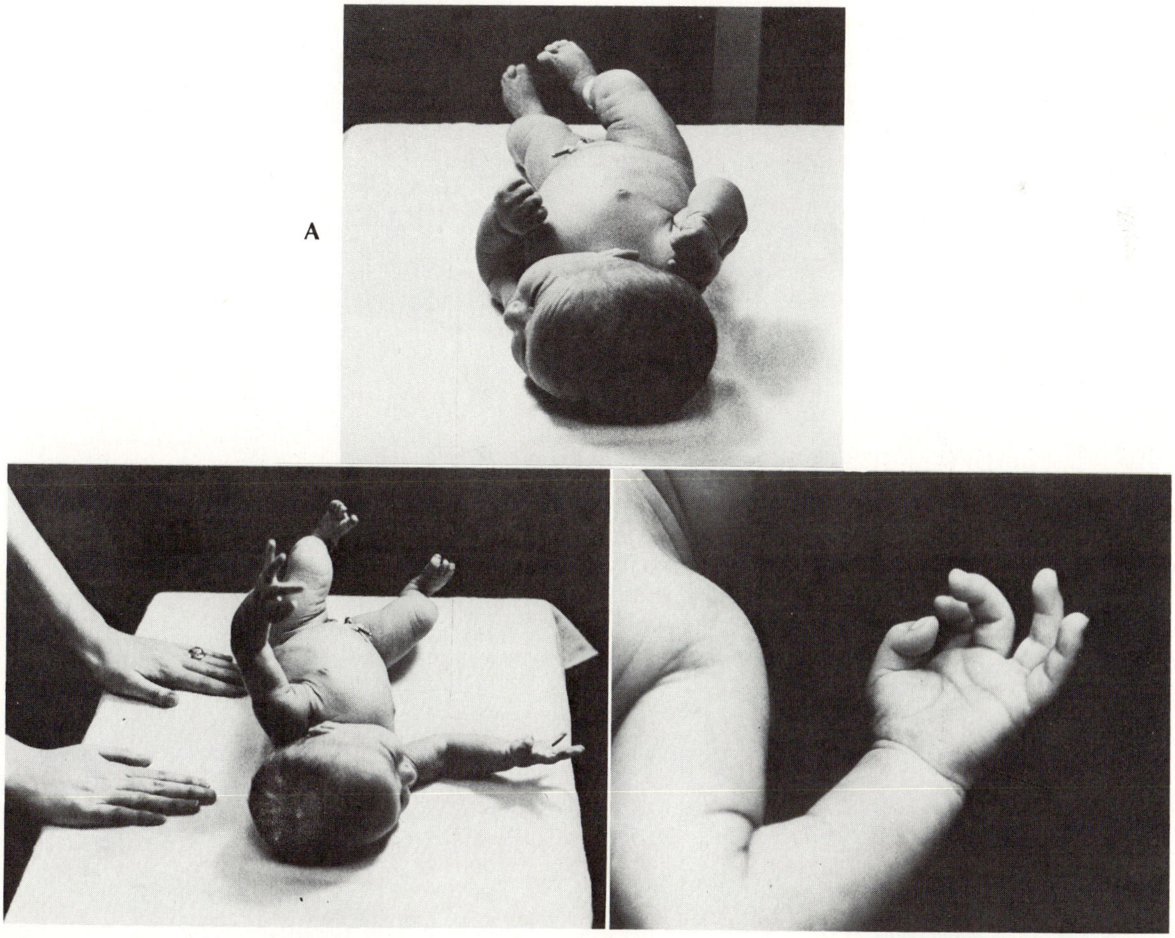

A

B

C

Fig. 28.26

Trunk incurvation reflex. In prone position, infant responds to linear skin stimulus (pin or finger) along paravertebral area by flexing trunk and swinging pelvis toward stimulus. With transverse lesions of cord, there will be no response below that level. Complete absence of response suggests general depression or nervous system abnormality. Response may vary but should be obtainable in all infants, including premature ones. If not seen in the first few days, it is usually apparent by 5 to 6 days. (Courtesy Mead Johnson & Co., Evansville, Ind.)

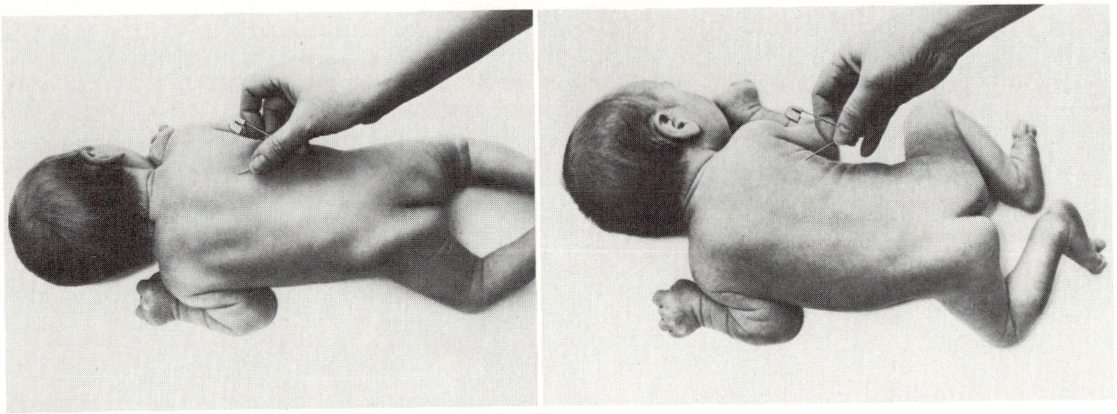

Fig. 28.27

Magnet reflex. With child in supine position and lower limbs semiflexed, light pressure is applied with fingers to both feet. Normally, while examiner's fingers maintain contact with soles of feet, lower limbs extend. Absence of this reflex suggests damage to spinal cord or malformation. Weak reflex may be seen following breech presentation *without* extended legs or may indicate sciatic nerve stretch syndrome. Breech presentation *with* extended legs may evoke an exaggerated response. (Courtesy Mead Johnson & Co., Evansville, Ind.)

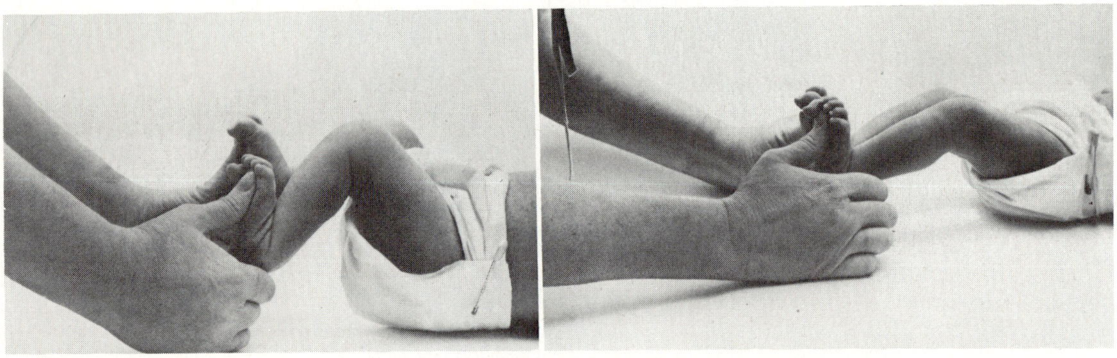

Fig. 28.28

Crossed extension reflex. With child in supine position, examiner extends one of infant's legs and presses knee down. Stimulation of sole of foot of fixated limb should cause *free* leg to flex, adduct, and extend as if attempting to push away stimulating agent. This reflex should be present during newborn period. Absence of response suggests a spinal cord lesion; weak response suggests peripheral nerve damage. (Courtesy Mead Johnson & Co., Evansville, Ind.)

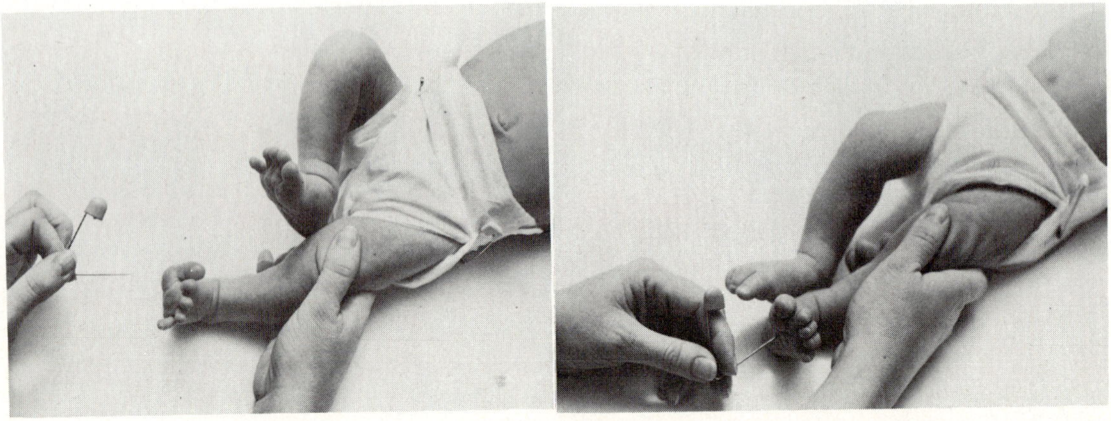

Table 28.2—cont'd
Assessment of Newborn's Reflexes

Reflex	Eliciting the Reflex	Characteristic Response	Comments
Trunk incurvation (Galant) (Fig. 28.26)	Infant should be prone on flat surface; run finger down back about 4-5 cm (1½-2 in) lateral to spine, first on one side, and then down other	Trunk is flexed and pelvis is swung toward stimulated side	Response disappears by fourth wk
Magnet (Fig. 28.27)	Infant should be supine; partially flex both lower extremities and apply pressure to soles of feet	Both lower limbs should extend against examiner's pressure	
Crossed extension (Fig. 28.28)	Infant should be supine; extend one leg, press knee downward, stimulate bottom of foot; observe opposite leg	Opposite leg flexes, adducts, and then extends	
Babinski's sign (plantar) (Fig. 28.29)	On sole of foot, beginning at heel, stroke upward along lateral aspect of sole, then move finger across ball of foot	All toes hyperextend, with dorsiflexion of big toe	Absence requires neurologic evaluation; should disappear after 1 yr of age
Stepping or "walking" (Fig. 28.30)	Hold infant vertically, allowing one foot to touch table surface	Infant will simulate walking, alternating flexion and extension of feet; term infants walk on soles of their feet, and premature infants walk on their toes	Normally present for 3-4 wk
Neck righting	Place neonate in supine position and turn head to one side	Shoulder and trunk and then pelvis will turn to be in alignment with head	Disappears at 10 mo of age; absence: implications same as for absent tonic neck reflex

Continued.

Fig. 28.29
Babinski reflex (line drawing). **A,** Direction of stroke. **B,** Dorsiflexion of big toe. **C,** Fanning of toes. **D,** Babinski reflex (neonate). (From Whaley, L.F., and Wong, D.L.: Essentials of pediatric nursing, St. Louis, 1982, The C.V. Mosby Co.)

A

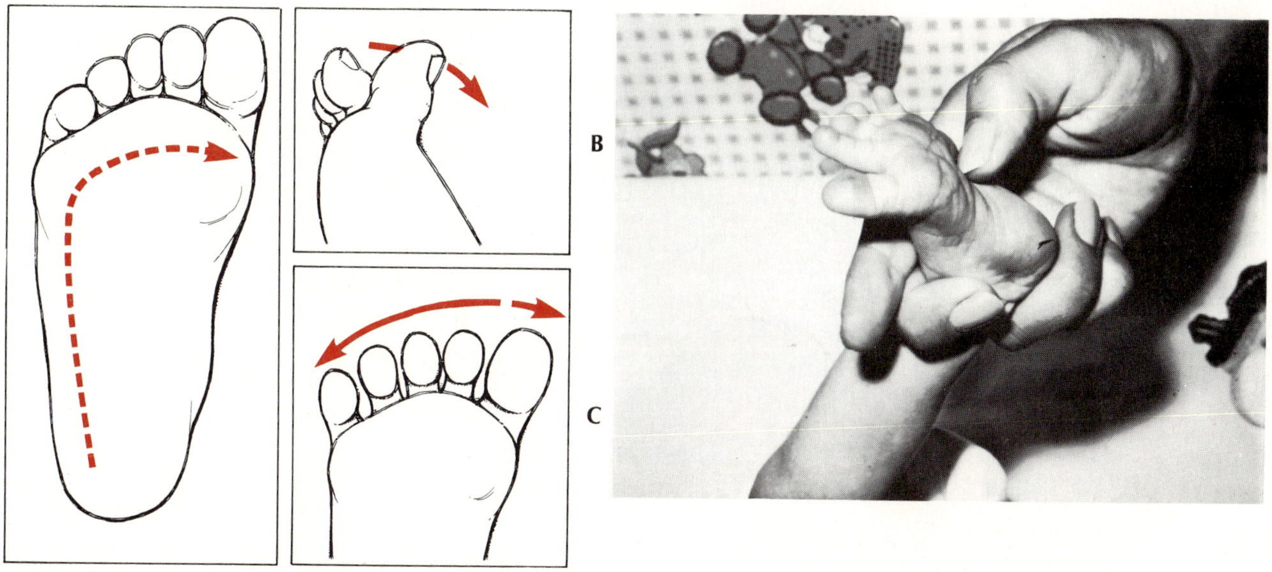

B

C

D

Fig. 28.30
A, Standing. **B,** Placing. **C,** Automatic walking reflex is phase of neuromuscular maturity from which infant normally graduates after 3 to 5 weeks. If infant is held so that sole of his foot touches table, reciprocal flexion and extension of leg occur, simulating walking. (Courtesy Joan Edelstein.)

A

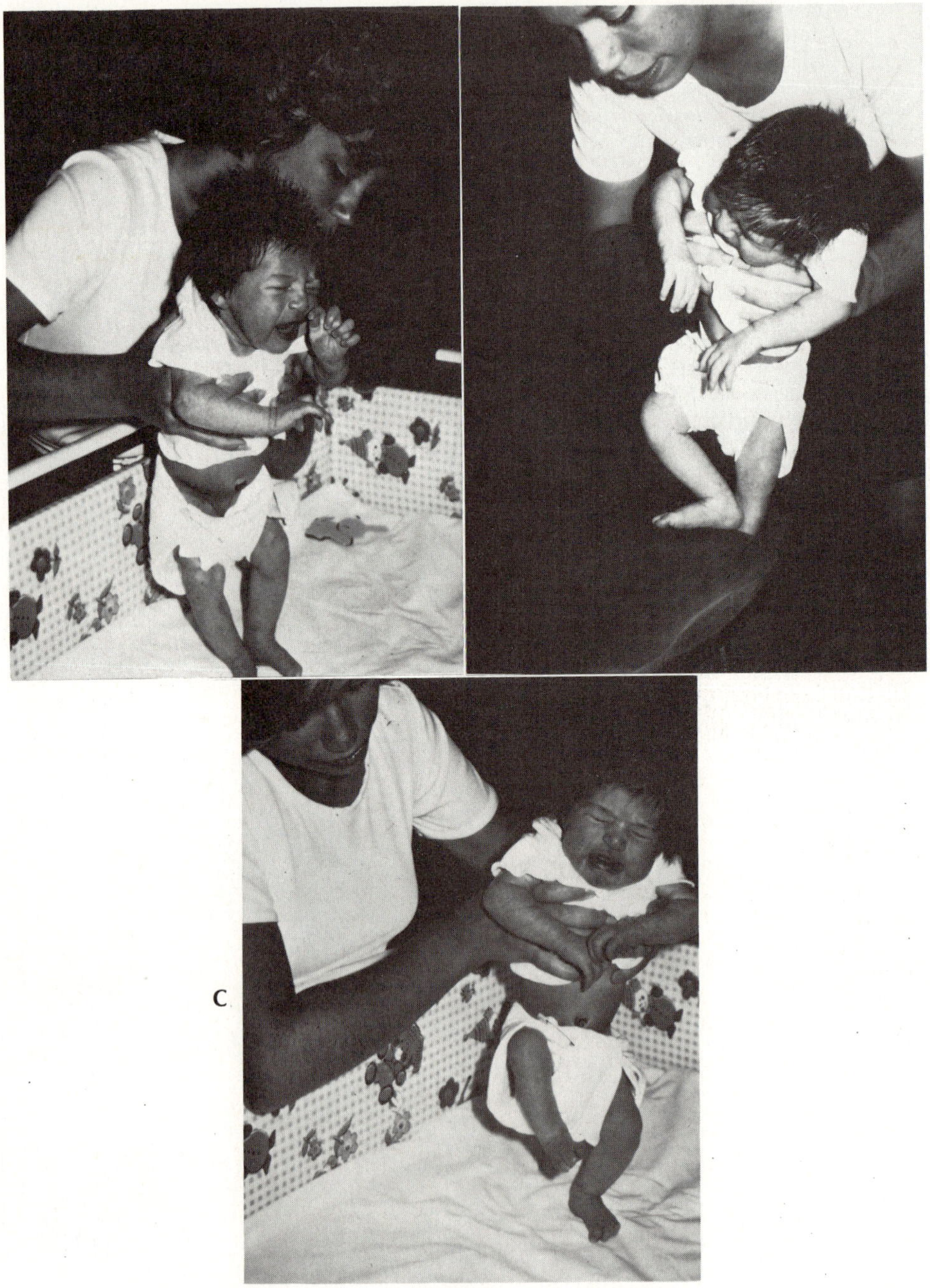

B

C

Table 28.2—cont'd
Assessment of Newborn's Reflexes

Reflex	Eliciting the Reflex	Characteristic Response	Comments
Otolith righting	Hold neonate erect and tilt body	Head returns to erect, upright position	Absence: implications same as for absent tonic neck reflex
Crawling (Fig. 28.31)	Place neonate on abdomen	Neonate makes crawling movements with arms and legs	Should disappear about 6 wk of age
Deep tendon	Use finger instead of percussion hammer to elicit patellar, or knee jerk, reflex; neonate must be relaxed	Reflex jerk is present; even with neonate relaxed, nonselective overall reaction may occur	
Landau	Over a crib or a table, using two hands, suspend infant in prone position	Infant attempts to hold spine in horizontal plane	Absence suggests need for neurologic examination
Yawn, stretch, burp, hiccup, sneeze	Spontaneous behaviors	May be slightly depressed temporarily because of maternal analgesia or anesthesia, fetal hypoxia, or infection	Parental guidance Most of these behaviors are pleasurable to parents Parents need to be assured that behaviors are normal Sneeze is response to lint, etc., in nose and (usually) not an indicator of a cold
Sweat	Usually not present in term newborn	Sweat response usually not present in term infant; may be seen in infants with cardiac distress	Parental guidance Amount of clothing for infant: indoors, outside Room temperature
Shiver	Usually not present in term newborn	Shiver response usually not present in term infant; if seen, check infant for postmaturity	See above
Kernig's sign	Flex thigh on hip and extend leg at knee	Procedure should be accomplished easily and without inflicting pain	Pain and resistance to extension of knee suggest meningeal irritability
Brudzinski's sign	Place infant in supine position; flex neck and observe knees	Infant does not move legs when neck is flexed	Spontaneous flexion of knees suggest meningeal irritability
Paradoxic irritability	Ascertain that infant is not hungry; hold and cuddle infant	Infant usually responds by quieting down	Infant cries when touched and held; response suggests meningeal irritability

Fig. 28.31
Crawling. (Courtesy Joan Edelstein.)

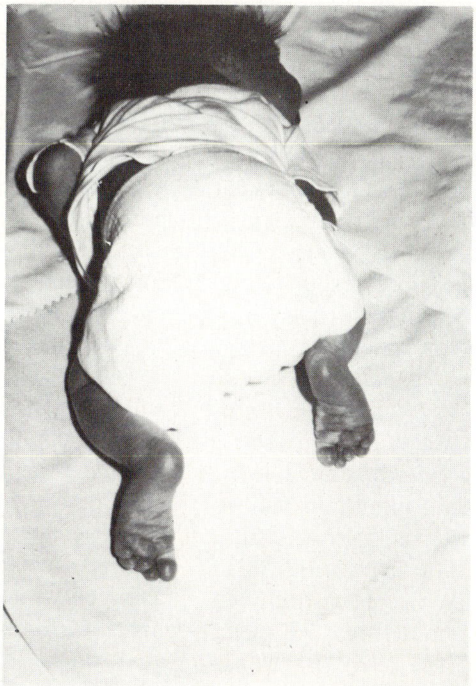

BEHAVIORAL ASSESSMENT

There are few tools to assess, with dependable accuracy, the neonate's capability, either physical or mental. Two tools are presented here: a neurologic assessment and reflex reactivity and the Brazelton Neonatal Behavioral Assessment Scale. The reflex reactivity tool (Table 28.2) is a limited indicator of the child's potential in either physical or mental capacity. The neonatal behavioral assessment scale developed by Brazelton provides a psychologic assessment of a neonate's capabilities that are relevant to later personality development. The most important element in the evaluation of the assessment is the infant's state of consciousness (Table 27.2). The assessment measures the ability of the infant to control his response as he moves from the sleep state to the waking state. Brazelton notes that the infant's use of a particular sleep or wake state to control or modify his reactions to external and internal stimuli reflects his potential for organization of his behavior. The scale also assesses the newborn's response to animate vs. inanimate stimulation.

The range of the infant's responses may impress the examiner with the newborn's formidable neurologic capacity, because the newborn's innate ability is truly amazing.

Brazelton Neonatal Behavioral Assessment Scale. Brazelton (1973) devised the Brazelton Neonatal Behavioral Assessment Scale (BNBAS) to determine individual characteristics of each infant. The scale assesses the infant's state of consciousness and ability to calm himself when upset (e.g., bringing his hand to his mouth to comfort himself by sucking) and includes an examination of reflexes to assess the neurologic adequacy of the infant. Brazelton has suggested the use of this scale in clinical research to predict the interaction the infant may set up in his environment.

Although the main focus of the BNBAS is interactive behavior, it includes a neurologic assessment of 17 items. The reflex reactivity of the neonate provides useful information on the normal infant's nervous system and neurologic maturity. Some reflex behaviors are necessary for survival, such as sucking and rooting. Others, such as gagging, coughing, and sneezing, act as safety mechanisms. In addition, many reflexes are necessary predecessors of later activity, such as walking, crawling, and grasping. For many reflexes the persistence of the reflex, rather than its disappearance, is of concern. For example, a persistent tonic neck, or "fencing," reflex (arm and leg extend on the side toward which the head is turned and opposite arm and leg flex) will interfere with the infant's ability to feed himself because feeding becomes difficult when the head turns away as the arm flexes. Base-line data is provided by the neurologic assessment of the BNBAS, and useful information regarding the neurologic status of the infant may be elicited. See Table 28.2 for a complete assessment of the newborn reflexes, including those assessed in the BNBAS.

The BNBAS comprises 27 behavioral responses and 20 elicited responses. The 27 behavioral items are scored on a nine-point scale, most of which are set so that the midpoint on the scale is considered the norm. According to Brazelton (1973, p. 4):

> The mean is related to the expected behavior of an "average" 7+ pound, full term (40 weeks gestation), normal Caucasian infant whose mother has had not more than 100 mg of barbiturates and 50 mg of other sedative drugs prior to delivery, whose Apgar scores were no less than 7 at 1, 8 at 5, and 8 at 15 minutes after delivery, who needed no special care after delivery, and who had an apparently normal intrauterine experience (i.e., normal hydration, nutrition, color and physiological responses).

Since the infant has often not adequately adapted to the environment because of immaturity of the CNS, the BNBAS is usually administered on the third day of life. In the case of an infant whose mother has been medicated for pain during labor or immediately before delivery, one should take the effects of the medication on the infant into consideration since it may take up to 5 days for the infant to recover from those effects.

The infant's score on the BNBAS is based on his best response rather than his average performance. Therefore it is up to the examiner to provide the optimal stimulation in order to elicit the best possible response. The examiner must be particularly adept in assisting the infant into the alert state in order to complete the assessment. This includes use of comforting measures such as rocking, talking, cooing, and cuddling, all of which serve to enhance the infant's performance.

The assessment should take place midway between feedings with the infant asleep, dressed, and covered (Fig. 28.32). Continuous observation of the state of the infant throughout the 20- to 30-min examination period provides information about the pattern of this infant's sleeping and waking states and movement from one state to another. The predominant two or three states the infant is in during the examination are also noted.

Assessment begins with the infant's ability to shut down responses to aversive stimuli, such as light and noise, in a quiet state (Figs. 28.33 to 28.37). The infant's responses provide particularly helpful information to parents, as is demonstrated by the following comment of one parent observing the assessment: "After watching the shut-down response for eyes and ears I realized I could lead a more normal life at home—in terms of being able to make some noise and leave on lights, etc., without hurting or bothering him."

Table 28.3
Behavioral Evaluation

Item	Parameters of Normal	Deviation from Normal: Probable Conditions
Behavioral patterns	Cortical control and responsiveness	CNS disorders
Feeding	Variations in interest, hunger; usually feeds well within 24 hr of birth	Lethargic, tires easily or may perspire while attempting to feed; poor suck, poor coordination with swallow, cyanosis, choking
Social	Cry is lusty, strong; soon indicative of hunger, pain, attention seeking	Weak or absent; high pitched
	Smiling, focusing evident within first week	Absence; no focusing on person holding him; unconsolable
	Responds by quietness and increased alertness to cuddling, voice	
Sleep-wakefulness	Transitional period with 2 periods of reactivity: at birth and 6-8 hr later	Lethargy; drowsiness
	Stabilization with wakeful periods about every 3-4 hr	Disorganized pattern
Elimination	Develops own pattern within first 2 wk:	See "Elimination behaviors"
	Stooling: see "Elimination behaviors"	
	Urination:	Diminished number: dehydration
	First few days: 3-4 times daily	
	End of first week: 5-6 times daily	
	Later: 6-10 times daily with adequate hydration	
Reflex response	Brain stem development and musculoskeletal intactness	Present in anencephalic neonates also
	See "Reflexes"	Absence; hyperreactive; incomplete; asynchronous
Sensory capabilities		
Vision	Limited accommodation with clearest vision within 18-20 cm (7-8 in)	Absence of these responses may be caused by absence of or diminished acuity or by sensory deprivation
	Detects color by 2 mo but attracted by black-white pattern at 5 days or less	
	Focuses and follows by 15 min of age	
	Prefers patterns to plain surfaces	
	Prefers changes in patterns by 2 mo	
	At birth, can gaze intently	
Hearing	By 2 min of age, moves eyes in direction of sound	Absence of response: deafness
	Responds to high pitch by "freezing," followed by agitation; to low pitch (crooning) by relaxation	
	Can hear beginning in last trimester of fetal life	
Touch	Sensitivity to pain may be diminished (because of beta-endorphins present prenatally)	
	Soothed by massaging, warmth, weightlessness (as in warm water bath)	Unable to be comforted; possible drug dependence
Smell	By fifth day can distinguish between own mother's breasts and those of another	
Taste	By 3 days of age, can distinguish between sucrose and glucose and grimaces in response to drop of lemon juice on tongue	
Motor	Coordinates body movement to parent's voice and body movement; imitates parent's actions by 2 wk of age	Absence

Fig. 28.32
Assessment begins with infant asleep, dressed, and covered. (Courtesy Joan Edelstein.)

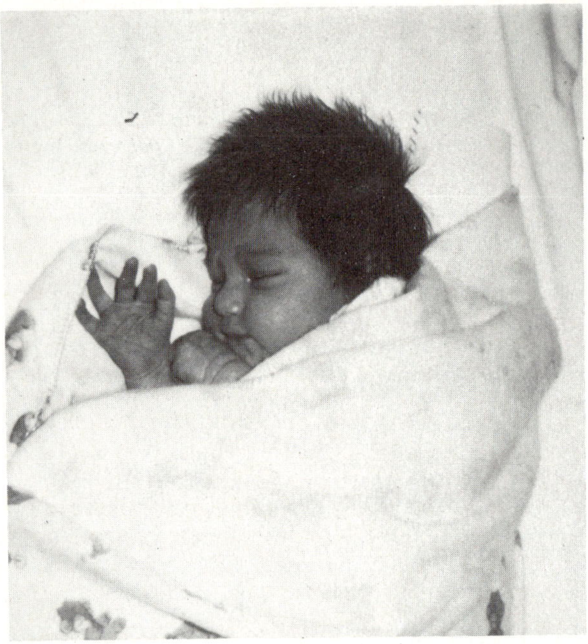

Fig. 28.33
Response decrement to light (states 1, 2, and 3). (Courtesy Joan Edelstein).

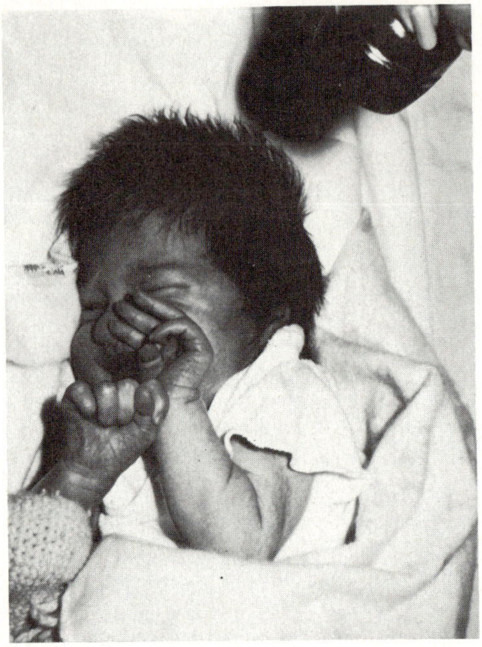

Fig. 28.34
Response decrement to rattle (states 1, 2, and 3). (Courtesy Joan Edelstein).

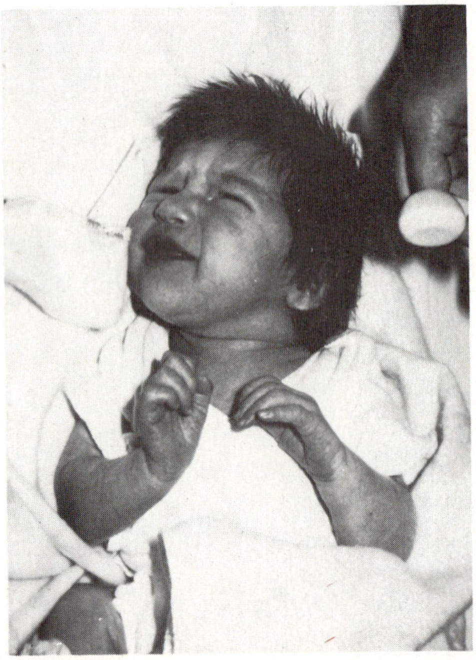

Fig. 28.35
Response decrement to bell (state 1, 2, and 3). (Courtesy Joan Edelstein.)

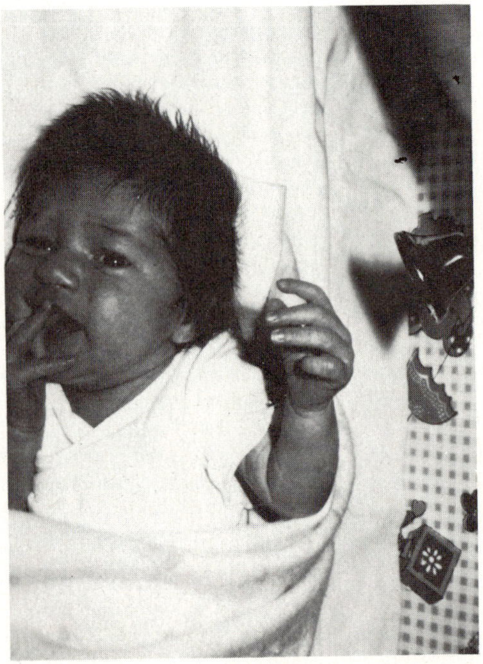

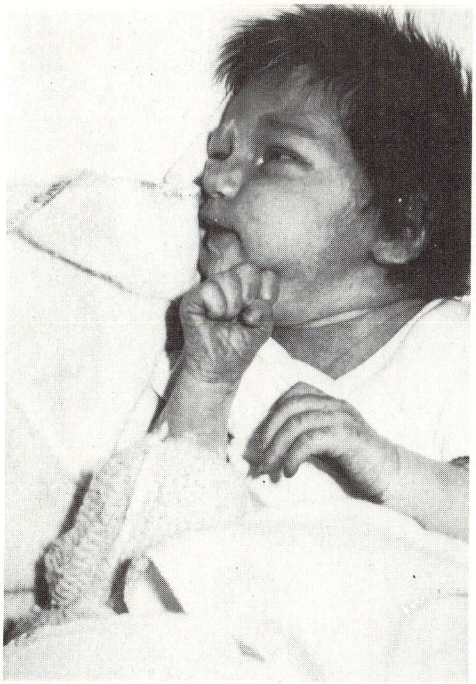

Fig. 28.36
State 3 (drowsy). Note position of booties—this infant had a cesarean birth because of frank breech position. At 10 days of age the position persists. (Courtesy Joan Edelstein.)

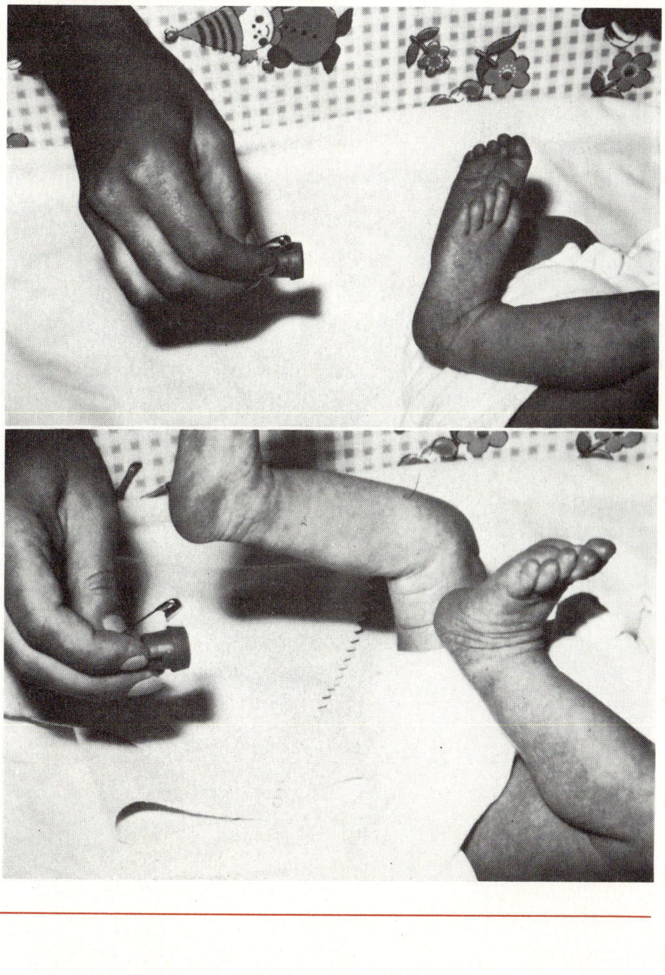

A

B

Fig. 28.37
A, Response decrement to pinprick (states 1, 2, and 3). Note that both feet are withdrawing together.
B, Response decrement to pinprick (states 1, 2, and 3). Note that response is localized to stimulated leg. (Courtesy Joan Edelstein.)

Fig. 28.38
Orientation—inanimate visual (state 4 only). Note brightening response—widened eyes and change in facial expression. (Courtesy Joan Edelstein.)

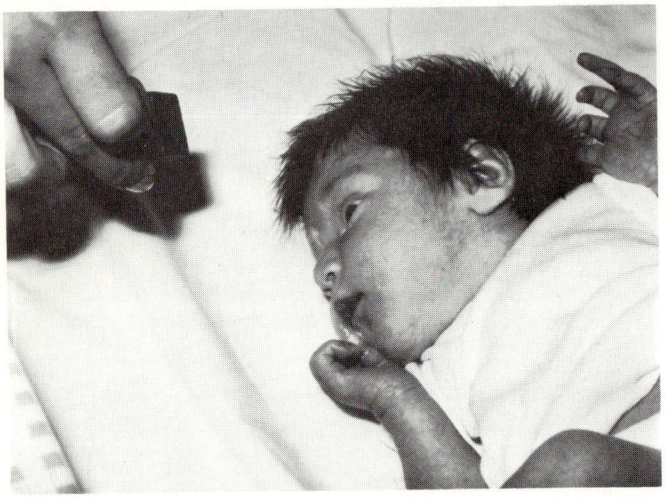

The auditory and visual responses to inanimate objects determine the infant's response to a nonsocial stimulus (Figs. 28.38 and 28.39) while in an alert state, and the three items following assess the response to the examiner's social cues (Fig. 28.40). Periods of alertness, or brightening and widening of the eyes, are assessed in state 4 only to determine the infant's capacity for responsiveness. The frequency of the best periods of alertness are scored over the entire examination period.

Muscle tone and motor maturity (Fig. 28.41) are determined followed by the infant's cuddliness, or response to being held (Fig. 28.42). This is a particularly important area of assessment, especially in working with parents. It is not unusual to find that infants respond differently to being held at various times. While it may be delightful for a parent to experience the feeling of an infant nestling and cuddling, it may be distressing to feel the infant push away. The nurse may assist parents at such times by identifying any stimulus (problem) in the environment (e.g., wet diaper, loud noises, neonate's excessive fatigue or hunger) that may

Fig. 28.39
Orientation response—inanimate auditory (states 4 and 5). This infant turned her head to stimulus. Persistence in position caused by frank breech presentation. (Courtesy Joan Edelstein.)

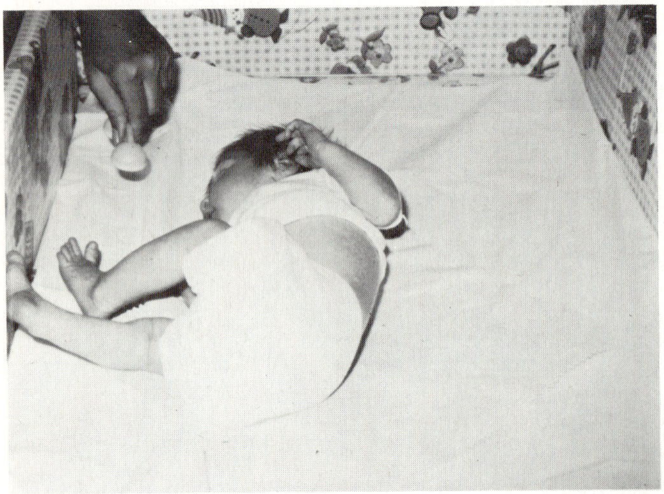

Fig. 28.40
Animated orientation—visual and auditory (state 4 only). Note change in facial expression and intense attention to examiner's face. (Courtesy Joan Edelstein.)

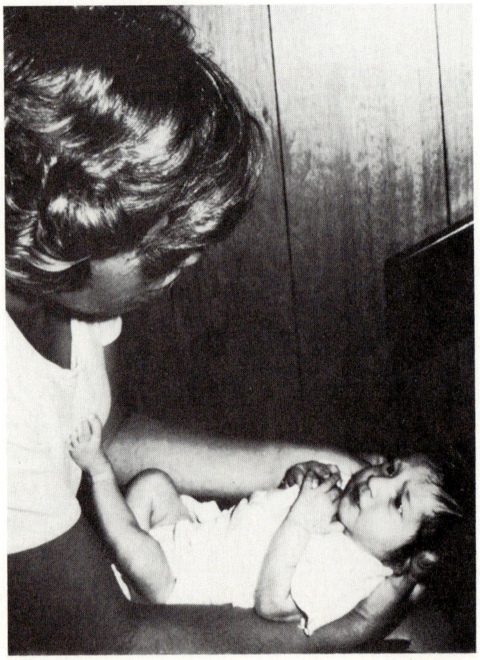

be contributing to an infant's lack of response to being held. Identification of the problem and of ways for dealing with it helps to relieve the parent's anxiety at this time, prevents feelings of rejection, anger, and resentment toward the infant and promotes parental sensitivity and understanding of neonatal behavior.

The infant's response to an aversive stimulus partially occluding the nose is assessed (Fig. 28.43), and the effect on the infant is assessed. Other items assessed during the examination are done on a continuous basis, including the infant's attempt to console himself when upset, the amount of consoling needed by the examiner to quiet the infant (Fig. 28.44), overall motor and crying activity (peak of excitement), the kind of stimuli that makes the infant cry, the amount of activity, tremulousness, and startle during the examination, and whether such activity is spontaneous or in response to stimuli. Changes in skin color (Fig. 28.45), changes in state, number of smiles, and ability to bring the hand to the mouth are also assessed.

Results of the examination may be used as part of the parent-teaching program. Examples of comments of parents involved in such teaching about their infants include the following (Edelstein, 1975):

> After the examination I seemed to notice the various things that were pointed out. Also, I myself tested the baby once we

Fig. 28.41

Pull-to-sit. **A,** States 3, 4, and 5. **B,** Infant attempts to right head. **C,** Infant unable to maintain head up. (Courtesy Joan Edelstein.)

A

B

C

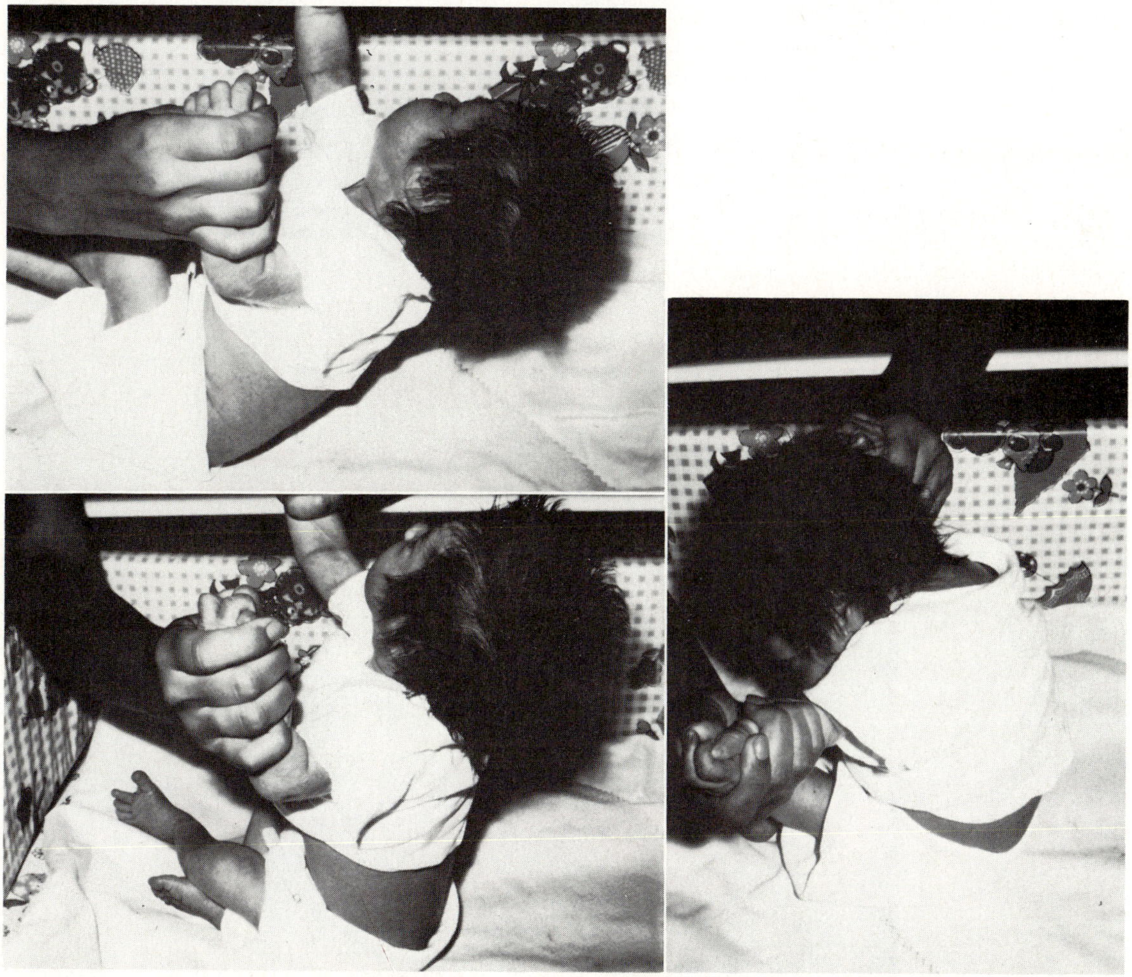

Fig. 28.42

A, Cuddliness (states 4 and 5) up on shoulder. **B,** Cuddliness. Infant has nestled head in crook of neck of examiner. (Courtesy Joan Edelstein.)

A 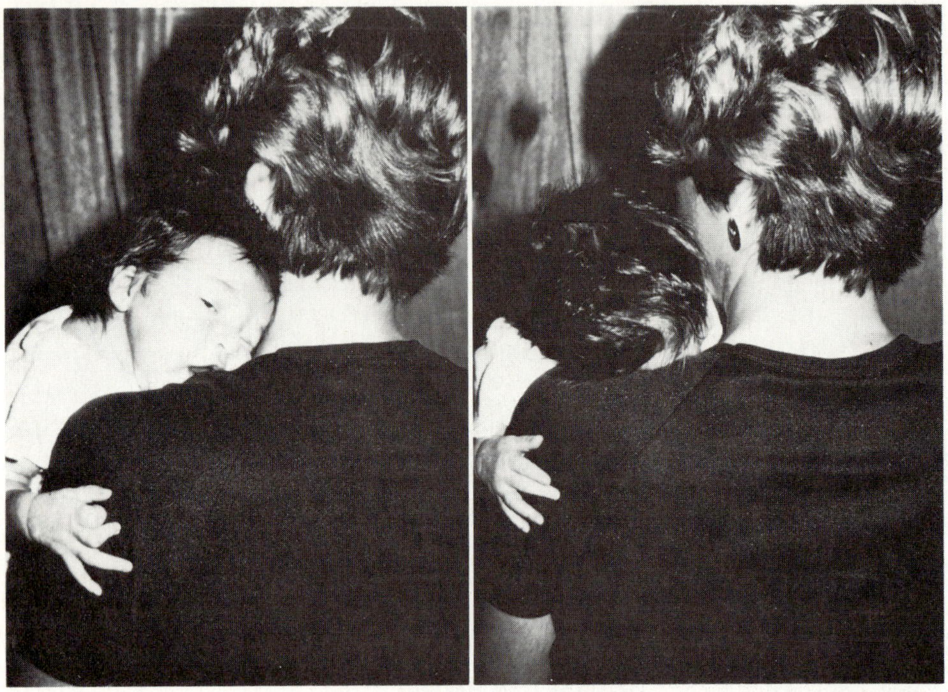 B

Fig. 28.43

Defensive movements (states 3 and 5). Note directed swipes at cloth. (Courtesy Joan Edelstein.)

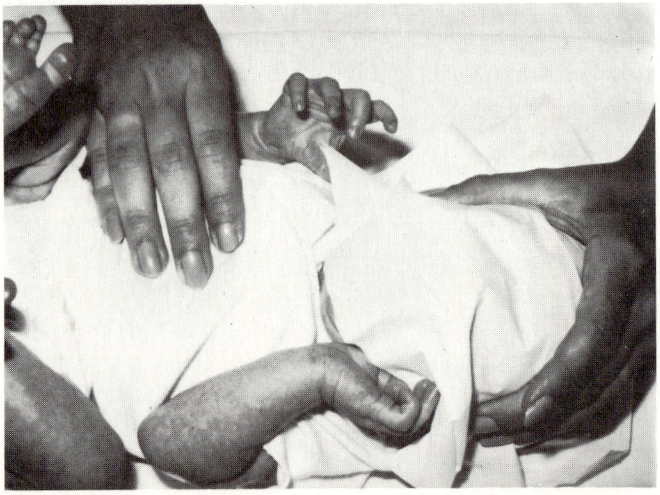

Fig. 28.44

A, Consolability with intervention (states 6 to 5, 4, 3, 2): examiner's face and voice. Note hand-to-mouth effort in attempt to quiet self. **B,** Consolability: hand on belly. **C,** Consolability: holding, rocking, and talking. (Courtesy Joan Edelstein.)

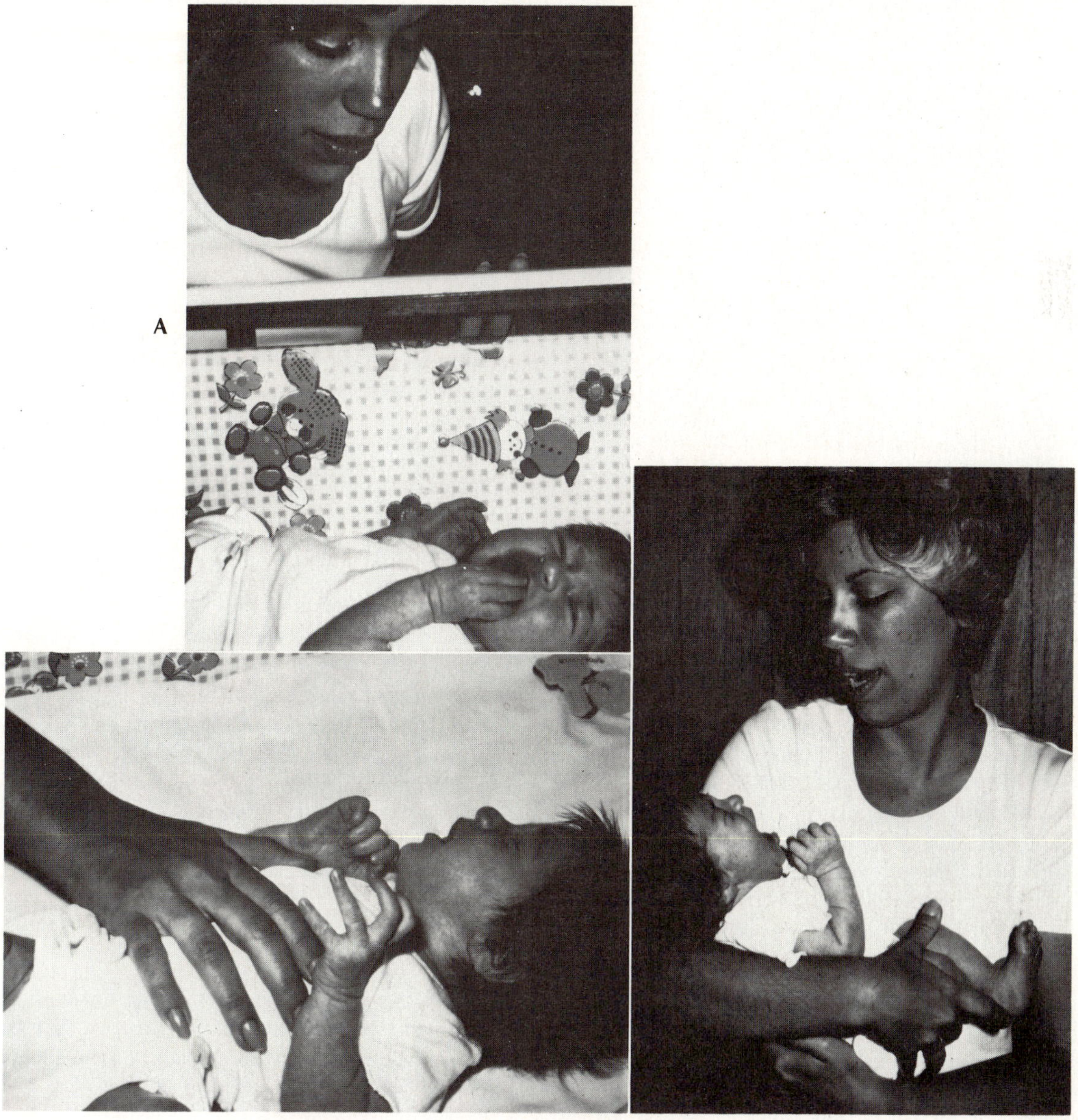
A B C

Fig. 28.45
Lability of skin color after undressing. Note mottling. (Courtesy Joan Edelstein.)

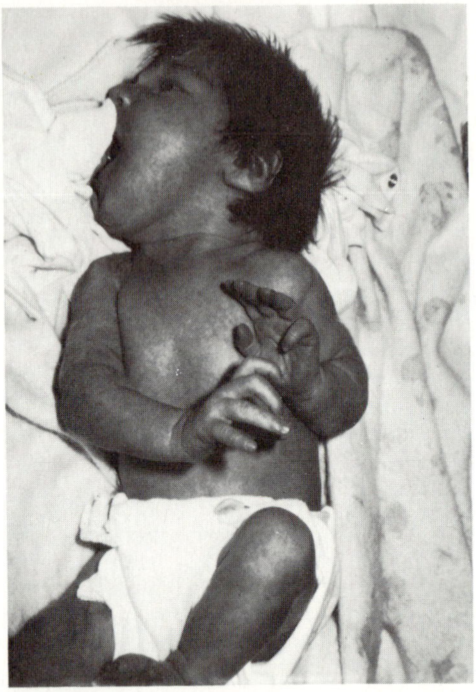

were home. Through the testing I realize more so now that the baby is quite aware of what goes on around him, and since, I've noticed I talk to the baby more now.

It helped me feel confident that she was a normal, healthy baby and that her reflexes and responses were good.

The test examination in the hospital made me more aware of various responses to expect from my baby. It also made me more aware of just how much more an infant can do than I had ever known before.

I was reassured that my baby was normal and healthy. Also, it was fascinating to discover all the things he was already aware of. I learned more about him (and babies in general) from participating in the test.

Factors influencing behavior of the newborn. Gestational age of the infant will affect observed behavior. Level of CNS maturity will be reflected in the behavioral assessment. An infant with an immature CNS will tend to have an entire body response to a pinprick of the foot. CNS immaturity will also be reflected in reflex development and sleep-wake cycles.

Time. Length of time to recuperate from labor and delivery will affect the behavior of the infant as he attempts to become internally organized. Time since the last feeding and time of day may influence the infant's responses.

Stimuli. Environmental events and stimuli will affect the behavioral responses of infants. Nurses in intensive care nurseries often observe infants' responses to loud noises, bright lights, monitor alarms, and tension in the unit. It has been well documented that infants are affected by nonverbal behavior in the environment. Infants of mothers who are tense have more muscle activity and their heart rates change parallel to their mothers during feeding.

Medication. For infants of mothers who were medicated for pain during labor or close to delivery, the effects of the medication seem to be strongest on the first day with recovery noted by the fifth day. Nonetheless, infants of mothers who were given medications may continue to demonstrate poor state organization beyond the fifth day (Murray et al., 1981). Other prenatal variables have been considered as well. A correlation has been found between maternal blood pressure at delivery and level of infant irritability as measured by the BNBAS.

Culture. One of the most interesting findings has been the differences in infant behavior on the BNBAS across cultures. Freedman and Freedman (1969) found that Chinese-American infants had more self-quieting activities, fewer state changes, and more rapid responses to consoling activities than white infants. The Zinacanteco Indians in southern Mexico demonstrated greater motor maturity and increased ability to maintain quiet alert states for longer times than U.S. infants (Brazelton et al., 1969).

Coll and co-workers (1981) determined that Puerto Rican infants had lower scores on habituation and higher scores on both orientation and maintaining organization than black and white infants.

Interestingly, studies done on infants delivered by the Leboyer method have not revealed any differences in behavior from those infants delivered by conventional methods (Nelson et al., 1980; Saisal et al., 1981).

ASSESSMENT STRATEGIES AND TOOLS FOR NORMAL NEWBORN: FIRST DAY (2 TO 24 HOURS)

Knowledge of characteristics of the newborn serves as the theory base for the nursing process. Assessment strategies and tools provide guidelines for methods and timing of assessments.

Respirations

1. Check and record infant's respiratory effort every 15 minutes for 4 hours, then every hour until breathing is stable.
   a. Count respirations by observing the chest wall. Note whether sternum retracts or nares flare on inspiration.

b. Note whether infant is a normal nose breather (i.e., sleeps with mouth closed, does not have to interrupt feedings to breathe).
c. Note abnormal sounds (grunting or wheezing) during inspiration or expiration.
d. Note efficiency of gagging, sneezing, and swallowing reflexes related to maintaining clear airway.

2. Be alert for bouts of rapid and irregular respirations, gagging, and regurgitation of mucus and so on during "reactivity periods" following birth and again after 4 to 6 hours of life.
3. Assess infant's color. Color over head, trunk, and mucous membrane is indicative of adequate oxygenation. Feet and hands may remain slightly cyanotic for 48 hours, especially when they are cold.

Temperature

1. Timing. Take and record infant's temperature on admission to unit and then every hour until it is stabilized. After that, take infant's temperature every 4 hours for remainder of first 24 hours by one of the following methods:
   a. Rectal temperature (usually once, to establish patency of anus)*
   b. Axillary temperature
   c. Skin temperature by sensor probe
2. Techniques for assessing body temperature. Before using a clinical thermometer, check it for intactness, and then shake the mercury down. For rectal temperatures, lubricate the tip well, immobilize the neonate (Fig. 28.12), insert it *gently (never force it),* and hold it in place for 5 minutes. For axillary temperatures, hold thermometer firmly in axilla (Fig. 28.11) for 5 minutes. When taking axillary temperatures, it is good technique to place the thermometer in the infant's axilla, wrap the infant snugly, and prop on his side for the 5 minutes; never leave an infant alone with a rectal thermometer in place, however. The technique for taking and maintaining the infant's temperature using a sensor probe is discussed under Procedures, p. 630.

Cardiovascular system. Check infant's heart rate every 4 hours. Note its regularity and presence of any heart murmurs. The apical beat is assessed for a full minute to determine rate and rhythm. The sounds should be clearly audible, 120 to 160 beats/min, and once the transition period is over, the sounds should be regular in rhythm. Functional murmurs are common for the first 48 hours after birth.

Integumentary system. Assessment of the integumentary system involves observation and palpation of the skin.

Color of skin. Development of *hyperbilirubinemia* (jaundice) before 24 hours of age may indicate a blood dyscrasia (e.g., Rh or ABO incompatibility) and requires immediate medical investigation (see Chapter 40). Jaundice may be expected to occur between 24 and 48 hours after birth as a consequence of the normal physiologic breakdown of fetal red blood cells (RBCs) and relative immaturity of the liver in clearing that bilirubin. Rarely does the circulating bilirubin derived from this source reach levels that result in brain damage (kernicterus, see p. 959).

Neonates who have received an extra infusion of blood from the placenta or who have an inadequate fluid intake may be particularly susceptible to hyperbilirubinemia. The neonate can get up to 100 ml of extra blood if the physician "milks" the umbilical cord toward the baby or holds the baby below the level of the placenta before the cord is clamped. Early feeding is relatively new; it was customary to give neonates nothing by mouth (NPO) for 24 hours after birth. This delay led to inadequate fluid intake and delayed bowel activity (bilirubin is also excreted along with stool); both of these sequelae led to an increase in neonatal bilirubin levels.

Cyanosis of the hands and feet (acrocyanosis, or "mitten and bootie" cyanosis) is not pathologic and is replaced by normal skin coloring by days 7 to 10. Circumoral pallor and cyanosis may be noticeable during crying or feeding. Report this finding to the physician. It may indicate cardiopulmonary problems, generalized infection, or hypoglycemia. If the infant appears pale or ruddy (plethoric), this should be reported to the physician also. *Paleness* may be due to anemia; *plethora* or ruddiness is a markedly red color that may be caused by an excess number of red blood cells (polycythemia).

Evidence of adequate hydration. Dehydration in the neonate is best assessed by *weight loss.* Lack of skin turgor is rare in the presence of dehydration and can be expected only when dehydration is extremely severe. The same can be said about depression of the fontanels and softness of the eyeball. These are clinical signs of extreme dehydration in older infants; they are not reliable indicators of dehydration in the neonate.

Evidence of increased intracranial pressure. Bulging of the fontanels when the infant is at rest may indicate increased intracranial pressure. Increased intracranial pressure also causes separation of the sutures: mastoid, sphenoid, and coronal especially (Fig. 20.2). Bulging

*Rectal temperature taking is discouraged in the neonatal period. It irritates rectal mucosa and exposes the neonate to tissue trauma; it stimulates a bowel movement; it can mislead the nurse regarding the neonate's progress (even if the infant is exposed to cold stress, a normal core temperature may exist for a while).

of the fontanels occurs normally when the infant cries or strains at stool because intracranial pressure is increased at these times.

Bruises or other evidence of trauma. A bruise on the cheek can result from forceps pressure. Note whether forceps were applied during delivery. Two small puncture wounds on the scalp may be from the electrode attached to the scalp for fetal monitoring during labor, or they may indicate the site where a specimen of blood was taken from the scalp. NOTE: In the nurses' notes, the cuts are listed as "two puncture wounds."

Bruises of the scalp and *petechiae* on the face are sometimes found on infants who have sustained great and prolonged pressure during passage through the birth canal or when the umbilical cord has been tightly wound around the neck before birth. Petechiae on the trunk and lower extremities are abnormal and must be reported immediately.

Bruising and swelling of the genitalia and buttocks are common findings in those infants born in breech presentation. They may be expected to subside by the end of the first week of life.

Rashes. A rash over the genitalia and buttocks may appear by the second day of life. Meconium is not irritating to the skin, but the transitional and later stools of bottle-fed infants are irritating. Although urine is sterile, urine of all infants is irritating. Cleansing with water is indicated with each diaper change. Diaper rash can vary from mild to severe. The mild form resembles chafing, with reddened, nonraised areas; exposure to air and frequent changing of diapers usually will clear the condition. A more severe type, called *ammoniacal diaper rash,* is characterized by bright red papules (well-defined, solid, elevated lesions of the skin, up to 5 mm in diameter) that erupt and continue to form craterlike ulcers. For treatment, see Chapter 29.

Mouth. The inside of the mouth can be inspected when the infant is crying. If white, curdy deposits are noted, give the infant some water to drink and see whether the white plaques are washed away. If they do not, do not attempt to remove them; notify the physician because the infant may have developed thrush (candidiasis or moniliasis) (see Chapter 36). Sucking calluses (milk blisters) may eventually form on the lips (not during the nursery period). These are not injurious and need no treatment. Note the shape of the infant's mouth when crying. If it is relaxed on one side, it may indicate facial paralysis and should be reported to the physician. The infant's tongue appears large in comparison with his mouth. Its growth is forward from the base, the frenulum. Tongue-tie (the inability to lift the tip of the tongue because of a too short frenulum) is a rare condition.

Cord and circumcised penis. Assessment of both the cord and the circumcised penis is the same.

1. Check every 30 minutes for 4 hours for excessive bleeding.
2. Check healing process. By 24 hours, cord appears dry (becomes black and stiff, like a twig), with no bleeding or signs of inflammation (odor, discharge, reddened skin at base), and clamp or cord tie may be removed. Incised area of penis should appear clean, with no odor or discharge.

Defecation

1. Note evidence of meconium passage (yellow-stained vernix, meconium-stained amniotic fluid, or passage of meconium at birth) before infant's admission to nursery.
2. Record passage of meconium; may be anticipated by 4 to 6 hours or at beginning of waking periods and after feedings. Eating stimulates movement of the bowel, a response known as the gastrocolic reflex. Patency of lower (but not of upper) gastrointestinal tract can be assumed if the infant passes meconium.
3. If there is a delay in passage of meconium (24 hours or more), check for patency of the anus, abdominal distention, and bowel sounds; assess amount of fluid intake; and notify physician of findings. About 6% of healthy infants do not defecate for 48 hours.

Urination

1. Note evidence of voiding before infant's admission to the nursery; that is, ask delivery room nurse if the infant voided at birth or if nurse changed a wet diaper.
2. Record voiding when noted. Some infants void as part of the delivery process; most void by 12 hours; about 8% may not void for 2 to 3 days, depending on amount of fluid in bladder at birth and fluid intake after birth.
3. After 24 hours, if infant has not voided, check bladder for distention and note whether infant is restless or appears in pain as pressure is applied to the bladder; assess fluid intake; and notify physician of findings. Physician may aspirate bladder to ascertain if urine is present. Position infant as for circumcision. Suprapubic area is exposed and cleansed. Physician will require sterile gloves, syringe (30 ml), and long needle.
4. Note presence of urates, which appear as rustish (copper dust) staining on diaper; these dissolve and disappear when diaper is placed in water and are not significant. Note also presence of blood, which does not disappear when diaper is soaked in water. Blood may result from pseudomenstruation in females, bleeding after circumcision, or too forceful retraction of foreskin in males. If blood on diaper is not from these sources, report this to the physician immediately.

Physical assessment

1. The physician or nurse-practitioner performs an assessment before 2 hours after birth for gestational age determination and another (complete) assessment before the twenty-fourth hour of life.
2. Nursery personnel do assessments during caretaking activities.
3. In the assessment for growth the infant is weighed daily while in the hospital, and the results are recorded. A total weight loss of more than 10% in the first 3 or 4 days indicates the need for clinical reappraisal. The head and chest circumference and body length are measured at birth and again in the 4-wk follow-up visit; these measurements are compared with established norms.

Neurologic assessment. The neurologic assessment of the normal newborn is discussed earlier in this chapter.

Behavioral assessment. The behavioral assessment of the normal newborn is discussed earlier in this chapter.

Newborn nutrition. For a discussion of newborn nutrition, see Chapter 30.

Parenthood. For a discussion of parenthood, see Chapter 32.

SUMMARY OF ASSESSMENT STRATEGIES AND TOOLS FOR NORMAL NEWBORN: DAYS 2 TO 14

1. While the infant is in the hospital, assess respirations and apical heart rate and rhythm and record every 8 hours.
2. While infant is in the hospital, take and record the temperature every 8 hours. Temperature is not a reliable indicator of infection in the neonate; infant may be septic and show a reduced temperature. If infection is suspected, check other signs and symptoms (e.g., poor feeding, poor muscle tone).
3. Perform tests on blood obtained by heel stick (for heel-stick procedure, see p. 637) for the following disorders*:
   a. Phenylketonuria (PKU) test 48 hours after ingestion of protein—milk or breast milk
   b. Galactosemia
   c. Hypothyroidism
4. If hyperbilirubinemia is suspected, alert the physician to order laboratory tests for bilirubin levels.
5. While infant is in hospital, note and record changes in stool color and consistency and in pattern the infant established (e.g., four times every day, every 2 days) for defecation.
6. While infant is in hospital, note and record color and concentration of urine and number of voidings.
7. Note changes in skin (color and rashes).
8. Note healing of circumcised penis and cord. When cord drops off (usually several days after discharge from the hospital), small beads of blood may appear for 1 or 2 days when infant cries or strains at stool. Navel may be protuberant.
9. Weigh daily while infant is in hospital; weigh at end of the second week.
10. Perform hearing tests before discharge.
    a. Note infant's failure to stir or be aroused by noises when asleep, startle to loud noises, or become quiet when spoken to. These indications of lack of response may indicate a sensorineural loss.
    b. Note infant's failure to respond to soft sounds (but has a good response to loud sounds) because these behaviors may indicate a conductive loss.

SUMMARY OF ASSESSMENT STRATEGIES AND TOOLS FOR NORMAL NEWBORN: DAYS 15 TO 28 (FIRST WELL-BABY VISIT)

1. Weigh infant.
2. Measure infant's height and head circumference.
3. Assess all body systems, using the techniques of inspection, palpation, auscultation, and percussion.
4. Assess infant's motor development: neurologic status (reflexes and behavior), including hearing and sight (the infant follows a moving object, raises his head, and looks about the room); and nutritional status.
5. Laboratory tests (hemoglobin or hematocrit, urinalysis, intradermal tuberculin test) are usually left until the infant is 10 to 12 months of age.
6. Assess general condition of infant (he is alert; skin is soft and clear; there are no rashes or evidence of trauma).
7. Assess parents' relationship with child and their knowledge of normal growth and development and symptoms of disease.

*These tests are mandated by the state of California. If on religious or moral grounds the parent objects to the tests, the tests will not be done. The parent will be asked to sign a statement relieving the hospital and physicians of liability for damages resulting from lack of early detection and treatment for these disorders. Even if the parent refuses the tests while the infant is in the hospital, the parents can request them from the physician or community health nurse at a later date. However, serious damage can occur within the first few weeks of life in an affected infant.

Nursing Diagnoses

Nursing diagnoses lend direction to types of nursing actions needed to implement a plan of care. Before establishing nursing diagnoses, the nurse analyzes the significance of findings collected during assessment:

1. The mother's prenatal record
2. The record of events during the mother's labor, during the neonate's birth, and during the neonate's first hours and days of life

Analysis of findings results in the identification of nursing diagnoses. The following are lists of possible nursing diagnoses. These lists are not exhaustive.

Possible nursing diagnoses *for the neonate* are as follows:

1. Ineffective breathing pattern because of obstructed airway
2. Alterations in comfort because of pain of circumcision
3. Impaired gas exchange because of hypothermia (cold stress)

Possible nursing diagnoses *for the parent or parents* are as follows:

1. Potential alterations in parenting because of parental lack of understanding of their neonate's muscle tone and motor maturity
2. Potential alteration in parenting because of parental lack of understanding of factors influencing neonatal behavior
3. Potential disturbance in self-concept in the parent because of lack of understanding of the characteristics of the neonate

Planning

Planning for nursing actions that assist in meeting goals for care is essential if goals are to be met. Planning is essential for the implementation of the following:

1. Continuous, comprehensive assessment of the neonate and the parent-child relationship
2. Coordination of the efforts of the health care team
3. Rapid identification of and intervention in medical-surgical conditions of the newborn
4. Support of the family's efforts to learn about and develop a relationship with the neonate
5. Formulation of nursing diagnoses individualized to specific neonates and their families

• • •

The implementation and evaluation of the nursing care of the neonate are presented in Chapter 29.

References and Readings

Albright, G.: Neurobehavioral assessment—a prospective, J. Cal. Perinat. Assoc. **1**(1):60, 1981.

Anderson, C.J.: Enhancing reciprocity between mother and neonate, Nurs. Res. **30**(2):89, 1981.

Brazelton, T.: Neonatal behavioral assessment scale, Philadelphia, 1973, J.B. Lippincott Co.

Chinn, P.L., and Leitch, C.: Child health maintenance: a guide to clinical assessment, St. Louis, 1979, The C.V. Mosby Co.

Coll, C.G., Spekoski, C., & Lester, B.M.: Cultural and biomedical correlates of neonatal behavior, Dev. Psychobiol. **14**(2):147, 1981.

Crockenberg, S.B.: Infant irritability, mother responsiveness and social support influences on the security of infant-mother attachment, Child Dev. **52**(3):857, 1981.

Edelstein, J.: The effect of nursing intervention with the Brazelton Neonatal Behavioral Assessment Scale on postpartum adjustment and maternal perception of the infant, unpublished masters thesis, 1975.

Eoff, M., et al.: Temperature measurements in infants, Nurs. Res. **23:**457, 1974.

Eoff, M., and Joyce, B.: Temperature measurements in children, Am. J. Nurs. **81**(5):1010, 1981.

Freedman, D.: Ethnic differences in babies, Hum. Nature, p. 4, Jan. 1979.

Freedman, D.G., and Freedman, N.: Behavioral differences between Chinese-American and European-American newborns, Nature **224:**1227, 1969.

Leijon, I., and Finnstrom, O.: Studies on the Brazelton neonatal behavioral assessment scale, Neuropediatrics **12**(3):242, 1981.

Lowrey, G.: Growth and development of children, ed. 7, Chicago, 1978, Year Book Medical Publishers.

Murray, A.D., et al.: Effects of epidural anesthesia on newborns and their mothers, Child Dev. **52**(1):71, 1981.

Nelson, N.M., et al.: A randomized clinical trial of the Leboyer approach to childbirth, N. Engl. J. Med. **302**(12):655, 1980.

Reid, T.: Newborn cyanosis, Am. J. Nurs. **82**(8):1230, 1982.

Rosner, B.S., & Doherty, N.E.: The response of neonates to intrauterine sounds, Dev. Med. Child Neurol. **21**(6):723, 1979.

Saco-Pollitt, C.: Birth in the Peruvian Andes: physical and behavioral consequences in the neonate, Child Dev. **52**(3):839, 1981.

Saisal, S., et al.: A comparison of infants delivered by the Leboyer and conventional methods, Am. J. Obstet. Gynecol. **139**(6):715, 1981.

Schachter, J., et al.: Heart rate and blood pressure in black newborns and white newborns, Pediatrics **58:**283, 1976.

Simkin, P., et al.: "Physiologic" jaundice of the newborn, Birth Fam. J. **6**(1):23, 1979.

Slumek, M.: Screening infants for hearing loss, Nurs. Outlook **19:**115, 1971.

Whaley, L.F., and Wong, D.L.: Essentials of pediatric nursing, St. Louis, 1982, The C.V. Mosby Co.

Whaley, L.F., and Wong, D.L.: Nursing care of infants and children, ed. 2, St. Louis, 1983, The C.V. Mosby Co.

29

Planning, Implementing, and Evaluating Care of the Newborn

- Plan and Implementation
  - General care of the neonate
    - Maintenance of respirations and adequate oxygen supply
    - Maintenance of neonate's temperature
    - Positioning and holding the infant
    - Cleansing infant
    - Umbilical cord care
    - Diaper rash
    - Clothing the infant
    - Care of infant's linens
  - Circumcision
    - Historic perspective
    - Current views
    - Parental decision
    - The procedure
    - Care of the newly circumcised penis
    - Care of the uncircumcised penis
  - Anticipatory guidance of parents: before discharge from hospital
  - Anticipatory guidance of parents: at first well-baby visit
- Procedures
  - Monitoring and recording of infant responses
  - Heat support: controlling the environment
    - Overhead radiant heater
    - Servo-Control incubator
    - Warming the hypothermic infant
  - Suctioning the newborn
  - Upper airway aspiration: mouth and nose
  - Midairway (nasopharynx, oropharynx) and stomach aspiration
  - Mouth-to-mouth resuscitation
  - Cardiopulmonary resuscitation
  - Positioning the newborn
  - Oxygen therapy
    - Hypoxemia
    - Regulating oxygen dosage
    - Methods of oxygen administration
  - Heel stick
  - Intramuscular injection
  - Therapy for hyperbilirubinemia
    - Phototherapy
  - Restraining neonate
    - Mummy
    - Extremity restraints
    - Towel support
    - Restraint without appliance
  - Assisting with collection of blood specimen: venipuncture
  - Using urine specimen collectors
  - Birth certificate
- Evaluative Criteria for Nursing Actions
  - Normal newborn: first day of life
  - Days 2 to 14
  - Days 15 to 28

Goals assist the nurse in the development of a plan for nursing actions. The goals of care of the newborn relate to the neonate and to the care-taking person. While meeting the goals for care of the neonate, the nurse models the role of caretaker for the parent. To meet goals for the care-taking person, the nurse acts as teacher, counselor, and support person.

Goals for the baby are (1) physiologic homeostasis following transition to extrauterine life, (2) freedom from trauma such as injury and infection, and (3) initiation of the child-parent relationship.

Goals for the parents are (1) development of motherliness and fatherliness, (2) knowledge and skill in parent craft (i.e., child-care activities), (3) confidence, and (4) initiation of the parent-child relationship.

Growth and development of the neonate are rapid. Changes in the neonate are measured in minutes and hours since birth. The plan includes care of the neonate and anticipatory guidance for the parents that reflect this time frame. Parents need to know the child's behavioral characteristics and needs for today and tomorrow. Although the rate of growth continues to proceed rapidly, by the end of the neonatal period (28 days), it has slowed enough to talk about the child's appearance and needs in terms of weeks and months.

The focus of care changes between birth and 28 days. During the first 2 hours of life, the main focus is on the neonate's physiologic adaptation. At the end of the neonatal period, socialization with the baby assumes equal importance with the infant's physiologic needs.

The discussion of nursing actions for the baby and parents is divided into those actions implemented early in the neonatal period* (generally within a hospital setting) and those implemented at the end of the neonatal period (generally outside the hospital setting). General care of the neonate and parents is followed by detailed descriptions of procedures and techniques that the nurse or physician may be required to utilize. Evaluative criteria appear at the end of the chapter. The criteria can serve as a check list in the neonate's progress notes. The student can use the criteria for a quick review (or reference) of the neonate's changing characteristics and evolving needs.

Plan and Implementation

The nursing care of the neonate involves carrying out certain *child care activities* and *procedures*. The child care activities are performed by anyone who takes care of newborns, such as nurse or parent. One of the nurse's responsibilities is to help parents become skilled in these activities. Some of the procedures discussed are usually performed by a nurse or physician. In addition to developing skill in the procedures, the nurse is prepared to explain them to parents.

GENERAL CARE OF THE NEONATE

Included in the general care† of infants are activites related to assessing the infant's condition, maintenance of respirations and temperature, hygiene, clothing and holding the infant, and care of the circumcision, if one had been performed. Much of the mother's knowledge concerning this care will stem directly from previous experience with infants, folkways learned from her ethnic or social group, and teaching by professionals during parent-craft classes. For the new parent with little skill in child care, these activities may cause much anxiety. Support from the nursing staff in the mother's beginning efforts can be an important factor in her seeking and accepting help in the future.

Maintenance of respirations and adequate oxygen supply. The first consideration is maintaining an open airway (see p. 439). The infant may be turned to the side and supported in this position with a rolled blanket at the back to facilitate drainage (Fig. 29.1). If there is excessive mucus present, in addition to maintaining a side-lying position, elevate the foot of the crib and suction the oral pharynx with a catheter and DeLee mucus trap (see p. 633).*

All parents need instruction in the care of an infant having a gagging or choking episode. The neonate is turned onto his stomach (prone) with the head lowered to permit drainage of mucus or milk. A bulb syringe may be used to aspirate the mouth and nose. Once the episode is resolved, the infant needs cuddling and reassuring. Following a demonstration of working with a gagging or choking infant, the nurse supervises the mother and father in the technique. Learning to meet this emergency in the hospital increases parental self-confidence and self-esteem as well as prepares the parent for this activity at home.

Maintenance of neonate's temperature. The temperature may be taken either by axilla or rectum every hour until stabilized (Fig. 29.2). Initial temperatures as low as 36° C (96.8° F) are not uncommon. By the twelfth hour the temperature should stabilize at 36.5° C (97.6° F). The nurse may assist the neonate to stabilize body temperature by one of the following methods:

1. Checking the temperature in the nursery. Ambient temperature of nursery unit should be maintained at 24° C (75° F).
2. Keeping the neonate dry and wrapped in warmed blankets (care is taken to keep head well covered) (Fig. 29.3) while being held by the parent. Check body temperature at least every hour until the neonate's temperature is stabilized and to prevent hyperthermia.
3. Placing the thoroughly dried neonate under radiant heat panel without clothing until the temperature is stabilized.

*The first 2 hours of life are discussed in Chapter 22.

†For nutritional care see Chapter 30.

*Take neonate back to nursery and administer oxygen by mask if the neonate shows excessive mottling or has cyanosis of the face.

Fig. 29.1
Infant is turned to side and supported in this position to facilitate drainage from mouth.

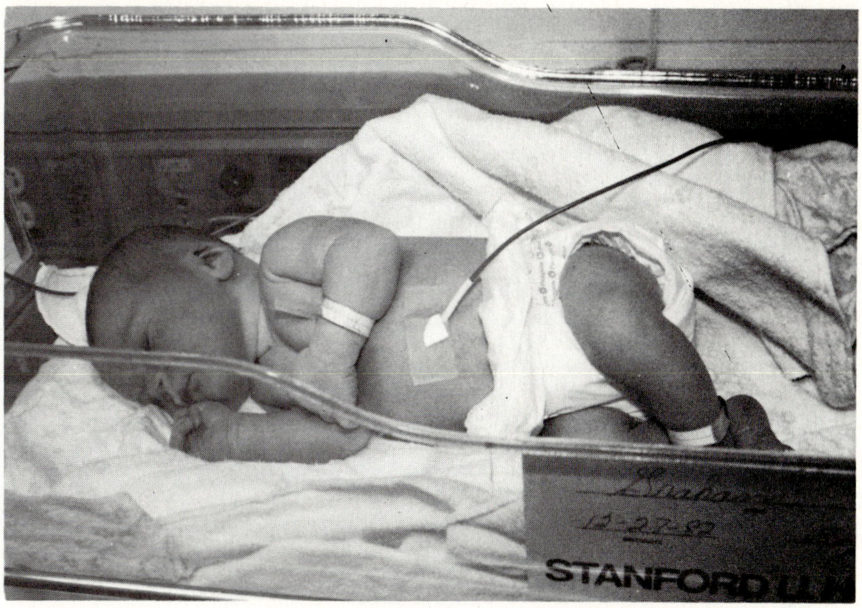

Fig. 29.2
A, Rectal temperature. Note how nurse stabilizes neonate's legs. Thermometer is lubricated and then inserted *gently*. **B,** Axillary temperature. Nurse is holding thermometer in place while counting his apical pulse. Baby is under radiant heat panel.

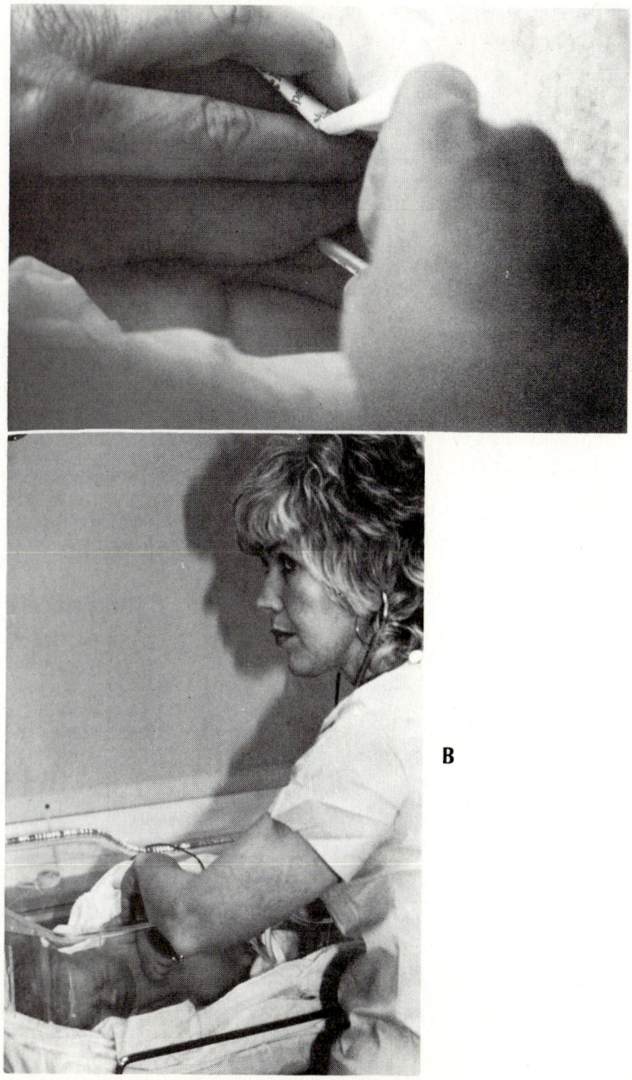

A

B

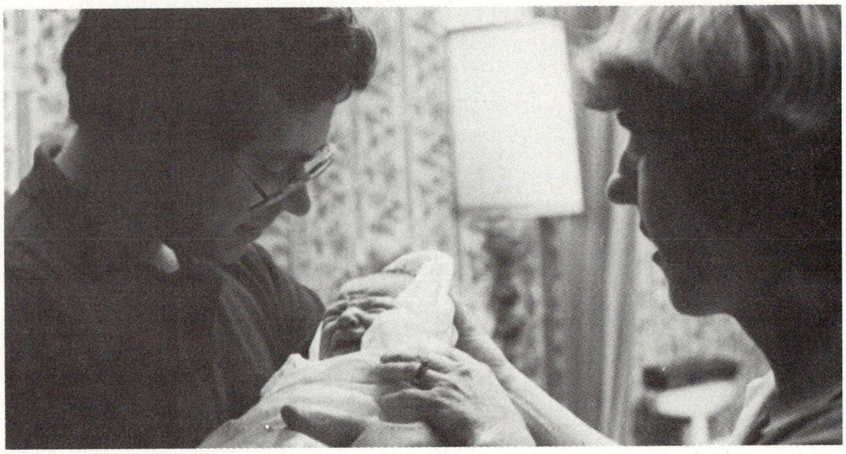

Fig. 29.3
Parent holding neonate who is wrapped to maintain body temperature.

Fig. 29.4
Holding baby securely with support for head. **A,** Holding baby while moving him from one place to another. Baby (whose temperature is well stabilized in a warm nursery) is undressed to show his posture. Note lack of curvature in normal neonate's spine and flexion of his extremities. **B,** Holding baby upright in "burping" position.

A

B

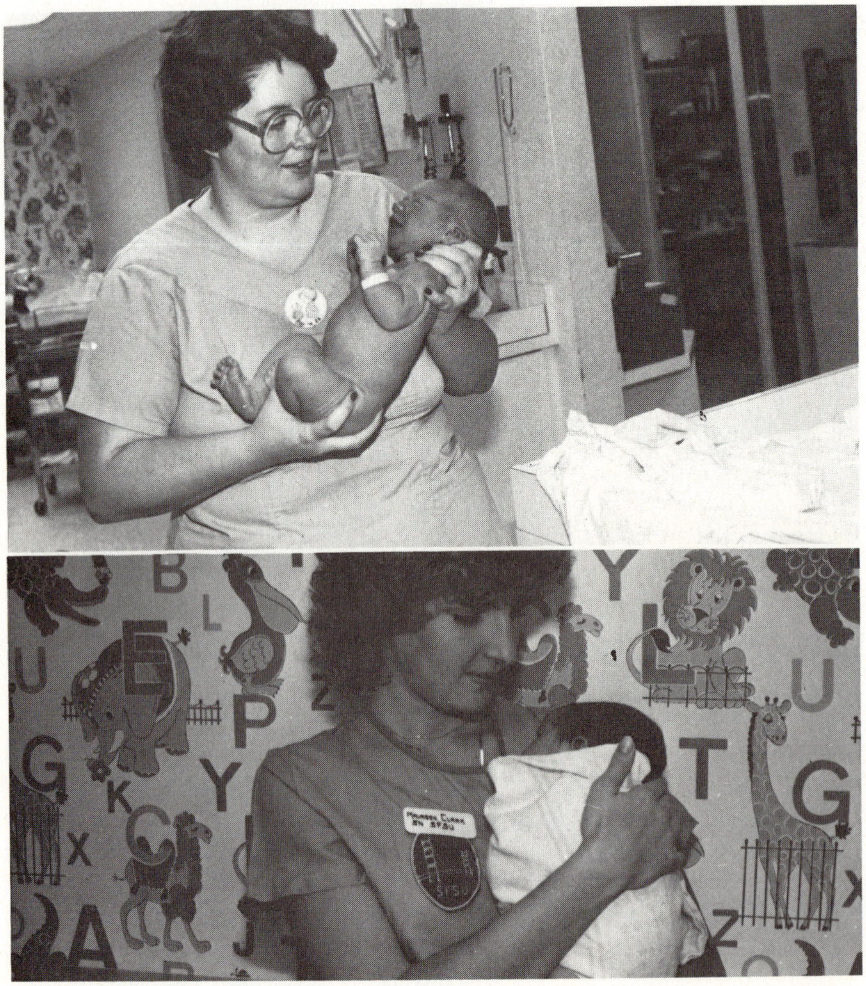

4. Minimizing heat loss by doing examinations or other activities with the neonate under a heat panel and by postponing the initial bath until the neonate's temperature reaches 36.5° C (97.6° F).

Positioning and holding the infant. Positioning the infant in the crib on his side permits drainage of mucus from the mouth and applies no pressure to the cord or the sensitive circumcised penis. Anatomically, the infant's shape—barrel chest; flat, curveless spine—makes it easy for him to roll. A folded or rolled blanket against the spine will prevent rolling to the supine position and add a feeling of security. Care must be taken to prevent the infant from rolling off flat unguarded surfaces; if the attendant must turn away from the infant even for a moment, the attendant must keep one hand securely on the infant. Infants must never be left alone on the bath table or in water, not even for a second. If the attendant has to leave, either the infant should be taken along or put back into the crib. If left on the parent's bed, the infant should be walled in with pillows. Changing the infant's position from side to side may be done after the feeding period to assist in developing even contours of the head, as well as easing pressure on other parts of the body.

An infant must be held securely with support for the head because he is unable to maintain erect head posture for more than a few moments. Fig. 29.4 illustrates various positions for holding an infant with adequate

Fig. 29.4, cont'd
C, "Football" hold. **D,** Cradling hold.

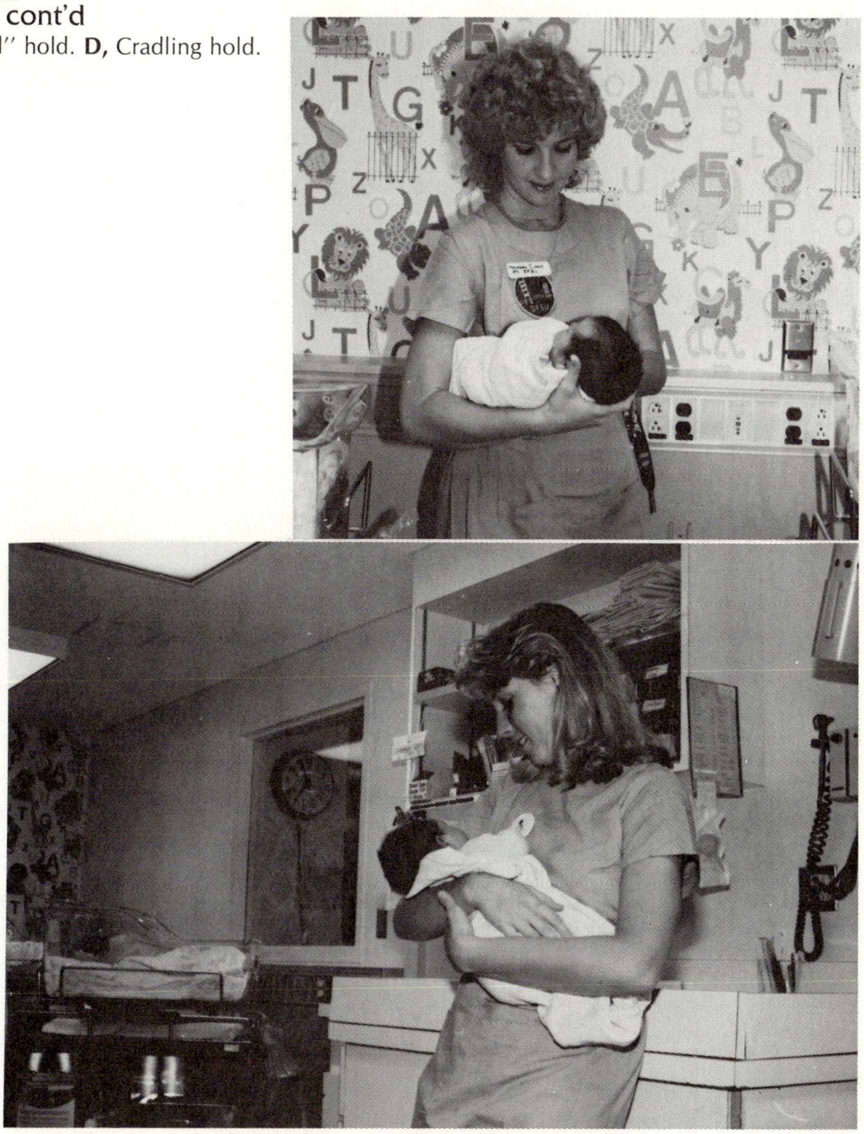

C

D

support. Too much stimulation is avoided after feeding and before a sleep period. After feeding, positioning the infant on the right side or prone promotes gastric emptying into the small intestine (Fig. 29.5).

Cleansing infant. Bathing (Fig. 29.6) serves a number of purposes. It provides opportunities for (1) a complete cleansing of the infant, (2) observing the infant's condition, (3) promoting comfort, and (4) parent-child-family socializing. The initial bath is postponed until the infant's temperature stabilizes at 36.5° C (97.6° F). Heat loss in the infant is disproportionate to heat loss in the adult because of the relatively large ratio of skin surface to body mass in the neonate. Heat loss must be controlled during the bath period to conserve the infant's energy. The ambient temperature of the room should be 24° C (75° F), and the bathing area should be free of drafts. Bathing the infant quickly, exposing only a portion of the body at a time, and thorough drying are therefore part of the bathing technique. After the initial bath, a daily bath may be given at any time convenient to the parents but not immediately following a feeding period, since the increased handling may cause regurgitation of the feeding. In some hospitals the infant is given an initial bath, and then cleansing of the genitalia as necessary is deemed sufficient for the first 3 or 4 days.

The infant's fragile skin can be traumatized by too vigorous cleaning. Gentleness, patting dry rather than rubbing, and use of a mild soap* without perfume or coloring are recommended. Coloring and perfume chemicals can cause rashes in sensitive skin.

If stool or other debris has caked and dried on the skin, soak the area to remove it. Do not attempt to rub it off, because abrasion may result. *Creases* under the chin and arms and in the groin need daily cleansing. Vernix may be left on for 48 hours; if it persists beyond that time, it may be washed off. The crease under the chin may be exposed by elevating the infant's shoulders 5 cm (2 in) and letting the head drop back. The *scalp* is washed daily with water and a mild soap, and it must be rinsed well. Scalp desquamation, called *cradle cap*, can often be prevented by removing any scales with a fine-toothed comb or brush after washing. If the condition persists, the physician may order an ointment to massage into the skin.

Cleanse the *eyes* from the inner canthus outward, using a clean washcloth. For the first 2 or 3 days there may be a discharge from the reaction of the conjunctiva to the substance (silver nitrate; erythromycin) used as a prophylactic measure against gonorrheal infection. Any

*If a documented staphylococcal skin infection outbreak occurs in a nursery, the newborn may be bathed with dilute hexachlorophene detergent (pHisoHex) (less than 3%), followed by thorough rinsing of the skin. pHisoHex is a potential neurotoxin, particularly for infants who weigh less than 2000 g, and it is no longer used in many areas.

Fig. 29.5
Right side-lying position after feeding. (From Whaley, L.F., and Wong, D.J.: Nursing care of infants and children, ed. 2, St. Louis, 1983, The C.V. Mosby Co.)

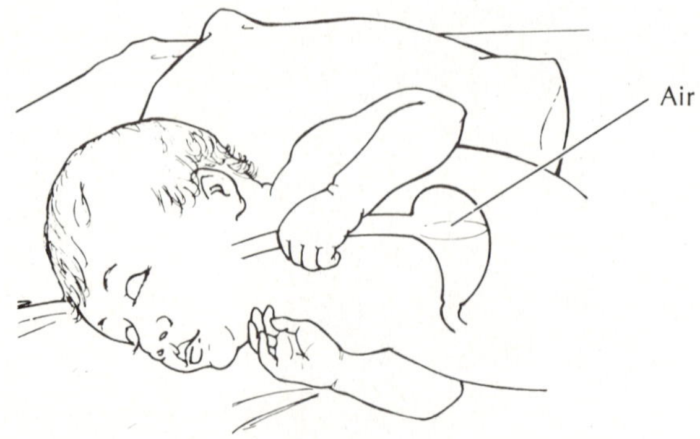

Fig. 29.6
Moro reflex during bath. Note mother's hand providing safety and comfort.

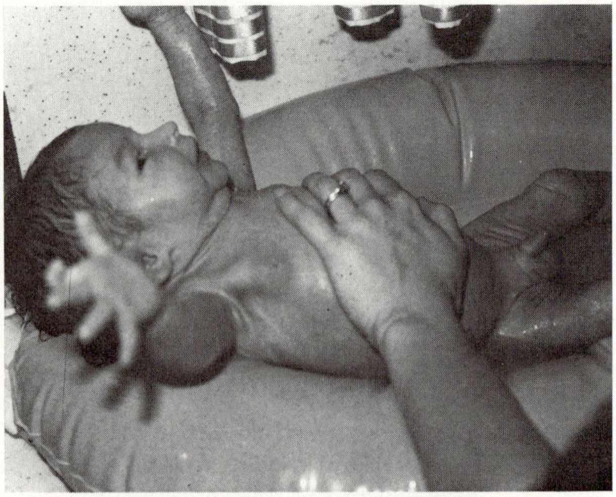

discharge should be considered abnormal and reported to the physician.

When removing eye discharge, avoid contamination of one eye with the discharge from the other by using a separate cotton swab and water source (running water from a tap is best) for each eye.

Cleanse the *ears* and *nose* with twists made of moistened cotton.

Fingernails and toenails are not cut immediately after birth. The nails have to grow out far enough from the skin so that the skin is not cut by mistake. Before the nails can be cut, if self-inflicted scratches bother the parent, the parent can use the fine side of an emery board to smooth the nails and can apply loosely fitted mitts over each hand.* When the nails have grown, the *fingernails* and *toenails* can be cut more readily with manicure scissors (with rounded tips preferably) when the infant is asleep. Hold the skin back from the nail and cut straight across. The nails are kept short; otherwise, they can be snagged by clothing, and the infant can scratch himself during normal random hand and leg movements. Wash and dry between the fingers and toes daily.

The *genitalia* of both boy and girl infants need at least daily cleansing. For uncircumcised boys complete retraction of the foreskin may not be possible for weeks, months, or even years (see p. 567). Do not use force either in trying to retract the foreskin or in washing the genitalia of the newborn male or female. Cleanse the glans penis with soap and water to remove smegma. For girls, daily cleansing of the genitalia may be done by separating the labia and gently washing from the pubic area to the anus.

Umbilical cord care. The care of the umbilical cord is the same as that for any surgical wound. The goal of care is prevention or early identification of hemorrhage or infection. If bleeding from the blood vessels of the cord is noted, the nurse checks the clamp (or tie) and applies a second clamp next to the first one. If bleeding is not stopped immediately, the nurse calls for physician assistance at once.

Hospital protocol directs the timing and technique for routine cord care. The nurse cleanses the cord and skin area around the base of the cord with the prescribed preparation (i.e., erythromycin solution, Triple Blue, or alcohol). The nurse or parent diapers the infant so that drying of the cord is facilitated by exposure to air. The diaper should not cover the cord. A wet or soiled diaper will slow or prevent drying and foster infection. The nurse or parent notifies the physician of any odor, discharge, or skin inflammation around the cord. The clamp is removed when the cord is dry (about 24 hours) (Fig. 29.7).

Diaper rash. Treatment of diaper rash involves exposure of the rash to warmth as well as to air and an immediate washing and drying of the wet and soiled area and change of the diaper after voiding or defecating. The warmth can be achieved with a 25-watt bulb placed 45 cm (18 in) away from the affected area. Avoid excessive heat (e.g., positioning the baby to have the sun shine in through a window and resulting in a sunburn) and drafts if the baby is partially uncovered. The most severe type of diaper rash occurs when the area becomes infected, indurated (hardened), and tender. Medical advice should be sought and a specifically ordered medication applied. A rash on the face may result from the infant's scratching (excoriation) or may be caused by rubbing his face against the sheets, particularly if regurgitated stomach contents are not washed off promptly.

Clothing the infant. Frequently parents ask about how warmly to dress the newborn infant. A simple rule of thumb for parents is to dress the child as they dress themselves, adding or subtracting clothes and wraps for the child as they do for themselves. A shirt and diaper may be sufficient clothing for the young infant. A bon-

Fig 29.7
Removal of cord clamp when cord is dry

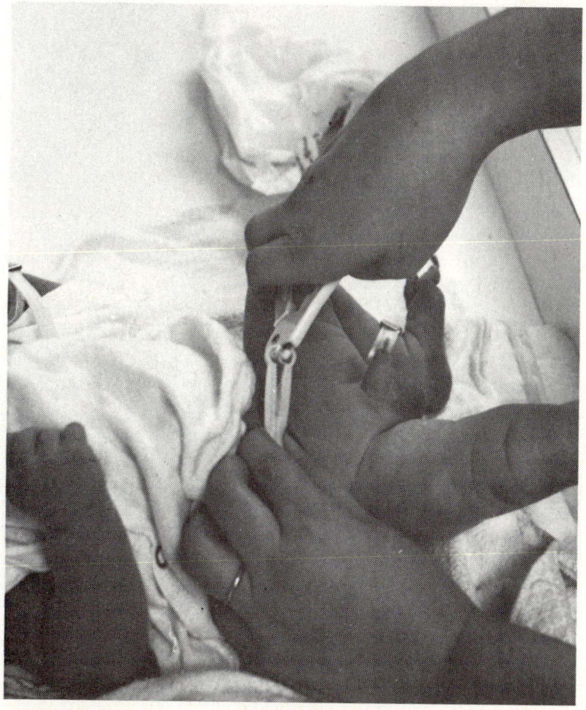

*This is done as a last resort because it interferes with baby's ability to console self.

net is needed to protect the scalp and minimize heat loss (if it is cool) or to protect against sunburn and shade the eyes if it is sunny and hot. Wrapping the infant snugly in a blanket serves to maintain body temperature and to give a feeling of security. Overdressing in warm temperatures can cause discomfort and prickly heat; underdressing in cold temperatures can also cause discomfort. Cheeks, fingers, and toes can readily become frostbitten.

A nurse was called to make a home visit to see an infant because the "baby just sleeps and sleeps and doesn't have any energy." In the apartment the thermostat was set for 33° C (92° F) because the mother "thought that babies need it warm." The mother was wearing a sleeveless dress because she could barely tolerate the extreme heat. The baby was found heavily wrapped in blankets. Lowering the thermostat and

Fig. 29.8
A, Gathering up shirt to enlarge neck opening. **B,** Placing neck opening to avoid dragging it across face.

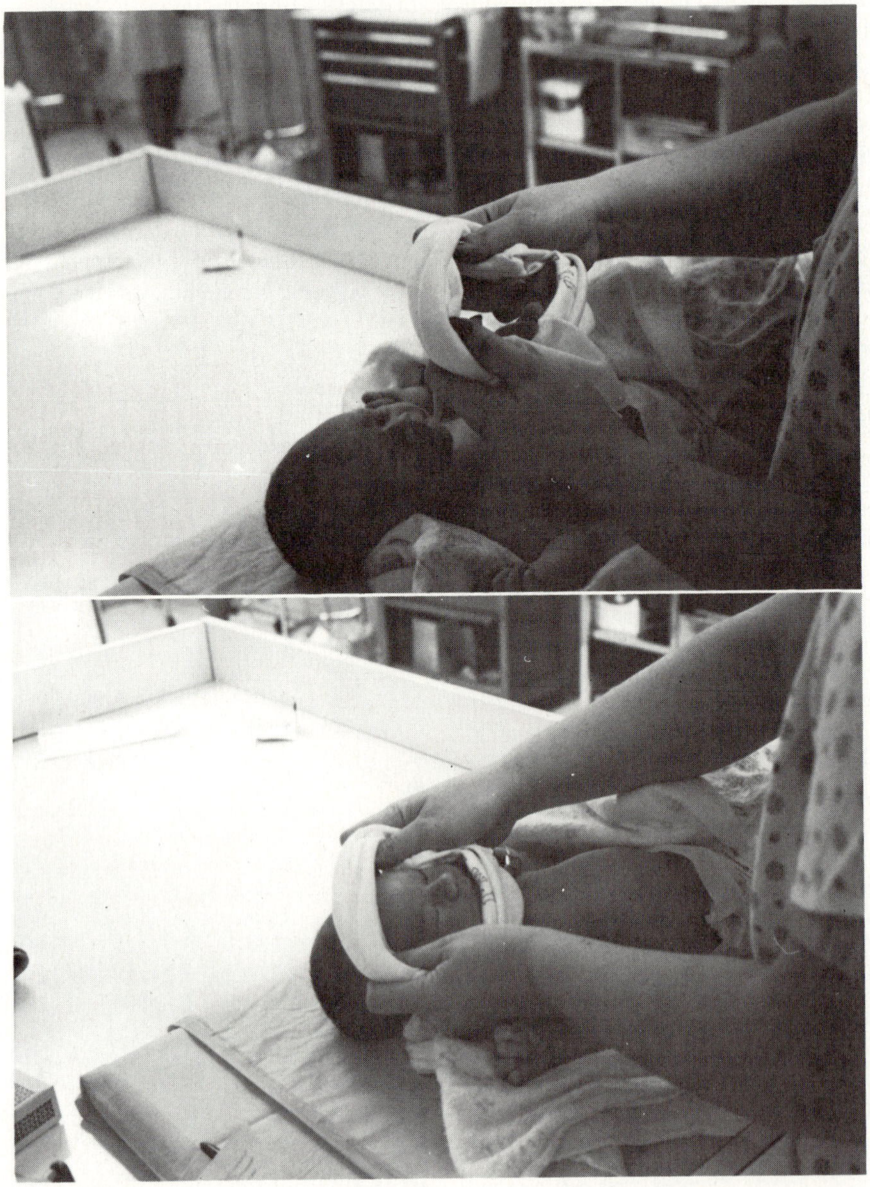
A

B

dressing the infant to match the temperature resulted in normal newborn behavior.

When dressing the child, avoid pulling shirts roughly over the face and catching fingers in shirt sleeves. Bunch up the shirt in both hands and expand the neck opening before placing the neck opening over the face first. Then slip the shirt over the rest of the head. Or, form a mask with your fingers over the baby's face as the shirt is pulled on or off (Fig. 29.8).

Diapering the infant may be done before and after feeding (Fig. 29.9). It is not necessary to wake the infant for changing because the above routine means about 12 changes per day. If cloth diapers are used, absorbency can be increased by bring the bulk of the diaper to the front area for boys and to the back for girls. This will help absorb urine so that the skin surface is protected. The diaper between the infant's legs should not be bulky because it can cause outward dis-

Fig. 29.8, cont'd
C, Drawing shirt down over back of head still avoiding face. **D,** Reaching into shirt's sleeve to grasp neonate's hand to pull arm through without snagging fingers.

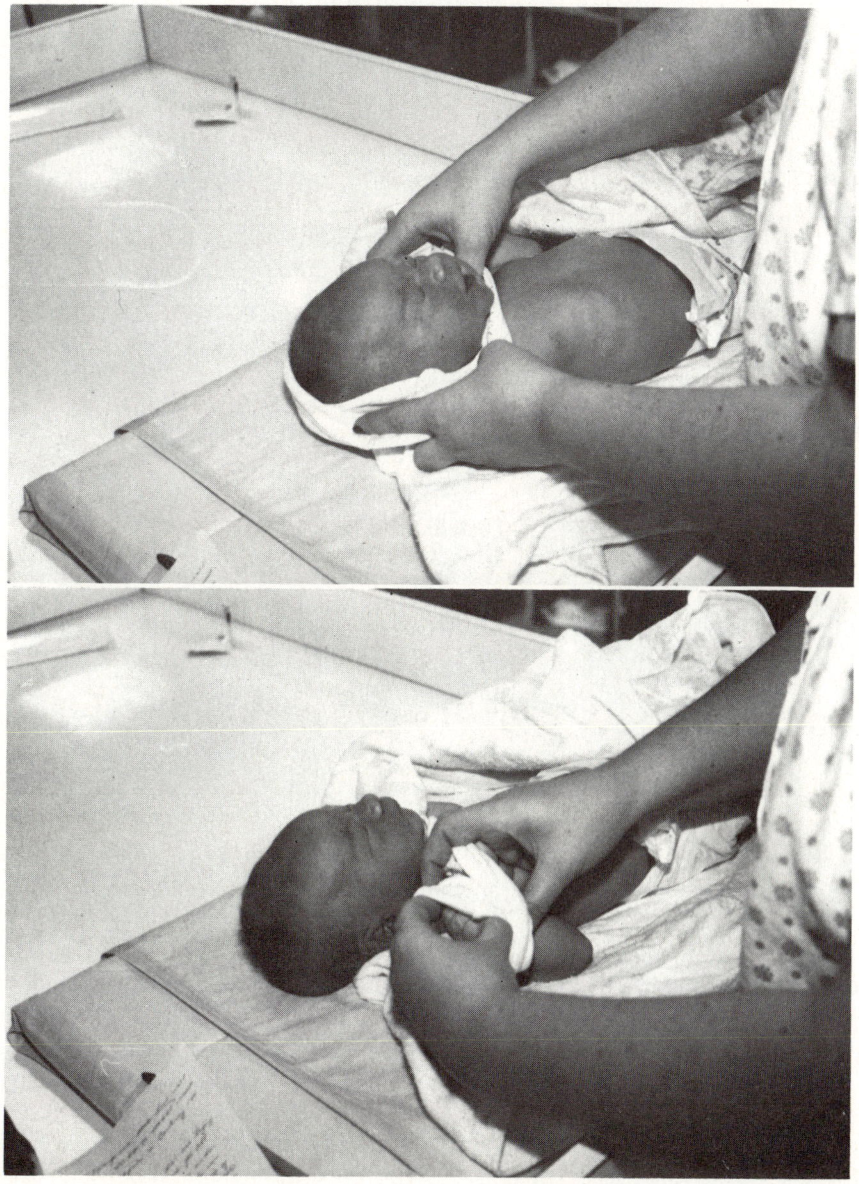

C

D

Continued.

Fig. 29.8, cont'd
E, Pulling left arm through. **F,** Pulling shirt down to cover trunk.

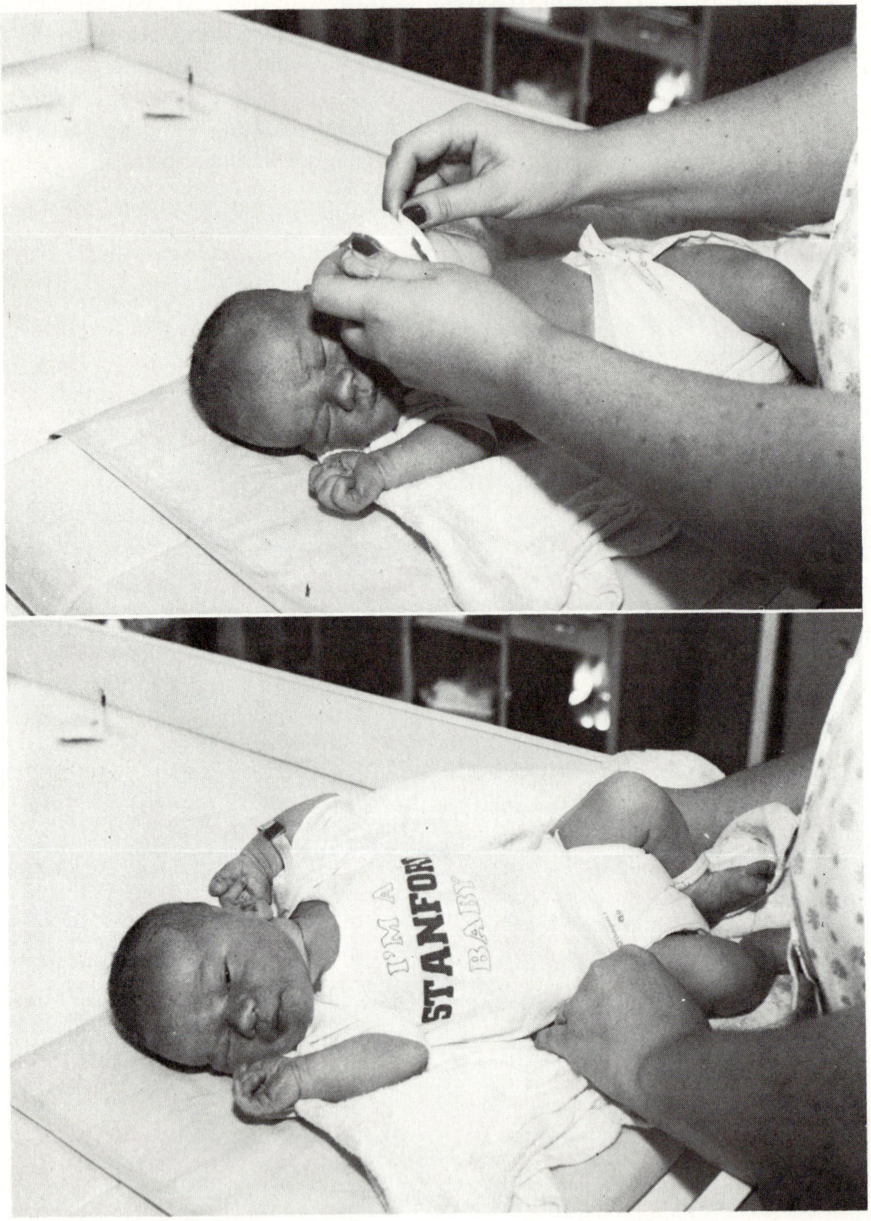

E

F

placement of the hips. A soaker pad can be placed under the infant as a protection for the blanket. The continued use of rubber or plastic pants may lead to diaper rash.

Care of infant's linens. Care of the infant's clothes and bedding is directed toward minimizing cross infection and removing residues from soap, feces, or urine that may irritate the infant's skin. In the hospital, clothing and bedding are washed separately from other linen and are autoclaved. Some hospitals use disposable shirts and diapers. At home, the baby's clothes should be washed separately, with a mild detergent or soap and hot water. A double rinse usually removes traces of the potentially irritating cleansing agent or acid residue from the urine or stool. If possible, dry the clothing and bedding in the sun to neutralize residues. Parents who

Fig. 29.9
Diapering infant. Dotted lines indicate folds. For kite type, start with large, regular diaper if single thickness is thin.

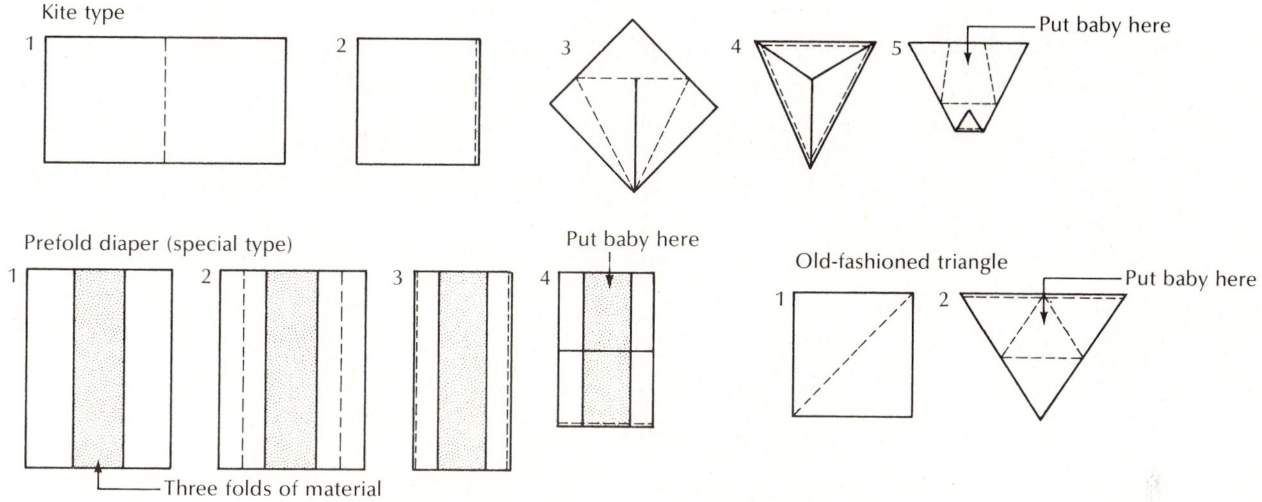

have to use coin-operated machines to wash and dry clothes may find it very expensive or almost impossible to wash and rinse the baby's clothes well.

Bedding requires frequent changing. The plastic-coated, firm mattress must be washed daily and the crib or bassinet damp dusted. A pillowcase makes an efficient bottom sheet for a bassinet.

The infant's toilet articles may be kept separate and convenient for use in a box or basket.

CIRCUMCISION

Historic perspective. Circumcision has been a rite in many cultures for centuries and continues to be a ritual in the Jewish and Moslem religions. Within the United States circumcision became a common practice in the early 1870s. From that time until the 1930s, people thought masturbation was harmful and that the removal of the foreskin would discourage this harmful activity by making it less pleasurable. In addition, circumcision was credited with preventing or curing a number of conditions such as epilepsy, syphilis, asthma, mental illness, and tuberculosis. At the present time, about 25% of the world's population circumcises its males sometime between birth and young adulthood.

Current views. Today the health-related reasons given most frequently are (1) to avoid phimosis, a painfully tight nonretracting foreskin; (2) to facilitate hygiene; (3) to prevent cancer (male: penile or prostatic cancer, and in a female partner: cervical cancer); (4) to decrease the chance of acquiring sexually transmitted diseases; and (5) to alleviate premature ejaculation.

Phimosis is a *rare* condition that can interfere with or impede the flow of urine (if the foreskin opening is tiny) and predispose to infection between the foreskin and glans.

In the majority of neonates the inner layer of the foreskin adheres to the glans. By the age of 3 years, in 90% of male children, the foreskin can be retracted easily without pain or trauma.

Recent studies do not support the connection between circumcision and cancer of the penis or prostatic gland or cervical cancer in the female partner. The coexistence of three non-circumcision-related factors is linked with cervical cancer: (1) the female who becomes sexually active before age 17 years, (2) the immature mucosal covering of the cervix of the female who is under 17 years that is exposed to sperm from a variety of different males, and (3) the cervix that has been infected with herpes virus.

There is no evidence to support the claim that circumcision decreases the risk to the male for sexually transmitted diseases. Because the foreskin contains numerous nerve endings that respond rapidly and intensely to sexual arousal, it was thought that eliminating the foreskin would cure premature ejaculation. Premature ejaculation is now known to be primarily caused by emotional problems and not physical conditions.

Fig. 29.10
A, Proper positioning of infant in Circumstraint. **B,** Physician performing circumcision. Note baby is completely covered to prevent cold stress.

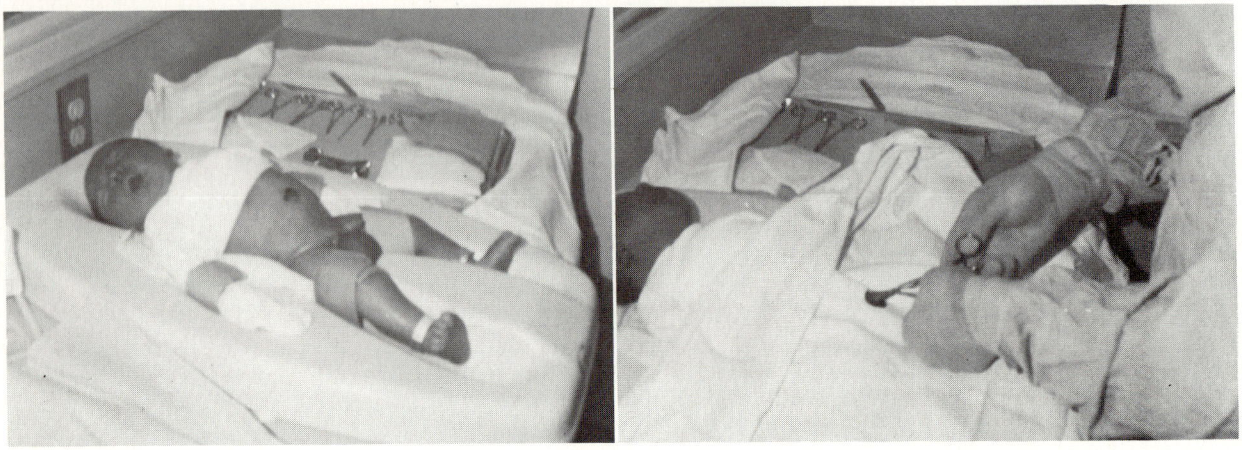

Fig. 29.11
Technique of circumcision. **A** to **D,** Prepuce is stripped and slit to facilitate its retraction behind glans penis. **E,** Prepuce is now clamped and excessive prepuce cut off. **F** and **G,** Suture material used is plain 00 or 000 catgut in very small needle, but some physicians prefer silk.

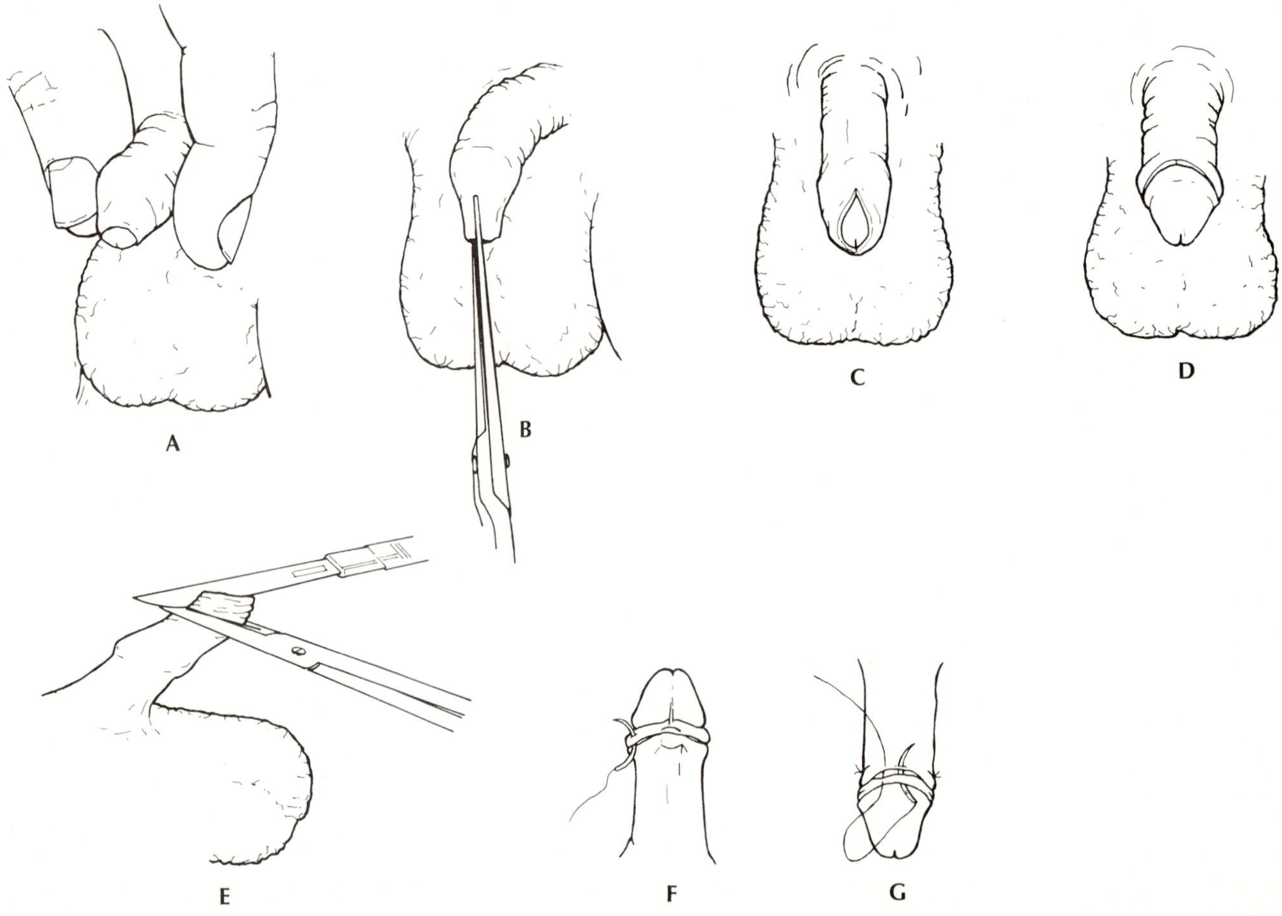

Parental decision. Circumcision is an *elective* surgical procedure and as such is a matter of personal choice. Parents' decision to have their newborns circumcised is usually based on one or more of the following factors: hygiene, religious conviction, tradition, culture, or social norms. Some people do not like to touch infant's genitalia. For those parents, circumcision may be the wisest choice.

Regardless of the reason for the decision, it should be made only after parents have the available facts and sufficient time to review their options. The American Academy of Pediatrics (1975) recommended that physicians provide parents with information about the risks of circumcision as well as options regarding this surgical procedure well in advance of delivery. Parents need to begin learning about circumcision during the prenatal period. However, circumcision often is not discussed with the parent or parents before labor. In many instances, it is on admission to the hospital or labor unit that the mother confronts the decision regarding circumcision. The stresses of the labor period make this a difficult time for parental decision making. Although consenting to their boy's circumcision is ultimately the parents' personal choice, the fact that there are no medical indications for the procedure should be emphasized.

The procedure. In circumcision the prepuce (foreskin) of the glans penis is excised to expose the glans. The operation is performed in the hospital before the infant's discharge with the parent or parents. The procedure is no longer done immediately after birth because the amount of cold stress has proved detrimental to the infant. Clotting factors drop somewhat immediately after birth and return to prebirth levels by the end of the first week. Therefore performing the circumcision after the baby is 1 week old has a firmer physiologic basis. The circumcision of a Jewish male infant is performed on the eighth day after birth unless the infant

Fig. 29.12

Circumcision with Yellen clamp. **A,** Prepuce drawn over cone. **B,** Pressure onto prepuce between cone and device for 3 to 5 minutes produces hemostasis. **C,** Prepuce (over cone) is cut away. **D,** Glans penis appears deep red during healing.

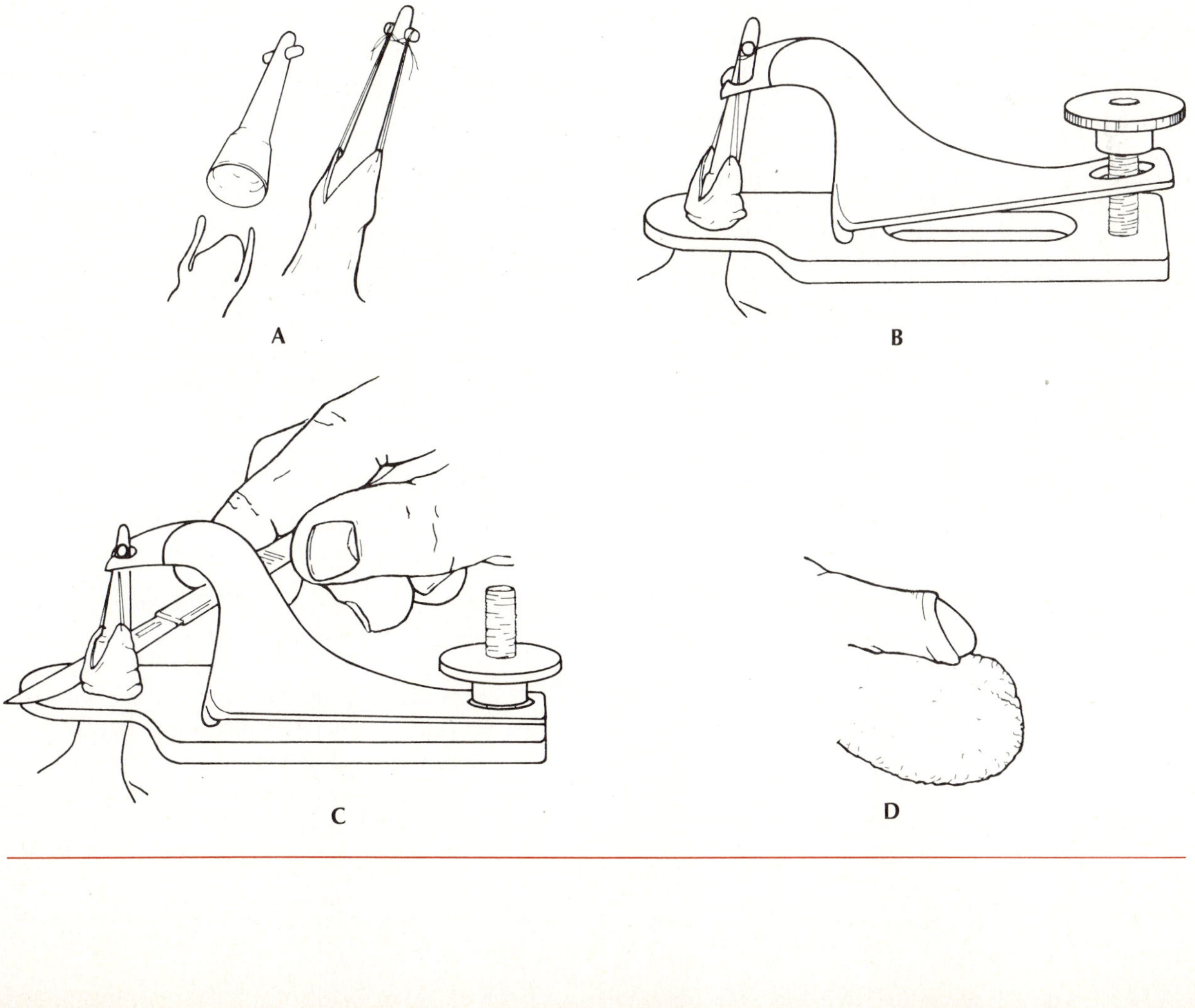

is unwell. To assist the neonate with clotting during the first week of life, vitamin K_1 (Aquamephyton) is administered to normal neonates as a routine measure in many institutions. Selection of the site for injection is very important (procedures, p. 637 and Fig. 29.18).

For the circumcision procedure the infant is positioned on a plastic restraint form so that his movements are restricted (Fig. 29.10). The penis is cleansed with soap and water. The infant is draped to provide warmth and a sterile field. The sterile equipment is readied for use.

Numerous instruments have been designed for circumcision (Figs. 29.11 and 29.12). The Yellen clamp, for instance, may make this an almost bloodless operation. Once the operation, which takes only a few minutes, is completed, a small petrolatum gauze dressing may be applied for the first day to prevent adherence of the cloth diaper. A cloth diaper is used because bleeding absorbed by cloth is easier to see than if absorbed by a disposable diaper.

Discomfort of the procedure. If the neonate has undergone this surgery without anesthesia, he is dressed and comforted until he is quieted. Then he is returned to his crib. These infants usually are fussy for about 2 to 3 hours and may refuse a feeding.

In the Jewish ritual, the neonate is given a few drops of wine to relax him in preparation for the surgery. In an article advocating dorsal nerve block for the circumcision, Kirya and Werthmann (1978) wrote:

> Anyone who circumcises a neonate using any of the available techniques, senses the pain and stress that the manipulative stages of this procedure generate. During the procedure when the prepuce is clamped with the forceps, the infant cries vigorously, trembles, and tries to wiggle out of the restraint. He may eventually become plethoric [flushed], dusky, and mildly cyanotic because of prolonged crying. Occasionally this results in respiratory pauses or regurgitation of feedings.

Pain may not end when the operation is over because the wound takes up to a week to heal.

Potential complications. Occasional occurrences of infection, hemorrhage, and injury to the penis are complications of circumcision that all parents should consider before deciding to have this surgery for their child. The healing process may result in distortion of the penis by scar tissue.

Care of the newly circumcised penis. The nurse observes the neonate for bleeding. If bleeding is noted from the circumcision, the nurse applies gentle pressure to the site of bleeding with a folded 4-in × 4-in gauze pad. If bleeding is not easily controlled, a blood vessel may need to be ligated. One nurse notifies the physician and prepares equipment (circumcision tray and suture) while the other nurse maintains pressure *intermittently* until the physician arrives. The penis is checked hourly for bleeding for 12 hours; if the parents take the neonate home before the end of 12 hours, they have to be taught the actions described above. Before discharge, the nurse checks to see that the parents have the physician's phone number.

Nursing actions are planned and implemented to prevent infection. The nurse washes the penis gently with water to remove urine and feces and reapplies a fresh (sterile) petrolatum gauze around the glans after each diaper change. The glans penis, normally dark red in appearance, becomes covered with a yellow exudate in 24 hours. This is part of the normal healing process, not an infective process. No attempt is made to remove the exudate, which persists for 2 to 3 days. Cloth diapers are applied loosely for 2 to 3 days because the incised area at the base of the glans penis remains tender for 2 to 3 days. Cloth diapers are used for about 1 week or until the glans is completely healed.

If a plastic bell is used to cover the glans, petrolatum gauze is not needed. The plastic bell remains firmly applied to the glans, preventing hemorrhage and contamination. The bell falls off when the glans is healed.

The nurse provides anticipatory guidance for the parents related to the older infant who had been circumcised. Parents need to know that the purpose of the foreskin is thought to be protection against irritation and injury. For the male infant, diapers and urine can be very irritating to the unprotected glans. For the male adult, clothing may be a source of irritation. Continual rubbing against clothing may adversely affect sexual response (Preston, 1970).

Care of the uncircumcised penis. The nurse teaches the parents of *uncircumcised* males to pull the foreskin back *gently* during bath time but to stop when they feel resistance. The parent washes the glans with mild soap and warm water and replaces the foreskin over the glans. The nurse warns the parent that the foreskin must be returned to its original position to prevent constriction and swelling. By late puberty, the foreskin is completely separated from the glans so that retraction can occur easily.

ANTICIPATORY GUIDANCE OF PARENTS: BEFORE DISCHARGE FROM HOSPITAL

Whether or not this is the couple's first child, new parents appreciate anticipatory guidance regarding the care of the child. Depending on the parents' needs, the nurse may choose to do any or all of the following within the first few days after the child is born:

I. Discuss normal growth and development and changing needs of infant (e.g., for stimulation, exercise, and social contacts).

II. Demonstrate and supervise practice in bathing

and cleansing, changing diapers, using thermometer, and holding infant.

III. Discuss pertinent information relating to following:
   A. Temperature
      1. Review causes of elevation in body temperature (e.g., exercise, cold stress with resultant vasoconstriction, minimal response to infection) and the body's response to extremes in environmental temperature.
      2. Review symptoms to be reported, such as high or low temperatures with accompanying symptoms of fussiness, stuffy nose, lethargy, irritability, poor feeding, and crying.
      3. Review interventions for reducing body temperature, such as giving a cool tub bath, dressing infant appropriately in relation to ambient temperature, protecting infant from long exposure to sunlight, and using warm wraps in cold weather.
   B. Respirations
      1. Review normal variations in rate and rhythm.
      2. Review reflexes, such as sneezing to clear air passage.
      3. Review need for protection of infant from the following:
         a. Individuals with upper respiratory tract infections (an efficient mask can be made from toilet paper if parent or another has a cold)
         b. Pollution from smoke-filled environment
      4. Review symptoms of common cold: nasal congestion, coughing, sneezing, difficulty in swallowing (sore throat), minimal fever. Advise parents on measures to help infant: for example, feed infant smaller amounts, but more frequently to avoid overtiring him; hold him in an upright position to feed; offer extra sterile water; for sleeping, raise mattress 30 degrees (do not use pillow) to raise infant's chest and head; avoid drafts; do not overdress; use only medications prescribed by physician (do not use nose drops, since aspiration may result in lung involvement); cover upper lip with light film of petrolatum to minimize excoriation.
   C. Elimination
      1. Review changes to be expected in color of stool and in number of bowel evacuations plus odor of stools for breast- or bottle-fed infants.
      2. Review color of normal urine and number of voidings to expect each day.
   D. Bathing
      1. Give sponge bath as indicated. Wash scalp every day. If soap is used, use mild, nonperfumed variety. Baby lotion may be used in small amounts, but parents should avoid powder and oil.
      2. Tub bath may be substituted for sponge bath when cord drops off.
      3. Select an area for bathing infant that is warm and free of drafts, with a surface large enough so that infant will not roll off.
      4. Complete preparations for bathing before bringing infant to area; have clothing organized and available.
      5. Form a habit of keeping instruments, pins, scissors, and so on closed and well out of reach of infant.
      6. Nails may be cut using manicure or special infant nail scissors when nail grows well beyond fingertips and infant is soundly asleep. Advise parents to cover neonate's hands if self-inflicted scratches bother them.
      7. Provide care for genitalia.
         a. Change diapers when they are soiled, but do not rouse infant from sleep to change them.
         b. Rashes over buttocks may appear by second or third day. Wash and dry area, expose buttocks to air, and use a heat lamp if rash is severe. Position light source (25 watts) at least 61 cm (24 in) above the infant; secure infant so that he cannot move and come into direct contact with light source.
         c. Wash female's genitalia *gently* to remove urine, feces, and smegma.

IV. Inform parents about whom to contact if assistance is needed, what community agencies are available, what symptoms require medical attention (e.g., fever persisting beyond 24 hours; infant rubbing his ear, coughing up purulent material, or vomiting; refusal of feedings; diarrhea; lethargy), and what to report (e.g., specific symptoms and how long they have persisted, temperature reading, what corrective measures have been undertaken and with what effect).

V. Refer parents to a class on cardiopulmonary resuscitation (CPR) after explaining that every adult needs to know this technique for use with anyone's child.

ANTICIPATORY GUIDANCE OF PARENTS: AT FIRST WELL-BABY VISIT

Anticipatory guidance and support of parents continue at the neonate's first well-baby visit at 1 month of age (approximately 28 days). The nurse is expected to do the following:

1. Welcome parent and infant.
2. Explain routine to be followed (e.g., physical assessment, discussion of changes to be expected, and assistance with problems).
3. Have parent undress infant and help with examination (this provides an opportunity to assess parental approach to infant).
4. Review plan of well-baby supervision (e.g., at 2 to 4 weeks of age, then every 2 months until 6 to 7 months of age, then every 3 months until 18 months, and then at 2 years, 3 years, preschool, and every 2 years thereafter*).
5. Give information about changes in growth and development to be expected over next 2 months.
6. Give information about disease processes and what to report to physician or community health nurse.
7. Counsel the mother regarding the neonate's temperature. By the fourth week the baby's temperature is maintained at 36.5° to 37° C (97.6° to 98.6° F). Although the method is not exact, the mother can determine whether the baby is too warm or too cold by placing her hand on his abdomen. If the abdomen feels moderately warm to the touch, the infant may be considered to be comfortable. If the parent does not know the technique for axillary temperature taking and reading the thermometer, the nurse demonstrates and then supervises the parent during the parent's return demonstration.
8. Review schedule for immunizations.
9. Assist parent or parents in coping with their perceived problems. (A general statement such as "Tell me how you and the baby spend your day" is preferable to "Are you having any problems?" which can be answered by a flat "no" or to "Are you bathing the baby every day?" which can place parent on the defensive.)

*Committee on Standards of Health Care: Standards of health care, ed. 2, Evanston, Ill., 1972, American Academy of Pediatrics.

Procedures

During the performance of all procedures* the nurse continuously assesses the neonate's responses. Until skill is gained, it is difficult for the learner to focus on both the mechanics of the procedure and the neonate. Until proficiency is achieved, arrange to have a skilled person present.

MONITORING AND RECORDING OF INFANT RESPONSES

The following parameters are assessed and recorded:

1. Respiratory rate, rhythm, and effort (If apnea monitor is used, set at 10 seconds.)
2. Heart rate (If cardiac monitor is used, set lower level at 80 to 100 beats/min.)
3. Skin color
4. Activity level and muscle tone
5. Feeding behavior

HEAT SUPPORT: CONTROLLING THE ENVIRONMENT

Overhead radiant heater (Fig. 29.13). The heater thermostat must be kept plugged into an electric outlet at all times. It is set to maintain an abdominal skin temperature of 36.5° C (97.7° F). The set point of 36.4° C (97.5° F) is usually chosen for activation of the heater.

Technique	Rationale
1. Dry newborn infant with warm absorbent blanket and place him under radiant heat shield.	1. Reduces heat loss by evaporation, conduction, convection, and radiation.
2. Adjust bassinet in head-down position (about 10 degrees).	2. Allows for gravity drainage of mucus in respiratory tract.†
3. Remove gross soiling (meconium, blood).	3. Facilitates observation of skin coloring and any changes.
4. Check the thermostat setting for accuracy.	4. Avoids overheating or underheating.

*For ease of use of the text as a resource for student learning, this section on procedures is included. Learning new skills is emotionally draining, a concept worth remembering when teaching new parents new skills.

†If the infant is suspected of having intracranial hemorrhage, keep his head on the same level as his body or slightly elevated if mucus is not excessive.

Fig. 29.13
Overhead radiant heater. Also note neonate has individual supplies readily available: suction equipment, clothes, diapers, bathing supplies. Cribs are clear plastic to permit easier visualization of neonate.

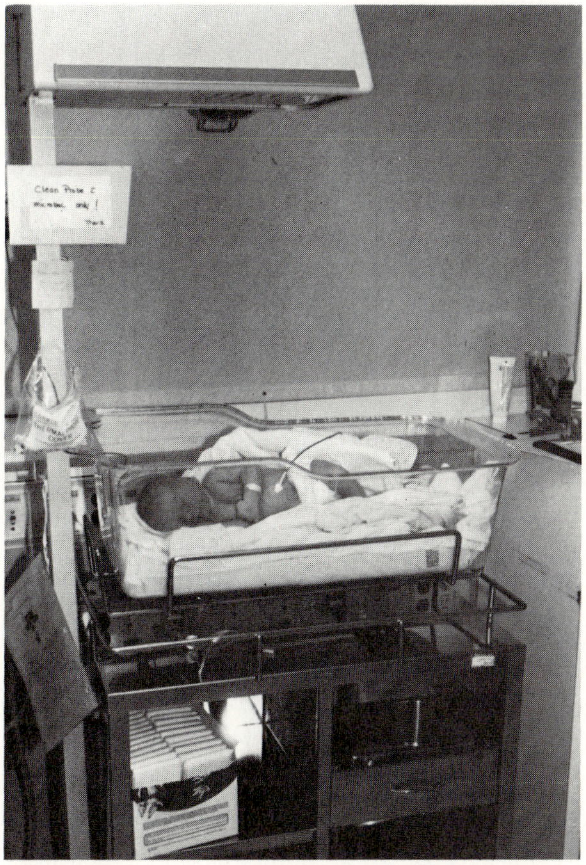

Technique	Rationale
5. Apply thermistor probe (metal side next to infant) with paper tape or nonirritating plastic tape (e.g., Hy-tape) to anterior abdominal wall between navel and xiphoid process; avoid placement over bony rib cage.*	5. Improves accurate reading of skin temperature. Sensors in skin respond more quickly to change.
6. Check frequently to ensure that probe retains skin contact.	6. Avoids overheating or underheating.
7. Observe infant for color change; crying, restlessness; increased respiratory rate.	7. Determines if abnormal behavior is caused by cold stress or other factors (debility, sepsis).
8. Note previous symptoms; recheck probe, thermostat setting, and heater contact.	8. Rules out equipment malfunction.
9. Record findings.	9. Effects communication with other caretakers.

*The thermistor, after it is taped to the abdominal wall, must be covered by a small plastic-foam square insulator. Optimally it should have a cover of aluminum foil. The foam insulation of the thermistor is essential to prevent the radiant heat from directly warming the thermistor more quickly than the baby himself is warmed. The response of the mechanism would be to a heated probe rather than to a warmed baby.

Servo-Control incubator. Servo-Control incubators or equivalents utilize the same principle as the thermostat in maintaining an even temperature in an oven or a room. The infant's skin temperature, as opposed to the circulating air, provides the point of control.

The skin is a very sensitive indicator of the infant's thermal state. Receptors note even minor changes resulting from peripheral vasoconstriction, dilatation, or increased metabolism long before a change in deep (core) body temperature develops. Therefore measurements of skin temperature provide a more reliable indicator of the energy exchange between the infant and his environment.

For automatic control of temperature using Servo-Control incubators, the following measures are necessary:

1. Set the incubator control panel at the physician-ordered predetermined level, usually between 36° and 37° C (96.8° and 98.6° F) to maintain skin temperature of 36.5° C (97.6° F).
2. Tape a thermistor probe (automatic sensor) from the control panel to the right upper quadrant of the abdomen immediately below the right infracostal margin.
3. Check the sensor periodically for its continued firm application to skin; check and record the core temperature (rectal) with a clinical thermometer; record incubator temperature readings.
4. Record the skin temperature reading and the ambient temperature within the incubator every 2 to 4 hours after the infant's temperature is stabilized.
5. Record the infant's general appearance and behavior.

The abdominal skin temperature of 36.5° C (97.6° F) is considered optimal because at that temperature, oxygen consumption (and metabolic rate) is minimal. When the skin temperature increases to 37.2° C (98.9° F), the oxygen consumption increases by 6%; a drop in skin temperature to 35.9° C (96.6° F) is accompanied by an increase in oxygen consumption of 10%.

Even a normal full-term neonate in good health can become hypothermic. Birth in a car on the way to the hospital, a cold delivery room, or inadequate drying and wrapping immediately after birth may cause the neonate's temperature to fall. Warming the hypothermic baby is accomplished with care.

Warming the hypothermic infant. Rapid warming or cooling may cause apneic spells and acidosis in an infant. Therefore the warming process is monitored to progress slowly over a period of 2 to 4 hours.

The nurse places the infant in a Servo-Control incubator (or other type) and proceeds as follows:

1. Set incubator temperature on control panel at 1.2° C (2° F) above skin temperature even if the skin temperature is lower than normal.
2. Tape thermistor probe to skin of anterior abdominal wall (not over bone).
3. When skin temperature reaches predetermined, set incubator temperature, repeat process until abdominal skin temperature of 36.5° C (97.6° F) is reached.

SUCTIONING THE NEWBORN

For the normal or distressed infant, the nurse's knowledge and skill in suctioning may be critical in assisting him to establish or maintain adequate respirations.

The equipment includes the following:

1. Bulb syringe (intact and fairly firm)
2. DeLee mucous-trap catheter (available in reusable glass or disposable plastic), with a two-holed tip
3. Catheters (external suction source and container of sterile water are needed also)
   a. French, rubber (moderately firm): size 10, 12, and 14; whistle tip; two-hole tip
   b. French, plastic disposable: sizes 8, 10, and 12; finger control; two-hole tip

The bulb syringe, catheters, and all tubing are sterile and wrapped.

During all procedures the infant's heat loss must be avoided or minimized by drying and wrapping the infant and placing him in a warmed Kreiselman or comparable crib or under overhead radiant heat or another source of heat. In addition, a humidified oxygen source and equipment for the administration of oxygen must be readily available.

Upper airway aspiration: mouth and nose. A clear airway is fundamental to establishing adequate ventilation. Generally the normal full-term infant born vaginally has little difficulty in clearing his air passages. Most secretions are drained by gravity, propelled to the oropharynx by the cough reflex to be drained or swallowed. However, in premature infants swallow and cough reflexes may be absent or not well developed.

To assist gravity drainage, the nurse supports the wrapped infant on the arm or on the hip (in the football hold), positioning his head downward. *Do not* hold him by his ankles in the head-down position, because this raises cerebral venous pressure, increases the risk of accidentally dropping the infant, hyperextends and stretches the spine, and is painful to the baby.

Mucus from the mouth and nose is easily removed with a bulb syringe. The technique and rationale for suctioning with a bulb syringe are as follows:

Technique	Rationale
1. Suction mouth first.	1. Sensitive receptors around nares respond to stimuli by initiating gasp. Any mucus present could be pulled into lower airway.
2. Compress the bulb *before* insertion, creating suction.	2. Prevents blowing secretions deeper into mouth and nose.
3. Insert syringe into space between cheek and gums, and release compression gradually (to suck out mucus).	3. Prevents tissue trauma and removes secretions.
4. Remove from mouth. Compress syringe to empty it and to create new vacuum to repeat procedure.	
5. Repeat steps 2 and 3 as needed in mouth, then in nose. Stop suctioning when cry is clear (infant does not sound like he has mucus or bubbles in his mouth).	

Midairway (nasopharynx, oropharynx) and stomach aspiration. Catheters are necessary for deeper suctioning. Position the infant for resuscitation as follows:

1. Place the infant on his back.
2. Place a folded towel under the head to move it slightly forward from the neck (as in sniffing) to (a) separate tongue from pharyngeal wall and (b) prevent obstruction from newborn's normally low palate and macroglossia. (Some physicians prefer to work with the neonate on a flat surface with no towel.)

Several precautions must be taken when suctioning with catheters:

Precaution	Rationale
1. Keep deep suctioning to minimum.	1. Hazards. a. Direct trauma to mucosa with edema formation, bleeding, or increased secretions. b. Stimulation of vagal reflex: bradycardia, cardiac arrhythmias, laryngospasm, and apnea, especially if this type of suctioning is done within first few minutes of infant's birth.
2. Limit suctioning to 10 seconds or less.	2. Prolonged suctioning stimulates laryngospasm and reduces air (O_2) content in airway.
3. Suction is *off* as tube is put into position.	3. Prevents direct tissue trauma.
4. Avoid forcing catheter.	4. Hazard; direct tissue trauma or perforation in presence of congenital anomalies such as choanal, esophageal, or intestinal atresia.
5. Apply suction only as tube is being withdrawn.	5. Prevents direct tissue trauma.
6. Rotate catheter when suctioning.	6. Prevents tissue trauma consequent to tissue's being drawn into eye of catheter.
7. Observe infant's response. Withdraw tube to suction posterior nasopharynx.	7. Gagging indicates entrance into esophagus; coughing indicates entrance into trachea.

Suctioning with DeLee mucous-trap catheter (Fig. 29.14). Catheter suction is supplied by the operator: no extra equipment is necessary; excess negative pressure is not attained. The mucous trap can be detached and the enclosed specimen sent to the laboratory for examination and culture as necessary.

Aspirate the mouth and throat first, then the nose to prevent inhalation of pharyngeal contents.

Discontinue suctioning when (1) the cry is clear and (2) air entry into lungs is heard by stethoscope.

Use of nasopharyngeal catheter with mechanical suction apparatus. Negative pressure on portable and wall gauges should be adjusted to avoid excessive suction.

The technique and rationale for using a nasopharyngeal catheter with suction apparatus are as follows:

Technique	Rationale
1. Lubricate catheter in sterile water.*	1. Facilitates passage of tube and prevents infection.
2. Insert catheter. a. Orally along base of tongue. b. Nasally horizontally into nares, then raising it to advance it beyond bend at back of nares	2. Decreases risk of laryngeal spasm and reflex apnea.
3. With catheter in place, place thumb over finger control to create suction. Rotate tubing between fingers while withdrawing catheter.	3. Prevents direct trauma caused by drawing mucosa into eye of catheter.
4. Limit each suctioning to 10 seconds or less.	4. Prevents laryngospasm and oxygen depletion.
5. If infant is active, an attendant may be needed to stabilize infant's head. Or if there is time, "mummy" infant before this procedure (see p. 643).	5. Prevents trauma and affects suctioning. Both hands are needed to manipulate catheter and finger control of suction pressure.

Additional comments. "Milking" the trachea is ineffective. This procedure may injure cartilage and will often delay effective suctioning.

In addition, if the infant is premature or is suspected of having intracranial hemorrhage, his head is kept level with his body to prevent increasing intracranial pressure and possible bleeding as a result of gravity.

MOUTH-TO-MOUTH RESUSCITATION

The emergency procedure of mouth-to-mouth resuscitation requires no equipment and can be initiated at a moment's notice. All personnel should be trained in this technique:

Technique	Rationale
1. Clear airway of any mucus or debris.	1. Prevents impelling debris down airway.

*A 120 ml (4 oz) bottle of sterile water for feeding is convenient, already comes in a sterile container, and decreases risk of contamination possible with large stock bottles.

Fig. 29.14
DeLee mucous-trap catheter.

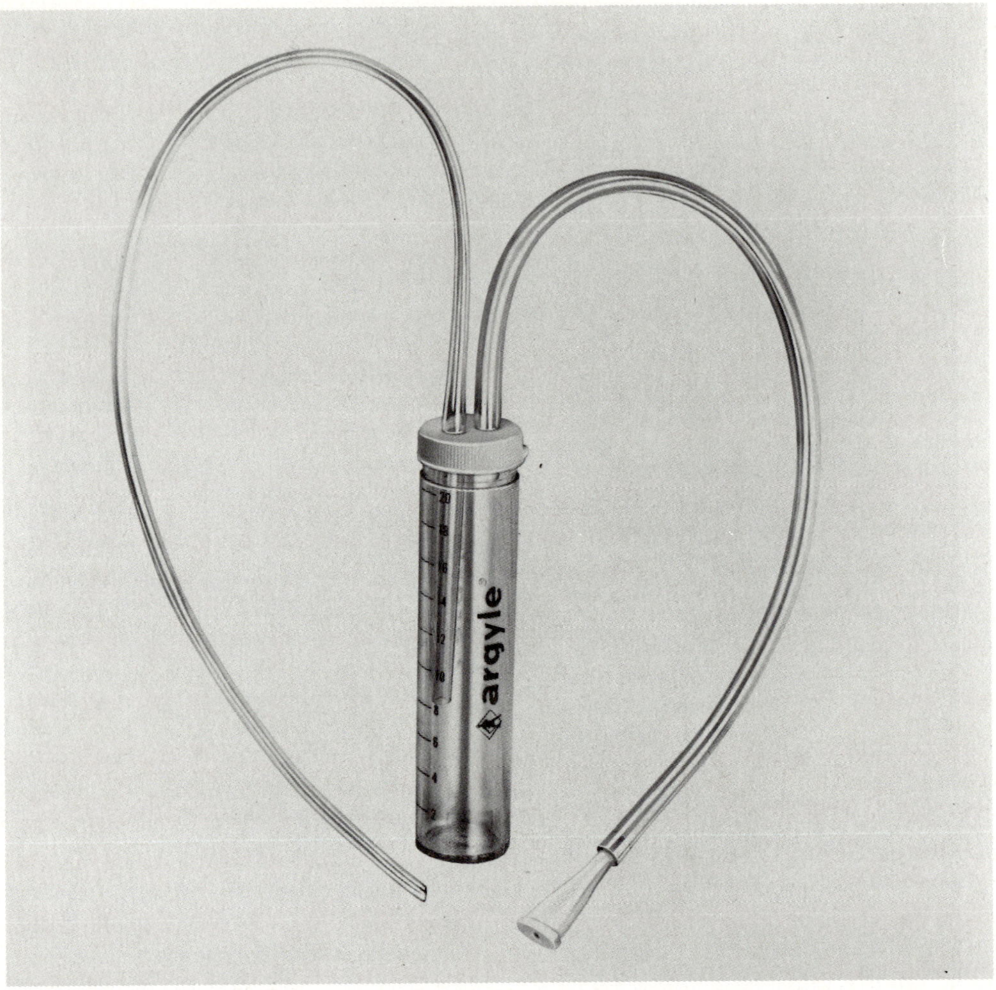

Technique	Rationale
2. Position infant. Place small rolled towel under the head to move it slightly forward from the neck ("sniffing position"), or leave neonate on flat surface.	2. Opens airway by straightening trachea and permitting back of tongue to fall away from posterior pharynx.
3. Insert plastic airway if available.	3. Provides unobstructed airway (especially from tongue if infant is flaccid).
4. Place your mouth over infant's nose and mouth to create a seal.	4. Permits insufflation under pressure.
5. Repeat the word *ho* as you gently puff volume of air *in your cheeks* into infant. *Do not* force air.	5. Prevents injury to lung tissue (e.g., pneumothorax, pneumomediastinum).
6. Repeat puffs at rate of 30/min.	6. Approximates normal respiratory rhythm.
7. Infant's chest should rise slightly with each puff; keep fingers on chest wall to sense air entry.	7. Determines if air is reaching alveolar level.
8. Allow chest to fall by passive recoil.	8. Allows removal of insufflated air.
9. If available, place tubing of O_2 in your mouth as you inhale quickly between puffs.	9. Increases O_2 content in insufflated air.

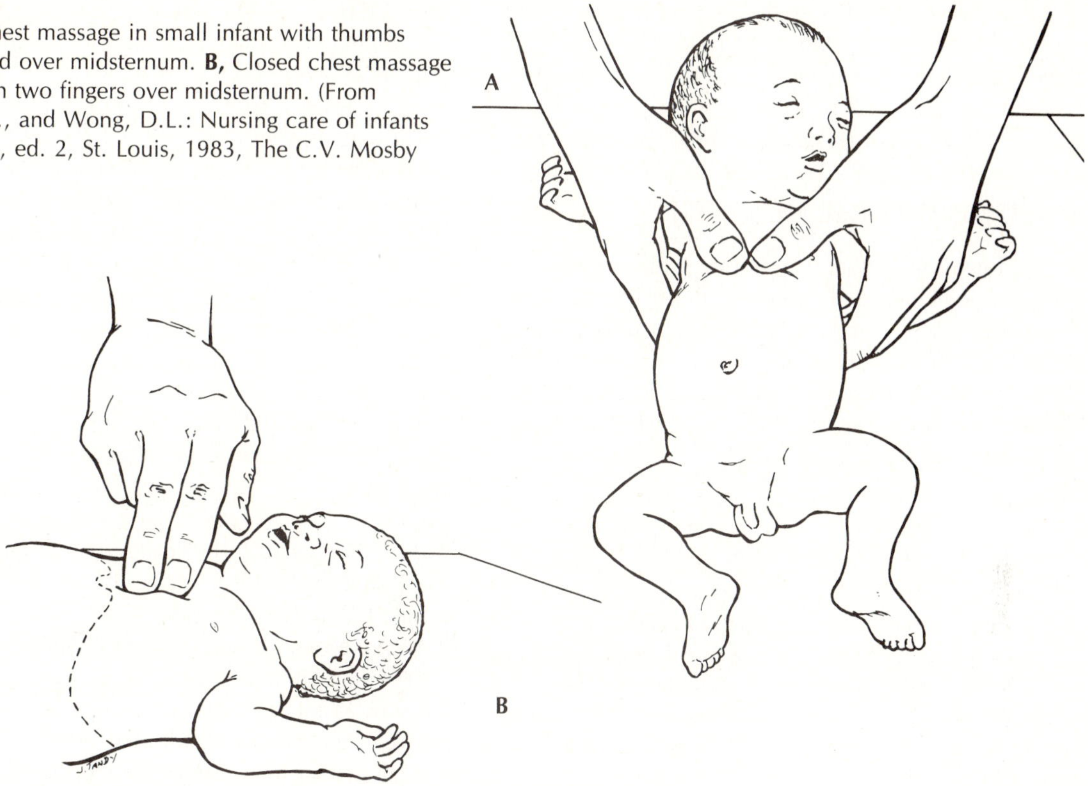

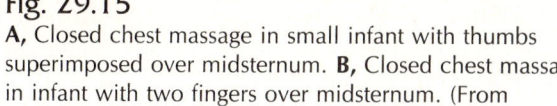

Fig. 29.15
A, Closed chest massage in small infant with thumbs superimposed over midsternum. **B,** Closed chest massage in infant with two fingers over midsternum. (From Whaley, L.F., and Wong, D.L.: Nursing care of infants and children, ed. 2, St. Louis, 1983, The C.V. Mosby Co.)

If chest wall does not rise and infant's vital responses do not improve in 30 seconds, consider airway obstruction. Infant may need laryngoscopy–endotracheal intubation aspiration.

CARDIOPULMONARY RESUSCITATION

Complete apnea signals the need for rapid and vigorous action to prevent cardiac arrest. In such situations nurses must be prepared to initiate action immediately. In anticipation, emergency equipment should be readily available in areas in which respiratory arrest might take place, and the status of this resuscitation equipment should be checked regularly (at least once daily). Regardless of the cause of the arrest, some very basic procedures are carried out, modified somewhat according to the size of the child (Fig. 29.15).

The initial step after cessation of respiration is to palpate peripheral pulses and quickly check the heartbeat. Absence of carotid or temporal pulse is considered sufficient indication to begin external cardiac massage. However, two essential elements determine the safety and efficacy of external cardiac massage: (1) the infant's spine must be supported during compression of the sternum, and (2) external pressure must be forceful but not traumatic.

After rapid ascertainment and restoration of a patent airway by removal of foreign material and secretions (if indicated), cardiac massage is initiated. Sternal compression is applied to small infants with both thumbs on the midsternum while joining the fingers of both hands behind the infant's back. It is best applied from the superior direction with the operator at the infant's head to minimize the chance of damage that might occur to the liver or spleen if applied from an inferior position. For an older infant a firm board is placed beneath the spine and pressure is applied with two fingers on the midsternum, exerting a sharp downward thrust. For children over age 5 years pressure is applied with the heel of one or both hands at the junction of the middle and lower two thirds of the sternum. The depth of compression is adapted to the size of the child—infants, 0.5 to 0.75 in; young children, 0.75 to 1 in; and older children, 1.5 to 2 in. The location, rate, and depth for adolescents are the same as for adults.

External massage is administered at a rate of 100 to 120 times/min in the newborn and 60 to 80 times/min in older children. Cardiac compression should be interspersed with ventilation, administered by the mouth-to-mouth method or artificial ventilator, at a ratio of one breath for five to eight compressions. Massage is continued unil there are signs of recovery as evidenced by palpable peripheral pulses, return of pupils to normal size, and the disappearance of mottling and cyanosis.

POSITIONING THE NEWBORN

Positioning the infant in respiratory distress must be carefully individualized in the nursing care plan. The infant's particular needs are considered: the amount of secretions; the maturity of gag, swallow, and cough reflexes; and the maturity of neuromuscular and skeletal systems. Following are the technique and rationale for positioning the infant:

Technique	Rationale
1. Flex and abduct infant's arms and place at his sides.	1. Weight of arms is kept off chest. Facilitates greater thoracic expansion.
2. Avoid use of diapers, or pin diapers on loosely.	2. Assists infant's efforts to utilize abdominal muscles for respirations.
3. Extend neck slightly to "sniffing" position or leave neonate flat.	3. Lessens tracheal obstruction by extending trachea. Prevents hyperextension obstruction from low palate or macroglossia. Overextension may make it difficult if not impossible for infant to swallow secretions. Hyperextension also causes apposition of vocal cords so that glottis is considerably smaller than otherwise. This impedes entry of air into larynx and from there to rest of respiratory tract.
4. Check towel placement frequently.	4. Obstruction may occur from flexion or overextension of neck (towel under head).
5. Turn from side to side every 1 or 2 hours.	5. Facilitates drainage of pulmonary secretions and prevents skin breakdown.

NOTE: There is no need to elevate the head of the mattress. Abdominal contents in a normal abdomen offer no difficulty to diaphragmatic movement. Furthermore, with the head elevated pulmonary secretions are more likely to pool if head of bed is elevated.

OXYGEN THERAPY

The administration of oxygen must be as carefully monitored as that of any drug. Oxygen overdosage results in tissue damage. The histologic change noted in pulmonary tissue is a thickening of the alveolar walls, epithelial lining, and basement membranes (bronchopulmonary dysplasia). In the retina, oxygen overdosage causes vasoconstriction and, later, ischemia. About 2 months after the cessation of oxygen therapy, these retinal vessels dilate, leading to edema, scarring, and detachment. Eyesight may be slightly to severely impaired, or total blindness (retrolental fibroplasia) may ensue.

Oxygen may be vital to an infant at birth for hypoxemia, to counteract acidosis, to promote pulmonary blood flow and closure of the ductus arteriosus, and to maintain capillary integrity.

Hypoxemia. An infant is presumed to be hypoxemic if he shows symptoms such as the following: cyanosis, the most frequent indication, and indirect indications, such as bradycardia—heart rate of less than 100 beats/min, hypothermia—temperature of less than 35.5° C (95.9° F), prolonged periods of apnea—apneic episodes of greater than 15 seconds, or anemia. Necrotizing enterocolitis (NEC) is a possible sequel if the infant survives.

Clinical measurements may be insufficient to determine oxygen need, since some noncyanotic (pink) infants are hypoxemic. Laboratory assessments are essential for accurate evaluation of blood gases and acid-base status.

Regulating oxygen dosage. Oxygen dosage should be sufficient to relieve cyanosis. If the infant has a cyanotic episode, the nurse may administer 100% oxygen by mask or bag for short periods. Blood is drawn for blood gas determination for accurate regulation of oxygen therapy. The only rational basis for oxygen therapy is the level of the arterial Po_2. No hospital should administer oxygen continuously to (premature) infants without the capacity to perform blood gas analyses. This capacity has become far more widespread in the last 5 years, even among smaller hospitals. Laboratory values used to determine dosage are the following:

1. Blood pH between 7.35 and 7.44
2. Arterial Po_2 between 50 and 70 mm Hg (For the very premature infant, 90 mm Hg may be too high and may expose him to sequelae of oxygen overdosage. Although the precise figure is unknown, an arterial Po_2 of 65 mm Hg should be safer.)

3. Arterial hemoglobin saturation between 85% and 90% (based on fetal maturity)

Newer methods of continuous monitoring of oxygen tension are available; these methods permit moment-to-moment changes in administration of oxygen.

Methods of oxygen administration

Incubator. The maintenance of a high and constant level of oxygen in an incubator is almost impossible because (1) the mechanism cannot achieve concentrations beyond 60% to 70% ambient oxygen and (2) opening of the incubator's portholes or lid rapidly dissipates oxygen into the room.

Plastic hood. The plastic hood is suitable for administering oxygen warmed to 31° to 34° C and humidified. In addition, it is useful within incubators. Portholes or lid can be opened without affecting oxygen levels within the hood (see Fig. 37.34).

Another advantage is that the plastic hood is practical outside the incubator when the infant is being treated. An overhead radiant heater maintains a thermoneutral environment for the infant at this time.

HEEL STICK

In some institutions, the nurse is responsible for performing the heel stick (Fig. 29.16) to obtain blood for the determination of the neonate's glucose level and hematocrit. The procedure is as follows*:

1. Cleanse heel by rubbing with 70% alcohol.
2. Dry with sterile cotton pledget or gauze square.
3. Using Bard-Parker no. 11 or Redi-Lance blade, puncture heel deep enough to get free flow of blood.
4. Discard first drop.
5. Quickly collect blood into appropriate capillary tubes.

The tests for phenylketonuria (PKU), galactosemia, and hypothyroidism are done on blood obtained by heel stick.

*Residual scars and corn formation may be sequelae if this procedure is not done in the proper area of the heel.

INTRAMUSCULAR INJECTION

The usual medication ordered for neonates is vitamin K_1 (Aquamephyton, 0.5 mg) (Fig. 29.17).

Injections must be placed in muscles large enough to accommodate the medication, yet major nerves and blood vessels must be avoided. The muscles of neonates may not tolerate more than 0.5 ml. The preferred site for neonates is the vastus lateralis, although the rectus femoris muscle can be used also. These two muscles are free of important nerves and blood vessels, with the exception of the femoral artery on the medial aspect of the thigh. The vastus lateralis muscle is the larger of the two and is well developed in the neonate.

NOTE: The posterior gluteal muscle is very small, poorly developed, and dangerously close to the sciatic nerve that occupies a larger proportion of space in infants than in older children. Therefore it is not recommended as an injection site until the child has been walking for at least a year. The gluteal musculature develops with locomotion. Fig. 29.18, *A*, illustrates the location of the preferred intramuscular injection site for neonates.

Neonates offer little, if any, resistance to injections. Although they squirm and may be difficult to hold in position if they are awake, they can usually be re-

Fig. 29.16

A, Puncture sites *(x)* on sole of infant's foot for heel-stick samples of capillary blood. (Adapted from Babson, S.G., and Benson, R.C.: Management of high-risk pregnancy and intensive care of the neonate, ed. 2, St. Louis, 1971, The C.V. Mosby Co.)

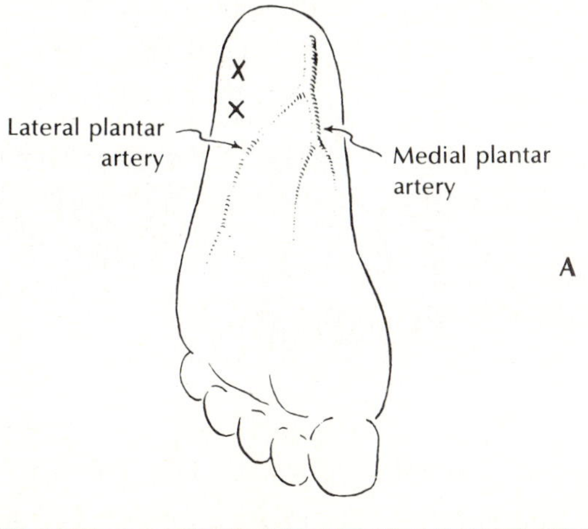

Continued.

Fig. 29.16, cont'd

B, Neonate with foot wrapped for warmth to increase blood flow to extremity before heel stick. Note his posture, linea nigra, and increased pigmentation of genital area caused by maternal hormones of pregnancy. He is smiling. **C,** Bandaid is applied to site of heel stick.

B

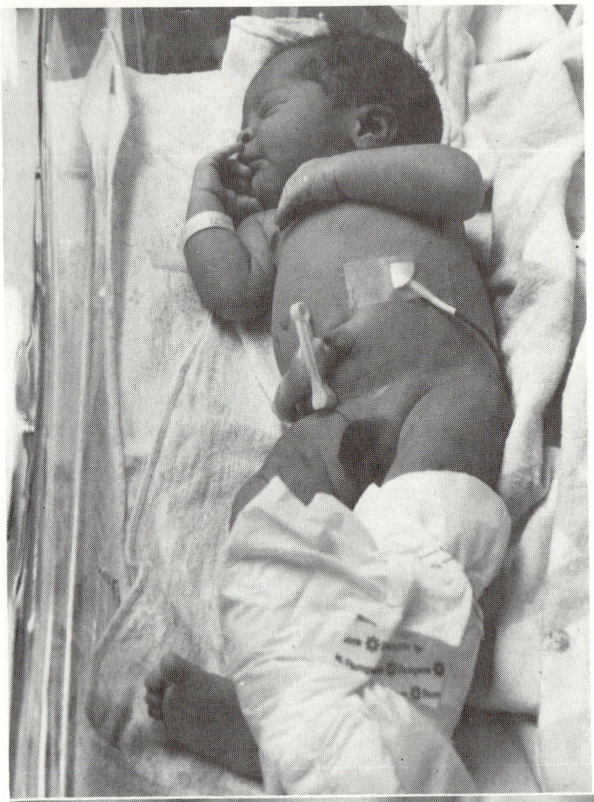

C

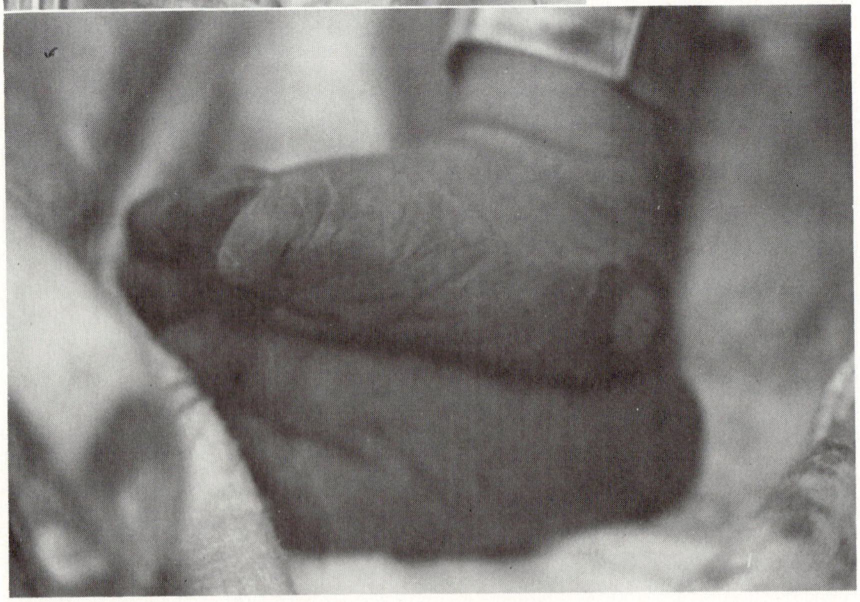

Fig. 29.17

A, Vitamin K (Aquamephyton) container is checked against physician's order. **B,** Nurse has shaken medication to bottom of vial. She protects her fingers as she snaps off top with a rapid wrist action. **C,** To avoid drawing small glass shards into syringe, nurse uses a filter needle to withdraw medication. **D,** Nurse replaces filter needle with short, small-gauge, tuberculin needle. **E,** Nurse records medication she has given on neonate's chart.

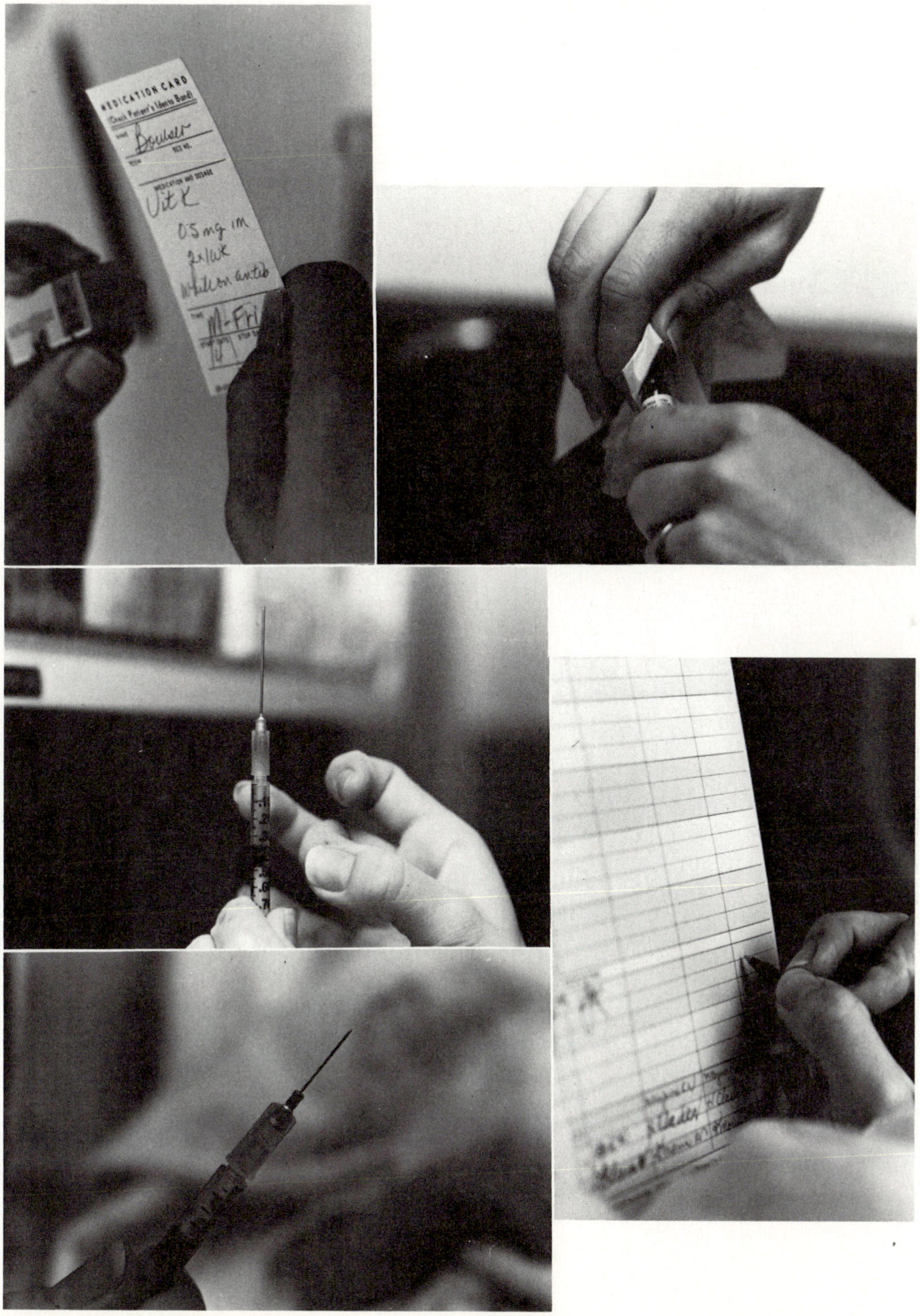

A

B

C

E

D

Fig. 29.18
A, Acceptable intramuscular site for children. *X,* Injection site; *Y,* alternate injection site.
B, Infant's leg stabilized for intramuscular injection. (From Whaley, L.F., and Wong, D.L.: Nursing care of infants and children, ed. 2, St. Louis, 1983, The C.V. Mosby Co.)

A

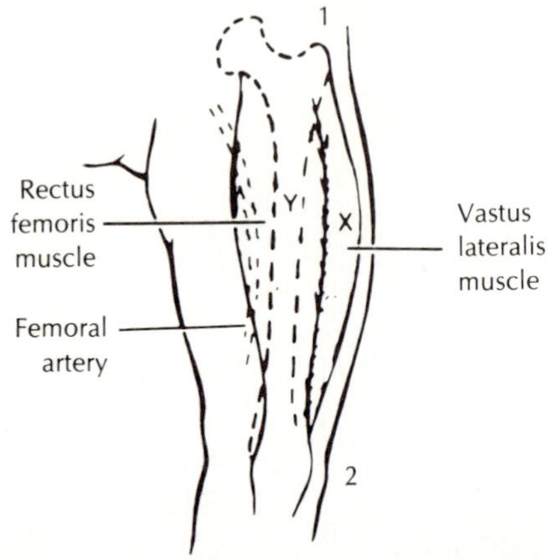

VASTUS LATERALIS MUSCLE
Landmarks
1 Greater trochanter
2 Knee
Injection site: lateral aspect of muscle mass in middle third of distance between landmarks; injected at 45 degree angle in direction of knee

B

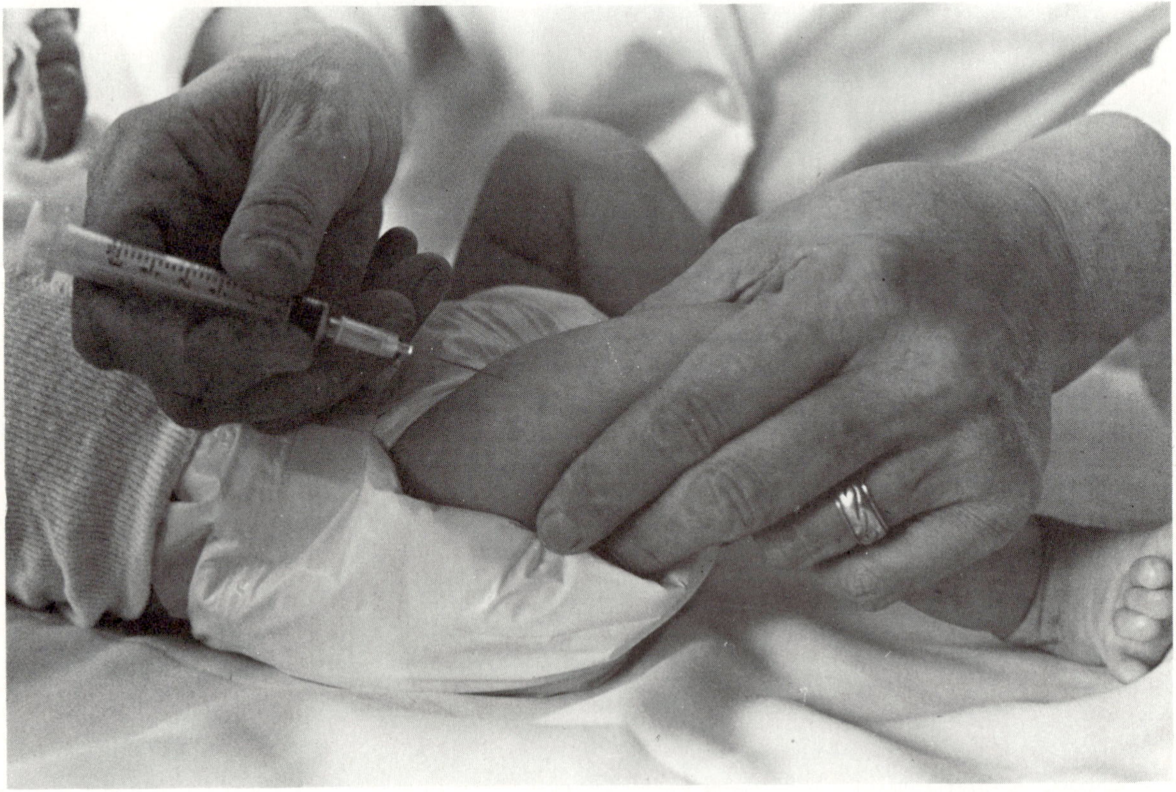

strained without assistance from a second person when the nurse is skilled. The muscle mass of the thigh to be injected is firmly grasped in one hand to stabilize the limb and compress the muscle mass for injection with the other hand (Fig. 29.18, *B*).

The dart method for injection is inappropriate when aiming at such a small target. The nurse poises the needle just over the site (without touching the skin) and then inserts the needle with a quick flexion of the wrist.

THERAPY FOR HYPERBILIRUBINEMIA

The goal of therapy for hyperbilirubinemia is to assist the neonate in reducing serum levels of unconjugated bilirubin. To be excreted by the liver, bilirubin must be conjugated (in water-soluble form). In the premature infant especially, body systems are functioning but immature. The conjugation system is overwhelmed, the serum levels of unconjugated bilirubin rise, and the risk of kernicterus increases.

There are two principal methods available to reduce serum bilirubin levels: phototherapy and exchange blood transfusion.

Exchange transfusion (see Chapter 40) is the treatment of choice in the presence of a hemolytic process (isoimmunization) to (1) remove bilirubin (primary purpose), (2) remove potentially hemolyzed red cells, (3) remove the antibodies responsible for hemolysis, and (4) correct anemia. However, the mere presence of the hemolytic process is not an indication for the procedure. Exchange transfusion is performed at various levels of serum bilirubin depending on birth weight or gestational age of the infant or both and on condition of the neonate.

Phototherapy. Bilirubin absorbs light energy that then acts on oxygen (O_2) to form singlet oxygen (O). Singlet oxygen then oxidizes bilirubin into several products, most of which are water soluble. The water-soluble and apparently nontoxic compounds can be converted by the liver for excretion in bile or urine. A newer theory suggests, however, that the singlet oxygen theory is incorrect. Instead, phototherapy is thought to cause photoisomerization of bilirubin in the skin. This photoisomerization changes the configuration of unconjugated bilirubin into stable new isomers that then rapidly bind to albumin and are quickly transported from the capillaries to the liver, where they are processed for excretion.

The distance of the light source from the baby is determined by the intensity of the light. The quantity of photoenergy that strikes the skin will vary inversely with the square of the distance between the skin surface and the light source. It is therefore best not to advise a specific distance. In one unit, for instance, a spotlight that provides an optimal dose of blue light at a distance between 60 and 75 cm (24 and 30 in) from the baby is used. Also, a blue light source has notable disadvantages. First, it is difficult to discern cyanotic or dusky color change. Second, during trials with blue light, a few of the nurses became light-headed and dizzy; one of them was nauseated. This experience is reported in the literature repeatedly. A point worth including is the need to measure with a photometer the quantity of light in the blue spectrum that strikes the skin surface. Stability of fluorescent lamps for 2000 hours is doubtful, the manufacturers' claims notwithstanding. Also, records of the duration of lamp use are notoriously inaccurate. The purchase of a photometer does not represent a large investment; it is extremely worthwhile.

For the hyperbilirubinemic infant, the procedure is as follows:

Technique	Rationale
1. Unclothe infant.	1. Exposes as much skin area as possible to light.
a. Protect infant's eyes with eye patches (Fig. 29.19, *A*).	a. Prevents possible injury to conjunctiva or retina.*
(1) Be sure eyes are closed.	(1) Prevents corneal abrasions.
(2) Check eyes for drainage each shift.	(2) Prevents or allows prompt treatment of purulent conjunctivitis, should it occur.
b. Cover head with stockinette.	b. This precaution is controversial and may differ from hospital to hospital.
c. For diapering, paper face mask may be used after removing the metal nose strip (Fig. 29.19, *B*).	c. This "string bikini" is scanty enough to allow skin exposure, yet sufficient to protect genitalia and bedding. Metal nose strip is heated by the light and can burn the neonate's skin.

*There is suggestive evidence that exposure of the eyes to the bright lights of phototherapy units may injure the retina. Exposure to light may alter biorhythms.

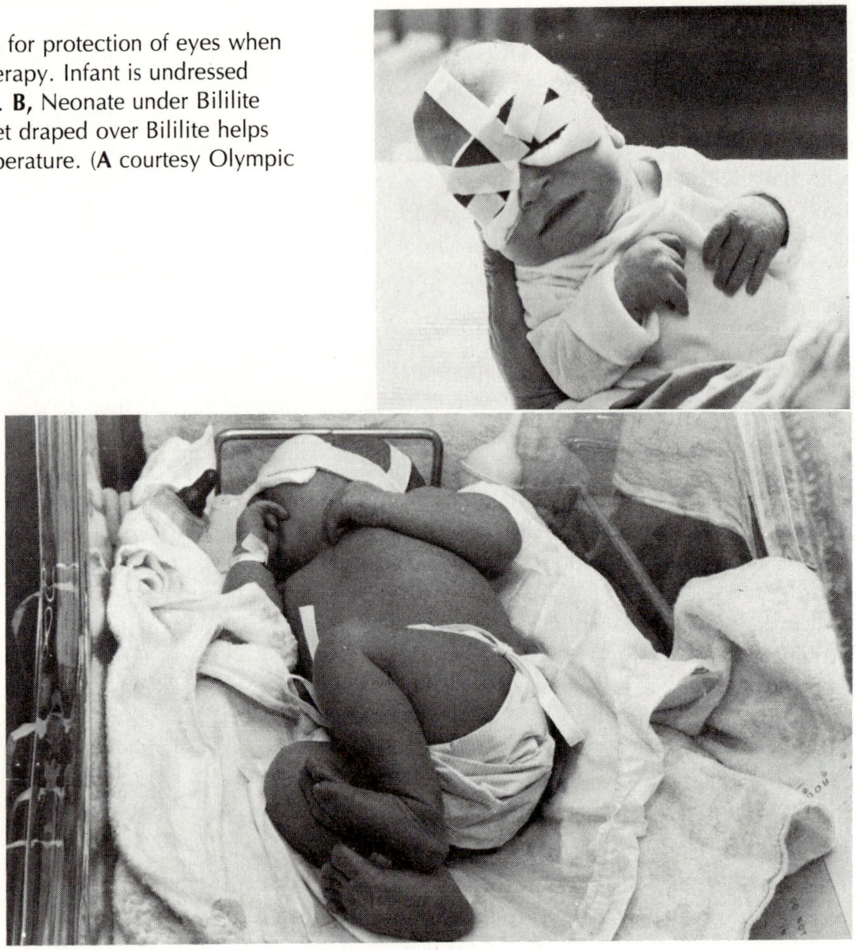

A

B

Fig. 29.19
A, Placement of eye patches for protection of eyes when infant is undergoing light therapy. Infant is undressed before being put under light. **B,** Neonate under Bililite wearing a face mask. Blanket draped over Bililite helps neonate maintain body temperature. (**A** courtesy Olympic Medical Corp., Seattle.)

Technique	Rationale
2. Monitor skin temperature. If infant is in incubator, temperature dial on control panel* may need to be turned to maintain proper temperature.	2. Prevents hyperthermia or hypothermia.
3. Periodically and especially with parents' visits discontinue phototherapy for few minutes and remove eye patches. Unwrap eyes and hold for feeding.	3. Necessary for normal psychosocial contact. Infant may visualize his contacts. Parent has opportunity to look into baby's eyes—a necessary activity to develop attachment to infant.
4. Observe infant's behavior a. Eating and sleeping patterns. b. Loose greenish stools, green urine. c. Priapism.	4. Effect of phototherapy on biologic rhythms is uncertain. Data base is needed to differentiate common side effects (loose greenish stools or green urine) from other problems that need appropriate treatment.
5. Replace fluid losses by increasing fluid volume offered to neonate by 25%; protect skin from excoriation.	5. Prevent dehydration; insensible and intestinal water loss is increased during phototherapy. Prevents infection of broken-down skin areas

*All electric equipment should be grounded, free of defects, and operationally sound to maximize therapeutic effectiveness and to prevent electric shock or burn to the neonate (or to the nurse).

Bronze baby syndrome has occurred in some neonates receiving phototherapy. The serum, urine, and skin turn bronze (brown-black) in color. The etiology is unclear. Almost all neonates recover without sequelae.

RESTRAINING NEONATE

The purpose of restraining an infant include (1) protecting the infant from injury and (2) facilitating examinations and limiting discomfort during tests, procedures, and specimen collections. When restraining an infant, there are special considerations one must keep in mind:

1. Check the infant frequently.
2. Apply restraints, and check them frequently to prevent skin irritation and circulatory impairment.
3. Maintain proper body alignment.
4. Apply restraints without use of knots or pins if possible. If knots are necessary, they are the kind that can be released quickly. Pins are used with care to prevent puncture wounds and pressure areas—and to prevent the infant's swallowing one of them.
5. If the infant is in an incubator, secure him to the mattress to protect his extremities, especially when the lid is raised or the mattress moved.

Restraining techniques include the following.

Mummy. The mummy technique is used for the stronger, more vigorous newborn. It is used for examinations, treatments, or specimen collections that involve the head and neck.

Equipment includes a blanket and one or two large safety pins (Fig. 29.20, *A*).

Fig. 29.20
A, Device to restrain infant during examination or treatments.

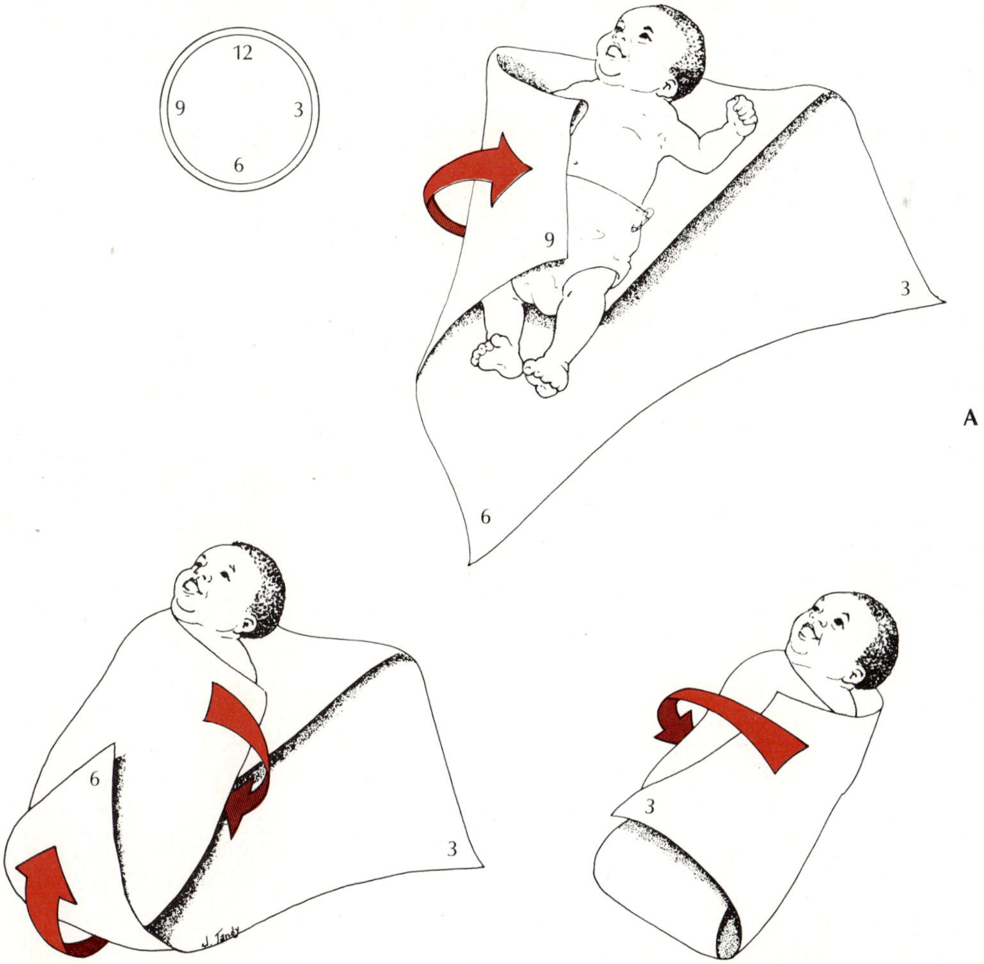

Continued.

Fig. 29.20, cont'd
B, Clove-hitch restraints in place. **C,** Clove-hitch device. This restraint does not tighten after its application. Apply padding before device. **D,** Position for lumbar puncture. **E,** Position of jugular venipuncture. Neonate is "mummied."

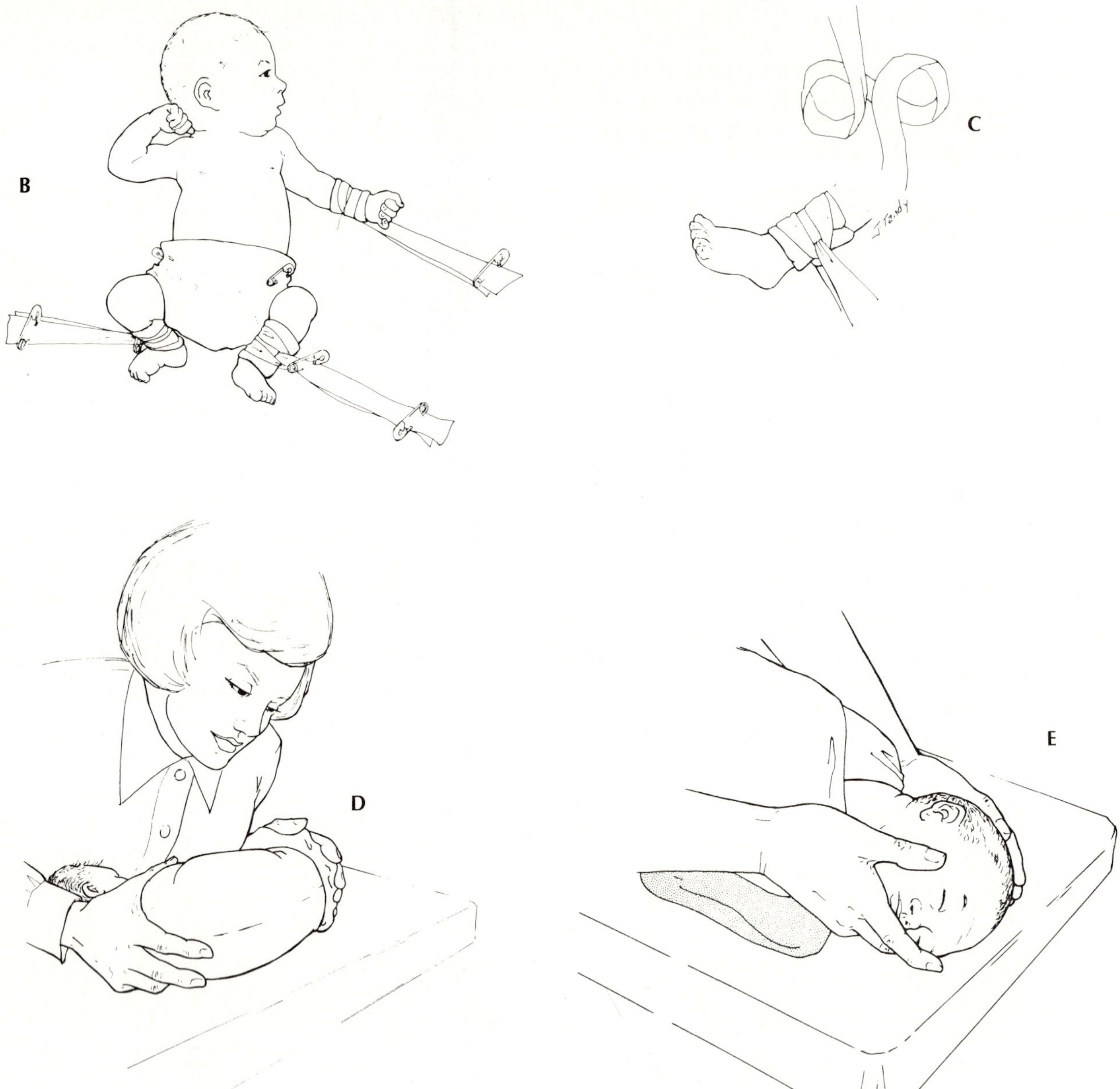

The procedure is as follows:

1. Spread blanket on flat surface; crib should suffice.
2. Fold over one corner (12-o'clock position).
3. Lay newborn on blanket so that neck is at fold.
4. Fold corner at 9-o'clock position over right shoulder; tuck that corner securely under infant's left side.
5. Bring corner at 6-o'clock position up over feet and tuck it either under infant's left side or, if long enough, fold over blanket, crossing it under infant's chin.
6. Swing corner at 3-clock position snugly over infant and fold under his right side. Pin this corner into place.

Extremity restraints. Restraining the infant's extremities is a technique used to control movements of his arms or legs.

Equipment includes gauze strips or wide strips of soft material and cotton wadding; pins are optional.

The procedure depends on which one of the many kinds of extremity restraints available is used. Examples are as follows:

1. *Pad extremity with cotton wadding*. Fold one end of gauze strip over the extremity and pin. Pin other end to mattress.

2. *Clove-hitch restraint*. Arrange strip of long, 5 cm (2 in) wide material as shown in Fig. 29.20, *B* and *C*. Loop device over extremity, which has been padded with cotton; pin loose ends to mattress. Clove hitch does not tighten even if infant's movements tug on restraint.

Towel support. Although the towel support is not a true restraint, it serves to control the infant's position and movement. The towel may be rolled and placed at the infant's back or sides or folded and placed under his neck or upper back. A towel support has the following advantages:

1. It provides comfort and security by stabilizing the infant's position.
2. It maintains positioning to assist respiratory effort and gastrointestinal functions and prevent skin breakdown.
3. It prevents the infant from rolling against the incubator wall, where he may lose heat by convection.
4. It prevents the infant from falling out of the incubator when the lid is lifted.

Restraint without appliance. The nurse may restrain the infant with the use of hands and body. Fig. 29.20, *D*, illustrates restraining the infant in position for lumbar puncture.

ASSISTING WITH COLLECTION OF BLOOD SPECIMEN: VENIPUNCTURE

Technique	Rationale
1. Position and restrain infant. a. Femoral venipuncture: Position child in frog posture; place hands over infant's knees. Avoid pressure of fingers over inner aspect of thigh because vein in this area may be occluded. b. External jugular venipuncture (Fig. 29.20, *E*): "Mummy" infant as necessary. Lower infant's head over rolled towel, edge of table, or your knee, and stabilize. c. Handle infant gently; talk quietly to him during procedure.	1. Facilitates venipuncture. Prevents tissue trauma. Prevents cold stress.
2. a. After venipuncture, apply pressure over area with sterile gauze for 1 to 3 minutes. b. If jugular vein was used, raise infant's head and shoulders while applying pressure. c. Comfort infant as necessary.	2. Prevents leakage of additional blood into tissues or formation of hematoma (later this may result in hyperbilirubinemia). If infant is vigorous, direct pressure, restraint, and comforting prevent activity that could initiate or prolong bleeding.
3. Observe infant for 1 hour.	3. Can detect further bleeding (oozing, hematoma). Enclosed bleeding can lead to hypovolemic shock, hyperbilirubinemia, or both.
4. Record site, amount of blood taken, reason for specimen, infant response.	4. Allows ongoing evaluation and adjustment of care plans.

USING URINE SPECIMEN COLLECTORS

A variety of urine specimen collection bags are available, usually with instructions accompanying them. Although the following directions are specific to the U-Bag (Hollister Inc., Chicago), they are generally applicable to many other types:

Technique	Rationale
1. Separate infant's legs. Make sure pubic and perineal area is clean, dry, and free from mucus. Do not apply powders, oils, or lotions to skin.	1. Ensures leak-proof seal. Decreases chance of contamination.
2. Remove protective paper, exposing hypoallergenic adhesive (Fig. 29.21, *A*).	2. Exposes adhesive. Decreases chance of allergic reaction.

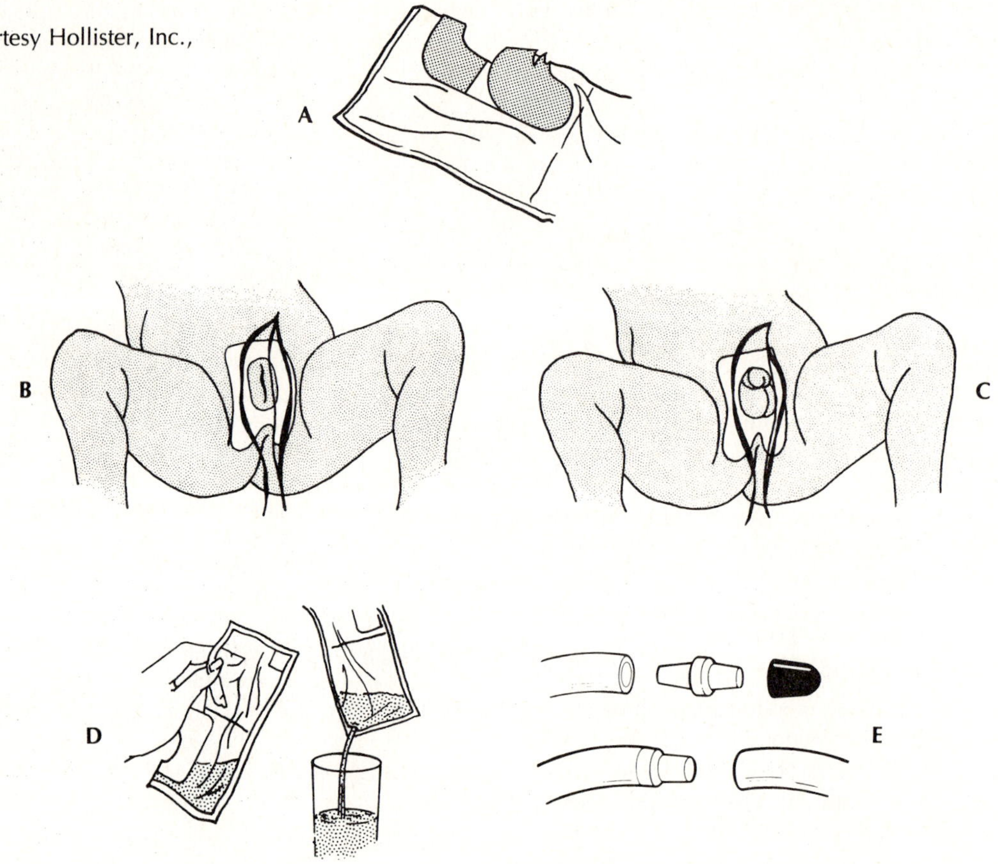

Fig. 29.21
Hollister U-Bag. (Courtesy Hollister, Inc., Chicago.)

Technique	Rationale
3. For girls, stretch perineum to flatten skin folds. Press adhesive firmly to skin all around urinary meatus and vagina. (NOTE: Start with narrow portion of butterfly-shaped adhesive patch.) *Be sure to start at bridge of skin separating rectum from vagina and work upward* (Fig 29.21, *B*). For boys, tuck penis and scrotum through aperture of collector before removing protective paper from adhesive. Fit bag over penis, and press flaps firmly to perineum, making sure entire adhesive coating is firmly attached to skin with no puckering of adhesive (Fig. 29.21, *C*).	3. Ensures leak-proof seal. Decreases chance of contamination from urine and stool.
4. To drain, hold bag in left hand. Tilt bag so that urine is away from blue tab. Remove tab and drain in clean receptacle (Fig. 29.21, *D*).	4. Facilitates emptying without use of scissors, which can contaminate or be contaminated.

Apply the 24-hour U-Bag in the manner just described. Direct the drainage into a receptacle. The collection tube can be shortened or capped (Fig. 29.21, *E*). See directions accompanying the bag.

BIRTH CERTIFICATE

For an example of a birth certificate, see Appendix M.

Evaluative Criteria for Nursing Actions

NORMAL NEWBORN: FIRST DAY OF LIFE

Physiologic adjustment to extrauterine existence on the first day of life* involves the following:

1. Respirations: airway is open, and respirations are stabilized at 30 to 60/min, with short periods of apnea by 6 to 10 hours. Breathing is quiet (no grunting or wheezing). Chest and abdomen rise and fall in synchronized motion, and there is no sternal retraction. Infant breathes through nose; nares do not flare on inspiration. Cyanosis may be present in hands and feet.
2. Temperature: infant's axillary temperature is stabilized by twelfth hour and maintained between 36.5° and 37° C (97.6° to 98.6° F).
3. Heart rate: heart rate (between 120 and 160 beats/min) and regularity in rhythm are stabilized by twelfth hour; rate may drop to 100 beats/min in deep sleep but returns immediately with activity. It increases with stress and activity. Most soft murmurs heard during neonatal period are functional and without pathologic significance.
4. Blood pressure: systolic pressure is 60 to 80 mm Hg; diastolic pressure is 40 to 50 mm Hg.
5. Feeding: acceptance and swallowing of nutrients and fluids are satisfactory by twelfth hour. Amount of regurgitation of mucus or nutrients and fluids is within normal limits by twenty-fourth hour.
6. Cord: there is adequate healing of cord (i.e., no oozing of blood or evidence of inflammation).
7. Penis: there is adequate healing of penis if circumcision was performed (i.e., no excessive bleeding or evidence of inflammation).
8. Defecation: meconium stool may be passed at birth or any time thereafter until twenty-fourth hour.
9. Urination: some infants void at birth; most void by twelfth to twenty-fourth hour after birth.
10. Appearance: infant's appearance and activity (reflexes and behavior patterns) are within normal limits.

Care-taking activities for the first day of life are as follows:

1. Plan of care
   a. Involves skilled personnel and adequate facilities to ensure continuous assessment, protection against infection or trauma, and care in case of emergency
   b. Reflects consideration of needs of particular infant with unique history, constitution, and membership in particular family group
   c. Includes complete medical and nursing records
2. Assessment of infant by twenty-fourth hour by professional personnel reveals satisfactory adjustment of infant and his physical status.
3. Initial feeding of infant is done by sixth hour. Mother begins breast feeding at birth (first wakeful period), or infant is given water by nursery personnel.
4. Initial bath is given once infant's temperature is stabilized, and routine of hygienic care is established.

Parenthood needs on the first day of life involve, initial and subsequent contacts between parents and infant to promote close parent-child ties (see Chapter 32).

DAYS 2 TO 14

Physiologic responses for day 2 to 14 are as follows:

1. Respirations: respirations are stabilized within normal limits (30 to 60/min). Mother is aware of normal variations in breathing rhythm and rate. Mother is able to keep infant's airway clear by positioning infant on his side in bassinet or crib to facilitate drainage or, if choking occurs, by turning infant onto his abdomen with his head down and removing mucus with bulb syringe.
2. Temperature: infant's temperature is maintained within normal limits. Mother becomes adept at using thermometer and is aware of influence of heat, cold, and dehydration on infant's temperature.
3. Blood pressure is maintained within normal limits.
4. Cord: healing of cord continues; cord drops off within first 2 weeks. There is no evidence of inflammation.
5. Penis: healing of circumcised penis continues. Yellowish exudate forms over glans penis; incised site remains tender for 2 or 3 days.
6. Defecation: number of stools varies on basis of the type of feeding—breast or bottle. Stools go through a transitional process from meconium to a greenish-yellow, curdy stool, to a yellow, more formed stool if mother is bottle feeding; or they remain golden yellow and loose if mother is breast feeding.
7. Urination: infant voids six to ten times in 24 hours; urine is pale and straw colored.
8. Weight: newborn loses up to 10% of birth weight in first few days (if birth weight was over 4256 g

*For a discussion of the first 2 hours of life, see Chapter 22.

[9 lb, 8 oz] neonate may lose up to 15%). Birth weight is regained by end of second week (tripled by end of first year, quadrupled by end of second year).

9. Appearance and behavior
   a. Molding of head lessens and head assumes a more rounded contour by second or third day.
   b. Icterus neonatorum begins 24 hours or later after (in ± 50%), reaches a peak on fourth or fifth day, and then subsides and disappears within 7 days of onset.
   c. Melanin in skin responds to light, and color tone changes from ruddy tones at birth to black, yellow, brown, or pink, depending on amount of melanin present.
   d. Rashes are of a transitory nature; skin may appear dry and may peel, especially in skin folds.
   e. Infant sleeps about 17 hr/day, wakens for feedings, and is alert and responsive. Neonate's cry is lusty, sustained, and demanding in tone. Neonate smiles and moves arms and legs in response to human voice. Muscle tone is good.

Care-taking activities for days 2 to 14 are as follows:

1. Sources of readily available emergency care are known to parents.
2. Protection is continued against infection and trauma.
3. Intake of nutrients and fluids is adequate for growth and hydration (see Chapter 30).
4. Parents are aware of and practice necessary activities of infant hygiene.
   a. Hygienic care and examination of infant are practiced as a daily routine. Mother (father) is aware of normal characteristics and responses of infant.
   b. Parent practices safe techniques for bathing and changing infant, including care of scalp, eyes, nose, mouth, cord, nails, body creases, buttocks, and genitalia.
   c. Parent is knowledgeable about dressing infant and about care of infant's clothing.
   d. Parent is aware of measures used to control discomforts (e.g., diaper rash, prickly heat rash).
5. Regular evaluation is made of degree to which desired outcomes have been attained and of tasks still to be accomplished.

Parenthood tasks for days 2 to 14 are as follows:

1. Parents become increasingly aware of infant's behavior as "cues" for type of care needed (food, fluids, easing of discomfort, reassurance, cuddling, exercise, changing, social contacts, and so on).
2. Parents become adept at care-taking activities.
3. Parents become knowledgeable as to normal vs. abnormal response of infant and where and how to seek assistance for infant problems and parenthood concerns.

DAYS 15 TO 28

Physiologic responses for days 15 to 28 are as follows:

1. Respirations are stabilized within normal limits, and lungs sound normal. Parents are aware of signs and symptoms of respiratory distress, whom to call, and what to communicate. Family practices protective measures to minimize respiratory tract infections.
2. Temperature: infant's temperature is maintained within normal limits—36.5° to 37° C (97.6° to 98.6° F). Parents are aware of signs and symptoms of fever, what measures to institute to reduce fever, and whom to contact for assistance.
3. Umbilicus: umbilicus may protrude slightly; parents are aware of its cause and effect. No treatment is necessary; however, culturally motivated care is accepted and supervised.
4. Defecation: infant establishes own pattern, varying from three to four times a day to once or twice a week. Stools are yellowish brown and of a soft consistency.
5. Urination: voiding six to ten times a day continues; urine is pale and straw colored.
6. Appearance and behavior
   a. Growth and weight are normal for infant's age and body structure.
   b. Vision and hearing are normal.
   c. Skin is soft with no evidence of bruising; there is no excoriation of buttocks or creases.
   d. Muscle tone is good.
   e. There is no evidence of malformation of or injury to bones or joints.
   f. Infant is alert and responsive (he smiles, may coo, follows people and objects with his eyes, and is desirous of stimulation and social contacts).
   g. Sleep pattern is established (infant is awake between one or two feedings; fussy period may be consistent).

Care-taking activities for days 15 to 28 are as follows:

1. Plan for periodic assessment of infant is established, with either a private physician or a well-baby clinic.
2. Protection against infection or trauma continues.
3. Parents are knowledgeable as to community sources of assistance for infant and for themselves (see Appendix C).

4. Routine observation of infant's growth and developmental needs is established as component of family's daily care of infant.
5. Child appears healthy and satisfied with nutritional intake.
6. Child appears clean, and skin is in good condition; routine of care has been established, and use has been made of these care-taking activities as modes of expression of parent-child relationships. There are opportunities for increasing socialization of infant with other family members and for verbal, tactile, and visual stimulation of infant.

Parenthood tasks for days 15 to 28 are as follows:

1. Child is accepted as an individual with persisting infantile dependency needs.
2. Child is also accepted as an integral part of the family unit.

References and Readings

American Academy of Pediatrics, Committee on Fetus and Newborn: Report of the Ad Hoc Task Force on Circumcision, Pediatrics, **56:**610, 1975.

Boyer, D.: Routine circumcision of the newborn: reasonable precaution or unnecessary risk? J. Nurs. Midwife. **25**(6):27, 1980.

Davis, V.: The structure and function of brown adipose tissue in the neonate, J.O.G.N. Nurs. **9**(6):368, 1980.

Ellison, S., et al.: Sucking in the newborn infant during the first hour of life, J. Nurs. Midwife. **24**(6):18, 1979.

Färdig, J.: A comparison of skin-to-skin contact and radiant heaters in promoting neonatal thermoregulation, J. Nurs. Midwife. **25**(1):19, 1980.

Gairdner, D.: The fate of the foreskin: a study of circumcision, Br. Med. J. **2:**1433, 1949.

Grimes, D.: Routine circumcision of the newborn infant: a reappraisal, Am. J. Obstet. Gynecol. **130:**127, 1978.

Hutton, N., and Schreiner, R.: Urine collection in the neonate: effect of different methods on volume, specific gravity, and glucose, J.O.G.N. Nurs. **9**(13):165, 1980.

Kaplan, L., et al.: Circumcision—an overview, Curr. Prob. Pediatr. p. 1, March 1977.

Kesselman, S.: Circumcision reconsidered: neither harmless nor healthful, routine circumcision no longer seems justified, Childbirth educator **1**(3):43, 1982.

King, L., et al.: Circumcision: rite, ritual or both? Patient Care 12:72, March 15, 1978.

Kirya, C., and Werthmann, M.: Neonatal circumcision and penile dorsal nerve block—a painless procedure, J. Pediatr. 92:998, June 1978.

Korones, S.G.: High-risk newborn infants: the basis for intensive care, ed. 2, St. Louis, 1976, The C.V. Mosby Co.

Lovell, J., and Cox, J.: Maternal attitudes toward circumcision, J. Fam. Pract. **9:**811, Nov. 1979.

McFadden, R.: Decreasing the infant's respiratory compromise during suctioning, Am. J. Nurs. **81**(12):2148, 1981.

Moore, M.: Newborn, family, and nurse, Philadelphia, 1981, W.B. Saunders Co.

Paige, K.: The ritual of circumcision, Hum. Nature **1:**42, 1978.

Patel, H.: The problem of routine circumcision? Can. Med. Assoc. p. 576, Sept. 10, 1966.

Perry, D.: The umbilical cord: transcultural care and customs, J. Nurs. Midwife. **27**(4):25, 1982.

Preston, E.: Whither the foreskin? A consideration of routine neonatal circumcision, J.A.M.A.,**213**(11):1853, 1970.

Strohback, M.E., and Kratina, S.: Diaper versus bag specimens: a comparison of urine specific gravity values, M.C.N. **7**(3):198, 1982.

Styer, G., and Freeh, K.: Feeding infants with cleft lip and/or palate, J.O.G.N. Nurs. **10**(5):329, 1981.

Tobiason, S.: Touching is for everyone, Am. J. Nurs. **81**(4):728, 1981.

Vanderzanden, E.: Anticipatory guidance for the first two months of life. J. Nurs. Midwife. **24**(5):28, 1979.

Wallerstein, E.: Circumcision: an American health fallacy, New York, 1980, Springer Publishing Co.

Wayland, J., and Higgins, P.: Neonatal circumcision: a teaching plan to better inform parents, Nurse Pract., **7**(6):26, 1982.

Whaley, L., and Wong, D.: Nursing care of infants and children, ed. 2, St. Louis, 1983, The C.V. Mosby Co.

Whitner, W., and Thompson, M.: The influence of bathing on the infant's body temperature, Nurs. Res. **19:**30, 1970.

Williams, C., and Oliver, T.: Nursery routines and staphylococcal colonization of the newborn, J. Pediatr. **44:**640, 1969.

Yu, V.: Body position and gastric emptying, Arch. Dis. Child. **50:**500, 1975.

30

Newborn Nutrition and Feeding

- **Infant Development and Its Relationship to Feeding**
  - Physical growth
  - Physiologic development
  - Neuromuscular development
  - Psychosocial development
- **Nutrient Needs of Infants**
  - Calories
  - Protein and amino acids
  - Fats
  - Carbohydrates
  - Water
  - Vitamins
  - Minerals
- **Breast Feeding**
  - Maternal nutritional needs
  - Impact of maternal diet on milk composition
  - Composition of human milk
  - Counseling the Breast-Feeding Mother
    - Preparation
    - The technique
    - Duration of breast feeding
    - Care of breasts
  - Common Problems and How to Avoid Them
    - Engorged breasts
    - Sore nipples
    - Plugged ducts
    - Infection
    - Leaking
    - Failure to thrive in the breast-feeding infant
    - Relactation and induced lactation
    - Breast pumping
- **Formula Feeding**
  - Types of commercial formulas
  - Evaporated milk formulas
  - Goat's milk
  - Soy formulas
  - Special formulas
  - Preparation of commercial formulas
  - Skim milk
  - Bottle-feeding techniques
    - Common problems
- **Introduction of Solids**
- **Selected Problems**
  - Overweight and obesity
  - Atherosclerosis
  - Hypertension
- **General Guidelines for Feeding the Normal Infant**
  - Initial oral feeding
  - First 6 months
  - After 6 months
- **Nutritional Screening and Assessment of Infants**
  - Children at nutritional risk
- **Nutritional Intervention in Clinical Practice**

Prenatal care is incomplete unless the expectant family is prepared to care for the infant. Infant feeding is one major task that will need attention immediately after birth. The first decision that parents need to make about feeding their infant is whether to breast feed, bottle feed, or combine the two. Early in pregnancy, information should be provided on all of these options; if this is done, an informed decision can be made.

The expectant parents need to understand that there is a relationship between food and health. They should be given basic information about their infant's nutritional needs and how these relate to breast milk, formula, or solid foods. The prenatal period is the best time to find out what opinions on infant feeding both mother and father already have so that appropriate attitudes can be reinforced and inappropriate ones can be corrected before it is actually time to feed the baby. After the baby is born, feeding practices should be examined, modified where necessary, and reinforced during visits for health care.

Infant Development and Its Relationship to Feeding

PHYSICAL GROWTH

While individual children have their own genetically predetermined growth patterns, growth proceeds in an orderly and predictable fashion. Parents are interested in their child's growth so discussion of this topic is often a good starting point for effective communication with parents.

A few basic facts about growth of full-term infants are worth remembering for clinical use (Pipes, 1981). The typical infant will generally double his birth weight by the age of 5 months and triple it in 1 year. Most infants regain their birth weight by 10 days after delivery after an initial small loss of weight associated with reduction in body fluids. Weight loss of up to 10% of birth weight is viewed as acceptable although smaller infants generally lose less than larger ones. Length increases about 50% during the first year but doubling of birth length does not occur until about 4 years of age. Head circumference also increases rapidly during the first year in conjunction with rapid growth of the brain.

Body composition gradually changes during the prenatal and postnatal periods. The fat content of the body increases slowly in the early fetal period and more rapidly in the last trimester. At birth the normal infant has a body composed of about 16% fat (by weight) (Widdowson and Spray, 1951). Between 2 and 6 months of age, the increase in adipose tissue is more than twice as great as the increase in muscle mass; fat deposition occurs at a steady pace until about 9 months of age. Throughout infancy, girls lay down a greater percentage of weight as fat than boys; this trend continues throughout the remaining developmental years.

Clinical evaluation of physical growth is essential in monitoring the health of children. This task is simplified by the use of growth standards that have been developed for height or length, weight, and head circumference. Normative data are also available for skinfold (fat-fold) thickness and skeletal maturation or bone age. The former is useful in estimating degree of overweight or underweight and the latter for evaluating physiologic maturity.

The National Center of Health Statistics (NCHS) compiled growth data on U.S. children in 1975. A series of percentiles was then established to reflect the growth of infants and children in contemporary society. From these percentiles, growth charts for boys and girls were developed. Comparison of the measurements for an individual child can be made against the NCHS percentiles. Measurements outside the extreme percentiles may indicate nutritional problems sufficiently severe to affect growth; marked changes in height-weight progress over time may also indicate that a problem is developing.

PHYSIOLOGIC DEVELOPMENT

The progress of gastrointestinal and renal development is relevant to a discussion of infant feeding. With regard to the digestive system, the stomach and small intestine of the newborn infant are sufficiently mature to support satisfactory breakdown of the substances found in human milk. The capacities of salivary, gastric, pancreatic, and intestinal digestion increase with age in accord with the natural pattern of introduction of solid foods. Major considerations about digestion in infancy and its effects on feeding are summarized in Table 30.1.

Kidney function of the full-term infant is not yet completely mature. Glomerular filtration is generally quite efficient, but the renal tubules are functionally less mature and limited in their ability to resorb water and some solutes. It is therefore wise to avoid a situation of excessive presentation of solutes (renal solute load) to the young infant. In terms of infant feeding this largely means avoidance of excessive dietary protein and salt (NaCl). This is especially important when the infant suffers from high fluid losses from diarrhea or perspiration. By about 6 to 8 weeks of age, the function of the renal tubules is reasonably mature so concern about a high renal solute load is obviously less.

NEUROMUSCULAR DEVELOPMENT

The normal development of feeding behavior is dependent on the maturation of the central nervous system. Acquisition of fine motor, gross motor, and oral motor skills is closely tied to the child's ability to effectively consume and manipulate food. Self-feeding is the ultimate goal, but this is only achieved after the child proceeds through an orderly sequence of developmental events. Assessment of the infant's developmental readiness should preceed the introduction of solid foods into the diet. While infants vary in their rate of maturation, few are developmentally prepared for the introduction of solid foods before 4 months of age. Early stages of neuromuscular development are outlined in Table 30.2.

Table 30.1
Digestion in Infancy

Location	Function	Effect on Feeding
Birth to 3 mo*		
Salivary	Lactose is not produced in salivary secretions; amylase not available in significant quantities.	Salivary enzymes play no role in digestion of milk.
Gastric	Hydrochloric acid (HCl) and pepsin precipitate casein into curds; separate and acidify whey protein.	Protein digestion begins; lactose ($C_{12}H_{22}O_{11}$) digestion partly begins; fat is not digested in stomach.
Intestinal	Pancreatic and intestinal enzymes digest proteins into amino acids, reduce carbohydrate to monosaccharides, and split fatty acids from triglycerides in the small intestine.	Protein from human milk is 95% digested, and a similar percentage of protein is digested from commercial formulas that are heat treated and sufficiently dilute to produce a soft curd.
	Disaccharidases are present in border of the intestinal mucosa.	Lactose in human milk and lactose or other carbohydrates in commercial formulas are digested in intestinal mucosa.
	Pancreatic amylase is present in small quantities.	Complex carbohydrates are poorly utilized.
	Pancreatic lipase is present in sufficient quantity.	A total of 80% of human milk fat is digested at birth, and almost 95% is digested by 1 month.
	Lipase, naturally found in human milk, is activated by bile salts.	Digestion of fats from commercial formulas equals that of human milk; fat from other sources (butterfat) is poorly digested.
4-6 mo†		
Salivary	Ptyalin aids digestion to starch.	As solid foods are added to diet, ptyalin plays a role in digestion of starches.
Gastric	Functions are already mature (occurs soon after birth), with HCl and pepsin for digestion of milk and nonmilk foods.	Pepsin and HCl aid in digestion of milk and nonmilk foods.
Intestinal	Enzymes previously lacking are produced in larger quantities and digest nonmilk food substances. More putrefactive bacteria occur in intestinal flora as solids foods increase amount of protein in lower gastrointestinal tract.	Amylase production increases and provides better utilization of starch-containing foods. Increased production of amylase coincides with observed increase in infant's utilization of iron from cereals and nonmilk foods.

Adapted from Willis, N.H.: Infant nutrition: birth to 6 months. A syllabus, Philadelphia, J.B. Lippincott Co.

*The capacities for salivary, gastric, pancreatic, and intestinal digestion increase with age, indicating what may be a natural pattern for the introduction of various solid foods.

†The major changes in digestive capacity that occur at 4 to 6 mo of age involve principally salivary and intestinal functions. Gastric capacities are usually adequate soon after birth and do not change significantly after the third month of life.

PSYCHOSOCIAL DEVELOPMENT

Early interactions between mother and infant may determine future aspects of the infant's personality; such interactions may also affect his relationships with his mother and others in his environment. Food and feeding are intimately involved in a number of the early mother-child situations that transpire. The infant learns that food is associated with warmth, tactile stimulation, and social interaction. The feeding situation is generally a time of pleasant contact between mother and child. If the infant's needs are satisfied through food, contact, and love, a sense of trust is developed between child and mother. Significant characteristics of psychosocial development in young infants are defined in Table 30.2.

Nutrient Needs of Infants

To support normal growth and development of infants, adequate nutrition must be provided in a manageable form. Since the growth rate is higher in infancy than it ever will be in later life, the amount of nutritional support demanded per kilogram of body weight is substantial. While nutrient needs are known to vary among infants in a normal population, recommended levels of nutrient intake for the "typical" infant have been established by the National Academy of Sciences (Table 30.3). It should be recognized, however, that wide ranges of nutrient intakes are appropriate for individual babies from day to day. There are *no* standards that can be arbitrarily applied to any child at any age period, no quantities of food that any baby should be urged to eat. Balanced studies have defined minimal acceptable levels of intakes of a few nutrients on which

Table 30.2
Neuromuscular and Psychosocial Development: Birth to 3 Months

Neuromuscular	Psychosocial	Implication for Feeding
Month 1		
Sucking and swallowing reflexes are present at birth; stimulus in mouth leads to rhythmic sucking and swallowing pattern; tongue protrusion predominates.	Early emotional, psychologic, and social attachment of mother and infant may determine future aspects of infant's personality. Mother's feeding practices determine exposure to tactile stimulation, which is essential to infant's physical and emotional growth.	Oral reflex is a definite adaptive food-seeking reflex for survival. On reaching satiety, infant withdraws head from breast or bottle and falls asleep. If infant's needs are satisfied through food and love, trust is developed between child and mother. Feedings are main means by which infant establishes human relationship with mother.
Month 2		
Corners of mouth are well approximated but not active in sucking; open gap separates lateral portions of lips. Tonic grasp is disappearing.	Strong emotional bond develops between mother and infant and can be viewed as beginning of social interaction of infant.	Infant is individual who shapes his own behavior and feeding schedule. Infant learns to equate mother with food. Infant eats about 5 times each day and sleeps through night.
Month 3		
Lip movement begins to refine; lower lip pulls in; infant may smack lips. Tongue protrusion still present, but infant may swallow with less protrusion. Infant can hold onto object without focusing on it. By end of third month, control of head and eyes is achieved.	More tactile stimulation exists with breast-fed infant. Basic trust factor (if established) is manifested in infant's responses to mother. Infant ceases to cry with hunger when mother approaches. Infant stares into mother's face while feeding and shows response to human voice.	Infant recognizes bottle or breast as source of food. Milk runs out of sides of mouth when nipple is withdrawn. Infant still does not readily accept cup.

Adapted from Owen, A.L., Pipes, P., and Lee, S.L.: Infant feeding guide, Bloomfield, N.J., 1980, Health Learning Systems, Inc.

Table 30.3
Recommended Dietary Allowances for Infants

	Age (mo)				Age (mo)		
Nutrient	**0-6**	**6-12**	**12-36**	**Nutrient**	**0-6**	**6-12**	**12-36**
Kilocalories	wt (kg) × 115	wt (kg) × 105	1130.0	Vitamin E (IU) (mg α-TE)†	3.0	4.0	5.0
Protein (g)	wt (kg) × 2.2	wt (kg) × 2.0	23.0	Ascorbic acid (mg)	35.0	35.0	45.0
Calcium (g)	0.36	0.54	0.8	Folacin (μg)	35.0	45.0	100.0
Iron (mg)	10.0	15.0	15.0	Niacin (mg NE)‡	6.0	8.0	9.0
Iodine (μg)	40.0	50.0	70.0	Riboflavin (mg)	0.4	0.6	0.8
Zinc (mg)	3.0	5.0	10.0	Thiamin (mg)	0.3	0.5	0.7
Magnesium (mg)	50.0	70.0	150.0	Pyridoxine (mg)	0.3	0.6	0.9
Vitamin A (μg RE)*	420.0	400.0	400.0	Vitamin B_{12} (μg)	0.5	1.5	2.0
Vitamin D (mg)	10.0	10.0	10.0				

From Food and Nutrition Board: Recommended daily dietary allowances, ed. 8, Washington, D.C., 1980, National Academy of Sciences–National Research Council.
*Retinol equivalents (1 retinol equivalent = 1 μg retinol or 6 μg carotene).
†α-tocopherol equivalents (1 mg D-α-tocopherol = 1 α-TE).
‡1 NE (niacin equivalent) is equal to 1 mg niacin or 60 mg dietary tryptophan.

recommendations for intake have been made. For most nutrients, however, observations of normal intakes of healthy children have served as a base for the establishment of guidelines presented in the Recommended Dietary Allowances Food and Nutrition Board (1980).

CALORIES

While total daily energy needs increase as a child proceeds through infancy and childhood, the number of calories required per kilogram of body weight decreases steadily in the early years of life. The National Research Council (National Academy of Sciences) recommends an intake of 115 (95 to 145) kcal/kg in early infancy, declining to 105 (80 to 135) kcal/kg at 6 to 12 months. Variation in needs for energy intake relate largely to the wide range of activity levels demonstrated by children (Beal, 1970). Placid infants, for example, may gain at an excessive rate, consuming 20 to 30 kcal/kg less than their peers who actively move about their cribs or other environments. If growth has been compromised by disease or malnutrition, 200 kcal/kg has been recommended to promote "catch-up" growth. The wide ranges of energy expenditure among children make it imperative that the recommended allowances for calories be used as guidelines for groups and not for individual children (Fig. 30.1).

The adequacy of a child's energy intake can best be monitored by observations of physical growth and deposition of adipose tissue. Heights and weights periodically plotted on growth charts help to assess rates of weight gain for individual children. Children who experience excessive increases in weight should be carefully monitored and parents should be encouraged to provide opportunities for increased activity whenever possible. Reduction in dietary sources of unnecessary calories may also be recommended; high-calorie, nutrient-poor solid foods should be major targets for reduction or elimination.

PROTEIN AND AMINO ACIDS

During the first year, the percentage of body protein increases from about 11% to 14.6%. This change reflects the gradual deposition of lean body mass that accompanies the progressive increase in size. The recommended daily allowance (RDA) for protein decreases from 2.2 g/kg during the first 6 months to 2 g/kg for the second half of the first year. Observations of children in the United States indicate that most consume more than recommended amounts (U.S. Department of Health, Education, and Welfare, 1972). However, kwashiorkor (protein-calorie malnutrition accompanied by edema) has been described in infancy and the early preschool years in families where one finds extreme poverty, parental alcoholism, child abuse, or an unorthodox life-style (Chase et al., 1980). Causes of inadequate intake of protein include excessive dilution of the formula, restrictive vegetarian dietary patterns, and infant's refusal of sufficient quantities of protein-containing food (Pipes, 1982).

FATS

Although no standards have been developed for intake of fat, the high concentration of calories in fats is an asset during early infancy when the volume of milk voluntarily consumed is limited. At least 15% of daily

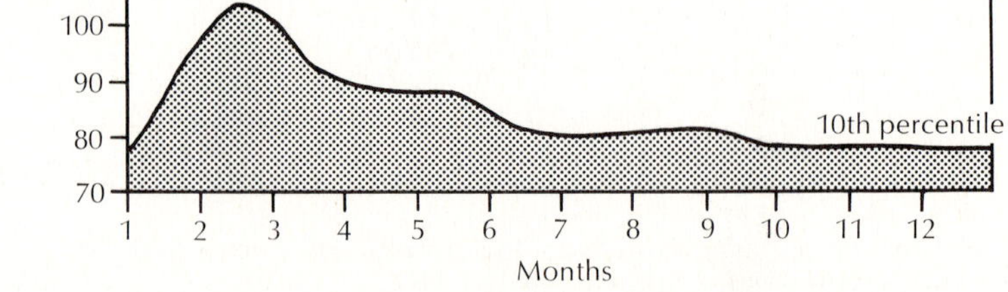

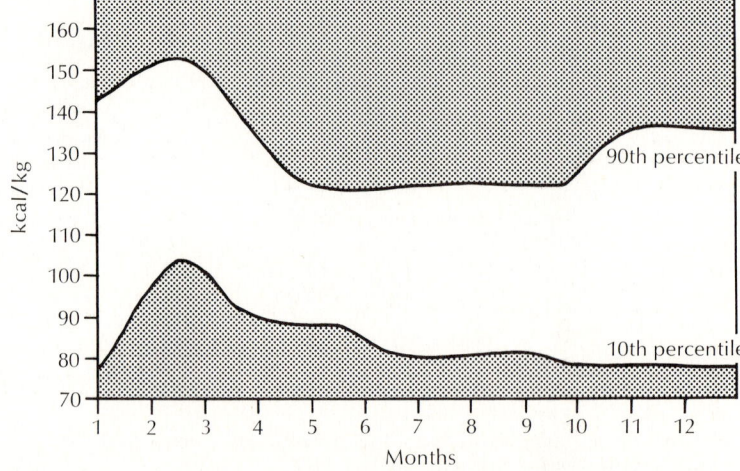

Fig. 30.1
Energy intake (10th and 90th percentiles) from human milk. (From Owen, A.L., Pipes, P., and Lee, S.L.: Infant feeding guide, Bloomfield, N.J., 1980, Health Learning Systems, Inc. Data from Beal, V.A.: Nutritional intake. In McCammon, R.W., editor: Human growth and development, Springfield, Ill., 1970, Charles C Thomas, Publisher.)

calories should derive from fat not only to ensure an adequate calorie intake but also to provide satisfactory amounts of the essential fatty acid, linoleic acid. The Committee on Nutrition of the Academy of Pediatrics (1976a) recommends that 2.7% of total calories should be provided by linoleic acid. Commercial infant formulas and human milk both satisfy the criteria for appropriate level and type of fat provided.

There is as yet no consensus as to whether children should limit their intakes of cholesterol to 300 mg/day and consume unsaturated rather than saturated fats in an effort to reduce the incidence of atherosclerotic heart disease in later life. The fact that human milk is a relatively rich source of cholesterol has led some to believe that it may be an essential nutrient in infancy and that there may be harmful effects from reducing its intake in the first year. In spite of this, infants who consume commercially prepared formula that is very low in cholesterol have not been found to have difficulties later. Serum cholesterol levels of 4- to 7-year-old children have been found to reflect current dietary intake. A cholesterol challenge in infancy by feeding human milk did not effect a reduced serum cholesterol level in preschool and school-age children (Friedman and Goldberg, 1976). Most of those who believe that modifications of the preschool and school-age child's fat intake are appropriate think that preventive measures must be applied in early childhood. Also, since food habits are formed at an early age, such regimens could be patterned into food habits. Others feel that the benefits of such a regimen remain unproven and that the inconveniences involved in changes in eating patterns are not necessary.

CARBOHYDRATES

Lactose is the major carbohydrate present in human milk, cow's milk, and most commercial formulas. This sugar provides calories in an easily available form, and its slow breakdown and absorption is thought to benefit calcium absorption. The percentage of calories from carbohydrates varies among milks but extends from 29% in cow's milk to approximately 42% in formulas. Complex carbohydrates may be provided to infants through solid food sources such as cereals and modified food starches, which are incorporated into some commercial infant foods. While the pancreatic amylase activity of the young infant is rather low, these foods, when provided at about 3 to 6 months of life, appear to be handled reasonably well. One might hypothesize, however, that some of the calories provided as complex carbohydrates will be recovered in the feces.

Honey is sometimes used as a sweetener for home-prepared infant foods or formula, and occasionally it is recommended for use on pacifiers to promote sucking in hypotonic babies. Use of honey for any of these purposes is currently discouraged since some sources contain spores of *Clostridium botulinum* (Arnon et al., 1979). These spores are extremely resistant to heat and therefore are not destroyed in the processing of honey. If ingested by a young infant, spores may germinate and lethal toxin may be released into the lumen of the bowel. Infant botulism may ultimately develop, and in some cases it is known to be fatal.

WATER

The percentage of body water decreases from 75% at birth to 60% at 1 year of age. This reduction is almost entirely in extracellular water, which decreases from 44% of body weight at birth to 26% of body weight at 1 year of age. The ability to retain body water through kidney function improves in the early months of life. To the infant this means that risk of dehydration decreases as renal concentrating capacity becomes better. The Food and Nutrition Board of the National Academy of Sciences (1980) suggests intakes of 1.5 ml/kcal of water for infants but only 1 ml/kcal for adults.

Human milk and properly prepared infant formulas provide sufficient water under normal environmental conditions. Infants who consume limited volumes of milk have episodes of vomiting or diarrhea, and those who receive improperly prepared formulas are vulnerable to water imbalance. Formulas that are concentrated because of improper preparation add a greater need for water; these infants may develop high blood sodium levels (hypernatremia) and ultimately demonstrate signs of dehydration. Such problems have been reported most often when powdered formula products have not been properly measured and the ratio of powder to water is greater than recommended. Similar problems have also occurred, however, when undiluted evaporated milk or concentrated formula were fed in early infancy. Infants who need more water express that need by crying. These cries may be interpreted as hunger. Continued feeding of concentrated formula further increases the need for water. A cyclic phenomenon occurs that may not only predispose an infant to dehydration but also set him up for development of obesity.

Water intoxication resulting in hyonatremia, weakness, restlessness, nausea, vomiting, diarrhea, polyuria or oliguria, and convulsions can result from excessive feeding of water to infants (David et al., 1981). This may also occur when water is fed as a replacement for milk (Partridge et al., 1981). In one reported case, water intoxication resulted from an infant swallowing much water while swimming in the home pool (Knopp and Schwartz, 1982).

VITAMINS

Adequate vitamin intake is especially important to support normal growth and metabolism. Many vitamins participate directly in energy and protein metabolism; some interact with other nutrients to promote growth of bones and mucous membranes and stimulate synthesis of hemoglobin. With only a few exceptions, the RDA for vitamins (Table 30.3) can be met by human milk or by commercially prepared cow's milk formula providing these are consumed at a rate of approximately 800 ml/24 hr. Relevant comments about specific vitamins include the following:

1. *Vitamin D*. Human milk contains relatively low levels of vitamin D and thus should be provided to the breast-fed baby in supplemental form at a level of 400 IU/day (Table 30.4). Commercial formulas are fortified with vitamin D and meet the daily needs of infants if consumed as the major source of nutrition. While exposure to sunlight may reduce the need for oral vitamin D, most infants in the United States do not spend a sufficient amount of time outside to capitalize on this potential vitamin D source.
2. *Ascorbic acid*. Commercial infant formulas and human milk from well-nourished mothers provide adequate levels of vitamin C for the young infant. Infants receiving evaporated milk formula (evaporated milk, Karo syrup, water), however, should receive a daily (20 to 50 mg) supplement of this vitamin (Table 30.4).
3. *Vitamin K*. It is recommended that every newborn infant receive a single parenteral dose of 0.5 to 1.0 mg of vitamin K soon after birth. This is especially important for breast-fed infants because human milk provides much less vitamin K than does cow's milk.
4. *Folacin*. Human milk, cow's milk, and commercial infant formulas provide adequate amounts of folacin for babies. Goat's milk, however, is low in this vitamin, and thus it should be provided as a supplement to infants who obtain a major portion of their nutrition from goat's milk.

MINERALS

Increases in the mineral content of the infant during growth result not only from increases in size but also from maturation of individual structures. The mineral content of the body increases from 3% of body weight in the newborn infant to 4.35% of body weight of the adult. Recommended intakes of specific minerals are defined in Table 30.3; specific comments of relevance include the following:

1. *Iron*. Because both human milk and cow's milk are poor sources of iron, breast-fed infants and those receiving whole cow's milk formulas need the early introduction of a bioavailable source of iron in their diets. Iron-fortified commercial infant formula meets the iron needs of infants who receive it as their major source of nutrition. Iron-fortified infant cereal may also fulfill iron needs of infants although introduction of cereal should be delayed until at least 4 months of age. Iron drops may also be used to fulfill iron needs of infants whose diets do not include iron-rich formula or foods (American Academy or Pediatrics, 1976b).
2. *Calcium*. Infants fed human milk consume less

Table 30.4
Suggested Supplements for Infants

	Type of Milk							
	Breast Milk		Commercial Infant Formula with Iron		Commercial Infant Formula without Iron		Evaporated Milk Formula	
Supplement	Newborn	4 Mo	Newborn	4 Mo	Newborn	4 Mo	Newborn	4 Mo
Vitamin C* (20 mg/day)							+	Continue
Vitamin D (400 IU/day)	+	Continue						
Iron† (7 mg/day)		+				+		+
Fluoride‡ (0.25 mg/day)	+	Continue	+	Continue	+	Continue	+	Continue

*Instead of a vitamin supplement, foods rich in vitamin C may be given.
†Instead of an iron supplement, infant cereal may be given.
‡Fluoride supplements are not needed for the formula-fed infant if the family's water supply is fluoridated.

calcium than infants fed cow's milk but they retain approximately two thirds of their intake in contrast to the formula-fed infant who retains 25% to 30% of intake. It is recommended that a calcium-to-phosphorus ratio of 1.5:1 be ingested by infants and 1:1 by older children. Rickets resulting from inadequate calcium intake has been noted in one full-term infant fed a lamb-base formula for 2 months and supplemented with vitamins but not calcium (Kooh et al., 1977).

3. *Zinc*. Normal newborn infants have no reserves of zinc but are born with tissue concentrations that approximate those of adults. Infants, therefore, are immediately dependent on food sources of this nutrient to meet their need for growth. Animal studies suggest the bioavailability of zinc in human milk to be 59%; of cow's milk, 43% to 54%; and of infant formula, 27% to 40% (Johnson and Evans, 1978).
4. *Iodine*. Concern about iodine deficiency in the United States has decreased substantially with the introduction of iodine not only into iodized salt but also into various major food sources (e.g., milk, commercial dough products). Soy-based formulas for infants are fortified with iodine to counteract the effect of goitrogens found in soy products.
5. *Fluoride*. The importance of fluoride in reducing the prevalence of dental caries has been well documented. When fluoridated water is consumed throughout life, the rate of formation of dental caries in permanent teeth is reduced by 50% to 60%. Current recommendations for supplementation are defined in Table 30.5; dosages should be adjusted to the fluoride content of the water supply (American Academy of Pediatrics, 1979).
6. *Sodium*. Concern about the role of sodium in the etiology of hypertension has provoked substantial changes in the production of commercial infant foods. In 1971 a subcommittee of the Food Protection Committee of the National Research Council reviewed the studies and concluded that although the level of salt added to infant foods was not harmful, neither was it beneficial (American Academy of Pediatrics, 1974). They suggested a reduction of added salt to 0.25% and manufacturers complied. Concern, however, continued, and salt is no longer added to commercially prepared infant foods. Families preparing their own infant foods, however, may utilize salt or salted foods in preparation. Under such circumstances, sodium content of homemade baby foods can reach very high levels. Salting of homemade baby foods should be discouraged.

Table 30.5
Supplemental Fluorine Dosage Schedule (mg/day*)

	Concentration of Fluoride in Drinking Water (ppm)		
Age	**< 0.3**	**0.3-0.7**	**> 0.7**
2 wk to 2 yr	0.25	0	0
2-3 yr	0.50	0.25	0
3-16 yr	1.00	0.50	0

From Committee on Nutrition: Fluoride supplementation: revised dosage schedule, Pediatrics **63**:150, 1979; copyright, American Academy of Pediatrics.

*2.2 mg of sodium fluoride contains 1 mg of fluoride.

Breast Feeding

Interest in breast feeding has increased significantly since the beginning of the 1970s. Before that time, formulas were preferred and in many areas were considered the "modern" method of infant feeding. As information about the apparent superiority of human milk has accumulated, enthusiasm for breast feeding has mounted. Currently more than 50% of U.S. mothers leave the hospital nursing (Martinez and Nalenzienski, 1979) and planning to continue the practice well into the first year of their infants' lives (Fig. 30.2). More than 15% of infants continue to breast feed well beyond 6 months of age (Fig. 30.3). While the advantages of nursing vary among mother-infant pairs, those features of breast feeding that are typically viewed as superior to formula feeding are listed below:

1. Breast milk is nutritionally superior to any alternative.
2. Breast milk is bacteriologically safe and always fresh.
3. Breast milk contains a variety of antiinfectious factors and immune cells.
4. Breast milk is the least allergenic of any infant feed.
5. Breast-fed babies are least likely to be overfed.
6. Breast feeding promotes good jaw and tooth development.
7. Breast feeding *generally* costs less than the commercial infant formulas currently available.
8. Breast feeding automatically promotes close mother-child contact.
9. Breast feeding is *generally* more convenient once the process is established.

The mammary glands prepare for lactation through a series of developmental steps that occur during adolescence and pregnancy (Worthington-Roberts et al.,

Fig. 30.2
In-hospital breast feeding in 1979 and 1978 to 1979 percentage point change. (From Martinez, G.A., and Nalezienski, N.P.: Pediatrics **67:**260, 1981. Copyright American Academy of Pediatrics, 1981.)

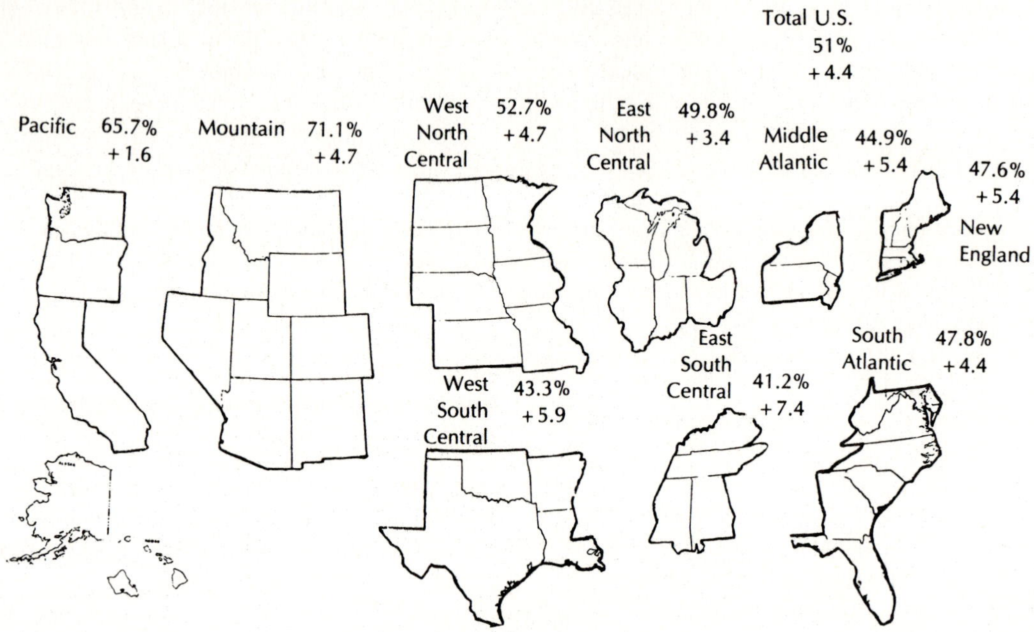

Fig. 30.3
Percent of infants in the United States breast feeding at different ages (from 1971 to 1978). (Data from Martinez, G.A., and Nalezienski, J.P.: Pediatrics **64:**686, 1979. In Worthington-Roberts, B., Vermeersch, J., and Williams, S.R.: Nutrition in pregnancy and lactation, ed. 2, St. Louis, 1981, The C.V. Mosby Co.)

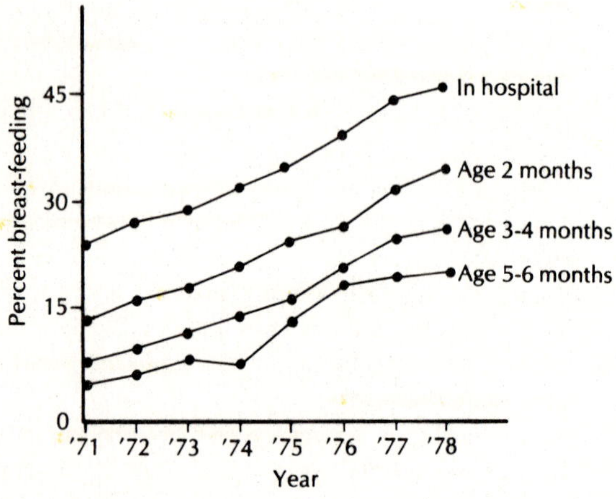

1981). Hormonal changes that take place before and during puberty markedly increase breast, areola, and nipple size. The major changes involve an increase in connective tissue and fat with limited development of the duct system and alveolar cells. The principal feature of mammary growth in pregnancy is a great increase in ducts and alveoli under the influence of many hormones. Late in pregnancy, the lobules of the alveolar system are maximally developed and small amounts of colostrum may be released for several months before delivery. Anatomic features of the human mammary gland are defined in Figs. 30.4, 30.5, and 6.22.

With delivery of the infant and placenta a dramatic change occurs in the hormonal pattern of the mother. A sudden drop in circulating levels of estrogen and progesterone (produced by the placenta) accompanies a rapid rise in secretion of prolactin. These and other changes set the stage for the formal onset of lactation.

The typical stimulus for milk production and secretion is the suck of the infant at the mother's breast. Nerves beneath the skin of the areola carry a nervous message to the spinal cord where it is transmitted to the hypothalamus; from the hypothalamus a message is sent to the pituitary gland where both the anterior and posterior areas are stimulated to release their respective hormones. Prolactin is released from the anterior pituitary for ultimate stimulation of mild production by alveolar cells in the mammary tissue (Fig. 30.6); oxytocin is released from the posterior pituitary for action on

Fig. 30.4
General anatomic features of human breast showing its location on anterior region of thorax between sternum and anterior axillary line. (From Worthington-Roberts, B., Vermeersch, J., and Williams, S.R.: Nutrition in pregnancy and lactation, ed. 2, St. Louis, 1981, The C.V. Mosby Co.)

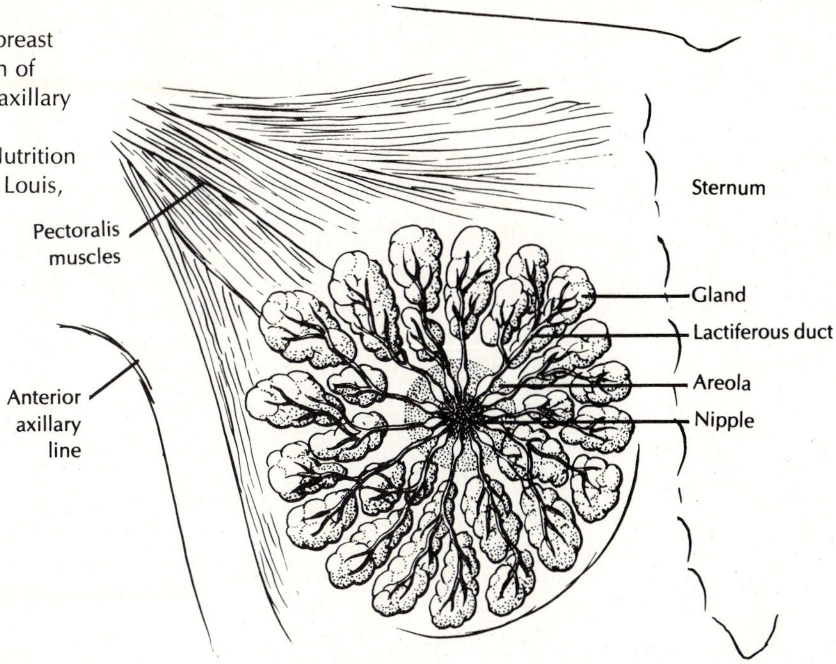

Fig. 30.5
Detailed structural features of human mammary gland showing terminal glandular (alveolar) tissue of each lobule leading into duct system, which eventually enlarges into lactiferous duct and lactiferous sinus. Lactiferous sinuses rest beneath areola and converge at nipple pore. (From Worthington-Roberts, B., Vermeersch, J., and Williams, S.R.: Nutrition in pregnancy and lactation, ed. 2, St. Louis, 1981, The C.V. Mosby Co.)

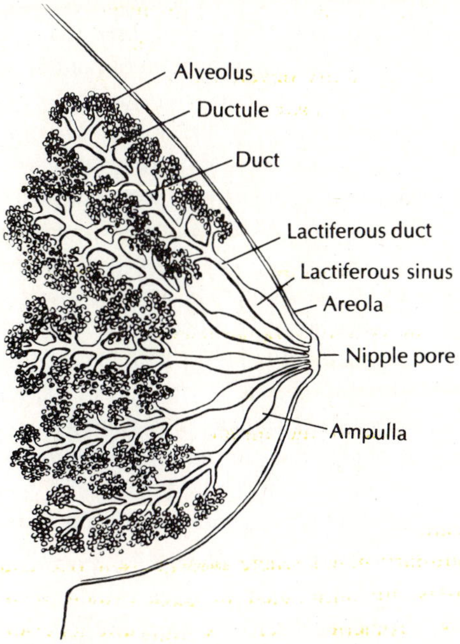

Fig. 30.6
Diagrammatic representation of basic physiological features of milk production. Sucking stimulus provided by baby sends a message to hypothalamus. Hypothalamus stimulates anterior pituitary to release prolactin, hormone that promotes milk production by alveolar cells of mammary glands. (From Worthington-Roberts, B., Vermeersch, J., and Williams, S.R.: Nutrition in pregnancy and lactation, ed. 2, St. Louis, 1981, The C.V. Mosby Co.)

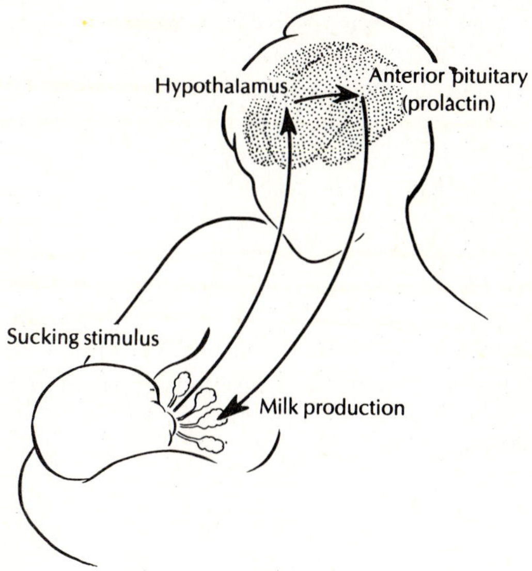

Fig. 30.7
Diagrammatic representation of basic features of "let-down reflex." Sucking stimulus arrives at hypothalamus, which promotes release of oxytocin from posterior pituitary. Oxytocin stimulates contraction of myoepithelial cells around alveoli in mammary glands. Contraction of these musclelike cells causes milk to be propelled through duct system and into lactiferous sinuses, where it becomes available to nursing infants. (From Worthington-Roberts, B., Vermeersch, J., and Williams, S.R.: Nutrition in pregnancy and lactation, ed. 2, St. Louis, 1981, The C.V. Mosby Co.)

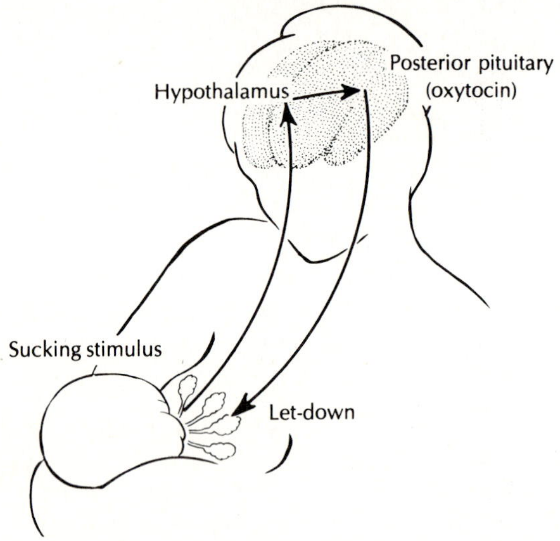

the myoepithelial cells of the mammary gland; these cells are stimulated to contract, causing movement of milk through the duct system and lactiferous sinuses for ultimate arrival in the mouth of the infant (Fig. 30.7). This latter process is referred to as *let-down* and is accompanied in the woman by a distinct sensation described as a tingling feeling. Since oxytocin also stimulates the muscle cells of the uterus to contract, lactation immediately following delivery is considered an aid in preventing postpartum hemorrhage.

The process of let-down appears to be sensitive to small changes in circulating oxytocin levels; minor emotional disturbances or environmental stresses may influence the ease with which breast milk is provided to the infant. The attitude of the mother toward breast feeding is a powerful factor in determining her success at lactation. The support of her husband, physician, nurse, extended family, and friends is also an important determinant of degree of satisfaction and success derived from the breast-feeding experience.

MATERNAL NUTRITIONAL NEEDS

The process of lactation is nutritionally demanding, especially for the woman who fully nurses for a number of months. Increased intake of all nutrients is reasonably advised as is indicated in the RDAs for the lactating woman (Table 30.6). Energy requirements vary in accord with the amount of milk produced. A typical woman synthesizing enough milk to meet all nutritional needs of a 5 kg (11 lb) infant must secrete about 850 ml of milk providing about 600 kcal daily. Since human milk is produced with close to 80% efficiency, the requirement for lactation is about 750 kcal/day. During the early months of lactation, the maternal fat stores accumulated during pregnancy may be drawn on to satisfy about one third of the daily calorie needs for lactation; the RDA for lactation is 500 kcal/day. When the maternal fat pad has been depleted, dietary calorie support for lactation must be increased if the mother intends to provide all or most of her infant's nutrition through breast milk alone.

The increased recommended intakes of specific nutrients in the diet largely represent the need to replace in the mother what is lost in her milk. With regard to protein, however, conversion of dietary protein to milk protein is not a process with 100 efficiency; thus intake of dietary protein must exceed the amount that is found in the daily milk supply.

IMPACT OF MATERNAL DIET ON MILK COMPOSITION

The influence of maternal diet on the composition of human milk reflects in part the nutitional status of the mother. If the mother's nutritional stores are substantial, consumption of a poor quality diet for a period of time may have a limited impact on the *quality* of the milk she produces; she will draw from her stores if her diet is suboptimal. However, this utilization of maternal stores has obvious limits; this is especially true for water-soluble vitamins, which are found in low levels in human milk if the maternal diet is low in these nutrients.

The major effect on lactation of maternal undernutrition is the production of a reduced *quantity* of milk each day. Such a consequence may be seen in the nursing mother who takes on a rigorous weight reduction diet while attempting to breast feed her young infant. A suboptimal *quantity* of milk production may also result from inadequate fluid intake on the part of the mother. Breast-feeding mothers should be discouraged from dieting and encouraged to consume 3 to 4 qt of fluid daily. They should also be advised that use of oral contraceptives may suppress lactation, especially in the first 6 to 10 weeks (Worthington-Roberts et al., 1981).

COMPOSITION OF HUMAN MILK

Human milk is ideally designed to satisfy the nutritional needs of human infants. Its composition varies

Table 30.6
Recommended Daily Dietary Allowances for Lactation

	Age			
	11-14 Yr	**15-18 Yr**	**19-22 Yr**	**23-50 Yr**
Body size				
Weight (kg)	46	55	55	55
(lb)	101	120	120	120
Height (cm)	157	163	163	163
(in)	62	64	64	64
Nutrients				
Energy (kcal)	2700	2600	2500	2500
Protein (g)	66	66	64	64
Vitamin A (RE*)	1200	1200	1200	1200
Vitamin D (μg)	15	15	12.5	10
Vitamin E activity (mg of alpha-TE)†	13	13	13	13
Ascorbic acid (mg)	90	100	100	100
Folacin (μg)	500	500	500	500
Niacin (mg)‡	20	19	19	18
Riboflavin (mg)	1.8	1.8	1.8	1.7
Thiamine (mg)	1.6	1.6	1.6	1.5
Vitamin B_6 (mg)	2.3	2.5	2.5	2.5
Vitamin B_{12} (μg)	4.0	4.0	4.0	4.0
Calcium (mg)	1600	1600	1200	1200
Phosphorus (mg)	1600	1600	1200	1200
Iodine (μg)	200	200	200	200
Iron (mg)	18§	18§	18§	18§
Magnesium (mg)	450	450	450	450
Zinc (mg)	25	25	25	25

Modified from Food and Nutrition Board, National Research Council, National Academy of Sciences: Recommended dietary allowances, ed. 9, Washington D.C., 1980, U.S. Government Printing Office.
*RE = Retinol equivalent.
†Alpha-tocopherol equivalents; 1 mg D-alpha-tocopherol = 1 alpha-TE.
‡Although allowances are expressed as niacin, it is recognized that on the average, 1 mg of niacin is derived from each 60 mg of dietary tryptophan.
§Iron needs during lactation are not substantially different from those of nonpregnant women, but continued supplementation of the mother for 2 to 3 months after parturition is advisable to replenish stores depleted by pregnancy.

considerably from that of cow's milk (Table 30.7). While commercial infant formulas provide satisfactory alternatives, none is comparable to human milk in its nutritional, antiallergic, or antiinfectious properties. In comparing human milk with the most common substitute, cow's milk, the following major features are relevant:

1. The *protein* content of human milk is lower than that of cow's milk; human milk contains far more lactalbumin in relation to casein, which reduces the amount of potential curd formation in the gut of the infant.
2. The *amino acid* composition of human milk is ideally suited to the newborn infant's metabolic capabilities. For example, phenylalanine and methionine levels are low and cystine and taurine levels are high.
3. *Fat* in human milk is easier to digest and absorb than that in cow's milk. This is due in part to the arrangement of fatty acids on the glycerol molecule, but it is also related to the natural lipase activity that is present in non-heat-treated human milk.
4. While the *iron* content of mammalian milk is low, its absorbability from human samples is approximately 50% compared to markedly lower levels from other sources (4% to 12%). *Zinc* in human milk is also more absorbable than that found in cow's milk alternatives. Human milk *calcium* is 65% to 70% absorbed, whereas formula-fed infants absorb 25% to 30%; in view of the fact that a higher concentration of calcium is found in cow's milk–based formulas than in human milk, the net uptake from these sources is about the same. In general, *most minerals* (e.g., sodium, potassium, phosphorus) are present in lower concentrations in human milk than in any of the alternatives. This feature is desirable in that the

Table 30.7
Nutrient Content of Human Milk and Cow's Milk

Constituent (per liter)	Human Milk	Cow's Milk
Energy (kcal)	690	660
Protein (g)	9	35
Fat (g)	45	37
Lactose (g)	68	49
Vitamins		
Vitamin A (IU)	1898	1025
Vitamin D (IU)	22	14
Vitamin E (IU)	2	0.4
Vitamin K (μg)	15	60
Thiamin (μg)	160	440
Riboflavin (μg)	360	1750
Niacin (mg)	1.5	0.9
Pyridoxine (μg)	100	640
Folic acid (μg)	52	55
Cobalamin (μg)	0.3	4
Ascorbic acid (mg)	43	11
Minerals		
Calcium (mg)	297	1170
Phosphorus (mg)	150	920
Sodium (mg)	150	506
Potassium (mg)	550	1368
Chlorine (mg)	385	1028
Magnesium (mg)	23	120
Sulfur (mg)	140	300
Iron (mg)*	0.56-0.3	0.5
Iodine (mg)	30	47
Manganese (μg)†	5.9-4.0	20-40
Copper (μg)	0.6-0.25	0.3
Zinc (mg)‡	4-5	3-5
Selenium (μg)	20	5-50
Fluoride (mg)	0.05	0.003-0.1

From Pipes, P.L.: Nutrition in infancy and childhood, St. Louis, 1981, The C.V. Mosby Co. Adapted from Hambreaus, L.: Pediatr. Clin. North Am. **24**:17, 1977; Siimes, M.A., et al.: Acta Paediatr. Scand. **68**:29, 1979; Vuori, E.: Acta Paediatr. Scand. **68**:571, 1979; Vuori, E., and Kuitunen, P.: Acta Paediatr. Scand. **68**:33, 1978, and Nayman, R., et al.: Am. J. Clin. Nutr. **32**:1279, 1979.
*Median values at 2 wk and 5 mo of lactation.
†Median values at 2 wk and 5 mo of lactation, after which time the manganese content of human milk tends to increase.
‡Median values at 2 wk and 37 wk of lactation.

renal solute load presented to the infant is small. With regard to *fluoride,* the low level of fluoride found in human milk is not optimal for enamel development of the teeth. Many clinicians therefore advise supplementing the breast-fed baby with fluoride until other fluoride sources enter the diet (Table 30.5).

5. The *lactose* content of human milk is significantly higher than that in cow's milk.
6. The *vitamin* content of human milk reflects to a significant degree the vitamin intake (and vitamin stores) of the mother. Vitamin D is somewhat unique in that its level in breast milk is particularly low (22 IU/L). If sunlight exposure of the breast-fed infant is limited, the child is at risk for development of vitamin D–deficiency rickets (Bachrach et al., 1979) if an appropriate supplement is not provided (Table 30.4).
7. *Antiinfectious factors* and *immune cells* are unique components of human milk. They include antibodies to intestinal microorganisms that may protect the infant from some enteric infections. Among the protective constituents that have been isolated from human milk are immunoglobulins, lactoferrin, lysozyme, lactoperoxidase, interferon, and macrophages. The presence of these factors is believed to explain the reduced incidence of illness in breast-fed babies not only in developing countries but also in the United States.

''*Contaminants*'' enter human milk as a result of planned or accidental maternal exposure. Most drugs taken by the nursing mother will be secreted in her milk although the degree of secretion varies in accord with the chemical characteristics of the compound. While many drugs, if taken in moderation, appear to produce no harm to the nursing infant, some have been identified as having adverse effects. While a complete list of these drugs has yet to be developed, some guidelines are provided in the box on p. 663 (see also Appendix J). Several drugs whose use contraindicates breast feeding include thiouracil, radioactive substances, and antineoplastic agents.

Other nonnutrients enter human milk from the bloodstream of the lactating mother. Such compounds include pesticide residues, polychlorinated and polybrominated biphenyls (PCBs and PBBs) and a variety of other *environmental pollutants*. Although levels found in typical milk are generally low in the United States, care should be taken to monitor human milk in regions where accidental water contamination or other such crises develop. Nicotine, marijuana, *caffeine,* and *alcohol* may also appear in human milk at levels related to the degree of maternal intake. Babies may demonstrate restlessness and diuresis from significant caffeine exposure. One infant exposed to substantial amounts of alcohol through his mother's milk developed a cushingoid appearance with obvious impairment in growth with excessive weight gain; the clinical picture was believed to relate to the ability of alcohol to increase circulating cortisol concentrations (Binkiewicz et al., 1978).

COUNSELING THE BREAST-FEEDING MOTHER

Preparation. Emphasis on the advantages of breast feeding should be presented early in pregnancy.

Abbreviated Guide to Drug Therapy in Nursing Mothers*

Drugs viewed as safe if used in moderation

- Aspirin
- Antidiarrheal agents
- Most antibiotics
- Most antihistamines
- Insulin
- Epinephrine

Drugs viewed as potentially harmful if used recklessly

- Sulfonamides†
- Oral contraceptives‡
- Chloramphenicol‡
- Lithium carbonate
- Reserpine
- Theophylline
- Narcotics (including codeine)
- Steroids
- Diazepam (Valium)
- Diuretics
- Nalidixic acid
- Barbiturates
- Phenytoin

Drugs contraindicated for nursing mothers

- Iodides
- Radioactive agents
- Anticoagulants
- Tetracycline
- Antimetabolites
- Ergot preparations
- Atropine
- Metronidazole (Flagyl)
- Bromides
- Propylthiouracil
- Dihydrotachysterol
- Most cathartics §

*A complete listing of drugs in human milk and suspected effects on infants is provided in Table F-1 in Lawrence R.: Breast-feeding: a guide for the medical profession, St. Louis, 1980, The C.V. Mosby Co.

†Probably contraindicated during the first month of the infant's life.

‡If utilized at all, the "minipill" is suggested, with observation of the baby for possible hormone effects.

§Milk of magnesia and nondigestible fibers are safe.

Women should be encouraged to express their opinions and feelings so that they can be discussed and any misinformation can be corrected. During the last months of pregnancy, counseling on the process of lactation should be made available to women who have decided to breast feed. Fathers should be encouraged to participate in counseling sessions since their encouragement and emotional support contribute to successful lactation. Many mothers have never seen a woman nursing an infant; they therefore find it especially helpful to have a woman who has successfully nursed an infant available to answer questions and provide reinforcement.

Fig. 30.8
Mother prepares for breast feeding; nightie is designed for breast feeding. Note appearance of breast. Lactation is established: nipples and areolar tissue are enlarged. (Courtesy Judy Bamber, San Jose, Calif.)

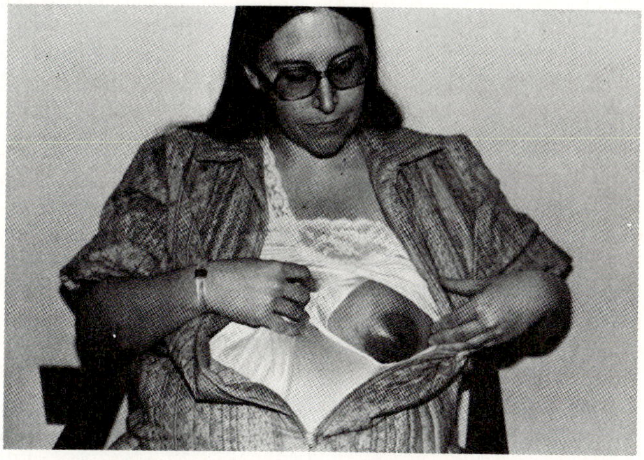

The technique. The baby should be put to the breast as soon after birth as the mother feels ready. It is not essential that suckling occur immediately after delivery, but some mothers wish this experience and if possible their wishes should be accommodated. Milk may be expected to flow within 48 to 96 hours after delivery. Before this time, however, the thin yellow fluid called colostrum should appear; colostrum is higher in protein and lower in fat and carbohydrate than mature milk; it provides approximately 15 kcal/oz along with a rich source of antibodies. As it becomes replaced by transitional and mature milk, the breasts become enlarged and firm as they fill with milk (Fig. 30.8). If the infant has not yet learned to suck vigorously by the third or fourth postdelivery day, the breasts may become so full and distended with milk that the nipples appear retracted, and the infant may be unable to nurse. The lag between the production of milk and the efficiency of the ejection reflexes often results in engorgement of the breasts for up to 48 hours after the milk comes in. The mother often complains that the breast is tender and that the tenderness extends into the axilla. The breasts usually feel firm, tense, and warm as a result of the increased blood supply, and the skin may appear shiny and taut. The unyielding areolae make it difficult for the infant to grasp the nipple. Hence nursing can be uncomfortable to the mother and frustrating for both mother and infant. Expression of milk manually or by using a breast pump generally will start the flow of milk and relieve the engorgement. In some instances, moist warmth (e.g., shower, cloths) will also start the flow. A mild analgesic may also be ordered for use before nursing. The mother should be encouraged to wear her supportive nursing brassiere most of the time. Careful attention to the general comfort of the mother during the nursing period is important. Selection of a comfortable position, use of pillows for support, and the presence of an attentive, unhurried nurse do much to help the mother weather these few days.

For breast feeding to be successful, it is important

Fig. 30.9
Feeding techniques: a series (may be used after vaginal or cesarean birth). **A,** Mother is seated comfortably in bed. Baby is supported in her arms and is resting on a pillow. **B,** Note mother makes a dimple in her breast so infant can breathe. **C,** Some mothers prefer a side-lying position. A pillow is placed at her back for support, her head is resting on a pillow. Baby is lying on bed beside her. **D,** "Football" hold is also a comfortable position. Baby is supported by one arm, her head resting in her mother's arm. (**A, B,** and **D** courtesy Judy Bamber, San Jose, Calif.)

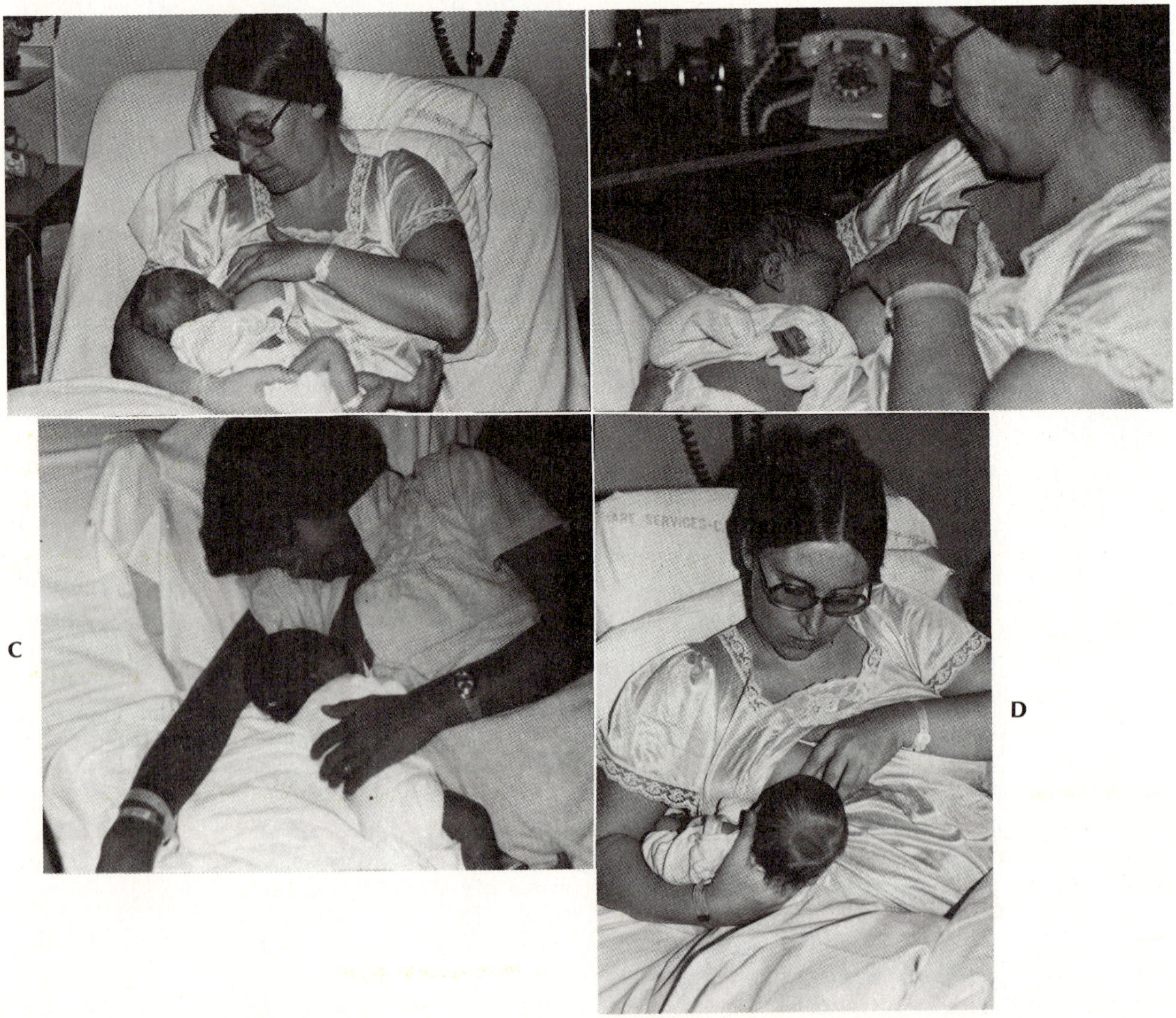

A B C D

that both mother and infant get into a comfortable position, either sitting or lying down (Fig. 30.9) The mother should hold the baby close, cradling him in her arm to support the head if she is sitting up. If the baby's cheek is touched, he will turn toward that side (the rooting reflex). The mother should hold her breast so that the brown areola and nipple are in the baby's mouth as much as possible. If the breast is very full, it helps to press the breast gently away from the baby's nose so that the infant can breathe more easily. The baby should be allowed to nurse from 5 to 10 minutes on each side initially and then longer if both mother and infant wish.

The *let-down reflex* is detected by a tingling sensation that is often accompanied by dripping from the opposite nipple and occasionally uterine cramps. It may take some time for the let-down reflex to become fully functional and conditioned. Some women never feel the let-down, but if the baby is swallowing, it has occurred. Rest, relaxation, or a hot shower before nursing may help initiate the let-down reflex.

The infant may start by sucking vigorously and, as the milk flows freely, develop a long, slow, rhythmic sucking. This may then change to a short, rapid sucking, with frequent rest periods. This behavior indicates a slowing of the flow of milk. Alternate massage of the breasts starts the milk flowing freely again, and the infant should revert to the slow, rhythmic sucking. As soon as sucking resumes, the massage is discontinued so that the infant will not be overwhelmed and choked by the milk's flowing too rapidly. If the woman has too much milk, the baby may need to nurse on only one side at a feeding for a while. This will reduce overall stimulation and reduce the milk supply.

To remove the baby from the breast, a finger is placed in the corner of the baby's mouth until the suction is broken. The breast can then be comfortably removed. Most babies need to be burped before feeding from the second breast; the need for burping, however, is highly individual among babies (Fig. 30.10).

Since breast milk is more easily digested than other infant feeds, breast-fed infants may wish to nurse more often than formula-fed babies. If the baby wants to nurse, there is no reason not to let him do so; breast-fed babies consume what they need and no more. Breast feeding whenever the baby is hungry is easy to do because the milk is always ready. Some babies may be hungry as frequently as every hour or two on some days, or it may not be any more often than every 4 hours for other babies on other days. The more often the baby nurses, the more milk the breasts produce; thus whenever a woman's supply is low (e.g., during or after an illness), she should nurse more often.

Parents should realize that crying does not always mean that the baby is hungry. He may be physically uncomfortable or just want to be held, burped, or changed. Mothers can be reassured that they are producing sufficient milk if the infant has six to ten voidings of pale, straw-colored urine in 24 hours. In time, parents learn to distinguish the meaning of their infant's cries.

The stools of breast-fed babies are very loose. Some infants have a bowel movement at each feeding, whereas others may go up to 5 days without one. Babies who are fed only breast milk do not become constipated, although they may strain considerably in passing the stool. The stool is not irritating to the skin.

If menstruation occurs, the mother can continue to breast feed. Although some babies may act fussy, the quality and quantity of the milk are not affected. No

Fig. 30.9, cont'd
E, Note how mother holds her breast to guide nipple into infant's mouth. Note molding on infant's head. Mother had cesarean delivery after a long labor. **F,** Another "football" position. Mother is sitting in a chair with infant supported on a pillow. (Courtesy Judy Bamber, San Jose, Calif.)

E

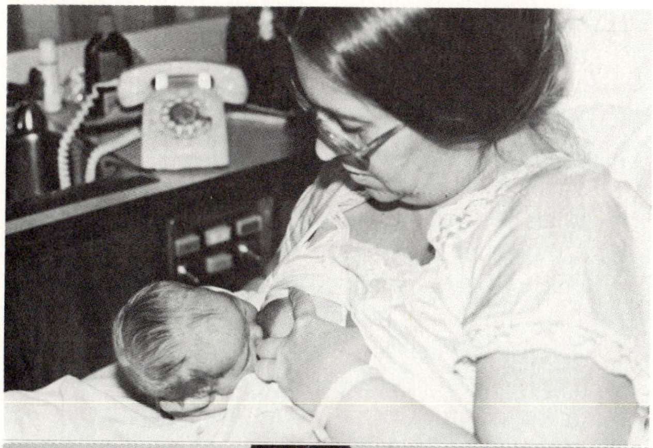

F

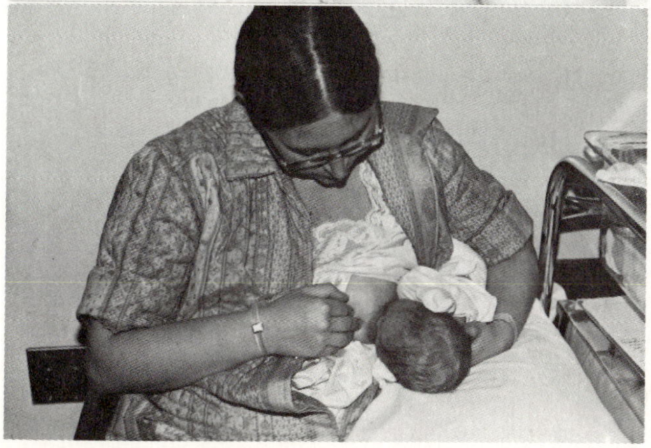

Fig. 30.10
Burping infant. **A,** Over-the-shoulder technique. Baby is held upright; back is gently rubbed upward. Cloth is in position to protect mother's gown. **B,** Sitting technique. Infant is held in a sitting position, and her back is gently patted or rubbed upward. (Courtesy Judy Bamber, San Jose, Calif.)

A

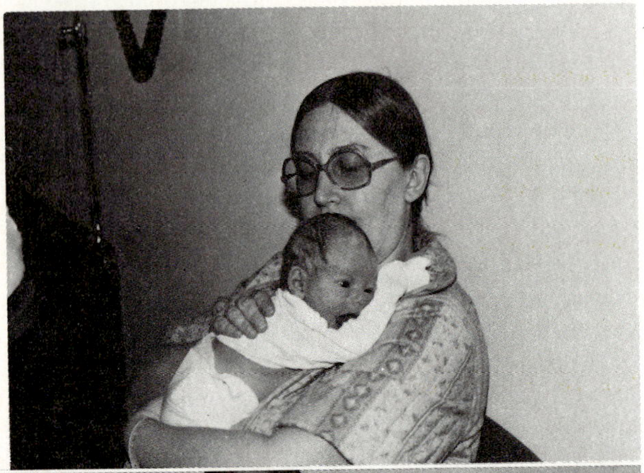

B

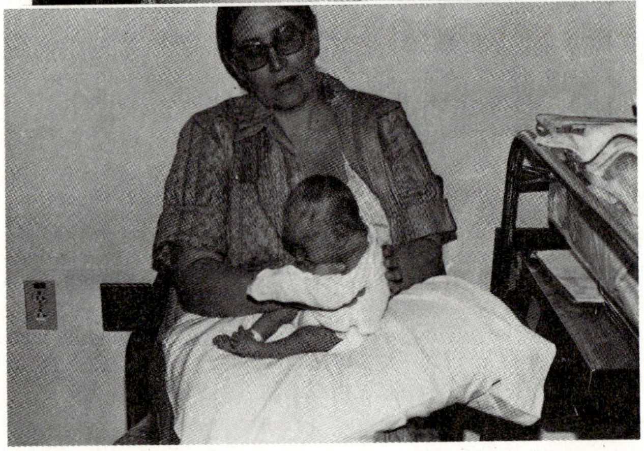

Fig. 30.11
Contented baby and mother following infant's feeding. (Courtesy Judy Bamber, San Jose, Calif.)

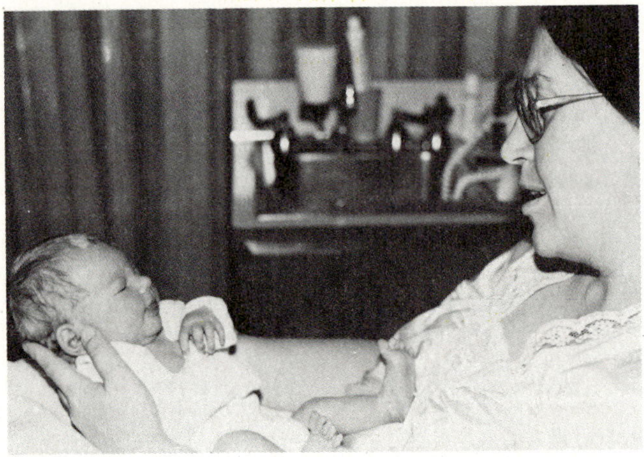

infant has been found to be allergic to breast milk itself, but a baby can react to certain foods that the mother eats. Avoidance of these foods is all that is necessary to curtail the reaction. The mother determines which foods to avoid primarily by means of trial and error.

Feeding time is perfectly suited for establishing and maintaining close parent-child interaction (Fig. 30.11). The mother, however, need not be tied to her infant all of the time. On occasions when she wants or needs to be away from the infant at the usual time of feeding, a bottle can be given. The bottle might contain formula or breast milk that has been expressed earlier. It is best to avoid supplemental bottles other than water until the woman is satisfied that her milk supply is well established and regulated, usually around 6 weeks postpartum. She should consider taking the baby with her instead. Whenever she wishes to nurse in a public place, she can do it unobtrusively if she is wearing an overblouse or sweater that can be pulled up and a nursing brassiere with a front opening.

Duration of breast feeding. The length of time a woman breast feeds her infant will depend on her own feelings and situation. If she is working, she can continue to breast feed, using bottles if necessary. Milk will continue to be produced as long as there is demand for it and it is taken from the breast, although a breast may be emptied at any given feeding.

Some mothers prefer to breast feed until the baby can be weaned to a cup (thus avoiding bottles altogether); this can be accomplished when the baby is about 9 or 10 months of age. Some mothers choose to breast feed much longer—for several years—letting the baby decide when to be weaned. There is a wide variability in ease of weaning, depending on the baby's overall interest in nursing, the relationship between mother and child, and the use of bottles. Babies who have had frequent supplemental bottles from birth are likely to wean themselves at an early age.

When a mother decides to wean her baby, it should be done gradually over a period of several weeks. At first, one feeding can be omitted for several days; two feedings may then be skipped until the baby is down to one feeding a day (usually the night or early morning feeding). Eventually this last feeding can be discontinued. Weaning in this gradual manner will be easier on the mother, avoiding engorgement of her breasts, and easier for the baby to adjust to the new routine.

Care of breasts. Daily washing of the breasts with water is sufficient for cleanliness. In addition, for the first 2 or 3 weeks the nipple and areolar tissue are washed and dried after each feeding, since the remaining colostrum or milk can contribute to the development of sore nipples. A lubricant such as liquid petrolatum or lanolin may then be massaged gently into the nipple area, and if feasible, the breasts can be exposed to the air for 20 to 30 minutes. The lubricant used should not contain alcohol, since the drying effects of the alcohol tend to encourage cracking of the tissue. Some infants object to either the taste or smell of ointments and will refuse to nurse until the breast has been washed.

The nursing brassiere needs to be well fitted, with broad shoulder straps and the flaps over the breasts large enough to release the breasts without discomfort.

COMMON PROBLEMS AND HOW TO AVOID THEM

The inexperienced nursing mother is likely to encounter major or minor problems in the course of adjusting to breast feeding. Some of the initial difficulties are summarized in Table 30.8 along with comments about counseling strategies. Success or failure at the breast-feeding effort may depend largely on the availability of help in the early weeks and the support of a clinician or friend who provides useful tips.

Engorged breasts. If nursing has been on demand since birth, painful engorgement of the breasts is not likely to occur. If the breasts do become engorged, the discomfort can be relieved by applying wet cloths as hot as can be endured to the whole breast and, at the same time, expressing milk from the nipple. This will help to relieve discomfort. As the wet cloth cools, replace it with another hot one.

To express milk by hand, the thumb and forefinger are placed on opposite sides of the breast just outside the areola, pressed into the rib cage, and then squeezed together and downward; the nipple should not be pulled outward. The procedure is repeated, moving the thumb and forefinger around the nipple until as much milk as desired has been expressed. Sometimes it helps to do breast massage before expressing the milk; this is done by putting the thumbs together on top of the breast and the remaining fingers under the breast (Fig. 30.12). Gentle traction is then exerted from around the breast toward the nipple. If the milk is to be used later, it should be expressed into a sterile bottle and refrigerated. Milk expression is not easy for some women at first, but persistence usually brings success if the mother takes the time.

Sore nipples. The nipples may become sore at the beginning of breast feeding. This problem may be min-

Table 30.8.
Common Problems and Their Solutions

Problem	Approaches to Management
Retracted nipple	Before feeding infant, roll nipple gently between fingers until erect.
Baby's mouth not open wide enough	Before feeding, depress infant's lower jaw with one finger as nipple is guided into mouth.
Baby sucks poorly	Stimulate sucking motions by pressing upward under baby's chin. Expression of colostrum often occurs and taste may stimulate sucking.
Baby demonstrates rooting but does not grasp nipple; eventually cries in frustration	Interrupt feeding, comfort infant; mother should take time to relax herself before trying again.
Baby falls asleep while nursing	If infant falls asleep early in feeding, he should be awakened by holding him upright, rubbing his back, talking to him, or providing similar quiet stimuli; another effort can then be made. If baby falls asleep again, feeding should be postponed.

Fig. 30.12
Manual expression of human milk. (Courtesy Health Education Associates, Inc., Glenside, Pa.)

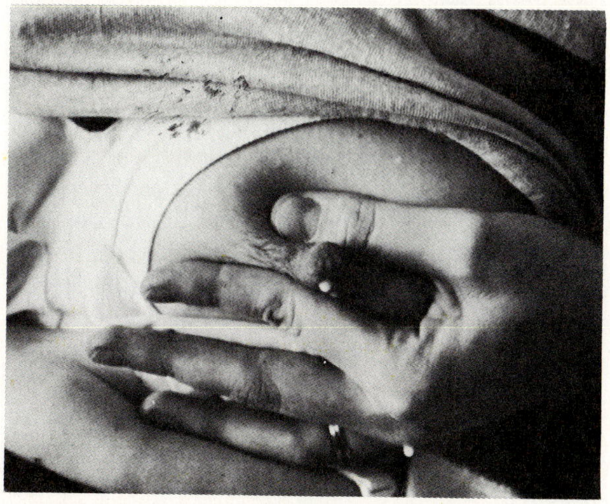

Fig. 30.13
Diagrammatic representation of proposed method for preparation of nipples for breast feeding. (From Worthington-Roberts, B., Vermeersch, J., and Williams, S.R.: Nutrition in pregnancy and lactation, ed. 2, St. Louis, 1981, The C.V. Mosby Co.)

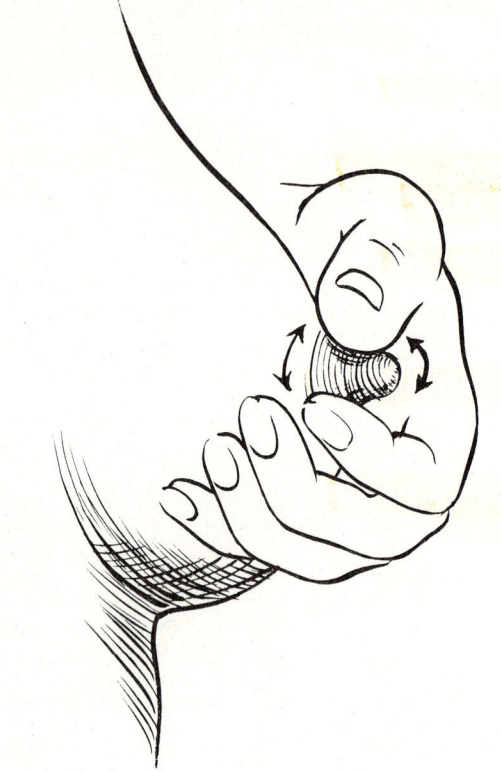

imized if the woman toughens the skin of the nipple and surrounding area by massage during the latter months of pregnancy. Nipple rolling is sometimes practiced (Fig. 30.13), or alternatively, frequent massage with a bath towel may be useful. During the early days of nursing, soreness may be limited by utilizing a correct nursing position and avoiding undue breast engorgement. If soreness occurs, it is always temporary and occurs until the nipples become accustomed to the baby's sucking. One of the ways to relieve the soreness is to expose the nipples to the air. This is done by removing the brassiere and wearing a loose cotton blouse or shirt. It is also helpful to briefly expose the bare nipples to a sunlamp or the sun. It may also help to apply a soothing ointment such as lanolin. Persistence in breast feeding is important because the soreness will be gone in several days. Until soreness subsides, nursing should be initiated on the side that feels the best. Limiting sucking leads to engorgement and increased soreness. Prolonged nursing, however, should be avoided while the soreness persists.

Plugged ducts. Occasionally a milk duct will become plugged, creating a tender spot on the breast, which may even appear lumpy and hot. This might result from inadequate emptying of the milk ducts or from wearing a brassiere that is too tight. Should a plugged duct develop, the following approaches might be taken:

1. Offer the sore breast first so that it will be emptied more completely.
2. Nurse longer and more often; if the breast gets too full, the plugged duct becomes worse and infection may develop.
3. Change positions at every feeding so that the pressure of the nursing will be applied to different places on the breast.
4. Apply warm compresses to the breasts between feedings to reduce the risk of infection by keeping the ducts open.

Infection. If breast tenderness is accompanied by fever and a general flulike feeling, a breast infection is probably present (see also p. 833). Treatment involves the following:

1. Bed rest
2. Continued nursing (offering the sore breast first)
3. Application of heat with a hot water bottle or heating pad
4. Supporting the breasts with a firm brassiere
5. Consulting a physician

There is generally no danger from the baby becoming ill from nursing the infected breast. He probably has the same bacteria in his nose and throat as those responsible for the infection of the mother. Breast infections are sometimes complicated by localized pus accumulation; this is referred to as a breast abscess and it may require surgical opening and draining in addition to antibiotics. Women are advised not to nurse on the affected side until the abscess heals. During the interval of not nursing, the milk should be frequently expressed by hand from the affected breast.

Leaking. Some mothers are bothered by leaking breasts either during or between feedings. Although this may help to relieve fullness in the early weeks of lactation, it soon becomes a nuisance. It can be stopped by simply pressing firmly with the palm of the hand against the leaking nipple. A less obvious way to stop both breasts from leaking is for the woman to cross her arms against her breasts and press firmly. Gauze pads with an outside plastic coat may be inserted inside the brassiere to catch any milk that may be released. Lining the brassiere cup with plastic material is not recommended, since moisture tends to soften the nipple and predispose to erosion. It is better to pad the brassiere with folded squares of soft cotton or a perineal pad cut in two.

Failure to thrive in the breast-feeding infant. Insufficient milk supply is rarely a problem for the well-fed mother. Since sucking stimulates the flow of milk,

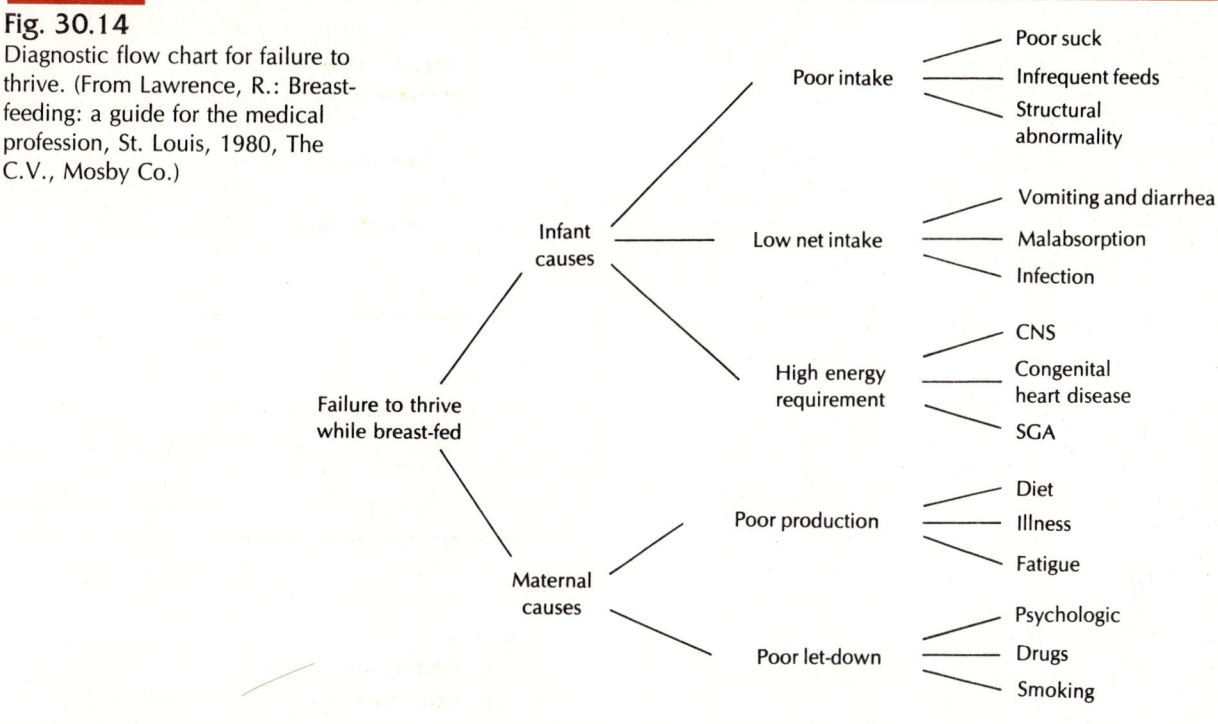

Fig. 30.14
Diagnostic flow chart for failure to thrive. (From Lawrence, R.: Breast-feeding: a guide for the medical profession, St. Louis, 1980, The C.V., Mosby Co.)

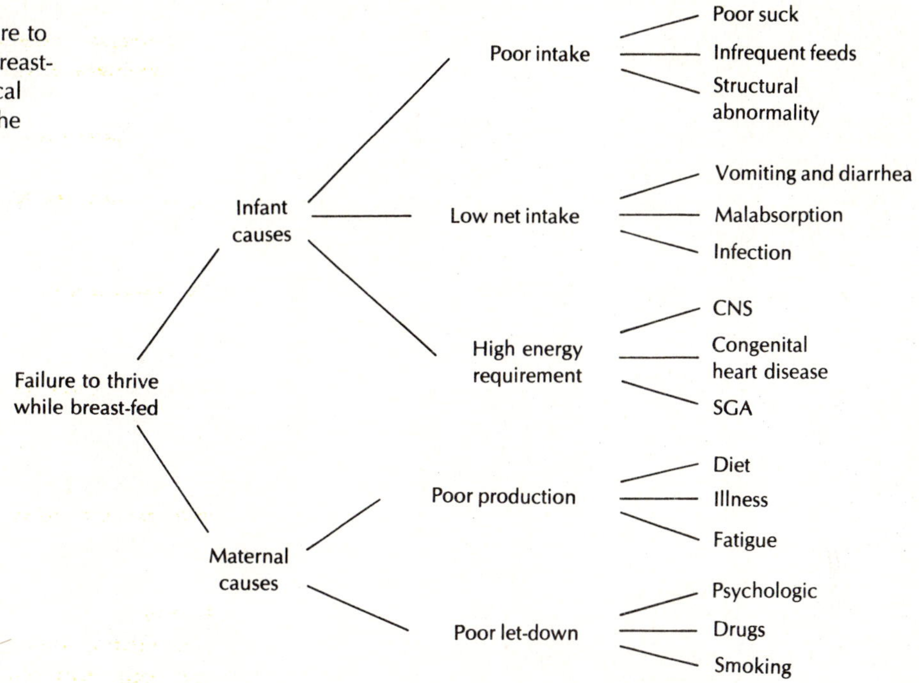

feeding on demand for adequate duration should supply ample amounts of milk. If the baby continues steadily to gain weight and length, has at least six wet diapers daily and normal stools, the milk supply is probably adequate.

Occasionally, however, an infant will fail to thrive while seemingly nursing properly. While diagnosis of the problem may sometimes be difficult, a variety of circumstances can be explored as likely bases for the unsatisfactory breast-feeding experience (Lawrence, 1980). Fig. 30.14 illustrates diagrammatically potential problems in the mother or in the infant that should be investigated during the course of evaluation. If the cause of the problem cannot be identified or the defined problem cannot be corrected, it may be necessary to encourage the mother to turn to commercial infant formula for at least partial nutritional support of the infant.

Relactation and induced lactation. Occasionally a mother starts breast feeding late or dicontinues nursing but decides at a much later date that she would like to begin again. She can attempt relactation through providing the infant substantial opportunities to suck at the breast. With much sucking stimulus over several days' time, many patient and persistent women can initiate the lactation process late or once again. Their volume of milk production may be less than the infant demands, in which case a supplemental feeding following nursing may be necessary. Alternatively, some women find the Lact-aid Nursing Trainer to nicely complement their own milk production (Fig. 30.15). While the baby

Fig. 30.15
Lact-Aid Nursing Trainer in use.

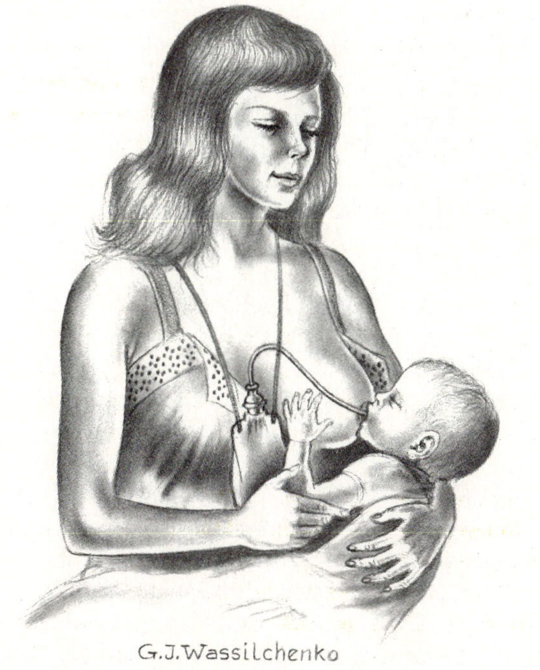

Fig. 30.16
Commonly used breast pumps. **A,** Swedish pump. **B,** Syringe pump. **C,** Electric pump.

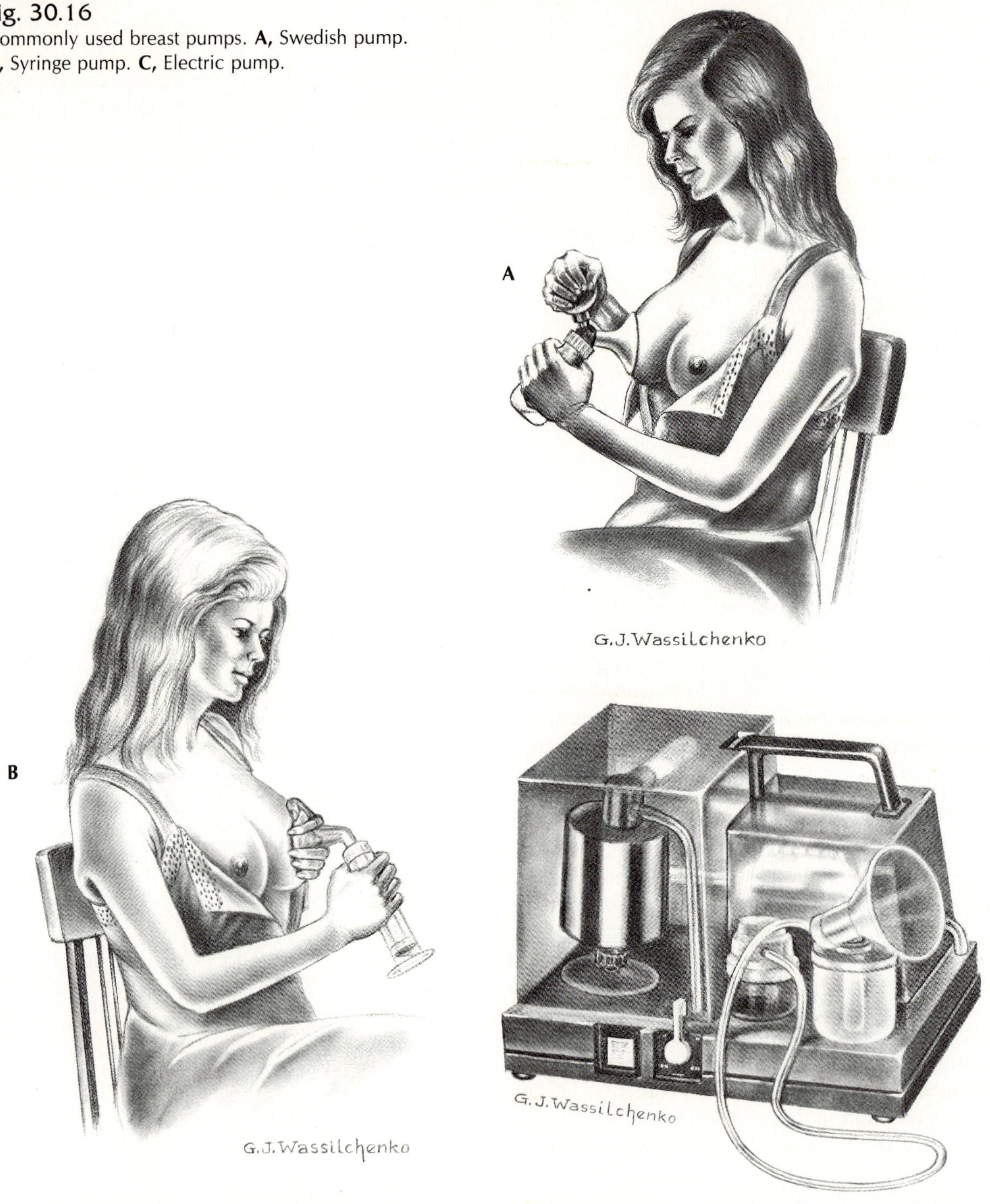

sucks at the breast, he also obtains milk via suction through a small tube leading to a bag of fresh formula that is clipped to the mother's brassiere. While the baby sucks, he simultaneously builds up the mother's milk supply but receives adequate nutrition through the Lact-aid feeding device.

After adopting an infant, a minority of women decide to attempt lactation even though they have never done so before or, at best, breast fed a previous baby of their own. With much sucking stimulus, lactation can be induced but only with great perseverance and in most cases only if a woman has once carried a pregnancy well into the second trimester. Since the mammary glands complete their development for lactation during the first 6 months of pregnancy, a woman who has never been pregnant or never carried a pregnancy beyond the first trimester is a poor candidate for successful induction of lactation.

Breast pumping. For a number of reasons, mothers may wish to remove milk from their breasts and save it for a later feeding, take it to their hospitalized neonate, or donate it to a milk bank. Under such circumstances, milk can be expressed by hand and for some women this method is satisfactory. For many women, however, a manual or electric breast pump provides a better stimulus for milk flow and a more efficient mode of milk collection (Fig. 30.16). Instructions for use of these pumps accompany each apparatus, but individual counseling by a skilled clinician or experienced nursing mother can greatly simplify the process of learning to pump.

Formula Feeding

A variety of formulas can be fed to infants as an alternative to providing human milk. Most commercial formulas provide 20 kcal/oz and are prepared from cow's milk that has been modified to reduce the solute load by reducing the protein and mineral content. The curd is made easier to digest through homogenization and heat treatment. Vegetable oils largely replace butterfat and carbohydrate; vitamins and minerals are added.

TYPES OF COMMERCIAL FORMULAS

Specific name brands of formulas are recommended by physicians. Most formulas are available in the following forms:

1. Concentrated: requires dilution with water
2. Ready-to-use: requires measuring into bottles
3. Ready-to-use: sold in disposable bottles
4. Dry powder form: requires mixing with water according to label instructions

The choice of a particular brand should be based on cost, convenience, and the mother's ability to prepare the formula accurately and safely (Pipes, 1981).

Instructions for mixing powdered or concentrated formulas should be followed accurately to prevent overdilution or underdilution. When formulas are underdiluted with water, the renal solute load is increased and may lead to dehydration of the infant. If overdilution occurs, inadequate calories and nutrients are provided and failure-to-thrive may result. When the safety of the community or home water supply is in doubt, sterile water is recommended for diluting formulas.

EVAPORATED MILK FORMULAS

Although home-prepared evaporated milk formula may be least expensive, it is not generally recommended because of the increased chance of improper measurement and bacterial contamination during preparation of the formula. Often the families who could benefit most by the savings are least able to understand the importance of sanitary precautions and accurate measurements in preparing the formula. Special counseling is needed for parents who choose to use evaporated milk formula; forunately, only about 1% of formula-feeding families opt for this alternative today.

To control growth of bacteria, single feedings should be prepared as needed rather than all feedings for a 24-hr period. A formula may be prepared as follows:

Evaporated milk: 3 oz
Water: 4.5 oz
Corn syrup: 2 tsp

An opened can of evaporated milk should be covered and refrigerated. Evaporated milk is fortified with vitamin D and forms an easily digested curd because of the heat processing it undergoes. Supplements of vitamin C (Fomon, 1979) and iron are needed for the infant fed with evaporated milk formula (Table 30.4). Fluoride supplements may be needed also (Table 30.5).

GOAT'S MILK

Occasionally a family will feed their infant goat's milk or a formula derived from it. There is no recognizable nutritional advantage for choosing goat's milk, and infants allergic to protein in cow's milk are often allergic to goat's milk protein as well. The high potassium chloride content of goat's milk makes it a less than optimal feed for the neonate, and metabolic acidosis has been reported in young infants provided goat's milk. Goat's milk is also deficient in folic acid, and a supplement of this vitamin should be provided along with supplements of vitamins D and C.

SOY FORMULAS

About 10% of infants in the United States are provided soy-based formulas instead of one derived from cow's milk. Most often this choice is made because the infant is suspected of demonstrating an allergy to cow's milk protein or proteins (Fomon, 1975). Sometimes, however, a family with a vegetarian–life-style orientation will select a soy formula for their infant. Commercial infant formulas prepared from soy protein isolate are designed to be nutritionally complete. Supplements may be recommended only for iron and fluoride when these nutrients are obviously missing from the daily food and water supply.

SPECIAL FORMULAS

When infants cannot tolerate commercial infant formulas made from cow's milk or soy protein isolate, another special formula may be selected. Some formulas provide the protein in broken-down form, such as casein hydrolysate. Other formulas are designed to be low in lactose, sodium, or phenylalanine. Several formulas provide the fat in easily digestible form (medium chain triglycerides); these products are especially useful for infants with severe fat malabsorption (Jelliffe, 1976; Barltrop, 1974). This array of special formulas meets the needs of a small fraction of infants in the United States; they are more expensive than the regular formulas and should only be chosen when a clear-cut justification exists.

PREPARATION OF COMMERCIAL FORMULAS

Although the formula labels still give instructions for sterilizing the water and bottles during formula preparation, this is no longer routinely recommended unless the sanitation conditions in the home require it. When the safety of a community or home water supply is in doubt, sterile water should be used to dilute the formula. Otherwise, this is not necessary. When the water supply is fluoridated, sterilizing the water will lower the fluoride content. Bottles, nipples, caps, and collars should be washed in soap and water and rinsed in hot water before using. The nipple hole should be checked for adequate flow; however, a heavy flow or a long nipple may prompt a choking response from the infant. If a nipple with a heavy flow or a long nipple is used over a long period of time, the infant could develop a deviant swallowing pattern or tongue thrust. Formula should be at room temperature before feeding although older infants may tolerate formula straight from the refrigerator.

SKIM MILK

Skim milk has about half the number of calories (10 kcal/oz) of breast milk, evaporated milk, or commercial infant formulas (20 kcal/oz). Research shows that infants fed skim milk have difficulty ingesting a volume sufficient to meet their energy needs (Fomon and Ziegler, 1977; Fomon et al., 1979). Measures of triceps skinfold thickness of infants fed skim milk show that body stores of fat are used to meet energy and growth requirements. It seems undesirable for fat stores to be depleted rapidly in the first months of life. The infant may not be able to withstand a serious illness should one occur.

Studies show that the rate of growth of infants fed skim milk is slower than infants receiving breast milk or formula (Fomon and Ziegler, 1977; Foman et al., 1979). In addition to being inadequate in iron and vitamin C, skim milk is insufficient in the essential fatty acids needed by young infants. It contains a relatively high percentage of calories from protein and large amounts of minerals, which increase the renal solute load. Although the normal healthy infant may be able to get rid of the increased waste products as long as his fluid intake is sufficient, this is of concern during illnesses associated with a decreased fluid intake, diarrhea, and increased renal output.

BOTTLE-FEEDING TECHNIQUES

For the first few feedings, until the baby becomes familiar with the process, the baby can be held slightly away from the mother's body while the nipple is being put into his mouth and he begins to suck. When the baby is held close to the mother, the rooting reflex is elicited, and the mother may find it more difficult to introduce the nipple.

The bottle-fed baby ingests more air while sucking than does the breast-fed baby; therefore it is important to hold the bottle at such an angle that the milk covers the neck of the bottle. The baby may be burped before beginning the feeding, especially if he has been crying, after about 30 ml (1 oz) of formula has been taken, and at the end of the feeding.

Once the baby begins sucking properly, the mother should hold him close so that he can relax against her warmth. Every infant needs physical contact with the mother, and the feeding period offers one of the most natural ways for infant and adult to share, to give, and to experience nurturing.

It is a dangerous practice to "prop the bottle" when feeding an infant. The nipple can lodge against the back of the throat and block the air passage, or if the infant regurgitates, the fluid may be aspirated, causing death or a lung infection. There is a higher incidence of otitis media in infants who are propped in the horizontal position. The eustachian tube orifice opens during swallowing, and mucus from the nose can drain into the duct and occlude it. The infant should never be left alone when feeding until he is old enough to hold the bottle and to remove it from his mouth by himself. After feeding, the infant is placed on his right side to permit the formula to flow toward the pyloric sphincter and to allow any swallowed air to rise above the fluid and out through the esophagus (Fig. 29.5).

Table 30.9
Guide for Formula Feeding

Age	Average Quantity Taken in Individual Feedings	Average No. of Feedings per 24 Hours
Birth to 3	2-3 oz	6-10
wk	5 oz	
2 wk to 2		5-8
mo	5-7 oz	
2-3 mo	6-8 oz	5-6
3-4 mo	8 oz	4-6
5-12 mo		3-4

Once the formula has been fed to the infant, any formula remaining in the bottle can be discarded or refrigerated for use by adults. It should not be left at room temperature; warm milk serves an an excellent medium for bacterial growth.

Most healthy babies are able to determine how much formula to consume. They should be allowed to stop eating at the earliest indication of a desire to stop. Table 30.9 gives some general ideas of amounts of formula to prepare. However, each baby has individual caloric requirements. You will note a decrease in actual amount of formula taken by the infant at 5 to 12 months since semisolid foods are added during this period.

Common problems. The following are common problems of mothers who are bottle feeding their infants, with suggestions for dealing with the problems:

1. The infant tires quickly and goes to sleep. The mother may try a softer nipple or may enlarge the hole in the nipple or both. To enlarge the hole, heat a needle stuck into a cork (used as a handle) and insert the hot needle into the nipple hole. New nipples may be softened by boiling for 5 minutes before using.

2. The infant takes ''forever'' to feed. This is not uncommon, particularly in smaller babies. Slow, patient feeding, keeping the infant awake, and encouraging him to suck by massaging upward under his chin may be necessary. Regardless of the time involved, the infant needs to consume approximately the total number of calories per day prescribed as normal for his weight.

3. The infant gulps down the formula, chokes, and regurgitates. The mother checks to see whether the hole in the nipple is too large. If the bottle is held upside down, the milk should come out in drops, not in a stream. Help the infant learn to drink more slowly by stopping the feeding after each ounce, burping and cuddling him, and then resuming the feeding.

4. The temperature of the warmed formula (place the bottle in a pan of hot water) can be checked by letting a few drops fall on the inside of the wrist. If the formula feels comfortably warm to the mother, it is the correct temperature. (Commercially prepared formula stored at room temperature does not need warming.)

5. Once a bottle of formula has been used for a feeding, the remaining formula should not be kept for the next feeding. It may be stored in the refrigerator and used as coffee or cereal cream by the adults in the family.

The stools of bottle-fed babies are soft but formed. They are light yellow and have a characteristic foul odor. The composition of the stool is irritating to the infant's skin; therefore the buttocks need frequent cleaning. By the end of the second week the number of stools has decreased from about five to one or two a day.

Introduction of Solids

Breast milk or infant formula provides all needed nutrition for the infant for at least 3 months of life. During this time, the infant is not developmentally ready for consumption of solid foods. When developmental readiness is apparent (about 3 to 5 months of age), the infant should be provided appropriate semisolids. By this time, food will be retained in the mouth when presented rather than being extruded by the tongue (Table 28.2). The jaw and tongue begin to move independently, and the head is held upright without support. The infant begins to model behavior in his environment and is ready to develop independent skills for self-feeding.

In deciding on a sequence for introduction of semisolid foods, the appropriateness of recommending any food group depends on its nutritional contributions to the total diet. Before recommending specific semisolids, one needs to know the type of milk or formula being consumed, the amount, and its contribution to the total daily energy needs. For example, the breast-fed infant has a greater need for foods rich in protein by the age of 6 months than the bottle-fed infant.

The semisolid food most often introduced first is infant cereal. Rice cereal is usually the first cereal fed since it is least likely to cause allergic reactions. Its smooth, silky texture is much like milk and will be somewhat familar. Gradually, barley, oats, and wheat cereals may be tried. The cereal selected should be an infant cereal since this is the kind that contains the greatest amount of available iron. A major reason for introducing semisolids is to provide a source of iron because infants' iron stores begin to dwindle at 4 to 6 months of age (Fomon et al., 1979).

Mild-flavored strained vegetables, fruits, and juices follow cereal. Plain vegetables and fruits are recommended rather than creamed vegetables, desserts, or puddings. Vegetables may be accepted more readily if

Table 30.10
Suggested Ages for Introduction of Semisolid Foods and Table Foods

Food	Age (mo) 4-6	6-8	9-12
Iron-fortified cereals for infants	Add		
Vegetables		Add strained	Gradually delete strained foods, introduce table foods
Fruits		Add strained	Gradually delete strained foods, introduce chopped, well-cooked, or canned foods
Meats		Add strained or finely chopped table meats	Decrease use of strained meats, increase varieties of table meats
Finger foods such as arrowroot biscuits, oven-dried toast		Add those that can be secured with a palmar grasp	Increase use of small-sized finger foods as pincer grasp develops
Well-cooked mashed or chopped table foods, prepared without added salt or sugar			Add
Juice by cup			Add

introduced before fruits, although there is no scientific evidence to support this idea. Home-prepared nitrate-containing vegetables, such as beets, spinach, turnips, mustard greens, and collard greens should not be offered first (Anderson 1977); plant nitrates can be converted into nitrites before consumption by the infant. This phenomenon is of concern since the nitrite ion can oxidize the iron contained in hemoglobin, resulting in the formation of another compound, methemoglobin. Since methemoglobin in incapable of binding molecular oxygen, a sufficient amount of methemoglobin in the blood will result in cyanosis. Commercially prepared baby foods have been found to contain only a trace amount of nitrite (Fomon, 1974). Strained meats and egg yolks should be introduced last since their higher protein and electrolyte content will increase the renal solute load. Egg white should not be fed during the first 10 months because it may cause allergic reactions. An outline of the recommended schedule for introduction of solids is provided in Table 30.10.

The introduction of solids to the diet of an infant can be achieved without problem for mother or infant. Some practical considerations, however, may simplify the process and prevent problems during this transitional period. Among the factors to consider are the following (Hinton and Kerwin, 1981):

1. Introduce only one new food at a time. Allow the infant to become familiar with that food before trying to give another. More importantly, if allergies are present, the cause can be more easily identified if new foods are introduced several days apart. Give mixed foods only after the infant has been given each food separately.

2. Give very small amounts of any new food—teaspoons or even less—at the beginning.

3. Use a very thin consistency when starting solid foods. A small spoon is put into the baby's mouth so that the food is placed on the middle of the tongue and swallowing is more readily accomplished. The fact that a baby spits out his first feedings of solid food may indicate that he has not yet learned the tongue movements or is not developmentally ready for the spoon.

4. Never force an infant to eat more of a food than he accepts willingly.

5. If, after several trials, it is apparent that a baby has an acute dislike for a food, omit that item for a week or two and then try it again. If the dislike persists, it is better to forget about that food for a while and substitute another.

6. It is not necessary to add salt, fat, or other seasonings to the baby's food.

7. Use foods of smooth consistency at first—strained fruits, vegetables, and meats.

8. When the baby is able to chew, gradually substitute finely chopped fruits and vegetables for pureed foods—usually at 7 to 8 months.

9. Infants may object to taking some foods by themselves but may take them willingly if they are mixed with another food. For example, egg yolk may be mixed with formula, cereal, or vegetable; vegetables may sometimes be made into a soup with a little formula until the baby becomes accustomed to the new flavor.

10. Semisolids should not be given by bottle. This may lead to excessive calorie consumption and does not contribute to the development of sound eating habits.

11. Variety in choice of foods is important. The baby, like older persons, may tire of the repetition of certain foods, especially cereals and vegetables. Including a variety of foods will more likely ensure an adequate nutritional intake also.

12. The mother or person feeding the infant must be careful to avoid showing in any way a dislike for a food that is being given.

13. Bottle-fed babies may accept semisolids only after first receiving 1 to 2 oz of formula. The formula quickly begins to satisfy their hunger and allows more patience for enjoying other foods.

The same safety rules apply to preparation and serving of baby food as to foods for adults. Since infants are more susceptible to illness and infections than adults, even more caution should be taken when handling their food. All utensils, work surfaces, cutting boards, and containers should be thoroughly washed with warm, soapy water and rinsed with hot water before and between usage. The person preparing the food should always wash his hands and nails and be careful not to touch the face, hair, other parts of the body, or other objects such as the telephone without washing his hands again before touching the food. Foods should never be left at room temperature longer than it takes to prepare them. Bacteria that cause food spoilage grow best between 40° and 60° C (104° and 140° F). The longer food remains in this temperature range, the greater the chance of spoilage.

When opening jars of commercially prepared baby food, listen for the "pop" of the hermetic seal. This sound lets you know that the product was safely processed and stored until the time it was opened. Unless the baby is consuming the contents of the entire jar, food should be spooned out of the jar and fed to the baby from a dish. Otherwise, saliva transferred to the jar may increase the likelihood of bacterial growth in the remaining food. Part of the food can be left in the jar and refrigerated up to 24 hours. Any food remaining in the baby's dish after feeding should be discarded.

The practice of preparing baby foods at home has become a very popular one. A considerable cost-saving benefit can result if economic food choices are made. However, sanitary conditions must prevail in the home, and safe food-handling procedures must be followed to prevent bacterial contamination that can cause mild or serious illness. Babies are more susceptible to intestinal upsets caused by bacterial growth than adults.

In preparing baby foods, high-quality fresh and frozen items should be selected. Several types of equipment can be used to change solid food to a semisolid state; these include mashers, sieves, food mills, and blenders. Salt, sugar, and spices should not be added. Babies are not born with an innate liking for spices or salt but develop their preferences over time. Preference for sweet tastes, is an inborn characteristic that does not need emphasis in the period of infancy. The caloric density of home-prepared meats and vegetables is likely to be greater than the commercial counterparts because of the higher total solids and fat content. Fruits and juices should be about equal in calories if no sugar is added to either. Mothers should be careful to adjust serving sizes if switching from commercial to home-prepared foods (Anderson, 1977).

When preparing baby food, it is often time saving and convenient to prepare several servings of baby food ahead of time for freezing. Ice cube trays are ideal for freezing foods in baby portions. Once the food is frozen, the cubes can be popped into a plastic bag or freezer container. Containers should be labeled and dated. One or more cubes can then be thawed at feeding time. Meat and protein foods should be thawed in the refrigerator; fruits and vegetables can be thawed at room temperature. Frozen foods can be immediately heated also. Thawed foods should not be refrozen.

Feeding of fruit juices by bottle should be avoided in that an infant may be left with the bottle for quite some time with constant coating of the teeth by sugary fluid. This practice may lead to *nursing bottle syndrome* and eventual destruction of the upper incisors. If juices are given to infants at this time, use of a cup will avoid any problem.

Selected Problems

Failure to follow proper feeding procedures for infants can compromise the normality of their growth and development. Both deficiencies and excesses of nutrients may be recognized, and these may accompany the early introduction of cow's milk, early introduction of solids, or inappropriate choice of formula or solid foods.

OVERWEIGHT AND OBESITY

Excessive body fatness may develop in infancy because of hereditary factors, overfeeding, underactivity, or a combination of these factors. Whether or not a strong genetic predisposition to obesity can be overcome by promotion of healthful eating and exercise patterns in infancy is still open to debate. It is certain, however, that obesity secondary to excessive food intake can certainly be avoided through support of appropriate feeding practices in the first year of life and thereafter.

Because the habits, attitudes, and unconscious feelings established early in infancy may be difficult to change, the parent and pediatrician are doing the infant no favor by inappropriately feeding excess calories in any form to show affection, promote sleep, or relieve irritation. Although it is a common belief that early feeding of semisolid foods causes infants to sleep through the night, careful studies have shown that this is not the case. Early feeding for behavioral rather than nutritional reasons or to demonstrate parental caring may contribute to the difficulty some older children, adolescents, or adults may have in restricting their diet when indicated. Those who advise young parents will recognize that a harried father or mother may be tempted to rely on an extra bottle, cookie, or other food to resolve the infant's fussiness or boredom. In some instances a parent may even resort to such practices out of his own desire to be a "good" parent, encouraging the infant to plumpness and precocious development by zealous overfeeding.

ATHEROSCLEROSIS

Atherosclerosis is a common problem in the United States and is characterized by lipid accumulation in arterial walls. Risk of development of this problem has been associated with a high-fat diet, but susceptibility to the disease appears to have a strong genetic component. Whether or not atherosclerosis begins in infancy is a question still open to debate; fatty streaks in the arterial walls may develop in early life but their progress to atheromatous plaques is unclear.

Although it appears rational to recommend that infants with diagnosed hyperlipidemias avoid foods containing high levels of saturated fats and cholesterol, it is not clear that such avoidance has any beneficial effect on the normal infant (Blumenthal, 1977). In fact, since human milk is rich in cholesterol and high in fat overall, one might speculate that the human infant profits from this fat-rich diet. Given the controversy, however, it seems well to advise that unnecessary sources of dietary fat and cholesterol should be limited in the diet by the end of the first year of life.

HYPERTENSION

High sodium intakes during the period of infancy have been suggested to be a predisposing factor in the development of hypertension. The causes of primary hypertension are many, however, and the contribution of specific factors is not well defined. Data derived from both animal models and human subjects support the notion that ingestion of a high-sodium diet by an individual genetically predisposed to hypertension may speed the onset of the disease and augment its severity. These data, however, do not establish a firm relationship between hypertension and sodium intake during infancy. Even if a relationship exists, 80% of infants are not at risk for development of the disorder. Since currently available clinical tools do not allow for the identification of the 20% of infants at risk for manifesting hypertension in later life, moderation in use of sodium in the diets of young children seems a reasonable strategy to support.

General Guidelines for Feeding the Normal Infant

Taking into account all that has been said and reviewing the recommendations of the American Academy of Pediatrics (1976a), an outline can be developed of basic strategies for feeding normal infants. The following points are relevant (Owen and Owen, 1981).

INITIAL ORAL FEEDING

When one prepares to give the initial feeding to any infant,* the following factors must be considered:

Factor	Rationale
1. Neonate's age in hours or infant's age in days	1. During reactivity periods, excessive mucus with gagging may occur. Feeding increases the danger of aspiration. In general, reactivity times occur at birth and at 4 to 6 hours of age.
2. Condition at birth	2. Infants with Apgar scores of 6 or less (depressed) or the infant with low birth weight (2500 g or less) may display a delayed reactivity. This may occur after 12 to 18 hours of age.

*If for any reason the infant cannot suckle (e.g., prematurity, maternal illness), the mother's supply of milk may be maintained by manual expression or by hand or electric pump. If milk is to be used for infant, cool and freeze immediately and transport in ice to infant.

Factor	Rationale
3. Possibility of congenital anomalies of gastrointestinal or respiratory tract*; incidence of congenital anomalies higher in preterm infants	3. With choanal atresia, neonate may be unable to breathe and feed simultaneously. With esophageal atresia, infant often will regurgitate and may aspirate. With tracheoesophageal fistula, feeding may enter trachea directly. With lower gastrointestinal tract obstruction (stenosis, atresia), regurgitation, vomiting, or abdominal distention may compromise respirations.
4. Gastric capacity	4. Limited stomach capacity dictates smaller feedings. To provide adequate nutrition, feedings are scheduled more frequently. For suggested initial amounts, see Table 30.9.
5. CNS maturity	5. Sucking and swallowing reflexes may not be well developed and synchronized (even in a term baby, the suck and swallow reflex may not be well coordinated during first few hours).
6. Energy level	6. Premature infant or infant with respiratory distress may not have sufficient energy to divert to the process of feeding. Use "preemie" nipple, or utilize gavage feedings (see below).
7. Type of feeding: plain sterile water	7. Until infant's ability to feed is assessed, danger of aspiration exists. Plain sterile water is least irritating to respiratory tree. a. Formula may cause aspiration pneumonia. b. Glucose water may cause inflammatory response in respiratory tree similar to response to aspirated formula.

*An infant with choanal atresia simply cannot breathe normally. The question of feeding will never arise in such deeply distressed infants. The infant with esophageal atresia or tracheoesophageal fistula will always regurgitate and may aspirate.

FIRST 6 MONTHS

1. Human milk should be used as the major source of nutrition.
2. The breast-fed infant should receive supplements of vitamin D, fluoride, and in some cases iron.
3. Infants fed commercially prepared iron-fortified formula require no supplements except fluoride (depending on the fluoride content of the local drinking water).
4. Infants receiving evaporated milk formulas should receive supplements of vitamin C and iron.
5. Solid foods should not be introduced before 4 to 6 months of age.

AFTER 6 MONTHS

1. Human milk or iron-fortified commercial infant formula should be used up to 1 year of age.
2. Between 4 and 6 months of age, the introduction of solids should begin. Iron-fortified infant cereal should be introduced first; rice or barley is least allergenic.
3. Other foods such as homemade or commercially prepared fruits and vegetables should then be introduced; no more than one or two new foods should be introduced each week.
4. If breast feeding is continued beyond 6 months of age, some good protein sources should be added.
5. Low-fat milks should not be fed during the first year of life.

Nutritional Screening and Assessment of Infants

The objective of screening is to identify infants who appear to have nutritional problems that require further evaluation. The interview with the family or caretaker is brief, and information sought is qualitative in nature. The nurse or the available paraprofessional is often in charge of preliminary discussions. An example of a 24-hr screening questionnaire that may be used in the initial contact is provided in the box on p. 678.

Screening Questionnaire for Infants

Infants (from birth to age 1 year) **Yes** **No**

1. Is the baby breast fed? ☐ ☐
   If yes, does he also receive milk or formula? ☐ ☐
   If yes, what kind? ______
2. Does the baby receive formula? ☐ ☐
   If yes ☐ Ready-to-feed
   ☐ Concentrated liquid
   ☐ Other: ______
   How is formula prepared (especially dilution)?
   ______
   ______
   Is the formula iron fortified? ☐ ☐
3. Does the baby drink milk? ☐ ☐
   If yes ☐ Whole milk
   ☐ 2% milk
   ☐ Skim milk
   ☐ Other: ______
4. How many times does he eat each day, including milk or formula? ______
5. Does the baby usually take a bottle to bed? ☐ ☐
   If yes, what is usually in the bottle? ______
6. If the baby drinks milk or formula, what is the usual amount in a day?
   ☐ Less than 16 oz
   ☐ 16 to 32 oz
   ☐ More than 32 oz
7. Please indicate which (if any) of these foods the baby eats and how often:

	Never or hardly ever (less than once a week)	**Sometimes (not daily but at least once a week)**	**Every day or nearly every day**
Eggs	☐	☐	☐
Dried beans or peas	☐	☐	☐
Meat, fish poultry	☐	☐	☐
Bread, rice, pasta, grits, cereal, tortillas, potatoes	☐	☐	☐
Fruits or fruit juices	☐	☐	☐
Vegetables	☐	☐	☐

8. If the baby eats fruits or drinks fruit juices every day or nearly every day, which ones does he eat or drink most often (not more than three)? ______
   ______
9. If the baby eats vegetables every day or nearly every day, which ones does he eat most often (not more than three)? ______
10. Does the person who cares for the baby have use of a
    Stove? ☐ ☐
    Refrigerator? ☐ ☐
    Piped water? ☐ ☐
11. Does the baby take vitamin or iron drops? ☐ ☐
    If yes, how often? ______
    What kind? ______
12. Is the baby on a special diet now? ☐ ☐
    If yes, what is the reason?
    Allergy—specify type of diet: ______
    Weight reduction—specify type of diet: ______
    Other—specify type of diet: ______
    Who recommended the diet? ______
13. Does the baby eat clay, paint chips, dirt, or anything else that is not usually considered food? ☐ ☐
    If yes, what? ______
    How often? ______
14. Do you think the child has a feeding problem? ☐ ☐
    If yes, describe: ______

From Fomon, S.J.: Nutritional disorders of children: prevention, screening, and follow up, pub. no. 76-5612, Rockville, Md., 1976, Department of Health, Education, and Welfare.

Anthropometric data plotted on growth charts are also valuable in screening. Growth charts defining the normal growth of American children have been developed by the National Center of Health Statistics; length, weight, head circumference, and weight-length relationship are defined for infant boys and girls while growth parameters of older boys and girls are provided on separate charts. Poor growth in height or weight should be evident to the clinician. Poor growth accompanied by evidence of inappropriately low food intake is justification for further nutritional assessment. Children who are at special nutritional risk have been defined by Pipes (1976) as follows.

CHILDREN AT NUTRITIONAL RISK

I. Infants or children who have an inappropriate rate of weight gain
   A. Insufficient weight gain: failure of the infant to gain at a rate in weight or length less than appropriate for an infant in his percentile since the infant's last clinic visit
   B. Very rapid rate of weight gain
   C. Gross discrepancy between length and weight

II. Infants whose parents feed them improperly prepared formulas
   A. Formulas that are prepared to yield more than or less than 20 cal/oz unless therapeutically prescribed; formulas are concentrated because of the following reasons:
      1. Parents do not understand concentrated vs. ready-to-feed formula
      2. Parents do not add sufficient water to concentrated formula
      3. Parents add additional formula powder to the water
   B. Calorically dilute formulas result from the following:
      1. Parents add additional water to formula
      2. Parents feed skim milk
      3. Parents feed sugar water rather than milk because they do not understand the need for milk in infancy

III. Infants or children who consume more than 40 oz or less than 16 oz of milk a day

IV. Infants whose parents lack skills in feeding technique or use equipment that makes it difficult for the infant to consume formula
   A. Infants who are fed at intervals of less than 2 hours or more than 5 hours on more than one or two occasions during the day
   B. Infants whose parents prop the bottle
   C. Breast-fed infants who nurse for inappropriately long periods at each feeding
   D. Infants who are not appropriately burped
   E. Young infants who consistently fall asleep before completing an acceptable caloric intake, whose parents are using bottles with firm nipples and have not adjusted the holes for the infant

V. Infants less than 60 days old who consume greater than 145 cal/kg or less than 90 cal/kg

VI. Infants of breast-feeding mothers who have the following problems:
   A. They restrict their intake of food or a group of foods that contributes appreciably to the increment for nutrients during lactation
   B. They have questions about scheduling and the use of supplementary feedings
   C. They have infants who refuse the breast
   D. They are concerned about not having sufficient milk for their babies

VII. Infants of parents who *appear* to have a lack of concern about feeding (e.g., they prop the bottle or do not know what to feed)

VIII. Children whose parents are anxious about what and how their children eat

IX. Infants or children who receive megadoses of vitamins

X. Children who consume inappropriate kinds of semisolids and table food because of the following reasons:
   A. Additions of semisolids to milk
   B. Unavailability of sufficient amounts of iron-containing foods at appropriate levels of growth
   C. Excessive use of semisolids, which distorts the milk intake
   D. Use of excessive quantities of high-carbohydrate foods or alcoholic beverages (e.g., beer, wine, carbonated beverages, cookies, crackers, potato chips, french fries)
   E. Additions of excessive quantities of high-calorie semisolids (e.g., meats, egg yolks, cookies)

XI. Children who refuse an entire group of foods

XII. Children of parents who have questions regarding what or how much to feed

XIII. Children whose parents do not use food to support developmental progression
   A. Progression to finger foods (when the in-

fant reaches out for food [at approximately 6 to 7 months of age], finger foods that will not splinter and cause choking should be added)

B. Appropriate progression in texture and consistency (when finger foods are introduced, the progression to soft mashed table foods can be begun; when strained meats are refused, finely chopped meat from the table can be offered)

C. Progression from bottle to cup (when the infant is developmentally 9 to 12 months of age, experience with a cup should be offered)

XIV. Children whose parents follow food fads or who have questions about food fads or diets

A. Feed sugar water or herb tea instead of milk

B. Feed raw cow's milk or goat's milk

XV. Infants or children with physical handicaps that influence the child's ability to ingest food (e.g., poor suck, cleft lip or palate, tongue thrust)

XVI. Children of parents who lack skill in home management

A. Time and money management

B. Housekeeping

C. Food procurement

XVII. Children of families who do not take advantage of the resources available to them to aid and improve the nutrition of their children (e.g., W.I.C. food program, school lunch)

XVIII. Children who have specific therapeutic dietary problems

When children have been identified with potential nutritional problems, more in-depth evaluation is in order (Christakis, 1973). Additional anthropometric measurements may sometimes be taken, and effort will be made to record any clinical signs of malnutrition (glossitis, cheilosis, enlargement of the costrochondral junctions, etc.). Selected biochemical measurements will be ordered which in most cases require the collection of a small sample of blood; iron status is routinely evaluated, but in some children additional information is desirable. Selection of additional biochemical tests is based on suspicions about deficiency deriving from dietary intake data as well as information about growth and clinical status.

Information about dietary intake is routinely collected through use of a 24-hr recall, a diet history, or a 3- or 7-day food record. The interview is the most important aspect of any of the tools used. The validity of the data obtained depends on the parents' understanding of the reasons for the interview and the information sought; the parents' comfort with the interviewer and the interviewer's skills at probing for and validating information are also important factors determining the quality of the data.

During the interview, the interviewer must be careful to avoid suggesting time, meals, food, or amounts consumed. For example, the question, "When does your baby first have something to eat or drink?" is appropriate, whereas the question, "Does he eat breakfast at 8 AM?" is inappropriate. The tone of the voice is also important. Neither approval nor disapproval should be expressed verbally or nonverbally by facial expression. Food preferences of the interviewer should never be indicated. Silences should be accepted with comfort, and the parents should be permitted time to formulate answers to questions and to present questions of their own.

At times it is desirable to obtain semiquantitative information about nutrient intake of infants. In these cases, the 3- or 7-day diet record or written diary of all foods and beverages consumed is a useful tool (see box below). Parents are carefully instructed to record accurately the name of the food and the amount consumed by the infant. Information accumulated in the record will be evaluated in accord with the strategy of the clinician. Average daily nutrient intake may be calculated such that comparisons can be made with available standards. In some instances, intake data may be compared with food groups; other times, knowledge of foods that are present or absent in the dietary history or record may give a sufficient indication of the presence or absence of problems of nutrient intake.

When parents are unwilling or unable to give information that can be quantitated, such as "two bites of cereal" or a "glass of juice," the analysis of food groups or foods as sources of nutrients seems appropriate. If, however, the child is underweight or overweight, or if food sources of a particular nutrient appear on the record only occasionally, calculations of nutrient intake are important. Several computer programs are available for rapid and efficient calculation of average daily nutrient intake.

When dietary data have been collected and summarized, assessment is made of the following:

1. Parental knowledge of nutrition and appropriateness of foods for infants
2. Adequacy of nutrients provided by the food offered to the baby
3. Adequacy of the diet consumed by the infant
4. Parental knowledge of and use of community resources to improve the nutritional status of the child
5. Delays in feeding skills that affect food and nutrients consumed

Food Diary for Infants

Instructions

1. Record *all* formula, milk, and food that the baby consumes immediately *after* each feeding.
2. If your baby is breast fed, record the time of day the baby is fed and how long the baby feeds.
3. If your baby is formula fed, record the time of day the baby eats, the kind of formula the baby is fed, and the amount he actually consumes.
   Infant formula preparation:
   Is the formula iron fortified?
   ☐ Yes ☐ No
   Formula (brand name): ____________
   _____ oz liquid *or*
   _____ tbsp powder
   Water
   _____ oz
   Other (describe): ____________
   _____ oz
   _____ tbsp
   Total prepared formula
   _____ oz
4. If the baby spits up or vomits, estimate the amount.
5. Measure the amounts of any other foods carefully in terms of ounces of liquid (e.g., 2 oz apple juice), level tablespoons (e.g., 2 tbsp dry rice cereal), or portions of commercially prepared foods (e.g., ½ of a 4.7-oz jar of strained peaches).
6. Does the baby take a vitamin supplement?
   ☐ Yes ☐ No
   If yes, what kind? ____________
   _____ ml per day

Day 1
Date ____________ Day of week ____________
Most recent weight ________ on (date) ____________.

Time	Food or formula	Amount	Time	Food or formula	Amount

From Pipes, P.: Nutrition in infancy and childhood, ed. 2, St. Louis, 1981, The C.V. Mosby Co.

6. Real or potential behavior patterns that can or do compromise a child's nutrient intake
7. Motivation of parents to modify the baby's pattern of food intake

If the assessment indicates that changes in current practices are needed, careful work with parents or other caretakers should proceed. In some cases, assistance from community sources is useful; the clinician should familiarize himself with food assistance programs such as the Supplemental Food Program for Women, Infants and Children, which provides foods such as iron-fortified formula, milk or cheese, eggs, iron-fortified cereals, and vitamin C–containing juices to pregnant women and their young children.

Nutritional Intervention in Clinical Practice

Nutritional intervention involves three components: nutrition counseling, nutrition education, and referral for additional services. Nutrition counseling is the process by which clients are helped to acquire more health-

Table 30.11
Guidelines for Population Groups in Community Nutrition: Infants and Children

			Intervention		
Determining Risk	**Standard Criteria (Technique/Equipment/ Standards)**	**Problem**	**General Guidelines**	**Sample Client Behavioral Objectives**	**Referral Sources**
Anthropometric assessment					
Height Weight Head circumference (to 2 yr old) Skinfold thickness (over 5 yr old)	Balance scales, steel measuring tape, infant measuring board, calipers; National Center for Health Statistics (NCHS) growth grids Triceps skinfold	Poor growth (ht/age < 5th percentile, wt/ht < 5th percentile, head circumference < 5th percentile) Failure to thrive (drop in position on growth grid)	Rule out child abuse or neglect Check diet for energy and nutrient adequacy Check feeding environment	Parent will plot and interpret screening values for height, weight, and head circumference on growth grids Parent will explain relationship between weight/ height and health problems	Private physician WIC Program Children and Youth Comprehensive Services Crippled Children's Services Regional center for high-risk newborns Title XIX (Early and Periodic Screening, Detection, and Treatment Program)
		Obesity (wt/ht > 95th percentile)	Aim for child to "grow in to ideal weight range" rather than lose weight	Parent will identify ideal weight for own infant	
Biochemical assessment					
Hemoglobin Hematocrit Serum cholesterol	Center for Disease Control standards; adjusted for altitude Cyanmethemoglobin method for hemoglobin Wybenga method on microsample	Anemia	Identify cause of anemia (malabsorption, dietary, bleeding)	Parent/participant will identify causes, symptoms, and consequences of anemia	Head Start Program National Center for Child Abuse and Neglect Food stamps Commodity foods
		Elevated serum cholesterol (> 160 mg/dl)	Investigate other cardiovascular disease risk factors	Client/parent will identify cardiovascular disease risk factors and state those that can be modified	
Clinical assessment					
Birth weight Blood pressure Dental caries	Sphygmomanometer with child-size cuff; quiet environment	Birth weight < 24.8 kg (5½ lb)	Monitor low–birth weight infant to determine catch-up growth rate	Parent explains meaning of systolic and diastolic readings	
		Diastolic blood pressure (children aged 3-12 yr) > 90 mm Hg	Caution should be exercised in labeling children as hypertensive because of psychosocial and economic implications; use of term "high normal blood pressure" is appropriate during evaluation and follow-up	Parent explains factors than contribute to hypertension	

From Frankle, R.T., and Owen, A.Y.: Nutrition in the community: the art of delivering services, St. Louis, 1978, The C.V. Mosby Co.

ful behavior. Nutrition education is the process by which beliefs, attitudes, environmental influences, and understanding about food are modified such that sound and practical dietary behaviors are promoted. Referral procedures provide an opportunity for individuals and groups to take advantage of services available from other sources. The skilled clinician will provide counseling, education, and referral when needed with the ultimate goal of optimizing nutritional status of the infant and his family.

To assist the nurse and other health care personnel in providing optimal nutrition services, a proposed guideline for nutrition services for infant and children has been developed by Frankle and Owen (1978). This guideline is summarized in Table 30.11, which defines the elements for determining risk, standard criteria, problems, and intervention strategies based on the elements of nutritional assessment.

References and Readings

American Academy of Pediatrics, Committee on Nutrition: Salt intake and eating patterns of infants and children in relation to blood pressure, Pediatrics **53:**115, 1974.

American Academy of Pediatrics, Committee on Nutrition: Commentary on breast feeding and infant formulas, including proposed standards for formulas, Pediatrics **57:**278, 1976a.

American Academy of Pediatrics, Committee on Nutrition: Iron supplementation for infants, Pediatrics **58:**765, 1976b.

American Academy of Pediatrics, Committee on Nutrition: Fluoride supplementation: revised dosage schedule, Pediatrics **63:**150, 1979.

Anderson, T.A.: Commercial infant foods: content and composition, Pediatr. Clin. North Am. **24:**37, 1977.

Arnon, S.S., et al.: Honey and other environmental risk factors for infant botulism, J. Pediatr. **95:**331, 1979.

Bachrach, S., Fisher, J., and Parks, J.S.: An outbreak of vitamin D deficiency rickets in a susceptible population, Pediatrics **64:**871, 1979.

Barltrop, D.: Artificial milks in neonatal nutrition, The Practitioner **212:**465, 1974.

Beal, V.A.: Nutritional intake. In McCammon, R.W.: Human growth and development, Springfield, Ill., 1970, Charles C Thomas, Publisher.

Binkiewicz, A., Robinson M.J., and Senior, B.: Pseudo-Cushing syndrome caused by alcohol in breast milk, J. Pediatr. **93:**965, 1978.

Blumenthal, S.: Infant nutrition and atherosclerosis. Dialogues in infant nutrition, vol. 1, no. 3, Bloomfield, N.J., 1977, Health Learning Systems, Inc.

Chase, H.P., et al.: Kwashiorkor in the United States, Pediatrics **66:**972, 1980.

Christakis, G., editor: Nutritional assessment in health programs, Am. J. Pub. Health **63**(suppl.):1, Nov. 1973.

Dallman, P.R., Siimes, M.A., and Stekel, A.: Iron deficiency in infancy and childhood, Am. J. Clin. Nutr. **33:**86, 1980.

David, R., Ellis, D., and Gartner, J.C.: Water intoxication in normal infants: role of antidiuretic hormone in pathogenesis, Pediatrics **68:**349, 1981.

Fomon, S.J.: Infant nutrition, Philadelphia, 1974, W.B. Saunders Co.

Fomon, S.J.: What are infants fed in the United States? Pediatrics **56:**350, 1975.

Fomon, S.J., et al.: Recommendations for feeding normal infants, Pediatrics **63:**52, 1979.

Fomon, S.J., and Ziegler, E.: Skim milk in infant feeding. U.S. Department of Health, Education and Welfare pub. no. (HSA) 77-5102, Washington, D.C., Aug. 1977, The Department.

Food and Nutrition Board: Recommended dietary allowances, Washington, D.C., 1980, National Academy of Sciences.

Frankle, R.T., and Owen, A.Y.: Nutrition in the community: the art of delivering services, St. Louis, 1978, The C.V. Mosby Co.

Friedman, G., and Goldberg, S.J.: An evaluation of the safety of a low-saturated fat, low-cholesterol diet beginning in infancy, Pediatrics **58:**655, 1976.

Harrison, H.L., et al.: Goat milk acidosis, J. Pediatr. **94:**927, 1979.

Hinton, S.M., and Kerwin, D.R.: Maternal, infant and child nutrition: a resource book for health professionals, 1981, Health Sciences Consortium, Inc., North Carolina Division of Health Services.

Jelliffe, D.B.: World trends in infant feeding, Am. J. Clin. Nutr. **29:**1227, 1976.

Johnson, P.E., and Evans, G.W.: Relative zinc availability in human milk, infant formulas, and cow's milk, Am. J. Clin. Nutr. **31:**416, 1978.

Kooh, S.W., et al.: Rickets due to calcium deficiency, N. Engl. J. Med. **297:**1264, 1977.

Knopp, R.M., and Schwartz, J.F.: Water intoxication from swimming, J. Pediatr. **101:**947, 1982.

Lawrence, R.: Breast-feeding: a guide for the medical profession, St. Louis, 1980, The C.V. Mosby Co.

Martinez, G.A., and Nalenzienski, J.P.: The recent trend in breastfeeding, Pediatrics **64:**686, 1979.

National Center for Health Statistics: NCHS growth charts. Vital Statistics Report 25(3), suppl. (HRA 76-1120) Rockville, Md., Health Resources Administration.

Owen, A.L., and Owen, G.M.: Infant nutrition. In Jensen, M.D., Benson, R.C., and Bobak, I.M.: Maternity care: the nurse and the family, St. Louis, 1981, The C.V. Mosby Co.

Owen, A.L., Pipes, P., and Lee, S.L.: Infant feeding guide, Bloomfield, N.J., 1980, Health Learning Systems, Inc.

Partridge, J.C., et al.: Water intoxication secondary to feeding mismanagement, Am. J. Dis. Child. **135:**38, 1981.

Pipes, P.: Assessing food and nutrient intake. In Erickson, M.: Assessment and management of development changes in children, St. Louis, 1976, The C.V. Mosby Co.

Pipes, P.: Nutrition in infancy and childhood, ed. 2, St. Louis, 1981, The C.V. Mosby Co.

Pipes, P.: Nutrition in infancy and childhood, Prim. Care **9:**497, 1982.

U.S. Department of Health, Education, and Welfare: Ten state nutrition survey 1968-70, pub. no. (HSM) 728132, Washington, D.C., July 1972, The Department.

Widdowson, E.M., and Spray, C.M.: Chemical development in utero, Arch. Dis. Child. **26:**205, 1951.

Willis, N.H.: Infant nutrition: birth to 6 months: a syllabus, Philadelphia, J.B. Lippincott Co.

Worthington-Roberts, B., Vermeersch, J., and Williams, S.R.: Nutrition in pregnancy and lactation, St. Louis, 1981, The C.V. Mosby Co.

Nursing Care During the Postpartum Period

31 Maternal Physiology and Nursing Care

32 Family Responses to the Birth of a Child and Nursing Care

UNIT SIX

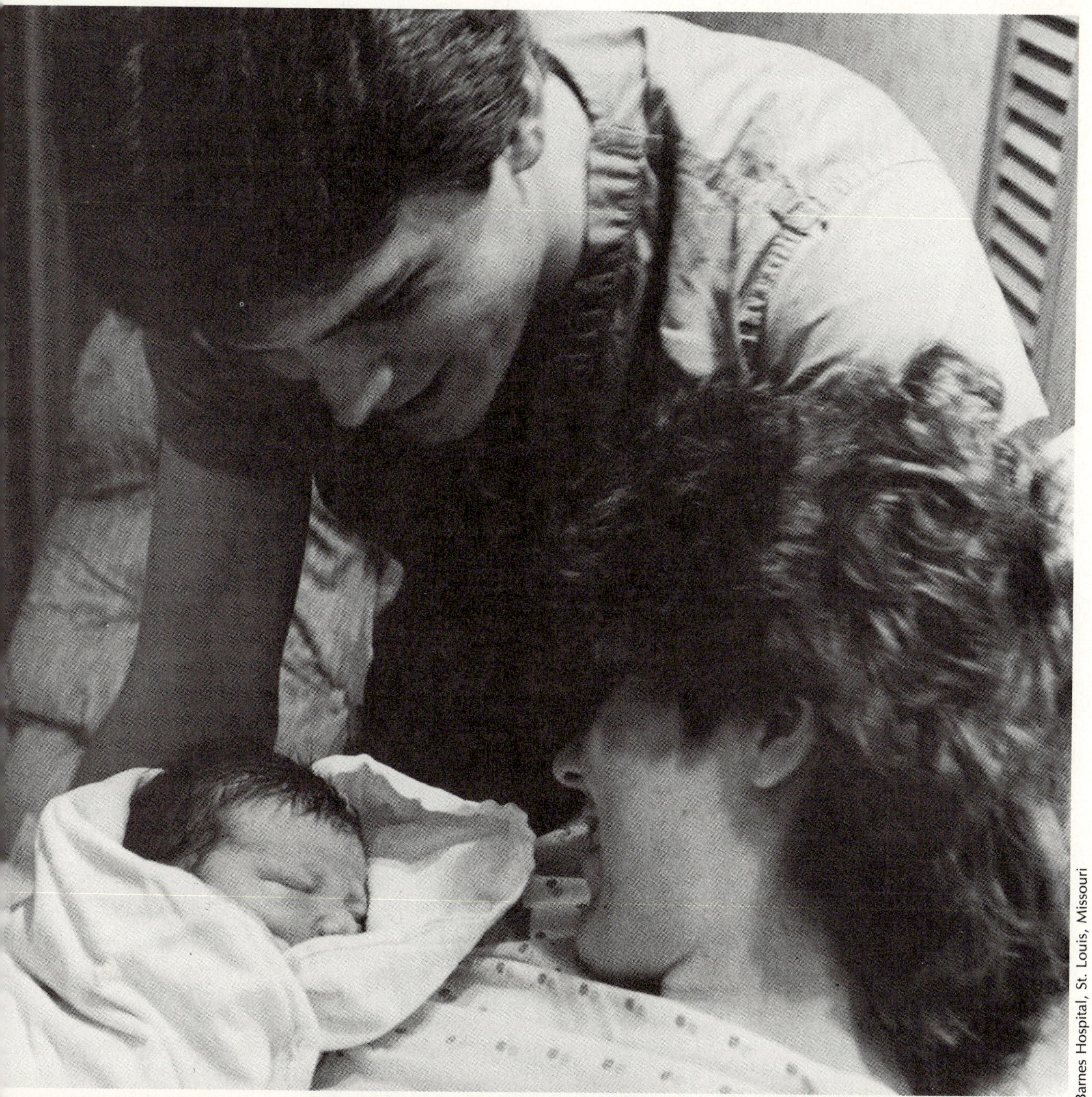

Barnes Hospital, St. Louis, Missouri

31
Maternal Physiology and Nursing Care

- Physiologic Changes
  - Vascular system
  - Reproductive system
  - Urinary system
  - Vital signs
  - Endocrine system
  - Gastrointestinal system
  - Abdominal musculature
- Postpartum Care
  - Assessment
    - Initial assessment
    - Subsequent assessment
  - Child care activities and response to birth of child
  - Examples of nursing diagnoses
  - Planning
  - Implementation
    - Goals
    - Nursing actions
  - Evaluation

The responses of the mother to the birth of her infant are influenced by many factors, for example, her energy level, freedom from discomfort, health of her newborn, and the care and encouragement supplied by professional persons. To provide care beneficial to the mother, the infant, and the family, the nurse synthesizes knowledge from maternal physiology of the recovery period, the newborn, his physical and behavioral characteristics and child care activities, and family responses to the birth of a child. The nurse, in short, uses a holistic approach to nursing care. For ease of presentation, however, the content of this chapter is limited to the physical recovery of the mother through the immediate puerperium to the final physical examination. The care associated with recovery, the physiologic changes, prevention of complications, and health teaching constitute an important part of postpartum nursing care. The care is necessary regardless of whether a mother has a normal newborn or is separated from her infant through infant prematurity, illness, death, or adoption, whether she is supported by family and friends or is alone, or whether she delivers in a traditional hospital setting or a birth center.

The postpartum period, or puerperium, is the period of recovery from childbirth. The postpartum period has been arbitrarily divided into the *immediate puerperium*, lasting from birth through 24 hours, the *early puerperium*, which extends through the first postpartum week, and the *late puerperium*, which lasts for 6 weeks. During this time repair of injury to the birth canal, involution of the uterus, and return of all systems to the prepregnant or nearly prepregnant state occur (also known as involution). The process is both anabolic (resulting in lactation) and catabolic (resulting in involution of the uterus). In nursing literature the term *fourth trimester* is used to encompass not only the physical recovery of the mother but also the early adjustment of all the family members to the birth of a child and is said to last approximately 3 months.

Physiologic Changes

VASCULAR SYSTEM

Pregnancy-induced hypervolemia (increase of at least 40% near term) allows most women to tolerate a considerable blood loss at delivery. Many women lose 300 to 400 ml of blood at vaginal delivery and about twice this amount at cesarean delivery. This influences the blood volume and hematocrit changes during the puerperium.

After vaginal delivery a declining blood volume usually is associated with a rise in hematocrit by the third to seventh day after delivery, suggesting that the loss of red blood cells is less than the reduction of vascular capacity (uterus and periphery) and that hemoconcentration results from the excretion of extracellular fluid.

After cesarean delivery a more rapid decline in blood volume and hematocrit occurs, but there is a tendency for the hematocrit to stabilize or even decline slightly in the early puerperium.

By the third week after delivery, the blood volume usually is back to prenatal values. There is no red blood cell destruction during the puerperium, but any gain will disappear gradually in accordance with the life span of the red blood cell. In uncomplicated cases the hematocrit will have returned to the normal, nonpregnant level by the fourth or fifth postdelivery week.

There is an extensive activation of blood-clotting factors after delivery. This activation, together with immobility, trauma, or sepsis, encourages thromboembolism (see Chapter 35). Avoidance of tissue damage and infection, early ambulation, and elimination of estrogen therapy for suppression of lactation should reduce the risk of thromboembolic complications.

REPRODUCTIVE SYSTEM

After delivery the cervix is soft, appears bruised, and has some small lacerations. It remains easily distensible; two fingers may still be introduced easily by the tenth hour after delivery. By the eighteenth hour the cervix has shortened, has a firm consistency, and has regained its form. By the end of the first week, recovery is almost complete. The external os, however, does not regain its prepregnant appearance; it is no longer shaped like a circle but appears as a jagged slit (see Fig. 6.12).

Estrogen deprivation of pregnancy is responsible for the thinness of the vaginal mucosa and the absence of rugae. The greatly distended, smooth-walled vagina gradually returns to its prepregnant condition by about the third or fourth week. Most rugae may be permanently flattened, and the mucosa remains atrophic in the lactating woman at least until such time as menstruation begins again. The torn hymen heals with the development of fibrosed nodules of mucosa called *hymenal caruncles*.

The uterus, which weighs about 11 times its prepregnant weight, rapidly involutes after delivery (Fig. 31.1). The uterus weighs approximately 1000 g (2.2 lb) immediately after delivery, 500 g (1.1 lb) 1 week after delivery, and 350 g (11 to 12 oz) 2 weeks after delivery. Estrogen-stimulated myometrial growth (hypertrophy and hyperplasia) is quickly reversed during the relative hypoestrogenism of the puerperium. Progesterone, which was responsible for much of the increased uterine weight and collagen formation during gestation, is not produced until the first ovulation, which is weeks or even months in the future. It is not surprising, then, that progesterone cannot be detected in serum after the first postdelivery week.

Withdrawal of estrogen and progesterone is followed by the release of proteolytic enzymes and the migration

Fig. 31.1
Immediately after delivery, fundus can be felt 2 cm below umbilicus; within 12 hours, fundus returns to 1 cm above umbilicus and then begins its descent of about 1 cm/24 hr. (From Ingalls, A.J., and Salerno, M.D.: Maternal and child health nursing, ed. 5, St. Louis, 1983, The C.V. Mosby Co.)

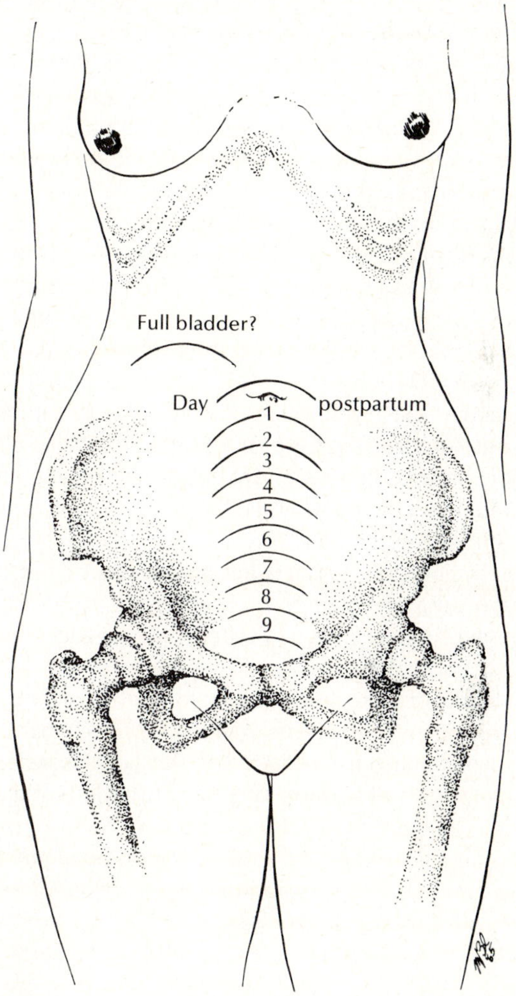

of macrophages into the endometrium and myometrium. Uterine involution within 4 to 6 weeks occurs principally by a decrease in the size of individual myometrial cells. However, the augmentation of connective tissue and elastin in the myometrium and blood vessels and the increase in the total uterine cell number are permanent. Hence the uterine size usually is increased slightly after each pregnancy.

Uterine contractions persist after delivery of the placenta. In primiparas the tone of the uterus is increased so that the fundus generally remains firm. Periodic relaxation and contraction are the rule for multiparas and may cause uncomfortable afterpains that persist for 2 or 3 days. Breast feeding frequently intensifies these afterpains because oxytocin is released by the posterior pituitary in response to stimulation of the nipple.

The placental site is partially obliterated by vascular constriction and thrombosis. The shedding of this mass of organized thrombi and obliterated arteries prevents scar formation. Endometrial regeneration of the area from stromal derivatives of the decidua basalis follows promptly, and regeneration of mucosal elements from vestiges of glands in the placental site also occurs. This unique healing process makes it possible for the endometrium to resume its usual cycle of changes and to permit implantation and placentation of future pregnancies. Endometrial regeneration is completed by the end of the third postpartum week except at the placental site, where regeneration is usually not complete until 6 weeks postpartum.

Failure of the placental site to heal completely is called *subinvolution of the placental site*. Women with this condition have persistent lochia and episodes of brisk, painless bleeding. Curettage usually is required (see p. 807).

Limitation of anesthesia, elevation of the uterus, and slight massage of the fundus usually will control excessive postdelivery blood loss. Long-lasting oxytocics such as ergonovine are useful if uterine relaxation and active bleeding resume. Oxytocin will not elevate the blood pressure, but ergot products may. Although ergot products are beneficial in the immediate treatment of uterine bleeding caused by hypotonia, it is unlikely that these drugs are of value after the first 1 or 2 days.

Immediately after delivery the nontender fundus should be about 2 cm *below* the umbilicus. On external palpation the uterus feels firm and about the size of a grapefruit. Within 12 hours, with the "take-up" and improved tone of the uterine supports, the fundus should be approximately 1 cm *above* the umbilicus (Fig. 31.1), although a distended bladder may obscure the level. From then on, involution progresses rapidly, and the fundus descends about 1 to 2 cm/24 hr. By the sixth postdelivery day the fundus normally will be one half the distance from the symphysis pubis to the umbilicus. The uterus should not be palpable abdominally after the ninth postdelivery day.

Initially, postdelivery vaginal discharge is blood *(lochia rubra)* and lasts about 3 days. The flow pales, becoming pink or brown after several days *(lochia serosa)*. About 10 days after delivery, the drainage should be yellow to white *(lochia alba)* because of the presence of numerous leukocytes and cellular debris.

Persistence of lochia rubra early in the postdelivery period suggests retained placental fragments. Recurrence of bleeding about 10 days after delivery indicates bleeding from the placental site, which is healing; however, after 3 or 4 weeks bleeding may be caused by infection or subinvolution of the placental site. Continued lochia serosa or lochia alba may indicate endometritis, particularly when fever, pain, or tenderness is associated with the discharge. Lochia should smell like normal menstrual flow; an offensive odor usually indicates infection. Lochia clots, but normal menstrual flow does not.

Ovarian activity remains suspended for differing periods of time after delivery. For lactating women, amenorrhea or anovulatory periods may persist until the infant is weaned. If menstruation does begin, there is no need to discontinue nursing. However, it should be remembered that ovulation precedes menstruation, and a woman may therefore become pregnant while lactating. Approximately 90% of nonlactating primiparas and 30% of lactating primiparas begin menstruating within 3 months of delivery. Multiparas often start to menstruate earlier. The first menstrual period is much heavier than normal and almost always anovulatory. Within 3 or 4 months the amount of flow has returned to normal.

For a discussion of breast changes associated with lactation, see Chapter 30.

URINARY SYSTEM

Kidney function returns to normal and ureteral dilatation gradually is reduced during the first month after delivery. Pelvic soreness as a result of the forces of labor, vaginal lacerations, or the episiotomy reduces or alters the voiding reflex. This alteration, together with postdelivery diuresis, may allow rapid filling of the bladder. Normally a marked diuresis begins within 12 hours after delivery. This mechanism, whereby the excess tissue fluid accumulated during pregnancy is eliminated, is often referred to as the *reversal of the water metabolism of pregnancy*.

Clean-catch or catheterized urine specimens after delivery often reveal hematuria from bladder trauma. Later, hematuria may be a sign of urinary tract infection. Mild proteinuria (+1) is a normal finding for 1 or 2 days in about 50% of women after delivery as a result of the catalytic processes of involution. However, proteinuria may persist for at least a week in women with preeclampsia-eclampsia (PIH). Acetonuria is common in diabetics and may even occur in women with uncomplicated deliveries after prolonged labor with dehydration.

The hormonal changes of pregnancy (high steroid levels) contribute to the increase in renal function, and so the diminishing steroid levels after delivery may partly explain the reduced renal function during the puerperium. The renal glycosuria induced by pregnancy disappears, and the creatinine clearance is generally normal at the end of the first postpartum week. The blood urea nitrogen (BUN) rises during the puerperium as autolysis of the pregnant uterus is accomplished; at the end of the first postpartum week, values of 20 mg/dl are reached, compared with 15 mg/dl in the late third trimester of pregnancy. Lactosuria may be expected in lactating women. However, it cannot be detected by use of the Clinitest, since this test is specific for the presence of glucose, not lactose, in the urine.

VITAL SIGNS

Maternal temperature during the first 24 hours after delivery may rise to 38° C (100.4° F) as a result of the dehydrating effects of labor. A diagnosis of puerperal sepsis is suggested, however, if a similar rise develops after the first 24 hours after delivery and recurs or persists for 2 days. Other possibilities may be mastitis, endometritis, urinary tract infections, or other systemic infections.

Bradycardia is a common finding for the first 6 to 8 days after delivery. A pulse rate of between 50 and 70 beats/min may be considered normal. Heart sounds return to the prepregnant state.

Blood pressure remains unchanged. A drop may indicate increased uterine bleeding. However, women are prone to develop orthostatic hypotension before the cardiovascular system readjusts to the loss of intrapelvic pressure after delivery. An increased reading may indicate pregnancy-induced hypertension. Therefore women who complain of headaches should be assessed for symptoms of pregnancy-induced hypertension before they are given any analgesia for relief of headache.

ENDOCRINE SYSTEM

During pregnancy hormonal production changes considerably. The placenta, adrenals, thyroid, and anterior pituitary act as major sources. Once delivery has occurred, there is a return to normal, with a reduction in some hormones (Table 31.1) and increases in the following:

1. Thyroid function: increased protein-bound iodine, butyl-extractable iodine, iodine uptake
2. Anterior pituitary gonadotropic hormones
3. Prolactin and oxytocin (in lactating women)

Table 31.1
Hormonal Reduction after Delivery

Day 1	Week 1	Weeks 2-3
HCG	Estrone	Estriol
Estrogen	Estradiol	
Aldosterone	Progesterone	
	Corticoids	
	17-Ketosteroids	
	11-Oxycorticosteroids	

GASTROINTESTINAL SYSTEM

The mother is usually hungry shortly after delivery and can tolerate a light diet. For a discussion of diet during lactation, see Chapter 30.

A spontaneous bowel evacuation may be delayed until several days after delivery. This can be explained by decreased muscle tone in the intestines, prelabor diarrhea or the predelivery enema, lack of food, dehydration, or perineal tenderness because of the episiotomy, lacerations, or hemorrhoids. For some women regular bowel habits must be reestablished after delivery. Attention to timing and to dietary and fluid intake is essential.

ABDOMINAL MUSCULATURE

The muscles of the abdominal wall and pelvic floor and their fascia regain their tone during the puerperium and approximate their original length after the stresses of pregnancy are over; therefore vigorous exercises are not recommended until 6 or 7 weeks after delivery (Fig. 31.9). Lacerations or overstretching at the time of delivery may weaken the pelvic floor and predispose the woman to development of a genital hernia. Marked distention of the abdominal wall during gestation may result in diastasis of the recti abdominis muscles.

Postpartum Care

The approach to care of women during the postpartum (puerperal) period has changed from one modeled on the concept of sick care to one that is health ori-

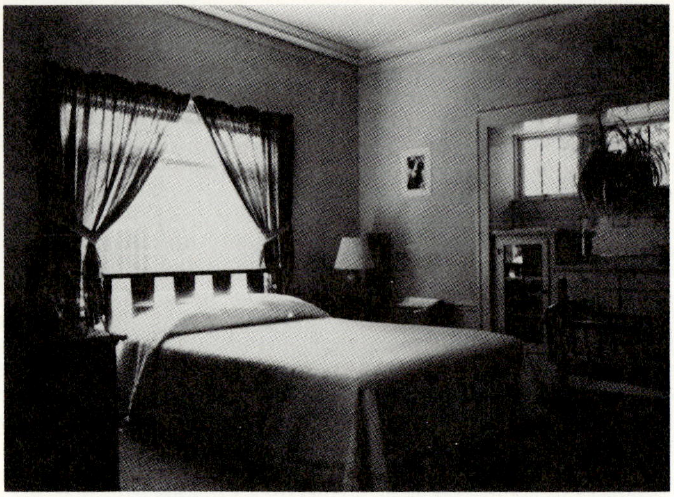

Fig. 31.2
A homelike setting for giving birth, for postdelivery recovery, and for fostering early parent-child relationships.

ented. Women are concerned about their comfort and recovery, desirous of having contact with their infants, motivated to learn about newborn care, and eager to share their experiences with their families. Their health care is now a collaborative effort on the part of all involved—mother, nurse, physician, and family—to prevent complications; to provide comfort, rest, and nourishment; to engage in teaching-learning activities related to self-care for the mother and the care of the newborn; and to foster parent-child relationships.

For those women who select a hospital birth it is often the first time that they have been in a hospital and experienced hospital routine. Although the care is concentrated in the first 3 to 5 days after delivery, health supervision should be continued for the 6-wk postdelivery period to ensure that adequate professional assistance is available during critical periods in child care and in readjustment to home and family.

The care of the woman and family begins with her admission to the postpartum unit (Fig. 31.2). The woman is admitted to the desired bed accommodation in the postdelivery unit, and if necessary, she is introduced to other mothers in the same room. If this is the first time she has been hospitalized, her anxiety will be further heightened. The admitting nurse is responsible for determining the woman's understanding of the use of the call bell; reviewing the routines of her care, the care of her newborn, and any visiting regulations; and ordering the diet according to the woman's preferences.

ASSESSMENT

Initial assessment. The initial assessment includes the report from the nurse in the labor unit. The admitting nurse is given a brief description of the type of labor, time of delivery, progress and care given during the first to fourth hours after delivery, including medications, plus any complicating conditions (e.g., postdelivery hemorrhage, preeclampsia, depressed emotional state). The woman's record is reviewed for information from the prenatal and labor records that is pertinent to plans for her care; for example, her need for rubella vaccination or $Rh_o(D)$ immune globulin (Table 31.2).

To complete the data base the nurse performs a complete assessment. Vital signs and blood pressure are taken (Fig. 31.3) and recorded. The uterus is then examined as follows. The woman is asked to empty her bladder if it appears distended on palpation. She assumes a supine position with her knees flexed to relieve tension on the abdomen. The uterine fundus is supported and assessed for firmness (contraction) and for its position relative to the midline and umbilicus (Fig. 31.4). Because this procedure can be uncomfortable, the nurse should explain the rationale for the examination, and as she massages the fundus, she should demonstrate to the woman how the woman can give intermittent, not constant, massage.

Next, the amount and character of the lochia are noted. It is very difficult to assess accurately the amount of lochia; therefore the terms *excessive, large, moderate,* and *scant* are used. Since the objective is to determine if there is postpartum hemorrhage, the nurse can use additional cues to determine the amount: (1) Lochia usually trickles from the vaginal opening; the steady flow is greater as the uterus contracts. However, if the lochia is seen to spurt from the vagina there may be cervical or vaginal tears or a relaxed uterus. (2) If

Table 31.2
Clinical Significance of Key Factors from Prenatal and Natal Periods and Associated Nursing Actions

Information	Clinical Significance	Nursing Action
Age	Immature mother may not be able to cope	Consider need for counseling or social service aid
Height, weight	Return to ideal weight desirable	Arrange for dietary advice
Parity, living children	One child adds about 20% to housework; two add 25-30%	Apply for homemaker assistance, if needed
Prenatal problem (e.g., diabetes, hypertension, urinary infection)	Disorder should have been cured or controlled	Reconsider problem; determine present status and therapy regimen
Birth: spontaneous; operative; complications	Operative delivery or complications may require longer convalescence	Assess uterine involution, wound healing, infection, and treatment
Infant: gestational age; problems; feeding	Special care needed for premature, sick, or birth-injured neonates	Obtain pediatric diagnosis and recommendations
	Proper diet needed for growth and development	Check adequacy of breast or formula feeding (see Chapter 30)
Laboratory tests	Evidence of infection, anemia, or hormone or other imbalance	Review laboratory reports: if abnormal, seek diagnosis and treatment
Mother's therapy	Is medication or contraception needed?	Request required drugs or contraceptive
Employment	Mother may be obliged to work for a living	Determine probable capability and likely date of mother's return to work place

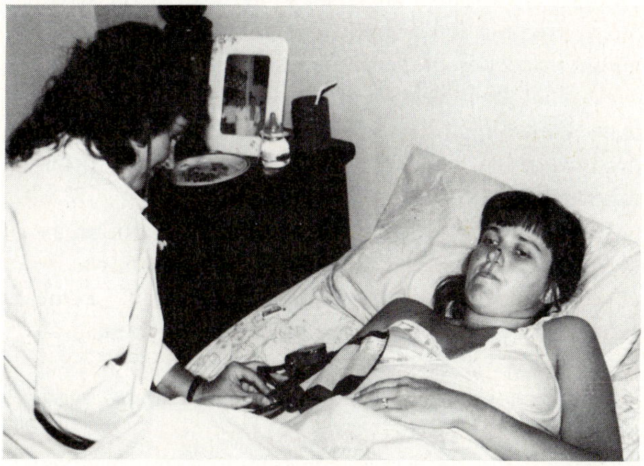

Fig. 31.3
Assessment of vital signs, blood pressure, and temperature.

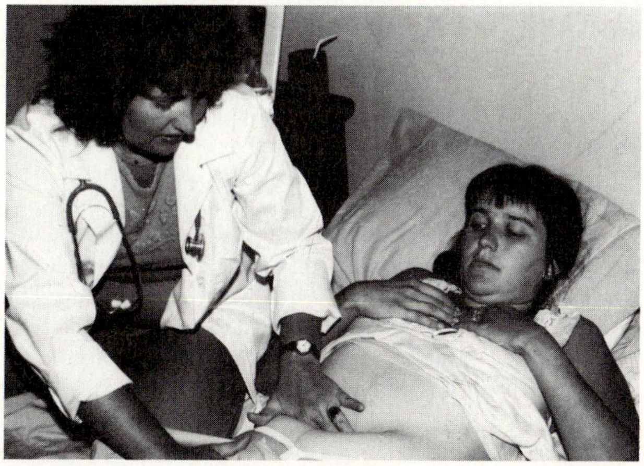

Fig. 31.4
Assessment of fundus for firmness and position.

the uterus is massaged at the same time the lochia is observed, a gush of lochia will result. If it is dark in color, it has been pooled in the relaxed vagina and the amount soon lessens to a trickle of bright red lochia. This is a clinically benign finding. If, however, the amount continues to be large and bright red in color, a tear or excessive bleeding from the placental site can be suspected. (3) If the woman has had an oxytocic, the flow of lochia is usually scant until the effect of the drug has disappeared. If the medication is administered intravenously, the effect persists for 30 minutes after the intravenous medication is discontinued; if the medication is administered intramuscularly, the effect persists for 30 to 60 minutes. If the woman is taking ergonovine maleate (Ergotrate), 0.2 mg by mouth three to four times a day for 2 days, lochia is usually scant. (4) If the pad is soaked through in 15 minutes or less, the flow is considered excessive.

If an episiotomy has been done, it is carefully examined for hematoma formation or signs of infection, and the woman is informed of the progress in healing. If the episiotomy is not readily visible in the lithotomy position, the woman is turned to the side of the episiotomy (right or left lateral), and her buttock is raised to permit inspection of the suture line. A good light source is essential for inspection of some episiotomies (e.g., in dark-skinned mothers). The rectum is checked for hemorrhoids at this time. The bladder is palpated to determine distention.

During the assessment, the nurse can determine the mother's emotional status, energy level, and knowledge concerning self-care and infant care (see Unit Five). Ethnic and cultural variations in care of the woman after delivery can be discussed and plans for modifying nursing actions made. An example of a cultural variation follows:

> A Vietnamese woman who had been in the United States for 4 years requested rooming-in facilities following delivery. Instead of participating in the care of her infant she refused to do so, remained in bed, wore a woolen cap, and appeared very distressed and angry. The staff were nonplussed by her behavior. One nurse decided to put newly learned concepts concerning cross-cultural nursing into effect. She began by praising the woman's ability to speak English and after eliciting a smile, remarked, "Every country has developed good ways to look after mothers and babies. Would you tell me about the care in Vietnam?" There was an immediate response. The woman explained that in her country, women remained in bed for 10 days after delivery, and the biggest danger to their health was getting a cold. The baby was kept in the room with his mother, but either a grandmother or nurse took complete charge of the care.

Evidently the woman was operating in tune with her cultural expectations, and the nurses were operating within theirs. This rather simple approach to resolving a nursing problem also proved successful in subsequent cases.

Subsequent assessment. Once the data base has been established, routine assessment is carried out, every 8 hours or more often if indicated, to detect complications, to evaluate the return of body systems to the prepregnant state, and to assess the mother's emotional status and extent of skill in self-care and infant care. On the basis of the findings, nursing diagnoses are established and nursing measures are instituted. The woman needs to understand the rationale for the procedures to be used in assessing her recovery from childbirth.

Vital signs. The temperature, pulse, respirations, and blood pressure are assessed every 8 hours. Except for the first 24 hours the woman should be afebrile and normotensive.

Vascular system

Hemorrhage. Assessment of the uterus as described above will be repeated routinely every 2 hours for the first 8 hours and then every 8 hours during the remainder of the hospital stay. (For a discussion of the care necessary should a postdelivery hemorrhage occur, see Chapter 35).

Hypertension. Since preeclampsia-eclampsia can persist into or occur first in the postdelivery period, routine evaluation of blood pressure is needed. If a woman complains of headache, hypertension must be ruled out as a cause before analgesics are administered. If the blood pressure is elevated, the woman is confined to bed and the physician notified. (See also Chapter 35).

Hypotension. Hypotension is a sign of hypovolemic shock; however, it is a late sign, and other symptoms of hemorrhage usually alert the staff. Orthostatic hypotension can develop in the first 48 hours as a result of the splanchnic engorgement occuring after delivery.

Thromboembolism. The woman's legs are examined daily for signs of thrombosis (pain, warmth, and tenderness; swollen reddened vein that feels hard or solid to touch). There may or may not be a positive Homans' sign (dorsiflexion of foot causes calf muscles to compress tibial veins and produce pain if thrombosis is present).

If a thrombus is suspected, notify the physician immediately; meanwhile, the woman should be confined to bed, with the affected limb elevated on pillows.

Hemorrhoids. If present, hemorrhoids are checked every 8 hours for size, number, and tenderness.

Reversal of water metabolism of pregnancy. Profuse diaphoresis, especially at night (night sweats), is not unusual for 2 or 3 days after delivery. Diaphoresis is a mechanism to reduce the retained fluids of pregnancy and usually is not a symptom of infection.

Reproductive system

Uterus. The fundus is assessed for consistency and position in the abdomen (see Figs. 31.1 and 31.4) every 30 minutes for 4 hours and then every 8 hours for 3 days (see p. 453 for care during fourth stage of labor).

Lochia. The lochia is assessed for amount, color, and odor every 8 hours for 3 days. A foul odor is an important symptom of uterine infection, and immediate therapy is indicated. A swab of vaginal contents may be ordered and sent to the laboratory for culture (routine nose or throat swab sticks may be used for this procedure).

Women need to be informed that they will note a consistent decrease in the amount of lochia for about 3 weeks. They usually have a ''small period,'' or an episode of painless bleeding from the placental site, about 3 weeks after delivery. If bleeding becomes profuse or prolonged, however, the woman should call her physician for advice.

Perineum. The perineum is inspected every 8 hours to detect any signs of infection or delayed healing in the episiotomy or repaired lacerations. The healing process of an episiotomy is the same as for any surgical incision. Signs of infection (pain, redness, swelling, or discharge) or loss of approximation (gaping) of the incision edges is reported immediately.

Breasts. The breasts are checked every 8 hours for the beginning of lactation and the presence of infection (mastitis) and masses (Fig. 31.5). The breasts feel generally nodular (in nonpregnant women they feel granular). The nodularity is bilateral and diffuse. As lactation is established, a mass (lump) may be felt; however, a filled milk sac will shift position from day to day. Before lactation begins the breasts feel soft and a yellowish fluid can be expressed from the nipples. After lactation begins the breasts feel warm to the touch and firm. Tenderness persists for about 48 hours. Milk, bluish-white in color (skim-milk appearance), can be expressed from the nipples. The nipples are examined for erectility as opposed to inversion, cracks, or fissures. The breast is then palpated to determine if there is an area of localized tenderness. The palpation technique used is the same as that women use for self-examination of the breasts. The nurse assesses the mother's knowledge of regular breast examination and observes the method the mother uses (Fig. 31.6).

Fig. 31.5
Assessment of breasts and nipples.

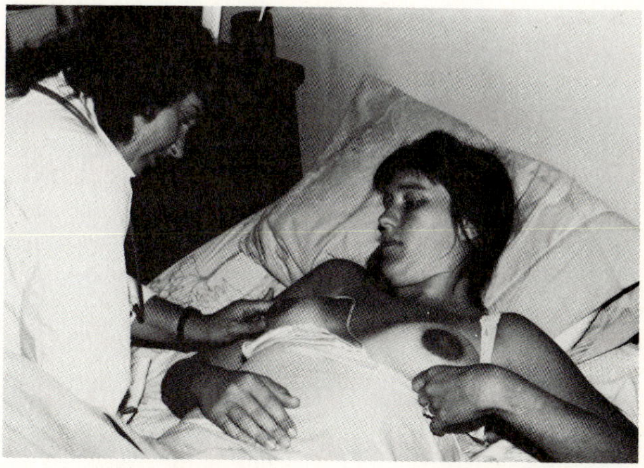

Urinary system. The bladder is checked for distention every 2 hours for 8 hours and then every 8 hours for 3 days. Urinary output is measured for 24 hours following delivery. Distention of the bladder can readily occur as the water metabolism of pregnancy is reversed and fluids are mobilized in the elimination of end products of protein catabolism. Overdistention can make the bladder more susceptible to infection as well as impede the resumption of normal voiding. The woman is encouraged to void at least every 3 or 4 hours during the day. She is requested to report if she (1) is experiencing pain or burning when she voids, (2) is voiding small amounts frequently, or (3) is unable to void every 4 hours.

Gastrointestinal system

Appetite. Appetite is usually very good. Women feel hungry and are able to tolerate regular meals.

Elimination. Most women do not have a spontaneous bowel movement for 2 or 3 days after delivery.

Immune system. The mother's need for rubella vaccination or for prevention of Rh isoimmunization is determined.

Rubella vaccination. For those women who have not had rubella (10% to 20% of all women) or women who are serologically negative (i.e., titer of 1:8 or less) rubella virus vaccine is recommended in the immediate postdelivery period to prevent fetal anomalies in future pregnancies. Seroconversion occurs in approximately 90% of women vaccinated after delivery. The live attenuated rubella virus is not communicable; therefore nursing mothers can be vaccinated. However, the live attenuated rubella vaccine is made from duck eggs, and so women who have allergies to these eggs may develop a hypersensitivity reaction to the vaccine, for which they will need adrenalin. A transient arthralgia or rash is common in vaccinated women but is benign. Since the vaccine may be teratogenic the client should sign an informed consent and should receive written information about the vaccine, its side effects and risks,

Fig. 31.6

Positions of client for breast examination. **A,** Supine, at rest. **B,** Seated, at rest. **C,** Seated, arms elevated. **D,** Seated, pectoral contraction. **E,** Seated, leaning forward. (From Malasanos, L., et al: Health assessment, ed. 2, St. Louis, 1981, The C.V. Mosby Co.)

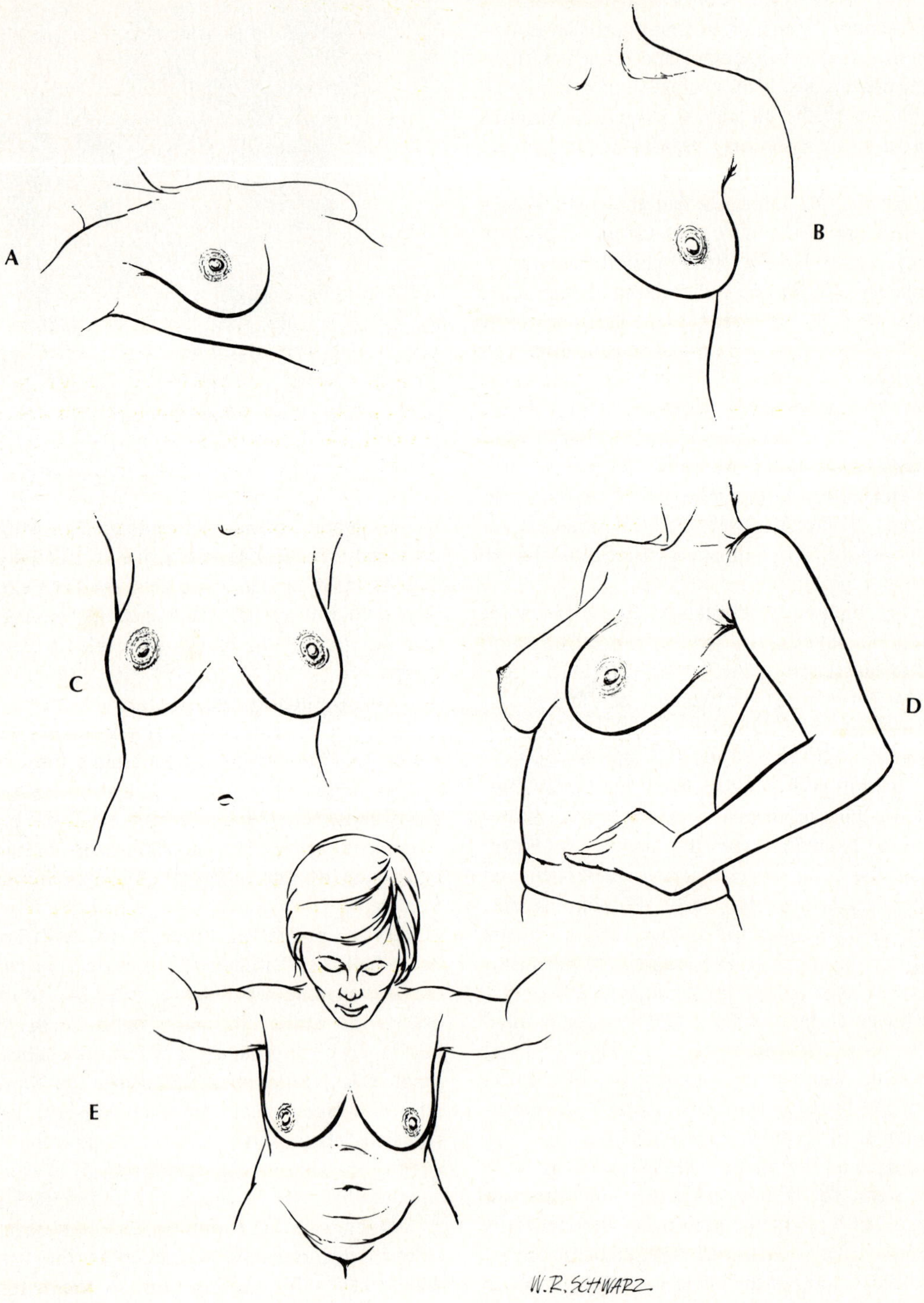

and the necessity for practicing contraception for a period of 2 to 3 months after vaccination.

Prevention of Rh isoimmunization. Injection of $Rh_o(D)$ immune globulin within 72 hours of delivery will prevent sensitization in the Rh-negative woman who has had a fetal-maternal transfusion of Rh-positive fetal red cells (see Chapter 40). The administration of 300 μg of $Rh_o(D)$ immune globulin is usually sufficient to prevent maternal sensitization by promoting lysis of fetal Rh-positive red blood cells circulating in the maternal bloodstream before the mother forms her own antibodies against them. If a large fetal-maternal transfusion is suspected, the dose needed can be assessed by either the Kleihauer-Betke smear or the D^u test, which detects 20 ml or more of Rh-positive fetal blood in the maternal circulation. The $Rh_o(D)$ immune globulin is administered after all known abortions (gestational age of 8 weeks or more) since the risk of sensitization after abortion is about half the risk after a full-term pregnancy.* It is administered after delivery to any woman who meets the following three criteria: (1) the mother must be $Rh_o(D)$-negative with no Rh antibodies (i.e., indirect Coombs' test is negative); (2) the infant must be $Rh_o(D)$- or D^u-positive; and (3) results of direct Coombs' test on the cord blood must be negative. If she meets these criteria, a 1:1000 dilution of $Rh_o(D)$ immune globulin is cross matched to the mother's red cells to ensure compatibility. The same precautions are followed when administering a blood transfusion to ensure that the immune globulin is administered to the correct woman. *If administered to an Rh-positive person, immune globulin will act to promote lysis of the Rh-positive red blood cells.* The dose is administered to the mother by intramuscular injection (*never* intravenously or to the infant).

CHILD CARE ACTIVITIES AND RESPONSE TO BIRTH OF CHILD

See Unit Five for details about child care activities and Chapter 32 for the family's response to the birth of a child.

EXAMPLES OF NURSING DIAGNOSES

To determine the nursing diagnoses that reflect the client's problems, the nurse reviews the client's records of the previous 24 hours for pertinent information and combines this data with information gained from ongoing assessments. Although women experience similar problems during the postpartum period, certain factors act to make each woman's experience unique; for example, the labor a woman experienced (whether it was long or short), whether she plans to bottle or breast feed, whether or not she had an episiotomy, and whether she has other children. To individualize the care for the client, the nurse begins by formulating nursing diagnoses; for example:

1. Sleep pattern disturbance because of discomfort of breast engorgement
2. Fluid volume deficit because of fluid restriction during labor
3. Self-care deficit because client avoids washing perineum because of "pain of stitches"

*For prenatal prophylaxis, see Chapter 40.

PLANNING

The nursing plan is used for the care of women postpartum as it is for other clients. Once the nursing diagnoses are formulated, the nurse decides what nursing measures would be appropriate and which are to be given priority. The organization of care has to take the newborn into consideration. The day actually revolves around the baby's feeding and care times (see box, "Nursing Care Plan").

The mother assumes increasing responsibility for her own self-care; however, the nurse is responsible for consistent assessment of actual or potential problems (Table 31.3). In some areas "couple nursing" (mother and baby) has been introduced. The nurse acts as the primary nurse for both mother and infant even if the newborn is kept in the central nursery (Fig. 31.7). This approach is a variation of rooming-in wherein mother and child room together and mother and nurse share the care of the infant.

The nursing care plan will include assessments to detect deviations from normal, comfort measures to relieve discomfort or pain, safety measures to prevent injury or infection, and teaching and counseling measures designed to promote a mother's (and father's) feeling of competence in the care of herself and the newly born child (see box, "Postpartum Teaching"). The nurse evaluates continuously and is ready to change the plan if indicated. The nurse's ability to adapt the care plan to specific diagnoses results in individualized care for clients.

IMPLEMENTATION

Goals. The goals of postpartum care are to maintain an environment that is conducive to the mother's physical recovery from childbirth and fosters family-child relationships and the learning of child care activities.

Nursing actions

Parent-child attachment and care of the newborn. Techniques for fostering parent-child attachment and

Text continued on p. 701.

Nursing Care Plan

Name:	Grav: Para: Ab: Stb:	Infant	Family
	Marital status:	Sex: Wt: Length:	Adults:
Room:	Occupation:	Time: Day: Date:	
		Pediatrician: Feeding:	
	Rh: Type:	Baby's Rh: Type: Coombs:	Siblings:
	Rubella antibody titer:	Condition of baby: Date:	

Short-term goal:	Long-term goal:

Emergency number: Person: Relationship: Address:

Date	Nursing diagnoses	Evaluative criteria	Nursing actions

Discharge planning:
Return visit:
Referrals: ( ) social work
( ) home care

Fig. 31.7
A, Nurse-midwife assesses newborn with mother watching. **B,** Nurse-midwife reviews assessment of newborn for older sister using sister's doll.

A

B

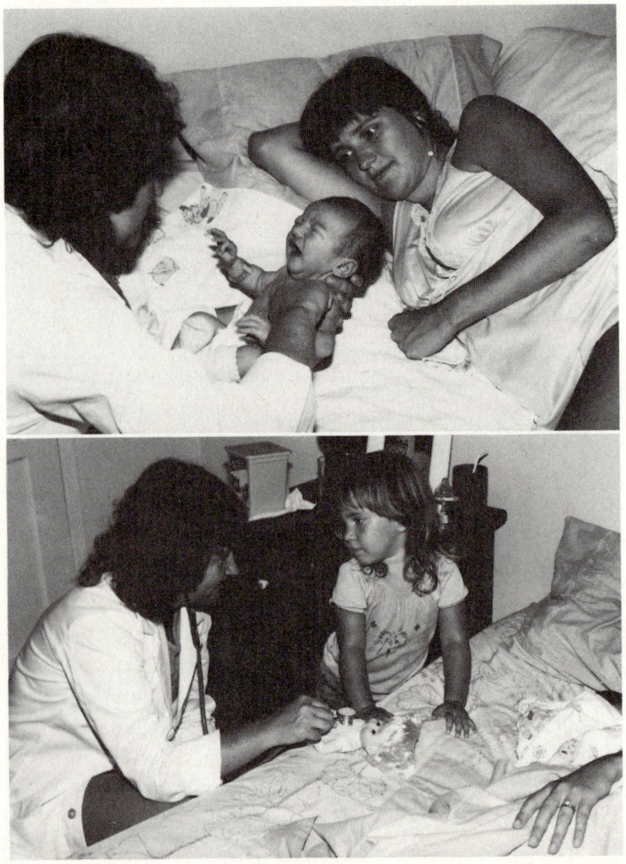

Postpartum Teaching: Assessment and Instruction

Date	Area	Instructed	Demonstrated by mother	Nurse's signature
	Mother Personal hygiene and care Breasts/examination Perineum			
	Lochia: amount, character			
	Comfort Peri care Tucks and Americaine Peri lamp Sitz bath			
	Sexual relations Birth control			
	Nutrition			
	Exercise			
	Rest			
	Emotional adjustments			
	Cesarean delivery			
	Tubal occlusion			
	Infant Bathing			
	Cord/circumcision care			
	Thermometer use			
	Bulb syringe			
	Safety/poison control Car seats			
	Breast feeding			
	Breast pumping			
	Storage of milk			
	Formula feeding			
	Formula preparation			
	Positioning/handling			
	Diapering			
	Clothing			
	Signs of illness			
	Family schedules			
	Special situations			

Table 31.3
Evaluative Criteria, Area Assessed, and Normal Findings

Area Assessed	First 2 Wk	By Wk 4-6
Temperature	Temperature is elevated to 38° C (100.4° F) in first 24 hr after delivery. This is not unusual, and if unaccompanied by other symptoms, e.g., pain in the calf or leg or a foul odor of lochia, it is considered to be caused by dehydration. If temperature elevation begins after 24 hr or persists for 48 hr, it is considered abnormal.	Returns to prepregnant level
Pulse	Pulse rate falls a short time after delivery (range of 50-70 beats/min), and bradycardia may persist for 6-8 days even in absence of stress.	Returns to prepregnant level
Respirations	Rate remains within normal limits.	Returns to prepregnant level
Blood pressure	Blood pressure remains in accord with previous normal readings.	Returns to prepregnant level
Breasts	For 2 or 3 days after delivery breasts secrete colostrum in increasing amounts. By second day in multiparas and by third day in primiparas, breasts become engorged, firm, tense, and tender. This is caused by venous or lymphatic stasis, and in 36-48 hr pain disappears as swelling spontaneously subsides. Fever does not accompany this process. Soon after onset of this engorgement, true milk is formed and let-down reflex in response to suckling of infant or manual manipulation causes expression of milk (see also Chapter 30).	Breasts do not reveal soreness, tenderness, or masses. If woman is not breast feeding, no milk or only a small amount of milk may be expressed.
Uterus	Involution of uterus progresses normally. Size of uterus diminishes. Immediately after delivery, uterus weighs about 1 kg; its size approximates that of pregnancy of 20 wk gestation; its position is at level of umbilicus, in midline or slightly to right of midline; it descends into pelvic cavity 1 cm per day. Uterine tone is maintained by contraction and retraction of uterine muscles. Uterus feels firm and contracts readily after massage; there is expulsion of clots and emptying of bladder or rectum. During first 12 hr after delivery contractions are strong, regular, and coordinated. Thereafter intensity, frequency, and regularity decrease. Afterpains occur for 2 or 3 days and are more noticeable in multipara than in primipara and during suckling of infant.	Uterus is only slightly larger than in prepregnant state and anteverted. If retroverted, it has developed free mobility.
Lochia	Color and consistency of lochia change. Lochia rubra contains blood, placental and decidual debris, and clots and is dark red. It persists from delivery through third day. Lochia serosa is thin, serous, and brownish and lasts from fourth to tenth day. Lochia alba, a yellowish-white discharge, contains an increased number of leukocytes and lasts from tenth day to as long as sixth week. Odor remains characteristically "fleshy" rather than foul. Amount of discharge is moderate for first 2 or 3 days and then is scant. Some women may have none after 2 wk; in others discharge persists until sixth wk.	Uterine bleeding (lochia) decreases until about fourth week and then ceases; vaginal discharge is minimal; a small period (menstruation) may have occurred during fourth or fifth week after delivery.
Cervix	Cervix regains its shape in a few days, and external os is contracted by end of first wk (introduction of a 1 cm probe is difficult) and cervical mucosa is restored.	Cervix is healed; external os has assumed typical transverse slit of parous woman. Occasionally glandular epithelium lining cervical canal can be visualized as a bright red area surrounding external os. Papanicolaou smear reveals normal estrogen pattern.

Table 31.3—cont'd
Evaluative Criteria, Area Assessed, and Normal Findings

Area Assessed	First 2 Wk	By Wk 4-6
Vagina	Vagina remains distensible; introitus gapes when intraabdominal pressure is increased by bearing-down effort or by coughing.	Pelvic floor has essentially regained its tone, permitting only a mild degree of uterine prolapse, cystocele, or rectocele. Vulva and perineal area show no evidence of infection. The episiotomy or laceration usually is healed without undue contraction, and introitus remains adequate to permit coitus without discomfort.
Abdomen	Abdominal wall is lax and weak in midline, where abdominal muscles may be widely separated. Muscles feel like masses on either side of abdomen and are not to be confused with fundus of uterus.	Muscles of abdomen reveal some degree of laxity, but tone is returning to prepregnant level.
Weight	There is an immediate weight loss of 4.5-5.1 kg (10-12 lb); then as excess tissue is eliminated, there is a further loss of 1.8-2.3 kg (4-5 lb) in first 3-4 days. Further decrease occurs as uterus involutes and plasma volume contracts.	Woman will retain about 60% of weight gained in excess of 11 kg (24 lb).
Urinary system	Most women void spontaneously by eight hr following delivery and thereafter void copious amounts frequently for 48 hr as retained tissue fluids are released.	There are no symptoms of urinary tract infection (e.g., frequency, urgency, dysuria, urinary incontinence). Urinalysis reveals normal findings; proteinuria has disappeared. Lactose may be present if woman is breast feeding, but no pus cells are present. Culture reveals no organisms.
Gastrointestinal system	Most women are hungry and have good appetities.	Appetite is good. Diet is adjusted for weight maintenance or weight loss (averages 2000-2500 cal/day). If woman is breast feeding, caloric intake is increased by 500 cal and fluid increased by 500 ml.
	Some women defecate spontaneously by third day. Others reestablish regular habits only with aid of laxatives or enemas in addition to added roughage in diet and fluids.	Regular bowel habits are reestablished without fecal incontinence or fistula formation.
Vascular system	Although a normal concentration of blood occurs as retained tissue fluids are released and tendency to clot increases as number of platelets increases, thrombi rarely develop. Hematocrit reading by third postdelivery day is within a normal range (42% ± 5%). There is no evidence of thromboembolism.	Hemorrhoids are reduced. Varicosities have disappeared. Woman wear support hose, if necessary. Hemoglobin level is 12 g/dl or greater, and hematocrit level is 37% ± 5%.
Pain or discomfort	Many women feel stress and strain of labor and delivery for 1 or 2 days, and discomfort associated with an episiotomy, hemorrhoids, engorgement of breasts, or other conditions may act to impede recovery for 3-5 days.	Discomfort from episiotomy is gone.
Emotional response	New mothers exhibit typical dependent behaviors for 24-48 hr. These usually are superseded by a mixture of dependent-independent behaviors, which in turn give way to interdependent behaviors. Depressive reactions may begin by end of second postdelivery day and persist for 1-3 days. Mother-child relationships may be positive immediately or show a "maternal lag," which may not interfere unduly with child care activities. Parents talk freely about their birthing experience (see also Chapter 32).	Emotional response has stabilized. Family roles are in the process of change through negotiation (see Chapter 32). Client is able to discuss client-centered problems.
Child care	Skill in child care activities increases with physical recovery and practice (see also Chapter 29).	Becoming skilled in child care activities, less apprehensive, able to ask questions (see also Chapter 32)

Continued.

Table 31.3—cont'd
Evaluative Criteria, Area Assessed, and Normal Findings

Area Assessed	First 2 Wk	By Wk 4-6
Health maintenance	Couple aware of contraception techniques available.	Couple has begun practicing their chosen method of family planning.
	Postdelivery immunization is completed (i.e., rubella vaccination and prevention of Rh isoimmunization), if appropriate.	Woman has established schedule for adequate rest and exercise.
	Woman is aware of need for rest, exercise, and nutrition.	Woman is aware of need for a medical reexamination in 6 mo.
	Couple is aware of danger signals, safety measures, and whom to contact: Hemorrhage Infection Thromboembolism Hypertension or hypotension Depressive states	Parents have chosen health care supervision for infant and have arranged for first examination.
	Couple is aware of need for medical examination by 4-6 wk.	
	Records are complete. Discharge summary is available for 4-6 wk examination.	Record keeping is completed to date.

Fig. 31.8
Initiation of family relationships. **A,** Mother and daughter observing newborn at breast. Mother's hand covers newborn; daughter's hand covers doll. **B,** Father tries to assist older sister to get acquainted. **C,** Older sister seeks comfort from her thumb. **D,** Older sister, thumb in mouth, places arm over baby but leans back to security of father's arm.

A B

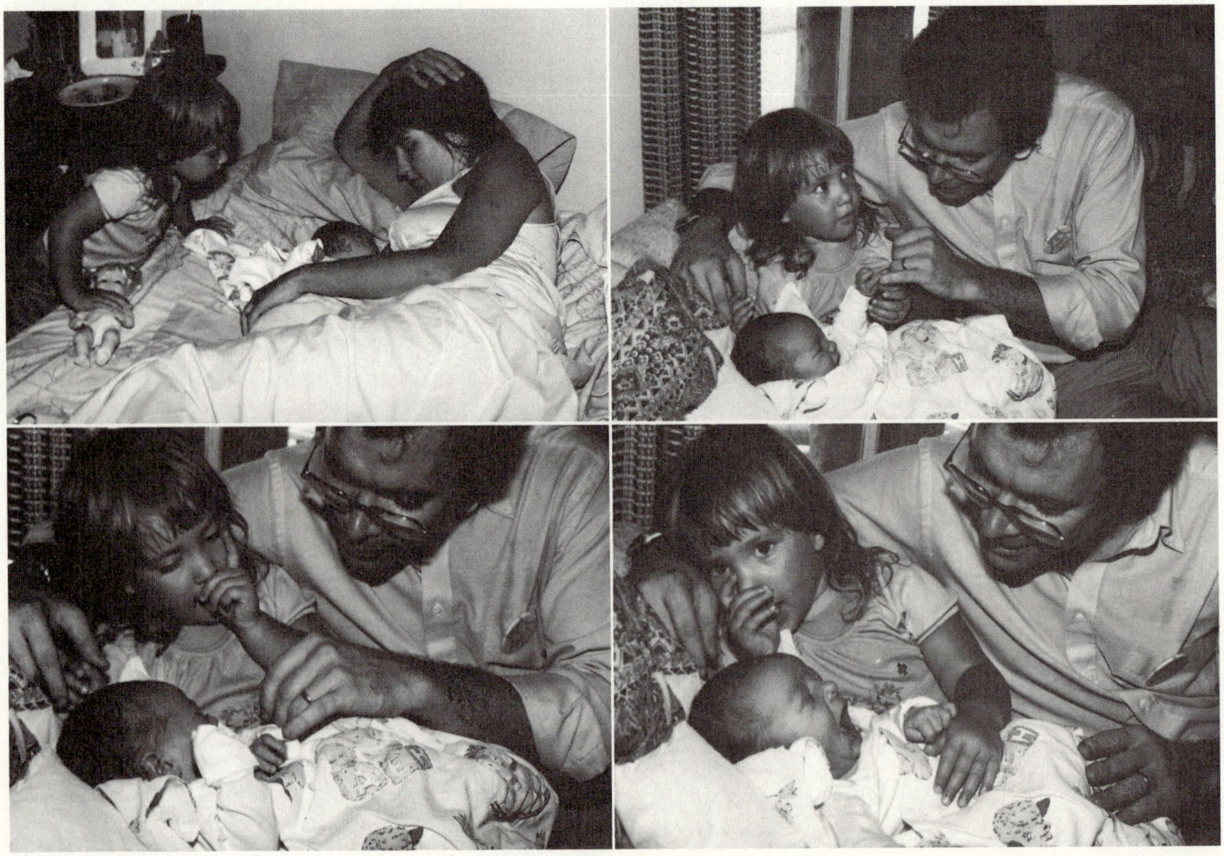

C D

care of the newborn (Fig. 31.8) are integral parts of the postdelivery care plan. A healthy, rested individual, free from discomfort, is more able to enter these crucial processes. (See Chapters 27 to 30 and 32 for more details.)

Facilities, supplies, and personnel. To prevent infection and promote recovery, attention to personal hygiene is important. Facilities and supplies (e.g., bathroom and bed units) must be kept scrupulously clean. Frequent changes of draw sheet and a daily change of linen are recommended. Supervision of use of facilities to prevent cross infection among women is necessary (e.g., common sitz bath must be scrubbed after each woman's use). Personnel must be conscientious about their hand-washing techniques to prevent cross infection. In many institutions the nurse is required to wear a face mask when carrying out perineal care. Personnel with colds, coughs, or skin infections (e.g., a cold sore on the lips [herpes simplex, type I]) must not be in contact with women during the puerperium.

Personal hygiene. A bed bath is given until the woman's condition permits use of shower or tub. She is instructed to use a fresh washcloth and towel and to begin her bath by washing the nipples and breasts. For the mother who is breast feeding, see Chapter 30 for further details. For the mother who elects not to breast feed, the daily bath provides all the cleaning necessary. Because orthostatic hypotension may cause a woman to faint, the first shower (or use of the bathroom) is carefully supervised. Use of a call bell in these areas is explained, and the woman is instructed to sit (on the floor, if necessary) should she feel faint.

Perineal care. Daily cleansing by bath or shower in addition to careful cleansing after voiding and defecating is sufficient unless the lochial flow is profuse. The woman may require encouragement to wash her perineum, including the episiotomy incision, with mild soap and warm water at least once daily. Fear of "breaking the stitches" or pain makes some women reluctant to do this. Soap and water or medicated wipes may be used for routine cleansing of the perineum after voiding or defecating. The woman is instructed to cleanse from symphysis pubis to anal area to prevent contamination of the vagina and urethra with fecal material and to use sterile perineal pads. She is instructed to wash her hands before and after changing her perineal pad. She is shown how to protect the inner surface of the pad from contamination and how to position the pad from front to back. Soiled pads are wrapped and placed in separate covered containers. She is instructed to change her pad at least four times a day.

Some women may require repeated instructions about frequent hand washing and the technique of keeping the sterile pad from being contaminated. Women need to be aware of the normal amount and appearance of lochia and to report if a foul odor should occur. The mother is cautioned to avoid placing her infant on the bedding (lower sheet) where she has been sitting to protect him from infection. The spread can be drawn up over this area and used as a base sheet for the baby.

Care of an episiotomy. Comfort measures are begun as soon as possible:

1. Moist heat (e.g., sitz bath) may be used once the woman is ambulating, twice a day or more often. The temperature of the water is maintained at 38° to 43.2° C (100° to 110° F). The call bell must be within reach in case the woman feels faint. She will need assistance in sitting down in some sitz baths. Instruct her to tighten her gluteal muscles until seated and then to relax them. If the gluteal muscles remain tightened, the perineal area may remain dry. A shower taken before use of a sitz bath helps to keep the bath clean. A sitz bath often *precedes* the use of the heat lamp.
2. Dry heat from a heat lamp positioned 50 cm (20 in) from the perineum may be used three times a day for 20-min periods. At home a desk lamp with a 40-watt bulb makes an effective heat lamp. In the hospital the extendible over-bed lamp has proved successful. If the over-bed lamp is used, the woman should be instructed to lie with her head at the foot of the bed, her perineal pad removed, and the lamp properly positioned; she should be draped for privacy and warmth. If a portable heat lamp is shared by several women, care must be taken to clean it between uses to prevent cross infection. However, the woman does not have to lie with her head to the foot of the bed.
3. Anesthetic sprays, ointments, or witch hazel pads (Tucks) may be applied directly to the sutured area.
4. Analgesics (e.g., oxycodone hydrochloride [Percodan], 1 or 2 tablets) may be offered for relief of pain. Some women will require medication every 4 hours for the first 2 postdelivery days.
5. Kegel exercises have proven effective (see p. 309). They can be repeated up to 10 times a day.

Since a mother who is free of discomfort is able to concentrate her energies on her child and child care, any needed medication should be administered 40 minutes before the infant's feeding period.

Care of hemorrhoids. Cold is effective in reducing hemorrhoidal swelling. A covered cold pack (rubber glove filled with small chips of ice works well) may be placed against the hemorrhoids soon after delivery, left in position no longer than 20 minutes, and repeated every 4 hours. Cold witch hazel compresses are also effective. Moist heat may also be used to reduce hemorrhoidal swelling. The woman may take a sitz bath with water temperature maintained at about 38° C (100° F) for 20-min periods. Careful observation of the woman for faintness is necessary. Show the woman how to replace the hemorrhoid in the anorectal canal by using a lubricated finger cot or rubber glove. Once the hemorrhoid is reduced, she should maintain digital pressure for 1 or 2 minutes, since an anal reflex will extrude the hemorrhoid. This reduction process must be repeated after bowel movements or as necessary. Judicious use of analgesics is indicated for the first postdelivery week. The woman can be advised that unless the rectal condition was present before pregnancy, it will correct itself once the increased blood supply and pressure symptoms of pregnancy are diminished and regular bowel habits are reestablished.

Elimination

Voiding. Every nursing measure to enhance the mother's ability to void spontaneously should be used. Some of these measures are (1) turning the tap on full because the sound of running water can act as a stimulus to voiding, (2) pouring warm water over the vulva, (3) having the woman void while using the sitz bath and then follow the bath with a shower, and (4) exposing the urinary meatus to fumes from peppermint spirits. (Woman should sit on bedpan. The fumes from peppermint spirits dropped into bedpan will cause relaxation of the urinary meatus, a local reaction.) If bladder distention occurs and she is unable to void, catheterization may be necessary. After delivery the urethra may be difficult to visualize because of swelling about the introitus; a dry sterile swab gently brushed upward from the vagina to the clitoris will cause the urethra to gape so that the catheter can be inserted. Because the catheterization procedure causes considerable discomfort and the possibility of causing a bladder infection is high, it is avoided unless adequate voiding cannot be induced by nursing measures by 6 hours postpartum. Intermittent catheterization, while still an infection-risky procedure, results in less infection than a closed system retention catheter. If the latter is used, it is removed in 48 hours and a urine specimen sent for culture and sensitivity. A urinary antibiotic may be ordered. The urinary antibiotic is continued for at least 1 week, when a clean-catch urine specimen is obtained for culture and sensitivity to assess effect of the medication.

Symptoms of bladder infection (pain and burning on voiding) or retention with overflow (small, frequent voidings) must be reported immediately to the physician, since treatment with antibiotics and a retention catheter may be indicated. A clean-catch specimen of urine should be obtained and sent to the laboratory for culture and sensitivity studies.

Defecation. Since the majority of women do not have a regular bowel movement for 2 or 3 days after delivery, oral laxative or stool softeners may be administered on the first or second postdelivery day. If a woman is unable to have a bowel movement by the third morning, a laxative suppository may be inserted and the woman given a hot drink. If this measure is unsuccessful, an enema usually is necessary.

Reestablishment of regular bowel habits may be assisted by exercise. roughage in diet (e.g., bran muffins, salads), and adequate fluid intake. Fear of discomfort because of the episiotomy or from hemorrhoids may hinder the woman from straining at stool; hence a stool softener may be ordered. An enema or laxative suppository is contraindicated for a woman with a third- or fourth-degree laceration until the suture line has healed, since the tip of the enema tubing or hard suppository may rupture the sutures. Oral stool softeners and laxatives may be administered, however.

Nutrition. Clear fluids may be offered immediately after delivery. The mother often wants either a light or regular diet with between-meal and bedtime nourishment. The use of protein, roughage, and ample fluid intake is to be encouraged. (See Chaper 18 for further details.)

Rest. The excitement and exhilaration experienced after birth of the infant may make rest difficult. The new mother, anxious about her ability to care for her infant or who is uncomfortable, may also have difficulty sleeping. Medication for sleep for the first few nights may be necessary.

Exercise. Most women can be ambulatory by at least 8 hours after normal delivery, assuming a local or light general anesthesia was used. Parturients who received *intrathecal subarachnoid spinal anesthesia* should remain flat in bed with one flat pillow to align the head with the shoulders for at least 8 hours before they are allowed to ambulate. This position prevents leakage of spinal fluid through the dural membrane at the site of the needle puncture (a potential fistula tract), which causes a severe headache (see Chapter 37). Since mothers automatically raise their heads to view their infants, the nurse needs to warn the mother to maintain the position of her head. The nurse then positions or holds the infant so the mother can see the child. Bathroom privileges are curtailed, and infant feeding by the mother may be delayed until she can sit up (check hospital protocol). Prevention of thrombosis is part of the nursing care plan. If a woman is confined to bed longer than normal (8 hours) (e.g., after spinal anesthesia or cesarean birth), exercise to promote circulation in the legs is indicated:

1. Alternate flexion and extension of feet.
2. Rotate feet.
3. Alternate flexion and extension of legs.
4. Press back of knee to bed surface; relax.
5. Do straight-leg raises.

If the woman is susceptible to thromboembolism, the physician may avoid use of estrogens to inhibit or suppress lactation. Women with varicosities are encouraged to wear support hose. The woman is encouraged to actively walk about for true ambulation, and she is discouraged from sitting immobile in a chair. If a thrombus is suspected, notify the physician immediately; meanwhile, the woman should be confined to bed, with the affected limb elevated on pillows.

Confinement to bed is not required for women who had *epidural* or *caudal anethesia* or for women who had local anesthesia such as cervical or pudendal block. Free movement is permitted once the anesthetic wears off unless an analgesic has been administered. After the first vital rest period is over (usually about 8 hours), the mother is encouraged to ambulate frequently.

Early ambulation has proved successful in reducing the incidence of thromboembolism and in the woman's more rapid recovery of strength.

Exercises may be started as soon as the mother's condition permits, usually by the first postdelivery day or when ordered by the obstetrician. They are helpful in trimming the figure and toning the musculature. If the woman is willing, calisthenics should be outlined; if she is not receptive, the exercise benefits of household activities, that is, bending and stretching, should be emphasized. The woman is instructed to begin with a single exercise performed five times and repeated three or four times a day. Additional exercises are added sequentially. See Fig. 31.9 for a description of the exercises and the plan for adding a new one each day.

Fig. 31.9
Postpartum exercise program. Do one new exercise each day. Begin by repeating exercise five times. Gradually increase to 10 times. Vigorous exercise is not recommended for 6 to 7 weeks. This allows abdominal muscles to regain their original length and tone.

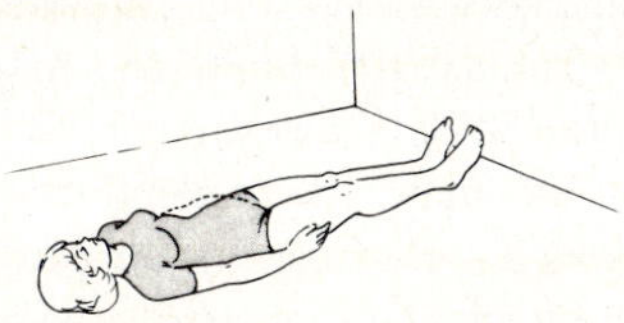

1st Day: Raise abdomen while inhaling deeply. Slowly exhale through pursed lips while contracting abdominal muscle forcibly.

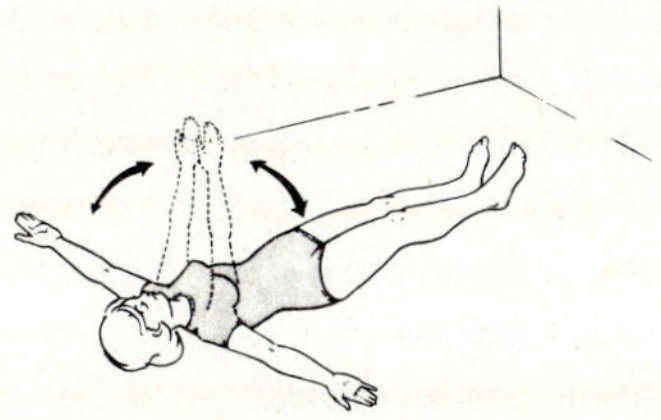

2nd Day: Lying on your back with your legs slightly parted, place your arms at right angles to your body and slowly raise them, keeping your elbows stiff. When your hands touch, lower your arms gradually.

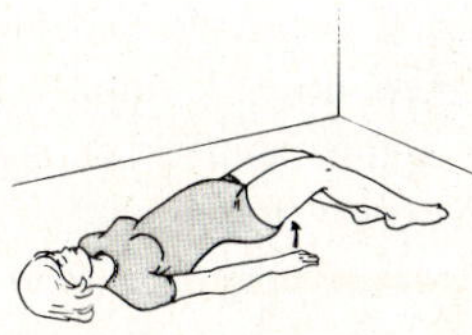

3rd Day: Lying with your arms at your sides, draw your knees up slightly, arch your back.

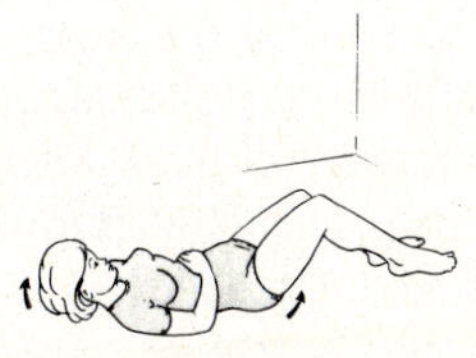

4th Day: Lying with your knees and hips flexed, tilt your pelvis inward and tightly contract your buttocks as you lift your head.

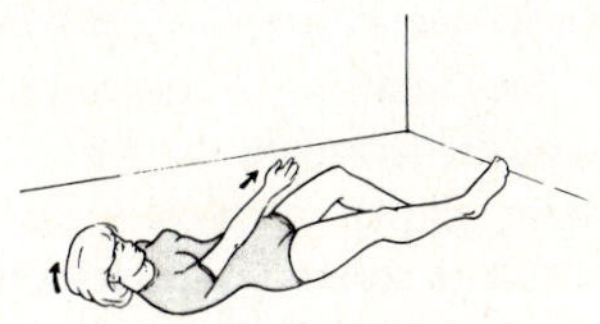

5th Day: Lying with your legs straight, raise your head and left knee slightly, then reach for (but do not touch) your left knee with your right hand. Repeat, using your right knee and left hand.

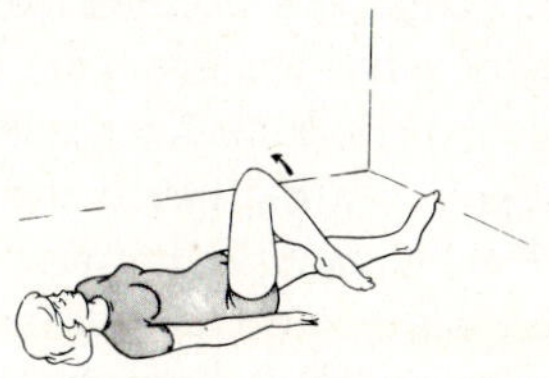

6th Day: Lying on your back, slowly flex the knee and then the thigh toward the abdomen; lower your foot toward your buttock, then straighten and lower your leg.

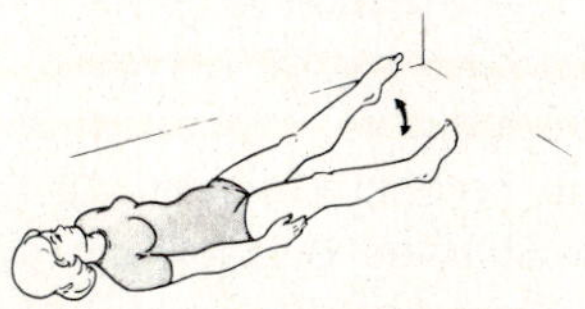

7th Day: Lying on your back, toes pointed and knees straight, raise one leg and then the other as high as possible, using your abdominal muscles but not your hands to lower your legs slowly.

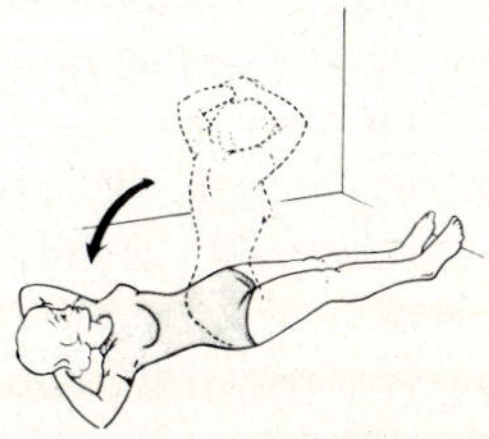

10th Day: Lying on your back with your arms clasped behind your head, sit up and lie back slowly. At first, you may have to hook your feet under furniture.

On the woman's return home, a gradual increase in ambulation about the house is suggested. Stairs offer few problems. Avoidance of fatigue should be the rule. Light housekeeping can be resumed after the first week. Moderate work can be done during the third week, but full activity should be delayed until after the postdelivery visit and examination. Most women can resume all but the most physically tiring employment 4 or 5 weeks after childbirth. An increase in the amount of lochia rubra or its reappearance may indicate too much activity.

Resumption of intercourse. The couple can safely resume intercourse by the third or fourth postdelivery week if bleeding has stopped and the episiotomy has healed. For the first 6 weeks to 6 months the vagina does not lubricate well because steroid depletion inhibits the vasocongestive response to sexual tension. A water-soluble gel or a contraceptive cream or jelly might therefore be recommended for lubrication. If there is some vaginal tenderness, the partner can be instructed to insert one or two fingers into the vagina and rotate them within the vagina to help relax it and to identify possible areas of discomfort. A coital position in which the woman has control of the depth of penile penetration is also useful. The side-by-side or female-superior position often is recommended.

Physiologic reactions to sexual stimulation for the first 3 postdelivery months are marked by a reduction in both rapidity and intensity of response. Vasocongestion of the labia majora and minora is delayed well into the plateau phase. The walls of the vagina are thin and pink, a condition similar to senile vaginitis. This results from the hormonal starvation of the involutional period. Finally, the size of the orgasmic platform and strength of orgasmic contractions are reduced.

The presence of the baby influences postdelivery lovemaking. Parents hear every sound made by the baby; conversely they may be concerned that the baby hears every sound they make. In either case any phase of the sexual response cycle may be interrupted by hearing the baby cry or move, leaving one or both of the couple frustrated and unsatisfied. The amount of psychologic and physiologic energy expended by the parents in child care activities may lead to fatigue. One newborn requires a great deal of attention and time; imagine caring for twins, triplets, or older children as well!

Some women have reported sexual stimulation to plateau and orgasmic levels when nursing their babies. It is interesting to note that although nursing mothers have a longer delay in ovarian steroid production, they are often interested in returning to sexual activity before nonnursing mothers. Nursing mothers also report higher levels of postdelivery eroticism.

In the event of fetal or newborn death or the birth of an infant who is small, sick, or deformed, the emotional energy required of the woman and her partner, the mother's depleted physical state, and the stress of burying the dead child or of visiting the hospitalized child strain all relationships. Because little definitive data are available, professional care givers can only speculate about the effect on sexual relationships during these stressful periods.

The woman should be instructed to follow the Kegel exercises to strengthen her pubococcygeal muscle. The pubococcygeal muscle is the major sphincter of the pelvis. It is associated with bowel and bladder function and with vaginal perception and response during intercourse.

Contraception. Contraception should be discussed and a tentative program outlined within the first week. Women neither menstruate nor do they conceive while they successfully nurse their infant because all ovarian functions are suppressed by a high level of serum prolactin. This hormone, which is responsible for milk production, rises slowly during pregnancy and increases rapidly to a plateau with suckling. Prolactin blocks the production of pituitary gonadotropin; hence the ovaries become inactive. Follicle formation is suspended, and ovulation does not occur. Consequently the secretion of estrogen is minimal, and no progesterone is produced. However, women who do not nurse or *who complement the infant's feeding* do not maintain an effectively high level of serum prolactin; follicle-stimulating hormone (FSH), luteinizing hormone (LH), and estrogen are secreted once more, and menstruation and ovulation resume. If these women do not employ contraceptives, they may conceive again, sometimes without having a period following the prior pregnancy.

If the mother is not nursing, she may resume use of oral contraceptives (after delivery) under the physician's directive. If she is nursing or wishes to use an intrauterine device (IUD) or diaphragm, temporary contraception, such as a condom, gel, or foam, should be provided until the first postdelivery examination, at which time the desired method can be instituted.

Laboratory tests. Explain rationale for repeating hemocrit on third day postpartum and for other tests.

Suppression of lactation. If the mother does not wish to suckle her infant or if this is medically contraindicated, lactation can be prevented by mechanical means. To do this, nursing the infant, expression of milk, or pumping of the breast must be discontinued. A tight compression "uplift" binder is applied for about 72 hours, after which use of a snug brassiere is advised. The breasts will become distended, firm, and tender, but after 48 to 72 hours lactation and discomfort will ease. Ice packs and analgesics may be used if necessary. It is also necessary to tell the mother to avoid immersion of her breasts in hot water when taking a bath or shower, since this will increase milk flow. Fluid restriction or laxatives are not helpful. Involution will be complete in about a month.

The administration of estrogens or androgens or both is not used often today and is not recommended to suppress lactation. Recent research has implicated the use of estrogen or other hormones as lactation-suppressant drugs in the etiology of endometrial cancer. The woman must give informed consent to the use of these drugs. Estrogens have also been implicated in the occurrence of thromboembolism after delivery, particularly after cesarean delivery or a complicated vaginal delivery. *Mechanical suppression of lactation is the treatment of choice.*

A drug that is an alternative to estrogens and other hormones in the prevention of postpartum lactation is bromocriptine mesylate (Parlodel). Bromocriptine mesylate acts to suppress lactation by preventing the secretion of prolactin. Since bromocriptine mesylate is known to cause hypotension in some women, *its use should not be initiated until the vital signs have been stabilized and no sooner than 4 hours after delivery.* The nurse needs to remain with the woman when she ambulates for the first time and to assess the blood pressure every 4 hours. Women receiving other medications to lower blood pressure are at risk for more severe hypotension. The recommended therapeutic dosage for prevention of lactation is one 2.5 mg tablet twice daily with meals. Therapy should be continued for 14 days or, if necessary, 21 days. Once bromocriptine mesylate therapy is stopped 18% to 40% of women experience a rebound of breast secretion, congestion, or engorgement, which is usually mild to moderate in severity. Therefore the nurse reviews the technique for mechanical suppression of lactation for use if this rebound occurs.

Hospitalization. The duration of hospitalization and the subsequent convalescence at home still are debated. Most women who do not experience complications can be dismissed from the hospital on the third postdelivery day. Some women who are carefully screened by the obstetrician and pediatrician leave much earlier—anywhere from 12 to 24 hours after delivery. Because this group is in particular need of follow-up care for themselves and their infants, hospitals have established early discharge programs to assist with such care. These programs provide an alternative mode of maternal-infant care. Planning for early discharge begins in the prenatal period. The families who participate should meet the following criteria: (1) live within a reasonable distance of the hospital, (2) have taken preparation-for-parenthood classes, (3) have someone at home to assist in the care of the infant and mother, and (4) have no major medical problems. If a family is interested, they are asked to notify the attending physician and nursing staff at the beginning of prenatal care. Opportunities are provided to meet the nurse who will be making home visits for health assessment and any teaching that is necessary; for example, infants must return for a phenylketonuria (PKU) test 48 hours after delivery, and the detection and care of neonatal hyperbilirubinemia need to be discussed (see Chapter 40). Women with complications, however, should be asymptomatic for at least 24 hours and capable of personal care before leaving the hospital.

Return visit. Since biblical times, the puerperium has been considered to last 6 weeks. Hence a return visit and examination have been scheduled traditionally 6 weeks after delivery. This is illogical because many problems, such as leukorrhea, may be identified and successfully treated earlier. Individualization is important, therefore, but a more logical date for return to the physician or clinic would be 3 or 4 weeks after delivery.

The nurse welcomes the woman and inquires about her general health and that of the child and other family members as indicated. A clean-catch urine sample for analysis and culture and a blood sample for Hct and VDRL are sent to the laboratory. The woman then undresses and puts on an examining gown. Once the blood pressure and vital signs are taken the nurse helps the woman position herself for examination of her breasts, abdomen, and legs. A vaginal examination is then done.

At this examination the physician, midwife, or nurse-practitioner assesses the progress of involution, discusses any physical problems, and institutes care if indicated (see Chapter 35). A Papanicolaou smear is taken and contraception is reviewed (see Chapter 13). The parents are encouraged to share their concerns over infant care-taking activities, and their responsiveness to their infant is noted (see Chapter 32).

EVALUATION

The nurse consistently evaluates the progress of the woman toward physical recovery and of the family toward skill in child care activities and attachment to the newborn. Table 31.3 presents the areas to be evaluated and normal findings. If there is a significant deviation from normal, remedial care is instituted (see Unit Seven).

References and Readings

Avery, M., et al.: An early postpartum hospital discharge program: implementation and evaluation, J.O.G.N. Nurs. **11**(4):200, 1982.

Benson, R.: Current obstetric and gynecologic diagnosis and treatment, ed. 3, Los Altos, Calif., 1980, Lange Medical Publications.

Brown, M.S., and Hurlock, J.T.: Mothering the mother, Am. J. Nurs. **77:**438, March 1977.

Carlson, S.E.: The irreality of postpartum: observations on the subjective experience, J.O.G.N. Nurs. **5:**28, Sept.-Oct. 1976.

Claypool, J.M.: Rubella protection for maternal child health care providers, M.C.N. **6:**53, Jan-Feb. 1981.

Cooke, I., et al.: The treatment of puerperal lactation with bromocriptine, Postgrad. Med. J. **52**(suppl.)75, 1976.

Danforth, D.N.: Textbook of obstetrics and gynecology, ed. 5, New York, 1982, Harper & Row.

Donaldson, N.E.: The post partum follow-up nurse clinician, J.O.G.N. Nurs. (4):249, July-Aug. 1981.

Edwards, M.: The crises of fourth trimester, Birth Fam. J. **1:**19, Winter 1973-1974.

Freda, V.J., et al.: Prevention of Rh hemolytic disease: ten years' experience with Rh immune globulin, N. Engl. J. Med. **292:**1014, 1975.

Gardner, S.: The mother as incubator—after delivery, J.O.G.N. Nurs. **8:**174, May-June 1979.

Greis, M.: Beyond maternity: post partum concerns of mothers. M.C.N., p. 182, May-June 1977.

Harr, B., and Hastings, J.: Parturition care planning, J.O.G.N. Nurs. **10**(1):54, 1981.

Hellman, L.M., and Pritchard, J.A.: Williams' obstetrics, ed. 15, New York, 1976, Appleton-Century-Crofts.

Ingalls, A.J., and Salerno, M.C.: Maternal and child health nursing, ed. 4, St. Louis, 1979, The C.V. Mosby Co.

Jiminez, M.H., and Niles, N.: Activity and work during pregnancy and the postpartum period: a cross cultural study of 202 societies, Am. J. Obstet. Gynecol. **135**:(2):198, 1979.

Klaus, M.H., and Kennell, J.H.: Parent-infant bonding, ed. 2, St. Louis, 1982, The C.V. Mosby Co.

LeMaster, E.E.: Parenthood as crisis. In Parad, H.J., editor: Crisis interventions: selected readings, New York, 1965, Family Service Association of America.

Ludington-Hoe, S.M.: Postpartum: development of maternity, Am. J. Nurs. **77:**1170, July 1977.

Nurses Association of the American College of Obstetricians and Gynecologists: Standards for obstetric gynecologic and neonatal nursing, ed. 2, Washington, D.C., 1981, The Association.

Rolland, R., and Schellekens, L.: A new approach to the inhibition of puerperal lactation, Br. J. Obstet. Gynaecol. **80:**945, 1973.

Strelinck, E.G.: Postpartum care: an opportunity to reinforce breast self-examination, M.C.N. **7**(4):249, 1982.

Warrick, L.: Femininity, sexuality and mothering, Nurs. Forum **8:**224, 1969.

Williams J.K.: Learning needs of new parents, Am. J. Nurs. **77:**1173, July 1977.

Willson, J.R., and Carrington, E.R.: Obstetrics and gynecology, ed. 6, St. Louis, 1979, The C.V. Mosby Co.

Zalar, M.K.: Human sexuality: a component of total patient care, Nurs. Dig. **3:**40, Nov.-Dec. 1975.

Zalar, M.K.: Sexual counseling for pregnant couples, M.C.N. **1:**176, May-June 1976.

Zuspan, F., and Quilligan, E.: Practical manual of obstetrical care, St. Louis, 1982, The C.V. Mosby Co.

32

Family Responses to the Birth of a Child and Nursing Care

- Part 1: Family Responses
  - Parenthood
    - Components
  - Parent-child attachment
  - Contact and attachment
  - Process of assuming parental role: reality phase
    - Parental tasks
    - Stages of development of parental role
  - Siblings
  - Grandparents
  - Factors influencing parental responses
    - Physical condition of mother
    - Physical condition of infant
    - Parental expectations
    - Parental age
    - Social and economic conditions
    - Interference with personal aspirations
    - Sensory impairment
- Part 2: Nursing Care
  - Assessment of parental responses
    - Assessment strategies
    - Assessment tools
  - Examples of nursing diagnoses
  - Planning and implementation
  - Evaluation

In this chapter Part 1 presents the responses of the family to the birth of a child and Part 2 presents the nursing care that such responses engender.

Part 1: Family Responses

PARENTHOOD

Biologic parenthood for both sexes begins with the union of ovum and sperm. During the prenatal (prebirth) period the mother becomes the primary agent in providing an environment in which the fetus may develop and grow. This close symbiotic union of mother and child ends with birth, and others may assume partial or complete involvement in the infant's care. Whoever assumes the parental role, whether it be a biologic or surrogate parent, woman or man, enters into a crucial relationship with a child that will persist throughout the lifetime of each. Men and women, of course, may exist without a child; thus, in essence, parenthood is optional. Parenthood may serve as a maturation factor in the life of a man or woman regardless of whether it is biologically based. For the child, parenthood is all important; his continued existence depends on the quality of care he receives.

Components. The tasks, responsibilities, and attitudes that make up this care have been designated by Steel and Pollock (1968) as the "mothering function," a process in which an adult (a mature, caring, capable, self-sufficient person) assumes the care of an infant (a helpless, dependent, immature person). They describe this process of parenting as one with two components: the first, being practical or mechanical in nature, involves cognitive and motor skills; the second, emotional in nature, involves cognitive and affective skills. The first component includes child care activities such as "feeding, holding, clothing, and cleaning the infant, protecting it from harm, and providing motility for it" (Steele and Pollock, 1968). The second component includes attitudes of tenderness, awareness, and concern for the child's needs and desires. This component influences the environment of the child and has a profound effect on the manner in which the practical aspects of child care are performed and on the emotional response of the child. Both components are essential to the infant's immediate well-being and future development.

Those components of the child's care that make up the practical, or mechanical, aspects do not appear automatically as efficient care-taking behaviors at the birth of one's child. The parent's ability in these respects has been altered by the effects of cultural and personal experiences. Many parents have to learn how to do these tasks, and this learning process can be a difficult one. If, however, the desire to learn is there and there are persons able and willing to support the parents' endeavors, the majority of parents become adept in care-taking activities.

The psychologic component in child care, motherliness and fatherliness, appears to stem from the parents' own earliest experiences with a loving, accepting mother figure. In this sense the parents may be said to *inherit* the ability to show concern and tenderness and to pass on this ability to the next generation by repeating the kind of parent-child relationship they experienced. Benedek (1950) describes a positive parent-child relationship as mutually rewarding and being fundamental to an individual's development of a feeling of confidence in the expectations that others will be willing to help and that he is worth helping. Erikson's concept (1959) of "basic trust" is similar in that he postulates that such a psychologic entity forms the basis for the adult's eventual relationships with others and his ability to look at others with a sense of trust. These persons tend to be social or outgoing in nature and able to seek and accept assistance from others. In contrast, those deficient in this sense tend to be alienated and isolated. They are more crisis prone because of their inability to make use of situational supports in times of stress.

Either parent may exhibit "motherliness"; it is now recognized to be a non-gender-related ability. As Josselyn (1956) maintains, the ability to show gentleness, love, and understanding and to place another's welfare above one's own is not limited to women—it is a human characteristic (Fig. 32.1)

PARENT-CHILD ATTACHMENT

Much research has been directed toward unraveling the process by which a parent comes to love and accept a child and a child comes to love and accept a parent. This process has been called the attachment process, and attachment has been defined as a unique emotional relationship between two individuals that is specific and

Fig. 32.1
Hands. (Courtesy St. Lukes Hospital, Kansas City, Mo.)

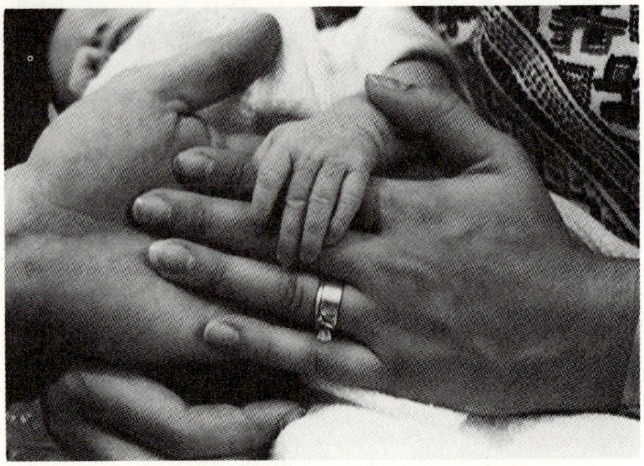

endures through time (Kenneth, 1982). In the infant's case the other individual is the primary caretaker, usually the mother. The end result of attachment behavior may be described as a successful attempt to be near certain people and to resist separation from them (McClinton and Meier, 1978).

Various theories have attempted to explain the basis for attachment behavior. Freudian psychoanalytic theory emphasized the development of the bond between child and mother as a result of the mother's satisfying the infant's innate needs related to the human need to socialize with another and the physical needs for survival. Social learning theory contributed the principles of reinforcement to the attachment process. As discomfort is reduced or removed by the mother (or other caretaker) and pleasure substituted, the mother eventually becomes associated with the pleasureable feeling of being satisfied. She becomes important to the infant, is loved, and can therefore act as a reinforcing agent or event. She becomes a *significant other* in the infant's life.

Bowlby (1958) and others (Ainsworth, 1969, 1970; Ainsworth and Bell, 1970; Brazelton, 1963, 1973a, 1973b) extended the concept of attachment to include *mutuality;* that is, the infant's behaviors and characteristics called forth a corresponding set of maternal behaviors and characteristics. The infant possesses a repertoire of behaviors that serve to initiate and maintain contact with the mother. *Signaling* behaviors, such as crying, smiling, and cooing, bring the mother into close proximity to the child. *Executive* behaviors, such as rooting, sucking, grasping, and postural adjustments, maintain the contact.

In addition to these responses, observers have noted

Fig. 32.2
Mother interacts with her daughter through touching. (Courtesy Judy Bamber, San Jose, Calif.)

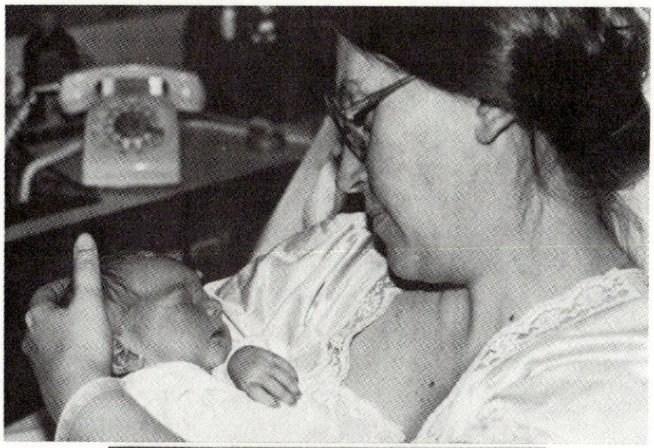

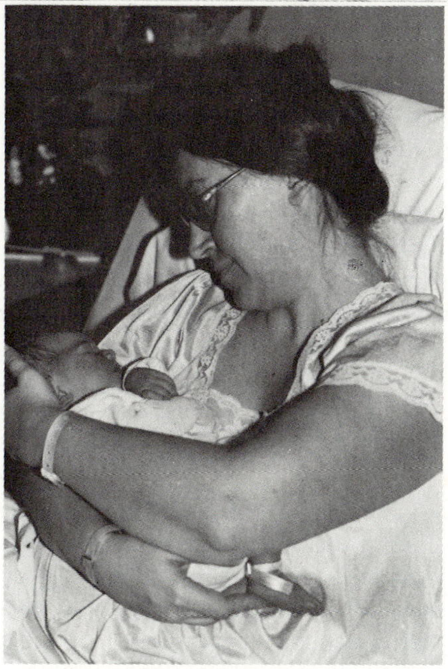

Fig. 32.3
Mother and her baby interact using eye contact. (Courtesy Judy Bamber, San Jose, Calif.)

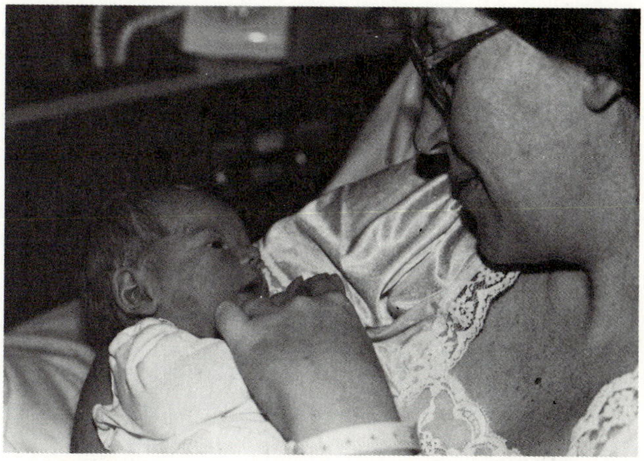

both partners in the parent-child interaction use sensual responses or abilities to strengthen attachment. (The infant is physiologically ready for the encounters; see Chapter 27.) The sensual responses and abilities include the following:

1. *Touch*. Studies have shown that in the first contacts a mother has with her infant, an orderly and predictable pattern of touch behavior ensues regardless of whether the mother is young or old, a primipara or multipara, wed or unwed (Klaus et al., 1970 Rubin, 1961). The mother begins with a fingertip exploration of the infant's head and extremities (Fig. 32.2). Within a short time the open palm is used to caress the trunk, and eventually the infant is enfolded in the mother's arms. Even after the initial period of interaction, gentle stroking motions are used to soothe and quiet the infant. Mothers pat or gently rub their infant's back after feedings. Infants pat the mother's breast as they nurse. The newborn infant will grasp a finger or a strand of hair and thereby attach himself to the parent. A father commented on his son's grasp reflex, "I put my finger in his hand, and he grabbed right on. It is just a reflex, I know, but it felt good anyway."

2. *Eye-to-eye contact*. Interest in having eye contact is demonstrated again and again. Some mothers remark that once their babies have looked at them, they feel much closer to them (Klaus et al., 1970). Others have also noted this response: "I was a mother and looked into his eyes so clear; fell into his eyes, and in love" (Lang, 1972). Parents spend much time getting babies to open their eyes and to look at them (the parents). Eye contact appears to have a cementing effect on the development of a beginning and trusting relationship and is an important factor in human relationships at all ages (Fig. 32.3).

As newborns become functionally able to sustain eye contact, parents and child spend much time mutually gazing at one another. We need to examine medical and nursing practices that thwart this exchange. Instillation of protective eye drops can be withheld until the infant and parents have a period of time together. Lights can be dimmed so that the child will open his eyes. The newborn can be held close enough to the parent's face so that he can see the parents.

3. *Odor*. Another behavior shared by parents and infant is responsiveness to each other's odor. Mothers comment on the smell of their babies when first born and have noted that each child has an odor of its own. As mentioned earlier, infants learn rapidly to distinguish the odor of their own mother's breast milk.

4. *Body warmth*. Parents and child seem to enjoy sharing each other's body warmth. Mothers will say, "I love her warm little body against mine." We all know the feeling when we pick up a baby who is still asleep, the warm, cocoonlike feeling he gives us. Research has demonstrated that the infant does not lose body heat if reasonable precautions are taken (e.g., if he is placed on the mother's abdomen after birth and dried thoroughly). The infant can be seen to relax completely against his mother's warm body.

5. *Voice*. The shared response of parents and infant to each other's voice is also remarkable. Parents wait tensely for the first cry. Once it has reassured them of the baby's health, they begin comforting behaviors. As the parents talk in high-pitched voices, the infant is alerted and turns toward them.

6. *Entrainment*. Newborns have been found to move in time with the structure of adult speech (Condon and Sander, 1974). This means that the infant has developed *culturally determined rhythms* of speech long before he uses the spoken language in communicating. There is a *carry-over* once he begins to talk (entrainment). This shared rhythm also acts to give the parent positive feedback and to establish a positive setting for effective communication.

7. *Biorhythmicity*. The fetus in utero can be said to be in tune with his mother's natural rhythms, such as heartbeats. After birth one of his tasks, as noted earlier, is to establish his own rhythm. Parents can help in this process by giving consistent loving care and by utilizing their infant's alert state to develop his responsive behavior and thereby increase social interactions and opportunities for learning. The more quickly parents can become competent in child care activities, the more quickly their psychic energy can be directed toward noting the communication cues the infant is giving them.

CONTACT AND ATTACHMENT

Research with mammals other than humans indicates that early contact between mother and offspring is important in developing future relationships. No scientific evidence to date has demonstrated that immediate contact after birth is essential for the human parent-child relationship. Seigel (1982) notes that findings from carefully controlled replicated investigations appear to document the following:

> that early contact, irrespective of its supplementation by extended contact, favorably affects maternal affectional behavior during the first postpartum days. The results are consistent across low and middle socio-economic status mother-infant pairs as well as in developed and less developed countries.

He also notes that early contact has a positive effect on the duration of breast feeding. However, long-range effects of early contact have yet to be documented (Lamb, 1982).

Early close contact may, however, *facilitate* the attachment process between parent and child. This is not to say a delay will negate this process (the human being is too resilient for that), but additional psychic energy may be needed to accomplish the same effect. For parents unable or unwilling to expend this energy the delay may be important to the infant's future well-being.

In one of the first texts on newborn disorders, Budin (1907) noted that "mothers separated from their young soon lost all interest in those whom they were unable to nurse or cherish." Subsequent investigators brought to light similar behaviors when interactions between parent and child met interference. Bowlby's work (1958, 1969) emphasized the attachment process between infant and mother and detailed the effects of loss of that attachment to the infant. Research in the area of child abuse documents the greater percentage of neglect, abuse, and failure to thrive among infants separated from parents for relatively long periods because of illness or preterm birth (Barnett et al., 1970; Hefler and Kempe, 1965; Klaus and Kennell, 1976; Leifer et al., 1972).

However, those parents who wish for but are unable to have early contact with their newborn infant *can be reassured that such contact is not essential for optimal parent-child interactions;* otherwise, adopted infants would not form the usual affectional ties with their parents. Nor does the mode of infant-mother contact after delivery (skin-to-skin vs. wrapped) appear to have any important effect. As far as is known the mode of infant-mother contact after delivery is just one of many variables affecting mother-infant attachment (Curry, 1979). The original study by Klaus and co-workers (1972) has been instrumental in making those in the health care system aware of the need to respect the early moments and hours after birth as a sensitive time for mother-infant interaction, and as a result, has facilitated the humanization of birthing practices. However, nurses need to counsel mothers to allay fears that their emotional bond to their infant might be weaker because they missed early contact or because the contact was not skin-to-skin (Curry, 1979).

The physiologic benefits of early contact between mother and infant have been documented (Klaus and Kennell, 1976). For the mother, levels of oxytocin and prolactin rise; for the infant, sucking reflexes are utilized early, and the process of developing active immunity begins as the infant inhales flora from the mother's skin.

The recent upsurge in demand by parents for home, rather than hospital, delivery is attributable in some measure to the parents' desire to share the birth process and to have immediate and continuous contact with their infant. The development in hospitals of family-centered maternity care units also reflects this demand. In December 1977 the American Medical Association adopted a policy on parent-newborn interaction that gives official medical sanction to efforts of groups identifying hospital practices that may frustrate family-oriented childbirth in America (see Appendix B).

One widely used method of family-centered care is the provision of rooming-in facilities for the mother and her baby. The infant is transferred to the area from the transitional nursery after evidencing satisfactory post-delivery adjustment. The father is encouraged to visit and to participate in the care of the infant (Fig. 32.4). Some hospitals are experimenting with alternate birth centers (see Chapter 26). The mother is accompanied by the father during the delivery of the infant, and all three may remain together until discharged. Medical and nursing personnel are available for any care necessary for the mother and child. Other hospitals arrange for the discharge of mother and infant anywhere from 2 to 24 hours after delivery if the condition of the mother and that of the child warrants it. Follow-up care with nursing personnel from a health agency is part of this plan.

Until recently, in our efforts to physically safeguard mothers and babies, the obstetric client and her newborn were restricted in contact with family members. This practice served a useful purpose earlier when infection was a persistent threat to hospitalized women and their newborns. Unfortunately, the practice persisted or was used inconsistently long after the need was no longer apparent. It took many years for the professional workers to concede that a father could scrub, gown, and observe good medical asepsis as well as they. As a result, much of the ritual of birth that acted as a ceremony to usher in parenthood and its many responsibilities was lost. Every child born depends for survival on the care given by concerned, loving adults. Any methods undertaken to enhance the quality of that care are worth serious consideration.

PROCESS OF ASSUMING PARENTAL ROLE: REALITY PHASE

Emotional adjustment in the postdelivery period pertains predominantly to recovery from the labor of birth and adaptation to the reality of the parental role. This adaptation involves mastery of the tasks and responsibilities inherent in the role and a modification of old behaviors or the addition of new ones. It involves the development of cognitive, motor, and affective skills;

Fig. 32.4
Family joy over birth of their child.

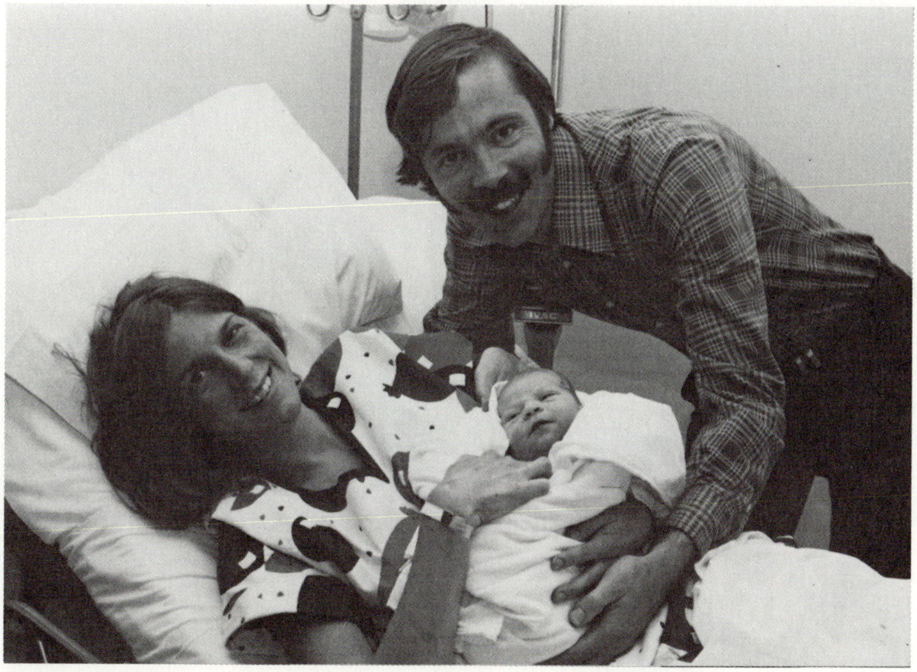

Fig. 32.5
Father and son share a day. **A,** Care of umbilical cord. **B,** Diapering. Note baby's facial expression and hands reaching out to father. **C,** Sharing mealtime. **D,** Sharing a smile: an example of synchrony. **E,** Studying together.

A

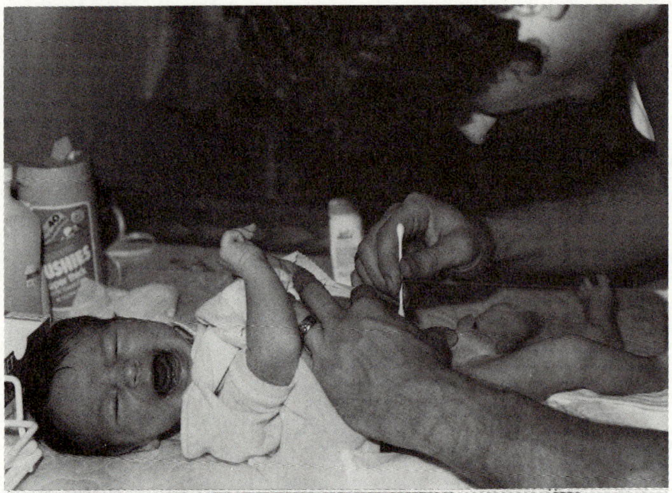

B

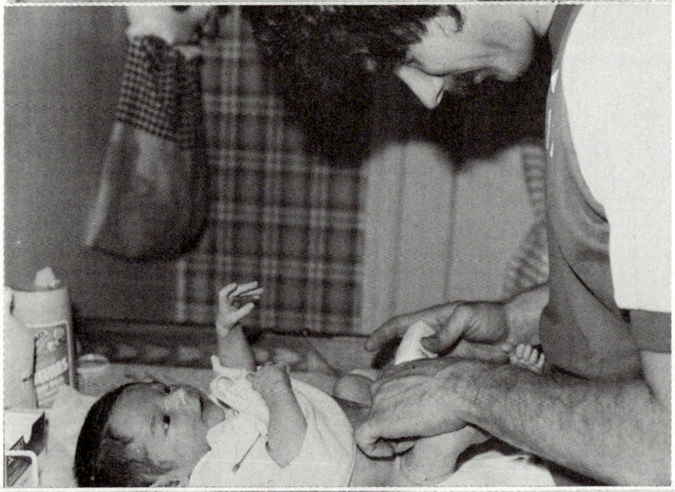

C

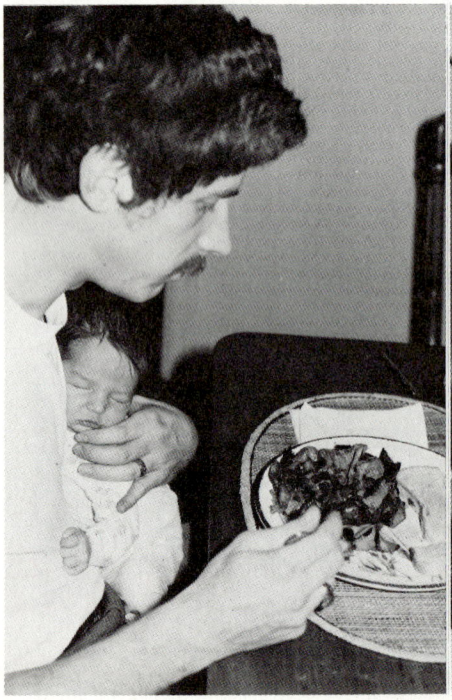

D, E

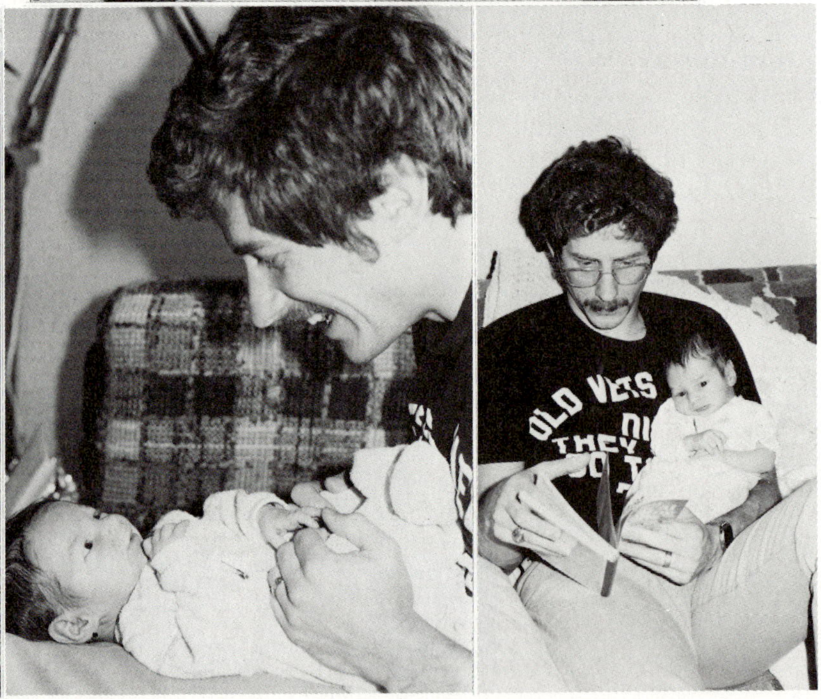

the goals of nursing are addressed to assisting parents to master these skills (Fig. 32.5).

The mother'a ability to master these skills and to advance through the developmental stages of dependent behavior, dependent-independent behavior, and finally interdependent behavior marks the success of attaining a new role in life. This developmental sequence is similar to any other; mastery of one step permits advancement to and mastery of the next step. Depending on their unique experiences, each parent will set an individual pace for progression.

Parental tasks

1. The parent needs to reconcile the actual child with the fantasy child. This means coming to terms with the infant's physical appearance, sex, innate temperament, and physical status. If the real child differs greatly from the fantasy child, acceptance may be delayed for a period of time, or in some instances the child is never accepted.
2. The parent needs to establish the newborn as a being separate from herself or himself, that is, as an individual having many dependency needs and requiring much nurturing.
3. The parent needs to become adept in the care of the infant. This includes the following:
   a. Care-taking activities
   b. Noting the communication cues given by the infant to indicate his needs
   c. Responding appropriately to the infant's needs
4. The parent needs to establish reasonable evaluative criteria to use in assessing the success or failure of the care given to the infant.
   a. Infant responses: parents are suprisingly sensitive to infant responses. One father told of his first attempt to give his child a kiss. At that moment, the child turned her head. The father felt hurt, although he understood that the baby was totally unaware of her own movements. How the infant responds to the parental care and attention is interpreted by the parent as a comment on the quality of the care being given. These responses may include crying, weight gain or loss, or sleeping at a designated time. Continued responses deemed negative by the parent can result in alienation of parent and child to the infant's detriment.
   b. Competence in care-taking activities: self-esteem grows with competence. Mothers of premature infants have noted that the adept handling of their infants by nurses was recognized as evidence of care yet at the same time was resented because it made *their* efforts to sustain their child appear inadequate. Mothers who have supplied breast milk for their infants comment that this makes them feel they are contributing in a unique way to the welfare of their child.
   c. Opinion of significant others: criticism, real or imagined, of new parents' ability to provide adequate physical care, nutrition, or social stimulation for their infant can prove devastating. These "critics" may need constructive direction. Assistance, including advice by husbands, wives, mothers, and mothers-in-law as well as professional workers, can be seen as either supportive or as an indication of how inept these persons have judged the new parent to be.
5. The parent must establish a place for the neonate within the family group. Whether the infant is the first or last of many, all family members must adjust their roles to accommodate the newcomer. An only child needs support to accept a rival to parental affections (Fig. 32.6). An older child needs support as he loses a favored position. It is usually the parents who are expected to negotiate these changes.
6. Parents need to establish the primacy of their adult relationships in order to maintain the family as a group. Since this includes reorganizing many roles, for example, sexual roles, child care roles, career roles, and community roles, time and energy must be provided for this vital task.

Fig. 32.6
Expectant mother helps her 4-year-old child prepare for new baby.

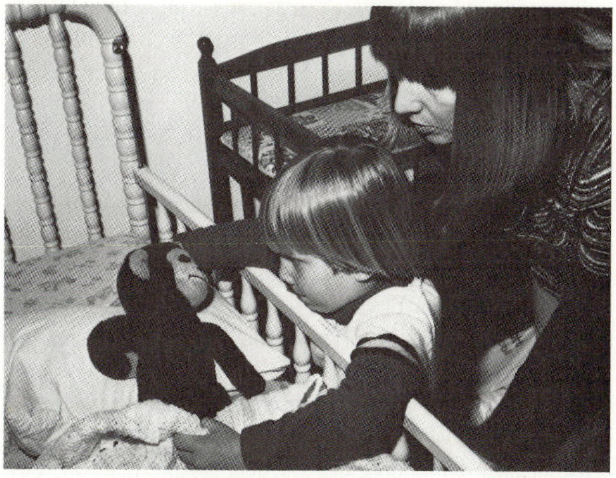

Stages of development of parental role

Stage 1: dependent behavior. During the 1- to 2-day

period after delivery, the mother's dependency needs predominate, and to the extent that these needs are met by others, the mother is able to divert her psychic energy to her child rather than to herself. She needs "mothering" in order to "mother." Rubin (1961) has aptly described these few days as the *taking-in-phase*—a time when nurturing and protective care are required by the new mother.

These mature and apparently healthy women appear to suspend involvement in everyday responsibilities and rely on others to respond to their needs for comfort, rest, nourishment, and closeness to their families and newborn.

Physical discomfort, arising from an episiotomy, sore nipples, hemorrhoids, aftercontractions, and occasionally a sprained coccygeal joint, can interfere with the mother's need for rest and relaxation. The judicious use of comfort measures and medication depends on the nurse. Many women hesitate to ask for medication, believing that any pain they experience is normal and to be expected; few have a knowledge of the use of heat or cold to relieve local pain.

Stage 1 is a time of great excitement, and most parents are extremely talkative. They need to verbalize all the happenings of pregnancy and their experience of birth to bring the pregnancy and birth into focus, analyze them, and accept them so that they can be put aside mentally and the parents can then move on to another phase. Some parents are able to use the staff or other mothers as an "audience"; others cannot, and for them, the opportunity to be with family or friends is imperative.

Since anxiety and preoccupation with her new role often narrow a mother's perceptual field, information may have to be repeated. The new mother may require reminders to rest or, conversely, to ambulate enough to promote recovery. Ward routine does not necessarily loom large in the new mother's order of priorities; showers are taken when the physicians are scheduled for examinations, and telephone conversations preclude "being ready" for the baby. Regulations seem cumbersome, and mothers and their families find it difficult at times to accept such rules when they interfere with their needs to share reactions about their child.

Stage 2: dependent ⇆ independent behavior. If the mother has received adequate nurturing in the first few days, by the third day her desire for independent action reasserts itself, and she responds enthusiastically to opportunities to learn and practice the care of the baby or, if she is an accomplished mother, to carry out or direct this care.

Professional care during this period of 4 or 5 weeks often is somewhat limited. The concept of the "naturalness of being a mother" deemphasizes the new parent's needs and problems. Regardless of the desire for a baby and the amount of prenatal preparation undertaken, the reality of parenthood has to be experienced to be understood fully on a personal level. One young mother expressed it as follows (Lang, 1972):

> But then in my second week, as my strength began to return, my energies began to focus on the overwhelming task of motherhood that stood before me. And I realized then that I faced that task alone. Not that my husband wouldn't stand by me, not that my friends would not share experiences with me, but I stood alone with the realization that only I could be the child's mother.

In this period the adjustments made to reality and the mastery of the tasks of parenthood are crucial for the subsequent functioning of the family as a unit. It has been found that those mothers who experience the most difficulty in adjusting are primiparas; women with careers; women who feel deeply the isolation of themselves with their babies and resent the endless coping with home responsibilities as well as those responsibilities associated with child care; women who miss the lack of outside stimulation, particularly if they are accustomed to a busy work environment; and women who lack friends or family members with whom to share delights and concerns. Unless some intervention is instituted, everyday problems may accumulate until a crisis situation develops.

Nursing must be aimed at increasing the mother's mastery of the "art of motherhood," thereby increasing or sustaining her self-esteem. These nursing interventions may be grouped under those pertaining to the crisis intervention theory, namely, perception, situational supports, and coping mechanisms (see Chapter 9).

Perception. One of the main concepts to be stressed repeatedly is that parenthood is a learned role. As any other learned role, it takes time to master, improves with experience, and evolves gradually and continually as the needs of the parents and child change.

The nurse's *teaching* should relate to the mother's prior knowledge and competence. For some mothers a simple review of points forgotten is all that is needed; others require detailed information, demonstrations done slowly and carefully to permit imitation, and supportive supervision. The need for repetitive teaching is to be expected if the mother's anxiety level distorts her ability to learn. As the mother's condition permits, she assumes more and more responsibility for her own hygienic care and the reporting of abnormalities in her progress. Therefore she will require careful explanation of what care is necessary and what symptoms would be considered abnormal (for women experiencing their first delivery, all symptoms are new and strange) and reportable.

Care of the newborn may be limited to feeding during the first few days. When the mother's strength returns, she may wish to bathe and change the infant also. Demonstrations of these techniques and supervision of her efforts are incorporated into the nursing care. Recognition of her successes and praise increase the mother's feeling of security in her ability to function.

Because of the sheltered environment provided after delivery, women may misjudge the actual amount of physical and psychic energy they possess. They may expect to resume tasks too soon and then feel discouraged when they are not able to do so. In addition, the baby's behavior does not always meet expectations. Sore nipples, worry about adequate milk supply, or even lack of sensations anticipated with breast feeding can lead to a mother's disappointment. Some babies cry more than expected or do not seem satisfied with their feedings. Many babies have fussy periods that do not respond to any ministrations (Lang, 1972):

> But my husband, too was disconcerted at first, for the intense, unending plaintive cries of our firstborn reached to the very depths of our hearts. And, we both had really believed that, somehow, a baby born naturally at home and never separated from its mother would not be so fretful. However, it becomes apparent that all babies cry.

Occasionally the mother becomes increasingly fatigued during the last month of pregnancy when sleep is interrupted by shortness of breath, urinary frequency, leg cramps, or inability to lie in a comfortable position. After delivery this fatigue is accentuated by the around-the-clock demands of the new baby.

Sibling rivalry may require parental time and attention to be handled successfully. Even if the children have participated in planning for the new baby, they may be unable to accept the reality of diminished parental attention; their behavior may reflect their feeling of frustration.

Forewarning about the possibility of such happenings even in the best-regulated homes permits the parents to judge themselves less harshly and to be better prepared to seek assistance, change routine, or accept the happening as a passing phase.

A young mother described such an experience to a nursing student on a postdelivery visit to the home:

> When you cautioned me that last day in the hospital about not getting involved with my clients too soon, I just didn't believe you. I felt so well and on top of things. But when we got home, everything seemed to fall to pieces. My episiotomy hurt dreadfully, and the baby never slept at night. I just had to phone and cancel out. If you hadn't said that, I would have figured I was a failure and I don't know what I would have done. Now everything is coming around.

Depressive states are not uncommon during this stage. Feelings of extreme vulnerability may arise from a number of factors. Psychologically the mother may be overwhelmed by the actuality of parental responsibilities, or she may feel deprived of the pregnant state, with its concomitant supportive care of family members and friends. Some mothers regret the loss of the mother-fetal relationship and mourn its passing. Still others experience a letdown feeling once labor and birth are complete. They had girded themselves for an elemental experience, a walk "through the shadows," and now it is safely over.

Once immediate tasks and adjustments have been undertaken and brought under control, a plateau is reached. At this time the lifelong effects of the parents' new responsibilities come into focus, and some parents experience a feeling of being trapped and of wondering what life is all about.

Such reactions are not necessarily expressed verbally, but the depressive state is signified by typical behaviors—withdrawal, loss of interest in surroundings, and crying.

Physiologically it has been suggested that a lowered level of circulating glucocorticoids or a condition of subclinical hypothyroidism may exist during the puerperium. This could explain some minor degrees of depression.

Whatever the cause, depressive reactions after delivery, often called "the baby blues," should not be dismissed lightly. Their prevalence has deprived many women of the support they need. Recognition of the state, helping the woman to verbalize her feelings, conveying warmth in touch and tone of voice, and setting up tasks she can accomplish easily and successfully are interventions that can help to counteract these feelings.

Situational supports. Because the U.S. culture has emphasized the instinctual components of motherhood, many parents hesitate to seek help from nurses, physicians, family, and friends. Gordon and Gordon (1960) found that long-term support by nurses or physicians was a positive factor in the ultimate adjustment of the family. Parents need to be encouraged to communicate openly with each other regarding their stresses. Relatives or friends can assist with housework and babysitting with older children and eventually the new baby. Being able to share experiences verbally with others who are interested and experienced also tends to reassure the new mother.

A mother, in discussing visits by the family to see the new baby, commented (Fig. 32.7):

> I want the family to come. You people praise him so and think he is the most wonderful baby. All my friends have their own babies and are too busy trying to get compliments for them to give us any. All babies need aunties and grandmothers!

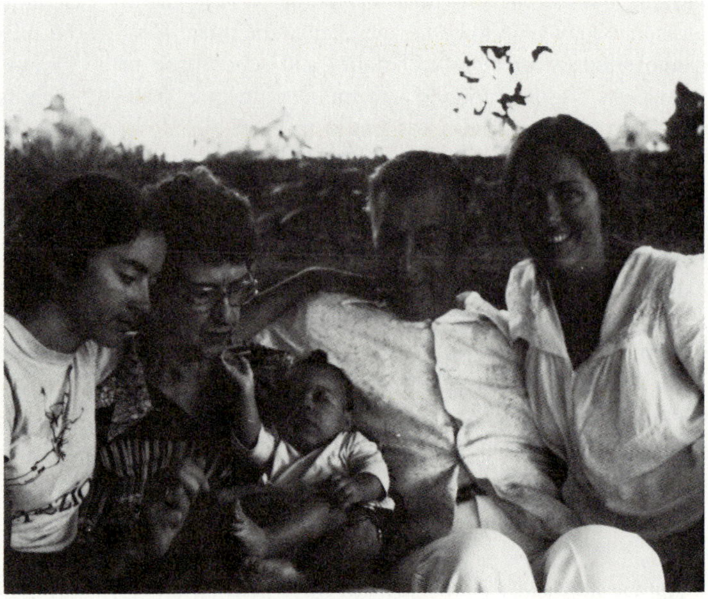

Fig. 32.7
Grandparents and an aunt provide reassurance to new mother as well as a caring group with whom to share experiences.

Being given information about the availability of health facilities and how to get in touch with the nurse or physician relieves new parents of feeling total responsibility for the health of the new baby. A physician reported one aspect of his plan for new mothers as follows:

> I make sure they have my phone number and ask them to call me day or night if they are worried. Since I've done this, the frantic calls have decreased to almost nothing. Knowing they can call seems to take the "steam" out of their concern. I feel it has worked both ways, for their benefit and mine.

Visits by nurses to the home may be spaced to take into account potential stress times, such as 2 or 3 days after coming home from the hospital and the third and sixth weeks at home. One woman, cared for throughout pregnancy and the postdelivery period by a nursing student, had anticipated a "kind of nervous breakdown." It did not materialize, and in the final visit with the student, she said, "You've been the best nerve medicine I've ever had."

The supportive care given at such times includes the entire family. Parents are as concerned with the ups and downs of other family members as they are with those of mother and child. The nurse may give supportive care by listening to (1) accounts of successes and failures, (2) individuals' feelings about the new baby, and (3) individuals' comments about what they expect of others (e.g., the new parents) in their new roles. One prime requisite is to set up a climate for the safe expression of doubts and anger, as well as happiness. The family will test the nurse's intent and knowledge, and she must recognize and accept this. The following dialogue is an example of this testing:

> Mother: I phoned the hospital and they said just what you said about the sitz bath.
>
> Nurse: Well, I'll give myself a star. [Both laughed.] Did it help any?

Coping mechanisms. In addition to new parents' learning the techniques for care of themselves and their babies, other suggestions have proved helpful to parents in coping with readjusting their lives. A list of these suggestions can be given to new parents, but discussion of specific ways of handling them is also necessary. Discussion with the parents should include the following points:

1. Set priorities for tasks. Many tasks can be left for a later period or done by others. Be adamant about not taking on extra tasks for family, friends, or community.
2. Do not become overconcerned with appearances—tidiness in the home is not as important as time spent with the family. Taking up the role of "super housekeeper" can be postponed until other adjustments are made; have others help with housework and cooking and leave yourself free to interact with your child.
3. Get plenty of rest and sleep; rearrange schedules if necessary. Since naps may not be possible if there are other children in the family, going to bed early is recommended; let friends know when to visit. Do not attempt to nurse another relative at this point; such responsibilities should be undertaken by other family members.

4. Try not to schedule a move to a new location soon after giving birth.

5. Arrange for some time away from the baby; enlist help of friends, family, or others for baby-sitting. Relaxation for both husband and wife is necessary.

6. Learn what health facilities are available and how to get in touch with the physician or nurse. If you have questions, remember the hospital is open all day and night, so you can call the emergency department.

7. Get out of the house at least once each day. Access to a car and being able to drive are assets, and taking the baby out for a walk or shopping breaks up the daily routine.

8. Be open in your communication with others. Share incidents of delight or of worry with others; give open indications of your needs for support and for sharing experiences.

It is to be hoped that toward the end of stage 2 the tasks and adjustments of daily routine will begin to follow a pattern. The new baby begins to take an established position in the family, and many of the feeding problems, whether related to breast feeding or bottle feeding, have been largely resolved. The mother's physical energy and strength return as the *taking-hold phase* (Rubin, 1961) is ending. By the fifth week the infant has been examined by the physician, and the mother has also been examined or has made arrangements for a checkup. The time for moving on to the next stage of adjustment has come.

Stage 3: interdependent behavior. In adjustment stage 3, interdependent behavior reasserts itself, and the family moves forward as a system with interacting members.

The relationship of husband and wife, although forever altered by the introduction of a child, resumes many of its former characteristics. A primary need is to establish a life-style that includes the child but is in some respects exclusive to him. Husband and wife must share interests and activities that are adult in scope. This time is often one of stress for the parental pair. Career patterns of men in their 20s and 30s show intensive activity centering around advancement in their profession or job. This often necessitates long hours away from the home or moving from one locality to another. Meanwhile, some women are engrossed in home activities directed toward the care of the young children, while others are attempting to combine the care of young children with careers. Interests and needs diverge, and there may be a gradual estrangement, which is glossed over for the time being because of the individual needs of each. A special effort must be undertaken to strengthen the adult-adult relationship as a basis for the family unit.

Most couples resume intercourse by the third or fourth week after the child is born, and some begin earlier, as soon as this can be accomplished without discomfort for the wife. This increases the man-woman aspect of the family, and the adult pair shares a closeness denied to the other family members. The resumption of marital relationships seems to bring the parents' relationship back into focus.

Many new fathers speak of the alienation experienced when they observe the intimate mother-child relationship, and some are frank in expressing feelings of jealousy toward the interloper. One father seemed anxious to talk about "this weird dream I had about a month ago" (the baby was 4 weeks old):

> I dreamed that we had a son and he was older already. Then I was preparing for a big wedding and I knew who was getting married . . . my son was marrying [my wife]. All the people came and congratulated me and everyone was happy. Then I was running around trying to find my son and [my wife] after the wedding because I realized that I would never see them again. This dream really frightened me. I was very upset for about 3 days afterwards.

As soon as intercourse is resumed, the possibility of pregnancy arises since in some women, ovulation and impregnation may occur as early as the sixth or seventh postdelivery week. Ovulation is delayed in women who are breast feeding, but this delay is not considered a phase of infertility, and pregnancy can occur. Planning for such a possibility is necessary before resumption of intercourse.

Baby-sitting, if at all possible, must be planned and a regular schedule developed. This includes time off for the mother during the day so that she can get away from the home and its responsibilities. In some localities church or other agencies have developed programs attuned to the needs of mothers. The young children are cared for while the mothers take part in activities with other mothers. This serves to help them establish relationships with others who are also involved in the care of young children. A mutual sharing of successes and failures in this regard helps the new mother maintain a feeling of equilibrium.

Most women are physically able to return to work by the end of the sixth week. If a woman plans to return to work, certain adjustments for child care must be made. Ideally a substitute parent would be one who could come to the home and provide love, as well as care, for the child. Some parents are fortunate enough to have grandparents or other relatives to fill such a role. Others must take the child to another person's home or a day-care center early in the morning and pick the child up at night. The care provided by day-care centers is needed by some children whose mothers must work to help support them or who are the sole support of the child. For those families who require this type of service, assistance in locating such help can be obtained from the local health department. Unfortunately there are not enough quality places for all children requiring day care.

Ideally parents make plans for care before the birth of the baby; however, if plans have not been made, medical personnel should be cognizant of the sources of assistance on a local level, and they must make sure that parents are aware of them also. There are many health services available to parents in most communities (e.g., well-baby centers and immunization clinics).

SIBLINGS

The baby's relationships with siblings take on more permanence as he assumes his position in the sibling hierarchy (Fig. 32.8). Many parents show ingenuity in

Fig. 32.8
A, First meeting of brother and sister. Brother seems overwhelmed: sucks thumb for comfort and withdraws from contact. **B,** First tentative touch—testing with fingertip. **C,** Relationship more secure—it is now okay to hold with whole hand. **D,** "Oh, she's holding my finger." (Courtesy Marjorie Pyle, Life Cycle, Costa Mesa, Calif.)

A B C D

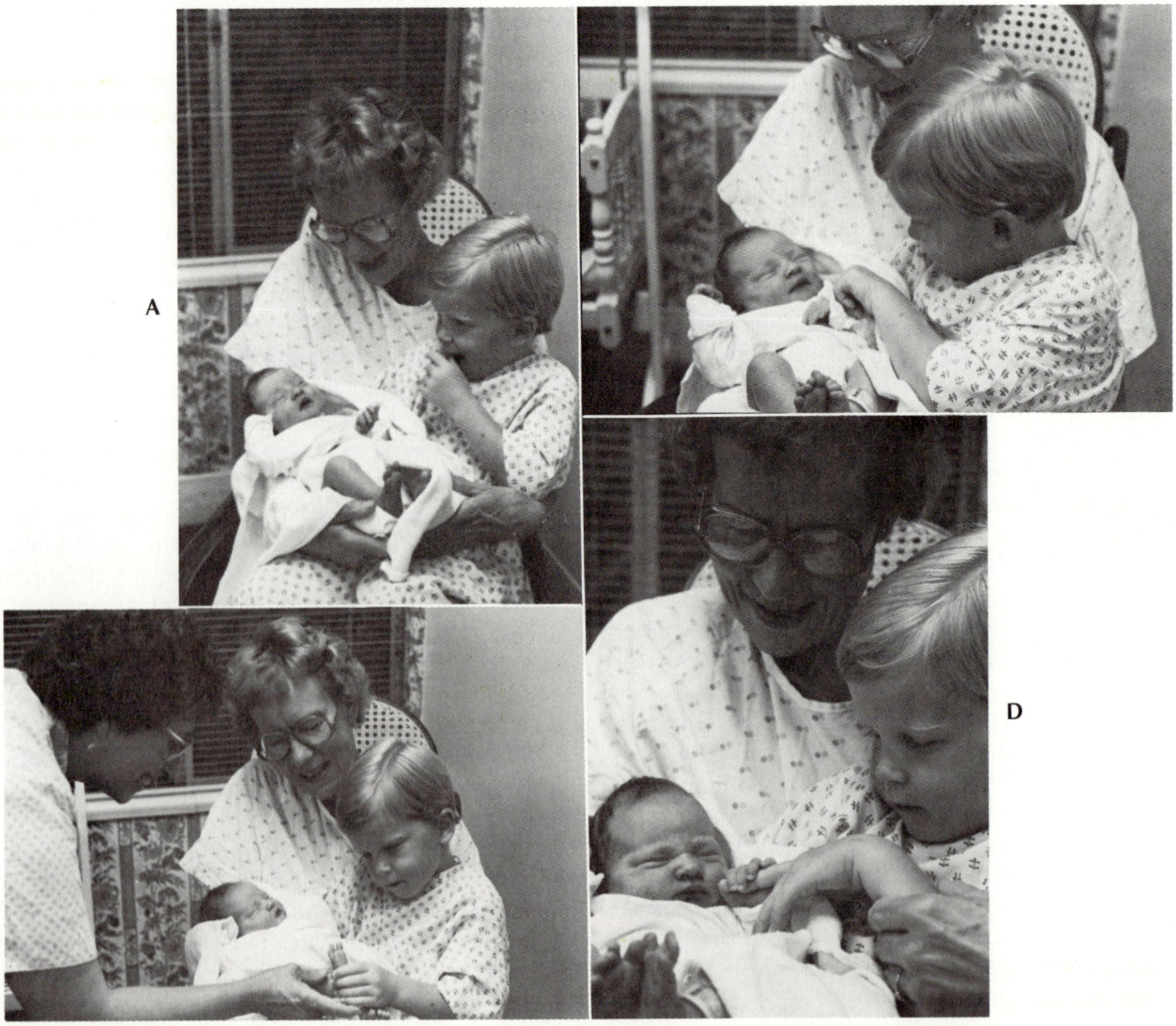

introducing the baby to brothers and sisters. Jealous reactions are to be expected once the initial excitement of having a new baby in the home is over, since the baby absorbs the time and attention of the significant persons in the other children's lives. The new parent can learn many innovative techniques by listening to other parents describe their efforts to ease the older siblings' acceptance of the new child.

Regression to an infantile level of behavior may be seen in the other children. Some will revert to bed-wetting, whining, or refusal to feed themselves. Much patience is required of parents to weather this phase. Lynch (1982) found in her study of second-time mothers that stress was caused not so much by regression of the older child but by a *difference* in the older child's behavior. The original mother-child relationship had changed, and this was seen as a reflection on the woman's mothering abilities. The mothers felt (self-concept) "they were not capable enough to mother two children."

The most consistent stressor for mothers, however, was the interval between the births, or the age of the older child. Children under 2 years, while moving toward independence, were still very dependent on the mother. The mother was the important person in the child's life, and competition for the attention of this individual was difficult for the toddler to handle. If the older child was 6 years or older, the mother's stress was less related to the older child's behavior than to her own reactions to the confinement caused by the care of the new baby. In this study children 4 to 6 years of age when a sibling was born apparently caused the least stress.

Plans must be undertaken to divert aggressive behavior directed toward the baby. A special time may be set aside for giving additional attention to older children when the baby is sleeping. For example, fathers can spend more time with older siblings and then can be attentive to the baby when older children are in bed at night.

Both girls and boys seem to enjoy helping in the care of the baby or a substitute baby (doll) (Fig. 32.9). Many parents relate difficulties with siblings when they are devoting attention to feeding the infant, either by breast or bottle. The other children seem to sense the closeness of the mother and child in this act and resent it. To counter these reactions some mothers have let the older children drink from a bottle or breast too. The tediousness and effort needed to obtain milk or fruit juice by this method often rapidly discourage them. One mother reported that her young son routinely "breast fed" his doll while she was breast feeding the new baby. They had conversations at this time, and she believed that by sharing this experience he seemed to take pride in his adult behavior of drinking from a cup.

Another difficulty arises when well-meaning relatives or friends concentrate on the new baby to the exclusion of the older children. Thoughtful adults often bring gifts to the older children and shower attention on them as well as paying attention to the baby.

To expect a young child to accept automatically and love a rival for parents' affection is assuming a too-mature response. Sibling love grows as does other love, that is, by being with another person and sharing experiences.

Fig. 32.9
Child enjoys caring for a substitute baby while mother is busy with his new baby sister.

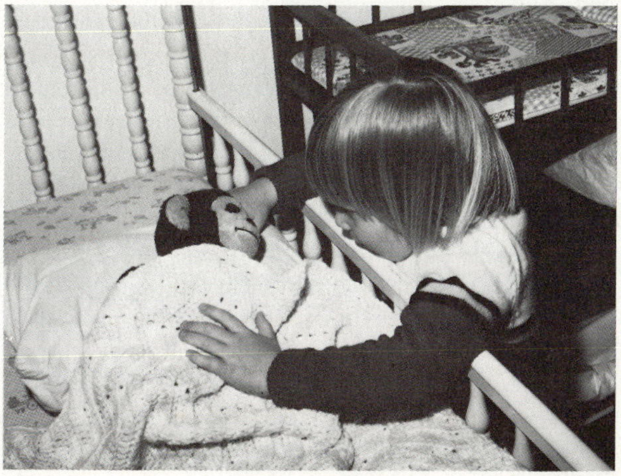

GRANDPARENTS

The amount of involvement of grandparents in the care of the child depends on many factors, for example, willingness of the grandparents to become involved, proximity of the grandparents, and ethnic and cultural expectations of the role grandparents play (Fig. 32-10) (Grosso, 1981). See also p. 355 for preparation for grandparenthood.

FACTORS INFLUENCING PARENTAL RESPONSES

Physical condition of mother. Women who have experienced long and difficult labors often are too exhausted to respond other than in a perfunctory way to the newborn. They may welcome the attention of others

Fig. 32.10
Grandparents can be a great help. **A,** Meeting new grandchild for the first time. **B,** Beaming grandfather.

A

B

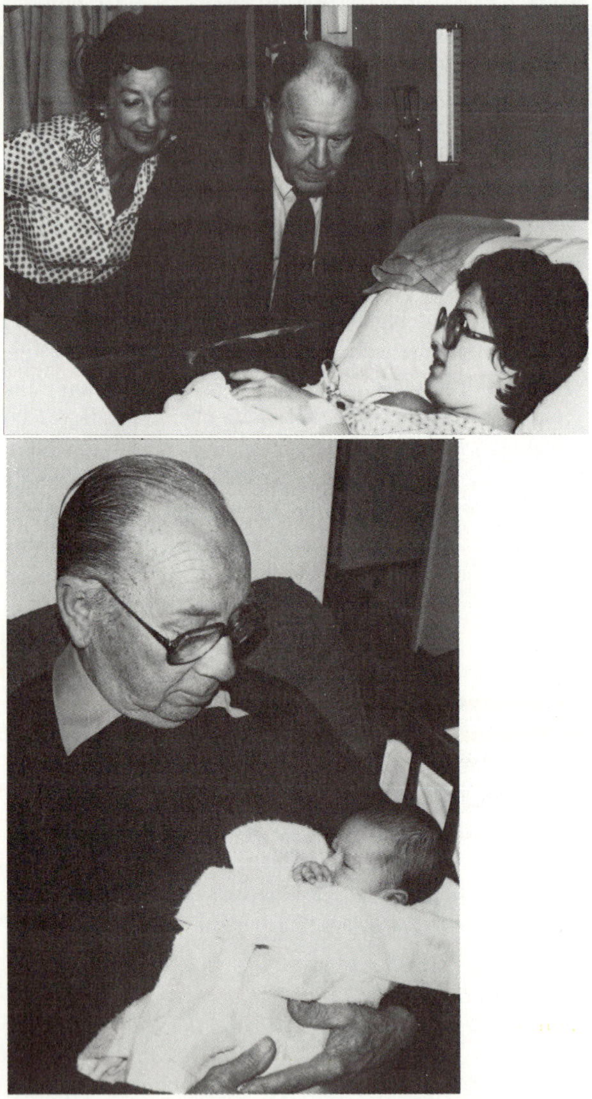

and be grateful that the infant is healthy, but their primary need centers on recovery from a physical and emotional ordeal.

Physical condition of infant. Those infants born at risk as a result of either fetal or maternal disabilities usually are transferred to the intensive care nursery as quickly as possible. Concerns for their need for intensive medical and nursing care supersede concerns about providing close contact between the infant and the mother or father. Opportunities to be with the infant in the intensive care nursery, to touch or hold him if at all possible, and to receive reports of the infant's progress must be part of the nursing plan.

Parental expectations. Some parents are startled by the appearance of the infant—size, color, molding of the head, or bowed appearance of the legs (see Chapter 27). Many parents have never seen or had contact with a newborn infant and find themselves disturbed by their feelings. Mothers and fathers may interpret the physical characteristics normal in all newborns as physical or mental deficiencies. Many fathers have commented that they thought the odd shape of the child's head (molding) meant the child would be mentally retarded (see Chapter 27).

Disappointment over the sex of the infant can take time to resolve. The mother or father may be able to give adequate physical mothering but may find it difficult to be sincerely involved with the infant until these feelings have been resolved. As one mother remarked:

> I really wanted a boy. I know it is silly and irrational, but when they said, ''She's a lovely little girl,'' I was so disappointed and angry—yes, angry—I could hardly look at her. Oh, I looked after her okay, her feedings and baths and things, but I couldn't feel excited. To tell the truth, I felt like a monster not liking my child. Then one day she was lying there and she turned her head and looked right at me. I felt a flooding of love for her come over me, and we looked at each other a long time. It's okay now. I wouldn't change her for all the boys in the world.

Nursing care plans need to include time for explanations about the child's appearance and opportunities for parents to discuss their lack of motherly feelings freely and without fear of censure or ridicule. Often the expression of doubts and concerns provides relief and makes it easier for parents to accept help with such feelings.

Parental age. Maternal age has a definite effect on pregnancy outcome. The fetus and the mother are at highest risk when the mother is at either extreme of age and parity although each age group has predominant problems (Table 32.1). The following discussion relates to the older client (over 30 years). Adolescent clients, both mother and father, are discussed in Chapter 38.

Parenthood after 30 years. There are two groups of older parents now discernible in the population of women having a child late in their childbearing years. One group is made up of multiparous women who have many children or who have a child during the menopausal period. The other group of older parents includes relative newcomers to maternity care. These are the persons who have deliberately delayed childbearing into their late 20s or early 30s.

1. *The first group* may have never used contracep-

Table 32.1
Age-related Pregnancy Problems

Age	Maternal	Fetal
Less than 20 yr		
Physical Emotional Development often incomplete	Nutritional deficiencies Hyperemesis gravidarum Chorea gravidarum Preeclampsia-eclampsia Fetopelvic dystocia Diabetes mellitus, class C or D Chronic nephritis	Highest incidence of growth retardation immature-premature birth Highest incidence of perinatal morbidity and mortality
20-30 yr		
Ideal period for conception Few serious problems	Diabetes mellitus, class B	Lowest perinatal morbidity and mortality
30-40 yr		
"Elderly" primipara, over 35 yr Age of appearance of many serious medical problems	Infertility Iron deficiency anemia Diabetes mellitus, class E Isoimmunization Ectopic pregnancy Placenta previa	Low–birth weight neonates after excessive smoking or excessive alcohol use Dizygous twins
40-50 yr		
Middle-age complications evident	Infertility (anovulation) Cardiovascular and other medical-surgical disorders Diabetes mellitus, class F Uterine or ovarian neoplasms Premature separation of placenta Rupture of uterus Postdelivery hemorrhage	High perinatal mobidity and mortality Increased frequency of Down's syndrome and other congenital anomalies (e.g., hydrocephalus, trisomy, Kleinfelter's syndrome)

tives either because of personal choice or lack of knowledge concerning contraceptives. Others may have used contraception successfully during the childbearing years. As menopause approaches they may cease to menstruate regularly, stop using contraception, and consequently become pregnant. Even after menstruation ceases, ovulation may continue for up to 1 year. Therefore contraceptive techniques must be continued for this time. Hogan (1979) relates the response of the older woman to pregnancy. She notes the displaced feeling the older woman experiences as pregnancy alienates her from her peer group and her age interferes with close associations with young mothers. Because the incidence of complicating conditions, such as hypertension, preeclampsia-eclampsia, and hemorrhage, increases in the mother of 40 years of age or older, many women do not see the pregnancy and childbirth as natural phenomena. Fortunately for some, anxiety concerning giving birth to an infant with a defect can be allayed through amniotic fluid analysis or ultrasonography (see Chapter 17). For mothers who learn they are carrying a fetus with a defect, abortion is an option. The percentage of older mothers who choose to terminate the pregnancy by abortion is relatively high. Many had assumed they would never have to make such a choice and report depression.

It is important to include the family in preparation for the birth. Because the other children in the family may be teenagers, women often welcome the professional's support and suggestions concerning how to best involve them. Measures designed to assist in regaining strength and muscle tone are stressed, for example, prenatal and postdelivery exercises. Some older mothers may find that the care of the new infant exhausts their physical capabilities, and if economic and social conditions are also adverse, neglect of the child can result. For others the unexpected infant is welcomed as evidence of a maternal (and paternal!) role still to be played, and because older siblings often assume aspects of the parental role, the child develops in a multiparent household.

2. *The second group* choose parenthood as opposed to the alternative, a child-free life-style. They often are

successfully established in a career and a life-style with a partner that includes time for self-attention, establishment of a home with accumulated possessions, and freedom for travel. Parents-to-be who belong to this emerging group are faced with having to resolve an important choice at a life stage when childbearing has increasing physical, psychologic, and social risks. The dilemma of choice includes recognition that being a parent will have both positive and negative consequences. Couples need to discuss the consequences of childbearing and child rearing before committing themselves to a lifelong venture. With this group there appears to be a sharing of preparation for parenthood, of planning for a family-centered birth, and of a desire to be a loving and competent parent. The reality of child care may prove difficult for these parents. The mother who is accustomed to the stimulation of and contact with other adults may find the isolation with her infant difficult to accept, and anger and resentment toward the father (or infant) can result. In the early infancy period, this group needs careful follow-up and supportive care, including opportunities to discuss alternative parenting approaches.* The nurse needs to be aware of community resources developed to meet the needs of this group. For example, *Parenthood after Thirty* is a project sponsored by the Foundation for Comprehensive Health Services and funded by grant no. 80-63575 from the Office of Family Planning, State of California Department of Health Services.

Social and economic conditions. Parents whose economic condition is made worse with the birth of each child and who are unable to use an acceptable method of family planning may find childbirth compounded by concern for their own health and a sense of helplessness. Mothers who are alone, deserted by husband, family, and friends, or who are in an untenable economic state may view the birth of the child with dread. The difficulties in which they find themselves may overcome any desire for mothering the infant.

Nursing measures designed to help such persons are directed toward involvement of social and economic community agencies as well as health agencies. Such problems often require long-term commitments from both the woman or couple and the community to effect satisfactory outcomes. Adequate situational supports need to be instituted in the prenatal period.

Interference with personal aspirations. The resentment some women feel toward parenthood (that it interferes with or curtails their plans for personal freedom or advancement in their career) may not have been resolved during the prenatal period. If this resentment is not resolved, it will spill over into care-taking activities and may result in indifference and neglect or, conversely, oversolicitousness and the setting of impossibly high standards by the mother for her behavior or the child's performance (Shainess, 1970).

Nursing intervention needs to include opportunities for parents (1) to vent their feelings freely to an objective listener; (2) to discuss measures to permit personal growth of the parent, for example, by part-time employment, volunteer work, and utilization of agencies that provide baby-sitting care or mother substitutes during parental vacations; and (3) to learn about care of the child.

Sensory Impairment. In the early dialogue between parent and child, all senses—sight, hearing, touch, taste, and smell—are used by both to initiate and sustain the attachment process. If a parent is deprived of one of those, for example, sight or hearing, an enriched use of the remaining sensory sources needs to develop.

Blindness. Although mothers who are blind will need the presence as well as the support of another responsible person, they can become adept in some of the child care activities, as the following report indicates:

> We had always planned to have a child. My family and Dick's both wanted us to have the happiness of children and were willing to help us with the baby care. First I bathed and changed a doll; then I practiced caring for my sister's baby. I would feel in all the creases with my finger to see they were clean and dry. We used Pampers that did not need pins. My mother made baby clothes with fastenings of press cloth so I would not have to fiddle with buttons. I feel really confident now. I know I can't do everything for her, but I can do enough to feel like a "mother" and I know she will have all the love she needs.

One of the major difficulties blind mothers experience is the skepticism, overt or covert, of the professional worker. Blind persons sense a reluctance on the part of others to concede that they have a right to be parents. One blind mother-to-be noted that the best approach by the nurse was to assess the mother's capabilities and her ideas of how to remedy gaps in knowledge and skills and from that basis to make plans to assist the woman (i.e., the same as for a sighted mother). Another mother talked about the shyness, fear, or reluctance she sensed in the nurse that resulted in being left alone or being involved in awkward conversations:

> I took it upon myself to put the nurses at ease. I was forthright about my condition and asked for specific help and supervision of my baby care efforts. Don't forget, I've had some 25 years' experience in dealing with the sighted public. I have considerable skill now in being blind.

Another mother expressed how sensitive the blind can become to other sensory input. She remarked that

*For further information contact Parenthood after Thirty, 451 Vermont, Berkeley, Calif. 94707, (415) 524-6635 (Lucy Scott, Ph.D., Project Director).

she could tell when her infant was facing her because she could feel his breath on her face.

Eye-to-eye contact is obviously missing from the blind parent–infant interaction. However, since the mother has no experience in using this strategy to promote relationships, she cannot be said to miss it. The infant will need other sensory input from the blind mother. It may be that the infant is not conscious that the eyes he looks into cannot see him. Other persons in the newborn's environment can participate in active eye-to-eye contact to supply this lack. Another possible problem may arise if the blind parent has an impassive facial expression. One observer noted an infant's making repeated attempts to engage his blind mother in face play. With repeated failure of his efforts he abandoned the behavior with his mother but intensified it with his father. This problem could be overcome by the blind person's learning to accompany talking and cooing to the infant with head nodding and smiling.

Deafness. The mother who has a hearing impairment faces another set of problems, particularly if the deafness dates from birth or early childhood. She and her partner are more likely to have established an independent household. There are a number of devices now on the market that transform sound into light flashes. The infant's room can be fitted with such a device so that crying can be readily detected. The vocalizing of the parent, even if he or she is not speech trained, can serve as both stimulus and response to the infant's early vocalizing. Parents can provide additional vocal training by use of records and television so that the child is aware from birth onward of the full range of the human voice. Sign language is acquired readily by the young child, and the first sign used is as varied as the first word. One mother reported her child first signed "good boy," and another reported "candy" as her child's first effort.

Section 504 of the Rehabilitation Act of 1973 requires that hospitals and other institutions receiving funds from the U.S. Department of Health, Education, and Welfare use varying communication techniques with the deaf, including staff who are proficient in sign language. The nurse who is bilingual is at an advantage in providing care for clients. Magelvy and co-workers (1979) point out that sign language is as complex as any spoken language and that deaf persons are linguistically and cognitively competent.

• • •

Much more research in the areas of sensory impairment and the parent-child attachment process should be undertaken.*

*We welcome information in this area. Address correspondence to I.M. Bobak, Department of Nursing, San Francisco State University, 1600 Holloway Ave., San Francisco, CA 94132.

Part 2: Nursing Care

ASSESSMENT OF PARENTAL RESPONSES

The quality of *motherliness* in the parent prompts nurturing, as opposed to neglect of the child, and protection, as opposed to abuse of the child. Cues indicating the presence or absence of this quality in parental behavior appear early in the postdelivery period as the parent reacts to the newborn child and then begins the process of establishing a relationship. Its presence is manifested by behavior indicative of the parent's realistic perception and acceptance of the infant's needs, limited abilities, immature social responses, and helplessness (Steele and Pollack, 1968). According to Morris (1966):

> Mother-infant unity can be said to be satisfactory when a mother can find pleasure in her infant and in the tasks for and with him; understand his emotional states and comfort him; read his cues for new experience and sense his fatigue points.

Those parents who are deficient in the quality of motherliness exhibit behavior that demonstrates their inability to respond appropriately to the needs of their infants. They expect responses from the infant far in excess of his ability to perform, and they interpret his inadequate responses as defiance or as negative judgment of parental capabilities. They obtain no pleasure from physical contact with their child, handle him roughly, let his head dangle without support, and do not cuddle him. The infant is seen as unattractive, and the tasks of bathing and changing the child are done with disgust or annoyance. There is a lack of discrimination in responding to the infant's signals relative to hunger, fatigue, need for soothing or stimulating speech, and need for comforting body or eye contact. These parents often show excessive concern over the health of their child and cannot distinguish between the expected minor illnesses of childhood and serious disabilities. It appears difficult for them to accept their child as healthy and happy (Morris, 1966).

Other typical behaviors have been described as the *claiming process*. The mother enfolds the child physically in her arms, points out characteristics that the child shares with other family members, and indicates recognition of a relationship between them by commenting on the infant's responses to her as a parent, as illustrated by the following: "Russ held him close and said, 'He's the image of his father,' but I found one part like me—his toes are shaped like mine. Look, he's smiling; he likes his mother's jokes."

On the other hand, some mothers react negatively. The infant is claimed, but this claiming is in terms of the discomfort or pain he caused his mother, and the infant's normal responses are interpreted as being derogatory to the mother. The mother reacts to her child with dislike or indifference. The child is not held close or touched in such a way as to comfort him; for example, "The nurse put the baby into Marie's arms. She promptly laid him across her knees and glanced up at the television. 'Stay still 'till I finish watching—you've been enough trouble already.' "

Many new mothers will experience *parenting difficulties* until their skills become established. Once they feel confidence in their skills, the increase in self-esteem promotes a positive affective response to the child. However, some parents will exhibit *parenting disorders* (a matter of degree) that place the child in jeopardy and at risk.

Although protocols for the physical screening of high-risk mothers and infants have been carefully developed and confirmed (see Chapter 16), tools predicting high-risk parenting behaviors are still relatively imprecise. Caretakers need to be alert to parents who have positive family circumstances, as opposed to those who exhibit warning signs during the postdelivery period. In terms of *disorders in parenting* the crucial event that seems to tip the scales toward neglect or abuse is an *abnormal pregnancy* or the *birth of an infant who is ill or premature*.

Assessment strategies. Nurses use numerous strategies for assessing parent-child relationships, for example, interviewing, observing, and listening. The nurse can select times such as feeding periods or when the mother or father is giving general care to the infant. These times present opportunities for assessing parental attachment behaviors as well as the mother's attitude toward herself and her new responsibility, her competency in child care, and the need for teaching or other support. The father's (family's) commitment to child care can also be noted as indications of motherliness or fatherliness, that quality that enriches and makes human the care activities.

During the *initiating phase* of the parent-child interaction the nurse may note behaviors such as the following:

1. Parental contact with the infant includes the following:
   a. Enfolding, massaging, and exploring with fingertips
   b. Scrutinizing infant's body carefully, noting variations in what parents deem normal and looking for reassurance
   c. Seeking eye contact
   d. Talking to the child
2. Parents' level of competence in handling and holding their child reflects their previous experience and level of anxiety.
3. Parents respond to the infant's eating, going to sleep, stopping crying, and so on with a lessening of tension and increased relaxation.
4. Parents' personal manner of reacting to emotional excitement (e.g., they may cry, laugh, talk, or remain silent) reflects interaction with their child.

As parents become more familiar with their child (the *phase of consolidation*) other behaviors become noticeable. The nurse can ask herself the following questions:

1. Do the parents seem to enjoy handling and touching, stroking and patting infant, or do they minimize any body contact? Is their touch gentle or rough? personal or impersonal?
2. Although it is difficult to assess modes of address used by parents to their infants, do parents' tones of voice indicate acceptance or rejection of the infant?
3. Do parents seek and maintain eye contact? Do they stare fixedly into infant's eyes?
4. Are they able to overcome a natural reluctance to handle excrement of infant?
5. Do they have rigid plans for infant routines and expectations of infant's fitting into these plans?

Later during the *phase of growth* in the parental role the nurse can assess parental behaviors during postdelivery visits to home, or during the 4-wk checkup of the infant at the pediatrician's office or well-baby clinic. The nurse's assessment would include such observations as the following:

1. How is child held by mother (or father)? Are parent's hand grasp and touch gentle? Does parent look at child's face or at examiner? Does parent participate in restraining and comforting child? Is parent overly concerned about child's health? Is child isolated except for necessary care-taking activities?
2. Does the physical examination show a healthy, developing child or evidence of neglect or abuse?
3. How is the mother handling her responsibilities, that is, how does the mother manage the child's crying, household chores, repetitive nature of child care, and inability to get unbroken rest? Does she feel isolated? Is she keeping up with her career?
4. Do the parents have knowledge of responses of the child (e.g., appetite, bowel movements, voiding, rashes)?
5. What coping mechanisms are being used (e.g., does mother get away from home responsibilities occasionally)? Do other family members help? Is there someone she can talk to? Can she express her feelings about her new responsibilities freely? Does she only allow expression of idealized mothering feelings?

In the postdelivery period three characteristics that

act as indicators of the quality of parenting have been documented: (1) the mother's degree of acceptance of her infant, (2) the mother's speed of response to her infant's needs, and (3) the quality and amount of verbal stimulation (Funke-Farber, 1978). The latter indicator is the best discriminator. It would seem from the examination of these three indicators that the maladaptive mothers may have been less able to identify their infant as independent and separate from themselves but requiring much nurturance than the adaptive mothers. The adaptive mothers were able to view their infants as independent, separate love objects and were therefore able to interact more positively with them.

Assessment tools. Stainton (1981) has devised scoring tools for assessing parent-child responses for use in the postpartum period (see box). The tools reflect the change in the mother's and father's responses as they move from first contact after delivery through the early puerperium. Days 4 and 5 were included because some mothers may remain in the hospital longer than the usual 2 or 3 days. The nurse may see the parents at 2 weeks, 4 weeks, or 6 weeks postpartum depending on hospital protocol.

The tools are concise enough for easy application and assess behaviors, similar to those noted above, that can prompt vigilance as to evidence of adaptation or maladaptation to the parental role. The information gained can be used to formulate nursing disagnoses.

If cues indicate the possibility of parenting disorders, development of extra support programs needs to be forthcoming.

Nursing care during the period of adaptation to the parental role is based on assessments such as the foregoing, as well as assessment of the mother's perceptual

Text continued on p. 729.

Parent Baby Interaction

Day one

Circle "M" and "F" for the best description in each of the five behavioral categories, to achieve a total score for Mother and Father.

Two (2) points		**One (1) point**		**Zero (0) points**	
Asks questions about baby's appearance and behavior, e.g., tries to relate baby's to familial characteristics	M F	Comments about baby's appearance and behavior	M F	Does not comment about baby's appearance or behavior	M F
Uses whole hand when touching baby's skin	M F	Uses fingertips when touching baby's skin	M F	Does not touch baby's skin	M F
Spontaneously speaks to baby using affectionate terms and/or tones	M F	Speaks to baby when prompted to do so	M F	Does not speak to baby	M F
Holds baby in "en face" position, maintaining eye contact	M F	Holds, baby close to body but makes little or no eye contact	M F	Holds baby away from her own body, with little or no eye contact	M F
Expresses feelings about the labor and delivery experience	M F	With assistance, vaguely discusses or describes the labor	M F	With assistance, reluctant to discuss the labor and delivery experience	M F

Mother's total score __

Father's total score __

8-10 requires *usual* nursing support for bonding
5-7 requires *extra* nursing support for bonding
0-4 requires *intensive* nursing support for bonding

Other observations ____________________

Day one (revised)

____
Signature

From Stainton, C.M.: Parent-infant interaction: putting theory into practice, Calgary, Alta., Canada, 1981, The University of Calgary Faculty of Nursing.

Day two

Two (2) points		One (1) point		Zero (0) points	
Seeks contact with baby	**M** **F**	Accepts contact with baby	**M** **F**	Avoids contact with baby	**M** **F**
With assistance, explores baby's whole skin surface, using both hands and arms	**M** **F**	Explores baby's body, avoiding some areas, e.g., genital area, back	**M** **F**	Avoids touching baby's skin	**M** **F**
Asks for interpretation of baby's appearance and behavior	**M** **F**	Interested when baby's appearance or behavior is interpreted but does not ask questions	**M** **F**	Shows little interest in the baby's appearance or behavior	**M** **F**
Consistently positions baby in "en face" position and seeks eye contact with baby	**M** **F**	Positions baby in "en face" position and makes intermittent eye contact	**M** **F**	Does not hold baby in "en face" position	**M** **F**
Describes feelings about infant and his responses	**M** **F**	Needs assistance in describing feelings about infant and his responses	**M** **F**	Does not express feelings about infant or his responses	**M** **F**

Mother's total score ___

Father's total score ___

8-10 requires *usual* nursing support for bonding
5-7 requires *extra* nursing support for bonding
0-4 requires *intensive* nursing support for bonding

Other observations ____________________

____

____

Day two (revised)

____
Signature

Day three

Two (2) points		One (1) point		Zero (0) points	
Holds baby close to body when feeding or cuddling, using both hands and arms	**M** **F**	Holds baby with a space between own and baby's body	**M** **F**	Unable, reluctant, or refusing to hold baby	**M** **F**
Spontaneously talks to baby, using name, son, or endearing terms and/or tones	**M** **F**	Speaks about baby but does not speak directly to baby	**M** **F**	Does not speak to baby	**M** **F**
Consistently positions baby in "en face" position and maintains eye contact	**M** **F**	Positions baby in "en face" position and makes intermittent eye contact	**M** **F**	Does not make eye contact with baby	**M** **F**
Describes some infant's characteristics to listener; i.e., "he's strong"	**M** **F**	Responds with interest when infant's characteristics are pointed out	**M** **F**	Does not express any interest in infant characteristics	**M** **F**
Seeks opportunities to carry out care taking of baby	**M** **F**	Needs prompting with all care taking of baby	**M** **F**	Unable, reluctant, or refusing to care for infant	**M** **F**

Mother's total score ___

Father's total score ___

8-10 requires *usual* nursing support for bonding
5-7 requires *extra* nursing support for bonding
0-4 requires *intensive* nursing support for bonding

Other observations ____________________

____

____

Day three (revised)

____
Signature

Day four

Two (2) points		One (1) point		Zero (0) points	
Engages infant's attention with voice and touch	M F	Uses voice and touch to engage infant when prompted	M F	Does not use voice or touch to engage infant	M F
Smiles, talks to, and kisses infant when holding or "en face"	M F	"En face" position maintained with intermittent or brief smiling	M F	Does not smile at baby	M F
Seeks clarification of the meaning of infant's behavior; i.e., "is he hungry?"	M F	Consistently needs infant's behavior interpreted	M F	Does not comment on infant's behavior	M F
Carries out care-taking activities with minimal anxiety or need for prompting	M F	Carries out care-taking activities with support of nurse	M F	Does not care for infant	M F
Requests information about infant's behavior, or needs anticipated after discharge	M F	Accepts information about ongoing infant's needs without comment or question	M F	Appears uninterested in future needs of infant	M F

Mother's total score __

Father's total score __

8-10 requires *usual* nursing support for bonding
5-7 requires *extra* nursing support for bonding
0-4 requires *intensive* nursing support for bonding

Other observations ____________________

Day four (revised)

Signature ____________________

Day five

Two (2) points		One (1) point		Zero (0) points	
Attempts to soothe infant with voice and touch	M F	Attempts to soothe infant by voice or touch	M F	Does not try to soothe infant	M F
Moves toward infant immediately when infant cries	M F	Interval of more than 30 seconds between infant's onset of crying and moving toward infant	M F	Interval of more than 1 minute between infant's onset of crying and moving toward infant	M F
Begins to interpret meaning of infant's behavior	M F	Seeks clarification of meaning of infant's behavior	M F	Does not comment on infant's behavior	M F
Seeks to elicit infant response when talking to infant	M F	Expresses wish to elicit infant response	M F	Does not attempt to elicit infant response	M F
Carries out care taking without prompting	M F	Carries out care taking only with prompting	M F	Does not carry out care taking	M F

Mother's total score __

Father's total score __

8-10 requires *usual* nursing support for bonding
5-7 requires *extra* nursing support for bonding
0-4 requires *intensive* nursing support for bonding

Other observations ____________________

Day five (revised)

Signature ____________________

Second week

Three (3) points		Two (2) points		One (1) point	
Maintains "en face" position and eye contact with infant unless speaking to observer	M F	Does not maintain "en face" position or eye contact for more than 15 seconds	M F	Unable or does not seek "en face" position or eye contact with infant	M F
Spontaneously touches infant—strokes skin with whole hand, caresses infant	M F	Touches infant with brief contact in response to infant's needs	M F	Unable or does not touch infant	M F
Stimulates infant to respond and can describe response expected	M F	When pompted, will attempt to elicit a response from infant	M F	Unable or does not seek infant response	M F
Describes care-taking activities, identifying specific questions or concerns about infant's needs	M F	Comments on care-taking activities anxiously; unable to specifically identify concern about infant's needs	M F	Comments on care-taking activities in relation to self only	M F
Expresses feelings about role of Mother/Father in positive or hopeful terms or tones	M F	Expresses feelings mainly in terms of own needs, acknowledging infant's needs	M F	Expresses negative feelings about parent role and/or infant	M F

Mother's total score ___

Father's total score ___

11-15 requires *usual* nursing support for bonding
6-10 requires *extra* nursing support for bonding
0-5 required *intensive* nursing support for bonding

Other observations ______________________________

____

Second week

____
Signature

Fourth week

Two (2) points		One (1) point		Zero (0) points	
Encourages infant to scan face in presence of observer, maintaining eye contact with infant when speaking to observer	M F	Maintains "en face" position and eye contact with infant unless speaking to observer	M F	Intermittent or absent eye contact or "en face" position with infant	M F
Consistently holds infant with chest and trunk touching parent; spontaneously strokes and caresses infant	M F	Holds infant close to, but not always touching parent; intermittent touching only	M F	Holds infant away from own body; infrequent or absent touching of infant's face	M F
Initiates demonstration of what infant response is, showing evidence of reciprocity	M F	When prompted, will demonstrate infant's response with little or no evidence of reciprocity	M F	Vague about infant's response patterns; no evidence of reciprocity	M F
Able to combine behaviors; i.e., care taking, stimulation with apparent ease, immediately responding to infant's cry (0-30 seconds)	M F	Finishes activity before responding to infant's cry; i.e., delay of 1 or 2 minutes	M F	Reluctant to respond to infant's cry; i.e., delay of more than 3 minutes	M F
Expresses increasing satisfaction with role of parent, infant behavior, and life-style	M F	Expresses two or more negative feelings about role of parent, infant behavior, or life-style	M F	Expresses mainly negative feelings about role of parent, infant behavior, or life-style	M F

Mother's total score ___

Father's total score ___

11-15 requires *usual* nursing support for bonding
6-10 requires *extra* nursing support for bonding
0-5 required *intensive* nursing support for bonding

Other observations ______________________________

____

Fourth week

____
Signature

Sixth week

Three (3) points		**Two (2) points**		**One (1) point**	
Maintains eye contact and "en face" position with infant, unless distraction occurs requiring immediate response	**M** **F**	Intermittent "en face" position and eye contact with infant	**M** **F**	Avoids or does not make eye contact or "en face" position with infant	**M** **F**
Usually holds infant on left side, using whole arm or hand, with infant's chest and trunk in contact with own body	**M** **F**	Undifferentiated side for holding infant, close to but not always touching own body	**M** **F**	Little or no evidence of holding infant	**M** **F**
Is able to describe at least two specific behaviors of infant with accurate perception of meaning of behavior	**M** **F**	Describes infant behaviors, needing assistance in clarifying meaning of behavior	**M** **F**	Unable to describe infant behavior clearly or identify meaning	**M** **F**
Carries out care-taking activities with ease, immediately moving toward crying infant (0 to 30 seconds)	**M** **F**	Anxious about care-taking activities; delay of 1 or 2 minutes before moving toward crying infant	**M** **F**	Care-taking activities inconsistently carried out; delay in moving toward crying infant of more than 3 minutes	**M** **F**
Expresses satisfaction with infant's behavior and role of parent	**M** **F**	Expresses feelings about infant's behavior and role of parent in vague terms	**M** **F**	Expresses dissatisfaction with infant and role of parent; concern mainly for self	**M** **F**

Mother's total score ___

Father's total score ___

11-15 requires *usual* nursing support for bonding
6-10 requires *extra* nursing support for bonding
0-5 requires *intensive* nursing support for bonding

Other observations ______________________________

____

____

Sixth week

____
Signature

acuity and the amount of physical and psychic energy she possesses. From these various assessments, plans of care may be developed that have as their desired outcomes enhancing the mother's physical recovery, increasing the parents' participation is successful care of themselves and their newborn, and encouraging a return to family commitments. These plans include strengthening the family's coping mechanisms, enlisting adequate situational supports, and role-modeling interaction with the newborn. This period is a crucial one with the potential for crisis for the family (Donner, 1972; Gordon and Gordon, 1960).

EXAMPLES OF NURSING DIAGNOSES

Before establishing nursing diagnoses the nurse correlates the observed maternal behaviors with such items as the following:

1. The mother's physical and psychic condition: fatigue, discomfort, and anxiety about assuming full responsibility for child and adverse social or economic factors should be taken into account, because they can affect manner and interest displayed toward child and can cloud true relationship.
2. Ethnic and cultural identity can dictate maternal behavior at the birth of a child. The nurse also correlates paternal behaviors with the father's shared cultural and personal concepts of fathering role and previous experience with infants. Both parental patterns are correlated against data collected earlier to establish evidence of a consistent pattern of reaction to child and parental roles.

The following are examples of nursing diagnosis:

1. Alterations in family dynamics because of unexpected birth of twins

2. Impaired verbal communication because of deafness
3. Alterations in parenting because of distress over sex of child (e.g., sixth boy)
4. Alterations in parenting because of fatigue of long, difficult labor

PLANNING AND IMPLEMENTATION

Nurses have played a leadership role in efforts to provide holistic client care in the postpartum period. The care encompasses both therapeutic and educational measures that encourage assertive self-reliant behaviors in family members. Research by Sullivan and Beeman (1981) indicates that parents express satisfaction with postpartum nursing care if efforts are made to facilitate parent-child relationships and to provide willing listeners for parental review of the birth process and instruction in the care of self and infant. The nursing actions presented below are designed to promote the above satisfactions.

In the early period contacts between parents and infant are as follows:

1. Timed to make use of infant's normal patterns of sleeping and waking: at birth, at about 4 to 6 hours, and every 2 to 5 hours thereafter
2. Provided at important times for parental attachment to take place (preferably at birth or as soon thereafter as the infant's and mother's conditions permit)
3. Long and often enough to permit parents to hold, examine, care for, and enjoy their child

The nurse reviews the normal characteristics of the newborn and gives the parent a report on the infant's initial physical examination. Later the nurse can examine or have infant examined in the parent's presence and review findings with them. Written instructions as to feeding, medications, and so on are provided. A daily report on the infant's progress and behaviors (e.g., eating, sleeping, voiding, defecating) is given.

The nurse provides a demonstration of infant care and explains hospital routines (e.g., when infant goes from nursery area to mother's bedside; discuss identification of infant, emergency care of infant if gagging or choking occurs, and protective measures used to minimize possibility of cross infection). Nursing personnel are available to give infant care as indicated, to reassure parents regarding normalcy of their infant, and to assist with care-taking activities and infant feeding techniques. Parents are encouraged to participate in infant care and, whenever possible, to use techniques developed by themselves.

As the family moves on to *consolidating* the parent-child relationship, the nurse encourages or initiates such discussions as the following:

1. *Focusing on the child*. The nurse and clients discuss the normal rhythms of the child and the parents' awareness of how the child communicates his needs. The parents are advised to take time to study their infant (e.g., what different types of crying mean; when he likes being awake—morning, afternoon, or evening). The nurse identifies problems experienced (e.g., infant crying, sleeping) and assists with solutions. Together, nurse and clients note successes and failures in care-taking activities and the nurse helps the parents with accumulating successful coping mechanisms and discarding unsuccessful ones.

2. *Focusing on the parents*. The nurse and clients discuss the normal responses of parents to the complex role of being a parent. The nurse provides an opportunity for safe revelation of feelings. Nurse and client discuss parental criteria for success in parenting skills (i.e., infant responses and competence in care-taking activities and opinions of significant others). Success is praised and parents are encouraged to be open minded about expectations of their role and that of others (e.g., siblings, grandparents) and of the infant's abilities.

The mother is encouraged to conserve her energy by having a rest period when the infant sleeps; by not becoming involved in ''perfect housekeeper'' image; by encouraging the infant to sleep through the night by waking him for a feeding at 10 or 11 PM; by enlisting the help of others, that is, relatives or friends, to help with household chores; and by accepting baby-sitting offers.

For some parents whose behavior indicates consistent rejection of the child's infancy and of his dependency needs, the above interventions apply; however, additional care is needed as follows:

1. Repeated contacts with parents are planned and carried out.
2. Other supportive personnel, such as a social worker, are enlisted to help.

At the time of the postpartum examination of mother and infant, *growth* in the parental role is usually evident. The infant is examined, and the findings are reviewed with the parent. Again the nurse initiates or encourages discussions.

1. *Focusing on the child*. The nurse reviews and assesses parental knowledge of the following:
   a. The signs and symptoms of illness and measures instituted to effect a cure or obtain medical assistance
   b. The infant's developmental needs as follows:
      (1) Accommodation to physical growth (e.g., introduction of solid foods into diet or weaning)
      (2) Use of longer wakeful periods to increase stimulation of infant and social interaction with siblings and other family members

(3) Adaptation to infant's persisting dependency and his inability to conform socially or show awareness of others' needs

c. The need for establishing routine pediatric care

2. *Focusing on the parents*. The nurse provides the opportunity for mother and family to discuss problems: parents' reactions to child, child's needs and demands, feelings of depression or helplessness and how such feelings affect care the parents can give the child. The nurse gives recognition to parental success in nurturing their child. If necessary, the family is helped to obtain further assistance (i.e., public health agency personnel or social workers) to develop more adequate coping mechanisms. Some communities have established round-the-clock telephone centers where parents can obtain help for emotionally based problems with the child. These are in addition to emergency medical services. If parenting disorders are noted, the parents are referred to follow-up agencies (e.g., the county public health department).

3. *Focusing on the family*. The nurse discusses balancing the infant's needs with those of other family members (e.g., jealousy of siblings (Fig. 32.11), husband's or wife's feelings of alienation), parents' need to modify infant's behavior to

Fig. 32.11
It is important to include siblings in new baby's arrival. **A,** Mother oversees older sibling's efforts to get acquainted with new brother. **B,** Mother focuses attention on son while father holds new daughter.

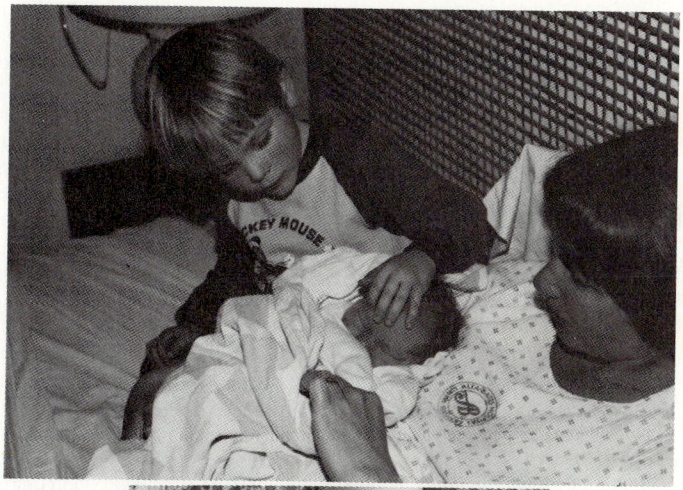

A

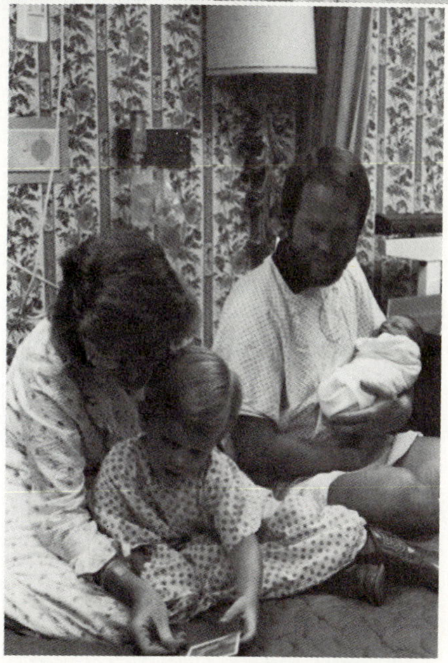

B

Table 32.2
Evaluation Criteria: Parent-Child Relationships

	Initiating the Relationship	Consolidating the Relationship	Growth in Parental Role
Infant growth and development	Parents are reassured of normalcy of infant's characteristics Appearance (e.g., molding of head, milia, lanugo, forceps marks) Behavior (e.g., sleeping, waking, crying, and sensory capabilities) Responses (e.g., eating, regurgitating, defecating, voiding, gaining weight)	Parents recognize infant's cues for interactions, meaning of types of cries; need for rest and privacy Parents can assess infant temperature and respirations, feeding, waking, and sleep patterns for normalcy	Parents become more knowledgeable about abnormal responses of infant and those responses for which professional consultation is required Knowledge of normal growth and development of infant increases Parents can anticipate change in infant's needs
Attachment process	Parents are assured of opportunity for attachment (bonding) with their infant (e.g., holding, touching, examining, establishing eye contact as soon after birth as possible, and either continuous contact [rooming-in or home birth] or protracted contact thereafter while in hospital)	Parents develop a satisfactory level of competence in routine care-taking activities of bathing, feeding, holding, and clothing infant Parents plan socializing periods with infant Parents recognize dual nature of parent-child relationship	Parents can adapt to the child to meet changing circumstances; necessity for rigid schedules lessens as competency increases
Infant identity	Infant's identity is established Claiming process: parents look for similarities or differences between their infant and other family members regarding size, weight, sex, appearance, behavior, and responses Identifying wristband is checked	Infant's identity expands with awareness of his particular rhythms of sleeping, waking, hunger, and satiety, as well as his cues for expressing his need for sleep, food, soothing, stimulation, socializing, and relief from pain or discomfort	Infant's identity continues to expand as he becomes part of a family group (e.g., he interacts with siblings)
Parental criteria	Parents are aware of following criteria they will use in assessing success or failure of care they give their child: Infant responses: parents may feel successful if infant snuggles against them, looks at them, stops crying when they hold him, or burps when feeding; they may feel unsuccessful if child persists in crying, is unable to breast feed, "frowns" at them, or will not wake up	Parents establish realistic criteria for use in evaluating their efforts in parenting relative to following: Infant responses: they accept a mixture of success and failure in control they can exert over such infant behaviors as crying, fussing, eating, sleeping, waking, growing, and gaining weight	Criteria for success in parenting are flexible with reference to following: Infant responses: infant's dependency needs are recognized and accepted as a beginning levels of development; parents are aware of parental actions as an important factor in behavior exhibited by infant; adaptation of parents' and infant's normal rhythms and responses begins as a process of mutual behavior modification
	Parental competence in care-taking activities: parents may feel inadequate to extent that they feel incompetent in handling or holding child	Parental competence in care-taking activities: Self-esteem grows as skill in care-taking activities increases Recognition develops as to what care is essential for well-being of infant as opposed to prior expectations of parents Flexible schedule for infant care is accepted	Parental competence in care-taking activities: parents recognize that skills required will change with child's growth and development and that it is reasonable to seek guidance and support as new needs arise

Table 32.2—cont'd
Evaluation Criteria: Parent-Child Relationships

Initiating the Relationship	Consolidating the Relationship	Growth in Parental Role
Opinions of significant others: parents may expect that others will be supportive and accepting of their beginning attempts or critical and intolerant of their less-than-perfect efforts; these expectations can prompt them to seek assistance or to avoid it	Opinions of significant others: assistance from others is accepted or rejected as knowledge and skill grow; parent is aware of vulnerability to praise or criticism of significant others (e.g., own mother, spouse, close relatives)	Opinions of significant others: parents recognize that this dependency will continue; but in its negative sense, it can be countered with mastery of parental tasks and growing self-esteem as a parent

meet their expectations (e.g., toilet training, sleeping patterns, stopping crying when admonished), and infant's ability to conform.

EVALUATION

Although the evaluation of the family's adjustment to the birth of an infant marks the completion of nursing care of the childbearing family, in reality it marks the beginning of the professional lifelong investment in the health of the family. Maternity nurses are privileged to be part of the beginning of a new family experience, of laying foundations for parental roles of the children just born. Table 32.2 presents criteria for assessing parental responses that indicate acceptance of and growth in a crucial social role.

References and Readings

Adams, M.: Early concerns of primigravid mothers regarding infant care activities, Nurs. Res. **12:**72, 1963.

Adamson, L., et al.: The development of social reciprocity between a sighted infant and her blind parents, J. Am. Acad. Child Psychiatry **16:**194, Spring 1977.

Aikens, R.M.: Hats and lamps in the prevention of neonatal hypothermia, Nurs. Mirror **144:**65, 1977.

Ainsworth, M.D.: Object relations, dependency, and attachment: a theoretical review of the infant-mother relationship. Child Dev. **40:**969, 1969.

Ainsworth, M.D.: The development of infant-mother attachment. In Caldwell, B.M., and Reccurti, H.N., editors: Review of child development research, vol. 3, New York, 1970, Russell Sage Foundation.

Ainsworth, M.D., and Bell, S.M.: Attachment, exploration and separation: illustrated by the behavior of one-year-olds in a strange situation, Child Dev. **41:**49, 1970.

Avanti, K.: Anxiety as a potential factor affecting maternal attachment. J.O.G.N. Nurs. **10**(6):416, 1981.

Barrett, C.R., et al.: Neonatal separation: the maternal side of interactional deprivation, Pediatrics **54:**197, 1970.

Bell, S.M., and Ainsworth, M.D.S.: Infant crying and maternal responsiveness, Child Dev. **43:**1171, 1972.

Bellugi, U., and Eischer, S.: A comparison of sign language and spoken language, Cognition **1:**173, 1972.

Benedek, T.: Adaptation to reality in early infancy, Psychoanal. Q. **7:**200, 1950.

Benedek, T.: Motherhood and nurturing. In Anthony, E.J., and Benedek, T., editors: Parenthood: its psychology and psychopathology, Boston, 1970, Little, Brown & Co.

Bernal, J.: Crying during the first ten days of life and maternal responses, Dev. Med. Child Neurol. **14:**362, 1972.

Blehar, M.C., Lieberman, A., and Ainsworth, M.D.: Early face-to-face interaction and its relation to later infant-mother attachment, Child Dev. **48:**182, 1977.

Bonvillian, J.D., Clarrow, V.R., and Nelson, K.E.: Psycholinguistic and educational implications of deafness, Hum. Dev. **16:**321, 1973.

Boston Women's Health Book Collective, Inc.: Ourselves and our children, New York, 1978, Random House.

Bowlby, J.: The nature of the child's tie to his mother, Int. J. Psychoanal. **39:**350, 1958.

Bowlby, J.: Attachment and loss, vol. 1, Attachment, New York, 1969, Basic Books, Publishers.

Brandon, H.K.: The blind mother, Am. J. Nurs. **75:**414, March 1975.

Brazelton, T.B.: The early mother-infant adjustment, Pediatrics **32:**931, 1963.

Brazelton, T.B.: Effect of maternal expectations on early infant behavior, Early Child Dev. Care **2:**259, 1973a.

Brazelton, T.B.: Neonatal behavioral assessment scale, London, 1973b, Spastics International Medical Publications.

Brazelton, T.B.: Behavioral competence of the newborn infant, Semin. Perinatol. **3:**35, Jan. 1979.

Brazelton, T.B., Koslowski, B., and Main, M.: The origins of reciprocity: the early mother-infant interaction. In Lewis, M., and Rosenblum, L.A., editors: The effect of the infant on its caregiver, New York, 1974, John Wiley & Sons.

Broussard, E.R., and Hartner, M.S.: Maternal perception of the neonate as related to development, Child Psych. Hum. Dev. **1:**16, Fall 1970.

Budin, P.: The nursling, London, 1907, Caxton Publishing Co.

Burnstein, I., et al.: Anxiety, pregnancy, labor and the neonate, Am. J. Obstet. Gynecol. **118:**195, 1974.

Carlsson, S.G., et al.: Effects of amounts of contact between mother and child on the mother's nursing behavior, Dev. Psychobiol. **11:**143, 1978.

Celotta, B.: New motherhood: a time of crisis, Birth Fam. J. **9**(1):21, 1982.

Cohen, R.: Maladaptation to pregnancy, Semin. Perinatol. **3:**79, Jan. 1979.

Condon, W., and Sander, L.: Neonate movement is synchronized with adult speech: interactional participation and language acquisition, Science **183:**99, 1974.

Curry, M.A.: Contact during the first hour with the wrapped or naked newborn: effect on maternal attachment behaviors at 36 hours and three months, Birth Fam. J. **6:**4, Winter 1979.

de Chateau, P.: The importance of the neonatal period for the development of synchrony in the mother-infant dyad—a review, Birth Fam. J. **4:**10, 1977.

de Chateau, P.: Effects of hospital practices on synchrony in the development of the infant-parent relationship, Semin. Perinatol. **3:**45, Jan. 1979.

Donaldson, N.E.: The post partum follow-up nurse clinician, J.O.G.N. Nurs. **10**(4):249, 1981.

Donner, G.J.: Parenthood as a crisis, Perspect. Psychiatr. Care **10:**84, April-June 1972.

Erikson, E.H.: Identity and the life cycle: selected papers. In Psychological issues, vol. 1, no. 1, New York, 1959, International Universities Press.

Fardig, J.A.: A comparison of skin-to-skin contact and radiant heaters in promoting neonatal thermoregulation, J. Nurs. Midwife, **25:**19, Jan.-Feb. 1980.

Funke-Farber, J.: Reliability and validity testing of maternal adaptive behavior, Edmonton, Alta., 1978, The University of Alberta, Faculty of Nursing.

Goldson, E., et al.: Child abuse: its relationship to birth weight, Apgar score and developmental testing, Am. J. Dis. Child. **132:**790, 1978.

Goodman, S., et al.: Bonding and attachment: theoretical issues, Semin. Perinatol. **3:**3, Jan. 1979.

Gordon, R., and Gordon, K.: Social factors in prevention of postpartum emotional problems, Obstet, Gynecol. **15:**453, 1960.

Gray, J., et al.: Prediction and prevention of child abuse, Semin. Perinatol. **3:**85, Jan. 1979.

Greis, M.: Beyond maternity: post partum concerns of mothers, M.C.N., p. 182, May-June 1977.

Grosso, C., et al.: The Vietnamese American family . . . and Grandma makes three, M.C.N. **6:**177, May-June 1981.

Hefler, R.E., and Kempe, C.H.: The battered child, Chicago, 1965, The University of Chicago Press

Hobbs, D.F.: Parenthood as crisis: a third study, J. Marr. Fam. **27:**367, 1975.

Hogan, L.R.: Pregnant again—at 41, M.C.N. **4:**174, May-June 1979.

Howley: The older primipara: implications for nurses, J.O.G.N. Nurs. **10**(3):182, May-June 1981.

Josselyn, I.M.: Cultural forces: motherliness and fatherliness, Am. J. Orthopsychiatry **26:**264, 1956.

Kennell, J.H., et al.: Maternal behavior one year after early and extended postpartum contact, Dev. Med. Child Neurol. **16:**172, 1974.

Kennell, J.: Evidence for a sensitive period in the human mother. In Klaus, M., Leger, T., and Trause, M., editors: Maternal attachment and mothering disorders, ed. 2, Skillman, N.J., 1982, Johnson & Johnson Baby Products Co.

Klaus, M., et al.: Maternal attachment: importance of the first postpartum days, N. Engl. J. Med. **286:**460, 1972.

Klaus, M.H., et al.: Human maternal behavior at the first contact with her young, Pediatrics **46:**187, 1970.

Klaus, M.H., et al.: Maternal attachment and mothering disorders. Pediatric Round Table 1, 1982, Johnson & Johnson Baby Products Co.

Klaus, M.H., and Kennell, J.H.: Maternal-infant bonding: the impact of early separation or loss on family development, St. Louis, 1982, The C.V. Mosby Co.

Klaus, M.H., and Robertson, M.: Birth, interaction and attachment. Pediatric Round Table 6, 1982, Johnson & Johnson Baby Products Co.

Lamb, M.: Early contact and maternal-infant bonding: one decade later, Pediatrics **70**(5):325, 1982.

Lang, R.: Birth book, Ben Lomond, Calif, 1972, Genesis Press.

Leifer, A.D., et al.: Effects of mother-infant separation on maternal attachment behavior, Child Dev. **43:**1203, 1972.

Lind, J., et al.: Psychosomatic medicine. In Morris, N., editor: Obstetrics and gynecology, Basel, 1973, S. Karger.

Lotas, M., and Willing, J.: Mothers, babies, perception, Image **11:**45, June 1979.

Lynch, A.: Maternal stress following the birth of a second child. In, Klaus, M., and Robertson, M., editors: Birth interaction and attachment, 1982, Johnson & Johnson Baby Products Co.

Magilvy, K., Pollard, B.L., and Harrison, L.L.: Stereotyping, words, and concepts (letter), M.C.N. **4:**254, July-Aug, 1979.

McClinton, B.S., and Meier, B.: Beginnings: psychology of early childhood, St. Louis, 1978, The C.V. Mosby Co.

McCrae, M.: Bonding in a sea of silence, M.C.N. **4:**29, Jan-Feb. 1979.

Meleis, A.I., and Sorrell, L.: Arab American women and their birth experiences, M.C.N. **6**(3):171, May-June 1981.

Morris, M.: Psychological miscarriage: an end to mother love, Transaction, p. 11, Jan-Feb, 1966.

Moss, J.R.: Concerns of multipares on the third postpartum day, J.O.G.N. Nurs. **10**(6):421, 1981.

Phillips, C., and Anzalone, J.: Fathering: participation in labor and birth, ed. 2, St. Louis, 1982, The C.V. Mosby Co.

Rubin, R.: Maternal behavior, Nurs. Outlook **9:**682, 1961.

Schiff, N.B.: Cummunication problems in hearing children of deaf parents, J. Speech Hear. Disord. **41:**348, Aug. 1976.

Seitz, S., and Marcus, S.: Mother-child interactions: a foundation for language development, Except. Child. **42:**445, May 1976.

Shainess, N.: Abortion is no man's business, Psychology Today, p. 18, March 1970.

Siegel, E.: A critical examination of studies of parent-infant bonding in birth, interaction and attachment (edited by Klaus, M., and Robertson, M.), Evansville, Ind., 1982, Johnson & Johnson Baby Products Co.

Smales, O.R., and Kime, R.: Thermoregulation in babies immediately after birth, Arch. Dis. Child. **53:**58, Jan. 1978.

Sroufe, L.A., and Waters, E.: Attachment as an organizational construct, Child Dev. **48:**1184, 1977.

Stainton, C.M.: Parent-infant interaction: putting theory into practice, Calgary, Alta., Canada, 1981, The University of Calgary, Faculty of Nursing.

Steele, B., and Pollock, C.: A psychiatric study of parents who abuse infants and small children. In Helfer, R.E., and Kempe, C., editors: The battered child, Chicago, 1968, The University of Chicago Press.

Sullivan, D., and Beeman, R.: Satisfaction with postpartum care: opportunities for bonding, reconstructing the birth and instruction, Birth Fam. J. **8:**3, Fall 1981.

Sussman, A.E., and Steward, L.G.: Counseling with deaf people, New York, 1971, New York Deafness Research and Training Center.

Sweet, P.T.: Prenatal classes especially for children, M.C.N. **4:**82, March-April 1979.

Tentoni, S., and High, J.: Culturally induced postpartum depression: a theoretical position, J.O.G.N. Nurs. **9:**246, July-Aug. 1980.

Vernon, M., and Mindel, E.D.: Psychological and psychiatric aspects of profound hearing loss. In Rose, D., editor: Audiological assessments, Englewood Cliffs, N.J., 1971, Prentice-Hall.

Wilbur, R.: The linguistics of manual languages and manual systems. In Lloyd, L.L., editor: Communication, assessments and intervention strategies, Baltimore, 1976, University Park Press.

High-Risk Mother and Neonate

33 Introduction to the High-Risk Mother and Neonate

34 Loss and Grief

35 Complications of Pregnancy

36 Major Complications Coincident with Pregnancy

37 Complications During Birth

38 Adolescent Parenthood

39 Psychosocial Risk Factors

40 Neonates with Hyperbilirubinemia and Congenital Disorders

41 Other Medical and Surgical Conditions

UNIT SEVEN

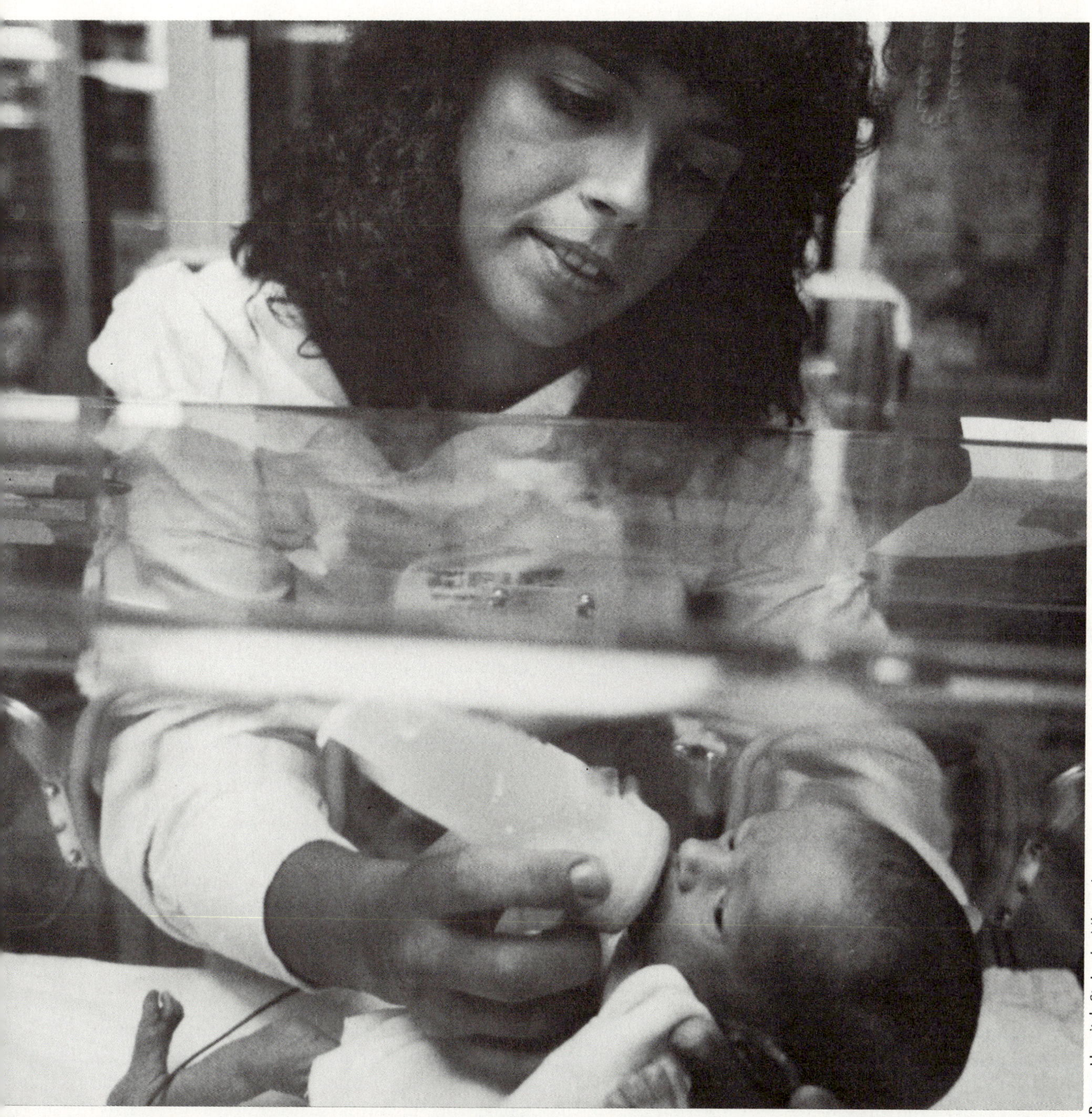

Barnes Hospital, St. Louis, Missouri

33

Introduction to the High-Risk Mother and Neonate

- Definition and Scope of the Problem
- Risk Factors
  - Maternal factors
  - Paternal factors
  - Fetal factors
  - Neonatal factors
- Goals for Care
- Regionalization of Health Care Services
- Maternal Health Problems
  - Statistical profile
- Fetal and Neonatal Health Problems
  - Statistical profile
    - Fetal death
    - Neonatal death
    - Perinatal death rate
    - Infant mortality
- General Care of the Infant at Risk
  - Nursing the neonate with respiratory distress
    - Goals of care
    - Assessment and analysis
    - Example of nursing diagnosis
    - Plan and implementation
    - Evaluation
    - Oxygen therapy
  - Temperature support and regulation
    - Goals of care
    - Assessment and analysis
    - Example of nursing diagnosis
    - Plan and implementation
    - Evaluation
  - Nutrition and elimination
    - General considerations
    - Nutritional requisites
    - Weight and fluid loss
    - Formula and feeding schedules
    - Goals of care
    - Assessment and analysis
    - Examples of nursing diagnoses
    - Plan and implementation
    - Evaluation
    - Nasogastric tube feeding
    - Monitoring parenteral fluid administration
    - Total parenteral nutrition
  - Emotional aspects of care
    - Neonate's emotional needs
    - Supportive care
  - Postmortem care: stillbirth
    - Definition of fetal death
    - Parents and child
    - Care of the child
    - Legal requirements for filing certificate of death (California)

Definition and Scope of the Problem

A high-risk pregnancy is one in which the life or health of the mother or offspring is jeopardized by a disorder coincidental with or unique to pregnancy. For the mother the high-risk status extends (arbitrarily) through the puerperium, that is, until 29 days after delivery. Postdelivery maternal complications are usually resolved within a month of birth, but perinatal morbidity may continue for months or years.

A better understanding of human reproduction has greatly reduced maternal morbidity and mortality. Knowledge of the fetus and neonatal disorders has increased dramatically in the last 10 to 15 years, and this has led to a gratifying drop in perinatal morbidity and mortality during this period.

Of the 5 to 10 million pregnancies that occur in the United States each year, 2 to 3 million terminate as spontaneous abortions. Many of these abortions are caused by genetic faults or infection. About 1 million early gestations end as elective abortions. Approximately 3.5 million pregnancies reach viability (24 to 28 weeks' gestational age), but of these at least 45,000 fetuses fail to survive. About the same number of neonates die during the first month of life. Another 40,000 babies have severe but perhaps correctable congenital anomalies. Pregnancy and delivery complications are responsible in part at least for approximately 90,000 mentally retarded individuals. In addition, these complications have partially handicapped more than 150,000 persons, who have difficulty coping in our complex society.

Even considering fetuses who have reached viability, perinatal mortality exceeds that of all other causes of death combined until 65 years of age. When viewed in this perspective, high-risk pregnancy presents one of the most critical and urgent problems of modern medicine.

A new social emphasis on the quality of life has developed. Family planning has reduced family size and the number of unwanted pregnancies. With these trends the wanted child has become increasingly important. As a consequence, periodic maternal and perinatal assessment is essential to emphasize safe delivery of normal infants who can develop to their maximal potential.

The experience of childbirth for each woman is influenced by many factors. Interaction of the various factors results in a holistic experience unique to each individual. At the start of this holistic view of the childbearing experience is the culture into which the woman was born (Fig. 33.1). As the young girl matures, she integrates cultural expectations (occasionally couched in folklore) and adds to these societal norms to which she is exposed. Her family and peers further direct and influence her expectations of herself as a member of the family, society, and community. Onto this structure of role definitions and expectations is the physiologic process of pregnancy that begins with conception and ends at childbirth. Between these two points there is an expected length of time—9 months—during which predictable events occur. Under optimal circumstances, even a normal pregnancy brings profound psychologic as well as physiologic changes (see Chapter 15). Even a normal pregnancy is a time of transient ego vulnerability for the woman and anticipated changes in the family unit.

It is well known that pregnancy is a *maturational* crisis in both the physiologic and psychologic sense. The diagnosis of high risk imposes another crisis, a *situational* crisis (e.g., the pregnancy terminates before the anticipated date; the woman develops gestational diabetes mellitus with its potential complications; a neonate is born who does not meet cultural, societal, or familial norms and expectations).

Fig. 33.1
Psychosocial expectations originating from every level are integrated by each woman into a unique pattern that individualizes her childbearing experience.

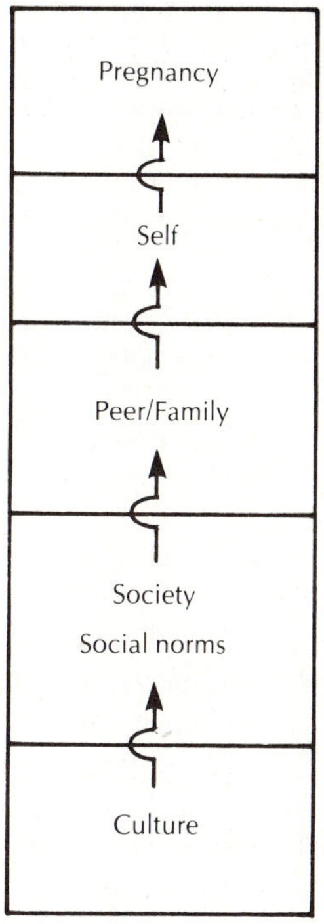

Risk Factors

Research and experience have led to the identification of factors that jeopardize the pregnant and postdelivery woman and the fetus-neonate (see boxes). This knowledge has permitted the development of increasingly effective preventive and therapeutic measures that could minimize the incidence of morbidity, disability, and death of the mother or infant. Frequently it is the alert nurse, conversant and familiar with deviations from normal, who notes and reports potential or real high-risk factors.

Psychosocial Factors that Place the Mother-Infant Dyad at Risk

Maternal, paternal, or familial history of vulnerability (e.g., child abuse)
Preexisting major health problem (e.g., mental illness, alcoholism, mental retardation)
Poverty (e.g., inability to comply with health care); lack of prenatal care
Insufficient support system (e.g., inadequate family support systems, systems prone to crisis, systems unable to fulfill family functions)
Family disruption or dissolution (e.g., absent parent because of divorce, death, military service, abandonment)
Role changes/conflicts (e.g., change in life-style, career, self, responsibilities, relationship; conflict about role expectations)
Maturational crisis (e.g., difficulty in or inability to accomplish maturational tasks; the "stigma" of being classified as high-risk)
Situational crisis (e.g., adolescent pregnancy; the "stigma" of being classified as high-risk)
Noncompliance with cultural norms (e.g., nonmarital pregnancy)
Dysfunctional behavior (e.g., anxiety, neurosis, depression psychosis)
Poor coping skills

From Fogel, C.I., and Woods, N.F.: Health care of women: a nursing perspective, St. Louis, 1981, The C.V.Mosby Co.

Serious biologic handicaps, health problems, obstetric disorders, and social deprivation may compromise the mother and the infant in subtle or more obvious ways. Early or late fetal damage may occur. The baby may be small for gestational (SGA), preterm, or postterm. Occasionally the infant may be preterm but of excessive size (large for gestational age [LGA]). In other instances the postterm infant may be large. Such hazards and their management constitute unique perinatal problems.

MATERNAL FACTORS

One must identify early those women who may have a greater likelihood of pregnancy complications. Careful continuing evaluation during pregnancy will minimize completely unexpected serious complications. If abnormal trends develop, disorders can be anticipated, and prompt treatment may eliminate or reduce the difficulty. Everyone in the health care system must work together as a team in the promotion of maternal and fetal health, particularly in stressful social situations or during illness that may compromise mother and infant.

High-risk factors that contribute to perinatal morbidity and mortality are numerous. The boxes above and on p. 741 present reasonably inclusive lists of associations that aid in the identification of high-risk women.

PATERNAL FACTORS

The father's influences in causing premature birth and other manifestations of high-risk pregnancy are largely speculative. What genetic damage is sustained by chronic alcoholism or other drug abuse is unknown, for example. SGA infants are often reported and the incidence of congenital anomalies may be slightly elevated when the father has diabetes mellitus or is a drug addict. Admittedly, the mother may suffer some impairment as well so that the responsibility may not be clear-cut.

FETAL FACTORS

Fetal factors that may jeopardize the infant include congenital anomalies, short umbilical cord, cord entanglement or compression, hydramnios, abnormal presentation or position, immaturity (Table 33.1), prematurity, response to exposure to chemicals (see Appendix H) or radiation, and fetal infection.

NEONATAL FACTORS

The period just after delivery, especially the first minutes, as exemplified by the 1- and 5-min Apgar scores, may be critical for the neonate who must quickly and effectively adapt to extrauterine life. Problems of resuscitation, especially the establishment of a patent airway and the reversal of narcotic overdosage by narcotic antagonists such as naloxone (Narcan), may be vital. The early diagnosis and proper management of congenital anomalies, such as tracheoesophageal fistula and meningomyelocele, may be important also. The incidence of cerebral palsy, mental retardation, and other neurologic disorders depends in large measure on the skillful management of the intranatal and immediate neonatal period.

Categories of High-Risk Pregnancy

1. Maternal age and parity factors
   a. Age 16 or under
   b. Nullipara 35 or over
   c. Multipara 40 or over
   d. Interval of 8 years or more since last pregnancy
   e. High parity (5 or more)
2. Nonmarital pregnancy
3. PIH, hypertension, kidney disease
   a. Preeclampsia with hospitalization before labor
   b. Eclampsia
   c. Kidney disease—pyelonephritis, nephritis, nephrosis, etc.
   d. Chronic hypertension, severe (160/100 or over)
   e. Blood pressure 140/90 or above on two readings 30 minutes apart
4. Anemia and hemorrhage
   a. Hematocrit 30% or below in pregnancy
   b. Hemorrhage (previous pregnancy)—severe, requiring transfusion
   c. Hemorrhage (present pregnancy)
   d. Anemia (hemoglobin below 10 g) for which treatment other than oral iron preparations is required (hemolytic, macrocytic, etc.)
   e. Sickle cell trait or disease
   f. History of bleeding or clotting disorder at any time
5. Fetal factors
   a. Two or more previous premature deliveries (twins = one delivery)
   b. Two or more consecutive spontaneous abortions (miscarriages)
   c. One or more stillbirths at term
   d. One or more gross anomalies
   e. Rh incompatibility or ABO immunization problems
   f. History of previous birth defects—cerebral palsy, brain damage, mental retardation, metabolic disorders such as PKU
   g. History of large infants (over 9 lb)
6. Dystocia (history of or anticipated)
   a. Contracted pelvis or cephalopelvic disproportion (CPD)
   b. Multiple pregnancy in current pregnancy
   c. Two or more breech deliveries
   d Previous cesarean delivery
   e. History of prolonged labor (more than 18 hours for nullipara; 12 hours for multipara)
   f. Uterine anomaly
7. History of or concurrent medical conditions
   a. Diabetic or prediabetic
   b. Hyperemesis gravidarum
   c. Thyroid disease (hypothyroidism or hyperthyroidism)
   d. Malnutrition or extreme obesity (20% over ideal weight for height; 15% under ideal weight for height)
   e. Organic heart disease
   f. Syphilis
   g. Rubella in first 10 weeks of *this* pregnancy
   h. Tuberculosis or other serious pulmonary pathologic condition (e.g., emphysema, asthma)
   i. Malignant or premalignant tumors (including hydatidiform mole)
   j. Alcoholism, drug addicition
   k. Psychiatric disease or epilepsy (documented)
   l. Mental retardartion
   m. Solitary ovary or tube (ectopic)
8. Those with previous history of
   a. Late registration
   b. Poor clinic attendance
   c. Home situation making clinic attendance and hospitalization difficult
   d. Mothers, including minors, without family resources (includes desertions, adoptions, injuries, separations, family withdrawals, sole support)

From Fogel, C.I., and Woods, N.F.: Health care of women: a nursing perspective, St. Louis, 1981, The C.V. Mosby Co.

Table 33.1
Immaturity and Resultant Problems

Developmental Immaturity	Physiologic Handicap
CNS	Sucking reflex; absent, poorly developed, or uncoordinated with swallowing reflex; constant danger of aspiration
	Poor gag reflex
Gastrointestinal tract	Small gastric capacity
	Variable food transit times through gastrointestinal tract, affecting digestion and absorption
	Poor tolerance for fats (especially saturated); fat lost in stool decreases calories available to neonate and is accompanied by loss of minerals and fat-soluble vitamins
	Lax abdominal musculature, ↓ HCl, weak cardiac sphincter
Metabolism (enzyme systems)	Inefficient handling of metabolic breakdown products (e.g., blood tyrosine levels from metabolism of protein rise, capable of causing positive PKU test even if baby does not have PKU)
Urinary system	Impaired water conservation
	Reduced selectivity in resorption of electrolytes
Limited glucose stores	Increased danger of hypoglycemia, hyperbilirubinemia, and protein catabolism and their sequelae (e.g., brain damage)

Kernicterus

Table 33.2
Factors that Place the Pregnancy and Fetus-Neonate at High Risk

Category	Factors that Result in Risk
First trimester	
Anatomic	Maternal
	Ectopic pregnancy
	Uterine abnormality
	Retroversion of uterus
Physiologic	Fetal
	Gross chromosomal defect
	Hydatidiform mole
	Multiple pregnancy
	Poor trophoblast invasiveness
	Folate deficiency
	Endocrine deficiency
	Hyperemesis gravidarum
	Defective sperm
Psychologic	Psychologic shock
	Drugs
Therapeutic	Social abortion (aspiration, saline, prostaglandin)
	Drug therapy
	X-ray therapy
Infections	Viral infection
Genetic	Sporadic mutation
	Inherited characteristics
	Sex-linked disease
Environmental	Poverty
	Drugs
	Tobacco
	Alcohol
	Nutrition, inadequate
Second trimester	
Anatomic	Maternal
	Uterine abnormality
	Incompetent cervical os
	Fetal
	Gross abnormality
	Acute hydramnios
	Multiple pregnancy
	Poor implantation
Maternal complications	Rh incompatibility
	Cyanotic heart disease
	Hypertension
	Renal disease
	Urinary tract infections
	Accidents
	Anoxia of eclampsia
	Anoxia of epilepsy
Infections	Viral infection
	Polio
	Hepatitis
	Syphilis
Genetic	Amniocentesis
Idiopathic	Genetic death
Environmental	Poverty
	Drugs
	Tobacco
	Alcohol
	Nutrition, inadequate
Third trimester	
Anatomic	Malpresentation
	Cord complications
	Placenta previa*
Maternal complications	Hypertension*
	Rh incompatibilities
	Diabetes
	Thyrotoxicosis
Infections	Viral infection*
	Pneumonia
Nutritional	Protein lack
	Iron deficiencies
	Abruptio placentae*
	Antibacterial drugs
Therapeutic to mother	Tetracycline
	Antithryoid drugs
	Corticosteroids
	Anticonvulsants
	Anticoagulants
Conditions peculiar to pregnancy	Hypertensive disease*
	Postmaturity
Fetal complications	Premature rupture of membranes
	Premature labor
	Hydramnios
Environmental	Poverty
	Drugs
	Tobacco
	Alcohol
	Nutrition, inadequate
Labor	
Anatomic	Fetal head compression
	Malpresentation
	Cord prolapse
	Breech presentation
	Placenta previa
	Abruptio placentae
	Rigid soft tissues
	Multiple pregnancy
	Fetal hemorrhage
	Placental or umbilical cord compression
	Excessive fetal size
Physiologic	Dehydration
	Ketosis
	Fetal acidosis
Maternal complications	Eclampsia
Iatrogenic	Sedative depression
	Hypotension of anesthesia
	Anoxia of labor
	Prolonged labor
	Forceps
	Oxytocin
Uterine and placental	Uterine hypotonicity, hypertonicity, inertia
	Placental insufficiency
Environmental	Drugs
	Poverty

Adapted from Fogel, C.I., & Woods, N.F.: Health care of women: a nursing perspective, St. Louis, 1981, The C.V. Mosby Co.
*Associated with intrauterine growth retardation.

Fig. 33.2
Summary of risk factors that may affect pregnancy outcome. (From Fogel, C.I., and Woods, N.F.: Health care of women: a nursing perspective, St Louis, 1981, The C.V. Mosby Co.)

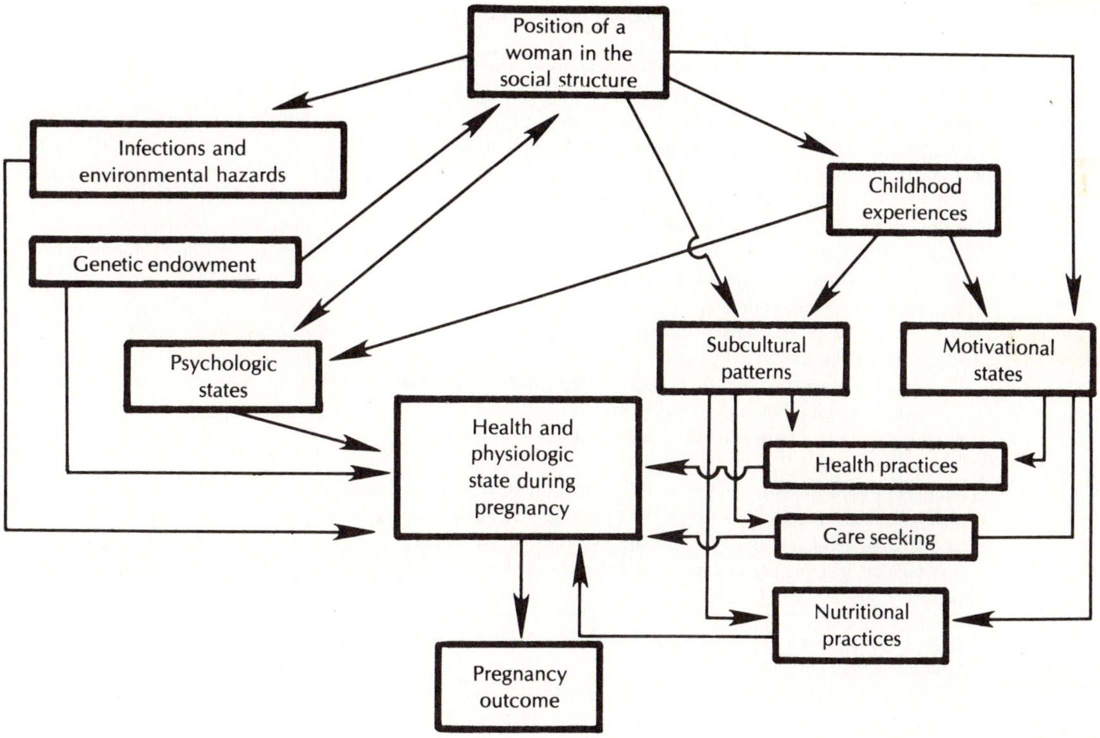

Factors that place the pregnancy and fetus-neonate at high risk are summarized in Table 33.2. The interrelationship of risk factors that influence pregnancy outcome are summarized schematically in Fig. 33.2.

Goals for Care

The goals for care (Table 33.3) are prevention, cure (includes detection), and rehabilitation of threatening maternal and fetal disorders (see Chapter 2). Therefore it is essential to screen those women who are jeopardized (high risk) from those who are not endangered (low risk). The system is only effective when it imposes a relentless search for problems that may threaten the pregnancy during the prenatal, natal, and postdelivery period.

The creative use of the nursing process (see Chapter 3) with childbearing families at high risk must be based on a comprehensive view of their experiences that takes into account the stresses of both the maturational and situational crises they face. *The nurse's actions can influence the health care team to keep the family's childbearing experience in focus rather than concentrate solely on the risk factors.*

Table 33.3
Goals for Care

Goal	Examples of Nursing Actions
Prevention	Health education of people: nutrition, general hygiene (rest, exercise, stress management, cleanliness), signs and symptoms of illness, community resources (clinics, etc.), environmental agents to avoid (drugs/chemicals, communicable disease, x rays)*
	Encouragement for women to keep scheduled appointments
	Development of a caring and trusting relationship with each client and her family
	Following assessment for level of knowledge and readiness to learn, health education regarding expected physical and psychologic changes and expected duration of those changes
Cure	Identification of family history or personal history of biophysical (e.g., genetic disorder), psychologic (e.g., recurrent depression), or social (e.g., poverty) risk factors
	Continuous assessment for detection of risk factors whenever nurse is in contact with childbearing family
	Education of childbearing family, supplemented by written information, regarding signs and symptoms of complications (e.g., visual disturbances, vaginal bleeding) and emergency telephone numbers
	Maintenance of client records
Rehabilitation	Rapid notification of appropriate health team member (e.g., physician, nutritionist, social worker)
	Assisting physician to Explain (and reexplain) problem and its management to woman and family Carry out prescribed therapy (Fig. 33.3) Encourage client cooperation during therapy and follow-up Maintain records
	Maintenance of a trusting and caring relationship with woman and family
	Assisting woman and family to cope with grief associated with being termed *high risk* (a term that some people see as a stigma) or having her fetus considered to be at risk; careful assessment of perceptions, coping mechanisms, and support systems permits nurse to utilize crisis theory (see Chapter 9) as a format for care (see Chapter 34 for details)

*In the broader sense, each nurse participates in prevention through working for legislation and with community efforts to reduce hazards in the environment and to educate the public regarding health maintenance.

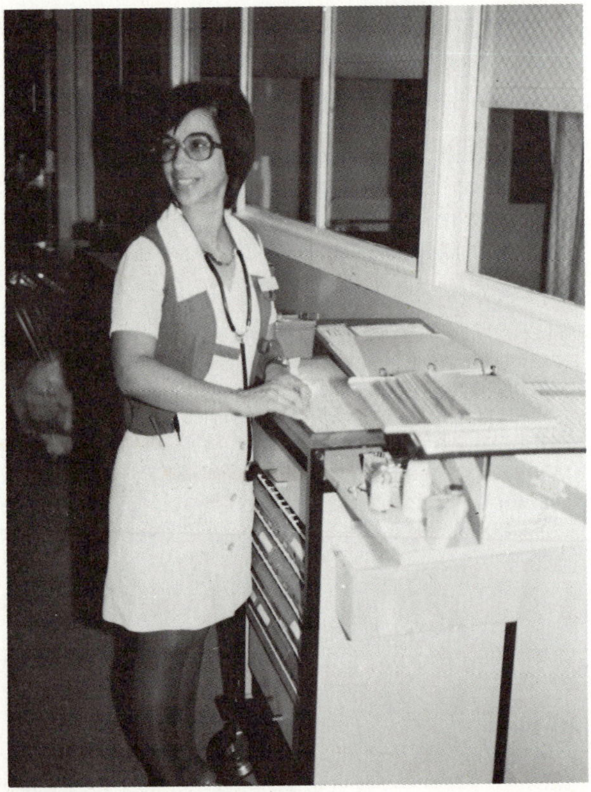

Fig. 33.3
Nurse carefully checks prescribed medication for correct dose per kilogram for 24 hours and route of administration and cross checks against client's known allergies. Following administration, nurse records data on appropriate records and later records client's response to the medication.

Regionalization of Health Care Services

Diagnostic and therapeutic advances during the past decade have resulted in the evolution of new types of facilities for the care of gravidas and neonates at high risk. Newly acquired understandings of pathophysiology of pregnancy-induced conditions and intercurrent disorders as well as of fetal and neonatal problems and the capacity to apply this knowledge clinically required an appropriate setting in which severely ill clients could be managed. Simultaneously, developments in electronics, biochemistry, genetics, and surgical procedures have resulted in the availability of practical methods of identification and monitoring of risk factors. These advances and developments have revolutionized the care of clients at high risk. The need was created for new facilities, reorganization of services, and specially trained personnel in several disciplines who must function together collaboratively if lives were to be saved.

There is excellent evidence that mortality decreases when high risk is identified and intensive care applied. In addition, follow-up studies have shown that serious residual handicaps (physical and mental) of surviving infants have been dramatically reduced.

It is not feasible nor reasonable for each hospital to develop and maintain the full spectrum of medical and nursing specialists, laboratory capabilities, and facilities with equipment. As a consequence, care is being regionalized. That is, all levels of care will be available within a given area, but facilities will be organized to provide different levels of care. A coordinated system within a region first requires the designation of certain hospitals for provision of levels of care based on their capacity to provide the care required. To provide appropriate services and continuity of care for each client, an effective pattern of communication for consultation and for transport of clients is mandatory. Fundamental to all these activities is a regional program for continuing education of personnel.

Ideally, a regionalized system includes primary care and three levels of facilities within a designated geographic area. Level I facilities have three main functions: (1) the management of normal pregnancy, labor, and delivery, (2) the earliest possible identification of high-risk pregnancy and high-risk neonates, and (3) the provision of competent care in the event of unanticipated obstetric or neonatal emergencies.

Level II facilities provide care for a number of maternal and neonatal complications as well as offer a full range of maternity and neonatal care in uncomplicated cases.

Level III facilities, the *regional centers,* have the capacity to manage uncomplicated maternity and neonatal cases and the most complex disorders. In addition, the regional centers provide outreach services, for example, consultation and continuing education for obstetricians, pediatricians, and nurses within the region.

Maternal Health Problems

STATISTICAL PROFILE

Maternal mortality is defined as the number of maternal deaths related to childbearing per 100,000 live births. The maternal mortality rates began to decline dramatically, beginning in the mid 1930s (see p. 11).

Year	Deaths/100,000 Live Births
1940	370.0
1951	82.7
1963	35.8
1974	15.0
1975	12.8
1978	9.6
1980	7.6

Complications of pregnancy, childbirth, or the puerperium account for 0.03 deaths per 1000 deaths.

Different parts of the world have different leading causes of death attributable to pregnancy, but in general the three major causes have persisted for the last 35 years: hypertensive disorders, infection, and hemorrhage.

Causes of Mortality	Percent
Hypertensive disorders	21
Infection	18
Hemorrhage	14
Other (cardiac, diabetes mellitus)	46

In the United States, maternal mortality among white women and all other women still differs, although the gap that existed 30 years ago has been narrowed dramatically. Today the mortality ratio for white women and all others is 2:3. This decline is attributed to changes in social and economic factors and availability of health care.

Many factors have contributed to the decrease in maternal mortality:

1. Advances in medical management (e.g., blood and plasma replacement, fluid and electrolyte balance, asepsis, chemotherapeutics to control infection, anesthesia, and surgical techniques)
2. Expansion of knowledge and capability to apply knowledge
3. Emergence of a philosophy of maternity care that recognizes the advantages of client participation in health care and that focuses on childbirth as a healthy event
4. Acceptance of prenatal care

Hypertensive disorders of pregnancy have replaced hemorrhage as the leading cause of maternal mortality. Chronic hypertension, probably caused by renal disease, makes up one third to one half of the cases of hypertension in pregnancy. Pregnancy-induced hypertension* may affect 6% to 7% of all pregnancies although accurate statistics are not possible at this time. It is discussed in Chapter 35.

Hemorrhage is no longer the major cause of maternal mortality. However, statistical data reflect only the direct cause of death but do not credit predisposing factors. Therefore maternal infection may be listed as the direct cause of death even though hemorrhage was the predisposing factor to the development of the infection. Deaths caused by hemorrhage and infection following abortion have declined significantly since 1973 when passage of federal legislation legalized abortion. Ectopic pregnancy is responsible for 1 out of 12 maternal deaths. Maternal hemorrhage is discussed in Chapter 35.

Puerperal infection (childbed fever) is defined as infection of the genital tract following delivery. Maternal infection throughout the childbearing cycle is the third leading cause of maternal death. Infection is discussed in Chapter 36.

Diabetes mellitus and cardiac disorders contribute to maternal mortality (see Chapter 36). Causes of death that are unrelated to pregnancy include suicide, accidents, and malignant diseases.

Although maternal mortality has decreased for vaginal and cesarean births, the rate for cesarean delivery is still greater (4:1 for primary cesarean delivery and 2:1 for repeat cesarean delivery). Nurses can take an active role in education of the public about the possibility and safety of vaginal delivery following low segment cesarean delivery. There has been no reference in the literature documenting maternal mortality directly attributed to rupture of a lower uterine segment scar. Women seeking vaginal delivery following cesarean delivery need to locate the hospital nearest them that has the staff and facilities to manage their high-risk labor.

Fetal and Neonatal Health Problems

STATISTICAL PROFILE

Fetal death. Fetal death (demise) is defined as the death in utero before complete expulsion of the product of human conception irrespective of the duration of pregnancy and not resulting from therapeutic or elective abortion; intrauterine death.

Neonatal death. Neonatal death is the death of a live-born neonate, that is, a neonate who shows any evidence of life after birth, even if only momentary (respiration, heartbeat, voluntary muscle movement, or pulsation within the umbilical cord), and who dies at 28 days or less.

Perinatal death rate. Perinatal death rate is defined as the sum of fetal and neonatal death rates. This statistic is considered the most sensitive indicator of the effectiveness of perinatal care.

Infant mortality. Infant mortality is defined as the death of a live-born neonate before the first birthday (see p. 11). Infant death rate is expressed as the number of deaths per 1000 live births. There has been a continuous decline in infant mortality:

Year	Rate/1000 Live Births
1940	47.0
1970	20.0
1975	16.1
1976	15.2
1977	14.1
1978	13.8
1979	13.0
1980	12.5
1981	11.7
1982	11.2

The incidence of each cause of infant mortality is expressed as the number of deaths per 100,000 live births. For 1979, the leading causes in the United States were congenital anomalies (257.7), respiratory distress syndrome (155.8), disorders related to preterm birth and low birth weight (100.5), intrauterine hypoxia and birth asphyxia (48.4), pneumonia and influenza (33.1), and birth trauma (31.7).

The infant mortality rate includes the neonatal death rate. Problems related to low birth weight and preterm birth are chiefly responsible for deaths during the first 4 weeks of life.

These statistics are utilized to determine health care needs for the general population. Resources such as funds and facilities are allocated to those segments of the population within a community or to the geographic location of the United States where the needs are the greatest. In addition, the identified causes of mortality are utilized in planning for (1) the type and distribution of health care services (e.g., research, location of regional centers) and (2) the development of curricula for educational programs for health care providers.

*Pregnancy-induced hypertension (PIH) may be referred to in the literature, especially the medical literature, as preeclampsia-eclampsia, toxemia, or acute hypertension.

General Care of the Infant at Risk

The high-risk infant is a sick baby whose intact survival is in jeopardy at the moment he is being considered high risk. Health care must support the high-risk newborn's basic functioning while compensating for his inadequacies and weaknesses. "Normal" values and parameters vary with the infant's level of maturity and his developmental problems. Assessment and therefore supportive care are complicated further by the infant's inability to speak and by his nonspecific, generalized responses to dysfunctional problems. Assessment rests heavily on historical data provided by the mother and obstetric team and on current levels of knowledge related to gestational age and disorders of the neonate. Plan and implementation of the nursing process with the high-risk infant focus on the physiologic maintenance of warmth, respiration, and nutrition.

The care of the high-risk neonate has become highly specialized and beyond the scope of this text.* The following discussion presents general content relevant to the care of the high-risk infant.

Care of infants with selected risk factors is discussed in greater detail in the chapters that follow (e.g., the premature infant is discussed in Chapter 37; the infant of a diabetic mother, Chapter 36; the infant suffering from hyperbilirubinemia and erythroblastosis fetalis, Chapter 40; the infant with a congenital anomaly, Chapter 40; the drug-dependent infant, Chapter 39; and the infant with infection, Chapter 36).

NURSING THE NEONATE WITH RESPIRATORY DISTRESS

Any neonate with respiratory difficulty is in jeopardy.† The infant's response to prompt, appropriate treatment bears a direct relationship to the cause, degree of maturity, and other medical problems.

Breathing is a new experience for the infant. In priority of care, it ranks second only to massive hemorrhage. Because of its high priority and its challenging nursing aspects, considerable space in the delivery room is devoted to the initiation and maintenance of respirations.

The alert nurse often is the pivotal point between functional and dysfunctional survival for the infant in respiratory distress. The nurse's alertness and informed observations place the nurse in a preventive, curative, and rehabilitative role.

*See References and Readings. Most facilities have developed modular study guides and manuals for procedures and for laboratory values and their management.

†See discussion on techniques for suctioning the neonate, oxygen therapy, and resuscitation in Chapter 29.

Goals of care

1. Respirations are maintained.
2. Bronchopulmonary dysplasia and retrolental fibroplasia do not develop.
3. Metabolism meets needs of repair, maintenance, and growth.
4. Respiratory needs of all tissues are met, (e.g., blood gases and acid-base balance are maintained within normal limits).
5. Congenital dysfunctions or anomalies are recognized early, and appropriate treatment is initiated.
6. Parents are able to cope constructively with the situation and to relate to the infant as a person.

Assessment and analysis. The infant in distress at birth is immediately identifiable. In addition, some infants who at birth appear pink and vigorous, with good muscle tone, and whose respiratory rates and rhythms are within normal range, become distressed soon afterward. Respiratory difficulty, with cyanosis and retractions such as occur after aspiration or tension pneumothorax, may appear suddenly. More commonly, respiratory difficulty follows a progressive sequential pattern:

1. The *respiratory rate* initially may increase without a change in rhythm. Flaring of the nares and expiratory grunt are also early signs of respiratory distress.
2. The *apical pulse* increases in rate.
3. *Retractions,* depending on the cause, may begin as subcostal and xiphoid and then progress upward to intercostal, suprasternal, and clavicular retractions (Fig. 33.4).
4. The *color* changes from pink to circumoral pallor, to circumoral cyanosis, and then to generalized cyanosis; acrocyanosis deepens.
5. *Respiratory effort* and deepening distress are indicated by the following (Fig. 33.5):
   a. Chin tug (chin is pulled down [and mouth opens wider] as auxiliary muscles of respiration are activated.)
   b. Abdominal seesaw breathing patterns (Figs. 27.3, 27.4, and 33.5)
   c. Increase in number of apneic episodes
6. If the neonate is hypoxic, the *temperature* may begin to drop. (Avoid rapid warming of the neonate because it may evoke apneic episodes.)

Example of nursing diagnosis. The following is an example of a nursing diagnosis for the neonate with respiratory distress: risk of respiratory distress caused by an obstructed airway.

Plan and implementation

Positioning. The neonate's respiratory efforts must be supported by careful positioning.

1. When the infant is on his back, his arms will be

Fig. 33.4
Retraction: substernal, subcostal, and intercostal retractions are evident. (Courtesy Ross Laboratories, Columbus, Ohio.)

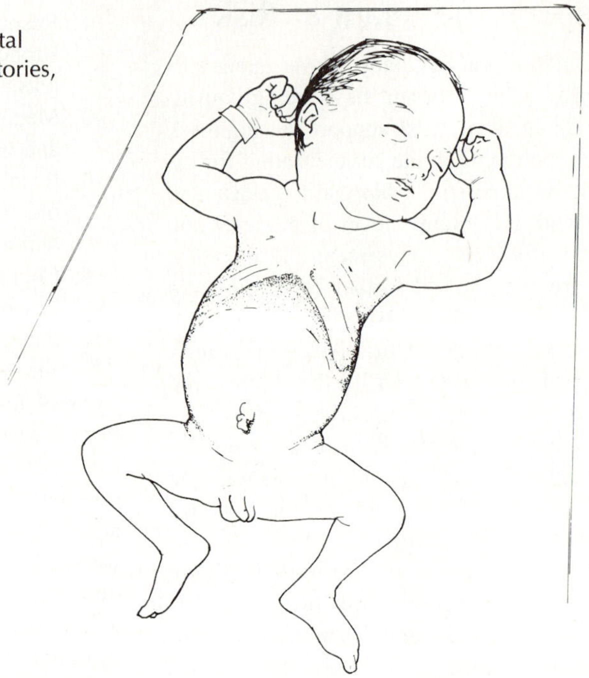

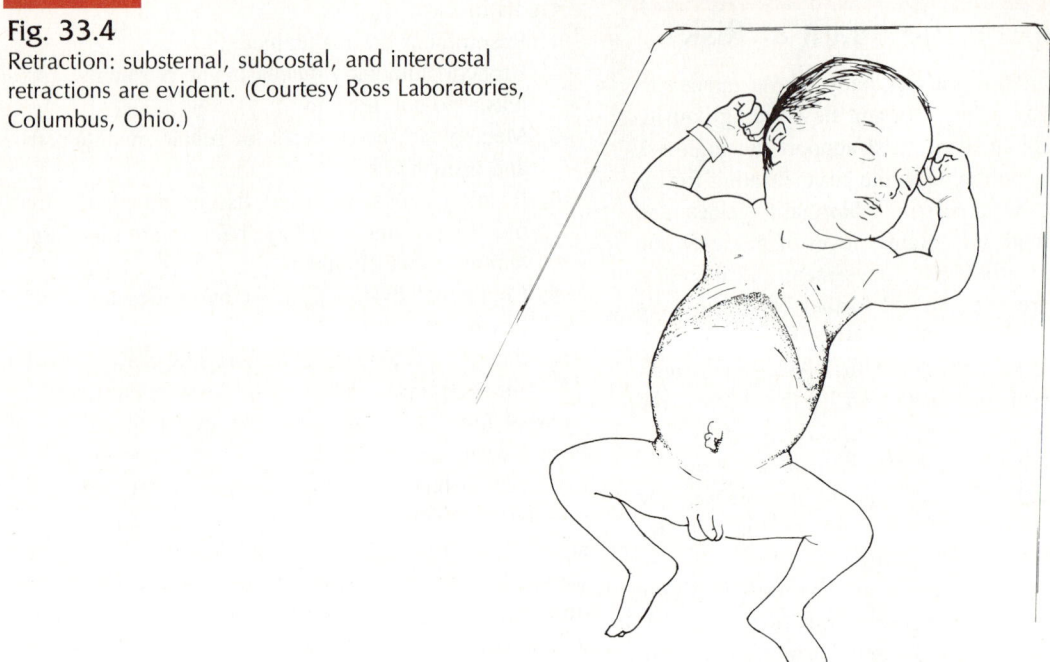

Fig. 33.5
Observation of retractions. Silverman-Anderson index of respiratory distress is determined by grading each of five arbitrary criteria: *grade 0* indicates no difficulty; *grade 1,* moderate difficulty; and *grade 2,* maximal respiratory difficulty. Retraction score is sum of these values; total score of 0 indicates no dyspnea, whereas total score of 10 denotes maximal respiratory distress. (Modified from Silverman, W., and Anderson, D.: Pediatrics **17:**1, 1956.)

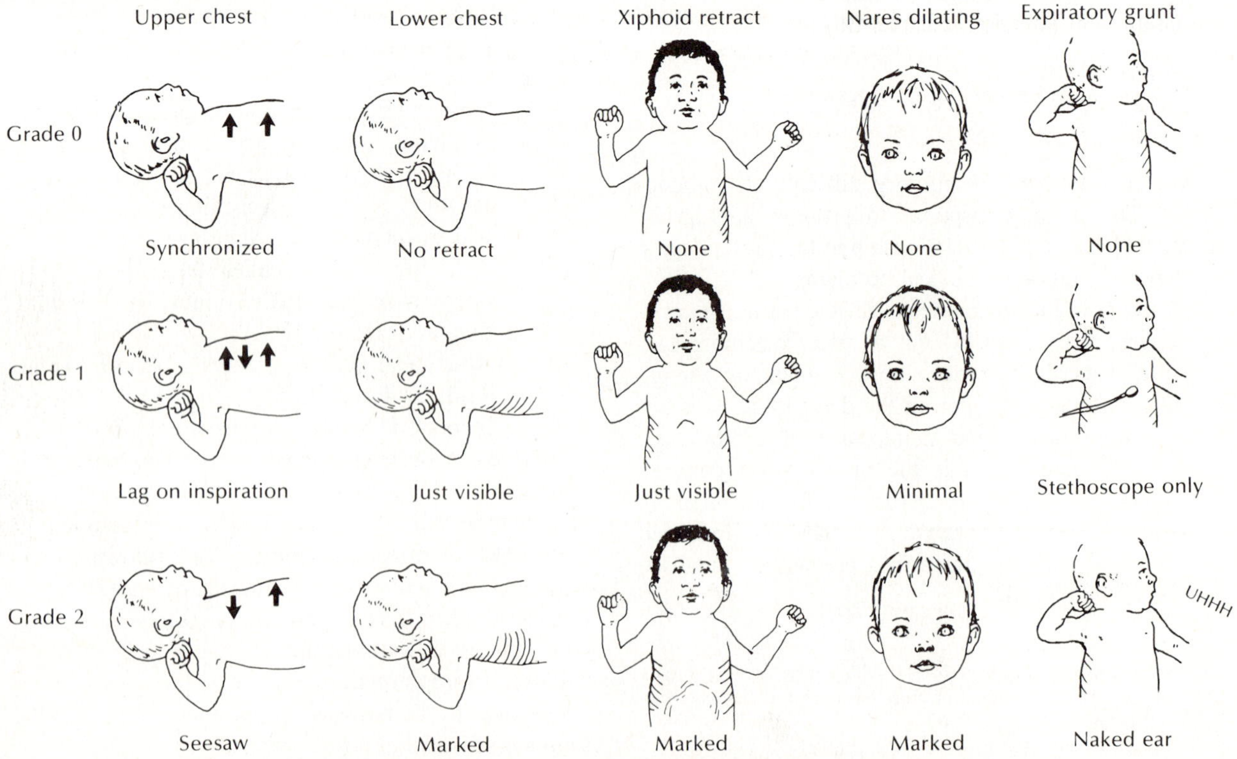

at his side, flexed and slightly abducted. Diapers, if used, must be pinned loosely. (For more detail, see Chapter 29.)

2. The prone position has recently been shown to improve respiratory effort, increase PaO_2, and diminish the work of respiration.

Suctioning. An open airway usually decreases the neonate's labored breathing by improving ventilation. (See discussion of suctioning procedures in Chapter 29.)

Oxygen needs and administration. Oxygen therapy may be lifesaving, but its administration must be carefully monitored as with any drug. Indiscriminate use of oxygen may be hazardous, resulting in retrolental fibroplasia and bronchopulmonary dysplasia. See the discussion on oxygen therapy (Chapter 29), retrolental fibroplasia and pulmonary dysplasia (Chapter 37).

Warmth. A thermoneutral environment is essential for metabolic homeostasis. Cold stress is detrimental to the well-being of any infant but especially the infant at risk. For a discussion of thermogenesis and the prevention of cold stress, see Chapters 27 and 29.

Nutrition. Nutrition of the infant in respiratory distress is as much a challenge for the nurse as for the infant. The extra work of breathing taxes his energy reserves and demands greater caloric input. Breast and bottle feeding are not appropriate for the neonate in distress.

The neonate in severe distress may require gavage feeding exclusively. Parenteral fluids or total parenteral nutrition (TPN) may be required for the neonate who cannot tolerate gavage feedings.

For the convalescent infant in no respiratory distress a softer nipple with an adequate opening is used (e.g., when the bottle is inverted, fluid should drip at 1 drop/sec) (Fig. 33.6). The airway must be cleared before and during feeding as necessary. Moreover, the infant is "bubbled" before feedings.

If the convalescent infant is feeding at the breast, the nurse remains at the bedside with a bulb syringe at hand. This provides reassurance for the mother and avoids a buildup of tension, which might be transferred from mother to infant. Should the infant gag or choke, the nurse can show the mother how to manage such a situation.

Evaluation. The nurse is assured that care was effective if the goals of care are met.

Oxygen therapy. Oxygen therapy seen frequently in the normal newborn nursery is discussed in Chapter 29.

Continuous positive airway pressure. Continuous positive airway pressure (CPAP) is most commonly administered through nasal prongs or an endotracheal tube (oral or nasal) (Fig. 33.7). The purposes of this technique include the following:

Fig. 33.6
Nurse offers prescribed formula in feeding method appropriate to neonate. Neonate's response to formula and feeding method is carefully assessed and recorded. This information is shared with parent or parents. Feeding also provides social interaction to be enjoyed by nurse as well as baby.

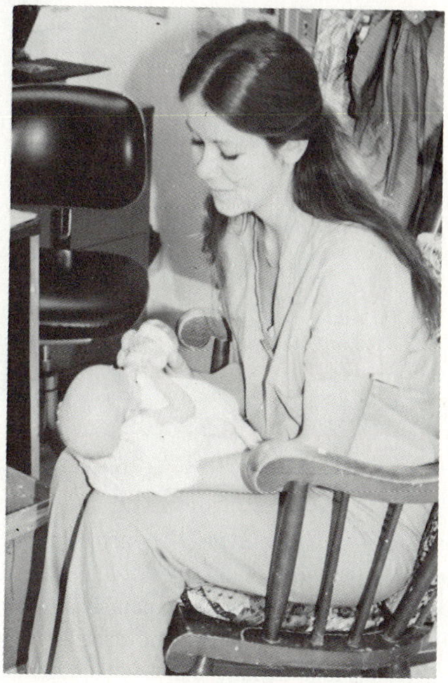

1. Employs same principle as the expiratory grunt (The expiratory grunt is a physiologic adaptation to trap air within the lungs, keeping alveoli open to prevent atelectasis on expiration.)
2. Increases functional residual capacity
3. Improves oxygenation
4. Decreases pulmonary shunting

Transcutaneous oxygen tension monitoring. Older methods of monitoring arterial oxygenation in the ill neonate involved such invasive techniques as umbilical artery catheterization and radial and temporal artery puncture or catheterization. Oxygen electrodes placed intravascularly to achieve continuous monitoring of arterial oxygenation did not meet with success in recent years.

Today accurate noninvasive transcutaneous (tc) oxygen tension ($tcPo_2$) monitoring is feasible on a continuous basis. The $tcPo_2$ electrode is applied according to the manufacturer's instructions. However, all electrodes are applied to a hairless and greaseless site, and an airtight contact with the skin is secured. The electrode ap-

Fig. 33.7
High-risk neonate (under heat lamp not shown). Note CPAP, eye patches (infant is receiving phototherapy), probe *(left)* for heartbeat, probe *(right)* for respirations, umbilical catheter from three-way stopcock, and syringe filled with heparinized saline. Note enlarged labia characteristic of premature neonate. Thermistor probe shown should not be near right shoulder. Thermistor probes for Servo-Control should properly be placed in right upper quadrant of abdomen just below inferior costal margin.

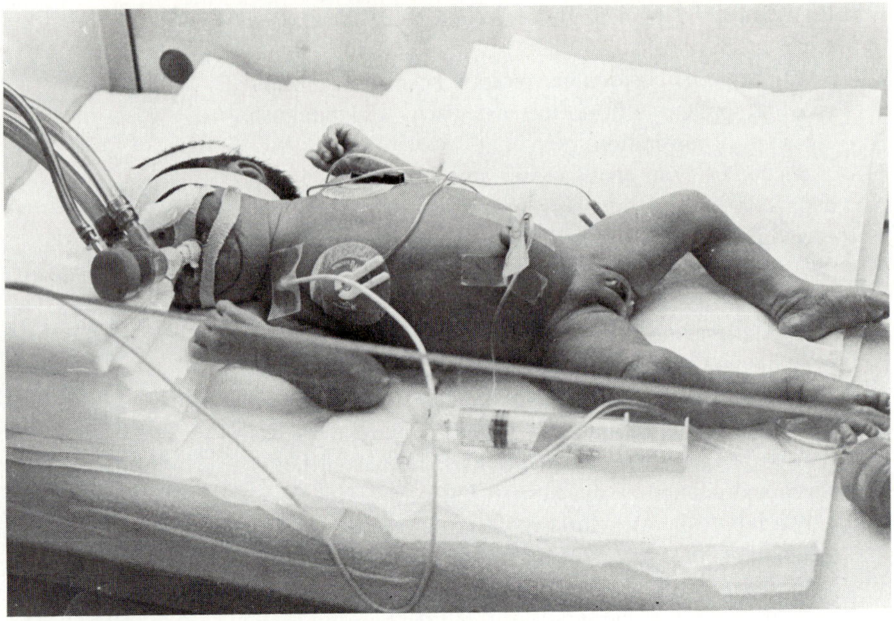

plication site is changed every 4 hours to avoid burns. The distinct advantage of this method is that the data are available on a moment-to-moment basis; for example, complications can be identified early, and the efficiency of respiratory therapy can be evaluated readily.

Weaning from oxygen therapy. The techniques and rationale for weaning the infant from oxygen therapy are as follows:

Technique	Rationale
1. Weaning process is gradual.	1. The hazards of sudden cyanosis and respiratory collapse become greater with increased time that infant has received O_2 therapy.
2. Decrease by 10% every 30 to 60 minutes (or 2 to 4 hours) as child improves.	2. Too rapid weaning with hypoxia can reopen right-to-left shunts: foramen ovale, ductus arteriosus.
3. Monitor laboratory values simultaneously: blood pH, PaO_2,* $PaCO_2$, arterial hemoglobin concentration.	3. Provides data for modifying rate of weaning process.
4. Observe infant closely for following: a. Pulse b. Respiratory effort c. Skin color If these symptoms occur, increase oxygen and proceed with slower weaning schedule.	4. Avoids adverse reactions to weaning. a. Pulse elevation b. Respiratory distress c. Cyanosis

*Blood gas values are given in Appendix I. Hospital intensive care units have protocols for care based on blood gas findings.

TEMPERATURE SUPPORT AND REGULATION

Goals of care

1. Skin temperature is maintained between 36.1° and 36.7° C (97° to 98° F).*
2. No apneic spells occur.
3. Adequate weight is gained.
4. Sequelae of cold stress (i.e., sclerema, oxygen deprivation to tissues, metabolic acidosis, hypoglycemia, abnormal blood gases, and dysfunction of CNS) do not develop.

Assessment and analysis

1. Monitor infant's temperature (see Chapter 29)
   a. Overhead radiant heat source with thermistor probe to skin

*See discussions on techniques for regulating warmth and humidity in infant's environment and for maintaining thermoneutral environment in Chapter 29.

b. Servo-Control incubator
   (1) Thermistor probe taped to skin
   (2) Thermometer on incubator wall
c. Anal (core) temperature
d. Axillary temperature
e. Coolness or warmth to touch of infant's body and extremities

2. Observe for physiologic signs of cold stress
   a. In stronger, more mature infant: increased physical activity, crying
   b. Increased respiratory rate
   c. Color change
      (1) Deepening acrocyanosis
      (2) Appearance of generalized cyanosis
      (3) Mottling of skin (cutis marmorata)
   d. In male with descended testes, activated cremasteric reflex (On exposure to cold, testes are pulled back up into inguinal canal.)

Example of nursing diagnosis. The following is an example of a nursing diagnosis relative to temperature support and regulation: risk of cold stress caused by physiologic immaturity of infant.

Plan and implementation

1. Nursing care should be planned and implemented to prevent or minimize cold stress.
   a. Quickly dry newborn infant in warm, absorbent blanket, taking particular care to dry and cover head (one fourth of body length). (If infant is of good weight and in good condition, he may be given to mother to hold.) Prevent cold air from blowing over face; receptors in facial skin are exquisitely sensitive to cold.
   b. Place the wrapped infant in a warm incubator, Kreiselman, or other heated carrier. Infant may be placed unwrapped under radiant heat source.
   c. All procedures and observations when infant is unwrapped are done in incubator, under radiant heat, on warm surface, etc.
   d. All surfaces and materials touching infant are warm.
   e. Caretakers' hands should be warm when handling neonate.
   f. O_2 or air administered to infant is warmed.
2. Maintain equipment in excellent operative condition. Know procedures and rationale for procedures.
   a. Maintain abdominal skin temperature at 36.1° to 36.7° C (97° to 98° F), axillary temperature at 36.5° C (97.8° F). Report any rise in temperature over 37.3° C (99° F) or a drop of 0.6° to 1° C (1° to 2° F).
   b. Equipment is plugged in and operative. Thermostat is set on control panel. Probe is in contact with skin. Portholes and lid are closed. Incubator is placed away from windows, air-conditioning units, etc.
   c. Know procedures for anal and axillary temperature taking (see pp. 580 and 611).
   d. Place bassinet away from drafts or sources of heat or cold. Take temperatures by thermometer periodically to check accuracy of equipment.
3. Alter environment to return infant to desired body temperature if infant's temperature is too low or too high.
   a. Check and readjust thermostat setting as necessary. Is equipment plugged into electrical outlet?
   b. Check and reapply probe as necessary. Wet or detached probe may lead to hyperthermia.
   c. Are portholes closed? open? Is sleeve off track (on incubators with plastic sleeve covers)?
   d. Increase or decrease amount of clothing and blankets as necessary.
   e. Lighting: If gooseneck lamp is directly over infant, it may increase his temperature.
   f. Check placement of incubators, cribs, etc.
   g. Use different thermometer.

Evaluation. The nurse can be assured that care was effective if the goals of care are met.

NUTRITION AND ELIMINATION

General considerations. Low–birth weight neonates make up the largest number of high-risk infants. Of these, about one third are small for gestational age (SGA) regardless of maturity, whereas about two thirds are preterm and appropriate for gestational age. SGA neonates may also be preterm.

The feeding and nutrition of the high-risk infant warrant careful consideration. The extent to which nutritional needs are met is directly related to the infant's immediate and long-range well-being. For example, if the full-term, low–birth weight (SGA) (dysmature) infant with low glycogen stores is not fed promptly, the resultant symptomatic or asymptomatic hypoglycemia may seriously damage his carbohydrate-dependent brain cells.

The preterm infant often suffers several physiologic handicaps that increase in severity as gestational age decreases (Table 33.1).

Early feeding. Early feeding, within 6 to 8 hours of birth of term, nonstressed neonates (earlier in preterm infants), either orally or parenterally, is necessary for the following reasons:

- To prevent dehydration
- To spare the available stores of glycogen

- To maintain blood glucose levels
- To lessen initial weight loss
- To keep serum bilirubin levels within normal limits
- To curtail protein catabolism that would result in metabolic acidosis, hyperkalemia, or elevated BUN levels
- To conserve energy for growth
- To stimulate sucking response

Early feeding is avoided if the neonate had low Apgar scores. Early feeding of asphyxiated neonates may be an important cause of necrotizing enterocolitis (NEC) (see p. 927).

Nutritional requisites. Caloric, nutrient, and fluid requirements of the infant at risk may be greater for many reasons, some of which follow:

1. Limited stores—preterm or dysmature (malnourished) neonate
2. Depleted stores—neonate who is stressed by one or a combination of the following factors:
   a. Birth asphyxia
   b. Increased respirations or respiratory effort
   c. Insensible fluid loss by evaporation when infant is under radiant heat or during phototherapy
   d. Hypothermic environment
3. Immature systems
   a. Gastrointestinal tract—losses through vomiting, diarrhea, dysfunctional absorption
   b. Kidneys—losses caused by inability to concentrate urine and maintain an adequate rate of urea excretion and by an inadequate response to antidiuretic hormone (ADH)
4. Growth demands—because preterm neonate's growth rate approximates fetal growth rate during the last trimester, which is two or more times that of an infant after delivery at term

Weight and fluid loss. Up to 85% of the preterm neonate's body weight consists of water, most of which occupies the extracellular fluid compartment. Even with early fluid and nutritional intake, the preterm infant's weight and fluid losses seem exaggerated. Factors predisposing to weight and fluid losses include the following:

1. Inadequate fluid intake (e.g., from delayed administration or insufficient volume) predisposes the infant to weight loss.

2. Insensible water loss (IWL) represents evaporative losses that occur largely through the skin. Approximately 30% of this IWL is from the respiratory tract, and most of this is prevented by humidified oxygen–enriched gases that are used for respiratory support in sick infants. Total IWL ranges anywhere from 1.75 to 3.6 ml/kg/hr. The quantity is influenced by gestational age, postnatal age, weight, and use of radiant warmer or incubator and other factors.

3. Greater fluid demands to meet increased cellular metabolic processes (e.g., from stress, repair, or growth) predispose the neonate to weight and fluid losses.

The limits of acceptable weight loss are as follows: During the neonate's first 3 days of extrauterine life, the preterm infant can lose 12% or less of birth weight. For the term infant, a weight loss of 10% or less is acceptable for neonates of normal weight for gestational age; weight loss of 15% or less is acceptable for infants weighing 4500 g (9 lb 14 oz) or more. For dysmature SGA infants, a loss of 5% or less of birth weight is acceptable.

After the first 3 days, a preterm neonate's loss or gain during each 24-hr period should not exceed 2% of the previous day's weight.

The following examples illustrate how to calculate weight loss and gain, suggesting causes and nursing actions for each case.

EXAMPLE 1

Day 4 1750 g
Day 5 1730 g
20 g loss

$$\frac{20}{1750} = \frac{x\%}{100\%}$$
$$1750x = 2000$$
$$1750\overline{)2000.00} = 1.1\%$$
$$x = 1.1\% \text{ weight loss}$$

Probable causes: Stool passage
Inadequate fluid: amount and type

Nursing actions: Record and report.
Observe infant.
Perform Dextrostix test.

EXAMPLE 2

Day 4 1750 g
Day 5 1790 g
40 g gain

$$\frac{40}{1750} = \frac{x\%}{100\%}$$
$$1750x = 4000$$
$$1750\overline{)4000.0} = 2.3$$
$$x = 2.3\% \text{ gain}$$

Probable causes: Overfeeding
Fluid retention

Nursing actions: Record and report.
Observe neonate for other symptoms.
Collect urine in bag: check amount, specific gravity.
Perform Dextrostix test.

EXAMPLE 3

Day 4 1750 g
Day 5 1715 g
35 g loss

$$\frac{35}{1750} = \frac{x\%}{100\%}$$
$$1750x = 3500$$
$$1750\overline{)3500.0} = 2.0$$
$$x = 2\% \text{ weight loss}$$

Probable causes: Excessive stooling, voiding
Excessive evaporative losses
Inadequate amount and type of fluid
Malabsorption problem

Nursing actions: Record and report.
Check incubator and infant for temperature; check incubator for humidity.
Observe neonate for other symptoms.
Collect urine in bag: check urine for amount and specific gravity; use Clinistix.
Perform Dextrostix test.

Formula and feeding schedules. The formula and feeding schedule of the infant at risk are based on the following criteria:

1. Infant's birth weight and pattern of weight gain or loss
2. Estimated gestational age
3. Physical condition: pharyngeal coordination (sucking, swallowing reflexes are present and coordinated), fatigability, malformations, amount of urine excreted per hour
4. Laboratory values: nitrogen balance, electrolyte imbalance, glucose level, serum bilirubin level, and other results

The following variants influence the feeding of the infant at risk:

1. Fluid volume given
2. Caloric requirements
3. Mode of feeding
4. Formula: predigested, breast milk, calories per ounce

Parenteral fluids and total parenteral nutrition. The very small neonate or the neonate who is unable to suck because of developmental or respiratory problems (especially the infant on assisted ventilation) is sustained by parenteral infusions. The electrolytes and nutrients per milliliter, as well as the milliliters of fluid per kilogram of body weight per hour, are carefully calculated by the physician. The nurse monitors the functioning of infusion equipment (tubing, infusion pump), ensures asepsis, secures and protects the needle (catheter) at the insertion site, and assesses and records the neonate's responses.

Weaning from parenteral therapy. As the infant's condition improves, the infant may be offered fluids by nipple. As the amount of feeding given orally is increased and tolerated, the amount given by infusion is decreased.

Oral preparations. The nurse assists in assessing the neonate's tolerance for oral feeding by noting the following:

- Pharyngeal coordination (suck and swallow reflexes present and synchronized)
- Presence and degree of respiratory distress or apneic episodes if any
- Presence of bowel sounds and absence of abdominal distention
- Gastric residual of 2 ml or less before feeding

Various milk formulas are available. These formulas vary in calories, protein, and mineral content (see p. 661). Formulas are fed by nipple, gavage, or both. Each neonate must be evaluated for his ability to handle solute and fluid load.

Oral feedings begin with sterile water. Feedings are advanced by increasing the amount of fluid *or* the number of calories per 30 ml (1 oz) at any one feeding, and the neonate's tolerance is observed. For infants weighing less than approximately 1800 g (4 lb) the feedings are advanced more slowly. Too rapid advancement may lead to the following:

1. Vomiting, diarrhea, abdominal distention
2. Apneic episodes
3. Residual feeding of 2 ml or more at the time of the next feeding
4. Retention of fluid with cardiopulmonary embarrassment or marked diuresis with loss of sodium (Na^+), leading to hyponatremia
5. Regurgitation—aspiration pneumonia

Goals of care

1. Feeding and nutrition of the high-risk neonate are accomplished with the following results:
   a. Minimal respiratory distress; no aspiration or aspiration pneumonia
   b. Minimal expenditure of energy
   c. Hypoglycemic reactions avoided
   d. Acceptable fluid-electrolyte balance maintained
   e. No abdominal distention
   f. No trauma to tissues of the gastrointestinal tract
   g. No diarrhea
2. Sucking satisfaction maximized
3. Nutrition sufficient to accomplish the following:
   a. Meet resting metabolic requirements
   b. Provide sufficient energy to perform physical activity
   c. Counter losses through gastrointestinal and urinary tracts
   d. Supply constituents for growth (The infant establishes a steady pattern of weight gain appropriate for him.)
4. Parent-child relationship fostered in the following ways:
   a. Parent: begins to participate in the feeding process in light of the infant's physical capabilities and the parent's desired degree of involvement
   b. Infant: begins to associate feeding and eating with pleasure as he develops a sense of trust
   c. At discharge: parents are comfortable with the feeding method needed by the infant, whether feeding is by breast, bottle, gavage, or gastrostomy

Assessment and analysis

1. Weight plotted on growth grid
   a. On admission
   b. Daily: weight loss or rate of weight gain
2. Elimination patterns
   a. Frequency of urination
   b. Amount, frequency, and character of stool
      (1) Obstipation or constipation or both
      (2) Diarrhea
      (3) Loss of fats (steatorrhea)
3. Oral feedings*
   a. Type of formula; calories/30 ml (1 oz)
   b. Volume
   c. Behavior during feeding
      (1) Attempts at sucking
      (2) Abdominal distention (Fig. 33.8)
      (3) Vomiting, regurgitation
      (4) Cyanosis
      (5) Amount of mucus
   d. Time necessary to feed
4. Gavage feedings*
   a. Observe as for oral feedings
   b. Order feeding tube of correct size; use nasogastric or orogastric route

*See discussions relevant to feeding, nutrition, and elimination in Chapter 30.

Fig. 33.8
Sudden abdominal distention. (Courtesy Ross Laboratories, Columbus, Ohio.)

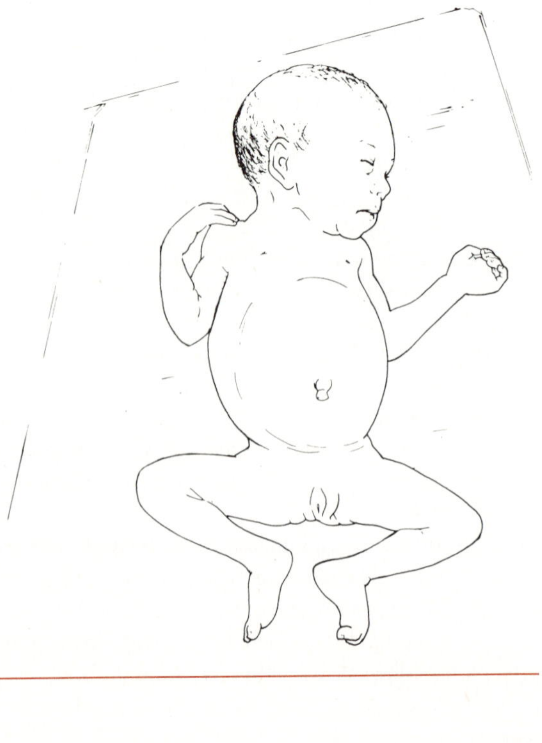

5. Abdominal distention
   a. Note time, degree, and effect on respiratory system
   b. Assist with x-ray examination
6. Vomiting or regurgitation or both
   a. Note color, amount, time in relation to feeding, and character (e.g., forceful? spill over?)
   b. Pass nasogastric tube for diagnosis as necessary
7. Parenteral fluids: type, rate per minute, infusion site
8. Total parenteral nutrition (TPN) (alimentation): assess per hospital protocol

Examples of nursing diagnoses

1. Risk of hypoglycemia because of low birth weight
2. Risk of respiratory embarrassment because of sudden abdominal distention

Plan and implementation

1. Readjust feeding (or infusion) to achieve acceptable weight gain.

2. Record observations accurately. Deviations from normal range in weight losses or gains guide future diagnostic evaluations to determine cause and treatment.

3. Readjust nursing care regarding continuation of gavage feedings, attempting oral feedings, providing simultaneous sucking satisfaction as soon as possible (before tenth day of life, gavage through nipple if necessary) (see p. 755), type and amount of formula, and frequency of feedings.

4. If infant is taking oral feeding, readjust nursing care regarding type of nipple (''preemie,'' regular, breast).

5. Avoid overfeeding: evaluate by checking amount of residual before subsequent feeding; refeed residual and subtract this amount from this feeding; decrease amount of feeding; feed more frequently.

6. Burp or ''bubble'' infant as necessary; readjust positioning during feeding.

7. Determine when to involve mother or father in actual feeding or when to teach parents how to give gavage feedings if child will need them after going home.

Evaluation. The nurse is assured that care is effective if the goals of care are met.

Nasogastric tube feeding. An indwelling nasogastric tube with continuous flow of formula supplied by an infusion pump is the method of choice for the infant who is (1) compromised by respiratory distress, (2) immature or has a weak suck or uncoordinated sucking-swallowing behavior, or (3) easily fatigued even when using a ''preemie'' nipple.

Necessary equipment for either the nasal or oral route includes the following:

1. Sterile feeding tube: rubber or plastic, rounded tip, sizes 5 to 10, infant lengths

2. Clearly calibrated syringe for feeding
3. Stethoscope and sterile medication syringe without needle
4. Sterile water for lubrication
5. Feeding formula
6. Medications

Tests for correct placement of feeding tube. Fortunately the infant's anatomy makes it difficult to enter his trachea. One or more of the following tests are done to determine correct stomach placement.

1. Use sterile syringe to inject 0.5 cc of air through catheter into stomach. Simultaneously, listen for sound of air bubbling or ''growling'' in stomach with stethoscope over epigastric region.

2. The most complete procedure involves listening with stethoscope first over the epigastrium and then on each side of the anterior chest. The sound of rushing air heard over the anterior chest should be of considerably diminished intensity compared to that heard over the epigastrium.

3. Aspirate small amount of stomach contents. Fill tube with stomach contents, and pinch off tube; add syringe containing feeding. This avoids allowing air into stomach with feeding.

Oral insertion: intermittent or indwelling catheter

Technique	Rationale
1. Position infant: head of mattress up one notch, folded towel under shoulders to slightly extend neck.	1. Opens oropharynx. Extends and straightens esophagus.
2. Select size 8 French feeding tube.	2. Is adequate size for feeding. Less apt to fold over or curl up.
3. Measure distance between bridge of nose and lower end of xiphoid process. Mark distance with 5 cm (2 in) thin strip of paper tape. Fold tape over tube, leaving two long ends with which to secure tube when it is in place.	3. Determines length necessary to reach into stomach without folding back on itself. Facilitates anchoring tubing, if it is to be indwelling. Paper tape is usually less irritating to skin.
4. Lubricate tube in sterile water.	4. Prevents trauma and infection.
5. Pass tube along base of tongue, advancing it into esophagus as infant swallows.	5. Offers less risk of vagal stimulation or of accidental entry into trachea. Stimulates esophageal peristalsis and opens cardiac sphincter.
6. Test placement of tube.	6. Avoids introduction of formula, vitamins, and medicines into trachea or esophagus.
7. Aspirate and measure any residual in stomach. If 1 ml or less, subtract same amount from this feeding. If more than 1 ml, physician may wish to have this feeding skipped.	7. Avoids overfeeding. Excessive fluid in stomach suggests intestinal obstruction.
8. Slowly pour warmed formula into syringe barrel and allow it to flow by gravity into stomach: hold reservoir 15 to 20 cm (6 to 8 in) above infant's head. If gravity flow is too rapid, lower syringe, or insert plunger into syringe, and inject *slowly*. Feeding time should approximate that of nipple feedings (20 minutes or about 1 ml/min).	8. Rapid entry of formula into stomach causes rapid rebound response with regurgitation, thus increasing danger of aspiration or abdominal distention, which compromises respiratory effort.
9. Do not allow level of formula to go below neck of syringe.	9. Prevents entry of air into stomach to minimize risks of regurgitation and distention.
10. Observe infant's response.	10. Prevents respiratory distress. Assists gastrointestional functioning.
11. Follow formula with specified amount of sterile water.	11. Gets all formula into stomach and clears tubing of formula.
12. Pinch tubing (or clamp it off) and withdraw it rapidly.	12. Prevents entry of air into stomach. Creates vacuum to hold fluid in tubing to prevent dripping it into trachea on withdrawal.
13. Burp or bubble infant. With left hand, support infant's head and shoulders.	13. Increases comfort. Prevents regurgitation.

Technique	Rationale
Raise to a sitting position and lean infant onto right hand. Right hand supports infant's chest with palm and his jaw with thumb and forefinger. Gently rub his back with left hand.	
14. Position on right side with small rolled drape or towel.	14. Facilitates stomach emptying.
15. Record following: a. Amount of residual b. Type and amount of feeding, medicine c. Time of feeding d. Infant response: fatigue, peaceful sleep, abdominal distention, respiratory distress, type and amount of vomiting or regurgitation; heart and respiratory rate	15. Provides basis for evaluation and readjustment of feeding regiman. Facilitates communication among personnel.

Nasal route: intermittent or indwelling catheter

Technique	Rationale
1. Position as for oral route (Fig. 33.9).	1. Opens oropharynx. Extends and straightens esophagus.
2. Select size 3½ to 5 French feeding tube.	2. Is adequate size for feeding and small enough to allow breathing space around it, since neonates are obligate nose breathers.
a. If indwelling, change every 2 or 3 days (48 to 72 hours) or more frequently if otitis is present, alternating sides of nares.	a. Prevents infection, irritation; excess mucus, ulceration, bleeding.
b. Observe infant for respiratory distress.	b. If tube causes distress, remove it. Use oral route.
c. May be preferred route for indwelling tube for continuous drip feeding.	c. Very small preterm infant often tolerates feeding better by continuous drip; stomach is not overloaded.
3. Measure distance from bridge of nose to xiphoid process (just beyond tip of sternum). Mark spot with 5 cm (2 in) thin strip of paper tape, and overlap tube, leaving ends free	3. Provides adequate length to reach stomach without curling. Facilitates anchoring of tubing. Decreases risk of skin irritation from tape.
4. Lubricate with sterile water.	4. Prevents tissue trauma.
5. Insert tube, holding it horizontally until it reaches back of nares; then lift tubing slightly and continue to advance. Allow infant to swallow tube down while it is being advanced.	5. Accommodates to bend in back of nares and minimizes direct tissue damage. Stimulates peristalsis and opens cardiac sphincter.
6 to 15. Same as for oral route.	6 to 15. Same as for oral route.

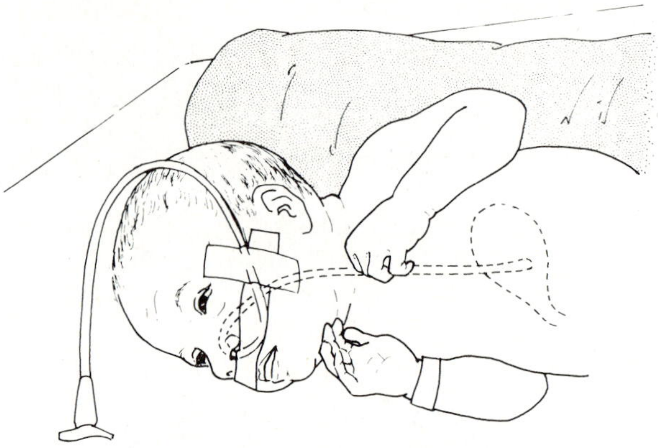

Fig. 33.9
Indwelling gavage tube: nasal route. Infant is propped on his right side to facilitate emptying of stomach. Note rolled towel for support.

Nursing care after feedings. Burp the infant gently after feedings. Turn his head or position him on right side after feeding and burping. In addition, postpone postural drainage and percussion for a minimum of 1 hour after feeding.

Avoid feeding the infant within an hour before a laboratory test for blood glucose.

Fig. 33.10
A, Venipuncture of scalp vein. **B,** With paper cup to protect venipuncture site.

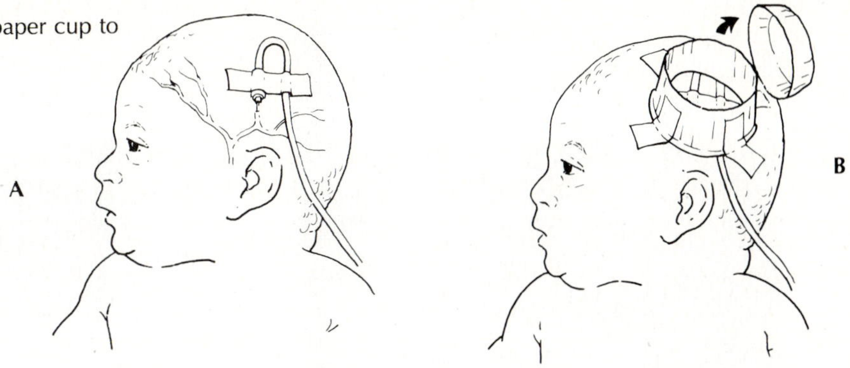

Monitoring parenteral fluid administration. For parenteral fluid administration one needs equipment to start and/or maintain intravenous therapy by way of a peripheral vein, venous cutdown, or umbilical catheter.

In addition, the following supplies are needed to prevent accidental overhydration:

1. Bottles containing 250 ml of infusion fluid
2. Administration sets with enclosed reservoirs and minidropper
3. Infusion pump with automatic alarm to signal an empty fluid chamber
4. Application of medicine cup (paper) or other applicance to protect insertion site (Fig. 33.10)

The technique and rationale of parenteral fluid administration follow:

Technique	Rationale
1. Prepare equipment.	1. Avoids searching for missing articles after procedure has begun.
2. Restrain infant.	2. For infant's safety and increased ease of starting parenteral fluids.
3. Provide pacifier to infant if appropriate.	3. Provides comfort for the infant who can handle a pacifier.
4. Continue care of intravenous infusion. Regulate rate of flow.	4. For adequate infusion.
a. Infusion pump: check setting; double-check by counting drops per minute every hour, and note amount infused every 4 hours.	a. Assures a more accurate and constant flow rate. Double-checks for equipment malfunction.
b. Reposition extremity or infant's head.	b. Assures proper body alignment and prevents breakdown of skin. Protects infusion site.
c. *Do not* make up deficiency or excess by changing rate of flow without consulting physician.	c. Fluid may overload infant's system. If infant has received more than prescribed amount for period, he must be assessed for overhydration and cardiac decompensation.
5. Check infusion site every hour.	5. Prevents trauma to tissues. Assures adequate hydration. Possible complications:
a. Check for tissue infiltration (swelling).	a. Infection
b. Check for tissue trauma: color, temperature.	b. Thrombophlebitis
c. If needle is in extremity, compare and contrast with other extremity.	c. Tissue and vein trauma (Fig. 33.11)
d. If needle is in scalp vein, check head and face for symmetry of contour and movement.	d. Needle out of vein with injection of fluid into surrounding tissues and possible tissue breakdown

Fig. 33.11
A, Intravenous infiltration in small infant can cause severe ischemia. **B,** Fortunately, preterm infant has remarkable regeneration abilities (same hand 1 week later). (Courtesy Mount Zion Hospital and Medical Center, San Francisco.)

A 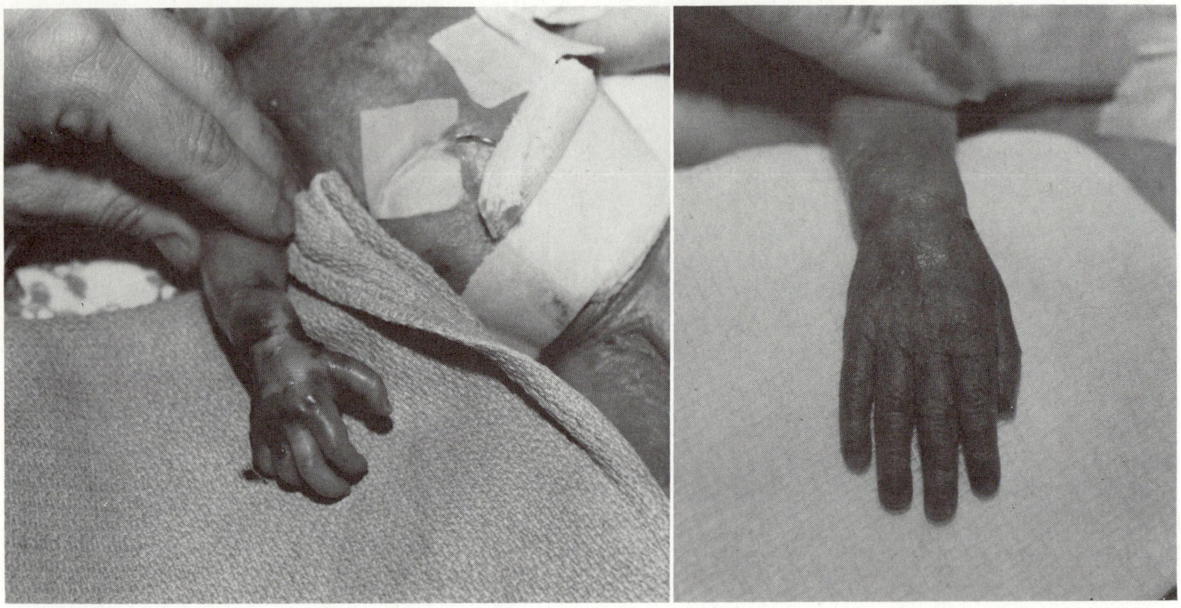 B

Technique	Rationale
6. Evaluate infant's hydration every hour.	6. Determines adequate rate of flow.
a. Urinary output: Collect or weigh diapers.	a. Assesses amount of urine excreted.
b. Specific gravity of urine (see p. 1027, Appendix I). See p. 645 for use of urine collectors.	b. Assists in assessing appropriate solute or fluid infant needs and kidney function.
c. Weight: Infant may be weighed every 8, 12, or 24 hours.	c. Weight gain or loss greater than 3% of body weight within a 24-hr period is cause for concern.
d. Urine: Check for glucose every 8 to 24 hours.	d. Presence of excess glucose in the urine would indicate an excessive glucose load in the intravenous fluid.
e. Other: tissue turgor; fever; sunken fontanels; soft, sunken eyeballs; or behavior changes may be present.	e. Assesses state of hydration.
7. Record the following:	7. Provides complete data.
a. Type of fluid being used	a. Evaluates treatment.
b. Amount of fluid absorbed every hour and amount scheduled to have been absorbed	b. Meets infant's changing needs.
c. Amount of fluid in bottle or fluid chamber	c. Identifies possible cause of any existing or new problem.
d. Flow rate	d. Provides base line for continuation at present rate or change in rate.

Technique	Rationale
e. Infant's condition	e. Indicates infant's response to this regimen and readiness for progression.
8. Change intravenous tubing and bottle every 24 hours.	8. Decreases possibility of infection.
9. Irrigate intravenously.	9. Maintains patency of system.
a. Three-way stopcock may be used to connect tubing to needle.	a. Facilitates flushing needle while decreasing chance of contamination and loss of blood during procedure.
b. Without three-way stopcock, clamp intravenous tubing and disconnect at junction with needle. Keep tubing end sterile. Attach syringe containing 1 to 3 ml of normal saline solution or heparinized saline solution to needle.	b. Clears out small occluding clots; prevents formation of clots.
c. *Slowly* inject fluid into vein. Disconnect syringe and reconnect to intravenous tubing. Unclamp intravenous tubing and regulate flow of infusion.	c. Prevents trauma to vein or dislodging the needle.
10. After intravenous fluid is discontinued:	10. Ensures adequate nutrition and hydration.
a. Observe infant for hypoglycemia for 24 hours.	a. Hypoglycemia often is seen after discontinuation of parenteral therapy.
b. Observe infant for adequacy of nutrition and hydration.	b. Assesses infant's ability to take and utilize nutrients and fluids by mouth or gavage.
c. Continue to assess infant for thrombophlebitis at previous insertion site and sloughing.	c. Begins definitive treatment and prevents tissue damage.

Total parenteral nutrition. Total parenteral nutrition (TPN; hyperalimentation) is designed to provide complete nutrition by the intravenous route for extended periods of time. The infusion solution consists of protein hydrolysate, glucose, electrolytes, minerals, and vitamins. The infusion is continuous at a prescribed rate through an indwelling catheter threaded into the vena cava (Fig. 33.12).

TPN is the method of choice for the infant who (1) requires several surgeries for repair of gastrointestinal anomalies or obstruction, (2) suffers from chronic diarrhea, or (3) has malabsorption syndrome.

Equipment necessary for TPN includes the following:

1. Instruments for starting intravenous infusion or a cutdown
2. Silastic catheter of appropriate size
3. Millipore intravenous filter
4. Constant infusion pump (Holter or other)
5. TPN solution (infusion fluid)
6. Pacifier and mobiles
7. Restraints as necessary

The procedure may be done in the operating room. Nursing actions are the same as those for the care of an infant receiving intravenous fluid therapy, except for the following notable additions:

1. Avoid using the cathether for purposes other than the infusion solution (e.g., not used for blood or medications).

2. Avoid making up excess or deficit by altering the drip rate without consulting the physician.

The procedure is as follows:

Technique	Rationale
1. Order prescribed mixture from pharmacy, or mix under aseptic conditions.	1. Ensures accuracy of amounts. Prevents microbial contamination.
2. Check on rate of flow.	2. Avoids overfeeding or underfeeding. Checks equipment for malfunction.
a. Check pump setting.	
b. Check amount given from calibrated, enclosed reservoir every 2 to 4 hours.	

Fig. 33.12
A, Total parenteral nutrition. **B,** Close-up to show infusion site and internal placement of catheter.

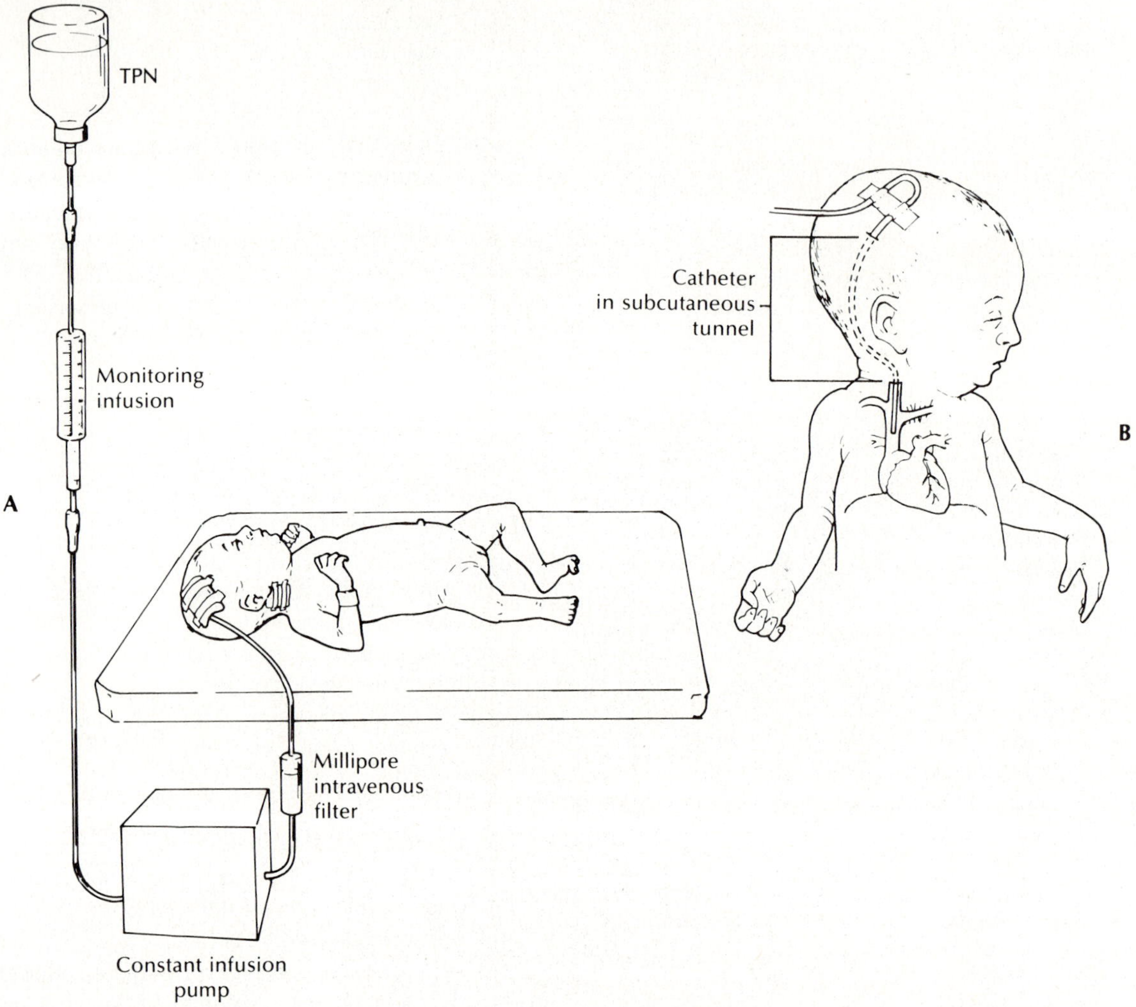

Technique	Rationale
3. Change bottle, tubing, and Millipore filter every 1 or 2 days. Culture filter after use.	3. Decreases risk of microbial contamination.
4. Change dressing around catheter.	4. Prevents infection and allows observation of area of needle insertion.
5. Monitor infant's weight daily at same times on same scales.	5. Provides index of response to this form of therapy.
6. Provide pacifier and mobiles.	6. Provides sucking satisfaction and some visual stimulation.
7. Observe infant for complications associated with hyperalimentation.	7. Facilitates prompt identification and treatment of problems.
a. Catheter and its insertion: local skin infection, septicemia, blood vessel thrombosis, obstructon or dislodgment of catheter, cardiac symptoms such as arrhythmia. *Candida* septicemia is quite common.	a. Fifty percent of complications from sepsis

Technique	Rationale
b. Infusion solution—type and amount: glucosuria, dehydration, acidosis, amino acid imbalance.	b. Metabolic complications

EMOTIONAL ASPECTS OF CARE

Neonate's emotional needs. Premature and sick infants who are not in acute distress or who are convalescing have at least the same emotional and developmental needs that the normal term infant has. It may be difficult for the infant at risk to meet his needs. The sick infant who needs intravenous therapy, nasogastric feedings, heel-stick samples, oxygen by plastic hood, or continuous positive airway pressure cannot be cuddled, fondled, or played with as can the term infant. Instead he must experience many painful stimuli, including numerous intrusive procedures such as having electronic leads taped to and removed from his chest wall. His view through the plastic walls of the incubator is blurred, a cacophony of sounds (e.g., motors, hiss of oxygen) penetrates his closed-in world, and overhead bright lights deny diurnal and nocturnal rhythms.

Without adequate attention to his emotional and developmental needs, the premature and sick infant, exposed to these life-support measures and separated from the constant presence of one mothering and comforting person, may begin to show signs of great anxiety and tension, including the following:

- Failure to thrive (slow or absent recovery, growth, weight gain)
- Looking away from or to the side of the people who are caring for him
- Absent, weak, or infrequent crying (as if to say, "What's the use?")

Supportive care. The infant's sense of trust develops when he learns the feel, sound, and smell of the same mothering person who comforts him and who removes uncomfortable stimuli (e.g., hunger, wet or soiled clothing). He even learns to anticipate these happenings. He soon learns that his cries bring this mothering person. These conditions cannot be duplicated in the nursery, but some modifications often can be made in the nursing care plan. In the technologic environment of a premature or sick baby nursery (Figs. 33.13 and 33.14), nursing's focus must be on people, not on

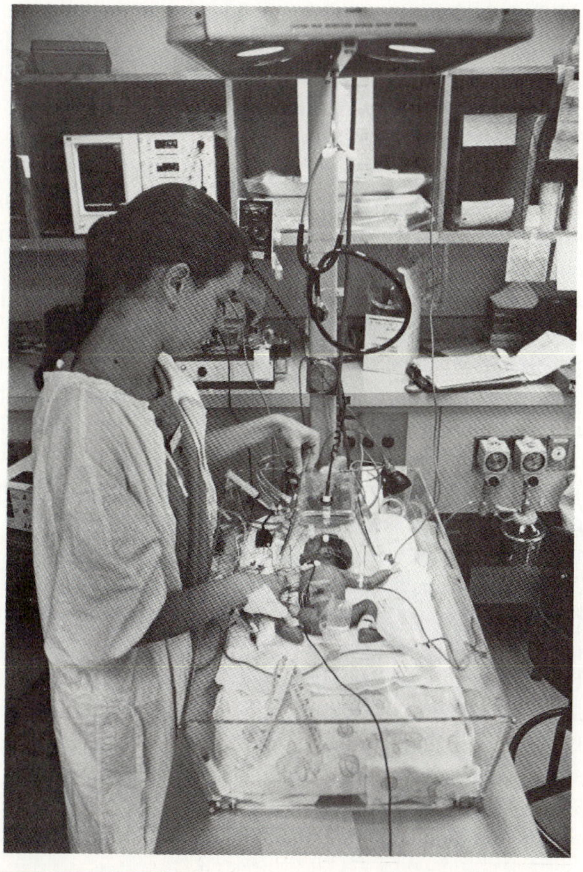

Fig. 33.13
Nursing the sick neonate. (Courtesy Linda Rae Rose, Children's Hospital, San Francisco.)

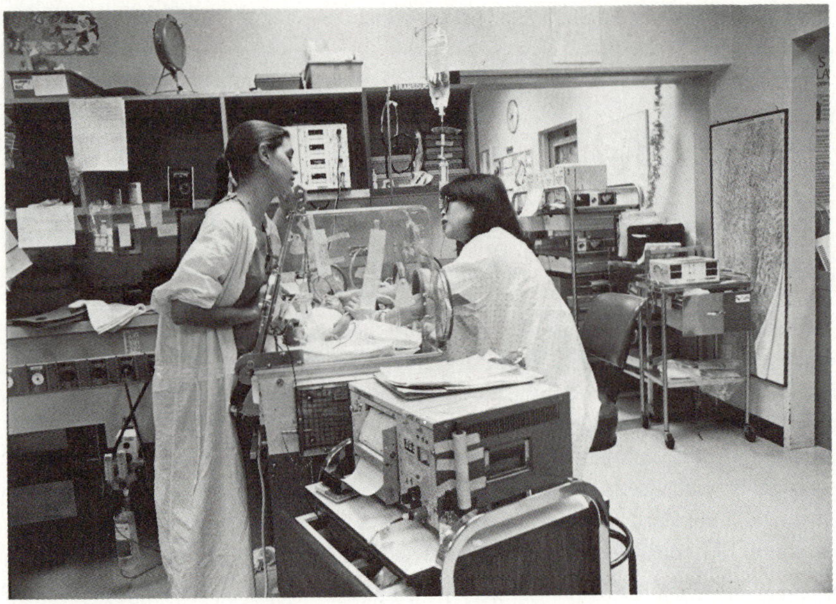

Fig. 33.14
The sick neonate nursery may be a frightening place for the parent. Note how the nurse is attending to the mother's questions. (Courtesy Linda Rae Rose, Children's Hospital, San Francisco.)

equipment. The possibilities are limited only by the parameters of human creativity. Following are some suggestions:

1. Assign nurses for continuity of nursing care.
2. Schedule time from treatments to stroke the infant's skin. The parents may touch the infant through portholes.
3. Insert mobiles and decals that can be changed frequently inside the incubator.
4. Respond to the infant's efforts to cry by reassuring him and offering a pacifier while stroking his skin and talking to him.
5. When the infant can tolerate being out of the incubator, even for short periods of time, remove him, cuddle and rock him, and sing to him, especially during his feedings—even when feeding by gavage or gastrostomy. If possible, take him out and hold him while helping him raise bubbles of air from his stomach. If the mother or father is able to visit frequently, both parent and infant will benefit immeasurably from this activity (Fig. 33.15).
6. If the infant must have feedings by gavage or gastrostomy, offer a pacifier during the feeding process (in the absence of respiratory distress). He will obtain sucking satisfaction and begin to associate this pleasant, self-gratifying, and self-initiated activity with the comforting feeling of a filling stomach.
7. Talk, sing, and hum to the infant whenever possible. Avoid loud talking and excessive discordant noise. Some nurseries permit the placement of windup muscial toys in the incubator or crib.
8. Hold the newborn so that he can see your face. Focus your eyes on his as you talk or sing to him.
9. Even if the infant is undergoing phototherapy, there can be some periods when he is not under the lamp. Remove his blindfold so that he can see your face or the parent's face during periodic, short comforting sessions.

POSTMORTEM CARE: STILLBIRTH

Definition of fetal death. According to Civil Code Section 1798.9 (California), fetal death is defined as follows:

1. Fetal death is death prior to the complete expulsion or extraction from its mother of a product of conception (irrespective of the duration of pregnancy); the death is indicated by the fact that after such separation, the fetus does not breathe or show any other evidence of life, such as beating of the heart, pulsation of the umbilical cord, or definite movement of voluntary muscles.
2. Fetal death is required to be registered if the twentieth week of gestation has been reached.

Parents and family. The death of any infant can prove very disturbing to the parents. The concerns expressed include both emotional responses and informational requests. The three questions most often raised by families pertain to feelings of personal guilt, uncertainty about heredity and its possible effect on the infant, and apprehension about the cause of death. These questions can be dealt with reasonably successfully on

Fig. 33.15
Parents participating in the care of their sick neonate. Note how mother is holding their infant's hand. (Courtesy Linda Rae Rose, Children's Hospital, San Francisco.)

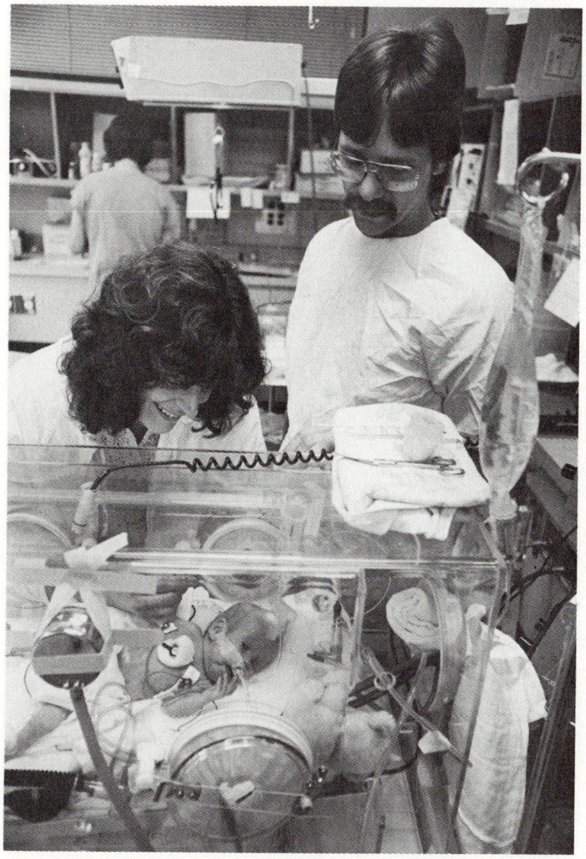

an informational level in the postmortem counseling session. The emotional problems of loneliness and depression seem less amenable to amelioration by counseling, however.

Parents who experience the death of an infant who has been transferred to an intensive care unit many miles from the home or hospital of delivery derive similar benefit from a follow-up phone call from the neonatologist.

Care of the child

1. Remove baby from the delivery area.
2. Remove all instruments from the baby. Occlude the cord with a tie or plastic clamp.
3. Baptize baby if so requested by parents or if not explicitly denied by parents.
4. Measure baby.
5. Weigh baby.
6. Identify baby with one baby band. Place other band on mother's wrist.
7. Attach completed stillborn card to baby.
8. Wrap baby in shroud.
9. Pin the second copy of stillborn card to shroud.
10. Take baby and placenta to designated area in the hospital.

Parents may request to see and hold baby (see Chapter 34). Follow hospital or community protocol for care of the stillborn and for legal requirements for filing certificate of death.

Legal requirements for filing certificate of death (California). Each death shall be registered with the local registrar of birth and death registration in the district in which the death was officially pronounced or the body was found, within 5 days after death and prior to any disposition of the human remains.

The medical and health section data and the time of death shall be completed and attested to by the physician last in attendance provided such physician is legally authorized to certify and attest to these facts or by the coroner in those cases in which he is required to complete the medical and health section data and certify and attest to these facts.

The medical and health section data and the physician's or coroner's certification shall be completed by the attending physician within 15 hours after the death or by the coroner within 3 days after examination of the body.

References and Readings

Babson, S.G., Pernoll, M.L., and Benda, G.I.: Diagnosis and management of the fetus and neonate at risk, ed. 4, St. Louis, 1980, The C.V. Mosby Co.

Benson, R.C., editor: Current obstetric and gynecologic diagnosis and treatment, ed. 4, Los Altos, Calif., 1982, Lange Medical Publications.

Behrman, R.E., editor: Neonatal-perinatal medicine: diseases of the fetus and infant, ed. 3, St. Louis, 1981, The C.V. Mosby Co.

Bowen, P.A.: Regional centers. I. A comparison of nursing responsibilities in level II and level III centers, Issues in Health Care of Women **2**(5-6):1, 1980.

Bowen, P.A.: Regional centers. II. The newborn transport system, Issues in Health Care of Women **2**(5-6):5, 1980.

Bowen, P.A.: Regional centers. III. Three regions' educational efforts and infant mortality rates, Issues in Health Care of Women **2**(5-6):19, 1980.

Chatterjee, M.S.: Paternal age and Down's syndrome, Contemp. Obstet. Gynecol. **21**(5):171, 1983.

Elliott, J.P., et al.: Helicopter transportation of patients with obstetric emergencies in an urban area, Am. J. Obstet. Gynecol. **143**(2):157, 1982.

Ferrara, A., and Harin, A.: Emergency transfer of the high-risk neonate: a working manual for medical nursing and administrative personnel, St. Louis, 1980, The C.V. Mosby Co.

Fogel, C.I., and Woods, N.F.: Health care of women: a nursing perspective, St. Louis, 1981, The C.V. Mosby Co.

Hein, H., and Brown, C.: Neonatal mortality review: a basis for improving care, Pediatrics **68:**504, 1981.

Jensen, M.D., Benson R.C., and Bobak, I.M.: Maternity care: the nurse and the family, ed. 2, St. Louis, 1981, The C.V. Mosby Co.

Johnson, S.H.: High risk parenting, Philadelphia, 1979, J.B. Lippincott Co.

Klaus, M.H., and Fanaroff, A.A.: Care of the high risk neonate, ed. 2, Philadelphia, 1979, W.B. Saunders Co.

Korones, S.B.: High-risk newborn infants: the basis for intensive nursing care, ed. 3, St. Louis, 1981, The C.V. Mosby Co.

Korones, S.B.: Personal correspondence, 1982.

Measel, C.P., and Anderson, G.C.: Nonnutritive sucking during tube feedings: effect on clinical course in premature infants, J.O.G.N. Nurs. **8:**265, Sept.-Oct. 1979.

National Center for Health Statistics: Annual summary for the United States, 1979. DHHS pub. no. (PHS) 81-1120, Monthly Vital Statistics Reports **30:**12, March 18, 1982.

National Summaries: Fetal deaths, U.S., 1954, National Office of Vital Statistics **44:**11, Aug. 1956.

Quilligan, E., and Keegan, K.: Cesarean section: some important considerations, Perinat. Press **5:**111, 1981.

Shirkey, H.C., editor: Pediatric therapy, ed. 6, St. Louis, 1980, The C.V. Mosby Co.

Shy, K.: Evaluation of elective cesarean section as a standard of care: an application of decision, Am. J. Obstet. Gynecol. **139:**123, 1981.

Statistical abstracts of the United States, 1981, Washington, D.C., 1981, U.S. Department of Commerce, Bureau of the Census.

United States Department of Health, Education, and Welfare: Characteristics of births: United States 1973-1975. DHEW pub. no. (PHS) 78-1908, Washington, D.C., Sept. 1980, The Department.

Varner, M.W., et al.: Maternal mortality in a major referral hospital, 1926 to 1980, Am. J. Obstet. Gynecol. **143**(3):325, 1982.

Vital Statistics of the United States, 1976, vol. 11. Mortality, part A, table 1-15, Washington, D.C., 1977, United States Department of Health, Education, and Welfare, Public Health Service.

Weil, S.G.: The unspoken needs of families during high risk pregnancies, Am. J. Nurs. **81**(11):2047, 1980.

Whaley, L.F., and Wong, D.L.: Nursing care of infants and children, ed. 2, St. Louis, 1983, The C.V. Mosby Co.

Zuspan, F.P., and Quilligan, E.J., editors: Practical manual of obstetrical care: a pocket reference for those who treat the pregnant patient, St. Louis, 1982, The C.V. Mosby Co.

34

Loss and Grief

- **The Grieving Process**
  - Shock and disbelief
  - Developing awareness and acute mourning
  - Resolution or acceptance
  - Pathologic mourning
- **Loss, Grief, and Maternity Nursing**
  - General goals of care
  - Assessment
  - Examples of nursing diagnoses
  - Plan and implementation
  - Evaluation
- **Psychosocial Role of Nurse in Care of Parents after Birth of Child with Disorder**
  - Mourning loss of perfect child
    - Early mother-child relationship
    - Continuing parent-child relationship
    - Families' grief reactions
  - Immediate diagnosis and management of child
  - Clinical evaluation and diagnosis of causes
  - Long-term management of child
  - Redefinition of parental role and social network
- **Premature Labor and Delivery: Psychologic Aspects**
  - Reactions to premature delivery
  - Giving birth too early
  - Mother-child relationship
  - Goals of care
- **Spontaneous Abortion and Ectopic Pregnancy: Psychologic Aspects**
- **Fetal Death: Psychologic Aspects**
- **Intranatal Fetal Death: Psychologic Aspects**
  - The nurse
  - The parents
- **Response of Family Members**
  - Sibling reaction to birth of a high-risk infant
  - Grandparents of high-risk infant

How often one hears that the "maternity ward is the happiest place in the whole hospital." This type of comment is most often expressed by those with no experience on a maternity service. However, experienced maternity nurses recognize the need to be prepared to meet the grief and grieving needs of women and their families.

Pregnancy and birth constitute an identity crisis situation in which everything is expected to proceed normally. During this natural transition in the woman's life cycle, she examines and actively relates to her femininity, sexuality, and capacity for motherhood. An unnatural or unexpected interruption in the process poses a potential threat to a woman's self-esteem and femininity. Possible threats to maternal mental health include abortion (spontaneous, elective, or therapeutic), nonmarital pregnancy, premature or postmature delivery, birth trauma, placing the baby for adoption, stillbirth, neonatal death, or the birth of a child with a defect.

When expectations of birth and joy are replaced by loss, the nurse's role is critical. The nurse must be able to cope constructively with her own response to loss and grief to meet the woman's needs. As in any crisis situation, the nurse's problems may be reactivated by those the woman and her family present; the nurse too becomes more vulnerable as these internal conflicts emerge in the face of the woman's problems. An understanding of loss and the normal grieving process is fundamental to the implementation of the nursing process.

The Grieving Process

In the face of a loss or the threat of a loss, the person's reactions usually follow a predictable pattern. Phases of mourning have been described by Lindemann (1944) and Kübler-Ross (1969) and may be compared as follows.

Lindemann (three phases)	Kübler-Ross (five stages)
1. Shock and disbelief	1. Denial and isolation: "No, not me!"
2. Developing awareness and acute mourning	2. Anger: "Why me?"
3. Resolution or acceptance	3. Bargaining: "If I . . ."
	4. Depression and acute grief: "How can I . . ."
	5. Acceptance: "I can, I must."

The phases of mourning according to Lindemann are explained further.

SHOCK AND DISBELIEF

During the period immediately after the loss the person struggles with the reality of the event and may even deny its existence. Mental symptoms may include restlessness, confusion, and apathy. The following somatic manifestations are common: dizziness, lightheadedness or syncope, pallor, perspiration, tachycardia, palpitations, nausea, and other gastrointestinal tract symptoms.

DEVELOPING AWARENESS AND ACUTE MOURNING

Reality of the loss begins to penetrate awareness; interest in daily affairs and activity diminishes. Feelings of sadness, self-depreciation, depression, guilt, helplessness, and hopelessness surface. Intense feelings of loneliness or emptiness, a strong urge to cry, and preoccupation with the loss are common. Blame may be internalized or projected onto others. Anger is a common characteristic in this phase. Exhaustion and shortness of breath may occur occasionally.

RESOLUTION OR ACCEPTANCE

Recovering from grief may take a year or longer, although the acute period lasts approximately 6 weeks. With resolution of the mourning process, the person gradually resumes daily activities, reestablishes precrisis relationships in light of the crisis event, forms new relationships, and becomes less preoccupied with the loss.

PATHOLOGIC MOURNING

The critical period for intervention is in the immediate crisis period. The goal of crisis intervention is to assist the woman and her family to begin *now* to mourn appropriately. The following signs *may* signal pathologic mourning:

1. Cheerfulness
2. Avoidance of the topic
3. Marked or persistent hostility toward the staff, her husband, or the maternal or parental family
4. Marked or persistent guilt feelings regarding the event
5. Viewing the sick or premature infant or the infant with a disorder as normal or as deceased

The nurse must be aware of possible individual differences and cultural prescriptions for mourning and the expression of grief when assessing the appropriateness of the grief response.

Loss, Grief, and Maternity Nursing

The repetition of some content in this chapter is deliberate. The intent is to present the nurse with quick complete reference packets for specific obstetric problems. Each packet can be used to add to the nurse's confidence and ability to initiate pertinent psychosocial care of the family immediately without the need to read extensively for general concepts and specific interventions.

GENERAL GOALS OF CARE

1. The woman retains a positive sense of self-esteem and self-worth as a woman, mother, and sexual being.
2. The woman and family appraise the situation realistically (e.g., ambivalent or negative feelings toward the pregnancy did not cause the loss).
3. The woman and family receive anticipatory guidance regarding components of grieving process and possible reactions of family and friends.

ASSESSMENT

1. Assess woman's responses to the loss, both verbal and nonverbal.
2. Assess woman's external support system—who they are, their availability, their effect on her (i.e., does she seem comforted by them).
3. Assess woman's and family's desire for spiritual support (e.g., baptism of the conceptus or neonate).

EXAMPLES OF NURSING DIAGNOSES

1. Potential loss of self-esteem because of lack of understanding of the grieving process
2. Potential impairment of parent-child relationship because of misunderstanding the older sibling's response to the loss
3. Potential inability to develop appropriate parent-

craft skills because of inadequate knowledge of developmental needs of the high-risk child

PLAN AND IMPLEMENTATION

The plan and implementation are individualized. Examples are presented for the following commonly encountered situations:

1. Birth of a neonate with a defect
2. Premature labor
3. Spontaneous abortion
4. Fetal death (before admission to hospital for delivery)
5. Intranatal death (stillbirth) or neonatal death

EVALUATION

The nurse can be assured that nursing care has been effective if the goals of care have been met.

Psychosocial Role of Nurse in Care of Parents after Birth of Child with Disorder

The birth of a child with an obvious defect is a shattering experience for parents and a disturbing experience for those who attend the birth. Parents feel devastated and inadequate; anticipated joy ends in despair and confusion. A flurry of activity often follows such a birth. The child may then be examined by specialists, often at a facility far from the mother's hospital. Physicians and others (e.g., clergy) may talk with the parents. The natural order of postdelivery psychologic tasks is disrupted, and the new parents are in crisis. The nurse is in a unique and critical position. Of all the members of the health team, the nurse alone can be available 24 hours a day. A nurse can help plan for discharge and postdischarge care. Although the nurse's clinical intervention will vary with each situation, in every case she must establish herself as a caring, knowledgeable, resourceful person.

Whether the child is premature, is ill, or has a defect, the parental responses and needs are similar in many respects. In general, the couple's needs can be summarized to include (1) mourning the loss of the fantasized perfect baby, (2) immediate diagnosis and management of the neonate, (3) clinical evaluation and diagnosis of the causes of the infant's disorder, (4) when appropriate, preparation and planning for the continued care of the affected newborn, (5) redefinition of their parental role in their social network (i.e., reentrance into their society), and (6) family planning and genetic counseling. Nursing management is planned to help parents meet these needs.

MOURNING LOSS OF PERFECT CHILD

Grieving is the first difficult task of the new parents of a child with a malformation or disorder. Psychologic shock, frequently coupled with the necessity of physical separation from the infant, makes this period trying and the parents vulnerable. Resolution of grief for the lost, assumed-perfect child precedes the development of acceptance or attachment to the real imperfect child or any decisions regarding his placement. The period of acute grief is usually about 6 weeks; however, in the continued presence of a child with a defect, grief may become chronic and persist for a lifetime.

The parents are profoundly affected by the manner and attitudes of those around them, especially the medical and nursing personnel. Parents are sensitive to and respond quickly to nonverbal cues from others that may connote nonacceptance, revulsion, or blame. Voice inflections, facial expressions, or the posture of the nurse who witnesses parental grief reactions or views the infant is quickly noted and internalized. Nurses also are representatives of society and may reflect society's reactions to them as parents of a child who is less than perfect.

Early mother-child relationship. Interaction between parent and child in the immediate postdelivery period is important in the development of potential maternal feelings. If a parent does not have the opportunity to see, hold, and fondle the child early and often after birth, parental feelings and the development of parenting skills are adversely affected. The very small premature infant, the sick infant, or a child with a serious congenital disorder may have to be taken to another institution immediately after birth, an event that can cause the mother to feel psychologically estranged from her infant.

Continuing parent-child relationship. The skilled medical and nursing care required by the infant in this period, which the parents cannot provide, may be overwhelming. In fact, they may focus on the gadgetry—the machines, tubes, and bottles—associated with the infant's care rather than on the infant.

Parents need to "keep in touch" with the infant somehow. This may be accomplished by viewing the infant frequently and at close range and hearing frequent progress reports and answers to their questions. At other times, parents may be permitted to touch, fondle, and stroke the infant when it is still not practical to involve them in actual feeding and bathing. During these initial contacts, and until parents gain self-confidence, the nurse should remain nearby, offering support as needed.

If the infant's hospitalization is prolonged, the nursing staff should keep the parents informed of the infant's progress with telephone calls and notes "from the baby."

Parents and nurse may feel frustrated, uncomfortable, and even helpless when faced with the birth of a child with a defect. However, parents and nurse can grow from this mutually shared experience. Touching and sharing another's experience of loss can be threatening but also rewarding.

Families' grief reactions. Grandparents may take this opportunity to blame the other parent's family, with remarks such as, "We've never had this happen in *our* family before—ever." Other comments that are frequently heard include, "The women in *our* family have never had problems having babies" and "I told him [her] that nothing good would come of this marriage [relationship]."

Comments such as these from members of the parents' families may mask hidden feelings of inadequacy about themselves, a deep concern for the young mother or couple, feelings of helplessness in the situation, concern by the grandparents that there may be no grandchild and therefore no "immortality" for them, and many other emotional reactions.

The nurse must avoid the pitfall of taking sides. Patience, tact, and warm sympathy coupled with efforts to help family members identify and explore feelings, clarify misconceptions, and provide simple, cogent explanations may contribute to the comfort, strength, and unity of the entire family.

IMMEDIATE DIAGNOSIS AND MANAGEMENT OF CHILD

Diagnosing the disorder and initiating appropriate therapy is the physician's responsibility; however, the nurse must be conversant with diagnostic techniques and rationale for therapy to reinforce and clarify the physician's explanations. If possible, the nurse should sit in with the parents and physician during their sessions to know what is being said. Open lines of communication between physician and nurse, always essential, are vital now. One nursing function is to assist parents to identify and verbalize their questions as well as their misgivings and fears. The nurse must deal with those questions and concerns within her realm of expertise and channel others to appropriate team members.

CLINICAL EVALUATION AND DIAGNOSIS OF CAUSES

The history taking and diagnostic procedures necessary to uncover the etiology are exacting. One is asked to look for disorders in ancestors, to explore prenatal acts of omission and commission (e.g., nutrition, drugs), and to seek out other environmental factors.

Parents may express feelings of shame and embarrassment lest they be carrying a "bad" gene or be responsible for exposure to a devastating environmental agent. Others are anxious to fix the blame somewhere. Many women remember transient (or persistent) negative feelings about the pregnancy or baby and interpret these feelings as punishment for their real or imagined transgressions.

The nurse's role must be supportive: preparing parents for what to expect and allowing for anticipatory worry, listening actively, and assisting with the formulation of questions and the ventilation of feelings.

LONG-TERM MANAGEMENT OF CHILD

Long-term management of a child with a disorder necessitates multidisciplinary planning and cooperation and a coordinated program of continual guidance and counseling of the parents. The emotional, physical, and financial status of the parents, available community resources, and the child's condition must be evaluated.

The nurse's role varies with the situation: Is the defect obvious? Is it curable? Is it treatable? How do parents perceive the disorder? Skillfully executed, the nurse's supportive function aids parents in decision making and in self-acceptance regarding their decisions (e.g., surgical procedures, institutionalization).

If the child requires medications, diet, or physical manipulation, the nurse should assist in teaching how, when, and why. Parents will benefit from supervised practice before discharge and frequent positive reinforcement of their ability to perform necessary tasks.

Community resources should be tapped to assist with the financial burden, equipment, drugs, and psychologic support (see Appendix C). For example, in the San Francisco Bay area, there is a group of parents of children with cleft lip and palate who meet to share feelings, problems, techniques, and new developments. A social worker may have the prime responsibility in this area of management, but the nurse should be cognizant of resources also, and visiting nurse associations may be involved in the follow-up care in the home.

Continued guidance and counseling are essential in helping the family and its members to live in harmony with each other, increasing their comfort and strengthening their unity. The child with a defect needs love, affection, and social and physical stimulation as much as or more than any other child. At the same time, his special needs and reactions must be considered. Other family members also need love, a sense of fulfillment, and recognition as worthwhile persons. Meeting all these needs requires much energy from each family member. The nurse can help family members understand the special dynamics of their situation and cope with the inevitable tensions and resentments.

REDEFINITION OF PARENTAL ROLE AND SOCIAL NETWORK

A society expects adults to produce healthy children to perpetuate that society. A social stigma is attached to bearing a defective child, a reality with which the parents must learn to cope.

After parents grieve and come to terms with their failure to produce a healthy offspring, they still face several hurdles. One is to make a decision regarding the disposition of the child—institution or home. If the child comes home, they must learn to meet his special needs and introduce him to society.

Another hurdle is facing others—the other children, family, friends, and strangers. Even during the hospital stay, parents experience society's adverse reaction. Subtle or blatant expressions of social isolation are evident. The cards, flowers, and other gifts of congratulation are sparse. Frequently the cheery forms of congratulations come only from those unaware of the "situation." Telephone conversations are guarded. Even medical personnel, unhappily, may shun these parents. Families may be insinuating blame on each other. At home, callers do not ask to see the baby. If they do, verbal response may be stilted, although nonverbal response is poignant.

The entire health team and community resources such as clergy must accept the task of helping parents reenter the outside world. Several of the techniques already discussed are helpful, but others may prove helpful also.

One simple technique is *role playing*. The anticipated meetings with the other children, family, and friends are acted out. Another approach is to discuss how parents will handle the curiosity of friends, acquaintances, and strangers. These techniques help in several ways. First, by anticipating the words and reactions of others, they verbalize their own. Second, the practice augments their store of coping strategies. Both techniques may uncover feelings that can be dealt with here and now, although resolution of these feelings may not come until much later. Each encounter may serve to strengthen coping mechanisms and bring the resolution of feelings a step closer.

Premature Labor and Delivery: Psychologic Aspects

Prematurity puts the infant and the family at risk. The parents face the threat of their infant's death. In the event that their infant may die, some parents pull away from any emotional attachment to this infant; anticipatory grieving is a protective mechanism. However, the danger inherent in grieving prematurely lies in the infant's recovery and subsequent relationship to the parents:

1. The parents may be unable to reestablish a positive relationship and therefore have difficulty developing effective parenting patterns.
2. The parents may continue to view the child as being at risk, vulnerable to disease and dysfunction, and only on temporary loan to them.
3. The parents may become overprotective and overindulgent or may place heavy demands or unrealistic expectations on the child's growth, development, and achievements.

Children of parents who grieved inappropriately after premature delivery and who have shown the behaviors just listed may demonstrate a variety of problems in psychosocial development such as the following:

- Difficulty with separation and dependency
- Sleep disturbances
- Failure to thrive
- School phobias
- Overconcern with body functions

REACTIONS TO PREMATURE DELIVERY

Grief reactions to the birth of a premature infant have been studied by Kaplan and Mason (1960) and others. The following four psychologic tasks must be faced and successfully resolved by the mother of a premature infant before effective relationships and parenting patterns can evolve:

1. *Anticipatory grief.* The mother withdraws from the normal process of bonding with her infant. She grieves in preparation for her infant's possible death, although she clings tenuously to the hope that the child will survive. This phase begins during labor and lasts until the infant dies or shows evidence of surviving.
2. *Confrontation and acknowledgment of her failure to deliver a normal full-term infant.* Grief and depression typify this phase, which persists until the infant is out of danger and is expected to survive.
3. *Resumption of the process of relating to the infant.* As the baby begins to improve—gains weight, feeds by nipple, and is weaned from the incubator—the mother should resume the process of developing the attachment or bonding to the infant that was interrupted by his precarious condition at birth.
4. *Learning how this baby differs in his special needs and growth patterns.* The mother's fourth task is to learn, understand, and accept this infant's care-taking needs and growth and developmental expectations. In most instances the special needs and developmental pattern differ only temporarily from those expected for normal full-term infants.

In the event that the infant survives, these psychologic tasks should be confronted and accomplished in the sequence given for the most successful outcomes for the mother and child.

If the infant dies during the neonatal period, the mother and her family are confronted with the mourning process.

GIVING BIRTH TOO EARLY

The mother whose pregnancy terminates before term (1) has not had time to develop her fantasized mother role with this child, (2) may not have reached the phase of wanting to be rid of the pregnancy, and (3) may not have come to the point of anxiously anticipating the infant. Many women are not ready to give up the pregnant state when premature labor begins.

In the labor unit the atmosphere surrounding the woman in premature labor is guarded, frequently tense. The focus is on the unborn:

1. Fetal status may be monitored electronically or frequently by fetoscope.
2. Decisions regarding analgesia and anesthesia are based on fetal tolerance.
3. Delivery is accomplished with episiotomy and forceps to minimize trauma to the infant.
4. The pediatrician is ready, and all the equipment has been assembled if the delivery is to occur at this hospital. Occasionally the mother may be transferred to another hospital (which may be a distance from her home and family) with facilities for premature care.
5. A subdued air of silent anticipation prevails as the infant is born and its status evaluated.

The mother may or may not see the infant before highly skilled specialists surround him for resuscitative and other life-sustaining measures. If the mother sees the infant, she may see a small, glistening, limp, and often nonpink body, and she may hear his silence, gasping, or weak cry. The infant's appearance does not project the ego-enhancing image proffered by a robust, healthy newborn. The mother is often disregarded as attention focuses on the baby. If it is not possible to give explanations concomitantly with the infant's care, remember to do so later.

MOTHER-CHILD RELATIONSHIP

As soon as possible the mother should see and touch the infant so that she may begin to acknowledge the reality of the event, reaffirm the infant's true appearance and condition, and begin working through the psychologic tasks imposed by premature delivery.

A nurse or physician should be present when the mother (or father) visits the infant for the following reasons:

1. To help her ''see'' the infant rather than focus on the equipment after hearing an explanation of the significance and function of the apparatuses that surround the infant
2. To provide the normal characteristics for an infant that age against which she can compare and contrast her infant instead of using norms for full-term infants for comparison
3. To encourage verbalization of feelings regarding the experience of pregnancy, labor, and delivery
4. To assess her perceptions of the infant to determine the appropriate time for her to become actively involved in his care

GOALS OF CARE

In addition to the general goals for care (see p. 766), the following goals are pertinent:

1. The mother
   a. Perceives the child as potentially normal (if this is medically substantiated).
   b. Provides the child with realistic care comfortably.
   c. Experiences pride and satisfaction in the care of the child.
2. The mother is able to organize her time and energies to meet the love, attention, and care needs of the other members of the family and herself as well.

Psychosocial Role of Nurse in Care of Parents Experiencing Premature Labor and Delivery

Assessment/analysis	Plan/implementation	Rationale
Premature labor (37 weeks' gestation or less)		
1. Assess woman's behavior. a. Angry or passive. b. Verbal or nonverbal. c. Crying, overtalkative, or quiet. d. Anxious. 2. Assess husband's (partner's) behavior. a. Supportive: positive response from woman. Verbal—coaching; nonverbal—stroking, looking. b. Nonsupportive: woman is distressed by his presence. Verbal—blaming, hostile to staff, and her; nonverbal—avoidance, distancing. 3. Check obstetric history. a. Length of this pregnancy; proximity to due date. b. Current symptoms: ruptured membranes, bleeding, degree of discomfort, in labor or not. c. Previous premature labors? Abortions?	1. Focus on mother's feelings. a. "All of this must leave you feeling confused and a little frightened." b. "You are probably wondering how your baby will be." c. "It's natural (OK) for you to ask for medication to stop the hurt. Let us see what we can do to help you with your discomfort." 2. Keep woman and husband informed of fetal and newborn status. 3. Inform woman of preparations for child (pediatrician is notified, etc.). 4. Stay with woman; coach her; give verbal and nonverbal support with each contraction. *Avoid* "think of the baby . . ." type of statements.	1. Woman is usually not tired of her pregnancy and not ready to let go of mother-fetus relationship. 2. Woman may feel guilty or be made to feel guilty by husband, personnel, and others for egocentric behaviors during labor. 3. In labor, women become self-centered. Reinforce normalcy of this to her (and to her family) during and after delivery. 4. Concern for infant should not distract nurse from mother's need to be reassured that she did well in labor, etc.
After delivery of premature infant (37 weeks' gestation or less)		
Tasks I and II 1. Assess mother's perception of situation. a. Realistic? b. Aware of problems or lack of problems? c. How she describes infant: "a plucked chicken," "a corpse-like thing," "he," "she," "such a tiny baby." 2. Is mother able to focus on infant as well as on herself? 3. Assess mother's support system. a. Family members: who, present or not. b. Religious. c. Cultural. 4. Assess mother's behavior. a. Denial. b. Hopeful. c. Ready to become involved in infant's care.	1. Keep mother informed of infant's status; reassure regarding infant's viability, lack of deformities, defects, if true. 2. Explain incubator, gadgetry, nursing procedures, and what mother can do if anything. 3. Describe any defects, surgery, etc., and encourage her to vent feelings regarding same. This is done to reinforce what physician has told her. Repeat as often as necessary. Reassure her that it is all right for her to ask same questions over and over if she expresses feelings about this. *Task I* 1. "It must be hard for you to let yourself love (get involved with) the baby when you are not sure he will make it." 2. "Some women feel it would be better if the baby died if there may be something wrong with him." (This statement is made after she makes some reference to subject herself.) 3. "At times, the whole thing doesn't seem real."	1. For the mother with an obstetric history of difficulty conceiving or many abortions, this child may be closest evidence of success so far, and parents may feel gratified that they could carry an infant this far along. 2. Working closely with mother (and her family) increases her sense of worth. 3. Knowledge of situation and what to expect are ego strengthening. Even if knowledge is "bad news," mother has a chance to do worry work or grief work at that time to prepare herself for next event.

Continued.

Psychosocial Role of Nurse in Care of Parents Experiencing Premature Labor and Delivery—cont'd

Assessment/analysis	Plan/implementation	Rationale
After delivery of premature infant (37 weeks' gestation or less)—cont'd		
	Task II 1. Encourage woman to verbalize feelings regarding this pregnancy, labor, and delivery and compare and contrast to previous experiences if any. 2. "Some women feel they may have caused an early labor themselves."	
Task III 1. Assess mother's behaviors. a. Muscle tension or relaxation. b. Perspiration or not. c. Skin color changes. d. Eye contact with infant. 2. Assess mother's verbal responses. a. Perception of infant: "he," "she," or "it"; human or animal characteristics; potential viability or "corpselike." b. Appropriateness to infant or to her care of infant.	1. Assist mother to regard infant as he really is. a. Show her wet or soiled diapers. b. Inform her of amount he eats and how he eats. c. Point out his behaviors: frowns, yawns, stretching. d. Go over infant with her from head to toe. 2. Describe any improvements. a. Respiratory activity. b. Weight gain. c. Change from gavage to nipple feeding. 3. Support her interactions with infant. a. Stroking, fondling, holding, etc. b. Feeding, burping, changing diapers. c. Eliciting grasp reflex. 4. Help her vent feelings regarding infant's behavior while she is providing care (he may not wish to burp; he may regurgitate, etc.). 5. Assist her with identification of infant. a. Whose eyes? Chin? Nose? b. Size of feet—who does he take after? c. Who else had a birthmark? etc.	1. Parents must release fantasy baby and see this baby as individual with his own physical and behavioral characteristics. Psychologic tasks once accomplished enable mother to see and meet this infant's special needs. 2. Mother needs substantive data to reassure her that now it is safe to invest emotional energy in developing relationship with this infant. 3. Tactile, visual, and auditory stimuli are needed to assist mother in knowing her baby. These activities increase her self-confidence and self-esteem as she learns to care for infant. 4. Parents are acutely aware of how others regard infant. Nurse acts as role model by giving infant a gender, calling him by name, using positive statements regarding his behavior ("he drank a whole ounce of formula today" vs. "he only drank half of his formula today"), handling him gently. 5. Parents can intellectualize that infant is as yet unaware of who is who (among his caretakers, including his parents), but they still feel rejected if infant does not look at them and pulls away from their touch, and they feel accepted if infant responds by rooting, grasping, burping, etc.
Task IV 1. As in Task III. 2. How often can mother come in to care for infant? How does mother (family) keep in touch? 3. Does mother have support of family members? Do others come in with her? 4. How much encouragement does mother need to take on tasks? 5. What are mother's comments as she interacts with infant?	1. Provide information and support as mother takes on care of infant. Allow her to pace herself. 2. Arrange for group meetings between mothers who share this experience; provide space, maybe even coffee, etc., and act as resource person as needed. 3. Arrange for home visit before infant's discharge and several afterward as circumstances allow. 4. Supply telephone numbers of those to call with questions. 5. Prepare mother for increase in anxiety as discharge date approaches. 6. Teach regarding expected growth and developmental patterns.	1. Mother's self-confidence may have been diminished by inability to carry to full term and by seeing that infant required highly trained professionals and complex equipment. 2. Supporting mother's successes increases her confidence and helps her build a positive concept of self as capable of caring for this infant.

Spontaneous Abortion and Ectopic Pregnancy: Psychologic Aspects

Conception affirms the woman's ability to initiate her biologic role. Any event that interferes with her ability to carry a normal fetus to term causes her to question her biologic intactness and may act as an assault to her self-concept and feelings of self-worth. She may feel cheated. Many women experience ambivalent feelings toward the idea of pregnancy; many harbor thoughts of self-abortion. Coincident loss of the pregnancy may precipitate a guilt reaction for real or imagined negative thoughts or actions.

For the woman who has a history of difficulty in conceiving and carrying a pregnancy to viability (24 to 28 weeks), negative feelings about herself as a complete woman may be expected. Nursing care of such a woman and her family should focus on helping them verbalize their feelings openly and honestly. Sympathetic, active listening by the nurse may assist the women in retaining or regaining her self-esteem and feelings of self-worth.

Psychosocial Role of Nurse in Care of Parents Experiencing Spontaneous Abortion or Ectopic Pregnancy

Assessment/analysis	Plan/implementation	Rationale
1. Assess the woman's behavior: a. Euphoric, talkative b. Quiet, nonverbal c. Denial or acknowledgement 2. Review her obstetric history: a. Was there difficulty conceiving?* b. Any previous abortions?† c. Was anything done to initiate abortion? 3. Assess the family's response.	1. Be available and indicate willingness to sit and listen to the woman and family. 2. Encourage and assist verbalization of: a. Feelings of loss, of being cheated b. The woman's fear of not being able to ever carry to term, of having something wrong with her c. Any feelings, actions, or lack of action that the woman or family may believe caused this d. Reflections on previous pregnancies, labors, etc. 3. Act as an advocate to the physician in regard to the woman's questions concerning cause and her biologic functioning capacity. 4. Make appropriate referrals: family planning, psychiatric social worker, genetic counselor, etc.	1. Verbal repetition of experience helps one cope with a situation and integrate experience into one's perception of self in a nonthreatening manner. 2. People experiencing loss may need to ask the same questions repeatedly from the same or other people. Answers may need to be given frequently, with patience and understanding. 3. People experiencing grief feel alienated from others, lonely, and helpless; they may exhibit anger in the presence of or toward an accepting, understanding, and caring other, such as the nurse.

*For a discussion of the grief response and infertility, see Chapter 12.

†For a discussion of the nurse's response and the woman's response to elective abortion, see Chapter 41.

Fetal Death: Psychologic Aspects

Fetal movements may cease before the onset of labor, that is, between 20 weeks and term. The mother may deny a lack of fetal activity: "Maybe he's just asleep . . . he's quiet sometimes." She may call the physician for reassurance that everything is all right. Subsequently she may be admitted to the hospital for tests of fetal status. Even in light of evidence from the tests and clinical symptoms, some women cling tenaciously to the hope that the infant will be born alive and well.

Other women acknowledge fetal death by a change in their behavior. One woman arrived on a maternity unit in active labor. A review of her chart showed that she had kept all her clinic appointments until 4 weeks before labor. She stated she was feeling well and described her labor so far. She said nothing as the nurse checked for the FHR. When none were heard, the nurse inquired about fetal activity. Quietly and unemotionally, the mother replied, "They stopped a month ago."

Occasionally it is the nurse who responds with denial. The nurse may rationalize the absence of FHR and funic and uterine souffles as "positional," "too much noise in the room," "defective fetoscope," and the like. The nurse may choose to avoid the woman or to avoid open communication on the subject. The nurse has several therapeutic alternatives available, however.

Psychosocial Role of Nurse in Care of Parents Experiencing Fetal Death

Assessment/analysis	Plan/implementation	Rationale
Prenatal		
1. Detection by gravida a. Determine time interval between first suspicion of cessation of fetal movements and calling physician. b. Note time when she stopped keeping appointments. 2. Detection by physician a. Pattern of increase in fundal height and weight gain not consistant with normal pregnancy. b. Tests for fetal status: estriol levels, sonography, amniocentesis, others. c. Test for maternal platelet levels. 3. Obstetric history a. Previous spontaneous abortion or fetal loss? b. Was she in high-risk category? c. Did she have any recent experiences with or is she now experiencing loss (other than this fetus)?	1. Arrange for immediate appointment. a. Call gravida who misses appointments. b. Schedule sufficient time to meet with physician or nurse, if situation is suspicious. 2. Help woman to express feelings of guilt or self-blame for any perceived acts of commission or omission. a. "Many women are unhappy when they first learn they are pregnant and wish they were not pregnant." b. "Are you thinking you may have done something to cause this?" c. "You are trying to find reasons . . . ?" 3. Help woman to express her feelings about carrying dead baby. a. "It isn't easy to know the baby is dead." b. "Do you wonder if you can stand it until delivery?" c. "Do you wonder if you will be hurt somehow?" d. "Are you wondering how to tell the other children, husband, grandparents, etc.?" 4. Fill in gaps in information and clarify misconceptions. Help woman formulate questions for physician; help her understand what physician tells her.	1. After mothers feel life, or quickening, most mothers begin to relate differently to child. Child is now real; there is, at least in fantasy, promise of child. 2. Generally, people feel uneasy about death. It is difficult for woman to realize that she is carrying within her something that is dead. 3. When medical and nursing staff are able to communicate comfortably and openly about fetal death and woman's possible reactions and feelings, she may be better able to face and cope with situation. 4. Knowledge about any situation helps dispel fear of unknown, misconceptions, fantasy. Knowledge supports ego strength. Woman needs to know following: a. When to expect labor and delivery. (Will it be induced, when, and how?) b. What to expect of her labor. c. What physiologic effect this may have on her. d. What may have caused fetal death. She has had sole responsibility for care and nurturance of embryo-fetus. She needs to be advised of possible causes well beyond her control. e. How to tell other children at

Psychosocial Role of Nurse in Care of Parents Experiencing Fetal Death—cont'd

Assessment/analysis	Plan/implementation	Rationale
Prenatal—cont'd		
	5. Prepare woman and family for procedures, tests for fetal status.	home. f. What reactions she may expect from others and some help with how to handle these.
Intranatal		
1. Assess maternal emotional response. a. Quiet, composed. b. Denial: "I just dont believe it"; euphoric, animated. c. Overtly upset, crying. d. Angry toward staff, others: "Why do I have to feel anything? Give me something now"; "If the doctor had only . . ."; "If I had only . . ."; sad, tearful. 2. Assess woman's external support system. a. Presence of relatives. b. Behavior of relatives. (Does she seem reassured by their presence and actions?) c. Family's interest and ability to stay with her, to provide comfort measures, etc. 3. Assess for desire to have fetus baptized.	1. Do not do Leopold's maneuvers or listen for FHR. Focus on woman (and family). 2. Introduce yourself and immediately indicate your awareness of situation. a. "This is a very difficult and sad time for you." b. If possible, keep father close by; he may feel awkward in "Dad's room." "This is hard for you, too. One feels so helpless. Can I help you?"	1. Focus remains on the woman and family. 2. Open communication and being available physically and psychologically helps in following ways: a. It fosters open communication between mother and significant others and between mother and staff. Energy does not have to be diverted to keeping up a front. b. It gives permission to grieve, validates appropriateness of grieving here and now in a manner acceptable to them, and gives permission to speak of death.
	3. Respect woman's choice of anesthesia. If she wishes to be awake or if couple wishes father to be present at birth, prepare them for following: a. Silence and tension at delivery. b. Sight of still, pale, or reddish infant; infant's peeling skin, and markedly molded head.	3. General anesthesia may keep experience unreal, dreamlike, thereby complicating efficient grieving.
	4. If mother, spouse, or relatives wish to see or hold infant: a. Prepare infant: bathe and wrap. c. Provide private space; physician, member of clergy, nurse, or other may stay close by for support. d. Give permission to cry by your actions, by giving tissues, by saying, "It's worth crying over." 5. Be cognizant of own nonverbal messages 6. Arrange for baptism and record event in progress notes.	4. Seeing and holding infant is useful in following ways: a. It validates reality of event. b. It allows identification of infant and eliminates fantasy of what woman or couple thought infant looked like (fantasy is frequently more horrifying than reality). c. It permits grieving process to begin. Even if event was anticipated, reality reactivates entire grief process. Steps in grieving process usually take less time when death has been diagnosed before beginning of labor.

Intranatal Fetal Death: Psychologic Aspects

Fetal heart rate (FHR) may be lost late in the first stage of labor or during the second stage. The atmosphere in the labor unit becomes tense and subdued. There is a sudden change from joyful anticipation to dread. Silence accompanies the birth. Resuscitative measures are attempted. All persons present focus on the newborn. Shock and disbelief are experienced by parent and staff alike.

THE NURSE

The nurse may undergo a period of self-recrimination relevant to her own behavior surrounding the incident, for example: Could the physician have been called earlier? Were the fetal heart tones really there and was the rate normal when they were last checked? Was it judicious to give that last medication at the time it was given? Were there any clues earlier? Did the nursing care (ability to assess labor and the maternal-fetal condition during labor, ability to resuscitate) cause the fetal or neonatal death? The nurse's self-examination can undermine self-confidence as a nurse. In her (their) search for answers and to vent angry feelings, the mother (couple) may also probe. The nurse may perceive the questioning as challenges to her capabilities as a nurse. At times like this even the most competent and self-assured nurse may need peer or other support to identify feelings and verbalize them and to regain perspective.

The nurse may be unaware that she is struggling with reactions to grief. She may resort to reassuring and comforting the grieving individual or individuals in a manner that does not foster a healthy grieving response. Some commonly heard responses given by physicians, nurses, and well-meaning friends are as follows:

- "There was a reason why God wanted this baby. Have faith."
- "It's God's will. We have to have faith that it was for the best."
- "It's probably better this way. This often happens when the baby has something wrong with it."
- "You are so young. There's time for more."
- "Be thankful you have those other lovely children at home. They'll be a solace and comfort to you."

This baby is important *now*. The mother needs to talk about *this* baby. She does not want or need to focus on her other children or any suggestions for substitutes for her loss.

THE PARENTS

Certain behaviors give the message that to face grief is "bad" for a person and to avoid facing it is better for all concerned, for example, avoiding talking about the infant, quelling tears, and forbidding the mother to see and hold the infant.

Somehow it is thought that to avoid an issue is the healthiest and easiest way. It does prevent "scenes." Out of sight is out of mind. But out of sight is not out of the mother's mind. The mother has felt life. She has developed a relationship with the infant through shared internal physical sensation and fantasy. If the child lives for a few hours or days after birth, the mother's relationship with the child has progressed even further. Even after delivery the hormones that sustain an attachment between mother and child are still present, as are the physical signs and discomforts that a delivery has occurred. At home are the baby clothes and furniture, family, and friends, awaiting the hoped-for new arrival. Resolution of grief is important *now* and can be a healthy growth-inducing process.

Mothers and family look to the hospital staff to meet their needs. Having had an unfortunate maternity experience, these mothers may suffer a severe blow to their sense of worth associated with the ability to give life and to their role concept, self-esteem, and femininity. Nursing interventions that may assist the grieving family in coping with this ego-threatening experience may foster a healthy mourning process and can be incorporated easily within the busiest nursing assignment.

Death is often equated with powerlessness, an end, and failure. However, the nurse need not be professionally and personally helpless. Preventive mental health measures are well within the scope of the nurse. Some therapeutic reactions and actions by the nurse are as follows:

1. Parents need an objective listener, one who is genuinely interested and willing to face true feelings and will not try to "talk them out of it." The nurse acts as a role model for open communication in facing grief and for feeling safe and comfortable in dealing with an unpleasant situation.

2. Parents need to feel that those around them know that it is natural for them to feel sad, weepy, and easily distracted.

3. Nurses should convey to parents that grieving takes time and that they may never really "get over it," although the pain does ease with time; good memories then tend to persist.

4. Nurses should be prepared for the anger and self-blame parents may feel and assist the parents to identify these feelings: "You may be wondering if you did or did not do something to cause this." Parents may not be able to work through their anger before discharge; some parents return or write many months later to apologize for their behavior and to thank those who were able to see beyond their anger and help them with their needs.

Psychosocial Role of Nurse in Care of Parents Experiencing Intranatal Fetal Death

Assessment/analysis

1. Assess mother's response: Does she show appropriate signs and symptoms of grieving process? (Her cultural background and past experiences with grief and the grieving process influence how she shows her grief and how she progresses through the grieving process.)
   a. Shock, disbelief, and anger.
   b. Developing awareness.
   c. Resolution or acceptance (may not be seen during short hospital stay).
   d. Occasionally mother must withdraw for a short while as if to take experience a small piece at a time. Signs that she is withdrawing are closing her eyes, drawing curtains around her bed (or shutting door), changing subject.
2. Assess mother's support system: husband, family, friends, culture, or religion.
3. Note mother's age—adolescent's needs are different from those of middle-aged woman.
4. Are there definite cultural (or religious) influences that help mother define death and direct her grieving process?
5. If possible, assess the older child's (children's) reactions. Assess the parent's reactions as they face the need to tell the older child or children, other family members, and friends.

Plan/implementation

1. Provide physical care and meet dependency needs in thoughtful and unhurried manner.
2. Make infant as attractive as possible, for example, clean him up, wrap him in pretty blanket. Allow time for the mother or couple to caress their dead infant if they choose to do so. Stay with mother or couple during this time.
3. Arrange for time for mother to talk over labor and delivery, to accomplish the following:
   a. Validate and assimilate experience.
   b. Work through shock and disbelief.
   c. Clarify events.
   d. Ease her need to search for reasons.
4. Assist woman (couple) to identify and verbalize feelings:
   a. "You must feel like you were cheated."
   b. "Somehow it just doesn't seem fair."
   c. "You seem so angry."
   d. "One feels so helpless, so powerless, in this type of situation."
   e. "There are times when your feelings may seem strange to you."
5. Do *not* minimize event with comments such as "You are still young" or "You have others."
6. Let mother (couple) share her (their) feelings without giving scientific reasons, referring to logic and so on.
7. Encourage mother (couple) to verbalize concerns (perhaps to role-play different approaches) regarding ways to inform the siblings, other family members, friends.

Rationale

1. Mother's postdelivery physical needs must be met.
   a. To revitalize after pregnancy and labor.
   b. To release energy for emotional work.
2. In her search for causes, mother reviews and rehashes events leading up to stillbirth.
   a. It is normal to look for answers. Nurse should not feel she must have all answers at her fingertips.
   b. Focusing in on event to exclusion of all other activities of daily living and interaction with other family members is normal now.
   c. It is normal to feel confused, indecisive, and a sense of unreality. Some grieving persons fearfully confide, "I think I must be going crazy."
3. Adolescent needs.
   a. Reassurance of her femininity. Adolescent who is unwed may have become pregnant to prove to herself her femininity and reproductive capacity.
   b. Reassurance that her conversations with nurse are confidential.
   c. "Safe" authority figure to whom to vent angry feelings. Bravado, defensiveness, and withdrawal may be signs of immaturity and struggles with autonomy, or she may use these behaviors to cover feelings that the stillbirth occurred as punishment for out-of-wedlock pregnancy.
   d. Support and empathy. Self-esteem and a sense of worth can be generated by including woman in planning for her care after discharge, providing information regarding her body after delivery, referring her to teenage rap sessions at family planning and adolescent clinics or other groups in area.

5. Coping with grief and recovering from childbirth exact a heavy toll on the mother's resources. Although the grieving process often makes sleep difficult and appetite nonexistent, adequate rest and diet must be assured to replenish the mother's vitality. Thoughtful nursing actions (e.g., back rubs, just sitting quietly with her) can meet very real, critical needs. Sleeping pills may delay the grieving process.

6. The nurse should prepare the parents for returning home, for example, what to expect of themselves emotionally and physically and what they can expect from the older children. Siblings may feel that the parent or parents lied to them about the coming of a new baby. The older child may feel that it is his or her fault that the baby died because he or she may not have wanted a new sibling now, or wanted a boy but got a girl, so that the girl then died. Older siblings may act out their feelings in other ways.

Physical symptoms that parents may experience include sleep problems with fatigue, anorexia, muscle aches and "knots," gastrointestinal symptoms, and palpitations.

Psychologic or emotional symptoms that parents may experience include an inability to concentrate for long on any one activity (i.e., their minds may wander or they may feel everything is whirling around in their heads) and pressure in the head. People frequently express the fear of "going crazy" when they experience reactions that they do not expect or understand. The mother may hold her abdomen and state she feels "empty" and that her arms "ache to hold a baby." Parents may fear being alone, wish to go away somewhere, or become overconcerned about or disinterested in their other children. Irritability with or disinterest in the other children may compound guilt feelings.

Reactions of the family, including older children, are also discussed on pp. 762 and 768.

Response of Family Members

SIBLING REACTION TO BIRTH OF A HIGH-RISK INFANT

As discussed earlier, preparation of parents of a high-risk infant begins long before the infant is discharged from the hospital. Preparation of the older children also needs to be undertaken before the infant's coming home. The very young child can easily "forget" the existence of a brother or sister in the hospital. If possible, visits to see the new baby should be encouraged. For the older child the idea of an imperfect baby can be clarified by seeing him and having a chance to discuss fears and misconceptions. One 8-year-old boy was given the job of "explaining" all about his premature sister to the visiting grandparents. He discussed the care of the baby and use of supportive equipment surprisingly well.

If, however, the infant dies, the older children will be affected as well as the parents. A small child who cannot understand verbal explanations needs demonstrations of love and affection to provide reassurance and security. He may be unable to express frightening thoughts that he is experiencing. Occasionally the small child may resort to misbehavior to draw attention or may cling excessively to his parents.

Older children need verbal explanations as well as assistance in voicing feelings and thoughts. Discussion about the fetal or newborn death as well as death in general should be an open subject in the family. The cause of the death should be openly presented so that the child may cope with any existing feelings of guilt.

Avoid references such as, "The baby went away [or to sleep]" or "God took him." These euphemisms are usually meant to help the child, but more often they can be threatening. Regardless of the way parents handle the reaction to the death, some children may manifest their inner disturbance in nightmares, bed-wetting, school problems, or other ways.

GRANDPARENTS OF HIGH-RISK INFANT

Grandparents are also touched by the birth of an infant at risk. Grandparents can be very supportive to the young family. For some, there is a natural response to protect their offspring from pain or grief. For others, the idea of their offspring's producing a child who is less than perfect seems to lower their own self-esteem. These grandparents may resort to blaming the young parents or their child's spouse for acts of omission or commission in precipitating the problem. A nursing care plan is incomplete without an assessment and plan for action regarding grandparental responses.

References and Readings

Backer, B., Hannon, N., and Russell, N.A.: Death and dying: individuals and institutions, New York, 1982, Wiley Medical Publication.

Kaplan, D.M., and Mason, E.A.: Maternal reactions to premature birth viewed as an acute emotional disorder, Am. J. Orthopsychiatry **30:**118, July 1960.

Klaus, M.H., and Fanaroff, A.A.: Care of the high-risk neonate, ed. 2, Philadelphia, 1979, W.B. Saunders Co.

Kübler-Ross, E.: On death and dying, New York, 1969, Macmillan Publishing Co.

Lindemann, E.: Symptomatology and management of acute grief, Am. J. Psychol. **101:**141, 1944.

Stewart, D.: Spiritual care of the neonate, Periscope (published by the California Perinatal Association), pp. 1-2, June 1980.

Whaley, L.F.: Genetic counseling in maternity nursing. In McNall, L.K., and Galeener, J.T., editors: Current practice in obstetric and gynecologic nursing, vol. I, St. Louis, 1976, The C.V. Mosby Co.

35 Complications of Pregnancy

- Hemorrhagic Disorders
- Early Pregnancy
  - Spontaneous abortion
  - Recurrent abortion
    - Etiology
    - Management
    - Incompetent cervix
  - Other categories of spontaneous abortion
    - Clinical classification
    - Clinical findings
    - Diagnosis
    - Prevention
    - Management
    - Prognosis
    - Summary of nursing actions
  - Ectopic pregnancy
    - Etiology
    - Clinical classification
    - Clinical findings
    - Diagnosis
    - Prevention
    - Management
    - Prognosis
    - Summary of nursing actions
  - Hydatidiform mole
    - Etiology
    - Clinical classification
    - Clinical findings and diagnosis
    - Prevention
    - Management
    - Prognosis
    - Summary of nursing actions
- Late Pregnancy
  - Premature separation of placenta
    - Incidence
    - Etiology
    - Clinical manifestations and differential diagnosis
    - Complications
    - Therapy
    - Prognosis
    - Summary of nursing actions
  - Placenta previa
    - Etiology
    - Pathology
    - Clinical manifestations and differential diagnosis
    - Clinical classification
    - Prevention
    - Management
    - Prognosis
    - Summary of nursing actions
  - Clotting disorders in pregnancy
    - Normal clotting
    - Clotting problems
    - Summary of nursing actions
    - Idiopathic thrombocytopenic purpura
    - Hemophilia
  - Management of hemorrhagic shock
    - Physiologic mechanisms
    - Assessment and interventions
    - Hazards of therapy
- Postdelivery Hemorrhage
  - Etiology
  - Clinical findings and differential diagnosis
  - Specific problems
    - Uterine atony
    - Lacerations of the birth canal
    - Retained placenta
    - Inversion of uterus
    - Subinvolution of uterus
- Postdelivery Anterior Pituitary Necrosis
- Neonatal Hematologic Conditions
  - Hematologic status: anemia and polycythemia
    - Anemia
    - Polycythemia
    - Summary of nursing actions
- Neonatal Hypovolemic Shock
  - Summary of nursing actions
- Hypertensive States in Pregnancy
  - Pregnancy-induced hypertension
  - Incidence
  - Maternal and fetal morbidity and mortality

Definitions
Preeclampsia
Eclampsia
Etiology
Pathologic findings
Medical diagnosis
Maternal prognosis
Fetal prognosis
Management
Mild preeclampsia
Moderate to severe preeclampsia

■ Hypertensive Cardiovascular Disease
Differential diagnosis
Prognosis
Medical and nursing management

Hemorrhagic Disorders

Hemorrhagic disorders in pregnancy are medical emergencies that require expert teamwork on the part of physician and nurse to minimize the deleterious effects. The *goals* of therapy are as follows:

1. To prevent or control severe hemorrhage
2. To establish a diagnosis
3. To sustain the pregnancy if possible or feasible
4. To provide emergency care
   a. Replace blood loss
   b. Perform cesarean delivery
   c. Treat compromised infant, whether premature or full term
5. To manage grief resulting from the loss of the infant or mother or to manage loss of positive self-concept of mother

The nurse must be alert to the symptoms of hemorrhage and shock and be prepared to obtain necessary blood replacement and complete laboratory orders. (If there is not time for typing and matching of blood, group O Rh-negative blood may be ordered.) The pregnant woman and her family need much supportive care during these times of stress, including prompt attention to needs, competent technical care, and information regarding the rationale for care and the progress of treatment. The woman's inability to carry a pregnancy to term or to maintain a normal sequence of development to delivery often causes her to question her femininity and capabilities as a woman.

Early in pregnancy, abortion or ectopic pregnancy is the most common cause of excessive bleeding. Later, premature separation of the normally implanted placenta or placenta previa may be the cause of hemorrhage.

Early Pregnancy

SPONTANEOUS ABORTION

Abortion is the termination of pregnancy before viability of the fetus. The abortion may be spontaneous, resulting from natural causes, or the pregnancy may be interrupted deliberately for medical reasons (therapeutic abortion) or for social reasons (elective abortion) (see p. 990).

Viability is reached at about the twenty-fourth week of gestation, when the fetus weighs 600 g or more. With excellent neonatal care, such an infant has at least a chance to survive. An early spontaneous abortion, or miscarriage, is one that occurs before 16 weeks' gestation; a late abortion is one occurring between 16 and 24 weeks' gestation. About three fourths of these abortions occur before the sixteenth week of pregnancy, and the majority of these take place before the eighth week. More than half of all spontaneous abortions, which account for an attrition rate of at least 15% of all pregnancies, are caused by fetoplacental development defects. Approximately 15% result from maternal causes; the reasons for the remainder are speculative. Many very early pregnancies are lost for unknown reasons before the diagnosis of pregnancy is even made.

RECURRENT ABORTION

Recurrent (habitual) spontaneous abortion is the loss of three or more previable pregnancies.

Etiology. Anomalies of the reproductive tract cause second- or third-trimester pregnancy loss. The causes of repeated early abortion may include (1) endocrine imbalance (e.g., hypothyoidism, diabetes mellitus, deficient endogenous progesterone), (2) infections (e.g., syphilis, bacteriuria, T mycoplasms, and *Chlamydia trachomatis*), (3) systemic disorders (e.g., lupus erythematosus), (4) psychologic factors (but proof is lacking), and (5) genetic factors (about 60% of early abortions display an abnormal chromosomal makeup).

Management. After the second consecutive abortion, a reasonably encouraging attitude should still prevail because at least 50% of those couples will achieve a normal pregnancy with the next gestation. Investigation for etiologic factors is usually begun: (1) genetic workup (e.g., history, karyotype of both the woman and her spouse) and (2) identification of infection.

After the third consecutive abortion or if the couple

Fig. 35.1
Top, Correction of incompetent internal cervical os: McDonald operation. *Bottom,* View of closed internal os (cross section).

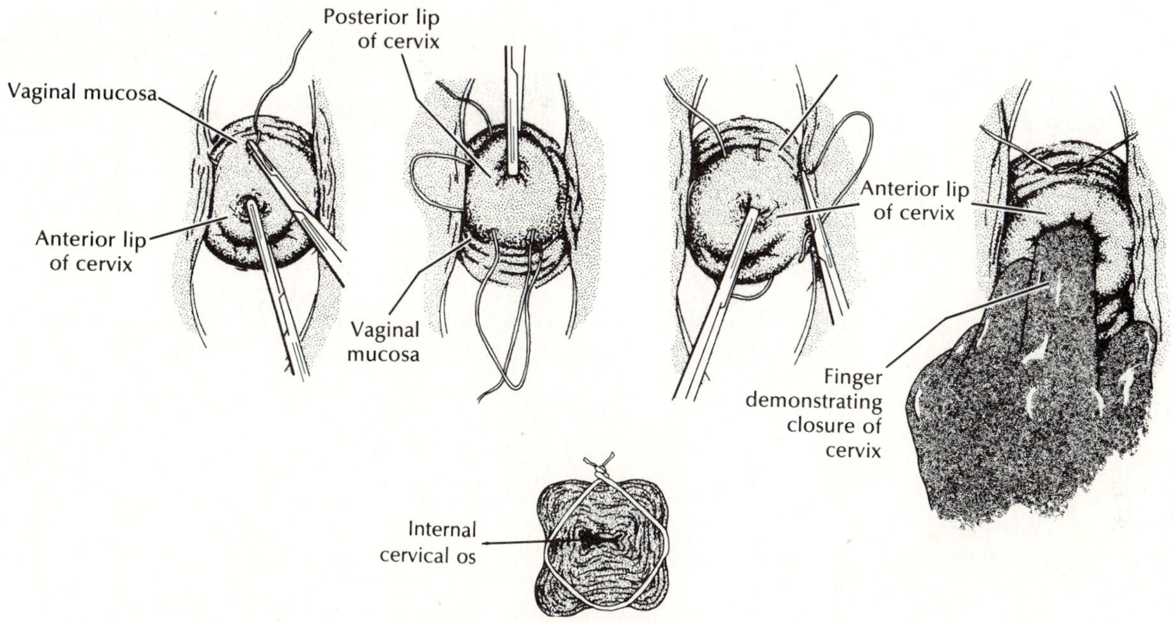

has had a child with a serious congenital abnormality, karyotypes of the parents are obtained. Amniocentesis during the second trimester of the next pregnancy should be planned for prenatal genetic assessment. Unfortunately little can be done to improve the prognosis when the inheritance of a serious genetic fault persists. However, if the man is the carrier, artificial insemination by donor (AID) or adoption may be acceptable options.

Incompetent cervix. Cervical incompetence is a condition characterized by painless dilation of the cervical os without labor or contractions of the uterus. Miscarriage or premature delivery may result. Etiologic factors include a prior traumatic delivery or forceful dilatation and curettage (D and C) of the cervix. Other instances may result from a congenitally short cervix or anomalous uterus.

Correction of the weakened cervix is possible by wedge trachelorrhaphy (removal of a wedge from the anterior segment of the cervix with closure) in the nonpregnant woman. During gestation, a cerclage, band of homologous fascia, or nonabsorbable ribbon (Mersilene) may be placed around the cervix beneath the mucosa to constrict the cervix (Fig. 35.1). Successful continuation of the pregnancy to viability or beyond occurs in the great majority of women, provided the membranes remain intact and that the cervix is not more than 3 cm dilated or more than 50% effaced at the time of correction.

OTHER CATEGORIES OF SPONTANEOUS ABORTION

Clinical classification. The diagnosis of the type of abortion a woman is experiencing is based on the signs and symptoms present (Table 35.1).

Complications of abortion include the following:

1. *Uterine lithopedion,* or *"womb stone."* A missed abortion is retained for months or years, during which time the products of conception have calcified.

2. *Hemorrhage* or *sepsis.* Hemorrhage and sepsis (e.g., salpingitis, peritonitis) occur especially in induced abortion under septic conditions and in instances of neglected care. Death may follow instrumentation and perforation of the soft, slightly enlarged uterus, or septicemia or septic emboli may follow spontaneous incomplete abortion. Even mild infection may be followed by tubal occlusion and infertility.

Clinical findings

Symptomatology. Signs and symptoms depend on the characteristic of the implantation site, which in turn is dependent on the duration of pregnancy. Three stages of the development of the implantation site are recognized.

Table 35.1
Assessing Abortion

Type of Abortion	Amount of Bleeding	Uterine Cramping	Passage of Tissue	Tissue in Vagina	Internal Cervical Os	Size of Uterus
Threatened	Slight	Mild	No	No	Closed	Agrees with length of pregnancy
Inevitable	Moderate	Moderate	No	No	Open	Agrees with length of pregnancy
Incomplete	Heavy	Severe	yes	Possible	Open with tissue in cervix	Smaller than expected for length of pregnancy
Complete	Slight	Mild	Yes	Possible	Closed	Smaller than expected for length of pregnancy
Septic	Varies; usually malodorous; fever present	Varies; fever present	Varies; fever present	Varies; fever present	Usually open; fever present	Any of the above with tenderness
Missed	Slight	No	No	No	Closed	Smaller than expected for length of pregnancy

From Gordon, R.T.: Emergencies in obstetrics and gynecology. In Warner, C.G., editor: Emergency care: assessment and intervention, ed. 2, St. Louis, 1978, The C.V. Mosby Co.

1. *Early,* or *decidual, stage.* Until the sixth week of pregnancy, the conceptus, which is virtually surrounded by decidua, is poorly attached to the uterus.

2. *Intermediate,* or *attachment, stage.* From the sixth to twelfth week of pregnancy, the anchor villi in the chorion frondosum (area of the basal plate) become moderately well attached to the myometrium.

3. *Later,* or *placental, stage.* The placenta is fully formed after the twelfth week and is firmly attached to the uterus.

Frequently the pregnancy will have been terminated for about a week before signs or symptoms of abortion become definite. For this reason it may be difficult to date the actual termination of pregnancy.

In the early, or decidual, stage of abortion, the symptomatology is not severe, and bleeding and cramping are minimal. During the intermediate, or attachment, stage of abortion, however, moderate discomfort and blood loss are expected because of the larger conceptus and adherence of portions of the placenta. The late, or placental, stage of abortion is typified by severe pain similar to that of labor, because the fetus must be expelled. Bleeding is less than that of women with an intermediate-stage abortion, because the placenta does not separate completely until after the fetus has been delivered. At this point uterine contractions generally are strong, checking any brisk bleeding.

Laboratory findings. The following laboratory findings are characteristic of abortion:

1. *Urine.* A negative or weakly positive urine pregnancy test is characteristic of abortion.

2. *Blood.* With considerable or persistent blood loss, anemia is likely (hemoglobin level less than 10.5 g/dl). Sepsis may develop with incomplete or missed abortion. Temperature is greater than 38° C (100.4° F), and white blood cell count (WBC) is greater than 12,000/cu mm. An increased sedimentation rate is the rule with pregnancy, anemia, or infection. Therefore it is not helpful for differential diagnostic purposes.

3. *Endocrine studies.* HCG, estrogen, and progesterone titers are minimal or absent in established abortions.

Diagnosis. An early spontaneous abortion is the uninitiated loss of a pregnancy of less than 16 weeks' duration. A late spontaneous abortion is one lost between 16 and 23 or 24 weeks (the beginning of viability).

Differential diagnosis. Abortion may be an obvious conclusion in pregnant women who are bleeding and in pain. In complicated cases or in those without accurate menstrual background information, however, the diagnosis may be obscure.

Ectopic pregnancy classically involves amenorrhea or menstrual changes, unilateral pelvic pain, uterine bleeding, and a sensitive adnexal mass. Decidua but no placental villi may be found on curettage.

In membranous dysmenorrhea the woman suffers pain, uterine bleeding, and the passage of tissue, but none of the usual symptoms of pregnancy can be identified. Moreover, the uterine scraping will contain secretory endometrium but no pregnancy decidua or chorionic villi.

Prevention. Although little can be done to avoid ge-

Table 35.2
Types of Spontaneous Abortion and Usual Management

Type of Abortion	Management
Threatened	Bed rest, sedation, and avoidance of stress and orgasm are recommended. Further treatment will depend on client's course.
Inevitable and incomplete	Prompt termination of pregnancy is accomplished usually by dilatation and curettage (D and C).*
Complete	No further intervention may be needed if uterine contractions are adequate to prevent hemorrhage and if there is no infection.
Septic	Immediate termination of pregnancy by method appropriate to duration of pregnancy (see Table 41.1). Cervical cultures and sensitivity studies are done and broad-spectrum antibiotic therapy (e.g., ampicillin) is started. Treatment for septic shock is initiated prn.
Missed	If spontaneous evacuation of the uterus does not occur within 1 mo, however, pregnancy is terminated by method appropriate to duration of pregnancy (see Table 41.1). Blood clotting factors are monitored until uterus is empty. Disseminated intravascular coagulation (DIC) and incoagulability of blood with uncontrolled hemorrhage may develop in cases of fetal death after twelfth week if products of conception are retained for longer than 5 wk (see p. 797 for discussion of DIC).

*For a discussion of dilatation and curettage, see Chapter 41.

netic causes of pregnancy loss, prepregnancy correction of maternal disorders, immunization against infectious diseases, proper early prenatal care, and treatment of pregnancy complications will do much to prevent abortion.

Cervical incompetence, a cause of second-trimester abortion, can be surgically corrected before or even during pregnancy in the majority of cases (Fig. 35.1).

Management. Management (Table 35.2) depends on the classification of spontaneous abortion. Therefore an early, accurate diagnosis of spontaneous abortion is vital.

General preoperative and postoperative care is appropriate for the woman experiencing therapeutic abortion. Before the procedure, a full history and a general and pelvic examination should be performed. Laboratory tests should include a complete blood count (CBC), blood typing for group and Rh factor and cross matching, and urinalysis. Chest x-ray films and electrocardiogram evaluation are obtained if necessary. Blood, fluid, and electrolyte imbalances are corrected as soon as possible.

Analgesics, or general or regional anesthesia appropriate to the procedure, or both are utilized. Intravenous administration of oxytocin, 1 ml (10 units) in 500 ml of 5% dextrose in water, may be needed to induce abortion, or following evacuation of the uterus, 10 to 20 units in 1000 ml of infusate may be given to prevent hemorrhage by contracting the uterine musculature. (See also Chapter 41.)

Ergot products such as ergonovine, which contract the uterus and cervix, are contraindicated until the uterus is emptied to avoid retention of fragments of tissue. Retained fragments of fetal or placental tissue predispose to uterine relaxation and puerperal infection. Three or four doses of ergonovine, 0.2 mg orally or intramuscularly every 4 hours, should be given if the woman is normotensive.

Antibiotics are given as necessary. Transfusion may be required for shock or anemia.

If the woman is Rh negative and has not developed isoimmunization, she is given an intramuscular injection of $Rh_0(D)$ immune globulin within 72 hours of the abortion (see p. 964).

Prognosis. Correction of maternal disorders that may cause abortion usually is followed by a normal pregnancy.

Summary of nursing actions

Goals of care

1. Severe hemorrhage is controlled or prevented.
2. Diagnosis is established and appropriate therapy instituted.
3. Reproductive function is maintained.
4. Sequelae (infection, anemia, DIC) are prevented or diagnosed and treated; Rh isoimmunization is prevented (anti-D immune globulin is administered to susceptible women).
5. The grief response (if any) progresses appropriately. The woman maintains a positive self-concept.

Examples of nursing diagnoses

1. In prenatal spontaneous abortion: potential loss of pregnancy caused by lack of understanding of rest.
2. In intranatal spontaneous abortion: potential spiritual distress caused by lack of knowledge of option to have clergy present.
3. In postnatal spontaneous abortion: potential for delayed recovery because of lack of knowledge of danger signs and symptoms.

Spontaneous Abortion

Assessment/analysis	Plan/implementation	Rationale
Prenatal		
1. Observe for signs of abortion: vaginal discharge or bleeding, abdominal cramps. Note time of onset. 2. Observe for additional symptoms: shock, amount and location of pain. 3. Observe woman's response to treatment. 4. Note previous obstetric history. 5. Take history of woman since last visit: drugs, activities, infections, etc.	1. Refer woman to physician immediately; alert physician. 2. Save all tissue or clots passed, so physician can institute appropriate treatment. 3. Give medications per order: sedatives, tranquilizers. 4. Requisition laboratory tests as ordered by physician. 5. Facilitate rest: physical rest by pain medication; emotional rest by encouraging expression of feelings, answering questions. 6. Avoid accusatory responses: verbal, nonverbal.	1. If woman to be treated is at home, teach about rest, diet, and avoidance of orgasm or straining at stool, signs and symptoms to report immediately, and the need for saving clots and tissue and bringing them to physician.
Intranatal		
1. Note woman's past obstetric history. 2. Note progress and duration of this pregnancy. 3. Observe current symptoms: vital signs; character of uterine consistency, cramping, vaginal discharge (save all bloodied material, keep pad count, save all vaginal discharge for physician to evaluate); note Rh factor. 4. Note if woman had cerclage for incompetent cervix. 5. Note woman's religious preference. a. Ask regarding baptism of products of conception. b. Ask regarding feelings about blood transfusions.	1. Maintain calm, confident, sympathetic manner. 2. Alert physician if cerclage had been done earlier. 3. Avoid accusatory verbal responses (e.g., "You and your man been fooling around, eh?") or nonverbal responses. 4. Stay with woman and provide comfort measures used with women in labor. 5. Comfort family members. 6. Assist with treatments and procedures (e.g., blood transfusion, antibiotic therapy). 7. Prepare woman and family if D and C is contemplated. 8. Have products of conception baptized or have clergy member there if desired.	1. Acquaint woman regarding treatments and procedures (e.g., what to expect during D and C). 2. Answer questions: some couples are interested in sex of fetus or wish to see fetus.
Postnatal		
1. Monitor physiologic responses: vital signs, bleeding, laboratory reports; response to blood transfusion, etc.	1. Administer physician-ordered medications and treatments. 2. Assist woman and family with emotional reactions. 3. Give Rh(D) immune globulin within 72 hours. 4. Notify clergy member to visit if woman and family desire.	1. Tell woman what to expect during recovery. 2. Teach woman about danger signs and symptoms (bleeding, fever, cramping, pain) and whom to call should they occur. 3. Provide information regarding contraceptives as appropriate.

Evaluation. The nurse can be assured that care was effective if goals of care are met.

ECTOPIC PREGNANCY

Ectopic pregnancy is a gestation implanted outside the uterine cavity (Fig. 35.2). Fully 90% of ectopic pregnancies occur in the fallopian tube, most of these on the right side, for undetermined reasons. Approximately 1 of every 200 pregnancies are ectopic, and at least three fourths of these become symptomatic and are diagnosed during the first trimester. Ectopic pregnancy is a significant cause of maternal morbidity and mortality even in developed countries.

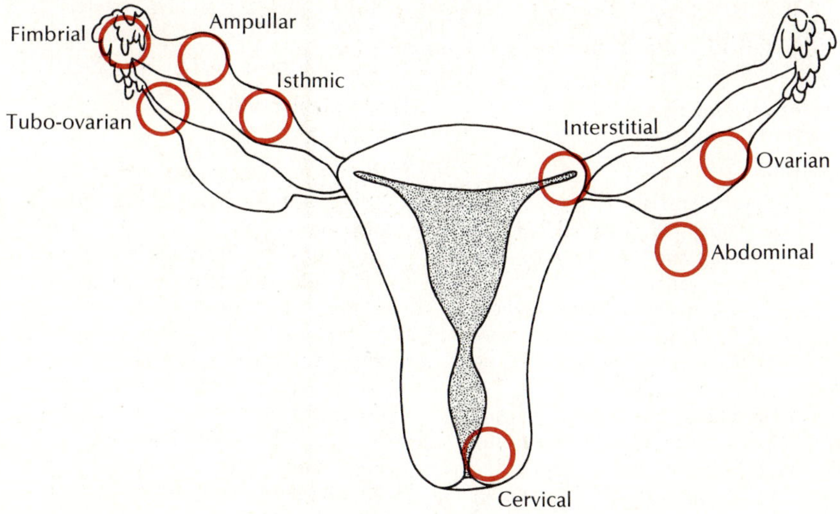

Fig. 35.2
Sites of implantation of ectopic pregnancies. In order of frequency of occurrence: ampulla, isthmus, interstitium, fimbria, tubo-ovarian ligament, ovary, abdominal cavity, and cervix (external os).

Etiology. The majority of extrauterine pregnancies result from abnormalities that impede or prevent the transit of the fertilized ovum through the fallopian tube (e.g., peritubal adhesions following pelvic inflammatory disease). On occasion, an ovum is fertilized within the ovary or soon after it has been ovulated.

Clinical classification. Ectopic pregnancy is classified according to the site of implantation (e.g., tubal, ovarian, etc.). The uterus is the only organ capable of containing and sustaining a term pregnancy. However, the rare abdominal pregnancy delivered by laparotomy, may result in a living infant.

Clinical findings. There are no signs or symptoms diagnostic of early ectopic pregnancy. A missed period, adnexal fullness, and tenderness may suggest an unruptured tubal pregnancy. In contrast, the following triad is associated with early ruptured extrauterine pregnancy in almost 50% of cases:

1. Amenorrhea or an abnormal menstrual period followed by slight uterine bleeding
2. Adnexal or cul-de-sac mass
3. Unilateral pelvic pain over the mass

Additional findings of *acute* rupture may include shock, referred shoulder pain, or evidence of acute blood loss in chronic ruptured tubal pregnancy.

Hysterosalpingography is contraindicated in suspected tubal pregnancy because it may initiate tubal rupture or hemorrhage. In possible advanced abdominal pregnancy, a sonogram showing a fetus high out of the pelvis, often in abnormal presentation, may be diagnostic.

In *chronic* ruptured tubal pregnancy, which represents slightly more than half the total of ectopic pregnancies, internal bleeding usually has been slow and the symptomatology atypical or inconclusive. In addition to slight dark vaginal bleeding, a sense of pelvic pressure or fullness, lower abdominal tenderness, flatulence, and a tense, sensitive, semicystic, perhaps crepitant, cul-de-sac mass may be felt. Slight fever, leukocytosis, and a falling hematocrit or hemoglobin level may be noted. An ecchymotic blueness of the umbilicus (Cullen's sign), which is indicative of hematoperitoneum, may develop in a neglected ruptured intraabdominal ectopic pregnancy.

Diagnosis. The following procedures are useful in the diagnosis of ectopic pregnancy:

1. A careful history with identification of a late LMP or an actual missed period followed by slight vaginal bleeding may be indicative.
2. Careful pelvic examination, under anesthesia if necessary, reveals an adnexal or cul-de-sac mass.
3. Culdocentesis may yield free blood that will not clot or is already clotted.
4. Culdotomy may release gross clotted blood, perhaps including the aborted products of an extrauterine pregnancy.
5. Laparoscopy may disclose an extrauterine pregnancy.
6. D and C will produce pregnancy endometrium, without chorionic villi in ectopic pregnancy. However, a uterine pregnancy or perhaps a threatened or incomplete abortion may be encountered.
7. Laparotomy will reveal the correct diagnosis and provide the best opportunity for treatment.

Differential diagnosis. The differential diagnosis of ectopic pregnancy involves a consideration of numerous

Ectopic Pregnancy

Assessment/analysis	Plan/implementation	Rationale
Prenatal		
1. Observe woman for symptoms: colicky pain on affected side, severe pain and shock (with rupture). 2. Note significant data on medical, surgical, and obstetric history: treatment for gonorrhea or other pelvic inflammatory disease, abdominal surgery, spontaneous or voluntary abortions, ectopic pregnancies. 3. Note woman's religious preference: ask woman (or family) regarding baptism of products of conception; blood transfusions. 4. Note woman's Rh factor to assess if candidate for Rh(D) immune globulin.	1. Refer woman to physician immediately; alert physician that woman is coming to hospital. 2. Alert laboratory and request blood work; type, cross match. 3. Set up for administration of intravenous fluids (use large-bore needle to accommodate blood if necessary), oxygen, and emergency medications, with appropriate equipment. (Frequently, women are admitted directly to surgery by way of emergency room.) Carry out preoperative procedures. 4. Arrange for conceptus to be baptized (or perform the rite).	1. Inform woman and family briefly of happenings. 2. Reexplain (clarify, simplify) physician explanations regarding cause, management, and postoperative recovery, including chances for subsequent pregnancies.
Postdelivery		
1. Assess woman's physiologic response: vital signs, bleeding, reaction to therapy, elimination, etc. 2. Assess woman's and family's emotional reactions to experience.	1. Give Rh$_0$(D) immune globulin, if indicated (see p. 964). 2. Facilitate grieving process. 3. Administer and monitor fluids, medications, treatments, and diet per physician's order and woman's preference and tolerance. 4. Inform woman and family if baptism was done (also record on nurses' notes). 5. Notify clergy member to visit if woman and family desire.	1. Acquaint woman with what to expect during recovery. 2. Alert woman to symptoms to report to physician immediately. 3. Reinforce woman regarding physician's explanations. 4. Encourage woman to return for follow-up care.

disorders that share many, perhaps all, of the same signs and symptoms. The physician must consider uterine abortion, ruptured corpus luteum cyst, appendicitis, salpingitis, ovarian cysts, torsion of the ovary, and urinary tract infection.

Prevention. Prevention of ectopic pregnancy per se is impossible. Early vigorous treatment of gonorrhea should prevent salpingitis or limit tubal disease. Prolonged bleeding or fever after supposedly complete abortion should be treated by D and C and antibiotic therapy to reduce the likelihood of postabortal salpingitis.

Management. The major problem in ectopic pregnancy is hemorrhage; bleeding must be quickly and effectively controlled. The physician must consider blood loss and impending shock. Blood transfusions must be available. Laparotomy may be effected immediately after the diagnosis of ectopic pregnancy is made. Blood and clots are evacuated, and bleeding vessels are controlled. Excision of the cornua and fallopian tube is recommended if the tube is grossly involved. The ovary should be conserved if possible. Hysterectomy usually is necessary for ruptured cornual or interstitial pregnancy.

Linear incision of the tube, salpingostomy, and evacuation of a small tubal pregnancy may be feasible in rare instances.

Ovarian pregnancy always requires loss of the ovary, and the tube if the latter is densely adherent.

Prophylactic appendectomy or other elective procedures are permissible only if the woman's general condition is good, the procedure is not difficult, and the woman has given informed consent.

Chronic or advanced ectopic pregnancy requires laparotomy as soon as the woman is fit for surgery. If the placenta of a second- or third-trimester abdominal pregnancy is attached to a vital organ, for example, the liver, no attempt at separation and removal should be made. The cord should be cut flush with the placenta and the afterbirth left in situ. Degeneration and absorption of the placenta usually occur without complications.

Prognosis. Maternal death from ectopic pregnancy is about 1 in 800 in North America. Maternal morbidity and secondary surgery are high, however, principally because of inaccurate or delayed diagnosis of ectopic pregnancy.

The perinatal mortality in ectopic pregnancy is virtually 100%.

Ectopic pregnancy recurs in approximately 10% of women, but more than 50% of women who have had an ectopic pregnancy achieve at least one normal gestation thereafter.

Summary of nursing actions

Goals of care

1. The woman's physiologic functions are restored. Shock is controlled.
2. The woman understands the anatomic and physiologic alterations in reproductive capacity resulting from the surgical intervention.
3. Sequelae (e.g., infection) are prevented or promptly diagnosed and treated; Rh isoimmunization is prevented; anemia is treated.
4. The woman retains a positive sense of self-esteem and self-worth.

Examples of nursing diagnoses

1. In an ectopic pregnancy: increased potential for anemia because of client's refusal of blood transfusion.
2. In a postdelivery situation: potential decrease in self-esteem because of loss of part of the reproductive tract.

Evaluation. The nurse can be assured that care has been effective if goals for care have been met.

HYDATIDIFORM MOLE

Hydatidiform (hydatid) mole is a developmental anomaly of the placenta; the fetus usually is absent. The fertilized ovum deteriorates, and the chorionic villi convert into a mass of clear, grapelike vesicles of tapioca consistency.

Etiology. The cause is unknown. Hydatidiform mole occurs in about 1 in 2000 pregnancies. It is much more common in the Orient, for unexplained reasons. Hydatidiform mole is more frequent after induction of ovulation by clomiphene. It is also more common in older women.

Clinical classification. The clinical classification of a hydatidiform mole reflects its localization or dissemination. A benign mole is well localized in the uterus, whereas a metastatic mole must be considered malignant.

Clinical findings and diagnosis

I. Symptomatology.
   A. The uterus becomes enlarged out of proportion to the duration of pregnancy. At 3 months it may be the size of a 5-mo pregnancy.
   B. There is excessive nausea and vomiting (hyperemesis gravidarum) (see p. 865).
   C. By the twelfth week there is an intermittent or continuous brownish red discharge.
   D. Uterine discomfort from overstretching may be reported. Rarely the uterus may rupture (Fig. 35.3).

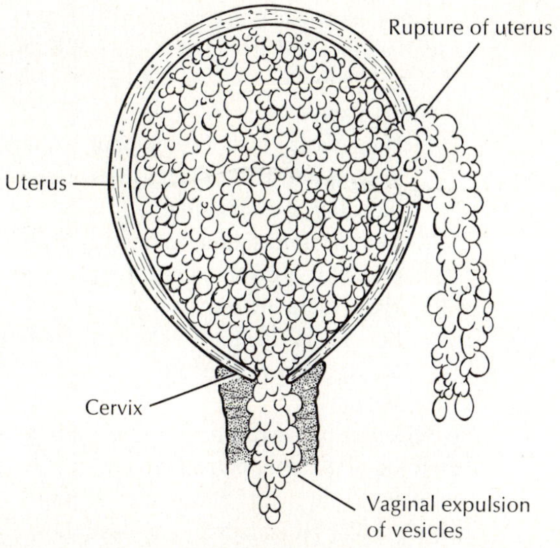

Fig. 35.3
Uterine rupture with hydatidiform mole. *1,* Evacuation of mole through cervix. *2,* Rupture of uterus and spillage of mole into peritoneal cavity (rare).

Hydatidiform Mole

Assessment/analysis	Plan/implementation
1. Observe for symptoms: excessive vomiting, hypertension, continuous or intermittent brown spotting or passage of grapelike vesicles, unusually rapid uterine enlargement. 2. Observe woman's response to medical induction of labor or surgical intervention: vital signs, pain, etc. 3. Observe for signs of grief and grieving by woman and family. Assess woman's support system.	1. Refer woman immediately to physician; alert physician to findings. 2. Prepare woman for diagnostic activities: sonography, serum HCG determination, induced abortion, possible D and C, or hysterectomy. 3. Assist physician with induction or other procedures. 4. Encourage woman and family to grieve by assisting them in the following ways: a. To cry and act out their grief b. To identify and explore feelings (inadequacy, guilt) regarding this event, one's responsibility for it, or delay in seeking treatment (should this exist) c. To talk of fears for future childbearing, possible surgery, and death from cancer 5. Provide simple, cogent explanations to woman and family, reemphasizing or repeating what physician has told her (them) regarding the following: a. Etiology b. Course of treatment for hydatidiform mole and any coexisting problems (e.g., hemorrhage, D and C, hysterectomy) c. Follow-up supervision for 1 year d. Need for contraception for 1 year

E. Fullness, softness, and thinning of the lower uterine segment can be detected.

F. In addition, symptoms of true preeclampsia-eclampsia (PIH) may occur even though it is well before the twentieth week of pregnancy (see p. 809).

II. Laboratory findings.

A. Routine urinalysis may reveal protein. (Pregnancy-induced hypertension [PIH] may occur in the *first* trimester as a result of this complication.)

B. Blood values.

1. Hematocrit and hemoglobin values as well as the RBC decrease as a result of bleeding and infection.
2. The sedimentation rate and WBC increase as a result of infection.
3. HCG titers are elevated up to 1 to 2 million IU in 24 hours. (Normal HCG titer at 10 weeks is approximately 400,000 IU.)

III. No FHR can be heard nor can fetal parts be discerned on abdominal palpation.

IV. Ultrasonography (the most useful tool) may identify molar pregnancy by the third month. No fetal skeleton is revealed.

Prevention. No prevention of hydatidiform mole is known.

Management. Management of hydatidiform mole involves evacuation of the uterus by carefully induced abortion or performance of a hysterectomy. Induced abortion may be followed by D and C in a few days after the friable (easily torn or perforated) uterine wall becomes firmer. Curetted tissue is examined for residual or proliferative trophoblastic tissue. Hysterectomy is often the procedure of choice, especially if the woman is 45 years of age or older or if the uterus appears to be ready to rupture. Blood loss is replaced.

Follow-up supervision for 1 year includes the following:

1. HCG is measured (a) once weekly until HCG titers are negative for 3 consecutive weeks, then (b) once monthly for 6 months, then (c) every 2 months for 6 months, and then (d) every 6 months.

2. Continued high titers or rising titers of HCG indicate a pathologic condition. D and C is done if the uterus is intact, and the tissue is examined. If malignant cells are found, chemotherapy for choriocarcinoma is begun: methotrexate and dactinomycin are the drugs of choice. Chemotherapy (methotrexate or dactinomycin or a combination of drugs) is administered if (a) HCG titers plateau for 3 consecutive weeks or double at any

time, or (b) HCG titers remain elevated at any level 3 to 4 months after termination of pregnancy. If chemotherapy is ineffective, the choriocarcinoma has a tendency toward rapid and widespread metastasis.

3. Chest x-ray studies are done every month until HCG titers are negative and then every 2 months for 1 year.

4. Oral contraceptive use is advocated to prevent another pregnancy (which would distort HCG titers) and to suppress endogenous pituitary luteinizing hormone (LH), which could distort HCG titer assays.

5. Another pregnancy is not advised until 1 year after tests are negative.

If HCG levels remain within normal limits for a year, the physician may assure the woman or couple that normal pregnancy can be anticipated, with a low probability of recurrence of hydatidiform mole if the woman is 40 years of age or younger.

Prognosis. The prognosis for hydatidiform mole is favorable if the chorionic gonadotropin titer does not persist at elevated levels or recur after elimination of the mole. The prognosis is unfavorable if a malignant mole is discovered and is untreated.

Summary of nursing actions

Goals of care

1. Pregnancy is terminated in a manner most conducive to the woman's health.
2. If invasive mole or choriocarcinoma develops, control and treatment with chemotherapy are successful.
3. The woman and family appreciate the seriousness of the condition and adhere to the treatment schedule; the couple postpones another pregnancy until a safe date.
4. The woman and family realize that the prognosis is excellent (almost 100%) if treatment is undertaken.

Example of nursing diagnosis. The following is a possible nursing diagnosis in hydatidiform mole: potential misdiagnosis of choriocarcinoma because of occurrence of pregnancy within 1 year after a molar pregnancy.

Evaluation. The nurse can be assured that care has been effective if goals of care are met.

Late Pregnancy

PREMATURE SEPARATION OF PLACENTA

Premature separation of the placenta, also termed *abruptio placentae,* is the separation of part or all of the placenta before the birth of the baby.

Premature separation of the placenta is a serious disorder and accounts for about 15% of all perinatal deaths. Approximately one third of infants of women with premature separation of the placenta will die. More than 50% of these die as a result of preterm delivery, and many others die of intrauterine hypoxia.

Incidence. Certain individuals seem predisposed to premature separation of the placenta. This problem is much more common in women with hypertension of any cause; 40% of women with diastolic pressures of 90 or more experience some degree of abruptio placentae. Premature separation of the placenta occurs about once in 150 late gestations. The incidence is three times greater in women with a gravidity of more than five than in primigravidas. Women with a history of reproductive loss (abortion, premature labor, prenatal hemorrhage, stillbirth, or neonatal death) experience premature separation of the placenta more than twice as often as the average population at risk. Between 15% to 20% of women who have had a previous premature separation of the placenta will have a recurrence. If the woman has had two prior premature separations, the chance in the next pregnancy is at least 25%.

Etiology. The cause of premature separation of the placenta is unknown in most cases, but a sudden decrease in uterine size (as can occur with rupture of the membranes) may be responsible. Precipitating factors include vascular engorgement during compression of the ascending vena cava, followed by sudden uteroplacental vasodilatation. Abdominal trauma is a factor in less than 5% of cases, and short cord is identified in less than 1%.

Clinical manifestations and differential diagnosis. The separation may be partial or complete, or only the margin of the placenta may be involved. Bleeding from the placental site may dissect (separate) the membranes from the decidua basalis and bleed out through the vagina; it may remain concealed (retroplacental hemorrhage); or it may do both. Clinical symptomatology varies with the degree of separation (Table 35.3).

I. Symptomatology
   A. *Uterine bleeding* with small to moderate amount of dark red vaginal bleeding in 80% of cases
      1. Hypovolemia: shock; oliguria, anuria
      2. Coagulopathy
   B. *Uterine hypertonicity* (mild to severe); possible Couvelaire uterus (see p. 792)
   C. *Pain:* mild to severe, localized over one region of the uterus or diffuse over uterus with a boardlike abdomen
II. Laboratory findings
   A. Apt test (see Glossary) of amniotic fluid: indicates presence of maternal blood
   B. Fall in hemoglobin and hematocrit: may appear later

Table 35.3
Summary of Findings: Abruptio Placentae and Placenta Previa

	Abruptio Placentae			
	Marginal Separation	Moderate Separation	Severe Separation* (more than 66%)	Placenta Previa
Bleeding: external, vaginal	Minimal	Absent to moderate	Absent to moderate	Minimal to severe and life threatening
Color of blood	Dark red	Dark red	Dark red	Bright red
Shock	Absent	Frequent	Very common; often sudden	Occasional
Coagulopathy	Rare	Occasional	Common	Rare
Uterine tonicity	Normal	Increased—may be localized to one region or diffuse over uterus; uterus fails to relax between contractions	Tetanic, persistent uterine contraction; boardlike uterus	Normal
Tenderness	Usually absent; if present, is localized	Increased—usually diffuse over uterus	Agonizing, unremitting uterine pain	Absent
Ultrasonographic findings				
Location of placenta	Normal—upper uterine segment	Normal—upper uterine segment	Normal—upper uterine segment	Abnormal—lower uterine segment
Station of presenting part	Variable to engaged	Variable to engaged	Variable to engaged	High—not engaged
Fetal position	Usual distribution†	Usual distribution	Usual distribution	Frequently transverse, breech or, oblique
Concurrent hypertensive state	Usual distribution	Frequently present	Frequently present	Usual distribution

*Onset is usually abrupt; fetus usually dies (see Fig. 35.6).
†Usual distribution refers to the usual variations or incidence seen when there is no concurrent problem.

C. Fall in coagulation factors: may appear later
D. Clot retraction increased

III. Sonography
A. Implantation site of placenta: normal
B. Initially, retroplacental blood clot may not be visible, but enlarging clot may be seen when sonogram is repeated
C. Fetal position: within usual distribution, (e.g., generally in vertical lie with head presenting)
D. Fetal station: within usual distribution (e.g., from high [−5 cm] to engaged [0 station] or deeper in the birth canal)

Complications. Most complications accompany moderate to severe abruptio placentae.

1. Hypovolemic shock
   a. Pituitary necrosis
   b. Renal failure
2. Fetal hypoxia, or anoxia with possible fetal death
3. Coagulopathy (DIC)
4. Couvelaire uterus
5. Hepatitis
   a. Sequel to blood transfusion
   b. Sequel to fibrinogen replacement

Hypovolemic shock may result from loss of blood from the maternal circulation. Prolonged hypovolemia results in ischemia (and hypoxia). Ischemia of the pituitary gland causes pituitary necrosis (Sheehan's syndrome) (see p. 807). Ischemia of the kidneys leads to renal failure: acute tubular necrosis that may be reversible or acute cortical necrosis that is not reversible.

Continued bleeding that cannot exit easily may rup-

Premature Separation of Placenta

Assessment/analysis

Prenatal

1. Assess all women for predisposing factors: hypertension, multiple gestation, vena cava syndrome, diabetes, multiparity, and advanced maternal age.
2. Observe woman for signs of premature separation (may occur during labor).
   a. Dark red vaginal bleeding or port-wine–colored amniotic fluid may be noted.
   b. Shock may occur, resulting in drop in blood pressure and increase in pulse rate, dyspnea, pallor, and syncope. Symptoms are often out of proportion to amount of bleeding seen.
   c. Uterine pain may be severe and sudden (if retroplacental) or painless (if separation is marginal and blood drains out through the vagina).
   d. During labor the uterus may not contract evenly or relax between contractions.
   e. Abdomen may or may not be rigid (if blood can exit, uterus is not rigid); myometrium becomes boardlike (Couvelaire uterus).
   f. Hyperactivity of fetus with onset of pain may be followed by loss of FHR. Use electronic monitor if available.
3. Observe woman for complications: shock, pulmonary emboli, coagulopathy, and acute renal failure.

Plan/implementation

1. Encourage left lateral position during labor to avoid compressing the vena cava. Instruct the couple in breathing and other techniques while the woman is in this position.
2. If symptoms are noted:
   a. Send for physician.
   b. Turn woman onto her side; administer oxygen at 10 to 12 L/min by means of face mask; start intravenous infusion or increase flow (if intravenous fluid does not have oxytocin in it!).
   c. Do not leave woman.
   d. Have someone request laboratory work: blood type and cross match, platelets, prothrombin time (PT), and partial thromboplastin time (PTT) (Table 35.5).
   e. Prepare for double setup examination to rule out placenta previa and for induction or augmentation of labor (e.g. amniotomy), abdominal surgery (cesarean birth, hysterectomy), or immediate vaginal delivery if cervix is dilated and presenting part is low.
3. Alert pediatrician and supporting nursing staff to be present for delivery. Infant may require attention for prematurity, hypoxia, or birth injury caused by interventions.
4. Briefly explain to woman's family what is occurring.

Assessment/analysis

Postdelivery or postsurgical

1. Determine:
   a. If hysterectomy was performed.
   b. If fetus died.
   c. If neonate is alive, its condition.
2. Assess woman's physiologic response: amount and source of bleeding, vital signs, gastrointestinal functioning, renal function. If uterus was retained, check height of fundus and its contractility; hemorrhage may occur in presence of "firm" fundus (Couvelaive uterus).
3. Observe for any reaction to cryoprecipitate, if this was given.
4. Assess for puerperal infection.
5. Assess for onset of lactation (a sign of pituitary function).
6. Assess woman's and family's emotional response to experience.

Plan/implementation

1. Institute care following cesarean or vaginal birth.
2. Administer medications per physician's order for discomfort, infection, anemia, or uterine atony. Monitor intravenous fluids.
3. Report oliguria, hematuria, or proteinuria so that therapy for acute renal tubular necrosis (may be reversible) or bilateral renal cortical necrosis (may be fatal) can be started promptly if either of these diagnoses is made.
4. Assist woman and family with grieving process.
5. Reinforce physician's explanation regarding cause, management, and prognosis.

---

ture through the fetal membranes or spread in between the muscle fibers of the myometrium. Pressure from the confined expanding volume of blood may rupture the amniotic sac; the blood imparts a port-wine color to amniotic fluid.

Extravasation of blood into the myometrium has several sequelae:

1. Myometrial tissue is damaged, necrosis results, and thromboplastin is released, thus initiating the clotting mechanism (see p. 796). Fibrinogen and platelet levels fall as these clotting factors are used to form the retroplacental clot, and coagulopathy (DIC) results.

2. Small amounts of blood in the myometrium cause ecchymosis and a localized increase in tonicity. The woman may or may not experience uterine tenderness.

3. Increasing amounts of blood in the myometrium increase uterine tonicity, irritability, and tenderness that spread over the entire uterus; the ability of the uterus to

relax between contractions diminishes or is lost. Electronic fetal monitoring reflects the increasing fetal distress that may finally end in fetal death.

4. After delivery, the uterus may feel firm because of the blood between the muscle fibers in the myometrium. However, uterine contractile efficiency and therefore its ability to close off bleeding sinuses are diminished or absent (Couvelaire uterus). Serious postpartum hemorrhage is a life-threatening sequel. Hysterectomy may be necessary to control bleeding.

Therapy. The nurse assists the physician in implementing the following therapeutic measures.

1. Restore blood loss.
   a. If shock is present or appears imminent *and* clotting mechanism is intact, central venous pressure (CVP) or pulmonary artery wedge pressure (PAWP) monitoring is started to monitor blood and fluid replacement accurately.
   b. A retention catheter is placed to monitor urinary output accurately for volume and proteinuria (oliguria and proteinuria are ominous signs).
2. Anticipate and correct coagulopathy.
3. Monitor fetal status.
4. Deliver the fetus.
   a. Fetal membranes are ruptured.
   b. Oxytocin infusion is begun if labor does not start spontaneously or if labor must be augmented.
   c. Cesarean delivery may be performed.
5. Perform hysterectomy if Couvelaire uterus occurs.
6. Provide emotional suppport for the woman and her family.

Prognosis. Maternal mortality approaches 1% in premature separation of the placenta; this condition remains a leading cause of maternal death. The mother's prognosis depends on the extent of the placental detachment, overall blood loss, degree of DIC, and time between the placental ''accident'' and delivery. Fortunately 80% to 90% of all premature separations of the placenta only involve two or three cotyledons, and therefore the prognosis generally is not grave.

Fetal prognosis is poor. At least 25% of babies of mothers with premature placental separation die before, during, or soon after birth. Of those who survive, there is an increase in the absolute numbers of neurologically damaged infants. Fetal depression occurs with at least twice the normal frequency. If the Apgar score at 5 minutes is less than 3, the infant may have sustained neurologic damage. If the 5-min Apgar score is 7 or greater, there is about a 90% chance of normal growth and development. Infants with premature separation of the placenta who weigh more than 2500 g and who have good Apgar scores usually develop normally. About 60% of infants with premature separation of the placenta who weigh less than 2500 g at birth develop normally.

Summary of nursing actions

Goals of care

1. Blood loss is minimized, and lost blood is replaced.
2. DIC is prevented or successfully treated.
3. Normal reproductive functioning is retained.
4. The fetus is safely delivered.
5. The woman retains a positive sense of self-esteem and self-worth.

Examples of nursing diagnoses

1. In premature separation of the placenta: potential hypovolemic shock because of abrupt, complete separation of the placenta.
2. In a possible postdelivery (or postsurgical) situation: potential hemorrhage because of inability of myometrium to contract (Couvelaire uterus).

Evaluation. The nurse is assured that care was effective if the goals of care are met.

PLACENTA PREVIA

In placenta previa the placenta is implanted in the lower uterine segment, where it encroaches on the internal os. All or a portion of the placenta may cover the internal os. The placenta completely covers the internal os in slightly more than 10% of the cases. Under these circumstances the placenta precedes the fetus in vaginal delivery.

Persistent excessive prenatal bleeding may seriously threaten the mother. The maternal (not fetal) circulation is the source of bleeding. Vaginal or rectal examination or attempts to deliver from below may lacerate or separate the placenta, and as a consequence, exsanguinating maternal or fetal hemorrhage (through a tear in the placenta) may occur. Placenta previa is a major cause of maternal and perinatal morbidity and mortality.

The incidence of placenta previa is about 1 in every 200 pregnancies and increases with parity.

Etiology. The cause of placenta previa is speculative. Reduced vascularity of the upper segment because of scarring from uterine surgery or tumor necessitating lower implantation of the placenta is a plausible theory.

Multiple gestation that requires a larger surface area for placental implantation may be a factor. Vessels of the endometrium involved in previous sites of implantation undergo changes that may reduce the blood supply to those regions thus predisposing to low implantation in subsequent pregnancies.

Pathology. The site of implantation and size of the placenta are related. Specifically, because the circulation of the lower uterine segment is less favorable than that of the fundus, placenta previa may have to cover a larger area for adequate efficiency. In placenta previa the surface area may be at least 30% greater than the averge placenta implanted in the fundus. The lower segment is relatively noncontractile, and bleeding can be considerable from open sinusoids. Ascending infection from the vagina may result in placentitis, especially in the area of exposure at or over the os.

Placenta previa or low-lying placenta may encourage oblique, breech, or transverse presentation and may prevent engagement of the presenting fetal part.

Clinical manifestations and differential diagnosis

Symptomatology. *Painless uterine bleeding,* especially during the third trimester, characterizes placenta previa (Table 35.3). Obviously placenta previa may occur in the first or second trimester also, but abortion generally occurs without knowledge of the site of placentation.

The bright red bleeding may be intermittent, in gushes, or, more rarely, continuous. It may start while the woman is resting or in the midst of any activity. Fortunately exsanguination almost never occurs unless vaginal or rectal examination initiates violent bleeding before or during early labor.

The detachment of placenta previa is painless. However, if the first bleeding coincides with the onset of labor, the woman may experience discomfort because of uterine contractions.

Abdominal examination usually reveals a soft (relaxed) uterus of normal tone and nontender. If the fetus is in a longitudinal lie, the fundal height is usually greater than expected for gestational age because the low placenta hinders descent of the presenting fetal part. Leopold's maneuvers may reveal a fetus in an oblique or breech position or transverse lie because of the abnormal site of placental implantation.

As a rule, fetal distress or fetal death occurs only if a significant portion of the placenta previa becomes detached from the decidua basalis or if the mother suffers hypovolemic shock.

Vaginal examination. Sterile vaginal examination by the physician will diagnose placenta previa as noted earlier, but examination should be postponed, if possible, until viability has been reached (preferably after the thirty-fourth week). Moreover, the examination should be a so-called *double-setup procedure.**

In a double setup a sterile vaginal examination is performed in an operating room with staff and equipment ready to effect an immediate vaginal or cesarean delivery. Since manipulation of the lower uterine segment or cervix may result in profound hemorrhage, preparation for immediate delivery is essential. Readiness implies an intravenous unit in place with a needle large enough to accommodate blood transfusion, two units of matched blood for the mother, sterile tables set up and open, anethetists present, at least one physician and one nurse scrubbed, and a pediatrician present. Amniotomy for anticipated vaginal delivery (if placenta is low lying, cervix is favorable, and presenting part is low) or cesarean delivery (if placenta encroaches on or covers the cervical os or fetus is in oblique or transverse lie) should be performed.

Laboratory findings. Laboratory findings are not diagnostic of placenta previa. Blood clots and blood may contain fetal red blood cells.

Ultrasonography. Ultrasonography is useful in that the two-dimensional B-scan can reveal the presence of a low-lying placenta, but whether the placenta overlays the cervix may be uncertain by this modality.

Clinical classification. Placenta previa (Figs. 35.4 and 35.5) often is described as *complete, total,* or *central* if the internal os is entirely covered by the placenta, when the cervix is fully dilated.

Partial placenta previa implies incomplete coverage. *Marginal placenta previa* indicates that only an edge of the placenta approaches the internal os. The term *low-lying (low) implantation* is used when the placenta is in the lower uterine segment but away from the os.

A better classification of placenta previa is the estimation of percentage coverage of the internal os *at full dilatation,* the diameter required for delivery of a mature fetus through the cervix (Fig. 35.6).

Prevention. Placenta previa cannot be prevented. The problem can be detected early, however, and with the avoidance of aggressive diagnostic methods, safe delivery after fetal viability has been reached usually is possible.

Management. Delivery by the most conservative means is the management of placenta previa. When fetal maturity is near, conservative management (e.g., bed rest in the hospital to extend the period of gestation) is usually possible, because initial spontaneous critical bleeding almost never occurs in placenta previa. When fetal lung maturity is achieved and survival is likely, then elective termination of pregnancy can be carried out.

After the diagnosis of placenta previa has been made, the woman should remain in the hospital under close supervision. At least two units of blood, typed and cross matched, must be available for emergency use. The duration of pregnancy should be confirmed and, except in an emergency, delivery postponed until after the thirty-sixth week.

If the woman has greater than a 30% placenta previa

*Sonography eliminates the need for examination under double-setup conditions in some instances.

Fig. 35.4
Types of placenta previa before onset of labor. **A,** Complete, or total. **B,** Incomplete, or partial. **C,** Marginal, or low-lying.

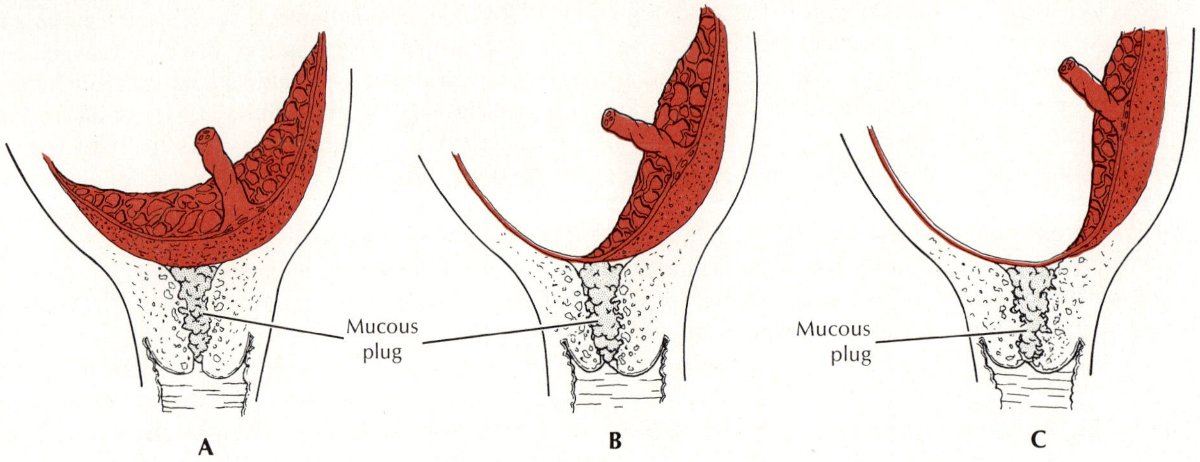

Fig. 35.5
Types of placenta previa after onset of labor. **A,** Complete, or total. **B,** Incomplete, or partial. **C,** Marginal, or low-lying.

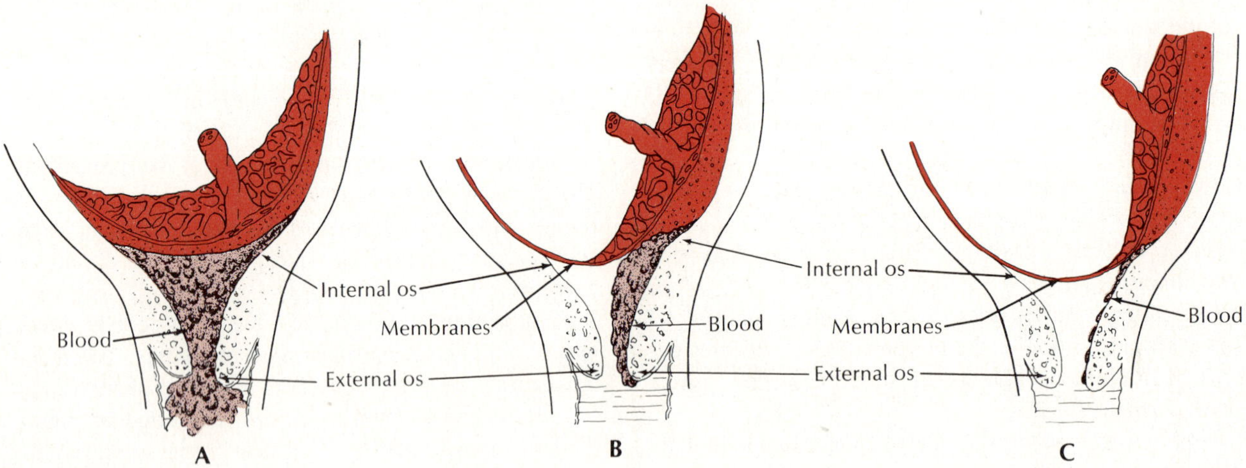

or if bleeding is excessive, cesarean delivery is indicated, preferably with the woman under light general inhalation anesthesia.

If hemorrhage is in progress and vaginal delivery is planned, the membranes are ruptured, if it is easy, permitting the presenting part to tamponade the edge of an incomplete placenta previa, thus checking brisk bleeding. If there is less than a 30% placenta previa, cautious stimulation of labor by continuous intravenous oxytocin drip is permissible unless bleeding is aggravated. If labor does not ensue within about 6 hours and if progress is not rapid, cesarean birth is indicated. The fetus may

Fig. 35.6
Classification of placenta previa. (Modified from Tatum, H.J., and Mule, J.G.: Am J. Obstet. Gynecol. **93:**768, 1965.)

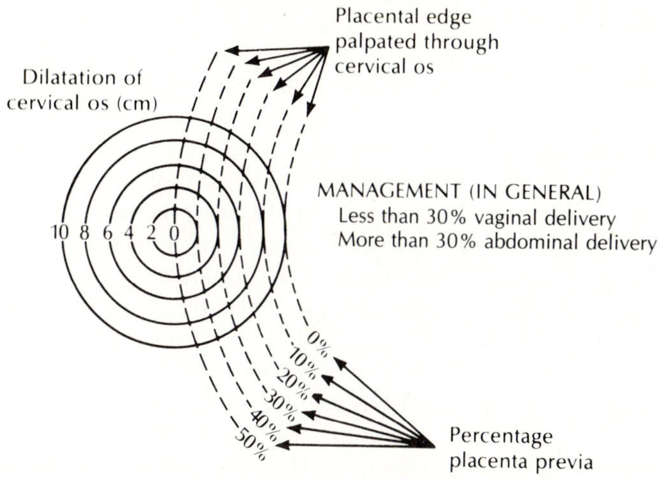

Placenta Previa

Assessment/analysis

Prenatal

1. Observe for and assess external blood loss: count pads and weigh pads and linen. Ask woman if bleeding ran down her legs and amounted to a "cupful" or a "tablespoonful." Bleeding is usually bright red (as opposed to dark, as in abruptio placentae).
2. Assess pain if present. Bleeding is generally painless, but women may be experiencing labor as well, or placenta previa may be complicated by abruptio placentae.
3. Assess uterine contractibility. Uterus should have normal tone and relax completely between contractions if abruptio placentae is not a complication.
4. Monitor FHR with ultrasound fetal pulse detector continuously. Otherwise, check every 5 to 10 minutes when woman is in active labor or more often if active bleeding is present.
5. Monitor maternal vital signs and CVP or PAWP.
6. Assess fetal lie; breech, transverse, or oblique position is frequent. Placental placement also hinders engagement of presenting part so that fundus is higher than expected.
7. Review chart for EDC, Rh factor, and history of this pregnancy. (Was there spotting earlier?)
8. Assess laboratory findings: hemoglobin and hematocrit values, Rh factor, urinalysis.

Postdelivery and postsurgical

1. Assess surgical response (if birth was cesarean).
2. Monitor height of fundus, uterine contractility, and amount of bleeding. (Lower uterine segment does not contract well; myometrial trauma may predispose it to atony.)
3. Observe woman for signs of infection. Woman is at increased risk for infection because abnormal placental site is slower to heal and closer to the vagina, and hemorrhage predisposes her to infection.

Plan/implementation

1. Utilize knowledge of position of placenta and amount of bleeding to guide management.
   a. Keep woman on NPO regimen.
   b. Do *not* perform rectal or vaginal examination; do *not* give enema.
   c. Institute bed rest with head of bed elevated 20 to 30 degrees (semi-Fowler's position). (This encourages fetal body to act as tamponade.)
   d. Start intravenous fluid administration with large-bore needle. (Ringer's lactated solution is a better volume expander than 5% dextrose in water.) Monitor drip rate.
   e. Throughout management, encourage verbalization of concerns and questions. Explain procedures to woman and family.
   f. If FHR is being monitored electronically and is good, turn audio on so couple can listen if they wish.
   g. Prepare woman for double-setup examination, ultrasonography, and placenta scan, as ordered.
   h. Assist with vaginal delivery if cervix is favorable, presenting part is low, and bleeding is minimal or contained.
   i. Prepare woman for cesarean birth if unable to deliver vaginally.
   j. Alert pediatrician and nursery staff to be present for delivery.

1. After vaginal delivery give usual postdelivery care, monitor blood transfusion, and administer antibiotics, oxytocics, and analgesics as ordered.
2. After cesarean birth give postoperative care.
3. If infant has died or is ill, provide emotional support.
4. Encourage verbalization and questions about this experience.
5. Reaffirm physician's explanations regarding cause, management, and expected recovery.

have bled through small tears in the placenta; hence the cord is clamped early at cesarean delivery.

Bipolar (Braxton Hicks, internal podalic) version should not be employed because of the serious risk of rupture of the lower uterine segment, cervical laceration, or hemorrhage.

Blood loss may not cease with the delivery of the infant. The large vascular channels in the lower uterine segment may continue to bleed because of the diminished muscle content of the lower uterine segment. The natural mechanism to control bleeding—the interlacing muscle bundles (the "living ligature") contracting around open vessels—so characteristic of the upper part of the uterus is absent in the lower part of the uterus. Therefore postpartum hemorrhage may occur even if the fundus is contracted firmly.

The location of the placental site close to the cervical os renders it more accessible to ascending infection from the vagina. Hemorrhage and anemia increase the predisposition to antenatal infection (placentitis) and postpartal (puerperal) infection.

If uterine bleeding cannot be controlled with oxytocic drugs, ligation of the internal iliac arteries or even hysterectomy may be necessary.

Hypovolemia must be treated without overtransfusion or overinfusion. Precise control of blood and fluid replacement necessitates continuous monitoring of central venous pressure or pulmonary artery wedge pressure (see p. 802).

Prognosis. Maternal morbidity may occur from the placenta previa itself, from the management, or from the birth. Antenatal hemorrhage may be fatal or nearly fatal. Prolonged hypovolemia and hypotension, more frequently associated with abruptio placentae, lead to cerebral or renal damage (see p. 807).

Complications associated with the management of placenta previa include sepsis, surgery-related trauma to structures adjacent to the uterus, anesthesia complications, blood transfusion reactions, or overinfusion of fluids.

Maternal mortality in placenta previa has dropped almost 50% to about 0.6% during the past decade in larger centers in North America because of conservative therapy. Regrettably, however, the perinatal mortality (due primarily to prematurity) still approaches 20% in most hospitals. This figure undoubtedly can be reduced by half with better management. Currently, placenta previa increases the likelihood of death of the neonate by about 10 times.

Summary of nursing actions

Goals of care

1. A viable neonate is delivered, or if infant dies, adequate emotional support is provided.
2. The woman sustains minimal hemorrhage or hypovolemia, and anemia is rectified.
3. The woman and family understand the cause of, management of, and expected recovery from the experience.
4. The woman maintains a positive sense of self-worth and self-esteem.

Examples of nursing diagnoses

1. In placenta previa: potential loss of self-esteem because of lack of knowledge of etiology of condition.
2. In a postdelivery or postsurgical situation: potential hemorrhage because of poor contractility of lower uterine segment.

Evaluation. The nurse can be assured that care was effective if the goals of care are met.

CLOTTING DISORDERS IN PREGNANCY

Normal clotting. Normally there is a delicate balance (homeostasis) maintained between two opposing systems, the hemostatic system and the fibrinolytic system. The hemostatic system is involved in the life-saving process of stopping the flow of blood from injured vessels, in part through the formation of insoluble fibrin that acts as a hemostatic plug. The fibrinolytic system refers to the process by which the fibrin is split into fibrinolytic degradation products (FDP) and circulation is restored.

Hemostatic system. When trauma occurs to a small vessel and there is an extravasation of blood, certain responses follow that assist in limiting the blood flow. (1) Vasoconstriction of the injured vessels reduces flow of blood to the area. (2) Escape of blood into the relatively rigid supporting extravascular tissue increases the pressure and collapses capillaries and venules. (3) Substances such as thromboplastin and adenosine diphosphate (ADP) necessary to the coagulation process are released from the injured tissue and enter the bloodstream. (4) The platelets are activated by the exposure to the collagen of the injured vascular wall (or by any intravascular contaminant) and aggregate to form a platelet plug.* This soft thrombus may provide temporary or complete hemostasis depending on the extent of the injury. (5) The coagulation process, which is essential for the formation of a firm thrombus, is initiated and proceeds through three phases: phase I, formation of a prothrombin activator; phase II, conversion of prothrombin to thrombin; and phase III, conversion of fibrinogen to fibrin. These phases involve an interaction of the coagulation factors (Table 35.4) in which each factor sequentially activates the factor next in line in the so-called "cascade effect" sequence.

Coagulation process. Phase I of the coagulation process can be initiated by one of two mechanisms: (1) the

*Aspirin inhibits platelet aggregation.

Table 35.4
Blood Clotting Factors

Factor	Synonyms
I	Fibrinogen
II	Prothrombin
III	Platelet factor 3, thromboplastin
IV	Calcium
V	Labile factor, proaccelerin, AC globulin (ACG)
VI	
VII	Serum prothrombin conversion accelerator (SPCA), proconvertin, autoprothrombin
VIII	Antihemotrophic factor (AHF), antihemophilic globulin
IX	Plasma thromboplastin component (PTC), Christmas factor, autoprothrombin II
X	Stuart-Prower factor, Stuart factor, Prower factor
XI	Plasma thromboplastin antecedent (PTA)
XII	Hagemen factor
XIII	Fibrin (protein) stabilizing factor

extrinsic mechanism—a rapid process in which the precoagulation material thromboplastin comes from damaged tissue into the blood or (2) the intrinsic mechanism—a slower process in which coagulation proteins that normally circulate in an inactive form are sequentially activated and platelets are induced to release a substance (platelet factor 3) into the blood. By either mechanism, several products, collectively called *prothrombin activator,* which are necessary to initiate clotting, form in plasma. Calcium is essential for this phase.

In *phase II* of the coagulation process prothrombin activator induces the conversion of prothrombin, a plasma protein, into thrombin. Prothrombin is formed in the liver by vitamin K induction. The rate of thrombin formation depends on the amount of prothrombin activator generated. Hence, an estimate of the level of prothrombin in the blood is an indirect assessment of the factors that make up the prothrombin couples, that is, for the extrinsic mechanism, factors II, V, VII, and X, or for the intrinsic mechanism the same factors plus IX and XII. Calcium is needed in this phase.

In *phase III* of the coagulation process thrombin and fibrinogen (which is formed in the liver like prothrombin) combine to form fibrin. Polymerization of the fibrin molecules then forms a mesh of long, fibrous threads, traps blood cells, and begins to shorten to form a clot. Factors I and XIII are necessary for phase III of the coagulation process.

The development of the clot that is attached to damaged blood vessels normally contracts further within minutes to close the open vessels and staunch the blood loss. Clot retraction requires an adequate number of platelets, which apparently provide the impetus for shortening of the fibrin strands. Thrombin has a proteolytic quality and can initiate additional clotting through the breakdown of prothrombin.

Fibrinolytic system. The formation of fibrin is, however, not a continuous process. The coagulation process can be limited by the presence in tissue and leukocytes of clotting antagonists, such as antithrombins, antithromboplastins, and inhibitors of prothrombin. The immunologic system also acts to rid the circulation of some of the activated coagulation factors.

The major physiologic means of disposing of fibrin once it is formed is in the activation of the fibrinolytic system. While some fibrinolysis is carried out by leukocytes, most is attributable to the presence of plasmin. Plasmin exists in normal plasma in the form of plasminogen, which can be activated by hypoxia, tissue extracts, bacterial enzymes, activated factor XII, thrombin, and hypoglycemia. Usually plasminogen has been deposited within the fibrin clot, and once activating substances penetrate the clot, the plasminogen is converted to its active form, bound plasmin, and localized secondary fibrinolysis begins. Plasmin splits fibrin and fibrinogen into progressively smaller units (FDP). These act as powerful anticoagulants, impairing the clumping of platelets and their release of substances necessary for clotting.

Just as there are inhibitors to the hemostatic system there are inhibitors of the fibrinolytic system. Excessive fibrinolytic activity would result in widespread destruction of fibrinogen and fibrin clots and place the woman in danger from hemorrhage. The degree of fibrinolytic activity may be determined by assessing the levels of plasminogen and FDP (a decrease in plasminogen and an increase in FDP result in marked fibrinolytic activity).

Clotting problems. A history of abnormal bleeding, inheritance of unusual bleeding tendencies, and a report of significant aberrations of laboratory findings indicate a bleeding or clotting problem (Table 35.5). The comprehension of useful tests of hemostasis is based on the usual mechanisms for the control of bleeding, that is, the function of platelets and the necessary clotting factors.

Disseminated intravascular coagulation. Disseminated intravascular coagulation (DIC, defibrination syndrome, defibrination coagulopathy), a pathologic form of clotting, (1) is diffuse rather than localized, (2) injures rather than protects the necessary site of coagulation, and (3) consumes clotting factors, such as fibrinogen, so avidly that widespread external and internal bleeding follows. Multiple factors are involved, including platelet and coagulation dysfunction. Unless DIC is treated immediately and effectively, death often results.

Stimuli likely to initiate DIC. The general categories of stimuli to DIC include infusion of tissue extract, endothelial damage, anoxia, bacterial debris or endotoxins

Table 35.5
Coagulation Tests

Test	Comments
Activated partial thromboplastin time (PTT; measures intrinsic system): 25-36 sec	Screening test of choice: very sensitive, relatively easy to perform, inexpensive. All coagulation factors except proconvertin are measured.
One-stage prothrombin time (PT; Quick test; measures extrinsic system): 9.5-11.3 sec	Test for proconvertin (VII), proaccelerin (V), Stuart-Prower factor (X), prothrombin (II), and fibrinogen deficiencies. Unfortunately, it does not measure factors necessary for earlier stages of coagulation.
Thrombin time (plasma): 10-15 sec	Test measures conversion of fibrinogen to fibrin and depends on concentration of fibrinogen or inhibitors such as fibrin split-products, antithrombins, and heparin.
Platelet count: 130,000-370,000/mm^3	Most reliable index for DIC.
Specific factor assays (e.g., plasma fibrinogen): 195-365 mg/dl	Each of coagulation factors can be assessed by indirect clotting method using natural or synthetic factor-deficient substrates and compared to activity of normal plasma (100%). However, fibrinogen is only factor that can be measured directly by chemical method.
Bleeding time Template: 2-8 min Ivy: 1-7 min Duke: 1-3 min	Finger or earlobe puncture 5 mm deep and 2 mm wide (Bard-Parker blade no. 11) is made after antiseptic preparation of skin. Note time of puncture; touch bleeding point gently with sterile filter paper to absorb blood every 30 sec until bleeding stops.

(bacteremic or septic shock), chemical and physical agents, hemolytic processes, immune reactions, and thrombocytopenia. DIC occurs in critical obstetric problems related to abruptio placentae, intrauterine dead fetus syndrome, amniotic fluid embolism, preeclampsia-eclampsia, hemorrhagic shock, saline abortion, hydatidiform mole, and ruptured uterus.

Unanticipated, profuse, locally uncontrollable uterine hemorrhage, bleeding from the episiotomy, lacerations or needle puncture sites, or shock often initiates the DIC syndrome in the woman (ecchymosis or bleeding from mucous membranes or gastrointestinal tract may be apparent in the infant).

Fragmented or distorted red blood cells, for example, schistocytes (helmet cells), and a form of hemolytic anemia (micropathic hemolytic anemia) may be recognized. Laboratory tests reveal reduced platelets, fibrinogen, proaccelerin, antihemophilic factor, and prothrombin (the factors consumed during coagulation). Other factors should be normal. Fibrinolysis is first increased but later severely depressed. Degradation of fibrin leads to the accumulation of fibrin split-products in the blood. Fibrin split-products have anticoagulant properties and thus prolong the prothrombin time.

One must distinguish DIC from other clotting abnormalities, such as vitamin K deficiency, primary fibrinolysis, and excessive anticoagulation therapy.

Treatment of the basic disorder, for example, sepsis or shock, is vital. Paradoxically, cautious intravenous heparin administration may stop the abnormal clotting and check bleeding. For marked fibrin deficiency, cryoprecipitate may be given.

Fresh frozen plasma is used to supply multiple clotting factors, volume replacement, and fibrinogen. The frozen plasma is thawed in the laboratory. It should be administered within 15 to 20 minutes, since the factors disintegrate as the plasma warms. If the platelets are decreased, a transfusion of platelets can be administered.

The prognosis is guarded. It depends on the degree and extent of the underlying disorder as well as the response of the woman to prompt and proper treatment.

Management. Because DIC in pregnancy may occur insidiously or with dramatic suddenness, constant vigilance on the part of the obstetric team is necessary. The diagnostic protocol will include the following observations and tests.

1. The woman is experiencing one or more predisposing conditions: pregnancy, abruptio placentae, eclampsia, retention of a dead fetus for more than 5 weeks, amniotic fluid embolism, sepsis, tumultuous or hypertonic labor, difficult delivery, oxytocin (Pitocin) induction.

2. The woman exhibits tachycardia, diaphoresis, restlessness with anxiety, or unusual bleeding.

3. Laboratory findings (see Appendix G: normal findings) are as follows. Platelet count *(the most reliable index)* shows a decreased number. In the presence of a healthy liver, low coagulation factors are not a reliable index, since increased consumption of these factors is matched by increased production. Bleeding time is normal; coagulation time shows no clot; clot retraction time shows no clot; prothrombin time is increased; and partial thromboplastin time (PTT) is increased.

Disseminated Intravascular Coagulation

Assessment/analysis	Plan/implementation
1. Establish and maintain an adequate data base to aid in identification. a. Be alert for predisposing conditions: abruptio placentae, retention of dead fetus for more than 5 weeks, eclampsia, amniotic fluid embolus, sepsis. b. Be alert for "typical" client profile: multipara who had hypertonic, tumultuous labor or difficult delivery; woman who had oxytocin induction or labor with meconium-stained fluid. 2. Note and report the following symptoms immediately: a. Spontaneous bleeding from gums or nose. b. Excessive bleeding from site of slight trauma (e.g., venipuncture sites, intrasmuscular or subcutaneous injection sites, nicks from shaving of perineum or abdomen, injury from insertion of urinary catheter). c. Sudden tachycardia, diaphoresis, or restlessness with anxiety.	1. Assist with medical or surgical management—order blood laboratory work; set up for intravenous infusion and CVP monitoring. 2. Monitor organ and system response for the following: a. Urinary output. b. CVP (see Management of hemorrhagic shock, p. 800). 3. Monitor for the following: a. Heparin* or other infusion. b. Woman's response to therapy. 4. Assist woman and family with grieving process. 5. Observe for most common sequelae: a. Minor hemorrhagic diathesis. b. Major hemorrhagic diathesis. c. Acute renal failure. d. Pituitary insufficiency (Sheehan's syndrome [see p. 807]). 6. Stress importance of adequate prenatal, intranatal, and postdelivery nursing and medical supervision. 7. Explain disease process and its management to woman and family.

*Heparin should be administered only after appropriate investigative studies, however, and usually in consultation with hematologist.

Treatment. The nurse assists the physician in the treatment of DIC, which includes the following measures:

1. Removal of causative factor, for example, delivery of dead fetus; treatment of existing infection or eclampsia; or delivery of fetus by cesarean birth and removal of abrupted placenta.
2. Establishment of support mechanisms (see Management of hemorrhagic shock, p. 800).
   a. Woman's right hip elevated to prevent hypotensive syndrome.
   b. Oxygen administered by tight-fitting mask at 10 to 12 L/min.
   c. Parenteral therapy begun (e.g., Ringer's lactated solution).
   d. CVP monitoring begun with attempt to maintain CVP within normal limits: 6 to 12 cm H_2O.
3. Treatment of the condition.
   a. Administer whole blood as needed at rate sufficient to maintain hematocrit (Hct) at 30% and urinary output at 30 to 60 ml/hr.
   b. Administer blood components as needed.
      (1) One unit of platelets raises adult level by 5000.
      (2) One unit of cryoprecipitate (fibrinogen and factor VIII) replaces depleted coagulation factors. Cryoprecipitate is more effective in restoring normal coagulation than lyophilized fibrinogen. In addition, it has the advantage of minimizing transmission of serum hepatitis (about 20% of people who receive fibrinogen acquire homologous serum hepatitis), *or*
      (3) Two units of fresh frozen plasma replace coagulation factors and fibrinogen.
   c. Heparin may be ordered. This is administered by constant infusion pump at 12.5 U/kg/hr to arrest coagulation and fibrinolysis.
4. Diagnosis and treatment of sequelae: minor or major hemorrhagic diathesis, acute renal failure, pituitary insufficiency (Sheehan's syndrome), compromised neonate (usually not affected, except indirectly through hypoxia).

Summary of nursing actions

Goals of care

1. The woman survives the disease with minimal or no damage to body organs or systems.
2. The woman's blood-clotting mechanism returns to normal.
3. The woman and her family understand the disease process and its management.
4. The neonate survives with no adverse sequelae.

Example of nursing diagnosis. The following is an example of a nursing diagnosis: potential occurrence of DIC because of oxytocin induction of labor.

Evaluation. The nurse can be assured that nursing care is effective if the goals of care are met.

Idiopathic thrombocytopenic purpura. Idiopathic thrombocytopenic purpura (ITP) is an autoimmune disorder in which antiplatelet antibodies decrease the life span of the platelets. The following results of tests are diagnostic: (1) thrombocytopenia, (2) capillary fragility, (3) increased bleeding time, and (4) a bone marrow smear showing a normal or increased megalocyte count with many young forms.

ITP may result in severe hemorrhage following cesarean delivery or from cervical or vaginal lacerations. The incidence of postdelivery uterine bleeding or vaginal hematomas is also increased in ITP. Neonatal thrombocytopenia occurs in about 50% of the cases and there is a high mortality. Platelet transfusions are given to maintain the platelet count at 100,000/cu mm. Corticosteroids are given if the diagnosis is made before or during pregnancy. (Splenectomy is deferred until after the puerperium.) The history taken during the initial prenatal visit should include reference to bleeding in the woman.

Hemophilia. At least nine types of congenital disorders of the clotting mechanism have been identified. These include hemophilia A, hemophilia A and C, and von Willebrand's disease. About 75% of hemophiliacs have the A variety, and about 15% have the B variety. These two types represent about 90% of all congenital hemorrhagic diseases caused by defective formation of a fibrin clot.

Classic hemophilia (A) is a bleeding disorder typified by a deficiency of factor VIII antihemophilic factor (AHF), an antihemophilic globulin that is essential in thromboplastin formation in phase 1 of blood coagulation. The source of factor VIII in the body is unknown. All degrees of severity of the disease have been reported. Bleeding occurs most often from the nasal or oral mucosa or from contusions or lacerations. Bleeding into the skin, muscles, or joints may also ensue. Hemophilia B, or Christmas disease, is caused by a genetically determined deficiency of factor IX and is clinically indistinguishable from hemophilia A.

Both hemophilia A and hemophilia B are transmitted as sex-linked recessive traits by the mother. Because they are expressed predominantly in the son and only rarely in the daughter (only in homozygous females), the major problem arising with pregnancy is the birth of an affected infant. Hematomas after injections and bleeding from circumcision are common. However, most affected newborns exhibit no clinical abnormalities. Recording and reporting of such incidences, if they occur, will aid in diagnosis at a later date.

The affected woman requires treatment with cryoprecipitate or fresh frozen plasma to replace factor VIII or factor IX to prevent hemorrhage during and after childbirth.

von Willebrand's disease. One type of hemophilia is von Willebrand's disease. It results from a factor VIII deficiency and platelet dysfunction. It is transmitted as an incomplete autosomal-dominant trait to both sexes; although von Willebrand's disease is rare, it is one of the most common congenital clotting defects in American women of childbearing age. The symptomatology includes a familial bleeding tendency, previous bleeding episodes, prolonged bleeding time (most important test), factor VIII deficiency (mild to moderate), and bleeding from mucous membranes. Since factor VIII increases during pregnancy, this increase may be sufficient to offset danger from hemorrhage during childbirth.

Treatment of von Willebrand's disease consists of replacement of factor VIII, if it is less than 30%, through administration of cryoprecipitate or fresh frozen plasma.

MANAGEMENT OF HEMORRHAGIC SHOCK

Hemorrhage* is a major threat to the mother during the childbearing cycle. Shock may result. Shock is an emergency situation in which the perfusion of body organs may become severely compromised and death may ensue. Vigorous treatment is necessary to prevent adverse sequelae (e.g., cellular death, fluid overload, shock lung [p. 802], and oxygen toxicity). A brief explanation of the physiologic mechanisms involved is provided to assist the nurse in implementing appropriate actions.

Physiologic mechanisms. Physiologic compensatory mechanisms are activated in response to hemorrhage (or other trauma such as cardiac arrest). The adrenals release catecholamines, causing arterioles and venules in the skin, lungs, gastrointestinal tract, liver, and kidney to constrict, thus diverting available blood flow to the brain and heart and away from other organs, including the uterus. If shock is prolonged, the continued reduction in cellular oxygenation results in an accumulation of lactic acid and acidosis (from anaerobic glucose metabolism). Acidosis (lowered serum pH) causes arteriole vasodilation; venule vasoconstriction persists. A circular pattern is established: decreased perfusion, increased tissue anoxia and acidosis, edema formation, and pooling of blood further decrease the perfusion. Cellular death occurs. Table 35.6 is an assessment guide to as-

*For a discussion of bacteremia (septic shock), see p. 835.

Table 35.6
Symptoms of Shock

	Mild	Moderate	Severe	Irreversible
Respirations	Rapid, deep	Rapid, becoming shallow	Rapid, shallow, may be irregular	Irregular, or barely perceptible
Pulse	Rapid, tone normal	Rapid, tone may be normal but is becoming weaker	Very rapid, easily collapsible, may be irregular	Irregular apical pulse
Blood pressure	Normal or hypertensive	60-90 mm Hg systolic	Below 60 mm H systolic	None palpable
Skin	Cool and pale	Cool, pale, moist, knees cyanotic	Cold, clammy, cyanosis of lips and fingernails	Cold, clammy, cyanotic
Urinary output	No change	Decreasing to 10-22 ml/hr (adult)	Oliguric (less than 10 ml) to anuric	Anuric
Level of consciousness	Alert, oriented, diffuse anxiety	Oriented, mental cloudiness or increasing restlessness	Lethargy, reacts to noxious stimuli, comatose	Does not respond to noxious stimuli
CVP	May be normal (6-12 cm H_20)	3 cm H_20	O-3 cm H_20	

Adapted from Royce, J.A.: Nurs. Clin. North Am. **8**:377, 1973; and Wagner, M.M., Clinical Nursing Specialist, University of Iowa Hospitals and Clinics.

sist the nurse in the observation and evaluation of the degree of shock.

Assessment and interventions. The following nursing interventions for the client in shock should be considered (Royce, 1973):

1. Stay with the woman. Send others to alert the physician and to obtain needed equipment. An emergency cart should be well supplied and available at all times and should include equipment to start intravenous fluid, to give oxygen, and to suction, retention catheter with urinometer, and blood pressure and CVP or PAWP apparatus.

Nurses should have standing orders to start intravenous fluids and know the type of infusion fluid to use and laboratory tests to order.

2. While waiting for the physician, the following procedures should be performed:
   a. Insert an airway to facilitate oxygen administration and suction.
   b. Start intravenous administration of 5% dextrose in water with 0.45% or 0.2% normal saline solution to maintain peripheral vascular circulation.
   c. Elevate the right hip (if woman cannot be in left side-lying position) to avoid vena cava syndrome. *Trendelenburg's position* (with head down and feet elevated) *is not advised*. This position may interfere with cardiac function. Use this position on physician request only.

3. Assist physician in instituting and monitoring measures to increase tissue perfusion. Monitor intravenous fluids. Too slow a rate (caused by slowing of drip rate or kinking or occlusion of tubing) may be inadequate to dilute blood viscosity or to maintain peripheral circulation. Too rapid a rate may result in fluid overload and pulmonary edema.

Fluids to increase blood volume include whole fresh blood, plasma, and albumin. Fluids to dilute hemoconcentration (viscosity) are dextrose in water and Ringer's lactated solution.

4. Monitor, assess, and record respirations, pulse, blood pressure, skin condition, urinary output, level of consciousness, and CVP to evaluate effectiveness of management (see Table 35.6):
   a. *Respirations*. The body rids itself of excess acids by increasing respiratory rate. Ventilatory assistance with oxygen or respirator or both may be needed.
   b. *Pulse*. The pulse rate increases and becomes irregular as shock progresses in severity.
   c. *Blood pressure*. In later stages of shock, the systolic pressure decreases.
   d. *Skin*. Perfusion of the skin is sacrificed in the body's attempt to maintain blood flow to the heart and brain. Therefore the condition of the skin is a valuable index to the severity of shock. The nurse assesses the degree of ischemia or cyanosis of the nail beds, eyelids, and skin inside the mouth (buccal mucosa, gums, tongue). The nurse then notes the degree of coolness and the degree of clamminess.
   e. *Urinary output*. Measure hourly output. Oliguria (50 ml/hr) may indicate worsening of shock or inadequate fluid therapy; an increased output indicates improvement in the woman's condition.
   f. *Level of consciousness*. The adequacy of cerebral perfusion may be estimated by an evaluation of

the woman's level of consciousness. In early stages of decreased blood flow, the woman may complain of "seeing stars," feeling dizzy, or feeling nauseous. She may become restless and orthopneic. As cerebral hypoxia increases, the woman may become confused and react slowly or not at all to stimuli. An improved sensorium is an indicator of improvement.

g. *Heart function.**
   (1) CVP: CVP readings measure the function (e.g., blood pressure) of the right side of the heart. Normal values range between 6 and 12 cm H_20. A low or falling value indicates inadequate blood volume or hypovolemia. A high or rising value indicates impaired contractility of the heart.
   (2) PA catheter: A multiple-lumen pulmonary artery (PA) catheter is used to measure both right- and left-side heart functions.
   (3) PAWP: A PA catheter when properly placed and when its flexible latex balloon is inflated is used to measure the pulmonary artery wedge pressure (PAWP), an indicator of left-side heart function.

Anxiety is contagious. The nurse's calm, confident manner, coupled with brief, simple explanations, is an important adjunct to the interventions just discussed.

Hazards of therapy. The 24 hours after the shock period are critical. Observe the woman for fluid overload, shock lung, and oxygen toxicity. *Fluid overload* results in pulmonary and peripheral edema. Alert the physician and decrease the drip rate if moist respirations, stridor, or dyspnea occurs. *Shock lung* may develop after the woman receives mechanical ventilatory assitance, especially if the ventilator is not maintained between 50 and 70 mm Hg. Tachypnea, dyspnea, anxiety, a rise in blood pressure, cyanosis, and harsh loud breaths follow alveolar capillary damage. *High concentrations of oxygen* are toxic to the adult as well as the neonate. Irritation of mucous membranes of the upper respiratory tract, substernal pain, and cough may occur. The first sign may be muscular twitching about the face, followed by convulsions resembling grand mal seizures. Later, neurologic symptomatology includes tinnitus, euphoria, confusion, and respiratory arrest.

The nurse-physician team's quick response and coordinated efforts are essential to institute, monitor, and continuously readjust therapy to the woman's changing needs. This collaboration, given the essential emergency apparatus and supportive services (e.g., laboratory tests), is requisite to meeting client care objectives.

*Techniques for measuring hemodynamic pressure are beyond the scope of this text. An excellent reference is *Nursing PhotoBook: Using Monitors*. Nurs. '81 Books, Horsham, Pa., 1981, Intermed Communications, Inc.

Postdelivery Hemorrhage

Hemorrhage is a leading cause of maternal death the world over. Postdelivery hemorrhage, traditionally the loss of 500 ml of blood or more after delivery, is the most common and most serious type of excessive obstetric blood loss. At least 5% of women suffer postdelivery hemorrhage.

A small woman is less able to withstand the loss of blood than a larger one. It has been noted that the average maternal blood loss can be as much as 10% of the woman's blood volume without immediate critical consequence. Therefore a more meaningful definition of postdelivery hemorrhage is the loss of 1% or more of body weight, a figure easily referable to blood volume because 1 ml of blood weighs 1 g.

Postdelivery hemorrhage may be sudden and even exsanguinating, or moderate but persistent bleeding may continue for days or weeks. Postdelivery hemorrhage may be early, within the first 24 hours after delivery, or late, from 24 hours after delivery until the twenty-eighth day.

Control of bleeding from the placental site is accomplished by prolonged contraction and retraction of interlacing strands of myometrium, the *living ligature*. A firm or contracted uterus does not bleed after delivery unless placenta previa had existed. Therefore careful assessment of uterine tone and the maintenance of uterine contractions through manual massage or oxytocic stimulation are important parts of postdelivery care.

ETIOLOGY

The causes of postdelivery hemorrhage, in approximate order of frequency, are as follows:

1. Mismanagement of the third stage of labor (e.g., incomplete placental separation)
2. Uterine atony caused by excessive analgesia or anesthesia, prolonged labor, overdistention of the uterus or urinary bladder
3. Lacerations of the birth canal
4. Hematologic disorders (e.g., DIC)
5. Complications of pregnancy (e.g., inversion of the uterus, placenta accreta)
6. Tumors of the cervix or uterus
7. Medical complications of pregnancy (e.g., hyperthyroidism, vitamin K deficiency)
8. Infections of the genital tract (e.g., endometritis)

Early postdelivery hemorrhage almost invariably is caused by uterine atony, lacerations of the birth canal, or DIC. *Late* postdelivery hemorrhage most commonly is the result of subinvolution of the placental site, retained placental tissue, or infection.

CLINICAL FINDINGS AND DIFFERENTIAL DIAGNOSIS

It is helpful to consider the problem of excessive bleeding with reference to the stages of labor. From delivery of the fetus until separation of the placenta, the character and quantity of blood passed may suggest excessive bleeding. For example, dark blood is probably of venous origin, perhaps from varices or superficial lacerations of the birth canal. Bright blood is arterial and indicates, for example, deep lacerations of the cervix. Spurts of blood with clots may indicate partial placental separation; the failure of blood to clot or remain clotted is indicative of coagulopathy (DIC).

The period from the separation of the placenta to its delivery may be when excessive bleeding occurs. Frequently this is the result of incomplete placental separation, often caused by poor management of the third stage of labor (e.g., undue manipulation of the fundus).

After the placenta has been recovered, persistent or excessive blood loss usually is the result of atony of the uterus (i.e., its failure to contract well or maintain its contraction) or prolapse of the uterus into the pelvis.

Late hemorrhage may be the result of partial involution of the uterus and unrecognized lacerations of the birth canal.

Complications of postdelivery hemorrhage are either immediate or delayed. Hypovolemic shock (see p. 800) and death may occur from sudden, exsanguinating hemorrhage. Delayed complications provoked by postdelivery hemorrhage include anemia, puerperal infection, and thromboembolism.

SPECIFIC PROBLEMS

Uterine atony. Uterine atony is marked hypotonia of the uterus. Uterine antony occurs in at least 5% of deliveries, particularly when the woman is a grand multipara; with hydramnios; when the fetus is large; or after the delivery of twins or triplets. In such conditions the uterus is ''overstretched'' and is poorly contractile. Uterine atony is the principal cause of postdelivery hemorrhage.

Placental separation and expulsion are facilitated by contraction of the uterus, which also prevents hemorrhage from the placental site. The corpus is, in essence, a basketwork of strong, interdigitating, smooth muscle bundles through which pass many large maternal blood vessels. If the uterus is flaccid after detachment of all or part of the afterbirth, brisk venous bleeding will occur and normal coagulation of the open vasculature will be impaired. In contrast, a firm, contracted uterus will not bleed because the myometrium will compress the vasculature and resolution of the placental site can occur.

Numerous preventable problems may be responsible for uterine atony. For example, undesirable side effects may follow the administration of ill-chosen drugs, of very potent analgesic agents (e.g., morphine) late in the first stage of labor, and of certain anesthetics (e.g., ethyl ether) that are especially efficient smooth muscle–relaxing drugs. Mismanagement of the third stage of labor, allowing only partial separation of the placenta or retention of placental fragments, may be associated with uterine atony. Moreover, the poorly contracting uterus may have slipped deep into the true pelvis to cause chronic passive congestion of the organ, an added cause of abnormal bleeding.

The first step in the treatment of uterine bleeding is to elevate and hold the uterus out of the pelvis and to massage the corpus to initiate and maintain a firmly contracted organ (Fig. 23.3). The physician orders oxytocin, 10 units administered intravenously, followed by ergonovine, 0.2 mg administered intravenously (well diluted), or its equivalent. Moreover, continuous intravenous administration of oxytocin solution (5 units/500 ml of 5% dextrose in water) should run for 3 or 4 hours. Blood transfusion for the treatment of shock and blood replacement may be urgently needed.

The accoucheur should hasten to palpate the interior of the uterus so that retained products of conception can be removed and possible rupture of the uterus diagnosed.

Lacerations of the cervix or of the birth canal should be repaired promptly. If the blood being lost fails to clot, a coagulopathy (e.g., DIC) may have developed, and prompt appropriate treatment may be lifesaving.

If the procedures outlined are ineffectual and normal clotting of blood is assured, bilateral ligation of the internal iliac arteries will usually stop the bleeding. Thus the uterus will be preserved for future childbearing. If this is not a serious consideration, if rupture of the uterus is confirmed, or if hemorrhage from uterine atony persists, hysterectomy may be required.

Lacerations of the birth canal. Lacerations of the birth canal are second only to uterine atony as a major cause of postdelivery hemorrhage. Therefore prevention, recognition, and prompt, effective treatment of birth canal lacerations are vitally important.

Continued bleeding despite efficient postdelivery uterine contractions demands inspection or reinspection of the birth passage. Continuous bleeding from so-called minor sources may be just as dangerous as a sudden loss of a large amount of blood, although often it is ignored until shock develops. Birth canal lacerations may include injuries to the labia, perineum, vagina, and cervix.

Factors that influence the etiology and incidence of obstetric lacerations of the lower genital tract encompass operative delivery; aseptic or unattended spontaneous delivery; congenital abnormalities of the maternal soft parts; contracted pelvis; size, presentation, and position of the fetus; relative size of the presenting part and the birth canal; prior scarring from infection, injury, or surgery; the presence of vulvar, perineal, and vaginal varices; and abnormalities of uterine action, for example, precipitate delivery. Other associated problems may be abnormal tissue elasticity or friability, the presence of tumors, the general condition of the mother (e.g., exhaustion, dehydration), and the presence of complicating diseases. All these factors may exist alone or in combination.

The diagnosis of birth canal lacerations requires (1) an inherent awareness of their possible occurrence and (2) an immediate routine, meticulous inspection of the entire lower birth canal after each delivery. Prerequisites for an adequate appraisal include aseptic technique (the woman for whom labor and birth has been precipitate must be prepared and draped), standard instruments for surgical repair, an assistant to provide exposure by retraction, and appropriate lighting.

Upward displacement of the cervix after its inspection by means of a "tailed" or "tagged" vaginal pack will greatly facilitate the inspection of the entire vaginal tract. Hence lacerations may be seen and repaired, and hematomas may be identified and treated before they reach serious proportions. A vaginal pack also serves to elevate the uterus, enhancing its contractility and limiting blood loss during repair.

Proper anatomic reapproximation of all tissues is performed immediately after delivery for the following reasons.

1. To ensure hemostasis and to prevent hematomas
2. To eliminate open sources of puerperal infection
3. To correct problems (e.g., a poorly repaired old laceration of the rectal sphincter may be revised when increased vascularity and physiologic hypertrophy of pregnancy may favorably influence healing)

Blood replacement and the administration of appropriate antibiotic agents, when indicated, are important. A retention urinary catheter may be required in specific cases.

Labial lacerations. Extreme vascularity in the labial and periclitoral areas often results in profuse bleeding. Immediate repair, by means of fine catgut such as no. 4-0 on an atraumatic needle, is required. Counterpressure with a gauze pad and a T binder may be required.

Perineal lacerations. Lacerations of the perineum are the most common of all injuries in the lower genital tract. These are classified as follows:

- *First degree:* involves the mucosa and skin with some fibers of the superficial musculature
- *Second degree:* also includes deeper structures of the perineum
- *Third degree:* involves all the structures of the vaginal wall, and the sphincter ani muscles are severed
- *Fourth degree:* involves all of aforementioned and the anal wall, so that the anus is laid open

An episiotomy may extend to become either a third- or fourth-degree laceration.

The care of the woman who has suffered lacerations of the perineum is similar to that advocated for episiotomies, that is, analgesia as needed for pain, and heat or cold applications as necessary. To avoid injury to the suture line, a woman with third- or fourth-degree lacerations is not given routine postdelivery rectal suppositories or enemas. Attention to diet and intake of fluids is emphasized, as well as oral stool softeners to assist her in reestablishing bowel habits.

Vaginal lacerations and hematomas. Prolonged pressure of the fetal head on the vaginal mucosa ultimately will interfere with the circulation and may produce ischemic or pressure necrosis. The state of the tissues, therefore, together with the type of delivery, may result in deep vaginal lacerations and may predispose to vaginal hematomas.

Vaginal hematomas occur more frequently in association with forceps rotation of a fetus in an occipitoposterior (OP) position; they are often found on the same side as the occiput, perhaps because of long-continued pressure of the fetal head in one posterior quadrant of the vagina.

A vaginal hematoma should be diagnosed at the incipient, or early, stage. Most hematomas can usually be detected by routine inspection after delivery. Many vaginal hematomas occur beneath the mucosa opposite the ischial spines in the plane of the midpelvis. Therefore the physician will palpate the vaginal walls to detect a full, crepitant, or fluctuant area that may not have become visible yet. The large masses will be purple, in contrast to the dark red of the remainder of the vaginal mucosa.

Many small hematomas undoubtedly go undetected and may even be self-limiting. The underlying principle of treatment is the prevention of a large hematoma, however, because all hematomas have a small start. The sequelae may include tissue devitalization, serious blood loss, shock, and infection.

During the postdelivery period, if the woman complains of persistent perineal pain or a feeling of fullness in the vagina, a careful inspection of the vulva is made.

The woman assumes a side-lying position, the upper buttock is raised, and she is asked to bear down. A large purplish mass may be seen at the introitus.

She is then returned to the delivery unit, where (after a suitable anesthetic has been administered) the hematoma is incised and evacuated, and deep sutures are placed for control of the bleeding.

If the hematoma is larger than 5 cm in diameter, a catheter is placed in the urinary bladder and a moderately tight vaginal pack inserted. A vaginal pack must be inserted carefully to avoid traumatizing the tissues. To facilitate insertion of the pack, an antibiotic ointment may be spread on the pack or applied within the vagina. The catheter and pack may be removed in 6 to 8 hours. Antimicrobial agents for systematic action are not required routinely.

Retained placenta

The nonadherent placenta. The obstetrician must recognize the completion of the third stage of labor, or complications may result. If the operator is hasty, for example, the placenta may not have an adequate opportunity to separate. If one waits too long, needless loss of blood may occur.

In the period after birth of the baby but before recovery of the placenta, some women may have only slight bleeding, but others may have considerable blood loss. If no marked bleeding occurs and with proper management, the normally implanted placenta separates with the first or second strong uterine contraction after delivery of the infant, within 15 minutes in about 90% of women.

Within 30 minutes after birth, an additional 5% of women will have a separated placenta. If one waits 45 minutes after delivery, only another 1% or 2% will achieve placental separation. Hence there is little to be gained by an extended wait-and-see attitude. If the placenta has not been recovered within 30 minutes of delivery, manual removal should be attempted.

If overly generous analgesia, such as morphine sulfate within 1 or 2 hours of delivery, or third-plane anesthesia with halothane or ether is given, prompt resumption of potent uterine contractions after the birth of the infant may be suppressed. Avoidance of sedation, administration of oxytocin intravenously (slowly) or intramuscularly immediately after delivery, and elevation of the uterus without manual stimulation should aid separation of the placenta and reduce blood loss.

If excessive bleeding develops, manual separation and removal of the placenta are carried out immediately.

Some obstetricians practice elective manual separation and extraction of the placenta to expedite the delivery sequence or to avoid abnormal bleeding, for example, after twin delivery. No supplementary anesthesia will be needed for parturients who have had block anesthesia for delivery. For other women, administration of light nitrous oxide and oxygen inhalation anesthesia or intravenous thiopental (Pentothal) will suffice for intrauterine exploration, placental separation, and recovery of the placenta.

If delivery occurs early (fifth or sixth month), either spontaneously or by induced abortion, placental retention is the rule because of poor separation of the afterbirth. This may be caused by an immature zone of separation, weak uterine contractions, or a relatively large placenta.

Retained placenta may be the result of one of the following:

1. Partial separation of a normal placenta
2. Entrapment of the partially or completely separated placenta by an hourglass constriction ring of the uterus (see Fig. 20.21) or by mismanagement of the third stage of labor, for example, massage of the uterus (Credé's method) before separation of the placenta or ill-timed administration of ergot products
3. Abnormal adherence of the entire placenta or a portion of the placenta to the uterine wall

In all instances postdelivery hemorrhage or infection may be a critical complicating factor.

Because of the possible complications, ergot preparations should be given only *after* recovery of the placenta, and they should always be given intramuscularly or orally, never intravenously.

The adherent placenta. Abnormal adherence of the placenta occurs for reasons unknown, but it is thought to be the result of zygote implantation in a zone of defective endometrium. Abnormal adherence of the placenta is diagnosed in only about 1 of every 12,000 deliveries. Approximately 90% of the mothers are multiparous, and many of them have also had abortions. The mother with an abnormally attached placenta is jeopardized mainly by postdelivery hemorrhage leading to hypovolemic shock. Firm placental attachment is associated with increased maternal morbidity and mortality. Moreover, prematurity caused by associated problems such as placenta previa accounts for increased perinatal loss.

Factors that predispose to abnormally firm placental attachment are (1) scarring of the uterus such as occurs after cesarean delivery, myomectomy, or vigorous curettage; (2) endometritis, associated with tuberculosis, for example; (3) abnormal site of implantation, such as the cervix or lower uterine segment; or (4) malformation of the placenta, for example, extrachorial placenta.

Unusual placental adherence may be partial or complete, and the following degrees of attachment are recognized.

- Placenta accreta (vera): slight penetration of myometrium by placental trophoblast (rare)
- Placenta increta: deep penetration by placenta (very rare)
- Placenta percreta (destruans): perforation of uterus by placenta (exceptional)

There are more cases of partial than complete placenta accreta.

In all types of abnormal adherence, placentation occurs in an area of deficient, sparse, or absent decidua. Thus the placenta develops on a surface partially or completely devoid of decidua (basalis). The uterine muscle is exposed, and invasion of the trophoblast and chorionic villi of the myometrium soon occurs. A dense fibrous area develops, together with hyalinization of neighboring uterine muscle. *There is no zone of separation;* no cleavage plane can be developed between the placenta and the uterine wall. Attempts to remove the placenta in the usual manner are therefore unsuccessful, and laceration or perforation of the uterine wall may result.

At least 15% of cases of abnormally adherent placenta (all types) are associated with placenta previa. Stated another way, about 3% of all cases of placenta previa are accompanied by placenta accreta, increta, or percreta. There are no sure signs of an abnormally adherent placenta during pregnancy.

Bleeding with complete or total placenta accreta does not occur unless separation of the placenta is attempted, but partial placenta accreta invariably is associated with excessive intranatal or postdelivery bleeding. The reason is that vessels adjacent to the adherent placenta remain open, and free bleeding prevents clotting.

When manual removal of a placenta accreta is attempted, damage to placental tissue and decidua, both rich in thromboplastin, occurs. When this substance is released in quantity into the circulation, DIC may develop.

At vaginal delivery the diagnosis of an abnormally adherent placenta generally is made when manual separation of a retained placenta is attempted. If the placenta will not separate readily (even a portion), immediate abdominal hysterectomy may be indicated. Persistent attempts at placental removal rarely will be successful, and fatal hemorrhage may result.

Placenta accreta or increta usually is diagnosed at cesarean delivery when an abnormally adherent placenta is discovered. In such cases, especially when surgery was indicated because of placenta previa, total hysterectomy may be the best treatment. If the woman wants to have another child and is in good condition, and if hemorrhage can be controlled, the risk of not removing the uterus may be justifiable. Small retained portions of the placenta may separate or be absorbed, but infection often is an added late complication. Reoperation may be necessary because of later hemorrhage. After a subsequent viable pregnancy, elective repeat cesarean delivery will be mandatory because another placenta accreta or increta is likely. Delivery should be followed immediately by total abdominal hysterectomy.

Inversion of uterus. Inversion of the uterus (turning inside out) after delivery is a critical obstetric complication. The inversion may be complete or partial. Traction applied to the fundus, especially when the uterus is flaccid, may result in inversion. More specifically the causes include straining (Valsalva's maneuver); traction on the cord before the placenta has separated; Crede's method, that is, kneading the uterine fundus in an attempt to separate an adherent placenta; and placental extraction under deep relaxing anesthesia. Occasionally a large uterine tumor may be responsible for inversion.

Profound shock follows complete inversion; postdelivery hemorrhage accompanies partial uterine inversion. Prompt assistance is imperative because maternal mortality may reach 30% without immediate corrective therapy.

Prevention. Prevention, always the easiest, cheapest, and most effective therapy, is especially appropriate in the avoidance of puerperal uterine inversion. *One must not pull on the umbilical cord unless the placenta has definitely separated.* The fundus should never be used as a piston to "push the placenta out." Crede's method is not used; it is harmful and not useful. Regional anesthesia is employed when feasible. An experienced attendant remains with the woman until the uterus is firm and rounded.

Physical findings. Complete inversion of the uterus is obvious; a large, red, rounded mass (perhaps with the placenta attached) protudes 20 to 30 cm outside the introitus. Incomplete inversion cannot be seen but must be felt; a smooth mass will be palpated through the dilated cervix, reducing the size of the uterine cavity by at least half.

Medical treatment. The nurse assists the physician in implementing the following:

1. Combat shock, which invariably is out of proportion to the blood loss. Give oxytocin intravenously to contract the uterus. (Ergot products are strictly contraindicated because the cervix, as well as the uterus, will contract, and replacement may be difficult unless the cervix is severed.)

2. Replace the uterus, after the woman is under deep ether or halothane anesthesia, by inserting and "working" first the lower uterine segment and then, finally, the fundus upward while applying traction to the cervix. Leave the placenta attached if it has not yet separated,

and then manually free the placenta. Give ergonovine maleate (Ergotrate) intramuscularly, and as the uterus and cervix contract, withdraw the placenta with the hand. Pack the uterus if inversion seems about to recur.

3. Abdominal or vaginal surgery may be necessary to reposition the uterus if successful manual replacement fails.

4. Give the woman a transfusion; initiate broad-spectrum antibiotic therapy; and insert a nasogastric tube to decompress the stomach and to minimize adynamic, or paralytic, ileus, a frequent sequela.

Prognosis. Successful, prompt vaginal replacement is likely in about 75% of women. Uterine inversion may recur in a subsequent delivery occasionally, despite the usual precautions.

Subinvolution of uterus. Late postdelivery bleeding may occur as a result of subinvolution of the uterus, which is defined as the delayed return of the enlarged puerperal corpus to normal size and function. The causes of subinvolution include reduced circulation because of malposition, myomas, retained products of conception, and infection.

Subinvolution may complicate the puerperium because of such symptoms as pelvic discomfort or backache, or there may be signs of abnormality such as leukorrhea or bleeding from an enlarged, boggy, perhaps tender uterus.

In the absence of frank bleeding, treatment is with ergonovine, 0.2 mg/4 hr for 2 or 3 days, antibiotic therapy, and warm acetic douches. With hemorrhage, dilatation and curettage (D and C) to remove retained placental secundines and to freshen the placental site for adequate healing generally is required, together with oxytocics and antibiotics.

The woman needs to be instructed to report symptoms to the physician. Although many women experience a short bleeding episode of up to 3 weeks after delivery, prolonged bleeding must be reported. After 3 to 4 weeks, bleeding may be caused by infection or subinvolution of the placental site.

Postdelivery Anterior Pituitary Necrosis

Postdelivery anterior pituitary necrosis (Sheehan's syndrome) follows hypovolemic shock and DIC in about 15% of survivors of severe postdelivery hemorrhage. Infarction of much or all of the anterior hypophysis causes partial or total loss of thyroid, adrenocortical, and gonadal functions. The degree of hormonal deficiency depends on the extent of gland destruction.

Women with Sheehan's syndrome fail to lactate, and there is a decrease in breast size. Loss of axillary and pubic hair, genital atrophy, and amenorrhea are the rule. Such women are apathetic and easily suffer fatigue.

The prognosis of Sheehan's syndrome depends on the degree of residual anterior pituitary function and the supplementary therapy required. Minimal treatment requires thyroid hormone, cortisone, and estrogen replacement. Infertility, reduced resistance to infection, proneness to shock, and premature aging are problems of women with pituitary cachexia.

Neonatal Hematologic Conditions

HEMATOLOGIC STATUS: ANEMIA AND POLYCYTHEMIA

Anemia. Neonatal anemia may be difficult to recognize by clinical evaluation alone. It is attributable to several causes, one of which is hypovolemia. The causes of hypovolemia include the following:

1. Placenta previa or abruptio placentae
2. Bleeding from the umbilical cord caused, for example, by holding the infant higher than the placenta before the cessation of pulsation in the cord
3. Iatrogenic factors, for example, incision of placenta during a cesarean delivery

Hemolysis is probably a more common cause of anemia. See the discussion of Rh and other blood incompatibilities and other conditions resulting in hemolysis in Chapters 36 and 40.

Polycythemia. Polycythemia is not fully understood. The most likely cause is iatrogenic, such as "milking" the cord before clamping and cutting the cord or holding the neonate below the level of the placenta before cessation of pulsation in the cord. Other possible causes are chronic fetal hypoxia (maternal hypertensive disease), maternal diabetes (or prediabetes), and cardiovascular anomaly. In addition to increasing the cardiac work load and possibly causing congestive heart failure, polycythemia causes respiratory distress and convulsions. Disseminated intravascular coagulation (DIC) may occur. Renal vein thrombosis may occur because of the thick blood.

Summary of nursing actions

Goals of care

1. There is adequate perfusion and ventilation of tissues.
2. Sequelae are avoided.

Anemia and Polycythemia

Assessment/analysis	Plan/implementation
Anemia: signs 1. Laboratory test: infant is anemic if hematocrit is below 50%. Watch this baby closely; note drop below 40%. 2. Skin color is pale.	1. Notify physician immediately. Assist with transfusion with fresh,* packed red blood cells, 10 ml/kg. If anemia is related to blood group incompatibility, exchange transfusion is performed.† 2. Observe for complications arising from transfusion (see Chapter 40). 3. Put neonate on constant cardiac and respiratory monitor, or monitor manually continuously. Assemble equipment for intubation, blood transfusion, and umbilical catheterization.
Polycythemia: signs 1. Venous (central) Hct is 60% or more; in severe polycythemia, Hct is 65% or more. 2. Hypoglycemia. 3. Plethora (deep red skin color) at rest or duskiness (cyanosis) when crying. 4. Episodes of apnea or respiratory distress. 5. Poor feeding. 6. Jaundice or hyperbilirubinemia.	1. Partial exchange transfusion with fresh frozen plasma may be done. 2. Phlebotomy with electrolyte and fluid replacement may be done, but phlebotomy alone is unacceptable. 3. Hypoglycemia with polycythemia is intractable (e.g., does not respond to therapy). 4. Feed by gavage if necessary. 5. Observe for apnea (use monitor); stimulate infant to breathe as necessary. 6. Assist parents in coping with situation.

*Enzyme 2, 3-diphosphoglycerate (2,3-DPG), which facilitates release of oxygen from red blood cells into tissues, is present in fresh blood; it is not present in infant blood or adult blood over 24 hours old.

†Exchange transfusion: volume of blood used is twice that of the infant's calculated blood volume (see Chapter 40).

Example of nursing diagnosis. The following is a possible nursing diagnosis: risk of polycythemia because of milking of cord toward neonate and delayed cutting of the cord.

Evaluation. The nurse can be assured that care was effective if the goals of care are met.

Neonatal Hypovolemic Shock

With the exception of a fall in blood pressure, hypovolemic shock may be asymptomatic. When present, signs of hypovolemic shock are similar to those of asphyxia. The infant who has suffered an acute hemorrhage generally has the following symptoms at birth:

- Fall in blood pressure (may be an unreliable indicator in some situations since normal blood pressure may be maintained until severe shock develops)
- Pallor with cyanosis
- Tachycardia
- Tachypnea
- Gasping breaths
- Retractions
- Feeble or absent pulses
- Weak cry
- Absent or diminished spontaneous movements
- Hypotonia

Blood pressure may be determined by the simple Doppler method or the more complex method involving direct measurements through an umbilical artery catheter.

Immediate transfusion is lifesaving. Proper treatment is predicated on correct diagnosis. Clinical differentiation often may be accomplished by assessing the three criteria shown below.

	Hypovolemic Shock	Asphyxia
Heart rate	160 beats/min (unless hypoxic)	Bradycardia
Cyanosis	Unrelieved by oxygen	Relieved by oxygen
Respiratory rate	Rapid	Slow

Neonatal Hypovolemic Shock

Assessment/analysis	**Plan/implementation**
1. Observe for symptoms listed under discussion of neonatal shock.	1. Monitor blood pressure—Doppler technique: 50 to 65 mm Hg.
2. Assess infant's response to administration of O_2.	2. Record observations accurately and thoroughly. If assessing infant at home, transfer to hospital immediately.
3. Observe infant's response to umbilical catheterization and transfusion (see Chapter 33).	3. Assist physician. a. Resuscitation: provide warmth, suction, O_2; accurately monitor and record neonate's responses. b. Transfusion. (1) Order blood typing and cross matching immediately. (2) Obtain transfusion equipment. (3) Assist with transfusion (see Chapter 40). (4) Maintain accurate record of transfusion and neonate's response.
4. Record amount of blood drawn for laboratory study.	4. Replace blood lost because of laboratory evaluations.
	5. Support parents: keep them informed, promote eye contact with and attachment to infant, and encourage expression of feelings and questions.

Summary of nursing actions

Goals of care

1. Neonate survives hypovolemic shock with no adverse sequelae.
2. Blood drawn for laboratory evaluation is replaced before hypovolemia occurs.

Example of nursing diagnosis. The following is a possible nursing diagnosis in neonatal hypovolemic shock: risk of anemia because of withdrawal of blood specimens for laboratory evaluation.

Evaluation. The nurse can be assured that care was effective if goals of care are met.

Hypertensive States in Pregnancy

Hypertension usually of vasospastic origin may complicate pregnancy. Hypertension may first appear during a well-established pregnancy (pregnancy-induced hypertension [PIH]), or hypertension may predate the pregnancy and be a manifestation of cardiovascular or renal disease.

PREGNANCY-INDUCED HYPERTENSION

Pregnancy-induced hypertension (PIH), a syndrome, is characterized by *hypertension* and *proteinuria* often accompanied by *edema*. It develops only during pregnancy or in the early puerperium. The syndrome usually appears between the twentieth and the twenty-fourth weeks of gestation and disappears after the forty-second postpartum day. The hypertensive state related to pregnancy is difficult to differentiate from chronic hypertensive states predating the pregnancy. Often the final diagnosis is based on whether or not the client's blood pressure returns to normal following pregnancy. If the blood pressure remains high, chronic hypertensive disease alone or with superimposed PIH may be the cause of the client's elevated blood pressure (Table 35.7).

Various terms have been and are being used to designate PIH. *Toxemia* is the term that originated when the cause of PIH was considered to be a circulating toxic substance. The presence of a circulating toxic substance has not been demonstrated. *Preeclampsia-eclampsia* is a term used widely today. ''Eclampsia'' is derived from the Greek word meaning ''shining forth,'' which is used to describe convulsions, a complication of severe PIH. The term means before convulsions (preeclampsia) and with convulsions (eclampsia).

INCIDENCE

About 5% of pregnant women in North America experience preeclampsia, and approximately 5% of these develop eclampsia. In lower socioeconomic groups in the United States and abroad, the incidence figures may be three to five times as high.

The following conditions are associated with PIH:

1. Primigravidity: approximately 65% of cases of

Table 35.7
Differential Diagnosis of Essential Hypertension and Preeclampsia

Features	Essential Hypertension	Preeclampsia
Onset of hypertension	Before pregnancy; during first 20 wk of pregnancy	After 20 wk of pregnancy (exception: trophoblastic tumors)
Duration of hypertension	Permanent; hypertension beyond 3 mo after delivery	Hypertension usually absent at 6 wk after delivery; always by 3 mo after delivery
Family history	Often positive	Usually negative; may be positive
Past history	Recurrent "toxemia"	Psychosexual problems common
Age	Usually older	Generally teenaged or in early 20s
Parity	Usually multigravida	Usually primigravida
Habitus	May be thin or brachymorphic	Usually eumorphic
Retinal findings	Often arteriovenous nicking, tortuous arterioles, cotton-wool exudates, hemorrhages	Vascular spasm, retinal edema; rarely, protein extravasations
Proteinuria	Often none	Usually present; absent at 6 wk after delivery

PIH occur with first pregnancies, especially if the primigravida is under 17 or over 35 years of age.

2. Multiple pregnancies: the incidence increases progressively with the number of fetuses.
3. Vascular disease particularly with essential hypertension, hypertensive renal diseases, or diabetes mellitus.
4. Hydatidiform mole (molar pregnancy): predisposes to development of PIH. *The disease often becomes manifest before week 20 of pregnancy*.
5. Dietary deficiencies, severe malnutrition: protein deficiencies and probably a deficiency in water-solubale vitamins may be associated with increased incidence of PIH.
6. Familial tendency: the family history may reveal relations who had the disease.

MATERNAL AND FETAL MORBIDITY AND MORTALITY

Preeclampsia-eclampsia is a *major* cause of maternal morbidity and mortality. About 8% of women with eclampsia die of the disease or its complications. Moreover, perinatal morbidity is high, because most women with preeclampsia-eclampsia deliver before the thirty-seventh week of gestation. A single maternal convulsion increases the prospect of perinatal death at least fivefold.

DEFINITIONS

Gestational hypertension during pregnancy is defined as an elevation of systolic and diastolic pressure equal to or exceeding 140/90 mm Hg. An alternative definition that is more sensitive to individual variations is a rise in systolic pressure of 30 mm Hg or a rise in diastolic pressure of 15 mm Hg. The latter definition is useful because blood pressure varies with age, race, physiologic state, dietary habits, and heredity. For example, average systolic/diastolic blood pressure values (in mm Hg) for nonpregnant females are 103/70 at age 10; 120/80 at age 20; 123/82 at age 30; 126/84 at age 40; and 130/86 at age 50. For the teenager a blood pressure of 130/85 may be indicative of hypertension. It is important therefore to determine the *base-line blood pressure* of a pregnant woman. It is preferable to determine the base-line pressure in the first trimester of pregnancy since the blood pressure is lower in the second trimester. The levels noted above must be present on two occasions 6 hours apart. Techniques of measurement must be standardized, for example, always taken with the woman sitting *or* supine *or* in a lateral position. The techniques must be noted in the client's record, to provide data to guide the interpretation of previous, present, and future readings.

Gestational proteinuria is the occurrence of proteinuria during pregnancy or the early puerperium. The protein must be in amounts greater than 300 mg/L in a 24-hr specimen or greater than 1 g/L in a random daytime urine collection on two or more occasions at least 6 hours apart (Table 35.8). The urine must be a midstream clean-catch or catheter-derived specimen (see p. 285).

Gestational edema is a generalized accumulation of interstitial fluid (face, hands, abdomen, sacrum, tibia, ankles) after 12 hours of bed rest or a weight gain in excess of 2 kg (4 to 4½ lb) per week. The presence of edema is of less significance than the rapidity of weight

Table 35.8
Protein Readings

Code	Milligrams per deciliter
0	—
Trace	—
+1	30 mg/dl (equivalent to 300 mg/L)
+2	100 mg/dl
+3	300 mg/dl
+4	Over 1000 mg (1 g)/dl

gain. While the amount of edema is difficult to quantitate, the following method may be used to record relative degrees of edema formation:

1+ Minimal edema of the pedal and pretibial areas
2+ Marked edema of the lower extremities
3+ Edema of the face and hands, lower abdominal walls, and sacrum
4+ Anasarca (generalized massive edema) with ascites

PREECLAMPSIA

Preeclampsia is the syndrome of hypertension with proteinuria or edema or both during pregnancy or within 48 hours of delivery. Preeclampsia is a disease with associated altered vascular reactivity, compromised metabolic function, notable sodium retention, and reduced renal function, together with a decrease in intravascular volume and increased central nervous system (CNS) activity. Preeclampsia develops after the twentieth week of gestation, but it may occur earlier in the presence of hydatidiform or choriocarcinoma. Preeclampsia may be divided into mild or severe degrees for treatment purposes.

Mild preeclampsia includes the following symptoms:

1. Hypertension with a rise in systolic blood pressure of 30 mm Hg or more or a rise in diastolic blood pressure of 15 mm Hg or more on two occasions at least 6 hours apart
2. Weight gain of more than 1.4 kg (3 lb)/wk during the second trimester, more than 0.5 kg (1 lb)/wk during the third trimester, or a sudden weight gain at any time
3. Slightly generalized edema
4. Proteinuria of 300 mg/L in a 24-hr specimen or greater than 1 g/L in a random daytime specimen on two or more occasions 6 hours apart

Severe preeclampsia includes the symptoms just listed, as well as the following:

1. Hypertension with a blood pressure of 160/110 mm Hg or more on two separate occasions 6 hours apart with pregnant woman at bed rest
2. Proteinuria of 5 g/24 hr or more
3. Oliguria of 400 ml/24 hr or less
4. Other signs or symptoms noted earlier and becoming more serious
   a. Severe generalized headache
   b. Visual problems
      (1) Blurred vision or other visual changes
      (2) Retinal arteriolar spasm on fundoscopy
   c. Epigastric pain or nausea and vomiting
   d. Irritability, emotional tension

ECLAMPSIA

Eclampsia includes the symptoms of severe preeclampsia and one or more of the following: (1) tonic and clonic convulsions or coma, with the coma possibly following an unobserved seizure unrelated to other seizure disorders, or (2) hypertensive crisis or shock.

The sensory symptomatology of preeclampsia-eclampsia (headache, epigastric pain, blurring of vision, lowered affect) may be caused by generalized edema of the brain or ischemia following vasoconstriction.

ETIOLOGY

Preeclampsia-eclampsia is defined in empirical clinical terms because its cause and pathogenesis are unknown. Preeclampsia-eclampsia has always been a subject of much speculation and has been called the "disease of theories." No known theory as yet accounts for all symptoms. Evidently preeclampsia is somehow related to the physiologic changes of pregnancy since it disappears after the termination of pregnancy. Therefore the gravid uterus, placenta, or fetus could be the central factor or factors in the condition. One current theory is that of uterine ischemia, which proposes that there is impaired uteroplacental circulation secondary to uterine distention. High myometrial tone in primigravidas, multiple pregnancy, hydramnios, and even a hydatidiform mole pregnancy may be responsible. As a consequence of slight relative hypoxia, placental or decidual metabolic products capable of causing sodium and water retention and vascular constriction may be released into the maternal circulation. It it hypothesized that this causes the development of preeclampsia-eclampsia in a sensitive or reactive woman. Nevertheless, none of the catabolites per se are toxic substances, and no toxin has ever been identified. Hence it is illogical to refer to the hypertensive syndromes of pregnancy as *toxemias*.

Another theory stresses the concept that pregnancy is a salt-losing state and that inadequate sodium intake in the face of increased loss leads to hypovolemia, which in turn results in compensatory vasospasm. According to this theory sodium intake should not be restricted and should, in fact, be increased.

A concept that is also gaining increased acceptance is that preeclampsia-eclampsia is a function of poor nutrition, especially of diets poor in protein. Proponents of this theory prescribe high-protein diets without caloric or sodium restriction in prevention and treatment of this disorder. In pregnancy—especially late pregnancy when the fetus has a high need of protein for body growth and functioning—the RDA for protein is greatly increased (from 46 to 76 g/day for a singleton pregnancy). If a woman begins pregnancy with a protein deficit (as teenagers might, or as women consuming a high carbohydrate diet secondary to low income or ignorance might), or if she has a multiple pregnancy (twins, etc.), then her RDA for protein in pregnancy is even greater. If the woman's life-style is associated with skipping meals or with "eating on the run" (e.g., the life-style of many "career-oriented women" or mothers of more than three or four children), then she is at risk for a deficient protein intake. All the women identified above are those who are at greatest risk for developing preeclampsia-eclampsia.

Recently researchers (Lueck et al., 1983, and Aladjem et al., 1983) have reported the presence of a microscopic organism previously unknown. The organism resembles a parasite and has been named *Hydatoci lualba*. It has been identified in the placental tissue and circulating blood of toxemic mothers. It may be that in the future, protective mechanisms can be developed against the parasites.

PATHOLOGIC FINDINGS

General arteriolar spasm is characteristic of preeclampsia-eclampsia. Whether this is a primary or secondary reaction is uncertain, however. In any event the arterial system becomes hyperresponsive to vasopressor drugs such as vasopressin and angiotensin II. With this lability of the vascular system, shock states may be rapid and profound especially with spinal anesthesia.

The general arteriolar spasm and the consequent increased peripheral resistance results in hypertension. Every organ in the body is affected. Cardiac output falls as a result of automatic reflexes arising in the carotid baroreceptors. Renal blood flow is affected. The glomerular filtration rate is reduced in preeclampsia-eclampsia. With the small volume of urine produced in this disorder, however, tubular reabsorption of sodium is more efficient. Sodium and water retention is also augmented by the increased secretion of antidiuretic hormone, corticosteroids, and aldosterone in many women with preeclampsia-eclampsia.

Because of degenerative changes in renal glomeruli, serum protein, largely albumin, is lost in the urine. As much protein as 1 g/dl urine (4+) may be passed by the preeclamptic-eclamptic woman.

As a result of hypoproteinemia the albumin-globulin (A-G) ratio is altered and even reversed. The colloid osmotic pressure, which acts to retain fluid in the intravascular system, is reduced even more than normally (through the relative hemodilution of blood; see p. 230). This reduction leads to increased accumulation of fluid in the interstitial spaces (edema). As the fluid leaves the vascular system, hemoconcentration of red blood cells occurs and the hematocrit rises.

It has been suggested that the perfusion of the placenta is decreased. Frequently the placenta is smaller than normal for the duration of pregnancy. Premature aging is apparent with numerous areas of broken syncytia. Ischemic necrosis (white infarcts) are numerous, and intervillous fibrin deposition (red infarcts) may be recorded.

A consequence of interference in placental circulation may be intrauterine growth retardation of the fetus of the mother with preeclampsia.

Blood chemistry changes include elevated serum uric acid, urea nitrogen, and creatinine levels. Low serum albumin and globulin levels, increased hematocrit, and reduced carbon dioxide combining power (particularly after convulsions) are notable in preeclampsia-eclampsia.

Women who die as a consequence of eclampsia have edema of the brain and lungs particularly. Many microfocal hemorrhages in the brain may be noted. Numerous small thrombi are present in the lungs. Slight enlargement of the blanched kidney is common. Microscopic examination usually discloses ischemic glomerular capillaries adherent to the thickened basement membrane. Degeneration of the endothelial cells is apparent. The tubular cells generally show hyaline degeneration. The dilated tubules contain protein and casts together with occasional red and white blood cells.

MEDICAL DIAGNOSIS

Onset of hypertension and proteinuria in any client after the twentieth week of gestation establishes a diagnosis of preeclampsia. The condition may develop suddenly with no prior symptoms or develop gradually with an increase in the severity of symptoms. The *roll-over test* is not a valid test* for diagnosing impending hypertension. False negative readings have been reported in 29.6% of clients and false positive readings in

*Controversy continues over the validity of this test.

74.5%. When a normotensive individual rolls from the left lateral recumbent position, there is often a rise in blood pressure. However, this rise cannot be related to subsequent preeclampsia (Kasser et al., 1980).

MATERNAL PROGNOSIS

Eclampsia, hemorrhage, and infection have been the three leading causes of maternal death for years in North America. Women with preeclampsia almost never die of this disorder, but in women who develop eclampsia maternal mortality may be as high as 10% to 15%. Should convulsions develop, the most common causes of death are intracranial hemorrhage or congestive heart failure. In addition, a woman who sustains eclamptic convulsions may bite her tongue or lips. Ribs or vertebras may be fractured while flailing during a convulsion. Retinal detachments may ensue.

With good therapy most women improve significantly in 24 to 48 hours. Rapid improvement follows early termination of pregnancy.

FETAL PROGNOSIS

The fetal outcome of maternal hypertension is questionable because of placental insufficiency. Generally the fetus is small for gestational age and may even die before delivery can be effected. However, these infants do better generally than preterm infants of the same weight and gestational age born of nonhypertensive mothers, probably secondary to intrauterine stress, which increases the rapidity of fetal lung maturation. In many parts of North America the perinatal mortality is at least 20% with eclampsia. This is mainly because of the effects of hypoxia, prematurity, or acidosis during maternal convulsions.

With correct and intensive therapy the need for early delivery will reduce perinatal mortality to about 10%.

MANAGEMENT

The management of the woman with PIH requires the coordinated efforts of medical and nursing personnel.

Pregnant women who do not receive regular prenatal care and consequent monitoring of their unborn child's condition are particularly vulnerable to the complications of preeclampsia-eclampsia. The first requisite of a successful health service is to make contact with childbearing families. Preventive measures include educational programs directed toward alerting pregnant women about (1) the symptomatology of the disease, (2) maternal and fetal nutritional requirements, and (3) when and where to go for treatment and advice. The care of the client with PIH depends on the degree of severity of the process. The client may remain at home or, if her condition warrants it, be cared for in a hospital. Modern therapy includes the following:

1. Protein intake is moderate or increased to maintain adequate protein levels. Protein levels that are deficient result in a decrease in oncotic pressure in the blood, which causes fluid to leave the vascular compartment and enter the interstitital compartment, manifested as edema. Concomitantly, with the fluid shift, there is a decreased blood flow to the kidneys and the uterus. The decrease in flow to the kidneys results in deficient renal perfusion, which triggers the release of angiotensin and renin (which increases blood pressure in the body in an effort to compensate for the noted decreased blood flow to the kidneys), and simultaneously it triggers inefficient kidney function (which yields the symptoms of albuminuria and, with marked disease, increased nitrogenous waste products in the blood serum). The decrease in blood flow to the uterus results in poor placental perfusion (which results in late deceleration patterns on the fetal monitor, and, with chronicity, small-for-gestational-age [SGA] infants who are rather severely compromised during labor and at birth).

2. Salt (sodium) intake up to 6 g/day is continued; however, excessively salty foods are to be avoided. Salt restriction and diuretics are no longer used as therapy for preeclampsia. Research (Danforth, 1982) now indicates that such therapy can be harmful by causing further disruptions in electrolyte balance, accumulation of purine metabolites, and impairment of placental production of estrogens and the normal expansion of the vascular volume.

3. Bed rest: the woman is placed on bed rest and encouraged to assume a *left* lateral (side-lying) position in order to increase the uterine perfusion by avoiding the compromised blood flow that results from compression of the vena cava. Bed rest also decreases the woman's basal metabolic rate, thereby decreasing her need for protein.

The overall goals for care during the maternity cycle are as follows:

1. Provision of early adequate prenatal care, including adequate nutrition specific to the needs of each woman to protect against preeclampsia-eclampsia
2. Prompt intensive therapy for preeclampsia to drastically reduce the incidence of eclampsia and the severity of its complications
3. Prompt initiation of corrective therapy for eclamptic convulsions to reduce maternal and perinatal morbidity and mortality

Mild preeclampsia. For the woman with mild preeclampsia, that is, the woman who has hypertension not exceeding 140/90 mm Hg, care is directed toward improving or stabilizing the condition. She may remain at home as long as edema and proteinuria are absent or slight.

Nursing care

Assessment

1. The woman is assessed by a physician or nurse-practitioner at least twice a week to note any change in condition. In anticipation of a possible urgent delivery, evaluations are made of fetal maturity, or cervical changes as term approaches, and of the adequacy of the maternal pelvis for vaginal delivery.

2. The woman is instructed to keep a daily record of her weight.

3. The woman and other family members are able to verbalize symptoms that require prompt reporting: edema, headache, unusual disturbances, undue irritability or reactivity, poor sleep, decreased urinary output, or epigastric pain.

Examples of nursing diagnoses

1. Disturbance in self-concept because of need to curtail normal daily activities
2. Alterations in parenting because of need for bed rest
3. Noncompliance with therapy because of feeling of well-being

Plan and implementation. The goal for care is preventive; that is, the condition does not progress. The woman spends most of the day in bed preferably lying on her left side (may be up for meals and to use bathroom). She should not go up and down stairs. Outings are restricted to visits to the physician's office. The diet is well balanced and includes 70 to 80 g of protein per day depending on assessed needs and sodium content up to 6 g/day. A low-sodium diet (less than 1 g/day) is ordered only if kidney damage exists; the woman can use a salt substitute for flavoring her food. The diet must include ample roughage and fluids, since restricted exercise can compound problems with constipation.

Such a regimen, although therapeutic, can be very boring and stressful. The family needs to be included in the care plan. The care of children and the house must be undertaken by another family member. Diversion for both mother and young children in the family is essential. Preschoolers find it hard to understand why their mother stays in bed all day and cannot pick them up. Friends and relatives can help by assuming the children's care for part of each day and arranging for outdoor activity during that period.

Evaluation. The therapy is considered successful if the following conditions are met:

1. The disease process remains stable or improves.
2. The woman continues to seek medical or nursing supervision.

Symptoms of Pregnancy-Induced Hypertension (to be reported immediately)

1. A rapid rise in blood pressure
2. A rapid gain in weight
3. Marked hyperreflexia (see p. 820) and, especially, transient or sustained ankle clonus
4. Severe headache
5. Epigastric pain
6. Visual disturbances
7. A quantitative increase in proteinuria
8. Oliguria, with urinary output of less than 30 ml/hr
9. Drowsiness, listlessness (dulled sensorium)

3. The woman complies with the regimen for rest, exercise, and diet.

4. The woman can verbalize the signs and symptoms requiring immediate care and how to report them.

5. The woman is able to maintain a positive outlook about herself and her baby.

Moderate to severe preeclampsia. If the woman's condition changes from mild to moderate or severe preeclampsia, hospitalization is recommended. The criteria for hospitalization are the following:

1. Hypertension of 150/100 mm Hg or more *or* proteinuria of 1 g/24 hr or more
2. Lesser degrees of hypertension but with any of the following:
   a. Proteinuria of 1+ or more
   b. Increasing edema
   c. Oliguria or anuria
   d. Persistent or severe headache
   e. Blurred vision
   f. Nausea and vomiting
   g. Epigastric pain

Medical management. For *moderate* preeclampsia a plan of care similar to that for the home will be instituted. However, additional assessment of both maternal and fetal health will be undertaken (see Chapter 33).

The management of *severe* preeclampsia is largely maternal. The *goals* of therapy are as follows:

1. Prevention or control of convulsions
2. Survival of mother with minimal morbidity (e.g., stroke)
3. Birth of an infant as mature as possible without significant postdelivery complications
4. Choice of a therapy that is beneficial for both mother and fetus and minimizes the dangers to each

Medical care. The medical care will include directives such as the following:

1. Absolute bed rest in left side-lying position, a quiet room with emergency supplies available (Table 35.11), minimal stimulation, and dimmed lighting are required.

2. Assessment of respirations, blood pressure, the level of consciousness, and reflex irritability and determinations of levels of serum electrolytes, urine protein, hematocrit, and plasma or urinary estriols are made at frequent intervals. The woman is weighed daily.

3. Fundoscopic examination is performed daily to note arteriolar spasm, edema, hemorrhages, arteriovenous nicking, and exudates.

4. A high-carbohydrate, low-fat, and moderate- or high-protein diet with moderate sodium is ordered.

5. If urinary output is above 700 ml/24 hr, the output plus other fluid loss is replaced with 100 ml of salt-free fluid (including parenteral) each day. If the output is less than 700 ml/24 hr, no more fluid than 2000 ml/24 hr, including intravenous fluids, is allowed. If renal failure exists, total fluid intake is not to exceed 500 ml/24 hr.

6. Sedatives, antihypertensives, and anticonvulsants are to be readily available and administered as indicated (Table 35.9). If diuretics are used, the physician must be ready to justify their use.

7. Monitoring is done for signs of hyperreflexia or hyporeflexia and for signs of labor and fetal heart rate (FHR).

Prevention and control of convulsions in eclampsia. Eclampsia is an awesome, frightening sequence to observe. Increased hypertension precedes the tonic-clonic convulsions; hypotension and collapse follow. Stertorous breathing and coma are the aftermath of a seizure. Nystagmus and muscular twitching persist for a time. Disorientation and amnesia cloud the immediate recovery. Oliguria and anuria are notable. (A more detailed description of tonic-clonic convulsions is given in the box below.)

The immediate care during a convulsion is to assure a patent airway. Once this has been attained adequate oxygenation must then be provided. Various drugs and equipment are used in the prevention or control of convulsions (Table 35.9).

Magnesium sulfate. Magnesium sulfate is an excellent anticonvulsant for the prevention or control of eclampsia. It may be given intravenously or intramuscularly. Various dosage schedules are used. For example, an initial dose of 4 g magnesium sulfate in 250 ml of 5% dextrose in water may be given intravenously (injected *slowly* at a rate of 5 ml/30 sec); this may then be followed by 4 to 5 g intramuscularly in each buttock (1% procaine can be added to the solution to reduce the pain of injection). This can be followed at 4-hr intervals with intramuscular doses of 4 to 5 g. When magnesium sulfate is given intravenously, the effect is immediate and lasts for about 30 minutes. When it is given intramuscularly, the onset of action occurs in 1 hour and the effect lasts 3 to 4 hours.

Magnesium sulfate has a CNS-depressant effect; because it reduces blood pressure by splanchnic vasodilatation, severe hypotension can occur. Therefore the woman's blood pressure should be monitored continuously while the drug is being administered intravenously and every 15 minutes at other times. The drug also increases the retention of sodium. The drug is excreted by the kidneys; therefore her urinary output must total 100 ml or more every 4 hours. If the urinary output is less than 25 ml/hour and the doses of magnesium sulfate are repeated, toxic levels of the drug can occur with severe diminution or absence of the patellar reflex and respiratory depression.

An indwelling catheter is inserted, and an hourly urometer is attached to ensure careful monitoring of urinary output and to minimize stress to the woman. If the output is not maintained, the drug should not be repeated.

Adverse effects of magnesium sulfate also include respiratory paralysis. *Maternal toxicity has been reached when the respirations are fewer than 16/min or when knee, biceps, or ankle jerks are no longer present.* It is imperative that these reflexes be checked before and after each injection and that the drug be withheld if the respirations are fewer than 16/min or there is hyporeflexia (see box, Table 35.10, and Figs. 35.7 and 35.8).

Description of Convulsions

Stage of invasion: 2 to 3 seconds; eyes fixed; twitching of facial muscles.

Stage of contraction: 15 to 20 seconds; eyes protrude and are bloodshot; all body muscles in tonic contraction (e.g., arms flexed, hands clenched, legs inverted).

Stage of convulsion: Muscles relax and contract alternatively. Respirations are halted and then begin again with long, deep, stertorous inhalation. Coma ensues (2 to 3 minutes to hours).

Occurrence: During prenatal, natal, or postdelivery period.

Recurrence: Within minutes of first convulsion or never.

Table 35.9
Pharmacologic Control of Hypertension and its Sequelae in Pregnancy and Labor

Medication	Target Tissue	Effects of Medication: Maternal	Effects of Medication: Fetal/Neonatal	Nursing Actions
Anticonvulsants				
Magnesium sulfate IV or IM Dosage: Pritchard (1980)—first dose: 4 g 20% IV at 1 g/min and 10 g 50% IM, subsequently: 5 g 50% IM q 4 hr; Zuspan (1966)—first dose: 6 g 20% IV, subsequently: 10-24 g/L of 5% D/W at 1 g/hr (or see p. 815)	Myoneural junction: decreases acetylcholine, thereby depressing neuromuscular transmission Thyroid: decreases parathormone secretion, resulting in increased urinary excretion of calcium Placental perfusion dynamics not altered	Minimal hypotensive effect Minimal if any direct effect on CNS because of blood-brain barrier to magnesium Hypocalcemia CAUTION: Do not give excessive dosages that tend to decrease urinary output and to depress DTRs DANGER: Muscular paralysis (cardiopulmonary) Antidotes: calcium gluconate, neostigmine, pentylenetetrazol (Metrazol)	Mild depression in small number (6%) Neonatal hypermagnesemia easily treated: calcium; exchange transfusion with citrated blood	Notify perinatal staff Decrease CNS irritability Arrange environment to promote rest Provide continuous nursing care Encourage kidney perfusion with left side-lying position and insert indwelling urinary catheter; monitor urinary output every hour Under 25 ml/hr—do not repeat dose Diuresis—good prognostic sign Repeat dose per order if: DTRs present (Figs. 35.7 and 35.8) Respirations of 12/min or more Urinary output over 1 dl/4 hr Assess maternal condition Hydration Affect Other signs or symptoms of preeclampsia Keep 20 ml of 10% calcium gluconate at bedside; with linen/equipment for delivery, eclamptic tray, oxygen, and suction equipment
Diazepam (Valium)	Thalamus and hypothalmus: direct depressant effect	Effective in initial management of eclamptic convulsions	Flattens fetal heart rate (FHR) base line (loss of beat-to-beat variability), an important criterion in assessing fetal oxygenation High levels in newborn: Depressed sucking ability Hypotonia Temperature instability (decrease) Decreased respiratory rate	Notify perinatal staff Assess DTRs, respirations, signs of labor Monitor labor: see Normal labor
Barbiturates (rapid-acting) Sodium phenobarbital: 0.2-0.3 mg IV Sodium amobarbital: 0.25-0.5 g IV	CNS: depressant effect	Controls seizures	Depressant effect on fetus May minimize hyperbilirubinemia	See Diazepam

Antihypertensives*				
Hydralazine (Apresoline, Neopresol)	Peripheral arterioles: decreases muscle tone, thereby decreasing peripheral resistance Hypothalamus and medullary vasomotor center: minor decrease in sympathetic tone	Headache Flushing Palpitation Tachycardia Some decrease in uteroplacental blood flow	Minimal effects: some decrease in P_{O_2}	Assess for effects of medications Alert mother (family) to expected effects of medications Assess blood pressure (precipitous drop can lead to shock and perhaps to abruptio placentae) and urinary output Maintain bed rest with side rails
Methyldopa (Aldomet) (used if maintenance therapy is needed): 250-500 mg orally q 8 hr	Postganglionic nerve endings: interferes with chemical neurotransmission to reduce peripheral vascular resistance CNS: sedation	Sleepiness Postural hypotension Constipation Rare: drug-induced fever in 1% of women and positive Coombs' test in 20%	After 4 mo of maternal therapy, positive Coombs' test in infant	See Hydralazine
Diuretics†				
Thiazides	Arteriolar smooth muscles: reduces responsiveness to catecholamines	Ineffective in preventing preeclampsia Further reduces already-present decreased plasma volume of preeclampsia Complications Fluid and electrolyte imbalance Pancreatitis Decrease in CHO intolerance Hyperuricemia	Hyponatremia Thrombocytopenia	Arrange to have blood drawn to measure levels of Na, Cl, H_2O, K, and H+ to prevent hyponatremia, hypokalemia, hypochloremia, metabolic acidosis
Furosemide (Lasix): 40 mg IV	Loop of Henle	Relieves pulmonary edema Excessive use results in hypokalemia and hyponatremia	No abnormalities noted	See Thiazides
Ethacrynic acid (Edecrin)	Similar to furosemide	Similar to furosemide	Deafness	See Thiazides
Mannitol (for impending renal failure, oliguria, DIC): 12.5-25 mg IV	Osmotic diuretic: pulls fluid into vascular bed (therefore not recommended for persons with congestive heart failure)	Increases renal plasma flow and urinary output Flushes out kidneys Reduces swelling in ischemic cells in kidney and myocardium	No known effect	See Thiazides
Blood volume expanders				
(salt-poor, serum albumin‡)	Intrasvascular volume	Increases blood volume		

*By midpregnancy, diastolic and systolic blood pressure normally falls by 10-15 mm Hg. If diastolic blood pressure is 75 mm Hg or more in second trimester and 85 mm Hg or more in third trimester there is a statistical increase in fetal mortality.

NOTE: For the obese woman, use a thigh cuff to obtain accurate readings (or use ultrasound).

†For control of chronic hypertension, pulmonary edema, renal oliguria, acute renal failure, chronic nephrotic syndrome. If used, physician must be ready to justify action.

‡May not be appropriate for the woman with severe preeclampsia-eclampsia.

Fig. 35.7

Elicitation of patellar reflex. **A,** With the legs hanging freely over end of examining table, or **B,** with the client in a supine position. A blow with the percussion hammer is dealt directly to patellar tendon, inferior to patella. The normal response is extension or kicking out of the leg. **C,** Elicitation of biceps reflex. A downward blow is struck over the thumb, which is situated over the biceps tendon. The normal response is flexion of the arm at the elbow.

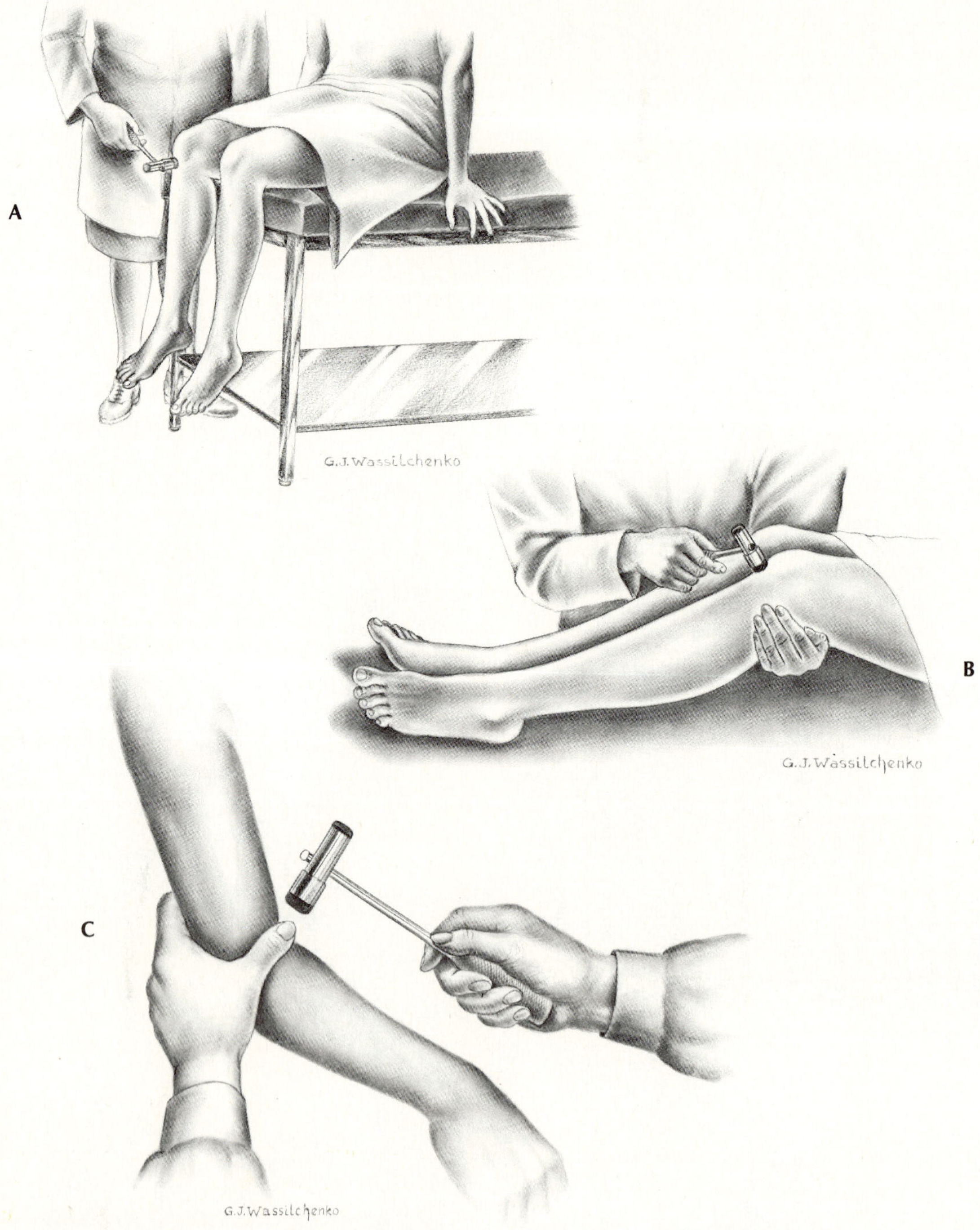

Fig. 35.8

A, Assessment for hyperreactive reflexes (clonus) at ankle joint. Support the leg with the knee flexed. With the other hand, sharply dorsiflex the foot, and maintain the dorsiflexed position for a moment, then release the foot. **B,** Normal (negative clonus) response: While foot is held in dorsiflexion, no rhythmic oscillations (jerking) are felt. When foot is released, no oscillations are seen as foot drops to plantar flexed position. **C,** Abnormal (positive clonus) response: Rhythmic oscillations are felt when foot is in dorsiflexion and are seen as foot drops to plantar flexed position.

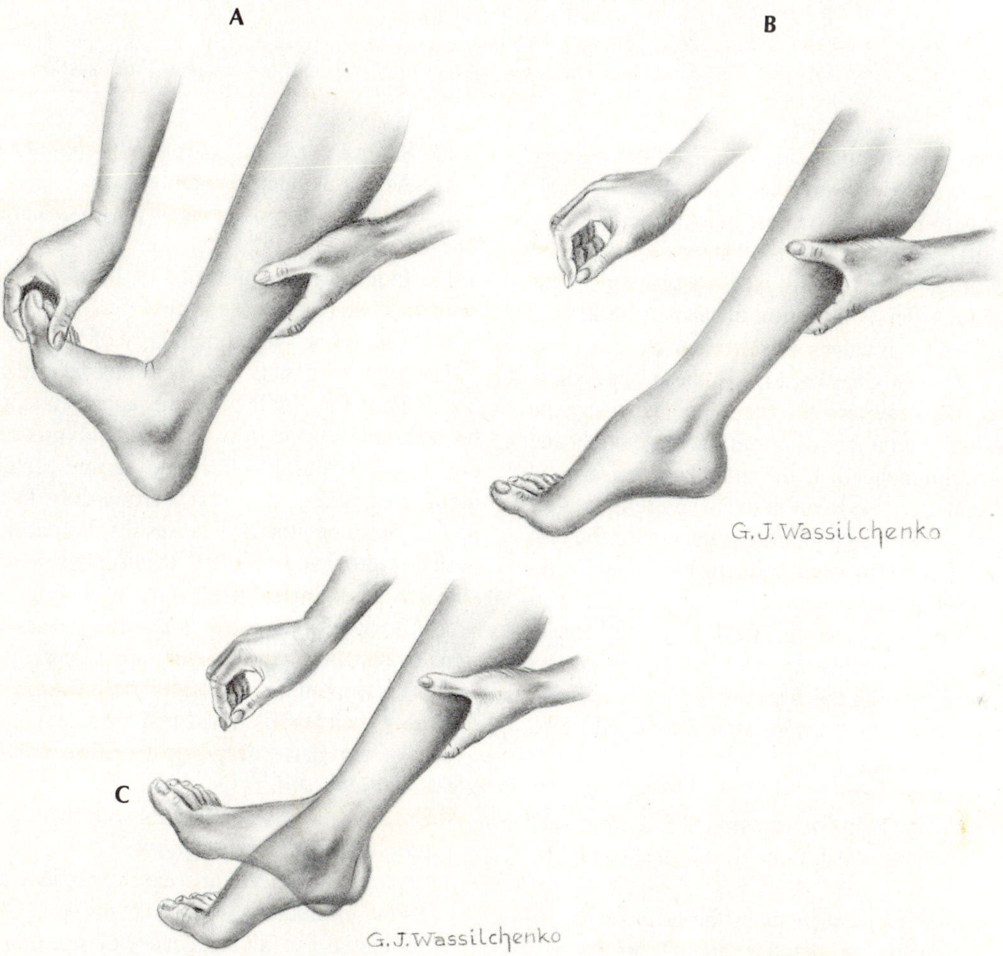

Magnesium Sulfate Monitoring

Response to rise in serum levels:

4 mg/dl or more	Prevents convulsions
10 to 12 mg/dl	Reflexes disappear
12 to 15 mg/dl	Respirations slow (below 16) or absent
15+ mg/dl	Cardiac arrest possible

Toxic levels may occur if urinary output is less than 100 ml in preceding 4 hours.

Toxic levels in fetus cause marked slowing of respirations and hyporeflexia in newborn.

The antidote is a calcium salt such as calcium gluconate. A 20 ml vial of a 10% aqueous solution of calcium gluconate should be kept at the bedside. If needed, it is administered slowly intravenously and repeated every hour until the respiratory, urinary, and neurologic depression has been alleviated. The maximal number of injections of a calcium salt is 8 injections in a 24-hr period.

Since magnesium salts cross the placenta the fetus may be affected. The drug should not be administered intravenously in the 2 hours preceding delivery (intramuscular magnesium does not seem to have adverse effects on the neonate), and the newborn should be assessed for hyporeflexia and for respiratory problems.

Table 35.10
Assessing Deep Tendon Reflexes (DTRs)

Degree	Grading	Clinical Significance and Nursing Actions
Hyperactive response	4+	Woman not responding to medications as desired; may be accompanied by apprehension, restlessness, excitability; notify physician
More than normal	3+	Woman responding; however, important to assess frequently
Normal	2+	Safe dosage level, therapeutic effect
Low response	1+	Notify physician for medical directives
No response	0	Turn off magnesium sulfate drip; change to "keep open" solution; notify physician for immediate care; prepare antidote (20 ml vial of 10% calcium gluconate) for injection

The woman receiving magnesium sulfate therapy *should never be left unattended* because magnesium sulfate toxicity with respiratory arrest may occur.

Delivery. If preeclampsia fails to improve within 24 to 48 hours in response to care, elective delivery is initiated (see discussion of induction of labor, p. 886).

Ultimate therapy involves fetal testing by nonstress and stress tests (see Chapter 24). If these tests show fetal deterioration, the termination of pregnancy by the method that will be the least harmful to the mother and the fetus is recommended. If the gravida is not a good subject for induction, cesarean delivery, preferably after the thirty-sixth week of pregnancy (to decrease the risk to the infant of superimposed prematurity), may be required. A delay of more than 2 weeks in severe preeclampsia is poor policy because fetal death may ensue. Estriol levels are generally observed closely to determine serious changes in the fetal condition. If delivery is still awaited 4 weeks or more after fetal death, DIC may result (see p. 797).

Intranatal nursing care

Assessment. The need for assessment is continuous; therefore these clients need a one-to-one staff-client ratio (see box).

The physical assessment includes the following:

1. Check woman's temperature every 4 hours.
2. Check blood pressure frequently during acute phase and every 2 to 4 hours thereafter.
3. Auscultate FHR (rate and rhythm) when blood pressure is obtained if fetal monitor is not being used.
4. Inspect and palpate woman's face, extremities, and sacrum (dependent area when woman is in bed) for edema.
5. Assess 24-hr fluid intake and hourly (and 24-hr) urinary output.
6. Check urine specimen for protein every 4 hours.
7. Auscultate chest for signs of pulmonary edema; listen for moist respirations or cough.
8. Test deep tendon reflexes: brachial, wrist, *knee*, ankle (clonus).
9. Observe for hyperactivity, signs of convulsion, coma, or cyanosis.
10. Record results of daily fundoscopic examination.
11. Assess woman's affect.
12. If labor begins, assess progress carefully (see Chapter 21).
13. Inquire about presence of headache, visual disturbances, or midepigastric pain.
14. Assess for symptomatology of DIC.

The physician will order various laboratory evaluations. The nurse will send the appropriate specimens, for example, urine for analysis and protein content; blood for serum electrolytes, serum protein, serum blood urea nitrogen (BUN), carbon-dioxide–combining power, and hematocrit. The results are checked against normal values and reported to the physician. The psychologic assessment includes the following:

1. The woman's affect is carefully assessed. Symptoms of restlessness or anxiety are recorded.
2. The woman's response to the presence or absence of family members is noted and recorded.
3. The woman's response to labor contractions is noted and recorded.

Record keeping is continuous with therapy.

Examples of nursing diagnoses

1. Potential fluid volume excess because of lessened urine production (≤100 ml in 4 hours)
2. Potential for injury because of sedation
3. Self-care deficit because of need for absolute bed rest

Plan and implementation. The goals for care are to maintain the functioning of the woman's body systems and to keep her as quiet and nonstimulated as possible. Careful planning is necessary if the care that is needed for the woman's hypertensive state, for her labor and delivery, and for care during emergencies is to be accomplished.

1. General care: The woman is admitted to a single darkened room; usually no visitors are permitted. The anxiety of family members can be "contagious." Careful explanation of the purpose for isolating the woman is given, and the family is kept informed of progress. Efforts are made to reduce family anxiety so that they may act as support persons. *For some women the pres-*

Clinical Assessment Guide: Preeclampsia

Assessment of client's environment

Criteria	Present	Absent	Comments
Environment			
Quiet			
Nonstimulating			
Lighting subdued			
Seizure precautions			
Oral airway (or padded tongue blade) near head of bed			
Padded side rails			
Suction equipment tested and ready to use			
Oxygen administration equipment tested and ready to use			
Call button within easy reach			
Emergency medication tray immediately accessible			
Magnesium sulfate in or adjacent to woman's room			
Calcium gluconate immediately available			
Emergency delivery pack accessible			

Assessment of client

Subjective

Write what the woman states when you ask her to describe how she feels.

Objective

Record what you see.
Describe facies.
Describe affect.
Observe and note location of edema.
Record temperature, blood pressure, weight.
Auscultate FHR; assess rhythm and quality.
Assess fetal activity.
Check urine for amount and protein.
Auscultate chest; listen for moist respirations or cough.
Test and record deep tendon reflexes.
Assess onset of labor.
Record amount of fluid intake and urinary output in past 24 hours.
Record drug, dosage, and time of medication during the past 24 hours.

ence of the supportive partner is essential. The woman is placed on absolute bed rest, on her left side, with side rails up. If she insists on lying on her back, the headrest is raised and a wedge (rolled towel) is placed under her right hip to prevent vena cava syndrome. She is only disturbed for essential procedures (e.g., no baths). The blood pressure cuff is placed on her arm and left in position. Intravenous fluids are begun at a "to keep open" rate. An indwelling catheter is inserted, and the amount of urine is recorded at 1- to 2-hr intervals.

Emergency equipment and drugs are kept in the room. These include plastic airway or tongue depressor bite stick, padded tongue blade, oxygen and suction equipment, ophthalmoscope, and medications such as magnesium sulfate, calcium gluconate, and cardiac stimulants, and hypertensive controls such as hydralazine and 50% glucose (Table 35.11). An emergency delivery pack is also kept in the room. The nurse maintains a matter-of-fact and calm attitude and approach; the rationale of treatment is explained briefly. NOTE: A plastic airway is preferred over a padded tongue blade because it permits passage of a tube for suction and for administration of oxygen.

2. Emergency care of convulsions is as follows:
   a. If convulsions occur, turn the woman onto her left side to avoid aspiration of vomitus and to prevent vena cava syndrome.

Table 35.11
Drugs and Equipment for Preventive Treatment of Convulsions of Eclampsia

Drugs	Supplies
Magnesium sulfate: 2 ampules, 10 ml/ampule (5 g, 50%); 500 mg (4 mEq)/ml	Emergency delivery pack
Sodium bicarbonate: 50 ml (7.5%) (44.6 mEq)	Ophthalmoscope
Hydralazine: 5 ampules, 20 mg/ampule	Reflex hammer
Heparin sodium: 10 ml, 5000 USP units/ml	Fetal monitor
Diazepam: 2 ml, 5 mg/ml	Padded tongue blade
Chlordiazepoxide: 5 ml, 20 mg/ml	Plastic airway
Epinephrine: 1:1000, 1mg/ml	Oxygen and suction
Atropisol, 1% (mydriatic)	Tourniquets
Atropine sulfate: 0.4 mg/0.5 ml	Syringes: 2, 10, and 50 ml
Sterile water ampules	Cutdown tray
Sterile normal saline ampules	
Calcium gluconate: 10%, 1 g/10 ml; 97 mg (4.8 mEq)/10 ml Ca++	
Phenytoin: 2 ml, 50 mg/ml	
Propranolol: tablets 40 mg	
Intravenous barbiturates	

b. Insert a folded towel, plastic airway, or padded tongue blade into side of mouth to prevent biting of lips or tongue and to maintain an airway. Do not put fingers into woman's mouth as she may bite them involuntarily.

c. Aspirate food and fluid from glottis or trachea.

d. Give magnesium sulfate as ordered.

e. Administer oxygen by means of face cone or tent after convulsion ceases (masks and nasal catheters cause excessive stimulation). O_2 rate may be up to 10 L/min (as opposed to 3 L/min advocated for continuous O_2 in chronic conditions).

f. Record time and duration of convulsions; include description (see box, p. 815).

g. Note any urinary or fecal incontinence.

3. Transfusion: Have the woman's blood typed and matched. Keep the blood available for emergency transfusion. (Women with eclampsia often develop premature separation of the placenta, hemorrhage, and shock.)

4. Diet and fluids: Give as directed; record time and amount and woman's response. Hospital protocols vary.

a. Permit nothing by mouth if the woman is convulsing.

b. Insert retention catheter for accurate measurement of urinary output.

c. Assist physician with intravenous infusion of 200 to 300 ml of 20% glucose solution, two to three times a day during critical period to support liver function, aid nutrition, and replace fluid; 50% glucose is rarely used since it often will sclerose veins.

d. To correct hypovolemia, crystalloids (0.9% saline or Ringer's lactated solution) are infused intravenously.

e. If woman is oliguric or if serum protein level is low, physician may order salt-poor albumin (25 to 50 ml) or 250 or 500 ml of plasma or serum to be administered intravenously.

f. Note and record maternal response (see Assessment).

5. Medications: Give as directed; monitor and record woman's response. Record drugs, dosages, and times given.

a. Diuretics are *no longer* advocated (Table 35.9).

b. Sedatives such as phenobarbital, 0.05 g, are given orally or intramuscularly on admission to the hospital and repeated to maintain moderate sedation until the woman's condition improves. Monitor for start of labor since woman may be unaware of sensation.

c. Magnesium sulfate (intravenous or intramuscular) may be ordered as necessary. Before repeating magnesium sulfate, check the following:

(1) Deep tendon reflexes (DTRs) are present.

(2) Respirations are at least 12/min.

(3) Urinary output is at least 100 ml/4 hr or greater.

6. Maintain body hygiene. The vulvar area may be washed with warm, soapy water.

7. Psychologic support: Physician or nurse explains procedures briefly and quietly. Woman is never left alone if condition is severe or she is receiving magnesium sulfate therapy. Family is also kept informed of management, rationale, and woman's progress.

8. Delivery: Preeclampsia-eclampsia and severe hypertensive or renal disease are intensified by continuing pregnancy. Termination of gestation is the only practical treatment. Fetus may therefore be premature or otherwise compromised.

a. Eclampsia is controlled before induction of labor is attempted; then labor is induced by amniotomy.

b. Oxytocin may be used cautiously to stimulate labor.

c. Nitrous oxide (70%) and oxygen (30%) may be given with contractions, but 100% oxygen should be given between contractions.

d. Vaginal delivery with pudendal block anesthesia is preferred. However, if labor cannot be induced readily, if the woman is bleeding, or if there is fetal distress, cesarean delivery should be effected, preferably with procaine (or equivalent) local infiltration of abdominal wall. Thiopental (Pentothal) may be given after delivery of infant for incisional closure.

e. A pediatrician and nurse are present for the delivery.

Evaluation

1. Within 24 to 48 hours:
   a. The condition improves.
      (1) CNS irritability is reduced.
      (2) Convulsions (if any) are terminated.
      (3) Hypertension is reduced (normal values usually return by 7 weeks after delivery, always by 3 months).
      (4) Water imbalance, acid-base imbalance, and other electrolyte imbalances are corrected.
      (5) Proteinuria is reduced, and serum protein level is increased.
      (6) Fetal well-being continues.
      (7) Placental complications are absent or controlled, and the delivery can proceed as previously planned whether vaginal, induced, or cesarean.
   b. If the condition does not improve the nurse assists in the care for elective delivery, that is, induction of labor or cesarean birth (see Chapter 37).
2. The woman and family are aware of the need for care, the cause of the symptoms, and the prognosis. Informed consent forms are completed.
3. Records are complete at all times.

Postpartum nursing care

Assessment

1. Check the blood pressure every 4 hours for 48 hours or more frequently as the woman's condition warrants. Even if no convulsions occurred before delivery, they may occur within this period.

2. Ask the woman to report headaches, blurred vision, etc. Assess her affect, alertness, or dullness. Check blood pressure before giving analgesic for headache. NOTE: No ergot products are given because they increase blood pressure.

3. Assess the woman's and family response to labor.

4. Continue regular assessment.

Plan and implementation. The postpartum care for the woman with PIH is basically the same as for all women. The woman and her family need opportunities to discuss their emotional response to having this complication. The nurse also provides information concerning the following:

1. Prognosis (i.e., preeclampsia-eclampsia does not necessarily recur in subsequent pregnancies, but careful prenatal care is essential)
2. Necessity for careful evaluation during postdelivery examination to rule out chronic hypertension
3. Family planning information (i.e., next pregnancy should be delayed for 2 years; woman is not a candidate for oral contraceptive use)

Evaluation. The nurse uses the following criteria to evaluate the plan of care:

1. Recovery from PIH is complete *or* the woman begins therapy for underlying cause of hypertension not related to pregnancy.

2. The woman's self-concept is not impaired.

3. The infant is healthy *or* has minimal impairment.

Hypertensive Cardiovascular Disease

Hypertension is considered to be present in women during the childbearing years when the blood pressure is maintained at or above 140/80 at rest. Hypertensive disorders during pregnancy make up an extremely important group that accounts for a high maternal and perinatal morbidity and mortality.

The vascular complications of hypertension, such as intracranial hemorrhage, are the consequence of increased arterial pressure and related ateriosclerosis.

Hypertension without apparent impairment of the heart is termed *hypertensive vascular disease,* in contrast with *hypertensive cardiovascular disease,* in which left ventricular hypertrophy, coronary artery disease, or heart failure has developed.

Primary (essential) hypertensive disease, in which no cause can be determined, is the diagnosis in about 85% of nonpregnant premenopausal hypertensive women. The remaining 15% of women with hypertension will have secondary hypertensive vascular disease, caused by disorders such as chronic pyelonephritis or glomerulonephritis, renal artery stenosis, or coarctation of the aorta.

Why primary hypertension occurs is still undetermined, but abnormalities in the regulation of blood pressure, including increased vascular resistance or activity of the sympathetic nervous system, may be at least partially responsible. Moreover, hypertension may be produced in ways difficult to explain by adrenal glucocorticoids, aldosterone, deoxycorticosterone, or other hormones.

The cardiac output and blood volume continue to be maintained until heart failure or severe edema develops. Obviously the increased load associated with even normal pregnancy increases the work of the heart and adds to the stress on the vasculature. When obstetric complications such as preeclampsia-eclampsia, diabetes mellitus, or multiple pregnancy ensue, vascular complications, including even heart failure, may develop.

When hypertension is sustained for years, the initially reversible arteriolar constriction becomes permanent as a result of intimal thickening, hypertrophy of vascular muscular coats, and hyaline degeneration. Left ventricular hypertrophy follows eventually. Coronary and cerebral artery atherosclerosis usually develop, often leading to myocardial infarction, cerebral hemorrhage, or infarction.

The person with mild to moderate essential hypertensive vascular disease may enjoy apparently normal health for years. Eventually, complaints typical of progressive, now symptomatic, disease may include suboccipital headaches, especially those that occur in the early morning but subside during the day, lightheadedness, tinnitus, and palpation of the heart. With more progressive disease, signs of heart failure, renal incompetence, or CNS complications develop.

DIFFERENTIAL DIAGNOSIS

The differential diagnosis of hypertension begins with the past history of disease, for example, nephritis. The woman's health and progress over the years may disclose advancing symptomatology of hypertensive disease, perhaps worsened by pregnancy. Careful evaluation of the woman's endocrine and cardiovascular-renal systems, as well as other possible causes of hypertension, may disclose the cause, independent of pregnancy-induced hypertension. Occasionally, when the hypertensive woman is seen initially late in pregnancy, studies after the puerperium may be required before the cause of hypertension can be determined. Often the etiology will be obscure and the tentative impression may be one of "essential hypertension" (Table 35.7).

PROGNOSIS

The prognosis for the pregnant woman with hypertension depends on the cause, the degree of hypertension, the woman's symptomatology, and her response to treatment. Whatever the cause, the fetus may be severely affected by hypertension and its sequelae. Early delivery may be lifesaving for the mother and the fetus.

MEDICAL AND NURSING MANAGEMENT

With chronic hypertensive disease, the physician treats the symptomatology during pregnancy. The pregnancy is usually permitted to continue if the woman responds to therapy. Frequent estriol determinations after the thirty-second week will be ordered in an attempt to carry the fetus to 34 to 36 weeks. Protracted therapy is futile if the woman is unresponsive. Fetal death or maternal CNS, cardiac, or renal complications may develop. If the woman's blood pressure reaches 200/110, immediate medical attention is necessary. The physician will usually order antihypertensive drugs, for example, hydralazine (Apresoline), and assess the need for a prompt delivery (Table 35.9).

The nursing care of women with chronic hypertensive disease is the same as that of women with hypertension attributable to pregnancy. If and when cardiac involvement is diagnosed, the nursing care of the woman with cardiac disease is superimposed on the original plan (see pp. 867-871). The woman and her family must be aware of the possibility of premature delivery and of the need for careful and continuous supervision during the prenatal, natal, and postdelivery periods.

References and Readings

Acker, D., et al.: Abruptio placentae associated with cocaine use, Am. J. Obstet. Gynecol. **146**(2):220, 1983

Aladjem, S., et al.: Experimental induction of a toxemia like syndrome in the pregnant beagle, Am. J. Obstet. Gynecol. **145**(1):27, 1983.

Brewer, G.S., and Brewer, T.: What every pregnant woman should know, New York, 1977, Random House.

Burke, S.R.: The composition and function of body fluids, ed. 3, St. Louis, 1980, The C.V. Mosby Co.

Clough, D.H., and Higgins, P.G.: Discrepancies in estimating blood loss, Am. J. Nurs. **81**(2):331, 1981.

Coco, C.D.: Intravenous therapy: a handbook for practice, St. Louis, 1980, The C.V. Mosby Co.

Curet, L.B., and Olson, R.W.: Evaluation of a program of bed rest in the threatment of chronic hypertension in pregnancy, Obstet. Gynecol **53:**336, 1979.

Danforth, D.: Obstetrics and gynecology, ed. 4, Philadelphia, 1982, Harper & Row.

de Alvarez, R.R.: Preclampsia-eclampsia and other gestational edema-proteinuria-hypertension disorders (GEPH). In Benson, R., editor: Current obstetrical and gynecologic diagnosis and treatment ed. 4, Palo Alto, Calif., 1982, Lange Medical Publications.

Dennis, E.J., et al.: The preeclampsia-eclampsia syndrome. In Danforth, D., editor: Obstetrics and gynecology 1982, ed. 4, New York, Harper & Row.

Gahart, B.L.: Intravenous medications: a handbook for nurses and other allied health personnel, ed. 3, St. Louis, 1981, The C.V. Mosby Co.

Gant, N.F., and Worley, R.J.: Hypertension in pregnancy: concepts and management, New York, 1980, Appleton-Century Crofts.

Hill, M.N.: Hypertension: what can go wrong when you measure blood pressure, Am. J. Nurs. **80:**942, 1980.

Jacobs, P.A., et al.: Mechanism of origin of complete hydatidiform moles, Nature **286:**714, 1980.

Jennings, B.M.: Improving your management of DIC, Nurs. '79 **9**(5):60, 1979.

Jones, M.B.: Hypertensive disorders of pregnancy, J.O.G.N. Nurs. **8:**92, 1979.

Kajii, T., and Ohama, K.: Androgenic origin of hydatidiform mole, Nature **286:**633, 1977.

Kasser, N.S., et al.: Roll over test, Obstet. Gynecol. **54:**411, 1980.

Kelley, M., and Mongiello, P.: Hypertension in pregnancy, labor, delivery and postpartum, **82**(5):813, 1982.

Lindheimer, M.D., and Katz, A.I.: Pathophysiology of preeclampsia, Kidney Int. **18:**259, Aug. 1980.

Lueck, J., et al.: Observation of an organism found in patients with gestational trophoblastic disease and in patients with toxemia of pregnancy, Am. J. Obstet. Gynecol. **145**(1):15, 1983.

McKay, D.G.: Chronic intravascular coagulation in normal pregnancy and preeclampsia, Contrib. Nephrol. **25:**108, 1981.

Moore, L.G., et al.: The incidence of pregnancy induced hypertension is increased among Colorado residents at high altitude, Am. J. Obstet. Gynecol. **144**(14):423, 1982.

Nursing photobook. Dealing with emergencies. Nurs. '81 Books, Horsham, Pa., 1981, Intermed Communications, Inc.

Nursing photobook. Managing I.V. therapy. Nurs. '82 Books, Springhouse, Pa., 1982, Intermed Communications, Inc.

Nursing skillbook. Giving emergency care competently. Nurs. '78 Books, Horsham, Pa., 1978, Intermed Communications, Inc.

Nursing skillbook. Monitoring fluid and electrolytes precisely. Nurs. '79 Books, Horsham, Pa., 1979, Intermed Communications, Inc.

Pritchard, J.A.: Management of preeclampsia and eclampsia, Kidney Int. **18:**259, Aug. 1980.

Pritchard, J.A., and MacDonald, P.C.: Williams obstetrics, ed. 16, New York, 1980, Appleton-Century-Crofts.

Programmed instruction. Nursing care of patients in shock. I. Pharmacotherapy, Am. J. Nurs. **82**(6):943, 1982.

Programmed instruction. Nursing care of patients in shock. II. Fluids, respiratory care, and the intra-aortic balloon pump, Am. J. Nurs. **82**(9):1401, 1982.

Programmed instruction. Nursing care of patients in shock. III. Evaluating the patient, Am. J. Nurs. **82**(11):1723, 1982.

Purcell, J.A.: Shock drugs: standardized guidelines, Am. J. Nurs. **82**(6):965, 1982.

Royce, J.A.: Shock: emergency nursing implications, Nurs. Clin. North Am. **8:**377, 1973.

Sehgal, N.N., and Hitt, J.R.: Plasma volume expansion in the treatment of preeclampsia, Am. J. Obstet. Gynecol. **138:**165, Sept. 15, 1980.

Sonstegard, L.: Pregnancy induced hypertension: prenatal nursing concerns, M.C.N. **4:**90, 1979.

Zuspan, F.P.: Treatment of severe preeclampsia and eclampsia, Clin. Obstet. Gynecol. **9:**954, 1966.

36 Major Complications Coincident with Pregnancy

- **Infection**
  - Prenatal infection
    - Suggested symptomatic management for woman with genital herpes
    - Assessment for syphilis
  - Postnatal infection
    - Puerperal infection
  - Mastitis
  - Urinary tract infections
  - Vaginal infections
    - Trichomonas vaginitis
    - Monilial vaginitis
    - Simple vaginitis
    - Vaginal douche procedure
  - Bacteremic shock
  - Summary of nursing actions: infections
    - Goals of care
    - Evaluation
- **Neonatal Sepsis**
  - Clinical findings
  - Incidence
  - Prognosis
  - Sequelae
  - Modes of transmission
  - General nursing care
  - Rubella
  - Herpesvirus type 2 infection
    - Prognosis
  - Gonorrhea
    - Prognosis
  - Syphilis
    - Clinical findings
    - Diagnosis
    - Medical management
    - Prognosis and sequelae
  - Chlamydial disease
  - Cytomegalovirus infection
  - Acquired immune deficiency syndrome (AIDS)
  - Oral thrush
  - Summary of nursing actions: neonatal infection
    - Goals of care
    - Example of nursing diagnosis
    - Evaluation
- **Endocrine and Metabolic Disorders**
  - Diabetes mellitus
    - Definitions
    - Significance
    - Incidence
    - Pathogenesis
    - Classification
    - Normal pregnancy: maternal metabolic adaptations
    - Gestational diabetes mellitus (type I, class A)
    - Insulin-dependent diabetes mellitus (type II and all other classes)
    - Effects of diabetes on pregnancy
    - Prognosis
    - Goals of management
    - Management
    - Summary of nursing actions: the diabetic mother
    - Effects of diabetes on the embryo-fetus-neonate
    - Neonatal hypoglycemia
  - Neonatal hypocalcemia
    - Definition
    - Clinical manifestations
    - Infants at risk
    - Summary of nursing actions: neonatal hypocalcemia

■ Hyperemesis Gravidarum
Definition
Clinical manifestations
Summary of nursing actions: hyperemesis gravidarum
Goals of care
Evaluation

■ Hyperthyroidism

■ Heart Disease
Effects of pregnancy on heart disease
Effects of heart disease on pregnancy
Symptoms
Diagnosis
Classification
Medical management
Class I
Class II
Class III
Class IV
Nursing actions
Prenatal care
Natal care
Postdelivery care
Evaluation

Infection

PRENATAL INFECTION

Pregnancy confers no immunity against infection. Women are becoming more sensitive to factors such as infections, which can jeopardize fetal development. The large number of infections, the varying responses of the fetus or neonate, and the range of nursing and medical actions necessitate a readily available source. Table 36.1 provides this information.

Suggested symptomatic management for woman with genital herpes

1. Take warm sitz baths for 15 minutes at a time with a drying agent such as Domeboro (two packets or tablets to a shallow tub of warm water) three to five times daily. Keep the genital area dry and clean. Drying the genital area with a blow dryer after showering is useful. Avoid strong deodorant soaps, creams, and ointments. Wash hands after using the toilet; and do not touch the face after genital contact. Urinating through an empty toilet paper tube is helpful in preventing pain during urination.
2. Wear 100% cotton underwear. Avoid tight-fitting jeans, pants, and pantyhose with nylon inserts.
3. If this is the first herpes infection, woman may experience headache, backache, and pain or tingling in the legs. Recurrences are sometimes preceded by itching, a burning sensation in the genital area, tingling in the legs, or a slight increase in vaginal discharge.
4. Taking care of one's physical and mental health is important. Being run down makes the woman more vulnerable to infection.
5. Yearly Papanicolaou smears are advisable. If the woman becomes pregnant, she should inform the physician that she has herpes.
6. Avoid *any* sexual contact during the entire time that lesions are present. Using condoms and spermicides will help prevent the spread of herpes.

Assessment for syphilis. Several methods of assessment of syphilis are available:

1. Dark-field microscopic examination or direct fluorescent antibody staining of material from lesions or umbilical cord
2. Assessment of clinical signs
3. Roentgenographic evidence of characteristic bone involvement
4. Serologic testing for antibodies known as reagins

Any test for antibodies may be negative in the presence of active infection because it takes time for the body's immune system to develop antibodies to any antigen.

Nonspecific Serologic Tests. Nonspecific serologic tests for nontreponemal antigens used for screening purposes are of two types: complement fixation—Kolmer, Wasserman; and flocculation—Kahn, RPR (rapid plasma reagin), VDRL (Venereal Disease Research Laboratories). The VDRL test is positive in 10 to 90 days after infection; that is, 50% are positive in 3 weeks, 90% in 6 weeks, and 100% in 13 weeks. Therefore infection may exist in the presence of a negative result from the VDRL test. If the antibodies have been acquired from the mother, titers should drop to zero by 3 months. False positive results may occur if the neonate has an acute infection of any kind or a collagen disease. Even in the presence of a syphilitic infection a false negative result may occur, for example, if the mother became infected late in pregnancy. A false positive result may occur in the presence of heroin dependence.

Specific Tests for Syphilis. Specific tests for treponemal antigen are more expensive, require special laboratory equipment, and are therefore used for differential diagnosis. These tests include TPI (*Treponema pallidum* immobilization), FTA-ABS (fluorescent treponemal antibody absorption), and FTA-ABS IgM. The FTA-ABS IgM is most specific for neonatal syphilis; a

Text continued on p. 832.

Table 36.1
Maternal Infections: Effects on Pregnancy and Fetus or Neonate

Infection	Maternal Effects	Fetal or Neonatal Effects	Counseling: Prevention, Identification, and Management
Chlamydia trachomatis (intracellular bacterium)	Mild infection usually; may be asymptomatic; symptoms similar to gonorrhea: discharge and bleeding from or an infection of the cervix; conjunctivitis; premature labor	Stillbirth and neonatal death 10 times more common than in noninfected women; preterm birth; neonatal conjunctivitis appears after 3-4 days; pneumonia	STD; three times more common than gonorrhea; high incidence in teen-age girls; usually controlled with antibiotics, but *not* by penicillin; tetracycline is the drug of choice; untreated, can lead to pelvic inflammatory disease (PID), with painful infection of fallopian tubes; in males, it is linked to nongonococcal urethritis (NGU); neonate may acquire disease by direct contact with infected birth canal
Chickenpox (varicella) (a herpes virus)	Herpes zoster (shingles)	Abortion; fetal death; defects of skin, bone, and muscle; chorioretinitis; hydrocephalus	Severe disseminated epidemic type of varicella during pregnancy may be fatal for mother (and fetus) because of necrotizing angitis (inflammation of blood and lymph vessels); zoster immune globulin (IM) may be given prophylactically to exposed gravidas
Corynebacterium vaginale vaginitis (*Hemophilus vaginalis* vaginitis)	Low virulence; mild illness	Chorioamnionitis; septicemia; fetal or neonatal death	
Coxsackie B virus	Mild illness	Fetal death; cardiovascular anomalies; myocarditis; meningoencephalitis	
Cytomegalovirus (CMV) (a herpes virus)	Respiratory or sexually transmitted asymptomatic illness or mononucleosis-like syndrome; may have a cervical discharge	Fetal or neonatal death or severe, generalized disease—hemolytic anemia and jaundice; hydrocephaly or microcephaly; pneumonitis; hepatosplenomegaly	Virus may be reactivated and cause disease in utero or during delivery in subsequent pregnancies; fetal infection may occur during passage through infected birth canal; disease is frequently progressive through infancy and childhood
Gonorrhea ("clap, drip") *Neisseria gonorrhoeae* (gonococcus bacterium) Genitourinary Anorectal Oropharyngeal Systemic	Lower urogenital tract (UG) (early stage): dysuria, frequency , heavy purulent vaginal discharge; cervical tenderness; vulvovaginitis; bartholinitis Upper UG tract (later stage) (10-15% of cases): lower abdominal pain, cervical tenderness; fever, nausea, vomiting; adnexal abscess, tenderness (PID); ectopic pregnancy; chronic pelvic pain Anorectal: inflammation, burning, pruritus Oropharyngeal: asymptomatic or inflammation, sore throat Systemic: gonococcemia, skin rashes, arthritis, pericarditis, meningitis	Gonococcal ophthalmia neonatorum, pneumonia; neonatal sepsis with temperature instability, hypotonia, poor feeding, and jaundice	Transmitted by sexual contact and fomites such as underwear, bedding, towels Both (all) partners treated to prevent reinfection; couple should use condoms and avoid orogenital sex until posttreatment cultures are negative at two consecutive follow-up visits Incubation period: 2-5 days; in females, early stage may be asymptomatic 5% of clients also have syphilis Gravid women allergic to penicillin can be given erythromycin or spectinomycin; nongravid clients can be given the cephalosporins and kanamycin During postnatal period, infection may reappear as gonococcal endometritis
Group B streptococcus	Septicemia; cellulitis (erysipelas); fever; puerperal infection; impetigo; scarlet fever	Neonatal death within 2-12 hr; blindness, deafness, spinal meningitis, mental retardation, learning or behavior problems in survivors	
Hepatitis A (virus)	Abortion—a cause of liver failure during pregnancy	Exposure during first trimester: fetal anomalies; fetal or neonatal hepatitis; premature birth; intrauterine fetal death	Usually spread by droplet or hand contact especially by culinary workers; Gamma-globulin can be given as prophylaxis for hepatitis A
Serum hepatitis (hepatitis B)	May be transmitted sexually	Infection occurs during birth	

			Generally passed by contaminated needles, syringes, or blood transfusions; can also be transmitted orally or by coitus, however, but incubation period is longer; hepatitis B immune globulin can be given prophylactically after exposure
Herpes genitalis (herpes simplex virus; HSV II)—poses same threat to neonate as does HSV I	Symptomatology more pronounced with first infection; painful blisters that rupture, leaving shallow ulcers that crust over and disappear after 2-6 wk; vaginal discharge if cervix or vaginal mucosa involved; fever, malaise, anorexia; painful inguinal lymphadenopathy Ascending infection of fetus occurs from lesions in birth canal after rupture of fetal membranes; therefore abdominal delivery is indicated before rupture of membranes	Abortion; premature birth Transplacental infection (rare): microcephaly; mental retardation; retinal dysplasia; patent ductus arteriosus; intracranial calcification; with intranatal infection, symptoms appear in 4-7 days: lethargy, poor feeding; jaundice; bleeding; pneumonia; convulsions; opisthotonus; bulging fontanels; skin, mouth lesions Neonatal infection with disseminated disease results in 82% mortality; survivors suffer central nervous system (CNS) or ocular sequelae and face recurrence in first 5 yr of life	If cervical lesions are acquired, infection initiates chain of events that leads to invasive carcinoma in middle age (cervical cells are more vulnerable just after puberty, when they change from columnar to squamous); age 17 yr, frequency of intercourse, and number of different partners are factors Transmitted primarily by sexual contact but also possibly by fomites Incubation period: 2-4 wk. Remains in body cells indefinitely; therefore infection recurs throughout lifetime—triggered by infection, fever, menstruation, emotional upset; lies dormant in sensory nerve ganglia; more severe during pregnancy Drug therapy: *acyclovir (Zovirax)* is first FDA drug approved for treatment of HSV II infection; effective in selected cases (see current literature); symptomatic therapy: see p. 827; researchers are seeking a herpes vaccine—*glycoprotein D* is under investigation
Influenza (virus)	Serious prognosis if complicated by pneumonia; abortion; premature labor	Abortion; fetal death; prematurity; occasionally anencephaly or meningomyelocele	Polyvalent influenza virus (attenuated live virus) vaccine contraindicated for pregnant women
Listeriosis (bacterium, *Listeria monocytogenes*)	Harbored in vagina and/or cervix by 4% of pregnant women; may exhibit influenza-like symptoms, most commonly in summer or fall; vaginitis; urinary tract infection (UTI); enteritis	Abortion Amniotic fluid may appear dirty brown in color Neonatal infection: generalized skin rash, meningitis, pneumonia (50% mortality) Meningitis (most often in term males) may appear later in neonatal period High rate of morbidity and mortality	Treatment with penicillin or erythromycin usually successful; unfortunately diagnosis of listeriosis often is obscure or delayed; hence prognosis for fetus generally is poor
Malaria (*Plasmodium falciparum,* protozoan)	Chills and fever; infertility; abortion, premature labor; labor may be prolonged, hazardous; fatiguing, and end in cesarean birth; recurrence in puerperium	Malarial infection in 10% of neonates of infected women Extensive involvement of placenta; small-for-gestational-age (SGA) neonates, stillbirth, abortion	Quinine (chloroquine phosphate; Aralen) may be fetotoxic; in severe cases of malaria, however, employment of appropriate medications may be an acceptable calculated risk
Mumps (virus)	Parotitis (rare); abortion; premature labor	Fetal death; congenital malformation (e.g., endocardial fibroelastosis [?])	Prophylaxis of epidemic parotitis possible with administration of hyperimmune mumps gamma-globulin.
Poliomyelitis (virus)	Increased susceptibility to poliomyelitis during pregnancy; if paralyzed, labor progresses normally; increased mortality	First trimester: abortion, possible anomalies, intrauterine growth retardation (IUGR) Flaccid paralysis; may contract poliomyelitis during passage through birth canal	Prophylaxis for poliomyelitis (polio) has almost eradicated this disorder in some countries; however, it is still prevalent and potentially devastating in parts of Asia and Africa Prophylaxis for pregnant women possible with Salk vaccine (killed virus) but *not* Sabin vaccine (attenuated live virus); Salk vaccine confers an immunity of about 2 yr; Sabin vaccination is followed by permanent immunization
Pyelonephritis (bacteria)	Acute UTI: frequency, urgency, dysuria, chills, fever, backache, tenderness over affected kidney May be asymptomatic	Prematurity with its hazards; sulfonamides may cause icterus, hemolytic anemia, kernicterus, growth retardation (?), or thrombocytopenia Nitrofurantoin therapy for mother may lead to megaloblastic anemia, G6PD deficiency in neonate	Most vulnerable: primigravidas; women with difficult labors; women with diabetes or sickle cell disease

Continued.

Table 36.1—cont'd
Maternal Infections: Effects on Pregnancy and Fetus or Neonate

Infection	Maternal Effects	Fetal or Neonatal Effects	Counseling: Prevention, Identification, and Management
Rubella (3-day German measles, virus)	Rash, fever, mild symptoms; suboccipital lymph nodes may be swollen; some photophobia Occasionally arthritis or encephalitis Abortion	Incidence of congenital anomalies: first month, 50%; second month, 25%; third month, 10%, fourth month, 4% Exposure during first 2 months: malformations of heart, eyes, ears, or brain; abnormal dermatoglyphics Exposure after fourth month: systemic infection, hepatosplenomegaly, IUGR, rash At 15-20 yr of age, may experience deterioration of intellect and development or develop epilepsy	Vaccination of pregnant women contraindicated, however, and pregnancy should be prevented for 2 mo after vaccination; hemagglutinin-inhibition-antigen–negative parturients can be safely vaccinated after delivery
Rubeola (2-week measles, virus)	Rubeola uncommon during pregnancy because most women have had the disease and are immune	Abortion or premature labor; neonate may be born with a rash but generally survives without developmental anomalies	Prophylactic gamma-globulin may prevent disease; measles vaccination of susceptible women before (but never during) pregnancy recommended
Syphilis ("lues") *Treponema pallidum* (spirochete) Chancre Condylomata lata "The great imitator" Cardiovascular disease Neurologic disease Congenital syphilis	Incubation period: several weeks—asymptomatic Primary stage: chancre (red base with firm, rolled edges); painless; local lymphadenopathy clears without treatment in 4-6 wk Secondary stage: symmetric, nontender rash anywhere over body, including palms of hands and soles of feet; on scalp, causes loss of hair Moist papular lesions, condylomata, on any moist skin surface Systemic: malaise, fever, headache Clears without treatment in 2-6 wk Latent stages: Early: up to 4 yr after infection, lesions reappear Late: for 50-70%, lasts a lifetime, no outward evidence of disease	Syphilis probably continues to be major cause of late abortion throughout the world, despite widespread success of diagnosis and treatment of this disease. Primary and secondary stages of untreated syphilis lead to stillbirth Latent, tertiary stages of untreated syphilis lead to secondary syphilis (congenital syphilis) in neonate Congenital syphilis: spirochetes cross placenta after sixteenth to eighteenth week of gestation with the following sequelae: snuffles (rhinitis), rhagades (scars around mouth), hydrocephaly, and corneal opacity; later: saddle nose, saber skin, Hutchinson's teeth (notched, tapered canines), and diabetes; not residual fetal-newborn effects if mother is treated adequately before fifth month	Transmitted through sexual contact from infected lesion of one person through intact mucosa or break in skin of other person, into blood and lymphatic systems to all parts of the body within a few hours Spirochetes are numerous in lesions in primary, secondary, and early latent stages, and in blood during late latent and tertiary stages If the gravida is treated with penicillin by the fifth month of gestation, congenital syphilis probably will not occur; erythromycin does not cure intrauterine syphilis; woman with untreated syphilis in labor should receive 3 million units intramuscularly and 2 million units every other day for a total of 7 million units; infant should be treated also NOTE: Yaws, a nonvenereal, contagious disease, is caused by the spirochete *Treponema pertenue,* closely related to the causative organism of syphilis; yaws is spread by contact with secretions or sores from an infected person; both syphilis and yaws give a positive result in the STS test; yaws is a common disease in equatorial Africa, Hawaii, South America, and the East and West Indies; it is effectively treated with antibiotics, especially penicillin See p. 827 for description of assessment for syphilis

	Tertiary: clinical evidence of disease seen throughout body; obliterative endarteritis leading to cell damage and death and to gumma nodules of dead tissue. The acronym "paresis" summarizes possible sequelae seen in changes in the following: Personality Affect Reflexes Eye function Sensorium Intellect Speech		
Toxoplasmosis (protozoa)	Maternal symptoms vague: headache, lethargy, rash, myalgia Acute infection (rare) is most hazardous to one third of exposed fetuses	Enters fetal tissues or transmitted through mother's milk: microcephaly, chorioretinitis, hydrops, hydrocephaly, hepatosplenomegaly, delayed CNS problems in childhood. Congenital infections are acquired during primary infections. Fetal damage is more severe when transplacental infection occurs before the third trimester; latent fetal infection of varying severity frequently occurs with maternal disease in third trimester.	Primary exposure to organism may be minimized by avoidance of cat and dog feces and of ingesting undercooked beef, lamb, or pork Treatment of toxoplasmosis during pregnancy is problematic; pyrimethamine currently is the first choice drug against *T. gondii;* however, it may be teratogenic, especially during first trimester; sulfonamide therapy is effective, but drug must be discontinued before delivery and even-exchange transfusion of newborn may be necessary to avoid kernicterus—may occur because sulfa drugs have a greater albumin-binding affinity than bilirubin, which may rise after delivery to critical levels; however, newborn may be treated with pyrimethamine, but folinic acid supplement will be required to reduce toxicity of the drug. In congenital toxoplasmosis, maldevelopment or neurologic damage will not be affected by treatment; however, progression of disease can be controlled by appropriate therapy; regrettably, encysted (intramuscular) forms of *T. gondii* cannot be eradicated by any therapy and may cause recurrence of disease
Tuberculosis (gram-negative, acid-fast bacillus)	Pregnancy does not affect pulmonary tuberculosis adversely Avoid pregnancy until tuberculosis is inactive for 2 yr	Outcome depends on stage of tuberculous infection Congenital tuberculosis rare Streptomycin may result in congenital nerve deafness	Contraception is most important for women with active tuberculosis; all pregnant women should be evaluated for tuberculosis (tine test) early in pregnancy and again later if suspicion of disease exists Once infant has been delivered, he should have no intimate contact with mother or others who may have the disease until contagion is no longer a problem
Typhoid fever		Intrauterine fetal death: abortion; premature birth	

positive result is especially valuable in diagnosis of the condition in the asymptomatic child. Results of the FTA-ABS IgM test may be negative, however, in the presence of active disease if infection occurred late in pregnancy and the fetus or neonate had insufficient time for an IgM response. In questionable cases the test is repeated.

POSTNATAL INFECTION

Puerperal infection. Puerperal infection (puerperal sepsis or "childbed fever") is any clinical infection of the genital canal that occurs within 28 days after abortion or delivery. Infections may result from bacteria commonly found within the vagina *(endogenous)* or from the introduction of pathogens from outside the vagina *(exogenous)*. Lacerations of the vagina or cervix may open avenues for sepsis. Even more formidable, however, may be the large placental site. Here the denuded endometrium (decidua basalis) and residual blood after parturition make the uterus an ideal site for a wound infection. The virulence of infecting organisms, the woman's resistance to them, and the rapidity and specificity of therapy determine the efficacy of treatment. Puerperal sepsis occurs after about 6% of deliveries in the United States, but fortunately body defenses generally limit the disease in most instances. Puerperal infection probably is the major cause of maternal morbidity and mortality throughout the world.

Pathogenesis. Only occasionally, perhaps after a traumatic delivery, does endogenous infection occur. Self-inoculation of bacteria—from pyogenic skin lesions or unclean bedding, for example—may be the means of contamination. Most puerperal infections, however, are exogenous and are caused by contamination by attendants who have respiratory or other infections or who have inadvertently carried pathogens from another infected person. Introduction of pathogens may be by respiratory droplet inoculation (poor masking), by hand or other contact (unsterile gloves or instruments, unwashed hands), or occasionally by contact with dust or insect vectors.

The most common infecting organisms are the numerous streptococcal and anaerobic organisms. Fulminating epidemic puerperal sepsis classically is caused by the hemolytic streptococcus. The less virulent anaerobic streptococci may be responsible for other puerperal infections, however, *Staphylococcus aureus,* gonococci, coliform bacteria, and clostridia are less common but serious pathogenic organisms causative of puerperal infection.

Frequently the infection is complicated by medical disorders such as anemia, malnutrition, or diabetes mellitus. Obstetric problems, including prolonged rupture of the membranes, a long, exhausting labor, instrument delivery, hemorrhage, and retention of the products of conception, increase the likelihood and severity of puerperal sepsis.

Pathosis. A variety of possible inflammatory sites are obvious. An episiotomy or laceration of the birth canal may be the primary focus, leading to parametritis, pelvic cellulitis, or thrombophlebitis. An endometritis, usually at the placental site, permits infection to begin. Localized infection may be followed by salpingitis, peritonitis, and pelvic abscess formation. (Tubal occlusion after salpingitis is a common cause of infertility.) Septicemia may develop, and secondary abscesses may arise in distant sites such as the lungs or liver. Pulmonary embolism or septic shock, often with disseminated intravascular coagulation (DIC), from any serious genital infection may prove fatal. Postdelivery femoral thrombophlebitis ("milk leg") may result in a swollen, painful leg.

Clinical findings. The symptomatology of puerperal infection may be mild or fulminating. Any fever, that is, a temperature of 38° C (100.4° F) or more on 2 successive days, not counting the first 24 hours after delivery must be considered caused by puerperal infection in the absence of convincing proof of another cause, for example, tracheobronchitis or pyelonephritis.

General malaise, anorexia, chills, or fever may begin as early as the second postdelivery day. Perineal discomfort or lower abdominal distress, nausea, and vomiting may soon develop. Foul or profuse lochia, hectic fever, tachycardia, ileus, pelvic pain, and tenderness characterize critical puerperal sepsis. Without improvement, bacteremic shock or death may ensue.

General physical examination to identify nonpuerperal infection should be carried out. Careful abdominal evaluation is made, and uterine or adnexal pain is noted. Examination of the perineum, episiotomy, and sutured lacerations and speculum visualization of the vagina and cervix, together with careful rectovaginal examination, are next in order.

Laboratory findings. Considerable leukocytosis, a shift to the left of the differential white blood cell count (WBC), and a markedly increased red blood cell (RBC) sedimentation rate are typical of puerperal infections. Anemia, often an accompaniment, is evidenced by reduced RBC, hemoglobin, and hematocrit values. Gram-stained smears of the lochia from within the cervix or uterus may suggest the type of infection; that is, gram-negative cocci may be streptococci or staphylococci, and gram-positive, long bacilli may be clostridia. Intracervical or intrauterine bacterial cultures (aerobic and anaerobic) should reveal the offending pathogens within 36 to 48 hours.

X-ray findings. Rarely do x-ray films aid in the diagnosis of puerperal infection, but they may be invaluable in identifying nonpuerperal sepsis, for example, pneumonia.

Differential diagnosis. One must distinguish nongenital from genital sepsis. For example, mastitis, respiratory and urinary tract infections, and enteritis must be considered in that order of probability.

Management. The most effective and cheapest treatment of puerperal infection is prevention, with measures such as good prenatal nutrition to control anemia and intranatal control of hemorrhage. Good maternal hygiene is essential. Strict adherence by all medical personnel to the best aseptic techniques during the entire hospital and delivery period is mandatory. Coitus after rupture of the membranes is contraindicated. Dystocia or prolonged labor should be avoided, especially after leaking of amniotic fluid. Traumatic vaginal delivery must be avoided, blood loss replaced, and fluid-electrolyte balance maintained.

Prognosis. The virulence of the organisms, the resistance of the woman, and her likely response to treatment are the intangibles of prognosis. Prevention, supportive therapy, and prompt massive antibiotic administration have reduced the maternal mortality in the United States to less than 0.4%. Regrettably, in underdeveloped countries, the death rate may be more than 10 to 20 times this figure.

The medical care would include measures such as the following:

1. Determination of source of infection; for example, specimens (urine, blood, cervical, throat) sent to laboratory for culture and sensitivity reactions
2. Maintenance of fluid and electrolyte balance
3. Institution of antibiotic therapy with broad-spectrum antibiotics administered intravenously until infecting organism is identified. (Then organism-specific antibiotic therapy is instituted.)
4. Separation of the mother and infant during the febrile period (Other family members should be encouraged to nurture the neonate.)
5. Surgical measures: dilatation and curettage (D and C) (to remove retained products of conception); hysterectomy (may be lifesaving in septic shock resulting from uterine rupture with infection); colpotomy (often necessary for drainage of pelvic abscess); ligation or clipping of the vena cava and ovarian veins (may be required in septic embolism)

MASTITIS

Mastitis, or breast infection, affects about 1% of recently delivered women, most of whom are primiparas who are nursing. Mastitis is almost always unilateral and develops well after the flow of milk has been established. The infecting organism generally is the hemolytic *staphylococcus aureus*. An infected nipple fissure usually is the initial lesion, but the ductal system is next involved. Inflammatory edema and engorgement of the breasts soon obstruct the flow of milk in a lobe, and regional, then generalized, mastitis follows. If prompt resolution of the septic process does not occur, a breast abscess is virtually inevitable.

Chills, fever, malaise, and local breast tenderness are noted first. Eventual localization of sepsis and axillary adenopathy are delayed developments.

Intensive antibiotic therapy (e.g., cephalosporin and vancomycin, which are particularly useful in staphylococcal infections), support of breasts, local heat (or cold), and analgesics are required. Lactation is maintained (if desired) by emptying the breasts every 4 hours by manual expression or breast pump. If an abscess develops, wide incision and drainage must be effected. Most women respond to treatment, and an abscess can be prevented.

Almost all instances of acute mastitis can be avoided by proper nursing technique and the limitation of nursing time (see Chapter 30) to prevent cracked nipples. Missed feedings, waiting too long between feedings, and abrupt weaning may lead to clogged nipples, followed by mastitis. Cleanliness practiced by all who have contact with the neonate and new mother also reduces the incidence of mastitis.

URINARY TRACT INFECTIONS

Postdelivery urinary tract infections, usually caused by coliform bacteria, are common because of trauma to the base of the bladder and urethra and catheterization during or after labor.

Suprapubic or costovertebral angle pain, fever, urinary retention, hematuria, dysuria, or urinary frequency often signifies urinary tract infection and indicates the need for urinalysis, urine culture, bacterial sensitivity tests, and probable wide-spectrum antibiotic therapy. Substitution of a specific antibacterial drug must await an assessment of the woman's history and response to initial therapy and of the sensitivity report.

Prompt treatment of definite urinary tract infections is indicated, but prophylactic therapy rarely is warranted. Most cases yield to treatment within a week; urologic consultation is indicated if symptoms persist.

VAGINAL INFECTIONS

Any irritating vaginal discharge should be evaluated promptly and appropriate treatment initiated immediately for maternal and fetal well-being.

Management of vaginal infections becomes more complicated if multiple organisms or agents are involved. Pediculosis pubis, threadworm, varicosities, and allergic response to perineal deodorants may obstruct the differential diagnosis and management. The discomforts imposed by these conditions challenge the woman's emotional as well as her physical well-being.

Infections must be distinguished from the normal vaginal discharge, leukorrhea. *Leukorrhea* is a whitish discharge consisting of mucus and exfoliated vaginal epithelial cells secondary to hyperplasia of the vaginal mucosa such as occurs during pregnancy, at the time of ovulation, and just before menstruation. If it is copious, it can cause discomfort from maceration.

Vaginal infections may be sexually transmitted. *Trichomonas vaginitis* and *monilial vaginitis* are considered to be sexually transmitted, but simple vaginitis may be attributed to faulty hygiene, tight clothing, or emotional stress.

Trichomonas vaginitis. *Trichomonas vaginalis* is a hearty protozoan that thrives in an alkaline milieu. Of all pregnant women, 20% to 30% harbor this organism, usually with no symptoms. The profuse, bubbly, white leukorrhea characteristic of this infection causes irritation, hyperemia, edema of the vulva, and dyspareunia. Urinary frequency and dysuria may occur. In the male partner the protozoan may be harbored in the urogenital tract (without symptoms) and remain a source of reinfection for his mate.

Objectives of management are the same as for simple vaginitis. Interventions include the following:

1. Maintain scupulous cleanliness, especially after elimination.
2. Douche with a weak acid solution (the same as for simple vaginitis).
3. Observe chemotherapy regimen as follows:
   a. Metronidazole (Flagyl), one dose of 2 g. (Metronidazole is contraindicated during the first half of gestation even though there is no evidence of fetotoxicity.)
   b. If metronidazole is not well tolerated by mouth, vaginal suppositories such as furazolidone (Tricofuron) or Vagisec should be used.
   c. The male partner should be treated with metronidazole and informed that intercourse should be avoided until the infection is cured.

Relief should be noted in 1 to 2 weeks. Rarely is a second course of treatment necessary.

Monilial vaginitis. *Candida albicans,* a fungus (yeast) normally found in the intestinal tract, contaminates and infects the vagina. (It is present in about one out of four women at term.) This infection is commonly seen in women with poorly controlled diabetes mellitus, since the organism thrives in a carbohydrate-rich milieu. Antibiotic or steroid therapy may be a causative factor by reducing the number of Döderlein's bacilli.

The thick vaginal discharge is irritating and pruritic. Frequently dysuria and dyspareunia are common complaints. Speculum examination reveals thick, white, tenacious cheeselike patches adhering to the pale, dry and sometimes cyanotic vaginal mucosa.

Objectives of treatment are the same as for simple vaginitis with one exception: women with recurrent infection should be checked for diabetes mellitus and control of diabetes should be instituted if required.

Interventions are as follows:

1. Maintain scrupulous cleanliness, especially after elimination.
2. Observe chemotherapy regimen; for example:
   a. Clotrimazole (Gyne-Lotrimin). Use as directed.
   b. Nystatin (Mycostatin) vaginal tablets, 100,000 units twice each day for 14 days, or suppositories, 0.5 g twice each day for 10 days, should be inserted.
   c. Gentian violet (2%) swabs may be administered to the vaginal mucosa with an applicator every 2 to 3 days until the vaginitis is cured. (The woman should wear a perineal pad to prevent permanent staining of clothing.)
3. Abstain from intercourse or use a condom until the infection is cured.
4. Gently bathe the vulva with a weak solution of sodium bicarbonate to relieve discomfort.

Candida albicans also causes thrush in the newborn. Infection may occur by direct contact with an infected birth canal or from the contaminated hands of those who take care of the infant.

Simple vaginitis. Infectious organisms such as *Escherichia coli,* staphylococci, and streptococci change the normal acidity of the vagina. A pH of 3.5 to 4.5 is needed to support Döderlein's bacilli, the vagina's main line of defense. The proximity of the urethra to the vagina predisposes the woman with vaginitis to a concurrent urethritis.

Burning, pruritus (itching), redness, and edema of surrounding tissues are characteristics. The symptoms are particularly discomforting during voiding and defecating.

Objectives of management of simple vaginitis are to relieve discomfort, to foster growth of Döderlein's bacilli, to eradicate offending organisms, and to prevent recurrence. Interventions include the following:

1. Maintain scrupulous cleanliness, especially after eliminating.

Fig. 36.1
Vaginal douche should be done with woman lying in bathtub. Douche pan may be placed under woman if desired. Douching is not recommended during pregnancy.

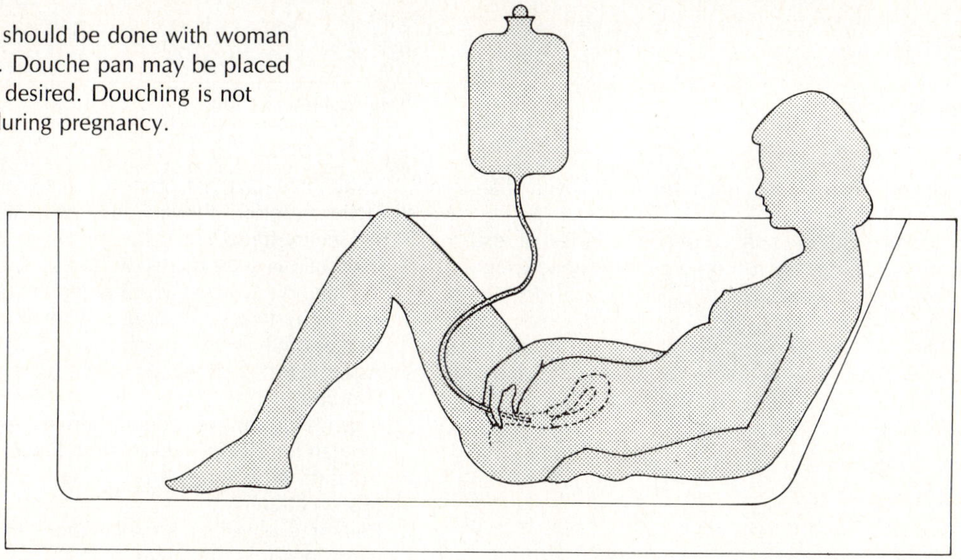

2. Douche with a weakly acid solution such as 15 ml (1 tbsp) white vinegar to 1000 ml (1 qt) water.
3. Insert a β-lactose suppository (to enhance growth of Döderlein's bacilli).
4. Observe chemotherapy regimen specific for organisms by inserting suppository into the vagina with an applicator or applying cream locally to the area as directed.

Vaginal douche procedure (Fig. 36.1)

Purpose. A vaginal douche is used to cleanse the vagina and to apply local medication or heat.

Procedure. The woman is instructed as follows:

1. Void and wash hands before douching.
2. Use the following position:
   a. The optimal position is semirecumbent in a clean tub (after a bath) or in bed. (Fig. 36.1). A douche pan may be used in the tub as well.
   b. The woman can douche while seated on the toilet; however, the labia should be held together to permit solution to fill the entire vaginal vault.
3. Prepare solution. The temperature should be 40° to 43° C (105° to 110° F), comfortably warm to the inner aspect of the wrist. Allow some solution to flow out of nozzle to lubricate tip, or lubricate with K-Y jelly or other water-soluble lubricant.
4. Hold or place solution container 60 cm (2 ft) above the hips (avoid greater heights, which increase the pressure of the flow). Do *not* use a bulb syringe; water or air embolus followed by death may ensue.
5. Insert nozzle up and backward for 7.6 cm (3 in).
   a. Rotate nozzle so that fluid flushes entire mucosa, including that of the posterior fornix. Rotation of nozzle also reduces the chance of forcing fluid into the cervix.
   b. When douching seated on a toilet, hold labia together to fill vaginal vault, then allow fluid to exit rapidly to flush out debris. Repeat until solution is used up.
   c. Hold labia together for specified period of time if the objective of the douche is to expose the mucosa to medication or moist heat.
6. If the woman is in the semirecumbent position for douching, sitting up and leaning forward aid in emptying the vagina.
7. Wash douche equipment with warm soap and water, dry, and store in well-ventilated place away from extremes of temperature.
8. Wash hands!

BACTEREMIC SHOCK

Critical infections, particularly by bacteria that liberate endotoxin, for example, enteric gram-negative bacilli, may cause bacteremic (septic) shock. Pregnant women, especially those with diabetes mellitus, or women who are receiving immunosuppressive drugs are at increased risk of having this disorder.

Decreased capillary resistance, activation of arteriovenous shunts, leakage of plasma into the interstitial tissues, reduced blood volume, and diminished cardiac

Infection

Assessment/analysis	Plan/implementation
Prenatal	
1. Observe for any signs of infection: rash, fever, gland enlargement. 2. Viral studies: culture and sensitivity studies of exudates, blood, urine; microscopic (fluoroscopic) examination for causative agents.	1. Viral infections are treated symptomatically. Prophylactic antibiotic therapy may be instituted to prevent secondary infection. 2. If woman is to be treated at home, assist her and family in planning how she will implement prescribed care. 3. Assist physician and support woman and family during tests and when hearing results. 4. Assist with counseling before proposed therapeutic abortion. 5. If genital lesions are found (herpesvirus type 2) prepare woman for elective cesarean delivery. 6. Isolation techniques (institute and prepare woman for this situation). 7. Reinforce physician's explanations of cause, management, possible outcomes. 8. General care. a. Adequate hydration. b. Rest. c. Adherence to medication regimen (if on oral antibiotics,, woman may prevent gastrointestinal upset by taking Lactinex or eating yogurt between doses). d. Temperature should be kept down with acetaminophen (Tylenol), fluids, cool sponge baths.
Postdelivery	
1. Assess effects on fetus or neonate. 2. Obtain cultures from mother and infant; send specimens. 3. Monitor vital signs. 4. General postdelivery care: evaluate findings.	1. Provide nursing-medical care for high-risk infant. 2. Isolate infant and mother if indicated. 3. Assist woman and family with grieving if indicated. 4. Ensure bed rest and proper diet. 5. Answer questions regarding infection, cause, management, expected prognosis.

output are important factors in the development of this type of shock. DIC may develop, causing abnormal bleeding. Hypoxia is the major problem, however, and this is especially noxious to the CNS, myocardium, and lungs.

High spiking fever and chills are evidence of serious sepsis. Anxiety and then apathy ensue. Concomitantly the temperature often falls to slightly subnormal levels. The skin then becomes pale, cool, and moist. The pulse will be rapid and thready. Marked hypotension and peripheral cyanosis develop. Oliguria ensues.

Laboratory studies should reveal marked evidence of infection (blood culture may reveal bacteremia later). Hemoconcentration, acidosis, and DIC may develop. Central venous pressure (CVP) generally is low; an electrocardiogram (ECG) may reveal changes indicative of myocardial insufficiency. Evidence of cardiac, pulmonary, and renal failure will be notable.

The physician will initiate antishock therapy. Massive doses of antibiotics and corticosteroids are given intravenously if possible. The woman may be given digitalis. Heart function and urinary output are monitored closely. The infected area is drained or the focus of infection is removed, for example, by hysterectomy or abortion if the woman's condition will permit.

Prompt diagnosis and intensive treatment afford a fairly good prognosis. Encouraging signs include increasing alertness and the establishment of good urinary flow.

SUMMARY OF NURSING ACTIONS: INFECTIONS

Goals of care

1. Infection is prevented.
2. Infection is treated promptly with no or minimal sequelae for mother and infant.

3. Parent or parents learn about prevention, identification, and management of infection.

Evaluation. The nurse can be assured that care was effective if the goals of care have been met.

Neonatal Sepsis

Sepsis refers to a generalized infection in the bloodstream. Inadequate immunity accounts for the neonate's increased susceptibility and is expressed in diminished phagocytic response, delayed chemotaxis (response to chemical stimuli), absent or minimal IgA and IgM, and inadequate serum complement levels. (Serum complement [C1 through C6] is involved in immunologic reactions, some of which act to kill or lyse bacteria and enhance phagocytosis.) Sepsis of the newborn may begin in the prenatal or postdelivery period. Fulminating or persistent sepsis generally is apparent at birth; other infections may be obscure and become manifest later.

CLINICAL FINDINGS

Clinical findings in sepsis may include lethargy, restlessness, or poor weight gain. Fever may be recorded; there may be leukocytosis; C-reactive protein may or may not be elevated. Vomiting, diarrhea, or CNS signs, such as convulsions, may be apparent, Examination usually reveals hyperbilirubinemia, hepatomegaly, or splenomegaly—notable after well-established sepsis. Hemorrhage may be an associated sign in sepsis.

INCIDENCE

Sepsis occurs about twice as often in males as it does in females and results in a higher mortality in males. The incidence of sepsis for all neonates remains unchanged but is highest among those classified as high risk. Frequency increases with prematurity and in bottle-fed neonates.

Protective mechanisms exist in breast milk. Colostrum contains agglutinins that are active against gram-negative bacteria. Human milk contains iron-binding protein that exerts a bacteriostatic effect on *Escherichia coli;* it also contains macrophages and lymphocytes that encourage a local inflammatory reaction.

PROGNOSIS

Before the advent of antibiotics, 90% of neonates with sepsis died. Antibiotic therapy decreased mortality to between 13% and 45% depending on the causative organism.

SEQUELAE

Sequelae to septicemia include meningitis, pyarthrosis, and septic shock.

Meningitis, a frequent sequela, may be evidenced by a bulging anterior fontanel (see discussion of signs of increased intracranial pressure, p. 909). Systemic antibiotics may not diffuse into cerebrospinal fluid (CSF). Intrathecal infusion of a drug such as polymyxin may be initiated.

Pyarthrosis, which may affect any joint, usually localizes in the hips. Limitation in joint movement is one of the few signs of this condition.

Septic shock results from the toxins released into the bloodstream. The most common sign is a drop in blood pressure—a vital sign frequently overlooked in the care of the neonate. Other signs are rapid, irregular respirations and pulse (similar to septicemia in general).

MODES OF TRANSMISSION

Sepsis may occur by one or more modes of transmission. The mother, the neonate, and the neonate's environment are all sources of infective agents. The fetus acquires the infection by (1) aspiration of infected amniotic fluid, (2) transplacental transmission, and (3) direct contact with an infected birth canal.

Two thirds of infections acquired during passage through the birth canal are caused by *Escherichia coli;* other organisms include *Neisseria gonorrhoeae, Candida albicans,* herpes virus type 2, *Listeria, cytomegalovirus (CMV),* and group-B β-hemolytic streptococci *(Streptococcus agalactiae).*

The neonate may acquire infections through (1) the umbilical stump; (2) skin and mucosa of the eye, ear, nose, and throat; and (3) body systems, such as respiratory, urinary, and gastrointestinal tracts and the CNS. The environment is an important source of infection. Water bugs thrive in humidifiers, sinks, and respiratory-assistance equipment. Direct contact with infected persons or their infected excrement or fomites is another environmental hazard.

GENERAL NURSING CARE

Nursing care of infants with sepsis should follow these guidelines:

1. Actions to minimize or eliminate environmental sources of infectious agents include careful and thorough housecleaning, frequent replacement of used equipment (e.g., changing intravenous tubing each day), hand washing, and disposal of excrement and linens in an appropriate manner.
2. Monitoring intravenous infusion rate and adminis-

tering antibiotics are the nurse's responsibility. It is important to administer the prescribed dose of antibiotic within 1 hour after it is prepared to avoid loss of drug stability. If the intravenous fluid the infant is receiving contains electrolytes, vitamins, or other medications, *do not* add antibiotics. The antibiotic (or other medication) may be deactivated or may form a precipitate. Instead, piggyback another bottle of the prescribed fluid to be infused and attach its tubing with a three-way stopcock to the needle at the infusion site. Remember to include the number of milliliters of fluid used from the piggyback bottle when calculating the neonate's intake.

3. Follow isolation procedures according to hospital policy as indicated.

RUBELLA

The congenital rubella syndrome frequently results in spontaneous abortion, congenital cataract, microcephaly, nerve deafness, or cardiac anomalies when infection occurs between 5 and 10 weeks of pregnancy. Rubella acquired later in gestation may lead to intrauterine growth retardation or premature delivery (Table 36.1).

Fig. 36.2
Newborn with congenital rubella syndrome, showing multiple purpuric lesions over face, trunk, and upper arm. (From Fanaroff, A.A., and Martin, R.J., editors: Behrman's neonatal-perinatal medicine: diseases of the fetus and infant, ed. 3, St. Louis, 1983, The C.V. Mosby Co.)

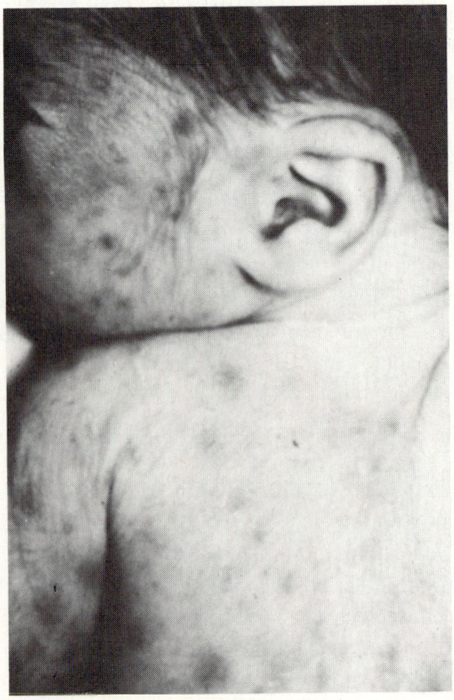

Numerous infants whose mothers had rubella during gestation are born alive with active viral infection (Fig. 36.2). This so-called extended rubella syndrome is typified by one or more of the following disorders: encephalitis, ocular abnormalities, pneumonitis, cardiac maldevelopment, hepatosplenomegaly and hyperbilirubinemia, and thrombocytopenic purpura. A tendency for infants born with rubella syndrome to develop leukemia during childhood has been noted.

Although many babies with active rubella die in early infancy, others survive longer. Because the rubella virus has been cultured in babies for 1 to 1½ years after delivery, these infants are a serious source of infection to susceptible individuals, particularly potentially or actually pregnant women. Extended pediatric isolation is mandatory until the noncontagious stage of rubella has been reached. (Isolate neonate until pharyngeal mucus and urine are free of virus).

For maternal vaccination in the puerperium, see p. 693.

HERPESVIRUS TYPE 2 INFECTION

Neonatal infection with herpesvirus type 2 is relatively rare, occurring in an estimated 1 in 3500 to 1 in 30,000 live births. Infection is often fatal (Fig. 36.3). The neonate may acquire the virus by any of four modes of transmission:

- Transplacental infection
- Ascending infection by way of the birth canal
- Direct contamination during passage through an infected birth canal
- Direct transmission from infected personnel or family

Fetal infection *may* be prevented if the following conditions are obtained:

1. Active cases of genital tract herpetic lesions are diagnosed before labor and the mother delivers by cesarean birth.

2. Amniotic membranes remain intact.

Genital herpes should be ruled out before artificial rupture of membranes or application of fetal scalp electrodes.

Fetal infection is almost certain if the mother has viremia, which occasions transplacental viral transfer, or in the presence of active genital herpes, if the amniotic membranes have been ruptured.

The nurse should note that this disease is highly contagious. Although herpesvirus type 2 is responsible for herpetic infections primarily occurring in the genital

Fig. 36.3
Neonatal herpesvirus infection. (From Fanaroff, A.A., and Martin, R.J., editors: Behrman's neonatal-perinatal medicine: diseases of the fetus and infant, ed. 3, St. Louis, 1983, The C.V. Mosby Co.)

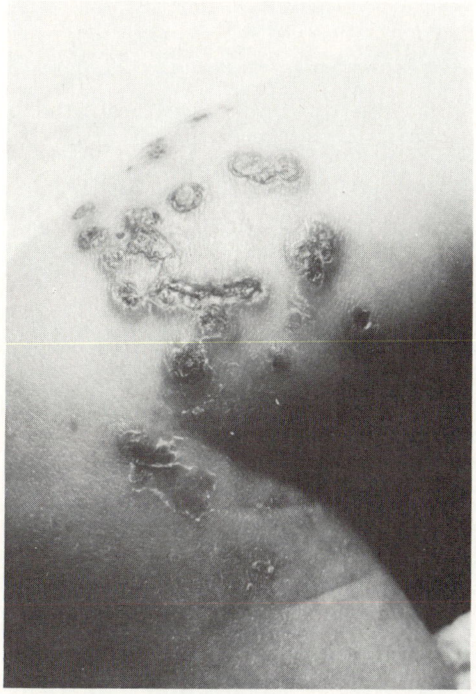

area, the nurse's ungloved hands may pick up the virus through breaks in the skin when infected lesions are touched.

Prognosis. Prognosis is grave in severe herpesvirus type 2 infections. Ocular or neurologic damage is a significant sequelae in survivors.

GONORRHEA

Gonorrheal infection (Table 36.1) other than ophthalmia neonatorum is an infrequent but significant cause of neonatal morbidity.

Endocervical cultures for *Neisseria gonorrhoeae* should be obtained routinely during pregnancy and appropriate treatment instituted when necessary to prevent fetal-neonatal infection.

Prognosis. The neonate with a mild infection often recovers completely with appropriate treatment. Occasionally infants die in the early neonatal period from overwhelming infection or pneumonia.

SYPHILIS

Congenital and neonatal syphilis (Table 36.1) has reemerged in recent years as a significant health problem. Fetal infestation with the spirochete *Treponema pallidum* is blocked by Langhans' layer in the chorion until this layer begins to atrophy, namely, between 16 and 18 weeks' gestation. If spirochetemia is untreated, it will result in fetal death by midtrimester abortion or stillbirth in one out of four cases. All neonates in whom the infection occurs before 7 months' gestation are affected; only 60% are affected if the infection occurs late in pregnancy. If maternal infection is adequately treated before the eighteenth week, neonates seldom demonstrate signs of the disease. Although treatment after the eighteenth week may cure fetal sphirochetemia, pathologic changes may not be prevented completely.

Because the fetus becomes infected after the period of organogenesis (first trimester), maldevelopment of organs does not result; however, any or all tissues and organ systems may be affected. Congenital syphilis may stimulate premature labor, but there is no evidence that it causes intrauterine growth retardation (IUGR). Stigmas of congenital syphilis (Fig. 36.4) may include inflammatory and destructive changes in the placenta, in organs such as the liver, spleen, kidneys, and adrenal glands, in bone covering and marrow, in the CNS, in teeth, and in the cornea of eyes. Disorders of the CNS, teeth, and cornea may not become evident until several months after birth.

Clinical findings. The most severely affected neonates may be *hydropic* (edematous) and *anemic,* with enlarged liver and spleen. Hepatosplenomegaly is probably secondary to extramedullary hematopoietic activity stimulated by the severe anemia.

In some cases signs of congenital syphilis do not appear until late in the neonatal period. In these newborns early signs, such as poor feeding, slight hyperthermia, and snuffles, may be nonspecific. *Snuffles* refers to the copious clear serosanguineous mucous discharge from the obstructed nose.*

By the end of the first week of life, in untreated cases, a copper-colored maculopapular *dermal rash* appears that is characteristically first noticeable on the palms of the hands, soles of the feet, and diaper area, and around the mouth and anus. The maculopapular lesions may become vesicular and confluent and extend over the trunk and extremities. *Condylomas* (elevated wartlike lesions) may be seen around the anus. Rough,

*NOTE: A mucopurulent discharge indicates secondary infection, usually by streptococci or staphylococci.

Fig. 36.4
Early congenital syphilis apparent at birth, which corresponds to secondary syphilis in the adult. (Late congenital syphilis, corresponding to tertiary syphilis, becomes apparent after 2 years of age.) **A,** Cutaneous lesions of congenital syphilis. Lines drawn on body indicate hepatosplenomegaly. No destruction of bridge of nose (common finding in congenital syphilis) is noted on this infant. **B,** Rhinitis (snuffles) resulting in rhagades and excoriation of upper lip. Red-colored rash is around mouth and on chin. (From Shirkey, H.C., editor: Pediatric therapy, ed 6, St. Louis, 1980, The C.V. Mosby Co.)

A 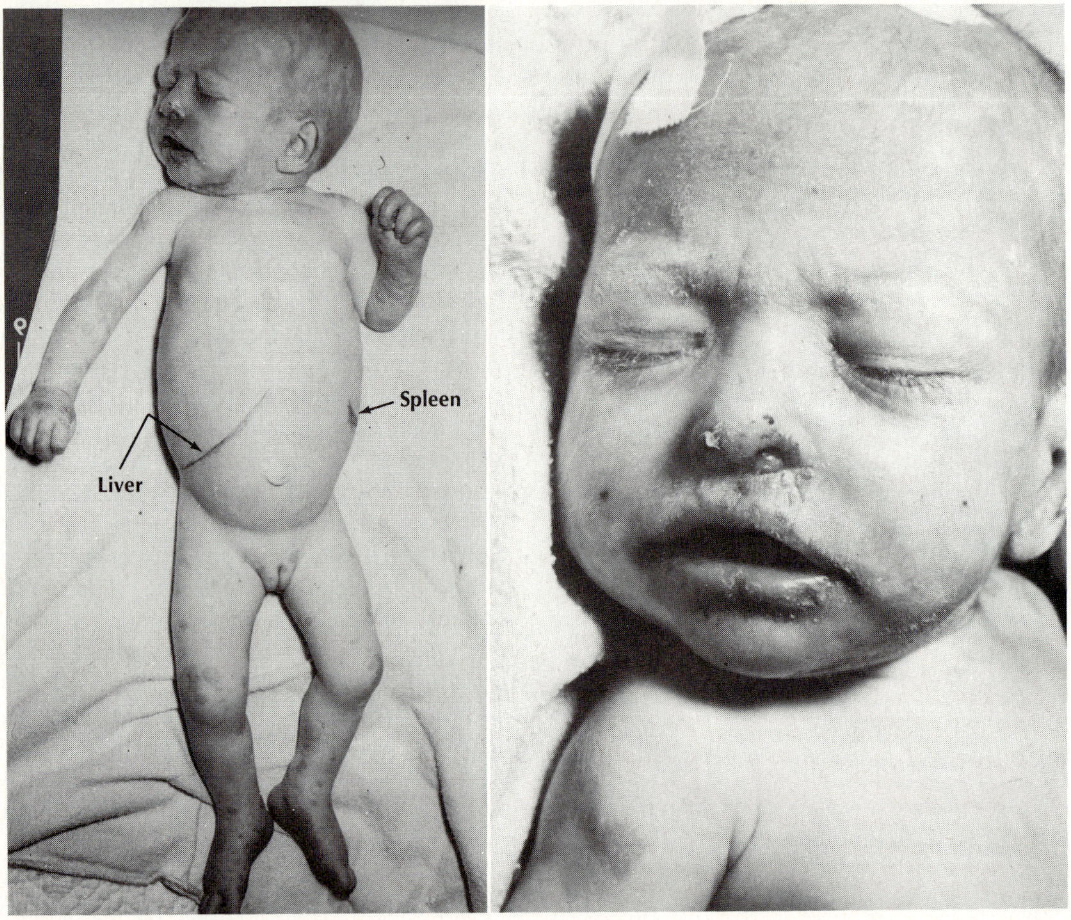 B

cracked mucocutaneous lesions of the lips heal to form circumoral radiating scars known as *rhagades*.

Other dermal involvement results in exfoliation (separation, flaking) of nails and loss of hair. Iritis and choroiditis are characteristic of infection of the eyes. Nephrotic syndrome secondary to renal infection, hepatitis with *jaundice*, lymphadenopathy, inflammation of the pancreas, testes, and colon, and a pseudoparalysis of the extremities may be noted. Laboratory tests may show a pleocytosis (usually lymphocytosis) and elevated CSF protein levels.

By 3 months of age, in 90% of infants (treated or untreated), periostitis and metaphyseal osteochondritis may be demonstrated by roentgenography. These bone lesions generally disappear by 10 months of age whether or not the infant receives antibiotic treatment.

Diagnosis. After the physician determines that congenital syphilis is possible, the CSF (obtained by lumbar puncture) is examined with the FTA-ABS test (p. 827). If results are inconclusive, the physician will probably opt to treat the child as if the disease existed.

Medical management. If the mother had been adequately treated before delivery and serologic testing of the neonate does not show syphilis, generally the neonate is not treated with antibiotics. In this case the neonate is checked for antibody titer (received from the mother via the placenta) every 2 weeks for 3 months, at which time the test result should be negative. Some physicians recommend antibiotic therapy for asymptomatic or inconclusive cases.

For antibiotic treatment to be effective, an ''adequate'' blood level must be maintained for an ''adequate'' period of time. Suggested medication protocol in the presence of symptomatic systemic disease differs from author to author and physician to physician. After 12 hours of antibiotic therapy, the child is not considered contagious.

It is generally accepted that erythromycin is the substitute antibiotic of choice for neonates sensitive to penicillin.

Prognosis and sequelae. In general, treatment of syphilis is more effective if it is begun early rather than late in the course of the disease. However, a recurrence rate of 5% can be expected. Even adequate treatment of congenital syphilis after birth does not always prevent late (5 to 15 years after initial infection) complications: neurosyphilis, deafness, Hutchinson's teeth (notched incisors), saber shins, joint involvement, saddle nose (depressed bridge), gummas (soft, gummy tumors) over the skin and other organs, and interstitial keratitis (inflammation of the cornea). The failure of therapy with the persistence of spirochetes in the eyes is not unusual. Antibiotics penetrate ocular tissue poorly.

Mortality from congenital syphilis during early childhood is uncommon.

CHLAMYDIAL DISEASE

Chlamydia trachomatis is an intracellular bacterium that causes *neonatal conjunctivitis* and *pneumonia*. The conjunctivitis is first noted about 3 or 4 days after birth. If chlamydial disease is not treated, chronic follicular conjunctivitis with conjunctival scarring and corneal neovascularization may result.

If prenatal screening reveals infection with *Chlamydia trachomatis,* treatment of the mother is deferred until the early postnatal period to avoid exposing the fetus to the therapy. After delivery the mother is treated with tetracycline, 500 mg orally four times each day for 7 to 14 days. The neonate is also treated with tetracycline, 6 mg/kg/24 hr for 7 days, and ointment or solution of tetracycline is instilled into the conjunctival sac every 2 to 4 hours for 2 to 4 days. Sodium sulfacetamide (10%) drops or ointment may be used instead.

Prognosis is generally good if the condition is diagnosed and both mother and neonate are treated in the early neonatal period.

CYTOMEGALOVIRUS INFECTION

The neonate with classic, full-blown infection is SGA and has microcephaly. He has a petecheal rash, jaundice, and hepatosplenomegaly. Anemia, thrombocytopenia, and hyperbilirubinemia are to be expected. Intracranial, periventricular calcification often will be noted on x-ray films. Inclusion bodies (''owl's eyes'' figures) in cells sedimented from freshly voided urine or in liver biopsy specimens are typical. The virus can be recovered from saliva or urine. Despite the extensive, endemic nature of the disease in women and men and its potential for havoc in perinatal life, critically affected neonates are only occasionally delivered. Milder forms of the disease may often result when the fetus is affected late in pregnancy.

Differential diagnosis includes other causes of jaundice: syphilis (positive VDRL), toxoplasmosis, hemolytic disease of the newborn (positive Coombs' test), or coxsackie virus infection (culture).

No reasonable prevention or specific therapy exists for mother or infant. Severe mental and physical handicaps mark virtually all infants who survive.

ACQUIRED IMMUNE DEFICIENCY SYNDROME (AIDS)

Severe depression of the cellular immune system characterizes this condition. Therefore the individual with AIDS is susceptible to a variety of other illnesses and ''opportunistic'' infections to which the normal population has resistance. Although the underlying etiology of AIDS is unknown, there is some evidence that a virus may be implicated.

In addition to pneumocystosis and Karposi's sarcoma, illnesses commonly seen in this syndrome include disseminated fungal infections caused by *Mycobacterium avium and M. intracellulare* and *Candida albicans;* viral infections caused by the cytomegalovirus (CMV), hepatitis B, and herpes simplex; and immunologic manifestations such as thrombocytopenic purpura.

According to University of California (San Francisco) guidelines (November 1982) treatment precautions by health care providers are the same as those for the care of people with hepatitis B. These precautions for health care providers and the nonpregnant people who come in contact with AIDS sufferers are as follows: when handling needles and syringes, avoid accidental needle sticks; dispose of needles and syringes in puncture-proof containers; use meticulous handwashing at all times; use gown and gloves when in contact with blood, secretions, and enteric excretions; wear masks if the client has pneumocystosis and is coughing.

About one half of AIDS sufferers have elevated CMV titers. Because CMV inclusion disease poses a serious hazard to the fetus, **pregnant women are advised to avoid direct contact with AIDS sufferers.**

AIDS may be sexually transmitted among homosexual or bisexual males. Some AIDS cases have been reported among women whose sexual partners have AIDS or are from the group identified as high risk for AIDS (Center for Disease Control, 1983). There have been some reports of infants born to women at risk for AIDS who have developed unexplained cellular immunodeficiencies and "opportunistic" infections, e.g., CMV. In addition, there seems to be a possibility of acquiring AIDS through transfusions of blood or blood products.

ORAL THRUSH

Oral thrush, or mycotic stomatitis, is caused by *Candida albicans*. This infection results from direct contact with a contaminated birth canal, hands (mother's or other's), feeding equipment, breast, or bedding. The appearance of white plaques on the oral mucosa, gums, and tongue is characteristic. The white patches are easily differentiated from milk curds; the patches cannot be removed and tend to bleed when touched. In most cases the infant does not seem to be discomforted by the infection; a few newborns seem to have some difficulty swallowing.

Infants who are sick, debilitated, or receiving antibiotic therapy are more susceptible. Those with conditions such as cleft lip or palate, neoplasms, and hyperparathyroidism seem to be more vulnerable to mycotic infection.

The objectives of management are to eradicate the causative organism, control exposure to *Candida albicans*, and improve the infant's resistance. Interventions include the following:

1. Maintain scrupulous cleanliness to prevent reinfection (nursing personnel, parents, others).
   a. Use good hand-washing technique.
   b. Provide clean surfaces for neonates (newborn is never placed directly on sheets on which the mother has been sitting).
   c. Clean and store feeding equipment well.
2. Support the compromised neonate's physiologic function (see Chapter 33).
3. Administer chemotherapy.
   a. Apply aqueous solution of gentian violet (1% to 2%) with swab to oral mucosa, gums, tongue. (Guard against permanent stain on skin, clothes, equipment. Warn parents about purple staining of baby's mouth.)
   b. Instill nystatin (Mycostatin) into mouth with a medicine dropper. Give infant sterile water to wash out milk before giving nystatin. Nystatin may also be swabbed over mucosa, gums, or tongue.

To give medication (vitamins) by medicine dropper, position the infant's head to the side or support the infant in a semi-Fowler position. Insert the dropper into the oral cavity so that the tip rests against the cheek, alongside the tongue. Wait until the infant begins to suck on the dropper, and then squeeze the rubber end slowly until the dropper is empty.

SUMMARY OF NURSING ACTIONS: NEONATAL INFECTION

Goals of care

1. Sepsis is prevented.
2. Early signs of sepsis are recognized, and appropriate therapy is instituted.
3. If therapy is necessary, no harmful sequelae result.
4. Pathophysiologic sequelae to septicemia are avoided.
5. Parents are able to form attachment to neonate.
6. Parents' self-esteem is maintained.

Reminders

Care of specimens following collection

1. Place container on paper towel at bedside or sink area until after you have removed isolation gown and gloves.
2. Cleanse outside of container with alcohol swipe.
3. Place container on paper towel on isolation cart.
4. Affix addressographed sticker labled "Isolation." (Do *not* lick label!)
5. Place specimen in a *single* plastic bag, marked "Isolation."
6. Attach requisition (also labeled "Isolation") with paper clip to outside of bag.
7. Send to appropriate laboratory.

Leaving isolation room

1. Untie lower strings of gown.
2. Remove gloves and discard in trash container; if gloves have not been used, wash hands.
3. Untie upper strings of gown, remove, place in laundry or trash container.
4. Wash hands.
5. Use paper towel to turn off faucet and open door.
6. Remove mask and discard in trash container. Mask shall not be worn around neck or reused.
7. If there are hand washing facilities immediately outside the door, wash hands there rather than in isolation room—use paper towel to turn faucet.
8. Wash hands in utility room before continuing duties.

Neonatal Infection

Assessment/analysis

1. Review of prenatal record
2. Age at onset
3. Clinical manifestations
   a. Nonspecific: "doesn't look right"; "not doing well"; "poor weight gain"
   b. Organism-specific
      (1) *Pseudomonas aeruginosa:* purple necrotic skin lesions
      (2) Group-B beta-hemolytic streptococci: severe respiratory distress, apnea
      (3) Herpesvirus II: fever, coryza, tachycardia, hemorrhage, often evidenced by hemoptysis, bloody stools
      (4) Gonorrhea: conjunctivitis, unstable temperature, hypotonia, poor feeding behavior
      (5) Syphilis: rash, lesions of skin and bone, rhinitis, hepatosplenomegaly
   c. Systemic signs
      (1) Respiratory system: apnea; irregular, grunting respirations with retractions
      (2) Gastrointestinal system: vomiting; bile-stained diarrhea; abdominal distention; paralytic ileus with no stools; poor suck
      (3) Skin: cyanosis, pallor, mottling, jaundice, local lesions
      (4) CNS: similar to signs of hypocalcemia, hypoglycemia; that is, lethargy, irritability, tremors, convulsions, coma (increased intracranial pressure if meningitis develops)
      (5) Temperature: normal or low or unstable
      (6) Hepatomegaly or splenomegaly: notable after well-established sepsis
      (7) Hemorrhage
4. Laboratory studies
   a. Cultures: blood, umbilical stump, nasooropharynx, ear canals, skin, CSF, stool, urine
   b. Bilirubin: increased direct (conjugated) bilirubin level, especially if organism is gram negative
   c. Blood studies: for anemia, increased WBC, decreased RBC (an ominous sign)
5. Drug side effects
   a. Penicillin: urticaria, skin rash, pruritus, vomiting, diarrhea, convulsions
   b. Kanamyin (Kantrex): WBCs, RBCs, protein in urine
   c. Polymyxin: proteinuria, irritability
6. Signs of infection with antibiotic-resistant and fungal organisms
7. Sequelae
   a. Meningitis
   b. Pyarthrosis
   c. Septic shock

Plan/implementation

1. Medical management
   a. Antibiotics
      (1) Penicillin, ampicillin, or kanamycin (Kantrex) for treatment of 90% of all organisms; treat for 10 days via intravenous infusion
      (2) Gentamicin: especially for gram-negative organisms, such as *Pseudomonas aeruginosa*
   b. Support of physiologic systems
      (1) Oxygen
      (2) Fluids and electrolytes
      (3) Warmth
   c. Isolation procedures according to hospital protocol
2. Nursing management
   a. Recognize signs.
   b. Institute preventive measures to block modes of transmission.
   c. Calculate dosage of medications accurately.
   d. Recognize side effects of medications.
   e. Monitor intravenous infusion rate, infusion site; change tubing and dressings at least every day.
   f. Monitor optimal thermal environment.
   g. Report symptoms of meningitis.
3. Facilitate parents' understanding of neonate's condition, medical and nursing management, expected results of therapies.
   a. Clarify misinterpretations or misinformation.
   b. Repeat explanations as often as needed.
   c. Prepare parents for possible prolonged hospitalization.
4. Care of parents (see Chapter 34).
   a. Encourage parents to express feelings.
   b. Encourage parents to visit frequently and participate in neonate's care.
   c. Keep parents informed of neonate's progress.
5. Instruct parents about hygiene measures: hand washing, especially after voiding or defecating.
6. Give parents written instruction on the following:
   a. Clinical manifestations
   b. What to report and whom to call
7. Teach use of and reading of thermometer, if necessary.
8. Support parents.
   a. Avoid blaming parents for infant's condition.
   b. Educate parents regarding transmission, treatment, prevention.
   c. Assist parents with communication with pediatricians.
   d. Involve parents with care if possible. Facilitate early and frequent parent-child contact. Acknowledge positive parent involvement (e.g., interest, cooperation, care of infant).
   e. If nurse feels unprepared or hesitant to provide necessary sexual counseling, as needed for sexually transmitted diseases, parents should be referred to someone else. Avoid critical attitude toward parents.

7. Staff establishes caring relationship with parents to foster their trust and to encourage continuing, active, positive interactions of family with members of health care system.

Example of nursing diagnosis. The following is a possible nursing diagnosis in neonatal infection: risk of inaccurate assessment of infection because of vague and nonspecific signs of infection in the neonate.

Evaluation. The nurse can be assured that care was effective if the goals of care are met.

Endocrine and Metabolic Disorders

DIABETES MELLITUS

Definitions

diabetes mellitus A complex disorder of carbohydrate, fat, and protein metabolism due primarily to a relative or complete lack of insulin secretion by the beta cells of the pancreas.

overt diabetes Elevation of plasma glucose (hyperglycemia) and presence of classic symptoms (polyuria, polydipsia, polyphagia, nocturia, weight loss).

type I diabetes mellitus Formerly called juvenile-onset diabetes or insulin-dependent diabetes; onset in people 40 years or *younger;* etiology: genetic, immunologic, viral.

type II diabetes mellitus Formerly called maturity-onset diabetes or non-insulin-dependent diabetes; onset in people 40 years or *older;* etiology: primarily genetic.

gestational diabetes Intolerance to glucose with onset during pregnancy with return to normal glucose tolerance after delivery.

impaired glucose tolerance Formerly known as chemical diabetes, this type of disorder is characterized by a normal fasting blood glucose, but an abnormally elevated blood glucose following food intake or injection of glucose.

secondary diabetes Refers to abnormalities in glucose tolerance following pancreatic disease, endocrine disorders (Cushing's syndrome), drug ingestion (oral contraceptives), cirrhosis, and the like.

glucose intolerance Inability of the body to metabolize carbohydrates resulting in high plasma (and urine) levels of glucose.

endogenous insulin Insulin produced by the person's own pancreas.

exogenous insulin Insulin injected into the body.

insulin reserve Ability of the pancreas to increase supply of insulin as needed. In type I there is little or no insulin reserve; in type II there is some insulin reserve.

excursion Movement or range in levels from one moment to another, that is, blood glucose levels or changing insulin requirements.

macrovascular disease Vascular disease resulting in problems such as myocardial infarction, angina, vascular accidents (stroke), and peripheral vascular disease of large and small vessels.

microvascular disease Renal and ophthalmologic complications resulting from thickening of the lining of blood vessels.

glucose tolerance test (GTT) A test to see how well the pancreas can respond to a load of glucose.

glycohemoglobin (HbA_{1c}) The hemoglobin to which glocuse attaches. If the person is producing and breaking down RBCs at a normal rate, the percent of HbA_{1c} at the time the blood is drawn for this test accurately reflects the average level of blood glucose *over the preceding 4 to 8 weeks;* normal values are between 6% and 8.8%.

Significance. Diabetes mellitus as a complication of pregnancy was a rare occurrence before the discovery of insulin. Before insulin therapy was available many diabetic females died before or during puberty; many were amenorrheic and therefore infertile or sterile. When pregnancy did occur, the maternal mortality rate was 25%; fetal-neonatal loss was 50%. Today the incidence of insulin-dependent diabetes mellitus among school children is increasing (American Diabetes Association, 1979). Improved techniques for diagnosing and managing this disorder in children have increased the numbers of females who reach childbearing age and who have normal ovulatory menstrual cycles. As a result, the number of pregnancies complicated by type I (including gestational) diabetes is expected to increase yearly. Only 25% of all diabetics develop the condition before the age of 40; however, the disorder is far more serious for this group.

Incidence. Diabetes mellitus is a complication in about 1 to 2 in 100 pregnant women. The incidence of diabetes mellitus increases with age; about 3.8 in every 100 women will eventually become diabetic. Many of these cases will be diagnosed during pregnancy. There is a 30% to 40% chance for the gestational diabetic to develop diabetes mellitus within 1 to 25 years. To prevent potential damage to the mother and the fetus, investigation for defective carbohydrate metabolism is an essential part of good medical and nursing management of every mother and embryo-fetus neonate. Although there is an overall improvement in the perinatal outcome of the well-managed *diabetic* pregnancy, there is still a significant risk for neonatal morbidity.

Pathogenesis. Diabetes mellitus is regarded primarily as a genetically determined disorder, usually inherited as a recessive trait, but occurring as a dominant trait in some families. If the B cells of the islets of Langerhans (pancreas) are deficient either in number or function, the production of endogenous insulin falls short of the need, glucose is poorly utilized, and abnormalities of carbohydrate and fat metabolism appear.

When glucose is poorly utilized it accumulates in the blood. This results in a hypertonicity of the blood. The body compensates by attempting to dilute the heavy concentration of carbohydrates by transferring fluids from the cellular and interstitial compartments into the vascular compartment. Thus, the person becomes *dehydrated* at the cellular and tissue level while having an excess volume in the vascular compartment. The kidney then functions to excrete large volumes of urine (resulting in *polyuria*) in an attempt to regulate the excess vascular volume and to excrete the unusable glucose. Hence hypertonic glucose serves as a diuretic and results in even more body dehydration with excessive thirst *(polydipsia)*.

In the absence of sufficient insulin, the body compensates for its inability to convert carbohydrate into energy by burning proteins and fats. Unfortunately the end products of this metabolism are ketones and fatty acids, which in excess quantity produce *acidosis* and *acetonuria*.

Inheritance of the genetic trait (genotype) for diabetes mellitus does not necessarily mean that the individual will demonstrate diabetic glucose intolerance (phenotype). Many people with the genotype do not show any evidence of diabetes until they experience one or more of a variety of precipitating factors. Examples of stressors include the following:

1. Increase in chronologic age
2. Normal developmental periods of rapid hormonal change (Rapid normal hormonal changes occur during menarche, pregnancy, and menopause.)
3. Obesity
4. Infection
5. Surgery
6. Pregnancy
7. Emotional factors
8. Tumor or infection of the pancreas (tumor or infection may damage the beta cells so that diabetes occurs secondary to the trauma.)

Classification. White's commonly used classification of pregnant diabetics considers age at onset, duration, and vascular or renal changes, if any.

1. *Class A:* abnormal GTT caused by diabetes mellitus. This class includes gestational diabetes.
2. *Class B*: frank (overt) diabetes with onset over 20 years of age; duration, 0 to 9 years; no vascular disease.
3. *Class C:* onset of diabetes between 10 to 19 years of age; duration, 10 to 19 years; no vascular disease.
4. *Class D:* onset under 10 years of age; duration, 20 years or more; vascular disease (retinitis; calcification in leg muscles).
5. *Class E:* diabetes with calcified pelvic vessels.
6. *Class F:* same as class E plus retinopathy and nephropathy (often Kimmelstiel-Wilson intercapillary nephrosclerosis).

Although even milder forms of diabetes pose a threat to mother and infant, the incidence of perinatal death increases with the presence and degree of vascular or renal pathologic changes (classes D, E, and F).

Normal pregnancy: maternal metabolic adaptations. Among the normal adaptations to pregnancy are alterations in metabolism. Metabolic changes must occur so that (1) the conceptus will have an adequate supply of glucose, its main energy fuel, for development and growth; and (2) the woman can meet her own energy needs for pregnancy and lactation.

Insulin resistance. The placenta is developed by the eighth to the tenth week of gestation. As it continues to develop and increase in size, there is a gradual increase in the production of placental hormones: *human chorionic somatomammotropin (HCS), estrogen, progesterone, and the placental enzyme insulinase*. HCS and estrogen gradually cause maternal tissue to become resistant to insulin. Insulin resistance is defined as the inability of tissue to utilize glucose at the cellular level. Insulin resistance is further increased as the woman's adrenal cortex increases its production of *cortisol*. Insulin resistance reaches its peak between weeks 18 and 20, when the levels of estrogen, HCS, and cortisol reach their peaks. Insulinase breaks down maternal insulin.

Changing insulin needs *(Fig. 36.5)*

First trimester. During the first trimester, the developing embryo-fetus siphons glucose across the placenta from the mother; *maternal insulin does not cross the placenta*. By the eighth week of gestation, the conceptus secretes its own insulin at levels adequate to utilize the glucose obtained from the mother. As maternal glucose is utilized by the fetus, maternal insulin needs, and therefore, insulin production decrease (Fig. 36.5).

Second and third trimesters. The development of maternal resistance to insulin keeps pace with the increasing levels of placental hormones, insulinase, and cortisol. Insulin resistance is a glucose-sparing mechanism that assures an abundant supply of glucose to the fetus. The mother responds by increased gluconeogenesis and production of insulin. The size and number of islets of Langerhans in the normal, healthy pancreas increase to meet increased maternal demands. Fetal insulin production matches the amount of glucose received from the mother.

Postnatal period. Delivery of the placenta brings about an abrupt drop in levels of circulating placental hormones, insulinase, and cortisol. Maternal tissues quickly regain their prepregnancy sensitivity to insulin, the maternal pancreas rapidly decreases its production of insulin, and the mother's CHO-insulin balance returns to the prepregnant state.

Gestational diabetes mellitus (type I, class A). When the mother's pancreas is challenged by the normal adaptations to pregnancy and the pancreas cannot respond appropriately to the increased demands for insulin, gestational diabetes mellitus* results. The follow-

*Pregnancy-induced glucose intolerance.

Fig. 36.5
Changing insulin needs during pregnancy caused by the properties of placental hormones and enzyme (insulinase) and cortisol.

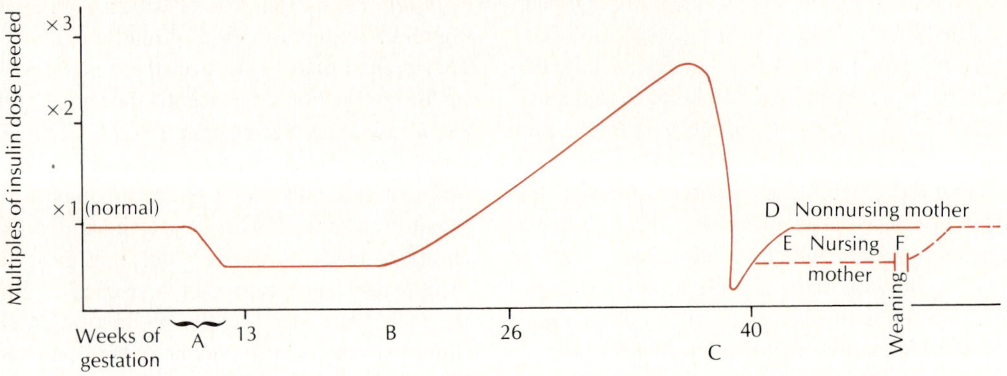

ing discussion shows the process leading to the exposure of pancreatic inadequacy during pregnancy.

First trimester. During the first trimester, maternal insulin needs decrease so that the mother's diabetic state remains hidden to routine surveillance.

Second and third trimesters. Between weeks 18 and 20, the maternal insulin requirements return to the prepregnancy level. Starting about weeks 18 to 20, the maternal pancreas is challenged to increase (endogenous) insulin production; pancreatic response is sluggish or incapable of meeting the challenge. Signs (e.g., glucosuria) and symptoms (e.g., thirst) of the developing diabetic condition appear. Exogenous insulin therapy may be started at or soon after the twentieth week.

Insulin-dependent diabetes mellitus (type II and all other classes). Many insulin-dependent women are capable of conceiving and maintaining a pregnancy today (as opposed to the low fertility of diabetic women in preinsulin days). They too must make the normal maternal adaptations to pregnancy. The following discussion describes the changes that occur during pregnancy.

First trimester. During the first trimester, maternal insulin needs decrease. The woman must decrease the dosage of exogenous insulin to prevent episodes of hypoglycemia and the resultant ketoacidosis.

Second and third trimesters. Throughout the pregnancy, the woman is supervised closely to prevent wide fluctuations in blood glucose—hypoglycemia and hyperglycemia. Carbohydrate and insulin balance is maintained in the following ways:

1. Careful assessment of blood and urine glucose
2. Management of woman's diet, exercise, insulin dosage, and avoidance of other stressors, for example, infections, emotional upheaval

Oral hypoglycemic agents, for example, tolbutamide (Orinase) and chlorpropamide (Diabinese), are never used in pregnancy. These drugs (1) may be teratogenic, (2) stimulate increased production of insulin by the fetus, and (3) exaggerate neonatal hypoglycemia.

A summary of maternal response to fetal glucose demands and the woman's changing insulin requirements is presented in Table 36.2.

Effects of diabetes on pregnancy. Conditions associated with diabetes increase maternal morbidity and mortality. Associated conditions vary slightly with the class of diabetes: For classes A to C (mild diabetes) there is a greater incidence of the following:

1. Intensification of preexisting diabetic condition
2. Pregnancy-induced hypertension (PIH; preeclampsia)
3. Hydramnios
4. Intranatal fetal death
5. Macrosomia (large for gestational age [LGA])
6. Large placenta

For classes D to F (more advanced diabetes) there is a greater incidence of the following:

1. Spontaneous abortions
2. Intrauterine growth retardation (small for gestational age [SGA])
3. Intrauterine fetal deaths and neonatal deaths
4. Complications associated with mild diabetes (above): occur but are less common

Insulin dosage per day does not reflect the severity of diabetes; the age of onset and the duration of diabetes are more important to pregnancy outcome.

Table 36.2
Summary: Maternal Response to Fetal Glucose Demands and Her Changing Insulin Requirements

	"Normal" Pregnancy	Gestational Diabetic Woman	Insulin-Dependent Diabetic Woman
First trimester	Glucose siphoned by embryo-fetus. Insulin requirement and production decreases.	Glucose siphoned by embryo-fetus. Insulin requirement and production decreases.	Glucose siphoned by embryo-fetus. Insulin requirement decreases—must decrease dosage.
Second trimester	Insulin resistance increases gradually. By week 18-20, insulin needs return to prepregnant requirement.	Insulin resistance increases gradually. Woman remains asymptomatic until 18-20 wk when her insulin needs return to and surpass her prepregnant requirement.	Insulin resistance increases gradually. Woman and physician need to be vigilant to her changing needs so that insulin dosage is increased to meet requirement. Some women may be started on a constant insulin infusion pump.
Third trimester	Insulin production by islets of Langerhans keeps pace with requirements.	Islets of Langerhans cannot respond adequately. If mother cannot maintain blood glucose within acceptable range with diet and exercise, she may require insulin therapy, starting anytime after wk 20 and continuing through delivery.	Insulin dosage must be carefully titrated to maternal blood levels.
Intranatal period	There are no special precautions for woman's fluid and food needs.	Woman requires careful monitoring of fluids, calories, insulin, and blood glucose.	Woman requires careful monitoring of fluids, calories, insulin, and blood glucose.
Postnatal period	There are no special precautions regarding food, fluids: ("as tolerated").	Monitor for blood and urine glucose. Woman may need no insulin injection after first 24-48 hr. Counsel her regarding need for follow-up because frank diabetes may develop in 1-25 yr.	Monitor for blood and urine glucose, insulin and caloric intake. May need to remain in hospital until insulin-CHO balance is reestablished.
Neonate	There are no special precautions.	Assess for signs of adverse effects of maternal condition: congenital anomalies, LGA, birth trauma, hypoglycemia, hypocalcemia, respiratory distress syndrome, hyperbilirubinemia (see p. 958).	

Dystocia. Dystocia (Chapter 37) is a possible complication because of hydramnios or macrosomia.

Hydramnios. Hydramnios (polyhydramnios) occurs about 10 times as often in diabetic pregnancies as in nondiabetic pregnancies. Hydramnios (amniotic fluid in excess of 2000 ml) increases the possibility of compression of abdominal blood vessels (vena cava and aorta) leading to supine hypotension. Hydramnios also causes maternal dyspnea because of upward pressure on the diaphragm. Hydramnios has been associated with premature labor (see p. 909), perhaps because of overstretching of the uterus.

Macrosomia. There is a greater likelihood of large fetuses (macrosomia) (see below). Large fetuses are associated with dystocia (difficult labor and delivery), often requiring the following (see Chapter 37):

1. Operative vaginal delivery (episiotomy and forceps)
2. Trauma to the mother's soft tissues or to the baby
3. Cesarean delivery

Infections. Infections are much more common and serious in diabetic women who are pregnant (e.g., pyelonephritis, monilial vaginitis).

Vascular damage. In the presence of type I diabetes mellitus, vascular lesions are of great concern. During pregnancy, preexisting vascular lesions may cause angina (followed by myocardial infarction) or other vascular lesions throughout the body including the retina. Fetal-neonatal (perinatal) mortality is related directly to the amount of vascular damage. During pregnancy, especially where diabetes is poorly controlled, there is a rapid progression in vascular damage that results in increasing retinopathy, uremia (nitrogen retention), and ketoacidosis. The severity of preeclampsia (occurring in 10% to 20% of pregnant diabetic women) is associated directly with the degree of renal vascular involvement. Severe vascular involvement has the following results:

1. Deterioration of the placenta and intrauterine growth retardation or death
2. The need to deliver the baby prematurely because of the risk to the mother in continuing the pregnancy
3. Possible abruptio placentae (premature separation of the normally implanted placenta; (see Chapter 35)

Prognosis. The outcome for both the mother and the

conceptus-neonate is determined in large measure by the degree to which diabetes is controlled. If there are no complications of pregnancy, and diabetes is well controlled, mortality for the woman with diabetes is about the same as that for any other woman.

Prognostically bad signs in diabetic pregnancy. Perinatal mortality increases by three fold to four fold for a diabetic pregnancy during which the following conditions become evident: pyelonephritis, severe acidosis, PIH, poor compliance by the woman, or poor diabetic control. Perinatal mortality of 50% follows an acute onset of hydramnios or a rapid drop in insulin requirements.

Goals of management. The goals of management are several: (1) minimize the risk to the mother; (2) minimize the need for antepartum hospitalization to maintain or restore diabetic control; (3) educate the woman and her family about diabetes mellitus and its control; and (4) prevent perinatal morbidity and mortality.

Euglycemia. Euglycemia (blood sugars within normal range) is the key to achieving the goals of management for the following reasons:

1. Maternal hyperglycemia early in pregnancy adversely influences embyogenesis resulting in major congenital anomalies such as caudal regression syndrome.
2. Fetal hyperglycemia and hyperinsulinism later in pregnancy are associated with (a) intrauterine fetal death; (b) delayed pulmonary maturation leading to respiratory distress syndrome in the neonate; and (c) neonatal illness, regardless of gestational age, such as hypoglycemia, hypocalcemia, and nonhemolytic hyperbiliubinemia.
3. Poorly controlled diabetes places the woman at increased risk for (a) pregnancy complications such as preeclampsia-eclampsia (and therefore abruptio placentae) and pyelonephritis and (b) permanent vascular damage.

To achieve the primary focus of management—euglycemia—the woman needs to become a member of the health team.

The diabetic gravida as a member of the health team. As an active participant, the woman's self-esteem is maintained or enhanced and her self-confidence in being able to care for herself and for her baby is developed. The responsive, reliable, self-assured woman, who has learned to assess her own blood glucose and maintain euglycemia and who communicates openly and frequently with the physician and nurse, often can be seen at the clinic or the office on the same schedule as the nondiabetic gravida (i.e., once per month until week 32; every 2 weeks until week 36; and then every week until labor begins). The need for hospitalization during pregnancy to control diabetes and the need for early delivery are minimized.

Under this type of team management, the nurse-clinician or nurse-practitioner is the primary educator for the woman and her family.

Management

Prenatal period

Diagnosis of diabetes mellitus. Early identification of glucose intolerance is essential so that prompt, appropriate therapy can be initiated. Factors in a woman's *history* that are associated with the risk of pregnancy-induced glucose intolerance include (1) family history of diabetes (first-degree relatives only [i.e., parents, siblings], (2) poor obstetric history (e.g., spontaneous abortion, unexplained stillbirth, hydramnios, unexplained prematurity or low birth weight) (3) birth of a previous neonate weighing 4000 g or more, and (4) previous neonate with major congenital anomalies.

Findings in the current pregnancy that alert the physician to the possibility of gestation-onset diabetes include (1) maternal age of 25 years or older, (2) obesity (weight of 90.7 kg [200 lb] or more), (3) recurrent monilial (Candida albicans or ''yeast'') vaginitis that is not responding to therapy, (4) glycosuria, (5) hydramnios, and (6) fetus that is LGA. Glycosuria can be diagnosed with Tes-Tape or Clinistix, both of which depend on enzyme reactions *specific for glucose,* without confusion with fructosuria and lactosuria.

Laboratory tests are required to establish the diagnosis of diabetes mellitus. Two types of laboratory tests are available: tests to identify levels of glucose in blood (Table 36.3) and the test to determine the percent of hemoglobin that is glycosylated (HA_{lc}).

Some physicians suggest that *all* pregnant women should be screened for blood glucose using the *1-hr glucose screen* during the first prenatal visit. This test can be accomplished in a clinic or office setting on a woman who is not fasting. It is unfortunate that the test is not accurate before the seventh week of gestation when malformation from any preexisting abnormalities of the carbohydrate metabolic state occurs. If the value is greater than or equal to 140 mg/dl, then 3-hr glucose tolerance test (GTT) is performed.

The *GTT* is abnormal if two more of the following values are found.

	Serum (mg/dl)	Venous whole blood (mg/dl)
Fasting blood sugar (FBS)	≥105	≥ 90
One hour	≥190	≥170
Two hours	≥165	≥145
Three hours	≥145	≥125

The above criteria are the same regardless of age, duration of pregnancy, or obesity.

The basis for the *HbA_{lc} test* is that glucose attaches to protein molecules (hemoglobin) in the red blood

Table 36.3
Blood Tests for Diabetes Mellitus in Pregnancy

Test	Instructions	Technique	Findings	Precautions
Fasting blood sugar (FBS): measures amount of glucose in blood when woman is fasting	No food for 12 hr before test, e.g., 8 PM to 8 AM; water is only fluid allowed	Blood drawn by venipuncture and sent to laboratory	Normal: 80-120 mg/dl serum Abnormal: 220 mg/dl or more, diagnostic of diabetes mellitus	None
Postprandial blood sugar: measures blood sugar following meal	None	Woman eats meal containing 100 g of carbohydrate; blood drawn by venipuncture 2 hr after meal and sent to laboratory	Normal: 80-120 mg/dl serum	None
Oral glucose tolerance test (GTT): measures woman's response to measured dose of glucose	High-carbohydrate diet (300 g of carbohydrates per day) for 3 days preceding test; no food for 12 hr before test or during test; no smoking, tea, coffee during test (alter body's response to carbohydrate); minimize activity (alters glucose metabolism); minimize stress (epinephrine and cortisone raise glucose levels by promoting gluconeogenisis)	Weigh woman, obtain fasting blood and urine specimens; administer 100 g of glucose orally in lemon juice; collect blood samples at 1, 2 and 3 hr; mark each specimen with time obtained and sent to laboratory	Plasma glucose level*: Normal fasting:<100 mg/dl 1 hr:< 200 mg/dl 2 hr:< 150 mg/dl 3 hr: <120 mg/dl Abnormal fasting: elevated or two other values lie outside normal range	Caution woman she may experience dizziness, sweating, weakness, nausea, vomiting, or diarrhea during second and third hr Diuretics, glucocorticoids, oral contraceptives may distort findings; do not use if FBS over 200 mg/dl
Intravenous glucose tolerance test: preferred test in pregnancy since absorption of glucose from intestinal tract is variable and may result in distorted findings in oral GTT	Same as oral GTT	Weigh woman; obtain fasting blood and urine specimen: administer 50 ml of 50% glucose in distilled water IV over a 4-min period and serial blood specimens obtained until 2 hr is reached, labeled as to time obtained, and sent to laboratory	Plasma glucose level Normal fasting: <100 mg/dl 2 hr: level not higher than fasting level	Caution woman she may experience facial flushing and dizziness as glucose is being administered Other precautions: same as for GTT
Tolbutamide response test not used since tolbutamide may have teratogenic effect on fetus				

Adapted from Luckmann, J., and Sorenson, K.: Medical-surgical nursing, Philadelphia, 1976, W.B. Saunders Co.
*Blood glucose readings lower.

cells. In the presence of normal carbohydrate metabolism in a healthy adult, 6% to 8.8% of hemoglobin is glycosylated. Values in excess of 8.8% indicate hyperglycemia over a period of time. The HbA_{1c} reflects the *mean blood sugar concentration over previous weeks to months.* A decreased incidence of congenital anomalies is associated with HbA_{1c} values that are within normal limits.

Diet. Dietary or insulin management must be based on blood glucose (not urinary glucose) values. The diet is individualized to allow for increased maternal and fetal metabolic requirements: calories, 35 to 40 kcal/kg ideal body weight*; protein, 1.5 g/kg ideal body weight; carbohydrates, 30% of total calories; fat, to make up remainder. Distribution should be two sevenths for each of three meals and one seventh for an evening snack. Women with brittle diabetes may require six small meals a day. The obese woman may need more food to prevent ketoacidosis. Sodium is not restricted; however, excesses are discouraged.

An average weight gain of 27.5 lb (12.5 kg) is associated with the lowest incidence of preeclampsia and perinatal mortality.

Exercise. Exercise must be regular, and the woman must be capable of making necessary adjustments to diet and insulin intake if the exercise pattern alters.

Insulin. Prenatal insulin requirements increase after the eighteenth to twentieth week; before that time hypoglycemic episodes may occur because of fetal drain and the low level of hormone antagonists to insulin. Insulin reactions are therefore common.

Monitoring blood glucose. The woman requires instruction as to the relevance of testing urine for glucose levels in pregnancy. By midpregnancy, trace to 1+ glucose is acceptable.

Blood glucose levels need monitoring by fasting blood sugar (FBS) and 2-hr postprandial tests (Table 36.4).

A recently developed technique using a color-graph machine (glucose reflectance meter) reduces or eliminates the necessity of obtaining venous blood samples and thereby "saves" accessible veins. The woman can perform the test at home. Using a micro lance,† the woman obtains a blood sample from the side of a finger (all the fingers are used in rotation). The drop of blood is placed on a glucose reagent strip. After the strip is rinsed in water and placed in the machine, the color graph is read. The results are recorded and reported to the physician. If blood glucose levels measure less than 100 mg/dl, it has been found that the infant is normosomic and has few hypoglycemic problems after delivery.

The advent of glucose reflectance meters has been credited with increasing the person's feeling of control over self, and decreasing or eliminating hospitalizations and therefore separation from family.

Continuous insulin infusion. Continuous insulin infusion systems (Fig. 36.6) simplify insulin administration for those women who need multiple injections per day. The system infuses insulin at a set basal rate with a bolus dose to cover meals. The infusion tubing from this portable, battery-operated pump can be left in place

Fig. 36.6
Continuous insulin infusion regulated closely with home monitoring of glucose makes tighter control of diabetes mellitus possible.

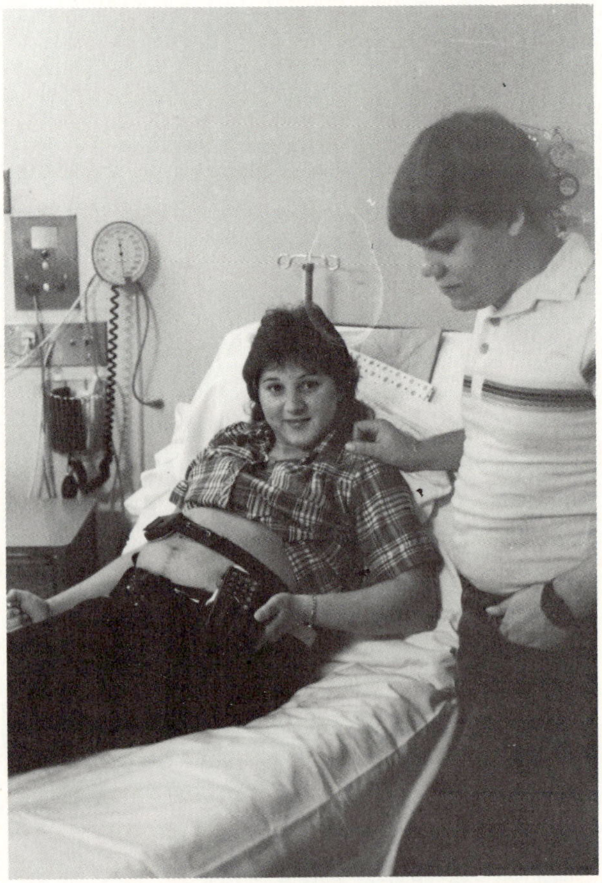

*The actual number of kilocalories the individual woman should receive varies. The woman needs sufficient kilocalories to achieve optimal weight gain and to prevent acidosis.

†The Autolet facilitates finger sticks. It consists of a disposable lancet on a springboard arm.

Table 36.4
Differentiation of Hypoglycemia, Ketoacidosis, and Hyperglycemic Hyperosmolar Nonketotic Coma (HHNK)

GOAL: Prevention or early recognition of these complications in order to establish and maintain good control in diabetic woman

	Hypoglycemia (insulin reaction)	**Ketoacidosis (diabetic coma)**	**Hyperglycemic Hyperosmolar Nonketotic Coma**
Causes	Too much insulin Not enough food (delayed or missed meals) Excessive exercise or work Indigestion, diarrhea, vomiting	Too little insulin Too much or wrong kind of food Infection, injuries, illness Insufficient exercise	Abnormally high glucose levels without ketoacidosis in mild or suspected diabetic—pancreatic disorders that lower production of insulin Complication of extensive burns, excess steroids (i.e., with steroid therapy), acute stress, TPN,* hemodialysis, peritoneal dialysis
Onset	Sudden (regular insulin) Gradual (modified insulin or oral agents)	Slow (days)	Rapid if woman dehydrated
Symptomatology	Hunger Sweating Nervousness Weakness Fatigue Blurred or double vision Dizziness Headache (especially with NPH or PZI insulin) Pallor, clammy skin Shallow respirations Normal pulse Laboratory values Urine: negative for sugar and acetone Blood glucose: 60 mg/dl or less	Thirst Nausea or vomiting Abdominal pain Constipation Drowsiness Dim vision Increased urination Headache Flushed, dry skin Rapid breathing Weak, rapid pulse Acetone (fruity) breath odor Laboratory values Urine: positive for sugar and acetone Blood glucose: greater than 250 mg/dl	Polyuria Thirst (intracellular dehydration) Hypovolemia Blood serum levels Fasting blood sugar (FBS): 600-3000 mg/dl Acetone level: normal or slightly elevated Dry skin Coma, death
Nursing actions	Notify physician Give orange juice Obtain blood and urine specimens for laboratory testing	Notify physician Keep woman flat in bed and warm Record intake and output Check and record vital signs	Administer insulin in line with blood glucose levels Monitor IV therapy (sodium and water deficits corrected without extreme shift of fluid into intracellular compartment with no reduction of hyperosmolarity of blood) Monitor woman for dehydration; record intake and output Check and record vital signs Notify physician of changes in symptomatology

Adapted from form used at Santa Clara Valley Medical Center, San Jose, Calif.
*TPN (total parenteral nutrition) replaces the term hyperalimentation.

for several weeks without local complications. Several biochemicals in addition to glucose are also maintained within normal limits, thus decreasing the risk of developing diabetes-related complications.

Supervision. Visits are scheduled a minimum of every 2 weeks for the first 32 weeks and then weekly until delivery. Fetal well-being is monitored closely. For example, after week 32, three estriol determinations per week (see Chapter 17) and one fetal activity determination (FAD) per week (see Chapter 24) may be scheduled. Procedures for estimating gestational age (include the use of ultrasound), fetal lung maturity (see

Fig. 36.7
Family in hospital for weekly NST. Nonstress testing for fetal status. A term pregnancy with a healthy mother and child is possible when the couple participates actively in the management of the pregnancy complicated by diabetes mellitus.

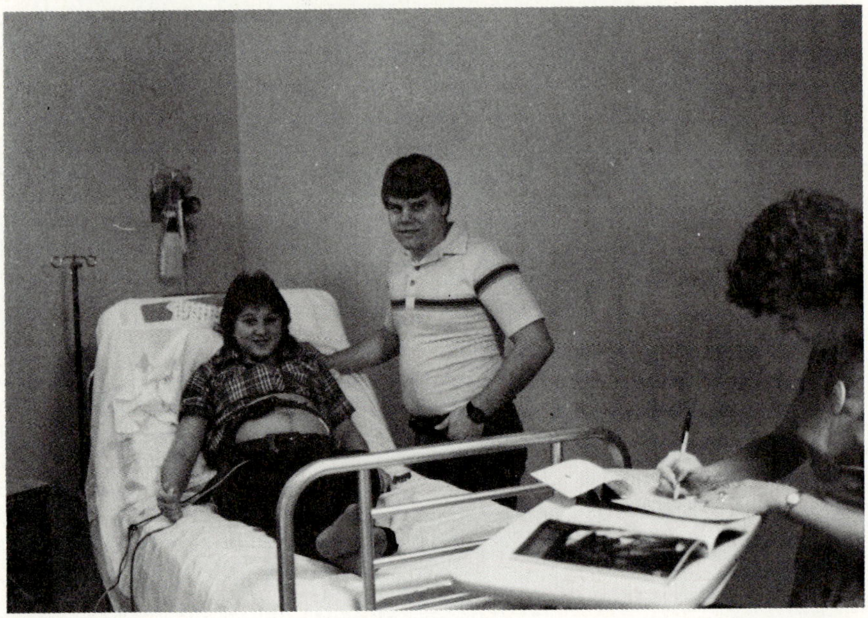

Chapters 14 and 17), and fetal response to labor contractions (nonstress tests Fig. 36.7 and stress tests [see Chapter 24] are appropriate.

Hospitalization. The woman may require regulation of insulin. Before pregnancy she may have been taking tolbutamide, and during pregnancy she may change to regular insulin. She may have poor control (''brittle diabetes'') so that daily evaluation is necessary. If she develops an infection, intravenous antibiotic therapy may be indicated. Close monitoring of fetal health may be required as a basis for early termination of the pregnancy.

Complications. The diabetic pregnant woman is provided with written instructions as to the need for prompt reporting of nausea, vomiting, and infections. Women having poor control need to be carefully assessed for infection; for example, asymptomatic urinary tract infections may significantly change a woman's insulin requirements. Mycotic vaginitis in the diabetic pregnant woman is more common and difficult to control.

Intranatal period

Determination of delivery date. The infants of class A diabetic women generally do well, and these mothers may be allowed to go to term unless complications develop.

The best time for delivery of the infant is when the intrauterine environment is not yet overwhelmingly hazardous and the fetus has developed sufficiently to exist outside of the uterus. The delivery date (by cesarean delivery or by induction) is frequently chosen on the basis of statistics of perinatal mortality: at 32 to 34 weeks there is a 19% mortality, primarily related to hazards of prematurity; at 36 weeks, the mortality is the lowest, at 11%; and at 37 to 40 weeks, the mortality is the highest, at 26%, primarily because of intrauterine death from acidosis or placental insufficiency. It is unclear whether the placenta is inadequate to meet the nurturing needs of the oversized infant or whether diabetes-induced vascular changes contribute to placental dysfunction.

Because fetal death is much more prevalent with diabetics in classes B through F, planned delivery about the thirty-seventh week has become accepted policy in most maternity centers; however, estimation of the gestational age is always subject to error. Monitoring the maternal serum or urinary estriol level during the last trimester provides some indication of developing placental insufficiency. A steady decline in estriol level is one indication for termination of the pregnancy.

Insulin therapy. Intranatal insulin requirements involve a prescribed dose of insulin added to 100 ml of 10% dextrose in water for intravenous solution. NOTE:

Insulin, a protein, is attracted chemically to the plastic in the intravenous tubing. It leaves the solution and adheres to the lining of the tubing. Therefore a sufficient quantity of the solution must be cleared through the tubing to completely coat the lining (usually 150 to 200 ml). Then the remaining solution of insulin will remain stable. (A protein [albumin]* may be added to the solution; however, it is more expensive.)

General care. The mother should assume a side-lying position during bed rest in labor to prevent supine hypotension because of a large fetus or polyhydramnios. If strong labor and good progress do not ensue within 6 to 8 hours, cesarean delivery should be carried out. Poorly controlled diabetes or obstetric indications such as fetopelvic disproportion, positive oxytocin challenge test (OCT), change in estriol levels, or preeclampsia-eclampsia are also indications for a cesarean delivery. A pediatrician should be present at delivery to initiate proper neonatal care.

Postnatal period

Insulin requirements. The woman must be closely monitored. She may require only one half to two thirds of her prenatal dosage on the first postnatal day if she is eating a full diet. It takes several days to reestablish carbohydrate homeostasis following the delivery of the placenta.

Complications. Possible complications include preeclampsia-eclampsia, hemorrhage, and infection.

Preeclampsia occurs in one fourth of all diabetic new mothers and in one third of all diabetic new mothers, class C or D. *Hemorrhage* is a possibility if the mother's uterus had been overdistended (hydramnios, macrosomic fetus), or overstimulated (oxytocin induction). Monilial *infection* of the vagina or nipples or other infections are more likely to occur in a person suffering from diabetes.

Breast feeding. Breast feeding is encouraged. Advantages of breast feeding include (1) maternal satisfaction and pleasure and (2) its antidiabetogenic effect. Breast feeding decreases the dosage for insulin-dependent women. The insulin dosage must be readjusted at the time of weaning.

Counseling. The insulin-dependent woman must realize that *she must eat on time* even if the baby is needing to be fed or other demands are pressing.

The new mother needs information for family planning and contraception. To assist in their decision making, couples need to be appraised that if the mother has type I diabetes, the offspring have a 22% chance of developing diabetes; if she has type II diabetes, the offspring have a 4% chance.

If contraception is chosen, the woman is advised to use the diaphragm with spermicide. Oral hormonal contraceptives are contraindicated because of their effect on carbohydrate metabolism. IUDs are associated with an increased risk of infection.

In the presence of severe renal disease and proliferative retinopathy, sterilization may be advised.

Summary of nursing actions: the diabetic mother

Goals of care

1. The woman and family understand the disease process and are informed about and willing to participate actively in its management.
2. Adverse effects of associated problems (i.e., changes in glucose tolerance, alterations in insulin metabolism, and utilization and increased tendency to ketosis) have a minimal effect on the mother and fetus.
3. The woman suffers no sequelae of diabetes (e.g., nephropathy, retinopathy) or worsening of preexisting complications.
4. The woman suffers no related complications during pregnancy: hyperemesis gravidarum, preeclampsia-eclampsia, hydramnios, postdelivery hemorrhage, or unresolved dystocia because of the infant's size.
5. Parent-neonate attachment occurs; or if neonate exhibits a disorder or dies, the grieving process is initiated.

Examples of nursing diagnoses

1. Failure of newly diagnosed gestational diabetic woman to comply with medical regimen (e.g., checking blood and urine glucose; diet; exercise; hygiene; keeping appointments) because of inadequate understanding of the condition
2. Potential negative perceptions (by the mother) about her female biologic function because of inadequate understanding of neonate's condition
3. Noncompliance with diet because of insufficient funds or lack of transportation to grocery store

Evaluation. The goals of care are met.

Effects of diabetes on the embryo-fetus-neonate. Wide fluctuations of blood glucose below and above the normal range adversely affect embryonic and fetal development. Good diabetic control during critical embryonic development is possible for the woman whose glucose intolerance was known *and* well controlled before pregnancy. However, gestational diabetes is diagnosed after the crucial period of organogenesis is over. Consequently, the risk for hydramnios and congenital anomalies is greater for the woman with gestational diabetes. The mechanism of the process leading to embryonic-fetal-neonatal problems is as follows.

Text continued on p. 859.

*Insulin does not have to be mixed with expensive albumin (more than $50 per bottle) to prevent loss of insulin by its sticking to the tubing. Sticking to the tubing can be prevented by flushing the line first with 100 ml of normal saline and 10 units of insulin.

The Diabetic Mother

Assessment/analysis	Plan/implementation
First half of pregnancy 1. Prenatal record is scanned for historical and clinical factors associated with risk of gestation-onset diabetes. 2. Perform urinalysis for glucose and acetone at each prenatal visit. 3. If woman had been diagnosed before pregnancy, assess for diabetic control and signs and symptoms related to her clinical classification.	1. Elicit woman's and family's cooperation in management of diabetes and pregnancy; make sure she keeps appointments and follows up on missed appointments, performs daily urine tests and/or blood glucose determinations accurately, maintains strict dietary control, gets adequate rest and exercise, and receives early treatment for infection and symptoms of insulin shock (Table 36.4). 2. Reinforce need for keeping the urine test at 1+ sugar level (to be assured of mild hyperglycemia and therefore of a control over hypoglycemia and hyperinsulinemia, which is very dangerous to the embryo and fetus). (Urine should be freshly voided.) 3. If complications develop, refer woman to physician. 4. Encourage woman to join community diabetic groups to help maintain motivation and follow diet. 5. Utilize "Patient Care Guidelines: Diabetic Teaching" (Table 36.5).
Second half of pregnancy 1. Observe woman for diabetic complications: hypoglycemia, hyperglycemia, ketosis, ketoacidosis, glycosuria (Table 36.4). 2. Observe woman for obstetric conditions complicating diabetes (e.g., preeclampsia). 3. If woman is hospitalized, make assessments appropriate to procedures performed (e.g., urinary estriols, NST, therapy for infection, readjustment of insulin dosage). 4. Assess maternal signs, fetal heart rate (FHR), fundal height, signs of onset of labor, weight, urinary output, dietary intake, exercise, and insulin requirements.	1. Encourage visits every week to supervise management. 2. Keep woman and family informed; reinforce physician's explanations (e.g., that insulin needs are usually higher during the third trimester). a. Maintenance: NPH until delivery. b. Fractional urine specimens tested four times daily as necessary. Woman's diet may need adjustment for rapid growth needs of fetus. Prepare for tests (Table 36.3). 3. Observe the woman closely during teaching sessions to see how well she is dealing with what is being taught. Encourage woman's and family's expression of feelings regarding self and infant. 4. If the woman is hospitalized, provide care as appropriate to reason for hospitalization (e.g., NST). Provide diversional activities for woman if appropriate.
Following diagnosis of diabetes mellitus 1. Assess woman's knowledge of diabetes and its management. 2. Assess woman's and family's reaction to situation; assess her support system and her self-care ability. 3. Assess woman's and family's need for referral to social services (housekeeping aid, financial assistance, peer support group, etc.).	

The Diabetic Mother—cont'd

Assessment/analysis

Intranatal period

1. Observe woman for hypoglycemia: palpitation, tachycardia, hunger, weakness, sweating, tremor, pallor.
2. Observe woman for preeclampsia (see Chapter 35 for symptomatology).
3. Monitor urine for amount and presence of protein and glucose.
4. Monitor intravenous infusions: insulin, oxytocin.
5. Culture urine following clean-catch collection for asymptomatic urinary tract infection.
6. Monitor labor.
   a. Monitor induction: maternal fetal responses.
   b. Use electronic fetal monitor if available.
   c. Assess amount and character of amniotic fluid.

Postnatal period

1. During first 24 to 48 hours after delivery insulin requirements fluctuate rapidly. Termination of pregnancy reverses gestation-induced endocrine changes: high serum blood glucose level, elevated levels of human growth hormone (HGH) and its potentiator, human placental lactogen (HPL).
   a. Do frequent fractional urine tests.
   b. Monitor foods and fluids taken.
   c. Assess woman for clinical manifestations of high or low serum glucose levels.
2. Monitor vital signs, amount of bleeding, uterine contractility, output, and so on as per usual postdelivery routine.
3. Assess woman's and family's reaction to experience, especially if fetal-neonatal death occurs or infant is malformed or at risk.

Plan/implementation

Intranatal period

1. The physician and nurse keep woman and family informed of treatment and fetal status.
2. Keep woman NPO. Monitor intravenous fluids per order for the following:
   a. For induction (with oxytocin [Pitocin]).
   b. 10% dextrose in water and insulin to meet woman's caloric and insulin needs for work of labor.
3. Provide supportive labor nursing, which is especially important to prevent hypoglycemia and acidosis from anxiety.
4. Prepare for induction or cesarean birth (e.g., in case of fetal distress, fetopelvic disproportion, or lack of response to induction).
5. Alert pediatrician and nursery personnel.

Postnatal period

1. Adjust insulin intake (usually regular insulin) according to protocol ordered. Woman may need no insulin for first 24 hours to 48 hours. Progress to NPH according to physician's orders. Allow woman to take over insulin injections when she desires.
2. Provide postdelivery nursing care (after vaginal or cesarean birth) according to routine.
3. Provide supportive care for woman and family after fetal-neonatal death or if neonate is malformed or at risk (see Chapter 33).
4. Keep woman and family informed of her status and infant's condition.
5. Give instruction on breast feeding:
   a. Caloric intake and insulin requirements will need adjusting; for example, women requiring large doses of insulin may need to triple caloric intake and decrease insulin by one half because of antidiabetogenic action (free glucose is utilized in production of lactose).
   b. If mother develops acetonuria, discontinue breast feeding (pump breasts and discard milk) and contact physician for supervision.
   c. If mother becomes hypoglycemic from lack of food or anxiety or other reason, her epinephrine level increases, which decreases her milk supply and letdown reflex.
6. Counsel woman regarding personal care: she *must* eat on time even if it means that others must wait; it will take more energy to add care of the new baby to her previous routine.
7. Couple may request genetic counseling. Infant will not necessarily acquire the disease (see p. 853).
8. Counsel couple on contraception, sterilization, and planning for future pregnancies (see Chapters 13 and 41).

Table 36.5
Patient Care Guidelines: Diabetic Teaching

Name of RN assuming primary care/teaching: ____

IIC code if necessary. Discuss with physician expected length of hospital stay.
Provide pamphlets (obtain from pharmacy): (1) *A Guide for the Diabetic* (Lilly), (2) *What Is Diabetes?* (Lilly), (3) *An Instructional Aid on Juvenile Diabetes* (Travis). Assign reading as appropriate.
RN to review specifics to teach. Have patient obtain Medic-Alert bracelet.

Potential Areas Needing Instruction	Expected Patient Outcomes	Target Dates	RN Initials and Date Done Satisfactorily	Nursing Orders
Ability to cope with diagnosis	Verbalizes reaction to diagnosis and expectations and verbalizes level of comprehension about diabetes			Ascertain level of understanding and knowledge of client and family and receptiveness to teaching Assess feelings about diabetes Have client fill out client information sheet
Pathophysiology of disease Urine testing	Verbalizes knowledge of normal and altered utilization of insulin and glucose in body Verbalizes reasons for testing and significance of results Demonstrates accurate testing of urine ac and hs or as ordered (second voiding) Records results and interprets each test; follows urine testing schedule without being reminded (keep at bedside) Demonstrates correct care of equipment			Discuss pathophysiology with client or significant other Check with physician about S/A method client will do at home ☐ Clinitest ☐ Acetest ☐ Ketodiastix ☐ Other ___ During morning the RN teaches, demonstrates techniques, interprets results (second voiding), and records results Supervise client or significant other Clinitest tablets—emphasize the following: Pass-through phase: 20 ml (4 tsp)—orange→muddy brown→orange Wait 15 sec before shaking for final reading Do not touch tablets Store tablets in cool, dark place Ketodiastix—emphasize the following: Read acetone after 15 sec Read sugar after 30 sec
Insulin administration (if appropriate) ☐ U100* ____ units ☐ U80* ____ units ☐ U40* ____ units ☐ NPH REG. ☐ Lente Other ____ ☐ How often ____	Defines insulin and states its action on body function States peak action of insulin Verbalizes importance of using correctly calibrated syringe with correct strength of insulin; e.g., U100 insulin with U100 syringe Demonstrates correct withdrawal and administration of insulin to self Verbalizes importance of site rotation and identifies sites used Verbalizes proper techniques of insulin storage			Determine correct injection technique (check angle used) ☐ 45-degree angle ☐ 90-degree angle Teach strict aseptic technique for withdrawing and administration of insulin Stress importance of giving and drawing up accurate dose Stress importance of using correct syringe with correct insulin Have client or significant other practice drawing up with normal saline and giving injection to an orange for a day

From Stanford University Hospital, Stanford University Medical Center, Stanford, Calif.
*To decrease errors, soon all insulin will be measured in *U100* dosages.

Table 36.5—cont'd
Patient Care Guidelines: Diabetic Teaching

Potential Areas Needing Instruction	Expected Patient Outcomes	Target Dates	RN Initials and Date Done Satisfactorily	Nursing Orders
Insulin administration—cont'd	Patient gives own injection daily with RN supervision			Teach importance of rotation and sites available Patient to give own injection with RN supervision remainder of hospital stay Use U100 insulin unless ordered otherwise Stress that current bottle of insulin being used can be stored at room temperature; unused bottle in refrigerator
Oral hypoglycemics	Verbalizes mode of action of prescribed oral agent and possible side effects and drug interactions			Discuss prescribed medication's action and side effects with client or significant other Review signs and symptoms and reasons for ketosis
Hyperglycemia and ketoacidosis	Lists four precipitating factors causing ketosis Describes potential signs and symptoms of ketoacidosis Verbalizes rationale for seeking medical attention for illness, infection Verbalizes need to continue testing urine and taking insulin during periods of illness			Stress sick day rules: take insulin, do S/A, notify physician if urine sugar levels run 4+M 2 days or if vomiting *Point out that illness, especially infection, vomiting, and diarrhea, may precipitate ketoacidosis*
Hypoglycemia	Explains causes and dangers of insulin (hypoglycemia) reaction Lists signs and symptoms of insulin reaction Describes care and treatment of and prevention of insulin reaction; verbalizes importance of treating immediately Lists foods to take during insulin reaction and amount to take Significant other verbalizes what to do in case of insulin coma; e.g., *glucagon injection* Verbalizes that increased exercise may induce hypoglycemia Relates importance of carrying diabetic identification			Review causes and dangers of insulin reaction with client or significant other Stress importance of carrying fast-acting sugar and consuming extra carbohydrate before exercise and importance of bedtime snacks Stress relationship of exercise and diet Stress seeking medical care immediately with onset of hypoglycemic reaction Stress importance of client or significant other to learn to recognize signs and symptoms of precipitating factors leading to hypoglycemic reaction Discuss glucagon action and injection technique with client or significant other Give Medic-Alert information
Diet management; calorie count; other restrictions; type of diet ordered for discharge	Verbalizes what is meant by carbohydrate, fat, protein, and nutrient needs for basic good nutrition Verbalizes interrelationship of energy expenditure, food intake, and weight control			Ascertain type of diet client is to follow at home RN informs dietitian that client is on diabetic protocol Dietitian (with reinforcement from nurse) performs the following

Continued.

Table 36.5—cont'd
Patient Care Guidelines: Diabetic Teaching

Potential Areas Needing Instruction	Expected Patient Outcomes	Target Dates	RN Initials and Date Done Satisfactorily	Nursing Orders
Diet management—cont'd	Correctly selects foods and exchanges for three meals for 2 days (to be done with dietitian) Verbalizes need to maintain or achieve normal body weight			Teaches role diet plays in disease management Assesses client's dietary habits and develops prescribed diet management within this framework Provides resource material to show equivalent food values RN to check with dietitian to see if client selects correct foods
Susceptibility to multiple system complications Skin; feet Arteriosclerosis; neurologic changes Sick day rules	Verbalizes understanding of good skin and foot care Demonstrates proper care of skin and feet Verbalizes potential changes in sensation and circulation and appropriate action Importance of exercise Avoidance of restrictive clothing Extremes in temperature Verbalizes what to do on sick days and why			Discuss with client importance of good foot and skin care Washing daily and drying Avoidance of temperature extremes Good-fitting shoes Inspection of feet and skin daily Trim toenails straight across Discuss possible complications of diabetes Neurologic changes Arteriosclerosis and importance of observing for and reporting symptoms to physician Discourage use of heating pads and hot water bottles if complications are already present Stress sick day rules: take insulin, do S/A, notify physician Stress that blood glucose is elevated with temperature, chills, etc.
Exercise considerations	Verbalizes understanding of relationship between exercise, insulin, and glucose utilization Discusses realistically exercise and activities to be maintained and reason for regular exercise Demonstrates ability to perform toe and ankle exercises Verbalizes understanding reason for eating extra carbohydrate before strenuous exercise and need to carry fast-acting sugars			Stress that exercise enhances utilization of glucose and decreases need for insulin Stress importance of regular exercise of any kind within client's limits Teach toe and foot exercises that help to increase peripheral circulation Stress importance of eating a little extra carbohydrate before engaging in strenuous exercise and stress that fast-acting sugars should be carried
Travel considerations	Verbalizes importance of consultation with a physician before travel and obtaining necessary supplies Verbalizes reason for carrying insulin on self			Stress importance of seeing physician before traveling for prescriptions for insulin syringes, where to seek medical assistance, and a written statement that client is diabetic *Stress carrying of insulin, syringes, and fast-acting sugars on self, not in glove compartments or nonpressurized cabins of planes or trains*

Table 36.5—cont'd
Patient Care Guidelines: Diabetic Teaching

Potential Areas Needing Instruction	Expected Patient Outcomes	Target Dates	RN Initials and Date Done Satisfactorily	Nursing Orders
Travel considerations—cont'd				Stress carrying an exchange list for dietary needs; call airlines, etc., to arrange for necessary meals Stress wearing of ID bracelet, learn how to say "diabetes" in foreign language
Discharge plans	Client or significant other verbalizes confidence and ability to cope with disease at home Discusses need for follow-up on discharge and other concerns Verbalizes importance of follow-up with physician and whom to contact for problems			Discuss need for follow-up, i.e., home referral Discuss with physician several days before discharge any necessary prescriptions and progress of client; ask physician to write any necessary orders Order needed equipment or discuss with client where she can obtain needed items Write referrals, complete diabetic teaching flow sheet, and discuss with discharge coordinator any referrals necessary Write summary in nurses' progress notes and on diabetic teaching flow sheet regarding client's or significant other's need for follow-up and comprehension of diagnosis

Wide fluctuations in blood glucose and episodes of ketoacidosis, present before the stress of pregnancy exposes the woman's glucose intolerance, are thought to cause congenital anomalies. Later in pregnancy, when the mother's pancreas cannot release sufficient insulin to meet increased demands, maternal hyperglycemia results. The high levels of glucose stimulate the fetal pancreas to release insulin to meet the high demand. For the fetus, insulin acts as a growth hormone. The combination of the increased supply of maternal glucose and fetal insulin results in excessive fetal growth called macrosomia. Hyperinsulinemia and macrosomia account for most of the problems seen: fetal hypoxia, fetal death, macrosomia (LGA), birth injury, asphyxia neonatorum, problems related to congenital anomalies, delayed appearance of lung maturity (regardless of gestational age and body weight) resulting in respiratory distress syndrome, hypoglycemia, hypocalcemia, polycythemia and hyperviscosity, and nonhemolytic hyperbilirubinemia.

Additional hazards are imposed on the fetus and neonate if the mother's pregnancy is further complicated by pregnancy-induced hypertension.

Maternal episodes of hypoglycemia and acidosis, consequences of poor diabetic control or superimposed infection, adversely affect the fetus. Normally, maternal blood has a more alkaline pH than does fetal blood (with its excess of CO_2). This phenomenon encourages exchange of O_2 and CO_2 across the placental membrane. When the maternal blood is more acidotic than the fetal blood, no CO_2 or O_2 exchange occurs at the level of the placenta, and the fetus becomes asphyxiated and dies.

Clinical picture of infants of diabetic mother (IDM) and infants of gestational diabetic mother (IGDM)

Macrosomia. At birth, the typical infant who is LGA has a round, cherubic, or cushingoid face, chubby body, and plethoric appearance (Fig. 36.8). This infant is macrosomic; for example, the infant has enlarged viscera (hepatosplenomegaly, splanchnomegaly, cardiomegaly) and increased body fat. The placenta and umbilical cord are larger than average. The brain is the only organ that is not enlarged. With good prenatal care and control of diabetes mellitus, the incidence of macrosomia can be decreased.

The excessive size of these infants can and often does lead to dystocia because of fetopelvic disproportion. These infants, who may be born vaginally or by cesarean delivery after a trial of labor, may incur birth trauma (see Chapter 37).

Fig. 36.8
"During their first 24 or more extrauterine hours they lie on their backs, bloated and flushed, their legs flexed and abducted, their tightly closed hands on each side of their head, the abdomen prominent and their respiration sighing. They convey a distinct impression of having had so much food and fluid pressed upon them by an insistent hostess that they desire only peace so that they may recover from their excesses."
A, Factors contributing to neonatal jeopardy of infant of diabetic mother (IDM). **B,** Infant of diabetic mother. (**B** from Shirkey, H.C., editor: Pediatric therapy, ed. 6, St. Louis, 1980, The C.V. Mosby Co.)

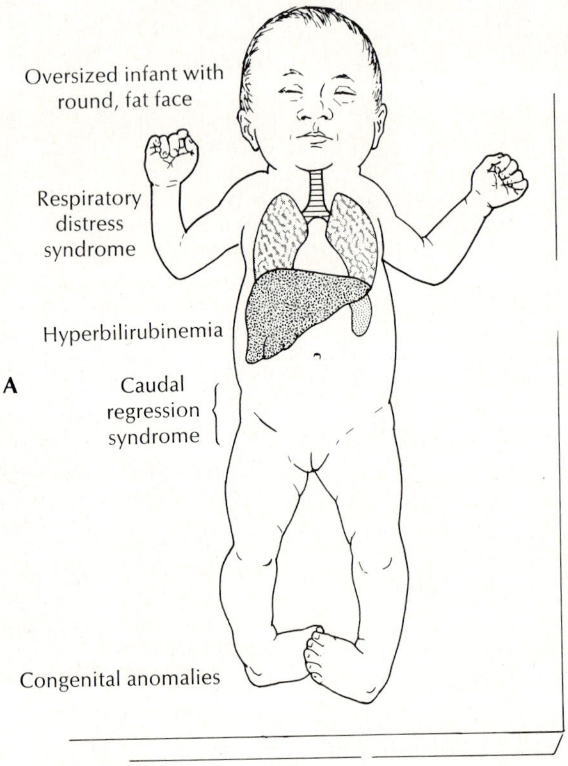

A

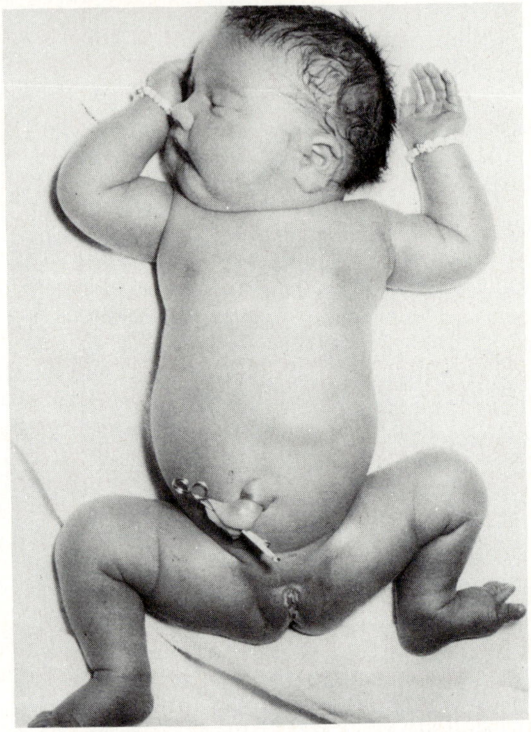

B

Hypoglycemia and hypocalcemia. Separation of the placenta interrupts the constant infusion of glucose. The high level of circulating glucose at the time the umbilical cord is severed falls rapidly in the presence of fetal hyperinsulinism. *Asymptomatic* or symptomatic hypoglycemia occurs within the first 1 to 3 hours after birth. Symptoms of hypocalcemia, a prevalent finding in IDM and IGDM, are similar to those of hypoglycemia, but they occur between 24 and 36 hours of age. However, hypocalcemia must be considered if therapy for hypoglycemia is ineffective.

Lung immaturity. IDM or IGDM manifest a greater incidence of respiratory distress syndrome (RDS) than is found in normal infants of comparable gestational age. Synthesis of surfactant may be delayed because of the high fetal serum level of insulin. Fetal lung maturity as evidenced by a lecithin-sphingomyelin (L-S) ratio of 2:1 is not reassuring if the mother has diabetes mellitus or gestation-induced diabetes mellitus. For the infants of such mothers, an L-S ratio of 3:1 or more or the presence of phosphatidylglycerol in the amniotic fluid is more indicative of adequate lung maturity.

Management. No single physiologic or biochemical event can explain the diverse clinical manifestations seen in the IDM or IGDM. For the conditions described below, the same principles of management pertain, whether they occur in the IDM or any other neonate:

1. Hypoglycemia (see p. 863).
2. RDS (see Chapter 37).
3. Hyperbilirubinemia. Fifty percent of neonates of 32 to 34 weeks' gestation develop hyperbilirubinemia; 15% of infants born at 37 weeks' gestation manifest this condition. Many neonates are plethoric bcause of polycythemia. This increased number of red blood cells to be hemolyzed increases the potential bilirubin load that the neonate must clear. The excessive red blood cells are produced in extramedullary foci (liver and spleen) in addition to the usual sites in bone marrow. Therefore both liver function and bilirubin clearance may be adversely affected.

4. Blood hyperviscosity. Polycythemia increases blood viscosity and thereby impairs circulation.

5. Hypocalcemia occurs in 30% of IDM. In addition, hypocalcemia is associated with preterm delivery, birth trauma, and perinatal asphyxia.

6. Birth trauma and perinatal asphyxia occur in 20% of IGDM and 35% of IDM (for nursing actions, see Chapter 37). Examples include the following:
   a. Cephalhematoma
   b. Paralysis of the facial nerve (seventh cranial nerve)
   c. Fracture of the clavicle
   d. Brachial plexus paralysis, usually Erb-Duchenne (upper right arm) paralysis
   e. Phrenic nerve paralysis, invariably associated with diaphragmatic paralysis

7. Congenital anomalies occur in about 6% of IDM. The incidence is greatest among the SGA neonates (for nursing actions, see Chapter 40). The most frequently occurring anomalies include the following:
   a. CNS—anencephaly, encephalocele, meningomyelocele, hydrocephalus
   b. Caudal regression syndrome—sacral agenesis with weakness or deformities of the lower extremities, malformation and fixation of the hip joints, and shortening or deformity of the femurs (Fig. 36.9)
   c. Tracheoesophageal fistula
   d. Congenital heart malformations

There is some indication that some neonatal conditions—macrosomia, hypoglycemia, hypocalcemia, hyperbilirubinemia, and perhaps fetal lung immaturity—may be eliminated or the incidence decreased by maintaining control over maternal glucose levels within narrow limits.

Summary of nursing actions: IDM and IGDM

Goals of care

1. Physician goals:
   a. A live-born infant is delivered.
   b. Infant suffers no birth trauma such as from cephalopelvic disproportion secondary to macrosomia.
2. Physician-nurse shared goals:
   a. Infant is delivered as near to term as possible.
   b. Hypoglycemia must be presented or recognized early and then minimized.
   c. Congenital anomalies or disorders are identified promptly, and appropriate treatment is instituted.
   d. Parents exhibit an understanding of the disease process and its effects on the fetus-neonate by compliance with medical and nursing care during the prenatal and neonatal period.
   e. Parent-neonate attachment occurs; or if neonate exhibits a disorder or dies, grieving process is initiated.

Fig. 36.9
Infant of diabetic mother with caudal regression syndrome (sacral agenesis). (From Fanaroff, A.A., and Martin, R.J., editors: Behrman's neonatal-perinatal medicine: diseases of the fetus and infant, ed. 3, St. Louis, 1983, The C.V. Mosby Co.)

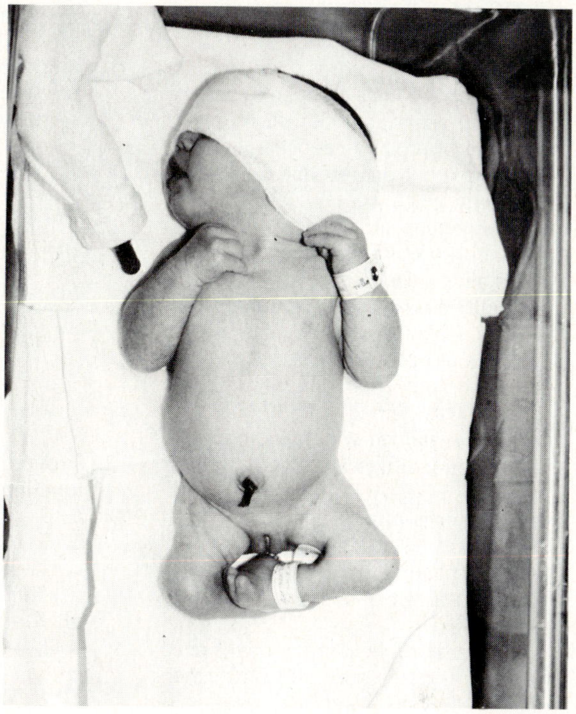

Example of nursing diagnosis. The following is a possible nursing diagnosis: potential fall in blood glucose below 45 mg/dl for the normal term neonate because of persistent neonatal hyperinsulinism.

Evaluation: The goals of care have been achieved if the following conditions have been met:

1. The neonate's airway has remained patent, and respiratory distress is prevented or treated quickly.
2. The neonate did not experience cold stress, and the neonate's temperature stabilized within 8 to 10 hours after birth.
3. The neonate experienced no hypoglycemic episodes (below 30 mg/dl), and blood glucose levels stabilized in the physiologic range (approximately between 45 and 130 mg/dl).
4. The neonate experienced no hypocalcemic episodes.

Neonate of a Diabetic Mother

Assessment/analysis*

1. Review prenatal records.
2. Assess the neonate frequently for the following associated clinical problems (in order of probable appearance):
   a. Respiratory distress and ventilatory adequacy
   b. Congenital anomalies or disorders (incidence is 6% compared to 2% in all deliveries)
   c. Birth trauma (e.g., cephalhematoma, paralysis of the facial nerve, fracture of the clavicle)
   d. Meconium aspiration (if amniotic fluid was stained or if skin, nails, or cord is stained with meconium)
   e. Gestational age and degree of maturity (LGA, AGA, SGA)
   f. Hypoglycemia (within the first 3 hours)
   g. Polycythemia (by 6 hours of age)
   h. Hypocalcemia (within 24 to 36 hours)
   i. Hyperbilirubinemia (on day 2 or 3)
3. Weigh neonate soon after birth, then daily. Measure head and chest circumference.
4. Assess parent-neonate interaction.

Plan/implementation

1. Maintain airway patency (see Chapter 29).

At birth:

1. Maintain equipment and ensure adequate oxygen and other supplies for resuscitative measures.
2. Assist with resuscitation as necessary.
3. Protect neonate against loss of body heat by drying, wrapping in warmed blankets, and positioning under a heat source.

Subsequent care:

1. Position neonate on the side, with head slightly elevated and neck slightly extended.
2. Observe, report, and record signs of respiratory distress.

2. Support physiologic function.
   a. Respiration
   b. Temperature
   c. Glucose requirement
   d. Fluid requirement
   e. Maintenance of low bilirubin levels

3. Treat as if infant is premature, regardless of weight, until gestational age and respiratory maturity are established.
   a. Place in incubator that has been set between 32° and 36° C (90° and 97° F) (depending on infant's maturity, size).
   b. Attach thermistor probe or take axillary temperature every 15 minutes until stabilized and then hourly. Temperature should stabilize at 36.5° C (97.7° F).
   c. Check respiratory rate every 15 minutes for 6 hours; place neonate on respiratory monitor if respirations are irregular.
   d. Have 0_2 and resuscitative equipment available.
4. Feed as necessary (glucose, calcium). Monitor parenteral fluid therapy. (See care of neonate with hypoglycemia, p. 863.)
5. Carry out orders for decreasing bilirubin levels (see Chapters 29 and 40).
6. Promptly report and record any signs of anomalies, dysfunction, or disorder.

3. Support parents.

7. Keep parents informed. Nurse is available to parents for their questions (e.g., explain that infant's condition is reflection of maternal condition rather than infant diabetes), discussion of feelings, and so on.

*Assessment of the neonate of a diabetic mother by the physician and nurse is the key to quality care of the neonate.

Neonatal Hypoglycemia

Assessment/analysis	Plan/implementation
1. Note if neonate comes under the categories of those at risk for hypoglycemia. 2. Do heel-stick test: Dextrostix, Clinistix.* a. Determine frequency of test by assessing condition of neonate: (1) For normal term infant, test is done at 45 minutes, 2 hours, and 6 hours of age. (2) For infant at risk, do test at following intervals: 30 minutes of age, 1½ hours of age, 4 hours of age, 9 hours of age, 12 hours of age, 24 hours of age, and then once daily for 8 days. b. If blood sugar is 45 mg/dl or less in term infant or 20 mg/dl or less in premature infant, order blood sugar test by laboratory immediately. 3. Observe for symptoms of hypoglycemia. 4. Assess for coordination of suck-swallow reflex.	1. If suck-swallow reflex is well coordinated, feed the neonate according to hospital protocol. Term infants may be fed at 4 hours of age or earlier, as necessary. Small neonates or those born of diabetic mothers may need to be fed at 1 hour of age. Because neonate's stomach capacity is small, the amount should be small and the feedings frequent. 2. If neonate cannot take fluids by mouth or if blood glucose is below 25 mg/dl, physician will administer 10% glucose in water intravenously.

*Do not confuse tests.

5. Bilirubin levels have been maintained below toxic levels.
6. Fluid and electrolyte balance has been maintained.
7. A positive relationship has been established between parent and neonate.
8. Parents understand the care provided to the neonate.
9. Discharge planning has been adequate:
   a. Parents feel ready to provide care to the neonate.
   b. Public health referral has been made, if appropriate.
   c. Referral to other community resources has been made, if appropriate.
   d. Parents state motivation to carry out follow-up care.

Neonatal hypoglycemia

Definition. Blood glucose concentration levels below 30 mg/dl during the first 72 hours of life or below 45 mg/dl after the first 3 days in the full-term infant constitute hypoglycemia. In premature neonates a blood sugar level below 20 mg/dl constitutes hypoglycemia.

Clinical manifestations. Most hypoglycemic infants are asymptomatic. The following symptoms may be seen, however:

1. Feeding difficulty, hunger
2. Apnea
3. Irregular respiratory effort
4. Cyanosis
5. Weak, high-pitched cry
6. Jitteriness, twitching, eye rolling, convulsions
7. Lethargy

Infants at risk. Those infants who are more vulnerable to hypoglycemia include the following:

1. Low–birth weight infants
2. Dysmature infants
3. Infants of diabetic or prediabetic mothers
4. Infants of preeclamptic-eclamptic mothers
5. Polycythemic infants
6. Cold infants
7. Infants with severe erythroblastosis fetalis
8. Infants with congenital heart disease

Summary of nursing care: neonatal hypoglycemia

Goals of care

1. Neonate suffers no hypoglycemic episodes.
2. Neonate suffers no brain damage.
3. Parents understand the condition and are able to establish a positive relationship with the neonate.

Evaluation. See also ''Summary of Nursing Care of the Infant with Hypocalcemia, Hypoglycemia, and Sepsis,'' p. 865.

NEONATAL HYPOCALCEMIA

Definition. Hypocalcemia is confirmed with serum electrolyte determinations. Normal values in the full-term neonate range from 8 to 10 mg/dl (4 to 5 mEq/L); with hypocalcemia the serum calcium level is below 7 mg/dl (3.5 mEq/L). About one third of premature neonates under 2000 g have serum calcium levels below 7 mg/dl for the first 24 hours of life.

Neonatal Hypocalcemia

Assessment/analysis	Plan/implementation
1. Note if neonate comes under the categories of those at risk for hypocalcemia. 2. Observe for clinical manifestations of hypocalcemia.	1. Medical therapy: acute care for hypocalcemia consists of calcium gluconate, 10% solution (100 to 150 mg/kg body weight) by intravenous infusion slowly; rapid infusion may cause flushing, vomiting, and circulatory collapse. Extravasation into surrounding tissue precipitates the calcium, causing necrosis and sloughing. Vitamin D_2 (ergocalciferol) every 24 hours for 2 or 3 weeks may be ordered. 2. The nurse assists in medical management by monitoring the calcium gluconate infusion and the newborn's heart rate. If the heart rate is below 100 beats/min, the infusion is discontinued. A scalp vein is not used; the needle is taped securely at the site, and firm pressure is exerted over the site when the needle is removed to prevent seepage of the calcium gluconate into surrounding tissues. The needle should be changed every 12 hours for the same reason. Supportive nursing care includes the following: a. Maintenance of normal temperature, hydration, and oxygenation b. Reduction of environmental stimuli (e.g., nursing care organized to minimize handling of infant) c. Observation for and precautions against seizures d. Keeping parents informed of care and progress; providing time for parents to express feelings; encouraging parents to visit frequently and to participate in care of infant (see Chapter 33)

High serum phosphorus values, that is, over 8 mg/dl, coexist with hypocalcemia in neonatal tetany. Normal serum phosphorus levels range between 4.0 and 6.5 mg/dl, although values approaching 8 mg/dl are considered normal in the full-term neonate.

Clinical manifestations. Within the first 48 hours, hypocalcemia may be expressed as edema, apnea, intermittent cyanosis, and abdominal distention, but classic symptoms of tetany are absent. Note that these symptoms are similar to those of other neonatal disorders, for example, hypoglycemia and sepsis. Therefore the infant's history must be taken to assist in the correct diagnosis.

Infants at risk. Hypocalcemia may occur from exchange transfusion of blood containing anticoagulant citrate. Citrate combines with calcium, thus depleting ionizable calcium needed for the coagulation process. To anticipate and replace this loss, 10% calcium gluconate is given. Other conditions that predispose an infant to hypocalcemia include the following:

- Perinatal asphyxia (33% of asphyxiated neonates)
- Use of bicarbonate to treat acidosis
- Diabetic mother (50% of neonates born to insulin-dependent mothers)
- Prematurity (33% of neonates born at 37 weeks' gestation or sooner regardless of birth weight)
- Preeclamptic-eclamptic mother treated before delivery with magnesium sulfate (a competitive antagonist to calcium)
- Infants who have had an exchange transfusion of blood to which the anticoagulant citrate has been added (see Chapter 40)

Tetany of the newborn was formerly a frequent occurrence, when 5- to 10-day-old infants were fed cow's milk.*

Summary of nursing actions: neonatal hypocalcemia

Goals of care

1. Neonate suffers no episodes of hypocalcemia.
2. Neonate has no episodes of tetany.
3. Parents understand the condition and are able to establish a positive relationship with the neonate.

Evaluation. The goals of care are achieved. See also, ''Summary of Nursing Care of the Infant with Hypocalcemia, Hypoglycemia, and Sepsis, p. 865.

*For a discussion of neonatal tetany from cow's milk, see Whaley and Wong (1983).

Summary of Nursing Care of the Infant with Hypocalcemia, Hypoglycemia, or Sepsis

Goals	Responsibilities
Recognize early signs of pathophysiologic state	Assess each system for signs and symptoms suggestive of each condition; correlate findings with general impression of progress of infant (feeding, weight gain, response to stimuli, and sleeping patterns)
Prevent or decrease potential side effects of medical intervention	
Hypocalcemia	Administer calcium gluconate slowly; if heart rate falls below 100 beats/min, stop infusion
	Prevent extravasation of calcium gluconate into tissues:
	Avoid scalp vein
	Ensure placement of needle before administering drug
	Tape needle securely at site of insertion
	Apply pressure to puncture site after removal of needle
	Counsel mother regarding infant feeding (breast feeding or appropriate formulas)
Hypoglycemia	Begin oral feeding as soon as possible after birth
	Administer glucose infusion carefully; avoid overloading the system by speeding up intravenous administration
	Observe for signs of hyperglycemia (acidosis) and possible need for insulin
	Decrease intravenous administration of glucose slowly to avoid hypoglycemia from physiologic hyperinsulinemia.
Sepsis	Observe for side effects of antibiotics
	Regulate infusion carefully to allow for antibiotic to be administered within 1 hour
	Use piggyback setup if main intravenous solution has added drugs
Monitor environment to decrease factors that will complicate recovery from each condition	Maintain thermoregulation, hydration, and oxygenation of infant
	Monitor vital signs and correlate with infant's progress
Hypocalcemia	Reduce environmental stimuli
	Organize care to ensure minimal handling of infant
	Discuss with parents reasons for minimal holding
	Institute seizure precautions
Sepsis	Institute appropriate isolation techniques
Observe for complications of disease	
Hypocalcemia	Observe for tetany and convulsions
Hypoglycemia	Check heel blood with Dextrostix
	Check urine for glycosuria
Sepsis	Observe for signs of meningitis, especially bulging anterior fontanel
	Observe for pyarthrosis, usually evidenced by limited movement of affected joint
	Observe for signs of shock, especially fall in blood pressure
Provide emotional support for parents	Allow parents the opportunity to express their feelings
	Keep parents informed of infant's progress
	Encourage frequent visiting and participation in care to foster parent-child attachment

From Whaley, L.F., and Wong, D.L.: Nursing care of infants and children, ed. 2, St. Louis, 1983, The C.V. Mosby Co.

Hyperemesis Gravidarum

DEFINITION

Hyperemesis gravidarum (pernicious vomiting of pregnancy) is defined as excessive vomiting during pregnancy, leading to dehydration and starvation.

Many pregnant women suffer nausea and vomiting at some time during early gestation. The indisposition is mild in most cases, but in about 1 of every 1000 pregnant women, severe intractable emesis will require hospitalization and perhaps even therapeutic abortion.

The cause of hyperemesis during pregnancy is still debated. Psychologically unstable women whose established reaction patterns to stress involve gastrointestinal disturbances often are affected. In some women, however, psychologic etiology cannot be elicited. Other causes could be multiple pregnancy, hormonal abnormalities (elevated T_4), or trophoblastic disease (hydatidiform mole).

Hyperemesis Gravidarum

Assessment/analysis

1. Assess amount of vomiting.
2. Assess dietary progress and daily weight, fluid intake, and urinary output.
3. Assess woman's affect and response to home environment and pregnancy.
4. Save and send any specimen to laboratory.
5. Monitor FHR and growth of fetus.
6. Observe for jaundice (a rare occurrence).
7. Observe for abnormal bleeding, for example, from mucosal surfaces (a rare occurrence).
8. Monitor intravenous line for infiltration, etc.

Plan/implementation

1. Management of hyperemesis gravidarum includes hospitalization in a pleasant, well-ventilated room.
2. Parenteral fluids, electrolytes, sedatives, and vitamins will be required. For the first 48 hours parenteral fluids are used to maintain hydration and restore fluid and electrolyte balance. Cautious resumption of a dry diet in six small feedings with clear liquids an hour after meals generally is acceptable.
3. Accept woman's behavior in gentle, nonjudgmental manner.
4. Encourage woman to discuss her feelings, emphasizing her complete recovery. Keep conversational topics pleasant.
5. Keep family informed as to progress. (Family may feel anger or hurt at being excluded from visiting, as well as contempt for wife and mother.)
6. Maintain excellent daily hygiene.
7. If additional psychotherapy is indicated, the physician will give woman referrals.
8. Report and record FHR abnormalities, maternal jaundice, and bleeding from mucosal surfaces.
9. Change intravenous tubing per hospital protocol to prevent infection. Reinsert intravenous line at another site if infiltration or venous thrombosis occurs.

CLINICAL MANIFESTATIONS

In extreme cases dehydration leads to fluid-electrolyte complications, particularly acidosis. Rarely does vomitus contain only gastric acid fluids. Most vomiting involves loss of contents (alkali) from deeper within the gastrointestinal tract, leading to development of metabolic acidosis. Starvation causes hypoproteinemia and hypovitaminosis. Degenerative changes produce characteristic symptomatology. Jaundice and hemorrhage secondary to vitamin C and B-complex deficiency and hypothrombinemia lead to bleeding from mucosal surfaces. The embryo or fetus may die, and the mother may die from irreversible metabolic alterations.

SUMMARY OF NURSING ACTIONS: HYPEREMESIS GRAVIDARUM

Goal of care. Hyperemesis gravidarum will be resolved with no adverse effects on mother and fetus and family unit.

Evaluation

1. Severe vomiting episodes are resolved; fluid and electrolyte homeostasis is achieved, and weight gain occurs.
2. No adverse sequelae, maternal or fetal, develop as a result of condition.
3. If medical treatment is unsuccessful, surgical intervention to terminate pregnancy is undertaken.
4. Woman comes to terms with self, pregnancy, and life situation.

In most cases hyperemesis gravidarum will respond to therapy; hence the prognosis is good. The woman is discharged home when fluid and electrolyte balance is restored and weight gain begins.

Hyperthyroidism

Hyperthyroidism, which affects about 1 of every 1500 pregnant women, may seriously complicate gestation or endanger the fetus. Hyperthyroidism may be responsible for anovulation and amenorrhea, but the disease is not a cause of abortion or fetal anomaly. Hyperthyroidism is associated with an increased incidence of premature labor and delivery. Symptoms include weakness, sweating, weight loss (or poor gain), nervousness, loose stools, and heat intolerance. Warm, soft, moist skin, tachycardia, stare with exophthalmos, tremor, and goiter with a bruit are characteristic. Laboratory findings, particularly the free T_4 index, will be elevated.

Radioactive iodine must not be used in testing or in therapy because it may destroy or compromise the fetal thyroid. Other antithyroid drugs such as iodine or the thiouracils may be employed to control the overactive maternal thyroid, provided the free T_4 index remains normal and that leukopenia does not develop.

Partial thyroidectomy, also an acceptable treatment for toxic goiter, requires preoperative preparation by antithyroid medication, usually Lugol's solution. Hypothyroidism, which occurs in at least 20% of hyperthyroid women postoperatively, must be treated promptly to spare the fetus. A free T_4 index determination on the cord blood at birth should be run to aid in determining the status of the infant.

Heart Disease

Every pregnancy taxes the cardiovascular system. The heart rate is accelerated, and the blood volume and the cardiac output increase 30% to 50%. The normal heart can compensate for these and associated burdens so that pregnancy and delivery are generally well tolerated. If myocardial or valvular disease develops or if a congenital heart defect is large, cardiac decompensation is likely.

Heart disease affects 0.5% to 2% of pregnant women. In North American congenital heart disease is now more frequently noted with pregnancy than rheumatic carditis. Syphilis and arteriosclerosis, as well as pulmonary and renal disorders, are responsible for cardiac complications, and some of these develop during pregnancy. Heart disease is of considerable importance for the expectant woman because a maternal mortality of 1% to 3% is likely with severe heart disease. It ranks fourth as a cause of maternal deaths. A perinatal mortality of up to 50% must be expected with persistent cardiac decompensation.

Rheumatic fever attacks the mitral, aortic, or tricuspid valves. Congenital maldevelopment involves the septa, valves, and conduction system, and persistently patent fetal cardiovascular communications may reduce the efficiency of the heart. Syphilis and arteriosclerosis alter the aortic valves and the conduction system principally.

Operations for the correction of congenital or acquired heart disease should be done before pregnancy if possible.

Closed cardiac surgery such as release of a stenotic mitral orifice can be accomplished with little risk to mother or fetus. Open heart surgery, on the other hand, requires extracorporeal circulation, and under these circumstances, hypoxia may develop. As a consequence the risk of fetal damage or loss rises to almost 30%. If anticoagulant therapy is required during pregnancy, heparin should be used, because this large molecular drug does not cross the placenta. Oral anticoagulants, such as warfarin (Coumadin) compounds, cross to the fetus and may cause anomalies or hemorrhage in the infant. Valvuloplasty clients should receive penicillin or other antibiotic prophylaxis against bacterial endocarditis during gestation, however.

EFFECTS OF PREGNANCY ON HEART DISEASE

The effects of pregnancy on heart disease involves an altered heart rate, trimester fluctuations in blood pressure, increased cardiac output, a 30% to 50% increase in blood volume, and other changes requiring compensation during pregnancy, labor, and postdelivery readjustments.

EFFECTS OF HEART DISEASE ON PREGNANCY

One effect of heart disease on pregnancy is chorea gravidarum, ascribed to rheumatic fever often associated with rheumatic heart disease. In addition, spontaneous abortion is increased, and premature labor and delivery are more prevalent with heart disease. A growth-retarded fetus, probably because of the low Po_2 level, is frequently seen as the offspring of the pregnant woman with cardiac problems.

SYMPTOMS

Symptoms of cardiac decompensation may appear abruptly or gradually. Medical intervention must be instituted immediately to correct cardiac status.

The *pregnant woman* notes the following *subjective symptoms:* increasing fatigue or dyspnea or both with her usual exertion; a feeling of smothering or difficulty in breathing; the need to cough frequently (coughing may be accompanied by hemoptysis); and periods of palpitation and tachycardia.

The *examiner* notes the following *objective symptoms:* progressive, generalized edema; rales at the base of the lungs; pulse irregularity.

DIAGNOSIS

The differential diagnosis of heart disease involves ruling out respiratory problems, primarily arrhythmias.

The diagnosis of heart disease depends on the history, physical examination, x-ray films, and ultrasonograms when required.

CLASSIFICATION

The degree of dysfunction (disability) of the woman with cardiac disease is often more important in the treatment and prognosis of cardiac disease complicating pregnancy than the diagnosis of the valvular lesion per se. The New York Heart Association's functional classification of organic heart disease, a widely accepted standard, is as follows:

1. Class I: persons with cardiac disease who have no limitation of physical activity
2. Class II: persons with cardiac disease who have a slight limitation of physical activity
3. Class III: persons with cardiac disease who have considerable limitation of activity, with even ordinary activity producing symptoms
4. Class IV: persons unable to undertake any physical activity without discomfort; symptoms of cardiac insufficiency occurring even at rest

No classification of heart disease can be considered rigid or absolute, but this one offers a basic practical guide for treatment, assuming frequent prenatal visits, good client cooperation, and proper obstetric care.

MEDICAL MANAGEMENT

Medical therapy is conducted as a team approach with a cardiologist. The functional class of the disease is determined at 3 months and again at 7 or 8 months. The maximal period of stress is between the fourteenth and thirty-second weeks of gestation. The therapy includes the following:

1. Treatment of anemia, hyperthyroidism, or obesity as necessary to reduce those risk factors that increase the work load of the cardiovascular circulation
2. Treatment of any infections promptly, since respiratory, urinary, or gastrointestinal tract infections can complicate the condition by accelerating heart rate and by direct spread of organism (as *Streptococcus*) to the heart structure
3. Restriction of sodium intake with careful monitoring for hyponatremia (The sodium ion, with its ability to attract and hold fluid, affects the quality and the amount of the circulating volume.)
4. Monitoring the woman's intake of potassium to avoid hypokalemia, which is associated with heart and other muscular weakness and dysfunction
5. Monitoring anticoagulant therapy, if used

Other therapy is directly related to the functional classification of heart disease.

Class I. The pregnant woman with class I heart disease should limit stress to protect against cardiac decompensation. Additional rest at night and after meals, frequent evaluations, and the early and effective treatment of respiratory and other infections should be stressed. Therapeutic abortion is never medically warranted. If there are no obstetric problems, vaginal delivery using pudendal block anesthesia with prophylactic forceps or shortening of the second stage is recommended.

Class II. A program similar to that for class I should be followed for the pregnant woman with class II heart disease. However, the woman should be admitted to the hospital near term (if signs of cardiac overload or arrhythmia develop) for evaluation and treatment.

Penicillin prophylaxis of nonsensitized pregnant women against bacterial endocarditis in labor and during the early puerperium is advised. Mask oxygen and pudendal block anesthesia are important. Ergot products should be avoided because of increases in blood pressure, but dilute intravenous oxytocin immediately after delivery may be employed to prevent postdelivery hemorrhage. Tubal sterilization may be carried out, but surgery should be delayed several days at least to ensure homeostasis. If sterilization is not accomplished, effective contraception must be provided.

Class III. Bed rest for much of each day is necessary for pregnant women with class III cardiac disease. Cardiac decompensation occurs during pregnancy in about 30% of class III women. With this possibility, hospitalization of the woman for the remainder of pregnancy and the early puerperium is advised. Early therapeutic abortion may be warranted, particularly after a previous episode of cardiac failure. Therapeutic abortion and elective sterilization may be feasible. Breast feeding is contraindicated. Sterilization should be postponed until a later date, but explicit contraceptive advice must be given.

Class IV. Because persons with class IV cardiac disease are decompensated even at rest, a major initial effort must be made to improve the cardiac status of pregnant women in this category. Early therapeutic abortion, although not innocuous, may be feasible with regional anesthesia in some cases. Prophylactic antibiotic therapy should cover the procedure. Vaginal delivery of women with class IV lesions is the safest approach if abortion is not done. The maternal mortality approaches 50% in class IV heart disease, and the perinatal mortality is even higher.

NURSING ACTIONS

The goals for care of the woman whose pregnancy is complicated by a cardiac problem are (1) to minimize stress associated with pregnancy and (2) to support cardiac function. The care begins in the prenatal period and continues until the mother has recovered from the birth.

Prenatal care

Assessment. The woman is seen at weekly intervals if at home or on a continuous basis if she is hospitalized. The nurse assesses for factors that would increase stress on the heart, such as anemia, infection, or a home situation that includes responsibility for the house, other children, or extended family members. The client is observed for signs of cardiac decompensation, that is, progressive generalized edema, rales at the base of the lungs, or pulse irregularity. The routine monitoring for the prenatal period, weight gain and pattern of weight gain, edema, vital signs, discomforts of pregnancy, urinalysis, and blood work continues. The nurse keeps careful check of the side effects and interactions of all medications—including supplemental iron—that the woman is taking, and she reports them to the physician in charge as well as documents their use on the client's record. For example, if a woman is being given anticoagulant therapy and is taking dicumarol, the drug will need to be changed to heparin because dicumarol causes fetal hemorrhage.

Examples of nursing diagnoses

1. Increased fatigue because of care of elderly grandmother who fell and injured her hip
2. Anxiety over money problems because of loss of work (enforced bed rest)

Plan and implementation. The plan of care must take into consideration the woman's social situation. The woman may be concerned with the welfare of other family members at the expense of her own welfare and that of the fetus. The care will include the following:

1. Reinforcing the physician's explanation for need for close medical supervision.
2. Reviewing (give the woman written as well as verbal instructions) symptoms of cardiac decompensation: increasing fatigue or dyspnea with the woman's usual exertion, feeling of smothering, need to cough frequently (hemoptysis at times), periods of palpitations and tachycardia.
3. Promoting adequate rest: The woman should sleep 8 to 10 hours every day and ½ hour after meals. Activities are restricted, for example, if at home, no housework, no shopping, no laundry.
4. Teaching regarding nutrition (especially difficult when someone else shops and cooks): The woman needs a diet high in iron and protein, and adequate calories to gain 10.8 kg (24 lb) during pregnancy.
5. If heparin is ordered in place of dicumarol, the woman is taught to give it to herself. If she is taking heparin, caution her to avoid foods high in vitamin K, such as raw, deep green, leafy vegetables. Vitamin K counteracts the effects of heparin; therefore she will require a substitute source of folic acid.
6. Teaching regarding the danger of infection: She should notify the physician at the first sign of infection or when she is exposed to infection.
7. Reviewing the information pertaining to management of the woman's labor and her early postdelivery period.

Natal care

Assessment. The assessment includes the routine assessments for all laboring women as well as assessments for cardiac decompensation. The latter include taking vital signs at least every 10 to 30 minutes. The physician is alerted if the pulse rate is 100/min or greater or if respirations are 25/min or greater. Respiratory status is checked constantly for developing dyspnea, coughing, or rales at base of lungs. The color and temperature of the skin are noted. Pallor, cooling, and sweating may indicate cardiac shock. The woman is carefully watched for symptoms of emotional stress.

Examples of nursing diagnoses

1. Anxiety increased because of fear for infant's safety
2. Fear of dying because of perceived inability to control stress of labor

Plan and implementation. These clients require a one-to-one staff ratio. The collaborating internist is notified of the woman's labor. Close cooperation between members of the obstetric team is mandatory. A pediatrician and nurse from the intensive care unit are present at the birth for the immediate care of the newborn.

Nursing actions include the following:

1. Making sure the woman does not take heparin if on anticoagulant therapy.
2. Administering prophylactic antibiotics as ordered to prevent infection, which could cause further valvular damage, and promoting cardiac function by the following measures:
   a. Alleviating anxiety through maintaining calm atmosphere and keeping the woman and the family informed.
   b. Placing the woman in a side-lying position with her head and shoulders elevated and body parts supported (with pillows, etc.).
   c. Mediating for discomfort and sedating as needed.
   d. Assisting the physician with anesthesia—saddle block (low spinal), caudal, or lumbar epidural—to minimize discomfort, eliminate bearing-down reflex, and decrease peripheral resistance, venous return, and cardiac output. Prevent, recognize, and/or report and treat hypotension, which may follow anesthesia.
3. Assisting the physician if evidence of cardiac de-

compensation appears. *(pulse rate is 100/min or greater; respirations are 25/min or greater; dyspnea).* Administer medications and record what has been given. These may include the following:

a. Deslanoside (Cedilanid-D) (fast acting, for digitalization).
b. Oxygen by intermittent positive pressure (decreases chance of pulmonary edema).
c. Diuretics (furosemide [Lasix] is potent and fast acting).

4. Keeping family members informed of the woman's progress.

Delivery is accomplished with the woman in left side-lying position, or if placed in the supine position, a pad is placed on the left hip to minimize the danger of aortic compression (vena cava syndrome). The knees are flexed, and the feet are flat on the bed. Stirrups are not used to avoid compression of popliteal veins and to avoid an increase in blood volume in the chest and trunk secondary to the effects of gravity. Episiotomy and use of outlet forceps also decrease work of the heart.

Postdelivery care. The immediate postdelivery period is hazardous for a woman with a compromised heart. Cardiac output increases rapidly as extravascular fluid is remobilized into the vascular compartment.

At the moment of delivery, intraabdominal pressure is reduced drastically; pressure on veins is removed, the splanchnic vessels engorge, and blood flow to the heart is increased. Fluid begins to move from extravascular spaces into the bloodstream. Some physicians favor the application of the abdominal binder or alternating tourniquets on the extremities to minimize the effects of this rapid change in intraabdominal pressure.

Assessment. Cardiac monitoring for decompensation continues through the first postpartum weeks because it has been known to occur as late as the sixth postpartum day. Routine assessment as for any newly delivered woman is instituted, for example, vital signs, bleeding, uterine contractility, urinary output, pain, rest, diet, and daily weight. Laboratory results are noted and reported if indicated to the physician, for example, hemoglobin, hematocrit, and urinalysis. It is important to assess the woman's support systems since activity will be curtailed until the cardiac system is recovered. The family response to the birth and the infant need to be observed because the mother may not be directly involved in the infant's care for a period (prematurity of infant, health of mother).

Plan and implementation. The woman's hospital stay is extended to 7 days or more to permit continuous assessment for cardiac decompensation and to support cardiac and respiratory function. The latter is achieved by the following measures:

1. Proper positioning in bed with same position as for labor; that is, elevate head of bed and encourage the woman to lie on her side.
2. Providing bed rest with bathroom privileges as tolerated (nurse meets the woman's grooming and hygiene needs and may even assist her with turning in bed, eating, and other activities).
3. Assisting with progressive ambulation as tolerated; the nurse assesses the woman's pulse, skin, and affect before and after walking.
4. Promoting bowel movements without stress or strain (stool softeners, diet, and fluids plus mild analgesia and local anesthetic spray applied to the episiotomy may facilitate process).
5. Preventing overdistention of bladder (over 1000 ml) because:
   a. A distended bladder prevents contraction of the uterus (see Chapter 31), and this predisposes to hemorrhage.
   b. Rapid emptying of the distended bladder results in a precipitous drop in intraabdominal pressure, leading to splanchnic engorgement and generalized hypotension. The nurse institutes intake and output recording.
6. Isolating the woman from sources of infection: people, objects, and so on. A private room is appropriate for this client.
7. Initiating prompt and energetic prevention or treatment of hemorrhage or infection.
8. Every attempt is made to facilitate mother-infant interactions that do not stress the mother. She may direct care of the infant by a designated family member in lieu of the mother. The mother may nurse if her condition warrants; that is, classes I and II may nurse; for classes III and IV, nursing is not advised. The fed baby can be brought regularly to the mother, held at her eye level and by her lips, and brought to her fingers so that she can establish an emotional bond with her baby with a low expenditure of her energy. At the same time, involving the mother passively in her infant's care helps the mother to feel vitally important—as she is—to the infant's well-being. (e.g., "There is something no one else can do for your baby—to provide him with your sounds, touch, and rhythms that are such a comfort to him.") Perhaps the mother can be encouraged to make a tape recording of her talking, singing, or whispering, to be played for the baby in the nursery, to help him feel her presence and to be in contact with her voice.

Before discharge the nurse assesses the home support for the woman and infant. Preparation for discharge is planned with the woman and family as follows.

1. Provision of help in home for the mother by relatives, friends, and others. If necessary, the nurse makes referrals of the family to community resources (e.g., for homemaking services).
2. Planning of rest and sleep periods, activity, and diet by mother.
3. Provision of information to couple regarding reestablishment of sexual relations, contraception, sterilization of the man or the woman (usually advocated for women in classes II, III, and IV), and medical supervision.

Evaluation. The nurse uses the following criteria as overall indications for the success of therapy:

1. The woman is able to tolerate the stresses imposed by pregnancy (i.e., increase in cardiac output by more than one third, increase in pulse rate by 10 beats/min, expansion of blood volume by 25%, and psychic stress common to pregnancy and related to the heart condition).
2. Congestive heart failure (the primary cause of maternal mortality in women with cardiac disease) is prevented.
3. The home situation is controlled, with assistance provided as necessary.

References and Readings

American Diabetes Association: Principles of nutrition and dietary recommendations for individuals with diabetes mellitus, Diabetes Care **2:**520, 1979.

Baker, D., et al.: The effect of prostaglandins on the multiplication and cell-to-cell spread of herpes simplex virus type 2 in vitro, Am. J. Obstet. Gynecol., **144**(3):346, 1982.

Baker, D.A.: The dangers of varicella-zoster in pregnancy, Contemp. Obstet. Gynecol. **20**(2):71, 1982.

Barden, T.P., and Knowles, H.C.: Diagnosis of diabetes in pregnancy, Clin. Obstet. Gynecol. **24:**3, 1981.

Bettoli, E.J.: Herpes: facts and fallacies, Am. J. Nurs. **82**(6):924, 1982.

Birch, G.E.: Heart disease and pregnancy, Am. Heart J, **93:**104, 1977.

Bohart, R.D., et al.: Continuous insulin infusion during the peripartum period: maternal and neonatal outcome, Calif. Perinatal Assoc. **2**(1):26, 1982.

Bonovich, L.: Participation: the key to learning for patients in antepartal clinics, J.O.G.N. Nurs., **10**(2):75, 1981.

Cabral, G.A., et al.: Expression of herpes simplex virus type 2 antigens in premalignant and malignant vulvar cells, Am. J. Obstet. Gynecol. **143**(6):611, 1982.

Campbell, C.E., and Herten, R.J.: VD to STD: redefining venereal disease, Am. J. Nurs. **81**(9):1629, 1981.

Carpenter, M.W., and Coustan, D.R.: Criteria for screening tests for gestational diabetes, Am. J. Obstet. Gynecol. **144**(7):768, 1982.

Claypool, J.M.: Rubella protection for maternal child health care providers, M.C.N. **6**(1):53, 1981.

Committee on Dietary Allowances, Food and Nutrition Board: Recommended dietary allowances, ed. 9, Washington, D.C., 1980, U.S. Government Printing Office, National Academy of Sciences.

Coustan, D.R.: Home glucose monitoring becomes more sophisticated, Contemp. Obstet. Gynecol. (special issue, Technology 1983) **20:**7, Oct. 1982.

Danforth, D., editor: Obstetrics and gynecology, ed.4, New York, 1982, Harper & Row.

Eder, J.M.: Genital herpes simplex virus infections during pregnancy, J. Calif. Perinatal Assoc. **2**(2):90, 1982.

Eilen, B., et al.: Aortic valve replacement in the third trimester of pregnancy: case report and reviews of the literature, Obstet. Gynecol. **57:**119, 1981.

Exrati, J.B., and Gordon, H.: Puerperal mastitis: causes, prevention, and management, J. Nurs. Midwife. **24**(6):3, 1979.

Fadel, H.E., et al.: Minor (glycosylated) hemoglobins in cord blood of infants of normal and diabetic mothers, Am. J. Obstet. Gynecol. **139:**397, 1981.

Fredholm, N.Z.: The insulin pump: new method of insulin delivery, Am. J. Nurs. **81**(11):2024, 1981.

Gabbe, S.G.: Optimal diabetes control = new techniques + physician enthusiasm + patient interest, Contemp. Obstet. Gynecol. **18**(special issue):105, Oct. 1981.

Gleicher, N., et al.: Eisenmenger's syndrome and pregnancy, Obstet. Gynecol. Surv. **34:**721, 1979.

Gorline, L.L., and Stegbauer, C.C.: What every nurse should know about vaginitis, Am. J. Nurs. **82**(12):1851, 1982.

Gothard, J.W.W.: Heart disease in pregnancy: the anesthetic management of a patient with prosthetic heart valves, Anaesthesia **33:**523, 1978.

Hare, J.W.: Diabetes control to reduce congenital malformations, Contemp. Obstet. Gynecol. **20**(2):85, 1982.

Hibbard, L.T.: Maternal mortality due to cardiac disease, Clin. Obstet. Gynecol. **18:**27, 1975.

Kitchener, H.C., et al.: Latency of herpes simplex in uterosacral ligaments, Am. J. Obstet. Gynecol. **143**(7):839, 1982.

Kitzmiller, J.L.: Diabetic ketoacidosis and pregnancy, Contemp. Obstet. Gynecol. **20**(1):140, 1982.

Kivelowitz, T.: Diabetes: a guide to self-management for patients and their families (client handbook), Englewood Cliffs, N.J., 1981, Prentice-Hall, Inc.

Laird-Meeter, K., et al.: Cardiocirculatory adjustments during pregnancy: an echocardiographic study, Clin. Cardiol. **2:**328, 1979.

Lipman, A.G.: Drugs that interfere with urine glucose tests, Mod. Med., p. 195, Aug. 15-Sept. 15, 1978.

Lumley, J., Owen, R., and Morgan, M.: Amniotic fluid embolism, Anaesthesia **34:**33, 1979.

Luta, D.J., et al.: Pregnancy and its complications following cardiac valve prosthesis, Am. J. Obstet. Gynecol. **131:**460, 1978.

Lynch, J.M.: Helping patients through the recurring nightmare of herpes, Nurs. '82, **12**(10):52, 1981.

Moore, D.S., et al.: Nursing care of the pregnant woman with diabetes mellitus, J.O.G.N. Nurs. **10**(3):188, 1981.

National Diabetes Data Group: Classification and diagnosis of diabetes mellitus and other categories of glucose intolerance, Diabetes **28:**1039, 1979.

Nemchik, R.: Diabetes today: the news about insulin (the latest in insulins, plus self-injection tips), R.N. **45**(12):49, 1982.

Nurses Assocation of the American College of Obstetricians and Gynecologists: Care of the infant of the diabetic mother, N.A.A.C.O.G. Tech. Bull., no. 11, Sept. 1981.

Nurses Association of the American College of Obstetricians

and Gynecologists: A sample teaching guide for the pregnant diabetic, N.A.A.C.O.G. O.G.N. Nurs. Pract. Resource, no. 5, Sept. 1981.

Oh, W.: Heading off problems in the diabetic's baby, Contemp. Obstet. Gynecol. **19**(6):91, 1982.

O'Sullivan, J.B.: Gestational diabetes, N. Engl. J. Med. **264:**1082, 1980.

Pass, M.A., et al.: Puerperal and perinatal infections with group B streptococci, Am. J. Obstet. Gynecol. **143**(2):147, 1982.

Pedersen, J.: The pregnant diabetic and her newborn, Baltimore, 1977, Williams & Wilkins Co.

Penticuff, J.H.: Psychologic implications in high-risk pregnancy, Nurs. Clin. North Am. **17**(1):69, 1982.

Plasse, N.J.: Monitoring blood glucose at home: a comparison of three products, Am. J. Nurs. **81**(11):2028, 1981.

Plauche, W.C., et al.: Phosphatidylglycerol and lung maturity, Am. J. Obstet. Gynecol. **144**(2):167, 1982.

Rafferty, E.G.: Chlamydial infection in women, J.O.G.N. Nurs. **10**(4):299, 1981.

Schneider, J.M., et al.: Ambulatory care of the pregnant diabetic, Obstet. Gynecol. **56:**144, 1980.

Stevens, D.: Monitoring blood glucose at home: who should do it and how, Am. J. Nurs. **81**(11):2026, 1981.

Surr. C.W.: Teaching patients to use the new blood-glucose monitoring products, Nurs. '83, **13**(1):42, 1983.

Taguchi, K.: Pregnancy in patients with a prosthetic heart valve, Surg. Gynecol. Obstet. **145:**296, 1977.

Vontver, L.A., et al.: Recurrent genital herpes simplex virus infection in pregnancy: infant outcome and frequency of asymptomatic recurrence, Am. J. Obstet. Gynecol. **143**(1):75, 1982.

Whaley, L.F., and Wong, D.L.: Nursing care of infants and children, ed. 2, St. Louis, 1983, The C.V. Mosby Co.

AIDS

California Nurses Association: UC sets guide on AIDS, Calif. Nurse **79**(2):1, July/August 1983.

Center for Disease Control (CDC): Morbidity and mortality weekly report, Atlanta, March 4 and July 14, 1983.

UCSF Task Force on AIDS: Report available from the office of Merle Sande, M.D., Chief of Medicine, San Francisco General Hospital, 1001 Potrero, Room 5H22, San Francisco, CA 94110.

USPHS AIDS information hotline: 800/342-AIDS.

37

Complications During Birth

- **Dystocia**
  - Definition and classification
  - Pelvic dystocia
    - Inlet contracture
    - Midpelvic contracture
    - Outlet contracture
  - Soft tissue dystocia
  - Dystocia of fetal origin
    - Fetopelvic disproportion
  - Uterine dystocia
    - Primary uterine inertia
    - Secondary uterine inertia
    - Complications of uterine dysfunction
  - Nursing care of dystocia
    - Assessment
    - Examples of nursing diagnoses
    - Plan and implementation
    - Evaluation
  - Therapies for dystocia
    - Trial of labor
    - Stimulation of labor
  - Obstetric operations
    - Episiotomy
    - Forceps delivery
    - Vacuum extraction
- **Cesarean Delivery**
  - Goal
  - Maternal indications
  - Fetal indications
  - Types of cesarean procedures
  - Postmortem cesarean delivery
  - Prognosis after cesarean delivery
  - Nursing care
    - Target population
    - Prenatal period: preparation for cesarean birth
    - Natal period: care in hospital
- **Infant Birth Trauma**
  - Classification of birth traumas
  - Goals for care
    - Soft tissue injuries
    - Skeletal injuries
    - Nervous system injuries
- **Preterm Birth**
  - Prognosis for infants
  - Obstetric management of premature labor
  - Prevention
  - Suppression of uterine activity (labor)
    - Outpatient management
    - In-hospital suppression of preterm labor
  - Pharmacologic stimulation of fetal lung maturity
  - Care during irreversible or acceptable preterm labor and delivery
  - Postpartum care
- **Care of Preterm Infants**
  - Definitions
  - Physiologic basis for problems
  - Nursing care
    - Admission to nursery
    - Classifications
    - Environmental support
    - Transfer from community (hospital or home) to regional neonatal care center
    - Examination for gestational age
    - Nursing actions
  - Complications of prematurity
    - Respiratory distress syndrome
    - Prematurity and oxygen toxicity
    - Neonatal necrotizing enterocolitis
  - Prognosis for preterm infants
    - Base-line examination
    - Favorable evaluative criteria
  - Psychologic aspects of preterm labor and delivery of a preterm infant
    - Child abuse and neglect
    - Baptism
  - Evaluation
- **Multiple Pregnancy**
  - Maternal problems
  - Fetal problems
  - Diagnosis
  - Management
    - Prenatal care
    - Natal care
    - Puerperal care

Fig. 37.1
Labor room. Equipment necessary for high-risk pregnancy: labor bed with side rails, oxygen flowmeter, call bell, blood pressure apparatus on wall behind bed, fetal monitoring equipment to left of bed, intravenous stand and drip meter to right of bed, and stethoscopes on overhead table. Clients and support persons need careful explanation of use of this equipment to reduce anxiety when seeing it for first time.

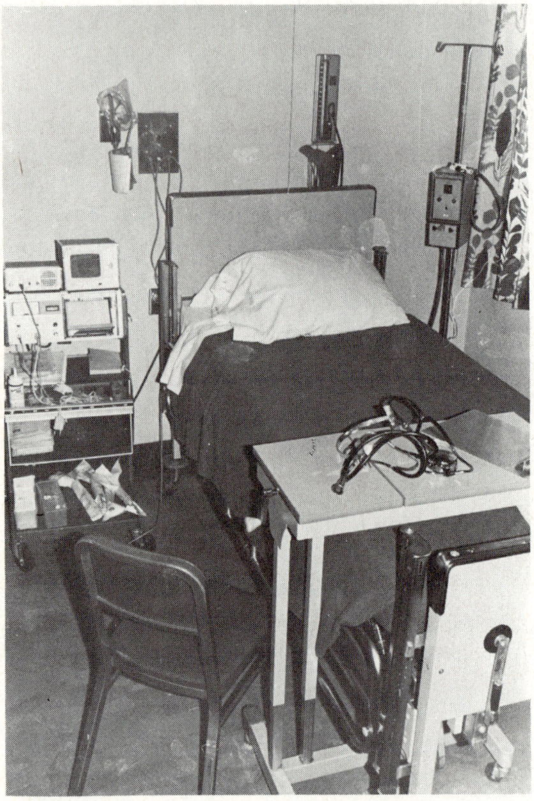

Complications *during the birth period* can cause death or injury to both mother and infant. Prevention and detection of complications and consequent institution of remedial measures require the concerted efforts of the obstetric team. Many of the complications can be diagnosed before the beginning of labor, and preparation can limit their effects. Others arise suddenly; thus only the critical judgment of those present safeguards the mother or infant, and the care afforded the expectant mother through normal labor must be adjusted to meet additional needs (Fig. 37.1).

The complications reviewed in this chapter include dystocia (difficult labor), preterm birth, and multiple birth.

Dystocia

DEFINITION AND CLASSIFICATION

Dystocia may be defined as difficult birth as opposed to easy (normal) birth, or eutocia. Dystocia results from deviations from normal interrelationships between any of the five *P's* of labor (see Chapter 20). The five *P's* are as follows:

1. The passage: the bones and soft tissues of the birth canal
2. The power: the uterine contractions
3. The passenger: the fetus, its size, presentation and position, and anomalies
4. The placenta: position and time and mode of expulsion
5. The psyche: the emotional response of the woman to labor

The interrelationship of these five factors determines the pattern of progress in labor (see Chapter 20).

The differences between dystocia and eutocia relate to changes in the pattern of progress in labor. Changes in the pattern of progress are reflected in the following aspects:

1. Alterations in the characteristics of uterine contractions
2. Lack of progress in effacement or dilatation of the cervix
3. Lack of progress in descent of the presenting part

The classification of dystocia refers to the areas or tissues involved, for example, pelvic dystocia, soft tissue dystocia, fetal dystocia, or uterine dystocia.

PELVIC DYSTOCIA

The size of the pelvis is more important that its architecture as far as the *outcome* of labor is concerned. However, the *mechanism* of labor depends on the configuration of the interior of the pelvis (see Chapter 20).

Pelvic dystocia may occur with significant shortening of one or more of the internal diameters of the bony pelvis. Such diminution in capacity is termed *pelvic contraction* (or *contracture*.)

Pelvic contraction generally is congenital, but malnutrition, neoplasms, pelvic fractures, or disorders of the spine or lower extremities may be responsible. Small pelvic measurements capable of causing dystocia are recorded in at least 15% of women in North America. Racial characteristics may influence the size and architecture of the pelvis greatly; for example, small pelvic measurements are common to the natives of Southeast Asia. The size of the bony pelvis is not complete until maturity, at approximately 20 years of age. Hence young teenagers may have dystocia, whereas several years later normal delivery of similar- or even larger-sized babies may be possible. Disease such as rickets or osteomalacia may cause serious bony deformity and narrowing of pelvic diameters.

Anticipation of possible pelvic dystocia and planning for a delivery, either vaginal or cesarean, that is safest for mother and child are important aspects of prenatal care. An experienced physician can predict accurately by clinical pelvimetry alone the course of labor in about two thirds of women before or early in labor. For the remaining one third the course of labor may differ from what was anticipated earlier. Previous successful performance is no guarantee of safe delivery. A woman who has delivered one or more average-sized babies without difficulty may produce an infant equal in size or larger or smaller who may present abnormally. The head may fail to engage or may arrest deep in the pelvis because of malposition or failure to rotate.

The diagnosis of pelvic *adequacy* generally is easy and accurate; the diagnosis of pelvic *inadequacy* is difficult and inaccurate. The cost of error in both is increased fetal and maternal morbidity and mortality.

The diagnosis of pelvic contraction requires measurement of the major pelvic diameters. Accurate clinical measurement of the bituberous (BT) and posterior sagittal (PS) diameters of the outlet should be obtained at the initial prenatal visit. Other necessary measurements and, perhaps equally important, the architecture of the bony pelvis require examination by radiography or ultrasonography (see Chapter 17).

In the pelvis there are three principal levels or planes of concern: the pelvic inlet, the midpelvis, and the pelvic outlet (see Chapter 20).

Inlet contracture. Inlet contracture occurs in 1% to 2% of pregnant women at term. A contracted pelvic inlet often prevents descent and engagement of the presenting part. Lack of pelvic accommodation of the fetus frequently results in malpresentation or malposition and prolapse of the cord.

The type and degree of pelvic inlet contraction, as determined by pelvic measurements, are the major factors pertaining to the mechanism of labor. The size and moldability of the head, as well as the contractile forces, also are important but less easily determined factors of the process.

Pseudo-overriding of the head above the inlet may be caused by acute flexion of the uterus, a pendulous abdomen, a low-lying placenta, or malpresentation or anomaly of the fetus. Therefore an attempt should be made to impress the presenting part into the pelvis (the DeLee-Hillis maneuver); the physician may allow a trial of labor but probably will order internal pelvimetry.

Midpelvic contracture. Midpelvic contracture is more difficult to recognize than inlet or outlet problems. Midpelvic dystocia occurs three or four times as frequently as inlet contraction. Midpelvic dystocia probably will occur at term with a normal-sized fetus when the midspinous measurement is less than 9 cm (normal, 10 cm) and the PS diameter is less than 4 cm. The physician orders ultrasonographic studies for a women with reduced intraspinous diameter or prominent spines.

Outlet contracture. Because the plane of the outlet is only 3 or 4 cm below the plane of the midpelvis, most women who have midpelvic narrowing have outlet constriction also, the best example being an android, or so-called funnel, pelvis (see Chapter 20). The usual cause of a contracted pelvic outlet is a long, narrow pubic arch. Ideally the subpubic arch should be rounded, low, and wide. This permits the fetal head to utilize the anterior pelvis and to come readily beneath the arch.

SOFT TISSUE DYSTOCIA

Soft tissue dystocia results from obstruction of the birth passage by an anatomic abnormality other than that of the bony pelvis. The causes may be congenital anomalies (e.g., bicornate uterus), tumors (e.g., myomas of the uterus), injury from previous delivery (e.g., healed cervical laceration or conization of cervix may prevent dilatation), pendulous abdomen (e.g., prevents descent of presenting part into pelvic cavity), or infection (e.g., scar tissue from lymphogranuloma venereum may prevent perineal dilatation). Other causes arise during labor. A *full bladder* may fill the pelvic inlet and prevent descent of the presenting part as the cervix dilates. Occasionally, *cervical edema* occurs in labor when the cervix is caught between the presenting part and the symphysis.

DYSTOCIA OF FETAL ORIGIN

Dystocia may be caused by fetal anomalies, excessive size, or malpresentation or malposition of the fetus. Although these conditions are uncommon, they constitute obstetric emergencies.

Fetal dystocia may be classified in accordance with the cause of the abnormality as follows:

1. *Large fetus.* Excessive fetal size is arbitrarily 4000 g (8 lb, 13½ oz) or more in North America. Such large fetuses represent about 5% of term births. Frequently, excessive size is a result of diabetes mellitus, obesity, maternal multiparity, or large size of one or both parents.
2. *Fetal anomaly* (e.g., hydrocephalus, conjoined twins, gross ascites or abdominal tumor, myelomeningocele).
3. *Fetal malpresentation or position* (e.g., breech

presentation, occiput posterior, transverse lie, or shoulder presentation.)

Fetopelvic disproportion. Fetopelvic disproportion caused by excessive size, abnormal development, and unusual presentation or position of the fetus almost always results in nonengagement. In vertex presentations a large head (e.g., hydrocephalus) may never enter the pelvis. The same applies to malpresentation from any fetal cause. In other instances the head or breech may engage, but obstructive labor follows because of gross abdominal enlargement (e.g., polycystic kidneys) or because the after-coming head is large and deformed. The type of arrest will depend on (1) the presentation and the type and degree of fetal deformity and (2) the mother's pelvic architecture and pelvic diameters.

Diagnosis. In fetopelvic dystocia with vertex (head) presentation the problem can usually be suspected within 6 hours of the onset of labor. It is suggested by the following signs:

1. Progress in the first stage is excessively slow.
2. The presenting part remains at a relatively high station and cannot be guided into the pelvis with external pressure.
3. Unusual size or contour of the uterus may be noted with a fetal anomaly.
4. Maternal pelvimetry and fetometry may reveal fetopelvic disproportion, an abnormal lie or position, or fetal skeletal maldevelopment. Soft tissue films or amniography may disclose unusual fetal contours.

Complications

Maternal complications. Frequently, premature rupture of the membranes and slow dilatation of the cervix are caused by the lack of engagement of the presenting part. Prolonged and often obstructed labor may give rise to secondary uterine inertia. Infection may develop. If strong labor persists, rupture of the uterus, perhaps after the development of a pathologic retraction ring, may ensue. Vaginal fistulas occur when impaction of the presenting part persists. Trauma, hemorrhage, and sepsis may occur, especially after attempts at delivery.

Fetal complications. Premature and often prolonged rupture of the membranes may result in amnionitis, omphalitis, placentitis, septicemia, or congenital pneumonia. Prolapse of the umbilical cord will cause hypoxia if occlusion develops. Severe molding of the head, often with excessive overlapping of the bones at the suture lines, may result in intracranial hemorrhage. Difficult forceps delivery can be critically traumatic.

Abnormal fetal presentations and positions. Two fetal presentations or positions are seen with some frequency in obstetric practice.* These are the breech presentation and posterior positions of a vertex presentation (see Figs. 20.7 and 37.5).

Breech presentation. During intranatal life breech presentation poses no hazards to either mother or fetus.

*Other abnormal fetal lies, presentations, and positions are rarely seen (see Chapter 20). The student is referred to appropriate texts.

Fig. 37.2
Types of breech presentation. **A,** Frank breech: thighs are flexed on hips; knees are extended. **B,** Complete breech: thighs and knees are flexed. **C,** Incomplete breech: foot extends below buttocks. **D,** Incomplete breech: knee extends below buttocks.

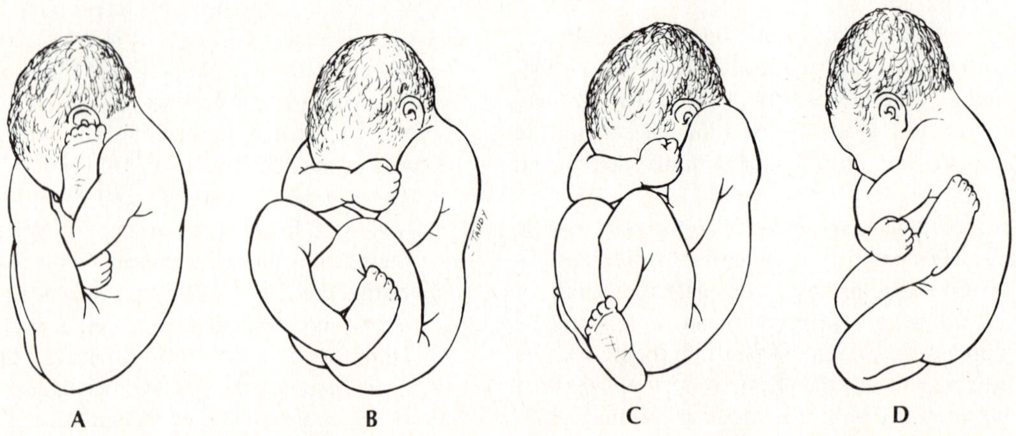

However, *breech delivery* is hazardous, especially for the infant. The fetus and neonate may sustain trauma, asphyxia, and prematurity. An ultraconservative attitude has gradually developed because the gross fetal mortality is 5% to 8% in breech delivery of infants over 2050 g, even in large well-staffed hospitals. Now breech presentation is an indication for cesarean delivery in nulliparas and in multiparas with fetuses larger than 3360 g (7¼ lb) (estimate) when labor is ineffective or when hazardous complications arise.

There are various types of breech presentation depending on the part that presents at delivery (Fig. 37.2). After the 34 weeks of gestation *external cephalic version* may be attempted in an effort to convert the breech to a cephalic presentation (Fig. 37.3). The procedure is preceded by ultrasound to confirm the presentation, to rule out multiple pregnancies, and to localize the placenta. The fetal heart rate (FHR) is monitored frequently, and the procedure is discontinued if FHR abnormalities appear and persist beyond 1 minute. The fetus may revert to a breech presentation even if the version is successful.

The mechanism of breech labor is reviewed in Fig. 37.4. The labor may be prolonged because the presenting part is soft and therefore does not help to dilate the cervix as efficiently.

The breech does not fill the pelvic cavity as completely as does the larger head; therefore *the danger of the cord's prolapsing with rupture of the membranes* is increased. Frank meconium draining from the introitus is a normal finding in breech presentations because the pressure on the fetal abdomen forces the meconium from the bowel. Its appearance thus is not necessarily an indication of fetal distress.

During delivery in cephalic presentation the delivery of the rest of the body follows delivery of the relatively larger head. With breech delivery, the sequence is reversed and the larger head must deliver after the shoulders are born. There is less time for the mechanisms of labor to occur, for example, flexion, rotation, and molding of the infant's skull. As a result the delay in delivery may prove hazardous to the infant, with brain damage or death the result.

The nursing care before delivery is unchanged from that of a vertex presentation because the complications arise as part of the delivery of the infant. However, the FHR is located above the umbilicus (see Fig. 20.24). Parents are more anxious if they are aware of the dangers to the fetus associated with delivery, and they need support from attending nurses and physicians. The use of cesarean delivery as the mode of delivery for questionable fetopelvic disproportion has lessened the fear for infant survival. Mothers in this situation will need the care outlined for cesarean delivery (see p. 895).

Postpartum care of the mother is dictated by the type of delivery. (For cesarean delivery see p. 901 and for

Fig. 37.3
External version of fetus from breech to vertex presentation. This must be achieved without force. **A,** Breech is pushed up out of pelvic inlet while head is pulled toward inlet. **B,** Head is pushed toward inlet while breech is pulled upward.

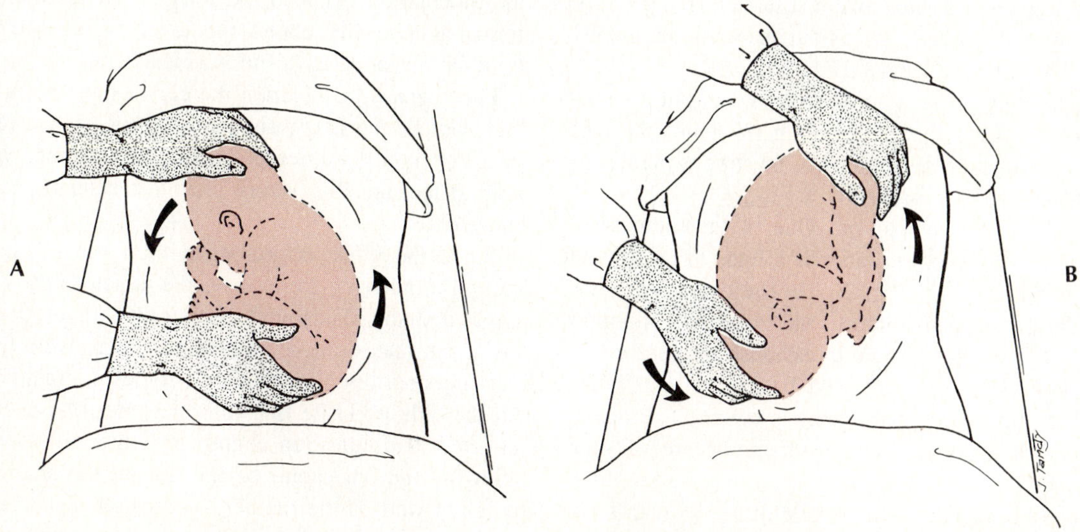

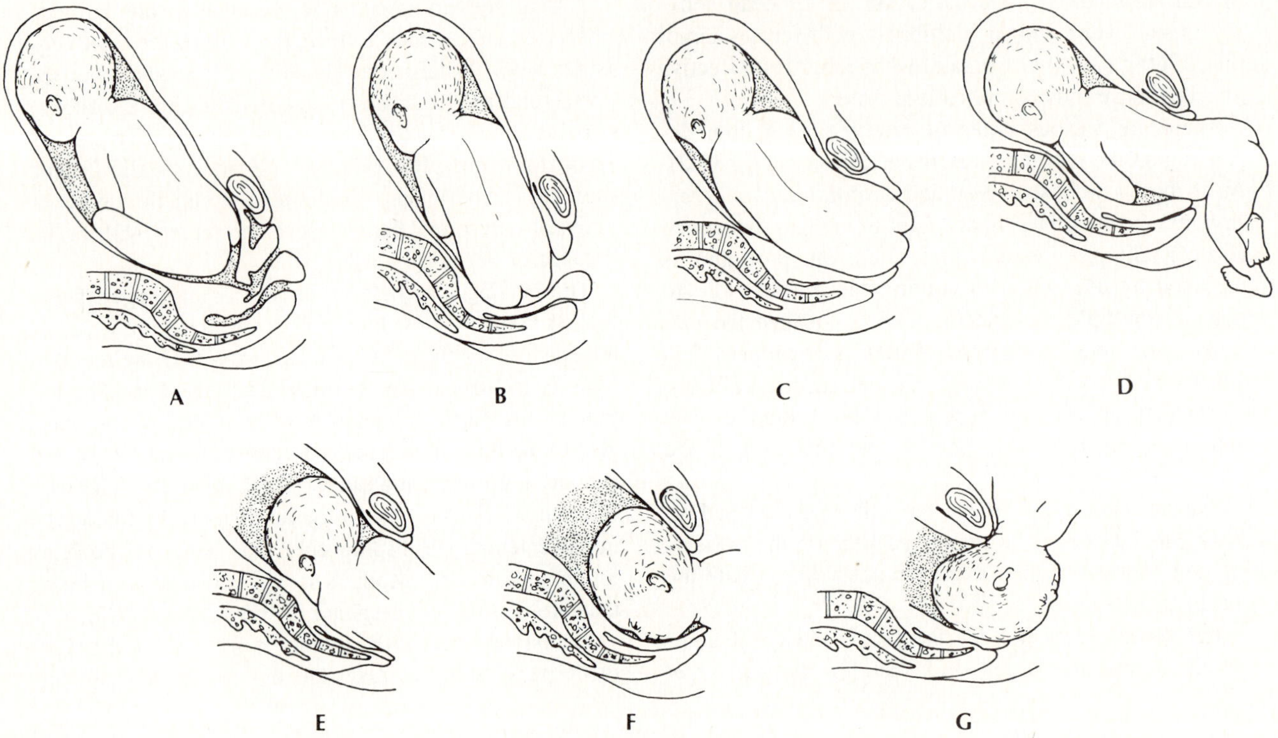

Fig. 37.4
Mechanism of labor in breech position. **A,** Breech before onset of labor. **B,** Engagement and internal rotation. **C,** Lateral flexion. **D,** External rotation or restitution. **E,** Internal rotation of shoulders and head. **F,** Face rotates to sacrum when occiput is anterior. **G,** Head is delivered by gradual flexion during elevation of fetal body.

vaginal delivery see Unit Six.) The care of the infant will be dictated by his gestational age (see p. 915) and whether trauma or hypoxia were sustained (see p. 906). If healthy and at term, the infant is cared for as any normal infant (see Chapters 27 to 30).

The infant has little molding of the head, but his resting posture, being that of a breech (if frank, the legs are straight up over the abdomen), must be explained to the parents (see Fig. 28.39).

Occiput posterior position. One of the more common causes of prolonged labor is a fetus in an occiput posterior position (see Fig. 20.7). The character of the labor, the abdominal contours, and the clinical findings on vaginal examination help to establish the diagnosis.

In labor there is accentuated backache, and in the second stage, gaping of the anus is common. Progress is slower than normal, and contractions are of poor quality.

There is a change in the outline of the woman's *abdomen* in the recumbent position (Fig. 37.5). In occiput posterior positions the contour from umbilicus to symphysis has a regular convexity. In posterior positions the indentation between the fetal chin and small parts forms a concavity above the level of the symphysis (may be obscured by a full bladder).

For *vaginal examination* the cervix must be fully dilated before the diagnosis can be made. If the fetus is in an occiput posterior position, the examiner will be able to feel the four suture lines that enter the anterior fontanel.

Since the *labor* is prolonged the woman will need careful monitoring for fatigue, the judicious use of sedatives and analgesics, and assessment of hydration. The physician may order an induction if there is no fetopelvic disproportion. The mother assumes a Sim's position on the side opposite that to which the fetal occiput is directed. This position encourages anterior rotation by allowing the fetal spine to fall toward the anterior abdominal wall of the mother. The hands and knees position (see p. 411) also encourages this rotation.

Fig. 37.5
Comparison of abdominal contours with fetus in, **A,** occiput anterior position and, **B,** occiput posterior position.

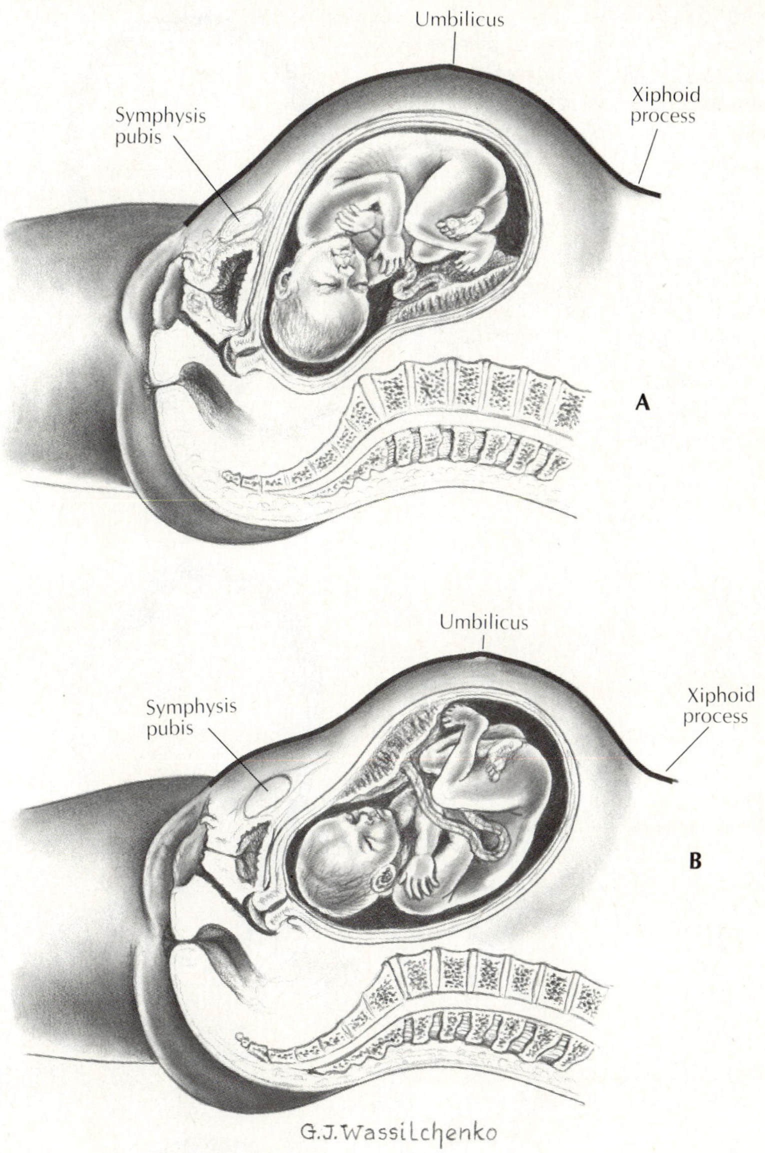

Approximately 70% of fetuses in the occiput posterior position rotate spontaneously to an anterior position, and therefore *delivery* is the same as for any occiput anterior position. If the posterior position persists, some infants may deliver in the face to pubes position. Others may be rotated either manually or with forceps to an anterior position.

UTERINE DYSTOCIA

Uterine dystocia or dysfunction is defined as an abnormality of the contractile pattern of the uterine muscles that prevents normal progress in labor. The uterine contractions may be too weak, too short, irregular, or infrequent (Fig. 37.6). Hence progressive cervical dilatation and effacement and descent of the presenting part do not occur.

Uterine dysfunction complicates almost 5% of all labors at term, and about 90% of the women are nulliparas. It is classified as follows:

1. Primary uterine inertia: inefficient contractions persist from the onset of labor.
2. Secondary uterine inertia: well-established, efficient contractions become weak and inefficient or stop altogether.

Primary uterine inertia. In primary uterine inertia, inefficient contractions persist from the onset of labor. The latent phase of the first stage of labor is usually prolonged, but inefficient contractions may continue

Fig. 37.6
Normal and dysfunctional uterine contraction types. *Black area,* strong contraction; *shaded area,* slight contraction; *white area,* atonic areas.

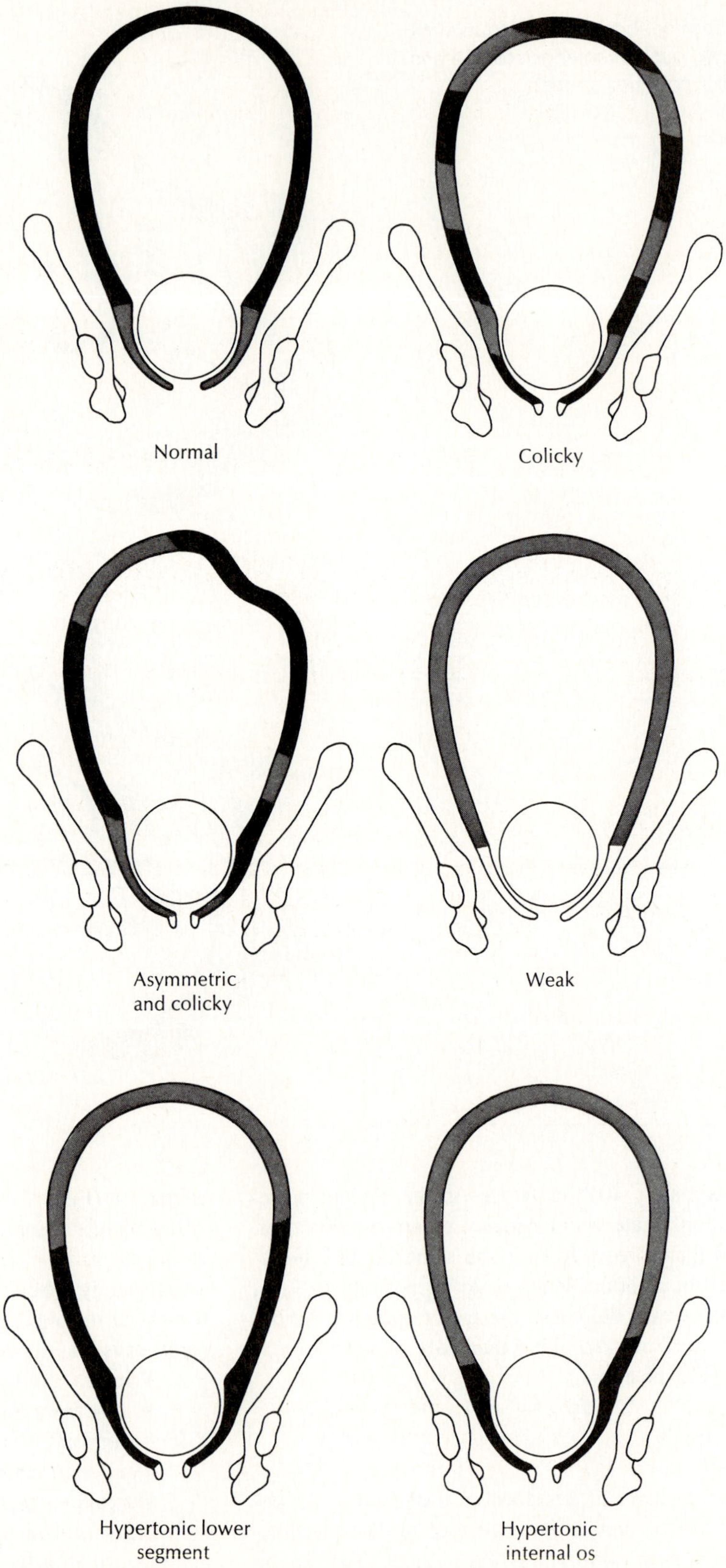

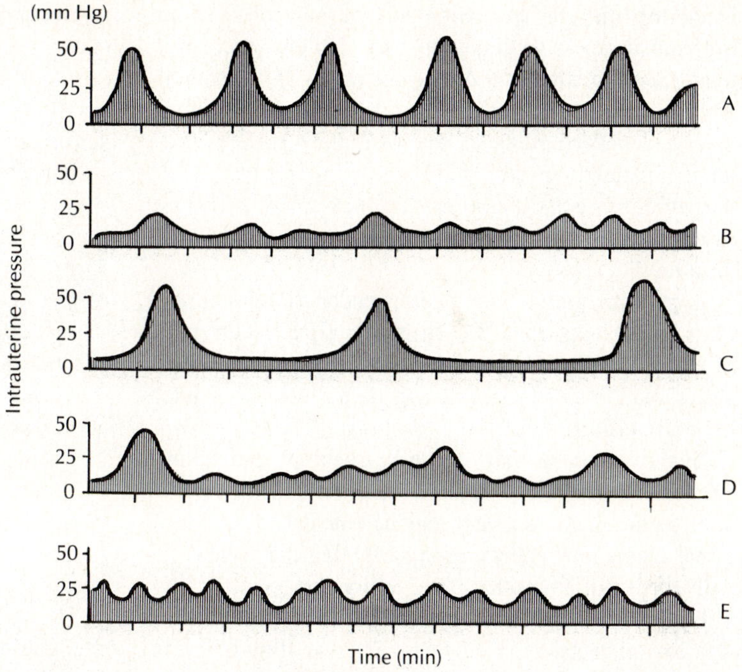

Fig. 37.7
Uterine contractility patterns in labor. **A,** Typical normal labor **B,** Subnormal intensity, with frequency greater than needed for optimal performance. **C,** Normal contractions, but too infrequent for efficient labor. **D,** Incoordinate activity. **E,** Hypercontractility.

into and even through the subsequent stages of labor (Fig. 37.7).

The normal pattern of uterine contractions is as follows:

1. Contractions are initiated simultaneously and bilaterally near each uterine horn.
2. They spread toward the center and downward to the cervix.
3. They increase in intensity, with maximal intensity first in the fundus, next in the midsection, and then in the lower uterine segment.

This pattern may be defined as two simultaneous contractions in each longitudinal half of the uterus, acting in a peristaltic manner and progressing toward the cervix.

Inefficient uterine contractions may be characterized as hypertonic, hypotonic, or dystonic (Figs. 37.6 and 37.7).

1. *Hypertonic*. Contractions are excessive in intensity and duration, with a diminished interval between contractions (least common problem).
2. *Hypotonic*. Contractions are weaker than normal and ineffective (most common problem).
3. *Dystonic*. Contractions are asymmetric or there is reverse peristalsis: contractions are painful but ineffective—very common in prelabor; associated with a tense, anxious, usually nulliparous woman, *or* a woman with a constriction ring dystocia (Fig. 20.21, *E*): the uterus contracts in segments and stays contracted almost continuously.

Although the periodic uterine contractions are of special significance, the resting tone or degree of uterine relaxation between contractions also is of great importance (normal = 8 to 15 mm Hg). When strong contractions are noted but with poor relaxation between them, the pattern is hypertonic. Moreover, a uterus that is flaccid between contractions rarely contracts strongly. Here the pattern is hypotonic. Occasionally the nurse encounters a woman whose uterus contracts irregularly, with one portion of the corpus more firm than the opposite side, for example. This is a dystonic pattern. Each of these abnormal sequences is inefficient, and if persistent, dystocia will result.

Occasionally, general irritability of the uterus results in numerous ectopic contractions (colicky uterus). These dysrhythmic uterine contractions are not productive, and progress of labor is poor.

Hypertonic uterine contractions are extremely painful. Normally a labor contraction is initiated in the myometrium near one cornu. It spreads rapidly over the uterus and to the lower segment, which has a low resting tone and is poorly contractile. In hypertonic uterine dystocia, the contractions may begin in the lower uterine segment and from there may spread upward (reverse polarity). If they are caused by reverse polarity, uterine discomfort and low backache are reported before the observer can palpate a contraction. Moreover, uterine irritability may be apparent, and one may observe an irregular firmness to the uterus as it tightens. Increased tone often prevails even during the phase of relaxation. Another type of hypertonic uterine contraction pattern involves well-coordinated but extremely strong, prolonged contractions with good relaxation between them. *A hypertonic contraction pattern may develop during oxytocic stimulation of labor*. Fetal and maternal distress may develop.

Hypertonic uterine contractions endanger mother and fetus because of their violence and rapid recurrence. Moreover, if there is reverse polarity, the lack of uterine relaxation also reduces placental perfusion and fetal hypoxia results.

Hypertonic labor may terminate in abrupt, precipitate delivery. Unless this eventuality is anticipated and preparations are made, delivery may be unattended, and maternal lacerations and excessive bleeding may result. If delivery is not controlled, fetal injury may occur.

Hypertonic uterine dysfunction demands heavy sedation and expectant management. Uterine stimulation is absolutely contraindicated. After morphine, 15 mg intramuscularly, and glucose, 5% to 10% solution intravenously, are given, tumultuous or dystonic labor usually will subside. After a period of sleep, a more normal pattern of labor may evolve.

Hypotonic uterine contractions display a normal gradient from each uterine horn to fundus to cervix, but the contractions are weak, brief, or irregular. Severe pain is not a problem, and fetal distress is rare.

Hypotonic uterine dystocia occurs in the following conditions:

1. False labor or the prodromal stage of true labor
2. Multiple pregnancy or hydramnios (uterine wall thinned or overstretched)
3. Missed or delayed labor, often after fetal death (altered hormonal status?)
4. Uterine abnormality (scarring, tumor anomaly)
5. Excessive analgesia (uterine contractions dulled)
6. High anxiety levels

Hypotonic and dystonic uterine dysfunction often recurs in subsequent labors.

Brief, weak (hypotonic) contractions may indicate, in some cases, that the woman is not yet in true labor or that she is only in the prodromal stage of labor. Mild sedation, for example, using phenobarbital (3 grains or 200 mg intramuscularly) or equivalent, may permit a period of rest after which a normal pattern of labor can be established.

In other cases ineffectual contractions may be the result of inanition (a pathologic state of the body resulting from lack of food and water) from debilitating systemic disease. Occasionally, after fetal death, labor may be ineffectual, presumably because of hormonal deficiencies.

Hypotonic uterine contractions increase the likelihood of the woman's experiencing prolonged labor, sepsis, and the need for operative intervention.

Secondary uterine inertia. Secondary uterine inertia results when well-established, effective uterine contractions become weak or brief or cease altogether (Fig. 37.8). Secondary uterine inertia may occur as a result of one of the following:

- Fetopelvic disproportion (e.g., contracted pelvis)
- Excessive analgesia or anesthesia (e.g., epidural block)
- Overdistention of the uterus (e.g., multiple pregnancy)
- Maternal exhaustion or extreme emotional tension

Although secondary inertia may be serious in one pregnancy, it need not recur in a subsequent normal gestation.

The treatment of secondary uterine inertia depends on the cause. Ultrasonographic or radiographic studies must be obtained to rule out disproportion. Overdistention of the uterus may be relieved by rupture of the membranes, provided the cervix is dilated at least 3 to 4 cm and the presenting part is at least beginning to engage. The effects of excessive analgesia-anesthesia will dissipate with time. Heavy sedation (sleep) restores the tense or tired mother.

Oxytocic stimulation of labor, after assurance of no obstructive pathosis and resolution of temporary difficulties, is in order. If, after a reasonable time, vaginal delivery seems unlikely or unduly hazardous, cesarean birth must be accomplished. Generally a low cervical cesarean delivery is most appropriate.

Complications of uterine dysfunction. The development of amnionitis is directly related to the length of labor and is more rapid and severe after rupture of the membranes. The incidence of instrument delivery is also increased in uterine inertia. If uterine atony complicates the third stage of labor, postdelivery hemorrhage may further jeopardize the mother.

A serious complication of neglected obstructed labor is the development of annular uterine strictures. In normal labor the cervix and the rather passive lower uterine segment are drawn upward by the strongly contracting uterine fundus. The juncture between the two segments blends evenly. With neglected obstructed labor, however, a narrow, depressed *pathologic retraction ring (Bandl's ring)* develops and rises as labor wears on (see Fig. 20.21, *E*). Bandl's ring, which holds the fetus in a powerful grip even with anesthesia, is a sign of impending uterine rupture, and fetal distress often is recorded.

Fig. 37.8

A, A partogram is a normal graphic appraisal of time factor in labor for primigravida. *Latent phase* includes that portion of first stage between onset of labor contractions and acceleration in rate of cervical dilatation. Upswing in curve denotes onset of *active phase* of first stage of labor, which includes *acceleration phase, phase of maximal slope,* and *deceleration phase.* Compare with **B, C,** and **D. B,** Partogram of primigravida with prolonged latent phase of labor. *S,* sedation; *P,* Pitocin; *A,* amniotomy. **C,** Partogram of primigravida with dysfunctional latent phase of labor and slow slope in active phase of labor. **D,** Anxious primigravida with tense, restless latent phase of labor. (Modified from Friedman, E.A.: Bull. Sloane Hosp. Wom. **1:**42, 1955.)

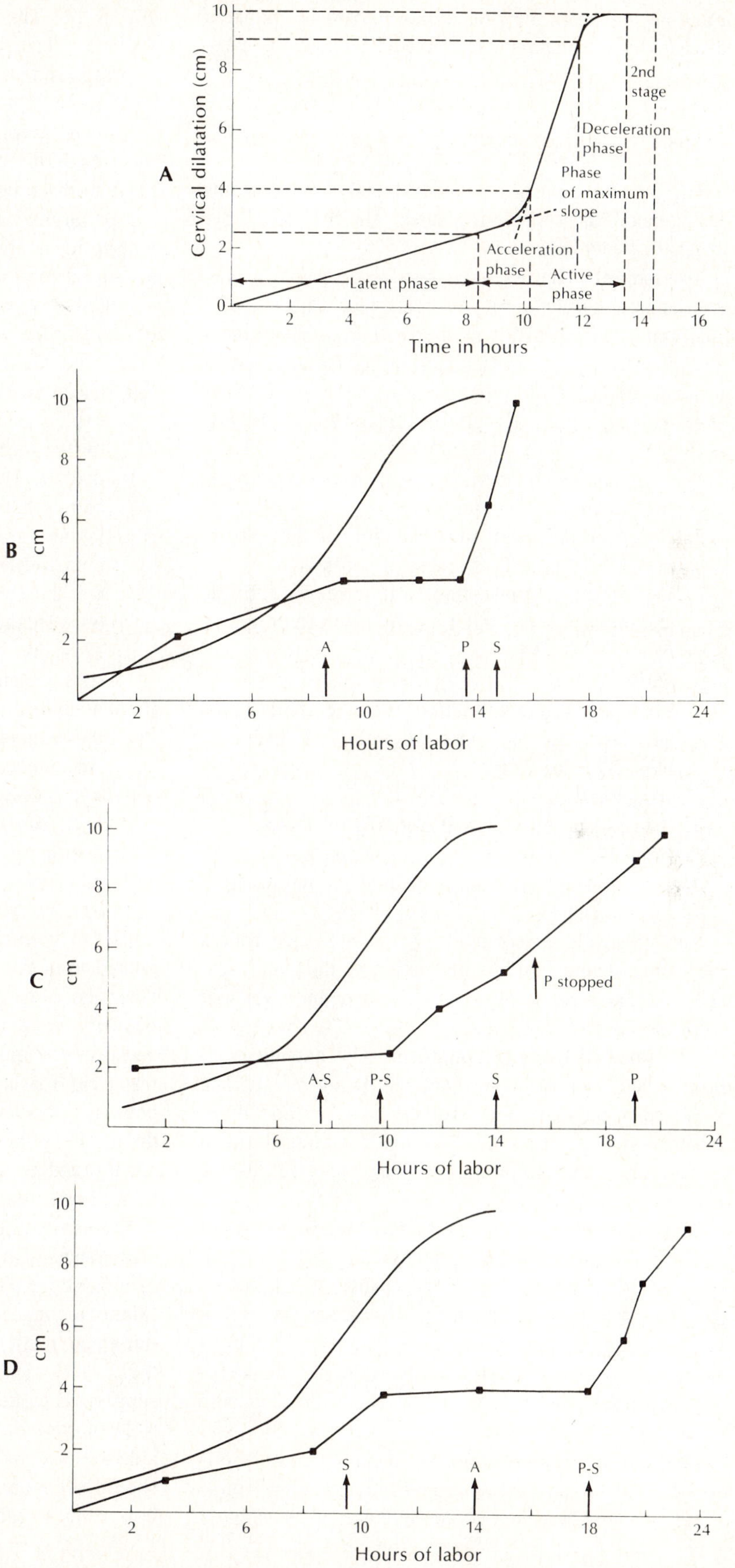

Bandl's ring may be felt from above if the woman is thin, but generally the ring is too high to be palpated vaginally. The treatment is immediate cesarean delivery.

NURSING CARE OF DYSTOCIA

The care of a woman with dystocial labor contains both general and specific measures. The following care is *generally* applicable.

Assessment. The assessment strategies used in normal labor are used during dystocia (see Chapter 21). Electronic monitoring of mother and fetus is initiated (see Chapter 24), and other monitoring is increased in amount, for example, the client-nurse ratio is 1:1. There is a systematic appraisal and recording of the following:

1. Contractions and their character, intrauterine pressure, relaxation interval
2. Cervix: effacement and dilatation of the cervix; presence of edema; firmness or softness
3. Descent of the presenting part: correlate with dilatation of cervix and time in labor (partogram) (see Fig. 21.4)
4. FHR
5. Membranes: intact, bulging; ruptured character of amniotic fluid, evidence of prolapsed cord (see Figs. 21.6 to 21.8)
6. Intake and output
7. Nutritional and fluid and electrolyte balance
8. Need for pain relief
9. Degree of exhaustion, including circumoral pallor, sunken eyes, and listless response

The nurse also systematically assesses and records the woman's and family's perception of the event (crisis) and the amount of support needed and available from the family.

Examples of nursing diagnoses. The nursing diagnosis related to maternal or fetal well-being will include those common to normal progress in labor and those arising as a result of the systematic appraisal noted above. The nurse may establish diagnoses such as the following:

1. Fearfulness for baby's safety because of labor prolonged beyond expectations
2. Alterations in self-concept because of inability to control unexpected changes in labor pattern or sensations (pain, pressure)

Such diagnoses can serve as the rationale for adapting a general plan of care to the needs of a specific client.

Plan and implementation. Dystocia represents a crisis in medical and nursing management. The nurse needs to plan for increased surveillance of the client's physical progress and for initiation of support measures (Fig. 37.9). The nurse works closely with the attending physician. The physician needs to be kept informed of progress, and the recording of information exchanged needs to be kept up-to-date. The woman and her family need to be prepared for any examination or tests. The nurse deals directly with the woman's problems in relation to the following areas:

1. *Prolonged labor*. Most women and families have definite ideas about how long the labor process should be. Any deviation in length causes anxiety levels to rise and doubts as to attending staff's interest and ability and as to their own capacity to cope. Nursing actions should include the following:

   a. Clear and repeated descriptions of progress and explanations for delay: "The baby's head needs to flex more on the chest [demonstrate on self] so that the head can fit through the pelvis." "The baby's head needs to turn from the side position [sutures transverse] until he is facing to the back; then the head can come down, and the back of the neck can come under the pubic bone" [show on woman].
   b. Provision of comfort measures (e.g., bath, back rubs, change in position, cool cloth to forehead, breathing and relaxation instructions). Stay with the woman; do not abandon her.
   c. Acceptance of the woman's frustration and hostility: "Yes, I know it's hard to take." "I'll try a back rub—tell me if it helps a little." "If the doctor gives medication now, it will slow up the labor even more."

2. *Unexpected pain sensations*. The uterine contractions can give rise to colicky, sharp pains if they are related to uterine dystocia. The contractions of induced labor are often more painful because they increase in intensity more rapidly, maintain acme (peak) longer, and decrease rapidly. Women often say, "It hits me so fast I can't control it." Low back pain is increased in posterior positions of the fetal head. The hard back of the head (occiput) is forced against the soft tissue of the sacrum and compresses the sensitive tissue against the sacral bone, thus intensifying pain.

Women who have attended preparation-for-childbirth classes and who want to control their responses to pain or experience a drug-free labor can develop feelings of failure or anger because of conflict between expectations and reality. (Some men become disappointed in their wives' inability to cope and can turn from being supportive to being actively hostile.) The nurse needs to keep complimenting the woman on any effort she is able to make and help her with coaching. Also, the staff should offer analgesia or anesthesia or both as though it were an expected result of a change in labor pattern

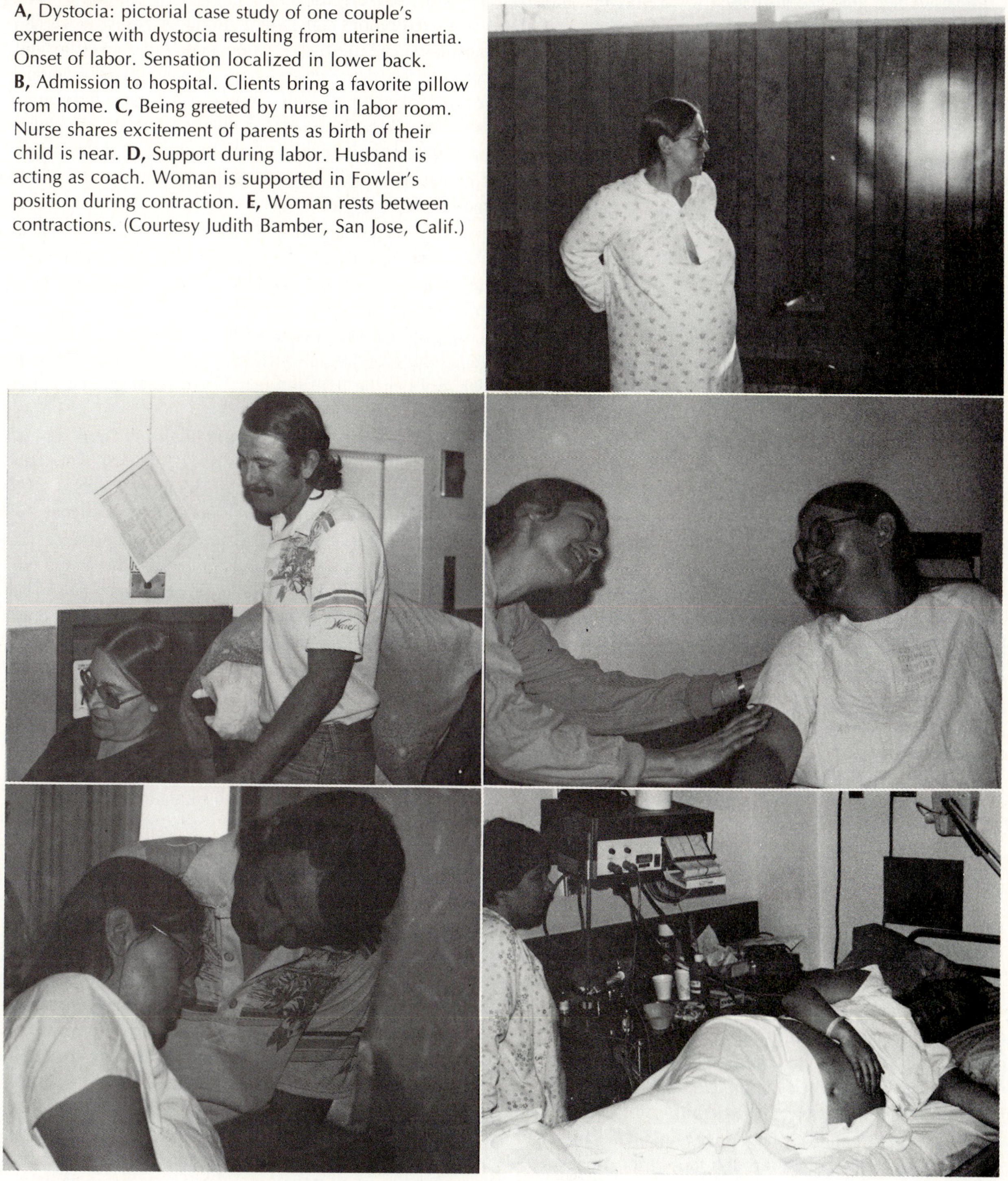

Fig. 37.9

A, Dystocia: pictorial case study of one couple's experience with dystocia resulting from uterine inertia. Onset of labor. Sensation localized in lower back. **B,** Admission to hospital. Clients bring a favorite pillow from home. **C,** Being greeted by nurse in labor room. Nurse shares excitement of parents as birth of their child is near. **D,** Support during labor. Husband is acting as coach. Woman is supported in Fowler's position during contraction. **E,** Woman rests between contractions. (Courtesy Judith Bamber, San Jose, Calif.)

and openly discuss what this may mean to the woman: "Some women are very distressed when they feel more pain than expected; they feel somehow they have failed."

3. *Fear for her own or baby's safety*. A frank but brief discussion of what the operative procedures entail should be given.

From a psychologic standpoint, surgery is a stressful situation wherein the woman fears a combination of three major imminent dangers: (1) possibility of suffering acute pain, (2) possibility of undergoing serious bodily damage, and (3) possibility of death. Since presurgical anxiety is rooted in fear of the unknown, relief from this anxiety may stem in part from information given as part of supportive care. The emergency nature of some conditions precludes any but the physical priorities of care, and this situation needs to be recognized. One nurse described such a situation: "As I was wheeling her down the corridor to the OR, I said, 'I can't explain much just now but tomorrow I'll come up and go over all the things we've been doing so you'll understand.' "

The nurse can use gentle touch, soft voice tones, attention to details, and explanations to convey caring and concern while carrying out procedures. The woman and family expect competent and efficient care.

There is no way to guarantee the infant's safety, and the nurse should indicate acceptance of parental concern: "I can appreciate how worried you must be." Again, the nurse's tone of voice and attitude convey the sincerity of her feelings to the woman and family.

Evaluation. The nurse evaluates the care given with respect to the following evaluative criteria:

1. Prompt detection of abnormal progress in labor permits diagnosis of the difficulty and the institution of remedial therapy.
2. Personnel utilize acceptable techniques to maintain the health of the mother and fetus (e.g., fluid and electrolyte balance is maintained; relaxation therapy, oxygen therapy, and positioning of the woman are used judiciously).
3. The woman and family accept the need for change from the expected labor pattern and outcome as being beyond their control.
4. The infant survives birth with no adverse sequelae, *or* if the death of the infant occurs, the family is supported through their grief process.

THERAPIES FOR DYSTOCIA

Many factors in modern maternity care continue to increase the margin of safety and comfort for both the mother and the infant. Improved methods for monitoring and assessing fetomaternal well-being have contributed to more effective prevention and treatment of the medical and surgical complications of childbirth. The use of antibiotics and blood products has reduced the morbidity and mortality associated with infection and hemorrhage. The judicious use of prostaglandins or injectable oxytocin for the stimulation or augmentation of labor has been lifesaving at times. Preventive surgical procedures (episiotomy, forceps delivery, and birth by cesarean delivery) have helped reduce the risk to the mother and the infant.

Some procedures in operative obstetrics are complicated, whereas others are so frequently used as to make them adjuncts or aids to normal delivery. Episiotomy and forceps delivery are included in such a category. Cesarean delivery is used with increasing frequency because the problems that signal the need for nonvaginal delivery can be detected earlier and with greater accuracy.

Trial of labor. If the fetus is clinically large and at term or past due or the mother has a "questionable pelvis," x-ray pelvimetry and fetal sonography are used to assess the possibility of a vaginal delivery. If there is no demonstrable fetopelvic disproportion and the cervix is soft and dilatable, a *trial of labor* may be instituted. A trial of labor is a reasonable period (4 to 6 hours) of good labor; that is, in conjunction with adequate contractions there is engagement and descent of the presenting part and progressive effacement and dilatation of the cervix. During this period it is essential to assess carefully the following:

- Strength, frequency, and character of uterine contractions
- Progressive effacement and dilatation of cervix
- Descent of head
- Fetal well-being

Trial of labor is seldom induced artificially. Once spontaneous labor has begun, heavy analgesia is avoided because it slows progress. Membranes are ruptured only when the cervix nears complete dilatation. If advancement of the fetal head fails to occur within 4 to 6 hours of strong labor (or 6 to 8 hours of moderate labor), cesarean delivery or repeat cesarean delivery is indicated. Any signs of significant maternal or fetal distress also make a cesarean birth mandatory.

Stimulation of labor

Prostaglandin. A prostaglandin gel for local application to the cervix has been formulated. The gel is used to soften or prime the cervix and induce labor. The cervix is assessed using the Bishop score (Table 37.1). For those women whose cervix is unfavorable, induction using prostaglandins is more efficient than using oxytocin.

Procedure. The client is admitted to the labor suite, and routine assessments are completed. The dilatation

Table 37.1
Bishop's Scale for Assessing Candidates for Induction of Labor

	Score*				
	0	**1**	**2**	**3**	**Subtotals**
Dilatation (cm)	0	1-2	3-4	5-6	
Effacement (%)	0-30	40-50	60-70	80	
Station (cm)	−3	−2	−1	+1	
Cervical consistency	Firm	Medium	Soft		
Fetal position	Posterior	Midline	Anterior		
				TOTAL	

*Parous woman can be induced at score of 5; nulliparous woman, at score of 7.

and effacement of the cervix are determined. A Bishop score of 5 or less is required. A 30-min electronic monitoring of the FHR and uterine contractions is done to establish base-line data. The physician instills 0.5 mg of PGE_2 gel intracervically using a plastic catheter. The catheter is then removed. The woman remains in bed for 30 minutes; then she may ambulate. The FHR, blood pressure, and pulse are monitored at least every 30 minutes. Ideally the monitoring is done electronically. Contractions usually begin a half hour after administration of the gel. The time of the beginning of contractions is recorded. An amniotomy is performed at 4 cm cervical dilatation, and internal fetal monitoring is applied. Progress of labor is then recorded as for other clients.

The local application of prostaglandins appears to minimize side effects. Any hypertonic contractions of the uterus are reported immediately. If the woman does not deliver within 24 hours, the cervix is reassessed using the Bishop score and an induction using oxytocin is done if indicated.

Oxytocin. Oxytocic stimulation of labor may be used either to induce the labor process or to augment a labor that is progressing slowly because of inadequate uterine contractions; it can also be used to assess fetal response to the stress of labor contractions (oxytocin challenge test [OCT]; see Chapter 24).

The indications for induction of labor include the following:

1. Slowing of progress of labor.
2. Management of abortion, to stimulate the uterus to pass the conceptus
3. Prolonged rupture of the membranes
4. Prolonged pregnancy (42 to 43 weeks)
5. Preterm delivery in diabetic mother or infant with severe isoimmunization
6. Severe preeclampsia, abruptio placentae, or fetal death necessitating termination of the pregnancy artificially
7. Multigravidas with a history of precipitate labor who live a long distance from the hospital

The management of stimulation of labor is the same regardless of indication. Because of the potential dangers associated with the use of injectable oxytocin in the prenatal and natal periods, the Food and Drug Administration has issued new restrictions on its use (FDA Drug Bulletin, 1978).

Contraindications. Contraindications to oxytocic stimulation of labor include the following:

1. Fetopelvic disproportion
2. Fetal distress
3. Previous uterine surgery (e.g., cesarean birth)
4. Overdistended uterus (hydramnios, multiple birth)
5. Grand multiparity (over four)

Hazards. The hazards to the mother include the following:

1. Tumultuous labor and tetanic contractions: may cause premature separation of placenta, rupture of uterus, laceration of cervix, or postdelivery hemorrhage
2. Sequelae to no. 1 above: complications of infection, disseminated intravascular coagulation (DIC), amniotic fluid embolism
3. Fear or anxiety: may be compounded if procedure is not successful (the woman must be aware of this possibility of what other techniques can be used)

The hazards to the fetus include fetal and neonatal hypoxia, physical injury, or prematurity if the estimated date of confinement (EDC) has been estimated inaccurately.

Procedure. The responsibility for initiating oxytocin stimulation of labor belongs to the physician, although the procedure is often administered by the nurse. The physician must determine the correct amount of oxytocin to be added to the infusion bottle, together with the number of drops per minute that will deliver a specific oxytocin dose in milliunits (mU) per minute (Table

Table 37.2
Oxytocin Administration

Drops per Minute (gtt/min)	10 Units Oxytocin in 1000 ml Fluid (mU/min)	5 Units Oxytocin in 1000 ml Fluid (mU/min)
15 gtt/ml tubing		
15	10.00	5.00
14	9.33	4.67
13	8.67	4.33
12	8.00	4.00
11	7.33	3.67
10	6.67	3.33
9	6.00	3.00
8	5.33	2.67
7	4.67	2.33
6	4.00	2.00
5	3.33	1.67
4	2.67	1.33
3	2.00	1.00
2	1.33	0.67
1	0.66	0.33
10 gtt/ml tubing		
10	10	5.0
9	9	4.5
8	8	4.0
7	7	3.5
6	6	3.0
5	5	2.5
4	4	2.0
3	3	1.5
2	2	1.0
1	1	0.5

From Tucker, S.M.: Fetal monitoring and fetal assessment in high-risk pregnancy, St. Louis, 1978, The C.V. Mosby Co.

37.2). Natural oxytocin (Pitocin) or synthetic oxytocin (Syntocinon) is added to an intravenous infusion of 5% dextrose in water. The usual dose is 10 units/1000 ml of 5% dextrose in water. A piggyback setup with 500 ml of 5% dextrose in water is used so that the induction solution can be stopped and the vein kept open with the second solution. An infusion pump (IVAC) or standard pump (Harvard) is used.

The induction is begun at 1 mU/min, and the dose is increased arithmetically by 2-mU increments (e.g., 1, 3, and 5 mU/min) at 15-min intervals. When the intensity of contractions results in intrauterine pressures of 50 to 75 mm Hg (by internal monitor) or lasts 40 to 60 seconds (by external monitor) and contractions occur at 2½- to 4-min intervals, the oxytocin dose should not be increased. If fetal monitors are available, they are used during induction of labor. If they are not available, the FHR is assessed using a fetoscope every hour until contractions begin and then every 15 minutes.

If excessive uterine contractions occur (intrauterine pressure above 75 mm Hg, over 60 seconds' duration, or more often than every 2 or 3 minutes) or if there is fetal bradycardia, tachycardia, or heart irregularity, the oxytocin is stopped and the 5% dextrose in water is infused.

Continuous and careful assessment is necessary to safeguard mother and fetus because uterine rupture, placental separation, and fetal asphyxia may result from too frequent and prolonged uterine contractions. Magnesium sulfate (1 to 2 g intravenously, slowly) may be given for oxytocin-induced uterine tetany (see p. 815) for precautions for administering magnesium sulfate). Record the time the contractions begin or intensify, and then record the time of contractions concomitantly with assessment.

Nursing care. The following nursing care specific to induction of labor is added to the general care of the woman with dystocia (Fig. 37.10, *A*). The nurse (1) applies the fetal monitor for constant, accurate recording of FHR and contractions (A base-line reading is obtained before induction is begun [see Chapter 24]); (2) prepares the woman and her family by explaining the technique and rationale and by describing how the contractions can differ from expected ones; (3) positions the woman in a left lateral position; (4) prepares the solutions and administers according to prescribed orders with a pump delivery system; and (5) makes preparations for emergency delivery, vaginal or cesarean. The nurse monitors and records the following:

1. FHR: If signs of stress appear, change drip from oxytocin to plain solution and report immediately to physician.
2. Contractions
   a. Monitor every contraction. When regular, forceful contractions begin, turn off oxytocin drip and administer plain solution slowly.
   b. If hypertonic contractions occur, change drip from oxytocin to plain solution and report immediately to the physician.
3. Signs of complications (e.g., boardlike abdomen) are reported immediately to the physician. Turn off oxytocin drip and administer 5% dextrose in water solution slowly.

The woman and her family are kept aware of progress. The physician apprises the family of the chances of success; that is, if inertia is not overcome in 8 hours (5 units of oxytocin) or less, the chance of success is minimal.

Transcervical amniotomy or artificial rupture of membranes. For stimulation of labor by transcervical amniotomy or artificial rupture of the membranes (ARM), the cervix should be soft, partially effaced, and slightly dilated, preferably with the presenting part engaged or engaging. Simple rupture of the membranes using a

Fig. 37.10

A, Oxytocic stimulation of labor. Decision to stimulate labor has been made. Couple discusses change in plans. Note intravenous setup. A red flash label alerts personnel to bag containing oxytocic. **B,** Induction continues. Nurse assesses client: vital signs are checked. **C,** No progress in dilatation of cervix is discernible. Husband shares weariness of his wife. **D,** Nurse assesses fetal monitor. Husband supports his wife. **E,** Decision has been made to deliver infant by cesarean birth. Parents wait for transfer of mother to operating room. Indwelling catheter has been inserted; note catheter over leg. Scar on woman's abdomen is old appendectomy scar. (Courtesy Judith Bamber, San Jose, Calif.)

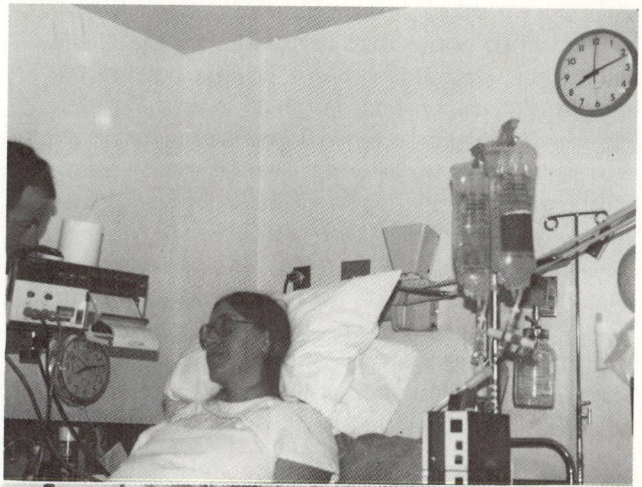

A

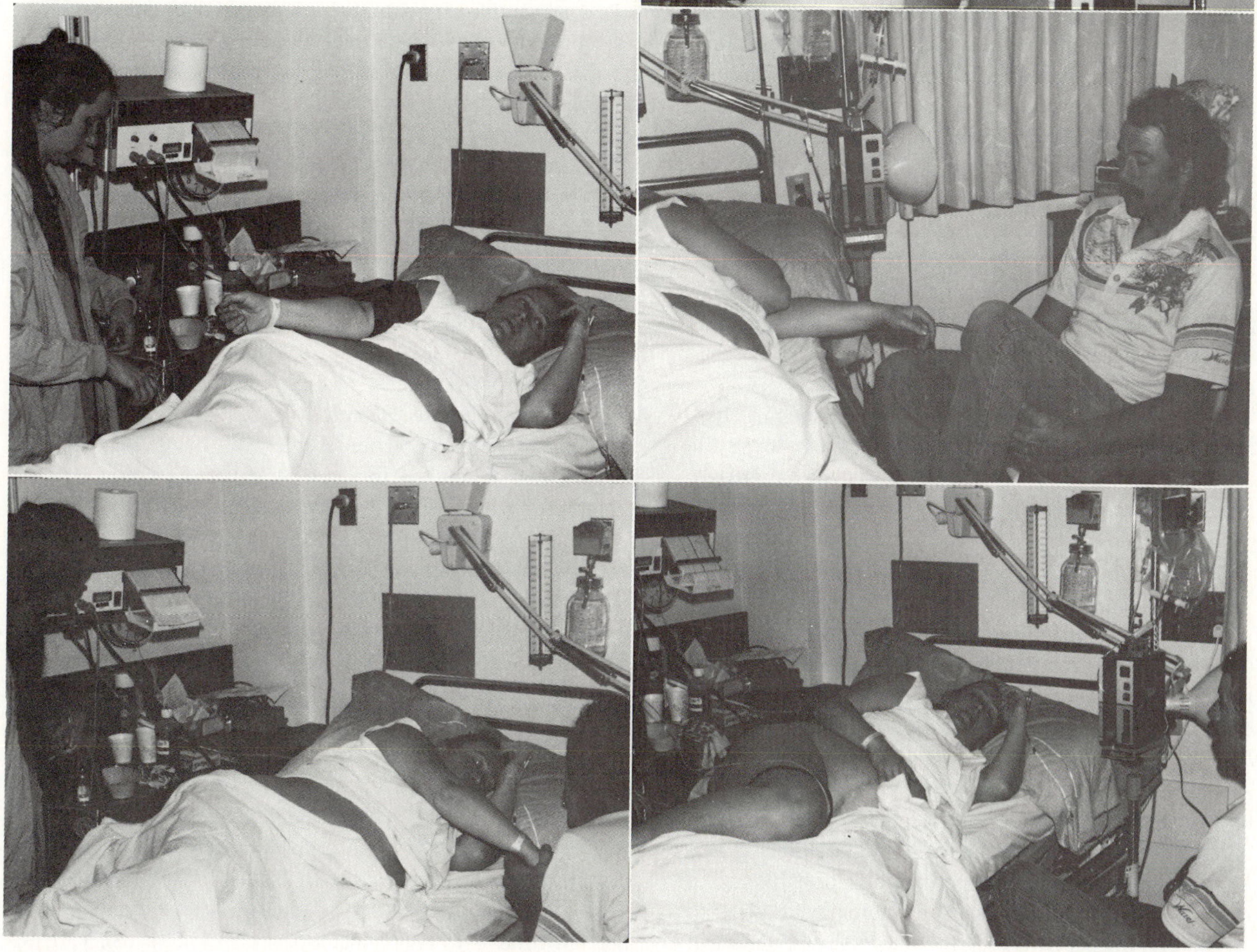

B

C

D

E

hook or other sharp instrument passed over a finger into the cervix will allow the drainage of amniotic fluid. The mother can be assured that neither she nor the infant will feel any pain. Within 6 to 8 hours, labor may be under way. Some obstetricians prefer to first stimulate the uterus with intravenous oxytocin and, as soon as good contractions are evident, rupture the membranes. Others prefer merely to rupture the membranes, knowing that oxytocin stimulation is often unnecessary.

Methods not recommended for stimulation of labor. The following methods are not recommended for stimulation of labor:

1. Intramuscular or intranasal oxytocin is condemned because of the physician's inability to control the effects of the drug, which may suddenly cause tetanic, prolonged uterine contractions.

2. "Stripping of the membranes" before or instead of rupture of the membranes is a dangerous procedure. It consists of the physician's inserting a finger through the soft, dilatable cervix at term and stripping the fetal membranes off the uterine wall in and around the internal os. It may cause rupture of the membranes, displacement of the presenting part, or prolapse of the cord, or it may initiate bleeding or sepsis. Rarely it may predispose the mother to amniotic fluid embolism.

3. Insertion of a bougie or packing the cervix may result in labor. However, these procedures are condemned because of the dangers of trauma, bleeding, and infection.

4. Intraamniotic injection of hypertonic sodium chloride is lethal for the infant and cannot be employed for induction of labor unless the fetus is dead or grossly abnormal (see Chapter 41).

OBSTETRIC OPERATIONS

Episiotomy. An episiotomy is an incision made in the perineum to enlarge the vaginal outlet. Episiotomies are performed more frequently in the United States and Canada than in Europe. The use of the side-lying position for delivery is routinely used in Europe while the supine position with legs in stirrups is more commonly used in the United States and Canada. With the side-lying position there is less tension on the perineum and a gradual stretching of the perineum is possible. As a result the indications for use of episiotomies are less.

The proponents of use of the episiotomy maintain it serves the following purposes:

1. Prevents tearing of the perineum: The clean and properly placed incision heals more promptly than does a ragged tear. Some conditions that predispose a woman to perineal tearing and are therefore indications for episiotomy are a large infant, rapid labor in which there is not sufficient time for stretching of the perineum to take place, a narrow suprapubic arch with a constricted outlet, and malpresentations of the fetus (e.g., face).
2. May prevent prolonged and severe stretching of the muscles supporting the bladder or rectum, which may later lead to stress incontinence or vaginal prolapse.
3. Reduces duration of the second stage, which may be important for maternal reasons (e.g., a hypertensive state) or fetal reasons (e.g., persistent bradycardia).
4. Enlarges the vagina in case manipulation is needed to deliver an infant, for example, in a breech presentation or for application of forceps.

Those who are opposed to the *routine* use of episiotomies mantain that:

1. The perineum can be prepared for delivery through use of the Kegel exercises (see p. 309), and use of the exercises in the postpartum period would improve and restore the tone of the perineal muscles.
2. Lacerations may occur even when the use of an episiotomy. (Benyon, 1974; Harris, 1970) Studies indicate a 13% to 22% occurrence of lacerations following episiotomies.
3. Pain and discomfort from episiotomies can interfere with mother-infant interactions (see p. 701) and the reestablishment of parental intercourse (see p. 704).
4. Episiotomies *are indicated* (a) for shortening the second stage of labor if the well-being of the mother or fetus is in jeopardy (b) if the infant is preterm and cerebral hemorrhage is a possibility because of capillary fragility, or (c) if the infant is large (greater than 4000 g [9 lb]).

Types of episiotomies. The type of episiotomy is designated by site and direction of the incision (Fig. 37.11).

Median episiotomy is the one most commonly employed. It is effective, easily repaired, and generally the least painful. Occasionally there may be an extension through the rectal sphincter (third-degree laceration) or even into the anal canal (fourth-degree laceration). Fortunately primary healing and a good repair usually will be followed by good sphincter tone.

Mediolateral episiotomy frequently is employed in operative delivery when posterior extension is likely. Although a fourth-degree laceration may thus be avoided, a third-degree laceration may occur. Moreover, as compared with a median episiotomy, blood loss is greater and the repair more difficult and painful. For nursing care related to episiotomies, see p. 701.

Forceps delivery. Two double-curved, spoonlike articulated blades make up the obstetric forceps that are

Fig. 37.11
Types of episiotomies.

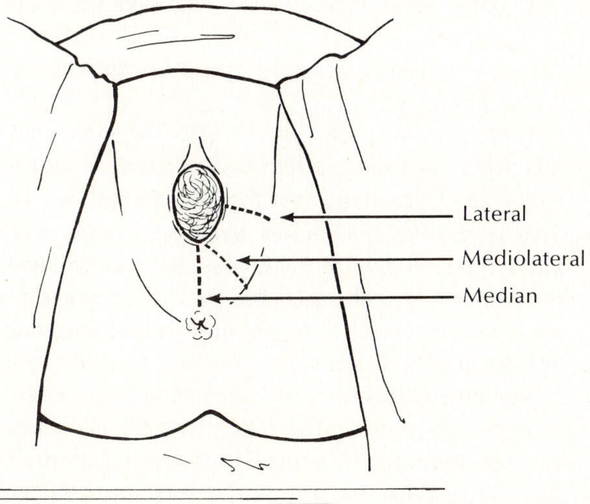

used to extract the fetal head, whether it be fore-coming (vertex presentation) or after-coming (breech presentation). This instrument, regarded by many as one of the greatest inventions of all time, was devised by Peter Chamberlen about 1625. Different *locks* (articulations) and varied curvature or length of the blades distinguish most obstetric forceps, which may have solid or fenestrated blades (Figs. 37.12 and 37.13). Some forceps are used for ordinary delivery (e.g., occiput anterior [OA] position); others are used for rotation of the vertex (e.g., left occiput posterior position [LOP] to OA position).

The commonly employed forceps have a cephalic curve shaped to that of the head and a pelvic curve that conforms to the pelvic axis. The blades are joined by a pin, screw, or groove arrangement.

Fig. 37.12
Types of forceps.

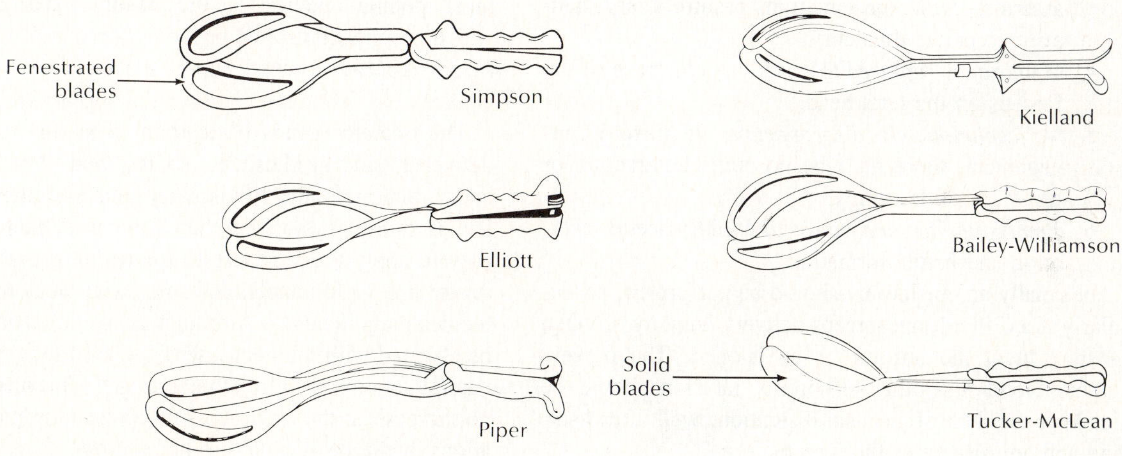

Fig. 37.13
Types of forceps locks.

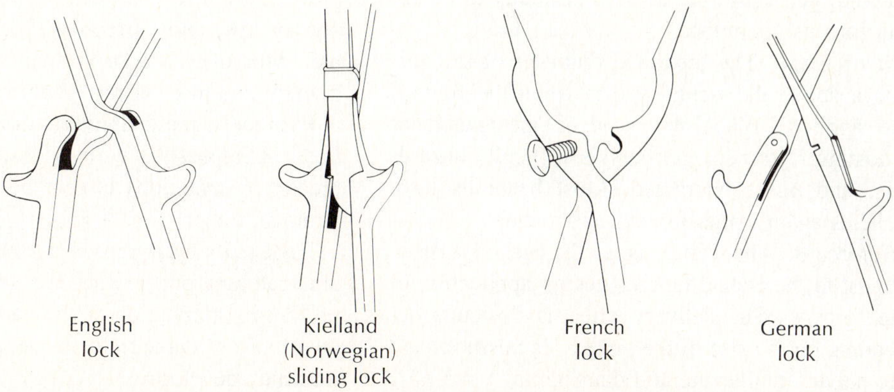

Possible indications for forceps delivery are as follows:

- Maternal: to shorten the second stage in dystocia (difficult labor) or when the mother's expulsive efforts are deficient (e.g., she is tired or she has been given spinal anesthesia) or when the woman is endangered (e.g., cardiac decompensation)
- Fetal: to rescue a jeopardized fetus (e.g., premature labor or fetal distress close to delivery)

The incidence of forceps delivery depends on the proportion of simple to complicated cases treated at a particular hospital, whether light or heavy analgesia is popular, and whether general or local infiltration anesthesia is favored.

Prerequisites for forceps operations. The following conditions must apply for successful forceps delivery:

1. *Fully dilated cervix.* Severe lacerations and hemorrhage may ensue if a rim of cervical tissue remains.
2. *Head engaged.* The extraction of a mature fetus with a "high" (unengaged) head usually is disastrous.
3. *Vertex presentation or face presentation* (mentum anterior). Other presentations require wider-than-average pelvic diameters.
4. *Membranes ruptured* to ensure a firm grasp of the forceps on the fetal head.
5. *No cephalopelvic disproportion.* If there is engagement, there must be no outlet contracture or gross sacral deformity.
6. *Empty bladder and bowel* to avoid visceral laceration and fistula formation.

Normally an episiotomy should be performed, particularly if a difficult midforceps delivery is likely or when a snug fit at the introitus is envisioned. The prevent undue blood loss, the episiotomy incision should be made at the time of perineal distention, well after locking and adjustment of the forceps.

Forceps designation relative to station of head. The station of the head determines the level of forceps application and, generally, the relative difficulty to be expected in forceps operations.

1. *High forceps.* The biparietal diameter of the vertex is above the ischial spines when the forceps are applied. When the head is unengaged or "floating," forceps delivery is difficult, hazardous, and never warranted. Most hospitals have policies against high-forceps application.
2. *Midforceps.* The vertex is at the ischial spines, almost to the ischial tuberosities on application of the forceps. The delivery often is difficult, depending on the size of the vertex, its position, and the pelvic architecture and diameters.
3. *Low forceps.* The vertex is distending the introitus with outlet forceps. This should be an "easy" forceps delivery. The blades are applied principally to provide control and guidance of the head.

Before forceps are applied, an attendant checks, reports, and records FHR. The physician will ask for the forceps by name (see Fig. 37.12). The nurse can tell the mother that they fit like two tablespoons around an egg. The blades come over the baby's ears.

After forceps application and before traction is applied, the attendant rechecks the FHR. Compression of the cord between the fetal head and the forceps would cause a drop in FHR. The physician would then remove and reapply the forceps.

Vacuum extraction. Vacuum extraction is delivery of a fetus in vertex presentation with the use of a cup-suction device that is applied to the fetal scalp for traction. Indications for use of the vacuum extractor, or ventouse, are similar to those for simple forceps delivery. This rather expensive instrument, widely used in Europe, often speeds labor and delivery, obviating difficult forceps procedures or even cesarean delivery. The most popular device is the Malmstroöm extractor, which permits controlled negative pressure of 0.6 to 0.8 kg/cm^2 beneath a metal cup available in various diameters.

The operator needs basic training in this method of delivery, and anesthesia is not required. The ventouse adds traction to the involuntary and voluntary efforts and is more physiologic than forceps extraction. It is easy to apply the ventouse to the occiput (away from a suture line or fontanel), and the device does not distort the head significantly. Although planned rotation cannot be effected with the ventouse because of lack of torque, natural rotation usually is encouraged. Because there is no increase in the volume of the presenting part, lacerations of the birth canal are uncommon.

The vacuum extractor cannot replace the obstetric forceps, however, because rotation (occiput posterior [OP] position to OA position) may be impossible without forceps, and correction of asynclitism is not feasible. Moreover, for a difficult midpelvic arrest, axis traction is almost always required.

Extremely rapid delivery (for fetal or maternal distress) is impossible with a vacuum extractor. Face and breech presentations cannot be delivered with this instrument either.

Fetal scalp ecchymoses must be expected; even cephalhematomas occur with the ventouse. When there is prolonged application of the vacuum extractor (30 minutes), severe damage to the scalp or subgaleal hematomas may develop.

Cesarean Delivery

Delivery of a fetus through a transabdominal incision of the uterus is an operative procedure known as cesarean section. Although the myth persists that Julius Caesar was delivered in this manner, the derivation of the term is more likely from the Latin word *caedo* meaning "to cut." Whether cesarean delivery is planned (elective) or unplanned (emergency), the loss of the experience of delivering a child in the traditional manner may have a negative effect on a woman's self-concept. In an effort to help maintain the focus on the *birth* of a child rather than the operative procedure, the term *cesarean delivery* or *cesarean birth* is coming into common usage; that is, the mother experiences abdominal rather than a vaginal birth.

GOAL

The basic purpose or use of cesarean delivery is to preserve the life or health of the mother and her fetus. The rate for this type of delivery has increased dramatically since 1965. The number of cesarean deliveries done in the United States rose from 160,000 in 1965 to 353,000 in 1975, an increase of 193,000. Although more research is indicated to produce definitive evidence in assigning reasons for this increase, there does appear to be a link between the increase in cesarean deliveries and the advent and widespread use of electronic fetal monitoring (EFM). Concomitantly, indications for cesarean delivery have been expanded; for example, in many areas it is routine practice to deliver all fetuses in a breech presentation by cesarean birth. Cephalopelvic disproportion (CPD) is the most common indication for cesarean delivery. The need for this mode of delivery is highest in areas where contracted pelvis, tumors, and other such difficulties are more prevalent. Repeat cesarean deliveries, correctly or incorrectly justified on the basis of possible or probable rupture of the uterus, represent at least 30% of all cesarean births in North America.

MATERNAL INDICATIONS

In addition to fetopelvic disproportion, maternal indications for cesarean delivery include a questionably weak or defective uterine scar (after cesarean delivery, myomectomy, or unification operation), preeclampsia-eclampsia, placenta previa or premature separation of the normally implanted placenta, dystocia, pelvic tumors, maternal gonorrhea, herpesvirus type 2 infections, or serious maternal conditions that might be complicated by labor and delivery, such as recent fractures of the pelvis.

FETAL INDICATIONS

Fetal distress (caused by hypoxia or blood loss), insulin-dependent diabetes mellitus, prolapse of the cord in labor, hydrocephalus, compound presentations, breech presentations, and shoulder presentations are indications for cesarean delivery. When infertility, marriage late in life, or other factors place a high social premium on the baby, elective cesarean delivery may be warranted.

TYPES OF CESAREAN PROCEDURES

There are five principal types of abdominal cesarean procedures (Fig. 37.14):

1. *Classic cesarean incision*. Classic cesarean incision is the simplest of all cesarean procedures. It is used when rapid delivery is necessary, in shoulder presentation, and in placenta previa when the placenta is implanted on the anterior wall. Classic cesarean delivery is useful when general anesthesia is unavailable, since this operation can be carried out under local infiltration anesthesia. A vertical incision is made through the visceral peritoneum and the contractile portion of the uterus above the bladder reflexion. Maternal bleeding may be considerable, especially if placenta previa is present, but no fetal blood loss usually occurs. The potential for rupture of the scar (1% to 2%) with a subsequent pregnancy and the frequent occurrence of small bowel adhesions to the anterior suture line have limited use of this type of cesarean delivery.

2. *Low cervical* or *lower segment cesarean delivery*. Low cervical or lower segment cesarean delivery is possible by means of a transverse (preferred method) or vertical incision through the visceral peritoneum at the bladder reflexion and downward displacement of the bladder. A flap of peritoneum is used to cover the myometrial closure, and intraperitoneal drainage is minimized; adhesions are uncommon. Blood loss is rarely excessive unless placenta previa is present. Good healing is the rule. Rupture of the scar with a later pregnancy occurs in about 0.5% of cases. This is the cesarean delivery most commonly employed.

3. *Peritoneal exclusion cesarean delivery*. Peritoneal exclusion cesarean delivery is useful when the intraperitoneal spill of infected fluid and blood should be avoided. The operation is merely a low cervical cesarean delivery with suture of the parietal peritoneum to the transversely incised visceral peritoneum before incision through the lower uterine segment. Drainage

Fig. 37.14
Cesarean delivery: skin and uterine incisions. **A,** Classic: vertical incisions of skin and uterus. **B,** Low cervical: horizontal incision of skin; vertical incision of uterus. **C,** Low cervical: horizontal incisions of skin and uterus.

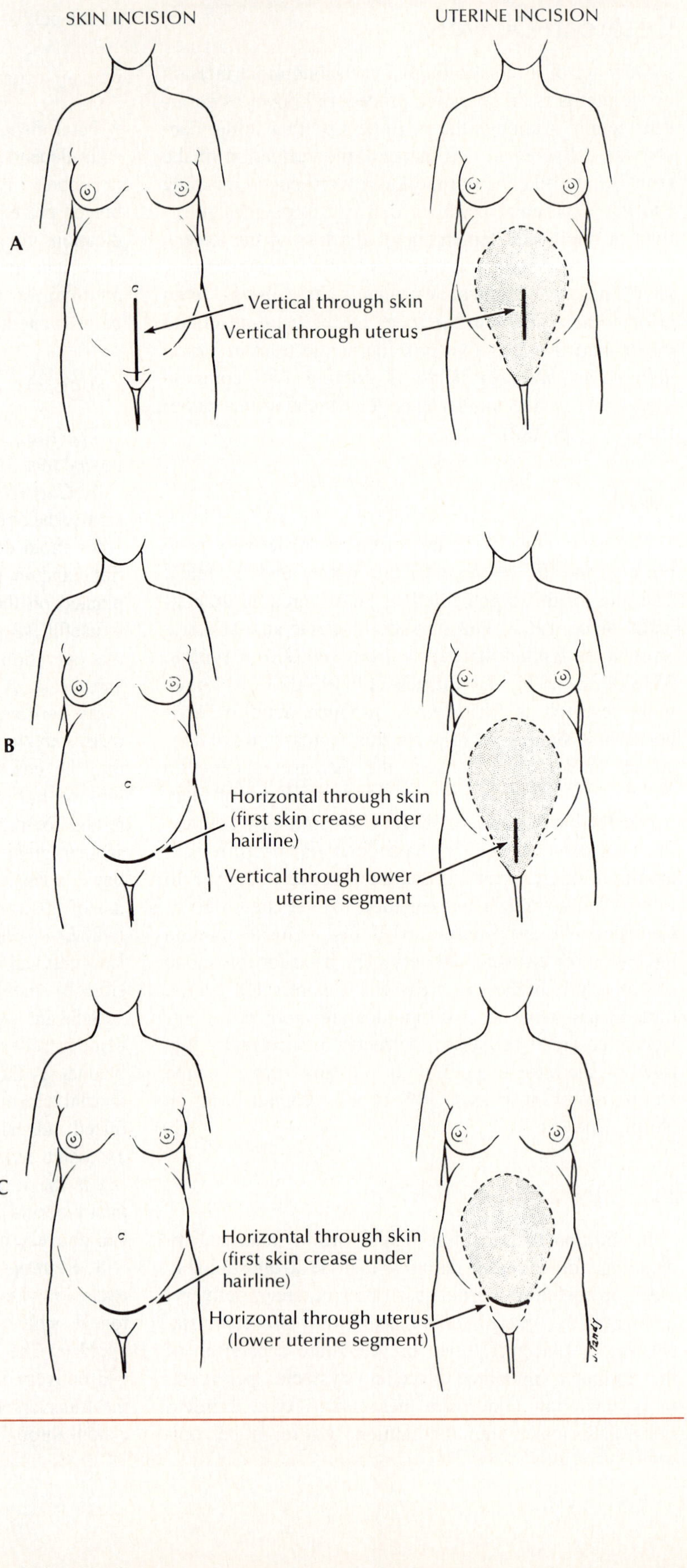

fluid has easy access to the surface, and the likelihood of peritonitis because of spill is greatly reduced. Although peritoneal exclusion cesarean delivery is not diffcult and is theoretically valuable, avoidance of delay and intensive antibiotic therapy have reduced the need for this operation.

4. *Extraperitoneal cesarean delivery*. Extraperitoneal cesarean delivery may be the procedure of choice in neglected, grossly infected cases. The operation is technically difficult, the peritoneum is often lacerated, and the bladder or ureter is often injured. The peritoneal exclusion operation and intensive, broad-spectrum antibiotic therapy probably will serve as well as the extraperitoneal cesarean delivery in most cases.

5. *Cesarean hysterectomy*. Total or subtotal hysterectomy may be elected, usually after classic cesarean delivery. The indication may be uterine pathosis, such as large uterine myomas. Placenta previa accreta, prenatal bleeding, and palpable placental tissue at the internal os may be reasons for cesarean delivery. When the placenta will not separate at operation, the uterus must be removed. If severe amnioitis is present, it may be best to remove the uterus after delivery of the fetus from above.

The disadvantages of cesarean hysterectomy include considerable blood loss and injury to the bladder or ureters. Hence its acceptability as a mode of sterilization remains in question.

• • •

Vaginal cesarean delivery, which is actually an extended anterior vaginal hysterectomy, may be appropriate to terminate an advanced pregnancy when the transabdominal approach is rejected, for example, in cases of fetal death and amnionitis at 34 weeks. Poor exposure, bleeding, bladder damage, and a limited area in which to work make this operation difficult and rarely feasible near term.

POSTMORTEM CESAREAN DELIVERY

Assuming a definitely viable fetus, a cesarean delivery within 5 to 10 minutes of the mother's death theoretically should result in a living fetus. Careful preparations for such a delivery are important, including permission for the operation. However, few babies have survived postmortem cesarean delivery, principally because of hypoxia related to the maternal death or to immaturity.

PROGNOSIS AFTER CESAREAN DELIVERY

Maternal morbidity and mortality are related to the indication for cesarean delivery, type of operation, duration of rupture of the membranes and labor, and blood transfusion and antibiotic therapy given. In large hospitals in North America the maternal mortality with cesarean delivery is 0.1% to 0.2%. In communities where good maternity care is lacking, it may be five times higher.

Perinatal mortality depends principally on fetal maturity, the problem for which cesarean delivery was done, the anesthetic used, and the immediate postoperative support given. It is the complications, for example, premature separation of the placenta, rather than the cesarean delivery, that results in the perinatal death of at least 1% to 2% of infants born in this way. In elective repeat cesarean delivery, however, a term perinatal mortality of 0.8% to 0.9% is achievable.

NURSING CARE

Target population. Women who must undergo cesarean delivery as the mode of delivery may be categorized in three groups. The first two are made up of women who will have elective cesarean deliveries, and for them there is time for psychologic preparation. The psychic response of women in these groups may differ in that those scheduled for a repeat surgery may have disturbing memories of the conditions preceding the initial surgical delivery, their experiences in the postoperative recovery period, and the added burden of care of an infant while recovering from a surgical operation. Those facing elective cesarean delivery for the first time share with other surgical patients the same apprehensions concerning surgery coupled with the uncertainty of being able to cope with child care.

The third group is made up of those women who face an emergency cesarean delivery as a result of a fetal or maternal response that suddenly necessitates changes in plans for vaginal delivery, postdelivery care, and care of self and infant at home. This may be an extremely traumatic experience. The woman approaches surgery usually tired and discouraged from a fruitless labor, worried and fretful about her own and the child's condition, and perhaps dehydrated and with low glycogen reserves. All preoperative procedures must be done quickly and competently. The time for explanation of procedures and of the operation is short, and since anxiety levels are high, much of what is said is forgotten or perhaps misconstrued. Postoperatively, time must be spent reviewing the events preceding the operation and the operation itself to ensure that the woman understands what has happened. Fatigue is often noticeable in these women, and they need much supportive care.

Many women who experience a cesarean birth speak to the feelings that interfere with their maintaining an adequate self-concept. These feelings range from fear, disappointment, or frustration at losing control, to anger (the "why me" syndrome), to loss of self-esteem as their body image is not sustained. Success in mothering activities and in the recovery process can do much to restore these women's self-esteem. Some women see the scar as mutilating, and worry concerning sexual attractiveness may surface. Some men are fearful of resuming sexual intercourse because of the fear of hurting their mates.

The separation of mother and child may prove detrimental to the establishment of parent-child bonds, particularly if other negative factors are present.

> One mother in discussing the impact of an unexpected cesarean delivery regarding her self-concept said, "At first I was despondent over not being able to deliver vaginally but then I comforted myself with the thought, you were a good mother for 9 months, no 12-hour period (delivery) can alter that.' My baby and I have our whole lives to be mother and daughter."

Professional staff can expect some anger directed toward them. Parents will wonder if it was absolutely necessary for them to have a cesarean dlivery. Cohen (1977) notes that such feelings may surface even years later. Support of the philosophy of family-centered birth in terms of offering prenatal and postdelivery education in the community and of minimizing separation of mother, father, and child at the time of birth will do much to mitigate such parental responses. Concerned professional and lay groups in the community have established councils for cesarean birth in an attempt to meet the needs of these women and their families. Such groups advocate including preparation for cesarean birth in all parenthood preparation classes even if parents-to-be "tune out" such discussions and feel later that they have been betrayed by not having been made aware of this eventuality. No woman can be guaranteed a vaginal delivery, even if she is in good health and there is no indication of danger to the fetus before the onset of labor. Every woman needs to be aware of and prepared for this eventuality. The unknown and unexpected is ego weakening. Each woman or couple needs accurate data to build new coping abilities or to strengthen old ones. "Walking through," role playing, or worry work before a crisis situation increases one's sense of control in that situation and serves to minimize the sense of loss experienced.

Childbirth educators stress the importance of emphasizing the similarities as well as differences between cesarean and vaginal births. Also, in support of the philosophy of family-centered birth, many hospitals have changed policies to permit fathers to share in these births as they have in vaginal ones (Fig. 37.16, *B*). Women undergoing cesarean birth stress that the continued presence and support of their partners have helped them to experience a positive response to the whole process:

> Knowing that he would be there and that he would be among the first to hold and nurture our baby made a tremendous difference to me. Even though "I" as the woman couldn't participate as directly as I had anticipated, "we" as the family could. I felt a sense of control, not a sense of being a passive . . .well . . .organ.

Prenatal period: preparation for cesarean birth

Characteristics of a group leader. The information pertaining to a cesarean delivery may be offered as an integral part of the regular childbirth preparation classes or as classes for a separate group. The characteristics of the group leaders of these classes are very important to the success of teaching. The leader of this type of prenatal group must be clear about her own attitude toward a surgical or abdominal route of delivery. Women who give birth by this method are not biologic deviants, the objects of injustice, or "poor souls" deprived of "natural" vaginal birth experiences. The woman or couple is entitled to a positive maternal or paternal experience, a maturing encounter that results in growth of self-esteem, expanded self-concept, and increased mutuality as a couple, and a mutually satisfying relationship with the newborn. These concepts serve as the nurse's evaluative criteria when working with this type of expectant parent group.

A *working knowledge of the concept of crisis* (loss or threat of loss) and of crisis intervention is a prerequisite of the nurse's ability to function therapeutically. One generally assumes that one's body is able to function or perform in a certain manner to achieve an expected goal. Thus, when confronted with the loss or threat of loss of control of body function, that person perceives the event as the loss or threat of loss of self. The domino effect may be set into motion; that is, a negative self-concept and loss of self-esteem may lead to a sense of unworthiness, which may lead to a poor concept of oneself as a parent and thus compromise the relationship to the child. The end result may be an abused child and a scared parent.

Negative unresolved feelings may have been simmering since a previous disappointing experience. Until this oppressive burden of angry and depressing feelings is confronted and resolved, it is difficult to develop skills and tools to cope effectively when the experience is repeated.

The group leader's effectiveness is increased if she is aware of the prevailing mood and thinking in the community. The "natural childbirth" and the "earth mother" orientations, beneficial to the struggle toward humanization of the childbearing experience, may inadvertently create a crisis situation for some women; that is, those whose preferences or experiences differ may feel shamed, confused, biologically deficient, and stigmatized. Occasionally women who are scheduled for or have experienced surgical delivery hear comments such as "Oh, you are having [have had] it the easy way!" Other women are exposed to remarks such as "Oh, my dear, how dreadful!" or "I'm so sorry!" Although these statements may be intended to express caring or concern, the woman or couple seldom perceives them positively.

The group leader should have a knowledge *of prenatal testing for fetal well-being and lung maturity.* From the nursing and medical perspectives, prenatal testing for fetal well-being and lung maturity provides a means of communication with the unborn and of evaluation of his living conditions. The expectant parents' rate of compliance increases significantly if they are given (1) factual data about the purpose and anticipated results of the tests in the form of written or verbal explanation of what is expected and (2) an opportunity to discuss their feelings and questions.

The group leader should have a *knowledge of content discussed in the usual prenatal classes:* anatomy and physiology, psychologic changes, discomforts, and their relief, fetal development, danger signs, relaxation techniques and other measures to increase comfort during procedures and labor, signs of labor, puerperal changes, parenting, and so forth. Each group leader needs to become acquainted with the local hospitals' policies concerning admission, regulation, protocol of care for the woman or family in labor, and nursery and postdelivery protocols for care. Generally, expectant parents appreciate assistance in assessing the physician's or midwife's orientation to the childbearing experience and how to proceed in negotiating for the type of care they would like to receive.

For many women, giving birth by cesarean delivery will be their first experience with surgery. The group leader must have *an awareness of the fears of pain, mutilation, and death that people feel when they face surgery.* When given concrete information regarding preoperative and postoperative care and the procedure itself, the expectant couple will be less likely to be surprised by sensations, sights, sounds, and smells common to surgical intervention. Knowledge permits anticipatory worry work to occur, allowing time to mobilize defenses and develop coping skills before the event. The involved individual retains a sense of control over the situation.

Well-developed communication skills are an invaluable asset, especially to the group leader of a population labeled as high risk. Without intrusive probing, the group leader must guide the expectant parents gently to identify and verbalize feelings, some of which may be uncomfortably hostile, angry, or sad. The leader needs skill to listen actively to the messages behind "jokes" and to recognize messages in body language or silence. Verbalization of feelings is cathartic if it is not carried to an extreme. The leader needs to be skilled in pacing; for example, the leader should not allow parents to wallow in self-pity but should encourage them to move on and come to terms with the new experience they will be facing soon.

The skilled leader avoids becoming trapped in the "injustices" experienced or perceived by group members. Instead, the leader focuses on the persons' feelings at the time by comments that acknowledge their right to have feelings, that impart support for them as people, and that give form and substance to an identifiable and solvable problem. Therapeutic comments include statements such as "It sounds as if you had a difficult time." "How did that make you feel when it happened to you?" and "When you think about it now, how does it make you feel?"

A sense of timing or pacing is also necessary to teach effectively. Learning occurs only when the learner is ready. Since any degree of stress impedes learning, repetition is an appropriate teaching method.

Course content. The content of classes varies with the composition of the group. Based on (1) the nurse's knowledge of the needs of women who experience surgical intervention and cesarean delivery and (2) an assessment of the population, the group leader may use the following suggestions in the group discussion. Overall course content emphasizes giving birth rather than fixation on any one "right" route or method of delivery.

1. Exploration and catharsis of feelings surrounding the expectant parents' situation
2. Content that is presented in usual prenatal classes, including clinical manifestations of labor; encouragement of each woman or couple to have the phone numbers of persons to contact in the event of onset of labor (physician, midwife, police, support persons, others)
3. Prenatal testing: rationale for testing, what tests can determine, what is expected of the woman or couple for the test, and the woman's (couple's) right to a full explanation of the results
4. Techniques to increase comfort or to cope with discomfort
   a. Relaxation breathing techniques: to be used during physical examinations, pelvic examination, prenatal tests, drawing of blood specimens, and insertion of intravenous lifelines and urinary catheters
   b. Abdominal tightening exercises: may be bene-

ficial in minimizing postsurgical discomfort from distention and gas formation

c. Splinting techniques: decrease discomfort at the operative site while coughing, deep breathing, or changing position in bed

d. Alternative methods of positioning and holding the neonate that facilitate breast feeding by minimizing stress on the incision line

5. Local hospitals' policies and procedures regarding preregistration and admission
6. Surgical procedure

a. Preoperative preparation

(1) Informed consent for surgery and anesthesia and for father in operating room

(2) Admission procedure: history and physical examination

(3) Laboratory hematologic evaluation: complete blood count, hemoglobin and hematocrit determinations, type and cross match for two units of blood; results of Coombs' test, if necessary

(4) Laboratory evaluation of urine for protein, sugar, specific gravity, and complete urinalysis

(5) Scrub and shave of operative site (There is now some question whether shaving the abdomen really does decrease the incidence of infection.)

(6) Sonographic location of placenta as necessary

(7) Options regarding preoperative medication (pharmacologic or psychologic tranquilizer), atropine or other drying agent, anesthetic (general inhalation or regional anesthetic, such as spinal or epidural block)

(8) Insertion of intravenous line and urinary catheters (In some hospitals, these procedures are done in operating room.)

b. Giving birth: equipment and lights of operating room, draping, where father of baby will sit and what he can do, what sensations (fundal pressure, pulling), sights, sounds (suction, hiss of oxygen), and smells to expect; time frames (how long between being "prepped" and giving birth); when to expect to see baby

c. Postoperative recovery: different rates of recovery with varying amounts of pain; pain control; early ambulation (when, why, how); normal variations in pacing early mother-child relationship; breast feeding; birth control; resumption of sexual relationship; sibling rivalry; grandparents' response; care of newborn infant: layette, normal physical and behavioral response, attachment, touching, and stimulation

Teaching methodology. Teaching methods vary from leader to leader and with the composition of the group:

1. Lecture and discussion paced to match parents' readiness to learn (repetition as needed)
2. Slides: surgical procedure, breast feeding (use as catalyst to stimulate questions and dicussion)
3. Slides: various persons interacting with pregnant woman; persons of differnt ages holding a newborn to trigger discussion about rivalry with and reactions of older siblings, family, friends
4. Films: giving birth by cesarean delivery with father of baby present; exploring postdelivery experience
5. Tours of hospital units: see preoperative and postoperative beds or maternity unit, labor room with monitors, operating room, nursery facilities; meet some of the staff
6. Visits to group by parents who have delivered by abdominal surgery

Subsequent deliveries. Data (Meier and Porreco, 1982) is gradually accumulating as to the safety of vaginal delivery following cesarean delivery. In the past, once a woman had a cesarean delivery, all future deliveries were elective cesarean deliveries. Often the woman was counseled to limit the number of pregnancies to three. The type of subsequent delivery is a decision to be made by the woman after full consultation with her physician. Danforth (1982) states that in general suitable candidates for future vaginal deliveries are (1) those women whose operation was of the low cervical (not classic) type; (2) those women who begin labor before the EDC; and (3) those women who enter the labor suite with the fetal head well engaged and the cervix soft, anterior, effaced, and dilated at least 3 cm.

If the original indication for the cesarean delivery is still present in a subsequent pregnancy, for example, a grossly contracted pelvis, repeat cesarean delivery is indicated. Moreover, for women who had a classic cesarean incision or any cesarean delivery marred by a septic course wherein questionable healing of the scar may result in rupture during labor a cesarean delivery is recommended.

When the original complication for which a cesarean delivery was initially done has not recurred (e.g., fetal distress caused by cord compression at term during labor), a trial of labor is recommended; this occurs under close observation with equipment for immediate cesarean delivery available in an emergency and with equipment for an elective low forceps delivery available if full dilatation is achieved. The alternative would be another cesarean delivery because of concern for the strength of the uterine scar. Unless the woman is in a center with emergency surgical, anesthesia, and blood transfusion facilities available, a trial of labor and vaginal delivery are too great a risk for mother and fetus.

A major physical hazard in performing elective repeat cesarean delivery is miscalculating the EDC and the consequent delivery of a premature infant.

Natal period: care in hospital

Preparation for surgery. The preparation of the woman for cesarean birth is the same for either elective or emergency surgery.

Assessment. The assessment strategies include the following aspects:

1. Careful and continuous monitoring of maternal and fetal response to labor and to the stress of labor (see Chapter 24).
2. Sending specimens to the laboratory for analysis, that is, blood is sent for typing and cross matching. Two units of matched blood are kept in reserve for 48 hours after surgery. Urine is sent for routine analysis.
3. Assessing vital signs, including blood pressure and FHR. They are evaluated and recorded.

The woman is examined by the anesthesiologist to determine the type of anesthesia to be used and the general condition of her cardiorespiratory system.

Examples of nursing diagnoses. Many of the nursing diagnoses will be the same as for the woman with dystocia. In addition there may be client or partner problems in relation to fear of surgery, disappointment over having to change their concept of birth, or fear for their infant's safety. The following are possible nursing diagnoses:

1. Disturbance in self-concept of father because of change in locus of control from parents to professionals
2. Fear expressed regarding injury to infant
3. Exhaustion because of long, difficult labor

Plan and implementation. The goal for preparation for surgery is to complete the care competently and quickly and to provide emotional support through a caring attitude, calm manner, and technical competence. The obstetrician or anesthesiologist discusses the operation and the choice of anesthesia with the woman or family and obtains informed consent to the procedures.

Preoperative preparation of the abdomen is completed. The abdomen is shaved beginning at the level of the xiphoid process and extending to the flank on

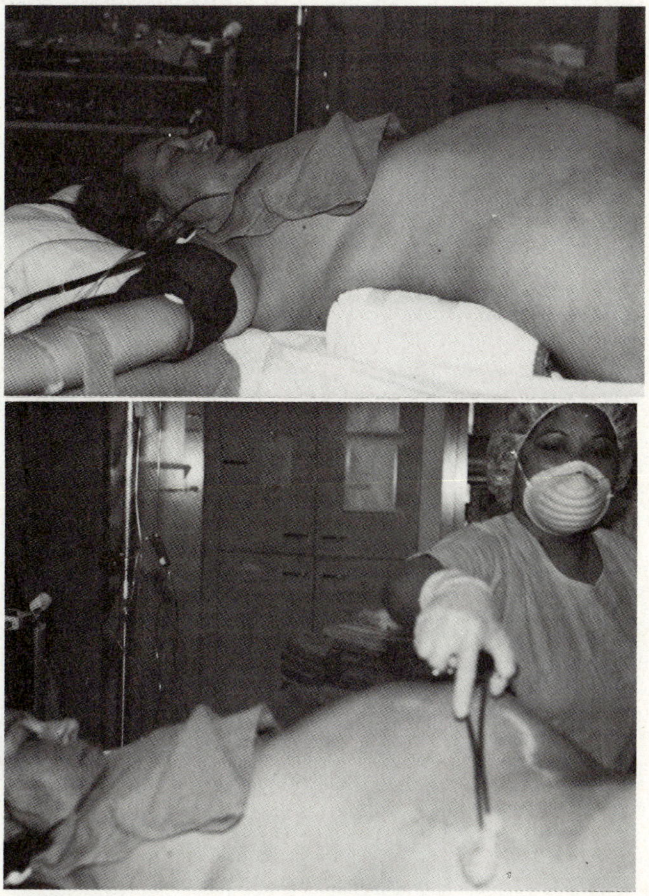

Fig. 37.15
A, Preparation for cesarean birth. Note pad under hip to tilt abdomen and avoid vena cava syndrome. **B,** Scrub nurse prepares abdomen for surgery. (Courtesy Judith Bamber, San Jose, Calif.)

Fig. 37.16
A, Surgical team continues preparing woman for surgery. Note father, wearing checked cap, at lower right. **B,** Surgery in progress. **C,** A time to be born: by cesarean birth. (**A** and **B** courtesy Jose Mercado. From News and Publication Service, Stanford University, Stanford, Calif. **C** courtesy Marjorie Pyle, R.N.C., Lifecircle, Costa Mesa, Calif.)

A

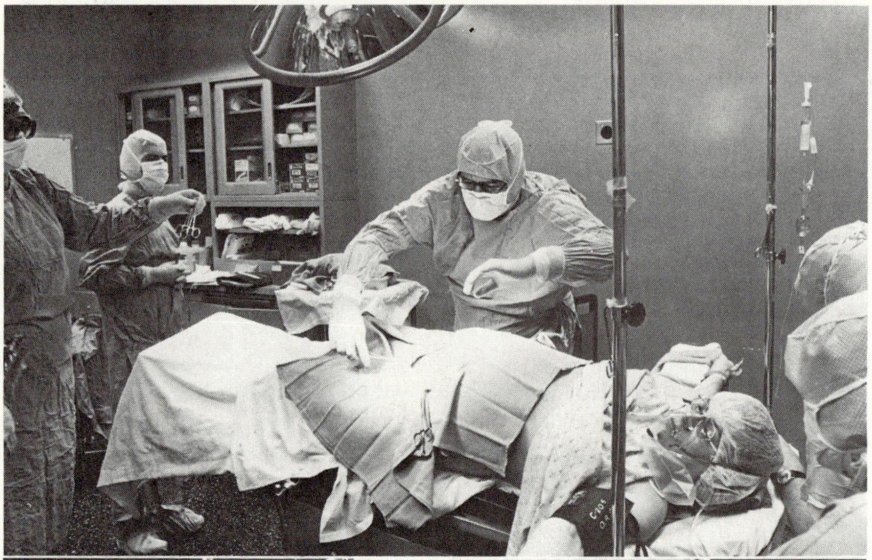

B

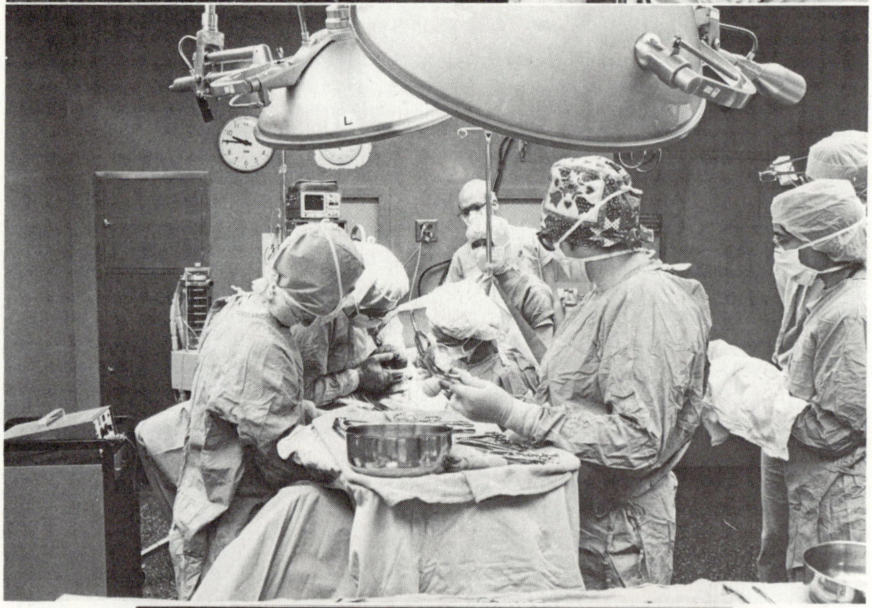

C

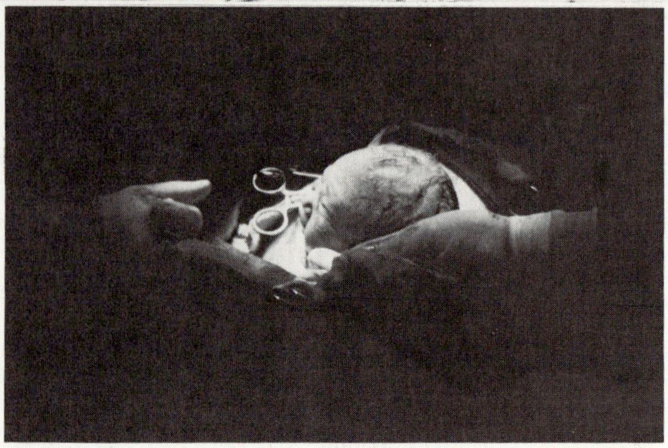

both sides and down to the pubic area (Fig. 37.15). A retention catheter is inserted to ensure that the bladder remains empty during the operation. It is attached to a continuous drainage system. Since the urethra is 7.6 cm (3 in) long (in nonpregnant women it is 3.8 cm [1.5 in] long), care must be taken to see that the catheter is properly placed and draining adequately. Preoperative medications are administered as ordered, for example, Maalox or other antacids, an analgesic, and atropine. An intravenous infusion (e.g., 1000 ml Ringer's lactated solution or 5% dextrose in water) is started. Routine preoperative care is completed including removal of dentures, contact lenses, rings, and fingernail polish. Valuables are put into safekeeping. The woman's chart is readied for use in surgery and is checked to see whether permission forms for care of the mother and infant are signed. If the woman has received analgesia or anesthesia, the responsible adult accompanying the woman signs the necessary forms.

Operative process. Once the woman has been taken to surgery her care becomes the responsibility of the obstetric team, surgeon, anesthesiologist, pediatrician, and nursing staff (Fig. 37.16). If possible, the father, gowned appropriately, accompanies the mother to the surgical unit and remains close to her.

Care of the infant. Care of the infant is delegated to a pediatrician and a nurse because these infants are considered to be at risk until there is evidence of physiologic stability after delivery (Fig. 37.17). A crib with resuscitative equipment is readied before the surgery, and those responsible for care are expert in resuscitative techniques, as well as in observational skills for detecting abnormal infant responses. After birth, if the infant's condition permits, he is given to the father to hold and to show to the mother (Fig. 37.18). The attachment process can continue uninterrupted. Some mothers are able to nurse the infant in the recovery room area; however, many are not ready for this direct participation and need to be reassured that the parent-child attachment process will not be impaired.

If the infant is compromised, he is transported immediately to the infant intensive care unit. Personnel need to keep the family informed of the infant's progress and begin father-child contacts as soon as possible.

If the family-oriented approach is not feasible, the family is directed to the surgical waiting room, where the physician reviews the condition of the mother and child after the birth is completed. Family members may accompany the infant as he is transferred to the nursery and have an opportunity to see and admire him (Fig. 37.19).

Postdelivery and postsurgical care. The care of the woman following cesarean delivery combines surgical and obstetric nursing. Once surgery is completed, the mother is transferred to the recovery room for intensive care until her condition stabilizes. Then she is moved to the postdelivery unit.

Assessment. The nurse sets a regular schedule to assess the following:

1. Assess for hemorrhage.
    a. Check the fundus gently but firmly. Since the uterus is sutured securely, the procedure may cause discomfort but will not rupture the incised uterus.
    b. Check amount and character of the lochia (see p. 688).
    c. Check the skin incision for signs of excessive bleeding or formation of hematomas.
    d. Check vital signs for evidence of shock. (NOTE: A newly delivered woman can lose a considerable quantity of blood before signs or symptoms of shock appear.)
2. Intake and output are recorded. Note whether the catheter is draining freely. Note and record the character of the drainage. Palpate gently for bladder fullness.
3. Assess her need for pain medication by noting facial expression, rigidity of body, uncomfortable-appearing posture, or circumoral pallor. Question the woman about the nature of the pain and where it is located.
4. Assess for signs of infection in the (a) incised area, (b) chest (for evidence of congestion), and (c) lochia.
5. Note the woman's and family's response to change in birth expectations.
6. Assess the family's knowledge of procedures used and the recovery needed.
7. Determine what teaching and support are necessary.

Examples of nursing diagnoses. Client problems most frequently noted by the nurse relate to discomfort from the incisional site, flank pain from manipulation of the incision and stretching of abdominal muscles with retractors during the surgery, afterpains (particularly if the woman is a multigravida), muscle fatigue and ache because of immobility, and "gas pains" because of decreased or absent gastric intestinal peristalsis related to anesthesia, manipulation of abdominal organs during surgery, immobilization and restricted diet, or pain from a distended urinary bladder. An example of a nursing diagnosis could be *inability to sleep because of incisional pain.* Other client problems revolve around separation from her infant, inability to hold the infant to breast feed, or anxiety concerning the well-being of the child. An example of a nursing diagnosis could be *alteration in self-concept because of inability to feed and care for the infant.*

Fig. 37.17

A, Care of newborn: pediatrician and nurse give immediate care to newborn. **B,** Newborn lies in relaxed position since muscle tone is decreased following stress of labor. **C,** Pediatrician administers oxygen. Note mask is held above infant's face; oxygen is heavier than air and will sink to face level. Nurse is assessing fetal heart rate. Infant is crying; note muscle tone now. Arms and legs are flexed and not resting on bed. **D,** Nurse inserts penicillin ointment in eyes. Note position of hand opening eye: fingers rest on forehead and cheek bone. Finger of hand holding penicillin tube rests on forehead so that movement is controlled. **E,** Infant rests quietly. Note she is sucking her finger. Her identity band is in place. (**A** courtesy Jose Mercado. From News and Publications Service, Stanford University, Stanford, Calif. **B** to **D** courtesy Judith Bamber, San Jose, Calif.)

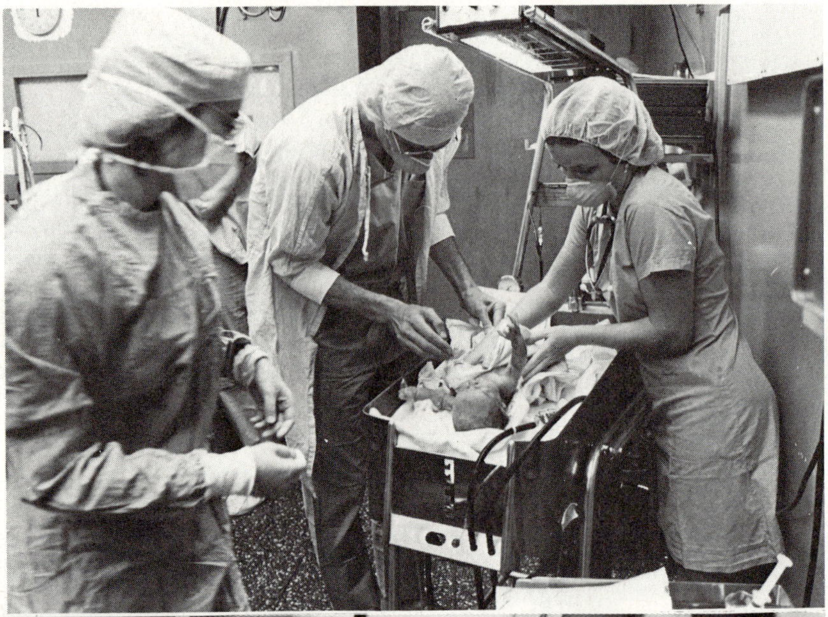

A

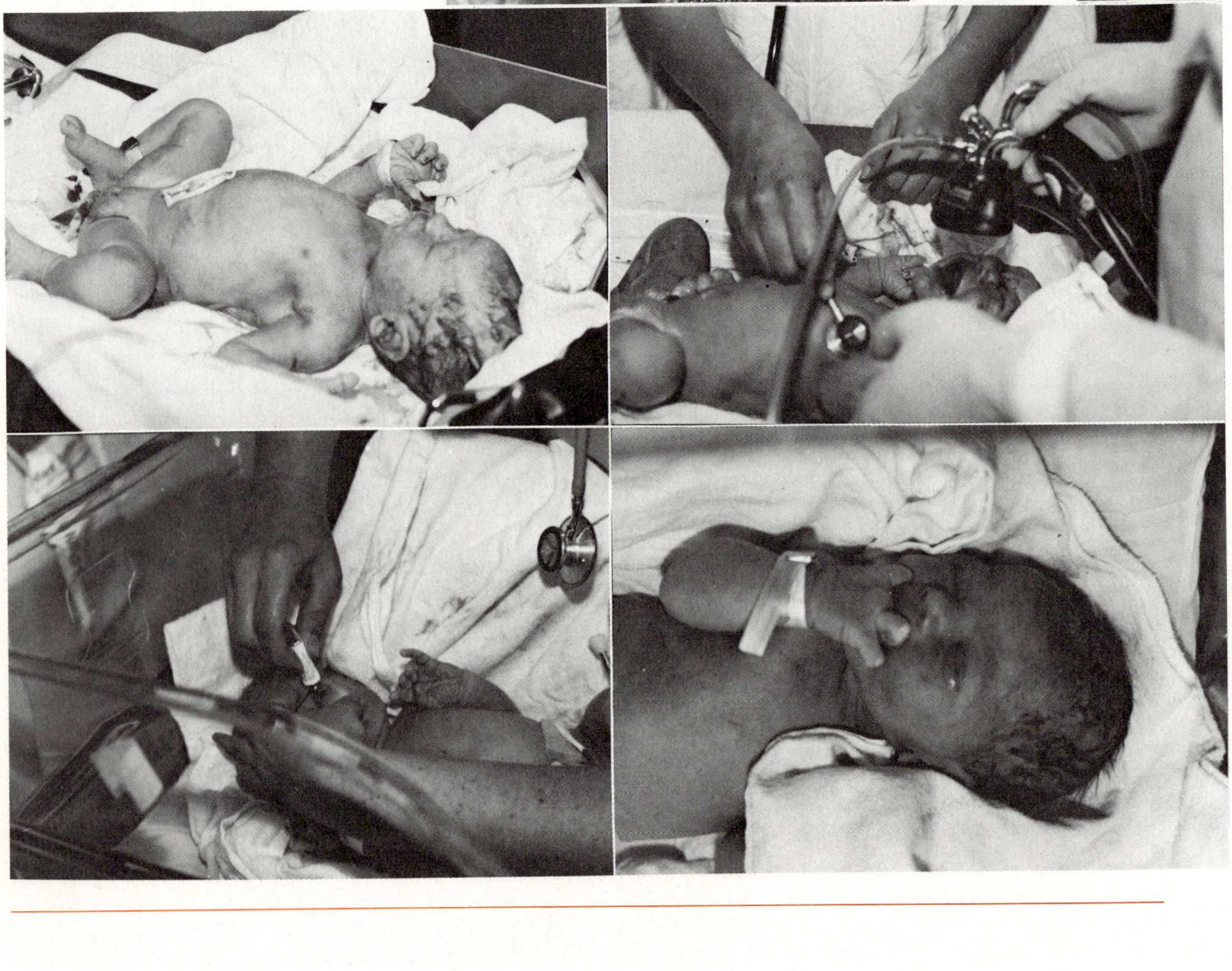

B

C

D

E

Fig. 37.18

A, Parents and their newborn. Father holds child. **B,** Father shows infant to mother. **C,** Mother holds and examines infant. (Courtesy Jose Mercado. From News and Publications Service, Stanford University, Stanford, Calif.)

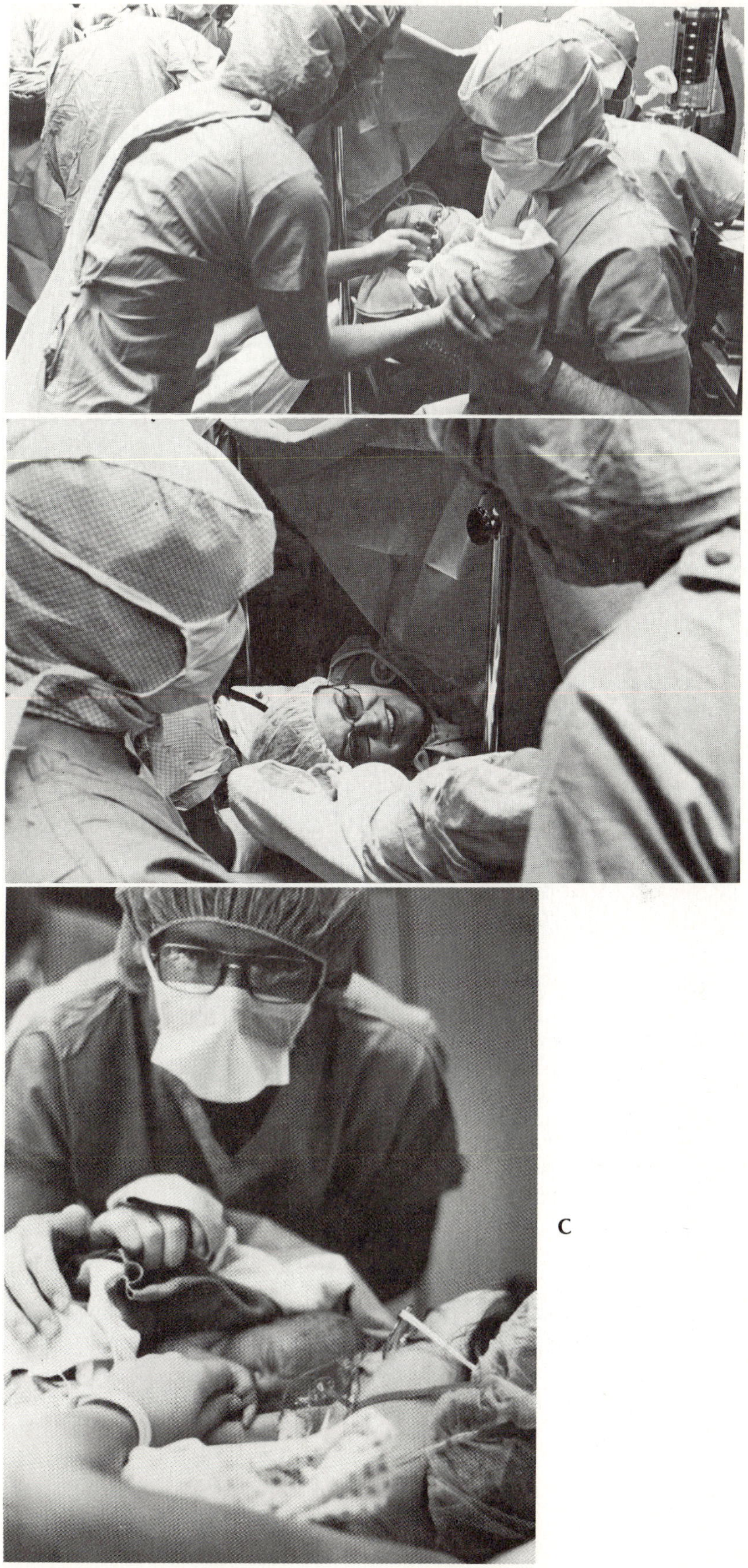

Fig. 37.19

A, Family and friends welcome baby: grandmother and father. **B,** Nurse and friends who shared labor with clients. (Courtesy Judith Bamber, San Jose, Calif.)

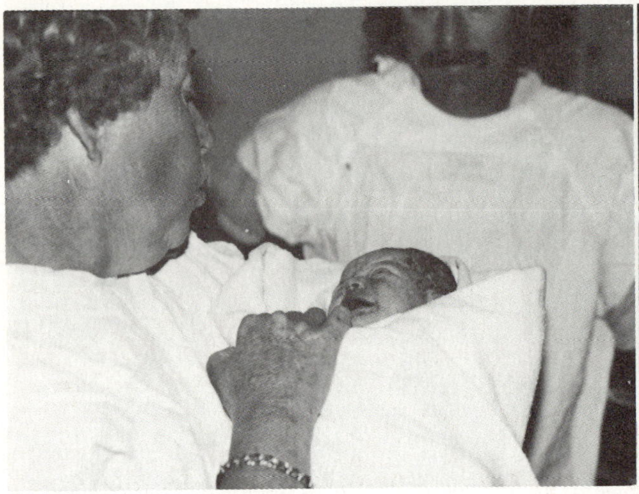

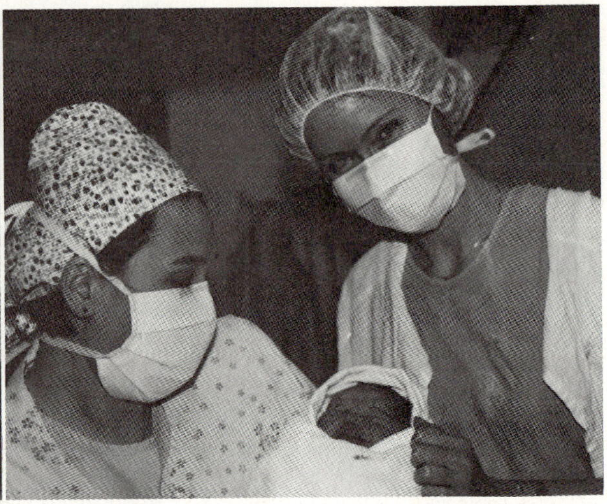

Fig. 37.20

Typical incision for cesarean birth. Note "skin clips" used to suture incision.

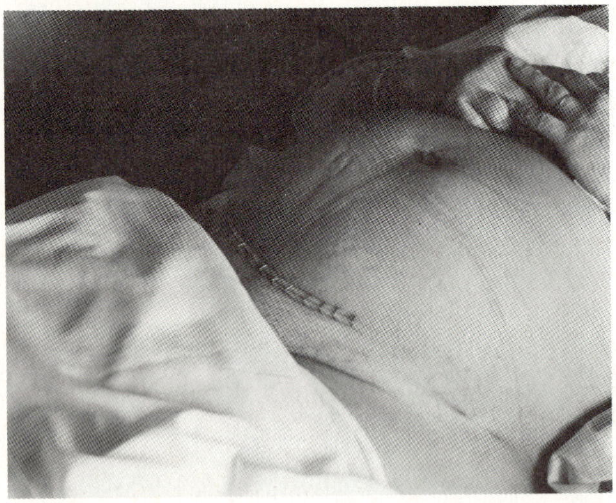

Plan and implementation. The woman is often reluctant to move about freely in bed and will require bed care for at least the first postoperative day. For prevention of hemorrhage, oxytocin may be administered by intravenous infusion for 4 hours or longer postoperatively. Prophylactic antibiotic therapy is usually ordered for administration via infusion (e.g., cephalothin [Keflin]). Postoperative pain and discomfort are controlled with judicious use of medication, positioning the woman in bed, and splinting of the incision while she does deep breathing exercises. Pain arises from the stretching of uterine musculature and supporting tissues, as well as from the incision site (Fig. 37.20). Coughing, deep breathing, paddling feet, and turning routines are instituted as for any postoperative client. The woman may be allowed out of bed after 8 hours or after the anesthesia has completely worn off. The woman must be carefully watched for fainting episodes as a result of hypotension and use of analgesic drugs.

Post-spinal-puncture headache, caused by a leakage of cerebrospinal fluid (CSF) through the hole in the dura, usually occurs within 24 to 72 hours of a subarachnoid block. Occasionally the dura is inadvertently punctured during attempted epidural block anesthesia.

Preventive measures include the use of a small-gauge needle by the anesthesiologist to pierce the dura, adequate hydration during anesthesia and during the postpartum period, and remaining flat in bed (supine, sidelying, but preferably prone to slow down leakage of CSF) for the time specified by the anesthesiologist (8 to 12 hours) (see Chapter 31, p. 703).

To provide care to the woman who develops a post-spinal-puncture headache, the nurse may use any of the following measures: ensure continuous hydration (by intravenous route if necessary); advise woman to remain on bedrest with her head flat or on a flat pillow; apply a tight abdominal binder when the woman wishes to be in an upright position; administer analgesics as necessary; and reinforce the fact that the headache inevitably resolves.

If the headache is incapacitating or if analgesics do not relieve symptoms or cannot be used, an *epidural blood-patch* may produce relief by stopping the leak of CSF through the puncture site. The hole in the dura is sealed by an injection of the woman's own blood (or serum) into the epidural space over the original puncture site.

Surgical liquids may be given orally when tolerated, within 4 to 6 hours. Intravenous infusion (1000 ml/8 hr) is usually continued for at least 24 hours until liquids are tolerated and bowel sounds heard. Once bowel sounds are heard, the diet is gradually increased. If gas pains are not relieved by increased ambulation, a Harris flush may be ordered to relieve the flatulence. With the Harris flush or return-flow enema the intestine is alternately filled with normal saline or water and drained to help remove flatus by stimulation of peristalsis.

Routine care for woman who has given birth is maintained, including sedation for afterpains or engorged breasts, breast care, perineal care for cleanliness, and temperature and blood pressure taken every 4 hours; showers may be taken by the second postoperative day if a spray dressing is used. Discharge of lochia will follow the same pattern as for a vaginally delivered woman.

The mother is shown her infant as soon as possible and given time to handle and examine the child. If the infant is in the intensive care unit, she may be taken by wheelchair. The mother can participate in infant care as soon as she feels able (often after 24 hours). If feeding is attempted, the infant can be supported on pillows to relieve pressure on the mother's abdomen. Some mothers find the side-lying position most comfortable (Fig. 30.9).

Most women remain in the hospital 5 to 7 days. In preparation for returning home the same teaching is done as is done for any newly delivered woman (see Chapter 31). In addition, instruction is given concerning the following:

1. *Discomfort*. Analgesics such as propoxyphene (Darvon) may be taken. This does not adversely affect the nursing infant.
2. *Exercise*. Progressive exercises may be started after abdominal discomfort has eased. Lifting objects heavier than the infant should be avoided for about 2 weeks.
3. *Complications*. Immediately report fever, dysuria, and frequency suggestive of urinary tract infection (may be secondary to use of catheters).
4. *Intercourse*. Intercourse may be resumed as soon as it is comfortable for the woman. Contraceptive information is provided as needed.
5. *Return examination*. This examination is planned for the third week; by that time the physical findings should be comparable to those of women who deliver vaginally.

Evaluation. The evaluation of the care given includes preoperative decisions as well as labor care and postdelivery care. Such criteria as the following may be used to evaluate the total care.

1. A joint decision (client-physician) regarding cesarean birth is made.
   a. Detection of abnormal condition or conditions during the prenatal period permits planning for cesarean birth, *or*
   b. Women who have had a cesarean birth are carefully screened so that those who may safely deliver vaginally do so and those who cannot are aware of the reasons for subsequent cesarean births, *or*
   c. Prompt detection of abnormal responses of mother or fetus to labor allows for institution of such remedial measures as cesarean delivery.
2. Personnel utilize acceptable techniques to maintain health of mother and fetus (e.g., fluid and electrolyte balance maintained, oxygen therapy instituted).
3. Mother and infant survive cesarean birth with no adverse sequelae, *or* the family is supported through the death or disability of the infant.
4. Personnel utilize acceptable techniques to maintain emphasis on birth of a child and family participation in the birth.
5. The woman and her family accept the change in expectations of birth and adjust their expectations to permit as satisfying an experience as possible.

Infant Birth Trauma

The forces of labor, in combination with the fetal presentation and position, the amount of resistance encountered during passage through the bony and soft birth canal, and the birth itself, may result in physical birth trauma. Many injuries are minor and readily resolve in the neonatal period without treatment. Other traumas require some degree of intervention. A few are serious enough to be fatal.

CLASSIFICATION OF BIRTH TRAUMAS

Birth traumas can be classified according to the following outline:

1. Soft tissue injuries
   a. Caput succedaneum
   b. Cephalhematoma
   c. Subcutaneous fat necrosis (pressure necrosis)
   d. Subconjunctival (scleral) hemorrhage
   e. Retinal hemorrhage
   f. Cyanosis, ecchymosis, and edema of buttocks and extremities
   g. Ecchymoses and petechiae of skin
   h. Hemorrhage into abdominal organs
2. Skeletal injuries
   a. Molding of fetal skull bones
   b. Fractures
      (1) Skull (depressed or linear)
      (2) Clavicle, humerus, or femur
3. Nervous system trauma
   a. Peripheral nervous system
      (1) Facial paralysis
      (2) Brachial paralysis (Erb-Duchenne, Klumpke's)
      (3) Phrenic nerve injury (diaphragmatic paralysis)
   b. Central nervous system (intracranial hemorrhage, spinal cord injury)

The nurse's critical contributions to the welfare of the newborn begin with early observation and accurate recording. The prompt reporting of signs indicative of deviations from normal permits early initiation of appropriate therapy.

GOALS FOR CARE

The overall goals for care of infants with birth trauma are as follows:

1. Anticipate and diagnose premonitory or early disease.
2. Minimize the effects of the disorder to avoid disability of the child.
3. Treat disease promptly and appropriately when possible.
4. Facilitate a positive parent-child relationship.

Soft tissue injuries. *Caput succedaneum* is a localized edematous swelling of the scalp that persists for a few days after birth and then disappears. It has no pathologic significance (see Figs 27.5, *A*).

Cephalhematoma is a collection of blood from ruptured blood vessels between the periosteum and surface of the parietal bone (see Fig 27.5, *B*, and discussion on p. 583). The swelling may appear unilaterally or bilaterally and disappears gradually in 2 to 3 weeks. Occasionally hyperbilirubinemia may result from breakdown of the accumulated blood.

Subcutaneous fat necrosis results from pressure against the pelvis or from forceps. The lesion is clearly defined and is a firm mass (size varies) fixed to the overlying skin but movable over underlying tissue. Skin over the lesion may be reddish purple. These lesions usually resolve spontaneously in a few days.

Subconjunctival (scleral) and *retinal hemorrhages* result from rupture of capillaries from increased intracranial pressure during birth. They clear within 5 days after birth and usually present no problems. However, parents need reassurance about their presence.

Cyanosis, ecchymosis, petechiae, and *edema* of buttocks and extremities may be present. Localized cyanosis may appear over presenting or dependent parts. Ecchymoses (and edema) appear as bruises anywhere on the body: over the presenting part, from the application of forceps, or as a result of manipulation of the infant's body during delivery. Petechiae, or pinpoint hemorrhagic areas, acquired during birth may extend over the upper trunk and face. These lesions are benign if they disappear within 2 days of birth and no new lesions appear. Ecchymoses and petechiae may be signs of a more serious disorder, such as thrombocytopenic purpura.

To differentiate hemorrhagic areas from skin rashes and discolorations, the nurse blanches the skin with two fingers. Because extravasated blood remains within the tissues, petechiae and ecchymoses do not blanch.

Hemorrhage into abdominal organs may occur following manipulation of the body during a difficult breech extraction. The liver is most susceptible to injury. The affected infant is pale, the liver enlarges progressively, and in some, a mass may be palpable. Rupture of the liver capsule occurs eventually, and the infant appears cyanotic and in shock. Surgical repair and blood transfusions are lifesaving.

Skeletal injuries

Molding. The shaping of the head as it passes through the bony pelvis during labor is discussed in Chapter 20.

Skull fracture. The newborn's immature, flexible skull can withstand a great degree of deformation (molding) before fracture results. Considerable force is required to fracture the newborn's skull. Location of the fracture determines whether it is insignificant or fatal; for example, if an artery lying in a groove on the undersurface of the skull is torn, subdural hemorrhage may occur. Symptoms of increased intracranial pressure will ensue. Unless a blood vessel is involved, linear fractures (which account for 70% of all fractures for this age group) heal without special treatment. The soft skull may become indented without laceration of either the skin or the dural membrane. These depressions, or

"Ping-Pong ball" indentations, may occur during difficult deliveries from pressure of the head on the bony pelvis or injudicious application of forceps.

Fracture of clavicle. The clavicle is the bone most often fractured during delivery. Generally the break is in the middle third of the bone. Dystocia, particularly shoulder impaction, may be the predisposing problem. *Limitation of motion of the arm, crepitus of the bone, and no Moro's reflex on the affected side are diagnostic.* Except for use of gentle rather than vigorous handling, there is no accepted treatment for fractured clavicle. The figure-eight bandage appropriate for the older child should not be used for the neonate. The prognosis is good.

Fracture of humerus or femur. The humerus and femur are other bones that may be fractured during a difficult delivery. Fractures in newborns generally heal rapidly. Immobilization is accomplished with slings, splints, swaddling, and other devices. The parents need support in handling these infants because they are often fearful of hurting them. Parents are encouraged to practice in the nursery under the guidance of personnel, handling, changing, and feeding the affected newborn so that their confidence and knowledge are assured and attachment is facilitated. A plan for follow-up therapy is developed with the parents so that the times and arrangements for therapy are workable and acceptable to them, as well as to those persons providing the therapy.

Nervous system injuries

Peripheral nerves

Brachial paralysis: upper arm. Erb-Duchenne paralysis (upper arm brachial paralysis) is the most common type of paralysis associated with a difficult delivery (Fig. 37.21). Typical symptoms are a flaccid arm with the elbow extended and the hand rotated inward, negative Moro's reflex on the affected side, sensory loss over the lateral aspect of the arm, and an intact grasp reflex.

Treatment consists of intermittent immobilization, proper positioning, and exercise to maintain the range of motion of joints. Gentle manipulation and range of motion exercises are delayed until about the tenth day to prevent additional injury to the brachial plexus.

Immobilization may be accomplished with a brace or splint or by pinning the infant's sleeve to the mattress. He should be positioned for 2 or 3 hours at a time in the following manner: abduct the arm 90 degrees; externally rotate the shoulder; flex the elbow 90 degrees; supinate the wrist with palm directed slightly toward the face (Fig. 37.22). The arm should be free periodically for good skin care. About the tenth day, gentle massage and range of motion exercises are begun to prevent contractures.

Brachial paralysis: lower arm. Damage to the lower plexus, Klumpke's palsy, is less common. With lower arm paralysis, the wrist and hand are flaccid, the grasp

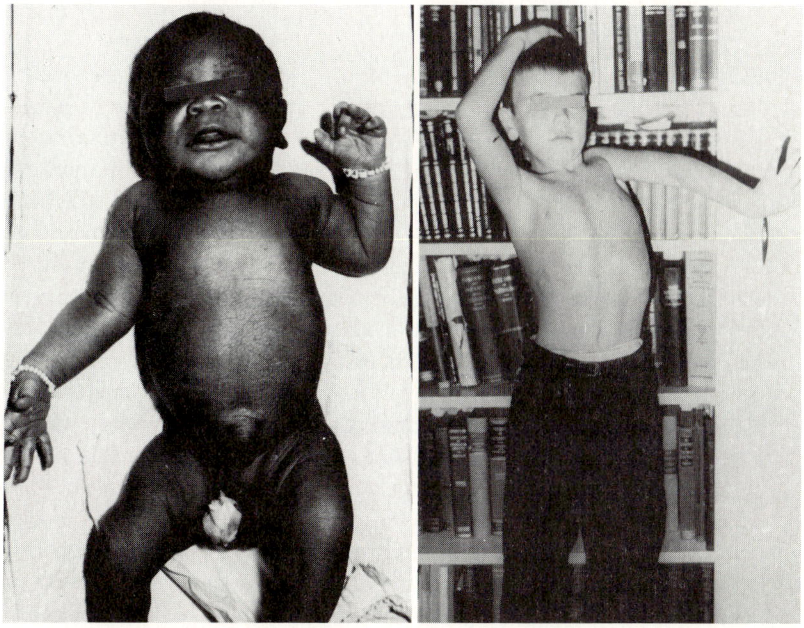

A B

Fig. 37.21
A, Erb-Duchenne paralysis in newborn infant. Right upper extremity failed to participate in Moro's reflex. Recovery was complete. **B,** Residual of Erb-Duchenne paralysis. Left arm was short; it could not be raised above level shown. (From Shirkey, H.C., editor: Pediatric therapy, ed. 6, St. Louis, 1975, The C.V. Mosby Co.)

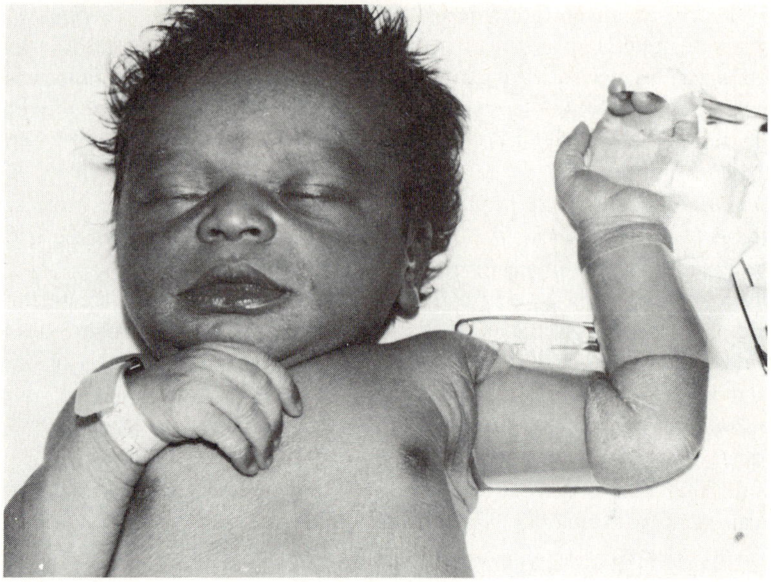

Fig. 37.22
Recommended corrective positioning for treatment of Erb-Duchenne paralysis. Note abduction and external rotation at shoulder, flexion at elbow, supination of forearm, and slight dorsiflexion at wrist. (From Behrman, R.E., editor: Neonatology: diseases of the fetus and infant, St. Louis, 1973, The C.V. Mosby Co.)

Fig. 37.23
A, Paralysis of right side of face 15 minutes after forceps delivery. **B,** Same infant 24 hours later. Recovery was complete in another 24 hours.

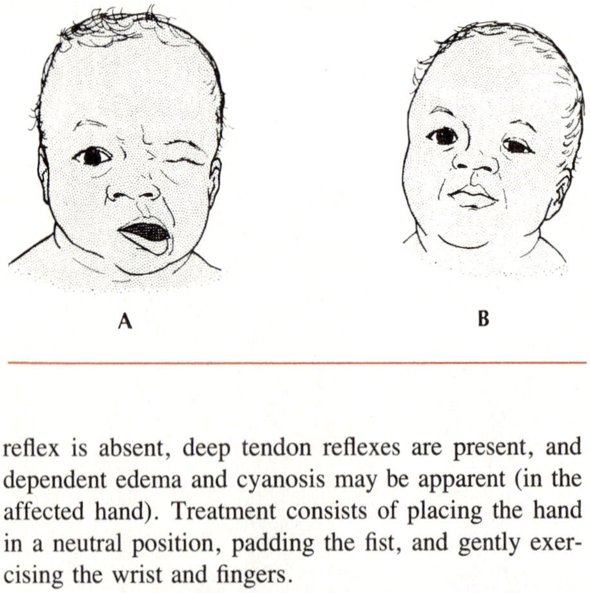

A B

reflex is absent, deep tendon reflexes are present, and dependent edema and cyanosis may be apparent (in the affected hand). Treatment consists of placing the hand in a neutral position, padding the fist, and gently exercising the wrist and fingers.

Parents are taught to position and immobilize the arm or wrist or both and to gently massage and manipulate the muscles to prevent contractures while the arm is healing. If edema or hemorrhage is responsible for the paralysis, the prognosis is good, and recovery may be expected in a few weeks. If laceration of the nerves has occurred and healing does not result in return of function within a few months (3 to 6 months or 2 years at the most), surgery may be indicated; little or no function will develop, however.

Facial paralysis. Facial paralysis (Fig. 37.23) is generally caused by misapplication of forceps and pressure by one blade against the facial nerve during delivery. The face on the affected side is flattened and unresponsive to the grimace of crying or stimulation, and the eye may remain open. Moreover, the forehead will not wrinkle. Often the condition is transitory, resolving within hours or days of birth. Permanent paralysis is rare.

Treatment involves careful, patient feeding, prevention of damage to the cornea of the open eye, and supportive care of the parents. Frequently the infant looks grotesque, especially when crying. Feeding may be prolonged, with the milk flowing out of the neonate's mouth around the nipple on the affected side. The mother may need understanding and sympathetic encouragement while learning how to feed and care for the infant, as well as how to hold and cuddle him.

Phrenic nerve injury. Phrenic nerve injury almost always occurs as a component of brachial plexus injury. Injury to the phrenic nerve results in diaphragmatic paralysis. Cyanosis and irregular thoracic respirations with no abdominal movement on inspiration are characteristic of paralysis of the diaphragm. Babies with diaphragmatic paralysis usually require mechanical ventilatory support, at least for the first few days after birth. Occasionally this support is essential for several weeks until corrective surgery can be performed.

Central nervous system

Intracranial hemorrhage. Intracranial hemorrhage as a result of birth trauma is more likely to occur in the full-term, large infant. The hemorrhage occurs into the brain substance or as a subdural hematoma. The latter is the principal manifestation of intracranial hemorrhage. The diagnostic signs arise from increased intracranial pressure and are (1) separation of the sutures and (2) bulging of the anterior fontanel. Subdural hematoma is seen with relative infrequency today because of the remarkable improvements in obstetric care in the last decade.

Hypoxia and hypovolemia are the most common causes of intracranial hemorrhage. Hemorrhage from hypoxia occurs in the subarachnoid space or in the ventricles of the brain. These intracranial hemorrhages, seen most frequently in premature infants, are not related to trauma. The symptomatology varies. Abnormal respiration with cyanosis, hypotonia, reduced responsiveness (lethargy), irritability, a high-pitched, shrill cry, tense fontanel, twitching, or convulsions may be noted.

General treatment consists of elevation of the head several inches higher than the hips, warmth, oxygen to relieve cyanosis, and administration of intravenous fluids or other suitable method of meeting the neonate's food and fluid needs. Minimal handling to promote rest should guide nursing care.

The treatment of subdural hemorrhage is aspiration or surgical removal of the blood collection. Repeated subdural taps for the evacuation of subdural blood is indicated whether or not the head size is increasing and the fontanel is bulging.

Spinal cord injuries. Spinal cord injuries may occur during manipulation of the neonate's body during breech extraction, when considerable traction force is required to deliver the shoulders or head or both. This injury is rarely seen today.

Preterm Birth

Preterm birth is that which occurs before the end of the thirty-seventh week of gestation, resulting in the birth of a premature infant usually weighing less than 2500 g. The overall incidence of prematurity in the United States is 6% to 7%; in blacks the incidence is 10% to 11%. Prematurity is responsible for almost two thirds of infant deaths. Maternal, placental, and fetal causes may be identified, but in approximately two thirds of cases, no definite cause can be identified. Thirty to fifty percent of premature labors occur after premature rupture of the membranes. Iatrogenic prematurity (delivery too early by induction or cesarean delivery) accounts for slightly less than 10% of preterm babies.

The importance of premature birth is that the infant is usually delivered too early for the growth and development necessary for uncomplicated adjustment to extrauterine life. Hence its prospects for survivial or good health may be severely compromised.

Although certain problems may be identified, many so-called causes of premature birth may be coincidental. The following associations or causes are prominent in premature labor.

1. *Maternal problems.* Debilitating disorders, trauma, abdominal surgery, maternal injury, preeclampsia-eclampsia, uterine anomalies or tumors, cervical incompetence, and sepsis often are preludes to premature labor.

2. *Placental disorders.* Gross placental abnormalities such as placental separation or extrachorial placenta are associated with premature labor.

3. *Fetal abnormalities.* Transplacental infections such as rubella, toxoplasmosis, or syphilis may be responsible for premature labor. Multiple pregnancy, hydramnios, and premature rupture of the membranes are also notable. Congenital adrenal hyperplasia is usually associated with premature labor.

4. *Iatrogenic causes.* Premature labor can result from elective delivery because of misjudgment of fetal maturity or miscalculation of the EDC.

The diagnosis of preterm birth may be difficult to distinguish from painful Braxton Hicks' contractions. Labor is progressive and associated with cervical dilatation, effacement, or both. It may be helpful to utilize external monitoring to record the frequency and intensity of contractions to be certain that labor is underway, as well as to monitor the FHR.

PROGNOSIS FOR INFANTS

Infants weighing more than 2500 g and delivered after 37 weeks of pregnancy have the best prospects of survival. There is a dramatic reduction in mortality in infants, regardless of weight, who are delivered after the thirty-sixth week of gestation. The prognosis for low–birth weight infants weighing more than 1800 g is more favorable than for those weighing 1500 to 1800 g. The mortality is less than 5% if pregnancy has progressed to 35 weeks and the fetus weighs more than 2000 g. With these guidelines it is illogical to try to stop labor if the duration of pregnancy is 37 weeks or longer. The hazardous zone is 34 to 37 weeks, but the fetus should weigh more than 1800 g.

OBSTETRIC MANAGEMENT OF PREMATURE LABOR

Obstetric management of prematurity may involve (1) preventing the onset of preterm labor; (2) suppressing uterine activity; and (3) improving intrapartum care of the fetus destined to be born early.

PREVENTION

Over the past 25 years, little if any progress has been made in preventing preterm birth, and the incidence of low–birth weight babies has remained unchanged. At the present time, the United States ranks sixteenth among industrialized nations in perinatal mortality, mainly because of the high incidence of preterm birth. Consequently, it is unlikely that this ranking will improve substantially unless this high incidence is lowered.

Prevention has played a minor role because the mechanisms responsible for preterm labor are unknown. However, conditions predisposing women to preterm birth are recognized. Indications such as the following emphasize the importance of early and continuous prenatal care.

1. Many women are unaware of the danger of preterm delivery and need to be informed of how they might reduce the risk. For example, there is an increased incidence of low–birth weight infants among the very young and among older nulliparas.
2. The presence of major medical or surgical illness should be identified whenever a woman contemplates pregnancy. The risk of preterm birth associated with hypertension, cardiac disorders, renal disease, and severe anemia should be pointed out.
3. Multiple gestation can result in preterm birth. Drugs taken for infertility can increase the risk of multiple gestation as can conception soon after discontinuation of oral contraceptives.
4. Occult cervicitis or amnionitis has been associated with premature labor. Intrapartum infection in women delivering low–birth weight infants increases with or without premature rupture of membranes (PROM), suggesting that infection might precede preterm labor and PROM.

SUPPRESSION OF UTERINE ACTIVITY (LABOR)

Because preterm labor is associated with an extremely high perinatal loss, one might think it best to try to quell uterine contractions in all women who threaten to deliver early. This is not reasonable, however, because many serious disorders cannot be diagnosed before labor. Moreover, early labor may spare the mother and infant. In some cases the diagnosis of anomalies indicates that the mother should not have to carry the pregnancy to term.

Attempts to arrest labor are justified only if the following conditions are present:

1. Labor is diagnosed: there are three or more contractions of moderate intensity and duration per 20 minutes; the cervix is dilated no more than 4 cm or effaced no more than 50%; but the membranes must be intact with no bulging.
2. The fetus must be live and viable (some hospitals specify 20 to 36 weeks; others, 27 to 37 weeks' gestation inclusive). Estimation of gestational age by ultrasonography is the preferred technique.
3. There are no signs of fetal distress or disease.
4. There must be no medical or obstetric disorder or clinically significant abnormalities in laboratory findings that are a contraindication to the continuation of pregnancy.
5. The woman is both willing and capable of giving an informed consent. She should be able to comply with the prescribed regimen of medication (on an outpatient basis) and weekly visits until delivery and to return for the 6-wk postdelivery examination.

Outpatient management. Preterm labor may be treated by bed rest and sedation in the home. The nurse assists the woman or couple in an understanding of "bed rest." Physical rest is facilitated by peace of mind, that is, someone to watch the other children, lack of guilt for not cooking supper, and so on. Bed rest is intended to keep the pressure of the fetus off the cervix and to enhance uterine perfusion. Kneeling or sitting in bed does not keep the fetus from pressing on the cervix. The woman is advised to lie on her left side with her head flat or raised on a small pillow. Coitus is contraindicated also because (1) prostaglandins in semen can stimulate labor in a susceptible woman and (2) touching the cervix may stimulate Ferguson's reflex (the increase in myometrial contractility that follows mechanical stretching or touching of the cervix).

The woman is instructed and given written instructions (for herself and her family) regarding the following areas:

1. The prescription for sedation, including dosage, times for administration, and side effects
2. What to do and whom to notify in case of onset of labor or rupture of membranes
3. Maintaining personal hygiene if membranes have ruptured earlier and assessing for signs of infection (e.g., odor of vaginal discharge, increase in body temperature)

In-hospital suppression of preterm labor. Various drugs have been used to suppress labor. They are known as tocolytic drugs. The term is derived from tocology, which refers to care during childbirth or labor.

Magnesium sulfate. The precautions taken during administration of magnesium sulfate are the same regardless of whether the rationale for therapy is the suppression of labor or the prevention of eclampsia (see p. 815). For example, before repeating a dose of magnesium sulfate, patellar and other reflexes must be present, respirations must be at least 16/min, and urinary output must be at least 100 ml every 4 hr. Magnesium sulfate toxicity is manifested by severe CNS depression. Therefore in addition to assessing for the above findings the nurse is alert to and reports (1) the subjective symptoms: the woman states she "feels hot all over" and is very thirsty and (2) the objective signs: flaccid paralysis, hypothermia, circulatory collapse, or depressed cardiac function. The *antidote* (calcium gluconate, 10 to 20 ml of a 10% solution) is kept at the bedside.

Ritodrine hydrochloride. Ritodrine hydrochloride (Yutopar) (Ueland, 1981) is the first β-sympathomimetic drug approved in the United States for use in preterm labor (Food and Drug Administration, 1980). The administration of ritodrine must be closely supervised by persons having knowledge of the pharmacology of the drug and qualified to identify and manage complications of drug administration or pregnancy.

Drug action. Ritodrine exerts a preferential effect on $beta_2$ adrenergic receptors such as those located in the uterine smooth muscle, vascular smooth muscle, and bronchial smooth muscle. Stimulation of $beta_2$-receptors causes relaxation of smooth muscle. Ritodrine, although exerting its predominant effect on $beta_2$-receptors, also stimulates $beta_1$-receptors, which are located in the heart and small intestines. Stimulation of these receptors causes excitation resulting in tachycardia or diarrhea. The clinically effective oral dose of ritodrine is not known. It is probably between 10 and 20 mg every 2 hours. The clinically effective half-life of ritodrine is between 1½ and 2 hours. Therefore it must be given every 2 hours.

Toxic effects. Maternal pulmonary edema has been reported in women treated with intravenous and oral ritodrine. This is a late manifestation usually occurring 12 to 48 hours after the initiation of therapy. In rare cases clients have developed cardiac arrhythmias and myocardial ischemia. If symptoms of chest tightness and pain or dyspnea occur, careful cardiopulmonary evaluation is imperative.

Contraindications for use

1. Antepartum hemorrhage that demands immediate delivery
2. Eclampsia or severe preeclampsia
3. Intrauterine fetal death or fetal anomaly incompatible with survival
4. Chorioamnionitis
5. Cardiovascular disease including hypertension
6. Hyperthyroidism
7. Uncontrolled diabetes mellitus
8. Any obstetric or medical condition in which prolonged pregnancy is contraindicated
9. Known drug hypersensitivity

Administration. The drug may be administered either intravenously or orally. *Intravenous administration* precedes the oral administration. The initial recommended dose is 50 to 100 μg (0.05 to 0.1 mg)/min. An infusion pump is used to control the dosage. The infusion solution is normal saline. The woman is not prehydrated and fluid intake is maintained at a minimum of 2500 ml/day to ensure adequate hydration. The dosage may be increased by 50 μg (0.05 mg)/min every 10 minutes until contractions cease or a maximal of 350 μg (0.35 mg)/min is attained. The infusion is continued for at least 12 to 24 hours at the lowest effective dose capable of inhibiting all uterine activity. The oral dose (20 mg) is begun 30 minutes before discontinuing the intravenous infusion. During the first 24 hours the oral dose should be 20 mg (two tablets) every 2 hours. Thereafter, the maintenance dose is 10 to 20 mg every 2 hours, titrating the dose against uterine activity. The dose at night may be spaced every 4 hours, that is, 22:00 hours, 02:00 hours, and 06:00 hours, if there are no contractions.

Management. Because of the possible cardiopulmonary effects an electrocardiogram is necessary before the treatment. The woman is encouraged to assume a left lateral position during the treatment. Monitoring of uterine activity and FHR is begun before medication is given and is continued throughout the treatment. Accurate and repeated assessment of maternal vital signs is necessary. *Hypotension* is among the expected side effects. Because the blood pressure may change rapidly during the initial intravenous treatment, it is recorded as frequently as every 10 minutes. An arteriosound increases accuracy in monitoring blood pressure. Several measures may be employed to minimize hypotension: absolute bed rest, Trendelenburg's position, side-lying position, TED stockings, and adequate hydration (at least 2500 ml/day).

A cardiac monitor for the mother may be indicated to maintain continuous assessment for *tachycardia* and *arrhythmia*. An electrocardiogram will be ordered by the physician for any pulse irregularity.

If tachycardia (110 beats/min or greater) or hypotension (diastolic pressure of 60 mm Hg or less) occurs, lower or withhold the next dose and notify the physician. If tachycardia and hypotension persist despite left side-lying position and adequate fluid therapy, the physician may order an *antidote,* propranolol (Inderal), a beta-blocking agent that reverses uterine inhibitory response and cardiovascular effects. Propranolol is given immediately intravenously in doses of 0.25 mg and repeated at 5-min intervals three times, as needed. A blood sample is sent for analysis for glucose, potassium, and hematocrit every 3 to 6 hours during the intravenous infusion. Intake and output are assessed and recorded every 4 hours.

The evaluation of drug therapy of premature labor is complicated by the inherent difficulty of diagnosing true vs. false labor, the clinical variables that influence the onset of premature labor, the beneficial effect of bed rest alone, and the variety of ways that success or failure may be judged. However, it is now estimated that 75% to 80% of women in premature labor may be prevented from delivering for at least 48 hours by treatment with tocolytic drugs, and any delay of premature delivery is potentially beneficial to the fetus. In addition, the tocolytic agents currently available are usually able to delay delivery long enough for the use of glucocorticoids to effect fetal pulmonary maturation.

PHARMACOLOGIC STIMULATION OF FETAL LUNG MATURITY

Respiratory distress syndrome (RDS), formerly known as hyaline membrane disease of the newborn (HMD), is especially common in small premature infants and often can be prevented or lessened by giving the mother a potent glucocorticoid to accelerate fetal lung maturity. Although research findings are not definitive there is a reduction in the incidence and severity of RDS if glucocorticoids are administered to the mother at least 24 to 48 hours before the delivery. The fetus must be less than 34 weeks' gestation, and the administration is made at least 24 hours before delivery and no longer than 7 days before delivery. Follow-up studies have shown that children who have been exposed to the stated levels of glucocorticoids in utero grow and develop normally during the early years of life. Hence most authorities consider that the chance of benefit to the fetus far outweighs the chance of harm. For these reasons the drug should not be withheld for fear of fetal damage from glucocorticoid exposure. Although the long-term effects are unknown, the following are contraindications to glucocorticoid therapy:

1. ''Prophylaxis'' for RDS, for example, in multiple pregnancy
2. Maternal infection, for example, tuberculosis, viral keratitis
3. Imminent delivery
4. Hypertensive disorders of pregnancy; peptic ulcer

CARE DURING IRREVERSIBLE OR ACCEPTABLE PRETERM LABOR AND DELIVERY

The labor is conducted in accordance with the principles that apply to a low–birth weight (easily compromised) fetus. If vaginal delivery is chosen, the analgesia is limited and continuous FHR monitoring is applied. Artificial rupture of membranes (ARM) if done is delayed until the cervix is more than 6 cm dilated to achieve maximal cervical dilatation and effacement and sufficient descent of the presenting part to avoid prolapse of the cord.

If the augmentation of labor is advisable, as it is in the presence of chorioamnionitis, a low concentration of oxytocin is administered continuously in an intravenous solution. Pudendal block anesthesia is desirable. An episiotomy is done to limit the length of the second stage and excessive pressure on the fragile fetal head. Outlet forceps are utilized for delivery unless easy spontaneous birth is likely. A pediatrician and a nurse from the infant intensive care unit are present at the birth so that resuscitative and supportive care for the infant can be initiated immediately if necessary (see Chapter 33). The neonate is permitted several breaths before clamping the cord; if resuscitation is required, however, the cord is clamped and cut immediately.

POSTPARTUM CARE

Parental concern for the well-being of the infant is apparent during labor. Parents need to be aware of the interest and support of the staff although false reassurance of fetal health must be avoided. However, for some parents the reality of the situation is not appreciated until they see their son or daughter in the intensive care unit. For others who experience fetal or neonatal death, the loss intensifies once the stress of labor and delivery is over (see Chapter 34).

The physical care of the mother is similar to that required for any vaginal delivery. However, the family will be very anxious concerning the health and prognosis of their infant. Nursing care of the preterm infant involves not only medical and nursing personnel but also the active participation of the parents.

Care of Preterm Infants

DEFINITIONS

The term *preterm,* or *premature,* refers to the neonate born before completion of 37 weeks' gestation, regardless of birth weight. *Term* refers to the neonate born between the beginning of the thirty-eighth week and the end of the forty-second week. *Postterm* infants are those infants born after the end of the forty-second week.

	Parameters in weeks of gestation
Preterm	Conception to end of week 37
Term	Start of week 38 to end of week 42
Postterm	Start of week 43

The weight of the infant has a normal range for each gestational week (Fig. 37.24 and 37.25). If at any week the weight is above the 90th percentile (or two or more standard deviations above the norm), the infant is said to be *large for gestational age (LGA)* or *large for dates*. If the weight is below the 10th percentile (or two or more standard deviations below the norm), it is termed *small for gestational age (SGA)*, or *small for dates*.

Fig. 37.24
Three babies of same gestational age, with weights of 600, 1400, and 2750 g, respectively, from left to right. Their weights are plotted on Fig. 37.25 at points *A, B,* and *C*. (From Korones, S.B.: High-risk newborn infants: the basis for intensive nursing care, ed. 3, St. Louis, 1980, The C.V. Mosby Co.)

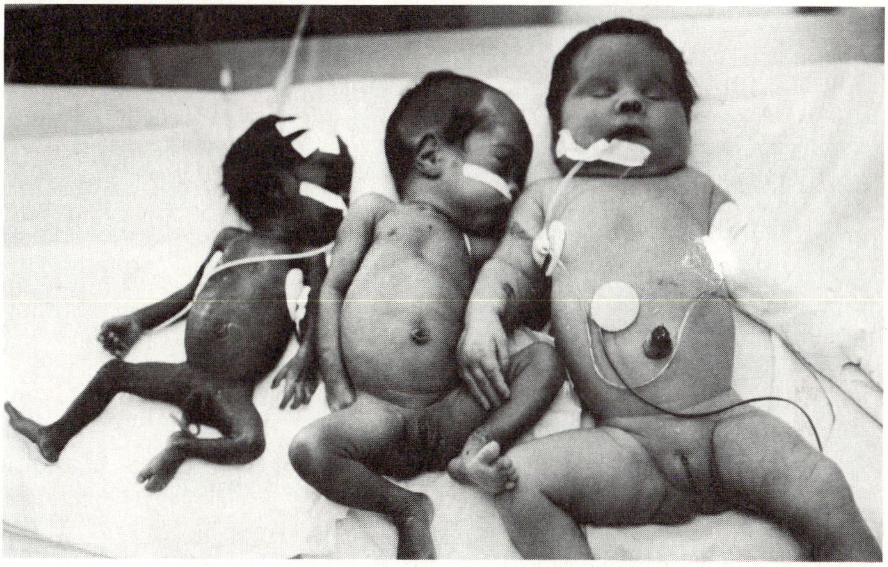

Fig. 37.25
Intrauterine growth status for gestational age and according to appropriateness of growth. Weights of infants shown in Fig. 37.24 are plotted at points *A, B,* and *C*. (Courtesy Mead Johnson & Co., Evansville, Ind. Adapted from Battaglia, F.C., and Lubchenco, L.O.: J. Pediatr. **71**:59, 1967.)

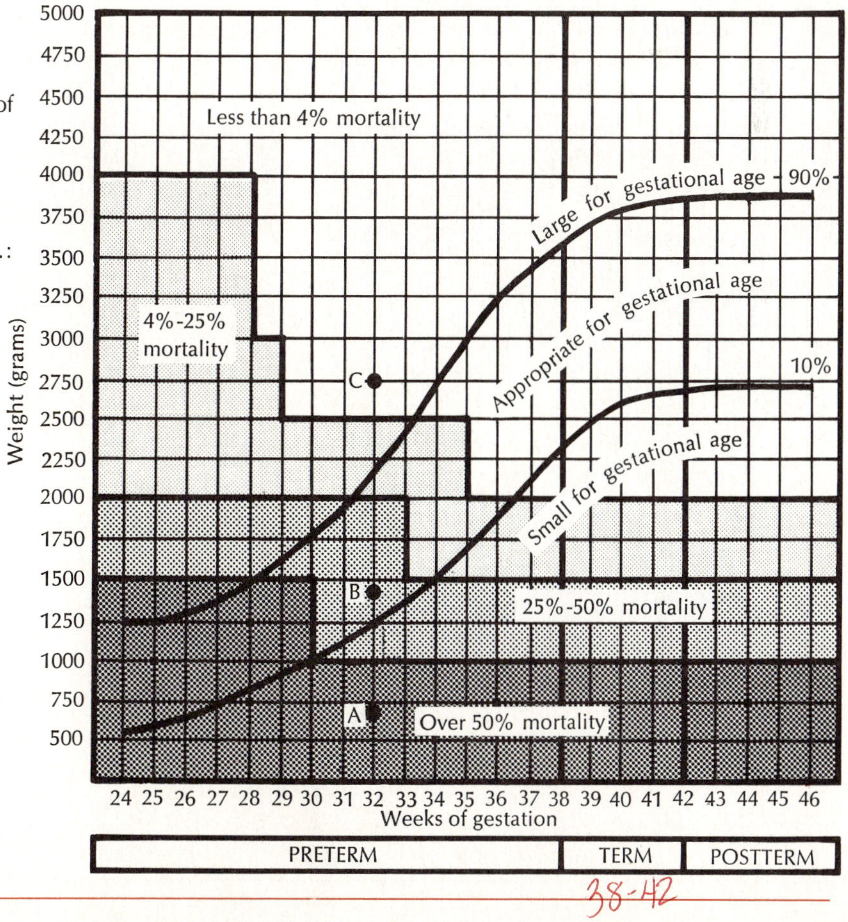

Fig. 37.26

Classification of newborns based on maturity and intrauterine growth. (Courtesy Mead Johnson & Co., Evansville, Ind. Adapted from Lubchenco, L.C., Hansman, C., and Boyd, E.: Pediatrics **37:**403, 1966; Battaglia, F.C., and Lubchenco, L.C.: J. Pediatr. **71:**159, 1967.)

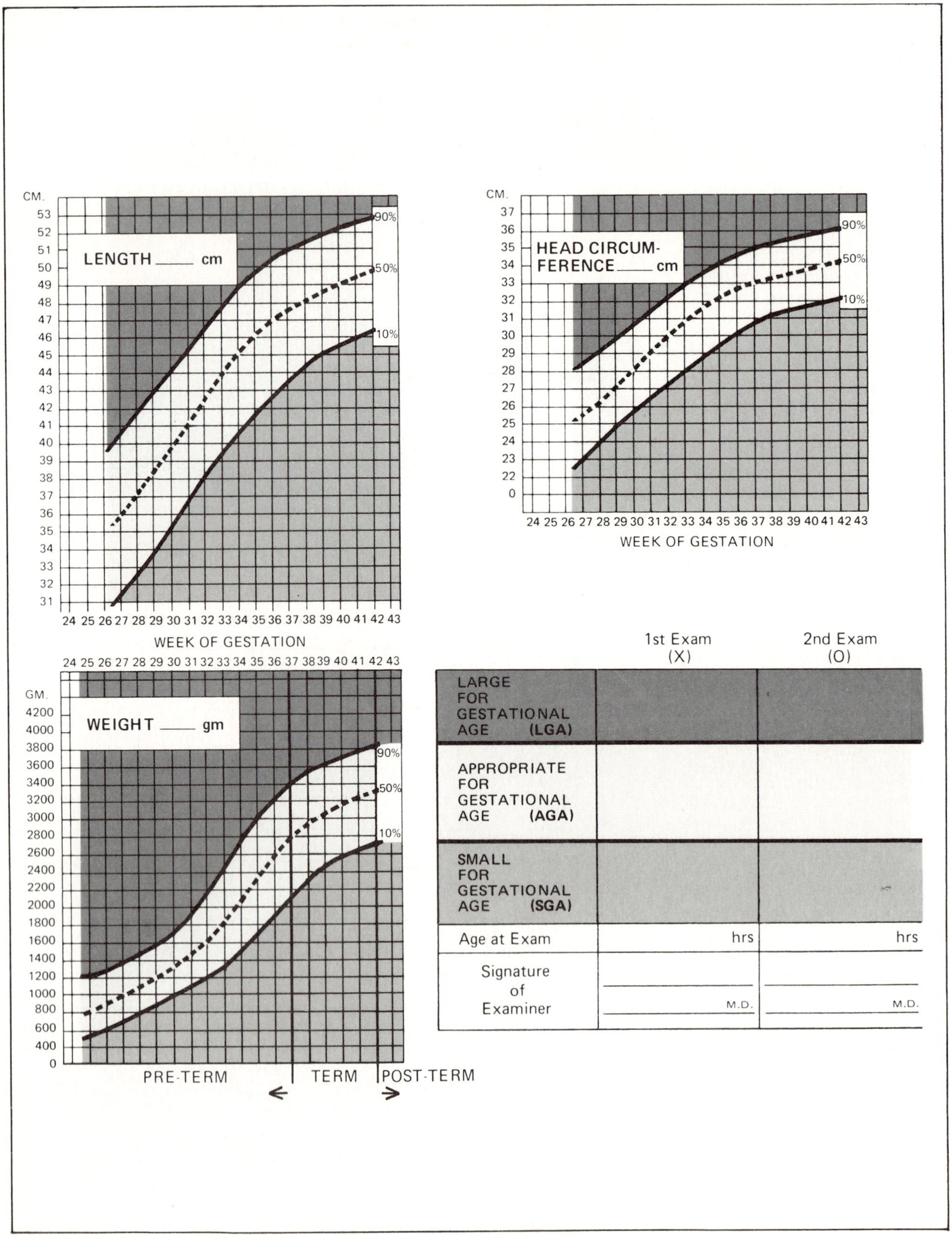

If weight falls between the 10th and 90th percentile for age, the infant is termed *appropriate for gestational age (AGA)*. The risks for morbidity and mortality vary not just with gestational age at birth but also with whether the infant is AGA, LGA, or SGA.

LGA neonates may be preterm, term, or postterm. Common causes of LGA neonates include gestational or true maternal diabetes mellitus, maternal overnutrition, and heredity. SGA neonates may also be preterm, term, or postterm. Often SGA neonates are born of mothers who smoke or mothers with hypertensive states (preeclampsia-eclampsia), maternal undernutrition (inadequate intake, depleted stores because of excessive number of or close spacing of pregnancies), anemia, or nephritis. In addition, the birth of an SGA neonate may be associated with multiple gestation, a discordant twin pregnancy, or congenital anomalies. High altitude, rubella, or intrauterine infection may predispose a woman to the birth of an SGA neonate. Fetal malnutrition, intrauterine growth retardation, and chronic fetal distress are other processes that may result in the birth of neonates who are SGA.

PHYSIOLOGIC BASIS FOR PROBLEMS

The morbidity and mortality rates occurring with preterm infants are higher by three to four times than those of older infants of comparable weight. The actual potential problems of the preterm infant of 2000 g differ from those of the term or postterm infant of equal weight.

The premature infant is at a distinct disadvantage when he faces the transition from intrauterine to extrauterine life. *The degree of disadvantage depends primarily on his level of maturity*. Physiologic disorders and anomalous malformations affect his response to treatment as well. In general, the closer he is to the normal term infant in gestational age and weight, the easier will be his adjustment to the external environment (Fig. 37.26).

The optimal environment for fetal growth and development is within the uterus of a healthy, well-nourished woman for 38 to 42 weeks. The extrauterine environment of the preterm neonate must approximate a healthy intrauterine environment for the normal sequence of growth and development to continue. Provision of such an environment is the basis for care of the preterm infant.

NURSING CARE

Prematurity implies some immaturity of physiologic functioning and a paucity of reserves. Physiologic problems of immature body systems govern the plan of care of these infants. Medical and nursing personnel and respiratory therapists work as a team to provide the intensive care needed. The nurse acts as a constant in the infant's support system.

Nursing actions are based on knowledge of the *physiologic problems* (Table 37.4) *imposed on the preterm infant and on his need to conserve energy for repair, maintenance, and growth.* Assessment and reassessment of the infant's condition are prerequisites to nursing care. The infant is faced with many emergency treatments and procedures. During these emergency treatments and procedures, the nurse must assess and record the signs and symptoms that may reveal the infant's condition and his response to therapy.

Admission to nursery. Admission of a premature newborn to the nursery usually is an emergency situation. A rapid initial evaluation is needed to ascertain the need for lifesaving treatment. Resuscitative measures should be instituted in the delivery room. The neonate's need for warmth and oxygen must be ensured during his transfer from the delivery room to the nursery.

Classifications. The preterm infant is classified according to the degree of supportive care required and the staff assigned to the infant on that basis:

- Class A: severely compromised infant: 1:1 nurse/infant ratio
- Class B: moderately compromised infant: a 1:2 nurse/infant ratio
- Class C: recovery and progress: a 1:4 nurse/infant ratio satisfactory
- Class D: ready for normal: a 1:8 nurse/infant ratio; newborn nursery

Environmental support. The premature infant's external environmental support consists of the following:

1. Incubator control for body temperature
2. Air or oxygen administration, depending on the infant's color and respirations
3. Electronic monitors as needed for the observation of respiratory and cardiac functions and blood gases

Metabolic support consists of measures such as the following:

1. Parenteral fluids to assist in supporting normal blood gas and acid-base homeostasis
2. Parenteral fluids to facilitate antibiotic therapy if sepsis is a concern
3. Blood specimen analyses to monitor blood gases, pH, hypoglycemia, and sepsis

Transfer from community (hospital or home) to regional neonatal care center. Hospitals that are not staffed or equipped to care for high-risk infants arrange for their immediate transfer to specialzed centers. During transport to a center, the following are necessary to meet the infant's needs (see Fig. 40.4).

Fig. 37.27
Newborn maturity rating and classification. (Courtesy Mead Johnson & Co., Evansville, Ind. Scoring section adapted from Ballard, J.L., et al.: Pediatr. Res. **11**:374, 1977. Figures adapted from Sweet, A.Y.: Classification of the low-birth-weight infant. In Klaus, M.H., and Fanaroff, A.A.: Care of the high-risk infant, Philadelphia, 1977, W.B. Saunders Co.)

NEWBORN MATURITY RATING and CLASSIFICATION

ESTIMATION OF GESTATIONAL AGE BY MATURITY RATING

Symbols: X - 1st Exam O - 2nd Exam

NEUROMUSCULAR MATURITY

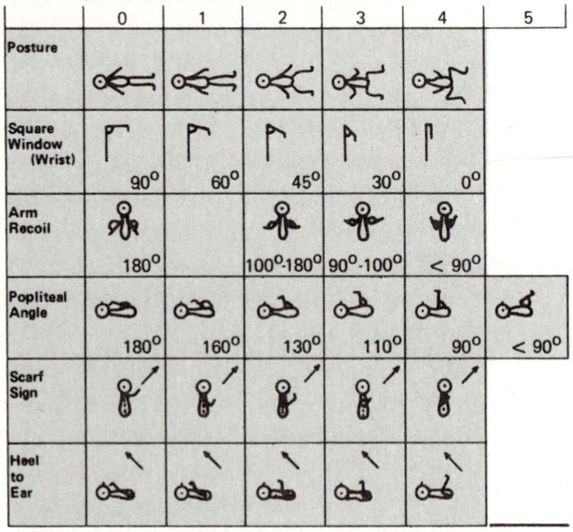

	0	1	2	3	4	5
Posture						
Square Window (Wrist)	90°	60°	45°	30°	0°	
Arm Recoil	180°		100°-180°	90°-100°	< 90°	
Popliteal Angle	180°	160°	130°	110°	90°	< 90°
Scarf Sign						
Heel to Ear						

PHYSICAL MATURITY

	0	1	2	3	4	5
SKIN	gelatinous red, trans-parent	smooth pink, visible veins	superficial peeling &/or rash, few veins	cracking pale area, rare veins	parchment, deep cracking, no vessels	leathery, cracked, wrinkled
LANUGO	none	abundant	thinning	bald areas	mostly bald	
PLANTAR CREASES	no crease	faint red marks	anterior transverse crease only	creases ant. 2/3	creases cover entire sole	
BREAST	barely percept.	flat areola, no bud	stippled areola, 1–2 mm bud	raised areola, 3–4 mm bud	full areola, 5–10 mm bud	
EAR	pinna flat, stays folded	sl. curved pinna, soft with slow recoil	well-curv. pinna, soft but ready recoil	formed & firm with instant recoil	thick cartilage, ear stiff	
GENITALS Male	scrotum empty, no rugae		testes descend-ing, few rugae	testes down, good rugae	testes pendulous, deep rugae	
GENITALS Female	prominent clitoris & labia minora		majora & minora equally prominent	majora large, minora small	clitoris & minora completely covered	

Gestation by Dates ____________ wks

Birth Date ____________ Hour ____________ am / pm

APGAR ____________ 1 min ____________ 5 min

MATURITY RATING

Score	Wks
5	26
10	28
15	30
20	32
25	34
30	36
35	38
40	40
45	42
50	44

SCORING SECTION

	1st Exam=X	2nd Exam=O
Estimating Gest Age by Maturity Rating	______ Weeks	______ Weeks
Time of Exam	Date ______ Hour ______ am / pm	Date ______ Hour ______ am / pm
Age at Exam	______ Hours	______ Hours
Signature of Examiner	______ M.D.	______ M.D.

Fig. 37.28

A, In prone position, premature infant lies with pelvis flat and legs splayed like a frog's. **B,** Normal full-term infant lies with his limbs flexed, pelvis raised, and knees usually drawn under abdomen. (Courtesy Mead Johnson & Co., Evansville, Ind.)

A

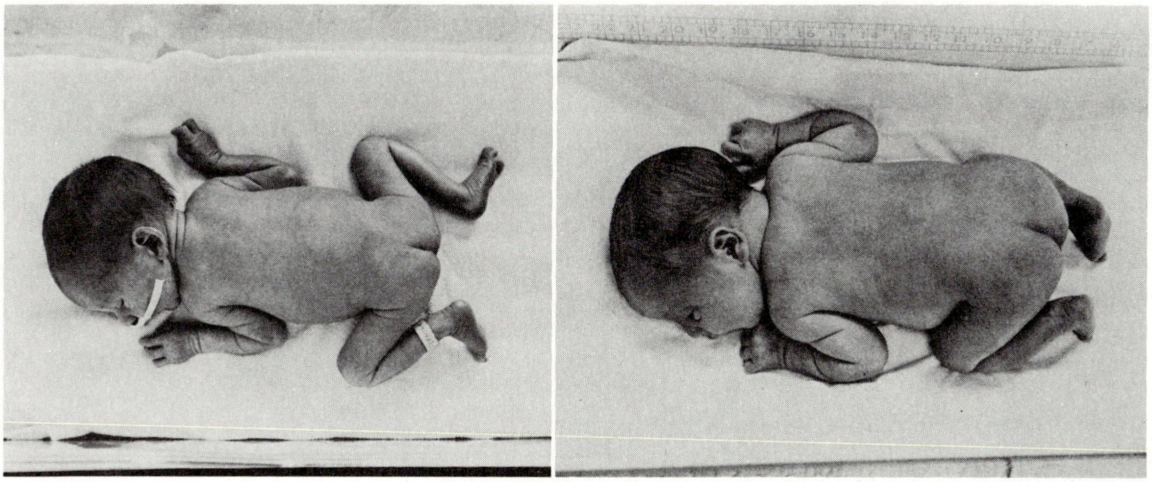

B

Fig. 37.29

A, Normal sole creases of full-term newborn. **B,** Sole of foot of premature infant. As infant loses interstitial fluid after birth, creases become apparent even in preterm infants. Therefore assessment needs to done in first 8 hours after birth.

A

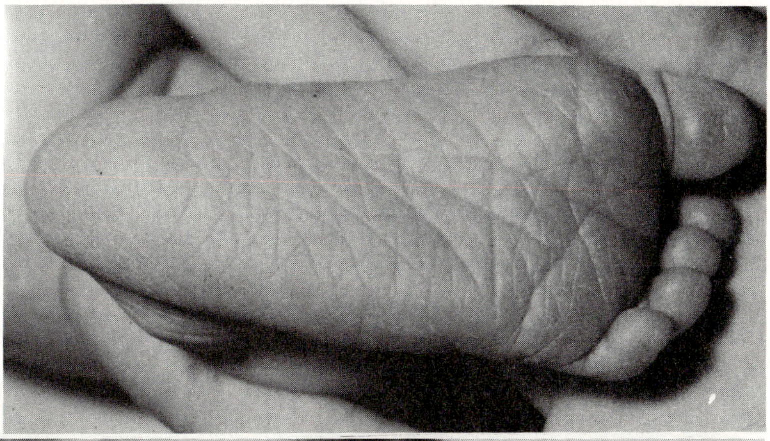

B

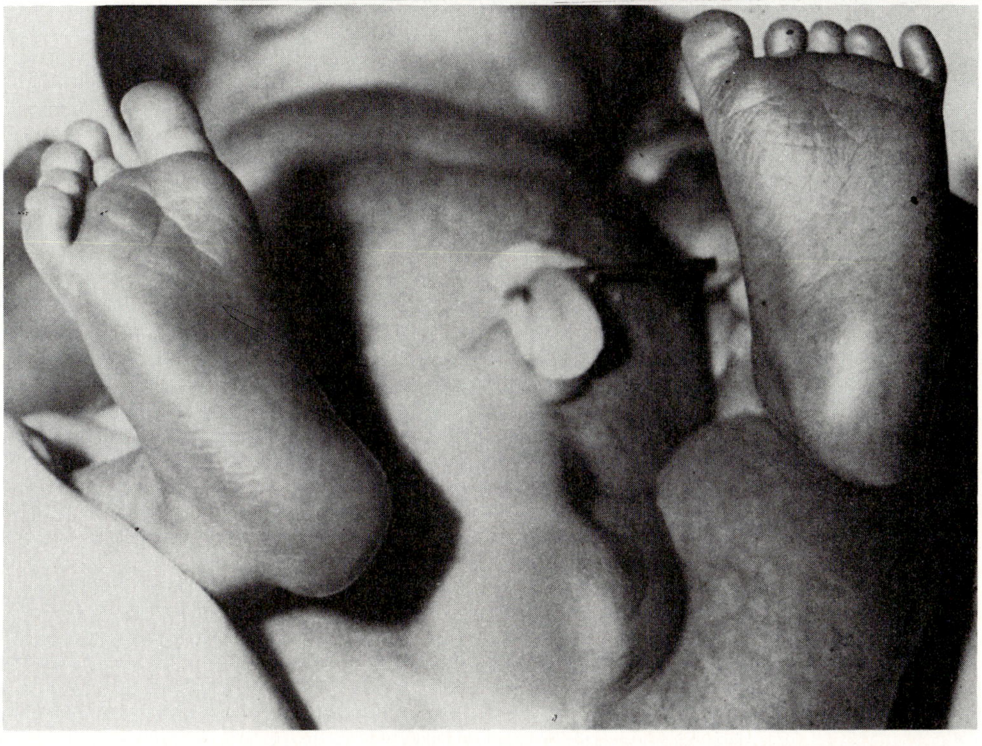

1. Prewarmed blankets, prewarmed incubator, or improvise: surround the infant with hot-water bottles at a distance of 5 to 10 cm from his body
2. Portable oxygen and suction apparatuses
3. Bulb syringe or DeLee mucous trap catheter
4. Intravenous setup with a battery-powered infusion pump
5. Medications as ordered by physician
6. Appropriate attendant or attendants

Once emergency care has been initiated, the infant's gestational age is estimated.

Examination for gestational age. The determination of gestational age by physical examination is a procedure that is appropriately done by the nurse. The most

Fig. 37.30
Assessment of gestational age in, **A,** term newborn and, **B,** preterm newborn.

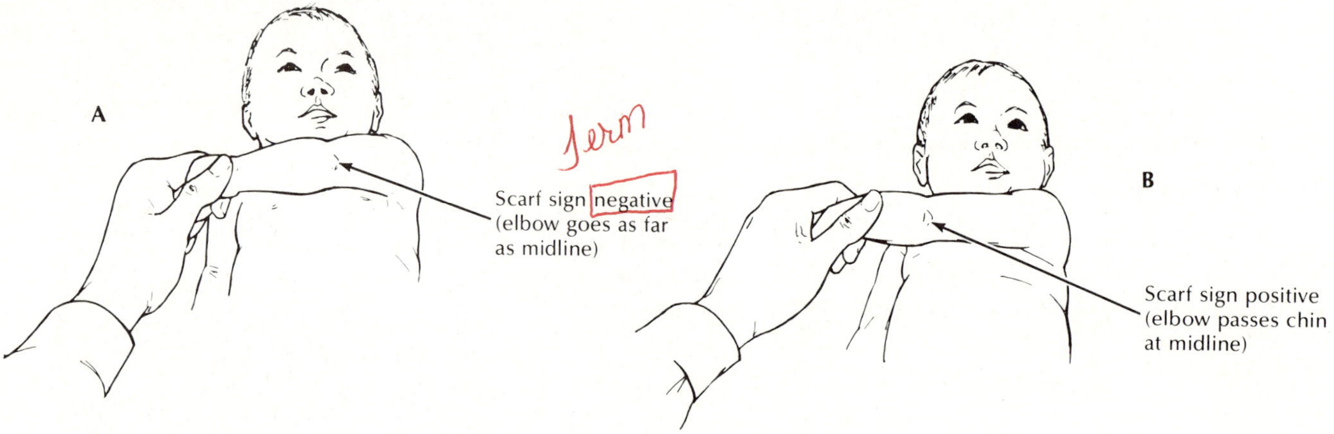

Fig. 37.31
Ankle dorsiflexion. **A,** Angle of 0 degrees in term newborn. **B,** Angle of 20 degrees, or 90%, in preterm newborn.

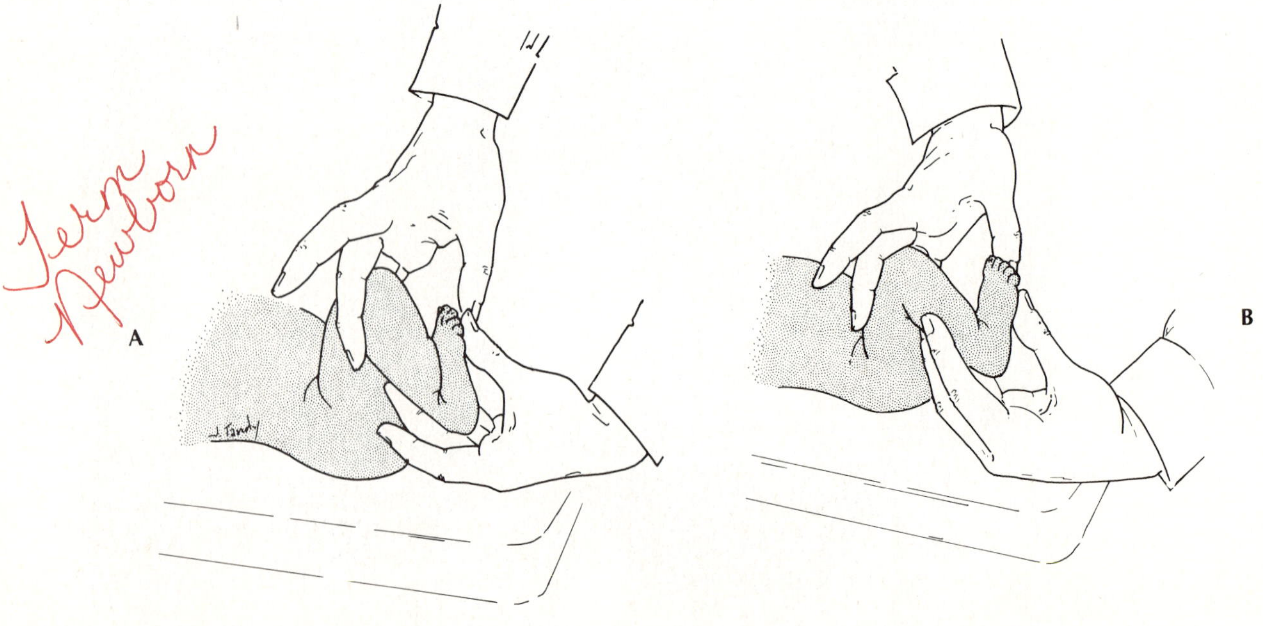

frequent procedure is the one described by Dubowitz and Dubowitz (1977). The nurse's correct knowledge of the indicators for gestational age and maturity and the methods of evaluation will increase her therapeutic potential at the crib site of all newborns, preterm or otherwise. These tests are performed ideally between 2 and 8 hours of age. For the first hour the infant is recovering from the stress of birth; for example, the arm recoil is slower in the fatigued infant. After 48 hours some responses change significantly; for example, the plantar creases on the soles of the feet appear to increase in number and become visible as the skin loses fluid and dries. See Figs. 37.27 to 37.32 and Table 37.3 for the clinical estimation of gestational age.

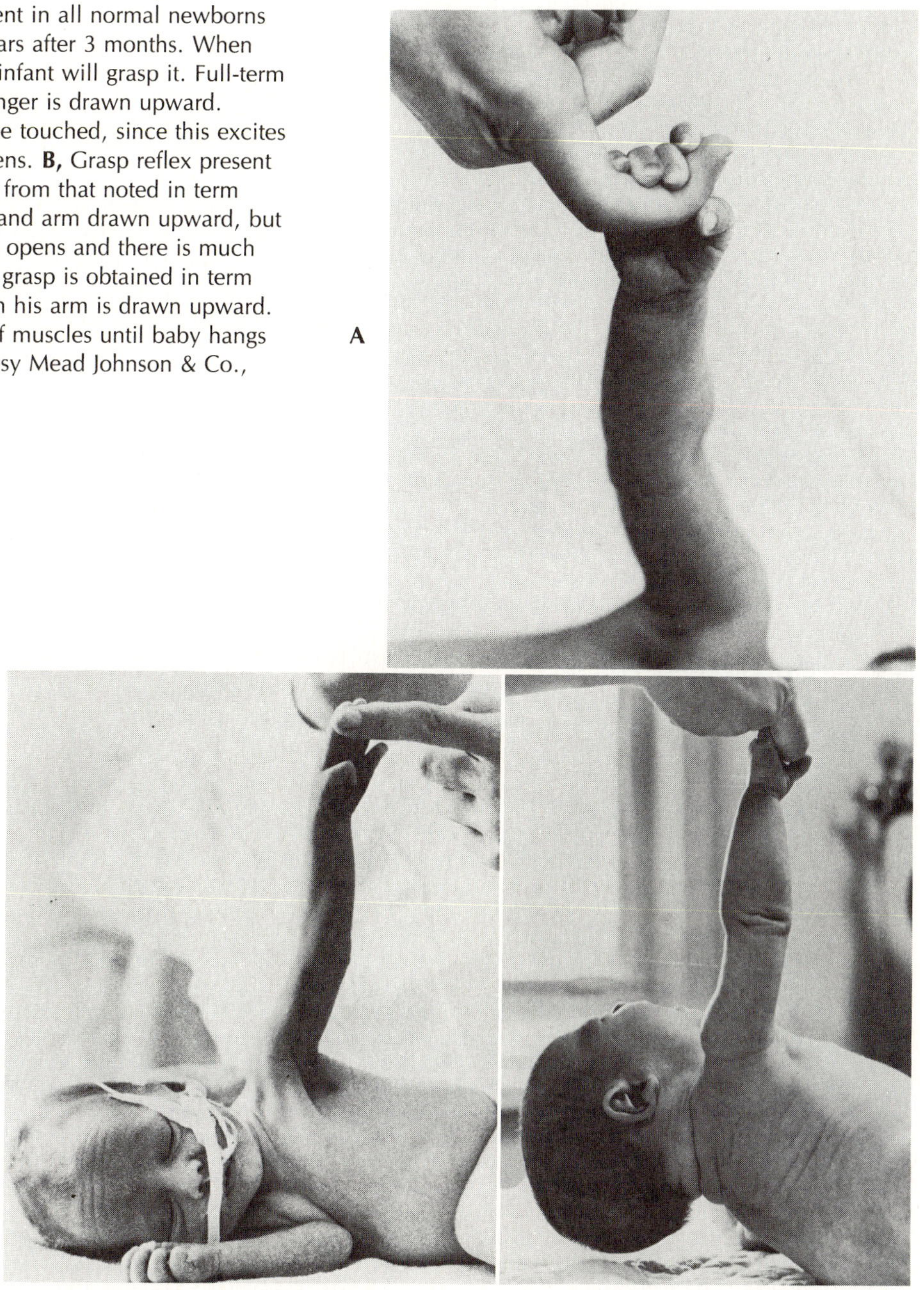

A

B

C

Fig. 37.32

A, Primitive grasp reflex present in all normal newborns usually weakens and disappears after 3 months. When palm is stimulated by finger, infant will grasp it. Full-term infant reinforces his grip as finger is drawn upward. Dorsum of hand should not be touched, since this excites opposite reflex, and hand opens. **B,** Grasp reflex present in premature infant is distinct from that noted in term infant. Grip can be obtained and arm drawn upward, but when traction is applied, grip opens and there is much less muscle tension. **C,** Once grasp is obtained in term infant, grip is reinforced when his arm is drawn upward. There is progressive tensing of muscles until baby hangs momentarily. (**B** and **C** courtesy Mead Johnson & Co., Evansville, Ind.)

Table 37.3
Elaboration of Neuromuscular Maturity Scales*

Criterion	Method of Assessment	0
Posture (Fig. 37.28)	Position: supine Activity: quiet Assessment: extension and flexion of arms, hips, legs	Complete extension 
Square window (wrist)†	Position: supine Method: with thumb supporting back of arm below wrist, apply gentle pressure with index and third fingers on dorsum of hand; do not rotate infant's wrist Assessment: angle formed between hypothenar eminence and forearm	Very premature (<30 wk)  90°
Arm recoil‡	Position: supine Method: flex forearms on upper arms for 5 sec; pull on hands to full extension and release Assessment: degree of flexion	No recoil; arms remain extended  180°
Popliteal angle	Position: supine; pelvis on flat, firm surface Method: flex leg on thigh; then flex thigh on abdomen; holding knee with thumb and index finger, extend leg with index finger of other hand behind ankle Assessment: degree of angle behind knee	Complete extension; very premature  180°
Scarf sign (Fig. 37.30)	Position: supine Method: support head in midline with one hand; pull hand to opposite shoulder Assessment: position of elbow in relation to midline	Elbow to opposite arm like scarf around neck 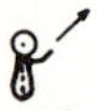
Heel to ear	Position: supine; pelvis is kept flat on surface Method: pull foot up toward ear on same side; do not hold knee Assessment: distance of foot from ear and degree of extension of knee	Toes touch ear; leg completely extended (180°) 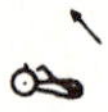

*Compare combined scores for physical and neuromuscular maturity to the "maturity rating" scores and read estimated weeks of gestational age. Estimate entered on appropriate graphs. All three measurements should fall within same approximate range, e.g., all within SGA, LGA, or AGA. If one measure **O,** second examination.

†Counterpart: ankle dorsiflexion (see Fig. 37.31).

‡Counterpart: leg recoil.

Finding and Assigned Scores					**Infant Score**	
1	**2**	**3**	**4**	**5**	**X**	**0**
Extension of arms; slight flexion of hips, legs 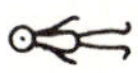	Extension of arms 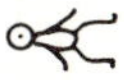	Slight flexion, arms full, with abduction of legs, hips 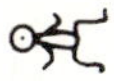	Complete flexion 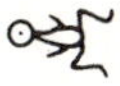	—	______	______
Premature (30-35 wk)  60°	Premature (30-35 wk)  45°	Maturing (35-38 wk)  30°	Term: hand lies flat on ventral surface of forearm 0°	—	______	______
—	Some recoil; sluggish response  100°-180°	Maturing (35-38 wk)  90°-100°	Brisk recoil to complete flexion  < 90°	—	______	______
Premature (30-35 wk)  160°	Premature (30-35 wk)  130°	Maturing (35-38 wk)  110°	Maturing (35-38 wk)  90°	Extension is resisted  < 90°	______	______
Elbow beyond midline of thorax 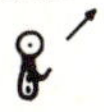	Elbow just beyond midline 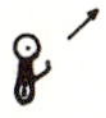	Elbow at midline 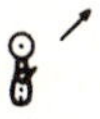	Elbow does not reach midline 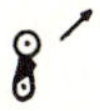	—	______	______
Toes almost reach face (130°) 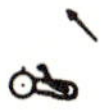	Knees flexed (110°) 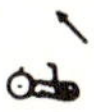	Knees flexed (90°) 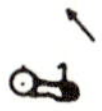	Knees flexed; popliteal angle is less than 90° 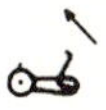	—	______	______
				NEUROMUSCULAR MATURITY TOTALS	______	______
				PHYSICAL MATURITY TOTALS	______	______
				COMBINED SCORE	______	______

of gestational age obtained is accurate only to plus or minus 2 wk. After gestational age is estimated, infant's length, weight, and head circumference are ment is excessively large (falling into LGA range) and other two fall into SGA range, growth deviation should be assessed. **X,** First examination;

Nursing actions. The nurse formulates plans for the specific needs of the premature infant based on the nursing diagnoses derived from a continuous assessment of the child's condition. Table 37.4 presents an overall plan for care. It includes the goals for care for the preterm infant, the physiologic problems, and the nursing actions relevant to assessment and implementation of a plan of care.

Table 37.4
Care of the Preterm Infant: Goals, Physiologic Problems, and Nursing Actions—Assessment and Implementation

		Nursing Actions	
Goals for Care	**Physiologic Problems**	**Assessment**	**Implementation**
Initiation and maintenance of respirations	Paucity of functional alveoli; incomplete aeration of lungs caused by deficient surfactant Smaller lumen and greater collapsibility or obstruction of respiratory passages Weakness of respiratory musculature Insufficient calcification of bony thorax Absent or weak gag reflex Immature and friable capillaries in brain and lungs Few functional alveoli in infants less than 28- wk gestational age (usually nonviable); marginal function in infants at 29-30 wk	Check respiration rate, depth, regularity Periodic breathing Apnea Respiratory rate after apneic episode: same, increased, or decreased Seesaw respirations Expiratory grunt Chin tug Retractions Flaring of alae nasi Cry: feeble, whining, high pitched Check heart rate Cyanosis When it occurs Where (circumoral, generalized) Relieved by O_2 or not; amount of O_2 needed Accompanied by pallor Check reflexes: presence and condition of gag, swallow Prebirth history Was mother treated with betamethasone? Preeclampsia? (Sedatives, magnesium sulfate, diuretics?)	Maintain respirations Respirations of 40 breaths/min at birth without significant fluctuations Respirations of 60/min after first hour of life, followed by no significant increase or decrease (e.g. ± 15 breaths/min) Periods of periodic breathing must not exceed 10 sec Apneic episodes must not exceed 15 sec Maintain warmth to decrease 0_2 consumption and sequelae of cold stress Suction as needed Administer warmed and humidified compressed air and 0_2 at levels to relieve cyanosis and dyspnea Analyze 0_2 concentration every 1-4 hr Blood gases and electrolytes: order, assist with, record time, procedure, amount of blood drawn, infant's response Position infant to assist ventilatory effort (Chapters 29 and 33) Feeding technique appropriate for this infant (see Chapters 30 and 33) Keep on respiratory monitor until infant weighs 1800 g (4 lb) or condition stabilizes; check rate every 1 or 2 hr and when necessary
Maintenance of body temperature	Large surface area in relation to body weight (mass) Absent or poor reflex control of skin capillaries (no shiver response) Small, inadequate muscle mass activity; absent or minimal flexion of extremities on body	Check for variations in body temperature Thermistor probe to skin Axillary temperature Rectal method (not recommended) Temperature of extremities should feel warm to touch	Maintain temperature Skin: 36.5° C (97.6° F) Axillary: 36.5° C (97.6° F) Incubator: usually 33.5° to 35° C (92° to 95° F) Keep incubator away from windows, air conditioners Ensure warmth during all procedures

Table 37.4—cont'd
Care of the Preterm Infant: Goals, Physiologic Problems, and Nursing Actions—Assessment and Implementation

Goals for Care	Physiologic Problems	Nursing Actions: Assessment	Nursing Actions: Implementation
Maintenance of body temperature—cont'd	Meager insulating subcutaneous fat Immature temperature-regulating center in brain plus friable capillaries in brain (The smaller the infant, the more difficulty it is for him to maintain normal body temperature.)	Check for dehydration Early sign: loss of weight Late signs Soft, sunken eyeball Depressed fontanel Poor skin turgor over abdomen, inner thigh Observe for apneic pauses Number Duration Whether accompanied by cyanosis or not Respiratory rate after apneic episode: same, increased, or decreased	Ambient warm air, draft-free Warmed blankets and equipment Blood transfusion warmed by passing tube through warm bath Nurse's hands warm Incubator lid and portholes closed Warm air or O_2 to infant Conserve infant's energy whenever possible; handle as little and as gently as possible
Maintenance of adequate nutrition	Mechanical feeding problems Absent or weak sucking and swallow reflexes; unsynchronized Absent or weak gag and cough reflexes Small stomach capacity Immature cardiac sphincter (stomach) Lax abdominal musculature Absorption and assimilation problems Paucity of stored nutrients: vitamins A and C; calcium, phosphorus, iron; glycogen; fat, protein; loss of fat and fat-soluble vitamins in stool Immature absorption, decreased amount of HCl Impaired metabolism (enzyme systems) or enzyme pathology	*Feeding* Check reflex maturity Suck and swallow Gag and cough Assess energy level Length of time needed to eat Degree of fatigability Observe for following: Diarrhea Dehydration Vomiting or regurgitation Gastric residual Color, amount, character of stools Plot daily weight on growth grid Measure for growth every week Head circumference Body length	Institute appropriate method for this infant Oral Gavage Nipple not used if respirations $\geq$ 60/min Feed early: To prevent depletion of reserves To support biochemical homeostasis Start feedings with sterile water, then proceed to glucose, then to formula if feeding by oral route Timing of feedings Infant under 1250 g (2 lb, 12 oz), feed every 2 hr Infant between 1500-1800 g (3½-4 lb), feed every 3 hr Infants in good condition and with active peristalsis, start first feeding between 6 and 12 hr after birth Infant with respiratory distress, given parenteral fluids
		Absorption and assimilation Observe for following: Steatorrhea (ordinarily not observable to naked eye) Activity level: active or lethargic? Color: pallor? Symptoms of hypoglycemia Test for hypoglycemia with Dextrostix ($\leq$20 mg/dl blood for preterm infant); may be otherwise asymptomatic Assess for edema	As above Administer and record vitamins and minerals per physician order (vitamins A, C, D, E; iron) Adjust formula, feeding method, etc., to infant's responses and changing needs
Support of CNS function	Birth trauma: damage to immature structures Fragile capillaries and impaired coagulation process; prolonged prothrombin time	Observe for symptoms of increased intracranial pressure Observe for convulsions Twitching and myoclonic jerks	Maintain adequate oxygenation to relieve cyanosis Maintain open airway Prevent or promptly identify and relieve hypoglycemia, hypocalcemia

Continued.

Table 37.4—cont'd
Care of the Preterm Infant: Goals, Physiologic Problems, and Nursing Actions—Assessment and Implementation

		Nursing Actions	
Goals for Care	**Physiologic Problems**	**Assessment**	**Implementation**
Support of CNS function—cont'd	Recurrent anoxic episodes Tendency toward hypoglycemia	Increased chewing movements Eye rolling Observe for behavior changes Infection	
Prevention of infection	Paucity of stored nutrients from mother Paucity of stored immunoglobulins from mother Impaired ability to synthesize antibodies Thin skin and fragile capillaries near surface Impaired ability to muster white blood cells	Note following: Feeding behavior Skin: irritations, rashes, jaundice Drainage from eyes, umbilicus; nasal congestion Frequency of stools Body temperature (unreliable) Behavior change: "just not right," lethargic, listless Respiratory rate increase or decrease (persistent) for 24 hr Check prenatal record Maternal temperature Maternal infection Premature rupture of membranes: length of time before delivery, color, odor, culture, amount of fluid	Meticulous hand washing is imperative; check personnel's health Use aseptic technique for anything puncturing skin and for umbilical catheterization Prevent skin breakdown Under monitor leads, tapes, restraints Over bony prominences (use flotation pad or sheepskin) Gentle insertion of orogastric or nasogastric tubes Supervise parents' hand washing and gowning when visiting Monitor administration of medications Restrict visitors, repairmen, equipment change, etc.
Maintenance of renal function	Impaired renal clearance of metabolites, drugs Inability to maintain acid-base, fluid, and electrolyte homeostasis Impaired ability to concentrate urine	Note following: Urinary output Diaper saturation; number of diapers each day Collect and measure; check specific gravity Edema Tachypnea Vomiting Abdominal distention	Assist kidney function by decreasing demands on that system Provide formula with right concentration of solute Support respirations, normal body temperature, nutrition, fluid balance Prevent infection Prevent hypovolemia
Minimization of hematologic problems	Increased capillary friability and permeability Low plasma prothrombin levels (increased tendency to bleed) Relatively slowed erythropoietic activity in bone marrow Relatively increased rate of hemolysis Loss of blood for laboratory specimens	Fragile capillaries and impaired coagulation process; prolonged prothrombin time Note following: Skin manifestations: ecchymoses, petechiae, jaundice, pallor Increased bleeding or oozing around cord, injection sites, etc., Symptoms of cerebral irritation (or increased intracranial pressure from hemorrhage)	Handle infant gently and as little as possible Give intramuscular injection of vitamin K (one dose) if not being given antiboitics that hamper its synthesis in gastrointestinal tract; if being given these antibiotics, more doses will be needed Treat to reduce hyperbilirubinemia with phototherapy or assist with exchange transfusions Monitor withdrawal of blood for laboratory examinations and evaluations; assist with blood replacement as necessary

Table 37.4—cont'd
Care of the Preterm Infant: Goals, Physiologic Problems, and Nursing Actions—Assessment and Implementation

		Nursing Actions	
Goals for Care	**Physiologic Problems**	**Assessment**	**Implementation**
Prevention of trauma to immature musculoskeletal system	Weak, underdeveloped muscles Immature skeletal system (bones, joints) Meager subcutaneous fat with its cushioning effect	Molding of cranial bones noted Also note following: Unnatural rotation or extension of joints Asymmetric contours of body Muscle tone, muscle mass Pressure area over body prominences	Position infant Change position frequently Place in correct body alignment; watch position of feet If diapers are used (infant under 1500 g should not be diapered), cut to size; pin or tape with posterior flap overlapping anterior flap Pad areas over bony prominences (sheepskin, bubble pads, other)
Maintenance of retinal integrity	Immature vascular structures in retina Need for oxygen therapy	Monitor following: Blood gas values O_2 concentration of inspired air Note and record respiratory distress and amount and duration of O_2 therapy required to relieve distress	Supervise collection of blood for study; method, time, amount Monitor amount and duration of O_2 therapy to keep Pao_2 between 50-70 mm Hg or better

COMPLICATIONS OF PREMATURITY

Respiratory distress syndrome (RDS), also know as hyaline membrane disease (HMD), retrolental fibroplasia, and bronchopulmonary dysplasia are seen almost exclusively in preterm neonates. RDS claims a significant number of lives, and the impaired vision or blindness resulting from retrolental fibroplasia places a serious burden on the survivors and their families.

Respiratory distress syndrome

Incidence. RDS is a leading cause of morbidity and mortality among preterm infants, affecting about 20,000 infants each year in North America. Generally the smaller the preterm infant, the higher the mortality. Occasionally a full-term neonate is affected.

Pathophysiology. The central problem in RDS is atelectasis. The *membrane* is composed in part of fibrin derived from the pulmonary circulation and is not the result of aspirated fluid or an irritant. Accompanying problems such as hypoxia, metabolic and respiratory acidosis, and pulmonary hypoperfusion with right-to-left shunting are secondary to atelectasis.

Cause. The development of a hyaline membrane within the terminal bronchial tree, that is, the alveolar ducts and the alveoli, of neonates within a few hours after birth still is unknown. The role of surfactant in preventing alveolar collapse at the end of expiration has been established. A deficiency in surfactant production may be the basis for RDS.

Onset. RDS may be apparent in the infant at birth. This neonate has a low Apgar score and frequently requires resuscitation and ventilatory assistance. Other symptoms generally appear within the first 6 hours. Initially expiratory grunting and nasal flaring are evident. As the disease progresses, tachypnea (60 breaths/min or more), retractions, and even cyanosis in room air may be noted. Hypotension and shock may be evident. Apneic pauses replace the expiratory grunting. An arterial Po_2 of 40 mm Hg or less in room air is a constant finding. Symptoms often peak in 48 to 72 hours.

Diagnosis. The diagnosis is confirmed by x-ray films, blood tests for pH, serum nonprotein nitrogen (NPN), potassium, and phosphorus, and tests for arterial blood gases.

Prognosis. Formerly if the infant with RDS survived the first 48 to 72 hours, his clinical condition improved slowly until recovery at about 10 to 12 days. Although newer methods and equipment may sustain the severely affected infant beyond 72 hours, death still may occur several weeks after birth. Therefore a guarded prognosis is given for several weeks.

Treatment. The following measures are important in the treatment of the infant with RDS:

1. A thermoneutral environment is provided so that

the infant's body temperature is maintained at 36.5° C (97.6° F).

2. Gentle handling of the neonate is necessary. This infant is disturbed as little as possible.
3. Caloric intake is sufficient to prevent catabolism (40 kcal/kg/24 hr or more).
4. Replace blood if excessive amount is lost, usually as a result of samples taken for laboratory analysis.
5. Control serum bilirubin levels by phototherapy (Fig. 37.33), exchange transfusion, or both. Low serum albumin levels, hypoxia, and acidosis interfere with the albumin's binding to bilirubin and therefore subject these infants to kernicterus at low serum bilirubin levels (10 mg/dl or less; see Chapters 27, 29, and 40).
6. Oxygen therapy, for example:
   a. Administer the oxygen (60% or less) by means of a hood (Fig. 37.34).
   b. Continuous positive airway pressure (CPAP) may be administered by means of an intratracheal tube, face mask, nasal prongs, or hood (see Chapter 33).
   c. Continuous negative airway pressure (CNAP) is a respirator that works in the same manner as CPAP but exerts negative pressure on the neonate's body while his head is exposed. The neonate may breathe room air or an air-oxygen mix by means of a mask or prongs.
   d. Intermittent positive end expiratory pressure (PEEP) may be used.

Prematurity and oxygen toxicity. Retrolental fibroplasia and bronchopulmonary dysplasia are diseases of prematurity secondary to oxygen therapy. Both conditions are relatively "new" disorders, recognized since the advent of methods of administering high concentrations of oxygen beginning in the 1940s. Although oxygen therapy may be lifesaving and occasionally must be given in high concentrations for extended periods of time, it is also potentially hazardous and must be administered judiciously.

Bronchopulmonary dysplasia. Bronchopulmonary dysplasia is a possible sequela to treatment with positive pressure ventilation (rarely found in neonates supported by negative pressure apparatuses). The levels of inspired oxygen concentration associated with bronchopulmonary dysplasia are no longer thought to be 60% or greater. It has been reported to occur at 40% and perhaps lower. The current concept is that there is little relationship to an exact level of inspired oxygen. It may be that any concentration of oxygen over room air, given for a sufficiently protracted period of time, will cause bronchopulmonary dysplasia.

Changes in the lung fields result in focal areas of emphysema. Symptoms of respiratory distress, tachypnea and increased effort, appear. It is difficult to wean the infant from the positive pressure ventilator. This finding may be the first indication of the disease process.

Prognosis. The first sign that the infant is recovering from bronchopulmonary dysplasia is a decreasing dependence on oxygen therapy. Recovery may take several months. Mortality is between 30% and 50%.

Retrolental fibroplasia. The retinal changes in retrolental fibroplasia were first described in 1942. The occurrence of this condition has been found to be related to the following factors:

- Vascular channels that may be functionally immature until 34 weeks
- Incomplete retinal differentiation and vascularization
- High arterial oxygen tension levels
- Prolonged duration of oxygen therapy

Pa_{O_2} between 50 and 70 mm Hg may be within safe limits. (The recently developed transcutaneous oxygen tension monitor [tcP_{O_2}] is a noninvasive device that provides continuous oxygen tension values.) The most crucial period for toxic levels to occur is during the recovery phase from RDS and other respiratory distress. The exact toxic level of arterial oxygen tension associated with retrolental fibroplasia is unknown.

Oxygen tensions that are too high for the level of retinal maturity initially result in vasoconstriction. Subsequently, after oxygen therapy is discontinued, neo-

Fig. 37.33
Intensive care nursery. Students are giving care to an infant receiving phototherapy, often administered prophylactically to preterm infants. Note eye patch protection.

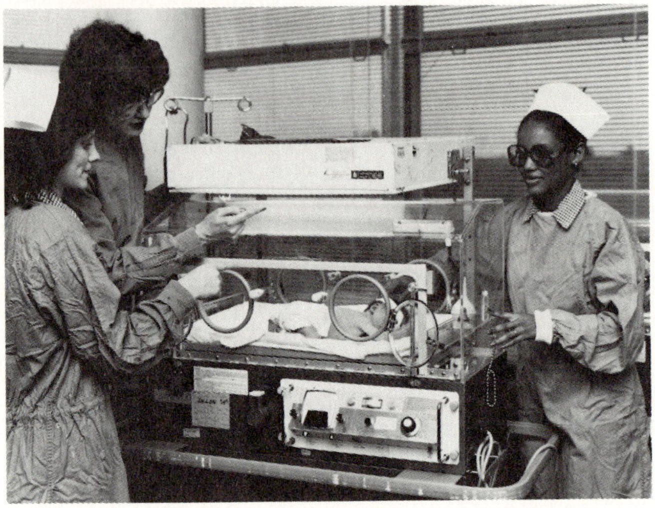

Fig. 37.34
Mother interacting with her baby. Oxygen hood and overhead warmer are being used in place of incubator.

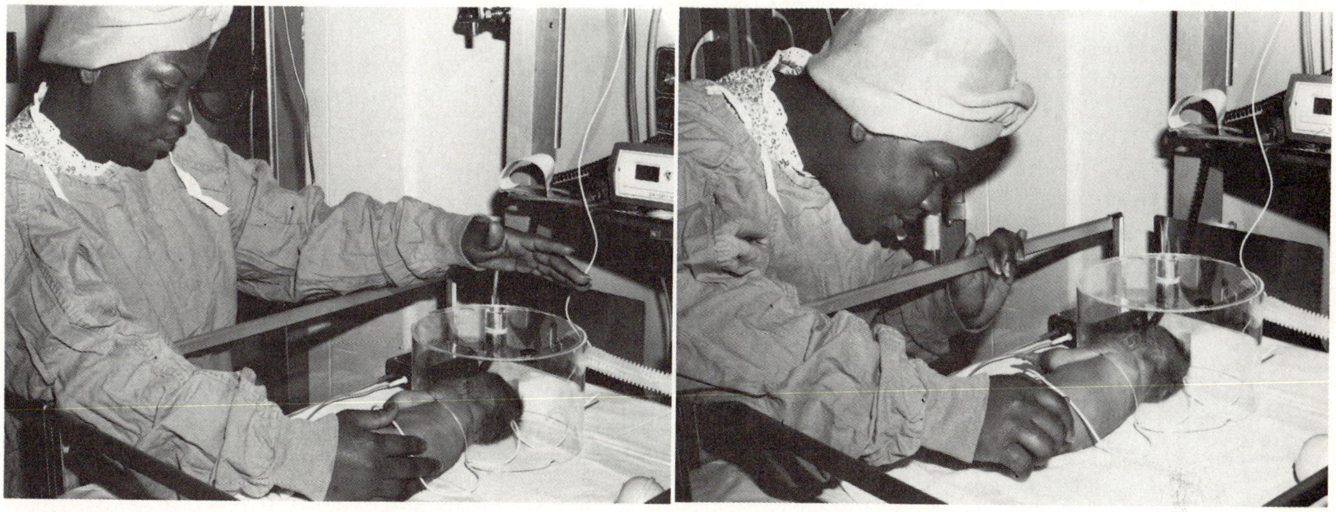

vascularization in the retina and vitreous occurs, with capillary hemorrhages, fibrotic resolution, and possible retinal detachment. Cicatricial (scar) tissue formation and consequent visual impairment may be mild or severe. The entire disease process in severe cases may take as long as 5 months to evolve. Examination by an ophthalmologist before discharge and a schedule for repeat examinations thereafter are recommended for guidance of parents.

Neonatal necrotizing enterocolitis. Necrotizing enterocolitis (NEC) is an inflammatory disease of the gastrointestinal mucosa, frequently complicated by perforation. This often fatal disease appears in about 5% of neonates in intensive care nurseries. Although its etiology is unknown, several possibilities are suspect:

1. Immaturity
2. Hypoxemia (postdelivery)
3. High-solute feedings
4. Excessive amounts of feedings
5. Perinatal asphyxia (frequent historical antecedent)

Recent research suggests that reversal of asphyxia within 30 minutes may prevent gastrointestinal tract insult and so prevent the initiation of NEC pathophysiology. After 30 minutes, distribution of cardiac output tends to be directed more toward the heart and brain and away from the abdominal organs. Therefore prompt delivery of the intrauterine asphyxiated fetus or ventilation of the asphyxiated neonate may be beneficial to the gastrointestinal tract as well as to other organs.

Septicemia may follow the initial intestinal events that are associated with NEC.

Signs of developing NEC are nonspecific, which is characteristic of many neonatal disease processes. Abdominal distention is probably the most frequent and regularly encountered sign. The infant's color is poor. Apneic periods increase in number. Frequently, there are gastric residuals of 2 ml or more before feedings. The stool may show occult blood (positive guaiac test). Diagnosis is confirmed by x-ray examination.

Treatment is supportive. Oral or tube feedings are discontinued to rest the gastrointestinal tract. Parenteral therapy (often by total parenteral nutrition [TPN]) is begun. Antibiotic therapy may be instituted. Surgery is performed when necessary. Therapy may be prolonged, since recovery may be delayed by adhesions, complications of bowel resection (malabsorption), and intolerance for oral feedings.

PROGNOSIS FOR PRETERM INFANTS

Base-line examination. An examination is performed to provide base-line data. From these data, handicapping conditions may be identified early and appropriate treatment begun. In addition, the infant's progress may be plotted and a tentative prognosis made. Suggested evaluative tests include growth grids adjusted to gestational age, the Denver Developmental Screening Test, and a neurologic examination.

Favorable evaluative criteria. Although it is impossible to predict with complete accuracy the growth and developmental potential of each premature neonate, some findings support an anticipated favorable outcome. The growth and development landmarks are corrected for gestational age.

The age of a preterm neonate is corrected by adding the gestational age and the postdelivery age. For example, if an infant was born at 32 weeks' gestation a month ago, today she is 36 weeks of age according to her gestational life (age since her mother's LMP). Six months after her birth date, the child's corrected age is 4 months. Her responses are evaluated against the norm expected of a 4-month-old infant.

Favorable findings that support the prediction of a growth and development pattern within the norm include the following:

1. At discharge from the hospital, which usually occurs between 37 and 40 weeks after the LMP the infant is assessed for the following characteristics:
   a. When prone, the infant can raise his head. He is able to hold his head parallel with his body when tested for head lag response. (When pulled up by the hands, the infant's head lags, but then his head and chest will be in line as he reaches the upright position. This alignment will be held momentarily before the head falls forward.)
   b. When the infant is hungry, he cries with vigor.
   c. The growth grid shows appropriate weight gain and pattern of weight gain.
   d. The neurologic examination reveals appropriate responses for age. The retinas appear normal.
2. At 39 to 40 weeks since the LMP, the infant is able to focus on the examiner's or parent's face and is able to follow it with his eyes.
3. At the corrected ages of 6 and 12 months, the infant is assessed again for age-appropriate responses.

The infant may have continued problems if he displays any of the following behaviors:

- Was and continues to be a poor eater
- Is irritable
- Displays sensory, perceptual, intellectual, or motor deviations as he matures
- Displays or develops hypertonia or hypotonia

These behaviors must be interpreted with caution and the infant reevaluated by an interdisciplinary team at frequent intervals. Parents will need continued support and attention should these signs appear. Minor behavioral deviations should be diagnosed also so that the parents can be assisted in their understanding and acceptance of the child. Deviations such as clumsiness, varying degrees of incoordination, slowness in reading and writing, and similar problems may be distressing to the child, parents, and other family members.

PSYCHOLOGIC ASPECTS OF PRETERM LABOR AND DELIVERY OF A PRETERM INFANT

Prematurity puts the infant and the family at risk.

Child abuse and neglect. The incidence of physical and emotional abuse is three times greater toward the infant who by virtue of prematurity or illness was separated from his mother for a period of time after his birth. Physical abuse includes varying degrees of poor nutrition and poor hygiene; emotional abuse ranges from subtle to outright dislike of the child; there may be preferential treatment for siblings, nagging, extremely high expectations of the child, and various other types of overt or covert negative responses by one or both parents.

Factors surrounding the birth, such as parental pain and anxiety, heavy financial burden for the infant's care, unresolved anticipatory grief and threat to self-esteem, and unwanted pregnancy, may predispose parents to subconsciously or overtly reject the child. The goal of the helping professionals is to reduce the incidence of child abuse and neglect.

A carefully devised medical-nursing care plan may help to reduce this threat to the infant born at risk. Parents who have negative feelings about the pregnancy or the infant at risk need support. Their feelings can be acknowledged as valid, including the burden they are experiencing financially and emotionally and their understandable feelings toward the infant. Parents are prepared for the procedures and gadgetry of the intensive care unit. Soon after delivery, the parents, especially the mother, should have the opportunity to meet the infant in the en face position, to touch him, and to see his favorable characteristics (Figs. 37.35 and 37.36). As soon as possible, depending primarily on the mother's physical condition, the mother is allowed to visit the nursery at will and assist with the infant's care. When she is not able to be physically present, the staff devises appropriate methods to keep the family in almost constant touch with the neonate (see Chapter 33). Some hospitals have instituted a parents' club for parents of infants in intensive care nurseries. These clubs encourage those who are experiencing the same anxiety and grief to share their feelings. An "older" member

Fig. 37.35
Father interacts with his baby. He is stroking baby's back.

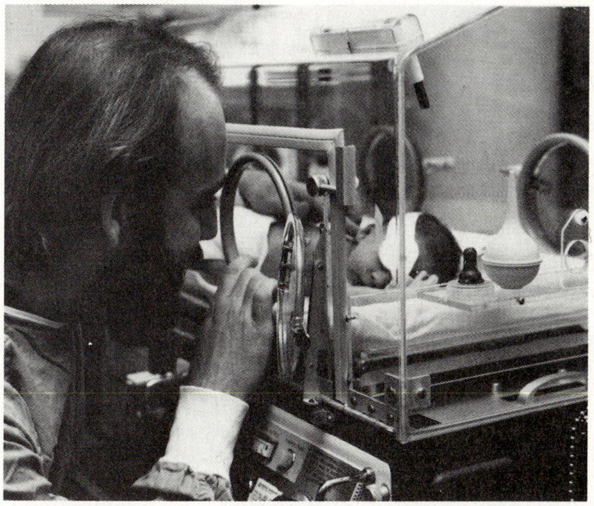

Fig. 37.36
Father admires newborn. Note father's finger tip touch.

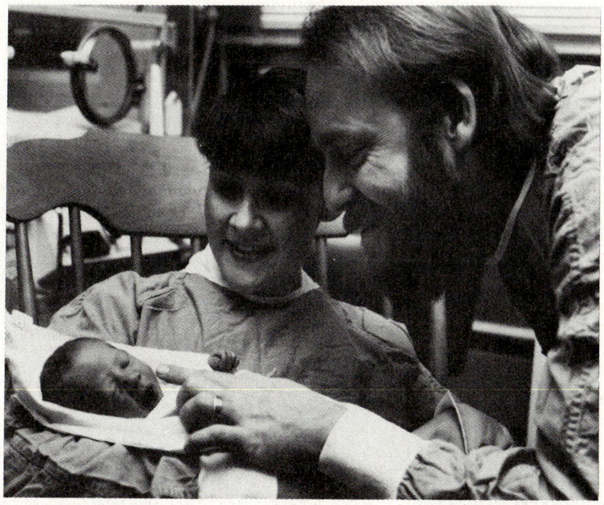

often takes over a "new" member and provides additional support. Incorporating these actions into the infant's care plan acknowledges and supports nature's design by engaging and maintaining a bond between the mother and infant that assures the infant of the continued care he needs for physical and emotional survival at the optimal level.

Baptism. The rite of baptism is particularly significant to Roman Catholic, some Episcopalian, and Greek Orthodox religious groups. If death of a preterm infant appears inevitable, the clergy should be notified according to the family's wishes. If death is imminent, any adult, preferably of the same faith, may baptize the infant. Water is poured down the head or other skin surface and the following words spoken: "I baptize you, in the name of the Father, of the Son, and of the Holy Spirit." (If an abortion or fetal death occurs, the expelled products of conception are baptized.)

The parents and the priest or minister should be notified of the baptism and a notation made on the record.

EVALUATION

The evaluation of the care given preterm infants and their families has to be multidimensional. For some families death of their infant happens in spite of all medical and nursing knowledge and skill. For other families, the sequelae of prematurity result in infants who will face lifetime disability. For these families evaluation criteria relate to the concepts of loss, grief, and self-concept (see Chapter 34).

For many other infants and families the immediate threat to well-being is overcome by intensive neonatal care. The criteria for evaluating the physical aspects of the care are:

1. Respirations are initiated and maintained.
2. Body temperature is maintained.
3. The infant is adequately nourished.
4. CNS trauma is prevented or minimized.
5. Infection is prevented.
6. Renal function is supported.
7. Hematologic problems are prevented or minimized.
8. Musculoskeletal problems are prevented or minimized.
9. Retinal damage is prevented or minimized.

The criteria for evaluating the psychosocial aspects of care include the following:

1. The mother retains a positive self-concept as a woman, mother, and sexual being.
2. The mother, father, and family (Figs. 37.37 to 37.39):
   a. Perceive the child as potentially normal (if this is medically substantiated).
   b. Provide the child with realistic care comfortably.
   c. Experience pride and satisfaction in the care of the child.

Fig. 37.37
Parents and child are united.

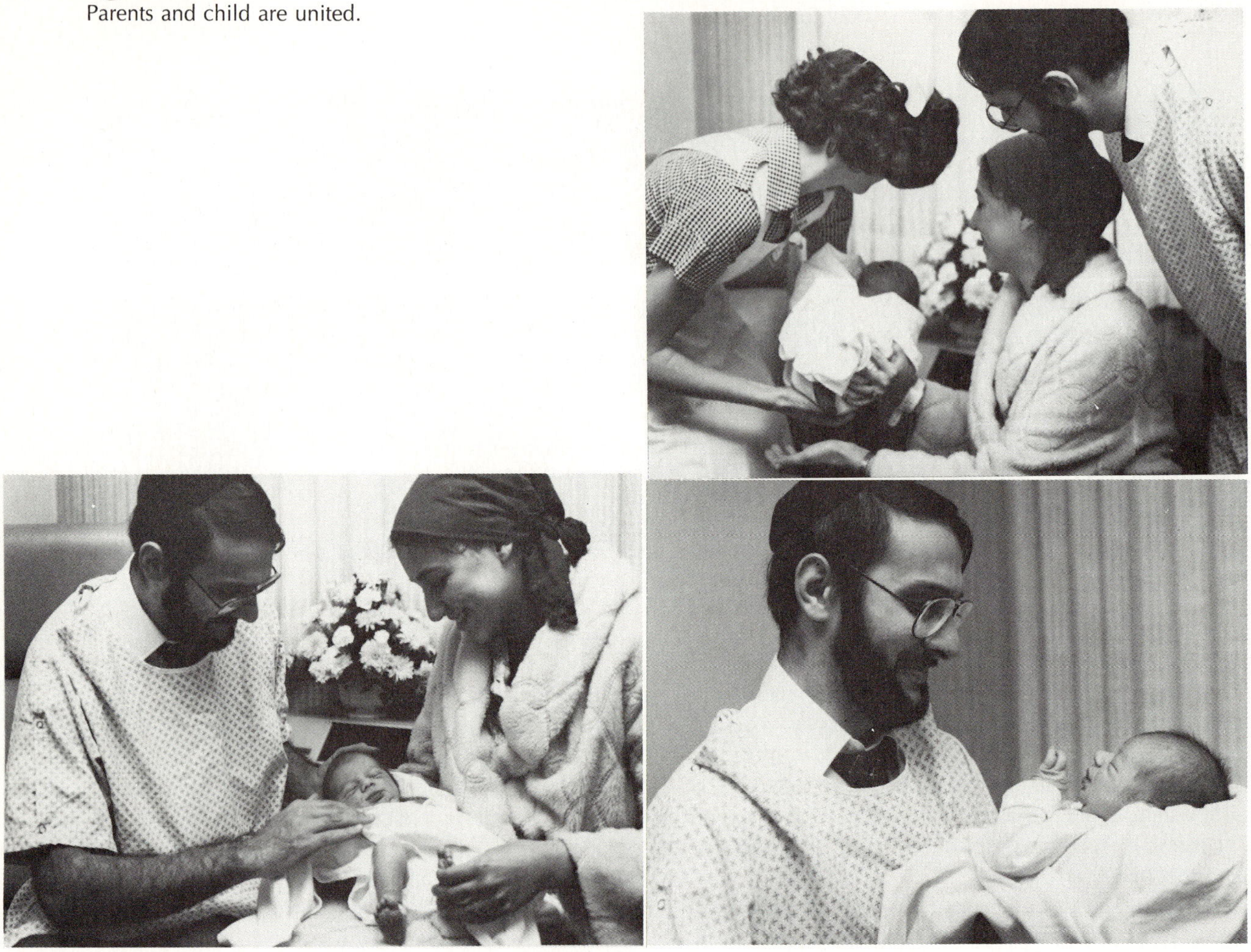

3. The parents are able to organize their time and energies to meet the love, attention, and care needs of the other members of the family and themselves as well.

Multiple Pregnancy

Multiple pregnancy is the gestation of twins, triplets, quadruplets, or more infants. Twins produced from a single ovum are termed monozygotic, or identical, and the sibling is always of the same sex (Fig. 37.40). Those produced from separate ova are dizygotic, or fraternal, and may be of the same or opposite sex (Fig. 37.41). Monozygotic twinning is a random occurrence. Dizygotic twinning (multiple ovulation), on the other hand, is an autosomal-recessive trait carried by the daughters of mothers of twins and occurs more frequently as maternal age at conception increases. Triplets can develop from one, two, or three ova (Fig. 37.42).

Infants of multiple pregnancies account for 2% to 3% of all viable births. Of twins, more than 15% weigh less than 2500 g, and most of these are preterm. Twins occur about once in 99 conceptions; triplets and quadruplets occur much less often. Multiple pregnancy is most common in blacks, least common in Orientals, and of intermediate occurrence in whites. Almost 30% of twins are monozygotic; nearly 70% are dizygotic. Fewer males than females are born in multiple pregnancies. Maternal morbidity and perinatal morbidity and mortality are greatly increased in multiple pregnancy by comparison with single pregnancy because of medical and obstetric complications. The prenatal diagnosis of

Fig. 37.38

Dressed for visitors: mother and father. Note hat (knitted by grandmother) to prevent heat loss through scalp.

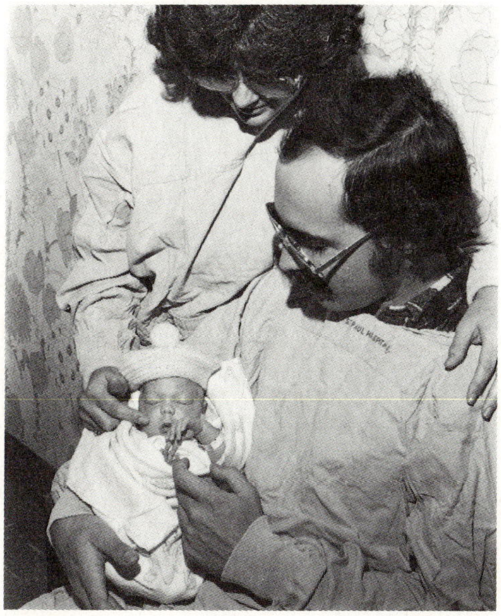

Fig. 37.39

Introduction of new baby born 4 weeks prematurely to new sister and grandmother.

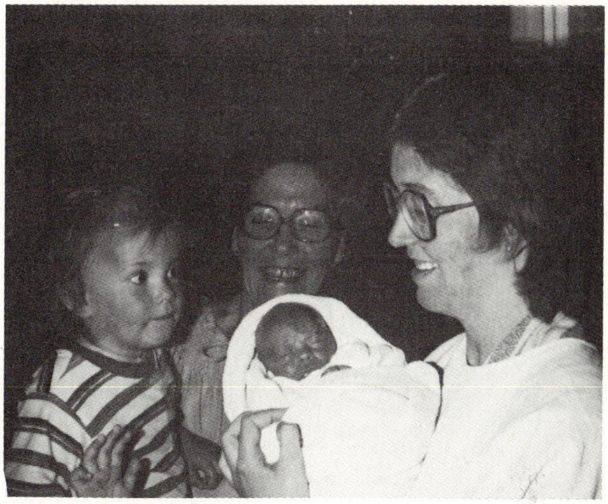

Fig. 37.40

Formation of monozygotic twins. **A,** One fertilization: blastomeres separate, resulting in two implantations, two placentas, and two sets of membranes. **B,** One blastomere with two inner cell masses, one fused placenta, one chorion, and separate amnions. **C,** Later separation of inner cell masses, with fused placenta and single amnion and chorion. (From Whaley, L.F.: Understanding inherited disorders, St. Louis, 1974, The C.V. Mosby Co.)

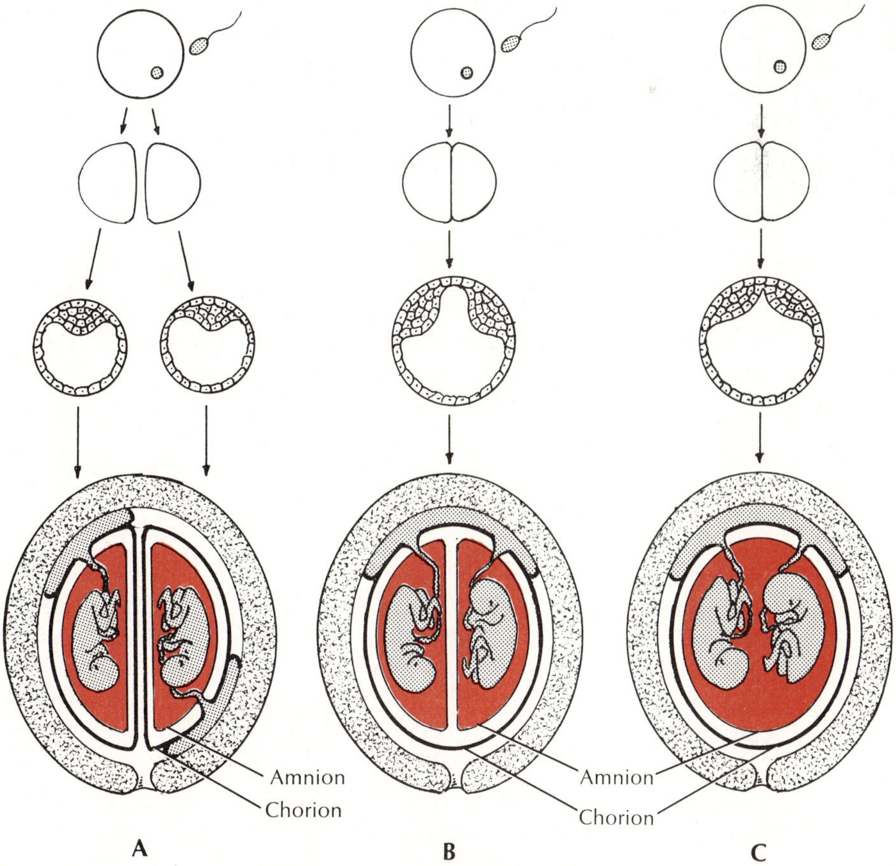

Fig. 37.41
Formation of dizygotic twins. There is fertilization of two ova, two implantations, two placentas, two chorions, and two amnions. (From Whaley, L.F.: Understanding inherited disorders, St. Louis, 1974, The C.V. Mosby Co.)

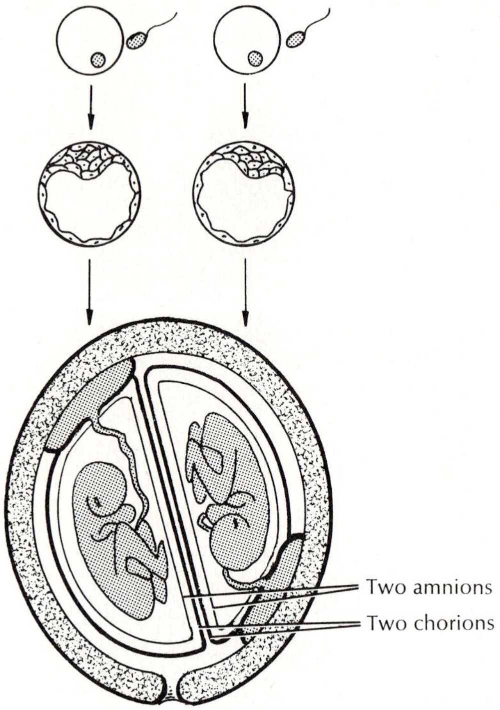

Fig. 37.42
Formation of triplets and quadruplets, indicating variety of mechanisms that can produce multiple births. Quadruplets can be formed from one to four ova. (From Whaley, L.F.: Understanding inherited disorders, St. Louis, 1974, The C.V. Mosby Co.)

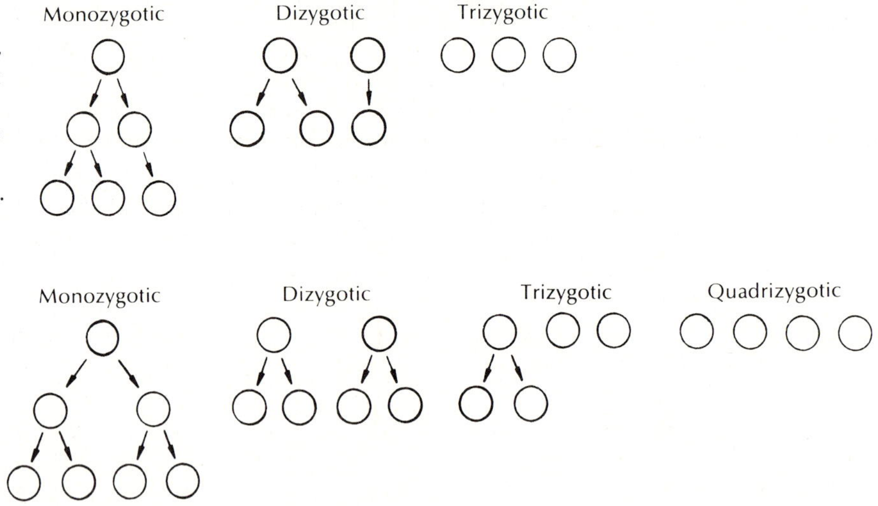

multiple pregnancy is made in only about 75% of cases and often late in gestation. This is regrettable, since much can be done for the mother and her infants if treatment is established early.

MATERNAL PROBLEMS

The maternal blood volume is increased in multiple gestations. As a result there is an increased strain on the maternal cardiovascular system.

Anemia often develops because of greater demand for iron by the fetuses.

Marked uterine distention and increased pressure on the adjacent viscera and pelvic vasculature occur in multiple pregnancy. Diastasis of the two recti abdominis muscles (in the midline) may occur.

Placenta previa develops more frequently in multiple pregnancies because of the large size of the placentas (see Figs. 35.4 and 35.5 and note placement of placentas). Premature separation of the placenta may occur before the second and subsequent fetuses are born.

FETAL PROBLEMS

Each twin and his placenta usually weigh less than the infant and placenta of a singleton pregnancy after the thirtieth week, but the aggregate weight is almost twice that of a singleton near term. The mean weight of twins in the United States is more than 2270 g (5 lb).

Congenital malformations are twice as frequent in monozygotic twins as in singletons, but there is no increase in the incidence of congenital anomalies in dizygotic twins.

Two-vessel cords, that is, cords with a single umbilical artery, occur more often in twins than in singletons, and this abnormality is most common in monozygotic twins.

The most serious problem for the fetus is a local shunting of blood between placentas (twin-to-twin transfusion). The *recipient* twin is larger, however, this twin may develop congenital heart failure during the first 24 hours after birth. The *donor* twin will be small, pallid, dehydrated, malnourished, and hypovolemic. A serious problem for the neonate is prematurity.

DIAGNOSIS

Clinical diagnosis of multiple pregnancy is accurate in only about three fourths of cases. With a high degree of suspicion and careful examination, a correct diagnosis of twins may be possible in most instances by the twenty-fourth to twenty-sixth week based on the following:

1. History of dizygous twins in the female lineage
2. Abnormally large maternal weight gain (inconsistent with diet or edema)
3. Polyhydramnios
4. Palpation of excessive number of small or large parts
5. Asynchronous fetal heart beats or more than one fetal electrocardiographic (ECG) tracing
6. Radiographic or ultrasonographic (B-scan) evidence of more than one fetus

In twin pregnancy, both fetuses will present by the vertex in about one half of cases; one will present by the vertex and one by the breech in approximately one third of the total. Other combinations are uncommon.

MANAGEMENT

Prenatal care. Prenatal visits by the mother with multiple pregnancy are scheduled no less than every 2 weeks in the second trimester and weekly thereafter.

The mother's diet and weight control are supervised to allow weight gain of about 50% more than the average woman with a singleton pregnancy (as much as 18 kg [40 lb] above the woman's ideal nonpregnant weight). Iron and vitamin supplementation is desirable. Attempts are made to prevent preeclampsia-eclampsia and vaginitis; if they do develop, they are treated early and properly.

Because of considerable uterine distention and, perhaps, backache, a well-fitted maternity girdle may be welcomed. Elastic stockings or leotards may control leg varices.

The woman with multiple pregnancy may go into preterm labor; the couple is advised to abstain from coitus or masturbation to the point of orgasm during the last trimester. Enforced rest periods, with the mother lying down on her side, begun as soon as pregnancy begins, may help to avoid untimely early labor; delivery after the thirty-sixth week increases the likelihood of survival of the neonates.

Natal care. Delivery in a maternity center where specialty care is always available is advisable when there is a multiple pregnancy.

The woman is admitted to the hospital at the first sign of labor.

First stage. The woman is placed on bed rest in a left lateral position. Her blood is typed and cross matched, and several units of bank blood are kept available in the delivery room for emergency transfusion. Parenteral infusion of 5% dextrose in water (or other infusate) is started through a no. 16 or 18 needle (that can accommodate blood if needed) in the first stage of labor and continued until the fourth stage is completed. Blood or drugs, if indicated, are administered intravenously slowly. Analgesia must be limited drastically since the infants often are premature.

If no complications occur, the management of the first stage of labor in multiple pregnancy does not differ from the single pregnancy with the same presentation.

Cesarean delivery is done only for accepted obstetric reasons. Multiple pregnancy itself is not an indication, but disproportion (e.g., conjoined twins), fetal distress, or monoamniotic twins (diagnosed by amniography) are.

Second stage. A physician-nurse team for each neonate is scrubbed, gowned, and gloved for the delivery of a woman with multiple pregnancy. After the first twin is born the cord is clamped promptly to prevent the second twin of a monozygotic pregnancy from partially exsanguinating through the first cord.

The time of birth is noted, and the infant is labled Baby A. The optimal time for delivery of the second child is 5 to 20 minutes after delivery of the first child. The physician's objective is to deliver the second child without difficult operative procedures. Some physicians prefer to deliver this fetus by cesarean birth. The second child is labeled Baby B and so on.

Third stage. The third stage of labor must be managed with care. Excessive blood loss is common to multiple pregnancy. Oxytocin (Pitocin), 1 ml intravenously, is administered immediately after delivery of the last child; the intravenous oxytocin *infusion is restarted.* The fundus is elevated but not massaged until after the uterus contracts and expels the separated placenta; then an ergot preparation, such as ergonovine (Ergotrate), 0.1 mg intravenously, is given, if the woman is not hypertensive. Gentle massage and elevation of the fundus are continued for 15 to 30 minutes. If separation of the placenta is delayed or bleeding is brisk, the physician manually separates and extracts the placenta.

Puerperal care. The mother with a multiple pregnancy requires the same physical care as any other parturient. She is more prone to develop postdelivery hemorrhage because of excessive uterine distention and therefore must be carefully assessed.

Psychologically, however, even the most willing of mothers can find their coping mechanisms overwhelmed by both the idea and reality of caring for two or more infants. Maternal-child attachment takes longer because she attaches first to one newborn and then to the other. Parents must organize simplified and flexible plans of care. The almost constant attention required until the infants' schedule of care can be synchronized may prove exhausting. If possible, help is obtained, particularly to guarantee sufficient rest for the mother. The added expense can also be burdensome to a young family. One mother expressed anger at the surprise birth of twins. The explanation of such errors did not placate her. She needed time to vent these feelings before she could be helped with changing her anticipated plan of care.

Most parents are anxious to know if their children are identical or fraternal. Since gross examination of the placenta at birth cannot prove whether or not twins are identical, it is best to tell parents differentiation in the type of twinning cannot be made at this time.

If the infants are born prematurely or are small for gestational age, their prolonged hospital stay can cause parental separation anxiety. If this is the case, the mother may be encouraged to visit or care for the infants in the hospital and to utilize this waiting time to recover as much physical strength as possible, as well as to prepare for the infants' homecoming. Introduction of multiple siblings into a family can also result in intense rivalry as all children compete for the mother's attention. Substitute mothering by interested relatives can do much to ease the strain.

Nursing twins takes planning and patience. If the mother elects the rooming-in regimen, the added care of two infants may prove too taxing to her strength, although many mothers have stated that the early adjustment made going home easier. It is suggested that these mothers remain longer in the hospital unless there is help at home. It is important to establish a feeding schedule as soon as possible. The mother may use a modified demand schedule, that is, feeding the first baby who wakes up and then awakening the second baby, or she may awaken both and nurse them simultaneously. A record of the feeding times, which breast was used by which baby, and which side was used first is essential during the early weeks. If one twin nurses more readily than the other, an effort should be made to have that twin nurse on alternate breasts so as to equalize stimulation. If feeding simultaneously, the mother should experiment with positions; for example, each baby may be supported on pillows and in the football hold, or one may be held in the football hold and the other in the cradle hold. Obviously the mother with twins will need extra assistance from her family, extra nourishment, and extra rest if she is to have sufficient energy not only to care for and nurse each baby but also to provide the mothering each needs.

However, having twins or triplets can be a most rewarding experience. As the children develop, they experience a closeness unique for siblings. One twin, when asked how many brothers and sisters she had, answered, "three sisters and Pam (her twin)."

References and Readings

Dystocia

Banta, D., and Thacker, S.: The risks and benefits of episiotomy: review, Birth **9:**(1):25, 1982.

Beynon, C.: Midline episiotomy as a routine procedure, J. Obstet. Gynaecol. Br. Commonw. **81:**126, 1974.

Buchan, P.C. and Nicholls, J.A.J.: Pain after episiotomy—a comparison of two methods of repair, J.R. Coll. Gen. Pract. **30:**297, 1980.

Cohen, N.W.: Minimizing emotional sequelae of cesarean childbirth, Birth Fam. J. **4:**114, Fall 1977.

Cranley, M., et al.: Women's perceptions of vaginal and cesarean deliveries, Nurs. Res. **32**(1):11, 1983.

Danforth, D.N.: Operative delivery. In Benson, R., editor: Current obstetric and gynecologic diagnosis and treatment, Los Altos, Calif., 1982, Lange Medical Publication.

Gibbs, C.E.: Planned vaginal delivery following cesarean section, Clin. Obstet. Gynecol. **23**(2):507, 1980.

Harris, R.: An evaluation of the median episiotomy, Am. J. Obstet. Gynecol. **106:**660, 1970.

Kelin, R.P., et al.: A study of father and nurse support during labor, Birth Fam. J. **8**(3):16, 1981.

Meier, P.R., and Parreco, R.P.: Trial of labor following cesarean section: a two year experience, Am. J. Obstet. Gynecol. **144**(6):671, 1982.

Newsletter: Cesareans/Support Education and Concern (C/SEC, Inc.), Vol. 8, no. 34, 1982.

Seitchik, J., and Ramakrishna, V.R.: Cesarean delivery in

nulliparous women for failed oxytocin-augmented labor: route of delivery in subsequent pregnancy, Am. J. Obstet. Gynecol. **143**(4):393, 1982.

Shearer, E.C.: NIH consensus development task force on cesarean childbirth: the process and the result, Birth Fam. J. **8**(2):25, 1981.

Shearer, E.C.: Education for vaginal birth after cesarean birth, J. Obstet. Gynecol. Nurs. **9**(1):31, 1982.

Shy, K.K., LeGufo, J.P., and Karp, L.E.: Evaluation of elective repeat cesarean section as a standard of care: an application of decision and analysis, Am. J. Obstet. Gynecol. **139**(2):123, 1981.

Toney, L.: The effects of holding the newborn at delivery on paternal bonding, Nurs. Res. **32**(1):17, 1983.

U.S. Department of Health and Human Services: Cesarean childbirth, Report of a consensus development conference, Sept 22-24, 1980, Oct. 1981. Available free on request from NIH pub. no. 82-2067.

U.S. Department of Health and Human Services: Cesarean childbirth. Conference summary, 1980. Available free on request from NIH.

Winer, E., et al.: Four to seven year evaluation in two groups of small-for-gestational-age infants, Am. J. Obstet. Gynecol. **143**(4):425, 1982.

Preterm Birth

Barden, T.P., Peter, J.B., and Merkatz, I.R.: Ritodrine hydrochloride: a betamimetic agent for use in preterm labor. I. Pharmacology clinical history, administration, side effects, and safety, Obstet. Gynecol. **56**(1):1, 1980

Bracken, M.B.: Oral contraception and twinning: an epidemiologic study, Am. J. Obstet. Gynecol. **133**:432, 1979.

Cavanagh, D., and Talisman, M.R.: Prematurity and the obstetrician, New York, 1969, Appleton-Century Croft.

Fuch, S.R.: Prevention of prematurity, Am. J. Obstet. Gynecol. **126**:809, 1976.

Kaltreider, D.F., and Koho, S.: Epidemiology of preterm delivery. In Johnson, J.W.C., Editor: Clinical obstetrics and gynecology, New York, 1980, Harper & Row.

Klaus, M.H., and Kennell, J.H.: Parent-infant bonding, St. Louis, 1982, The C.V. Mosby Co.

Merkatz, I.R., Peter, J.B., & Barden, T.P.: Ritodrine hydrochloride: a betamimetic agent for use in preterm labor. II. Evidence of efficacy, Obstet. Gynecol. **56**(1):7, 1980.

Morris, N.M., et al.: Reduction of low birth weight birth rates by the prevention of unwanted pregnancies, Am. J. Pub. Health **63**:935, 1973.

O'Conner, M.C., et al.: The merits of special antenatal care for twin pregnancies, Br. J. Obstet. Gynecol. **88**:222, 1981.

Ueland, K.: Ritodrine hydrochloride (Yutopar) for treatment of preterm labor, Periscope, p. 4, April 1981.

Preterm Infant

Babson, S.G., Pernoll, M.L., and Benda, G.I.: Diagnosis and management of the fetus at risk: a guide for team care, ed. 4, St. Louis, 1979, The C.V. Mosby Co.

Behrman, R.E., editor: Neonatal-perinatal medicine: diseases of the fetus and infant, ed. 2, St Louis, 1977, The C.V. Mosby, Co.

Bresadola, C.: Neonatal intensive care: one infant/one nurse/one objective: quality care, Denver General Hospital, Colo. I. M.C.N. **2**:286, Sept.-Oct. 1977.

Christensen, A.: Coping with the crisis of premature birth—one couple's story, M.C.N. **2**:24, Jan.-Feb., 1977.

Dubowitz, L.M.S., and Dubowitz, V.: Gestational age of the newborn, Menlo Park, Calif., 1977, Addison-Wesley Publishing Co.

Eager, M.: Long-distance nurturing: the family bond, M.C.N. **2**:293, Sept.-Oct. 1977.

Eager, M., and Exoo, R.: Parents visiting parents for unequaled support, M.C.N. **5**:35, Jan.-Feb. 1980.

Erdman, D.: Parent-to-parent support: the best for those with sick newborns, M.C.N. **2**:291, Sept.-Oct. 1977.

Ferrara, A., and Harin, A.: Emergency transfer of the high-risk neonate: a working manual for medical, nursing, and administrative personnel, St. Louis, 1980, The C.V. Mosby Co.

Gennaro, S.: Necrotizing enterocolitis: detecting it and treating it, Nurs. '80 **10**:52, Jan. 1980.

Glassanos, M.R.: Infants who are oxygen dependent—sending them home, M.C.N. **5**:42, Jan.-Feb. 1980.

Gluck, L.: Evaluating functional fetal maturation, Clin. Obstet. Gynecol. **21**:547, June 1978.

Hardgrove, C., and Warrick, L.H.: How shall we tell the children? Am. J. Nurs. **74**:448, 1974.

Harper, T.L.: Observation on unrestricted parental contact with infection in the NICU, Pediatrics **89**:441, 1976.

Henderson, K.J., and Newton, L.D.: Helping nursing mothers maintain lactation while separated from their infants, M.C.N. **3**:352, Nov.-Dec. 1978.

Johnson, S.H.: High risk parenting, Philadelphia, 1979, J.B. Lippincott Co.

Klaus, M.H., and Fanaroff, A.A.: Care of the high-risk neonate, ed. 2, Philadelphia, 1979, W.B. Saunders Co.

Korones, S.: High-risk newborn infants: the basis for intensive nursing care, ed. 3, St. Louis, 1981, The C.V. Mosby Co.

Mangurten, H., et al.: Parent-parent support in the care of high-risk newborns, J.O.G.N. Nurs. **8**:275, Sept.-Oct. 1979.

Measel, C.P., Porter, C., & Anderson, C.G.: Nonnutritive sucking during tube feedings: effect on clinical course in premature infants, J.O.G.N. Nurs. **8**:254, 1979.

Price, E., and Gyotoku, S.: Using the nasojejunal feeding technique in a neonatal intensive care unit, M.C.N. **3**:361, Nov.-Dec. 1978.

Rauch, P.: Effects of tactile and kinesthetic stimulation on premature infants, J.O.G.N. Nurs. **10**(1):34, 1981.

Rice, R.D.: Caressing and cuddling helps a baby grow, Psychol. Today **101**:46, 1976.

Scanlong, J.W., et al.: A system of newborn physical examination, Baltimore, 1979, University Park Press.

Schraeder, B.D.: A creative approach to caring for the ventilator-dependent child, M.C.N. **4**:165, May-June 1979.

Schraeder, B.D.: Attachment and parenting despite lengthy intensive care, M.C.N. **5**:37, Jan.-Feb. 1980.

Shirkey, H.C., editor: Pediatric therapy, ed. 6, St. Louis, 1980, The C.V. Mosby Co.

Silverman, W.A.: Dunham's premature infants, New York, 1961, Paul A. Moeker.

U.S. National Institute of Child Health and Human Development, Department of Health, Education & Welfare: Little babies, born too soon, born too small. Office of Research Reporting, pub. no. (NHIH) 77-1079, Washington, D.C., 1977, The Department.

Vidyasagar, D., and Asonye, U.O.: Critical care problems of

the newborn: practical aspects of transcutaneous oxygen monitoring, Crit. Care Med. **4:**149, April, 1979.

Whaley, L.F., and Wong, D.L.: Nursing care of infants and children, ed. 2, St. Louis, 1983, The C.V. Mosby Co.

Whaley, P.A., et al.: Relieving parental anxiety: a booklet for parents of an infant in NICU, J.O.G.N. Nurs. **8:**49, Jan.-Feb. 1979.

Winer, E., et al.: Four-to-seven year evaluation in two groups of small-for-gestational-age infants, Am. J. Obstet. Gynecol. **143**(4):425, 1982.

Multiple Pregnancy

Benson, R.C., editor: Current obstetric and gynecologic diagnosis and treatment, ed. 3, Los Altos, Calif., 1980, Lange Medical Publications.

Elwood, J.M.: Maternal and environmental factors affecting twin birth in Canadian cities, Br. J. Obstet. Gynaecol. **85:**351, 1979.

Danforth, D., editor: Obstetrics and gynecology, ed. 4, New York, 1982, Harper & Row.

Gromada, K.: Maternal-infants attachment: the first step toward individualizing twins, M.C.N. **5**(2):129, 1981.

Jiminez, S., and Jungman, R.: Supplemental information for the family with a multiple pregnancy, M.C.N. **5**(5):320, 1981.

Kamaromy, B., and Lampe, L.: The value of bed rest in twin pregnancies, Obstet. Gynecol. **15:**262, 1977.

Medearis, A.L., et al.: Perinatal deaths in twin pregnancy: a five-year analysis of statewide statistics in Missouri, Am. J. Obstet. Gynecol. **134:**413, June 15, 1979.

Pettersson, F., et al.: Outcome of twin birth: review of 1,636 children born in twin birth, Obstet. Gynecol. Surv. **32:**79, Feb. 1977.

Theroux, R., and Tingley, J.: The care of twin children: a common-sense guide for parents (edited by D.M. Keith and L.G. Keith), Chicago, 1978, The Center for Study of Multiple Gestation.

38

Adolescent Parenthood

- Adolescent Mother
  - Trends
  - Factors
  - Pregnancy at risk
  - Dynamics
  - Adolescent developmental tasks
  - Developmental tasks of pregnancy
  - Developmental tasks of parenthood
  - Nursing care
    - Adolescent clinics
    - Characteristics of personnel
    - Prenatal period
    - Labor period
    - Postdelivery period
- Adolescent Father
  - Trends
  - Factors
  - Nursing

Adolescent Mother

Adolescent pregnancy, a worldwide phenomenon, represents one of the most critical problems for persons engaged in maternity care. Although the period of adolescence varies somewhat depending on the culture, the World Health Organization (1975) defines it as follows:

1. The individual progresses from the point of the initial appearance of the secondary sex characteristics to that of sexual maturity.
2. The individual's psychologic processes and patterns of indentification develop from those of a child to those of an adult.
3. A transition is made from the state of total socioeconomic dependence to one of relative independence.

TRENDS

The following trends (MacDonnell, 1981) have been identified in adolescent pregnancy and childbearing in the United States and Canada. Proportionately fewer adolescents are bearing children; however, of all children born, a greater percentage of the infants are being born to adolescent mothers. Birth to an adolescent is more likely to be out of wedlock, to a mother who has less than a high school education and who received inadequate prenatal care. Young, single mothers are choosing to keep and raise their children alone. They also are making this choice without seeking advice or help from any of the traditional agencies, for example, children's aid societies or maternity homes. To a great degree these young mothers are dependent on public services and welfare agencies for financial support.

FACTORS

Factors contributing to adolescent pregnancy are physically and culturally interrelated. Sexual maturity is now occurring at an earlier age, although marriage is taking place at a later age. The now-traditional patterns of sexual activity, ranging from dating in the early teens to living together in late adolescence, lack the stabilizing effect of known expectations or norms. In addition, studies indicate that although teenagers with unplanned pregnancies have an adequate level of knowledge of contraceptives, they do not practice contraception consistently. Moreover, there is a lack of explicit education in sexuality both in the home and at school.

PREGNANCY AT RISK

In every sense—physically, emotionally, and socially—these young persons and their offspring are at risk (see Table 32.1) and the society shares that risk. For the adolescent who becomes pregnant the life consequences are far reaching; her future opportunities are restricted in every aspect. Education may be terminated or at best interrupted, and as a result her contributions to the well-being of herself and the society are limited. She may, in fact, be relegated to a low socioeconomic status for life, with an attendant lowering of her self-esteem and of her ability to contribute to society.

Although one third of adolescents give birth outside of wedlock, those who are married are often abandoned either before or shortly after the birth of the infant. If not supported by community resources, the children of these adolescents are prominent targets for child abuse and neglect.

Health and social factors are more important to poor fetal outcome among nulliparous mothers than adolescent status. The adolescent facing socioeconomic and social handicaps is much more likely to have a low-birth weight infant than is her more secure counterpart.

Twice as many infants weighing less than 1500 g are born to teenage mothers as to older mothers, especially if conception occurred less than 2 years after menarche. For gravidas under 15 years old, the prematurity rates are double those for any other age. For the infant, prematurity and low birth weight are associated with an increased incidence of physical and mental disability.

Other obstetric hazards for the adolescent have been documented. They include increased mortality and increased incidence of anemia, vaginitis, gonorrhea, urinary tract infections, and preeclampsia-eclampsia. Young teenagers may have dystocia as a result of cephalopelvic disproportion (CPD), whereas several years later, as the pelvis reaches adult size, normal delivery of similar-sized or even larger babies may be possible. For pregnant adolescents the duration of labor, however, is similar to that of the adult woman.

The incidence of congenital abnormalities is only a trace higher, but it is still higher than that for infants born to older women for all disorders except hydrocephalus. The following chart shows the incidence (per 100,000 population) of birth disorders among gravidas of three age groups:

	Under 20 years	25 to 30 years	40 years or over
Anencephaly	3.5	2.0	3.3
Spina bifida	1.7	0.9	1.5
Occipital meningocele	0.35	0.2	0.35
Hydrocephalus	0.28	0.32	0.70

DYNAMICS

On a personal level the reasons adolescents give for becoming pregnant vary widely. For some there may be faulty relationships within the family. It may be that in mother-daughter conflicts the daughter uses pregnancy to act out her rebellion or as a statement of her growing sexuality as opposed to her mother's declining sexuality. For others there may be a search for nurturance from a mother or father who failed to provide it. Pregnancy can serve as a rite of passage into adulthood and irrefutable evidence of sexual identity and attractiveness.

If human behavior is purposeful (even if the purpose is obscure), cues to the young girl's behavior may sometimes be gained by having her assess where she is now and where she was before pregnancy. For young girls living in poverty, having babies is one form of economic survival. The allotments of money, food stamps, medical and dental care, and special schooling provided by the government establish their economic as well as personal independence. In reality, however, the adolescent's concept of wealth is usually distorted, and a cycle of poverty can be established or perpetuated.

Sometimes an unwanted partner is removed or tested: "Somehow I sensed that if I got pregnant, he wouldn't stand by me. Was I ever right! He abandoned me in a foreign country—just took off. I'm glad I found out his true colors."

Researchers have found a significant love relationship between some teenage couples. They report that a crisis during the pregnancy often arose in the relationships of the putative father and the girl's parents. Of those adolescents who keep their children, a substantial number eventually marry; the premarital sexual relationship was part of a longer commitment to one another.

Some adolescents living in multigenerational families know that their offspring will become family members. In a few instances the pattern for early adolescent pregnancy out of wedlock is a familiar and accepted one. There appears to be a warm, supportive relationship, which, once the initial shock to the family system is resolved, results in supportive and nurturing care for the adolescent and her infant.

Some adolescents view the child to be born as an ally for themselves, someone who will love them in spite of adversity and who will act as a supportive person. The infant's need to be dependent, to be nurtured, and to be viewed as a person apart is not recognized. The young mother's disappointment and bewilderment over her infant's normal behavior can lead to bitterness and eventual neglect.

Other adolescents become pregnant as a result (1) of experimentation with genital sex or (2) of sexual intercourse that the teenager assumes is a normal part of peer activity. Still other tenagers seem to have little or no respect for themselves or their bodies.

The young parents also need career and education counseling. Because many of these young women have not completed their basic education, programs for continuing education are being developed across the nation. These programs attempt to combine learning self-care (including contraceptive care), prenatal preparation for labor and delivery, and child care activities with the traditional classroom subjects. Some school districts provide separate schooling, whereas others stress maintenance of the young parent in her original environment among existing friends. Counselors and teachers hope to provide these young people with alternate methods of coping with life relationships and of meeting the need for closeness to and acceptance by another person that are appropriate for their age levels and resources.

A comprehensive health program for the adolescent will also include family planning services and interconceptional care, such as screening for and treatment of gynecologic problems.

One student who worked with school-age mothers remarked:

> I was appalled by their passivity. They seemed to feel that another person had every right to do things to their bodies. I feel what is needed most is for them to value themselves, to see the beauty of their own bodies, and not to allow themselves to be destroyed.

A large number of unplanned pregnancies could have been prevented since the young mothers had adequate knowledge of contraception. However, they were not motivated to continue use of these contraceptives. Technical knowledge needs to be combined with knowledge relating to adult sexuality, its responsibilities, and its repercussions.

ADOLESCENT DEVELOPMENTAL TASKS

The developmental tasks of adolescents are interrupted by pregnancy. As with other developmental sequences, there are critical periods when interference can have traumatic effects. Obviously the younger the adolescent, the greater will be the effects. For the 12- to 14-year-old girl, pregnancy can be a fearful experience. Because of the extreme youth of these younger adolescents, society tends to respond in a more protective way, and there seems to be a generalized effort to minimize the trauma. The 15- to 17-year-old girl, with her mixture of childlike and adult behavior and her more overt conflicts wth parents, seems to arouse more societal anger and resentment, perhaps because both family and society must respond in a responsible way to behavior they are at a loss to control. The 18- to 20-year-old girl is viewed somewhat as an adult who, with a modicum of support, can fend more adequately and who can assume the major responsibility for her offspring.

The following developmental tasks may be interrupted by pregnancy in adolescence:

TASK: *Achievement of new and more mature relations with age mates of both sexes*

The pregnant adolescent may find herself isolated from her peer group. Within some social groups, parents will try to prevent contact between their teenagers and the one who has become pregnant—an attempt to proclaim societal condemnation of adolescent behavior. In some areas regular school attendance must be discontinued, which effectively limits meetings with peers. The pregnant adolescent has contact largely with other pregnant teenagers, her boyfriend if he remains faithful, and relatives. Thus the practice time for developing social relationships is curtailed.

TASK: *Achievement of a feminine social role*

In one sense pregnancy confers overt adult sexuality on the teenager, but in another sense it limits the feminine role to one of procreation. Opportunities for social development of feminine potential are either abandoned or are set aside until early or middle adulthood.

TASK: *Acceptance of one's physique and effective use of the body*

Adolescents are experiencing a period of rapid change in physical growth and become acutely conscious of their bodies and body sensations.

The symptoms of pregnancy can cause the teenager much dismay. Elimination, for example, is not necessarily talked about openly, and the need for care in the area is equated with being infantile or elderly. The frequent urination of early and late pregnancy may be "treated" by restricting fluid intake. This restriction increases the likelihood of severe constipation or bladder infections.

The increase in melanin causes deepening of color in the areolar tissue of the breasts, the formation of the mask of pregnancy, and the appearance of the linea nigra. These changes may be viewed by the adolescent as stigmas. The increased mucoid vaginal secretions may be thought to be caused by infection, and if the adolescent resists care, they may increase her anxiety and fear. Increased sensitivity of the breasts can be a source of discomfort and anxiety. The fatigue of early pregnancy, compounding the fatigue experienced by many adolescents, can cause the adolescent to assume that she is ill.

Until late adolescence, body image is still formative. By midpregnancy the enlarging abdomen and the increasing size of breasts and buttocks may prompt the teenager to try to control her appearance by dieting, with adverse consequences for fetal health and her own growth needs. The shift in the center of gravity as body posture changes to accommodate the protuberant abdomen causes back strain and lack of balance. These are aggravated by the disparity between the rate of growth of the skeleton and the muscles supporting it; the muscles are not strong enough (even in the nonpregnant state) to maintain correct posture. The effects may be severe if the teenager feels compelled to compete in strenuous activities (including dancing) or to wear nonsupportive shoes because of her need to belong to her peer group. Symptoms of abnormalities, vaginal bleeding, and dizziness are sometimes concealed until serious conditions develop.

It is one thing for a woman who is knowledgeable and secure to accept and cope with the symptoms of pregnancy. She may feel compensated by the feeling that the child she is creating will be wanted and loved. For the adolescent whose pregnancy is condemned and whose baby most often will not be welcomed, the discomforts of pregnancy can assume major proportions. Unfortunately to some they are seen as punishment for their illicit or ''sinful'' behavior.

TASK: *Achievement of independence from parents and other adults*

For the teenager who becomes pregnant, her move toward independence comes to an end, and she is compelled to turn to her family for nurturance just as she did as a young child. Even with the support provided by social agencies, the school-age mother-to-be finds it almost impossible to separate herself from her family. With that support comes a reestablishment of family dominance and dependency.

For example, a 15-year-old girl cannot make a decision relative to the continuing care of her infant without family concurrence. She is not able to provide such care for her child unless some adult is willing to provide shelter and assistance for them both. If this support is not forthcoming, the young teenager must examine other options (e.g., foster care or giving the child up for adoption). However, the pregnancy may act as a catalyst to force the family to examine its relationships. In many instances the pregnancy has been a means of resolving parent-child conflicts in a more growth-responsive way.

Although certain areas of independence are curtailed, others may be substituted. The teenager who assumes responsibility for attendance at prenatal care classes, follows an adequate dietary regimen, and participates in parent-craft groups may emerge from this life experience as one who can function in an interdependent manner with adults.

In some adolescents the forced contact with a caring individual during pregnancy may have a dramatic effect and provide a role model. As one 16-year-old girl expressed it:

> The only thing that was okay with it all was that I met F_______ (nursing counselor). She likes me—well, I know she does. Even when I got rough, she'd be there. I never knew grown people were like that, that they cared about me. I would like to be like her, not a nurse, but like someone who loves people.

TASK: *Establishment of a life-style that is personally and socially satisfying*

A prerequisite of a satisfying life-style is the opportunity to make thoughtful and informed choices in the areas of career, sexual relationships, marriage, family interdependence, and parenthood.

Because of interruptions in schooling, many teenagers who might realistically have had other career goals are relegated to occupations that are not commensurate with their capabilities and temperament. Some never overcome this disadvantage; others must postpone any formal preparations until much later in life.

Precipitate marriage by the older adolescent does not have a good success rate. Unprepared for the give-and-take of such a close relationship, beset by economic problems, living in inadequate housing (often with inlaws), and having no time for the ''fun'' of growing up, participants in early marriage tend to experience desertion or divorce, intensifying their sense of alienation and defeat. For the early adolescent, pregnancy and parenthood seem not to be recognized as possible consequences of sexual behavior; pregnancy comes as a surprise. Parenthood is something that happens to parents, from whom the younger teenager is seeking to establish independence, not a state in which giving of oneself to another will be required.

The older adolescent, being less egocentric and more capable of problem solving, often is able to face the reality of pregnancy and parenthood in an adult manner. She can seek assistance from social agencies in her own right. She may find, however, that the care of a child without the emotional and economic support of another caring adult means altering career plans.

TASK: *Acquisition of a set of values (an ethical system) that will serve as a guide to socially responsible behavior*

Becoming pregnant and producing a child who will not receive the concerned parenting that is his due cannot be said to be socially responsible behavior. However, by assuming adult responsibilities associated with pregnancy and parenthood, some adolescents emerge as stronger, other-centered individuals. For those who are unable to be helped or who are not helped to use this experience as a time of maturation, pregnancy may become a coping mechanism, albeit an inadequate one, to solve the problems of the moment. For this group recidivism is more prevalent, and the adolescent who sought to become independent through sexual activity remains a dependent person.

DEVELOPMENTAL TASKS OF PREGNANCY

In common with the older pregnant woman, the adolescent faces certain developmental tasks directly related to becoming a parent.* Her response to the implications and challenges of these tasks reflects her cognitive level (see Chapters 2 and 7). Adolescents are in the period of transition between the inductive reasoning of late childhood (concrete operations) and the deductive reasoning of the older individual (formal operations). For an adolescent whose thoughts are circumscribed by the "here and now" and "seeing is believing," movement toward the "there and then" and predictions of the future may be very limited. The old saying that "you cannot put an old head on young shoulders" holds true.

TASK: *"I am pregnant."*

The usual response of the adolescent is denial. Anxiety about the response of her family or boyfriend will often delay the seeking of outside support. Adolescents have reported that sharing their suspicions of pregnancy with their parents was the most difficult part of their pregnancy and assumed crisis proportions. Many parents also have reported how emotionally distraught their daughter became. Evidently the idea of being pregnant comes with a sense of surprise and disbelief: "I can't believe it is happening to me," "I didn't think I could get pregnant, I'm too young," "I keep thinking it is some awful dream and I will wake up." The sense of denial is so profound that the girl experiences genuine shock at the consequences of her sexual behavior.

Suspicions of pregnancy may be first discussed with a girlfriend, and fantasies about what will happen when the mother is told will be reviewed. Some adolescents leave clues that they hope will be noticed by their mothers. Containers of pills are left in accessible places, diaries previously locked and secreted away are left open, or letters to girlfriends are placed so that they can easily be read. The parent is expected to note the repetitive nausea, vomiting, and weight loss in early pregnancy, and perhaps the changing body shape of midpregnancy as well, and to bring up the subject of possible pregnancy. The girl expects anger, recriminations, and, depending on the family culture, perhaps physical abuse; in a sense she is suprised by the support and nurturing that are often forthcoming. If the pregnancy were not such a tragic event, the components of the drama resemble many adolescent-adult confrontations. The girl speaks in her adolescent language and expects the all-wise and all-knowing adult to understand.

The end result of the denial of the reality of pregnancy is the postponement of medical care, to the detriment of both the adolescent and her fetus. Abortion as an option may have to be ruled out because of the advanced stage of pregnancy. Infection, drug ingestion, and inadequate nutrition may have already traumatized the fetus. Those who have contact with school-age adolescents need to be particularly alert to changes in their behavior patterns. Often the teacher, school counselor, or school nurse is the first to note symptoms suggestive of pregnancy and to broach the possibility of pregnancy to the girl. In many instances the professional acts as her support in telling her parents of her condition and in initiating medical and social care.

The older adolescent will often seek professional confirmation of her pregnancy before seeking parental or societal help.

Once the pregnancy is confirmed and care has been initiated, the adolescent, whatever, her age, needs help in assuming the responsibility for continuing the care.

TASK: *"I am going to have a baby."*

The second task relating to acceptance of the fetus develops in the same manner with the adolescent as with the older woman. The idea of a happy, cuddly baby who will love and obey the parent seems a common fantasy. The young adolescent can be enthusiastic about how she will dress her baby, take her baby out for walks, and bathe and play with the baby. In fantasy, the infant acquires a doll-like form. The realities of infant care taking and the problems with alleviating crying, feeding the infant, and washing clothes are not faced, nor is the concept of the infant projected into the future—the baby is not visualized as a growing child.

TASK: *"I am going to be a parent."*

The third task, in which the adolescent moves from the idea of having a baby to being a parent—a loving, concerned adult who is capable of providing the nurturing care an infant needs—is the most difficult task for adolescents, as it is for many adult pregnant women. The desire for knowledge about child care activities, nutritional needs of infants, and infant growth and development is evidenced in this group as in any other. One is impressed by the *desire* of the adolescent to be a good mother.

However, the young adolescent's meager life experiences, her own need to grow and develop, and her inability to cope with abstractions and to solve problems on the basis of inference and projection limit the reality of her commitment to her child. The need for continued assessment of her parenting abilities during the postdelivery period is essential if needed support is to be forthcoming. Although the nurse may be responsive to cues of parenting ability evidenced in the prenatal period, these findings are not as predictive as the cues noted during the reality phase of parenthood.

The older adolescent, being able to project herself into the future, can see herself and her infant more readily as separate entities with differing needs. She is more able to fantasize about her child as a preschooler or even a teenager. However, in spite of her greater

*Students are encouraged to review Chapter 16.

ability to propose solutions to problems and follow through on suggestions, the family she will create will remain one of the most vulnerable in our society. (see p. 132).

DEVELOPMENTAL TASKS OF PARENTHOOD

The developmental tasks of parenthood*—that is, reconciling the fantasy with the actual child, becoming adept in care-taking activities, being aware of the infant's needs and source of support as well as one's own, and establishing oneself and one's infant as a family—will be as important to the new adolescent parent's schema as to the adult's.

The adolescent who has a prematuely born infant or small-for-gestational-age (SGA) infant may find it extremely difficult to reconcile this tiny, scrawny infant with her fantasized baby. Her feelings of helplessness when she contemplates the care of a healthy term infant are compounded when she is introduced to her child in the intensive care unit. It may be impossible for her to perceive herself as mothering such an infant. The additional care needed can overwhelm the coping mechanisms she had built up so trustingly in the prenatal period. The consequent alienation of mother and infant may never be overcome.

Intensive teaching and continuous support programs are essential if both the young mother and her vulnerable infant are not to be overwhelmed.

As noted earlier, the young adolescent is not able to establish a family unit for herself or her child. The interdependence possible in such a unit is denied her. If the young mother and her child are incorporated into the older family unit, the process in which she was moving from dependent to interdependent behavior must be adjusted to accommodate an essentially dependent individual. Persons who provide counseling that involves the parents of the young mother seek to set realistic goals for developing the independence of the adolescent. Topics for open discussion among all persons concerned should include infant care responsibilities, the teenager's need to continue her education and her need to work toward maturity. The adolescent's parents will need support as well since they face a new set of responsibilities and tasks. They, too, in a sense, must adjust a fantasy to an actual child.

Professionals who work with young parents stress the need to recognize the maturational differences within the chronologic age groups. The following descriptions of three 17-year-old girls illustrate the differing attitudes, acceptance of the pregnancy, readiness for parenthood, and amount and kind of outside support available.

Case 1. Sharon, 17 years old and with an attractive, outgoing personality, was married 3 months before the birth of her baby. She was enthusiastic about attending parent-craft classes, and her husband, Bob, came to those relating to support in labor. She stated that he was to finish high school in June, 2 months before the baby was born, and she expected him to go to work immediately in a local gas station. Their parents were going to help them for 6 months by paying the rent on a small, three-room apartment, but they were expected to provide for other necessities. Bob made a cradle for the baby, and she made most of the baby clothes. They were using old furniture, but the baby had a new crib. Both familes were excited about the baby and nonjudgmental in their attitudes toward Sharon and her husband.

Sharon had a normal pregnancy and delivery. She was pleased and happy with her baby and found caring for the child rewarding. Bob did well in his job and accepted his new responsbilities. When they began to feel too confined to home and child care, the young couple decided that Sharon could supplement the family income by caring for neighbor's children rather than Bob's getting a second nighttime job, since they needed the time to be together. The additional money would be spent on recreation for themselves.

Case 2. Mary Lou, 17 years old, was a small, fragile-looking young woman. Mary Lou was the youngest of four sisters, all of whom were married and away from home. She had numerous relatives—aunts, uncles, and cousins—in the vicinity. Both her mother and father worked.

Mary Lou never divulged the name of the father of her child. She had no intention of giving the baby up for adoption; she intented to stay home and care for it herself. She refused to attend group classes but was eager and willing for the nurse to teach her individually. When she was taken on a tour of the hospital facilities, she clung to the nurse and needed much reassurance and mothering. The birth was normal, and she had a baby boy. This was an occasion for great family rejoicing, since there had not been a boy for three generations, and her sisters had had girls. Mary Lou came to the hospital with a suitcase containing pretty clothes for herself and lovely baby clothes. The extended family accompanied her to the hospital and were there to greet the new baby. On the first visit to the home, the nurse was extremely aware of the overwhelming presence of the family, particularly Mary Lou's father. Mary Lou was feeding the baby his bottle in a correct but perfunctory manner. Subsequent visits found her increasingly trying to isolate herself. The nurse encouraged Mary Lou to seek additional counseling because she was concerned with Mary Lou's lack of affective response. Mary Lou refused, and within a week ran away from home, leaving the baby boy behind.

Case 3. Betty, 17 years old, was an overweight young woman. She refused to wear maternity clothes and bought herself an overlarge dress in a dark-brown material with small red flowers. She took no other interest in her appearance. She talked repeatedly about how the father of the child had taken

*Students are encouraged to review Chapter 32.

advantage of her, that she was a good girl, and that "he was bad." The baby was to be put up for adoption. She refused to discuss her relationships with her parents, who lived in another city.

Betty had a long, difficult labor. At one time she struck the nurse who was caring for her and screamed for the nurse to "get this monster out of me." She refused to see the baby or to talk about the child. She appeared to deny the whole experience. When the time came for her to return to her home, the nurse accompanied her to the bus. She boarded the bus, an overweight girl in an unattracive, dark-brown dress. The bus pulled away; the nurse waved, but Betty did not look back.

It is obvious that to each of these teenagers, pregnancy had a different meaning; their perceptions of themselves varied, as did their needs. A stereotyped approach to the young pregnant woman is no more successful than a similar approach to the older one.

NURSING CARE

The goals for care of the pregnant adolescent parallel those of all pregnant women, namely, to assist her in experiencing a physically safe and emotionally satisfying pregnancy and to promote optimal health in her offspring. Many interacting biologic and social factors will affect the quality of human reproduction, and these in turn are influenced by the preconceptional, maternity, and neonatal care that is made available. The adolescent and her offspring are particularly vulnerable to the risks inherent in pregnancy and parenthood because of circumstances characteristic of her age group, such as physiologic immaturity, economic dependency, poor nutritional status, lack of education, inadequate or delayed medical care, and political ineffectiveness.

Adolescent clinics. Because of the circumstances of adolescent pregnancy, programs specifically addressed to the problems of the adolescent are being developed across the country. Separate clinics for adolescents are better equipped to provide health services that are responsive to the teenager's unique needs. They also provide for supportive associations with the father of the child and with the girl's parents or other authority figures. They utilize a multidisciplinary team of nurse-midwives, physicians, nurses, nutritionists, and social workers. The outcomes of lower recidivism and increased birth weights are two indications of their effectiveness (Chanis et al., 1979; Doyle and Widhalm, 1979; Peoples and Barrett, 1979).

Characteristics of personnel

Personal qualities. The characteristics of persons who work with this population are very important. They need to have come to terms with their own sexuality to be able to maintain a nonjudgmental approach. They must be genuinely interested in the adolescent, as well as being enthusiastic, warm, caring individuals who are able to view adolescents as young persons involved in an exciting growth period, who are willing to respond to a concerned adult, and who basically want to be accepted and successful. Nurses need to be able to listen and to respond with honest answers, to be available when needed, and to be capable of accepting repeated "testing" by the adolescent. They need to be able to create a safe and stable environment that engenders trust. Such an environment will enable the professional to determine the adolescent's real problems and to set realistic goals.

Knowledge. Nurses who work with pregnant adolescents need to be knowledgeable concerning (1) the physical attributes of the adolescent and her developmental needs, (2) the adolescent's maturational level relative to personality and cognitive development, (3) maternal responses to pregnancy and the adolescent's interpretation of them, and (5) the cues that indicate stress in the adolescent and difficulties in parenting.

Teaching ability. Persons working with adolescents need to be adept in using a variety of teaching strategies. Group discussions are effective because adolescents have a strong need for peer contact and acceptance. However, because of the immaturity of the participants, the nurse will need to act as leader. Question boxes and anonymous pretests are devices that reveal gaps in knowledge or belief in myths. Demonstrations by the nurse, with group members demonstrating the same skill, are effective in assessing the teenager's ability.

Counseling ability. As counselers, nurses are concerned with the adolescent's ability to make decisions, to explore the risks and consequences of her actions, and to assume responsibility for her behavior. Some of the techniques used to encourage growth in these areas include having the adolescent set up a discussion group, decorate a child care space, select a menu, plan a day for herself and her infant, and talk over solutions to problems. Independent function is encouraged; the nurse acts as a catalyst in solving problems, but the problem solving belongs to the adolescent.

Another area in which the adolescent requires assistance is in helping her separate herself from her baby so that she can see its unique needs. Information relative to child development and to infant care-taking activities is basic to this goal.

Prenatal period. The adolescent is considered to be at risk during her pregnancy. There is an increase in scheduled prenatal visits. Effort is expended to prompt attendance at the clinic; lapses in attendance are followed by telephone calls or personal contacts.

Prenatal classes. The content of prenatal classes is

chosen with the adolescent's needs in mind. Content relating to maternal adaptations during pregnancy should be presented in terms of how the adolescent can adjust to changes. For example, exercises to promote posture, the care of skin, hair, and nails, and hygiene for increased perspiration and vaginal secretions are discussed. Concrete examples of "what to do" and "what not to do" are needed.

Information about what happens during labor and delivery and how pain is controlled requires considerable emphasis. Opportunities to discuss feeling and fears with other adolescents who have experienced birth are welcome.

Basic information about sex and reproduction is needed to ensure accuracy of the adolescent's knowledge in this area. Birth control information should be included in prenatal classes and presented realistically and nonjudgmentally.

Adolescents welcome information about infant care but need help to see the usefulness of information given about child growth and development.

Nutritional needs. Adolescence (ages 13 to 18 years) presents its own special nutritional problems. Most adolescent girls attain physiologic maturity at 17 years of age; pregnancy before that age presents certain biologic hazards. The course and outcome of pregnancy of women between 18 and 20 years of age are comparable to those of mature women 20 to 24 years of age.

The orderly sequence of growth and skeletal maturation is related to sexual maturation. Sexual maturity may be attained before musculoskeletal maturation is complete. Dietary surveys among adolescents have revealed that this group receives less than two thirds of the recommended daily intake of iron, calcium, and vitamins A and C (Food and Nutrition Board, 1970). About one in ten adolescents who become pregnant is obese. Since weight-conscious adolescents may consume less than 2000 kcal/24 hr, the recommended allowance of iron (18 mg/24 hr) is deficient. Female adolescents who are anemic and underweight at a time when their body growth needs are at a peak (17 years of age or younger) are more vulnerable to skeletal problems, communicable diseases, and infections. Pregnancy at this time superimposes metabolic demands for nutrients on the dietary requirements for the adolescent's own growth. Weight gain during pregnancy must be evaluated in light of her normal growth (anabolism) during that period. Her need for increased protein, calories, and iron will exceed that of the pregnant woman over 20 years of age.

The outcome for the fetus may not be reflected in lowered birth weight alone. Research indicates that brain growth takes place in an orderly sequence, as does growth of other organs. The first-phase hyperplasia (growth by increase in the number of cells) takes place prenatally, and the second-phase hypertrophy (growth by increase in cell size), in combination with hyperplasia, is the growth pattern noted in the first 6 months of life. Maternal malnutrition may therefore contribute to a reduced complement of brain cells in the fetus, and the mother's lack of knowledge of the nutritional requirements of her newborn compounds the problem.

Adolescence is a period of developing independence. Symbols of home—milk, fresh fruits and vegetables, and a "square meal"—if these were present, are associated with dependency and as such may be threatening (e.g., "peanut butter is for children"). Often there is the desire to "be free," to choose "forbidden" foods. Peers congregate at the hamburger stand; soda, hamburgers, and french fries may be supplemented with candy bars.

The young married adolescent may have just learned how to cook. This achievement, as well as her desire to please her husband and cater to his preferences, must be considered in nutrition conseling. Supporting her inner desire to assert independence during nutrition counseling sessions lends support to the overall developmental task of this period: movement from the role of child to that of adult. Listen, and allow her to talk. Build on what she and her family already know and practice. Reinforce sound dietary patterns and acknowledge adaptations that are willingly made. Promote the idea that it is adult sometimes to do what one must, even if one does not wish to do so. When appropriate to meet the health needs of the mother and fetus, set some limits. Elicit help from the mother's parents or parent substitute in identifying these limits. In planning a teaching strategy to meet the objectives of nutrition counseling, the nurse must first set realistic goals such as the following:

1. To support the pregnant adolescent's psychosocial move toward independence
2. To increase her knowledge of nutrients and daily allowances
3. To teach her how to plan diets for herself and her family
4. To teach her how to select foods to meet nutritional needs, personal preferences, budget requirements, and seasonal availability
5. To teach her how to prepare foods to ensure optimal nutritive value

Of necessity these goals go beyond the immediate objectives of a healthy pregnancy, an uneventful labor, and a full-term, healthy infant whose weight and maturity are appropriate for gestational age and who subsequently grows and develops normally. Recent animal research has disclosed that two generations are required to counteract the mental and physical retardation resulting from protein deficiency during pregnancy. The young mother who improves her own and her family's dietary patterns is building the foundation for a healthier beginning for generations to follow.

The relationship between sound nutrition and physical appearance can be used to gain the attention of adolescents (and perhaps older women as well) for nutrition education. Frequently the condition and appearance of the skin, hair, and nails are uppermost in the minds of adolescents. Body contours in both the male and female adolescent and muscular development in the male teenager are selling points for good nutrition.

Labor period. The adolescent in labor should have the support of a knowedgeable coach, whether husband, boyfriend, parent, or nurse. Many teenagers come to labor lacking preparation; they are fearful and often alone. If they are admitted early in the first stage, teaching about relaxation with contractions, ambulation, side-lying positions, and comfort measures can be accomplished (see Chapter 21).

If the adolescent is giving her baby up for adoption, she may or may not wish to see the baby after birth or to know its sex. It is generally agreed that releasing a child is facilitated if one grieves for an actual loss rather than a fantasy one; however, the mother has the right to make her own choice. She can be given the information about the infant's health (e.g., "your baby is healthy and strong") since it may affect her response to her own feelings of self-worth.

Placing an infant for adoption may be accepted by young parents with varying emotional responses. For some, it may be another episode in a "bad" experience. With others, the birth of the child and the arrangement for his care are undertaken with little or no apparent understanding of a child's needs, as indicated by the following:

> The baby, whom the couple will call ________, is under county care at the ________ and will probably be given to foster parents—although the couple would like to see their daughter live with in-laws.
>
> The couple are now staying with friends in a small apartment above a garage in ________ but talked happily about the rush of events that brought them a daughter last Saturday night.
>
> "We're happy to have a baby, even though the doctors at the hospital told us it wasn't a very good idea," said the young mother.
>
> "I was so happy that I bought her $50 worth of new clothes," said her husband, tugging at his wife's burgundy double-knit slacks.
>
> ________, the mother, smiled, puffed on her cigarette, and said she could hardly recall much of her moments during childbirth.
>
> "I remember the patient's helping me walk. I remember there were some nurses and technicians and a doctor at the end. And I remember a baby too. That was nice," she said.*

On the other hand, giving a baby up for adoption may be attended by all the symptoms of grief one would expect at the death of a newborn: "She is only 15 years old, but she loves the baby. Her parents won't take it, so she has to give it up. Her grief was heartbreaking. On the day she went home she came into the nursery to hold her baby for one last time." The grief of the young parent at her loss has to be balanced with the need of her infant for continued care and nurturing. If the infant is born at risk, the parent will need professional support, as reviewed in Chapters 33 and 34.

Many adolescents keep their infants and are responsive to the staff's sharing in their delight and joy. For these young parents, efforts to promote parent-child attachment are particularly important.

Postdelivery period. If possible, the young mother and child should be in a rooming-in accommodation so that the process of mothering the child can be started as early as possible. This support needs to be sustained after the mother and child return home. The process of continued care should include home visiting and group sessions for discussion of infant care or parenting problems. Research indicates that outreach programs that are concerned with parent-child interactions, child injuries, and instances of failure to thrive and that provide prompt, effective community intervention prevent more serious subsequent problems (Gray et al., 1979).

Efforts are made to determine the young mother's feeling toward her infant, the quality of the interaction between mother and infant, her knowledge of and attitude toward infant care-taking activities, and her understanding of her infant's growth and developmental needs. Jarrett (1982) found that the young parents expected too much of their children too soon (Table 38.1). Many of these mothers pattern their practice on what they themselves had experienced. It is vital, therefore, to determine the kind of support those close to these young mothers are able or prepared to give and the kinds of community aid that can supplement this support. The box on p. 946 developed by Poole (1976), gives sample interview questions that the nurse may use to obtain information, which then serves as the data base for the care of the adolescent parent and her child.

*From San Francisco Chronicle, No. 17, 1976, p. 24.

Table 38.1
Ages at which Mothers Expect Children to Accomplish Specific Behaviors

Behavior	Norm for Mastery	Mother's Expectations			
		<12 mo	12-18 mo	18-24 mo	>36 mo
Bladder control	18-24 mo	43%	43%	14%	0%
Bowel control	24-36 mo	26%	30%	30%	14%
Obedience training	>24 mo	80%	14%	6%	0%
Recognition of right from wrong	30-36 mo	78%	20%	2%	0%

Sample Interview Questions

Often girls your age, when they become mothers, find their lives to be very different from what they had planned themselves. They sometimes must drop out of school, and it may be hard for them to find a job they like. Plans they once had for themselves may just seem like unreachable dreams. Let's talk about how you feel regarding these things.

1. Are you going to school now?
   What do you feel about that?
   If necessary: Are you glad that you are?
   or Do you wish that you were?
2. Do you have any kind of job right now?
   what do you feel about it?
   If necessary: Do you like your job?
   Does it seem adequate to meet your needs?
   Do you wish you were working?
3. What would you most like to be doing with your life right now if you could do anything that you wished?
4. What would you most like to do in the future if you had the choice of doing anything that you wanted to do?
   Is this a possible goal for you?
   What do you feel about that?

Young mothers often find their lives totally filled with school, job, and caring for their babies. Often they do not have time to do the things they like to do, such as visit with their friends, make new friends, or be with their husband or boyfriend. Sometimes their own mothers seem to use the baby as a means of controlling what their daughters do and do not do. This can sometimes be very frustrating.

5. Do you seem to be able to find time to be by yourself?
   What do you feel about that?
   What do you usually do when you have free time for yourself?
   What would you most like to do during this time?
6. Do you find time to be with your friends?
   Are you able to see them as often as you would like?
   What do you feel about that?
   Have you made any new friends since you had the baby?
   If unmarried: Have you been able to be with your boyfriend or meet and date new guys since you had the baby?
   What do you feel about that?
7. Do you feel that your mother puts a lot of pressure on you to do the things that you should do?
   What do you feel about that?

Husbands or boyfriends sometimes get involved with the baby, and sometimes they do not. Young mothers often feel isolated and alone and resent the fact that the father is not helping much with the baby. Sometimes mothers feel that they do not get along with the husband or boyfriend as well as they did before the baby came.

8. Does your baby's father seem to enjoy the baby?
   What type of things does he do with him (her)?
   Change diapers?
   Bathe?
   Feed?
   Play?
   Other?
   Do you get enough help from him?
   What do you feel about that?
   Do you seem to be closer, less close, or about the same as you were before the baby was born?
   What do you feel about that?

It is important what some people think about us, but with other people we do not really care what they think. I'm going to give you a list of people and I want you to tell me whether or not they would agree with the way you take care of your baby and how you feel about whether they agree or not.

9. mother
   father
   baby's father
   baby's father's parents
   teacher
   employer
   friends
   nutritionist
   social worker
   nurse
   doctor
   church members
   minister or priest
   neighbors
   relatives

> Some things about caring for the baby are fun, but others may be very irritating to a mother. I'm going to ask you about different things you do in caring for your baby and about what your baby does. Tell me what you feel about them.

10. First, feeding your baby?
    What do you feel about this?
    How much time does it usually take?
    Does it seem to take a lot out of you?
11. Now let's consider changing your baby's diapers.
    What do you feel about that?
12. How about bathing your baby?
13. How about playing with your baby?
    What do you feel about that?
    Do you find time to play with your baby often?
    Do you feel that it is important for you to play with him (her)?
14. Does your baby try to annoy you sometimes?
    What does he do that really annoys you?
    What do you feel about that?
    What do you usually do about it?
    Do you ever find that you need to punish your baby?
    What types of things does he do that he needs to be punished for?
    How do you usually punish him (her) when he (she) needs it?

Adolescent Father

TRENDS

The National Center of Health Statistics reported that in 1979, of the infants born to adolescent mothers, 20% had fathers under 20 years of age. Of all infants born in the United States in 1979, 135,581 infants had fathers less than 20 years of age. The majority of these were in their late teens. It is estimated that there are approximately three times as many adolescent mothers as fathers.

FACTORS

The effect of pregnancy and parenthood on adolescent fathers has recently become an area of nursing concern. Three major factors have prompted interest in the problems of these young parents.

1. The critical role of the father in the development of a child has been demonstrated (Frodi and Lamb, 1978; Lamb, 1976; Lamb, 1981; Parke and O'Leary, 1975; Parke et al., 1980).

2. Health programs have been developed that consider the needs of both the adolescent mother and father.

3. The role of the father in the birth process has changed. Fathers are now encouraged to be participants in birth. Responsibilities and rights of fathers are more accepted. For example, the federal government expects the unwed mother to attempt to gain child support from the father of the child before granting financial assistance (Moore, 1981). The unwed father has the legal right to petition for custody of his child if the mother wishes to place the baby for adoption (Panner and Evans, 1975).

NURSING CARE

The adolescent father as well as the adolescent mother is faced with immediate developmental crises, that is, completing the developmental tasks of adolescence and making a transition to parenthood. If the young couple marry a third stress is added—transition to marriage. The long-range effects of premature parenthood are related to delayed educational and vocational attainment and to lack of stability in marriage.

If at all possible the father is approached through his pregnant partner. Some clinics make clear that the pregnant adolescent will bring her partner to the clinic and that he will take an active interest in the birth process. At other times the father needs to be contacted directly. In order to provide data for inclusion of the young father in all aspects of the care, four areas need to be assessed: (1) the future of the couple together, (2) the adequacy of coping, (3) educational and vocational goals, and (4) the adequacy of health education knowledge (Elster, 1982).

Adolescent fathers (as all fathers) need support to discuss their emotional responses to the pregnancy. These include pleasure, ambivalence, or anger. Counseling needs to be reality oriented. Topics such as child care and expense, parenting skills, and knowledge of the father's role in the birth experience need to be explored. The teenage father also needs knowledge of reproductive physiology and of birth control options.

The adolescent mother's boyfriend, as well as her family, have an impact on how she will deal with her pregnancy, labor, and delivery, and subsequent parenthood. The adolescent partner has usually been involved in an ongoing relationship with the young mother. In many instances he plays an important role in the decisions she is faced with in pregnancy, that is, to continue the pregnancy or have an abortion and to keep the child or place the child for adoption.

The nurse supports the young father by helping him develop realistic perceptions of his role of "father to a child." She encourages his use of coping mechanisms that are not detrimental to his, his partner's, and his child's well-being. The nurse enlists support systems, parents, and professional agencies on his behalf.

References and Readings

Aiman, J.: X-ray pelvimetry of the pregnant adolescent, Obstet. Gynecol. **48:**281, 1976.

Ambrose, L.: Misinforming pregnant teenagers, Fam. Plan. Perspect. **10:**51, Jan.-Feb. 1978.

Baldwin, W.: Adolescent pregnancy and childbearing—an overview, Semin. Perinatol. **5:**1, Jan. 1981.

Battaglia, F., Frazier, T., and Hellegers, A.: Obstetric and pediatric complications of juvenile pregnancy, Pediatrics **32:**902, 1963.

Baum, D.J.: Teenage pregnancy: a handbook for teachers, parents, counselors, and kids, New York, 1980, Beaufort Books.

Baumrind, D.: Clarification concerning birthrate among teenages, Am. Psychol. **36:**528, May 1981.

Bolton, F.G., Jr.: The pregnant adolescent: problems of premature parenthood, Beverly Hills, Calif., 1980, Sage Publications.

Bracken, M.B., Klerman, L.V., and Bracken. M.: Abortion, adoption or motherhood: an empirical study of decision-making during pregnancy, Am. J. Obstet. Gynecol. **130:**251, 1978.

Burchinal, L.G.: Trends and prospects for young marriages in the United States, J. Marr. Fam. **27:**243, 1965.

Burst, H.V.: Adolescent pregnancies and problems, J. Nurs. Midwife. **24:**19, March-April 1979.

Card, J.J., and Wise, L.L.: Teenage mothers and teenage fathers: the impact of early childbearing on the parents' personal and professional lives, Fam. Plan. Perspect. **10:**199, 1978.

Catano, J.W.: Teenage pregnancy: a resource kit. Halifax, Nova Scotia, The Prepared Childbirth Association of Nova Scotia, 1979.

Chanis, M., O'Donohue, N., and Stanford, A.: Adolescent pregnancy, J. Nurs. Midwife. **24:**18, May-June 1979.

Chilman, C.S.: Adolescent pregnancy and childbearing: findings from research, Washington, D.C., 1980 U.S. Department of Health and Human Services.

Copeland, D.A.: Unwed adolescent primigravidas identify subject matter for prenatal classes. J.O.G.N. Nurs. **8:**248, July-Aug. 1979.

Corkum, T.: Adolescent pregnancy outcomes in Halifax-Dartmouth since 1970. Paper presented at Sexuality and the Family Conference, Halifax, Nova Scotia, June 1979.

Daniel, W.: Adolescents in health and disease, St. Louis, 1977, The C.V. Mosby Co.

DeLissovoy, V.: High school marriages: a longitudinal study, J. Mar. Fam. **35:**245, 1973.

Doyle, M.B., and Widhalm, M.V.: Midwifing the adolescent at Lincoln Hospital's teen-age clinics, J. Nurs. Midwife. **24:**27, July-Aug. 1979.

Duenholter, J., Jimenez, J., and Baumann, G.: Pregnancy performance of patients under fifteen years of age, Obstet. Gynecol. **46:**49, 1975.

Edwards, M.: Teenage parents, Seattle, Wash., 1978, The Pennypress.

Elster, A.L.: Effects of pregnancy and parenthood on adolescent fathers and implications for clinical intervention, J. Calif. Perinat. Assoc. **2**(2):44, 1982.

Fischman, S.J.: Delivery or abortion in inner-city adolescents, Am. J. Orthopsych. **147:**127, 1977.

Food & Nutrition Board: Recommended daily dietary allowances, Washington, D.C., 1970, National Academy of Science–National Research Council.

Foster, S.: The one girl in ten: a self-portrait of the teenage mother, Claremont, Calif., 1981, Arbor Press.

Frodi, A.M., and Lamb, M.E.: Fathers' and Mothers' responses to the faces and cries of normal and premature infants, Dev. Psychol. **14:**490, 1978.

Furstenberg, F.F., Lincoln, R., and Menken, J., editors: Teenage sexuality, pregnancy and childrearing, Philadelphia, 1981, University of Pennsylvania Press.

Gallas, H.B., special issue editor: Teenage parenting: social determinants and consequences, J. Soc. Issues **36:**1, Winter 1980.

Gray, J.D., et al.: Prediction and prevention of child abuse, Semin. Perinatol. **3:**85, Jan. 1979.

Hendricks, L.E., Howard, C.S., and Caesar, P.P.: Help-seeking behavior among select populations of black unmarried adolescent fathers: implications for human service agencies, Am. J. Pub. Health **71:**733, 1981.

Hibbard, B.M.: The effectiveness of antenatal education, Health Educ. J. **38:**39, 1979.

Higgins A.C.,: Nutritional status and the outcome of pregnancy, J. Can. Diet. Assoc. **37:**17, 1976.

Hutchins, F.L., Jr., Kendall, N., and Rubino, J.: Experience with teenage pregnancy, Obstet. Gynecol. **54:**1, July 1979.

Inselberg, R.M.: Marital problems and satisfaction in high school marriages, Mar. Fam. Liv. p. 74, Feb. 1962.

Jarrett, G.E.: Childrearing patterns of young mothers: expectations, knowledge, and practices, M.C.N. **7:**119, March-April 1982.

Kerckhoff, A.C., and Parrow, A.A.: The effect of early marriage on the education attainment of young men, J. Mar. Fam. *41:*97, 1979.

Lamb, M.E.: Interaction between two-year-olds and their mothers and fathers, Psychol. Rep. **38:**447, 1976.

Lamb, M.E.: The father's role in the facilitation of infant mental health, Inf. Ment. Health J. **1:**140, 1980.

Lamb, M.E.: Fathers and child development: an integrative overview. In Lamb, M.E., editor: The role of the father in child development, New York, 1981, Wiley-Interscience.

Lorenzi, M.E., Kerman, L.V., and Jekel, J.F.: School-age parents: how permanent a relationship? Adolescence **45:**13, Spring 1977.

MacDonnell, S.: A teenage pregnancy epidemic? Can. Nurs. *75:*22, Nov. 1979.

Mac Donnel, S.: Vulnerable mothers, vulnerable children: a follow-up study of unmarried mothers who kept their children, Halifax, Nova Soctia, 1981, Policy, Planning and Research Division, Nova Scotia Department of Social Services.

March of Dimes–Birth Defects Foundation, Committee on Perinatal Health: Toward improving the outcome of pregnancy, White Plains, N.Y., 1979, The Foundation.

McAnarney, E.R., and Friedman, S.B.: Experience with an adolescent health care program, Pub. Health Rep. **90:**412, 1975.

McAnarney. E.R., et al.: Teenagers evaluate their own health care, Pediatrics **55:**290, 1978.

Mednick, B.R., Baker, R.L., and Sutton-Smith, B.: Teenage pregnancy and perinatal mortality, J. Youth Adolesc. **8:**343, 1979.

Mercer, R.: Becoming a mother at sixteen, M.C.N. **1:**44, Jan.-Feb. 1976.

Moore, K.A.: Government policies related to teenage family formation and functioning: an inventory. In Ooms, T., editor: Teenage pregnancy in a family context: implications for policy, Philadelphia, 1981, Temple University Press.

Moore, K.A., and Waite, L.J.: Early childbearing and educational attainment, Fam. Plan. Perspect. **9**:220, 1977.
Panner, R., and Evans, B.W.: The unmarried father revisited, J. School Health **45**(5):271, 1975.
Parke, R.D., and O'Leary, L.: Father-mother-infant interaction in the newborn period: some findings, some observations, and some unresolved issues. In Riegel, K.F., and Meacham, J., editors: The developing individual in a changing world, vol 2. Social and environmental issues, The Hague, 1975, Mouton.
Parke, R.D., Power, T.G., and Fisher, T.: The adolescent father's impact on the mother and child, J. Soc. Issues **36**:88, 1980.
Pederson, F.A., Rubinstein, J. and Yarrow, L.J.: Infant development in father-absent families, J. Gen. Psych. **135**:51, 1979.
Peoples, M.D., and Barrett, A.E.: A model for the delivery of health care to pregnant adolescents, J.O.G.N. Nurs. **8**:339, Nov.-Dec. 1979.
Petrella, J.: Caring for the unwed adolescent, J.O.G.N. Nurs. **7**:22, July-Aug. 1978.
Poole, C.: Adolescent mothers: can they be helped? Pediatr. Nurs. **2**:7, March-April 1976.
Sumner, G., and Fritsch, J.: Postnatal parental concerns: the first six weeks of life, J.O.G.N. Nurs **6**:27, May-June 1977.
Surr, C.W.: Student nurses teach pregnant teens, J.O.G.N. Nurs. **2**:44, March-April, 1973.
Tankson, E.: The adolescent parent: one approach to teaching child care and giving support, J.O.G.N. Nurs. **5**:9, 1976.
Theirreu, M.E.: Evaluating empathy skill training for parents, Social Work **9**:417, Sept. 1979.
World Health Organization: Pregnancy and abortion in adolescence, tech. rep. series no. 583, Geneva, 1975, The Organization.
World Population Growth and Response: 1965-1975, Washington, D.C., April 1976, Population Reference Bureau, Inc.
Zuckerman, B. et al.: Neonatal outcome: is adolescent pregnancy a risk factor, Pediatrics **71**:(4), 1983.

Resources for Providers Working with Teens

Teenage parent self development program
Group exercises in decision making on becoming sexually active, using birth control, pregnancy, marrying, relationships with men, parenting, and an education career.
Armsworth, J.A., et al.
600 Nol Mound St.
Macogdoches, TX 75961
Cost: $20

Teenage pregnancy: a new beginning
Photo essay instruction book on pregnancy, birth, breast feeding. Exercise, breast feeding, and student study guide may be ordered separately for 50¢ each.
Barr, L., et al.
New Futures School
110 Broadway NE
Albuquerque, MN 87102
Cost: $4.95

Teenage parents
Overview of teenage pregnancy, with many resource listings and case histories. Good for professional who wants to begin but does not know where to start. Includes birth preparation techniques in high school setting and model for infant care.
Edwards, M.
Pennypress
1100 23rd Ave. East
Seattle, WA 98112
Cost: $5.00

Teenager's guide to childbirth
Pamphlet for handout that covers labor, hospital admission, and childbirth, at sixth-grade reading level. Part of Pennypress' Better Baby Series.
Edwards, M.
1100 23rd Ave. East
Seattle, WA 98112
Cost: 50¢

Hi, I'm Yolanda
Sixteen-page-comic book about breast feeding, written on a fourth-grade reading level. Multiracial drawings.
Gonzales, C., et al.
24920 Pine Hills Drive
Carmel, CA 93923
Cost: $1.00

How to reduce teenage pregnancy
Move teens to commitment to nonparenthood during adolescence through school newspapers and other youth-oriented publications.
Scales, P.
National Organization for Non-Parents
3 No. Liberty Street
Baltimore, MD 21201
Cost: $1.50

Every child and family matters: tender loving care
Curriculum outline for mother-baby and maternity centers, and community outreach. Target group: low-income teenager. Good for middle-class provider. Salvation Army also uses Education for Parenthood programs, DHEW pub. no. (OHDS) 77-30125.
Salvation Army
120 W. 14th St.
New York, NY 10011

39 Psychosocial Risk Factors

- **Childbearing Psychosis**
  Manic-depressive psychosis
  Schizophrenia
- **Drug Dependence**
  Fetal alcohol syndrome
  Narcotic drug dependence
- **Poverty**
  Reproductive experience
  Complications
  Prenatal care

Not all complications during childbearing have a physical condition as the basic element. Complications that have implications for the health of the mother and child and of other family members may arise from a variety of psychosocial factors. This chapter addresses a number of these factors: childbearing psychosis, sensory impairment, substance abuse, and poverty.

Childbearing Psychosis

The incidence of major psychiatric complications in pregnant women is about 3:1000. So-called "nervous breakdowns" during the prenatal period occur in only about 15% of women; almost 60% of these develop manic-depressive or schizophrenic reactions in the first 2 weeks after delivery. The remainder will require psychiatric care and treatment during the last several weeks of the puerperium.

Pregnancy per se is not a cause of psychiatric illness, but psychologic and physical stresses relating to pregnancy or to the formidable new obligations of motherhood may precipitate an emotional crisis.

The principal psychoses complicating gestation are manic-depressive psychosis and schizophrenia. Toxic deliriums, associated with drug addiction, excessive analgesia, or serious metabolic disorders, are not common. Rarely, psychosis secondary to alcoholism or syphilis may complicate both prenatal and postdelivery progress.

MANIC-DEPRESSIVE PSYCHOSIS

Although the etiology of manic-depressive psychosis is unknown, the family history may record one or more adults who have had this problem. Moreover, women who have psychiatric complications during the course of pregnancy often have had similar crises previously.

Over 50% of pregnancy-related psychoses are affective reactions. Of these, about 10% are predelivery manic or depressive states; the remainder disturb the postdelivery period. Younger women seem more prone to manic reactions, but depression is the more common problem for most women.

Rejection of the infant, often caused by abnormal jealousy, is a prominent feature of manic-depressive psychosis. The mother may be obsessed by the notion that the offspring may supplant her in her husband's affections. In other instances, guilt regarding aversion to pregnancy, attempted abortion, or other personal conflicts may be the basic problem. *Manic reactions* often occur during the first or second week of the puerperium, perhaps, after a brief depression. Agitation, excitement, and volubility, often with rhyming or punning, develop. The woman becomes disinterested in personal care and food. Since dehydration or exhaustion may ensue, prompt and effective supportive treatment is essential.

Psychiatric therapy may include a tranquilizer with a prominent sedative effect, for example, promethazine hydrochloride (Phenergan). Lithium carbonate may be given later for more prolonged control. Electroshock treatment is beneficial, but this modality is contraindicated in pelvic sepsis. Psychotherapy is essential. The usual duration of the manic state is 1 to 3 weeks. The prognosis for mother and infant is good after initial separation and gradual reunion.

Depressive reactions, far more common than manic reactions, may begin as a mild feeling of discouragement (the "baby blues") during the first week after delivery. However, anxiety, anorexia, and exaggerated fatigue soon color the despondency. The woman seems helpless; she is self-accusatory and often expresses strange or inappropriate thoughts or feelings. Occasionally a disconsolate mother may kill her infant and herself.

Depression may continue for weeks or months. Amphetamines are not helpful and may add to agitation. However, a tranquilizer with a prominent stimulatory effect, such as trifluoperazine (Stelazine), should be beneficial. Electroshock therapy may result in striking improvement, but relapses are common. Psychotherapy must be intensive and often prolonged. Meanwhile, separation of mother and infant will be necessary. If the depression lifts within several weeks, the prognosis is good. However, women who have been depressed previously, especially those who have had even longer depressions, have a poor prognosis.

SCHIZOPHRENIA

Schizophrenia, now suspected of being a disorder of cerebral metabolism, affects adolescents and younger adults rather than older persons. Abnormal personality features are common. Unusually shy, retiring, hypersensitive, or overly suspicious women are prone to schizophrenic break. A sudden onset of delusions or hallucinations may alter a seemingly well-accepted normal pregnancy, indicating the woman's inability to adjust to and cope with her new obligations as a mother.

The husband and infant are totally rejected. Hostility toward the spouse and the medical staff is obvious. Often the excited, confused woman believes hers to have been an immaculate conception, or she may believe that she is being influenced by the Deity. The women abandons reality and retreats completely into her own world of unreality. The mother totally neglects her infant but rarely harms it. Suicide is unlikely. A phenothiazine type of tranquilizer, for example, chlorpromazine (Thorazine), will be useful. Transfer of the woman to a psychiatric hospital usually is necessary. Electroshock therapy and psychotherapy usually are effective.

A good prognosis is likely with the first psychotic episode, especially if it occurs unexpectedly during the puerperium. The child probably will never suffer from schizophrenia, despite speculation regarding hereditary tendencies.

Drug Dependence

The adverse effects of exposure of the fetus to drugs varies from transient behavioral changes such as fetal breathing movements to irreversible effects such as fetal death, intrauterine growth retardation, structure malformations, or mental retardation. Maternal use of drugs may be for the pharmacologic control of disease processes (e.g., insulin) or for symptomatic relief of be-

Fig. 39.1
Critical periods in human embryogenesis. (From Fanaroff, A.A., and Martin, R.J., editors: Behrman's neonatal-perinatal medicine: diseases of the fetus and infant, ed. 3, St. Louis, 1983. The C.V. Mosby Co.)

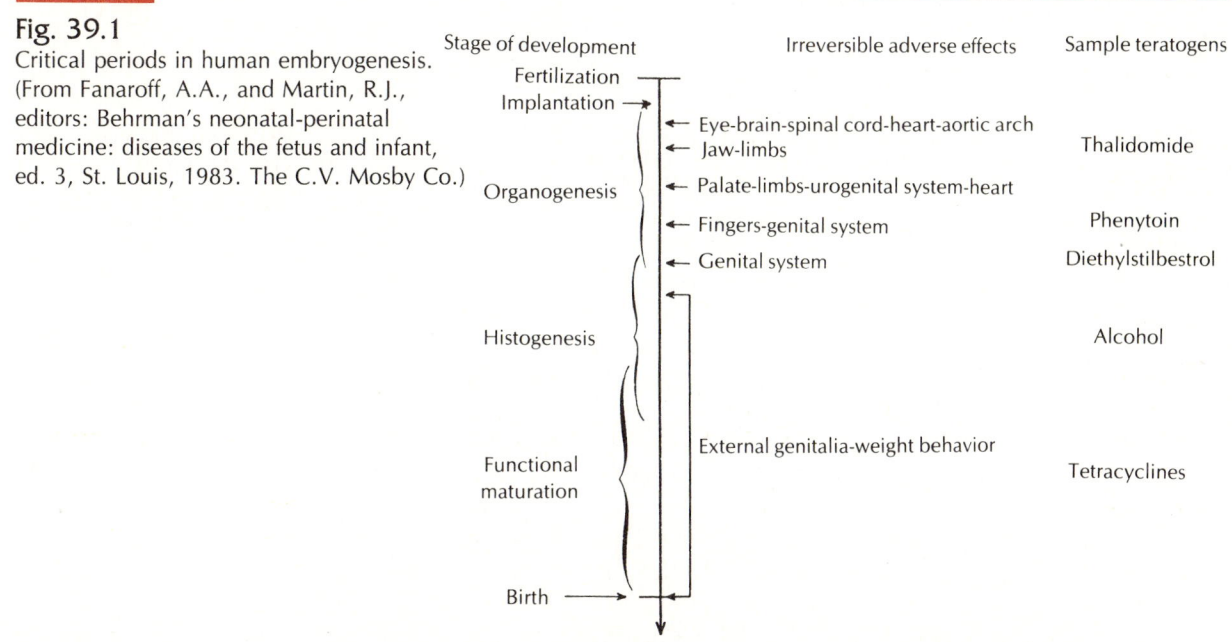

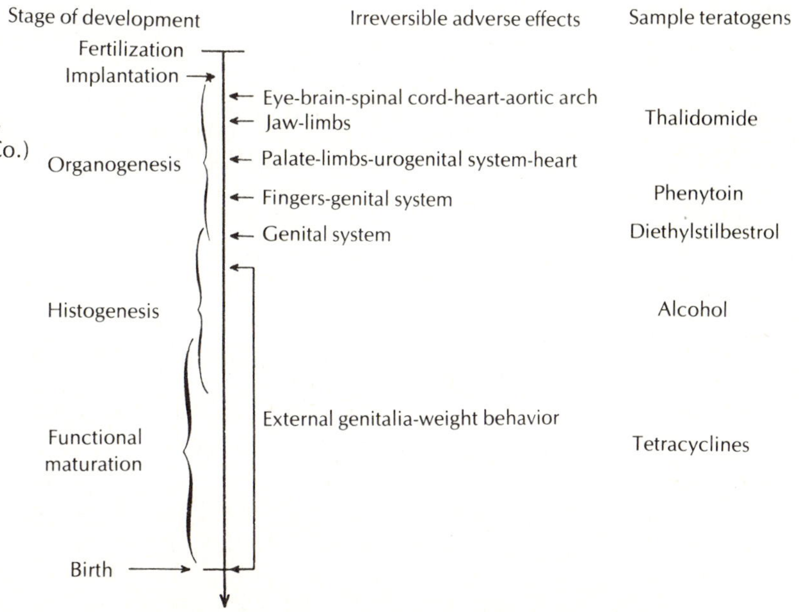

nign problems (e.g., aspirin). It has been shown that 92% to 100% of all obstetric clients took at least one physician-prescribed drug, and 65% to 80% also took self-prescribed drugs. In addition to the therapeutic use of drugs, the nontherapeutic use of drugs, for example, alcohol or narcotics, poses threats to fetal well-being. Critical determinants of the effect of the drug on the fetus include the specific drug, the dosage, the route of administration, the genotype of the mother or fetus, and the timing of the drug exposure. Fig. 39.1 shows critical periods in human embryogenesis and the teratogenic effects of drugs.

FETAL ALCOHOL SYNDROME

Reference to the association between fetal malformation and maternal alcoholism can be found in Greek and Roman mythology. Laws in Carthage and Sparta forbade consumption of alcohol by couples on their wedding night to prevent the conception of children with defects. Documentation of the fetal alcohol syndrome (FAS) can be found in the literature since the early part of the eighteenth century.

Predictable patterns of fetal and neonatal dysmorphogenesis are attributed to severe, chronic alcoholism in women who continue to drink heavily during pregnancy. The pattern of growth deficiency begun in prenatal life persists after delivery, especially in the linear growth rate, rate of weight gain, and growth of head circumferences.

Ocular structural anomalies, such as short palpebral fissures, ptosis, strabismus, and occasionally microphthalmia, are frequent findings (Fig. 39.2). Limb anomalies, such as altered palmar creases and joint dis-

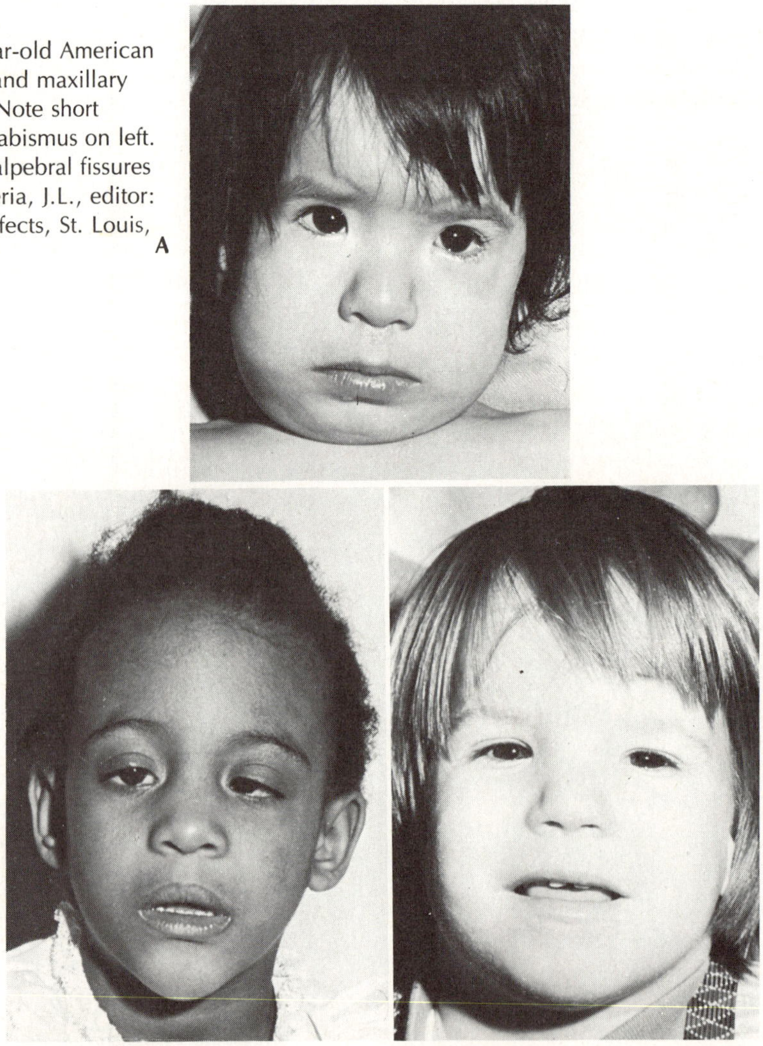

A

B

C

Fig. 39.2
Fetal alcohol syndrome (FAS). **A,** One-year-old American Indian girl. Note short palpebral fissures and maxillary hypoplasia. **B,** Three-year-old black girl. Note short palpebral fissures, bilateral ptosis, and strabismus on left. **C,** Two-year-old white boy. Note short palpebral fissures and maxillary hypoplasia. (From Rementeria, J.L., editor: Drug abuse in pregnancy and neonatal effects, St. Louis, 1977, The C.V. Mosby Co.)

orders, a variety of cardiocirculatory anomalies, especially ventricular septal defects, mental retardation (IQ of 79 or below at 7 years of age), and fine motor dysfunction (poor hand-to-mouth coordination, weak grasp) add to the handicapping problems that maternal alcoholism can impose. Genital abnormalities are seen in daughters of alcoholic mothers. Two thirds of neonates with fetal alcohol syndrome are girls; the cause of this altered sex birth ratio is unknown.

Severe and chronic alcoholism (ethanol toxicity), not maternal malnutrition, is responsible for the severity and consistency of postdelivery performance problems (e.g., growth deficiency, mental retardation, fine motor dysfunction). Regardless of maternal nutritional status, high alcohol levels are lethal to the developing embryo; lower levels cause brain and other malformations. Long-term prognosis (no studies are available as yet) is discouraging even in an optimal psychosocial environment, when one considers the combination of growth failure and mental retardation.

NARCOTIC DRUG DEPENDENCE

Drug abuse implicates many preparations, including alcohol. However, the morphine derivatives or synthetic opium derivatives are the most serious for the newborn whose mother is an addict (Table 39.1). The perinatal mortality of these neonates is six to eight

Table 39.1
Nursing Care of the Addicted Infant

Infant Behavior	Nursing Observations	Nursing Intervention
High-pitched cry	Note onset. Note length of time the cry persists: is it continuous? Is it high pitched and piercing as though infant were in pain? Observe infant for other causes of abnormal crying patterns (meningitis, intracranial bleeding, etc.). Is anterior fontanel full or bulging? Are cranial sutures widely separated? Is head circumference increased? Does infant stare without blinking and exhibit adder's tongue? Is cry aggravated or alleviated when infant is picked up?	Soothe infant by wrapping him tightly in blanket (swaddling), holding him tightly and close to one's body, or both. Decrease feeding intervals or implement a demand-feeding schedule. Reduce environmental stimuli.
Inability to sleep	Note how long infant sleeps after feeding. Note general sleep and wake patterns. If drug therapy has been initiated, note changes in sleep patterns, ability to rest, and whether there is decreased activity, which may indicate drug overdose.	Decrease environmental stimuli. Swaddle. Feed small amounts at frequent intervals.
Frantic sucking of fists	Note onset and amount of sucking. Observe for blisters on fingertips and knuckles. If blistering occurs, observe sites for signs of infection.	Use infant shirts with sewn-in sleeves for mitts to prevent skin trauma. Keep skin area clean; use aseptic technique.
Yawning	Note onset and frequency.	None
Sneezing	Observe onset and frequency.	Aspirate nasopharynx.
Nasal stuffiness	Note severity of nasal stuffiness and determine whether it hinders feeding; if mucus is excessive, consider possibility of other underlying problems, such as esophageal atresia, tracheoesophageal fistula, and congenital syphilis.	Give frequent nose care. Allow more time for feeding with rest between sucking. Aspirate trachea if tracheal mucus is increased Check rate and character of respirations frequently.
Poor feeding	Note sucking pattern: is infant uncoordinated in his attempt to suck? Observe for other possible causes of poor feeding (sepsis, hypoglycemia, immaturity, bowel obstruction, pyloric stenosis).	Feed small amounts at close intervals. Maintain fluid and caloric intake required for infant's weight.
Regurgitation Vomiting	Note when regurgitation or vomiting occurs: is there a precipitating factor (medication, handling, manipulation, position, etc.)?	Measure intake and output closely and correlate with infant's general condition, progress, and therapy.

Modified from Finnegan, L.P., and Macnew, B.A.: Am. J. Nurs. **74:**685, 1974. Copyright © 1974, American Journal of Nursing Co. Reprinted with permission.

Continued.

Table 39.1—cont'd
Nursing Care of the Addicted Infant

Infant Behavior	Nursing Observations	Nursing Intervention
Loose stools	Observe for signs of dehydration. Poor skin turgor Sunken anterior fontanel Sunken orbits around eyes Marked weight loss Note time, color, consistency, and quantity of vomit and stool. When stools are loose, estimate amount of water loss with stools. Note whether vomiting is nonforceful or projectile. Observe for electrolyte imbalance.	Offer supplementary fluids if signs of dehydration appear. Weigh frequently if weight loss, vomiting, and diarrhea persist. Maintain IV fluid at prescribed rate. Maintain infant in side-lying position to prevent aspiration of vomit. Give skin care to prevent excoriation of neck folds, buttocks, and perineum.
Tachypnea	Note onset of respiratory heart rate over 60/min. If tachypnea worsens, note heart rate and report if more than 180/min. Note retractions, their severity (mild, moderate, severe), and location (subcostal, intercostal, sternal, suprasternal, supraclavicular). Note presence of nasal flaring. Note infant's color: pallor or cyanosis? If cyanosis is present note location (extremities, circumoral, generalized) and degree (mild, moderate, severe). Observe for other possible underlying pathophysiologic causes (anemia, aspiration pneumonia, congenital heart disease, etc.)	Maintain infant in semi-Fowler's position. Hyperextend head slightly to ensure patent airway. Minimize handling and manipulation. Correlate respiratory rate, heart rate, retractions, and color with infant's progress, general condition, and blood gas levels. If infant is receiving O_2 and is premature, observe color closely, correlate with blood gases, and reduce O_2 if Po_2 exceeds 85-90. Maintain warmth since hypothermia or hyperthermia increases O_2 consumption. Place infant on cardiac-apnea monitor. If apnea occurs, resuscitate
Mottling	Is mottling precipitated or intensified by factors such as handling, hypothermia? Watch closely for apnea.	
Hyperactive Moro's reflex	Is reflex moderately or markedly exaggerated? If drug therapy has been started, note a diminished or absent Moro's reflex. Is there asymmetry of the reflex? Asymmetry may indicate underlying pathophysiology: Erb's paralysis, fractured clavicle, intracranial hemorrhage.	
Hypertonicity	Note degree (mild, moderate, or severe) of increased muscle tone by the following assessments: Attempt to straighten arms and legs and record degree of resistance. Pick up infant by hands and note body rigidity with degree of head lag. (Withdrawing infant often exhibits trunk rigidity and holds his head on a plane with his body for a prolonged time.) Raise infant by arms and let him stand. (Withdrawing neonate exhibits marked leg rigidity and can support his body's weight for considerable periods.) Correlate mother's obstetric history and delivery with infant's condition and observe baby for other pathophysiology: hypocalcemia, hypoglycemia, meningitis, asphyxia neonatorum, and intracranial hemorrhage. Observe for reddened areas over heels, occiput, sacrum, and knees. Observe temperature frequently; increased activity may cause pyrexia.	Change infant's position often, since prolonged or marked rigidity predisposes him to develop pressure areas. Use sheepskin garments and bedding to reduce pressure, pad crib sides, cover hands with mitts. Decrease environmental temperature if infant's temperature goes above 37° C (98.6° F).

Table 39.1—cont'd
Nursing Care of the Addicted Infant

Infant Behavior	Nursing Observations	Nursing Intervention
Tremors Convulsions	Note if tremors occur when infant is disturbed or undisturbed. Note location of tremors Upper extremities Lower extremities Generalized Note whether degree of tremoring is mild, moderate, or severe. Observe skin over nose, elbows, fingers, toes, knees, heels for excoriation. Observe face for scratches. Observe for underlying pathologic conditions under Hypertonicity above. Check temperature often for pyrexia. Observe for seizures. If they occur, note onset, length, origin, body involvement, whether tonic, clonic, or both, eye deviation, and infant's color.	Change position frequently to prevent excoriation. Give frequent skin care (cleansing, ointment, and exposure to air and/or heat lamp). Use sheepskin garments and bedding. Observe excoriations for healing, worsening, infection. If skin is excoriated, apply zinc oxide ointment, karaya powder; expose to air and/or heat lamp. Decrease environmental temperature if infant exhibits pyrexia. If infant convulses, maintain patent airway and prevent self-trauma. If infant is apneic after seizure, begin resuscitation. Decrease environmental stimuli.

times higher than that of a control group. Abortion, premature birth, stillbirth, and neonatal complications are the major reasons.

The nurse is frequently the first to observe the symptoms of drug dependence in the neonate. Typical signs, which are caused by withdrawal rather than narcosis, appear soon after birth or after several hours, depending on the length of maternal addiction, the amount of drug taken, and time of injection before birth. The newborn may be depressed initially.

The nurse's observations serve to assist the physician in differentiation between drug dependence and other conditions: tracheoesophageal fistula, CNS disorder, sepsis, hypoglycemia, and electrolyte imbalance.

The onset of withdrawal signs in the neonate generally begins within 24 hours after birth. The neonate may be jittery and hyperactive. Frequently his cry is shrill and persistent. The infant may yawn or sneeze frequently. The tendon reflexes are increased, but the Moro reflex is decreased. If withdrawal is not treated, the infant may develop fever, vomiting, diarrhea, dehydration, apnea, and convulsions and die.

Therapeutic programs that have been effective include the following:

1. Phenobarbital, 6 mg/kg/24 hr intramuscularly or 2 mg orally four times a day for 3 or 4 days, and then reducing the dose by one third every 2 days but continuing to treat for about 2 weeks
2. Compound tincture of opium (paregoric), 2 to 4 drops/kg orally every 4 to 6 hours initially to as much as 20 to 30 drops/kg orally every 4 to 6 hours, depending on the symptomatology

Methadone should not be given to the newborn, even if the mother is on methadone maintenance, because of possible addiction.

Reports on observations of methadone-dependent neonates indicate that withdrawal symptoms may occur more frequently and be more prolonged than in heroin-dependent neonates; however, most infants are asymptomatic and normal by 10 days of age. Crib death has been linked to methadone dependence. Further study of the short-term and long-term effects of methadone on the neonate and young child is needed.

With treatment, the prognosis for the neonate is good; without treatment, at least one third of infants of narcotics addicts will die.

Drug dependence in the neonate is physiologic, not psychologic, so that there is no predisposition to dependence later in life. However, the psychosocial environment in which the infant is raised may predispose to addiction.

If the infant is to be discharged to the care of his mother, several nursing actions may be employed:

1. Keep mother informed. Involve her with decision making when possible.
2. Involve mother with infant care if she is willing. Promote mother-child attachment.
3. Avoid angry, argumentative encounters with mother. Respond with patience and sympathy.
4. Support mother's positive maternal responses and

feelings, even if she is relinquishing her infant.

5. Involve infant's father if possible.
6. Refer to social worker.

Poverty

The differences in pregnancy outcomes related to socioeconomic class have been well documented for over half a century (Fig. 39.3). Studies have consistently demonstrated a relationship between economic class and maternal and infant morbidity and mortality. These discrepancies have been of major concern to nursing groups as they have attempted to improve the health and well-being of all individuals in society. Researchers have repeatedly identified two recurrent factors that predispose low-income women to poor pregnancy outcomes (Osofsky and Kendall, 1973). The first relates to reproductive experience of the women and the second to the specific obstetric and neonatal complications involved.

REPRODUCTIVE EXPERIENCE

Low-income individuals tend to begin reproducing at an earlier age and to end at a later age than women generally. In addition, they have many pregnancies and these are adversely affected by the close spacing of the gestations. Birch and Gussons (1970) describes this phenomenon as "too young, too old, and too often." Maternal age and parity are implicated in perinatal mortality. As discussed earlier, there is increased risk to the fetus, infant, and mother when the mother is at either extreme of age or parity (see Table 32.1). Prematurity and its complications remain the chief causes in perinatal mortality. Low-income mothers are more likely to give birth to premature infants than are mothers in the population at large.

Fig. 39.3
Poverty influences on pregnancy outcomes. (From Fogel, C.I., and Woods, N.F.: Health care of women, St. Louis, 1983, The C.V. Mosby Co.)

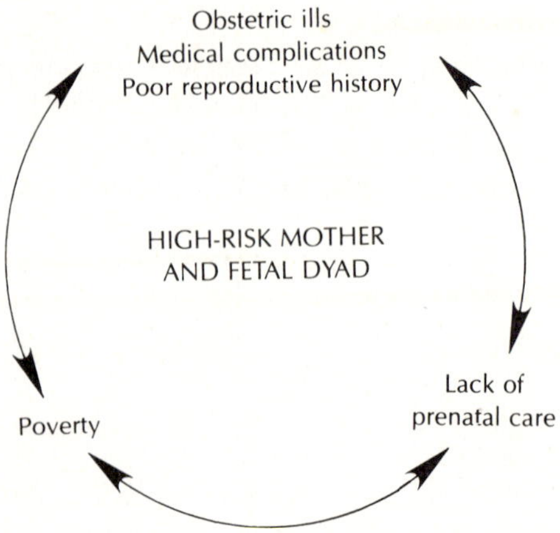

COMPLICATIONS

Low-income mothers are also more predisposed to intercurrent illness and obstetric complications during pregnancy. Obstetric complications such as placenta previa, abruptio placentae, and placental insufficiency often result in preterm births or small-for-dates babies and subsequent infant difficulties. Many obstetric complications have life-threatening consequences for the mother as well as the infant, for example, hemorrhage, cardiac disease, or uncontrolled infection.

The problems faced by low-income mothers have direct implication for nursing service. At present much of our current knowledge could be used to ameliorate or to prevent the occurrence of many of these problems. One of the prerequisites to providing assistance to the low-income mother is to bring her into the health system.

PRENATAL CARE

The vulnerability of economically and socially deprived persons in our society to health problems is apparent across the spectrum of health care from prevention to rehabilitation.

Preventive health is more than the prevention of disease states. It involves those factors in an individual's life that protect the individual and allow for growth and development of potential. Adequate clothing and shelter, proper nutrition, education, a safe environment, all taken for granted by the economically advantaged, are noticeably lacking in the health experience of many low-income groups.

In addition, the concept of preventive health is often missing. The development of a concept of preventive health begins in childhood as the child is directed and encouraged to "eat your dinner and grow up to be a strong boy," "clean your teeth," "go to the doctor for a check-up," and "get enough sleep." These repeated admonitions eventually result in a concept of health care that includes prevention as well as cure. For women who have experienced this indoctrination, acceptance of the necessity for prenatal care comes more readily. For those women who have only gone to a physician when they were very ill, the relative health of the pregnant state precludes full utilization of care available. For some low-income women a choice between prenatal care (preparation for birth) and providing their families with necessities results in their foregoing prenatal care.

A study (Curry, 1983) presently being conducted in Oregon highlights the dilemma facing such individuals. The preliminary reports show the effects of government funding cuts on access to prenatal care for low-income women. Of the 1458 women in the study, 10.2% were not receiving care and 6.3% in their third trimester were without prenatal care.

Preliminary data from another part of the study indicated that of 503 women admitted to the hospital for complications, only 59% had received adequate prenatal care and 16% had received no prenatal care. The study is to be replicated in five eastern states and the District of Columbia by state nurses' associations and the Mid-Atlantic Regional Nursing Association (MARNA).

In some communities clinics have been established specifically for high-risk mothers and their infants. Adolescent mothers and prematurely born infants make up a large part of the client population at these clinics. Although prevention of the problem is probably the best approach, follow-up care is of great importance. Helping mothers to develop parenting skills will do much to promote the optimal growth and development of these disadvantaged children.

Nursing and nursing researchers are in the forefront of efforts to provide care for childbearing families as a fundamental basis for the health of our society.

References and Readings

Postdelivery Psychosis

Carmack, B.J., and Corwin, T.A.: Nursing care of the schizophrenic maternity patient during labor, M.C.N. **5:**107, March-April 1980.

Focusing on today's issues in perinatal care. Postpartum depression (with a commentary by Niles Newton), I.C.E.A. Review **4:**2, Aug. 1980.

Uddenberg, N., and Englesson, I.: Prognosis of postpartum mental disturbance: a prospective study of primiparous women and their 4.5-year-old children, Acta Psychiatr. Scand. **58:**201, 1978.

Drug Dependency

Bartlett, D. and Davis, A.: Recognizing fetal alcohol syndrome in the nursery, J.O.G.N. Nurs. **9**(4):23, 1980.

Bodendorfer, T.W., et al.: Obtaining drug exposure histories during pregnancy, Am. J. Obstet. Gynecol. **135:**490, 1979.

Finnegan, L.P., and Macnew, B.A.: Nursing care of the addicted infant, Am. J. Nurs. **74:**685, 1974.

Fricker, H.S., and Segal, S.: Narcotic addiction, pregnancy, and the newborn, Am. J. Dis. Child. **132:**360, April 1978.

Lindor, E., et al.: Fetal alcohol syndrome, J.O.G.N. Nurse. **9**(4):222, 1980.

Little, R.: Moderate alcohol use during pregnancy and decreased infant birth weight, Am. J. Pub. Health **67:**1154, 1977.

Rementeria, J.: Drug abuse in pregnancy and neonatal effects, St. Louis, 1977, The C.V. Mosby Co.

Robinson, R.: Fetal alcohol syndrome, Dev. Med. Child Neurol. **19:**538, 1977.

Rosett, H., et al.: Therapy of heavy drinking during pregnancy, Obstet. Gynecol. **51:**41, 1978.

Streissguth, A.: Maternal drinking and the outcome of pregnancy, Am. J. Obstet. Gynecol. **47:**422, 1977.

Poverty

Birch, H.G., and Gussons, J.D.: Disadvantaged children: health, nutrition, and failure, New York, 1970, Harcourt Brace & World, Inc.

Curry, M.A. (nurse researcher): Nurses study effects of cuts on access to prenatal care. As reported in Am. Nurs. **15**(3):1, 1983.

Osorsky, H.J., and Kendall, N.: Poverty as a criterion of risk, Clin. Obstet. Gynecol. **16:**103, 1973.

Miscellaneous References

Magil, B.: Cover story—operating on the fetus: the new frontier of perinatology, Contemp. Obstet. Gynecol. **21**(4):216, 1983.

McElroy, M.E., and Fitzmaurice, N.E.: The role of the area genetic nurse in California's newborn screening program, J. Calif. Perinat. Assoc. **11**(1):31, 1982.

Nakayama, D.D., et al.: The prenatal management of a fetus with a correctable congenital defect, J. Calif. Perinat. Assoc. **11**(1):21, 1982.

Swartz, J., and Schwartz, L.: Vulnerable infants, New York, 1977, McGraw-Hill Book Co.

40

Neonates with Hyperbilirubinemia and Congenital Disorders

- **Hyperbilirubinemia**
  - Definitions
  - Kernicterus
    - Pathosis
    - Symptomatology
  - Summary of nursing actions: hyperbilirubinemia
    - Goals of care
    - Example of nursing diagnosis
    - Evaluation
  - Isoimmune hemolytic disease of the newborn (erythroblastosis fetalis, Rh or ABO incompatibility)
    - RBC antigenicity
    - Rh incompatibility
  - Therapy for hyperbilirubinemia
    - Exchange transfusion
    - Intrauterine fetal transfusion
    - Umbilical catheterization
- **Congenital Anomalies**
  - Assessment of perinatal signs and factors
    - Amount of amniotic fluid
    - Respiratory tract
    - Neurologic system
    - Cardiovascular system
    - Gastrointestinal tract
    - Urogenital tract
  - General preoperative and postoperative care
  - Most common surgical emergencies
    - Diaphragmatic hernia
    - Tracheoesophageal anomalies
    - Omphalocele
    - Intestinal obstruction
    - Imperforate anus
  - Common malformations
    - Meningomyelocele
    - Congenital hydrocephalus
    - Anencephaly and microcephaly
    - Cleft-lip or palate
    - Musculoskeletal problems
    - Genitourinary tract anomalies
    - Teratoma
  - Disorders not apparent at birth
    - Diethylstilbestrol

Most infants move from intrauterine to extrauterine life with little difficulty. For some, however, birth is complicated by many factors, and survival is jeopardized. These high-risk infants' survival and well-being depend on advanced and often aggressive nursing and medical management and a suitably controlled environment. The parents of the high-risk infant may experience feelings of lowered self-esteem and self-worth and alienation from the infant. Thus the nurse plays a vital role in the care of both the high-risk newborn and his parents. In this chapter, hyperbilirubinemia and congenital anomalies are discussed.

Hyperbilirubinemia

DEFINITIONS

Elevated serum levels, especially of unconjugated (indirect) bilirubin, pose a grave danger to the neonate. Physiologic hyperbilirubinemia may become pathologic and require diagnostic tests and vigorous treatment.

Physiologic hyperbilirubinemia is characterized by a progressive increase in serum levels of unconjugated bilirubin from 2 mg/dl in cord blood to a mean peak of 6 mg/dl by 72 hours of age, followed by a decline to 5 mg/dl by day 5, and not exceeding 12 mg/dl. These serum values are within the normal physiologic limitations of the healthy term neonate who was not exposed to perinatal complications (e.g., hypoxia). No bilirubin toxicity develops (see Chapters 27 to 29).

Pathologic hyperbilirubinemia cannot be defined solely in terms of serum concentrations of unconjugated bilirubin. Pathologic hyperbilirubinemia refers to that level of serum bilirubin at which a particular neonate will sustain lesions in the brain tissue (kernicterus), renal tubular cells, intestinal mucosa, and pancreatic cells. Hyperbilirubinemia may result from any of the following factors:

1. Physiologic limitations of the newborn such as prematurity and low birth weight
2. Presence of conditions associated with increased red blood cell (RBC) destruction such as Rh_o, ABO, or other RBC-antigen incompatibility or neonatal sepsis
3. Maternal diabetes mellitus
4. Superimposed perinatal risk factors such as hypoxia, asphyxia, acidosis, hypothermia, or hypoglycemia

KERNICTERUS

Kernicterus refers to bilirubin encephalopathy that results from the deposit of bilirubin, especially within the brain stem and basal ganglia. The yellow staining (jaundice of the brain tissue) results from unconjugated bilirubin, which is readily capable of crossing the blood-brain barrier because of its high lipid solubility. Kernicterus may occur in certain newborns with no apparent clinical jaundice.

Pathosis. Staining and necrosis of neurons in the basal ganglia hippocampal cortex, and subthalamic nuclei result from the deposit of unconjugated bilirubin. Usually the cerebral cortex is not involved. Pathogenesis is complex and poorly understood. Only one sequela in survivors is specific: choreoathetoid cerebral palsy. Other sequelae, such as mental retardation and serious sensory disabilities, may reflect hypoxic, vascular, or infectious injury that is often associated with kernicterus. About 70% of newborns who develop kernicterus die in the neonatal period.

The perinatal events that enhance the development of hyperbilirubinemia also incease the likelihood that kernicterus will develop, perhaps even in the presence of

Hyperbilirubinemia

Assessment/analysis

1. Review prenatal chart and intranatal record for presence of risk factors.
2. Assess for hyperbilirubinemia:
   a. If any predisposing factors are present, check to see that cord blood has been sent to laboratory for blood type, Rh, hemoglobin, hematocrit, Coombs' test, or other values appropriate for that neonate. Obtain daily hemoglobin and hematocrit values until a stable state has been reached. Record results.
   b. Note appearance of jaundice during first 24 hours; and note degree of jaundice. Test for jaundice, preferably in daylight, because there is possible distortion of color from artificial lighting, reflection from nursery walls, and the like. (See also integument entry in Table 28.3.)
      (1) Blanch area over bony area (forehead) with thumb. Skin will look yellow before area is perfused again.
      (2) Check conjunctival sacs and buccal mucosa in darker-skinned infants.
   c. Note infant's behavior:
      (1) Changes in feeding and sleeping patterns
      (2) Color and consistency of stools; dark, concentrated urine
      (3) Pallor
      (4) Neurologic signs of kernicterus

Plan/implementation

1. Prevent occurrence of perinatal risk factors.
2. Prevent infection.
3. Provide early feedings.
4. Record and report jaundice immediately for prompt diagnosis and initiation of treatment.
5. Maintain phototherapy.
6. Assist with exchange transfusion.
7. Support parents.
   a. Keep parents informed.
   b. Reinforce explanations of physiologic and pathologic hyperbilirubinemia. Explain need for adequate fluid intake for neonate (e.g., offer water between feedings).
   c. Reinforce physician's explanations regarding disease, its treatment, infant's condition, and possible prognosis.
   d. Especially if mother is discharged with infant soon after delivery, teach her how to identify jaundice and when to call physician.
   e. Involve parents with infant's care when possible.

mild to moderate unconjugated hyperbilirubinemia. These perinatal events include hypoxia, asphyxia, acidosis, hypothermia, hypoglycemia, bacterial infection, certain medications, and hypoalbuminemia. These conditions interfere with conjugation or compete for albumin-binding sites.

Symptomatology. Clinical manifestations of kernicterus commonly first appear between 2 and 6 days after birth; kernicterus is never present at birth. Symptomatology changes as the disease process progresses. Four phases are recognized:

1. Phase one: the neonate is hypotonic and lethargic and exhibits a poor sucking reflex and depressed or absent Moro's reflex (some infants die during this phase).
2. Phase two: the neonate develops spasticity and hyperreflexia, often becomes opisthotonic, has a high-pitched cry, and may be hyperthermic. The neonate may convulse.
3. Phase three: at about 7 days of age, the neonate's spasticity lessens and may disappear.
4. Phase four: after the first month of life, the infant develops late sequelae (e.g., spasticity, athetosis, partial or complete deafness, or mental retardation).

SUMMARY OF NURSING ACTIONS: HYPERBILIRUBINEMIA

Goals of care

1. Hyperbilirubinemia and its sequela, kernicterus, are absent.
2. There are minimal or no sequelae from hyperbilirubinemia and its treatment.
3. Parents understand neonate's condition, therapies, and possible sequelae.

Example of nursing diagnosis. The following is a possible nursing diagnosis: Risk of neurologic damage from hyperbilirubinemia caused by hypoglycemia.

Evaluation. The nurse can be assured that care was effective if the goals for care were met.

ISOIMMUNE HEMOLYTIC DISEASE OF THE NEWBORN (ERYTHROBLASTOSIS FETALIS, RH OR ABO INCOMPATIBILITY)

RBC antigenicity. Isoimmune hemolytic disease of the newborn, or erythoblastosis fetalis, is a disorder of the blood and blood-forming organs of the fetus and neonate characterized by hemolytic anemia and hyperbilirubinemia. A transfer of RBC-destroying antibodies from the mother to her fetus causes erythroblastosis. Once the mother is sensitized, increasingly serious disease tends to develop in subsequent children who have a blood type or group that differs from hers.

ABO incompatibility. Fetal-maternal incompatibility of either ABO groups or the D factor of the Rh group may cause hemolytic disease. The blood type of a person who has RBCs without either the A antigen or the B antigen is designated as group O. Blood of group O individuals contains anti-A and anti-B antibodies. Therefore the group O mother who is carrying a fetus whose blood group is A, B, or AB has anti-A and anti-B antibodies that are transferred across the placenta to her fetus. In this situation even the firstborn infant may be affected.

Because fetal RBCs of groups A, B, or AB are not strongly antigenic, the maternal immune system is not stimulated to produce larger amounts of antibodies against the A and the B factors. The largest percentage of affected infants with ABO incompatibility occurs with a mother of blood group O and an infant of blood type A_1. (Type A_1 has greater antigenicity than types A_2, A_3, or B.)

Although similar to Rh disease, the clinical manifestations of fetal-maternal ABO incompatibility are generally milder and of shorter duration. However, severe hemolysis, jaundice, and kernicterus are possible.

Other RBC antigen incompatibilities. Other, less common red blood cell antigens also capable of transplacental isoimmunization include Kell, Duffy, and Kidd. Fortunately, serious fetal damage from these factors is unlikely.

Rh incompatibility. The more severe forms of isoimmune hemolytic disease result from Rh_oD^u group incompatibility. This form of hemolytic disease of the newborn occurred in 0.5% to 1% of all mature pregnancies in North America before prophylactic Rh_o(D) human immune globulin (RhoGAM) became available in the mid-1960s. Many children died or were seriously affected. Since immunization against this antigen began, however, the incidence of severe erythroblastosis has been drastically reduced.

Discovery of the Rh factor. During antibody studies in the 1940s, it was observed that the injection of RBCs of rhesus monkeys into rabbits caused the production of an antiserum that agglutinated the RBCs of these monkeys and of most humans as well. Consequently RBCs that could be agglutinated by this specific antiserum possessed the rhesus (Rh) antigen and were called *Rh positive,* whereas those that did not possess the Rh factor (antigen) could not be agglutinated and were called *Rh negative*. Subsequently it was discovered that the Rh factor is not a single antigen but a complex blood system with a number of variants.

Six common Rh (rhesus) antigens are identified as follows: C, D, E, c, d, e. Antibody formation results from the presence of one or more of these (and other less common) antigens. Because two chromosomes are present in every cell, one derived from each parent, the genetic constitution of an individual with reference to these antigens might be, for example, DD, dd, or Dd.

Different combinations allow eight Rh genotypes, each with a single Rh chromosome (e.g., CDE, cde, cDE). Actually, 36 different combinations (genotypes) are possible. The order of antigenicity potency of these antigens is D, C, E, c, e, and d.

Discovery of Rh isoimmunization. Soon after the Rh factor was reported, it was found that erythroblastosis fetalis, hydrops fetalis, and icterus gravis—variations of hemolytic disease of the newborn—were caused by the hemolysis of fetal RBCs by maternal antibodies. Later studies showed that slightly more than 90% of cases of clinically evident hemolytic disease of the newborn followed sensitization or isoimmunization of an Rh-negative woman by the presence of the Rh factor in the RBCs of her fetus inherited from an Rh-positive father. Also maternal isoimmunization (or sensitization) can result from a transfusion with Rh-positive blood.

Identification of population at risk. Between 10% and 15% of marriages of white persons will involve Rh-incompatible partners. About 5% of black couples will be Rh incompatible, but it is rare that an Oriental couple will be similarly affected.

Not all Rh-positive men are homozygous for the Rh factor, nor will all children of Rh-positive men married to Rh-negative women be Rh positive. About 50% of the progeny of Rh-positive men who are heterozygous will be Rh positive; the remainder will be Rh negative. Actually, approximately 65% of newborns of Rh-incompatible marriages are Rh positive.

The risk of maternal sensitization is less than expected; some women have a greater antigenic (immune) response to the Rh factor. In the first pregnancy only 0.1% of mothers will be sensitized. In the second and third pregnancies 11% will be affected, and 15% in the fourth or subsequent Rh-positive pregnancies will be affected. About 5% of Rh-incompatible matings produce affected infants.

Pathogenesis of hemolytic disease. Hemolytic disease of the newborn develops according to the following sequence (Fig. 40.1):

1. Isoimmunization of an Rh-negative woman (by the administration of Rh-positive blood or Rh-positive fetal RBCs) stimulates the production of anti-Rh antibodies.

2. Transplacental passage of the woman's anti-Rh antibodies to her fetus causes hemolysis of its RBCs together with other abnormal processes in utero and in neonatal life.

Sensitization during pregnancy. Sensitization of an

Fig. 40.1
Rh isoimmunization. **A,** Rh-negative woman before pregnancy. **B,** Pregnancy with Rh-positive fetus. Some Rh-positive blood passes into mother's blood. **C,** During separation of placenta, a massive inoculation of mother by Rh-positive red blood cells occurs. **D,** Approximately 72 hours after delivery, mother becomes sensitized to Rh-positive blood and develops anti–Rh-positive antibodies, shown as darkened squares. She now has titer, or positive Coombs test. **E,** During subsequent pregnancy with Rh-positive fetus, maternal anti–Rh-positive antibodies enter fetal circulation, attach to fetal Rh-positive red blood cells, and subject them to hemolysis.

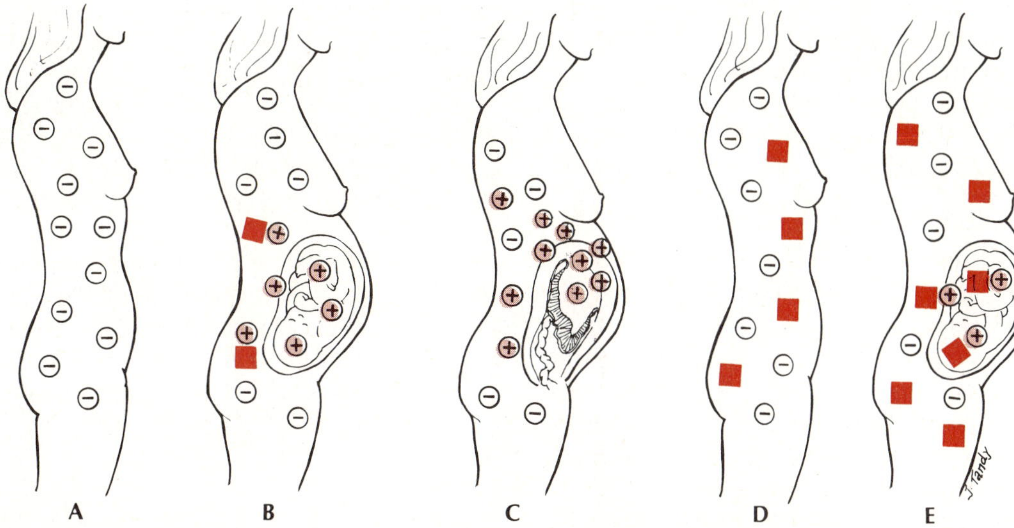

Rh-negative woman must precede intrauterine transfer of antibodies and fetal damage. Hematopoiesis (formation and development of blood cells) begins in the live embryo during the sixth week after conception (i.e., during the eighth week after the last menstrual period [LMP]). Therefore a woman who has experienced one or more abortions 2 months or more since her LMP or has given birth has received fetal transfusions generally at the time of placental separation.

Sensitization following blood transfusion. Sensitization of the mother occurs promptly after an incompatible blood transfusion (improperly typed [Rh-positive] blood) or after one or more pregnancies in which fetal erythrocytes have escaped into the maternal circulation.

Effects of sensitization on subsequent pregnancies. The placenta of the seriously affected fetus is larger than normal. Increased villous size, persistence of Langerhans' cells, and foci of erythropoiesis are apparent. Frequently the amniotic fluid is yellowish, that is, pigment stained (from the decomposition of bilirubin).

Severe Rh incompatibility results in marked fetal hemolytic anemia with erythroid hyperplasia of bone marrow and extramedullary (e.g., spleen) hematopoiesis. The placenta clears the released blood pigments fairly well, however, so that only in extreme cases (e.g., icterus gravis) is the fetus icteric (yellow, or jaundiced). The marked anemia leads to cardiac decompensation, cardiomegaly, hepatomegaly, and splenomegaly. Edema, ascites, and hydrothorax develop. Severe anemia may lead to hypoxia. Intrauterine or early neonatal death may occur.

Once delivery has occurred, the erythroblastotic newborn becomes icteric (in severe cases, within 30 minutes after birth) because it cannot excrete the considerable residue of RBC hemolysis. Yellowish pigmentation of cerebral basal nuclei, hippocampal cortex, and subthalamic nuclei often develops (kernicterus) when the serum bilirubin rises to levels toxic to that neonate, and serious CNS abnormalities may develop and persist (e.g., choreoathetoid cerebral palsy) if the infant survives. The most frequent sequela of kernicterus in the neonatal period is death.

Management

Assessment and analysis

I. Prenatal period
   A. Rh (and ABO) typing should be done early in pregnancy.
   B. Hemantigen test. The diagnosis of hemolytic disease of the newborn of the woman sensitized to the Rh_o(D) or other blood factors is likely when a Hemantigen test or its equivalent (cell pool containing antigens), done on maternal serum at about midpregnancy, is positive. If the test is negative initially, it should be repeated at 32 to 36 weeks.
   C. *Indirect* Coombs' test. In this test the *maternal blood* serum is mixed with RH_o-positive RBCs. The test is positive (e.g., maternal antibodies are present) if Rh_o-positive RBCs agglutinate (clump). The dilution of the specimen of blood at which clumping occurs (if it does occur) determines the titer (level of maternal antibodies). The titer determines the degree of maternal sensitization (isoimmunization). If the titer reaches 1:16, an amniocentesis for ΔOD analysis is performed after the twenty-sixth week of gestation.
   D. Delta optical density (ΔOD) analysis (Fig. 40.2). This test determines the amount of bilirubin in amniotic fluid.

II. Neonatal period
   A. Prenatal history
      1. Blood typing reveals Rh-negative mother.
      2. Maternal history reveals condition that could lead to sensitization in the mother (e.g., previous pregnancies that persisted beyond 8 weeks of gestation, blood transfusions).
   B. Postdelivery physical assessment
      1. Yellow-stained vernix or cord.
      2. Edema (hydrops fetalis), pleural and pericardial effusions, and ascites, all of which indicate cardiac failure (many of these neonates are stillborn).
      3. Placental enlargement. There is an alteration of the average ratio of placental to fetal weight at term. The weight of the placenta is generally one sixth that of the fetus. With hemolytic disease of the newborn, the placenta may weigh as much as one half to three fourths the neonate's weight.
      4. Hepatosplenomegaly.
      5. Cord blood studies.
         a. Blood typing reveals an Rh-positive neonate. (Occasionally an Rh-positive infant is wrongly typed as Rh-negative because of so-called blocking antibodies covering his RBCs.)
         b. Positive *direct* Coombs' test is performed with *neonatal cord blood*. The neonate's RBCs are "washed" and mixed with Coombs' serum. The test is positive (e.g., maternal antibodies are present) if the neonate's RBCs agglutinate (clump). The dilution of the specimen of blood at which clumping occurs (if it does occur) determines the titer of maternal antibodies in fetal serum. The titer determines the degree

Fig. 40.2

Transabdominal amniocentesis: spectrophotometric analysis of amniotic fluid surrounding erythroblastotic fetus. Amniocentesis was performed at 31½ and 32½ weeks. Spectral absorption curve was obtained by plotting optical densities at various wavelengths on two-cycle semilogarithmic graph paper. Tangential line joining lowest portions of this curve approximates unstained amniotic fluid and is baseline for calculations. Difference between involved and uninvolved curves is measured at 450 nm. (Maximum absorption by bilirubin or bilirubin-like products occurs at 450 nm.) This difference is plotted at appropriate number of weeks of gestation *(dotted line)*. Case illustrated shows rapid progression from moderate to severe disease. Under such conditions fetal death is often imminent. Prompt delivery usually must be accomplished if gestational age will permit; otherwise, intrauterine fetal transfusion may be considered. (From Babson, S.G., Pernoll, M.L., and Benda, G.I.: Diagnosis and management of the fetus at risk: a guide for team care, ed. 4, St. Louis, 1980, The C.V. Mosby Co.)

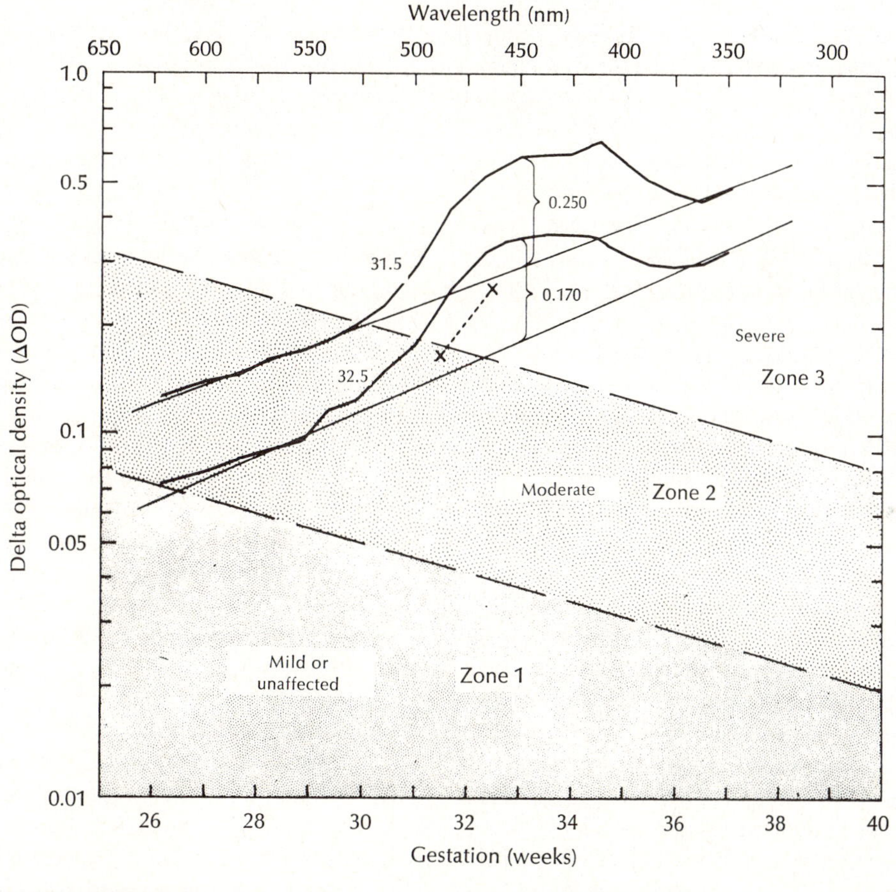

of maternal sensitization. If the titer is 1:64, and exchange transfusion is performed.

c. Hemolytic anemia of a progressive type is present, with increased erythropoiesis (many nucleated RBCs are seen).
d. Hypoglycemia may be present.
e. Indirect or occasionally direct serum bilirubin is present.
f. There is a reduced capacity for albumin binding of bilirubin.

6. There is neonatal pallor with jaundice, generally appearing during the first 24 to 36 hours after birth.
7. There are CNS signs if kernicterus develops.

Plan and implementation. For management of *pathologic hyperbilirubinemia,* see the discussion presented earlier in this chapter.

Prophylaxis for Rh isoimmunization involves the use of Rh immune globulin as a preventive measure against Rh isoimmunization. It is not a treatment for women who are already sensitized, because it has no effect against antibodies already present in the maternal bloodstream. $Rh_o(D)$ immune globulin provides **passive immunity,** which is transient and therefore will not affect a subsequent pregnancy. $Rh_0(D)$ immune globulin (RhIG) prepares RBCs containing the Rh antigen for lysis by phagocytes, before the recipient's immune system is activated to produce antibodies (develops **active immunity**). Antibodies formed by an active immune response remain within the individual's bloodstream, presumably for life. RhIG given to an $Rh_o(D)$-negative woman who is already sensitized would accomplish no purpose. Therefore it is recommended only for nonsensitized Rh-negative women at risk of developing Rh isoimmunization.

Given to any Rh-positive person, an injection of RhIG would result in hemolysis of the RBCs.

The United States Public Health Service recommendations are as follows:

1. Rh immunoglobulin (RhIG) is given only to a woman after delivery or abortion who is $Rh_o(D)$ negative and D^u (allelomorph variant) negative and whose fetus is $Rh_o(D)$ positive or D^u positive. It is *never* given to an infant or father.

2. RhIG is not useful in a woman who has Rh antibodies.

3. RhIG should be given intramuscularly, not into fatty tissue or intravenously.

Prevention of isoimmunization of an Rh-negative woman to the Rh factor in her fetus is now possible in over 95% of cases by RhIG administered within 72 hours of evacuation of the uterus (by abortion or more advanced pregnancy).

Antenatal administration of $Rh_0(D)$ immune globulin (human). Rh sensitization is possible during pregnancy if the cellular layer separating fetal and maternal circulations is disrupted and fetal blood enters the maternal bloodstream. The cellular layer may be disrupted during amniocentesis or by placental abruption. For the woman who is $Rh_0(D)$ negative, D^u negative, and Coombs' negative, RhIG administered during the antenatal period at about 28 weeks gestation and again within 72 hours following delivery can reduce the incidence of maternal isoimmunization further.

Prognosis. In the United States Rh hemolytic disease of the newborn occurs once in approximately 150 to 200 full-term deliveries. At least 200,000 children are affected by Rh isoimmunization each year, of which 5000 are stillborn. If severe hemolytic disease of the newborn is untreated, about 10% of infants will develop kernicterus. With intrauterine (fetal) transfusions, about 40% of these children can be saved despite maternal and fetal hazards of the procedures. Amniocentesis studies, early delivery of affected fetuses, and exchange as well as replacement transfusions save many more.

Complete recovery may be expected in most infants who do not develop kernicterus. If hyperbilirubinemia is treated promptly and effectively, most infants recover without residua or sequelae.

THERAPY FOR HYPERBILIRUBINEMIA

Phototherapy for hyperbilirubinemia is discussed in Chapter 29.

Exchange transfusion. The purposes of exchange transfusion are as follows:

- To reduce serum bilirubin levels.
- To remove red cells that are destined for hemolysis by circulating antibodies
- To correct the anemia
- To remove antibodies (or other causative agents) responsible for hemolysis

The nurse is alert to the fact that a significant risk for morbidity and a mortality risk of 0.1% to 1.0% exist with this procedure. It is time consuming and expensive as well.

An exchange transfusion is accomplished by alternately removing a small amount of the infant's blood and replacing it with a like amount of donor blood. Depending on the infant's size, maturity, and condition, amounts of 5 to 20 ml are slowly exchanged at a time. The total amount of blood exchanged approximates 170 ml/kg of body weight (80 ml/lb) or between 75% and 85% of the infant's total blood volume.

This procedure is done under conditions that prevent cold stress to the infant, as with other procedures. The following equipment is necessary.

1. Disposable exchange transfusion set
2. Fresh donor's blood (under 3 days old and heparinized), two units on hand in case of error or contamination
3. Monitoring equipment
4. Transfusion record
5. Water bath (38° C [100 F]) to warm the blood
6. Medications: **calcium gluconate** in 5 ml syringe with no. 24 needle; 50% glucose solution in 10 ml syringe with no. 24 needle; sodium bicarbonate in 10 ml syringe with no. 24 needle
7. Sterile gowns, drapes, gloves, caps, and masks
8. Cleansing solution with sterile cotton pledgets or gauze sponges
9. Adequate lighting
10. Heat source to keep the infant warm

The exchange transfusion procedure is as follows:

Technique	Rationale
1. Prepare and adjust heat lamps or overhead radiant heat shield; have warmed blankets available for infant.	1. Prevents cold stress.

Technique	Rationale
2. Infant is given nothing orally for 3 or 4 hours, or stomach contents are aspirated by gastric tube.	2. Prevents aspiration.
3. Assemble resuscitative equipment: O_2 source, masks, breathing bag, airways, laryngoscope (extra batteries), endotracheal tube with obturator, suction, medication.	3. Is readily available if needed for immediate supportive therapy.
4. Position infant on back and restrain. Take and record vital signs.	4. Facilitates treatment. Prevents dislodging catheter and tissue trauma. Provides base line to evaluate change.
5. Assemble electronic monitoring equipment or stethoscope. Attach electrodes, or keep stethoscope over apex of heart. Monitor and record results continuously during procedure.	5. Hazards of procedure include apnea, bradycardia (100 beats/min or less), cardiac arrhythmia or arrest.
6. Physician *and* nurse check donor blood: type, Rh, age, and free of sickle cell trait.	6. Minimizes chance of error. Provides donor RBCs that are not affected by maternal antibodies present in the fetal system. Acts as precaution against fatal intravascular sickling.
7. Run tubing from bottle (bag) through warm water bath to infant.	7. Avoids cold stress, ventricular fibrillation, vasospasm, or decrease in blood viscosity.
8. Before starting transfusion, assist physician as necessary.	8. Prevents microbial contamination.
a. Cleanse site of cutdown (jugular or femoral artery) or umbilical stump (umbilical vein).	
b. Drape.	
c. Put on gown and gloves.	
9. During transfusion:	9. During transfusion:
a. Physician measures central venous pressure (CVP) before initiating transfusion.	a. Acts as precaution against heart failure from volume overload. Change from 10 to 12 cm pressure is indication to stop and reassess infant's status.
b. Nurse notes and records time exchange is begun.	b. Maintains accurate record.
c. For *each* successive withdrawl of infant's blood *and* injection of donor's blood, nurse records time, amounts in and out, cumulative amounts in and out.	c. Maintains accurate, continuous record to assist with ongoing procedure and provides index of infant response.
d. After 100 ml has been exchanged, physician gives calcium gluconate; nurse monitors heart and respiratory rates and records them.	d. Possibility of cardiac arrhythmias or arrest is minimized.
e. Nurse records pertinent comments.	e. Maintains accurate record.
f. Nurse records medications: time, type, amount, infant response.	f. Maintains accurate record.
10. After transfusion (catheter may be removed or left in place with dressing):	10. Infant is observed to prevent hemorrhage from site and to detect and treat promptly any complications of blood transfusion such as heart failure, hypocalcemia, acute hypercalcemia, hyperkalemia, hypernatremia, hypoglycemia and acidosis,* sep-
a. Nurse finishes charting.	
b. Nurse continues to observe and record infant's behavior closely for 24 to 48 hours.	

*Red blood cells continue anaerobic glycolysis with production of acid metabolites after removal from donor. Blood stored for longer than 2 days is likely to contain potentially dangerous levels of potassium and to be more readily subjected to hemolysis.

Technique	Rationale
(1) Vital signs: heart rate, respirations, temperatures, pedal pulses (2) Lethargy, jitteriness, convulsions (3) Dark urine (4) Edema	sis, shock thrombus formation, transfusion mismatch reaction.

Intrauterine fetal transfusion. The transfusion is accomplished in the following manner: An ultrasonogram is used to locate the placenta. Then a needle is passed transabdominally into the amniotic sac, and radiopaque dye is injected. The fetus swallows the amniotic fluid. The radiopaque dye in the fetal gastrointestinal tract can be visualized by x-ray film. Then the physician injects packed RBCs directly into the fetal peritoneal cavity. The packed RBCs (about 10 ml) are cross matched with maternal serum, and the type used is Rh_o(D) negative and (usually) group O. The fetus is able to absorb these RBCs into the fetal circulation via the lymphatic vessels and great veins and to utilize them to counteract the anemia; cardiac decompensation is thus forestalled. Results of this procedure are encouraging. Transfusions may be required every 2 weeks until delivery.

Umbilical catheterization. The only valid purpose of umbilical artery catheterization is to obtain blood samples for frequent determinations of blood gases. The umbilical artery catheter is not recommended solely for parenteral fluid therapy or for exchange transfusion. The umbilical vein is the portal of choice for exchange transfusion. It also is not recommended for parenteral fluid therapy except in emergency circumstances. The lengthy indwelling of umbilical venous catheters is associated with a high incidence of infection. This is not apparently true of umbilical artery catheters.

The dangers of umbilical catheterization include the development of emboli, thrombi, and sepsis.

A heat source is necessary to prevent cold stress (e.g., acidosis, apnea). Emergency drugs and oxygen, suction, and resuscitation equipment should be available if needed. It is also necessary to check that all electric equipment is grounded to prevent electric shock or burn to infant.

The technique and rationale are as follows:

Technique	Rationale
Physician	
1. Prepare area; drape neonate.	1. Sterile procedure.
2. Insert catheter into artery; location of catheter confirmed by x-ray film.	2. Placement must be accurate. If in vein, may cause thrombosis and liver damage. Arterial lines may be left in place for up to 2 weeks.
3. Apply organic iodine jelly over area.	3. Prevents infection: redness, edema, drainage, elevated temperature.
Nurse	
1. Monitors vital signs every 10 to 15 minutes until stable, after procedure.	1. Assesses neonatal tolerance of procedure.
2. If bleeding from site occurs, apply direct pressure.	2. Prevents blood loss.
3. Observe color and warmth of legs and peripheral pulses.	3. Catheter may have entered femoral artery, or thrombus may have formed.
4. Maintain patency of line per order (e.g., heparinized solution).*	4. Prevents clogging and emboli.
5. Record. Keep physician informed.	5. Is legal record and facilitates communication among staff. Provides base line to evaluate change.

Congenital Anomalies

Each year 250,000 infants are born with significant structural and functional disorders. The seriousness of this community health problem is reflected in the more than 6 million hospital days and $200 billion a year allocated to the care and treatment of these neonates. Prevention and detection procedures are being improved continuously; methods of promoting the availability of these services to populations at risk challenge the community health care systems. An interdisciplinary team approach is imperative to provide holistic care: surgery, rehabilitation, and education of the child and social, psychologic, and financial assistance to the parents. Parental disappointment and disillusion and the nurse's own negative feelings toward (or stigmatization of) the infant's disorder add to the complexity of nursing care.

When studying and utilizing this content, the student

*In many intensive care units heparinized solution is no longer used to maintain the patency of an umbilical artery catheter. Apparently there is no higher incidence of thrombi or occlusions in the catheter when heparin is omitted. In addition, omission of heparin avoids the danger of (relative) heparinization of the infant.

is asked to keep an open mind. New data are constantly being identified. Some of the appropriate procedures and treatments of the recent past are considered ineffective and even hazardous today. To support the goal of intact survival, therapy must be continuously reviewed and improved in light of advancing progress.

Many congenital anomalies require intervention soon after birth. Careful assessment alerts the medical-nursing team to the infant's need for therapy.

ASSESSMENT OF PERINATAL SIGNS AND FACTORS

Assessment for congenital anomalies begins with a general assessment (see Table 28.3). Any deviations from normal are reported to the physician immediately.

Amount of amniotic fluid. An excessive amount of amniotic fluid, hydramnios, is frequently associated with congenital anomalies in the neonate. The infant should be examined closely at the earliest possible time. In the presence of hydramnios, any of the following may be suspected:

1. Cephalocaudal malformations, such as, hydrocephalus, microcephaly, anencephaly, and spina bifida
2. Orogastrointestinal malformations, such as, cleft palate, esophageal atresia with or without a tracheal fistula, pyloric stenosis, volvulus, and imperforate anus
3. Miscellaneous conditions, such as Down's syndrome, congenital heart disease, deformed extremities, and infants of diabetic or prediabetic mothers
4. Prematurity

Oligohydramnios is primarily associated with those anomalies of the urinary tract that preclude normal micturition in utero. As a rule, renal agenesis or renal dysplasia is involved. Urethral stenosis has also been reported to be associated with oligohydramnios. Anomalies of the earlobes, rather than agenesis of the ear, are sometimes associated with renal abnormalities and are not direct results of oligohydramnios. Potter's syndrome (renal agenesis) is the classic example of an association between oligohydramnios and renal anomalies. It includes a typical facies that involves abnormal earlobes.

Respiratory tract. Screening for congenital anomalies of the respiratory tract is necessary even for the infant who is apparently normal at birth. Respiratory distress (see Chapter 33) at birth or shortly thereafter may be the results of lung immaturity (see Chapter 37) or anomalous development. Congenital laryngeal web and bilateral choanal atresia (Fig. 40.3) are readily apparent at birth. Both require emergency surgery.

Fig. 40.3

Choanal atresia. Posterior nares are obstructed by membrane or bone either bilaterally or unilaterally. Infant becomes cyanotic at rest. With crying, neonate's color improves. Nasal discharge is present. Snorting respirations are often observed with increased respiratory effort. Neonate may be unable to breathe and eat at same time. Diagnosis is made by noting inability to pass small feeding tube through one or both nares. (Courtesy Ross Laboratories, Columbus, Ohio.)

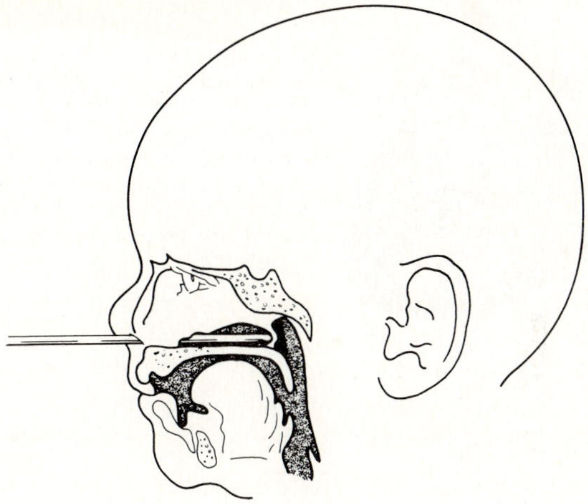

Neurologic system. Neurologic signs may reflect hidden congenital anomalies as well as numerous other conditions. Many neonatal responses are nonspecific. Each sign, such as high-pitched cry, hypotonia, jitteriness, low-set ears, and microcephaly or hydrocephaly, must be evaluated carefully before appropriate therapy can be instituted.

One of the therapeutic contributions the nurse can make is the identification of the neonate who is "just not right," even when there is a negative prenatal history or unreported laboratory or other data. This feeling that something may be wrong is the beginning of the statement of a hypothesis. The nurse thus alerted can mobilize and initiate further diagnostic procedures to institute corrective or palliative therapy.

Cardiovascular system. Severe congenital cardiovascular disorders often are evident immediately after birth, for example, severe cyanotic heart disease (Fig. 40.4). These infants usually are transferred directly to special nurseries or pediatric units. Some problems, such as a small patent ductus arteriosus or a minimal coarctation of the descending aorta, become apparent only as the infant is exposed to stresses such as growth-demands of later infancy and early childhood, or infec-

Fig. 40.4
Congenital heart abnormalities. (Courtesy Ross Laboratories, Columbus, Ohio.)

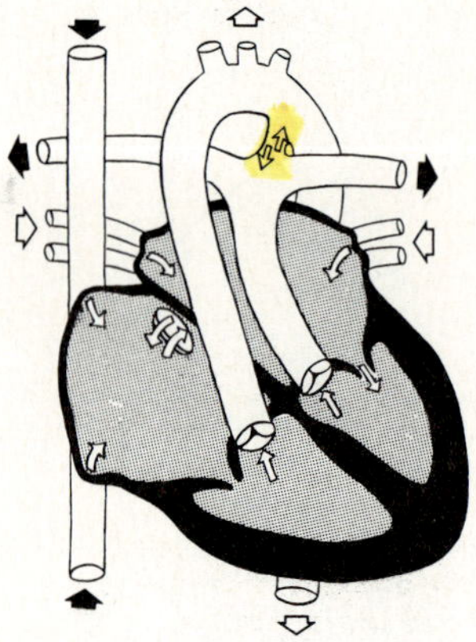

Complete transposition of great vessels

The anomaly is an embryologic defect caused by a straight division of the bulbar trunk without normal spiraling. As a result, the aorta originates from the right ventricle, and the pulmonary artery from the left ventricle. An abnormal communication between the two circulations must be present to sustain life.

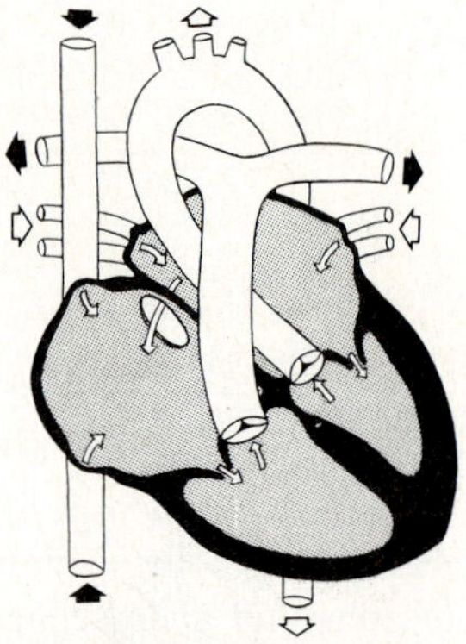

Atrial septal defects

An atrial septal defect is an abnormal opening between the right and left atria. Basically, three types of abnormalities result from incorrect development of the atrial septum. An incompetent foramen ovale is the most common defect. The high ostium secundum defect results from abnormal development of the septum secundum. Improper development of the septum primum produces a basal opening known as an ostium primum defect, frequently involving the atrioventricular valves. In general, left to right shunting of blood occurs in all atrial septal defects.

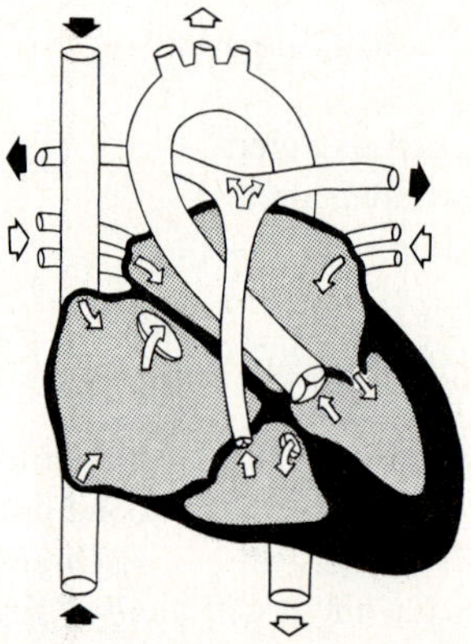

Tricuspid atresia

Tricuspid valvular atresia is characterized by a small right ventricle, large left ventricle, and usually a diminished pulmonary circulation. Blood from the right atrium passes through an atrial septal defect into the left atrium, mixes with oxygenated blood returning from the lungs, flows into the left ventricle, and is propelled into the systemic circulation. The lungs may receive blood through one of three routes: (1) a small ventricular septal defect, (2) patent ductus arteriosus, (3) bronchial vessels.

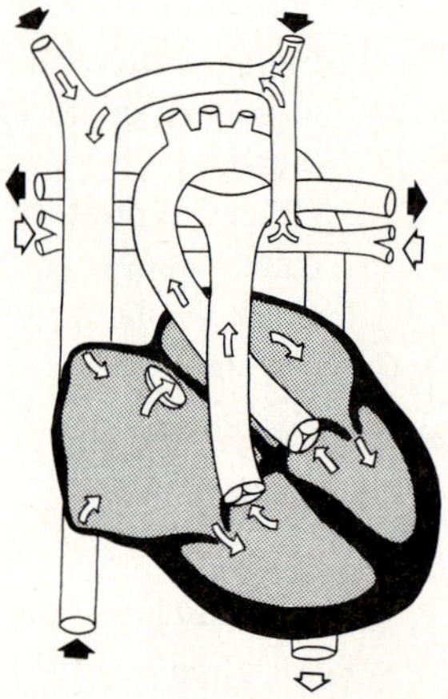

Anomalous venous return

Oxygenated blood returning from the lungs is carried abnormally to the right heart by one or more pulmonary veins emptying directly, or indirectly, through venous channels into the right atrium. Partial anomalous return of the pulmonary veins to the right atrium functions the same as an atrial septal defect. In complete anomalous return of the pulmonary veins, an interatrial communication is necessary for survival.

Continued.

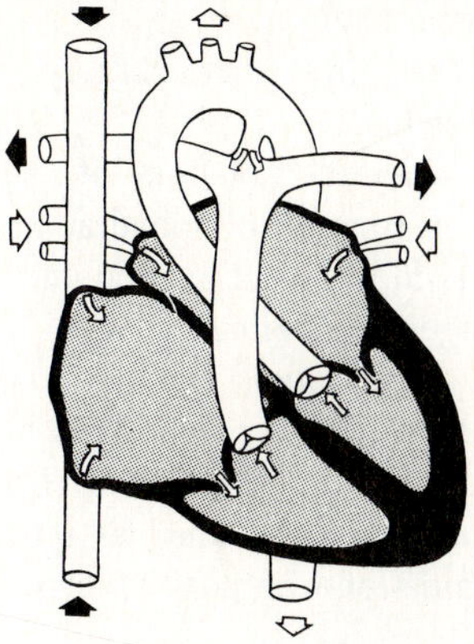

Patent ductus arteriosus

The patent ductus arteriosus is a vascular connection that, during fetal life, short circuits the pulmonary vascular bed and directs blood from the pulmonary artery to the aorta. Functional closure of the ductus normally occurs soon after birth. If the ductus remains patent after birth, the direction of blood flow in the ductus is reversed by the higher pressure in the aorta.

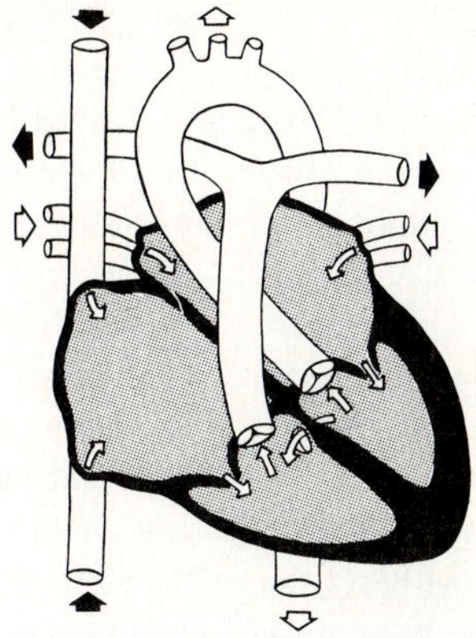

Ventricular septal defects

A ventricular septal defect is an abnormal opening between the right and left ventricle. Ventricular septal defects vary in size and may occur in either the membranous or muscular portion of the ventricular septum. Due to higher pressure in the left ventricle, a shunting of blood from the left to right ventricle occurs during systole. If pulmonary vascular resistance produces pulmonary hypertension, the shunt of blood is then reversed from the right to the left ventricle, with cyanosis resulting.

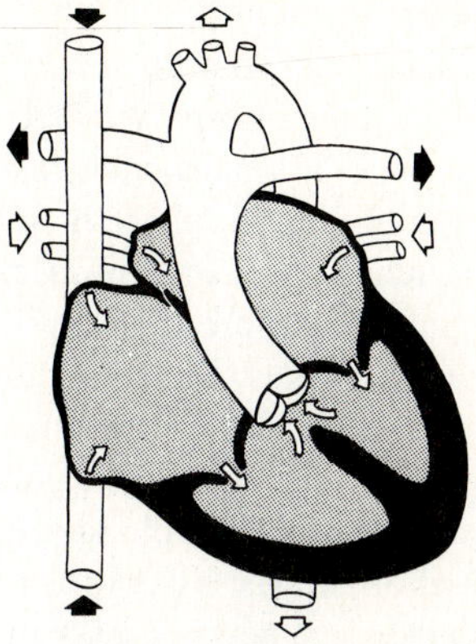

Truncus arteriosus

Truncus arteriosus is a retention of the embryologic bulbar trunk. It results from the failure of normal septation and division of this trunk into an aorta and pulmonary artery. This single arterial trunk overrides the ventricles and receives blood from them through a ventricular septal defect. The entire pulmonary and systemic circulation is supplied from this common arterial trunk.

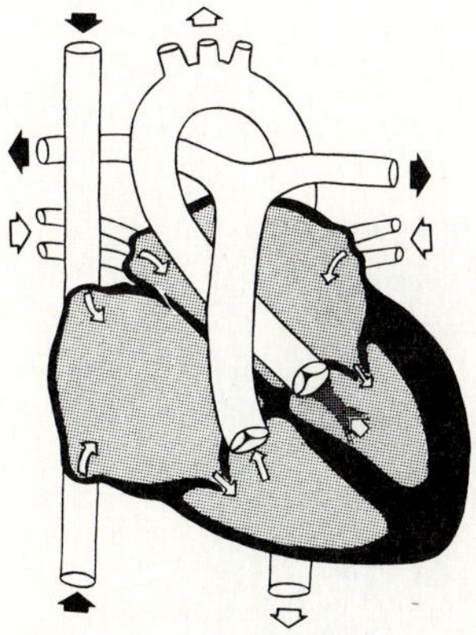

Subaortic stenosis

In many instances, the stenosis is valvular with thickening and fusion of the cusps. Subaortic stenosis is caused by a fibrous ring below the aortic valve in the outflow tract of the left ventricle. At times, both valvular and subaortic stenosis exist in combination. The obstruction presents an increased work load for the normal output of the left ventricular blood and results in left ventricular enlargement.

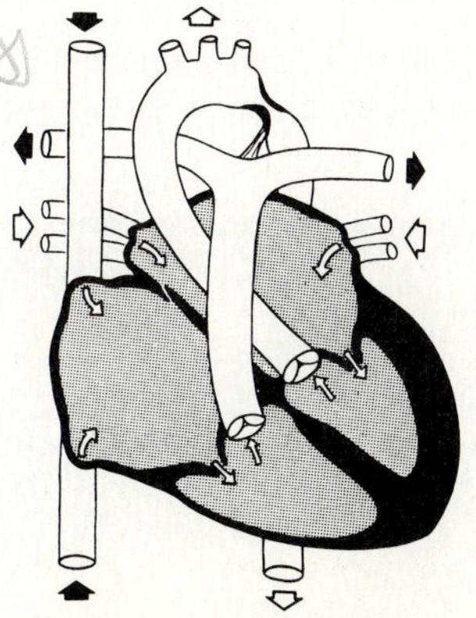

Coarctation of the aorta

Coarctation of the aorta is characterized by a narrowed aortic lumen. It exists as a preductal or postductal obstruction, depending on the position of the obstruction in relation to the ductus arteriosus. Coarctations exist with great variation in anatomic features. The lesion produces an obstruction to the flow of blood through the aorta causing an increased left ventricular pressure and work load.

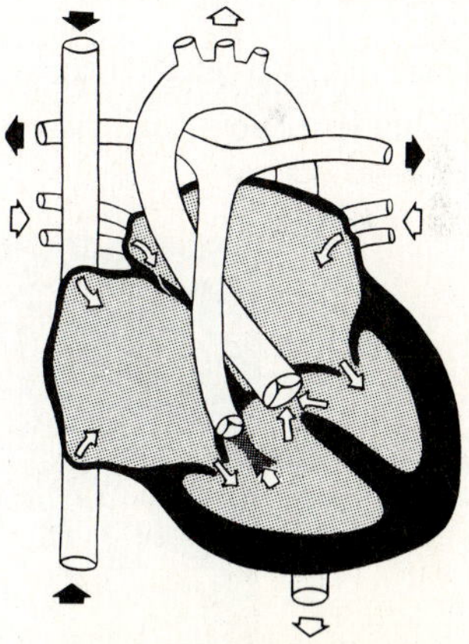

Tetralogy of Fallot

Tetralogy of Fallot is characterized by the combination of four defects: (1) pulmonary stenosis, (2) ventricular septal defect, (3) overriding aorta, (4) hypertrophy of right ventricle. It is the most common defect causing cyanosis in patients surviving beyond two years of age. The severity of symptoms depends on the degree of pulmonary stenosis, the size of the ventricular septal defect, and the degree to which the aorta overrides the septal defect.

tion. In about 75% of cases the cardiovascular anomalies are unexpected.

Cardiovascular defects occur in 3 of every 1000 births; congenital heart disease is implicated in approximately 50% of deaths from malformations during the first year of life. Etiology is still unclear, although a familial tendency is evident in many cases. Coexisting congenital defects are frequent in neonates with cardiovascular anomalies. Maternal disease during pregnancy has been implicated. Symptoms characteristically are first evident after the umbilical cord is severed.

Gastrointestinal tract. Screening for gastrointestinal tract malformations is performed on a routine basis for all infants. Obstruction occurs in about 1 in 3000 newborns. The following findings are reported immediately:

1. A scaphoid (sunken) abdomen usually indicates a diaphragmatic hernia.
2. Inability to pass tube into stomach suggests esophageal atresia (Fig. 40.5).
3. Inability to pass thermometer or failure of meconium passage within the first 24 hours of life suggests imperforate anus (Fig. 40.8) or probable obstruction; with abdominal distention, probable meconium ileus.

The distended abdomen is particularly noteworthy in H-type tracheoesophageal fistula.

These conditions require immediate surgery and are discussed later in this chapter.

Urogenital tract. Careful notation of perinatal events and observations such as oligohydramnios and absence of voiding aids in the identification and confirmation of existing congenital anomalies.

In cases of ambiguous genitalia (Fig. 40.14), there is an urgent association between the parent-child relationship and the identification of the infant's sex. The identity of the neonate must be established as quickly as possible to facilitate initiation of a positive parent-child relationship (see p. 32).

GENERAL PREOPERATIVE AND POSTOPERATIVE CARE

The neonate withstands the stress of surgery surprisingly well, provided it is done as soon after birth as feasible and the facilities available for care are adequately equipped and staffed. The medical-nursing team must be specially trained to anticipate and meet the neo-

Fig. 40.5
Transport incubator. Compartments contain medications and equipment to administer oxygen and to suction. Unit ensures thermoneutral environment. (Courtesy Air-Shields, Inc., Hatboro, Pa.)

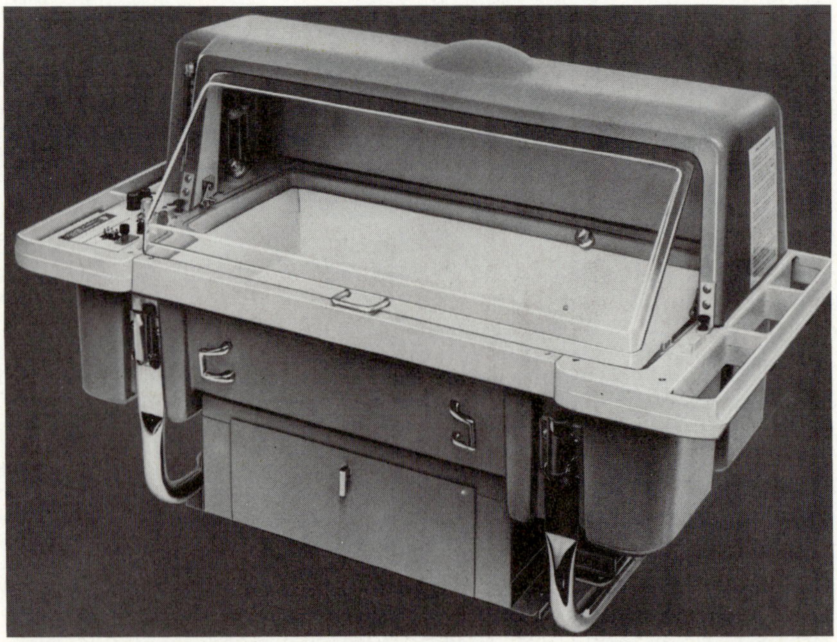

nate's physiologic needs. The surgical team consists of the radiologist, surgeon, anesthesiologist, and nurse. Diagnostic studies are kept to a minimum, and consideration of the neonate's immaturity is kept in mind. For example, air may be used rather than standard radiopaque materials for diagnostic x-ray examinations to reduce the danger of regurgitation and aspiration, and microtechniques are utilized for the necessary blood chemistry studies (e.g., preoperative hemoglobin levels) to minimize blood loss.

The infant is transported to the operating room in an incubator with a self-contained power pack for the continuous provision of warmth (Fig. 40.5) and is accompanied by an intensive care nursery nurse. Preanesthesia preparation includes hydration, administration of preoperative medications, usually minute amounts of atropine, insertion of an endotracheal tube, and gastric emptying.

During the operation, blood loss is constantly monitored, and blood is replaced milliliter by milliliter because the neonate's remarkable ability to maintain blood circulation through vasoconstriction means that vital signs remain unaltered until sudden and complete collapse occurs as the compensatory system is overtaxed. Temperature is maintained by positioning the infant on a thermal mattress and draping suitably.

Once the operation is completed, the infant is returned to the intensive care nursery. The first hour after the procedure is a crucial one, and constant surveillance of recovery from the anesthesia is imperative. Body temperature is maintained between 36.1° and 36.7° C (97° and 98° F); optimal temperature is 36.5° C (97.7° F). An open airway is maintained by means of positioning of the head, suctioning, and use of high humidity. (If the respiratory rate increases, suctioning is indicated.) Oxygen dosage is prescribed on the basis of arterial blood gas values (e.g., Po_2). Fluid-electrolyte balance is monitored, and intravenous replacement is given as ordered. Postural drainage and percussion are ordered as necessary. The infant is turned from side to side to equalize pressure areas. An indwelling gastric catheter attached to intermittent suction removes gastric secretions to prevent their possible aspiration because the cough reflex is inadequate.

MOST COMMON SURGICAL EMERGENCIES

The following five congenital anomalies account for more than 90% of surgical emergencies of the neonate:

1. Diaphragmatic hernia
2. Tracheoesophageal anomalies
3. Omphalocele
4. Intestinal obstruction
5. Imperforate anus

Diaphragmatic hernia. Diaphragmatic hernia is the most urgent of the neonatal emergencies. Incomplete embryonic development of the diaphragm allows herniation of abdominal viscera into the thoracic cavity. The defect and herniation may be minimal and easily reparable or so extensive that the viscera present in the thoracic cavity during embryonic life precluded the normal development of pulmonary tissue. Most cases involve a posterolateral defect, usually on the left. The extent of the defect and the severity and timing of the symptomatology determine the seriousness of the problem.

Signs that are suspicious of extensive diaphragmatic herniation include the following: constant respiratory distress from birth that becomes increasingly severe as bowels fill with air, large or asymmetric chest contour, dullness to percussion on affected side, bowel sounds heard in thoracic cavity, and breath sounds diminished.

Prompt surgical repair is imperative after correction of acidosis, insertion of a nasogastric tube and aspiration, and oxygen therapy.

The prognosis depends largely on the degree of pulmonary development and the success of diaphragmatic closure. Prognosis in severe cases is guarded.

Tracheoesophageal anomalies. Esophageal atresia is an urgent congenital anomaly. Various types are recognized, depending on the presence or absence of an associated tracheoesophageal fistula, the site of the fistula, and the point and degree of esophageal obstruction (Fig. 40.6). The most common variety is associated with moderate hydramnios.

The following signs are suspicious for tracheoesophageal fistula: excessive oral secretions with drooling; progressive respiratory distress as unswallowed secretions spill over into trachea; and feeding intolerance. In feeding intolerance, choking, coughing, and cyanosis follows even a small amount of fluid taken by mouth; there is regurgitation of unaltered formula (unmixed with stomach secretions or bile) soon after first feeding is initiated.

Nursing actions are supportive. In the presence of excesive oral secretions and respiratory distress, *do not feed* infant orally before consulting physician. In the presence of abdominal distention, place neonate in semi-Fowler's position and raise his head 30 degrees or more (infant seat may be used). This position facilitates respiratory efforts and discourages reflux (spillage) of stomach secretions into respiratory tree, with resultant chemical bronchitis and pneumonitis. On physician's order or per standing orders, insert suction tube into blind pouch. Connect to low, intermittent suction.

Immediate surgical correction of the anomaly is mandatory. The prognosis depends on the degree of maturity of the neonate and the presence of a fistula or pneumonia. Cardiac and other gastrointestinal anomalies commonly are associated with esophageal atresia.

Omphalocele. Omphalocele is a herniation noted at birth in which part of the intestine protrudes through a defect in the abdominal wall at the umbilicus (Fig. 40.7). Failure of migration of the midgut in embryonic development probably is responsible for omphalocele. The protruding bowel is covered only by a thin, transparent membrane composed of amnion.

Prompt closure of defects of less than 5 cm in diameter usually is successful. Larger defects may require

Fig. 40.6
Congenital atresia of esophagus and tracheoesophageal fistula. **A,** About 87%. Upper segment of esophagus ends in blind pouch; lower segment connects with trachea by small fistulous tract. **B,** About 8%. Upper and lower segments of esophagus end in blind sac. **C,** About 4%. Esophagus is continuous but connects by fistulous tract to trachea; known as *H-type.* **D,** Less than 1%. Both segments of esophagus connect by fistulous tracts to trachea. Infant may drown with first feeding. **E,** Less than 1%. Upper segment of esophagus ends in atresia and connects to trachea by fistulous tract. Infant may drown with first feeding.

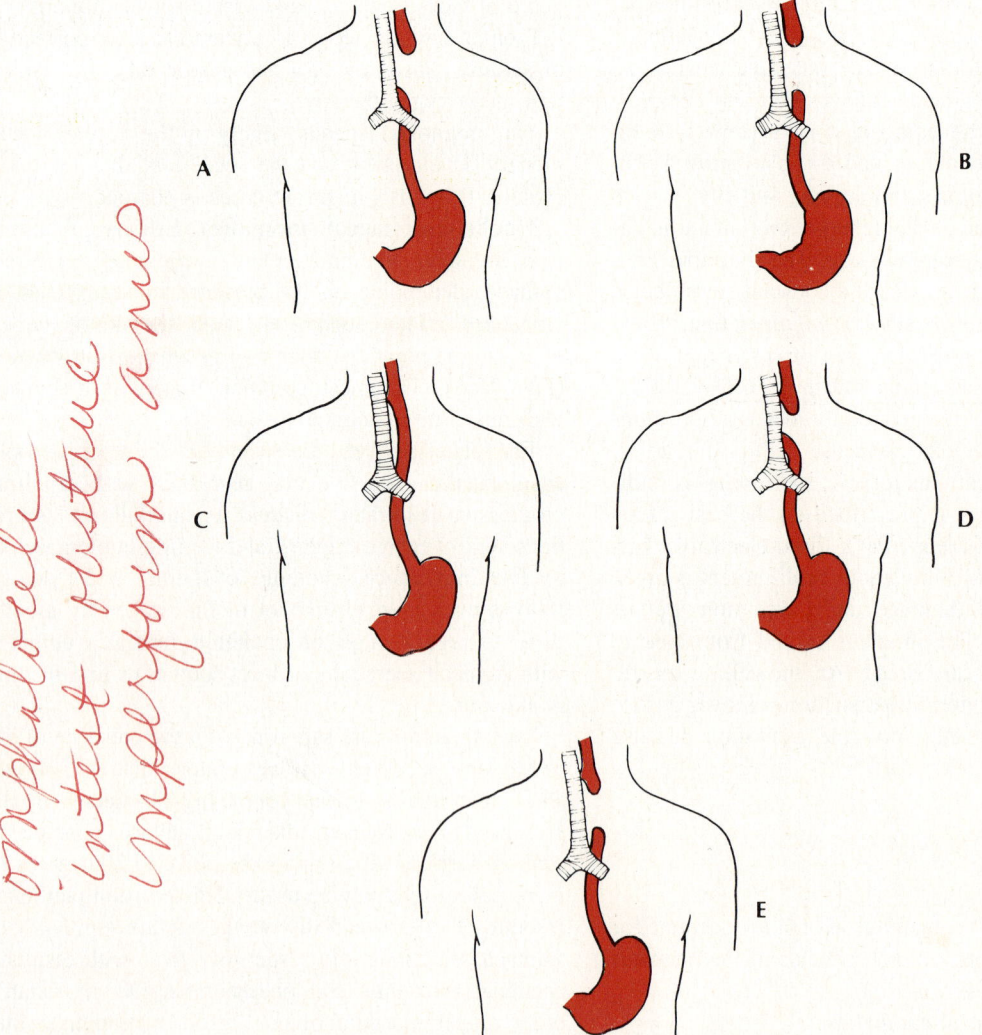

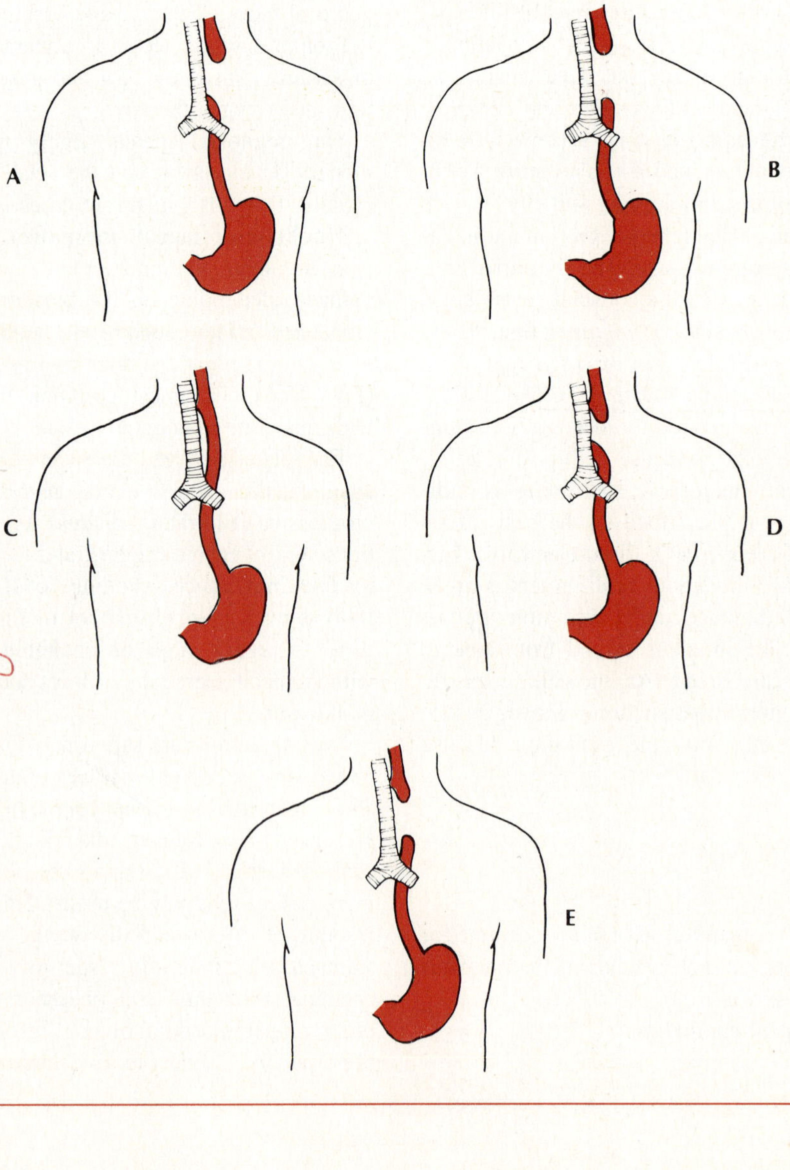

closure in stages. The general prognosis is related to associated anomalies.

There is usually only a short span of time between the neonate's birth and surgical intervention. In addition to the usual preoperative orders, preparation of the infant for surgery includes protecting the defect from infection, rupture, and drying. The physician prescribes that the omphalocele be protected by one of the following:

1. Sterile towels or sponges kept moist with sterile saline solution that has been warmed to body temperature
2. Protective sterile petrolatum dressings and a firm plastic or metal covering

Planning for the provision of support to the parents is an essential aspect of nursing care.

Intestinal obstruction. Congenital jejunal or ileal obstruction is suspected when distention and bile-stained or fecal vomiting occur in a newborn in the first 24 to 48 hours of life. Although this condition is uncommon, premature infants and those with other anomalies may be affected.

Nursing care is supportive: stop oral feedings and monitor intravenous therapy (see p. 757); prevent aspiration and suction gastric contents on physician's order (Indwelling catheter to low, intermittent suction may be ordered.); and place infant in semi-Fowler's position to facilitate respiration.

X-ray films of the abdomen usually show a dilated small bowel without gas in the colon. A barium enema may be helful in determining the cause of the obstruction. Hirschsprung's disease, ileus secondary to sepsis, meconium ileus, and volvulus must be considered in the differential diagnosis (Fig. 40.8). Prompt surgery usually provides a good result.

Fig. 40.7.
Omphalocele containing liver. (Courtesy John R. Campbell, M.D., University of Oregon Health Sciences Center, Portland, Ore.)

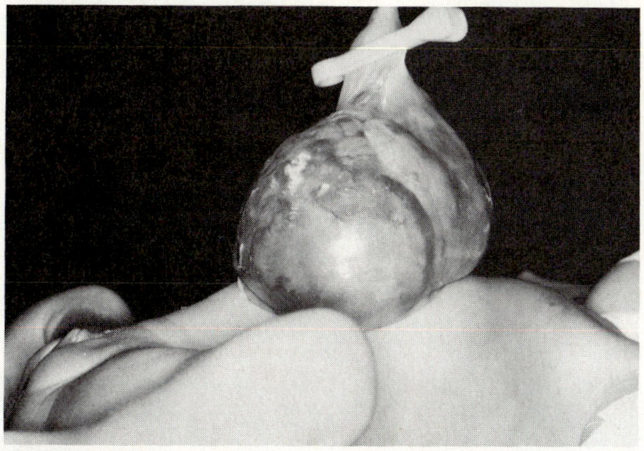

Fig. 40.8
Meconium ileus with midgut volvulus. Meconium ileus is frequently associated with cystic fibrosis. Normal meconium stool is not passed, and abdomen distends progressively. Treatment is directed at removal of mechanical obstruction and at prevention of complications of cystic fibrosis. (Courtesy John R. Campbell, M.D., University of Oregon Health Sciences Center, Portland, Ore.)

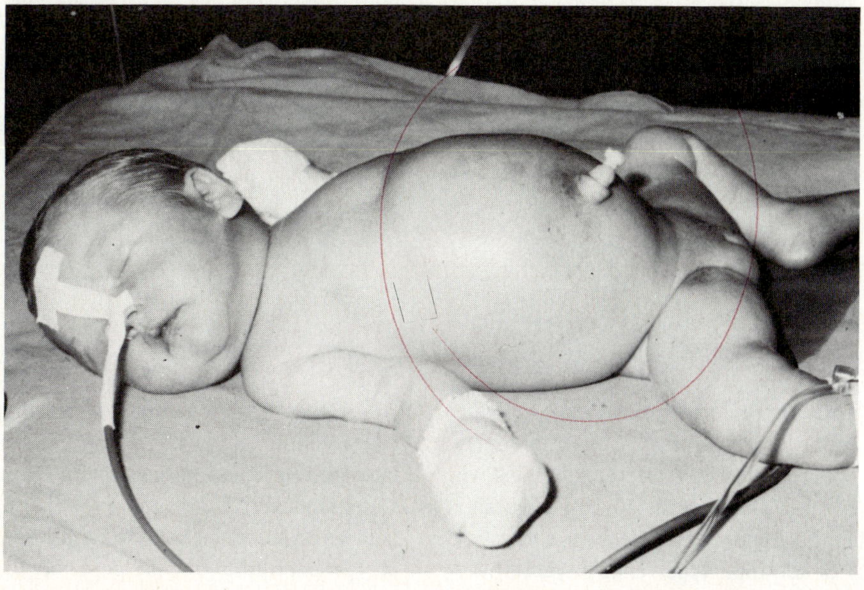

Fig. 40.9
Types of imperforate anus. Anal sphincter muscle may be present and intact. **A,** High lesion opening onto perineum through narrow fistulous tract. **B,** High lesion ending in fistulous tract to urinary tract. **C,** Low lesion in bowel passes through puborectal muscle. **D,** High lesion ending in fistulous tract to vagina.

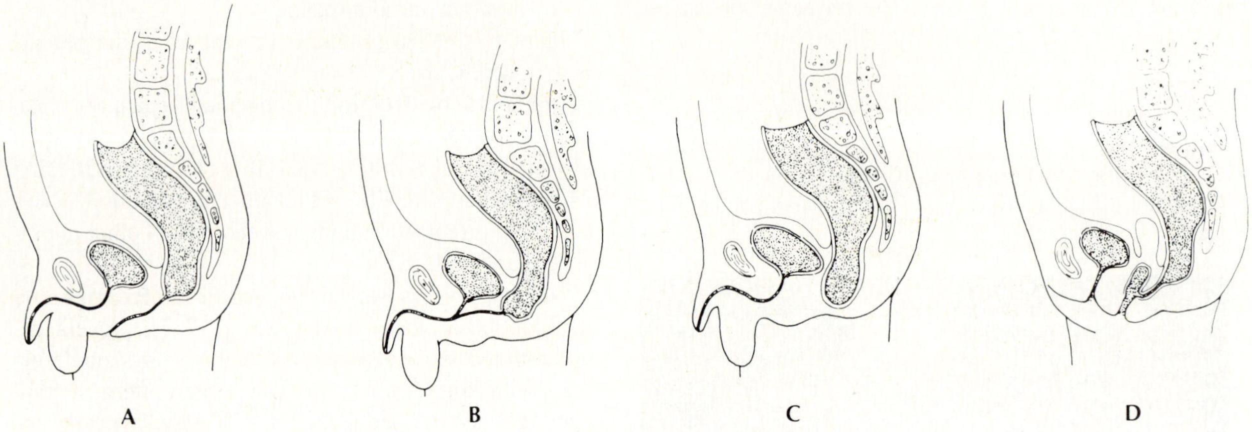

Fig. 40.10
Imperforate anus: fourchet fistula. Note meconium draining through fistula. Arrow indicates meconium exiting via fistulous tract. (Courtesy John R. Campbell, M.D., University of Oregon Health Sciences Center, Portland, Ore.)

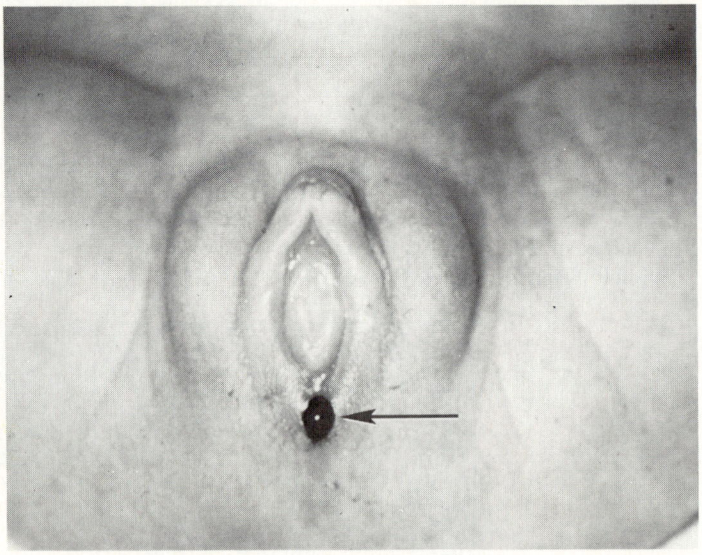

Imperforate anus. Imperforate anus is a congenital disorder that is more common in male than in female infants (Fig. 40.9). About 85% of affected females will have developed a small fistula (Fig. 40.10), but this is rare in males. The obstruction may be of the low type (anal membrane) or the high type (anal or rectal atresia). Because some anomalies are not apparent by direct visualization, initial insertion of probe (thermometer) into the anal canal is done with *extra* caution until patency is established.

Since continence for a lifetime may be dependent on the proper corrective surgery, a pediatric surgeon is consulted at once. Surgery may be as simple as an incision of an anal membrane, but with anorectal agenesis, a prompt colostomy will be necessary.

Survival is expected. Continence, on the other hand, is dependent on several factors, including sacral anomalies and proper surgery.

COMMON MALFORMATIONS

Meningomyelocele. Meningomyelocele, a neural tube defect, is a herniation of part of the meninges (containing cerebrospinal fluid [CSF] and CNS tissue) through a defect in the vertebral column or skull. The defect often occurs in the lower back. In the accompanying spinal malformation, *spina bifida,* the meningomyelocele extrudes through the opening of the spinal column, which is caused by a congenital absence of one or more vertebral arches. Occasionally a familial history (5% recurrence rate) of this anomaly is identified, but most cases are of unknown (infectious?) origin. A *meningocele* is also a herniation of the meninges and contains CSF but does not contain CNS tissue (cord or nerve roots).

Prenatal diagnosis of neural tube defects (meningomyelocele, meningocele, anencephaly) is now possible. Three methods are available:

1. Since the levels of alpha-fetoprotein in the maternal serum and amniotic fluid increase in the presence of neural tube defects, serum assays may be utilized for screening. Amniotic fluid determinations are needed for definitive diagnosis.
2. Ultrasound.
3. Amniography.

The couple may be advised of the existence of the defect and assisted in arriving at their own decision regarding the affected pregnancy.*

If the neonate is born with a large defect, the nurse aids in preventing its rupture and infection before surgery by the following actions:

1. Position with care.
   a. Position prone or side-lying with rolled towels to prevent pressure or injury to defect, thereby providing portal of entry for infectious agents.
   b. Change position every hour to prevent pressure areas.
   c. If physician permits infant to be held, exercise caution to avoid injury to defect.
2. Provide skin care: Skin around defect is cleansed and dried carefully to prevent breakdown, which would establish portal of entry for infectious agents. Apply physician-ordered dressings, ointments, and so on.

*In utero surgery may be possible.

The nurse assists in the diagnosis of a hidden defect by assessing neurologic function and noting the following:

1. Paralysis of lower extremities
2. Flaccidity and spasticity of muscles below defect
3. Sphincter control: character and number of voidings and stools; leakage of urine and stool

Surgical repair often can be done in the neonatal period. If other anomalies, such as hydrocephalus, are present, delayed correction may be elected. Permanent impairment of neuromuscular function below the level of the defect depends on the amount of CNS tissue involved. In severe cases, voluntary and involuntary functions are absent. The prognosis is guarded. Only about 60% of cases are operable, and many of these children die or achieve only partial function. Hydrocephalus ultimately develops in virtually all infants.

The parents will need considerable support and instruction regarding the infant's care (see Chapter 34). In some instances parents may require assistance in placing the child in a special care facility.

Congenital hydrocephalus. Congenital hydrocephalus is macrocephaly caused by abnormal enlargement of the cerebral ventricles and skull as the result of increased intraventricular CSF pressure. This condition is accompanied by enlargement of the head, prominence of the forehead, "setting sun" sign of the eyes, atrophy of the brain, weakness, and convulsions as the condition worsens.

Congenital hydrocephalus is encountered in approximately 1 in 2000 fetuses (about 12% of all malformations). Several types are known.

External hydrocephalus is caused by an abnormal accumulation of fluid between the brain and the dura mater. Obstruction of the CSF anywhere along its course may be responsible. Maldevelopment, infection, hemorrhage, neoplasia, or unknown causes must be considered. A history of maternal (and possibly fetal) bacterial or viral infection may be elicited. The most common lesion is atresia of the aqueduct between the third and fourth ventricles (Arnold-Chiari syndrome).

In *internal hydrocephalus* an excessive amount of CSF accumulates in the ventricular system of the brain. Rarely, oversecretion of CSF by a choroid plexus papilloma, rather than an obstruction, may result in internal hydrocephalus.

The fetus with hydrocephalus frequently assumes the breech presentation in utero. Severe dystocia caused by cephalopelvic disproportion (CPD) is encountered; cesarean delivery is usual. When vaginal delivery is attempted, puncture of the fetal head and drainage of the excess fluid may be necessary before the head can be delivered. Fetal mortality after this procedure is approximately three deaths out of every four deliveries. Regardless of the route of delivery, the experience is emotionally traumatic for the parents and family.

X-ray films should confirm widening of the fontanels and sutures. Intracranial calcifications caused by cytomegalic viral (CMV) inclusion disease or toxoplasmosis (a protozoal infection) may be revealed.

Subdural aspiration or transillumination of the head may disclose a subdural hematoma or tumor. The location and extent of obstruction usually can be identified by pneumoencephalography or ultrasonography.

Spina bifida occurs in approximately one third of neonates born with hydrocephalus.

Surgery is usually performed soon after birth. If surgical shunting is not accomplished, **increasing intracranial pressure,** evidenced by palpably widening fontanels and sutures, lethargy, irritability, or vomiting, will eventuate in irreversible neurologic damage. A period of observation is necessary, however, to determine the type of operation required. Meanwhile, nursing care is individualized.

Assessment for hydrocephalus includes notations describing the following typical signs:

1. Changes in head size every day
   a. Width of sutures
   b. Size and tension of anterior fontanel
   c. Head circumference
2. Facial appearance
   a. Flat, broad bridge of nose
   b. Bulging forehead
   c. "Setting-sun" effect as eyes are displaced downward by pressure from accumulating fluid
3. Neurologic signs
   a. High-pitched, shrill cry
   b. Irritability or restlessness
   c. Poor feeding or changes in feeding pattern from good to poor
   d. Behavior changes
   e. Spina bifida

Nursing actions appropriate to the needs of a neonate with hydrocephalus include the following.

1. Carefully note and report observations and changes.
2. Provide skin care to prevent infection.
   a. Prevent pressure areas. Use lamb's wool, sheepskin, flotation mattress, frequent position changes.
   b. Keep clean and dry.
3. Support head carefully when holding or turning infant.
4. Initiate feeding.
   a. Choose method, amount, and frequency of feeding to accommodate infant's tolerance and energy level.
   b. Be alert for vomiting and possible aspiration.
5. Meet infant's touching and cuddling needs.
6. Nurture parent: provide support and information regarding defect and treatment (see Chapter 34).

Restoration of damaged or destroyed brain tissue cannot be achieved. Spontaneous arrest of hydrocephalus may occur, but often surgical shunting may be required to eliminate excess CSF. Despite arrest of the process, serious mental retardation and neurologic sequelae are common.

Anencephaly and microcephaly. Anencephaly and microcephaly are congenital fetal deformities in which the head is considerably smaller than normal. In anencephaly there is complete or partial absence of the brain and of the overlying skull. Because the pituitary gland is absent or vestigial, the adrenal cortex is diminutive (for lack of ACTH stimulation). About 70% of anencephalic infants are female. This condition is frequently accompanied by hydramnios. The cause of anencephaly is unknown, but multiple environmental factors have been postulated. A 3% recurrence rate in familial histories has been noted.

In microcephaly the head generally is well formed but small. X-ray exposure of the woman has been followed by microcephaly in the child she was carrying at the time. Rubella, cytomegalic inclusion disease, and perhaps other infectious processes are the causes in some cases.

Anencephaly is incompatible with life; warmth and fluid are provided until the neonate's death, which is usually before the end of the first 24 hours after birth. Microcephalic infants require specific nursing care and medical observation to appraise the extent of psychomotor retardation that almost always accompanies this abnormality. The nurse's supportive role with parents is considerable.

Cleft-lip or palate. Cleft lip or palate is a common congenital midline fissure, or opening, in the lip or palate; one or both deformities may occur. The incidence is approximately 1 in 700 white neonates and 1 in 2000 black neonates. Polygenetic factors are causative in some cases, but fetal viral infection, maternal corticosteroid therapy, radiation, dietary influence, and hypoxia have been associated factors. The combination of cleft lip and palate affects more male than female infants.

Treatment requires special feeding techniques, for example, the use of uniquely designed nipples.

Cleft lip repair may be done soon after delivery if the neonate is free of infection, in good condition, and weighs 2500 g (5 lb, 9 oz). Cleft lip repair is best done when the infant weights 4500 g (10 lb) or more, however, since there is more tissue to work with. Advantages of earlier labial repair include facilitating a positive parent-child relationship and permitting the infant to learn to use and strengthen musculature around the mouth. Infants with palatolabial fissues often look grotesque and repulsive to the parents. After repair and with collaborative health team support, the mother frequently is able to assume responsibility for the newborn's care until palatal repair is feasible, between 16 and 24 months of age (9 kg [20 lb] body weight or more). The plastic surgeon, pediatrician, orthodontist, hospital and community nurses, speech therapist, and social worker make up the collaborative health team that has made possible the effective treatment available today. Until repair of the palate is performed, a prosthesis is fitted to aid the infant's feeding and speech development and to reduce respiratory tract infections.

The grief reaction to have a child with this and other disorders and the nursing care involved are discussed in Chapter 34. Parents also benefit from seeing before and after pictures of other babies born with this defect. Coupled with other verbal and nonverbal supportive care, this visual reassurance is effective. Parents can be referred to other parents (or organizations of parents such as the Cleft Palate Club) for continuing mutual support.

Musculoskeletal problems. The two most common musculoskeletal deviations seen in the neonatal period are congenital dysplasia of the hip and congenital clubfoot. Both conditions are easily recognized. Early detection and definitive treatment are mandatory for successful correction; delay makes repair more difficult and prognosis less favorable.

Congenital hip dysplasia (congenital dislocation of the hip). This often hereditary disorder occurs more commonly in female infants (Fig. 40.11) because of the structure of the pelvis. Because the acetabulum is abnormally shallow, the head of the femur becomes dislocated upward and backward to lie on the dorsal aspect of the ilium, where a false acetabulum may be formed. A stretched joint capsule results, and ossification of the femoral head is delayed.

Before dislocation occurs, reduced movement, splinting of the affected hip, limited abduction, and asymmetry of the hip may be noted. After dislocation, all these signs will be present, together with the external rotation and shortening of the leg. A clicking sound may be noted on gentle forced abduction of the leg (Ortolani's sign), and a bulge of the femoral head is felt. X-ray films will reveal a deformity in congenital dysplasia of the hip.

Treatment involves pressing the femoral head into the acetabulum to form an adequate socket before ossification is complete. The following methods are possible:

1. Thick diapers to abduct and externally rotate leg and flex hip (pin anterior flaps of diapers under posterior flaps) or the
2. Frejka pillow (apply diapers and plastic pants, and then apply pillow). Later this appliance will be followed by a spica cast in most instances to maintain abduction, extension, and internal rotation, usually with the infant in a "frog-leg" position.

Fig. 40.11

Congenital dysplasia of hip. **A,** Normal gluteal and popliteal skin creases. **B,** Abnormal skin creases and asymmetry of skin folds. **C,** Apparent shortening of femur. Femur head is displaced. (Courtesy Ross Laboratories, Columbus, Ohio.)

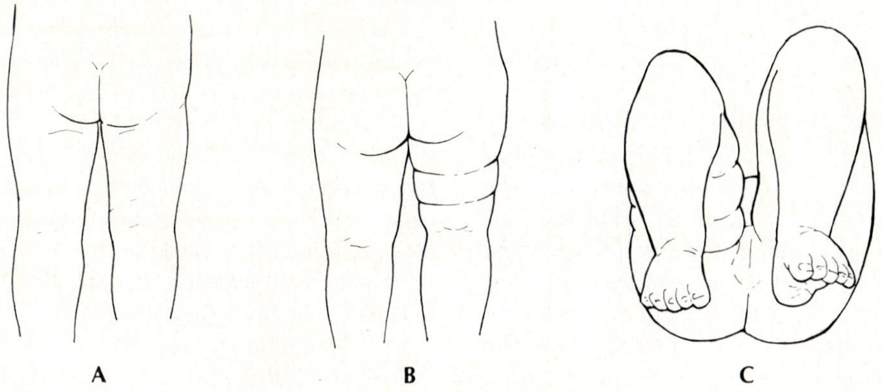

Talipes equinovarus. Talipes equinovarus, or clubfoot, is a congenital fixed postural deformity in which the foot is twisted out of shape or position. The heel is turned inward from the midline of the leg, the sole of the foot is flexed at the ankle joint, and the Achilles tendon is shortened.

Before the infant is 2 months old, often during his nursery stay, successive plaster casts are applied first to correct the heel inversion and adduction of the forefoot and later, the equinus deformity. Special shoes with lower leg braces will be necessary when the child learns to walk, and surgery may even be required in childhood if correction is incomplete. The prognosis depends on the extent of the deformity and the response to progressive orthopedic treatment.

Phocomelia. Phocomelia, or "seal-like limbs," is a developmental anomaly typified by absence of the arms or legs, or both, or stunting of the extremities. In the early 1960s the drug thalidomide was implicated as the causative agent for the limb deformities of many thousands of infants, especially in Germany. As a result the United States Food and Drug Administration tightened its regulations governing drug approval. Painfully apparent was evidence that drugs ingested during pregnancy may have tragic implications for fetal development. Thalidomide (and perhaps imipramine [Tofranil]) is a cause of this condition; sporadic cases of congenital amputation or stunting are of unknown etiology.

The child born with these deformities requires special care as follows:

1. Rehabilitative problems are often complex. The prostheses require frequent refitting as the child grows. The child requires careful guidance and training in achieving the optimal level of functioning possible. Approximately 15 child amputee centers are located throughout the United States.

2. Psychosocial developmental problems are significant. The kinesthetic satisfaction derived from kicking the legs and waving the arms is not possible. The hand-to-mouth movement behavior pattern, necessary for self-gratification and exploration of one's environment, is missing. The child learns about his environment by pushing the trunk up by the arms; a pillow prop under the infant's chest will compensate somewhat. The child's concerns about body image and obvious differences from others will require attention in later years. Any child reflects the attitudes and sentiments of those around him; if that child senses positive attitudes toward him and his defect, he will incorporate these into a positive self-concept.

3. Supportive care of the parents must begin at the birth of the child and continue for years. After the initial grief reaction, the parents need information regarding the rehabilitative and psychosocial components of their child's care.

Fig. 40.12
Polydactyly: supernumerary digit of right hand. Most common congenital anomaly of upper extremity and is occasionally seen in conjunction with other congenital malformations. (Courtesy Mead Johnson & Co., Evansville, Ind.)

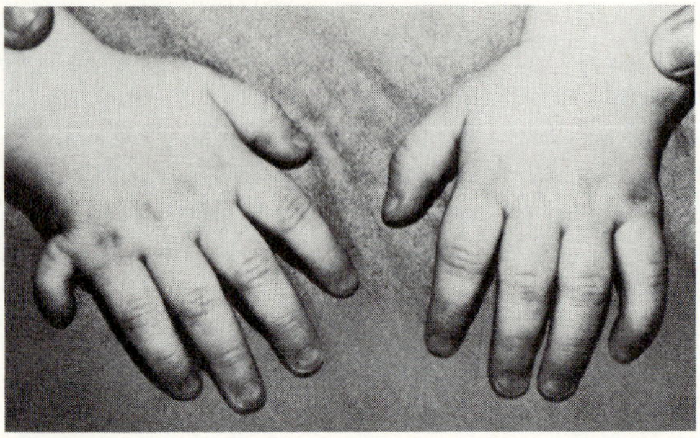

Polydactyly. Extra digits on the hands or feet occur occasionally (Fig. 40.12). In some instances polydactyly is hereditary. If there is little or no bone involvement, the extra digit is tied with silk suture soon after birth. The finger falls off within a few days, leaving a small scar. When there is bone involvement, surgical repair is indicated.

Genitourinary tract anomalies. Abnormally low-set or misshapen ears my indicate other, often genitourinary, anomalies (e.g., renal agenesis) (Fig. 40.13).

Exstrophy of the bladder In exstrophy of the bladder (Fig. 40.14), which is a congenital anomaly of unknown etiology, a separation of the symphysis pubis and anterior abdominal wall structures results in exterioration of the bladder trigone and surrounding mucosa. The exposed mucosa is deep red, has numerous folds, and is sensitive to touch. A direct passage of urine to the outside occurs. Associated anomalies, such as undescended testes, inguinal hernia, absence of the vagina, or bowel defects, should be sought. Surgical correction, often elimination of the bladder and construction of an ileal conduit, is rarely justified in the neonatal period. A prosthesis for collection of the urine and protection of the bladder may be employed.

Nursing management in the presence of exstrophy of the bladder involves the following:

1. Prevent urinary tract infection.
2. Prevent ulceration of adjacent skin from the constant seepage of urine.
3. Meet the infant's touching and cuddling needs.
4. Support parents.
5. Teach parents to care for the defect if surgery is

Fig. 40.13

Abnormally low-set ears characterize many syndromes and may indicate abnormality of internal organs, especially bilateral renal agenesis (Potter's syndrome). **A,** In normal infant, insertion of ear to scalp falls on extension of line drawn across inner and outer canthi of eye. **B,** If ear is twisted or rotated, it may give false impression of being low set. **C,** True low-set ear. (Courtesy Mead Johnson & Co., Evansville, Ind.)

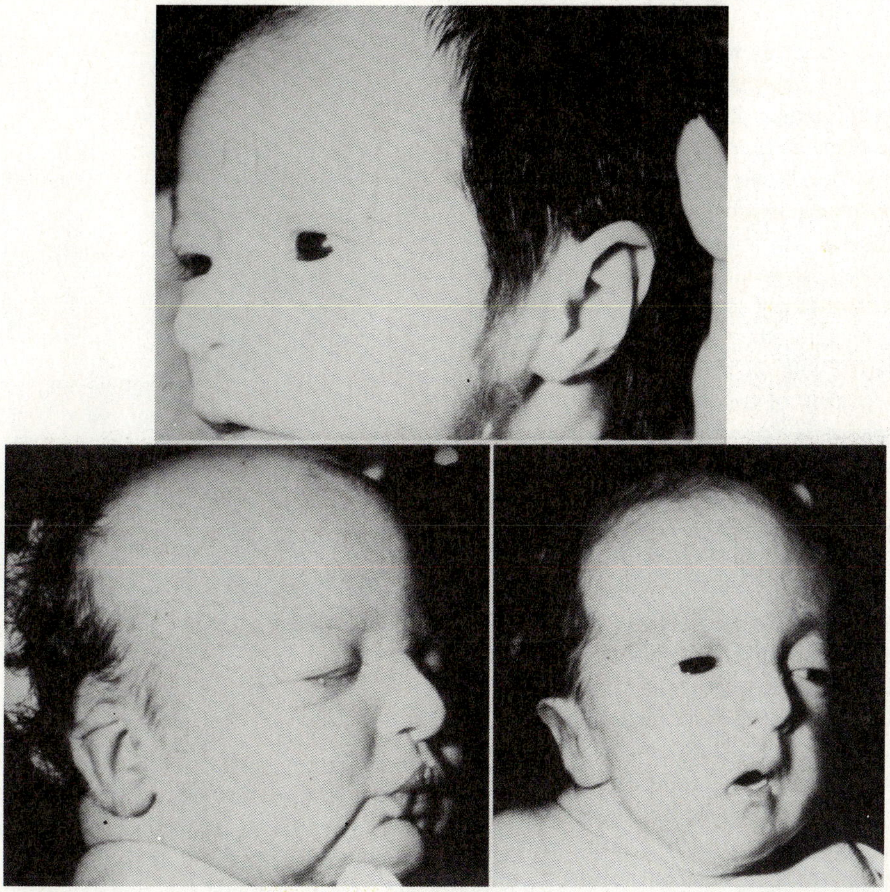

Fig. 40.14

Exstrophy of bladder. (Courtesy Edward S. Tank, M.D., Division of Urology, University of Oregon Health Sciences Center, Portland, Ore.)

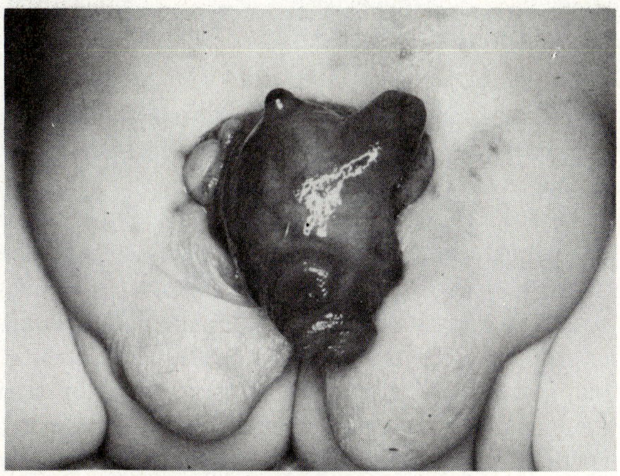

scheduled when the infant is several weeks or months of age.

Hypospadias and epispadias. Hypospadias is a developmental anomaly of the urethral meatus. In the male infant the meatus opens in the midline of the undersurface of the penis or on the perineum. In the female infant the meatus opens into the vagina. This condition tends to be hereditary.

Epispadias, also occurring in both sexes but predominating in males, is a congenital absence of the upper urethral wall. In the female it is often associated with exstrophy of the bladder. In the male the meatal opening is located anywhere along the dorsum of the penis.

Most instances of hypospadias are minor and require no corrective surgery. Pronounced defects require extensive urethroplasty. If needed, surgery is completed before the boy enters school so that he can urinate from a standing position like other boys. The more serious defects often coexist with other, multiple anomalies.

Nursing management of the physical care of the infant with hypospadias is the same as that for the normal infant. Should urethroplasty be required, no circumcision is done, since the foreskin is used in the surgical procedure. The parents are taught how to care for the urethral meatus and foreskin to prevent infection and promote cleanliness.

Sexual ambiguity. Sexual ambiguity in the neonate often is discovered by the nurse, who has more time and perhaps a better opportunity to examine the infant than the obstetrician, who may be concerned with maternal complications (Fig. 40.15).

Erroneous or abnormal sexual differentiation may be a genetic aberration (e.g., congenital adrenal hypoplasia), or it may be caused by maternal problems (e.g., steroid sex hormone therapy for threatened abortion). It is imperative to establish the genetic sex and the sex of rearing as soon as possible, not only to save embarrassment for reporting the birth of a (genetic) male who in fact is a female or the opposite, but to permit the surgical correction of anomalies before an individual or social pattern is set.

Prompt consultation with a surgeon who is experienced in the area of intersexuality should be arranged without delay. Meanwhile parents need supportive care as they await the decision.

Teratoma. Teratoma, a solid or semisolid neoplasm, is composed of the three embryonal tissue types (ectoderm, mesoderm, entoderm). A teratoma in the newborn may occur in the skull, mediastinum, or abdomen, but a solid or semisolid tumor in the sacral area also may prove to be a teratoma. It is protected by sterile dressings before surgical removal. Many teratomas diagnosed in the newborn are malignant. If the lesion cannot be entirely removed by surgery, x-ray therapy and chemotherapy are used. Long-term survival rate for infants with sacrococcygeal teratoma is 85% after surgical removal in the neonatal period but only 50% if surgery is delayed until the infant is more than 1 month old. Rectal and anal function can always be perserved.

Fig. 40.15
Ambiguous external genitalia (e.g., structure can be an enlarged clitoral hood and clitoris or a malformed penis). (Courtesy Edward S. Tank, M.D., Division of Urology, University of Oregon Health Sciences Center, Portland, Ore.)

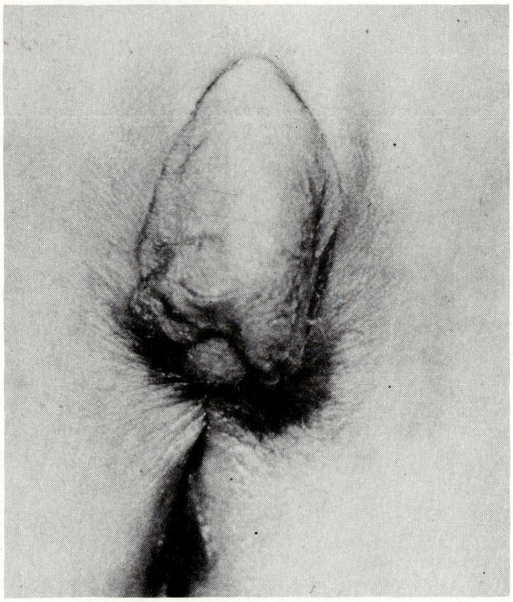

• • •

Neonatal conditions in which the mother is implicated for hereditary reasons (Rh-negative or O blood type) are ego threatening for the mother. Nursing care to meet the physical needs of the neonate born with an anomaly requiring immediate surgical intervention presents a challenge. The neonate's physiologic functioning must be supported, infection prevented, and a protective environment provided (pediatric unit, neonatal intensive care nursery). To meet the psychosocial needs of parents whose child is born with a disorder, sensitive nursing care is required (see Chapter 34).

DISORDERS NOT APPARENT AT BIRTH

Some disorders do not appear until some time after birth. The severity of the psychologic impact varies with the disorder and the time it appears. Together the parents and the affected child, if he is old enough, experience mourning, restructuring of self-image, and the reaction to stigmatization by society. Parents who had other children before the appearance of a disorder in an older child fear for the younger children. The middle-aged individual who develops Huntington's chorea, perhaps even after he has become a grandfather, fears for two generations of descendants. In many cases, affected individuals may experience anger and resentment toward the offending parents, just as parents of a child with a disorder feel resentment toward the child who "did this to us." If the mother unwittingly accepted therapy now shown to have adverse effects on her children (e.g., DES), she may feel betrayed, angry, and afraid.

Diethylstilbestrol. Administration of diethylstilbestrol (DES) or another nonsteroidal estrogen to the mother may be followed by developmental or functional genital problems in both female and male progeny. The abnormalities are rare, when one considers the estimate that about 500,000 pregnant women received DES between 1940 and 1970. Single or multiple abnormalities may be noted; some develop or are recognized after puberty. Curiously, most individuals who were exposed prenatally appear to have been unaffected. Hence, an association rather than an actual cause-and-effect relationship is likely and a trigger factor or factors are being sought.

In DES-exposed females, the following developmental or functional disorders have been described: circumferential vaginal ridges; cervical deformity, for example, "cock's comb" cervix, hooding, clefts, pseudopolyps; hypoplastic or T-shaped uterus; constricting bands within the uterus; tubal anomalies; vaginal or cervical adenosis, dysplasia, or cervical incompetence. There appear to be an increased frequency of oligomenorrhea and a lower incidence of pregnancy in these women also. Most critical is the assessment that 3 or 4 out of 1000 women exposed to DES prenatally develop vaginal or cervical clear-cell carcinoma, usually during adolescence.

In DES-exposed males the most common gross lesions reported are epididymal cysts, hypotrophic testes, or testicular capsular thickening. In addition, sperm analyses have revealed low volume of ejaculate, oligospermia, diminished sperm density, and lower motile sperm count per milliliter. No equivalent of female clear-cell carcinoma or increase in male genitourinary cancer has been noted, however.

References and Readings

Babson, S.G., Pernoll, M.L., and Benda, G.I.: Diagnosis and management of the fetus at risk: a guide for team care, ed. 4, St. Louis, 1979, The C.V. Mosby Co.

Behrman; R.E., editor: Neonatal-perinatal medicine: diseases of the fetus and infant, ed. 2, St. Louis, 1977, The C.V. Mosby Co.

Bowman, J.M., et al.: Rh isoimmunization during pregnancy: antenatal prophylaxis, Can. Med. Assoc. J. **118:**623, 1978.

Bowman, J.M., and Pollock, J.M.: Antenatal prophylaxis of Rh isoimmunization: 28 weeks' gestation service program, Can. Med. Assoc. J. **118:**627, 1978.

Gottesfeld, I.B.: The family of the child with congenital heart disease; M.C.N. **4:**101, March-April 1979.

Henry, G., Wexler, P., and Robinson, A.: Rh-immune globulin after amniocentesis for genetic diagnosis, Obstet. Gynecol. **48:**557, 1976.

Klaus, M.H., and Fanaroff, A.A.: Care of the high-risk neonate, ed. 2, Philadelphia, 1979, W.B. Saunders Co.

Korones, S.B.: High-risk newborn infants: the basis for intensive nursing care, ed. 2, St. Louis, 1976, The C.V. Mosby Co.

Lozoff, B., et al.: The mother-newborn relationship: limits of adaptability, J. Pediatr. **91:**1, 1977.

Pierog, S.M., and Ferrara, A: Medical care of the sick newborn, ed. 2, St. Louis, 1976, The C.V. Mosby Co.

Shirkey, H.C., editor: Pediatric therapy, ed. 6, St. Louis, 1980, The C.V. Mosby Co.

Smith, K.: Recognizing cardiac failure in neonates, M.C.N. **4:**98, March-April 1979.

Tovey, L.A., and Taverner, J.M.: A case for the antenatal administration of anti-D immunoglobulin to primigravidae, Lancet **1:**878, 1981.

Waechter, E.H.: The birth of an exceptional child, Nurs. Forum **9:**202, 1970.

Whaley, L.F.: Understanding inherited disorders, St. Louis, 1974, The C.V. Mosby Co.

Whaley, L.F., and Wong, D.L.: Nursing care of infants and children, ed. 2, St. Louis, 1983, The C.V. Mosby Co.

41

Other Medical and Surgical Conditions

- Medical Problems Complicating Pregnancy
  - Anemia
    - Iron deficiency anemia
    - Folic acid deficiency anemia
    - Sickle cell hemoglobinopathy
    - Thalassemia
  - Urinary problems
    - Urinary tract infection
    - Glomerulonephritis
    - Nephroureterolithiasis
  - Pulmonary complications
    - Bronchial asthma
    - Adult respiratory distress syndrome
    - Pulmonary embolus
    - Aspiration pneumonia
  - Gastrointestinal problems
    - Hyperemesis gravidarum (pernicious vomiting of pregnancy)
    - Peptic ulcer
    - Cholelithiasis and cholecystitis
    - Ulcerative colitis
  - Dermatologic problems
  - Neurologic disorders
    - Epilepsy
    - Multiple sclerosis
    - Myasthenia gravis
  - Disseminated lupus erythematosus
  - Nursing management of medical complications
- Surgical Conditions Coincident with Pregnancy
  - Appendicitis
    - Management
    - Prognosis
  - Gynecologic problems
  - Abdominal hernias
  - Carcinoma of the breast
  - Intestinal obstruction
  - Varices and hemorrhoids
  - Nursing management of surgical conditions coincident with pregnancy
- Surgical Interruption of Pregnancy
  - Early abortion
    - Potential complications
  - Second- and third-trimester abortions
  - Nurse's role
- Surgical Termination of Fertility
  - Motivation for sterilization
  - Laws and regulations
  - Sterilization procedures
  - Female sterilization
    - Timing of female sterilization
    - Tubal occlusion
    - Hysterectomy
  - Male sterilization: vasectomy
  - Nurse's role
    - Counselor
    - Preoperative preparation
    - Postoperative care
    - Discharge planning

Some complications of pregnancy stem from the pregnant condition. Others are preexisting or represent pathologic conditions that affect the population in general. In this chapter the pathologic basis for understanding the effects of selected clinical complications on pregnancy and the nursing care that can lead to early detection and effective management are presented.

Some clients of reproductive age seek health care services related to the surgical interruption of pregnancy and to the surgical termination of fertility. These surgical procedures and the related nursing role are discussed in the latter part of this chapter.

Medical Problems Complicating Pregnancy

ANEMIA

Anemia, the most common medical disorder of pregnancy, affects at least 20% of pregnant women. These women have a higher incidence of puerperal complications such as infection than do pregnant women with normal hematologic values.

Anemia results in reduction of the oxygen-carrying capacity of the blood. An indirect index of the oxygen-carrying capacity is the packed red blood cell volume (PCV), or hematocrit level. The normal hematocrit range in nonpregnant women is 38% to 45%. However, normal values for pregnant women with adequate iron stores may be as low as 34%. This has been explained by hydremia (dilution of blood), or the *physiologic anemia of pregnancy*.

About 90% of cases of anemia in pregnancy are of the iron deficiency type. The remaining 10% of cases embrace a considerable variety of acquired and hereditary anemias, including folic acid deficiency and hemoglobinopathies.

Normal values during pregnancy. Normal and abnormal changes confuse the hematologic profile during pregnancy. The blood values of pregnant women differ significantly from those of nonpregnant women. All the constituents of blood normally increase during pregnancy; plasma volume, by 30% to 35%; red cell volume, by 20% to 30%; and hemoglobin mass, by 12% to 15%. The dilution of red blood cells and hemoglobin resulting from the relatively greater increase in plasma volume does not significantly change cell indices such as the mean corpuscular volume (MCV). However, this dilution does affect red blood cell count (RBC), hemoglobin, and hematocrit values; laboratory values drop progressively to a low between the thirtieth and thirty-fourth weeks of pregnancy.

Definition of anemia during pregnancy. At or near sea level, during the *first* trimester, the pregnant woman is anemic when her hemoglobin level is less than 11 g/dl or her hematocrit level falls below 37%. She is anemic in the *second* trimester when the hemoglobin level is less than 10.5 g/dl or the hematocrit level falls below 35%; and she is anemic in the *third* trimester when the hemoglobin level is less than 10 g/dl or the hematocrit level is less than 33%. Much higher values are indicative of anemia in areas of high altitude; for example, at 1500 m (5000 ft) above sea level, a hemoglobin level less than 14 g/dl indicates anemia.

Iron deficiency anemia

Iron needs during pregnancy. The demand for iron during pregnancy is about 1000 mg (250 mg for the fetus and 750 mg for the mother). Maternal needs are approximately as follows: placenta, 150 mg; blood volume increases, 300 mg; and blood loss at delivery and during the puerperium, 300 mg. If the demand for iron were constant through pregnancy, the average daily requirement (18 mg) would have to be increased by at least 3 mg. Actually the demand is not constant. During the first half of pregnancy, the additional demand for iron is small and usually met by iron conserved because menstruation has ceased, but during the last 20 weeks, a serious deficiency is likely.

Maternal adaptations to meet increased need for iron. In response to the inceased requirements, the maternal organism adjusts to increased daily absorption by improved iron binding, from about 1.5 mg in the second trimester to less than 4 mg in the third trimester. Despite this improvement, the balance is tenuous. If iron deficiency anemia mars the onset of pregnancy and iron supplement is not given, anemia usually ensues.

Iron therapy. Even the normal pregnant woman who has enjoyed excellent nutrition will conclude pregnancy with a deficit in iron storage. Inadequate nutrition will most certainly mean iron deficiency anemia during late pregnancy and the puerperium. A woman cannot replace gestational iron losses merely from dietary sources.

Successful iron therapy during pregnancy can be carried out in the vast majority of cases with oral iron supplements (e.g., ferrous sulfate, 0.3 g three times a day). Some pregnant women cannot tolerate or fail to take the prescribed oral iron. In such cases the woman should receive parenteral iron such as the iron-dextran complex (Imferon).

Folic acid deficiency anemia. Folic acid deficiency anemia occurs in at least 2% of pregnant women in North America, an incidence much higher than that suspected even 5 years ago. Many of these women have urinary tract infections because of their anemia.

Poor diet, cooking with large volumes of water, or canning of food may lead to a folate deficiency. Also, malabsorption or increased folate utilization may play a part in the development of anemia caused by lack of folic acid.

Macrocytic (megaloblastic) anemia, hypersegmented (multinucleate) neutrophils, thrombocytopenia, markedly elevated lactic dehydrogenase (LDH), or low serum folate levels are diagnostic of folate deficiency anemia. Many of these woman also show abnormalities in vaginal or cervical cytology that may suggest a folate lack.

It is important to recall that iron deficiency or hemoglobinopathy anemia may be associated with folate deficiency.

During pregnancy the recommended daily intake is

150 μg of folic acid. In folate deficiency a dosage of about 5 mg/24 hr orally for several weeks should ensure a remission. A generous maintenance dose each day should prevent a relapse. Because iron deficiency anemia may also accompany folate deficiency, augmented iron intake should also be provided.

Sickle cell hemoglobinopathy. Sickle cell trait (SA hemoglobin pattern) is sickling of the red blood cells but with a normal RBC life span. Pregnant women with sickle cell trait are susceptible to urinary tract infection. Hematuria is common.

With the sickle cell test, induced sickling of abnormal hemoglobin-containing red blood cells, which occurs at a low Po_2, especially at a low pH, may be demonstrated by observing a sealed drop of blood under the microscope after constriction of the finger by a rubber band or by adding a drop of 2% sodium bisulfite to the blood and viewing the sealed, moist preparation.

Sickle cell anemia (sickle cell disease) is a recessive, hereditary, familial hemolytic anemia peculiar to those of black or Mediterranean ancestry. These individuals usually have abnormal hemoglobin types (SS or SC). Persons with sickle cell anemia have recurrent attacks (crises) of fever and pain in the abdomen or extremities beginning in childhood. These attacks are attributed to vascular occlusion (from abnormal cells), tissue hypoxia, edema, and red blood cell destruction. Crises are associated with normochromic anemia, jaundice, reticulocytosis, positive sickle cell test, and the demonstration of abnormal hemoglobin (usually SS or SC).

Almost 10% of blacks in North America have the sickle cell trait, but less than 1% have sickle cell anemia, often complicated by iron and folic acid deficiency.

Pregnant women with sickle cell anemia are prone to pyelonephritis, leg ulcers, bone infarction, and cardiopathy. (Oral contraceptives are contraindicated.) An aplastic crisis may follow serious infection. Medical therapy, including transfusions to maintain the hematocrit level at at least 30% is essential, but cesarean delivery is warranted only on obstetric indications.

Pregnancy may impose critical complications in sickle cell disease. Maternal mortality often ranges between 5% to 10%, and the perinatal mortality may reach 30%. Therapeutic abortion is not medically indicated, but the limitation of pregnancy, often by sterilization, will be beneficial.

Thalassemia. Thalassemia (Mediterranean or Cooley's anemia), a relatively common anemia in which an insufficient amount of hemoglobin is produced to fill the red blood cells, is a hereditary disorder that involves the abnormal synthesis of the α- or β-chains of hemoglobin. β-thalassemia is the more common variety in the United States and is often diagnosed in individuals of Italian, Greek, or southern Chinese descent. The unbalanced synthesis of hemoglobin leads to premature red blood cell death resulting in severe anemia. Thalassemia major is the homozygous form of the disorder, thalassemia minor is the heterozygous form.

Thalassemia major may complicate pregnancy. Preeclampsia is more frequent in women with thalassemia major. Thalassemia major may be associated with low–birth weight infants and increased fetal wastage. Placental weight often is increased, perhaps secondary to maternal anemia. The frequency of fetal distress from hypoxia is greater than in control women. Therefore pregnant women with thalassemia major should be monitored more closely than normal pregnant women.

Regular transfusion may be necessary. Folic acid should be given to avoid folate deficiency. Aggressive therapy, for example, partial exchange transfusion, may be warranted in severe thalassemia. Splenectomy may be necessary if enlargement and pain occur.

Women with thalassemia major may die of chronic infection or progressive hepatic or cardiac failure, the result of excessive iron deposition.

Persons with *thalassemia minor* have a mild but persistent anemia, but the RBC may be normal or even elevated. However, no systemic problems are caused by the anemia that is a part of the minor form of the disease. Thalassemia minor must be distinguished principally from iron deficiency anemia.

Pregnancy will neither worsen thalassemia minor nor will it be compromised by the disease. The anemia will not respond to iron therapy, and prolonged parenteral iron can lead to harmful, excessive iron storage. Infants born to parents with thalassemia will inherit the disorder. Persons with thalassemia minor should have a normal life span despite a moderately reduced hemoglobin level.

URINARY PROBLEMS

Urinary tract infection. Urinary tract infection affects about 10% of pregnant women, most of these in the prenatal period. Those who have had previous urinary tract infections are especially prone to develop them again during pregnancy. Cervicitis, vaginitis, obstruction of the flaccid ureters (particularly on the right because of pressure by the pregnant uterus against the slightly dilated flaccid ureters), vesicoureteral reflux, and the trauma of delivery predispose the pregnant woman to urinary tract infection, generally from *Escherichia coli*. Asymptomatic bacteriuria (100 colonies/ml or more) occurs in about 5% of all pregnant women. If untreated, pyelonephritis during gestation will develop in approximately 30% of these women. Premature labor and delivery may be more frequent also.

Urine culture and sensitivity tests should be obtained early in pregnancy, preferably at the first visit, from a clean-catch urine specimen. Catheterization should be avoided if possible. If infection is diagnosed, treatment with an appropriate antibotic drug for 2 to 3 weeks, together with forced fluids and urinary tract antispasmodic medication (e.g., belladonna derivatives) is recommended. Infections caused by the colon aerogenic organisms generally respond well to sulfisoxazole or nitrofuratoin. Treatment should be continued for 2 to 3 weeks until two negative cultures are obtained, and the infant should be observed for hyperbilirubinemia (see Chapter 40). Retreatment of the mother may be necessary if there is a recurrence. Acute pyelonephritis may be confused with appendicitis, cholecystitis, or premature labor.

If persistent or recurrent infection is noted, urologic investigation will be necessary to identify contributory causes such as urinary tract obstruction, stone, diverticulum, tuberculosis, or poor personal hygiene.

Glomerulonephritis. Acute glomerulonephritis, generally caused by a respiratory infection from group A streptococci, is a rare complication of pregnancy. It is characterized by hematuria, edema, and hypertension. Treatment requires antibotic therapy, bed rest (in side-lying or semi- to high-Fowler's position to facilitate renal perfusion), and fluid-electrolyte and dietary control. Pregnancy does not seriously affect acute early glomerulonephritis. Severe or prolonged glomerulonephritis may be an indication for therapeutic abortion during the first trimester.

Women with mild, inactive glomerulonephritis generally can go through pregnancy safely. Women with progressive, chronic glomerulonephritis, that is, severe renal damage associated with proteinuria, hypertension, and an elevated blood urea nitrogen (BUN) level, do not tolerate pregnancy well. If pregnancy is not interrupted, spontaneous abortion is likely; preeclampsia-eclampsia often supervenes, and fetal death may result. Cardiac or renal failure generally is the cause of maternal death.

Nephroureterolithiasis. Pregnancy causes dilatation of the renal hilum and calyces so that small stones often are lodged, and most of these pass painfully. Whether urinary stones form more readily during pregnancy because of urinary stasis, hypercholesterolemia, or increased calciuria and vitamin D is still debated.

PULMONARY COMPLICATIONS

Bronchial asthma. Bronchial asthma is an acute, dramatic respiratory illness caused by allergens, marked change in ambient temperature, or emotional tension, but in many cases the actual cause may be unknown. A family history of allergy is likely in about 50% of all persons with asthma. Almost 2% of individuals in the United States have bronchial asthma, but less than 1% of pregnant women suffer from this disorder. The effect of pregnancy on asthma is unpredictable. Certainly, psychologic alterations induced by pregnancy do not make the pregnant woman more prone to asthmatic attacks. Asthma increases the incidence of abortion and premature labor, but the fetus per se is unaffected. However, in severe cases, asthma may be life threatening for the gravida.

Severe, prolonged asthma may cause progressive hypoxemia, hypercarbia, atelectasis, pneumothorax, or physical exhaustion. Few persons die in an asthmatic attack, but pulmonary emphysema or cor pulmonale may develop in individuals with chronic asthma.

Asthma causes wheezing, respiratory dyspnea, cough, and the production of excessive tenacious mucus from the upper respiratory tract. Many persons will give a history of allergy or previous asthmatic attacks. The wheezing must be distinguished from bronchitis, obstructive emphysema, congestive heart failure, and pulmonary embolism.

A careful medical evaluation and x-ray films of the chest should be obtained. In severe asthma, pulmonary function studies and measurement of the blood gases and electrolytes should be obtained.

Therapy for bronchial asthma has two objectives: (1) release of the acute attack and (2) prevention or limitation of later attacks.

In all asthmatics, known allergens should be eliminated and a comfortable home temperature maintained. Tranquilizers (but not sedatives) should be given to relieve apprehension. Respiratory infections should be treated and mist or steam inhalation employed to aid expectoration of mucus. The outline below details treatment of asthma and pregnancy, providing a basis from which to develop a nursing care plan:

1. Treatment of acute bronchial asthma
   a. Administer hydrocortisone sodium succinate and aminophylline as ordered.
   b. Employ oxygen freely by mask.
   c. Correct fluid-electrolyte imbalance.
2. Treatment of mild or moderate bronchial asthma
   a. Administer epinephrine (1:1000).
   b. Offer isoproterenol inhalation (1:200 aqueous solution) by nebulizer for one or two inhalations.
   c. Give phenobarbital, 30 mg orally three times daily, if necessary to counteract overstimulation by bronchodilator drugs. Except for this purpose, sedatives should be avoided in the treatment of persons with asthma.
3. Interim therapy of bronchial asthma

   a. Diagnose offending antigens and treat allergy properly—by desensitization, if feasible.
   b. Reduce emotional tension; avoid respiratory infections or treat if they occur.
4. Management of pregnancy
   a. Consider therapeutic abortion only in extremely severe cases of asthma recurrent during pregnancies.
   b. Deny morphine in labor, since it may cause bronchospasm. Meperidine (Demerol) usually will relieve bronchospasm.
   c. Avoid or limit ephedrine and corticotropins (pressor drugs) in preeclampsia-eclampsia.
   d. Opt for vaginal delivery under local or regional anesthesia, whenever possible.

The prognosis for both mother and fetus will be good except in the very rare situation in which abortion or premature delivery is mandatory.

Adult respiratory distress syndrome. Adult respiratory distress syndrome (ARDS, shock lung) occurs when the lungs are unable to maintain levels of oxygen and carbon dioxide within normal limits because of deficits in gas exchange and uneven distribution of blood flow to the lungs. Marked tachycardia, dyspnea, and cyanosis that does not respond to nasal oxygen or intermittent positive pressure breathing are the most noted signs. This condition may occur in women who have given birth vaginally or by cesarean delivery and after spontaneous or medically induced abortion. The chance of developing ARDS increases with the amount of trauma experienced during pregnancy or delivery. ARDS is not a condition specific to pregnancy; it can also result from chest trauma, drug ingestion, or pneumonia. When ARDS is associated with pregnancy, pulmonary embolism, disseminated intravascular coagulation (DIC) (see Chapter 35), and aspiration pneumonia are the precipitators.

It has been noted that during pregnancy there is an increase in some of the coagulation factors, and this results in shortening of the partial thromboplastin time (PTT). This state predisposes the woman to an increase in rapidity of blood clotting and an increased tendency to form blood clots (hypercoagulability).

Early recognition. Laboratory reports are important in identifying the origin of acute pulmonary problems. The important observations for the nurse to note are vital signs, signs of thrombophlebitis, and hemorrhage.

Vital signs. Temperature elevation may indicate the development of thrombophlebitis. The pulse rate increases to compensate for respiratory insufficiency of any origin. The severity of the pulmonary problem increases as the pulse rate rises. An initial rise in blood pressure occurs as cardiac output increases to try to supply the body tissue with oxygen. When lung damage is severe, the blood pressure drops. The most important indicator of ARDS is respiratory changes. The rate, depth, respiratory pattern, symmetry of chest movement, and use of accessory muscles should be noted. When the woman is at rest, changes may not be noted; therefore observation of respiratory characteristics after activity is important. If there is any indication of abnormality, count respirations for a full minute; an error of plus or minus four may be highly significant. During the postdelivery period, apprehension, distended neck veins, cyanosis, diaphoresis, or pallor may be clues to watch for. Also mental confusion or disorientation may be noted.

On auscultation of the lungs, rales, rhonchi, wheezes, or a pleural friction rub needs to be reported, especially when they have occurred since an earlier assessment. The pregnant woman should be positioned for breathing comfort, and oxygen and emergency equipment should be available while the physician is notified. Reassure the woman so that her anxiety is lessened.

Thrombophlebitis. The lower extremities need to be checked for swelling, pain, inflammation, venous distention, and Homans' sign. If thrombophlebitis is suspected, the woman should be kept on bed rest until the physician can be notified. Sudden movement or straining can dislodge a clot and lead to pulmonary embolism.

Postdelivery hemorrhage. Petechiae, ecchymosis, hematuria, and epistaxis are important indications of DIC. Replacement of clotting factors and heparin therapy may be required for DIC. Sources of trauma should be identified and eliminated so that outside causes of hemorrhage are avoided.

Pulmonary embolus. Pregnancy also brings about changes in the vascular system. Alterations in vein distensibility have been noted, possibly because of softening of collagen induced by humoral influences. The combination of vein distensibility and obstruction of venous blood return from the lower extremities (caused by fetal pressure on veins, especially in the last trimester) predisposes a woman to pooling of blood. In addition, hypercoagulation and pooling may lead to thrombophlebitis, which in turn can result in ARDS (emboli from thromboembolism cause obstruction in the pulmonary circulation).

Aspiration pneumonia. Aspiration pneumonia can be caused by changes in the gastrointestinal system during pregnancy. Progesterone has been known to relax smooth muscles. When the resting tone is lowered, the cardiac sphincter becomes weak and reflux of the stomach contents can easily occur. Increased intraabdominal pressure (because of fetal growth) further predisposes the mother to gastric reflux. Food eaten as long as 24 to 48 hours before labor can be vomited and then aspirated. Aspiration of solid foods and liquids may cause bronchial obstruction leading to bronchoconstriction, which in turn can result in ARDS. Large particles can be removed by coughing, suctioning, or bronchoscopy, but liquids are harder to remove. The hydrochloric acid in the aspirated stomach contents may cause an asthmatic-like syndrome with necrotizing bronchitis. For this reason an antacid is given preoperatively to women who are to have a cesarean delivery as a prophylactic measure.

GASTROINTESTINAL PROBLEMS

Compromise of gastrointestinal function during pregnancy is apparent to all concerned. There are psychogenic overtones generally admitted in nausea and vomiting of pregnancy. However, a capricious food choice is observed in many women during pregnancy. In addition, obvious physiologic alterations, such as the greatly enlarged uterus, and less apparent changes, such as hypochlorhydria, require understanding for proper diagnosis and treatment.

Hyperemesis gravidarum (pernicious vomiting of pregnancy). See Chapter 36 for a discussion of hyperemesis gravidarum.

Peptic ulcer. Peptic ulcer is less common in women than men, and this problem is even more uncommon during pregnancy. Moreover, women with a diagnosed peptic ulcer generally improve during gestation. Therefore hemorrhage and perforation are unlikely. Fortunately emergency surgery for peptic ulcer complications rarely jeopardizes the pregnancy. Postdelivery reactivation of the ulcer may occur. Medical therapy is similar to that recommended for nonpregnant individuals.

Cholelithiasis and cholecystitis. Women are more likely to have cholelithiasis than men, and pregnancy seems to play a part in its development. It is known that gallstones are more frequently diagnosed in women of advanced parity than in nulliparas of the same age and background. Increased biliary cholesterol and biliary stasis are probable causes. Cholecystitis does not commonly occur during pregnancy.

Generally, gallbladder surgery should be postponed until the puerperium, but impaction of a stone in the cystic or common duct during pregnancy may require cholelithotomy or cholecystectomy.

Meperidine (Demerol) or atropine alleviates ductal spasm and pain. Morphine may be given also.

Ulcerative colitis. The cause of ulcerative colitis is unknown, but its effect on pregnancy is minimal unless there is marked debilitation, whereupon spontaneous abortion, fetal death, or premature delivery may occur. In general, when pregnancy coincides with active ulcerative colitis, the great majority of women will experience a severe exacerbation of the disease. When pregnancy occurs during a period of inactivity of the disorder, a flare-up is unlikely.

There is no specific therapy for ulcerative colitis, but adrenocorticosteroids and antibiotics may be beneficial. Therapeutic abortion is justified in fulminating cases, and avoidance of pregnancy (see Chapter 13) is important because of chronic invalidism.

DERMATOLOGIC PROBLEMS

Dermatologic disorders induced by pregnancy (see Table 17.10) include melasma (chloasma), herpes gestationis, noninflammatory pruritis of pregnancy, vascular spiders, palmar erythema, and pregnancy granulomas (includng epulides).

Skin problems generally aggravated by pregnancy are acne vulgaris (in the first trimester), erythema multiforme, herpetiform dermatitis, granuloma inguinale, condylomata acuminata, neurofibromatosis, and pemphigus. Dermatologic disorders usually improved by pregnancy include acne vulgaris (in the third trimester), seborrhea dermatitis, and psoriasis.

An unpredictable course during pregnancy may be expected in atopic dermatitis, lupus erythematosus, and herpex simplex.

Therapeutic abortion or early delivery may be justified if the following dermatologic conditions occur: herpes gestationis, disseminated lupus erythematosus, and neurofibromatosis (von Recklinghausen's disease).

Explanation, reassurance, and common sense measures should suffice for normal skin changes (see Table 17.10). In contrast, disease processes during and soon after pregnancy may be extremely difficult to diagnose and treat.

NEUROLOGIC DISORDERS

Epilepsy. Epilepsy may result from developmental abnormalities or injury. Epilepsy seriously complicates about 1 of every 1000 gestations. Convulsive seizures may be more frequent or severe during complications of pregnancy, such as edema, alkylosis, fluid-electrolyte imbalance, cerebral hypoxia, hypoglycemia, and hypocalcemia. On the other hand, the effects of pregnancy on epilepsy are unpredictable.

The differential diagnosis of epilepsy vs. eclampsia may pose a problem. Certainly epilepsy and eclampsia can coexist, but a past history of seizures, the absence of hypertension, generalized edema or proteinuria, and a normal plasma uric acid level point to epilepsy. Electroencephalography (EEG) rarely is diagnostic.

Grand mal seizures can be controlled by intravenous

sodium amobarbital or magnesium sulfate. Phenytoin (Dilantin) and its analogues may be fetotoxic, but diazepam (Valium) or chlordiazepoxide (Librium) are safe analeptic drugs. Epilepsy is not an indication for therapeutic abortion or cesarean delivery. Diazepam and chlordiazepoxide both affect the newly delivered infant.

Multiple sclerosis. Multiple sclerosis, a patchy demyelinization of the spinal cord and CNS, may be a viral disorder. Multiple sclerosis frequently develops initially after a pregnancy and is more common during the childbearing years. Multiple sclerosis may occasionally complicate pregnancy, but exacerbations and remissions are unrelated to the pregnant state. For this reason medically indicated therapeutic abortion is illogical. The burden of pregnancy and subsequent care of the child may warrant early interruption of pregnancy and sterilization in extreme cases. Women with multiple sclerosis occasionally may have an almost painless labor. The character of uterine contractions is unaffected by the disease, however.

Myasthenia gravis. Myasthenia gravis, a motor (muscle) end plate disorder that involves acetylcholine utilization, affects the motor function at the myoneural junction. This causes muscle weakness, particularly of the eyes, face, tongue, neck, limbs, and respiratory muscles. The peak prevalence of myasthenia gravis is about 25 years of age, and pregnancy may complicate the disorder, although some women experience a remission during gestation. Pregnancies in women with this disease can be carried to safe delivery if certain precautions are taken. Moreover, congenital myasthenia gravis is rare. Therefore the disorder is not an indication for therapeutic abortion.

The nurse and physician should be alert to symptomatology, such as easy fatigue, intermittent double vision, upper eyelid drooping, facial muscle weakness, and, in more serious cases, upper arm weakness and breathing difficulty. Infections may precipitate the onset or relapse and must be treated aggressively during pregnancy.

Parturients with myasthenia gravis usually tolerate labor well, because they already have some degree of muscle relaxation. Meperidine is the obstetric analgesic of choice. Local anesthesia is preferred. If a general anesthetic is required, a combination of nitrous oxide, oxygen, and cyclopropane generally is best. Oxytocin may be given, but scopolamine and muscle relaxants are contraindicated.

After delivery, women must be carefully supervised, because relapses often occur during the puerperium.

An occasional neonate born to a mother with severe myasthenia gravis may also show myasthenic signs sufficient to require neostigmine treatment for 1 or 2 months. Complete recovery of the infant is the rule. Infants born with the disorder do not have as good a prognosis, however, as infants born without the disorder.

DISSEMINATED LUPUS ERYTHEMATOSUS

As with other collagen disorders, when lupus erythematosus is not severe, pregnancy usually can be undertaken without great risk to the mother or fetus, especially if the woman is in remission. Cortisone therapy may or may not be required. If renal or vascular complications develop or the disorder is active, pregnancy usually makes the disease worse, and early therapeutic abortion may be warranted. Fortunately, disseminated lupus erythematosus does not affect the fetus.

NURSING MANAGEMENT OF MEDICAL COMPLICATIONS

A careful intake history and assessment of the woman's symptomatology at each prenatal contact provide the data base needed to initiate diagnostic tests. After diagnosis, the nurse assists the woman in the following ways:

1. To understand the disorder, its management, and probable outcome
2. To understand her role in the management, including when and how to take medication, diet, and preparation for and participation in treatment
3. To cope with the emotional reactions to a pregnancy and infant at risk

If the woman is hospitalized, nursing care is governed by the medical problem diagnosed. In addition, the nurse must consider the pregnancy, including fetal heart rate (FHR) and fetal activity, uterine activity, vaginal discharge, and discomforts of pregnancy. Tests for fetal maturity and placental sufficiency may be necessary. The community health nurse, social worker, and pediatrician are some of the resource people whose services may need to be incorporated into the plan of care.

Surgical Conditions Coincident with Pregnancy

The abdomen requiring immediate surgery occurs as frequently among pregnant women as among nonpregnant women of comparable age. Diagnosis is more difficult in the pregnant woman, however. An enlarged uterus and displaced internal organs may prevent adequate palpation and alter the position of the surgical process.

Differential diagnosis includes consideration of obstetric complications, such as ectopic pregnancy and premature separation of the placenta, and the onset of labor.

Mild leukocytosis and increased serum values of alkaline phosphatase and amylase are characteristic of pregnancy, as well as surgical intraperitoneal processes. Rising or abnormally high laboratory values are suspect, however. X-ray evaluation, a valuable adjunct to diagnosis, is contraindicated, particularly in the first trimester, except in extreme cases. The surgeon is confronted with both a surgical and an obstetric problem.

Laparotomy or laparoscopy may be required. Hazards of these procedures include abortion and premature labor. Surgical or anesthetic intervention does not affect the incidence of congenital malformations, however.

APPENDICITIS

Acute suppurative appendicitis complicates about 1 in every 1000 pregnancies. This disorder poses the following special problems during gestation:

1. Appendicitis is more difficult to diagnose during pregnancy. The appendix is carried high and to the right, away from McBurney's point, by the enlarged uterus.
2. Appendiceal rupture and peritonitis occur two to three times more often in pregnant women than in nonpregnant women.
3. Maternal and perinatal morbidity and mortality are greatly increased when appendicitis occurs during pregnancy.

Most cases of acute appendicitis occur during the first 6 months of gestation, with decreasing frequency through the third trimester, labor, and puerperium.

The differential diagnosis of appendicitis during pregnancy is also difficult because of gastrointestinal or genitourinary problems that may be confused with appendicitis. A high level of suspicion is important in the diagnosis of appendicitis.

Management. Appendectomy before rupture is extremely important. Antibiotic therapy before rupture is of questionable value; after rupture it may be lifesaving. Therapeutic abortion is never indicated in appendicitis. Cesarean delivery at or near term may be justified in association with appendectomy.

Prognosis. Maternal mortality increases to about 10% in the third trimester and is about 15% when appendicitis develops during labor. Perinatal mortality is approximately 10% with unruptured appendicitis but is at least 35% with peritonitis.

GYNECOLOGIC PROBLEMS

Ovarian cysts and twisting of ovarian cysts or adnexal tissues may occur. Pregnancy predisposes a woman to ovarian pathoses, especially during the first trimester. Pathoses include retained or enlarged cystic corpus luteum of pregnancy, ovarian cyst, and bacterial invasion of reproductive or other intraperitoneal organs.

Laparotomy or laparoscopy is required to discriminate between ovarian pathoses and early ectopic pregnancy, appendicitis, or other infectious processes.

See p. 833 for a discussion of common vaginitis.

ABDOMINAL HERNIAS

The incidence of abdominal hernias and related incarceration of the bowel is reduced during pregnancy despite permanent enlargement of umbilical or incisional hernial rings. Displacement of nonadherent bowel by the enlarging uterus and its shielding of so-called weak areas of the abdominal wall are fortuitous. In fact, temporary spontaneous reduction of some abdominal wall hernias occurs during gestation. In contrast, however, the uncommon irreducible or adherent hernias may become incarcerated as pregnancy progresses.

Women with hernias should not strain or bear down during the second stage of labor. Therefore low forceps delivery should be planned. Abdominal hernia is not an indication for cesarean delivery; herniorrhapy should be done as an interval procedure (i.e., between pregnancies).

CARCINOMA OF THE BREAST

The obstetrician should carefully check for breast tumors. Although breast cancer is an uncommon complication of pregnancy or the puerperium, a malignant neoplasm may develop to considerable size, obscured by the increased breast fullness during childbearing. Contrary to popular belief, however, pregnancy does not accelerate the progress of breast cancer. Hence therapeutic abortion is not medically indicated. If breast cancer is diagnosed during gestation, prompt therapy, for example, lumpectomy or radiation, should be effected. The 5-yr arrest of stage I breast cancer (cancer confined to the breast without nodal spread) diagnosed and surgically treated during pregnancy is about 65%. In stage II (cancer confined to the breast but with metastases to the axillary nodes on the same side), the likelihood of 5-yr arrest with radical surgery and irradiation therapy is only about 10%.

INTESTINAL OBSTRUCTION

Although intestinal obstruction (dynamic ileus) is not common during pregnancy, any woman with a laparotomy scar is more likely to suffer intestinal obstruction during gestation because of adhesions, an enlarging uterus, and displacement of the intestines. A dynamic ileus can also occur with incarcerated hernia, volvulus, or intussusception, but such cases are seen rarely by the obstetrician.

Persistent, abdominal, cramplike pain, vomiting, auscultatory rushes within the abdomen, and ''laddering'' of the intestinal shadows on x-ray films aid in the diagnosis of intestinal obstruction. Immediate operation is required for release of the obstruction. Pregnancy is rarely affected by the surgery, assuming the absence of complications such as peritonitis. Cesarean delivery is not indicated in intestinal obstruction.

VARICES AND HEMORRHOIDS

See p. 304 and Table 17.10 for discussions of varices and hemorrhoids complicating pregnancy.

NURSING MANAGEMENT OF SURGICAL CONDITIONS COINCIDENT WITH PREGNANCY

Principles of maternity nursing are added to those of nursing care of the surgical client. The preoperative and postoperative plan of care incorporates consideration for the woman's concern for her infant as well as for herself, fetal vital signs and activity, uterine contractility (labor may have begun), and constant vigilance for symptoms of impending obstetric complications. The woman and her family may have heightened concerns regarding effects of the procedure and medication on fetal well-being and the course of pregnancy.

Surgical Interruption of Pregnancy

Therapeutic abortion is the purposeful interruption of a previable pregnancy (before 24 weeks' gestational age of a fetus weighing less than 500 g). Indications for therapeutic abortion are as follows:

1. Preservation of the life or health of the mother (e.g., class III or IV heart disease)
2. Avoidance of the birth of an offspring with a serious developmental or hereditary disorder (e.g., Tay-Sachs disease)
3. Voluntary abortion (e.g., because of inability of the parents to support or care for the child, rape, mental incompetence, or severe emotional problems)

The control of birth, dealing as it does with human sexuality and the question of life and death, is one of the most highly emotionalized components of health care. Abortion as one of the surgical alternatives to contraception is regulated in most countries, presumably to protect the mother from the complications of abortion or because of religious constraints. The U.S. Supreme Court set aside previous antiabortion laws in January 1973, holding that first-trimester abortion is permissible in this country inasmuch as the mortality from interruption of early gestation is now less than the mortality after normal term delivery. Second-trimester abortion was left to the discretion of the individual states. Roman Catholic hospitals and some of those maintained by strict fundamentalists forbid abortion (and often sterilization) despite legal challenge.

Before the legalization of abortion, many illegal abortions took place, with little-documented sequelae other than death from infection or hemorrhage or both. Although studies indicate that biologic sequelae do occur after abortion, rates of biologic complications tend to be low, especially if the woman aborts during the first trimester. Studies related to psychologic sequelae reveal that they are short lived and related to circumstances surrounding the abortion, such as rape or the attitudes reflected by friends, family, and health workers. It must be remembered that the woman facing an abortion is pregnant and will exhibit the emotional responses shared by all pregnant women, including postdelivery depression.

In an attempt to regulate the conflict between professional responsiblities and personal ethics, the Nurses' Association of the American College of Obstetricians and Gynecologists (NAACOG) published a position paper on the nurse's role with the abortion client in May 1972, in which the simultaneous rights of each were described (Tyrer, 1973). Women have the right to expect and receive supportive, non-judgmental care, and nurses have the right to refuse to assist with abortions or sterilizations in keeping with their own moral or religious beliefs, unless the woman's life is in danger.

Compelling medical, surgical, or psychiatric indications for elective abortion are not numerous, but the following probably would qualify: class III coronary heart disease; fulminating (pelvic) Hodgkin's disease; stage 1B carcinoma of the cervix; and Marfan's syndrome with early aortic aneurysm.

The woman who is diagnosed as Rh negative must receive RhoGAM after an abortion.

The length of pregnancy and the condition of the woman determine the appropriate type of abortion procedure (Table 41.1).

Table 41.1
Interruption of Pregnancy: Basis for Counseling

Methods*	Advantages	Disadvantages and Side Effects	Effectiveness
First-trimester procedures			
Menstrual extraction: forced endometrial extraction through undilated cervix	Performed up to 14 days after missed period No legal proscriptions	Cervical trauma may occur, may lead to incompetence Hemorrhage	100% if implantation site is not missed
Prostaglandin: IV administration or injection into cul-de-sac of Douglas or by vaginal suppository or pessary	Stimulates smooth muscle Causes degeneration of corpus luteum	Requires about 24 hr to take effect May cause vomiting, diarrhea, chills, local tissue reaction Retained placenta necessitates D and C	100%
Vacuum (suction) curettage: cannula suction after cervical dilatation, under local anesthesia	Effective with relatively few complications: minimal bleeding, minimal discomfort 5-15 min duration Done on come-and-go basis	Pregnancy 12 wk or less Possibility of cervical trauma (decreased if dilatation accomplished by insertion of laminaria tent 4-24 hr before procedure): endometrial trauma possible Hazards: possible uterine perforation, hemorrhage, or infection	100% if implantation site is not missed and if other reproductive tract anomaly (double uterus) does not exist
Dilatation and curettage (D and C): cervix dilated, endometrium scraped with spoonlike instrument	Duration of 15 min Usually few complications	Pregnancy 12 wk or less Hazards: uterine perforation, infection (25%), effects of general anesthesia, cervical trauma	100% if implantation site is not missed
Second-trimester procedures			
Intraamniotic infusion: between wk 14 and 23 or 24 (uterus in abdominal cavity and sufficient amniotic fluid present)	Does not require laparotomy	Increase in complications proprotionately with weeks of gestation	Fetal death within 1 hr of injection; abortion completed within 36-40 hr
Transabdominal extraction: amniotic fluid extracted replaced with equal amount of saline solution (20%) (or 30% urea in 5% D/W)	Ambulation until labor starts (within 24 hr) and during early labor	Reaction to saline solution (hypernatremia): tinnitus, tachycardia, and headache Water intoxication: edema, oliguria (≤ 200 ml/8 hr), dyspnea, thirst, and restlessness Induced labor, occasionally explosive with an unripe cervix; fetus passes out of posterior vault of vagina and forms fistula Hazards requiring hospitalization (6% readmitted for complications): Hemorrhage and possible D and C May require postabortal D and C or vacuum extraction as well Fever with sepsis	Two thirds of fetuses aborted within 24 hr
Instillation of 40-45 mg $PGF_{2}\alpha$, E_2	Labor usually shorter than with saline solution Avoids complications of water intoxication and hypernatremia	May cause vomiting, diarrhea, nausea Fetus may be born alive D and C may be required to remove placental fragments	100%

Adapted from Bobak, I.M.: Nursing during the reproductive years. In Lagerquist, S., editor: Addison-Wesley's graduate nurse review, Menlo Park, Calif., 1982, Addison-Wesley Publishing Co.

*Prophylaxis against Rh isoimmunization, $Rh_o(D)$ immune globulin, is given within 72 hr to every Rh-negative, Du-negative, unsensitized (Coombs' negative) woman.

Continued.

Table 41.1—cont'd
Interruption of Pregnancy: Basis for Counseling

Methods	Advantages	Disadvantages and Side Effects	Effectiveness
Dilatation and evacuation (D and E)	Hospitalization shortened With skilled operator, complication rate lower than intraamniotic injection methods	24 hr before procedure, 2 or 3 laminaria tents required to dilate cervix to required 2 cm Fetus possibly born alive	100%
Second- and third-trimester procedures			
Hysterotomy: cesarean incision	Preferred method if woman wishes tubal ligation or hysterectomy to follow	Complications after major surgery—hemorrhage and infection Fetus possibly born alive, opening ethical, moral, religious, and legal problems Mortality risk—combination hysterotomy-hysterectomy 10% greater than with D and C	100%
Hysterectomy: at or before 24 wk without first emptying uterus	As above	As above	100%

EARLY ABORTION

Methods for performing early therapeutic abortion include the following:

1. Menstrual extraction—early aspiration of the endometrium in women who have not yet missed a period
2. Surgical dilatation and curettage (D and C) when newer aspiration equipment is unavailable
3. Uterine aspiration after one or two missed periods

The insertion of a small laminaria tent* retained by a vaginal tampon for 4 to 24 hours usually will facilitate the purposeful interruption of a first-trimester pregnancy by dilating the cervix atraumatically.

On removal of the moist, expanded laminaria, the cervix will have dilated two or three times its original (dry) diameter. Rarely will further mechanical dilatation of the cervix be required, because the insertion of an adequate-sized aspiration cannula (8.5 to 10.5 mm) almost always is possible. Cervical laceration and bleeding are reduced by the use of laminaria. A disadvantage is the delay necessary and the need for an additional visit to the physician's office or clinic.

The suction procedure for accomplishing an early therapeutic abortion (ideal time is 8 to 10 weeks since last menstrual period) usually requires less than 5 minutes and can easily be effected under paracervical block anesthesia and single sedation (Fig. 41.1). Bleeding after the operation normally is about the equivalent of a heavy menstrual period, and cramps are rarely severe. Infection such as endometritis or salpingitis occurs in about 8% of women, and a subsequent D and C procedure for bleeding or sepsis caused by retained placental tissue is necessary in about 2% of women. With good counseling and proper selection of women, serious depression or other psychiatric problems are rare.

The woman comes to the clinic or physician's office the day before the abortion procedure. An antiseptic solution is used to prepare the pelvic area. A vaginal speculum is inserted, and the vaginal canal and cervix are cleansed. Injection of a local anesthetic agent into the cervix may follow. Again the area is cleansed, and the laminaria tent is inserted into the endocervical canal. Prophylactic use of an antibiotic is usually begun. Some women experience a mild cramping or have light spotting from the anesthetic injection. Discomfort can usually be controlled with analgesics.

Aspiration abortion may be performed in the physician's office or in the hospital setting. If the woman chooses a hospital setting, she is admitted the day following insertion of the laminaria tent and is given preoperative sedation. (Physician and nursing interventions for suction curettage in which a local anesthetic is used are given on p. 994.) The vaginal area is cleansed (shaving is not necessary). The anesthetic agent is ad-

*For a definition of the laminaria tent, see glossary.

Fig. 41.1

A, Suction (vacuum) curettage machine. **B,** Suction method of therapeutic abortion. **C,** Suction (vacuum) catheters. (**A** and **C** courtesy Berkeley Bio-Engineering, Inc., San Leandro, Calif.)

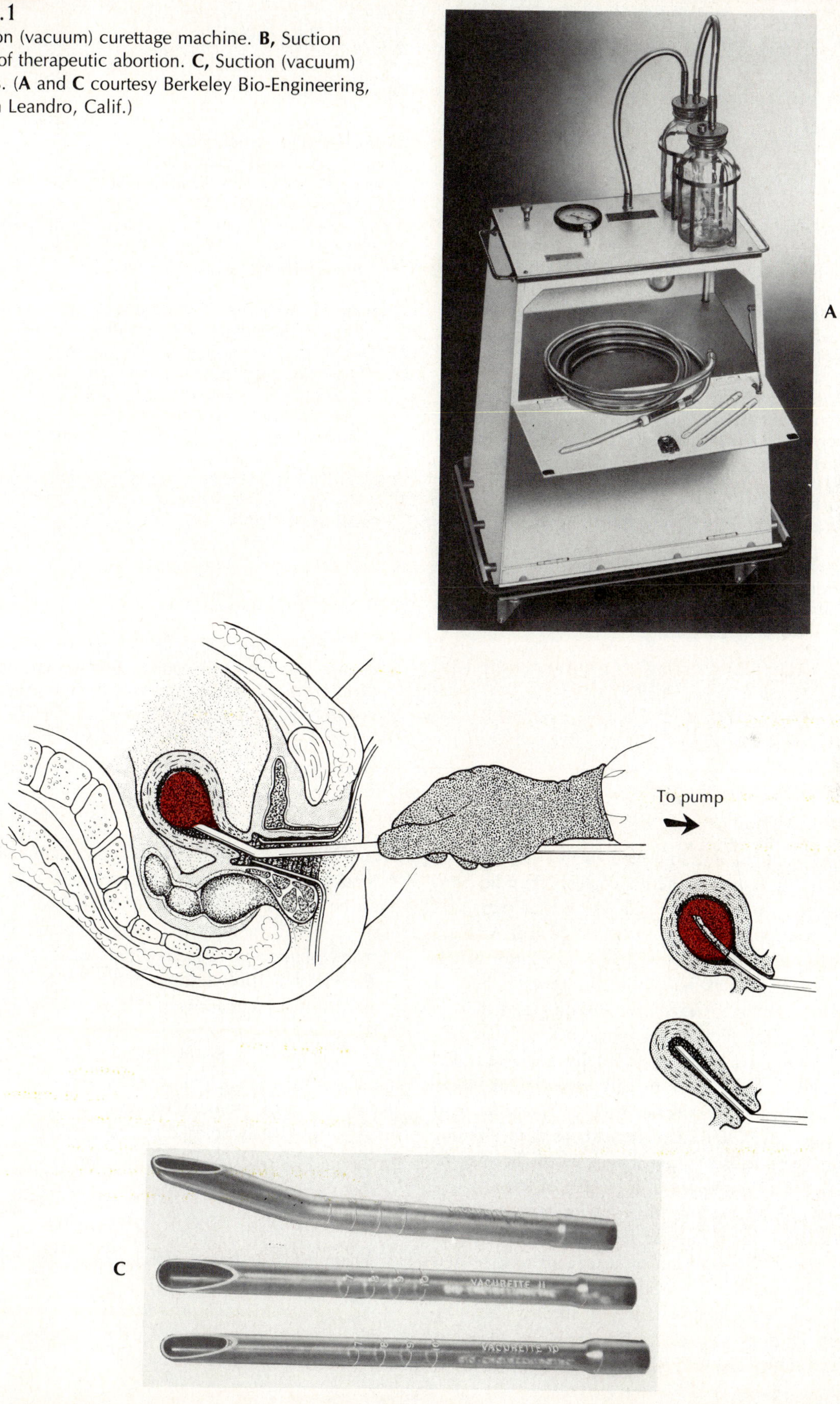

Suction or Vacuum Curettage Using Local Anesthetic

Physician interventions	Nursing actions
	Assess and encourage woman's support system.
	Assist woman to empty bowel and bladder.
	Prepare pelvic area with shave, if ordered. Wash pelvic area with antiseptic solution such as pHisoHex or povidone-iodine (Betadine).
Prepare woman for what to expect.	Prepare her for what to expect. Remain at head of table with her.
Insert sterile speculum and wash vaginal walls and cervix with antiseptic solution (cotton balls and ring forceps).	Explain: "The vagina is being washed. This will probably feel cold."
Inject local anesthetic agent (as for paracervical block) such as lidocaine (Xylocaine), and rewash vaginal vault with antiseptic.	Explain: "You will feel a needle stick as the anesthetic is injected. The vagina is being washed again."
Remove laminaria tent (if used) and sound size, depth, and position of uterus and configuration of cervix.	Tell her, "You may feel some cramping."
Dilate cervix until it is 1 mm greater than the number of weeks of gestation (e.g., for a gestation of 8 weeks, dilate to 9 mm).	As largest dilator is inserted, warn her, "You may feel some heavy pressure for 10 or 15 seconds now."
Insert vacuum tip (of same diameter as previous dilator or one size smaller) and rotate it around uterine cavity. Suctioning is accomplished within 30 seconds to 3 minutes.	Explain, "The noise you hear is the suction machine. This will last about 2 to 4 minutes. You may feel some menstrual-like cramping."
Examine aspirate to ensure that all products of conception have been removed.	
When indicated, gently scrape with sharp metal curette for any retained decidua.	
	Postprocedure care: Observe for vagal response and excessive cramping or bleeding. Check vital signs. If not done previously, during counseling interview that usually precedes the decision to have an abortion, counsel regarding birth control method she prefers.

ministered, and the dilatation and suction procedure is completed. The aspirated uterine contents must be carefully inspected to ascertain whether all fetal parts and adequate placental tissue have been evacuated. A single dose of oxytocin is usually sufficient to control bleeding. The woman may remain in the hospital 3 or 4 hours for detection of excessive bleeding and then is discharged. If the procedure is done in the physician's office, preoperative sedation is usually not given, and the anesthetic of choice is usually paracervical block. After the abortion the woman rests on the table until she is ready to get up. Then she remains in the waiting room until she feels she can travel, when she may be discharged in the company of a relative or friend.

Postabortal instructions differ with the institution (e.g., tampons may be denied for only 3 days or for up to 6 weeks, and resumption of sexual intercourse may be permitted within 1 week or discouraged for 6 weeks). The woman may bathe or shower daily. Instruction is given to watch for excessive bleeding, cramps, or fever and to avoid douches of any type. The woman may expect her menstrual period to resume 4 to 6 weeks from the day of the procedure. The woman must be strongly encouraged to return for her follow-up visit so that complications can be avoided and an acceptable contraceptive method prescribed.

Potential complications. Some conditions may be present in the pregnant woman that may result in hemorrhage with currettage or in missing the site of an implantation obscured by a submucous fibroid mass. Uterine abnormalities such as partially joined double uterus present a unique problem; for example, the wrong intrauterine cavity may be aspirated or curetted.

SECOND- AND THIRD-TRIMESTER ABORTIONS

There are four types of techniques used for second- and third-trimester abortions:

1. *Transabdominal intrauterine injection of hypertonic sodium chloride, used from the fourteenth week until the twenty-third or twenty-fourth week of preg-*

Table 41.2
Comparison of Prostaglandin and 20% Saline Solution Abortion Procedures

Prostaglandin	Saline Solution
No aspiration is necessary. The obstetrician injects 20-40 mg of $PGF_{2\alpha}$ into the amniotic sac.	The obstetrician inserts a needle into the intraamniotic sac, withdraws 200 ml of amniotic fluid, and injects 200 ml saline solution.
The procedure takes 1 or 2 min.	Duration of procedure is 15-30 min.
Contractions usually begin within the first half-hour after injection. Labor usually takes place within 24 hr.	Contractions usually begin approximately 12 hr after saline solution is injected; labor averages 36 hr.
It is not necessary to administer oxytocin IV; therefore woman's movements are not restricted.	To shorten labor, a continuous IV oxytocin drip is often administered. This restricts woman's movements for the reduced period of labor, approximately 24 hr.

nancy. The woman is admitted to the hospital for this procedure. Amniocentesis is performed. The physician determines where the needle (an 18-gauge, 7.5 cm [3-in] spinal needle) will be inserted. The area is cleansed, and if desired, a local anesthetic agent is given. Approximately 200 ml of amniotic fluid is withdrawn, and a similar amount of sterile 20% sodium chloride is injected. The woman is instructed to report when uterine contractions begin—generally within 8 to 48 hours. In most cases augmentation with oxytocin is necessary to effect uterine evacuation in a reasonable time. Occasionally reinjection is required. Labor begins, in theory at least, because the hypertonic saline solution releases the placental uterine progesterone blockade that normally prevents the onset of labor. The same careful monitoring of the contractions is as necessary as for a term delivery. Instruction in relaxation and breathing techniques is indicated, and analgesia can be administered for discomfort (see Chapter 25). The assistance of a supportive person at the time of birth of the dead fetus is essential. If the woman wishes to see the fetus, emotional support should be provided before and after the ordeal. Many women are relieved to find the fetus normal and frequently inquire as to its sex. After the delivery, the standard observations and care are carried out (see Chapter 31). Contraceptive counseling is given before discharge, and the woman is told to return should excessive bleeding occur.

Complications of hypertonic saline injection for second-trimester abortion, with the approximate frequency of their occurrance, are as follows:

- Postinjection infection (10%)
- Incomplete separation, requiring D and C (15%)
- Excessive bleeding, necessitating transfusion (2%)
- Disseminated intravascular coagulation (DIC)
- Potentially fatal hypernatremia caused by intravascular injection (rare)
- Uterine-vaginal fistula caused by unripe cervix and propulsion of fetus out of uterus through the uterine isthmus
- Severe hypotension or cardiac arrest (rare)
- Failure to abort (10%)

2. *Injection of urea solution after amniocentesis*. After the removal of about 200 ml of amniotic fluid, 200 ml of a 30% solution of urea in 5% dextrose in water is given by gravity drip. After 1 hour, a solution of 5 units of oxytocin in 500 ml of 5% dextrose in water is started. Fetal death occurs, and delivery ensues in most cases within 12 hours. Complications are less common and are less serious than with hypertonic saline solution.

3. *Transabdominal intrauterine injection of* $PGF_{2\alpha}$. The undesirable side effects of hypertonic saline solution, such as hypernatremia or DIC, do not occur with prostaglandins; therefore it has become the treatment of choice (Table 41.2). However, nausea and vomiting are common problems. Abortion usually takes place within 18 to 24 hours following injection. If it does not occur, the procedure is repeated, but only half the dosage is used.

The management of the three types of abortion just discussed is the same. Since anywhere from 1 to 4 days of hospitalization may be required, involvement of the family of the young teenage woman is almost inevitable. Measures taken to foster supportive relationships are part of nursing care.

4. *Abdominal or vaginal hysterotomy*. Hysterotomy may be chosen after more than 14 to 16 weeks of pregnancy, after failure of intrauterine injection of saline solution or $PGF_{2\alpha}$, and when sterilization is desirable. The vaginal approach is employed when transabdominal surgery should be avoided. The woman may remain in the hospital a week to 10 days. The management is comparable to that of cesarean delivery.

NURSE'S ROLE

The introduction of new members into cultural complexes has always been predominantly by birth. The need of a society to protect the welfare of these new members has prompted development of institutions, value systems, and rituals that regulate responsibility and dispense support. These become part of the fabric of a nation, its moral fiber, and changes are faced with reluctance and fear. International consensus for the necessity to limit population levels to those compatible with earth's resources and the subsequent legalizing of techniques for limiting the numbers of children precipitated moral dilemmas for persons such as nurses who have the knowledge and skills that are required for the safe use of these techniques. The values, beliefs, and moral convictions of the nurse are involved to the same extent as those of the pregnant woman. Since the conflicts and doubts of the nurse can be readily communicated to women who are already anxious and overly sensitive, health professionals need assistance to identify and come to terms with their own feelings.

It is not uncommon for confusion to arise as beliefs are challenged by the reality of care. A nursing student reacted to learning experiences associated with in-hospital abortions in the following manner:

> I really feel I believe in the rightness of therapeutic abortion, but when I watched the physician insert the needle and then inject the dose of prostaglandin, I felt an unreasoning rage sweep over me. I could have attacked him. Funny, I felt no anger toward the girl at all. I really need to rethink my beliefs.

Responses can also change with life experiences. A nurse who before her marriage had worked as counselor in a municipal clinic established a reputation as a supportive and concerned counselor of young persons with regard to birth control. Four years later she remarked:

> I've been trying to get pregnant for the past 3 years. I didn't realize how important it would be to me. You know I can't counsel about abortion any more. I can't be objective. I keep feeling, "Have your baby and please give it to me." I am more concerned about myself now, not them [the pregnant women], and counseling won't work that way.

Counseling about abortion includes help for the woman in identifying how she perceives the pregnancy; information about the choices available, that is, having an abortion or carrying the pregnancy to term and then either keeping the child or giving it up for adoption; and information about types of abortion procedures. The goal is to assist the woman in coming to a decision that is her own. She will need help to explore the meaning of the various alternatives and consequences to herself and her significant others. It is often difficult for a woman to express her true feelings (e.g., what abortion means to her now and in the future, and what support or regret her friends and peers may demonstrate). A calm, matter-of-fact approach on the part of the nurse can be helpful (e.g.: "Yes, I know you are pregnant. I am here to help. Let's talk about alternatives.") Listening to what the woman has to say and encouraging her to speak is essential. Neutral responses such as "Oh," "Uh-huh," and "Umm" and nonverbal encouragement such as nodding, maintaining eye contact, and use of touch are helpful in setting an open, accepting environment. Clarifying, restating, and reflecting statements, use of open-ended questions, and giving feedback are communication techniques that can be used to maintain a reality focus on the situation and bring her problems into the open. Once a decision has been made, she must be assured of continued support. Information about what is entailed in various procedures, how much discomfort or pain can be expected, and what type of care is needed must be given. If family or friends cannot be involved, scheduling time for the nursing personnel to give the necessary support is an essential component of the care plan.

Surgical Termination of Fertility

Since 1950, voluntary sterilization has grown rapidly in acceptance and is currently the most prevalent method of contraception in the world. Approximately 100 million couples choose voluntary sterilization, and the demand is expected to grow during this century. In the United States, voluntary sterilization is the most common choice of contraception for couples who are 30 years of age or older.

MOTIVATION FOR STERILIZATION

Motivation for elective sterilization includes (1) personal preference, (2) obstetric reasons, such as multiparity, (3) medical reasons such as hypertensive, cardiovascular, or renal disease in the woman or recurrent acute epididymitis in the man, and (4) diagnosis of inheritable disease.

Sterilization as a means of contraception may be requested by couples who have almost come to the end of their childbearing years and have the desired number of children or by young adults who have decided not to bear children. Persons in the first group are generally acceptive of the procedure even though there may be some feelings of regret because one of life's phases is over. Persons in the second group need the opportunity to explore the consequences of their choice.

LAWS AND REGULATIONS

All states have strict regulations for informed consent (see Chapter 5). Now many states in the United States permit voluntary sterilization of any mature, rational woman without reference to her marriage or pregnancy status. Although the partner's consent is not required, the client is encouraged to discuss the situation with her or his partner.

Sterilization of minors or mentally incompetent females is restricted by most states, and the operation often requires the approval of a board of eugenicists or other court-appointed individuals.

If federal funds are used, the person must be at least 21 years of age and mentally competent. Some state and federal regulations govern Medicaid funds for elective sterilization; for example, counseling and a waiting period following the decision are mandatory.

STERILIZATION PROCEDURES

Sterilization refers to surgical procedures intended to render the person infertile (Table 41.3 and Fig. 41.2). Most procedures involve the occlusion of the passageways (the oviducts [fallopian tubes] or sperm ducts [vas deferens]) for ova or sperm; however, only removal of the ovaries or uterus or both will result in absolute sterility for the woman. All other operations have a small but definite failure rate; that is, pregnancy may result.

FEMALE STERILIZATION

Timing of female sterilization. Female sterilization may be done immediately after delivery (within 24 to 48 hours), concomitantly with abortion, or as an interval procedure (during any phase of the menstrual cycle). Most sterilization procedures are performed immediately following a pregnancy, probably because of heightened motivation or increased practicality. Usually the woman is already in the hospital and all preoperative preparations (blood work, physical examination, etc.) have been completed.

However, all sterilization procedures have the lowest morbidity and failure rates when accomplished at a time other than immediately following a pregnancy perhaps because of the absence of tissue edema, which may permit the sutures to cut through the tubal wall.

Tubal occlusion. The operation used frequently is the laparoscopic tubal fulguration (Fig. 41.3). The woman is admitted the morning of surgery, having been NPO since midnight, and preoperative sedation is given. The procedure may be carried out with local anesthesia. A small vertical incision is made in the abdominal wall below the umbilicus. The woman may experience sensations of tugging but no pain, and the operation is completed within 20 minutes. She may be discharged 4 hours later if she has recovered from anesthesia. Any abdominal discomfort usually can be controlled with a mild analgesic (e.g., aspirin). Within 10 days the scar is almost invisible.

Complications. Major medical complications after elective sterilization are rare. Dysfunctional uterine bleeding or ovarian cyst formation may occur after tubal surgery, presumably because of disturbance of the uteroovarian circulation.

Tubal reanastomosis. Tubal continuity is not difficult to reestablish except after laparoscopic tubal fulguration, but the incidence of successful pregnancy after reanastomosis is only about 15%, probably because of

Table 41.3
Surgical Sterilization Procedures: Basis for Counseling

Occlusion Technique or Surgical Resection	Method of Gaining Access to Oviducts or Sperm Ducts
Female	
Ligation: with or without resection or with or without crushing	*Abdominal route:* in-hospital
Transection and burying of stumps into myometrium	Via laparoscopy
Fulguration (electrocoagulation) with resection of fulgurated portion	Minilaparotomy
Bands* (rings placed around the tubes, e.g., Falope ring)	Laparotomy (following cesarean delivery)
Clips* (placed over the tubes, e.g., Hulka-Clemens, Filshie)	*Vaginal route:* in-hospital
Chemical agents	Culdotomy
Removal of ovaries and/or uterus	*Abdominal route:* in-hospital
	Laparotomy or minilaparotomy
	Vaginal route: in-hospital
	Hysterectomy
Male	
Vasectomy: ligation and resection of small portion of each duct	Two small incisions in scrotum: physician's office or clinic
Clips (placed over tubes)	
Chemical agents	

*These occlusive devices have the theoretic advantge of possible reversibility.

Fig. 41.2
Sterilization. **A,** Tubal ligation. **B,** Vasectomy.

A

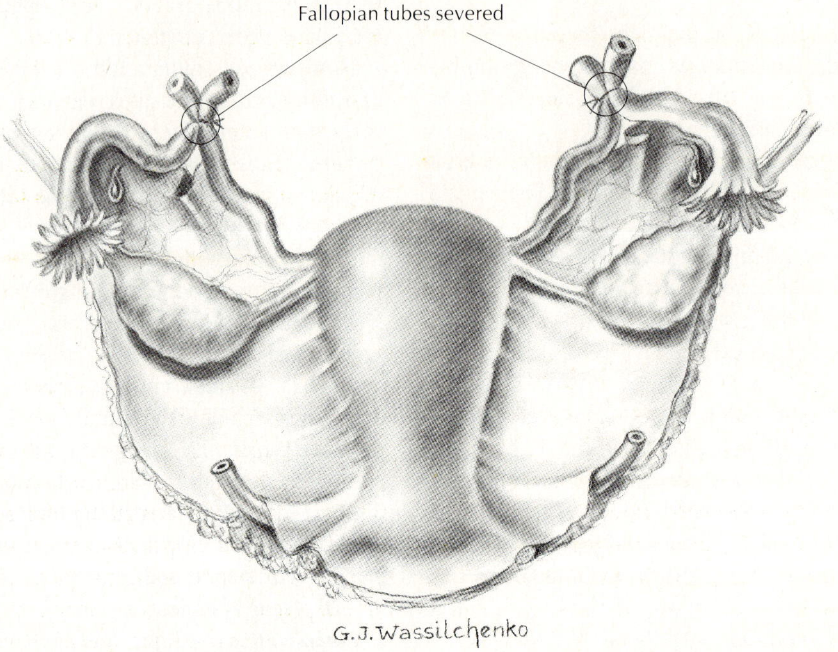

B

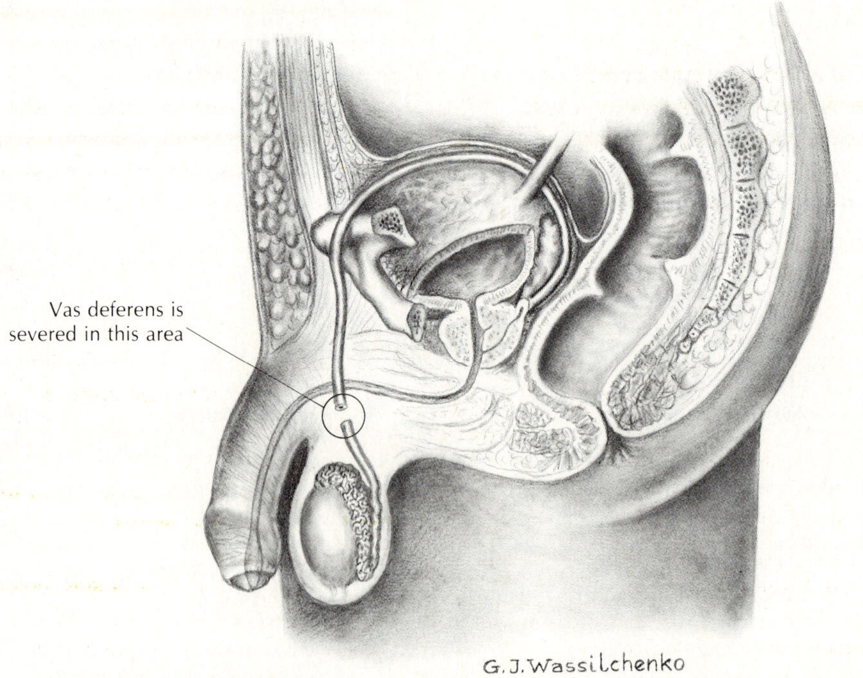

Fig. 41.3
Tubal ligation by minilaparotomy. Tenaculum is used to lift uterus upward *(arrow)* toward incision.

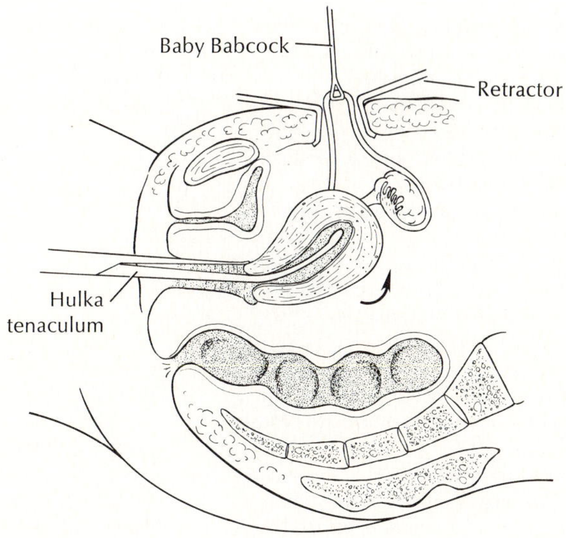

the loss of a segment of tube necessary for sperm capacitation and fertilization.

Hysterectomy. Hysterectomy, abdominal or vaginal, may be accomplished when pathosis such as in situ carcinoma of the cervix should be eliminated or for sterilization of the woman.

MALE STERILIZATION: VASECTOMY.

Vasectomy is the easiest and most commonly employed operation for male sterilization. In the United States since 1975, 1 million men undergo vasectomy each year. Vasectomy can be carried out with local anesthsia and on an out-patient basis.

In vasectomy, short right and left incisions are made into the anterior aspect of the scrotum above and lateral to each testis over the spermatic cord (Fig. 41.2). The vas is identified, doubly ligated with fine nonabsorbable sutures, and incised between the ligatures, or clipped. Occasionally, the surgeon fulgurates the cut stumps of the ducts. Many surgeons bury the cut ends into scrotal fascia to lessen the chance of reunion. Then the skin incisions are closed, generally with one nonabsorbable suture for each incision, and a dressing is applied.

To reduce swelling and relieve discomfort, ice packs are applied to the scrotum intermittently for a few hours postoperatively. A suspensory, or bandage, is applied to decrease discomfort by supporting the scrotum.

Moderate inactivity for about 2 days is advisable because of local scrotal tenderness. The skin suture can be removed 5 to 7 days postoperatively. Sexual intercourse may be resumed as desired.

Some sperm will remain in the proximal vas after vasectomy. At least 10 ejaculations and about 6 weeks are required to clear the tract of sperm.

Vasectomy has no effect on endocrine production or function of testosterone and on potency. Therefore secondary sex characteristics, potency (ability to have and maintain an erection), and volume of ejaculate are not affected. Men occasionally may develop a hematoma, discharge, or infection. Less common are painful granulomas from accumulation of sperm. Sperm production continues. Sperm unable to leave the epididymis are lyzed by the immune system. Some men develop antibodies against their own sperm (autoimmunization). Even if the procedure is reversed, many men may remain infertile because of this autoimmune reaction. Microsurgery to reanastomose the sperm duct can be accomplished successfully in 40% to 90% of cases.

Complications following bilateral vasectomy are infrequent and usually not serious: bleeding (usually external), suture reaction, and reaction to anesthetic agent.

Sterilization failures, usually due to a recanalization, are rare occurring in about 2 per 1000 men.

Table 41.4 summarizes sterilization methods, expected actions, advantages, disadvantages and side effects, and effectiveness and can serve as a basis for counseling.

NURSE'S ROLE

Counselor. The nurse plays an important role in assisting people with decision making so that all of the requirements for informed consent are met. Clients seek information about the various methods available and what to expect from the different methods of sterilization (Table 41.4). The nurse also provides information about alternatives to sterilization, for example, contraception.

The nurse acts as a sounding board for people who are exploring the possibility of choosing sterilization and their feelings about and motivation for this choice. The nurse records this information, which may be the basis for referral to a family planning clinic, a psychiatric social worker, or another professional health care provider.

Information about what is entailed in various procedures, how much discomfort or pain can be expected, and what type of care is needed must be given. Many individuals fear sterilization procedures because of the

Table 41.4
Summary of Sterilization Methods: Basis for Counseling

Method and Action	Advantages	Disadvantages and Side Effects	Effectiveness
Female			
Tubal occlusion: fallopian tubes ligated and severed, banded or clipped, or fulgurated, to prevent passage of egg	Abdominal surgery utilizing 2.5 cm (1 in) incision and laparoscopy. Ovaries and endometrium remain intact; menstruation continues	Major surgery with possible complications of anesthesia, infection, hemorrhage, and trauma to other organs Psychologic trauma in some women Sperm may enter peritoneal cavity if tubal ligature slips, and ectopic (abdominal) pregnancy may ensue	100% effective if ligatures, bands, or clips do not slip or cut through
Hysterectomy with salpingo-oophorectomy; no egg produced	No further menstruation	Abrupt loss of ovarian hormones, simulating menopause Possibility of major surgical complications Psychologic trauma in some perceived loss of femininity and sexuality	100% effective
Male			
Vasectomy: vas deferens ligated and severed or banded to interrupt passage of sperm	Relatively simple surgical procedure Does not affect endocrine production or function of testosterone Does not alter volume of ejaculate	Possibility of impotence in some men because of psychologic response to procedure Reversible in many cases Even if procedure is reversed, man may remain infertile if he has developed an autoimmune response (antibodies) to his sperm	100% effective after ejaculate is free of sperm that was in vas deferens (about 6 wks or 10 ejaculations)

imagined effect on their sexual life. They need reassurance concerning the hormonal and psychologic basis for sexual function and the fact that fallopian tube occlusion or vasectomy has no biologic sequelae in terms of sexual adequacy.

If federal funds are to be used for the procedure, the nurse assures that all of the legal requirements are met.

Preoperative preparation. Printed instructions are usually available for clients from the physician. The physician performs the preoperative health assessment, which includes a psychologic assessment and physical examination. The nurse assists with the health assessment, answers questions, and confirms the client's understanding of printed instructions (e.g., NPO after midnight). Ambivalence and extreme fear of the procedure are reported to the physician.

Postoperative care. Postoperative care depends on the procedure performed, for example, laparoscopy,* laparotomy, hysterectomy, or vasectomy. General care includes postanesthesia recovery, vital signs, fluid-electrolyte balance (intake and output, laboratory values), prevention of or early identification and treatment for infection or hemorrhage, control of discomfort, and assessment of emotional response to the procedure and recovery.

*See p. 172 for a discussion of laparoscopy, the procedure and postoperative care.

Discharge planning. Discharge planning depends on the type of procedure performed. In general, the client is given written instructions about observing for and reporting symptoms and signs of complications, the type of recovery to be expected, and the date and time for a follow-up appointment.

• • •

Personnel who function in birth control clinics or in hospitals must be carefully selected. Studies indicate that attitudes of personnel affect significantly the client's perception of the quality of care received (World Health Organization, 1971). This consideration is important in planning for the overall delivery of health services, since seeking help for fertility control is frequently the only contact young adults have with the health care system. Positive perceptions of the interest, concern, and technical skill of health workers in this instance may induce wider use of health facilities and care in the future.

References and Readings

Aby-Nielsen, K.: Physical sensations during stressful hospital procedures: a preliminary study of saline abortion, J.O.G.N. Nurs. **8**:105, March-April 1979.

Babaknia, A., et al.: Appendicitis during pregnancy, Obstet. Gynecol. **50**:40,1977.

Berger, J.M.: The relationship of age to nurses' attitudes toward abortion, J.O.G.N. Nurs. **8**:231, July-Aug. 1979.

Bishop, B.E.: The maternity cycle: one nurse's reflections, Philadelphia, 1980, F.A. Davis Co.

Buchsbaum, H.J.: Accidental injury in pregnancy, Contemp. Obstet. Gynecol. **20**(1):26, 1982.

Coughlan, B.M., and O'Herlihy, C.: Acute intestinal obstruction during pregnancy, J.R. Coll. Surg. Edinb. **23:**175, 1978.

Devees, C.B.: Hematologic disorders in pregnancy, Nurs. Clin. North Am. **17**(1):57, 1982.

Devore, N.E.: The relationship between previous elective abortions and postpartum depressive reactions, J.O.G.N. Nurs. **8:**237, July-Aug. 1979.

Executive Board of ACOG: Further ethical considerations in induced abortion, J.O.G.N. Nurs. **7:**53, May-June 1978.

Gibbs, C.E.: Sudden sensorium derangement during pregnancy, Contemp. Obstet. Gynecol. **20**(1):452, 1982.

Holbreich, M.: Care of the asthmatic during pregnancy, Contemp. Obstet. Gynecol. **21**(4):155, 1983.

Hyde, J.S.: Understanding human sexuality, New York, 1979, McGraw-Hill Book Co.

Johnston, W.G., and Baskett, T.G.: Obstetric cholestasis: a 14 year review, Am. J. Obstet. Gynecol. **133:**299, 1979.

Kjervik, D.K., and Martinson, I.M.: Women in stress: a nursing perspective, New York, 1979, Appleton-Century-Crofts.

Martin, J.N., and Morrison, J.C.: Sickle cell crisis: recognizing it and treating it, Contemp. Obstet. Gynecol. **20**(1):171, 1982.

Phipps, W.J., Long, B.C., and Woods, N.F.: Medical-surgical nursing: concepts and clinical practice ed. 2, St. Louis, 1983, The C.V. Mosby Co.

Ruff, C.C.: Childbearing in sickle cell anemia: a nursing approach, J.O.G.N. Nurs. **6**(3):23, 1977.

Tyrer, L.: The new morality, ethics, and nursing, J.O.G.N. Nurs. **2:**54, Sept.-Oct. 1973.

van Lith, D.A., Keith, L.G., and van Hall, E.V., (editors:). New trends in female sterilization, Chicago, 1983, Year Book Medical Publishers.

Wade, T.R., Wade, S.I., and Jones, H.E.: Skin changes and diseases associated with pregnancy, Obstet. Gynecol. **52:**233, 1978.

World Health Organization: Technical report series, Geneva, 1971, The Organization.

Wotring, K.E.: Adult respiratory distress syndrome as a complication of pregnancy, M.C.N. **4:**314, 1979.

Appendixes

A The Pregnant Patient's Bill of Rights

B Statements on Maternity Care and on Parent and Newborn Interaction

C Community Resources

D Nursing Magazines and Publications

E Nurse-Midwife Education

F Conversion Tables and Equivalents

G Standard Laboratory Values: Pregnant and Nonpregnant Women

H Human Fetotoxic Chemical Agents

I Standard Laboratory Values in the Neonatal Period

J Relationship of Drugs to Breast Milk and Effect on Infant

K Recommended Schedule for Active Immunization of Normal Infants and Children

L Brazelton Scale

M Birth and Death Certificates

N Standards of Care for Maternal-Child Nursing

APPENDIX A

The Pregnant Patient's Bill of Rights

The Pregnant Patient has the right to participate in decisions involving her well-being and that of her unborn child, unless there is a clear-cut medical emergency that prevents her participation. In addition to the rights set forth in the American Hospital Association's "Patient's Bill of Rights" (which has also been adopted by the New York City Department of Health), the Pregnant Patient, because she represents *two* patients rather than one, should be recognized as having the additional rights listed below.

1. *The Pregnant Patient has the right,* prior to the administration of any drug or procedure, to be informed by the health professional caring for her of any potential direct or indirect effects, risks or hazards to herself or her unborn or newborn infant which may result from the use of a drug or procedure prescribed for or administered to her during pregnancy, labor, birth or lactation.

2. *The Pregnant Patient has the right,* prior to the proposed therapy, to be informed, not only of the benefits, risks and hazards of the proposed therapy, but also of known alternative therapy, such as available childbirth education classes which could help to prepare the Pregnant Patient physically and mentally to cope with the discomfort or stress of pregnancy and the experience of childbirth, thereby reducing or eliminating her need for drugs and obstetric intervention. She should be offered such information early in her pregnancy in order that she may make a reasoned decision.

3. *The Pregnant Patient has the right,* prior to the administration of any drug, to be informed by the health professional who is prescribing or administering the drug to her that any drug which she receives during pregnancy, labor and birth, no matter how or when the drug is taken or administered, may adversely affect her unborn baby, directly or indirectly, and that there is no drug or chemical which has been proven safe for the unborn child.

4. *The Pregnant Patient has the right,* if cesarean section is anticipated, to be informed prior to the administration of any drug, and preferably prior to her hospitalization, that minimizing her and, in turn, her baby's intake of nonessential preoperative medicine, will benefit her baby.

5. *The Pregnant Patient has the right,* prior to the administration of a drug or procedure, to be informed if there is *no* properly controlled follow-up research which has established the safety of the drug or procedure with regard to its direct and/or indirect effects on the physiological, mental and neurological development of the child exposed, via the mother, to the drug or procedure during pregnancy, labor, birth or lactation (this would apply to virtually all drugs and the vast majority of obstetric procedures).

6. *The Pregnant Patient has the right,* prior to the administration of any drug, to be informed of the brand name and generic name of the drug in order that she may advise the health professional of any past adverse reaction to the drug.

7. *The Pregnant Patient has the right* to determine for herself, without pressure from her attendant, whether she will accept the risks inherent in the proposed therapy or refuse a drug or procedure.

8. *The Pregnant Patient has the right* to know the name and qualifications of the individual administering a medication or procedure to her during labor or birth.

9. *The Pregnant Patient has the right* to be informed, prior to the administration of any procedure, whether that procedure is being administered to her for her or her baby's benefit (medically indicated) or as an elective procedure (for convenience or teaching purposes).

10. *The Pregnant Patient has the right* to be accompanied during the stress of labor and birth by someone she cares for, and to whom she looks for emotional comfort and encouragement.

11. *The Pregnant Patient has the right* after appropriate medical consultation to choose a position for labor and for birth which is least stressful to her baby and to herself.

12. *The Obstetric Patient has the right* to have her baby cared for at her bedside if her baby is normal, and to feed her baby according to her baby's needs rather than according to the hospital regimen.

13. *The Obstetric Patient has the right* to be informed in writing of the name of the person who actually delivered her baby and the professional qualifications of that person. This information should also be on the birth certificate.

14. *The Obstetric Patient has the right* to be informed if

☐ From Haire, D. B.: The Pregnant Patient's Bill of Rights, J. Nurse Midwife. **20:**29, Winter, 1975. This article is not reproduced here in its entirety.

there is any known or indicated aspect of her or her baby's care or condition which may cause her or her baby later difficulty or problems.

15. *The Obstetric Patient has the right* to have her and her baby's hospital medical records complete, accurate and legible and to have their records, including Nurses' Notes, retained by the hospital until the child reaches at least the age of majority, or, alternatively, to have the records offered to her before they are destroyed.

16. *The Obstetric Patient,* both during and after her hospital stay, has the right to have access to her complete hospital medical records, including Nurses' Notes, and to receive a copy upon payment of a reasonable fee and without incurring the expense of retaining an attorney.

It is the obstetric patient and her baby, not the health professional, who must sustain any trauma or injury resulting from the use of a drug or obstetric procedure. The observation of the rights listed above will not only permit the obstetric patient to participate in the decisions involving her and her baby's health care, but will help to protect the health professional and the hospital against litigation arising from resentment or misunderstanding on the part of the mother.

APPENDIX B

Statements on Maternity Care and on Parent and Newborn Interaction

Joint Statement on Maternity Care (1971)

The American College of Obstetricians and Gynecologists, The Nurses Association and The American College of Obstetricians and Gynecologists and the American College of Nurse-Midwives recognize the increasing needs for general health care and, more specifically, the deficits in availability and quality of maternity care. The latter, which are not confined to any social class, can best be corrected by the cooperative efforts of teams of physicians, nurse-midwives, obstetric registered nurses and other health personnel. The composition of such teams will vary and be determined by local needs and circumstances. The functions and responsibilities of team members should be clearly defined according to the education and training of the individuals concerned.

To achieve the aims of providing optimal maternity care for all women the following recommendations are made:

1. The health team organized to provide maternity care will be directed by a qualified obstetrician-gynecologist.

2. In such medically directed teams, qualified nurse-midwives may assume responsibility for the complete care and management of uncomplicated maternity patients.

3. In such medically directed teams, obstetric registered nurses may assume responsibility for patient care and management according to their education, training and experience.

4. In such medically directed teams, other health personnel who have been trained in specific areas of maternity care may participate in the team functions according to their abilities and within the definitions of responsibility established by the team.

5. Written policies describing the specific functions of each of the team members should be prepared. They should be reviewed and revised periodically according to changing needs.

In endorsing the above statement, The American College of Obstetricians and Gynecologists, The Nurses Association of The American College of Obstetricians and Gynecologists and the American College of Nurse-Midwives recognize as their common goal the need for improvement and expansion of health services being provided for women.

In order to maintain a continuing evaluation of the health services being provided for women and to plan for needed improvements and expansion, a mechanism for continued communication between all the organizations responsible for their provision is being developed.

The American College of Nurse-Midwives
1012 14th St., N.W.
Suite 801
Washington, DC 20005

The American College of Obstetricians and Gynecologists
Suite 2700, Resource Center
One East Wacker Drive
Chicago, IL 60601

The Nurses Association of The American College of Obstetricians and Gynecologists
Suite 300, 60 Maryland Ave. S.W.
Washington, DC 20024

Supplementary Statement (1975)

Many questions have arisen concerning the meaning of the recommendation in the Joint Statement on Maternity Care (1971) that the health care team be "directed by a qualified obstetrician-gynecologist." These questions are justified and are accentuated by other developments in the speciality of obstetrics-gynecology which include the changing birth rate, formalization of new roles for personnel, emphasis on preventive care, HMOs, plans for national health insurance, PSROs, and regionalization of health services.

It is recognized that the obstetrician-gynecologist cannot under all circumstances be physically present to direct the health team; therefore it is essential that mechanisms of communication be clearly established for him or her to provide direction. Thus, the nature of the direction of the health team indeed becomes crucial.

The obstetrician-gynecologist working within a team giving health care to women has many responsibilities. These range from the direct provision of services to community health efforts and include:

a. The supervision of the medical care provided by all team members.
b. The direct provision of care for complications of pregnancy and for complex medical and surgical gynecological conditions.
c. The setting of medical care standards.
d. The provision of consultation to other team members.
e. The surveillance of task distribution within the team.
f. Participation in the ongoing educational activities of the team.
g. The introduction of new medical techniques as they become available.
h. The development of medical research.*

In view of the diversity of health care systems in which the obstetric-gynecologic health team currently functions, no universal systems model can be applied. Generally, however, the team is found in the following broad contexts:

1. Urban (intramural, on site, immediate referrals)
2. Rural (with institutional affiliation)
3. Rural (without institutional affiliation but with obstetric consultation available)
4. Private office (urban or rural)

The logistics of consultation and referral may vary with geographic and climatic conditions, but the following basic principles of team interaction are valid regardless of these conditions:

1. There must be a written agreement among members of the team clearly specifying consultation and referral policies and standing orders. The representatives of each practice discipline should participate in the development of and be signatory to the agreement.
2. The obstetrician-gynecologist, upon signing protocols, must accept full responsibility for direction of medical care rendered by the team in accordance with his or her orders.
3. In circumstances wherein the functions of the team leader are necessarily performed by physicians without specialty training in obstetrics-gynecology, medical direction should be provided through a formal consultative arrangement with a qualified obstetrician-gynecologist who is available to team members for continuing consultation and assurance of quality care.

*From "Medical Practice in the Obstetric-Gynecologic Health Care Team," Interorganizational Committee on Ob/Gyn Health Personnel, September, 1973.

Statement on Parent and Newborn Interaction (1977)*

Mothers separated from their young soon lost all interest in those whom they were unable to nurse or cherish.

Pierre Budin (1907)

Since the above 1907 statement of concern about the psychosocial cost of interference with parent and newborn interaction, increasing evidence has accumulated to support the concept of an "attachment and bonding" process in the human race. The major components of very early contact are touching, eye contact between mother and infant and parallel facial positioning (en face). Coincident with the development of that concept, the family-oriented birth process has received increasing acceptance by the providers of perinatal care. A more sophisticated public awareness, with emphasis on smaller families, has intensified the desire of mothers and fathers for greater involvement in all aspects of the birth and nurturing process in their families. Disruptions of the service and/or increased cross infection have not been reported when hospitals and professional staffs have encouraged early parent-newborn interaction.

It is timely to review all hospital procedures and professional practices for their appropriateness and thereby encourage the hospitals to reassess their policy in support of the bonding principle. Such a review should include: public health regulations, hospital admission policies, labor and delivery practices, and nursery and postpartum care. Reevaluation of existing practices must preserve the significant technological advances which have resulted in improved obstetrical and newborn care. Innovative alternative settings for birth in the hospital with adequate professional support should be explored and evaluated.

The Committee on Maternal and Child Care encourages medical staffs to continue to review hospital practices and, when necessary, to develop and formulate appropriate policies respecting all aspects of professional support for the birth and nurturing processes.

*American Medical Association House of Delegates, Chicago, December 4-7, 1977.

APPENDIX C

Community Resources

Alternative Birth Crisis Coalition
P.O. Box 48731
Chicago, IL 60648

American Academy of Husband-Coached Childbirth
P.O. Box 5224
Sherman Oaks, CA 91413
Teaches Robert A. Bradley's method of "Husband-Coached Childbirth," an offshoot of Grantly Dick-Read's method.

American Academy of Pediatrics
P.O. Box 1034
Evanston, IL 60204
Provides literature for families, parents, and health profession groups related to child health, illness, and welfare.

American Cancer Society
219 East 42nd St.
New York, NY 10017
Provides brochures on Papanicolaou (Pap) smears, smoking during pregnancy, and breast self-examination.

American College of Nurse-Midwives
1012 14th St., N.W., Suite 801
Washington, DC 20005

American College of Obstetricians and Gynecologists
Suite 2700
Resource Center
1 East Wacker Dr.
Chicago, IL 60601
Provides extensive lists of publications and resources.

American National Red Cross
17th and D St., N.W.
Washington, DC 20006
Provides service to the armed forces and their families; service to the veterans and their families; disaster services; blood services; health and community services.

American Society for Psychoprophylaxis in Obstetrics (ASPO)
1411 K St., N.W.
Washington, DC 20005
Teaches Lamaze technique of prepared childbirth to interested couples; prepares qualified people for teaching this method. Offers brochures, publications, teaching materials, and audiovisual aids.

Association for the Aid of Crippled Children
345 East 46th St.
New York, NY 10017
Devoted to the prevention of crippling diseases and conditions and to improvment in the care of disabled children and youth and their adjustment in society.

Association for Childbirth at Home, International
P.O. Box 1219
Cerritos, CA 90701

Boston Women's Health Book Collective, Inc.
Box 192
West Somerville, MA 02144
Publishes books concerning women's health.

Center for Family Growth
555 Highland Ave.
Cotati, CA 94928

Cesarean Birth Council
1402 Nilde Ave.
Mt. View, CA 94040

Cesarean/Support, Education, and Concern (C/SEC)
66 Christopher Rd.
Waltham, MA 02154
Provides informational pamphlets and slide presentations.

Channing L. Bete Co., Inc.
Greenfield, MA 01301
Publishes material regarding childbearing in cartoon form.

Child Study Association of America
9 East 89th St.
New York, NY 10028
Provides parent education materials.

Child Welfare League of America, Inc.
44 East 23rd St.
New York, NY 10010
Develops standards of service for the protection and care of children in their own homes or away from home through boarding home care, institutional care, adoption, day care, or homemaker service; and in community programs through the following means: cooperation with governmental departments of child welfare, publications, information exchange service, loan library and record forms, case record collection, and general information and education in the field service consultation and regional agencies.

Childbirth Without Pain Education Association
20134 Snowden
Detroit, MI 48235

Coalition for the Medical Rights of Women
4079A 24th St.
San Francisco, CA 94114
Provides classes (1) for expectant and new mothers and parents, (2) on health concerns of middle-aged women, (3) on lesbian health issues and self-health, (4) on fertility awareness, and (5) on natural birth control.

Cooperative Birth Center Network
Box 1, Route 1
Perkiomenville, PA 18074

Council of Childbirth Education Specialists, Inc.
168 West 86th St.
New York, NY 10024

Cybele Society
Suite 414, Peyton Building
Spokane, WA 99201

Ed-U-Press
760 Ostrum Ave.
Syracuse, NY 13210
Offers series of excellent cartoon books for adolescents and parenting classes.

Educational and Scientific Plastics, Ltd.
76 Holmethorpe Ave.
Holmethorpe, Red Hill Surrey, RH1, 2PF,
England
Offers numerous plastic models.

Family Service Association of America, Inc.
44 East 23rd St.
New York, NY 10010
Provides counseling and mental health services to families under stress, preventing family breakdown and promoting the development of family social work and wholesome family life through the following means: field service for family service agencies, assistance in development of qualified personnel in family casework, and information and research on family life.

Feminist Women's Health Centers
112 Crenshaw Blvd.
Los Angeles, CA 90005
Provides information regarding women's health.

Florence Crittenton Association of America
608 South Dearborn St.
Chicago, IL 60605
Unites in forming an effective and continuing organization; develops and maintains standards of service; in general, assists in bringing about a greater understanding of factors relating to unmarried mothers and adolescent girls with other problems in adjustment.

Holistic Childbirth Institute
1627 Tenth Ave.
San Francisco, CA 94122
Sponsors an educational program for teaching about childbirth.

Home Oriented Maternity Experience (HOME)
511 New York Ave.
Takoma Park, MD 20012

International Childbirth Education Association (ICEA)
P.O. Box 20048
Milwaukee, WI 55420
Assists individuals and childbirth groups who are interested in family-centered maternity. ICEA is a worldwide organization. Has an excellent film and record directory. Provides books and pamphlets (e.g., *Bookmarks* is an annotated catalogue of resources available that is published several times a year and is available free of charge).

La Leche League International, Inc.
9615 Minneapolis Ave.
Franklin Park, IL 60131
Provides support and brochures for nursing mothers and pattern for making a baby carrier.

Maternity Center Association, Inc.
48 East 92nd St.
New York, NY 10028
Publishes free brochure describing their many publications and pattern for knitted uterus.

National Academy of Sciences
2101 Constitution Ave.
Washington, DC 20418
Provides recommended dietary allowance and other nutrition resources.

National Association of Childbirth Education, Inc. (NACE)
3940 Eleventh St.
Riverside, CA 92501

National Association of Parents and Professionals for Safe Alternatives in Childbirth (NAPSAC)
P.O. Box 1307
Chapel Hill, NC 27514

National Childbirth Trust
9 Queensborough Terrace
London, W2, England
Offers books, films, and other aids for use in classes or in labor.

National Clearinghouse for Drug Abuse Information
P.O. Box 1701
Washington, DC 20013
Provides educational and informational materials related to drug use and abuse to professional and lay groups.

National Committee on Homemaker Services
1790 Broadway
New York, NY 10019
Promotes improvement in the quality of homemaker services and stimulates the extension of services under both voluntary and public auspices in communities throughout the country.

National Conference of Catholic Charities
1346 Connecticut
Washington, DC 20036
Gives particular emphasis to service for children and youth; i.e., foster care, counseling (unmarried parents), adoption services (statewide), short-term counseling to families and youth, emergency material assistance.

National Dairy Council
6300 N. River Rd.
Rosemont, IL 60018
Provides many teaching aids, including sets of food models pertaining to dairy foods and nutrition.

National Foundation/March of Dimes
1275 Mamaroneck Ave.
White Plains, NY 10605
Seeks to improve the level of care for all patients with arthritis and birth defects by national grant support of clinical study centers throughout the United States. Grants are made to teaching institutions to conduct clinical research and teaching and to provide patient care.

National SIDS Foundation
310 S. Michigan Ave.
Chicago, IL 60604
Dedicated to supporting medical research into the cause and prevention of sudden infant death syndrome (SIDS), helping parents of SIDS infants understand what is known about this mysterious disease, training health professionals to assist SIDS families, and educating the public and the professional community.

National Society for Crippled Children and Adults, Inc.
2023 West Ogden Ave.
Chicago IL 60612
Carries out the following three-point program: (1) education of the public, professional workers, and parents; (2) research to provide increased knowledge of the causes of handicapping conditions and their prevention and of improved methods of care, education, and treatment; and (3) direct services for crippled children and adults in the fields of health, welfare, education, recreation, rehabilitation, and employment; also charters and develops state and territorial societies to implement the program at the state and local levels.

National Society for the Prevention of Blindness, Inc.
16 East 40th St.
New York, NY 10016
Studies causes of blindness or impaired vision; advocates measures leading to the elimination of such causes.

National Tuberculosis Association, Inc.
1790 Broadway
New York, NY 10019
Studies tuberculosis and other respiratory diseases and disseminates information and stimulates the programs of its 2000 affiliated state and local associations for the prevention, treatment, and control of tuberculosis and other respiratory diseases.

National Women's Health Network
P.O. Box 24192
Washington, DC 20024
Provides information regarding women's health.

Nurses' Association of the American College of Obstetricians and Gynecologists
Suite 300, 60 Maryland Ave. S.W.
Washington, DC 20024
Provides numerous teaching aids and sponsors workshops for nurses.

Parents Without Partners, Inc.
80 Fifth Ave.
New York, NY 10011
Develops and provides a broad comprehensive program for the enlightenment and guidance of parents without partners and their children on the special problems they encounter and for assistance on the various readjustments involved.

Patient Counseling Library
Budlong Press Co.
5428 N. Virginia Ave.
Chicago, IL 60625
Provides videotapes (e.g., "A doctor discusses . . .") suitable for clinics or waiting rooms covering topics such as pregnancy, infant care, sexuality, breast feeding, and weight control.

Planned Parenthood Federation of America, Inc.
810 Seventh Ave.
New York, NY 10019
Provides leadership for universal acceptance of family planning as an essential element of responsible family life through education, service, and research.

Save the Children Federation, Inc.
345 East 46th St.
New York, NY 10017
Helps eliminate the causes of poverty among children in the United States and overseas while maintaining efforts to ameliorate the effects of poverty in those areas where the needs are greatest.

SIECUS
Human Science Press
72 Fifth Ave.
New York, NY 10011
Provides publications (e.g., ''Sexual relations in pregnancy and postpartum'') and teaching aids.

Trainex Corporation
Box 116
Garden Grove, CA 92642
Provides audiovisual aids suitable for childbirth and parent education.

Travelers Aid and International Social Services Association (TAISSA)
345 East 46th St.
New York, NY 10017
Assists youths and adults with problems related to travel, including returning to former residence, assistance in obtaining employment, and counseling for personal problems.

United Cerebral Palsy Associations, Inc.
321 West 44th St.
New York, NY 10036
Promotes research through a grant program; provides treatment, education, and rehabilitation of persons with cerebral palsy; subsidizes through grants-in-aid professional training programs of all types related to the problem of cerebral palsy; furthers, by professional and public education, information concerning all aspects of the problem of cerebral palsy; promotes better techniques and facilities for the diagnosis and treatment of persons with cerebral palsy; acts as a source of information on law and legislation in the field of the handicapped, including those disabled by cerebral palsy; cooperates with governmental and private agencies concerned with the welfare of the handicapped.

United States Government
Children's Bureau
U.S. Department of Health and Human Services
Washington, DC 20402
Consumer Product Safety Commission
Washington, DC 20207
Public Documents Distribution Center
Consumer Information
Pueblo, CO 81009
U.S. Government Printing Office
Washington, DC 20402
Provides information and publications on many aspects related to pregnancy.

The Women's Health Forum (Healthright)
175 Fifth Ave.
New York, NY 10010

For genetics clinics and treatment centers in area, contact the following organizations:

National Foundation/March of Dimes*
1275 Mamaroneck Ave.
White Plains, NY 10605

National Genetics Foundation, Inc.
250 West 57th St.
New York, NY 10019

Other resources include the following:

1. State Department of Public Health
2. Maternal and Child Health Services, Office of Economic Opportunity, Washington, D.C.
3. Local organizations: National Society for Crippled Children and Adults, Inc.; National Cystic Fibrosis Society; Muscular Dystrophy Association of America; organizations for parents of children with Tay-Sachs disease, sickle cell anemia, or crippling diseases; pediatric units in local hospitals and medical centers; city and county services (e.g., mental retardation).

*The National Foundation/March of Dimes publishes a directory of genetic services. It is involved in professional education, as well as research on genetic defects. The Foundation also sponsors programs for purchase of teaching and disseminating information to the general public.

APPENDIX D

Nursing Magazines and Publications

Behavioral Publications
72 Fifth Ave.
New York, NY 10011

Birth (formerly **Birth and Family Journal**)
110 El Camino Real
Berkeley, CA 94705
Quarterly publication, sponsored by International Childbirth Education Association (ICEA) and American Society of Psychoprophylaxis in Obstetrics (ASPO)

Bookmarks
ICEA Supplies Center
P.O. Box 20048
Minneapolis, MN 55420
Complimentary annotated catalogue of book reviews published several times per year

Briefs—Footnotes on Maternity Care
48 East 92nd St.
New York, NY 10028
Publication of the Maternity Center Association

Canadian Nurse
The Canadian Nurses' Association
50 The Driveway
Ottawa, Canada K2P1E2

Journal of the California Perinatal Association
16952 Ventura Blvd.
Encino, CA 91316

Journal of Obstetric, Gynecologic and Neonatal Nursing
Harper & Row, Publishers
Medical Department
2350 Virginia Ave.
Hagerstown, MD 21740
Journal of the Nurses' Association of the American College of Obstetricians and Gynecologists

Journal of Nurse-Midwifery
Mary Ann Shah (editor)
82 Willow Ln.
Tenafly, NJ 07670
or
American Elsevier Publishing Co.
52 Vanderbilt Ave.
New York, NY 10017
Official publication of the American College of Nurse-Midwives

Maternal/Newborn Advocate
The National Foundation/March of Dimes
P.O. Box 2000
White Plains, NY 10602
Complimentary quarterly publication of the National Foundation/March of Dimes

MCN The American Journal of Maternal Child Nursing
555 W. 57th St.
New York, NY 10019

Nurse Practitioner: A Journal of Primary Nursing Care
3845 42nd Ave. N.E.
Seattle, WA 98105

Nursing Research
555 W. 57th St.
New York, NY 10019

Perinatal Press
Perinatal Press Subscriptions
The Perinatal Center
Sutter Memorial Hospital
52nd and F St.
Sacramento, CA 95819

Sources for pamphlet and articles printed in various languages and for various ethnic groups may be obtained by checking with the local representatives of the following:

American Red Cross
17th and D St., N.W.
Washington, DC 20006

Merrell-National Laboratories
Division of Richardson-Merrell
Cincinnati, OH 45215
Offers informational publications regarding vaginal conditions and therapy and free loan of films such as "Vaginitis" and "Laparoscopy, the view within."

Ross Laboratories
Division of Abbott Laboratories
Columbus, OH 43216
Offers informational publications regarding nutrition for pregnant women and neonates and free loan of films such as "Amazing newborn" and "Death of a newborn."

Languages available in Ross Laboratories Instructional Materials*:

1. Spanish
2. Pictorial†
3. Vietnamese
4. Laotian
5. Korean
6. Cambodian
7. French/Haitian
8. Chinese
9. Hmong
10. Arabic
11. Japanese
12. Portuguese
13. Hebrew
14. Greek
15. Italian
16. Polish
17. German
18. Russian
19. Hindi‡
20. Thai‡

---

*Ranked according to number of items requested, July through December 1982.
†Formula preparation instruction sheets only.
‡First available in February 1983.

APPENDIX E

Nurse-Midwife Education

When a nurse-midwife is certified by the American College of Nurse-Midwives (ACNM), she is entitled to use the initials C.N.M. after her name.

Institutions offering ACNM-approved basic education in nurse-midwifery, internship programs, or refresher programs are listed below. Approval status is subject to change periodically. This information* is current as of August 1978.

American College of Obstetricians and Gynecologists
Nursing Division
1 East Wacker Dr.
Chicago, IL 60601

Booth Maternity Center R,I†
6051 Overbrook Ave.
Philadelphia, PA 19131 (215) 878-7800
in affiliation with
Maternity Center Association
48 E. 92nd St.
New York, NY 10028

College of Medicine and Dentistry of New Jersey CB
School of Allied Health Professions
Nurse-Midwifery Program
100 Bergen St.
Newark, NJ 07102 (201) 456-4249

Columbia University Graduate Program in Maternity Nursing and Nurse-Midwifery MB
Department of Nursing, Faculty of Medicine
Columbia-Presbyterian Medical Center
622 West 168th St.
New York, NY 10032 (212) 694-5755

*From ACNM-approved basic education in nurse-midwifery, J. Nurse-Midwife. **25**:44, March-April 1980.
†CB = Certificate basic program. Prerequisite is RN. Length is 8 months to 1 year.
MB = Master's basic program. Prerequisite is RN plus Bachelor's Degree. Length is 1 to 2 years.
R = Refresher program. For nurse-midwives who have not practiced in recent years and want to update their knowledge and clinical practice and/or take the National Certification Exam in order to become a Certified Nurse-Midwife. Length varies according to needs of individual but usually a minimum of 12 weeks is necessary to fulfill requirements for certification.
I = Internship. For recent gradutes of CB and MB programs who desire additional clinical experience. Length varies according to individual's needs.

Cuyahoga County Hospital I
3395 Scranton Rd.
Cleveland, OH 44109
ATT: Ms. Patricia J. Lupe, Education Program Director

Emory University MB
School of Nursing
Atlanta, GA 30322 (404) 329-7978

Frontier School of Midwifery and Family Nursing CB
Hyden, KY 41749 (606) 672-2901

Georgetown University School of Nursing CB
3700 Reservoir Rd., N.W.
Washington, DC 20007 (202) 625-7572

The Johns Hopkins University MB
School of Hygiene & Public Health
Nurse-Midwifery Program
Department of Maternal & Child Health
615 North Wolfe St.
Baltimore, MD 21205 (301) 955-3780

LAC/USC Medical Center I
Women's Hospital, Room 8K5
1240 North Mission Rd.
Los Angeles, CA 90033 (213) 226-3386

Medical University of South Carolina CB
Nurse-Midwifery Program, College of Nursing
171 Ashley Avenue
Charleston, SC 29403 (803) 792-2200

Meharry Medical College CB
Nurse-Midwifery Program
Department of Nursing Education
1005 18th Ave., N.
Nashville, TN 37207 (615) 327-6497

St. Louis University MB
Department of Nursing
Graduate Program in Nurse-Midwifery
3525 Carolina St.
St. Louis, MO 63104 (314) 664-9800

State University of New York CB
College of Health Related Professions
Nurse-Midwifery Program
P.O. Box 93
450 Clarkson Ave.
Brooklyn, NY 11203 (212) 270-1359 or 1360

United States Air Force CB
Nurse-Midwifery Program
Malcolm Grow USAF Medical Center
Andrews Air Force Base, MD 20331 (301) 981-6104

University of California at San Diego CB
Nurse-Midwifery Program
University Hospital
Primary Care Unit
225 W. Dickinson
San Diego, CA 92103 (714) 294-6113

University of California at San Francisco CB
San Francisco General Hospital
Room 6J5
1001 Potrero Avenue
San Francisco, CA 94110 (415) 821-5106 or 647-7828

The University of Illinois at the Medical Center MB
College of Nursing
Department of Maternal-Child Nursing
Nurse-Midwifery Program
P.O. Box 6998
Chicago, IL 60680 (312) 996-7935

University of Kentucky MB
College of Nursing
Lexington, KY 40506 (606) 223-5406

*Graduate credit offered.

University of Miami MB,R
School of Nursing
P.O. Box 248106, Main Campus
Miami, FL 33152 (305) 284-2830

University of Minnesota MB
3313 Powell Hall
500 Essex St., N.W.
Minneapolis, MN 55455 (612) 373-4199

University of Mississippi *CB
Nurse-Midwifery Program
2500 North State St.
Jackson, MS 39216 (601) 987-4823

University of Utah MB
College of Nursing
Graduate Major in Maternal and Newborn Nursing and Nurse-Midwifery
25 South Medical Drive
Salt Lake City, UT 84112 (801) 581-8274

Yale University School of Nursing *MB
Graduate Program in Maternal and Newborn Nursing and Nurse-Midwifery
855 Howard Ave.
New Haven, CT 06520 (203) 436-3673 or 3785

*Three-year program for non-nurse college graduates.

APPENDIX F

Conversion Tables and Equivalents

Metric system

The units of measurement in the metric system are as follows:

meter (m) for length
gram (g) for weight
liter (L) for capacity or volume
(NOTE: cubic centimeter [cc] also indicates volume.)

With these units the following prefixes are used:

micro 1/1,000,000 of a unit
milli 0.001 (1/1000) of a unit
centi 0.01 (1/100) of a unit
deci 0.1 (1/10) of a unit
deka 10 times the unit
hekto 100 times the unit
kilo 1000 times the unit
cubic the total area covered, measured in square lengths

Thus:

1 kilogram (kg) = 1000 grams (g)
1 gram (g) = 1000 milligrams (mg)
1 milligram (mg) = 1000 micrograms (μg or mcg)

Approximate metric and imperial equivalents

Useful approximate metric and imperial equivalents

1 cm = 0.39 in	1 in = 2.54 cm
1 meter = 1.1 yd	1 ft = 30.48 cm

To convert centimeters to inches

Divide the length in centimeters by 2.54.

Example: The average newborn infant measures 50.8 cm: = $\frac{50.8}{2.54}$ = 20 in

To convert inches to centimeters

Multiply the length in inches by 2.54.

Example: The average newborn infant measures 20 in: 20 × 2.54 = 50.8 cm

□ Adapted from Chinn, P. L., and Leitch, C. J.: Child health maintenance, St. Louis, 1974, The C. V. Mosby Co.

Avoirdupois and imperial systems

Weight

1 pound (lb) = 16 ounces (oz)
1 oz = 437.5 grains

Height

1 yard (yd) = 3 feet (ft)
1 foot (ft) = 12 inches (in)

Capacity

1 gallon (gal) = 4 quarts (qt) = 8 pints (pt)
1 qt = 2 pt
1 pt = 16 fluid ounces (fl oz)
1 fl oz = 8 drams (or drachm)
1 dram = 60 minims

Fluid volume

Useful approximate metric and imperial equivalents

1 L = 1.75 pt
1 oz = 30 ml
1 pt = 0.568 L, or 568 ml
1 gal = 4.55 L

Conversion table

LITERS		PINTS
0.28	0.5	0.88
0.57	1	1.75
1.14	2	3.50
1.70	3	5.28
1.28	4	7.04
2.85	5	8.80
3.42	6	10.50
3.99	7	12.30
4.55	8	14.08

To read the table: 3 L = 5.28 pt
3 pt = 1.70 L

Measurements

Domestic	Apothecary	Metric
1 teaspoon	1 dram	4 ml
1 tablespoon	½ fl oz	15 ml
1 teacup	4 oz	120 ml
1 tumbler	8 oz	240 ml

Temperature equivalents

Celsius	Fahrenheit	Celsius	Fahrenheit
34.0	93.2	38.6	101.4
34.2	93.6	38.8	101.8
34.4	93.9	39.0	102.2
34.6	94.3	39.2	102.5
34.8	94.6	39.4	102.9
35.0	95.0	39.6	103.2
35.2	95.4	39.8	103.6
35.4	95.7	40.0	104.0
35.6	96.1	40.2	104.3
35.8	96.4	40.4	104.7
36.0	96.8	40.6	105.1
36.2	97.1	40.8	105.4
36.4	97.5	41.0	105.8
36.6	97.8	41.2	106.1
36.8	98.2	41.4	106.5
37.0	98.6	41.6	106.8
37.2	98.9	41.8	107.2
37.4	99.3	42.0	107.6
37.6	99.6	42.2	108.0
37.8	100.0	42.4	108.3
38.0	100.4	42.6	108.7
38.2	100.7	42.8	109.0
38.4	101.1	43.0	109.4

To convert Fahrenheit to Celsius:
(Temperature minus 32) × $^5/_9$
Example: To convert 98.6 degrees Fahrenheit to Celsius:
98.6 − 32 = 66.6 × $^5/_9$ = 37 degrees
To convert Celsius to Fahrenheit
$^9/_5$ × temperature + 32
Example: To convert 40 degrees Celsius to Fahrenheit:
$^9/_5$ × 40 = 72 + 32 = 104 degrees

Converting French size into millimeters or inches*

French size†	Diameter (mm)	Diameter (inches)
1	⅓	0.013
2	⅔	0.026
3	1	0.039
4	1⅓	0.052
5	1⅔	0.065
6	2	0.078
7	2⅓	0.091
8	2⅔	0.104
9	3	0.118
10	3⅓	0.131
11	3⅔	0.144
12	4	0.157
13	4⅓	0.170
14	4⅔	0.183
15	5	0.196
16	5⅓	0.209
17	5⅔	0.223
18	6	0.236
19	6⅓	0.249
20	6⅔	0.262
21	7	0.275
22	7⅓	0.288
23	7⅔	0.301
24	8	0.314
25	8⅓	0.328
26	8⅔	0.341
27	9	0.354
28	9⅓	0.367
29	9⅔	0.380
30	10	0.393

*Courtesy Sterilon Corporation, Buffalo, N.Y.
†Since many catheters are labeled in French sizes, the above information is presented to aid the nurse in selecting the most appropriate size catheter for use.

Conversion of inches to centimeters

Inches	Centimeters	Inches	Centimeters
¼	0.635	14½	36.83
½	1.27	15	38.10
1	2.54	15½	39.37
2	5.08	16	40.64
3	7.62	16½	41.91
4	10.16	17	43.18
5	12.70	17½	44.45
6	15.24	18	45.72
7	17.78	18½	46.99
8	20.32	19	48.26
9	22.86	19½	49.53
10	25.40	20	50.80
10½	26.67	20½	52.07
11	27.94	21	53.34
11½	29.21	21½	54.61
12	30.48	22	55.88
12½	31.75	22½	57.15
13	33.02	23	58.42
13½	34.29	23½	56.69
14	35.56	24	60.96

Approximate weight equivalents

Apothecary	Metric
1/600 grain	0.1 mg
1/300 grain *or* 1/320 grain*	0.2 mg
1/200 grain *or* 1/210 grain	0.3 mg
1/160 grain	0.4 mg
1/120 grain	0.5 mg
1/100 grain	0.6 mg *or* 0.65 mg
1/60 grain *or* 1/64 grain	1.0 mg
1/32 grain	2.0 mg
1/20 grain	3.0 mg
1/16 grain	4.0 mg
1/12 grain	5.4 mg
1/10 grain	6.4 *or* 6.0 mg
1/8 grain	8.0 mg
1/6 grain	11.0 mg
1/4 grain	16.0 *or* 15.0 mg
1/3 grain	22.0 *or* 20.0 mg
3/8 grain	24.0 mg
1/2 grain	32.0 *or* 30.0 mg
3/4 grain	50.0 mg
1 grain	64.0 *or* 60.0 mg
1 1/2 grains	0.1 g (100 mg)
2 grains	0.128 or 0.12 g
2 1/2 grains	0.16 *or* 15.0 g
3 grains	0.2 g
4 grains	0.25 g
5 grains	0.32 g
7 1/2 grains	0.5 g
10 grains	0.64 *or* 0.6 g
15 grains	1.0 g
1 dram	4.0 g
1 ounce	30.0 g

*Discrepancy occurs because 1 grain = 60 mg, or 1 grain = 64 mg, depending on the source.

Conversion of pounds and ounces to grams for newborn weights*

Pounds \ Ounces	0	1	2	3	4	5	6	7	8	9	10	11	12	13	14	15	Pounds
0	—	28	57	85	113	142	170	198	227	255	283	312	430	369	397	425	0
1	454	482	510	539	567	595	624	652	680	709	737	765	794	822	850	879	1
2	907	936	964	992	1021	1049	1077	1106	1134	1162	1191	1219	1247	1276	1304	1332	2
3	1361	1389	1417	1446	1474	1503	1531	1559	1588	1616	1644	1673	1701	1729	1758	1786	3
4	1814	1843	1871	1899	1928	1956	1984	2013	2041	2070	2098	2126	2155	2183	2211	2240	4
5	2268	2296	2325	2353	2381	2410	2438	2466	2495	2523	2551	2580	2608	2637	2665	2693	5
6	2722	2750	2778	2807	2835	2863	2892	2920	2948	2977	3005	3033	3062	3090	3118	3147	6
7	3175	3203	3232	3260	3289	3317	3345	3374	3402	3430	3459	3487	3515	3544	3572	3600	7
8	3629	3657	3685	3714	3742	3770	3799	3827	3856	3884	3912	3941	3969	3997	4026	4054	8
9	4082	4111	4139	4167	4196	4224	4252	4281	4309	4337	4366	4394	4423	4451	4479	4508	9
10	4536	4564	4593	4621	4649	4678	4706	4734	4763	4791	4819	4848	4876	4904	4933	4961	10
11	4990	5018	5046	5075	5103	5131	5160	5188	5216	5245	5273	5301	5330	5358	5386	5415	11
12	5443	5471	5500	5528	5557	5585	5613	5642	5670	5698	5727	5755	5783	5812	5840	5868	12
13	5897	5925	5953	5982	6010	6038	6067	6095	6123	6152	6180	6209	6237	6265	6294	6322	13
14	6350	6379	6407	6435	6464	6492	6520	6549	6577	6605	6634	6662	6690	6719	6747	6776	14
15	6804	6832	6860	6889	6917	6945	6973	7002	7030	7059	7087	7115	7144	7172	7201	7228	15
Ounces	0	1	2	3	4	5	6	7	8	9	10	11	12	13	14	15	

*To convert pounds and ounces to grams, multiply the pounds by 453.6 and the ounces by 28.35; add the totals.
To convert grams into pounds and decimals of a pound, multiply the grams by 0.0022.
To convert grams into ounces, divide the grams by 28.35 (16 oz = 1 lb).

APPENDIX G

Standard Laboratory Values: Pregnant and Nonpregnant Women

	Nonpregnant	Pregnant
Hematologic values		
Complete blood count (CBC)		
Hemoglobin, g/dl	12-16*	10-14*
Hematocrit, PCV, %	37-47	32-42
Red cell volume, ml	1600	1900
Plasma volume, ml	2400	3700
Red blood cell count, million/cu mm	4-5.5	4-5.5
White blood cells, total per cu mm	4500-10,000	5000-15,000
Polymorphonuclear cells, %	54-62	60-85
Lymphocytes, %	38-46	15-40
Erythrocyte sedimentation rate, mm/hr	≤20	30-90
MCHC, g/dl packed RBCs (mean corpuscular hemoglobin concentration)	30-36	No change
MCH/(mean corpuscular hemoglobin per picogram [less than a micromicrogram])	29-32	No change
MCV/cu μm (mean corpuscular volume per cubic micrometer)	82-96	No change
Blood coagulation and fibrinolytic activity†		
Factors VII, VIII, IX, X		Increase in pregnancy, return to normal in early puerperium; factor VIII increases during and immediately after delivery
Factors XI, XIII		Decrease in pregnancy
Prothrombin time (protime)	60-70 sec	Slight decrease in pregnancy
Partial prothrombin time (PTT)	12-14 sec	Slight decrease in pregnancy and again decrease during second and after third stage of labor (indicates clotting at placental site)
Bleeding time	1-3 min (Duke) 2-4 min (Ivy)	No appreciable change
Coagulation time	6-10 min (Lee/White)	No appreciable change
Platelets	150,000 to 350,000 cu mm	No significant change until 3-5 days after delivery, then marked increase (may predispose woman to thrombosis) and gradual return to normal
Fibrinolytic activity		Decreases in pregnancy, then abrupt return to normal (protection against thromboembolism)
Fibrinogen	250 mg/dl	400 mg/dl

*At sea level. Permanent residents of higher levels (e.g., Denver) require higher levels of hemoglobin.
†Pregnancy represents a hypercoagulable state.

	Nonpregnant	Pregnant
Hematologic values—cont'd		
Mineral/vitamin concentrations		
Serum iron, μg	75-150	65-120
Total iron-binding capacity, μg	250-450	300-500
Iron saturation, %	30-40	15-30
Vitamin B_{12}, folic acid, ascorbic acid	Normal	Moderate decrease
Serum proteins		
Total, g/dl	6.7-8.3	5.5-7.5
Albumin, g/dl	3.5-5.5	3.0-5.0
Globulin, total, g/dl	2.3-3.5	3.0-4.0
Blood sugar		
Fasting, mg/dl	70-80	65
2-hour postprandial, mg/dl	60-110	Under 140 after a 100 g carbohydrate meal is considered normal
Cardiovascular determinations		
Blood pressure, mm Hg	120/80*	114/65
Peripheral resistance, dyne/sec-cm^{-5}	120	100
Venous pressure, cm H_2O		
Femoral	9	24
Antecubital	8	8
Pulse, rate/min	70	80
Stroke volume, ml	65	75
Cardiac output, L/min	4.5	6
Circulation time (arm-tongue), sec	15-16	12-14
Blood volume, ml		
Whole blood	4000	5600
Plasma	2400	3700
Red blood cells	1600	1900
Plasma renin, units/L	3-10	10-80
Chest x-ray studies		
Transverse diameter of heart	—	1-2 cm increase
Left border of heart	—	Straightened
Cardiac volume	—	70 ml increase
Electrocardiogram	—	15° left axis deviation
V_1 and V_2	—	Inverted T wave
V_4	—	Low T
III	—	Q + inverted T
aVr	—	Small Q

*For the woman about 20 years of age.
10 years of age: 103/70.
30 years of age: 123/82.
40 years of age: 126/84.

Continued.

Standard laboratory values: pregnant and nonpregnant women—cont'd

	Nonpregnant	Pregnant
Hepatic values		
Bilirubin total	Not more than 1 mg/dl	Unchanged
Cephalin flocculation	Up to 2+ in 48 hr	Positive in 10%
Serum cholesterol	110-300 mg/dl	↑60% from 16 to 32 wk of pregnancy; remains at this level until after delivery
Thymol turbidity	0-4 units	Positive in 15%
Serum alkaline phosphatase	2-4.5 units (Bodansky)	↑from wk 12 of pregnancy to 6 wk after delivery
Serum lactate dehydrogenase		Unchanged
Serum glutamic-oxaloacetic transaminase		Unchanged
Serum globulin albumin	1.5-3.0 g/dl 4.5-5.5 g/dl	↑slight ↓3.0 g by late pregnancy
A/G ratio		Decreased
α_2-globulin		Increased
β-globulin		Increased
Serum cholinesterase		Decreased
Leucine aminopeptidase		Increased
Sulfobromophthalein (5 mg/kg)	5% dye or less in 45 min	Somewhat decreased
Renal values		
Bladder capacity	1300 ml	1500 ml
Renal plasma flow (RPF), ml/min	490-700	Increase by 25%, to 612-875
Glomerular filtration rate (GFR), ml/min	105-132	Increase by 50%, to 160-198
Nonprotein nitrogen (NPN), mg/dl	25-40	Decreases
Blood urea nitrogen (BUN), mg/dl	20-25	Decreases
Serum creatinine, mg/kg/24 hr	20-22	Decreases
Serum uric acid, mg/kg/24 hr	257-750	Decreases
Urine glucose	Negative	Present in 20% of gravidas
Intravenous pyelogram (IVP)	Normal	Slight to moderate hydroureter and hydronephrosis; right kidney larger than left kidney
Miscellaneous laboratory values		
Total thyroxine concentration	5-12 μg/dl thyroxine	↑9-16 μg/dl thyroxine (however, unbound thyroxine not greatly increased)
Ionized calcium		Relatively unchanged
Aldosterone		↑1 mg/24 hr by third trimester
Dehydroisoandrosterone	Plasma clearance 6-8 L/24 hr	↑plasma clearance tenfold to twentyfold

Commonly used drugs that affect urine glucose determinations*

Drug	Clinitest	Testape, Keto-Diastix	Comments
Ascorbic acid (vitamin C)	False positive	False	Inhibits glucose-oxidase (Testape, Keto-Diastix); large doses produce false negative result with Clinitest
Cephalexin (Keflex)			
Cephaloridine (Loridine)	False positive		Confusing black-brown color
Cephalothin (Keflin)			
Chloral hydrate (Noctec)	False positive		Only with large doses
Chloramphenicol (Chloromycetin)	False positive†		
Isoniazid (INH)			False positive result with Benedict's; also has hyperglycemic activity and therefore may produce true glycosuria
Levodopa (L-dopa) (Dopar, Larodopa)			Small doses, either may result; doses 3.5-5 g, both result
Metaxalone (Skelaxin)	False negative		
Methyldopa (Aldomet)	False positive		One possible case reported
Nalidixic acid (NegGram)	False positive		
Probenecid (Benemid)	False positive		
Salicylates	False positive	False negative	Due to gentisic acid metabolite; occasional use of aspirin not likely to affect test significantly
Sulfonamides (Gantanol, Gantrisin, etc.)	False positive†		
Tetracycline	False positive		May be due to large amounts of ascorbic acid in parenteral product

*From Jensen, M. D., and Bobak, I. M.: Handbook of maternity care: a guide for nursing practice, St. Louis, 1980, The C. V. Mosby Co.; data from Drug Intell. Clin. Pharm. **8**(7):422-429, July 1974, and from Applied therapeutics for clinical pharmacists, 1975, pp. 229-232.
†Substantiating information not given.

APPENDIX H

Human Fetotoxic Chemical Agents

Maternal medication	Reported effect on fetus or neonate
Analgesics	
Indomethacin (Indocin)	Prolongs gestation (monkey); in neonates, used to close patent ductus arteriosus
Narcotics	70% of maternal level; death, apnea, depression, bradycardia, hypothermia
Salicylates	Death in utero; hemorrhage, methemoglobinemia, ↓ albumin-binding capacity, salicylate intoxication, difficult delivery, ? prolonged gestation
Anesthesia	
Conduction	Indirect effect of maternal hypotension; direct effect—convulsions, death, acidosis, bradycardia, myocardial depression, fetal hypotension, methemoglobinemia
General	Apnea, depression (prolonged inhalation by gravid (female), ? congenital malformations, chromosomal abnormality*; ether has direct narcotic effect on infant
Ether	
Halothane (Fluothane)	
Trichloroethylene (Trilene)	
Hypnosis	Indirect effect of maternal hyperventilation and excessive bearing down
Local	
Paracervical	Methemoglobinemia, fetal acidosis, bradycardia, neurologic depression, myocardial depression
Anticoagulants	
Coumarins	Fetal death, hemorrhage, calcifications
Anticonvulsant agents	
Barbiturates	Irritability and tremulousness 4-5 mo after delivery; hemorrhage, enzyme inducer
Paramethadione (Paradione)	CHD, microphthalmia, mental retardation, abortion
Phenytoin and barbiturate	Congenital malformations, cleft lip and palate, congenital heart disease (CHD), CNS and skeletal anomalies, failure to thrive, enzyme inducer, hemorrhage
Trimethadione (Tridione)	
Antidiabetics	*See* hypoglycemic agents
Antimalarial	
Quinine	? Congenital anomalies of CNS and extremities, thrombocytopenia, hypoplastic optic nerve, congenital deafness
Antimicrobials	All antimicrobials cross placenta
Ampicillin	↓ Maternal urinary and plasma estriol levels
Cephaloridine	Blood levels maintained for hours after delivery; ? false positive direct Coombs' test
Chloramphenicol	Crosses placenta with no reported effect; interferes with biotransformation of tolbutamide, phenytoin, biohydroxycoumarin (i.e., hypoglycemia may occur if used in combination)
Chloroquine	Death, deafness, retinal hemorrhage
Erythromycin	Possible hepatic injury
Nitrofurantoin	Megaloblastic anemia, G6PD deficiency
Novobiocin	Hyperbilirubinemia
Quinine, quinidine	Possible ototoxicity, thrombocytopenia
Streptomycin	Therapeutic levels reached, nerve deafness
Sulfonamides	
Long and short acting	Icterus, hemolytic anemia, kernicterus, ? growth retardation, thrombocytopenia
Tetracycline	Placental transfer after 4 months' gestation; enamel hypoplasia, delay in bone growth, ? congenital cataract

□ Modified from Babson, S. G., Benson, R. C., Pernoll, M. L., and Benda, G. I.: Management of high-risk pregnancy and intensive care of the neonate, ed. 3, St. Louis, 1975, The C. V. Mosby Co., p. 133; and Perinatal pharmacology, Mead Johnson Symposium on Perinatal and Developmental Medicine (no. 5), Vail, Colo., June 9-13, 1974.

*Pregnant nurses working in operating rooms have shown a higher incidence of abortion, stillbirths, and congenital anomalies for unknown reasons.

Maternal medication	Reported effect on fetus or neonate
Antituberculous	
Isoniazid	Toxic blood level in fetus; no reported effect; mother should be on pyridoxine supplement
Pyridoxine	*See* vitamins
Belladonna derivatives	
Atropine	Intrauterine tachycardia; dilated, nonreacting pupils
Scopolamine	? Delays labor, ? delays respiration, deleterious to premature infant
Cancer chemotherapeutic agents	
Aminopterin Busulfan Cyclophosphamide 6-Mercaptopurine Methotrexate	Abortion, congenital anomalies (first trimester); combination of drugs detrimental to fetus; skeletal and cranial malformations, hydrocephalus; questionable long-term effects = slow somatic growth; ovarian agenesis; ↓ immune mechanisms
Cardiovascular agents	
Digitoxin	Placental transfer, no reported effect
Propranolol	Indirect effect of delay in cervical dilatation
Cholinesterase inhibitors	Myasthenia-like symptoms for 1 wk; muscle weakness in 10% to 20% of infants
Cigarette smoking	Effect equal to number of cigarettes smoked; ↑ incidence of stillbirth; low birth weight; ? effect on later somatic growth and mental development; reduction in O_2 transport to fetus
Diuretics	
Ammonium chloride Benzothiazides Chlorothiazide Thiazide	Maternal and fetal acidosis; thrombocytopenia, hemorrhage, hypoelectrolytemia, convulsions, respiratory distress, death, hemolysis
Diazoxide	Hypertrichosis lanuginosa, alopecia, ? hypoglycemia
Drugs of abuse (usually multiple drugs consumed)	
Alcohol	Blood level equal to mother's; convulsions, withdrawal syndrome, hyperactivity, crying, irritability, poor sucking reflex, low birth weight; cleft palate, ophthalmic malformation, malformation of extremities and heart; poor mental performance; microencephaly, small-for-dates, growth deficiency
Barbiturates	Withdrawal symptoms, convulsions, onset immediately after birth or at 2 wk of age
Glutethimide	Small-for-dates, irritability
LSD (lysergic acid)	Chromosome breakage, limb and skeletal anomalies
Narcotics Heroin Methadone	Small-for-dates, 4% to 10% mortality, habituation, withdrawal symptoms, convulsions, sudden death, indirect effect of maternal complications (i.e., infection, hepatitis, venereal disease), ? permanent effect on somatic growth
Fluorine	Placental transfer—utilized for growth and development of bones and teeth of fetus
Hormones	
Androgens Estrogens Progestins	Labioscrotal fusion prior to wk 12; after 12 weeks', phallic enlargement; ? other anomalies; ?↑ bilirubin, vaginal cancer; cleft lip and palate; CHD; tracheoesophageal fistula; anal atresia; cancer of prostate, testes, and bladder
Corticosteroids	Adrenal insufficiency, cleft palate, small-for-dates infant
Ovulatory agents	? Anencephaly, ? chromosomal abnormalities in abortus, multiple pregnancy

Continued.

Human fetotoxic chemical agents—cont'd

Maternal medication	Reported effect on fetus or neonate
Hypoglycemic agents	
Chlorpropamide	Higher fetal mortality, prolonged hypoglycemia, competes for albumin-binding sites
Insulin	Insulin coma, ? increased fetal damage
Tolbutamide	? Potentiates hypoglycemia in newborn, thrombocytopenia
Hypotensive agents	
Hexamethonium	Paralytic ileus, perforation; death
Reserpine	1% to 15% of infants have symptoms; nasal stuffiness, bradycardia, respiratory distress, hypothermia, abnormal muscle tone (in mice, hyperactivity and increased emotionalism)
Insecticide and pesticides	
Organochlorine	Present in fetus, ? enzyme induction, ? premature labor
Intravenous alcohol	Hypoglycemia; abnormal bone marrow morphology in premature infant
Intravenous fluids	Excessive fluids—hyponatremia, seizures
Muscle relaxants	
Curare	Paralysis in utero (prolonged use), position deformities
Narcotic antagonist	
Nalorphine (Nalline)	Not effective unless large doses of narcotics administered to mother; act as respiratory depressant if cause of depression is other than narcotic
Levallorphan (Lorfan)	
Oxytocin	Thrombocytopenia, fetal bradycardia, water intoxication, ? ↑ bilirubin level; abortions (ergot)
Psychotropic drugs	
Antidepressants	
Aventyl	Withdrawal, coliclike syndrome, cyanosis, irritability, weight loss, hyperhydrosis, respiratory distress, craniofacial anomalies, CNS and skeletal anomalies; urinary retention
Chloropyramine	
Imipramine	
Nortriptyline	
Diazepam (Valium)	High fetal levels; hypotonia, poor sucking reflex, hypothermia; ↑ low Apgar score; ↑ resuscitation, ↑ assisted deliveries; dose related
Lithium carbonate	Neonatal serum levels reach adult toxic range; lethargy, cyanosis for 10 days; teratogenic—dose related
Phenothiazine	? Effect on eyes; withdrawal; extrapyramidal dysfunction; delay in onset of respiration; maternal hypotension, ? prolongs labor, ↓ effective uterine contraction; ? chromosomal breakage; hypotonia, hyperactivity
Radiation	Microencephaly, mental retardation, many unknown effects; nondisjunction of chromosomes
Radiopaque media	Elevated parathyroid hormone inhibition (PHI), depressed ^{131}I uptake
Sedatives	
Barbiturate	Apnea, depression, depressed EEG, poor sucking reflex, slow weight gain; concentration of drug in brain; enzyme inducer = lower bilirubin level
Bromides	Growth failure, lethargy, dilated pupils, dermatitis, hypotonia, ? effect on mental development
Magnesium sulfate	Neonatal blood level does not correlate with clinical condition; respiratory depression, hypotonia, convulsions, death; exchange transfusion may be required
Paraldehyde	Apnea, depression
Thalidomide	Administered between days 34-50 of gestation causes phocomelia, malformation of cord, angiomas of face, CHD, intestinal stenosis, eye defects, absence of appendix
Thyroid medications	
Iodine	Normal or goitrous; euthyroid, hyperthyroid, or hypothyroid; respiratory distress due to tracheal compression; thrombocytopenia
Thioureas	
^{131}I	Uptake by fetal thyroid after 12 weeks' gestation; exophthalmos, arrest of brain development
Toxins	
Carbon monoxide	Stillbirth, brain damage equal to anoxia
Heavy metals	
Arsenic	Concentrated in brain
Lead	Abortion, growth retardation, congenital anomalies, sterility
Mercury	Cerebral palsy, mental retardation, convulsions, involuntary movements, defective vision; mother asymptomatic
Naphthalene	Hemolysis
Vitamins	
A and D	Congenital anomalies
K (water-soluble analogs)	Icterus, anemia, kernicterus
Pyridoxine	Withdrawal seizures

APPENDIX I

Standard Laboratory Values in the Neonatal Period

1. Hematologic values		*Neonatal*
Clotting factors		2 min
Activated clotting time (ACT)		2 min
Bleeding time (Ivy)		1-8 min
Clot retraction		Complete 1-4 hr
Clotting time		
2 tubes		5-8 min
3 tubes		5-15 min
Fibrinogen		150-300 mg/dl*
Fibrinolysin (plasminogen)		Lysis of clot
Partial thromboplastin time (PTT)		<90-120 sec
Prothrombin time, one-stage (PT)		12-21 sec
Thromboplastin generation test (TGT)		8-24 sec in 6 min tube
	Term	*Preterm*
Hemoglobin (g/dl)	17-19	15-17
Hematocrit (%)	57-58	45-55
Sedimentation rate, erythrocytes (ESR) mm/hr	0-2	1-5
Reticulocytes (%)	3-7	Up to 10
Fetal hemoglobin (% of total)	40-70	80-90
Nucleated RBC/cu mm (per 100 RBC)	200 (0.05)	(0.2)
Platelet count/cu mm	100-300,000	120-180,000
WBC/cu mm	15,000	10,000-20,000
Neutrophils (%)	45	47
Eosinophils and basophils (%)	3	
Lymphocytes (%)	30	33
Monocytes (%)	5	4
Immature WBC (%)	10	16

2. Biochemical values		*Neonatal*
Ammonia		100-150 μg/dl
Amylase		0-1000 IU/hr
Antistreptolysin O titer, group B		
Normal		12-100 Todd units
Recent streptococcal infection		200-2500 Todd units
Bilirubin, direct		0-1 mg/dl
Bilirubin, total	Cord:	<2 mg/dl
	Peripheral blood: 0-1 day	6 mg/dl
	1-2 day	8 mg/dl
	3-5 day	12 mg/dl
Blood gases	Arterial:	pH 7.31-7.45
		P_{CO_2} 33-48 mm Hg
		P_{O_2} 50-70 mm Hg

☐ *1* to *6* from Pierog, S. H., and Ferrara, A.: Medical care of the sick newborn, ed. 2, St. Louis, 1976, The C. V. Mosby Co.
*dl refers to deciliter (1 dl = 100 ml); this conforms to the SI system: international measurements that have been standardized.

2. Biochemical values—cont'd

	Neonatal—cont'd
Blood gases—cont'd	Venous: pH 7.28-7.42
	P_{CO_2} 38-52 mm Hg
	P_{O_2} 20-49 mm Hg
Calcium, ionized	2.1-2.6 mEq/L
Calcium, total	4-7.0 mEq/L
Catecholamines (μg/24 hr)	
Neonatal: norepinephrine, 2-12; epinephrine, 1-2	
Newborn: norepinephrine, 2-4; epinephrine, 0-1	
Ceruloplasmin (p-phenylenediamine dihydrochloride, 37 C)	1-30 mg/dl
Chloride	95-110 mEq/L
Cholesterol, esters	42% to 71% of total
Cholesterol, total	45-170 mg/dl
Copper	20-70 μg/dl
Cortisol	
AM specimen	15-25 μg/dl
PM specimen	5-10 μg/dl
C-reactive protein (CRP)	0
Creatine	0.2-1 mg/dl (higher in females)
Creatine phosphokinase (CPK) (creatine phosphate, 30 C)	10-300 IU/L
Creatinine	0.3-1 mg/dl
Electrophoresis, total protein	Preterm: 4.3-7.6 g/dl Newborn: 4.6-7.4 g/dl
Preterm: albumin, 3.1-4.2; α_1-globulin, 0.1-0.5; α_2-globulin, 0.3-0.7; β-globulin, 0.3-1.2; γ-globulin, 0.3-1.4	
Newborn: albumin, 3.6-5.4; α_1-globulin, 0.1-0.3; α_2-globulin, 0.2-0.5; β-globulin, 0.2-0.6; γ-globulin, 0.2-1.2	
Fatty acids, free	0.4-1 mg/L
α_1-fetoprotein	0
Fibrinogen	150-300 mg/dl
Glucose, fasting (FBS)	
Hepatitis-associated (Australia) antigen	0
Immunoglobulin levels, serum, newborn	660-1.439 mg/dl
IgG 645-1.244	
IgM 5-30	
IgA 0-11	
Iodine, butanol extractable (BEI)	3-13 μg/dl
Iodine, T_4-by-column (thyroxine)	3-12 μg/dl
Iodine, T_4 (competitive protein-binding thyroxine)	3-12 μg/dl
Iodine, total serum organic (PBI)	4-14 μg/dl
Iron	100-200 μg/dl
Iron-binding capacity (IBC)	60-175 μg/dl
17-Ketogenic steroids (17-KGS)	2.4 mg/24 hr
17-Ketosteroids (17-KS)	0.5-2.5 mg/24 hr
Lactic dehydrogenase (LDH) (pyruvate, 30 C)	300-1500 IU/L
Lipids, total	170-450 mg/dl
Lipoproteins, newborn (mg/dl)	
Alpha 70-180	
Beta 50-160	
Chylo 50-110	
Magnesium	1.4-2.9 mEq/L
Malate dehydrogenase (MDH) (oxaloacetic acid, 37 C)	41-68 IU/L
Phosphatase, acid	10.4-16.4 IU/L
Phosphatase, alkaline	50-275 IU/L
Phospholipids	75-170 mg/dl
Phosphorus	3.5-8.6 mg/dl
Potassium	4-7 mg/L
Pregnanetriol	0 mg/24 hr
Protein, total	4.3-7.6 g/dl
Sodium	140-160 mEq/L
Transaminases, serum	
Glutamic-oxaloacetic (SGOT) (aspartate, 30 C)	5-70 IU/L
Glutamic-pyruvic (SGPT)	5-50 IU/L
Triglycerides	5-40 mg/dl
Urea nitrogen (BUN)	5-15 mg/dl
Vanillylmandelic acid (VMA)	0-1 mg/24 hr

Continued.

Standard laboratory values in the neonatal period—cont'd

3. Urinalysis

Volume: 20-40 ml excreted daily in the first few days; by 1 wk, 24 hr urine volume close to 200 ml
Protein: may be present in first 2-4 days
Casts and WBCs: may be present in first 2-4 days
Osmolarity (mOsm/L): 100-600
pH: 5-7
Specific gravity: 1.001-1.020

4. Cerebrospinal fluid

Calcium	2-3 mg/L
Cell count	WBCs/cu mm 0-15 RBCs/cu mm 0-500
Chloride	110-120 mg/L
Color	May be xanthochromic
Glucose	24-40 mg/dl
Lactate dehydrogenase (LDH)	5-80 IU/L
Magnesium	3-3.3 mg/dl
Pándy's test (for excess globulins)	Negative
pH (at 37 C)	7.33-7.42
Pressure	50-80 mm Hg
Protein, total	20-120 mg/dl
Sodium	130-165 mg/L
Specific gravity	1.007-1.009
Transaminase, glutamic-oxaloacetic (GOT)	2-10 IU/L
Volume	5 ml

5. Cardiorespiratory determinations

Blood pressure at birth
- Term: systolic, 78 mm Hg; diastolic, 42 mm Hg
- Preterm: systolic, 50-60 mm Hg; diastolic, 30 mm Hg

Respiratory rate: 30-60/min
Heart rate, fetus
- Baseline: 120-160/min
  - Tachycardia: >160 beats/min (with maternal complication)
  - Bradycardia: <120 beats/min (with maternal hypotension and hypoxia)
  - Acceleration: tachycardia >160 beats/min with uterine contraction—normal (usually)
- Beat-to-beat variability: disappears with fetal distress
- With uterine contraction
  - Early deceleration: bradycardia with onset of contraction—benign
  - Variable deceleration: bradycardia due to cord compression—usually benign
  - Late deceleration: bradycardia after lag period due to fetal hypoxia—ominous sign

Heart rate, term infant: 140 ± 20 beats/min

6. Urine screening tests for inborn errors of metabolism

Benedict's test: for reducing substances in the urine—glucose, galactose, fructose, lactose; phenylketonuria, alkaptonuria, tyrosyluria, and tyrosinosis *may* give positive Benedict's test.

Ferric chloride test: an immediate, green color for phenylketonuria, histidinemia, and tyrosinuria; a gray to green color for presence of phenothiazines, isoniazid; red to purple color for presence of salicylates or ketone bodies.

Dinitrophenylhydrazine test: for phenylketonuria, maple syrup urine disease, Lowe's syndrome.

Cetyltrimethyl ammonium bromide test: for mucopolysaccharides: immediate positive reaction in gargoylism (Hurler's syndrome); delayed, moderately positive reaction for Marfan's, Morquio-Ullrich, and Murdoch syndromes.

Metachromatic stain (of urine sediment): Granules (free or as inclusion bodies in cells) are seen in metachromatic leukodystrophy; may also be seen rarely in Tay-Sachs and other lipid diseases of the central nervous system.

Amino acid chromatography: Aminoaciduria may be normal in newborns; chromatography may be helpful to detect hypophosphatasia and argininosuccinicaciduria.

Diagnostic tests for phenylketonuria*

Test	Method	Use
Urine tests		
Diaper test	10% ferric chloride dropped on freshly wet diaper; green spot (positive): probable PKU	Inexpensive; useful in screening large groups of infants but not of value until infant is at least 6 wk of age
Phenistix† test	Prepared test stick pressed against wet diaper or dipped in urine; green color reaction: probable PKU	Simple; more accurate than diaper test; useful in screening large groups of infants but not of value until after infant is 6 wk of age
Dinitrophenyl-hydrazine (DNPH) test‡	0.5-1 ml of urine placed in test tube, equal amount of DNPH solution added; immediate pale yellow-orange color reaction: negative; gradual change to opaque bright yellow: positive, indicates probable PKU	Inexpensive; accurate but more complicated than diaper test or Phenistix; most useful in clinical setting to confirm these tests
Blood serum phenylalanine tests		
Guthrie inhibition assay methods§	Drops of blood placed on filter paper; laboratory uses bacterial growth inhibition test; phenylalanine level above 8 mg/dl blood: diagnostic of PKU	Effective in newborn period; used also to monitor PKU diet; blood easily obtained by heel or finger puncture; inexpensive; used for wide-scale screening
LaDu-Michael method‖	5 ml of blood; serum separated and tested for phenylalanine; level above 8 mg/dl blood: PKU; in persons with PKU, phenylalanine level above 8-12 mg/dl blood: loss of dietary control	Useful diagnostic tool and to monitor PKU diet; requires blood drawn from person; laboratory method difficult (test not available in many laboratories)
McCaman and Robins fluorometric method¶	5 ml of blood; serum separated and tested for phenylalanine; level above 8 mg: PKU or loss of dietary control	Diagnostic and diet monitoring tool; laboratory procedure more simple than LaDu-Michael method; test not available in many laboratories

*From Williams, S. R.: Nutrition and diet therapy, ed. 2, St. Louis, 1973, The C. V. Mosby Co., p. 427.
†Manufactured by Ames Co., Elkhart, Ind.
‡Centerwall, W., and Centerwall, S.: Phenylketonuria, U.S. Children's Bureau, pub. no. 338, Washington, D.C., 1961, U.S. Department of Health, Education, and Welfare.
§Guthrie, R.: Blood screening for phenylketonuria, J.A.M.A. **178**:863, 1961.
‖LaDu, B., and Michael, P.: An enzymatic spectrophotometric method for the determination of phenylalanine in blood, J. Lab. Clin. Med. **55**:491, 1960.
¶McCaman, M., and Robins, E.: Fluorometric method for the determination of phenylalanine in the serum, J. Lab. Clin. Med. **59**:885, 1962.

APPENDIX J

Relationship of Drugs to Breast Milk and Effect on Infant*

Drug	Excreted in milk	Amount in milk after therapeutic dose	Effect on infant
Analgesics and anti-inflammatory drugs (nonnarcotic)			
Acetaminophen (Datril, Tylenol)	Yes		Detoxified in liver. Avoid in immediate postdelivery period, otherwise no problems with therapeutic dose.
Aspirin	Yes	1-3 mg/dl†	Long history of experience shows complications rare. Can cause interference with platelet aggregation and diminished factor XII (Hageman factor) at birth. When mother requires high, continuing level of medication for arthritis, aspirin is drug of choice. Observe infant for bruisability. Platelet aggregation can be evaluated. Salicylism only seen in maternal overdosing. Mother should increase vitamin C and vitamin K intake.
Donnatal (phenobarbital, hyoscyamine sulfate, atropine sulfate, hyoscine hydrobromide)	Yes		Consider for its component parts. Can be given to children but can accumulate in neonate.
Flufenamic acid (Arlef)	Yes	0.50 μg/ml (mean)‡	No apparent effect on infant when maternal dosage was 200 mg, three times a day. Infant able to excrete via urine.
Indomethacin (Indocin)	Yes		Convulsions in breast-fed neonate (case report). Used to close patent ductus arteriosus. Insufficient data as to effect on other vessels. May be nephrotoxic.
Mefenamic acid (Ponstel)	Yes	Trace amounts§	No apparent effect on infant at therapeutic doses; infant able to excrete via urine.
Naproxen (Naprosyn, synaxsyn, naprosine, naxen, proxen)	Yes	1% of maternal plasma; binds to plasma protein	Less toxic in adults than some other organic derivatives.
Oxyphenbutazone (Tandearil)	Yes	In milk of 2 of 55 mothers, 10% to 80% of maternal plasma level	No known effect.
Pentazocine (Talwin)	No		Withdrawal in neonatal period from ingestion during pregnancy.
Phenylbutazone (Butazolidin)	Yes	0.63 mg ml 90 min after 750 mg given IM	Very potent drug; risk to infant not well defined but considerable. Not given directly to children; may accumulate in infant.

Continued.

*Adapted from Lawrence, R. A.: Breast feeding: a guide for the medical profession, St. Louis, 1980, The C. V. Mosby Co., pp. 316-330.
†Plasma level was 1-5 mg/dl.
‡Shown when mean maternal plasma level was 6.41 μg/ml. Mean level in infant's plasma was 0.12 μg/ml; in infant's urine, 0.08 μg/ml. (Maternal plasma level was 50 times that of infant.)
§0.91 μg/ml mean maternal plasma level showed 0.21 μg/ml mean milk level. Mean infant plasma level was 0.08 μg/ml and mean urine level, 9.8 μg/ml.

Relationship of drugs to breast milk and effect on infant—cont'd

Drug	Excreted in milk	Amount in milk after therapeutic dose	Effect on infant
Analgesics and anti-inflammatory drugs (nonnarcotic)—cont'd			
Propoxyphene (Darvon)	Yes	0.4% of maternal* dose	Only symptoms detectable would be failure to feed and drowsiness. On daily, around-the-clock dosage infant could consume 1 mg/day.
Antibiotics			
Amantadine (Symmetrel)	Yes	Not defined	Vomiting, urinary retention, rash. Contraindicated.
Ampicillin (Polycillin, Amcill, Omnipen, Penbritin)	Yes	0.07 μg/ml	Sensitivity due to repeated exposure; diarrhea or secondary candidiasis.
Carbenicillin (Pyopen, Geopen)	Yes	0.265 μg/ml 1 hr after 1 g given	Levels not significant. Drug is given to neonate.
Cefazolin (Ancef, Kefzol)	Yes	1.5 μg/ml (0.075% of dose)	Probably not significant.
Cephalexin (Keflex)	No		
Cephalothin (Keflin)	No		
Chloramphenicol (Chloromycetin)	Yes	Half blood level; 2.5 mg/dl	Gray syndrome. Infant does not excrete drug well, and small amounts may accumulate. Contraindicated. May be tolerated in older infant with mature glycuronide system.
Chloroquine (Aralen)	Yes	2.7 mg in 2 days†	Can be used to *treat* child under 6 mo of age who is wholly breast-fed.
Colistin (Colymycin)	Yes	0.05-0.09 mg/dl	Not absorbed orally.
Demeclocycline (Declomycin)	Yes	0.2-0.3 mg/dl	Not significant in therapeutic doses. Can be given to infants.
Erythromycin (Ilosone, E-Mycin, Erythrocin)	Yes	0.05-0.1 mg/dl; 3.6-6.2 μg/ml	Higher concentrations have been reported in milk than in plasma. Should not be given under 1 mo of age because of risk of jaundice. Dose in milk higher when given IV to mother.
Gentamicin	Unknown		Not absorbed from gastrointestinal tract, may change gut flora. Drug is given to newborns directly.
Isoniazid (Nydrazid)	Yes	0.6-1.2 mg/dl‡	Infant at risk for toxicity, but need for breast milk may outweigh risk.
Kanamycin (Kantrex)	Yes	18.4 μg/ml after 1 g given IM	Infant absorbs little from gastrointestinal tract. Infants can be given drug.
Lincomycin (Lincocin)	Yes	0.5-2.4 mg/dl	Not significant in therapeutic doses to affect child.
Mandelic acid	Yes	0.3 g/24 hr after dose of 12 g/day	Not significant in therapeutic doses to affect child.
Methacycline (Rondomycin)	Yes	½ plasma level; 50-260 μg/dl	Same precautions as with tetracycline.
Methenamine (Hexamine)	Yes		Not significant in therapeutic doses to affect child.
Metronidazole (Flagyl)	Yes	Level comparable to serum§	Caution should be exercised because of its high milk concentrations. Contraindicated when infant under 6 mo, may cause neurologic disorders and blood dyscrasia.
Nalidixic acid (Neggram)	Yes	0.4 mg/dl	Not significant in therapeutic doses beyond neonatal period. Hemolytic anemia in an infant attributed to nalidixic acid in G6PD deficiency or when mother has renal failure.
Nitrofurantoin (Furadantin)	Yes	Trace to 0.5 μg/ml	Not significant in therapeutic doses to affect child except in G6PD deficiency.
Novobiocin (Albamycin, cathomycin)	Yes	0.36-0.54 mg/dl	Infant can be given drug directly.
Nystatin (Mycostatin)	No	Not absorbed orally	Can be given to infant directly.
Oxacillin (Prostaphlin)	No		
Para-aminosalicylic acid	No		
Penethamate (Leocillin)	No	24-74 μg/dl	Animal study suggests it be avoided.

*Shown by animal experiments. Milk plasma ratio (M/P) = ½.
†Peaks in 6 hr.
‡Same concentration in milk as in maternal serum.
§Gives serum levels in infants of 0.05 to 0.4 μg/ml.

Drug	Excreted in milk	Amount in milk after therapeutic dose	Effect on infant
Antibiotics—cont'd			
Penicillin G, benzathine (Bicillin)	Yes	10-12 units/dl	Clinical need should supersede possible allergic responses.
Penicillin G, potassium	Yes	Up to 6 units/dl; 1.2-3.6 μg/dl	Infant can be given penicillin directly. Parents should be told to inform physician that infant has been exposed to penicillin because of potential sensitivity.
Pyrimethamine (Daraprim)	Yes	0.3 mg/dl (3% of dose)	Significant in therapeutic doses when infant under 6 mo and entirely breast-fed.
Quinine sulfate	Yes	0-0.1 mg/dl after maternal dose of 300-600 mg	In therapeutic doses, no effect on child except rare thrombocytopenia.
Sodium fusidate	Yes	0.02 μg/ml	Not significant in therapeutic doses to affect child.
Streptomycin	Yes	Present for long periods in slight amounts when given as dihydrostreptomycin	Not to be given more than 2 wk. Ototoxic and nephrotoxic with long use. Is given to infants directly.
Sulfanilamide	Yes	9 mg/dl after dose of 2-4 g/24 hr	Not significant in therapeutic doses; may cause a rash or hemolytic anemia. Should be avoided for first month after delivery.
Sulfapyridine	Yes	3-13 mg/dl after dose of 3 g/24 hr	To be avoided; has caused skin rash.
Sulfathiazole	Yes	0.5 mg/dl after dose of 3 g/24 hr	Not significant in therapeutic doses to affect child after 1 mo of age.
Sulfisoxazole (Gantrisin)	Yes	Concentration similar to plasma level	To be avoided during first month after delivery; may cause kernicterus.
Tetracycline HCl (Achromycin, Panmycin, Sumycin)	Yes	0.5-2.6 μg/ml after dose of 500 mg four times a day	Not enough to treat an infection in an infant. May cause discoloration of the teeth in the infant; the antibiotic, however, may be largely bound to the milk calcium. Do not give over 10 days or repeatedly.
Anticoagulants			
Coumarin derivatives Dicumarol (bishydroxycoumarin) Warfarin (Panwarfin)	Yes	Probably little but may be cumulative*	Monitor prothrombin time. Give vitamin K to infant. Discontinue if surgery or trauma occurs. Drug of choice if mother to continue nursing.
Ethyl biscoumacetate (Tromexan)	Yes	0-0.17 mg/dl†	Hemorrhage around umbilical stump and cephalhematoma reported. Prothrombin normal in infants with hemorrhage. Vitamin K has no effect. Contraindicated while nursing.
Heparin	No		Heparin ineffective orally.
Phenindione (Hedulin) (Dindevan)	Yes		Breast milk a major route of excretion. Reports of serious hemorrhage in infant. Prothrombin times prolonged in infant. Contraindicated while nursing.
Anticonvulsants and sedatives‡			
Barbital (Veronal)	Yes	8-10 mg/L after 500 mg dose	May produce sedation in infant. In general, barbiturates pass into milk but do not sedate infant. Watch for symptoms.
Carbamazepine (Tegretol)	Yes	60% of plasma level§	Animal studies show lack of weight gain, unkempt appearance.
Chloral hydrate (Noctec, Somnos)	Yes	Up to 1.5 mg/dl	No significant symptoms, can be given to infants directly.
Phenytoin (Dilantin)	Yes	1.5 to 2.6 μg/ml after 300 mg/24 hr dose	One case of hemolytic reaction reported. Other infants appear to tolerate the small doses. Therapeutic plasma level 10-20 μg/ml.
Mephenytoin (Mesantoin) (hydantoin homologue of mephobarbital)	Unknown		Detoxified in liver. No information.

*Reports conflict.
†No correlation with dosage, continues in milk after plasma clear.
‡All barbitals appear in breast milk.
§When plasma 13.0 μmoles/L, 7.5 μmoles/L in milk.

Continued.

Relationship of drugs to breast milk and effect on infant—cont'd

Drug	Excreted in milk	Amount in milk after therapeutic dose	Effect on infant
Anticonvulsants and sedatives—cont'd			
Pentobarbital (Nembutal)	Yes		Depends on liver for detoxification so may accumulate in first week of life until infant able to detoxify. No problem for older infant in usual doses.
Phenobarbital (Luminal)	Yes	0.1-0.5 mg when plasma level 0.6-1.8 mg	Sleepiness and decreased sucking possible. On usual analeptic doses infants alert and feed well. On hypnotic doses infant depressed and difficult to rouse.
Phensuximide (Milontin)			No specific data.
Primidone (Mysoline)	Yes		Causes drowsiness and decreased feeds. May cause bleeding due to hypoprothrombinemia. Infant needs vitamin K. Avoid drug during lactation.
Sodium bromide (Bromo-Seltzer and across-the-counter sleeping aids)	Yes	Up to 6.6 mg/dl	Drowsy, decreased crying, rash, decreased feeding.
Trimethadione (Tridione)			No specific data.
Antihistaminics Brompheniramine (Dimetane) Diphenhydramine (Benadryl) Methdilazine (Tacaryl) Tripelennamine (Pyribenzamine)	Yes	No specific data available. All pass into milk.	Drug is used in neonates. May cause sedation, decreased feeding, or may produce stimulation and tachycardia. Should avoid long-acting preparations, which may accumulate in infant. When combined with decongestants, may cause decrease in milk.
Autonomic drugs			
Atropine sulfate*	Yes	0.1 mg/dl	Hyperthermia, atropine toxicity, infants especially sensitive; also inhibits lactation. Infant dose 0.01 mg/kg.
Carisoprodol (Soma, Rela)	Yes	Two to four times maternal plasma	Blocks interneuronal activity in descending reticular formation and spinal cord; drowsiness, hypotonia, poor feed.
Ergot (Cafergot)	Yes	Unknown	90% of infants had symptoms of ergotism: vomiting and diarrhea to weak pulse and unstable blood pressure. Short-term therapy for migraine should not exceed 6 mg. Cafergot also contains 100 mg caffeine.
Mepenzolate bromide (Cantil)	No		Postganglionic parasympathetic inhibitor used to diminish gastric acidity and decrease spasm of colon. Oral absorption low.
Methocarbamol (Robaxin)	Yes	Minimum	Too little in milk to produce effect.
Neostigmine	No		No known harm to infant.
Propantheline bromide (Pro-Banthine)	No	Uncontrolled data indicate no measurable levels	Drug rapidly metabolized in maternal system to inactive metabolite. Mother should avoid long-acting preparations, however.
Scopolamine (hyoscine)	Yes		Usually given as single dose and of no problem to neonate. No data on repeated doses.
Cardiovascular drugs			
Diazoxide (Hyperstat)			Arteriolar dilators and antihypertensive, only given IV, not active orally.
Dibenzyline†			No data available.
Digoxin	Yes	0.96-0.61 ng/ml‡	Digoxin 20% bound to protein; infant receives <1/100 of dose. If mother at toxic level of 5 ng/ml, milk would have 4.4 ng/ml and infant would receive only 1/20 daily dose.
Guanethidine (Ismelin)§	Yes		Not significant in therapeutic doses to affect child.
Hydralazine (Apresoline)	Yes		Jaundice, thrombocytopenia, electrolyte disturbances possible.
Methyldopa (Aldomet)§	Yes		Galactorrhea. No specific data except as affects mother's milk production.

*Ingredient in many prescription and nonprescription drugs.

†α blocking agent.

‡Peak level occurs 4-6 hr after dose given. Maternal plasma level was higher, M/P = 0.9 and 0.8; infant's plasma level was 0.

§Adrenergic blocking agent.

Drug	Excreted in milk	Amount in milk after therapeutic dose	Effect on infant
Cardiovascular drugs—cont'd			
Propranolol (Inderal)*	Yes	40 ng/ml of maternal plasma†	Insignificant amount. Infants reported had no symptoms noted. Should watch for hypoglycemia and/or "β-blocking" effects.
Quinidine	Yes		Arrhythmia may occur.
Reserpine (Serpasil)‡	Yes		May produce galactorrhea, lethargy, diarrhea, or nasal stuffiness.
Cathartics			
Aloin	Yes	Low	Occasionally gave symptoms, caused colic and diarrhea in infant.
Anthraquinone laxatives such as dihydroxyanthraquinone (Dorbane and Dorbantyl)	Yes	High	Caused colic and diarrhea in infant.
Calomel	No	None	None.
Cascara	Yes	Low	Caused colic and diarrhea in infant.
Milk of magnesia	No	None	No effect.
Mineral oil	No	None	No effect.
Phenolphthalein	Unknown	Unknown§	Reported to cause symptoms in some.
Rhubarb	Unknown	None	None in syrup form. Fresh rhubarb may give symptoms of colic and diarrhea.
Saline cathartics	No	None	No effect.
Senna	No	None	None.
Stool softeners and bulk-forming laxatives	No	None	No effect.
Suppositories (for constipation)	No	None	Not absorbed.
Diagnostic materials and procedures			
Barium	No		Not absorbed.
Iopanoic acid (Telepaque)	Yes		Not sufficient to produce problem in infant on single dose. Does contain iodine radical.
Radioactive compounds			
Radioactive sodium	Yes	0.5% to 1.3% of dose/L‖	Diminished after 24 hr; discontinue nursing 24 hr.
[^{67}Ga] citrate	Yes		Discontinue nursing until ^{67}Ga has cleared, usually 24 hr.
^{125}I, ^{131}I	Yes	M/P = 0.13 μCi/0.002 μCi¶	^{131}I content in milk proportional to amount of milk. Most excreted in 24 hr. Discontinue nursing for 48 hr or check milk prior to resuming feeding if under 48 hr.
^{90}Sr	Yes	M/P = $^1/_{10}$	Less than in cow's milk. Bottle infant doubles stores in 1 mo.
^{99m}Tc	Yes		Reported to clear in 6-22 hr. Discontinue breast feeding 24 hr. ^{99m}Tc preferentially picked up by breast tissue.
Tuberculin test	No		Tuberculin-sensitive mothers can adoptively immunize their infants through breast milk, and that immunity may last several years.
X-ray films	No		No effect.
Diuretics			
Acetazolamide (Diamox)	Probable	No specific data available but probably similar to sulfonamide	Acts as enzyme inhibitor on carbonic anhydrase non-bacteriostatic sulfonamide. Observe only for dehydration and electrolyte loss by monitoring urine and turgor.
Furosemide (sulfamoylanthranilic acid) (Lasix)	No		Drug is given to children under medical management.
Mercurial diuretics (Dicurin, Thiomerin)	Yes		In addition to diuretic effect, there is risk of mercury deposition. However, drug not absorbed orally.

*β blocking agent.
†Total daily dose to infant via milk is 15-20 μg.
‡Adrenergic blocking agent.
§Reports differ.
‖Peak in 2 hr; detectable for 96 hr.
¶27% of dose in 48 hr.

Continued.

Relationship of drugs to breast milk and effect on infant—cont'd

Drug	Excreted in milk	Amount in milk after therapeutic dose	Effect on infant
Diuretics—cont'd			
Spironolactone (Aldactone)	Yes	Canrenone, a metabolite, appears	Acts as antagonist of aldosterone; causes sodium excretion and potassium retention. The metabolite apparently has some activity.
Thiazides (Diuril, Enduron, Esidrix, Hydrodiuril, Oretic, Thiuretic tablets)	Yes	>0.1 mg/dl*	Risk of dehydration and electrolyte imbalance, especially sodium loss, which would require monitoring. Watching weight and wet diapers and taking an occasional specific gravity reading of the urine and serum sodium would indicate status of infant. Risk, however, is extremely low. May suppress lactation due to dehydration in mother.
Environmental agents			
Aldrin	Yes	Varies by location	Not a reason to wean from breast. No need to test milk unless inordinate exposure.
Benzene hexachloride (BHC)	Yes	Varies by location	Not a reason to wean from breast. No need to test milk unless inordinate exposure.
Dichlorodiphenyltrichloroethane (DDT or DDE)	Yes	Varies by location	Not a reason to wean from breast. No need to test milk unless inordinate exposure.
Dieldrin	Yes	Varies by location	Also found in permanently mothproofed garments. Avoid these. Not a reason to wean.
Hexachlorobenzene (HCB)	Yes	Varies by location	Not a reason to wean from breast. No need to test milk unless inordinate exposure.
Heptachlorepoxide	Yes	Varies by location	Not a reason to wean from breast. No need to test milk unless inordinate exposure.
Methyl mercury	Yes	500-1000 ng/ml†	Infant blood level 600 ng/ml in heavy exposure. Only in excessive exposure is testing and/or weaning necessary.
Polybrominated biphenyl (PBB)	Yes	Varies by location	If mother at high risk from the environment or the diet, milk sample should be measured. If level in milk is high, then breast feeding should be discontinued. Those at risk are (1) workers who handle PBB/PCB and (2) individuals who eat game fish from contaminated waters. Crash diets mobilize fats and should be avoided especially if PBB or PCB present.
Polychlorinated biphenyl (PCB)	Yes	Varies by location	
^{90}Sr, ^{89}Sr (strontium)	Yes	1/10 of that in maternal diet	Cow's milk has six times as much as human milk. Cow's milk–fed infant doubles amount in body in 1 mo.
Heavy metals			
Arsenic	Yes	Can be measured for given woman	Can accumulate. Check infant's blood level if there is reason to suspect exposure.
Copper	Yes		
Fluorine	Yes		Monitor for excessive dose.
Gold thiomalate (Myocrisin)	Yes	0.022 μg/ml when mother given 50 mg/wk	No proteinuria or aminoaciduria observed.
Halothane	Yes	2 ppm	Nursing mothers who work in environment with halothane should be checked.
Iron	Yes		
Lead	Unknown		Nursing contraindicated if maternal serum 40 μg; conflicting reports, breast milk not always cause of lead poisoning in breast-fed infant.
Magnesium	Yes		Not sufficient to be toxic.
Mercury	Yes		Hazardous to infant.

*Linear relationship between plasma and milk. In 1 L of milk at 0.1 mg/dl there would be 1 mg/24 hr. Infant dose is 20 mg/kg/24 hr.
†M/P = 8.6% in heavy exposure.

Drug	Excreted in milk	Amount in milk after therapeutic dose	Effect on infant
Hormones and contraceptives			
Carbimazole (neo-mercazole)	Yes		Antithyroid effect may cause goiter.
Chlorotrianisene (Tace)	Yes		Has estrogenic effect although does not change consistency of milk. May have feminizing effect on infant.
Contraceptives (oral) Ethinyl estradiol Mestranol 19-Nortestosterone Norethindrone (Norlutin) Norethynodrel (Enovid)	Yes		May diminish milk supply. May decrease vitamins, protein, and fat in milk. One author showed no difference when mothers took norethindrone. Most significant concern is long-range impact of hormone on young infant, which is not certain. Reports of feminization of infant.
Corticotropin	Yes		Destroyed in gastrointestinal tract of infant. No effect.
Cortisone	Yes		Animal studies show 50% lower weight than controls and retarded sexual development and exophthalmos.
Dihydrotachysterol (Hytakerol)	Yes		May cause hypercalcemia; need monitoring of infant serum and urine calcium.
Epinephrine (adrenalin)	Yes		Destroyed in GI tract of infant.
Estrogen	Yes	0.17 μg/dl after 1 g	Risks as with oral contraceptives.
Fluoxymesterone (Halotestin, Ora-Testryl, Ultandren)	Yes		Suppress lactation; masculinizing
Insulin	Unknown		Destroyed in gastrointestinal tract.
Liothyronine (Cytomel)	No		Synthetic form of natural thyroid.
Medroxyprogesterone acetate (Provera)	No		
Phenformin HCl	Yes	Minimum	Not sufficient to cause symptoms in infant. Does not cause hypoglycemia in normal infants. No case reports available.
Prednisone	Yes	0.07-0.23% dose/L after 5 mg dose*	Minimum amount not likely to cause effect on infant in short course.
Pregnanediol	Yes		Unknown risk as with other female hormones over a long period of time.
Tolbutamide (Orinase)	Yes		Not recommended in the childbearing years.
Narcotics			
Codeine		0 to trace after 32 mg every 4 hr (6 doses)	No effect in therapeutic level and transient usage. Can accumulate. Individual variation. Watch for neonatal depression.
Heroin	Yes		13 of 22 infants had withdrawal. Historically breast feeding had been used to wean addict's infant. This is no longer recommended.
Marijuana *(Cannabis)*	Yes		Shown in laboratory animals to produce structural changes in nursling's brain cells; impairs DNA and RNA formation. Infant at risk of inhaling smoke during feeding or when held by person who is smoking.
Meperidine (Demerol)	Yes	>0.1 mg/dl†	Trace amounts may accumulate if drug taken around the clock when infant is neonate. Watch for drowsiness and poor feeding.
Methadone	Yes	0.03 μg/ml or 0.023-0.028 mg/24 hr‡	When dosage not excessive, infant can be breast-fed if monitored for evidence of depression and failure to thrive.
Morphine	Yes	Trace amount	Single doses have minimum effect. Potential for accumulation. May be addicting to neonate. Breast feeding no longer considered appropriate means of weaning infant of an addict.
Percodan (oxycodone [derived from opiate thebaine] aspirin, phenacetin, caffeine)	Yes		Consider for its component parts. In neonatal period sleepiness and failure to feed, which increase maternal engorgement and neonatal weight loss, have been observed, probably caused by oxycodone.

*0.16 μg/ml after 10 mg dose; 2.67 μg/ml after 2 hr.
†Plasma 0.07-0.1 mg/dl.
‡Mother received 50 mg/24 hr; M/P = 0.83. Peak level 4 hr after oral dose. Results obscured if addict also taking the herbal root golden seal.

Continued.

Relationship of drugs to breast milk and effect on infant—cont'd

Drug	Excreted in milk	Amount in milk after therapeutic dose	Effect on infant
Psychotropic and mood-changing drugs			
Alcohol	Yes	Similar to plasma level	Ordinarily no problem and can be therapeutic in moderation. Infants are more susceptible to effects. Chronic drinking reported to cause obesity in one infant. Ethanol in doses of 1-2 g/kg to mother causes depression of milk-ejection reflex (dose dependent). No acetaldehyde found in infants.
Amphetamine	Yes		Has caused stimulation in infants with jitteriness, irritability, sleeplessness. Long-acting preparations cumulative.
Benzodiazepines*			
Chlordiazepoxide HCl (Librium)	Yes		Not sufficient to affect infant first week when glucuronyl system needed for detoxification. May accumulate. Older infant, no apparent problem.
Diazepam (Valium)	Yes	90 μg/L†	Detoxified in glucuronyl system. In first weeks of life may contribute to jaundice. Metabolite active. Effect on infant: hypoventilation, drowsiness, lethargy, and weight loss. Single doses over 10 mg contraindicated during nursing. Accumulation in infant possible.
Pineazepam	Yes	Metabolite, 5-11.2 ng/ml; pineazepam, >1.0 ng/ml‡	No data, probably similar to diazepam.
Haloperidol (Haldol)	Yes	Unknown	A butyrophenone antidepressant; animal studies in nurslings show behavior abnormalities.
Lithium carbonate (Eskalith, Lithane, Lithonate)	Yes	⅓-½ maternal plasma level§	Measurable lithium in infant's serum. Infant kidney can clear lithium; however, lithium inhibits adenosine 3′:5′-cyclic monophosphate, significant for brain growth. Also affects amine metabolism. Real effects not measurable immediately. Report of cyanosis and poor muscle tone and ECG changes in nursing infant.
Monoamine oxidase (MAO) inhibitors (Eutonyl, Nardil)			Inhibits lactation.
Meprobamate (Miltown, Equanil)	Yes	2-4 times maternal plasma level	If therapy continued, infant should be followed closely.
Penfluridol‖	Yes	Unknown	Animal studies show learning abnormalities in sucklings. This is a potent long-acting oral neuroleptic drug.
Phenothiazines			
Chlorpromazine (Thorazine)	Yes	⅓ plasma level¶	Can be safely nursed; minimum in milk. Increases maternal prolactin. No symptoms in infants reported; 5 yr follow-up showed infants normal.
Mesoridazine (Serentil)	Yes	Minimum	
Piperacetazine (Quide)	Yes	Minimum	Probably no effect.
Thioridazine (Mellaril)	Yes	No information	Thioridazine is less potent in general than other phenothiazines. Probably quite safe.
Trifluoperazine (Stelazine)	Yes	Minimum	
Tricyclic antidepressants			Apparently no accumulation. No infants that have been observed showed symptoms. Watch for depression or failure to feed. Increases maternal prolactin secretion.
Amitriptyline HCl (Elavil)	Yes	Minimum amounts	
Desipramine HCl (Norpramin, Pertofrane)	Yes	Minimum amounts	
Imipramine HCl (Tofranil)	Yes	0.1 mg/dl#	

*Alcohol enhances effect of this group.

†10 mg or less yields 45 ng of diazepam/ml and 85 ng of metabolite/ml. P/M ratio is variable. Mean P/M ratio of diazepam is 6.14; of metabolite is 3.64. Effect lasts about 4 days.

‡Both drug and active metabolite appear for about 4 days after dose.

§0.030 mmol/L in infant's serum, 0.57 mmole/L in infant's urine. Milk level was half of maternal serum level in one case report.

‖Neuroleptic drug.

¶If dose <200 mg, milk contains bare trace. Dose of 1200 mg showed trace.

#Plasma level 0.2-1.3 mg/dl.

Drug	Excreted in milk	Amount in milk after therapeutic dose	Effect on infant
Stimulants			
Caffeine	Yes	1% of dose	Accumulates when intake moderate and continual. Causes jitteriness, wakefulness, and irritability. Caffeine present in many hot and cold drinks. Consider if infant very wakeful.
Theobromine	Yes	3.7-8.2 mg/L after 240 mg dose*	No adverse symptoms observed in the infants. Chocolate most common cause of exposure.
Theophylline	Yes	10% of maternal dose†	Irritability, fretfulness.
Thyroid and antithyroid medications			
Carbimazole (neo-mercazole)	Yes		May cause goiter.
Methimazole (Tapazole)	Yes	M/P > 1	Inhibits synthesis of thyroid hormone but does not inactivate existing thyroid. Can inhibit infant thyroid. ⅛ grain/day of thyroid can be given to infant simultaneously.
Potassium iodide	Yes	3 mg/dl‡	May alter thyroid function of infant; may cause goiter in infant.
Propylthiouracil	Yes	M/P > 1; 4.5-6% of dose	Risk of goiter and agranulocytosis. With present microtechniques for T_3, T_4 and TSH, close monitoring of infant is possible, as with methimazole.
Radioactive iodine ^{125}I, ^{131}I (as a treatment)	Yes	M/P > 1	*Treatment* doses are excreted via the breast for 1-3 wk. Milk can be checked by Geiger counter if there is a question. Breast feeding should be discontinued until milk is clear.
Thiouracil	Yes	9-12 mg/dl§	Same as for propylthiouracil.
Thyroid and thyroxine	Yes		Does not produce adverse symptoms on long-range follow-up. Noted to improve milk supply of hypothyroid mothers. No contraindication.
Miscellaneous			
Cyclophosphamide	Yes	Present‖	Antineoplastic agent. Any amounts contraindicated.
DPT	Yes	Minimum	Does not interfere with immunization schedule.
Methotrexate	Yes	Minor route of excretion: M/P = 0.08/1.0	Antimetabolite. Infant would receive 0.26 μg/dl, which researchers consider nontoxic for infant.
Nicotine	Yes	Mean 91 ppb (20-512 ppb)¶	Decreases milk production. No apparent effect on infant—perhaps a tolerance is developed in utero. Smoking may interfere with let-down reflex if smoking started prior to onset of a feeding.
Poliovirus vaccine	No		Live vaccine taken orally. Not necessary to withhold nursing 30 min before and after dose. Provide booster after infant no longer nursing.
Rh antibodies	Yes		Destroyed in gastrointestinal tract; not effective orally.
Rubella virus vaccine	Yes	Minimum	Will not confer passive immunity. Mother should not be given vaccine when at risk for pregnancy.
Smallpox vaccine	No		Exposure is by direct contact. Live virus. No longer given.

*113 g chocolate bar.
†M/P = 0.7.
‡Dose was 325-650 mg three times a day.
§Maternal plasma level was 3.4 mg/dl after a 1.0 g dose; M/P = 3.
‖Single 500 mg IV dose in milk at 1, 3, 5, and 6 hr after injection.
¶At ½-1½ packs/day. Large variation from single donor.

APPENDIX K

Recommended Schedule for Active Immunization of Normal Infants and Children

	Diphtheria-tetanus-pertussis	Polio (TOPV)	Measles	TB test	Rubella	Mumps	Tetanus-diphtheria
2 months	✓	✓					
4 months	✓	✓					
6 months	✓						
1 year				✓			
15 months			✓		✓	✓	
1½ years	✓	✓					
4 - 6 years	✓	✓					
14 - 16 years							✓

☐ From American Academy of Pediatrics: You and your pediatrician: common childhood problems, Evanston, Ill., 1977, the Academy.

APPENDIX L

Brazelton Scale

SUMMARY OF BRAZELTON SCALE SCORING DEFINITIONS*

1. Response decrement to light (states 1, 2, 3)†

1 No diminution in high responses over the 10 stimuli.
2 Delayed startles and rest of responses are still present, i.e., body movement, eye blinks, respiratory changes continue over 10 trials.
3 Startles no longer present but rest are still present, including body movement in 10 trials.
4 No startles, body movement delayed, respiratory and blinks same in 10 trials.
5 Shutdown of body movements, some diminution in blinks and respiratory changes in 9-10 stimuli.
6 —in 7-8 stimuli
7 —in 5-6 stimuli
8 —in 3-4 stimuli
9 —in 1-2 stimuli
NA No response; hence, no decrement.

2. Response decrement to rattle (1, 2, 3)

1 No diminution in high responses over the 10 stimuli.
2 Delayed startles and rest of responses are still present, i.e., body movement, eye blinks, respiratory changes continue over 10 trials.
3 Startles no longer present but rest are still present, including body movement in 10 trials.
4 No startles, body movement delayed, respiratory and blinks same in 10 trials.
5 Shutdown of body movements, some diminution in blinks and respiratory changes in 9-10 stimuli.
6 —in 7-8 stimuli
7 —in 5-6 stimuli
8 —in 3-4 stimuli
9 —in 1-2 stimuli
NA No response; hence, no decrement.

3. Response decrement to bell (1, 2, 3)

1 No diminution in high responses over the 10 stimuli.
2 Delayed startles and rest of responses are still present, i.e., body movement, eye blinks, respiratory changes continue over 10 trials.
3 Startles no longer present but rest are still present, including body movement in 10 trials.
4 No startles, body movement delayed, respiratory and blinks same in 10 trials.
5 Shutdown of body movements, some diminution in blinks and respiratory changes in 9-10 stimuli.
6 —in 7-8 stimuli
7 —in 5-6 stimuli
8 —in 3-4 stimuli
9 —in 1-2 stimuli
NA No response; hence, no decrement.

4. Response decrement to pinprick (1, 2, 3)

1 Response generalized to whole body, and increases over trials.
2 Both feet withdraw together. No decrement of response.
3 Variable response to stimulus. Response decrement but return of response.
4 Response decrement after 5 trials. Localized to stimulated leg. No change to alert state.
5 Response decrement after 5 trials. Localized to stimulated foot. No change to alert state.
6 Response limited to stimulated foot after 3-4 trials. No change to alert state.
7 Response limited to stimulated foot after 1-2 trials. No change to alert state.
8 Response localized and minimal. Change to alert state (4).
9 Complete response decrement. Change to alert state (4).
NA No response; hence, no decrement.

5. Orientation response—inanimate visual (4 only)

1 Does not focus on or follow stimulus.
2 Stills with stimulus and brightens.
3 Stills, focuses on stimulus when presented, brief following.
4 Stills, focuses on stimulus, following for 30° arc, jerky movements.
5 Focuses and follows with eyes horizontally for at least a 30° arc. Smooth movement, loses stimulus, but finds it again.
6 Follows for 30° arc, with eyes and head. Eye movements are smooth.
7 Follows with eyes and head at least 60° horizontally, maybe briefly vertically, continuous movement, loses stimulus occasionally, head turns to follow.

*From Brazelton, B.: Neonatal behavioral assessment scale, London, 1973, Spastics International Medical Publications.
†States and numbers 1 to 6 refer to sleep and wake states in Table 29-2.

Continued.

SUMMARY OF BRAZELTON SCALE SCORING DEFINITIONS—cont'd

5. Orientation response—inanimate visual—cont'd

8 Follows with eyes and head 60° horizontally and 30° vertically.
9 Focuses on stimulus and follows with smooth, continuous head movement horizontally, vertically, and in a circle. Follows for 120° arc.

6. Orientation response—inanimate auditory (4, 5)

1 No reaction.
2 Respiratory change or blink only.
3 General quieting, as well as blink and respiratory changes.
4 Stills, brightens, no attempt to locate source.
5 Shifting of eyes to sound, as well as stills and brightens.
6 Alerting and shifting of eyes, and head turns to source.
7 Alerting, head turns to stimulus, and search with eyes.
8 Alerting prolonged, head and eyes turn to stimulus repeatedly.
9 Turning and alerting to stimulus presented on both sides on every presentation of stimulus.

7. Orientation—animate visual (4 only)

1 Does not focus on or follow stimulus.
2 Stills with stimulus and brightens.
3 Stills, focuses on stimulus when presented, brief following.
4 Stills, focuses on stimulus, follows for 30° arc, jerky movements.
5 Focuses and follows with eyes horizontally for at least a 30° arc. Smooth movement, loses stimulus but finds it again.
6 Follows for two 30° arcs, with eyes and head.
7 Follows with eyes and head at least 60° horizontally, maybe briefly vertically, partly continuous movement, loses stimulus occasionally, head turns to follow.
8 Follows with eyes and head 60° horizontally and 30° vertically.
9 Repeatedly focuses on stimulus and follows with smooth, continuous head movement horizontally, vertically, and in a circle. Follows for 120° arc.

8. Orientation—animate auditory (4, 5)

1 No reaction.
2 Respiratory change or blink only.
3 General quieting, as well as blink and respiratory changes.
4 Stills, brightens, no attempt to locate source.
5 Shifting of eyes to sound, as well as stills and brightens.
6 Alerting and shifting of eyes, and head turns to source.
7 Alerting, head turns to stimulus, and search with eyes.
8 Alerting prolonged, head and eyes turn to stimulus repeatedly.
9 Turning and alerting to stimulus presented on both sides on every presentation of stimulus.

9. Orientation animate—visual and auditory (4 only)

1 Does not focus on or follow stimulus.
2 Stills with stimulus and brightens.
3 Stills, focuses on stimulus when presented, brief following.
4 Stills, focuses on stimulus, follows for 30° arc, jerky movements.
5 Focuses and follows with eyes horizontally for at least a 30° arc. Smooth movement, loses stimulus but finds it again.
6 Follows for two 30° arcs, with eyes and head.
7 Follows with eyes and head at least 60° horizontally, maybe briefly vertically, partly continuous movement, loses stimulus occasionally, head turns to follow.
8 Follows with eyes and head 60° horizontally and 30° vertically.
9 Repeatedly focuses on stimulus and follows with smooth, continuous head movement horizontally, vertically, and in a circle. Follows for at least a 120° arc.

10. Alertness (4)

1 Inattentive—rarely or never responsive to direct stimulation.
2 When alert, responsivity brief and generally quite delayed—alerting and orientation very brief and general.
3 When alert, responsivity brief and somewhat delayed—quality of alertness variable.
4 When alert, responsivity somewhat brief but not generally delayed though variable.
5 When alert, responsivity of moderate duration and response generally not delayed and less variable.
6 When alert, responsivity moderately sustained and not delayed. May use stimulation to come to alert state.
7 When alert, episodes are of generally sustained duration, etc.
8 Always has sustained periods of alertness in best periods. Alerting and orientation frequent and reliable. Stimulation brings infant to alert state and quiets infant.
9 Always alert in best periods. Stimulation always elicits alerting, orienting. Infant reliably uses stimulation to quiet self or maintain quiet state.

11. General tonus (4, 5)

1 Flaccid, limp like a rag doll, no resistance when limbs are moved, complete head lag in pull-to-sit.
2 Little response felt as he is moved, but less than about 25% of the time.
3 Flaccid, limp most of the time, but is responsive about 25% of the time with some tone.
4 Some tone half the time, responds to being handled with some tone less than half the time.
5 Tone when handled, lies in fairly flaccid state between handling.
6 Variable tone in resting, responsive with good tone as he is handled approximately 75% of the time.
7 Is on the hypertonic side approximately 50% of the time.
8 When handled, infant is responsive with hypertonicity about 75% of the time.
9 Hypertonic at rest (in flexion) and hypertonic all the time (abnormal).

12. Motor maturity (4, 5)
1 Cogwheellike jerkiness, overshooting of legs and arms in all directions.
2 Jerky movements and/or mild overshooting.
3 Jerky movements, no overshooting.
4 Only occasional jerky movements, predominantly 45° arcs.
5 Smooth movements predominate, arcs are predominantly 60° half the time.
6 Smooth movements, arcs predominantly 60°.
7 Smooth movements and arcs of 90° less than 50% of the time.
8 Smooth movements and unrestricted arms laterally 90° most of the time.
9 Smoothness, unrestricted (90°) all of the time.

13. Pull-to-sit (3, 5)
1 Head flops completely in pull-to-sit, no attempts to right it in sitting.
2 Futile attempts to right head but some shoulder tone increase is felt.
3 Slight increase in shoulder tone, seating brings head up once but not maintained, no further efforts.
4 Shoulder and arm tone increase, seating brings head up, not maintained but there are further efforts to right it.
5 Head and shoulder tone increases as infant is pulled to sit, brings head up once to midline by self as well, maintains position for 1-2 sec.
6 Head brought up twice after seated, shoulder tone increases as infant comes to sit, and maintained for more than 2 sec.
7 Shoulder tone increases but head not maintained until seated, then can keep it in position 10 sec.
8 Excellent shoulder tone, head up while brought up but cannot maintain without falling, repeatedly rights it.
9 Head up during lift and maintained for 1 min after seated, shoulder girdle and whole body tone increases as infant is pulled to sit.

14. Cuddliness (4, 5)
1 Actually resists being held, continuously pushing away, thrashing, or stiffening.
2 Resists being held most but not all of the time.
3 Does not resist but does not participate either, lies passively in arms and against shoulder (like a sack of meal).
4 Eventually molds into arms, but after a lot of nestling and cuddling by examiner.
5 Usually molds and relaxes when first held, i.e., nestles head in crook of neck and of elbow of examiner. Turns toward body when held horizontally; on shoulder he seems to lean forward.
6 Always molds initially with above activity.
7 Always molds initially with nestling, and turning toward body, and leaning forward.
8 In addition to molding and relaxing, he nestles and turns head, leans forward on shoulder, fits feet into cavity of other arm; i.e., all of body participates.
9 All of the above, and baby grasps hold of examiner to cling.

15. Defensive movements (4)
1 No response.
2 General quieting.
3 Nonspecific activity increase with long latency.
4 Same with short latency.
5 Rooting and lateral head turning.
6 Neck stretching.
7 Nondirected swipes of arms.
8 Directed swipes of arms.
9 Successful removal of cloth with swipes.

16. Consolability with intervention (6 to 5, 4, 3, 2)
1 Not consolable.
2 Pacifier in addition to dressing, holding, and rocking.
3 Dressing, holding in arms, and rocking.
4 Holding and rocking.
5 Picking up and holding.
6 Hand on belly and restraining both arms.
7 Hand on belly steadily.
8 Examiner's voice and face alone.
9 Examiner's face alone.

17. Peak of excitement (6)
1 Low level of arousal to all stimuli. Never above state 2, does not awaken fully.
2 Some arousal to stimulation—can be awakened to state 3.
3 Infant reaches state 4 briefly but predominantly is in lower states.
4 Infant reaches state 5 but is predominantly in state 4 or lower.
5 Infant reaches state 6 after stimulation once or twice but predominantly is in state 5 or lower.
6 Infant reaches state 6 after stimulation but returns to lower states spontaneously.
7 Infant reaches state 6 in response to stimuli but with consoling is easily brought back to lower states.
8 Infant screams (state 6) in response to stimulation, although some quieting can occur with consoling, with difficulty.
9 Infant achieves insulated crying state. Unable to be quieted or soothed.

18. Rapidity of buildup (from 1, 2 to 6)
1 No upset at all.
2 Not until tonic neck reflex (TNR), Moro's reflex, prone placement, and defensive reactions.
3 Not until TNR, Moro's reflex, prone placement, or defensive reactions.
4 Not until undressed.
5 Not until pulled to sit.
6 Not until pinprick.
7 Not until uncovering him.
8 At first auditory and light stimuli.
9 Never was quiet enough to score this.

Continued.

SUMMARY OF BRAZELTON SCALE SCORING DEFINITIONS—cont'd

19. Irritability (3, 4, 5)

Aversive stimuli

Uncover	*Pinprick*
Undress	*TNR*
Pull-to-sit	*Moro's reflex*
Prone	*Defensive reaction*

1 No irritable crying to any of the above.
2 Irritable crying to 1 stimulus.
3 Irritable crying to 2 stimuli.
4 Irritable crying to 3 stimuli.
5 Irritable crying to 4 stimuli.
6 Irritable crying to 5 stimuli.
7 Irritable crying to 6 stimuli.
8 Irritable crying to 7 stimuli.
9 Irritable crying to all stimuli.

20. Activity (alert states)

Score spontaneous and elicited activity separately on a 4-point scale: 0 = none, 1 = slight, 2 = moderate, 3 = much. Then add up the 2 scores.
1 = total score of 0.
2 = total score of 1.
3 = total score of 2.
4 = total score of 3.
5 = total score of 4.
6 = total score of 5.
7 = total score of 6.
8 = continuous but consolable movement.
9 = continuous, unconsolable movement.

21. Tremulousness (all states)

1 No tremors or tremulousness noted.
2 Tremors only during sleep.
3 Tremors only after Moro's reflex or startles.
4 Tremulousness seen 1 or 2 times in states 5 or 6.
5 Tremulousness seen 3 or more times in states 5 or 6.
6 Tremulousness seen 1 or 2 times in state 4.
7 Tremulousness seen 3 or more times in state 4.
8 Tremulousness seen in several states.
9 Tremulousness seen consistently in all states.

22. Amount of startle during examination (3-6)

1 No startles noted.
2 Startle as a response to the examiner's attempts to set off Moro's reflex only.
3 Two startles, including Moro's reflex.
4 Three startles, including Moro's reflex.
5 Four startles, including Moro's reflex.
6 Five startles, including Moro's reflex.
7 Seven startles, including Moro's reflex.
8 Ten startles, including Moro's reflex.
9 Eleven or more startles, including Moro's reflex.

23. Lability of skin color (as infant moves from 1-5)

1 Pale, cyanotic, and does not change during examination.
2 Good color, which changes only minimally during examination.
3 Healthy skin color; no changes except change to slight blue around mouth or extremities when uncovered, or to red when crying; recovery of original color is rapid.
4 Mild cyanosis around mouth or extremities when undressed; slight change in chest or abdomen, but rapid recovery.
5 Healthy color but changes color all over when uncovered or crying; face, lips, extremities may pale or redden, mottling may appear on face, chest, limbs; original color returns quickly.
6 Change in color during examination, but color returns with soothing or covering.
7 Healthy color at outset, changes to very red or blue when uncovered or crying; recovers slowly if covered or soothed.
8 Good color, which rapidly changes with uncovering; recovery is slow but does finally recover when dressed.
9 Marked, rapid changes to very red or blue, no recovery to good color during rest of examination.

24. Lability of states (all states)

The score corresponds to the frequency of swings:
1 = 1-2 swings over 30 min
2 = 3-5
3 = 6-8
4 = 9-10
5 = 11-13
6 = 14-15
7 = 16-18
8 = 19-22
9 = 23 or more

25. Self-quieting activity (6, 5 to 4, 3, 2, 1)

1 Cannot quiet self, makes no attempt, and intervention is always necessary.
2 A brief attempt to quiet self (less than 5 sec), but with no success.
3 Several attempts to quiet self, but with no success.
4 One brief success in quieting self for a period of 5 sec or more.
5 Several brief successes in quieting self.
6 An attempt to quiet self, which results in a sustained successful quieting, with the infant returning to state 4 or below.
7 One sustained and several brief successes in quieting self.
8 At least 2 sustained successes in quieting self.
9 Consistently quiets self for sustained periods.

26. Hand-to-mouth facility (all states)

1 No attempt to bring hands to mouth.
2 Brief swipes at mouth area, no real contact.
3 Hand brought to mouth and contact, but no insertion, once only.
4 Hand brought next to mouth area twice, no insertion.
5 Hand brought next to mouth area at least 3 times, but no real insertion, abortive attempts to suck on fist.
6 One insertion, which is brief, unable to be maintained.
7 Several actual insertions, which are brief, not maintained, abortive sucking attempts, more than 3 times next to mouth.
8 Several brief insertions in rapid succession in an attempt to prolong sucking at this time.
9 Fist and/or fingers actually inserted and sucking on them for 15 sec or more for several brief insertions.

27. Smiles (all states)

Record number observed.

BEHAVIORAL AND NEUROLOGICAL ASSESSMENT SCALE*

Infant's name ______________________ Sex ________ Age ________ Born: Date ________ Hour ________
Mother's age ________ Father's age ________ Father's S.E.S. ______________________
Apparent race ______________________
Examiner(s) ______________________ Place of examination ______________________
Conditions of examination: Date of examination ______________________
Birth weight ____________ Current weight ____________ Length ____________ Head circ. ____________
Time examined ____________ Time last fed ____________ Type of feeding ____________
Type of delivery ____________ Apgar score ____________
Length of labor ____________ Birth order ____________
Type, amount, and timing of medication given mother ______________________

Anesthesia? ____________
Abnormalities of labor ______________________

Initial state: observe 2 min

1	2	3	4	5	6
Deep	Light	Drowsy	Alert	Active	Crying

Predominant states (mark two)

1	2	3	4	5	6

Elicited responses

	O†	L	M	H	A‡
Plantar grasp		1	2	3	
Hand grasp		1	2	3	
Ankle clonus		1	2	3	
Babinski's sign		1	2	3	
Standing		1	2	3	
Automatic walking		1	2	3	
Placing		1	2	3	
Incurvation		1	2	3	
Crawling		1	2	3	
Glabella		1	2	3	
Tonic deviation of head and eyes		1	2	3	
Nystagmus		1	2	3	
Tonic neck reflex		1	2	3	
Moro's reflex		1	2	3	
Rooting (intensity)		1	2	3	
Sucking (intensity)		1	2	3	
Passive movement					
Arms R		1	2	3	
Arms L		1	2	3	
Legs R		1	2	3	
Legs L		1	2	3	

Descriptive paragraph (optional)

Attractive	0	1	2	3
Interfering variables	0	1	2	3
Need for stimulation	0	1	2	3

What activity does he use to quiet self?
- Hand to mouth
- Sucking with nothing in mouth
- Locking onto visual or auditory stimuli
- Postural changes
- State change for no observable reason

COMMENTS:

*From Brazelton, B.: Neonatal behavioral assessment scale, London, 1973, Spastics International Medical Publications.
†Response not elicited (omitted).
‡Asymmetry.

BEHAVIOR SCORING SHEET*

Initial state ____________

Predominant state ____________

Scale (note state)	1	2	3	4	5	6	7	8	9
1. Response decrement to light (2, 3)†	☐	☐	☐	☐	☐	☐	☐	☐	☐
2. Response decrement to rattle (2, 3)	☐	☐	☐	☐	☐	☐	☐	☐	☐
3. Response decrement to bell (2, 3)	☐	☐	☐	☐	☐	☐	☐	☐	☐
4. Response decrement to pinprick (1, 2, 3)	☐	☐	☐	☐	☐	☐	☐	☐	☐
5. Orientation inanimate visual (4 only)	☐	☐	☐	☐	☐	☐	☐	☐	☐
6. Orientation inanimate auditory (4, 5)	☐	☐	☐	☐	☐	☐	☐	☐	☐
7. Orientation animate visual (4 only)	☐	☐	☐	☐	☐	☐	☐	☐	☐
8. Orientation animate auditory (4, 5)	☐	☐	☐	☐	☐	☐	☐	☐	☐
9. Orientation animate visual and auditory (4 only)	☐	☐	☐	☐	☐	☐	☐	☐	☐
10. Alertness (4 only)	☐	☐	☐	☐	☐	☐	☐	☐	☐
11. General tonus (4, 5)	☐	☐	☐	☐	☐	☐	☐	☐	☐
12. Motor maturity (4, 5)	☐	☐	☐	☐	☐	☐	☐	☐	☐
13. Pull-to-sit (3, 5)	☐	☐	☐	☐	☐	☐	☐	☐	☐
14. Cuddliness (4, 5)	☐	☐	☐	☐	☐	☐	☐	☐	☐
15. Defensive movements (4)	☐	☐	☐	☐	☐	☐	☐	☐	☐
16. Consolability (6 to 5, 4, 3, 2)	☐	☐	☐	☐	☐	☐	☐	☐	☐
17. Peak of excitement (6)	☐	☐	☐	☐	☐	☐	☐	☐	☐
18. Rapidity of buildup (from 1, 2 to 6)	☐	☐	☐	☐	☐	☐	☐	☐	☐
19. Irritability (3, 4, 5)	☐	☐	☐	☐	☐	☐	☐	☐	☐
20. Activity (alert states)	☐	☐	☐	☐	☐	☐	☐	☐	☐
21. Tremulousness (all states)	☐	☐	☐	☐	☐	☐	☐	☐	☐
22. Startle (3, 4, 5, 6)	☐	☐	☐	☐	☐	☐	☐	☐	☐
23. Lability of skin color (from 1 to 6)	☐	☐	☐	☐	☐	☐	☐	☐	☐
24. Lability of states (all states)	☐	☐	☐	☐	☐	☐	☐	☐	☐
25. Self-quieting activity (6, 5 to 4, 3, 2, 1)	☐	☐	☐	☐	☐	☐	☐	☐	☐
26. Hand-mouth facility (all states)	☐	☐	☐	☐	☐	☐	☐	☐	☐
27. Smiles (all states)	☐	☐	☐	☐	☐	☐	☐	☐	☐

*From Brazelton, B.: Neonatal behavioral assessment scale, London, 1973, Spastics International Medical Publications.

†Refer to sleep and waking states in Table 29-2.

Birth and Death Certificates

104 -

STATE BIRTH CERTIFICATE NUMBER

CERTIFICATE OF LIVE BIRTH
STATE OF CALIFORNIA

LOCAL REGISTRATION DISTRICT AND CERTIFICATE NUMBER

THIS CHILD	1A. NAME OF CHILD—FIRST	1B. MIDDLE	1C. LAST	
	2. SEX	3A. THIS BIRTH, SINGLE, TWIN, ETC.	3B. IF MULTIPLE, THIS CHILD 1ST, 2ND, ETC.	4A. DATE OF BIRTH—MONTH, DAY, YEAR / 4B. HOUR—(24 HOUR CLOCK TIME)
PLACE OF BIRTH	5A. PLACE OF BIRTH—NAME OF HOSPITAL OR FACILITY	5B. STREET ADDRESS (STREET, NUMBER, OR LOCATION)		
	5C. CITY OR TOWN	5D. COUNTY		
FATHER OF CHILD	6A. NAME OF FATHER—FIRST	6B. MIDDLE	6C. LAST	7. STATE OF BIRTH / 8. AGE OF FATHER
MOTHER OF CHILD	9A. NAME OF MOTHER—FIRST	9B. MIDDLE	9C. LAST (BIRTH NAME)	10. STATE OF BIRTH / 11. AGE OF MOTHER
PARENT'S CERTIFICATION	I CERTIFY THAT I HAVE REVIEWED THE STATED INFORMATION AND THAT IT IS TRUE AND CORRECT TO THE BEST OF MY KNOWLEDGE	12A. PARENT OR OTHER INFORMANT—SIGNATURE	12B. RELATIONSHIP TO CHILD	12C. DATE SIGNED
ATTENDANT'S CERTIFICATION	I CERTIFY THAT I ATTENDED THIS BIRTH AND THAT THE CHILD WAS BORN ALIVE AT THE HOUR, DATE AND PLACE STATED	13A. PHYSICIAN OR OTHER ATTENDANT—SIGNATURE—DEGREE OR TITLE	13B. LICENSE NUMBER	13C. DATE SIGNED
	14.	13D. TYPED NAME AND ADDRESS		
LOCAL REGISTRAR	15. DEATH—ENTER DATE OF DEATH	16. LOCAL REGISTRAR—SIGNATURE	17. DATE ACCEPTED FOR REGISTRATION	

CONFIDENTIAL INFORMATION FOR PUBLIC HEALTH USE ONLY

FATHER	18. RACE/ETHNICITY	19. SPANISH/HISPANIC ☐ NO	20A. USUAL OCCUPATION	20B. KIND OF BUSINESS OR INDUSTRY
MOTHER	21. RACE/ETHNICITY	22. SPANISH/HISPANIC ☐ NO	23A. USUAL OCCUPATION	23B. KIND OF BUSINESS OR INDUSTRY
	24A. RESIDENCE (STREET, NUMBER OR LOCATION)			24C. COUNTY
	24D. CITY OR TOWN			24E. STATE / 24F. ZIP CODE
MEDICAL DATA	25A. DATE LAST NORMAL MENSES BEGAN MONTH | DAY | YEAR	25B. MONTH OF PREGNANCY PRENATAL CARE BEGAN (1ST, 2ND . . . 8TH, 9TH)	26. BIRTHWEIGHT GRAMS	27. PREGNANCY HISTORY (COMPLETE EACH SECTION) LIVE BIRTHS (DO NOT COUNT THIS CHILD): NOW LIVING (NUMBER) A; NOW DEAD (NUMBER) B. OTHER TERMINATIONS (EXCLUDE INDUCED ABORTIONS): BEFORE 20 WKS (NUMBER) C; AFTER 20 WKS (NUMBER) D
	ENTER THE APPROPRIATE CODE OR CODES FOR EACH ITEM 28 THRU 32 FROM THE VS 10A SUPPLEMENTAL WORKSHEET: IF NONE CHECK—NONE		28. CESAREAN SECTION ☐ NO	
	29. COMPLICATION OF PREGNANCY AND CONCURRENT ILLNESSES ☐ NONE		30. BIRTH INJURY TO CHILD ☐ NONE	DATE OF LAST LIVE BIRTH MONTH | DAY | YEAR E; DATE OF LAST TERMINATION MONTH | YEAR F
	31. COMPLICATIONS OF LABOR AND DELIVERY ☐ NONE		32. CONGENITAL MALFORMATIONS OR ANOMALIES OF CHILD ☐ NONE	
STATE REGISTRAR	A. B. C.	D. E.	F.	CENSUS TRACT

NOTICE: THE INFORMATION YOU PROVIDE IN COMPLETING THE BOTTOM HALF OF THE BIRTH CERTIFICATE WILL BE KEPT STRICTLY CONFIDENTIAL AND WILL BE USED FOR HEALTH AND MEDICAL PURPOSES ONLY.

VS 10 (REV.1-82) PENALTY FOR UNAUTHORIZED RELEASE. $500 FINE OR SIX MONTHS IMPRISONMENT

CERTIFICATE OF FETAL DEATH

STATE OF CALIFORNIA

STATE FILE NUMBER

LOCAL REGISTRATION DISTRICT AND CERTIFICATE NUMBER

THIS FETUS	1A. NAME—FIRST	1B. MIDDLE	1C. LAST	
	2. SEX	3A. THIS DELIVERY, SINGLE, TWIN, ETC.	3B. IF MULTIPLE, THIS FETUS 1ST, 2ND, ETC.	4A. DATE OF DELIVERY MONTH, DAY, YEAR / 4B. HOUR (24 HOUR CLOCK TIME)
PLACE OF DELIVERY	5A. PLACE OF DELIVERY—NAME OF HOSPITAL	5B. STREET ADDRESS (STREET, NUMBER, OR LOCATION)		
	5C. CITY OR TOWN	5D. COUNTY		

FATHER	6A. NAME OF FATHER—FIRST	6B. MIDDLE	6C. LAST	7. STATE OF BIRTH	8. AGE OF FATHER
MOTHER	9A. NAME OF MOTHER—FIRST	9B. MIDDLE	9C. LAST (BIRTHNAME)	10. STATE OF BIRTH	11. AGE OF MOTHER

CERTIFICATION	I CERTIFY THAT THIS FETUS WAS BORN DEAD AT THE HOUR, DATE AND PLACE STATED AND FROM THE CAUSES STATED.	12A. PHYSICIAN OR CORONER—DEGREE OR TITLE AND TYPED NAME	12B. DATE SIGNED
FUNERAL DIRECTOR AND LOCAL REGISTRAR	13. DISPOSITION	14. DATE (MONTH, DAY, YEAR)	15. NAME AND ADDRESS OF CEMETERY OR CREMATORY
	16. NAME OF FUNERAL DIRECTOR (OR PERSON ACTING AS SUCH)	17. LOCAL REGISTRAR—SIGNATURE	18. DATE ACCEPTED BY LOCAL REGISTRAR

CONFIDENTIAL HEALTH AND MEDICAL INFORMATION

CAUSE OF DEATH

19. **FETAL DEATH WAS CAUSED BY** — ENTER ONLY ONE CAUSE PER LINE FOR A, B AND C

FETAL OR MATERNAL CONDITION DIRECTLY CAUSING FETAL DEATH. — IMMEDIATE CAUSE (A)

FETAL AND/OR MATERNAL CONDITIONS, IF ANY, WHICH GAVE RISE TO THE IMMEDIATE CAUSE, STATING THE UNDERLYING CAUSE LAST. — DUE TO, OR AS A CONSEQUENCE OF (B) — DUE TO, OR AS A CONSEQUENCE OF (C)

20. OTHER SIGNIFICANT CONDITIONS OF FETUS OR MOTHER—CONTRIBUTION TO FETAL DEATH BUT NOT RELATED TO CAUSE GIVEN IN 19A — 21. AUTOPSY (SPECIFY YES OR NO)

FATHER	22. RACE/ETHNICITY	23. SPANISH/HISPANIC ☐ NO	24A. USUAL OCCUPATION	24B. KIND OF BUSINESS OR INDUSTRY
MOTHER	25. RACE/ETHNICITY	26. SPANISH/HISPANIC ☐ NO	27A. USUAL OCCUPATION	27B. KIND OF BUSINESS OR INDUSTRY
	28A. RESIDENCE (STREET, NUMBER OR LOCATION)	28B. CITY OR TOWN	28C. STATE / 28D. ZIP CODE	28E. COUNTY

MEDICAL DATA

29A. DATE LAST NORMAL MENSES BEGAN MONTH / DAY / YEAR — 29B. MONTH OF PREGNANCY PRENATAL CARE BEGAN (1ST, 2ND . . . 8TH, 9TH)	30. BIRTHWEIGHT GRAMS	31. PREGNANCY HISTORY (COMPLETE EACH SECTION) — LIVE BIRTHS (DO NOT COUNT THIS CHILD): NOW LIVING (NUMBER) A; NOW DEAD (NUMBER) B — OTHER TERMINATIONS (EXCLUDE INDUCED ABORTIONS): BEFORE 20 WKS (NUMBER) C; AFTER 20 WKS (NUMBER) D
ENTER THE APPROPRIATE CODE OR CODES FOR EACH ITEM 32 THRU 36 FROM THE VS 10A SUPPLEMENTAL WORKSHEET. IF NONE CHECK—NONE	32. CESAREAN SECTION ☐ NO	DATE OF LAST LIVE BIRTH MONTH / DAY / YEAR E — DATE OF LAST TERMINATION MONTH / YEAR F
33. COMPLICATION OF PREGNANCY AND CONCURRENT ILLNESSES ☐ NONE	34. BIRTH INJURY TO CHILD ☐ NONE	
35. COMPLICATIONS OF LABOR AND DELIVERY ☐ NONE	36. CONGENITAL MALFORMATIONS OR ANOMALIES OF CHILD ☐ NONE	

STATE REGISTRAR	A.	B.	C.	D.	E.	F.	CENSUS TRACT

VS 12 (REV 1-82) **PENALTY FOR UNAUTHORIZED RELEASE, $500 FINE OR SIX MONTHS IMPRISONMENT.** [illegible]

APPENDIX N

Standards of Care for Maternal–Child Nursing

American Academy of Pediatrics: Standards and recommendations for hospital care of newborn infants, Evanston, Ill., 1977, The Academy.

American College of Nurse-Midwives: Functions, standards, and qualifications, Washington, D.C., 1975, The College.

American College of Obstetricians and Gynecologists: Standards for obstetric-gynecologic services, Chicago, 1974, The College.

American Nurses' Association: Standards of maternal-child health nursing practice, 1973, The Association.

The American College of Obstetricians and Gynecologists and The Nurses Association of The American College of Obstetricians and Gynecologists: The obstetric-gynecologic nurse practitioner, Washington, D.C., 1979, The College.

Interprofessional Task Force on Health Care of Women and Children, The American College of Obstetricians and Gynecologists, The American College of Nurse-Midwives, and The Nurses Association of The American College of Obstetricians and Gynecologists: Joint position statement on the development of family-centered maternity/newborn care in hospitals, 1978.

Joint Commission on Accreditation of Hospitals: Accreditation manual for hospitals, Chicago, 1976, The Commission.

The National Foundation-March of Dimes Committee on Perinatal Health: Toward improving the outcome of pregnancy: recommendations for the regional development of maternal and perinatal health services, White Plains, N.Y., 1976, The Foundation.

The Nurses Association of The American College of Obstetricians and Gynecologists: Guidelines for childbirth education, Washington, D.C., 1981, The Association.

The Nurses Association of The American College of Obstetricians and Gynecologists: Obstetric, gynecologic and neonatal nursing functions and standards, Washington, D.C., 1975, The Association.

The Nurses Association of The American College of Obstetricians and Gynecologists: Standards for obstetric, gynecologic, and neonatal nursing, ed. 2, Washington, D.C., 1981, The Association.

Planning and evaluating nursing care, Wakefield, Mass., 1974, Contemporary Publishing, Inc.

U.S. Department of Health, Education, and Welfare, Public Health Service, Health Services Administration: Guidelines for review of nursing care at the local level, Washington, D.C., 1976, The Department.

Glossary

abdominal Belonging or relating to the abdomen and its functions and disorders.
- **a. delivery** Birth of a child through a surgical incision made into the abdominal wall and uterus; cesarean delivery.
- **a. gestation** Implantation of a fertilized ovum outside the uterus but inside the peritoneal cavity.
- **a. hysterectomy** Surgical removal of the uterus through an abdominal wall incision.
- **a. pregnancy** See *abdominal gestation.*

ablatio placentae See *abruptio placentae.*

abortion Termination of pregnancy before the fetus is viable and capable of extrauterine existence, usually less than 21 to 22 weeks' gestation (or when the fetus weighs less than 600 g).
- **complete a.** Abortion in which fetus and all related tissue have been expelled from the uterus.
- **criminal a.** Termination of pregnancy performed by unqualified people usually under septic conditions. Women may resort to this if therapeutic abortions are unavailable.
- **elective a.** Termination of pregnancy chosen by the woman that is not required for her physical safety.
- **habitual (recurrent) a.** Loss of three or more successive pregnancies for no known cause.
- **incomplete a.** Loss of pregnancy in which some but not all the products of conception have been expelled from the uterus.
- **induced a.** Intentionally produced loss of pregnancy by woman or others.
- **inevitable a.** Threatened loss of pregnancy that cannot be prevented or stopped and is imminent.
- **missed a.** Loss of pregnancy in which the products of conception remain in the uterus after the fetus dies.
- **septic a.** Loss of pregnancy in which there is an infection of the products of conception and the uterine endometrial lining, usually resulting from attempted termination of early pregnancy.
- **spontaneous a.** Loss of pregnancy that occurs naturally without interference or known cause.
- **therapeutic a.** Pregnancy that has been intentionally terminated for medical reasons.
- **threatened a.** Possible loss of a pregnancy; early symptoms are present (e.g., the cervix begins to dilate).
- **voluntary a.** See *abortion, elective.*

abortus Fetus usually less than 21 weeks' gestational age and under 600 g.

abruptio placentae Partial or complete premature separation of a normally implanted placenta.

abstinence Refraining from sexual intercourse periodically or permanently.

accreta, placenta See *placenta accreta.*

acculturation Process of adopting the cultural traits or social patterns of another group.

acetonuria Presence of acetone and diacetic bodies in the urine.

acidosis Increase in hydrogen ion concentration resulting in a lowering of blood pH below 7.35.
- **metabolic a.** Increase in hydrogen ion concentration caused by increased acids from (1) abnormal metabolism (too many acids produced), (2) renal malfunction (acids not being excreted), or (3) excessive loss of base (diarrhea).

acini cells Milk-producing cells in the breast.

acme Highest point (e.g., of a contraction).

acrocyanosis Peripheral cyanosis; blue color of hands and feet in most infants at birth that may persist for 7 to 10 days.

acromion Projection of the spine of the scapula (forming the point of the shoulder); used to explain the presentation of the fetus.

adenomyoma Type of tumor affecting glandular and smooth muscle tissue, such as uterine musculature.

adnexa Adjacent or accessory parts of a structure.
- **uterine a.** Ovaries and fallopian tubes.

adult respiratory distress syndrome (ARDS) Set of symptoms including decreased compliance of lung tissue, pulmonary edema, and acute hypoxemia. The condition is similar to respiratory distress syndrome of the newborn.

afibrinogenemia Absence or decrease of fibrinogen in the blood such that the blood will not coagulate. In obstetrics, this condition occurs from complications of abruptio placentae or retention of a dead fetus.

afterbirth Lay term for the placenta and membranes expelled after the birth or delivery of the child.

afterpains Painful uterine cramps that occur intermittently for approximately 2 or 3 days after delivery and that result from contractile efforts of the uterus to return to its normal involuted condition.

AGA Appropriate (weight) for gestational age.

agalactia Absence or failure of milk secretion after childbirth.

agenesis Failure of an organ to develop.

alae nasi Nostrils.

albuminuria Presence of readily detectable amounts of albumin in the urine.

alkalosis Abnormal condition of body fluids characterized by a tendency toward an increased pH, as from an excess of alkaline bicarbonate or a deficiency of acid.

allantois Tubular diverticulum of the posterior part of the embryo's yolk sac that passes into the body stalk, accompanied by the allantoic blood vessels that develop and become the umbilical vein and paired umbilical arteries; later, after fusing with the chorion, it helps to form the placenta.

allele One of two or more alternative forms of a gene at the same site on a chromosome; alleles determine alternative characters in inheritance. Alleles that occur at the same position, or locus, on a chromosome pair may produce different effects during development.

alveoli, fetal Terminal pulmonary sacs that in fetal life are filled with fluid. This fluid is a transudate of fetal plasma.

ambient Surrounding; around.

amenorrhea Absence or suppression of menstruation.

amnesia Loss of memory.

amnii, liquor See *liquor amnii.*

amniocentesis Procedure in which a needle is inserted through the abdominal and uterine walls into the amniotic fluid; used for assessment of fetal health and maturity and for therapeutic abortion.

amniography Procedure used primarily to detect placenta previa by x-ray examination, entailing injection of radiopaque dye into amniotic fluid.

amnion Inner membrane of two fetal membranes that form the sac and contain the fetus and the fluid that surrounds it in utero.

amnionitis Inflammation of the amnion, occurring most frequently after early rupture of membranes.

amniotic Pertaining or relating to the amnion.

- **a. fluid** Fluid surrounding fetus derived primarily from maternal serum and fetal urine.
- **a. sac** Membrane "bag" that contains the fetus before delivery.

amniotomy Artificial rupture of the fetal membranes (AROM).

anaerobic catabolism In the absence of free oxygen, the breakdown of organized substances into simpler compounds, with the resultant release of energy.

analgesia Lack of pain without loss of consciousness.

analgesic Any drug or agent that will relieve pain.

androgen Substance that produces masculinizing effects (e.g., testosterone).

androgynous personality Having some characteristics of both sexes.

android pelvis Male type of pelvis.

anencephaly Congenital deformity characterized by the absence of cerebrum, cerebellum, and flat bones of skull.

anesthesia Partial or complete absence of sensation with or without loss of consciousness.

anomaly Organ or structure that is malformed or in some way abnormal with reference to form, structure, or position.

anorexia nervosa Psychoneurotic disorder characterized by a prolonged refusal to eat, resulting in emaciation, amenorrhea, emotional disturbance concerning body image, and an abnormal fear of becoming obese.

anovular menstrual period Cyclic uterine bleeding not accompanied by the production and discharge of an ovum.

anovulatory Failure of the ovaries to produce, mature, or release eggs.

anoxia Absence of oxygen.

antenatal Occurring before or formed before birth.

antepartal Before labor.

anterior Pertaining to the front.

- **a. fontanel** See *fontanel, anterior*.

anteroposterior repair Operation in which the upper and lower walls of the vagina are reconstructed to correct relaxed tissue.

anthropoid pelvis Pelvis in which the anteroposterior diameter is equal to or greater than the transverse diameter.

antibody Specific protein substance developed by the body that exerts restrictive or destructive action on specific antigens, such as bacteria, toxins, or Rh factor.

anticipatory grief Grief that predates the loss of a beloved object.

antigen Protein foreign to the body that causes the body to develop antibodies. Examples: bacteria, dust, Rh factor.

Apgar score Numeric expression of the condition of a newborn obtained by rapid assessment at 1, 5, and 15 minutes of age; developed by Dr. Virginia Apgar.

apnea Cessation of respirations for more than 10 seconds associated with generalized cyanosis.

Apt test Differentiation of maternal and fetal blood when there is vaginal bleeding. It is performed as follows: Add 0.5 ml blood to 4.5 ml distilled water. Shake. Add 1 ml 0.25N sodium hydroxide. Fetal and cord blood remains pink for 1 or 2 minutes. Maternal blood becomes brown in 30 seconds.

areola Pigmented ring of tissue surrounding the nipple.

- **secondary a.** During the fifth month of pregnancy, a second faint ring of pigmentation seen around the original areola.

arthralgia Any pain that affects a joint.

articulation Fastening together or connection of the various bones of the skeleton; a joint. The articulations of the bones are classified as (1) immovable (synarthrosis), (2) slightly immovable (amphiarthrosis), and (3) freely movable (diarthrosis).

artificial insemination Introduction of semen by instrument injection into the vagina or uterus for impregnation.

Aschheim-Zondek test Pregnancy determination in which a woman's urine is injected into a mouse. After 5 days the animal is killed and its ovaries are examined. Enlarged ovaries and maturing follicles indicate pregnancy.

asphyxia Decreased oxygen and/or excess of carbon dioxide in the body.

- **fetal a.** Condition occurring in utero, with the following biochemical changes: hypoxemia (lowering of Po_2), hypercapnia (increase in Pco_2), and respiratory and metabolic acidosis (reduction of blood pH).
- **a. livida** Condition in which the infant's skin is characteristically pale, pulse is weak and slow, and reflexes are depressed or absent; also known as *blue asphyxia*.
- **a. pallida** Condition in which the infant appears pale and limp and suffers from bradycardia (80 beats/min or less) and apnea.

aspiration pneumonia Inflammatory condition of the lungs and bronchi caused by the inhalation of vomitus containing acid gastric contents.

aspiration syndrome See *meconium aspiration syndrome*.

asynclitism Oblique presentation of the fetal head at the superior strait of the pelvis; the pelvic planes and those of the fetal head are not parallel.

ataractic Drug capable of promoting tranquility; a tranquilizer.

atelectasis Pulmonary pathosis involving alveolar collapse.

atherosclerosis Common arterial disorder characterized by yellowish plaques of cholesterol, lipids, and cellular debris in the inner layers of the walls of large and medium-sized arteries, resulting in reduced circulation in organs and areas normally supplied by the artery.

athetosis Neuromuscular condition characterized by slow, writhing, continuous, and involuntary movement of the extremities, as seen in some forms of cerebral palsy and in motor disorders resulting from lesions in the basal ganglia.

atony Absence of muscle tone.

atresia Absence of a normally present passageway.

- **biliary a.** Absence of the bile duct.
- **choanal a.** Complete obstruction of the posterior nares, which open into the nasopharynx, with membranous or bony tissue.
- **esophageal a.** Congenital anomaly in which the esophagus ends in a blind pouch or narrows into a thin cord, thus failing to form a continuous passageway to the stomach.

attachment Relationship between two persons (e.g., a parent and a child).

attitude Body posture or position.

- **fetal a.** Relation of fetal parts to each other in the uterus (e.g., all parts flexed, all parts flexed except neck is extended, etc.).

auscultation Process of listening for sounds produced within the body.

autoimmunization Development of antibodies against constituents of one's own tissues (e.g., a man may develop antibodies against his own sperm).

autosomes Any of the paired chromosomes other than the sex (X and Y) chromosomes.

axis Line, real or imaginary, about which a part revolves or that runs through the center of a body.

pelvic a. Imaginary curved line that passes through the centers of all the anteroposterior diameters of the pelvis.

azoospermia Absence of sperm in the semen.

bacteremic shock Shock that occurs in septicemia when endotoxins are released from certain bacteria in the bloodstream.

bag of waters Lay term for the sac containing amniotic fluid and fetus.

ballottement (1) Movability of a floating object (e.g., fetus). (2) Diagnostic technique using palpation: a floating object, when tapped or pushed, moves away and then returns to touch the examiner's hand.

Bandl's ring Abnormally thickened ridge of uterine musculature between the upper and lower segments that follows a mechanically obstructed labor, with the lower segment thinning abnormally.

Barr body (sex chromatin) Chromatin mass located against the inner surface of the nucleus in females, possibly representing the inactive X chromosome.

Bartholin's glands Two small glands situated on either side of the vaginal orifice that secrete small amounts of mucus during coitus and that are homologous to the bulbourethral glands in the male.

basalis, decidua See *decidua basalis.*

Bell's palsy See *palsy, Bell's.*

bicornuate uterus Anomalous uterus that may be either a double or single organ with two horns.

biliary atresia See *atresia, biliary.*

bilirubin Yellow or orange pigment that is a breakdown product of hemoglobin. It is carried by the blood to the liver, where it is chemically changed and excreted in the bile or is conjugated and excreted by the kidneys.

Billings method See *ovulation method.*

bimanual Performed with both hands.

b. palpation Examination of a woman's pelvic organs done by placing one hand on the abdomen and one or two fingers of the other hand in the vagina.

biopsy Removal of a small piece of tissue for microscopic examination and diagnosis.

birthing chair Chair used in labor and delivery to promote the comfort of the mother and the efficiency of parturition. The chair may be specially designed, having many technical features, or it may be a simple three-legged stool with a high, slanted back and a circular seat with a large central hole in it.

blastoderm Germinal membrane of the ovum.

b. vesicle Stage in the development of a mammalian embryo that consists of an outer layer, or trophoblast, and a hollow sphere of cells enclosing a cavity.

bleeding diathesis See *diathesis, bleeding.*

blood-brain barrier Obstruction that prevents passage of certain substances from blood into brain tissue.

bloody show Vaginal discharge that originates in the cervix and consists of blood and mucus; increases as cervix dilates during labor.

body image Person's subjective concept of his or her physical appearance.

bonding See *attachment.*

born out of asepsis (BOA) Pertaining to birth without the use of sterile technique.

Bradley method Preparation for parenthood with active participation of father and mother.

Braxton Hicks sign Mild, intermittent, painless uterine contractions that occur during pregnancy. These contractions occur more frequently as pregnancy advances but do not represent true labor.

Braxton Hicks version One of several types of maneuvers designed to turn the fetus from an undesirable position to a more acceptable one to facilitate delivery.

Brazelton assessment Criteria for assessing the interactional behavior of a newborn.

breakthrough bleeding Escape of blood occurring between menstrual periods; may be noted by women using chemical contraception (birth control pill).

breast milk jaundice See *jaundice, breast milk.*

breech presentation Presentation in which buttocks and/or feet are nearest the cervical opening and are born first; occurs in approximately 3% of all deliveries.

complete b. p. Simultaneous presentation of buttocks, legs, and feet.

footling (incomplete) b.p. Presentation of one or both feet.

frank b. p. Presentation of buttocks, with hips flexed so that thighs are against abdomen.

bregma Point of junction of the coronal and sagittal sutures of the skull; the area of the anterior fontanel of the fetus.

brim Edge of the superior strait of the true pelvis; the inlet.

bronchopulmonary dysplasia Emphysematous changes caused by oxygen toxicity.

brown fat Source of heat unique to neonates that is capable of greater thermogenic activity than ordinary fat. Deposits are found around the adrenals, kidneys, and neck, between the scapulas, and behind the sternum for several weeks after birth.

bruit, uterine Sound of passage of blood through uterine blood vessels, synchronous with fetal heart rate.

cachexia Severe generalized weakness, malnutrition, and emaciation.

caked breast See *engorgement.*

calcemia See *hypercalcemia.*

Candida vaginitis Vaginal, fungal infection; moniliasis.

capsularis, decidua See *decidua capsularis.*

caput Occiput of fetal head appearing at the vaginal introitus preceding delivery of the head.

c. succedaneum Swelling of the tissue over the presenting part of the fetal head caused by pressure during labor.

carrier Individual who carries a gene that does not exhibit itself in physical or chemical characteristics but that can be transmitted to children (e.g., a female carrying the trait for hemophilia, which is expressed in male offspring).

catamenia Menses.

caudal anesthesia Type of regional anesthesia used in childbirth in which the anesthetic agent is injected into the caudal area of the spinal canal through the sacral hiatus, affecting the caudal nerve roots and thereby anesthetizing the cervix, vagina, and perineum. Medication does not mix with cerebrospinal fluid (CSF).

caul Hood of fetal membranes covering fetal head during delivery.

cautery Method of destroying tissue by the use of heat, electricity, or chemicals.

centesis suffix pertaining to a surgical puncture or perforation.

cephalhematoma Extravasation of blood from ruptured vessels between a skull bone and its external covering, the periosteum. Swelling is limited by the margins of the cranial bone affected (usually parietals).

cephalic Pertaining to the head.

c. presentation Presentation of any part of the fetal head.

cephalopelvic disproportion (CPD) Condition in which the infant's head is of such a shape, size, or position that it cannot pass through the mother's pelvis.
cervical amputation Removal of the neck of the uterus.
cervical cap (custom) Individually fitted contraceptive covering for the cervix.
cervical cauterization Destruction (usually by heat or electric current) of the superficial tissue of the cervix.
cervical conization Excision of a cone-shaped section of tissue from the endocervix.
cervical erosion Alteration of the epithelium of the cervix caused by chronic irritation or infection.
cervical mucus method See *ovulation method.*
cervical os "Mouth" or opening to the cervix.
cervical polyp Small tumor on a stem (pedicle) attached inside the cervix.
cervical stenosis Narrowing of the canal between the body of the uterus and the cervical os.
cervicitis Cervical infection.
cervix Lowest and narrow end of the uterus; the "neck." The cervix is situated between the external os and the body or corpus of the uterus, and its lower end extends into the vagina.
cesarean delivery Birth of a fetus by an incision through the abdominal wall and uterus.
cesarean hysterectomy Removal of the uterus immediately after the cesarean delivery of an infant.
Chadwick's sign Violet color of mucous membrane that is visible from about the fourth week of pregnancy; caused by increased vascularity of the vagina.
change of life See *climacteric.*
chemotaxis Response involving movement that is positive (toward) or negative (away from) to a chemical stimulus.
chloasma Increased pigmentation over bridge of nose and cheeks of pregnant women and some women taking oral contraceptives; also known as *mask of pregnancy.*
choanal atresia See *atresia, choanal.*
cholecystitis Acute or chronic inflammation of the gallbladder.
cholelithiasis Presence of gallstones in the gallbladder.
choreoathetoid cerebral palsy Condition characterized by both choreiform (jerky, ticlike twitching) and athetoid (slow, writhing) movements.
chorioamnionitis Stimulated by organisms in the amniotic fluid, which then become infiltrated with polymorphonuclear leukocytes.
chorioepithelioma Carcinoma of the chorion; rapid malignant proliferation of the epithelium of the chorionic villi.
chorion Fetal membrane closest to the intrauterine wall that gives rise to the placenta and continues as the outer membrane surrounding the amnion.
chorionic villi See *villi, chorionic.*
chromosome Element within the cell nucleus carrying genes and composed of DNA and proteins.
circumcision Excision of the male's prepuce (foreskin).
cleft lip Incomplete closure of the lip; harelip.
cleft palate Incomplete closure of the palate or roof of mouth; a congenital fissure.
climacteric (change of life) Period when the human body undergoes significant psychologic and physiologic changes, such as the termination of reproductive function in the woman.
clitoris Female organ analogous to male penis; a small, ovoid body of erectile tissue situated at the anterior junction of the vulva.
  prepuce of the c. see *prepuce of the clitoris.*
coccyx Small bone at the base of the spinal column.
coitus Penile-vaginal intercourse.
  c. interruptus Intercourse during which penis is withdrawn from vagina before ejaculation.
colostrum Yellow secretion from the breast containing mainly serum and white blood corpuscles preceding the onset of true lactation 2 or 3 days after delivery.
colpectomy Surgical excision of the vagina.
colporrhaphy (1) Procedure of suturing the vagina. (2) Procedure whereby the vagina is denuded and sutured for the purpose of narrowing the vagina.
colpotomy Any surgical incision into the wall of the vagina.
communicating hydrocephalus See *hydrocephalus, communicating.*
complement Naturally occurring blood component that is a factor in the destruction of bacteria.
complementary feeding Supplemental feeding given to the infant if he is still hungry after breast feeding.
complete abortion See *abortion, complete*
complete breech presentation See *breech presentation, complete.*
compliance, lung Degree of distensibility of the lung's elastic tissue.
conception Union of the sperm and ovum resulting in fertilization; formation of the one-celled zygote.
conceptional age In fetal development, the number of completed weeks since the moment of conception. Because the moment of conception is almost impossible to determine, conceptional age is estimated at 2 weeks less than gestational age.
conceptus Embryo or fetus, fetal membranes, amniotic fluid, and the fetal portion of the placenta.
concurrent sterilization Method of preparing formula in which all the ingredients and equipment are sterilized prior to mixing.
condom Mechanical barrier worn on the penis for contraception; "rubber."
condyloma Wartlike growth on the skin usually seen near the anus or external genitals. There is a pointed type, and there is the flat, broad, moist papule of secondary syphilis.
confinement Period of childbirth and early puerperium.
congenital Present or existing before birth as a result of either heredity or prenatal environmental factors.
conjoined twins See *twins, conjoined.*
conjugate
  diagonal c. Radiographic measurement of distance from *inferior border* of SP to sacral promontory; may be obtained by vaginal examination; 12.5 to 13 cm.
  true c. (c. vera) Radiographic measurement of distance from *upper margin* of symphysis pubis (SP) to sacral promontory; 1.5 to 2 cm less than diagonal conjugate.
conjunctivitis Inflammation of the mucous membrane that lines the eyelids and that is reflected onto the eyeball.
consanguinity Existing blood relationship between persons.
contraception Prevention of impregnation or conception.
contraction ring See *Bandl's ring.*
Coombs' test Indirect: determination of Rh-positive antibodies in maternal blood; direct: determination of maternal Rh-positive antibodies in fetal cord blood. A positive test result indicates the presence of antibodies or titer.
coping mechanism Any effort directed at stress management. It can be task oriented and involve direct problem-solving efforts to cope with the threat itself or be intrapsychic or ego defense oriented with the goal of regulating one's emotional distress.
copulation Coitus; sexual intercourse.

corpus Discrete mass of material.

c. cavernosum Term referring to one of two cylinders of spongy tissue within the penis or tissue within the clitoris that engorges with blood during sexual excitement resulting in erection.

c. luteum Yellow body. After rupture of the graafian follicle at ovulation, the follicle develops into a yellow structure that secretes progesterone in the second half of the menstrual cycle, atrophying about 3 days before sloughing of the endometrium in menstrual flow. If impregnation occurs, this structure continues to produce progesterone until the placenta can take over this function.

c. spongiosum One of the spongy cylinders of tissue within the penis; has a protective function.

cotyledon One of the 15 to 28 visible segments of the placenta on the maternal surface, each made up of fetal vessels, chorionic villi, and an intervillous space.

couvade Custom whereby the husband goes through mock labor while his wife is giving birth.

Couvelaire uterus See *uterus, Couvelaire*.

CPAP Continuous positive airway pressure.

cradle cap Common seborrheic dermatitis of infants consisting of thick, yellow, greasy scales on the scalp.

craniotabes Localized softening of cranial bones.

creatinine Substance found in blood and muscle; measurement of levels in maternal urine correlates with amount of fetal muscle mass and therefore fetal size.

Crede's method Obsolete method by which the placenta is expelled by downward manual pressure on the uterus through the abdominal wall. The thumb is placed on the posterior surface of the fundus of the uterus and the flat of the hand on the anterior surface. Pressure is applied in the direction of the birth canal.

Crede's prophylaxis Instillation of 1% silver nitrate solution into the conjunctivas of newborn infants immediately after birth to prevent ophthalmia neonatorum, particularly that caused by gonorrheal organisms.

crepitus (1) Noise produced when pressure is applied to tissues containing abnormal amounts of air. (2) Grating sound heard when broken bone ends are moved. (3) Noise of gas being expelled from the intestines.

crib death Unexpected and sudden death of an apparently normal and healthy infant that occurs during sleep and with no physical or autopsic evidence of disease. Also referred to as sudden infant death syndrome (SIDS).

cri-du-chat syndrome Rare congenital disorder recognized at birth by a kittenlike cry, which may prevail for weeks, then disappear. Other characteristics include low birth weight, microcephaly, "moon face," wide-set eyes, strabismus, and low-set misshaped ears. Infants are hypotonic; heart defects and mental and physical retardation are common. Also called cat-cry syndrome.

crowning Stage of delivery when the top of the fetal head can be seen at the vaginal orifice.

cryo- Prefix meaning cold, freezing.

cryosurgery Local freezing and removal of tissue without injury to adacent tissue and with minimum blood loss, done with special equipment.

cryptochidism Failure of one or both of the testicles to descend into the scrotum. Also called undescended testis.

cul-de-sac of Douglas Pouch formed by a fold of the peritoneum dipping down between the anterior wall of the rectum and the posterior wall of the uterus; also called *Douglas' cul-de-sac, pouch of Douglas,* and *rectouterine pouch*.

culdocentesis Use of needle puncture or incision to remove intraperitoneal fluid (blood, purulent material) by way of the vagina.

culdotomy Incision or needle puncture of the cul-de-sac of Douglas by way of the vagina.

Cullen's sign Faint, irregularly formed, hemorrhagic patches on the skin around the umbilicus. The discolored skin is blue-black and becomes greenish brown or yellow. Cullen's sign may appear 1 to 2 days after the onset of anorexia and the severe, poorly localized abdominal pains characteristic of acute pancreatitis. Cullen's sign is also present in massive upper gastrointestinal hemorrhage, ruptured ectopic pregnancy.

culture The total learned way of life of a society.

curettage Scraping of the endometrium lining of the uterus with a curet to remove the contents of the uterus (as is done after an inevitable or incomplete abortion) or to obtain specimens for diagnostic purposes.

cutis marmorata Transient vasomotor phenomenon occurring primarily over extremities when the infant is exposed to chilling. It appears as a pink or faint purple capillary outline on the skin. Occasionally it is seen if the infant is in respiratory distress.

cyesis Pregnancy.

cystocele Bladder hernia; injury to the vesicovaginal fascia during labor and delivery may allow herniation of the bladder into the vagina.

cytogenics Branch of genetics concerned primarily with the study of chromosomes and correlations with associated gene behavior.

cytology The study of cells, including their formation, origin, structure, function, biochemical activities, and pathology.

death Cessation of life.

fetal d. Intrauterine death. Death of a fetus weighing 500 g or more of 20 weeks' gestation or more.

infant d. Death during the first year of life.

maternal d. Death of a woman during the childbearing cycle.

neonatal d. Death of a newborn within the first 28 days after birth.

perinatal d. Death of a fetus of 20 weeks' gestation or older or death of a neonate 28 days old or younger.

decidua Mucous membrane, lining of uterus, or endometrium of pregnancy that is shed after giving birth.

d. basalis Maternal aspect of the placenta made up of uterine blood vessels, endometrial stroma, and glands. It is shed in lochial discharge after delivery.

d. capsularis That part of the decidual membranes surrounding the chorionic sac.

d. vera Nonplacental decidual lining of the uterus.

decrement Decrease or stage of decline, as of a contraction.

deletion Loss of a piece of a chromosome that has broken off.

delivery Expulsion of the child with placenta and membranes by the mother or their extraction by the obstetric practitioner.

abdominal d. See *abdominal delivery*.

ΔOD_{450} (read delta OD_{450}) Delta optical density (or absorbance) at 450 nm, obtained by spectral analysis of amniotic fluid. This prenatal test is used to measure the degree of hemolytic activity in the fetus and to evaluate fetal status in women sensitized to Rh(D).

deoxyribonucleic acid (DNA) Intracellular complex protein that carries genetic information, consisting of two purines (adenine and guanine) and two pyrimidines (thymine and cytosine).

dermatoglyphics Study of skin ridge patterns on fingers, toes, palms of hands, and soles of feet.

DES Diethylstilbestrol, used in treating menopausal symptoms. Exposure of female fetus predisposes her to reproductive tract malformations and (later) dysplasia.

desquamation Shedding of epithelial cells of the skin and mucous membranes.

developmental crisis Severe, usually transient, stress that occurs when a person is unable to complete the tasks of a psychosocial stage of development and is therefore unable to move on to the next stage.

developmental task Physical or cognitive skill that a child must accomplish during a particular age period in order to continue developing, as walking, which precedes the development of sense of autonomy in the toddler period.

diaphragmatic hernia Congenital malformation of diaphragm that allows displacement of the abdominal organs into the thoracic cavity.

diastasis recti abdominis Separation of the two rectus muscles along the median line of the abdominal wall. This is often seen in women with repeated childbirths or with a multiple gestation (triplets, etc.). In the newborn it is usually due to incomplete development.

diathesis Hereditary condition, tendency, or susceptibility of an individual to some abnormality or disease.

bleeding d. Predisposition to abnormal blood clotting.

DIC Disseminated intravascular coagulation.

Dick-Read method An approach to childbirth based on the premise that fear of pain produces muscular tension, producing pain and greater fear. The method includes teaching physiological processes of labor, exercise to improve muscle tone, and techniques to assist in relaxation and prevent the fear-tension-pain mechanism.

dilatation of cervix Stretching of the external os from an opening a few millimeters in size to an opening large enough to allow the passage of the infant.

dilatation and curettage (D and C) Vaginal operation in which the cervical canal is stretched enough to admit passage of an instrument called a *curet*. The endometrium of the uterus is scraped with the curet to empty the uterine contents or to obtain tissue for examination.

discordance Discrepancy in size (or other indicator) between twins.

disparate twins See *twins, disparate*.

disseminated lupus erythematosus Chronic inflammatory disease affecting many systems of the body. The pathophysiology of the disease includes severe vasculitis, renal involvement, and lesions of the skin and nervous system. The primary cause of the disease has not been determined; viral infection or dysfunction of the immune system has been suggested. Also called systemic lupus erythematosus (SLE).

diverticulum Pouch-like herniation through muscular wall of a tubular organ. A diverticulum may be present in the stomach, small intestine, or, most commonly, in the colon.

dizygotic Related to or proceeding from two zygotes (fertilized ova).

dizygous twins See *twins, dizygous*.

Döderlein's bacillus Gram-positive bacterium occurring in normal vaginal secretions.

dominant trait Gene that is expressed whenever it is present in the heterozygous gene state (e.g., brown eyes are dominant over blue).

Douglas' cul-de-sac See *cul-de-sac of Douglas*.

Down's syndrome Abnormality involving the occurrence of a third chromosome, rather than the normal pair (trisomy 21), that characteristically results in a typical picture of mental retardation and altered physical appearance. This condition was formerly called *mongolism* or *mongoloid idiocy*.

dry labor Lay term referring to labor in which amniotic fluid has already escaped. A "dry birth" does not exist.

Dubowitz assessment Estimation of gestational age of a newborn, based on criteria developed for that purpose.

ductus arteriosus In fetal circulation, an anatomic shunt between the pulmonary artery and arch of the aorta. It is obliterated after birth by a rising $P\bar{O}_2$ and change in intravascular pressures in the presence of normal pulmonary function. It normally becomes a ligament after birth but in some instances remains patent.

ductus venosus In fetal circulation, a blood vessel carrying oxygenated blood between the umbilical vein and the inferior vena cava, bypassing the liver. It is obliterated and becomes a ligament after birth.

Duncan's mechanism Delivery of placenta with the maternal surface presenting, rather than the shiny fetal surface.

dura (dura mater) Outermost, toughest of the three meninges covering the brain and spinal cord.

dynamic ileus Spastic ileus; intestinal obstruction characterized by recurrent and continuous spasms (sudden muscular contractions).

dys- Prefix meaning abnormal, difficult, painful, faulty.

dyscrasia Incompatible mixture (e.g., fetal and maternal blood incompatibility).

dysfunction, placental See *placental dysfunction*.

dysfunctional uterine bleeding Abnormal bleeding from the uterus for reasons that are not readily established.

dysmaturity See *intrauterine growth retardation (IUGR)*.

dysmenorrhea Difficult or painful menstruation.

dysmorphogenesis Development of ill-shaped or malformed structures.

dyspareunia Painful sexual intercourse.

dystocia Prolonged, painful, or otherwise difficult delivery or birth because of mechanical factors produced by either the passenger (the fetus) or the passage (the pelvis of the mother) or because of inadequate powers (uterine and other muscular activity).

placental d. Difficulty in the delivery of the placenta.

ecchymosis Bruise; bleeding into tissue caused by direct trauma, serious infection, or bleeding diathesis.

eclampsia Severe complication of pregnancy of unknown cause and occurring more often in the primigravida; characterized by tonic and clonic convulsions, coma, high blood pressure, albuminuria, and oliguria occurring during pregnancy or shortly after delivery.

ectoderm Outer layer of embryonic tissue giving rise to skin, nails, and hair.

ectopic Out of normal place.

e. pregnancy Implantation of the fertilized ovum outside of its normal place in the uterine cavity. Locations include the abdomen, fallopian tubes, and ovaries.

EDC Expected date of confinement; "due date."

effacement Thinning and shortening or obliteration of the cervix that occurs during late pregnancy or labor or both.

effleurage Gentle stroking used in massage.

ejaculation Sudden expulsion of semen from the male urethra.

elective abortion See *abortion, elective*.

electroshock (therapy) Induction of a brief convulsion by passing an electric current through the brain for the treatment of affective disorders, especially in clients resistant to psychoactive drug therapy. Also called electroconvulsive therapy (ECT).

embolus Any undissolved matter (solid, liquid, or gaseous) that is carried by the blood to another part of the body and obstructs a blood vessel.

embryo Conceptus from the second or third week of development until about the eighth week after conception, when mineralization (ossification) of the skeleton begins. This period is characterized by cellular differentiation and predominantly hyperplastic growth.

empathy Projection of one's own consciousness and awareness onto that of another so as to obtain an objective awareness of and insight into the emotions, feelings, and behavior of another person and their meaning and significance. Empathy may be distinguished from sympathy in that sympathy is usually nonobjective and noncritical, whereas the state of empathy includes relative freedom from emotional involvement.

endocervical Pertaining to the interior of the canal of the cervix of the uterus.

endocrine glands Ductless glands that secrete hormones into the blood or lymph.

endometriosis Tissue closely resembling endometrial tissue but aberrantly located outside the uterus in the pelvic cavity. Symptomatology may include pelvic pain or pressure, dysmenorrhea, dyspareunia, abnormal bleeding from the uterus or rectum, and sterility.

endometrium Inner lining of the uterus that undergoes changes caused by hormones during the menstrual cycle and pregnancy; decidua.

engagement In obstetrics, the entrance of the fetal presenting part into the superior pelvic strait and the beginning of the descent through the pelvic canal.

engorgement Distention or vascular congestion. In obstetrics, the process of swelling of the breast tissue brought about by an increase in blood and lymph supply to the breast, which precedes true lactation. It lasts about 48 hours and usually reaches a peak between the third and fifth postdelivery days.

engrossment Sustained involvement of a parent with an infant.

entoderm Inner layer of embryonic tissue giving rise to internal organs such as the intestine.

entrainment Phenomenon observed in the microanalysis of sound films in which the speaker moves several parts of the body and the listener responds to the sounds by moving in ways that are coordinated with the rhythm of the sounds. Infants have been observed to move in time to the rhythms of adult speech but not to random noises or disconnected words or vowels. Entrainment is thought to be an essential factor in the process of maternal-infant bonding.

epicanthus Fold of skin covering the inner canthus and caruncle that extends from the root of the nose to the median end of the eyebrow; characteristically found in certain races but may occur as a congenital anomaly.

episiotomy Surgical incision of the perineum at the end of the second stage of labor to facilitate delivery and to avoid laceration of the perineum. (See also *perineotomy*.)

epispadias Defect in which the urethral canal terminates on dorsum of penis or above the clitoris (rare).

Epstein's pearls Small, white blebs found along the gum margins and at the junction of the soft and hard palates. They are a normal manifestation and are commonly seen in the newborn. Similar to Bohn's nodules.

epulis Tumorlike benign lesion of the gingiva seen in pregnant women.

equilibrium A state of balance or rest owing to the equal action of opposing forces, as calcium and phosphorus in the body. In psychiatry, a state of mental or emotional balance.

Erb-Duchenne paralysis Paralysis caused by traumatic injury to the upper brachial plexus, occurring most commonly in childbirth from forcible traction during delivery. The signs of Erb's paralysis include loss of sensation in the arm and paralysis and atrophy of the deltoid, the biceps, and the branchialis muscles. Also called Erb's palsy.

ergot Drug obtained from *Claviceps purpurea,* a fungus, which stimulates the smooth muscles of blood vessels and the uterus, causing vasoconstriction and uterine contractions.

erythema toxicum Innocuous pink papular neonatal rash of unknown cause, with superimposed vesicles appearing within 24 to 48 hours after birth and resolving spontaneously within a few days.

erythroblastosis fetalis Hemolytic disease of the newborn usually caused by isoimmunization resulting from Rh incompatibility or ABO incompatibility.

erythropoiesis Erythrocyte (RBC) production, which involves the maturation of a nucleated precursor into a hemoglobin-filled, nucleus-free erythrocyte regulated by erythropoietin, a hormone produced by the kidney.

escutcheon Pattern of distribution of pubic hair.

esophageal atresia See *atresia, esophageal.*

estradiol An estrogen.

estrangement, psychologic Reaction to the birth of and subsequent separation from a sick and/or premature infant, whereby the mother is diverted from establishing a normal relationship with her baby.

estriol Major metabolite of estrogen that increases during the second half of pregnancy with an intact fetoplacental unit (normal placenta, normal fetal liver and adrenals) and normal maternal renal function.

estrogen Female sex hormone produced by the ovaries and placenta

estrus Cyclic period of sexual activity in mammals other than primates; state of being in heat.

ethnocentrism Belief in the inherent superiority of the race or group to which one belongs. Also a proclivity to consider other ethnic groups in terms of one's own racial origins.

eu- Prefix meaning normal, good, well, easy.

eugenics Science that deals with the improvement of the human race through control of hereditary (genetic) factors by voluntary social action.

euthenics Science that deals with the improvement of the human race through the control of environmental factors (pollution, drug abuse, malnutrition, and disease).

eutocia Normal or natural labor or birth.

exchange transfusion Replacement of 75% to 85% of circulating blood by withdrawing the recipient's blood and injecting a donor's blood in equal amounts, the purposes of which are to prevent an accumulation of bilirubin in the blood above a dangerous level, to prevent the accumulation of other by-products of hemolysis in hemolytic disease, and to correct anemia.

exocervix Outer layer of the portion of the cervix that protrudes into the vagina; ectocervix.

exostosis Benign cartilage-covered hump on the surface of a bone, often resulting from chronic irritation.

expulsive Having the tendency to drive out or expel.

e. contractions Labor contractions that are characteristic of the second stage of labor.

exstrophy Eversion; the turning inside out of a part.

extension Straightening of a body part; opposite of flexion.

extraperitoneal Occurring or located outside the peritoneal cavity.

extrauterine Occurring outside the uterus.

e. pregnancy Ectopic pregnancy in which the fertilized ovum implants itself outside the uterus.

facies Pertaining to the appearance or expression of the face; certain congenital syndromes typically present with a specific facial appearance.

FAD Fetal activity determination.

failure to thrive Condition in which neonate's or infant's growth and development patterns are below the norms for age.

fallopian tubes Two canals or oviducts extending laterally from each side of the uterus through which the ovum travels, after ovulation, to the uterus.

false labor Uterine contractions that do not result in cervical dilatation, are irregular, are felt more in front, often do not last more than 20 seconds, and do not become longer or stronger.

false pelvis The part of the pelvis superior to a plane passing through the linea terminalis.

familial Pertaining to a condition present in more members of a family than would be expected by chance.

fecundation Act of fertilization or impregnation.

fecundity Ability to bear children frequently and in large numbers.

Ferguson's reflex Reflex contractions of the uterus after stimulation of the cervix.

ferning (arborization) test The appearance of a fernlike pattern in dried smears of uterine cervical mucus, indicating the presence of estrogen.

ovulation f. t. Test in which cervical mucus, placed on a slide, dries in a branching pattern in the presence of high estrogen levels at the time of ovulation.

pregnancy f. t. Test in which cervical mucus, placed on a slide, does not dry in a branching pattern because of high levels of progesterone along with estrogen.

fertility Quality of being able to reproduce.

fertility rate Number of births per 1000 women aged 15 through 44 years.

fertilization Union of an ovum and a sperm.

fetal Pertaining or relating to the fetus.

f. alcholol syndrome Congenital abnormality or anomaly resulting from maternal alcohol intake above 3 oz. of absolute alcohol per day. It is characterized by typical craniofacial and limb defects, cardiovascular defects, intrauterine growth retardation, and developmental delay.

f. alveoli See *alveoli, fetal.*

f. attitude See *attitude, fetal.*

f. asphyxia See *asphyxia, fetal.*

f. death See *death, fetal.*

f. distress Evidence such as a change in the fetal heartbeat pattern or activity indicating that the fetus is in jeopardy.

f. lie Relation of the fetal spine to the maternal spine; i. e., in vertical lie, maternal and fetal spines are parallel and the fetal head or breech presents; in transverse lie, fetal spine is perpendicular to the maternal spine and the fetal shoulder presents.

f. presentation The part of the fetus that presents at the cervical os.

fetofetal transfusion See *parabiotic syndrome.*

α-fetoprotein (AFP) Fetal antigen; elevated levels in amniotic fluid associated with neural tube defects.

fetotoxic Poisonous or destructive to the fetus.

fetus Child in utero from about the eighth week after conception, until birth.

fibroid Fibrous, encapsulated connective tissue tumor, especially of the uterus.

fimbria Structure resembling a fringe, particularly the fringelike end of the fallopian tube.

FiO_2 (fraction of inspired oxygen) Percentage of oxygen a person is receiving.

fissure Groove or open crack in tissue.

fistula Abormal tubelike passage that forms between two normal cavities, possibly congenital or caused by trauma, abscesses, or inflammatory processes.

flaccid Having relaxed, flabby, or absent muscle tone.

flaring of nostrils Widening of nostrils (alae nasi) during inspiration in the presence of air hunger; sign of respiratory distress.

flexion In obstetrics, resistance to the descent of the baby down the birth canal causes the head to flex, or bend, so that the chin approaches the chest. Thus the smallest diameter (suboccipitobregmatic) of the vertex presents.

fluid, amniotic See *amniotic fluid.*

folic acid deficiency anemia Anemia caused by lack of folic acid in the diet.

follicle Small secretory cavity or sac.

graafian f. Mature, fully developed ovarian cyst containing the ripe ovum. The follicle secretes estrogens, and after ovulation, the corpus luteum develops within the ruptured graffian follicle and secretes estrogen and progesterone.

follicle-stimulating hormone (FSH) Hormone produced by the anterior pituitary during the first half of the menstrual cycle. Stimulates development of the graafian follicle.

fomites Nonliving material on which disease-producing organisms may be conveyed (e.g., bed linen).

fontanel Broad area, or soft spot, consisting of a strong band of connective tissue contiguous with cranial bones and located at the junctions of the bones.

anterior f. Diamond-shaped area between the frontal and two parietal bones just above the baby's forehead at the junction of the coronal and sagittal sutures.

mastoid f. Posterolateral fontanel usually not palpable.

posterior f. Small, triangular area between the occipital and parietal bones at the junction of the lambdoidal and sagittal sutures.

sagittal f. Soft area located in the sagittal suture, halfway between the anterior and posterior fontanels; may be found in normal newborns and in some neonates with Down's syndrome.

sphenoid f. Anterolateral fontanel usually not palpable.

footling (incomplete) breech presentation See *breech presentation, footling.*

foramen ovale Septal opening between the atria of the fetal heart. The opening normally closes shortly after birth, but if it remains patent, surgical repair usually is necessary.

foreskin Prepuce, or loose fold of skin covering the glans penis.

fornix Any structure with an arched or vaultlike shape.

f. of the vagina Anterior and posterior spaces, formed by the protrusion of the cervix into the vagina, into which the upper vagina is divided.

fossa Shallow depression.

fourchet Tense band of mucous membranes at the posterior angle of the vagina connecting the posterior ends of the labia minora.

Fowler's position Posture assumed by client when head of bed is raised 18 or 20 inches and individual's knees are elevated.

frank breech presentation See *breech presentation, frank.*

fraternal twins Nonidentical twins that come from two separate fertilized ova.

frenulum Thin ridge of tissue in midline of undersurface of tongue extending from its base to varying distances from the tip of the tongue.

Friedman's curve Labor curve; pattern of descent of presenting part and of dilatation of cervix; partogram.

Friedman's test Modification of the Aschheim-Zondek pregnancy test: the urine of a woman suspected of pregnancy is injected into a mature, unmated female rabbit. If at the end of 2 days of these injections, the ovaries of the rabbit contain fresh corpora lutea or hemorrhagic corpora, the test is positive, signifying that the woman is pregnant.

frigidity Archaic term designating a woman's inability to achieve orgasm; orgasmic dysfunction.

FSH See *follicle-stimulating hormone.*

fulguration Destruction of tissue by means of electricity.

fundus Dome-shaped upper portion of the uterus between the points of insertion of the fallopian tubes.

funic souffle See *souffle, funic.*

funis Cordlike structure, especially the umbilical cord.

galacto-, galact- Combining form denoting milk.

galactorrhea Excessive flow or secretion of milk.

galactosemia Inherited, autosomal recessive disorder of galactose metabolism, characterized by a deficiency of the enzyme galactose-l-phosphate uridyl transferase.

gamete Mature male or female germ cell; the mature sperm or ovum.

gastroschisis Abdominal wall defect at base of umbilical stalk.

gastrostomy Surgical creation of an artificial opening into the stomach through the abdominal wall, performed to feed a client when oral feeding is not possible.

gastrula Early embryonic stage of development that follows the blastula.

gate control theory Proposed in 1965 by Melzack and Wall, this theory explains the neurophysical mechanism underlying the perception of pain.

gavage Feeding by means of a tube passed to the stomach.

gender identity The sense or awareness of knowing to which sex one belongs. The process begins in infancy, continues throughout childhood, and is reinforced during adolescence.

gene Factor on a chromosome responsible for hereditary characteristics of offspring.

generative Capable of reproduction.

genetic Dependent of the genes. A genetic disorder may or may not be apparent at birth.

genetic counseling Process of determining the occurrence or risk of occurrence of a genetic disorder within a family and of providing appropriate information and advice about the courses of action that are available, whether care of a child already affected, prenatal diagnosis, termination of a pregnancy, sterilization, or artificial insemination is involved.

genetics Biologic science that deals with the genetic transmission of physical and chemical characteristics from parents to offspring, as well as the influence of environmental agents on genes and genetic expression.

genitalia Organs of reproduction.

genotype Hereditary combinations in an individual determining his physical and chemical characteristics. Some genotypes are not expressed until later in life (e.g., Huntington's chorea); some hide recessive genes, which can be expressed in offspring; and others are expressed only under the proper environmental conditions (e.g., diabetes mellitus appearing under the stress of obesity or pregnancy).

gestation Period of intrauterine fetal development from conception through birth; the period of pregnancy.

abdominal g. See *abdominal gestation.*

gestational age In fetal development, the number of completed weeks counting from the first day of the last normal menstrual cycle.

glabella Bony prominence above the nose and between the eyebrows.

glans penis Smooth, round head of the penis, analogous to the female glans clitoris.

glomerulonephritis Noninfectious disease of the glomerulus of the kidney, characterized by proteinuria, hematuria, decreased urine production, and edema.

glycosuria Presence of glucose (a sugar) in the urine.

gonad Gamete-producing, or sex, gland; the ovary or testis.

gonadotropic hormone Hormone that stimulates the gonads.

Goodell's sign Softening of the cervix, a probable sign of pregnancy, occurring during the second month.

gossypol Oral contraceptive produced from cotton plants; currently in experimental stage of use by males in the United States.

graafian follicle (vesicle) See *follicle, graafian.*

gravid Pregnant.

grieving process A complex of somatic and psychological symptoms associated with some extreme sorrow or loss, specifically the death of a loved one.

grunt, expiratory Sign of respiratory distress (hyaline membrane disease [respiratory distress syndrome, or RDS] or advanced pneumonia) indicative of the body's attempt to hold air in the alveoli for better gaseous exchange.

gynecoid pelvis Pelvis in which the inlet is round instead of oval or blunt; heart shaped. Typical female pelvis.

gynecology Study of the diseases of the female, especially of the genital, urinary, and rectal organs.

habitual (recurrent) abortion See *abortion, habitual.*

habituation An acquired tolerance from repeated exposure to a particular stimulus. Also called negative adaptation; a decline and eventual elimination of a conditioned response by repetition of the conditioned stimulus.

habitus Indications in appearance of tendency or disposition to disease or abormal conditions.

harlequin sign Rare color change of no pathologic significance occurring between the longitudinal halves of the neonate's body. When infant is placed on one side, the dependent half is noticeably pinker than the superior half.

Hegar's sign Softening of the lower uterine segment that is classified as a probable sign of pregnancy and that may be present during the second and third months of pregnancy and is palpated during bimanual examination.

hematocrit Volume of red blood cells per deciliter (dl) of circulating blood; packed cell volume (PCV).

hematoma Collection of blood in a tissue; a bruise or blood tumor.

hemoconcentration Increase in the number of red blood cells resulting from either a decrease in plasma volume or increased erythropoiesis.

hemoglobin Component of red blood cells consisting of globin, a protein, and hematin, an organic iron compound.

h. electrophoresis Test to diagnose sickle cell disease in newborns. Cord blood is used.

hemorrhagic disease of newborn Bleeding disorder during first few days of life based on a deficiency of vitamin K.

hereditary Pertaining to a trait or characteristic transmitted from parent to offspring by way of the genes; used synonymously with *genetic.*

hermaphrodite Person having genital and sexual characteristics of both sexes.

heterologous insemination Artificial insemination in which the semen specimen is provided by an anonymous donor. The procedure is used primarily in cases where the husband is sterile. Also called artificial insemination donor (AID).

heterozygous Having two dissimilar genes at the same site, or locus, on paired chromosomes (e.g., at the sites for eye color, one chromosome carrying the gene for brown, the other for blue).

high risk An increased possibility of suffering harm, damage, loss, or death.

hirsutism Condition characterized by the excessive growth of hair or the growth of hair in unusual places.

Homans' sign Early sign of phlebothrombosis of the deep veins of the calf in which there are complaints of pain when the leg is in extension and the foot is dorsiflexed.

homoiothermic Referring to the ability of warm-blooded animals to maintain internal temperature at a specified level regardless of the environmental temperature. This ability is not fully developed in the human neonate.

homologous Similar in structure or origin but not necessarily in function.

homologous insemination Artificial insemination in which the semen specimen is provided by the husband. The procedure is used primarily in cases of impotence or when the husband is incapable of sexual intercourse because of some physical disability. Also called artificial insemination husband (AIH).

homozygous Having two similar genes at the same locus, or site, on paired chromosomes.

hormone Chemical substance produced in an organ or gland that is conveyed through the blood to another organ or part of the body, stimulating it to increased functional activity or secretion. See specific hormones.

hour-glass uterus Uterus in which a segment of circular muscle fibers contracts during labor. The resultant "constriction ring" dystocia is characterized by lack of progress in spite of adequate contractions; by pain experienced prior to palpation of a uterine contraction and persisting after the observer feels the contraction end; and by recession of the presenting part during a contraction, instead of descent of the presenting part.

human chorionic gonadotropin (HCG) See *prolan*.

human chorionic somatomammotropin (HCS) Another term for human placental lactogen (HPL) and placental growth hormone.

hyaline membrane disease (HMD) Disease characterized by interference with ventilation at the alveolar level, theoretically caused by the presence of fibrinoid deposits lining alveolar ducts. Membrane formation is related to prematurity (especially with fetal asphyxia) and insufficient surfactant production (L/S ratio less than 2:1). Otherwise known as *respiratory distress syndrome (RDS)*.

hydatidiform mole Abnormal pregnancy characterized by a degenerative process in the chorionic villi that produces high levels of human chorionic gonadotropin (HCG), multiple cysts, and rapid growth of the uterus with hemorrhage. Signs and symptoms include vaginal bleeding, the discharge containing grapelike vesicles. Sequela may be chorioadenoma, a highly malignant neoplasm.

hydramnios (polyhydramnios) Amniotic fluid in excess of 1.5L; often indicative of fetal anomaly and frequently seen in poorly controlled, insulin-dependent, diabetic pregnant women even if there is not coexisting fetal anomaly.

hydremia Excess of watery fluid in the blood.

hydrocele Collection of fluid in a saclike cavity, especially in the sac that surrounds the testis, causing the scrotum to swell.

hydrocephalus Excessive accumulation of cerebrospinal fluid within the ventricles of the brain resulting from interference with normal circulation and absorption of the cerebrospinal fluid and especially from the destruction of the foramens of Magendie and Luschka because of congenital anomaly, infection, injury, or brain tumor. In infants, the increased head diameter is possible because the sutures of the skull have not closed.

- **communicating h.** Hydrocephalus in which normal communication between the fourth ventricle and the subarachnoid space is maintained, allowing cerebral fluid to circulate into the lumbar thecal space.
- **noncommunicating h.** Failure of the ventricular fluid to empty into the lumbar thecal space because of an obstruction.

hydropic Dropsical or pertaining to dropsy; abnormal accumulation of serous fluid in the body tissues and cavities.

hydrops fetalis Most severe expression of fetal hemolytic disorder, a possible sequela to maternal Rh isoimmunization; infants exhibit gross edema (anasarca), cardiac decompensation, and profound pallor from anemia and seldom survive.

hymen Membranous fold that normally partially covers the entrance to the vagina in the virgin.

hymenal caruncles Small, irregular bits of tissue that are remnants of the hymen.

hymenal tag Normally occurring redundant hymenal tissue protruding from the floor of the vagina that disappears spontaneously in a few weeks after birth.

hymenotomy Surgical incision of the hymen.

hyperbilirubinemia Elevation of unconjugated serum bilirubin concentrations.

hypercalcemia Excess of calcium in the blood.

hypercapnia Excessive arterial P_{CO_2} caused by inadequate ventilation. In greater degrees it acts as a respiratory depressant.

hypercarbia Greater than normal amounts of carbon dioxide in the blood. Also called hypercapnia.

hyperemesis gravidarum Abnormal condition of pregnancy characterized by protracted vomiting, weight loss, and fluid and electrolyte imbalance.

hyperesthesia Unusual sensibility to sensory stimuli, such as pain or touch.

hyperlipidemia Excessive amount of fats in the blood.

hypermagnesemia Excessive amount of serum magnesium; in obstetrics, it occurs in the mother or fetus or both after the mother is treated with magnesium sulfate for preeclampsia-eclampsia.

hyperplasia Increase in number of cells; formation of new tissue.

hyperreflexia Increased action of the reflexes.

hypertrophy Enlargement, or increase in size, of existing cells.

hyperventilation Rapid, shallow (or prolonged, deep) respirations resulting in respiratory alkalosis: a decrease in H^+ concentration and P_{CO_2} and an increase in the blood pH and the ratio of $NaHCO_3$ to H_2CO_3. Symptoms may include faintness, palpitations, and carpopedal (hands and feet) muscular spasms. Relief may result from rebreathing in a paper bag or into one's cupped hands to replace the CO_2 "blown off" during hyperventilation.

hypocalcemia Deficiency of calcium in the serum that may be caused by hypoparathyroidism, vitamin D deficiency, kidney failure, acute pancreatitis, or inadequate plasma magnesium and protein.

hypochlorhydria Diminished secretion of hydrochloric acid.

hypofibrinogenemia Deficient level of a blood clotting factor, fibrinogen, in the blood; in obstetrics, it occurs following complications of abruptio placentae or retention of a dead fetus.

hypogastric Pertaining to the lower middle of the abdomen or hypogastrium.

hypogastric arteries Branches of the right and left iliac arteries carrying deoxygenated blood from the fetus through the umbilical cord, where they are known as *umbilical arteries,* to the placenta.

hypoglycemia Less-than-normal amount of glucose in the blood, usually caused by administration of too much insulin, excessive secretion of insulin by the islet cells of the pancreas, or by dietary deficiency.

hypospadias Anomalous positioning of urinary meatus on undersurface of penis or close to or just inside the vagina.

hypotensive drugs Drugs that lower the blood pressure.

hypothalamus Portion of the diencephalon of the brain forming the floor and part of the lateral wall of the third ventricle. It activates, controls, and integrates the peripheral autonomic nervous system, endocrine processes, and many somatic functions, as body temperature, sleep, and appetite.

hypothenar Fleshy elevation on the ulnar (little finger) side of the palm of the hand. Also called *hypothenar eminence*.

hypotonia Reduced tension; relaxation of arteries. Also, loss of tonicity of the muscles or intraocular pressure.

hypoxemia Reduction in arterial Po_2 resulting in metabolic acidosis by forcing anaerobic glycolysis, pulmonary vasoconstriction, and direct cellular damage.

hypoxia Insufficient availability of oxygen to meet the metabolic needs of body tissue.

hysterectomy Surgical removal of the uterus.

abdominal h. See *abdominal hysterectomy*.

panhysterectomy Removal of entire uterus, but ovaries and tubes remain.

subtotal h. Removal of fundus and body of the uterus, but the cervical stump remains.

total h. Removal of entire uterus, including the cervix, but the ovaries and tubes remain.

hysterosalpingography Recording by x-ray of the uterus and uterine tubes after injecting them with radiopaque material.

hysterotomy Surgical incision into the uterus.

iatrogenic Caused by a physician's words, actions, or treatment.

icterus gravis Acute yellow atrophy of the liver with cerebral disorders.

icterus neonatorum Jaundice in the newborn.

idiopathic respiratory distress syndrome (hyaline membrane disease) Severe respiratory condition found almost exclusively in premature infants and in some infants of diabetic mothers regardless of gestational age. See also *hyaline membrane disease (HMD)*.

IDM Infant of a diabetic mother.

IgA Primary immunoglobulin in colostrum

IgG Transplacentally acquired immunoglobulin that confers passive immunity against the infections to which the mother is immune.

IgM Immunoglobulin neonate can manufacture soon after birth. Fetus produces it in the presence of amnionitis.

iliopectineal line Bony ridge on the inner surface of the ilium and pubic bones that divides the true and false pelvises; the brim of the true pelvic cavity; the inlet.

immature baby Infant usually weighing less than 1134 g (2½ lb) and who is considerably underdeveloped at birth.

implantation Embedding of the fertilized ovum in the uterine mucosa; nidation.

impotence Archaic term designating a man's inability, partial or complete, to perform sexual intercourse or to achieve orgasm; erectile dysfunction.

impregnate To fertilize, or make pregnant.

inanition Pathophysiologic condition of the body resulting from lack of food and water; starvation.

inborn error of metabolism Hereditary deficiency of a specific enzyme needed for normal metabolism of specific chemicals (e.g. deficiency of phenylalanine hydroxylase results in phenylketonuria [PKU]; a deficiency of hexosaminidase results in Tay-Sachs disease).

incompetent cervix Cervix that is unable to remain closed until a pregnancy reaches term, because of a mechanical defect in the cervix resulting in dilatation and effacement usually during the second or early third trimester of pregnancy.

incomplete abortion See *abortion, incomplete*.

increment An increase, or buildup, as of a contraction.

incubator Apparatus used for an infant in which the temperature may be regulated.

induced abortion See *abortion, induced*.

induction Artificial stimulation or augmentation of labor.

inertia Sluggishness or inactivity; in obstetrics, refers to the absence or weakness of uterine contractions during labor.

inevitable abortion See *abortion, inevitable*.

infant A child who is under 1 year of age.

infantile uterus Uterus that has failed to attain adult characteristics.

infertility Decreased capacity to conceive.

infiltration Process by which a substance such as a local anesthetic drug is deposited within the tissue.

inhalation analgesia Reduction of pain by administration of anesthetic gas. Occasionally given during the second stage of labor. Consciousness is retained to allow the woman to follow instructions and to avoid the adverse effects of general anesthesia.

inlet Passage leading into a cavity.

pelvic i. Upper brim of the pelvic cavity.

innominate Without a name.

i. bone The hip bone.

internal os Inside mouth or opening.

interstitial cell–stimulating hormone (ICSH) Hormone that stimulates production of testosterone; analogous to LH in the female.

intertuberous diameter Distance between ischial tuberosities. Measured to determine dimension of pelvic outlet.

intervillous space Irregular space in the maternal portion of the placenta, filled with maternal blood and serving as the site of maternal-fetal gas, nutrient, and waste exchange.

intrapartum During labor and delivery.

intrathecal Within the subarachnoid space.

intrauterine device (IUD) Small plastic or metal form placed in the uterus to prevent implantation of a fertilized ovum.

intrauterine growth retardation (IUGR) Fetal undergrowth of any etiology, such as deficient nutrient supply or intrauterine infection, or associated with congenital malformation.

introitus Entrance into a canal or cavity such at the vagina.

intromission Insertion of one part or object into another (e.g., introduction of penis into vagina).

intussusception Prolapse of one segment of bowel into the lumen of the adjacent segment.

in utero Within or inside the uterus.

in vitro fertilization Fertilization in a culture dish or test tube.

inversion Turning end for end, upside down, or inside out.

i. of the uterus Condition in which the uterus is turned inside out so that the fundus intrudes into the cervix or vagina, caused by a too vigorous removal of the placenta before it is detached by the natural process of labor.

involution (1) Rolling or turning inward. (2) Reduction in size of the uterus after delivery and its return to its normal size and condition.

iontophoretic pilocarpine test Sweat test, usually a diagnostic test for cystic fibrosis (mucoviscidosis).

ischium Lower lateral two fifths of the acetabulum and the short, stout column of bone that supports it.

isoimmune hemolytic disease Breakdown (hemolysis) of fetal/neonatal Rh-positive RBCs because of Rh antigens formed by an Rh-negative mother who had been previously exposed to Rh-positive RBCs.

isoimmunization Development of antibodies in a species of animal with antigens from the same species (e.g., development of anti-Rh antibodies in an Rh-negative person).

ITP Abbreviation for idiopathic thrombocytopenic purpura.

jaundice Yellow discoloration of the body tissues caused by the deposit of bile pigments (unconjugated bilirubin); icterus.

breast milk j. Yellowing of infant's skin from pregnanediol (in mother's milk) inhibition of enzyme (glucuronyl transferase) necessary for conjugation of bilirubin.

pathologic j. Jaundice noticeable within 24 hours after birth; caused by some abnormal condition such as an Rh or ABO incompatibility and resulting in bilirubin toxicity (e.g., kernicterus)

physiologic j. Jaundice usually occurring 48 hours or later after birth, reaching a peak at 5 to 7 days, gradually disappearing by the seventh to tenth day, and caused by the normal reduction in the number of red blood cells. The infant is otherwise well.

Kahn test Precipitation or flocculation test for the diagnosis of syphilis.

kalemia Presence of potassium in the serum.

karyotype Schematic arrangement of the chromosomes within a cell to demonstrate their numbers and morphology.

Kegel exercises Excises to stengthen the pubococcygeal muscles.

kernicterus Bilirubin encephalopathy involving the deposit of unconjugated bilirubin in brain cells, resulting in death or impaired intellectual, perceptive, or motor function, and adaptive behavior.

Kernig's sign Stiffness of the back; nuchal rigidity.

ketoacidosis Acidosis accompanied by an accumulation of ketones in the body, resulting from faulty carbohydrate metabolism.

ketonemia Acetone bodies in the blood, causing the characteristic fruity breath odor of ketoacidosis.

ketosis Increase in ketone bodies (acetone) from incomplete metabolism of fatty acids.

kin group People related by blood or marriage.

Klumpke's palsy Atrophic paralysis of forearm.

labia Lips or liplike structures.

l. majora Two folds of skin containing fat and covered with hair that lie on either side of the vaginal opening and from each side of the vulva.

l. minora Two thin folds of delicate, hairless skin inside the labia majora.

labor Series of processes by which the fetus is expelled from the uterus; parturition; childbirth.

laceration Irregular tear of wound tissue; in obstetrics, it usually refers to a tear in the perineum, vagina, or cervix caused by childbirth.

lactase Enzyme necessary for the digestion of lactose.

lactation Function of secreting milk or period during which milk is secreted.

lactogen Drug or other substance that enhances the production and secretion of milk.

lactogenic Stimulating the production of milk.

l. hormone Gonadotropin produced by anterior pituitary and responsible for promoting growth of breast tissue and lactation; prolaction; luteotropin.

lactose intolerance Inherited absence of the enzyme lactose.

lactosuria Presence of lactose in the urine during late pregnacy and during lactation. Must be differentiated from glycosuria.

Lamaze method Method of psychophysical preparation for childbirth developed in the 1950s by a French obstetrician, Fernand Lamaze. It requires classes, practice at home, and coaching during labor and delivery.

lambdoid Having the shape of the Greek letter lambda.

l. suture Suture line extending across the posterior third of the skull, separating the occipital bone from the two parietal bones, and forming the base of the triangular posterior fontanel.

laminaria tent Cone of dried seaweed that swells as it absorbs moisture. Used to dilate the cervix nontraumatically in preparation for an induced abortion or in preparation for induction of labor.

lanugo Downy, fine hair characteristic of the fetus between 20 weeks' gestation and birth that is most noticeable over the shoulder, forehead, and cheeks but is found on nearly all parts of the body except the palms of the hands, soles of the feet, and the scalp.

laparoscopy Examination of the interior of the abdomen by inserting a small telescope through the anterior abdominal wall.

laparotomy Incision into the abdominal cavity.

large for dates (large for gestational age [LGA]) Exhibiting excessive growth for gestational age.

lavage Washing out of a cavity such as the stomach.

lecithin A phospholipid that decreases surface tension; surfactant.

lecithin/sphingomyelin ratio Ratio of lecithin to sphingomyelin in the amniotic fluid. This is used to assess maturity of the fetal lung.

Leopold's maneuver Four maneuvers for diagnosing the fetal position by external palpation of the mother's abdomen.

let-down reflex Oxytocin-induced flow of milk from the alveoli of the breasts into the milk ducts.

leukorrhea White or yellowish mucous discharge from the cervical canal or the vagina that may be normal physiologically or caused by pathologic states of the vagina and endocervix (e.g., *Trichomonas vaginalis* infections).

LH See *luteinizing hormone (LH)*.

libido Sexual drive.

lie Relationship existing between the long axis of the fetus and the long axis of the mother. In a longitudinal lie, the fetus is lying lengthwise or vertically, whereas in a transverse lie the fetus is lying crosswise or horizontally in the mother's uterus.

ligation Act of suturing, sewing, or otherwise tying shut.

tubal l. Abdominal operation in which the fallopian tubes are tied off and a section is removed to interrupt tubal continuity and thus sterilize the woman.

lightening Sensation of decreased abdominal distention produced by uterine descent into the pelvic cavity as the fetal presenting part settles into the pelvis. It usually occurs 2 weeks before the onset of labor in nulliparas.

linea nigra Line of darker pigmentation seen in some women during the latter part of pregnancy that appears on the middle of the abdomen and extends from the symphysis pubis toward the umbilicus.

linea terminalis Line dividing the upper (false) pelvis from the lower (true) pelvis.

lingua Tongue or tonguelike structure.

l. frenata Tongue with a very short frenulum, resulting in tongue-tie, an extremely rare condition.

liquor Any fluid liquid.

l. amnii Amniotic fluid that surrounds the fetus within the amniotic sac.

lithotomy position Position in which the woman lies on her back with her knees flexed and abducted thighs drawn up toward her chest.

live birth Birth in which the neonate, regardless of gestational age, manifests any heartbeat, breathes, or displays voluntary movement.

livida, asphyxia See *asphyxia livida.*

lochia Vaginal discharge during the puerperium consisting of blood, tissue, and mucus.

l. alba Thin, yellowish to white, vaginal discharge that follows lochia serosa on about the tenth postdelivery day and that may last from the end of the third to the sixth postdelivery week.

l. rubra Red, distinctly blood-tinged vaginal flow that follows delivery and lasts 2 to 4 days after delivery.

l. serosa Serous, pinkish brown, watery vaginal discharge that follows lochia ruba until about the tenth postdelivery day.

L/S ratio (lecithin/sphingomyelin ratio) Test for fetal lung maturity.

lunar month Four weeks (28 days).

lutein Yellow pigment derived from the corpus luteum, egg yolk, and fat cells.

l. cells Ovarian cells involved in the formation of the corpus luteum and that contain a yellow pigment.

luteinizing hormone (LH) Hormone produced by the anterior pituitary that stimulates ovulation and the development of the corpus luteum.

luteotropin (LTH) Lactogenic hormone; prolactin; an adenohypophyseal hormone.

lysis of adhesions Operation to free adhesions (bands of scar tissue) that have caused organs to be abnormally drawn or tied to each other.

lysozyme Enzyme with antiseptic qualities that destroys foreign organisms and that is found in blood cells of the granulocytic and monocytic series and is also normally present in saliva, sweat, tears, and breast milk.

maceration (1) Process of softening a solid by soaking it in a fluid. (2) Softening and breaking down of fetal skin from prolonged exposure to amniotic fluid as seen in a postterm infant. Also seen in a dead fetus.

macroglossia Hypertrophy of tongue or tongue large for oral cavity; seen in some preterm neonates and in neonates with Down's syndrome.

macrophage Any phagocytic cell of the reticuloendothelial system including Kupffer cell in the liver, splenocyte in the spleen, and histocyte in the loose connective tissue.

macrosomia Large body size as seen in neonates of diabetic or prediabetic mothers; macrosomatia.

magnesemia Presence of serum magnesium.

malpractice Professional negligence that is the proximate cause of injury or harm to a client, resulting from a lack of professional knowledge, experience, or skill that can be expected in others in the profession or from a failure to exercise reasonable care or judgment in the application of professional knowledge, experience, or skill.

mammary gland Compound gland of the female breast that is made up of lobes and lobules that secrete milk for nourishment of the young. Rudimentary mammary glands exist in the male.

manic depressive psychosis Major affective disorder characterized by episodes of mania and depression. One or the other phase may be predominant at any given time; one phase may appear alternately with the other; or elements of both phases may be present simultaneously. Also called bipolar disorder.

mask of pregnancy See *chloasma.*

mastalgia Breast soreness or tenderness.

mastectomy Excision, or removal, of the breast.

mastitis Inflammation of mammary tissue of the breasts.

maternal mortality Death of a woman related to childbearing.

maturation (1) Process of attaining maximum development. (2) In biology, a process of cell division during which the number of chromosomes in the germ cells (sperm or ova) is reduced to one half the number (haploid) characteristic of the species.

maturational crisis Crisis that arises during normal growth and development, e.g., puberty.

meatus Opening from an internal structure to the outside (e.g., urethral meatus).

mechanism Instrument or process by which something is done, results, or comes into being; in obstetrics, labor and delivery.

meconium First stools of infant: viscid, sticky; dark greenish brown, almost black; sterile; odorless

m. aspiration syndrome Function of fetal hypoxia: with hypoxia, the anal sphincter relaxes and meconium is released; reflex gasping movements draw meconium and other particulate matter in the amniotic fluid into the infant's bronchial tree, obstructing the air flow after birth.

m. ileus Lower intestinal obstruction by thick, puttylike, inspissated meconium that may be the result of deficiency of trypsin production in the newborn with cystic fibrosis.

m.-stained fluid In response to hypoxia, fetal intestinal activity increases and anal sphincter relaxes, resulting in the passage of meconium, which imparts a greenish coloration.

megaloblastic anemia Hematologic disorder characterized by the production and peripheral proliferation of immature, large, and dysfunctional erythrocytes.

meiosis Process by which germ cells divide and decrease their chromosomal number by one half.

-melia Pertaining to a limb or part of a limb or extremity, as in amelia (absence of a limb) or phocomelia (absence of part of arms or legs).

membrane Thin, pliable layer of tissue that lines a cavity or tube, separates structures, or covers an organ or structure; in obstetrics, the amnion and chorion surrounding the fetus.

membrane rupture Tearing of the fetal membranes (amnion and chorion) with the release of amniotic fluid.

menarche Onset, or beginning, of menstrual function.

meningomyelocele Saclike protrusion of the spinal cord through a congenital defect in the vertebral column.

menopause From the Greek word *men* (month) and *pausis* (to stop), the actual permanent cessation of menstrual cycles.

menorrhagia Abnormally profuse or excessive menstrual flow.

menses (menstruation) Periodic vaginal discharge of bloody fluid from the nonpregnant uterus that occurs from the age of puberty to menopause.

mentum Chin, a fetal reference point in designating position (e.g., "Left mentum anterior" [LMA], meaning that the fetal chin is presenting in the left anterior quadrant of the maternal pelvis).

mesoderm Embryonic middle layer of germ cells giving rise to all types of muscles, connective tissue, bone marrow, blood, lymphoid tissue, and all epithelial tissue.

metabolic acidosis See *acidosis, metabolic.*

metritis Inflammation of the endometrium and myometrium.

metrorrhagia Abnormal bleeding from the uterus, particularly when it occurs at any time other than the menstrual period.

microcephaly Congenital anomaly characterized by abnormal smallness of the head in relation to the rest of the body and by underdevelopment of the brain, resulting in some degree of mental retardation.

micrognathia Abnormal smallness of mandible or chin.

midwife One who practices the art of helping and aiding a woman to give birth.

migration In obstetrics, the passage of the ovum from the ovary into the fallopian tubes and thence into the uterus.

milia Unopened sebaceous glands appearing as tiny, white, pinpoint papules on forehead, nose, cheeks, and chin of a neonate that disappear spontaneously in a few days or weeks.

milk-leg See *phlegmasia alba dolens.*

miscarriage Spontaneous abortion; lay term usually referring specifically to the loss of the fetus between the fourth month and viability.

missed abortion See *abortion, missed.*

mitleiden Suffering along with.

mitochondria Slender microscopic filaments or rods found in the cell cytoplasm; the principal sites of oxidative reactions by which the cell is provided with energy.

mitosis Process of somatic cell division in which a single cell divides, but both of the new cells have the same number of chromosomes as the first.

mittelschmerz Abdominal pain in the region of an ovary during ovulation, which usually occurs midway through the menstrual cycle. Present in many women, mittelschmerz is useful for identifying ovulation, thus pinpointing the fertile period of the cycle.

molding Overlapping of cranial bones or shaping of the fetal head to accommodate and conform to the bony and soft parts of the mother's birth canal during labor.

mongolian spot Bluish gray or dark nonelevated pigmented area usually found over the lower back and buttocks present at birth in some infants, primarily nonwhite. The spot fades by school age in black or Oriental infants and within the first year or two of life in other infants.

mongolism, See *Down's syndrome.*

moniliasis Infection of the skin or mucous membrane by a yeastlike fungus, *Candida albicans.* see *thrush.*

monitrice One trained in psychoprophylactic methods and who supports women during labor.

monosomy Chromosomal aberration characterized by the absence of one chromosome from the normal diploid complement.

monozygotic Originating or coming from a single fertilized ovum, such as identical twins.

monozygous twins See *twins, monozygous.*

mons veneris Pad of fatty tissue and coarse skin that overlies the symphysis pubis in the woman and that, after puberty, is covered with short curly hair.

Montgomery's glands tubercles Small, nodular prominences (sebaceous glands) on the areolas around the nipples of the breasts that enlarge during pregnancy and lactation.

morbidity (1) Condition of being diseased. (2) Number of cases of disease or sick persons in relationship to a specific population; incidence.

morning sickness Nausea and vomiting that affect some women during the first few months of their pregnancy; may occur at any time of day.

Moro's reflex Normal, generalized reflex in a young infant elicited by a sudden loud noise or by striking the table next to the child, resulting in flexion of the legs, an embracing posture of the arms, and usually a brief cry. Also called startle reflex.

mortality (1) Quality or state of being subject to death. (2) Number of deaths in relation to a specific population; incidence.

fetal m. Number of fetal deaths per 1000 births (or per live births). See also *death, fetal.*

infant m. Number of deaths per 1000 children 1 year of age or younger.

maternal m. Number of maternal deaths per 100,000 births.

neonatal m. Number of neonatal deaths per 1000 births (or per live births). See also *death, neonatal.*

perinatal m. Combined fetal and neonatal mortality. See also *death, perinatal.*

morula Developmental stage of the fertilized ovum in which there is a solid mass of cells resembling a mulberry.

mosaicism Condition in which some somatic cells are normal, whereas others show chromosomal aberrations.

muscous membrane Specialized thin layer of tissue lining certain cavities and passages that is kept moist by the secretion of mucus.

mucous-trap suction apparatus Device consisting of a catheter with a mucous trap that prevents mucus aspirated from the newborn infant's nasopharynx and trachea from being sucked or drawn into the operator's mouth.

mucus Viscid fluid secreted by the mucous membranes.

multigravida Woman who has been pregnant two or more times.

multipara Woman who has carried two or more pregnancies to viability, whether they ended in live infants or stillbirths.

multiple pregnancy Pregnancy in which there is more than one fetus in the uterus at the same time.

multiple sclerosis (MS) Progressive disease characterized by disseminated demyelination of nerve fibers of the brain and spinal cord.

mutation Change in a gene or chromosome in gametes that may be transmitted to offspring.

myasthenia gravis Abnormal condition characterized by the chronic fatigability and weakness of muscles, especially in the face and throat, as a result of a defect in the conduction of nerve impulses at the myoneural junction.

Naegele's rule Method for calculating the estimated date of confinement (EDC), or "due date."

natal Relating or pertaining to birth.

navel Depression in the center of the abdomen, where the umbilical cord was attached to the fetus; umbilicus.

necrotizing bronchitis Pathologic death of cells within the bronchi.

necrotizing enterocolitis (NEC) Acute inflammatory bowel disorder that occurs primarily in preterm or low-birth-weight neonates. It is charcterized by ischemic necrosis (death) of the gastrointestinal mucosa that may lead to perforation and peritonitis.

negligence Commission of an act that a prudent person would not have done or the omission of a duty that prudent person would have fulfilled, resulting in injury or harm to another person. In particular, in a malpractice suit a professional person is negligent if harm to a client results from such an act or such a failure to act, but it must be proved that other prudent persons of the same profession would ordinarily have acted differently under the same circumstances.

neonatal hypovolemic shock Cardiovascular collapse due to a diminished volume of circulating fluid in the cardiovascular system.

neonatal mortality Statistical rate of infant death during the first 28 days after live birth, expressed as the number of such deaths per 1,000 live births in a specific geographic area or institution in a given period of time.

neonatology Study of the neonate.

nephroureterolithiasis Stones in the kidneys and ureters.

neurofibromatosis Congenital condition transmitted as an autosomal dominant trait, characterized by numerous neurofibromas of the nerves and skin, by cafe-au-lait spots on the skin, and, in some cases, by developmental anomalies of the muscles, bones, and viscera.

neutral temperature range That grouping of environmental conditions in which the neonate's oxygen consumption is at a minimum and his temperature is within normal limits.

nevus Natural blemish or mark; a congenital circumscribed deposit of pigmentation in the skin; mole.

- **n. flammeus** Port-wine stain; reddish, usually flat, discoloration of the face or neck. Because of its large size and color, it is considered a serious deformity.
- **n. vasculosus (strawberry hemangioma)** Elevated lesion of immature capillaries and endothelial cells that regresses over a period of years.

nidation Implantation of the fertilized ovum in the endometrium, or lining, of the uterus.

nondisjunction Failure of homologous pairs of chromosomes to separate during the first meiotic division or of the two chromatids of a chromosome to split during anaphase of mitosis or the second meiotic division. The result is an abnormal number of chromosomes in the daughter cells.

nonshivering thermogenesis Infant's method of producing heat by increasing his metabolic rate.

nonstress test (NST) Evaluation of fetal response (fetal heart rate) to natural contractile uterine activity or to an increase in fetal activity.

nosocomial Pertaining to a hospital.

nucleotide Single segment of helical strand of DNA.

nulligravida Woman who has never been pregnant.

nullipara Woman who has not yet carried a pregnancy to viability.

nursing practitioner Registered nurse who has additional education to practice nursing in an expanded role.

nystagmus Constant, involuntary, rhythmic oscillation of the eyeball. The movements may be in any direction.

obstetrix Midwife; from *obstare,* to stand before.

occipitobregmatic Pertaining to the occiput (the back part of the skull) and the bregma (junction of the coronal and sagittal sutures) or anterior fontanel; the smallest diameter of the fetal head.

occiput Back part of the head or skull.

oligohydramnios Abnormally small amount or absence of amniotic fluid; often indicative of fetal urinary tract defect.

oliguria Diminished secretion of urine by the kidneys.

omphalic Concerning or pertaining to the umbilicus.

omphalitis Inflammation of the umbilical stump characterized by redness, edema, and purulent exudate in severe infections.

omphalocele Congenital defect resulting from failure of closure of the abdominal wall or muscles and leading to hernia of abdominal contents through the navel.

oocyesis Ectopic ovarian pregnancy.

oocyte Primordial or incompletely developed ovum.

oophorectomy Excision or removal of an ovary.

operculum Plug of mucus that fills the cervical canal during pregnancy.

ophthalmia neonatorum Infection in the neonate's eyes usually resulting from gonorrheal or other infection contracted when the fetus passes through the birth canal (vagina).

opisthotonos Tetanic spasm resulting in an arched, hyperextended position of the body.

oral GTT Test for blood sugar following oral ingestion of a concentrated sugar solution.

orchitis Inflammation of one or both of the testes, characterized by swelling and pain, often caused by mumps, syphilis, or tuberculosis.

orgasmic platform Congestion of the lower vagina during sexual intercourse.

orifice Normal mouth, entrance, or opening, to any aperture.

os Mouth, or opening.

- **external o. (o. externum)** External opening of the cervical canal.
- **internal o. (o. internum)** Internal opening of the cervical canal.
- **o. uteri** Mouth, or opening, of the uterus.

ossification Mineralization of fetal bones.

-otomy Combining form meaning cutting, incision, section.

outlet Opening by which something can exit.

- **pelvic o.** Inferior aperture, or opening, of the true pelvis.

ovary One of two glands in the female situated on either side of the pelvic cavity that produces the female reproductive cell, the ovum, and two known hormones, estrogen and progesterone.

ovulation Periodic ripening and discharge of the unimpregnated ovum from the ovary, usually 14 days prior to the onset of menstrual flow.

- **o. method** Evaluation of cervical mucus throughout the menstrual cycle; ovulation occurs just after the appearance of the peak mucus sign; Billings method.

ovum Female germ, or reproductive cell, produced by the ovary; egg.

oxygen toxicity Oxygen overdosage that results in pathologic tissue changes (e.g., retrolental fibroplasia, bronchopulmonary dysplasia).

oxytocics Drugs that stimulate uterine contractions, thus accelerating childbirth and preventing postdelivery hemorrhage. They may be used to increase the let-down reflex during lactation.

oxytocin Hormone produced by the posterior pituitary that stimulates uterine contractions and the release of milk in the mammary gland (let-down reflex).

- **o. challenge test (OCT)** Evaluation of fetal response (fetal heart rate) to contractile activity of the uterus stimulated by exogenous oxytocin (Pitocin).

$PaCO_2$ Partial pressure of carbon dioxide in arterial blood.

pallida, asphyxia See *asphyxia pallida*.

palpation Examination performed by touching the external surface of the body with the fingers or palmar surface of the hand.

- **bimanual p.** See *bimanual palpation*.

palsy Permanent or temporary loss of sensation or ability to move and control movement; paralysis.

Bell's p. Peripheral facial paralysis of the facial nerve (cranial nerve VII), causing the muscles of the unaffected side of the face to pull the face into a distorted position.

Erb's p. See *Erb-Duchenne paralysis*.

panhysterectomy See *hysterectomy*.

PaO_2 Partial pressure of oxygen in arterial blood.

Papanicolaou (Pap) smear Microscopic examination using scrapings from the cervix, endocervix, or other mucous membranes that will reveal, with a high degree of accuracy, the presence of premalignant or malignant cells.

para Term used to refer to past pregnancies that reached viability regardless of whether the infant was dead or alive at birth.

parabiotic syndrome Fetofetal blood transfer caused by placental vascular anastomoses occurring in a small plethoric twin (polycythemia) and one pale twin (anemia).

parametritis Inflamed condition of the cellular tissue or parmetrium of the uterus; pelvic cellulitis.

parametrium Flat, smooth muscle, and loose connective tissue lying around the uterus and extending laterally between the layers of the broad ligaments.

parenteral Administration or injection of nutrients, fluids, or drugs into the body by any way other than the digestive tract.

parity Number of pregnancies that reached viability.

parovarian Pertaining to the residual structure in the broad ligament between the fallopian tubes and the ovary.

parturient Woman giving birth.

parturition Process or act of giving birth.

patent Open.

pathogen Substance or organism capable of producing disease.

pathognomonic Characteristic or distinctive symptom or sign of a disease that facilitates recognition or differentiation from other conditions.

pathologic hyperbilirubinemia High (toxic) levels of serum bilirubin due to a disease process causing hemolysis (e.g., Rh incompatibility); jaundice apparent within first 24 hours.

pathologic jaundice See *jaundice, pathologic*.

pathosis A disease condition.

patulous Open or spread apart.

peak mucus sign Lubricative, cloudy-to-clear-egg white cervical mucus occurring under high estrogen levels close to time of ovulation; ferns; good spinnbarkeit.

pedigree Shorthand method of depicting family lines of individuals who manifest a physical or chemical disorder.

pelvic Pertaining or relating to the pelvis.

p. axis See *axis, pelvic*.

p. inlet See *inlet, pelvic*.

p. outlet See *outlet, pelvic*.

pelvimeter Device for measuring the diameters and capacity of the pelvis.

pelvimetry Measurement of dimensions and proportions of the pelvis to determine its capacity and ability to allow the passage of the fetus through the birth canal.

pelvis Bony structure formed by the sacrum, coccyx, innominate bones, and symphysis pubis, and the ligaments that unite them.

android p. See *android pelvis*.

anthropoid p. See *anthropoid pelvis*.

false p. Pelvis above the linea terminalis and symphysis pubis.

gynecoid p. See *gynecoid pelvis*.

platypelloid p. See *platypelloid pelvis*.

true p. Pelvis below the linea terminalis.

pemphigus An uncommon, serious disease of the skin and mucous membranes, characterized by thin-walled bullae arising from apparently normal skin or mucous membrane. The bullae rupture easily, leaving raw patches. The person loses weight, becomes weak, and is subject to major infections.

pemphigus neonatorum Neonatal impetigo.

penis Male organ used for urination and copulation.

perforation of the uterus Accidental puncture of the uterus, usually with a curet and occasionally by an intrauterine device (IUD).

peridural anesthesia Injection of anesthetic outside the dura mater (anesthetic does not mix with spinal fluid); epidural anesthesia.

perinatal Of or pertaining to the time and process of giving birth or being born.

perinatal period Period extending from the twentieth or twenty-eighth week of gestation through the end of the twenty-eighth day after birth.

perinatologist Physician who specializes in fetal and neonatal care.

perineorrhaphy Suture or operation used in repairing a laceration of the perineum, usually following labor.

perineotomy Surgical incision into the perineum. In obstetrics the perineotomy is usually called an *episiotomy* and is done at the end of the second stage of labor to avoid laceration of the perineum and to facilitate delivery. (See also *episiotomy*.)

perineum Area between the vagina and rectum in the female and between the scrotum and rectum in the male.

periodic breathing Sporadic episodes of cessation of respirations for periods of 10 seconds or less not associated with cyanosis commonly noted in premature infants.

peritoneum Strong serous membrane reflected over the viscera and lining the abdominal cavity.

pessary Device placed inside the vagina to function as a supportive structure for the uterus or a contraceptive device.

petechiae Pinpoint hemorrhagic areas caused by numerous disease states involving infection and thrombocytopenia and occasionally found over the face and trunk of the newborn because of increased intravascular pressure in the capillaries during delivery.

pH Hydrogen ion concentration.

phenotype Expression of certain physical or chemical characteristics in an individual resulting from interaction between genotype and environmental factors.

phenylketonuria (PKU) Recessive hereditary disease that results in a defect in the metabolism of the amino acid phenylalanine caused by the lack of an enzyme, phenylalanine hydroxylase, that is necessary for the conversion of the amino acid phenylalanine into tyrosine. If PKU is not treated, brain damage may occur, causing severe mental retardation.

phimosis Tightness of the prepuce, or foreskin, of the penis.

phlebitis Inflammation of a vein with symptoms of pain and tenderness along the course of the vein, inflammatory swelling and acute edema below the obstruction, and discoloration of the skin because of injury or bruise to the vein, possibly occurring in acute or chronic infections or after operations or childbirth.

phlebothrombosis Formation of a clot or thrombus in the vein; inflammation of the vein with secondary clotting.

phlebotomy Incision of a vein for the letting of blood, as in collecting blood from a donor.

phlegmasia alba dolens Phlebitis of the femoral vein with thrombosis leading to a venous obstruction, causing acute edema of the leg, and occurring occasionally after delivery; also called *milk-leg*.

phocomelia Developmental anomaly characterized by the absence of the upper portion of one or more limbs so that the feet or hands or both are attached to the trunk of the body by short, irregularly shaped stumps, resembling the fins of a seal.

phototherapy Utilization of lights to reduce serum bilirubin levels by oxidation of bilirubin into water-soluble compounds that are then processed in the liver and excreted in bile and urine.

physiologic hyperbilirubinemia Hemolysis of excessive fetal RBCs in the early neonatal period; jaundice not apparent during first 24 hours. Levels are nontoxic to the individual.

physiologic jaundice See *jaundice, physiologic*.

pica Unusual craving during pregnancy (e.g., of laundry starch, dirt, red clay).

pinna Ear cartilage.

placenta Latin, flat cake; afterbirth; specialized vascular disc-shaped organ for maternal-fetal gas and nutrient exchange. Normally it implants in the thick muscular wall of the upper uterine segment.

abruptio p. See *abruptio placentae*.

battledore p. Umbilical cord insertion into the margin of the placenta.

circumvallate p. Placenta having a raised white ring at its edge.

p. accreta Invasion of the uterine muscle by the placenta, thus making separation from the muscle difficult if not impossible.

p. previa Placenta that is abnormally implanted in the thin, lower uterine segment and that is typed according to proximity to cervical os: total—completely occludes os; partial—does not occlude os completely; and marginal—placenta encroaches on margin of internal cervical os.

p. succenturiata Accessory placenta.

placental Pertaining or relating to the placenta.

p. dysfunction Failure of placenta to meet fetal needs and requirements; placental insufficiency.

p. dystocia See *dystocia, placental*.

p. infarct Localized, ischemic, hard area on the fetal or maternal side of the placenta.

p. souffle See *souffle, placental*.

platypelloid pelvis Broad pelvis with a shortened anteroposterior diameter and a flattened, oval, transverse shape.

plethora Deep beefy red coloration (''boiled lobster'' hue) of a newborn caused by an increased number of blood cells (polycythemia) per volume of blood.

pneumomediastinum Accumulation of air around the heart and vena cava.

pneumothorax Escaped air from affected lung into the pleural space, displacing the heart and mediastinum toward the unaffected side of the chest.

podalic Concerning or pertaining to the feet.

p. version Shifting of the position of the fetus so as to bring the feet to the outlet during labor.

polycythemia Increased number of erythrocytes per volume of blood, which may be caused by large placental transfusion, fetofetal transfusion, or maternal-fetal transfusion, or it may be due to hypovolemia resulting from movement of fluid out of vascular into interstitial compartment.

polydactyly Excessive number of digits (fingers or toes).

polygenic Pertaining to the combined action of several different genes.

polyhydramnios See *hydramnios*.

polyuria Excessive secretion and discharge of urine by the kidneys.

position Relationship of an arbitrarily chosen fetal reference point, such as the occiput, sacrum, chin, or scapula on the presenting part of the fetus to its location in the front, back, or sides of the maternal pelvis.

positive sign of pregnancy Definite indication of pregnancy (e.g., hearing the fetal heartbeat, visualization and palpation of fetal movement by the examiner, sonographic examination).

posterior Pertaining to the back.

p. fontanel See *fontanel, posterior*.

postmature infant Infant born at or after the beginning of week 43 of gestation or later and exhibiting signs of dysmaturity.

postnatal Happening or occurring after birth.

postpartum Happening or occurring after birth.

Potter's syndrome Silicosis.

precipitate delivery Rapid or sudden labor of less than 3 hours' duration beginning from onset of cervical changes to completed birth of neonate.

preeclampsia Disease encountered during pregnancy or early in the puerperium characterized by increasing hypertension, albuminuria, and generalized edema; pregnancy-induced hypertension (PIH): toxemia.

pregnancy Period between conception through complete delivery of the products of conception. The usual duration of pregnancy in the human is 280 days, 9 calendar months, or 10 lunar months.

abdominal p. See *abdominal gestation*.

ectopic p. See *ectopic pregnancy*.

extrauterine p. See *extrauterine pregnancy*.

premature infant Infant born before completing week 37 of gestation, irrespective of birth weight; preterm infant.

premenstrual syndrome Syndrome of nervous tension, irritability, weight gain, edema, headache, mastalgia, dysphoria, and lack of coordination occurring during the last few days of the menstrual cycle preceding the onset of menstruation.

premonitory Serving as an early symptom or warning.

prenatal Occurring or happening before birth.

prepartum Before delivery; prior to giving birth.

prepuce Fold of skin, or foreskin, covering the glans penis of the male.

p. of the clitoris Fold of the labia minora that the glans clitoris.

presentation That part of the fetus which first enters the pelvis and lies over the inlet: may be head, face, breech, or shoulder.

breech p. See *breech presentation*.

cephalic p. See *cephalic presentation*.

presenting part That part of the fetus which lies closest to the internal os of the cervix.

pressure edema Edema of the lower extremities caused by pressure of the heavy pregnant uterus against the large veins; edema of fetal scalp after cephalic presentation (caput succedaneum).

presumptive signs Manifestations that suggest pregnancy but that are not absolutely positive. These include the cessation of menses, Chadwick's sign, morning sickness, and quickening.

preterm infant See *premature infant*.

previa, placenta See *placenta previa*.

priapism Continous erection of the penis, not usually accompanied by sexual feeling, which may appear in conjunction with leukemia, renal calculi, and spinal cord lesions.

primigravida Woman who is pregnant for the first time.

primipara Woman who has carried a pregnancy to viability without regard to the child's being dead or alive at the time of birth.

primordial Existing first or existing in the simplest or most primitive form.

probable signs Manifestations or evidence which indicates that there is a definite likelihood of pregnancy. Among the probable signs are enlargement of abdomen, Goodell's sign, Hegar's sign, Braxton Hicks' sign, and positive hormonal tests for pregnancy.

proband Individual in a family who comes to the attention of a genetic investigator because of the occurrence of a trait; the index case, or propositus.

prodromal Serving as an early symptom or warning of the approach of a disease or condition (e.g., prodromal labor).

progesterone Hormone produced by the corpus luteum and placenta whose function is to prepare the endometrium of the uterus for implantation of the fertilized ovum, develop the mammary glands, and maintain the pregnancy.

projectile vomiting Extremely forceful, expulsive vomiting.

prolactin See *lactogenic hormone.*

prolan Hormone produced by chorionic villi, now called *human chorionic gonadotropin (HCG),* that is found in the serum and urine of pregnant women and forms the basis of the biologic and immunologic pregnancy tests.

prolapsed cord Protrusion of the umbilical cord in advance of the presenting part.

proliferative phase of menstrual cycle Preovulatory, follicular, or estrogen phase of the menstrual cycle.

promontory of the sacrum Superior projecting portion of the sacrum at the junction of the sacrum and the L-5.

prophylactic Pertaining to prevention or warding off of disease or certain conditions; condom, or "rubber."

propositus See *proband.*

prostaglandin (PG) Substance present in many body tissues; has a role in many reproductive tract functions.

proteinuria Excretion of protein into urine.

pruritus Itching.

pruritus gravidarum Itching of the skin caused by pregnancy.

pseudocyesis Condition in which the woman has all the usual signs of pregnancy, such as enlargement of the abdomen, cessation of menses, weight gain, and morning sickness, but is not pregnant; phantom or false pregnancy.

pseudopregnancy See *pseudocyesis.*

pseudoprematurity See *intrauterine growth retardation (IUGR).*

psychologic miscarriage Absence or lack of love for one's infant.

psychoprophylaxis Mental and physical education of the parents in preparation for childbirth, with the goal of minimizing the fear and pain and promoting positive family relationships.

ptyalism Excessive salivation.

puberty Period in life in which the reproductive organs mature and one becomes functionally capable of reproduction.

pubic Pertaining to the pubis.

pubis Pubic bone forming the front of the pelvis.

pudendal block Injection of a local anesthetizing drug at the pudendal nerve root in order to produce numbness of the genital and perianal region.

pudendum External genitalia of either sex; Latin, "that of which one should be ashamed."

puerperal sepsis Infection of the pelvic organs during the postdelivery period; childbed fever.

puerperium Period of time following the third stage of labor and lasting until involution of the uterus takes place, usually about 3 to 6 weeks.

pulse pressure Difference between systolic and diastolic blood pressure.

pyloric stenosis Narrowing of the pyloric sphincter at the outlet of the stomach, causing an obstruction that blocks the flow of food into the small intestine.

quickening Maternal perception of fetal movement; usually occurs between weeks 16 and 20 of gestation.

rabbit test See *Friedman's test.*

radium insertion Introduction of metallic element radium (Ra) into the uterus or cervix to treat cancer.

rales Crackling sounds heard as air passes through the fluid present within the terminal bronchioles and alveoli.

raphe A line of union of the halves of various symmetrical parts, as the abdominal raphe of the linea alba or the raphe penis, which appears as a narrow, dark streak on the inferior surface of the penis.

RDS See *respiratory distress syndrome (RDS).*

recessive trait Genetically determined characteristic that is expressed only when present in the homozygotic state.

rectocele Herniation or protrusion of the rectum into the posterior vaginal wall.

rectovaginal ligament A posterior ligament.

reflex Automatic response built into the nervous system that does not need the intervention of conscious thought (e.g., in the newborn, rooting, gagging, grasp).

regional block anesthesia Anesthesia of an area of the body by injecting a local anesthetic to block a group of sensory nerve fibers.

regurgitate Vomiting or spitting up of solids or fluids.

residual urine Urine that remains in the bladder after urination.

respiratory distress syndrome (RDS) Condition resulting from decreased pulmonary gas exchange, leading to retention of carbon dioxide (increase in arterial PCO_2). Most common neonatal causes are prematurity, perinatal asphyxia, and maternal diabetes mellitus; hyaline membrane disease (HMD).

restitution In obstetrics, the turning of the fetal head to the left or right after it has completely emerged from the introitus as it assumes a normal alignment with the infant's shoulders.

resuscitation Restoration of consciousness or life in one who is apparently dead or whose respirations or cardiac function or both have ceased.

retained placenta Retention of all or part of the placenta in the uterus after delivery.

reticulocytosis Increase in number of reticulocytes in circulating blood.

retraction (1) Drawing in or sucking in of soft tissues of chest, indicative of an obstruction at any level of the respiratory tract from the oropharynx to the alveoli. (2) Retraction of uterine muscle fiber. After contracting, the muscle fiber does not return to its original length but remains slightly shortened, a unique attribute of uterine muscle that aids in preventing postdelivery hemorrhage and results in involution.

retroflexion Bending backward.

r. of the uterus Condition in which the body of the womb is bent backward at an angle with the cervix, whose position usually remains unchanged.

retrolental fibroplasia (RLF) Retinopathy of prematurity associated with hyperoxemia, resulting in eye injury and blindness.

retroversion Turning or a state of being turned back.

r. of the uterus Displacement of the uterus; the body of the uterus is tipped backward with the cervix pointing forward toward the symphysis pubis.

Rh factor Inherited antigen present on erythrocytes. The individual with the factor is known as *positive* for the factor.

rhonchi Coarse, snorelike sounds produced as air passes through the fluid in the large bronchi, frequently heard after aspiration of oral secretions or feedings.

rhythm method Contraceptive method in which a woman abstains from sexual intercourse during the ovulatory phase of her menstrual cycle and at least 3 days before and 1 day after the ovulation date.

ribonucleic acid (RNA) Element responsible for transferring genetic information within a cell; a template, or pattern.

risk factors Factors that cause a person or a group of people to be particularly vulnerable to an unwanted, unpleasant, or unhealthful event.

Ritgen maneuver Procedure used to control the delivery of the head.

role playing Psychotherapeutic technique in which a person acts out a real or simulated situation as a means of understanding intrapsychic conflicts.

rooming-in unit Maternity unit designed so that the newborn's crib is at the mother's bedside or in a nursery adjacent to the mother's room.

rooting reflex Normal response in newborns when the cheek is touched or stroked along the side of the mouth to turn the head toward the stimulated side, to open the mouth, and to begin to suck. The reflex disappears by 3 to 4 months of age but in some infants may persist until 12 months.

rotation In obstetrics, the turning of the fetal head as it follows the curves of the birth canal downward.

Rubin's test Transuterine insufflation of the fallopian tubes with carbon dioxide to test their patency.

rugae Folds of vaginal mucosa.

sac, amniotic See *amniotic sac*.

sacroiliac Of or pertaining to the sacrum and ilium.

sacrum Triangular bone composed of five united vertebras and situated between L-5 and the coccyx; forms the posterior boundary of the true pelvis.

saddle block anesthesia Type of regional anesthesia produced by injection of a local anesthetic solution into the cerebrospinal fluid intrathecal (subarachnoid) space in the spinal canal.

sagittal suture Band of connective tissue separating the parietal bones, extending from the anterior to the posterior fontanel.

salpingo-oophorectomy Removal of a fallopian tube and an ovary.

scaphoid abdomen Abdomen with a sunken interior wall.

schizophrenia Any one of a large group of psychotic disorders characterized by gross distortion of reality, disturbances of language and communication, withdrawal from social interaction, and the disorganization and fragmentation of thought, perception, and emotional reaction.

Schultze's mechanism Delivery of the placenta with the fetal surfaces (shiny in appearance) presenting (archaic).

sclerema Hardening of skin and subcutaneous tissue that develops in association with such life-threatening disorders as severe cold stress, septicemia, and shock.

scrotum Pouch of skin containing the testes and parts of the spermatic cords.

sebaceous glands Oil-secreting glands found in the skin.

secondary areola See *areola, secondary*.

secretory phase of menstrual cycle Postovulatory, luteal, progestational, premenstrual phase of menstrual cycle; 14 days in length.

secundines Fetal membranes and placenta expelled after childbirth; afterbirth.

segmentation Process of cleavage or division by which the fertilized ovum multiplies before differentiating into layers.

semen Thick, white, viscid secretion discharged from the urethra of the male at orgasm; the transporting medium of the sperm.

sensitization Development of antibodies to a specific antigen.

septic abortion See *abortion, septic*.

shake test "Foam" test for lung maturity of fetus; more rapid than determination of L/S ratio.

Sims' position Position in which the client lies on the left side with the right knee and thigh drawn upward toward the chest.

singleton Pregnancy with a single fetus.

situational crisis Crisis that arises suddenly in response to an external event or a conflict concerning a specific circumstance. The symptoms are transient, and the episode is usually brief.

Skene's glands Paraurethral glands situated on each side of urethral meatus.

small for dates (small for gestational age [SGA]) Refers to inadequate growth for gestational age.

smegma Whitish secretion around labia minora.

socioeconomic status Combined social and economic level of individuals or groups.

souffle Soft, blowing sound or murmur heard by auscultation.

- **funic s.** Soft, muffled, blowing sound produced by blood rushing through the umbilical vessels and synchronous with the fetal heart sounds.
- **placental s.** Soft, blowing murmur caused by the blood current in the placenta and synchronous with the maternal pulse.
- **uterine s.** Soft, blowing sound made by the blood in the arteries of the pregnant uterus and synchronous with the maternal pulse.

sperm Male sex cell. Also called spermatozoon.

spermatic cord Structure supporting the testis and containing blood vessels, nerves, muscle fibers, and the vas deferens.

spermatogenesis Process by which mature spermatozoa are formed, during which the diploid chromosome number (46) is reduced by half (haploid, 23).

spermicide Chemical substance that kills sperm by reducing their surface tension, causing the cell wall to break down by a bactericidal effect or by creating a highly acidic environment. Also called spermatocide.

spina bifida occulta Congenital malformation of the spine in which the posterior portion of laminas of the vertebras fails to close but there is no herniation or protrusion of the spinal cord or meninges through the defect. The newborn may have a dimple in the skin or growth of hair over the malformed vertebras.

spinnbarkeit Formation of a stretchable thread of cervical mucus under estrogen influence at time of ovulation.

splanchnic engorgement Excessive filling or pooling of blood within the visceral vasculature that occurs following the removal of pressure from the abdomen, e.g., birth of a child, removal of an excess of urine from bladder (1000 ml), removal of large tumor.

spontaneous abortion See *abortion, spontaneous*.

square window Angle of wrist between hypothenar prominence and forearm; one criterion for estimating gestational age of neonate.

station Relationship of the presenting fetal part to an imaginary line drawn between the ischial spines of the pelvis.

sterility (1) State of being free from living microorganisms. (2) Complete inability to reproduce offspring.

sterilization Process or act that renders a person unable to produce children.

stillborn Born dead.

striae gravidarum ("stretch marks") Shining reddish lines caused by stretching of the skin, often found on the abdomen, thighs, and breasts during pregnancy. These streaks turn to a fine pinkish white or silver tone in time in fair-skinned women and brownish in darker-skinned women.

stroma Supporting tissue.

subculture Group having social, economic, ethnic, or other traits distinctive enough to distinguish it from others within the same culture or society.

subinvolution Failure of a part (e.g., the uterus) to reduce to its normal size and condition after enlargement from functional activity (e.g., pregnancy).

subluxation Incomplete dislocation.

subtotal hysterectomy See *hysterectomy, subtotal.*

succedaneum See *caput succedaneum.*

superfecundation Successive fertilization of two or more ova formed during the same menstrual cycle by the sperm of the same father or different fathers.

superfetation Fertilization of an ovum when the woman is already pregnant.

supernumerary nipples Excessive number of nipples varying in size from small pink spots to the size of normal nipples and usually not associated with underlying glandular tissue.

supine hypotension Shock; fall in blood pressure caused by impaired venous return when gravid uterus presses on ascending vena cava, when woman is lying flat on her back; vena caval syndrome.

suppuration Process by which pus is formed.

surfactant Phosphoprotein necessary for normal respiratory function that prevents the alveolar collapse (atelectasis). See also *lecithin* and *L/S ratio.*

suture (1) Junction of the adjoining bones of the skull. (2) Operation uniting parts by sewing them together.

symphysis pubis Fibrocartilaginous union of the bodies of the pubic bones in the midline.

syndactyly Malformation of digits, commonly seen as a fusion of two or more toes to form one structure.

synostosis Articulation by osseous tissue of adjacent bones; union of separate bones by osseous tissue.

taboo Proscribed (forbidden) by society as improper and unacceptable.

tachypnea Excessively rapid respiratory rate (e.g., in neonates, respiratory rate of 60 breaths/min or more).

talipes equinovarus Deformity in which the foot is extended and the person walks on the toes.

telangiectasia Permanent dilatation of groups of superficial capillaries and venules.

telangiectatic nevi ("stork bites") Clusters of small, red, localized areas of capillary dilatation commonly seen in neonates at the nape of the neck or lower occiput, upper eyelids, and nasal bridge that can be blanched with pressure of a finger.

teratogenic agent Any drug, virus, or irradiation, the exposure to which can cause malformation of the fetus.

teratogens Nongenetic factors that cause malformations and disease syndromes in utero.

teratoma Tumor composed of different kinds of tissue, none of which normally occur together or at the site of the tumor.

term infant Live infant born between weeks 38 and 42 of completed gestation.

testis One of the glands contained in the male scrotum that produces the male reproductive cell, or sperm, and the male hormone testosterone; testicle.

tetany, uterine Extremely prolonged uterine contractions.

tetralogy of Fallot Congenital cardiac malformation consisting of pulmonary stenosis, intraventricular septal defect, dextroposed aorta that receives blood from both ventricles, and hypertrophy of the right ventricle.

thalassemia Hemolytic anemia characterized by microcytic, hypochromic, and short-lived red blood cells (RBCs) caused by deficient hemoglobin synthesis. It is an autosomal recessive, genetically transmitted disease occurring in two forms.

- **t. major** (homozygous form) evident in infancy, it is recognized by anemia, fever, failure to thrive, and splenomegaly and confirmed by characteristic changes in the RBCs on microscopic examination.
- **t. minor** (heterozygous form) it is characterized only by a mild anemia and minimal RBC changes.

therapeutic abortion See *abortion, therapeutic.*

thermogenesis Creation or production of heat, especially in the body.

thermoneutral environment Environment that enables the neonate to maintain a body temperature of 36.5° C (97.7° F) with minimum use of oxygen and energy.

threatened abortion See *abortion, threatened.*

thrombocytopenia Abnormal hematologic condition in which the number of platelets is reduced, usually by destruction of erythroid tissue in bone marrow owing to certain neoplastic diseases or to an immune response to a drug.

thrombocytopenic purpura Hematologic disorder characterized by prolonged bleeding time, decreased number of platelets, increased cell fragility, and purpura, which result in hemorrhages into the skin, mucous membranes, organs, and other tissue.

thromboembolism Obstruction of a blood vessel by a clot that has become detached from its site of formation.

thrombophlebitis Inflammation of a vein with secondary clot formation.

thrombus Blood clot obstructing a blood vessel that remains at the place it was formed.

thrush Fungal infection of the mouth or throat characterized by the formation of white patches on a red, moist, inflamed mucous membrane and is caused by *Candida albicans.*

toco- (toko-) Combining form that means childbirth or labor.

tocolytic drug Drug used to suppress premature labor.

tocotransducer Electronic device for measuring uterine contractions.

tongue-tie Congenital shortening of the frenulum, which, if servere, may interfere with sucking and articulation; a rare condition.

TORCH organisms Organisms that damage the embryo or fetus; acronym for *t*oxoplasmosis, *o*ther (e.g., syphilis), *r*ubella, *c*ytomegalovirus, and *h*erpes simplex.

torticollis Congenital or acquired stiff neck caused by shortening or spasmodic contraction of the neck (sternocleidomastoid) muscles that draws the head to one side with the chin pointing in the other direction; wryneck.

total hysterectomy See *hysterectomy, total.*

toxemia Term previously used for disorders occurring during pregnancy or early puerperium, known as *preeclampsia-eclampsia,* that are characterized by one or all of the following: edema, hypertension, proteinuria, and, in severe cases, convulsion and coma; pregnancy-induced hypertension (PIH).

tracheoesophageal fistula Congenital malformation in which there is an abnormal tubelike passage between the trachea and esophagus.

transition Last phase of first stage of labor; 8 to 10 cm dilatation.

translocation Condition in which a chromosome breaks and all or part of that chromosome is transferred to a different part of the same chromosome or to another chromosome.
trauma Physical or psychic injury.
Trichomonas vaginitis Inflammation of the vagina caused by *Trichomonas vaginalis,* a parasitic protozoon and characterized by persistent burning and itching of the vulvar tissue and a profuse, frothy, white discharge.
trimester Time period of 3 months.
trisomy Condition whereby any given chromosome exists in triplicate instead of the normal duplicate pattern.
trophectoderm See *trophoblast.*
trophoblast Outer layer of cells of the developing blastodermic vesicle that develops the trophoderm or feeding layer which will establish the nutrient relationships with the uterine endometrium.
tubal ligation See *ligation, tubal.*
tubercles of Montgomery Small papillae on surface of nipples and areolae that secrete a fatty substance that lubricates the nipples.
twins Two neonates from the same impregnation developed within the same uterus at the same time.
conjoined t. Twins who are physically united; Siamese twins.
disparate t. Twins who are different (e.g., in weight) and distinct from one another.
dizygous t. Twins developed from two separate ova fertilized by two separate sperm at the same time; fraternal twins.
monozygous twins. Twins developed from a single fertilized ovum; identical twins.

ultrasonography High frequency sound waves to discern fetal heart rate or placental location or body parts.
umbilical cord (funis) Structure connecting the placenta and fetus and containing two arteries and one vein encased in a tissue called *Wharton's jelly.* The cord is ligated at birth and severed; the stump falls off in 4 to 10 days.
umbilical vasculitis Inflammation of the umbilical cord and its blood vessels.
umbilicus Navel, or depressed point in the middle of the abdomen that marks the attachment of the umbilical cord during fetal life.
urachus Epithelial tube connecting the apex of the urinary bladder with the allantois. Its connective tissue forms the median umbilical ligament.
urethra Small tubular structure that drains urine from the bladder.
urinary frequency Need to void often or at close intervals.
urinary meatus Opening, or mouth, of the urethra.
uterine Referring or pertaining to the uterus.
u. adnexa See *adnexa, uterine.*
u. bruit Abnormal sound or murmur heard while auscultating the uterus.
u. ischemia Decreased blood supply to the uterus.
u. prolapse Falling, sinking, or sliding of the uterus from its normal location in the body.
u. souffle See *souffle, uterine.*
uterus Hollow muscular organ in the female designed for the implantation, containment, and nourishment of the fetus during its development until birth.
Couvelaire u. Interstitial myometrial hemorrhage following premature separation (abruptio) of placenta. A purplish-bluish discoloration of the uterus and boardlike rigidity of the uterus are noted.
inversion of the u. See *inversion of the uterus.*
retroflexion of the u. See *retroflexion of the uterus.*
retroversion of the u. See *retroversion of the uterus.*

vagina Normally collapsed musculomembranous tube that forms the passageway between the uterus and the entrance to the vagina.
vaginismus Intense, painful spasm of the muscles surrounding the vagina.
varices (varicose veins) Swollen, distended, and twisted veins that may develop in almost any part of the body but are most commonly seen in the legs, caused by pregnancy, obesity, congenital defective venous valves, and occupations requiring much standing.
vasectomy Ligation or removal of a segment of the vas deferens, usually done bilaterally to produce sterility in the male.
VDRL test Abbreviation for Venereal Disease Research Laboratory test, a serological flocculation test for syphilis.
venous Pertaining or relating to the veins.
vera, decidua See *decidua vera.*
vernix caseosa Protective gray-white fatty substance of cheesy consistency covering the fetal skin.
version Act of turning the fetus in the uterus to change the presenting part and facilitate delivery.
podalic v. See *podalic version.*
vertex Crown or top of the head.
v. presentation Presentation in which the fetal skull is nearest the cervical opening and born first.
vesicle Tiny blister; a small, thin-walled raised skin lesion containing clear fluid.
vesicle, blastoderm See *blastoderm vesicle.*
vestibule Area at the entrance to another structure.
v. of vagina Space between the labia minora where the urinary meatus and vaginal introitus are lcoated.
viable Capable of living, such as a fetus that has reached a stage of development, usually 24 to 28 weeks, which will permit it to live outside the uterus.
villi Short, vascular processes or protrusions growing on certain membranous surfaces.
chorionic v. Tiny vascular protrusions on the chorionic surface that project into the maternal blood sinuses of the uterus and that help to form the placenta and secrete HCG.
voluntary abortion See *abortion, elective.*
volvulus Twisting of the bowel on itself, causing intestinal obstruction.
vulva External genitalia of the female that consist of the labia majora, labia minora, clitoris, urinary meatus, and vaginal introitus.
vulvectomy Removal of the external genitalia of the female.

well-baby clinics Clinics that offer medical supervision and services to healthy infants.
Wharton's jelly White, gelatinous material surrounding the umbilical vessels within the cord.
witch's milk Secretion of a whitish fluid for about a week after birth from enlarged mammary tissue in the neonate, presumably resulting from maternal hormonal influences.
womb See *uterus.*

X chromosome Sex chromosome in humans existing in dupicate in the normal female and singly in the normal male.
X linkage Genes located on the X-chromosome.

Y chromosome Sex chromosome in the human male necessary for the development of the male gonads.

zero fluid balance Equality of amount of intake and amount of output.

zero population growth In a given year, live births equal to total number of deaths (i.e., no population increase for that year).

zona pellucida Inner, thick, membranous envelope of the ovum.

zygote Cell formed by the union of two reproductive cells or gametes; the fertilized ovum resulting from the union of a sperm and an ovum.

Index

A

AAHCC; *see* American Academy of Husband-Coached Childbirth
Abandonment, 47
ABCs; *see* Alternative Birth Centers
Abdomen
contour of, during uterine contractions, 381
enlargement of, as presumptive sign of pregnancy, 273
landmarks on, 69
mother's, quadrants of, and fetal position, 369
of neonate, assessment of, 588-589
in postpartum period, evaluative criteria for, 699
scaphoid, 970
Abdominal aorta and uterus, 66
Abdominal breathing for relaxation, 351
Abdominal discomfort during pregnancy, treatment of, 307
Abdominal distention, sudden, while feeding, 754
Abdominal electrocardiograph for fetal heart rate monitoring, 471, 475
Abdominal hernias complicating pregnancy, 989
Abdominal hysterectomy for therapeutic abortion, 992, 995
Abdominal musculature, changes in, in postpartum period, 689
Abdominal organs of neonate, hemorrhage into, 906
Abdominal orifice of fallopian tube, 60
Abdominal pain
and oral contraceptives, 193
during pregnancy, 242
Abdominal palpation to determine fetal presentation, position, and descent, 382-384
Abdominal wall, 68-69
Aberrations, 147
chromosomal, 147-150
disorders caused by, 149
ABO incompatibility, 960
ABO typing of mother, 962
Abortion
after amniocentesis, 44
complete, 782
management of, 783
congressional amendment restricting funds for, 45
counseling regarding, 112
elective; *see* Therapeutic abortion
ethical and legal issues of, 44-46
and fetal research, 44
habitual, from small uterus, 179
incomplete, 782, 783
inevitable, 782, 783
missed, 782, 783
multiple, 110
by older mother, 721
septic, 782, 783
spontaneous; *see* Spontaneous abortion
therapeutic; *see* Therapeutic abortion
threatened, 782, 783
Abruptio placentae; *see* Premature separation of placenta
Abscess
breast, 668
tubo-ovarian, and IUD, 196
Abstinence from intercourse in natural family planning, 188
Abstract thought, capacity for, in adolescence, 107
Abuse
child, 710
Abuse—cont'd
drugs of, effect of, on fetus or neonate, 1023
and neglect and premature infant, 928-929
Acceleration in fetal heart rate, 485, 486
Acceleration phase of cervical dilatation, 398
Acceptable preterm labor and delivery, care during, 912
Acceptance of grief, 766
Accessory reproductive tract glands of male, 82
Accommodation in cognitive development, 134
Accountability, 6
and decision making, 34
legal view of, 39-40
Acculturation, 115
Acetabulum, 70
Acetaminophen in breast milk, 1029
Acetazolamide in breast milk, 1033
Acetonuria
after delivery, 689
in diabetes mellitus, 845
Acetylsalicylic acid
in breast milk, 663, 1029
and neonatal platelets, 558
Achondroplasia, 146
Achondroplastic dwarfism, 142
Achromycin; *see* Tetracycline
Acid indigestion during pregnancy, 241, 303
Acid-base balance during pregnancy, 234
Acidity, gastric, of neonate, 560
Acidosis in diabetes mellitus, 845
Acinus of breast, 72, 73
Acne vulgaris, 238, 239, 273, 987
ACNM; *see* American College of Nurse-Midwives
ACOG; *see* American College of Obstetricians and Gynecologists
Acquired immune deficiency syndrome, 109, 841-842
Acrocyanosis of neonate, 564, 611
Acrodysesthesia, 306
Acroesthesia, 240
Acrosome of sperm, 80
Acrosome cap, 207
Acrosome reaction, 206
ACTH; *see* Adrenocorticotropic hormone
Acting and values clarification, 32
Activated partial thromboplastin time, 798
Active immunity of neonate, 562
Active immunization of normal infants and children, recommended schedule for, 1038
Active phase
of cervical dilatation, 398
of labor, 392
Active transfer across placenta, 215
Activity
fetal, determination of, 496
during pregnancy, 300
cultural views of, 118
energy needs for, 320
uterine; *see* Uterine activity
Actions, effect of values on, 29-33
Adaptation
in cognitive development, 134
to pregnancy and parenting, psychologic, maternal, assessment of, 294-295
Addicted infant, nursing care of, 953-955
Addiction, drug, as nutrition risk factor, 326
Adenohypophysis, 86
Adenomas, hepatic, and oral contraceptives, 194
Adenosine diphosphate, interference with release of, 558
ADH; *see* Antidiuretic hormone
Adherent placenta, postdelivery hemorrhage from, 805-806
Adhesions, tubal, 178
Administration of medications, routes of
intramuscular, 504
intravenous, 504, 505
Administrator role of nurse, 7
Admission
to labor unit, 409-410
to postpartum unit, 690
of preterm infant to nursery, 915
Adnexa, 60
Adolescence, 937
developmental tasks of, 939-940
personality development in, 136
sexual development in, 105-109
Adolescent clinics, 943
Adolescent father, 947
Adolescent mother, 937-947
adjustment of, to pregnancy, 135
postdelivery care of, 945
Adolescent parenthood, 937-947
Adolescent pregnancy, 937-947
dynamics of, 938-939
factors contributing to, 937
risks in, 937-938
trends in, 937
Adoption, placing infant for, 945
Adrenal cortex
fetal, 219
during pregnancy, 247
Adrenal glands, changes in, during pregnancy, 247
Adrenalin; *see* Epinephrine
Adrenergics causing increased uterine activity, 490
Adrenocorticosteroids for ulcerative colitis, 987
Adrenocorticotropic hormone, 86
Adult
sexual development in, 109-112
sexuality of, 109-112
Adult respiratory distress syndrome complicating pregnancy, 802, 986
disseminated intravascular coagulation and, 986
Adult responsibilities and pregnancy, 257
Adultery and artificial insemination, 43
Adulthood, personality development in, 136
Adverse reactions to childbearing, stresses causing, 284
Advocacy, client, by maternity nurses, 5-6, 7
Advocate, client, nurse as, 12, 30
After-birth classes, 342
Afterpains, 457, 688
AGA; *see* Appropriate for gestational age
Age
and fertility, 161
gestational; *see* Gestational age
menstrual, 208
of neonate and initial oral feeding, 676
parental, and response to infant, 720-722
Agenesis, sacral, 861
Age-related pregnancy problems, 721
Aggressive behavior by siblings toward baby, 719
Aging, fear of, 11
AID; *see* Artificial insemination by donor
AIDS; *see* Acquired immune deficiency syndrome

AIH, *see* Artificial insemination by husband
Air, exposure to, for sore nipples, 668
Airway
  for neonate, clearing, 440
  open, in neonate, maintenance of, 616
Airway pressure, continuous positive, for neonate with respiratory distress, 749, 750
Alarm system on fetal monitor, legal aspects of, 46
Albamycin; *see* Novobiocin
Albinism, 146
Albumin
  decrease in, during pregnancy, 316
  serum, tests to measure, 329
Albuminuria, 236
Alcohol, 215
  in breast milk, 1036
  for cord care, 621
  effect of, on fetus or neonate, 1023
  in human milk, 662
  intravenous, effect of, on fetus and neonate, 1024
  and male infertility, 182
  during pregnancy, 301
  as teratogen, 951
Alcoholism
  maternal, and fetal malformations, 952; *see also* Fetal alcohol syndrome
  as nutrition risk factor, 326
Aldactone; *see* Spironolactone
Aldomet; *see* Methyldopa
Aldosterone and nutrition, 316
Aldrin in breast milk, 1034
Alert inactivity by neonate, 569
Alienation
  of new father, 717
  toddler's experience of, 135
Alimentary canal, functional alterations in, during pregnancy, 316
Alkalinity of cervical mucus, 179-180
Allergy to iodine, 384
Aloin in breast milk, 1033
Alpha-fetoprotein levels, amniocentesis to determine, 288
Alpha-lipotropin hormone, 86
Alpha-melanocyte–stimulating hormone, 86
Alphaprodine
  for analgesia, 523
  causing decreased variability in fetal heart rate, 483
  causing pseudosinusoidal pattern in fetal heart rate, 483
Alterations in parenting, 20
Alternative Birth Center, 5, 532, 534-536
  high-risk factors excluding admission to, 536, 538
Alternative Birth Crisis Coalition, 1007
Alternative settings for childbirth, 529-549
Alveolar period of fetal lung development, 217
Alveolar ventilation, changes in, during pregnancy, 234
Alveolus of breast, 72
Amantadine in breast milk, 1030
Ambiguous genitalia, 970, 980
Ambivalence about pregnancy, 256
Ambulation, early, after delivery, 703
Amcill; *see* Polycillin
Amenorrhea
  after delivery, 688
  postpill, 194
  as presumptive symptoms of pregnancy, 269
  secondary, in young women, 177
  stressful emotional stimuli causing, 84
American Academy of Husband-Coached Childbirth, 346, 357, 1007
American Academy of Pediatrics, 531, 1007
American Cancer Society, 1007
American College of Nurse Midwives, 13, 14, 531, 541, 1007
American College of Obstetricians and Gynecologists, 13, 14, 46, 531, 1007
  ACNM-approved basic education in, 1013
American family, 122
American Indians
  food patterns of, 329
  handling of umbilical cord by, 123
  infant care by, 123
  use of contraceptives by, 124
  views on pregnancy of, 116-117
American Indian families, value of children in, 116
American Indian women, labor and delivery of, 119
American National Red Cross, 1007
  childbirth education classes of, 344
American Nurses' Association, 531
American Society for Psychoprophylaxis in Obstetrics, 346, 357, 531, 1007
Amino acid chromatography, 1027
Amino acids
  in human milk, 661
  for infant, 654
Aminophylline for acute bronchial asthma, 985
Aminopterin, effect of, on fetus or neonate, 1023
Amish communal family, 132
Amitriptyline hydrochloride in breast milk, 1036
Ammoniacal diaper rash, 612
Ammonium chloride, effect of, on fetus or neonate, 1023
Amnesia between contractions during second stage of labor, 425
Amnesics
  for analgesia, 508, 510, 523
  for anesthesia, 508, 510
Amniocentesis, 5, 216, 281-282, 287-291
  data-recording system for, 290
  to determine gestational age of fetus, 280, 281-282
  to diagnose fetal disorders, 152
  indications for, 152, 287-288
  injection of urea solution after, for therapeutic abortion, 995
  laboratory utilization of aspirant from, 289
  legal aspects of, 43-44
  preparation for, 288
  procedure for, 152, 153, 288-290
  risks of, 290-291
  selection of site for, 289
  summary of, 283
  transabdominal, in erythroblastosis, 963
Amniography, 152-153
Amnion
  and chorion, fusion of, and placenta, 214
  development of, 212
Amnioscopy
  to detect fetal disorders, 153
  to determine gestational age, 283
Amniotic fluid, 212, 215-216
  amount of, 402
    and congenital anomalies, 967
  assessment of, 401-402
  character of, 402
  color of, 401-402
  function of, 215-216
  increase in, during pregnancy, 287
  leakage of, 401
  meconium-stained, 401-402
    and fetal distress, 283
  port wine-colored, 402
  rupture of membranes and, 401-402
  yellow-stained, 401
Amniotomy, transcervical, 888, 890
Amobarbital
  for analgesia, 509
  causing decreased variability in fetal heart rate, 483
Amphetamine in breast milk, 1036
Ampicillin
  in breast milk, 1030
  effect of, on fetus or neonate, 1022
  and oral contraceptives, 195
Ampulla
  of breast, 72, 73
  of fallopian tube, 60, 61
Amylase
  and infant digestion, 652
Amylase—cont'd
  and neonatal digestion, 560
Amytal; *see* Amobarbital
Amytal Sodium; *see* Amobarbital
ANA; *see* American Nurses' Association
Anal intercourse, 110
  during pregnancy, 308
Anal sphincter
  external, 58, 61
  muscle fibers of, 57
  "wink" reflex of, 593
Anal varices, 223
Analgesia
  and anesthesia, pharmacologic, 508-509
  definition of, 501
  goals of nursing care in use of, 500-501
  informed consent for, 501
  inhalation, 508, 510-511
  modalities for, comparison of, 523
  narcotic, intravenous administration of, 505
Analgesics
  in breast milk, 1029-1030
  causing decreased variability in fetal heart rate, 483
  after delivery, 457-458
  effect of, on fetus or neonate, 1022
  and placenta, 215
  for relief of pain of episiotomy, 701
  for spontaneous abortion, 783
Analysis
  delta optical density, 962, 963
  diet history and, 331
  hormone, as fertility test, 171
Anaprox; *see* Maproxen
Anatomic and physiologic adaptations to pregnancy, 221-251
Anatomy and physiology of reproduction, 50-101
Ancef; *see* Cefazolin
Androgenic hormones and male development, 219-220
Androgens
  effect of, on fetus or neonate, 1023
  ovaries and, 68
Androgynous personalities, 103
Android pelvis, 378, 875
  women with, 372
Anectine; *see* Succinylcholine chloride
Anemia
  fetal, sinusoidal pattern in, 483
  folic acid deficiency, 983-984
  hemolytic, fetal sequelae of, 962
  iron deficiency, 983
  Mediterranean or Cooley's, 984
  neonatal, 807
    nursing care for, 807-808
  of pregnancy, 315, 326, 983-984
  sickle cell, 146
    screening for, 43
Anencephaly, 152, 976
  and hydramnios, 967
  prenatal diagnosis of, 975
Anesthesia
  and analgesia, pharmacologic, 508-509
  caudal, 524
    care after, 703
  for cesarean delivery, 515
  combination, for cesarean birth, 524
  conduction, effect of, on fetus or neonate, 1022
  definition of, 501
  effect of, on fetus or neonate, 1022
  epidural, 518-522
    care after, 703
  general, 508, 511
    effect of, on fetus or neonate, 1022
  goals of nursing care in use of, 500-501
  informed consent for, 501
  local, effect of, on fetus or neonate, 1022
  local infiltration, tray for, 515
  paracervical, effect of, on fetus or neonate, 1022
  regional, 508, 511, 513, 516
  spinal, intrathecal subarachnoid, care after, 702

Anesthesia—cont'd
for spontaneous abortion, 783
for vaginal delivery, 515
Anesthetic risks, 46
Anesthetics
general, causing decreased variability in fetal heart rate, 483
during labor and delivery, legal concepts regarding, 46
maternal, causing fetal bradycardia, 481
and placenta, 215
Anesthesiologist, 501
Aneurysm, aortic, elective abortion in, 990
Angiomas, spider, 238
Ankle dorsiflexion in neonate, 918
Annular hymen, 57
Annular uterine strictures from obstructed labor, 882
Anomalies
congenital; *see* Congenital anomalies
of earlobes, 967
of ears, 979
fetal, and dystocia, 875
Anomalous venous return, 968
Anovulation, 177
during pregnancy, 223
Anovulatory period after delivery, 688
Antabuse, 200
Antacid, preoperative, before cesarean section, 987
Anteflexion of uterus, 64, 65
Antepartum testing, 496-498
Anterior commissure, 54
Anterior fontanel of fetal skull, 363, 364
Anterior fornix, 68
Anterior ligament, 62, 65
Anterior pectoral nodes, 74
Anterior pituitary necrosis, postdelivery, 807
Anteroposterior diameter of pelvic outlet, 375
Anteversion of uterus, 64, 65
Anthraquinone laxatives in breast milk, 1033
Anthropoid pelvis, 372, 378
Antibiotic therapy for chorioamnionitis, 402
Antibiotics
and breast feeding, 663
in breast milk, 1030-1031
after cesarean delivery, 904
for congenital syphilis, 841
for glomerulonephritis during pregnancy, 985
for lower genital infection, 180
for mastitis, 833
for neonatal necrotizing enterocolitis, 927
and placenta, 215
after spontaneous abortion, 783
for tubal infections, 178
for ulcerative colitis, 987
for urinary tract infection during pregnancy, 985
and vaginal infection, 161
Antibody(ies), 562
humoral, 562
to sperm, 172
and male infertility, 181, 182
Anticipatory guidance of parents
before discharge from hospital, 628-630
at first well-baby visit, 630
Anticoagulants
and breast feeding, 663
in breast milk, 1031
effect of, on fetus or neonate, 1022
Anticonvulsants
in breast milk, 1031-1032
effect of, on fetus or neonate, 1022
Antidepressants, effect of, on fetus or neonate, 1024
Antidiarrheal agents and breast feeding, 663
Antidiuretic hormone, storage of, 86; *see also* Vasopressin
Antigen-antibody complex, 562
Antigen-antibody reaction, sperm immobilization, 172
Antigenicity, red blood cell, 960
Antigens, 562
Rh, 960-961
of sperm membrane, 80
Antihistamines
and breast feeding, 663
in breast milk, 1032
and placenta, 215
Antihypertensives for pregnancy-induced hypertension, 817
Antiinfectious factors in human milk, 662
Antiinflammatory drugs in breast milk, 1029-1030
Antimalarial, effect of, on fetus or neonate, 1022
Antimetabolites and breast feeding, 663
Antimicrobials, effect of, on fetus or neonate, 1022
Antineoplastic agents in human milk, 662
Antithyroid medications in breast milk, 1037
Antituberculous agents, effect of, on fetus or neonate, 1023
Anus, 54, 61
imperforate, 970, 974-975
and hydramnios, 967
of neonate, assessment of, 593
varicose veins of, 241
Anxiety
during first stage of labor, 403
during pelvic examination, 164
during pregnancy, 256-258
separation, 135
Aorta, 67
abdominal, and uterus, 66
coarctation of, 969
Aortic aneurysm, elective abortion in, 990
Apgar scoring chart, 441
Apical pulse in neonate, location of, 579
Apnea
in neonate, 558
treatment of, 635
Appearance of neonate, evaluative criteria for, 647, 648
Appendectomy during pregnancy, 989
Appendicitis complicating pregnancy, 242, 989
Appendix epididymis, 79
Appendix testis, 79
Appetite
changes in, during pregnancy, 241
after delivery, 693
Appliance, restraint without, 645
Appointments, missed or broken, and time sense, 29
Approach to cultural differences, 125
Appropriate for gestational age, 915
Apresoline; *see* Hydralazine
Aquamephyton; *see* Vitamin K_1
Arab women
male progeny of, 123
modesty of, 117
pain tolerance of, 120
views of motherhood of, 116
Arab-American women, views on pregnancy of, 117
Arachnoid in spinal cord, 512
Aralen; *see* Chloroquine
Arch
of foot of newborn, absence of, 592
subpubic, 70
angle of, estimation of, 375, 376, 378
female and male, contrast of, 72
ARDS; *see* Adult respiratory distress syndrome
ARENA, 184
Areola, 72, 73, 74
changes in, during pregnancy, 228
Arlef; *see* Flufenamic acid
Arm(s)
of neonate, assessment of, 591
paralysis of, from delivery, 907-908
Arnold-Chiari syndrome, 975
Arousal, optimal state of, 569-570
Arousal states of neonate, 569-570
Arrhythmia, sinus, in neonate, 555
Arsenic
in breast milk, 1031
effect of, on fetus or neonate, 1024
Art and science of nursing, 5
Arterial blood pressure, changes in, during pregnancy, 232, 233
Arteriolar spasm, general, in preeclampsia-eclampsia, 812
Artery
of clitoris, 67
hemorrhoidal, middle, 68
hypogastric, 66, 67
iliac, 66, 67
obturator, 67
ovarian, 66, 67, 68
perineal, 59, 67
pudendal, internal, 67, 68
superior vesical, 557
umbilical, 67, 213
changes in, at birth, 557
and fetal development, 216
uterine, 67, 68
vaginal, 59, 67
vesical, 67
Artificial insemination
after cervical procedures, 180
by donor, 43, 182-183
by husband, 43, 182
legal problems involved in, 43
Artificial rupture of membranes, 888, 890
Ascorbic acid
effect of, on glucose determination, 1021
for infant, 656
need for, during pregnancy, 323
supplements of, 323
Asian women, postpartal care of, 120, 121
Aspermatogenesis, 182
Asphyxia
neonatal, signs of, 808
and neonatal necrotizing enterocolitis, 927
perinatal, in infants of diabetic mother, 861
severe, results of, 218
Aspiration
midairway, 632-633
personal, interference with, and parental responses, 722
stomach, 632-633
upper airway, of neonate, 632
uterine, for therapeutic abortion, 992
Aspiration pneumonia complicating pregnancy, 986-987
Aspirin; *see* Acetylsalicylic acid
ASPO; *see* American Society for Psychoprophylaxis in Obstetrics
Assays
factor, specific, 798
immunologic, for human chorionic gonadotropin as pregnancy test, 277
Assessment, 18-20
of amniotic fluid, 401-402
of birth canal after delivery, 452
of bony pelvis, 370-373
for cardiac decompensation in postdelivery care, 870
cephalocaudal, 19
of deep tendon reflexes, 819, 820
dietary, during pregnancy, 329, 331
in first stage of labor, 395
initial, 395-397
of infants, nutritional screening and, 677-681
during labor, techniques for, 382-388
of maternal psychologic adaptation to pregnancy and parenting, 294-295
of mother
following delivery, general, 451-452
during fourth stage of labor, 454
of neonate, 439
behavioral, 602-610
neurologic, 594-601
nursing, and nursing diagnosis, 574-614
physical, 576-593, 613
timing for; *see* Timing for assessing neonate using Apgar score, 441-442
of neurologic functioning, 563
nutrition, 327-331
of parental responses, 723-729

Assessment—cont'd
of parent-child relationship
strategies for, 724-725
tools for, 725-729
physical, of nutritional status, 328
during pregnancy with evaluative criteria, 310-312
during prenatal period, 269-291
of presenting part, 383
in problem-oriented record, 23
for syphilis, 827, 832
of uterine contractions, 381-382
of women in postpartum period, 690-695
initial, 690-692
Assessment guide for preeclampsia, 821
Assessment sheet for cervical dilatation and descent of presenting part, 400
Assessment strategies, 21
for normal newborn, 610-613
Assessment tool
family, 293
for normal newborn, 610-613
Assimilation, 115
in cognitive development, 134
Association for Aid of Crippled Children, 1007
Association for Childbirth at Home, International, 1007
Assortment, independent, principle of, 145
Asthma, bronchial, complicating pregnancy, 985-986
Asymmetry, facial, in neonate, 577
Asynclitism, 389, 391
Ataractics
for analgesia during birth period, 510
causing decreased variability in fetal heart rate, 483
Atelectasis in respiratory distress syndrome, 925
Atherosclerosis and infant feeding, 676
Atony, uterine
causes of, 803
factors associated with, 452
postdelivery hemorrhage caused by, 803
prevention of, 456
Atopic dermatitis, 238, 987
Atresia
choanal, 677, 967
esophageal, 560, 970, 971, 972
feeding of infant with, 677
and hydramnios, 967
tricuspid, 968
Atrial septal defect, 968
Atropine
and breast feeding, 663
for cholelithiasis, 987
causing decreased variability in fetal heart rate, 483
effect of, on fetus or neonate, 1023
Atropine sulfate
in breast milk, 1032
to prevent convulsions of eclampsia, 822
Atropisol to prevent convulsions of eclampsia, 822
Attachment, parent-child, in postpartum period, 695, 701
Attachment behavior, 708
Attachment process, 708
Attachment stage of spontaneous abortion, 782
Attitude
fetal, 367-369
toward sex, changes in, 109
Auscultation, 20
to determine fetal presentation, position, and descent, 384
of fetal heart, periodic, 402
of intrauterine sounds, 225
Auscultatory changes during pregnancy, 229-230
Autoantibodies to sperm, reduction in, 182
Autoimmune disorders, 800
Autoimmunization to sperm, 172
and male infertility, 181
therapy for, 182
after vasectomy, 999
Automatic walking reflex, 600
Autonomic drugs in breast milk, 1032
Autonomic nerves of uterus, 66
Autonomy vs. shame and doubt in personality development, 135-136
Autosomal aberrations, 149
common, characteristics of, 150
Autosomal trait, 145
Autosomal-dominant inheritance, 146
Autosomal-recessive inheritance, 146
Autosomes, 80, 143, 207
Aventyl, effect of, on fetus or neonate, 1024
Avoidance reflex in fetus, 218
Avoirdupois system, units of, 1015
Awareness phase of grieving, 766
Axillary nodes, central, 74
Axillary temperature in neonate, 580
taking, 581, 617
Azoospermia from autoimmunity, 181

B

Babies, "test-tube," 43
Babinski reflex, 599
Babinski's sign, 599
"Baby blues," 715, 915
Baby foods, preparation and storage of, 675
Babylonia, humoral pathology and, 116
Back
fetal, and small parts, palpation of, 383
of neonate, assessment of, 592, 593
Back rubs during labor, 414
Backache, sacral, from endometriosis, 179
Bacteremic shock, 835-836
Bacteria, placental transfer of, 215
Bacterial tubal infection, 178
Bahamians, view on menstruation of, 124
Bailey-Williamson forceps, 891
Balance
acid-base, during pregnancy, 234
fluid and electrolyte, during pregnancy, 236-237
and harmony during pregnancy, 116
restoration of, after delivery, 120-121
sodium, during pregnancy, 236
water
in neonate, 559-560
during pregnancy, 236-237
Ballottement as probable sign of pregnancy, 274
Bandl's ring, 380, 882, 884
Baptism of premature infant, 929
Barbital in breast milk, 1031
Barbiturates
and breast feeding, 663
causing decreased variability in fetal heart rate, 483
effect of, on fetus or neonate, 1022-1024
and oral contraceptives, 195
for pregnancy-induced hypertension, 816
to prevent convulsions of eclampsia, 822
Barium in breast milk, 1033
Barr body, 149, 151
Barrier, placental, 215
Bartholin's duct, opening of, 54
Bartholin's glands, 54, 56
changes in, in response to sexual stimulation, 95
Basal body temperature
assessment of, 166, 167
and contraception, 189-190
elevation of, as presumptive sign of pregnancy, 272
thermometer for recording, 167
Basal layer of endometrium, 87, 88
Basal metabolic rate during pregnancy, 234, 320
changes in, 246
Basal temperature record, 168
Base-line fetal heart rate, 480-484
Bath, sitz, in care of episiotomy, 701
Bathing
of neonate, 620-621
parental guidance concerning, 629
in postpartum period, 701
cultural views on, 121
Bathing—cont'd
during pregnancy, 299
Battledore placenta, 214
Bearing-down efforts, 421, 425
voluntary, and expulsion of fetus, 382
Beat-to-beat changes in fetal heart rate, 480
Bed
borning, 533-534
labor, transfer to delivery table from, 425
Bed rest
for pregnancy-induced hypertension, 813
to suppress uterine activity, 910
Bedding of neonate, care of, 624-625
Behavior
aggressive, by siblings toward baby, 719
attachment, 708
cyclic trends in, in child, 135
dependent, by mother, 713-714
executive, of infant, 708
homosexual, prepubescent, 104-105
infant, age of accomplishment of, mothers' expectations of, 946
associated with infertility, 184
interdependent, by family, 717-718
of neonate
elimination, 572
evaluative criteria for, 648
factors influencing, 610
feeding, 571-572
sensory, 567-569
sleeping and waking, 569-571
social, 571
neuromuscular, fetal, 218
parenting, high-risk, 724
of parents and family, expected, among various cultures, 116-119
during pregnancy, 256
regression in, by siblings, 719
signaling, by infant, 708
Behavioral assessment of neonate, 602-610
Behavioral characteristics of newborn, 567-572
Behavioral evaluation, Brazelton, 603
Behavioral patterns of neonate, assessment of, 603
Behavioral Publications, 1011
Behavioral tasks of neonate, 554
Beliefs held by maternity nurses, 8-9
Bell
plastic, for circumcision, 628
response decrement to, 604
Belladonna derivatives
effect of, on fetus or neonate, 1023
for urinary tract infection during pregnancy, 985
Benadryl; *see* Diphenhydramine
Benedict's test, 1027
Benemid; *see* Probenecid
Benzene hexachloride in breast milk, 1034
Benzodiazepines in breast milk, 1036
Benzothiazides, effect of, on fetus or neonate, 1023
Beta scanner, 218; *see also* Ultrasonography
Beta-endorphins, 86
Beta-lipotropin hormone, 86
Beta-melanocyte–stimulating hormone, 86
BHC; *see* Benzene hexachloride
Biceps reflex, elicitation of, 818
Bicillin; *see* Penicillin G, benzathine
Bililite, 642
Bilirubin in neonate, 561; *see also* Hyperbilirubinemia
Bilirubinoid pigments, test for, and gestational age, 282
Bill of Rights, Pregnant Patient's, 1003-1004
Billings method of contraception, 190
Biochemical tests
to detect genetic disorders, 153-154
and nutrition assessment, 327, 329
Biochemical values for neonate, 1025-1026
Biographic data on client, 18
Biologic basis of inheritance, 141-145
Biologic characteristics of newborn, 555-567
Biologic parenthood, 707
Biologic system, review of, 19

Biomedical model
and nursing, 115
of prenatal care, 116
Biopsy, endometrial, as fertility test, 172
Biopsychosocial status of client, assessment of, 18-19
Biorhythmicity and parent-child attachment, 710
Biparietal diameter
fetal, to determine gestational age of fetus, 280, 281, 282
and fetal weight, correlations of, 297
Biphasic sexual response, 100
Biphasic temperature curve, 168
Birth, 1011
Birth; *see also* Delivery
cesarean; *see* Cesarean delivery
of child with disorder, 767-769
complications during, 873-934
conception to, period from, 206-220
condition of infant at, and prenatal diet of mother, 319
emergency, 447-449
of fetus in breech presentation, 449
of fetus in vertex position, 447-448
family adjustment to, 4-5
family responses to, 707-723
of handicapped infant, sibling's response to, 135
of high-risk infant, response of family members to, 778
home, 542-549
legal aspects of, 44
preterm, 449, 909-912; *see also* Premature infant; Prematurity
process of, seen through father's eyes, 415
relationship of husband and wife after, 717
of sibling
and "loss" of mother, 135
response of child to, 135
stressors on family caused by, 3
time of, 391-392
to unmarried women, 11
unusual occurrences during and after, 448-449
Birth canal
assessment of, after delivery, 452
axis of, 374
descent through, 378
during labor, 369-379
lacerations of, postdelivery hemorrhage from, 803-805
soft tissues of, 379
Birth center
alternative; *see* Alternative Birth Centers
freestanding, 538-541
Birth certificate, 1045
Birth choices, 532
Birth control; *see* Contraception; Contraceptives; oral contraceptives
Birth defects, 142; *see also* Congenital anomalies
Birth EZ Birthing Chair, 438
Birth and Family Journal, 1011
Birth period, 360-549
discomfort during, pharmacologic control of, 500-528
"Birth plan," 539
Birth process
anxiety about, 257-258
role of father in, 6
technology related to, advances in, 4, 5
Birth room, 5
Birth trauma
classification of, 906
infant, 905-909
in infants of diabetic mothers, 861
Birth weight, infant, and maternal nutrition, 318
Birthing chairs, 437, 438, 439
Birthing rooms, 120, 532-534
Birthmarks
food taboos and, 117-118
on neonate, 582-583
Birthrate, 11
Bisexuality, 110
Bishop's scale for assessing candidates for induction of labor, 886, 887
Bishydroxycoumarin; *see* Dicumarol
Bites, "stork," 565
Bivalve speculum examination, 286
Black infants, mortality for, 11
Black women
discomfort of labor in, 120
labor and delivery of, 119
pica among, 118
postpartal behavior of, 121
proscriptions during pregnancy for, 119
Blacks
family planning by, 124
food patterns of, 330
maternal mortality among, 12
pregnancy diets among, 117, 118
value of children to, 116
views of
on family, 123
on menstruation, 124-125
regarding sexual activity during pregnancy, 118-119
Bladder, 56, 58, 61, 67, 78
assessment of, after delivery, 693
distention of
after delivery, 456, 693
during labor, 410
exstrophy of, 978-980
full, and dystocia, 875
infection of, 702
midtract, 79
neck of, 56
during pregnancy, 235-236
Bladder muscle, 56
Blades, fenestrated, 891
Blastocyst, 210
Blastomeres, 210
Bleeding
after circumcision, 628
implantation, 210
with IUD, 197
midcycle, 87
from umbilical cord, 621
vaginal examination and, 384
withdrawal, 87
from oral contraceptives, 192
Bleeding gums
during pregnancy, 238-239
as presumptive sign of pregnancy, 273
Bleeding time, 798
Blind mother, response of, to infant, 722-723
Blisters, milk; *see* Sucking calluses
Block
caudal, 516
epidural, 513, 516
lumbar, 512
lumbar sympathetic, 512
nerve root, 513
paracervical, 512, 513
peridural nerve, 513, 516
peripheral nerve, 513
pudendal, 512, 513, 514
subarachnoid, 516
Blood
coagulation of, standard values for, pregnant and nonpregnant, 1018
cord, studies using, 962-963
extravasation of, into myometrium with premature separation of placenta, 791-792
fetal, sampling of, 491
hyperviscosity of, in infants of diabetic mother, 861
maternal, biochemical monitoring of, summary of, 283
in placental lakes, 214-215
Blood cells, red; *see* Red blood cells
Blood clot
chemical irritation from, 66
Blood clot—cont'd
menstrual, 87
Blood constituents, changes in, during pregnancy, 232, 233
Blood count, complete, and differential, 160
Blood flow
fetal, 216
during pregnancy, regional increases in, 230
renal, functional alterations in, during pregnancy, 316
uterine, during pregnancy, 225
Blood glucose, monitoring of, with diabetes mellitus during pregnancy, 850
Blood lipids, biochemical tests for, 329
Blood pressure
arterial, changes in, during pregnancy, 232, 233
after delivery, 452, 689
assessment of, 691
in neonate, 555, 557, 580
evaluative criteria for, 647
in postpartum period, evaluative criteria for, 698
in shock, 801
venous, changes in, during pregnancy, 233
Blood serum phenylalanine tests for phenylketonuria, 1028
Blood specimens, collection of, from neonate, 645
Blood sugar, fasting, 848, 849
Blood supply
to breast, 74
to ovaries, 68
of pelvis, 67
of perineum, 67
uterine, 66, 67
to vagina, 68
Blood transfusion, maternal sensitization to Rh factor after, 961, 962
Blood typing of mother, 962
Blood volume
and constituents during pregnancy, nutrition and, 315-316
after delivery, 687
increased, during pregnancy, 230
of neonate, 557
Blood volume expanders for pregnancy-induced hypertension, 817
Blood-clotting factors, 797
Blood-forming nutrients, tests to measure, 327
Blood-patch, epidural, of post-spinal-puncture headache, 905
Bloody "show," 309, 388
in first stage of labor, 397
during second stage of labor, 421
BMR; *see* Basal metabolic rate
BNBAS; *see* Brazelton Neonatal Behavioral Assessment Scale
Body
Barr, 149, 151
of clitoris, 54, 55
of infant, delivery of, 420
perineal, 57, 59
polar, 145, 207
of sperm, 207
double, 81
Body fluids of neonate, composition of, 559
Body image, 31
adolescent's, 106
and pregnancy, 255-256, 300
Body segment of neonate, assessment of, 584-593
Body systems, deviation of, during pregnancy, 9
Body temperature, basal elevation of, as presumptive sign of pregnancy, 272
Body warmth and parent-child attachment, 710
Body water
of infant, 655
total, during pregnancy, 316
changes in, 233
Bone
breast, lower border of, 69
of fetal skull, 363
hip, 70

Bone—cont'd
innominate, 70
pubic, 58, 70
Bony pelvis, 70-71
anatomy of, 69-71
assessment of, 370-373
measurement of, methods of taking, 371
relaxation of joints and ligaments of, 274
Bookmarks, 1011
Booth Maternity Center, ACNM-approved basic education in, 1013
Border, costal, 69
Borning Bed, 533-534
Borning 800 birth chair/childbearing bed, 437, 438
Borning room, 2
Boston Women's Health Book Collective, Inc., 1007
Bottle
"propping," 672
sterilizing of, 672
supplemental, 666
Bottle feeding
vs. breast feeding, 261
guide for, 673
problems with, avoiding, 673
techniques for, 672-673
Bottle-fed infant, stools of, 673
Bougie, insertion of, to induce labor, 890
Bowel movement
after delivery, 689, 693
in high-risk neonate, 751-761
of neonate, 572
assessment of, 612
evaluative criteria for, 647, 648
parental guidance concerning, 629
in postpartum period, 702
Bowel sounds in neonate, 560
Brachial nodes, 74
Brachial paralysis from delivery, 907-908
Bradley, R., 346
Bradley method, 348
classes in, 299
Bradycardia
after delivery, 689
fetal, 402-403, 480, 481
Brain
fetal development of, 218
growth of, 563
Brassieres, maternity, 299
Braun von Fernwald's sign, 272, 274
Braxton Hicks contractions, 214, 225
treatment of, 307
Braxton Hicks' sign, 275
Brazelton, T. B., on behavioral responses of neonates, 567
Brazelton Neonatal Behavioral Assessment Scale, 602-610, 1039-1044
Breach of duty, 40
Breast(s), 71-76
anatomy of, 72-74
assessment of, after delivery, 693
blood flow to, during pregnancy, 230
blood supply to, 74
carcinomas of, complicating pregnancy, 989
care of, 667
during pregnancy, 228
changes in
and breast feeding, 657-658, 659
during pregnancy, 228
as presumptive sign of pregnancy, 273
prevention and treatment of, 306
in response to sexual stimulation, 94
cross section of, 73
development and growth of, 74-76
effects of estrogen and progesterone on, 89
engorged, 667
examination of, positions of client for, 694
infection of, 833
treatment of, 668
leaking from, 668
Breast(s)—cont'd
location of, 71, 73
lymphatics of, 74
menstrual changes and, 76
neoplasms of, and oral contraceptives, 194
nodules in, and menstrual cycle, 76
physiology of, 74-76
in postpartum period, evaluative criteria for, 698
removing infant from, 665
sensitivity of, as presumptive symptom of pregnancy, 269
structure of, 72, 73
support for, 74
swelling of, in neonate, 567
tenderness of, coital position and, 309
Breast abscess, 668
Breast bone, lower border of, 69
Breast cup for inverted or retracted nipples, 300
Breast feeding, 5, 657-667
advantages of, over formula feeding, 657
vs. bottle feeding, 261
by diabetic women, 853
duration of, 666
maternal nutritional needs while, 660, 661
oral contraceptives and, 660
percentage of infants involved in, 658
preparation for, 662-663
problems with, avoiding, 667-671
questions about, 300-301
sexual stimulation from, 704
technique for, 663-666
of twins, 934
by women with heart disease, 870
Breast milk, 300-301
drugs in, and effect on infant, 1029-1037
pollutants in, 301
supplements for infant receiving, 656
Breast milk jaundice, 562
Breast pumps, 670, 671
Breast-feeding infant, failure to thrive in, 668-669
Breast-feeding mother, counseling of, 662-667
Breath
first, 558
panting, 349
to control urge to push, 382
shortness of
and oral contraceptives, 193
during pregnancy, 305
Breath sounds of neonate, 558
Breathing
abdominal, for relaxation, 351
while bearing-down, 421
in Dick-Read method, 347
expulsion, 349-350
in Lamaze method, 347
in neonate, 558
abnormal, 442
while pushing, 349-350
reflex, 558
during transition, 348-349
Breathing capacity, maximal, during pregnancy, 234
Breathing techniques during labor and delivery, 348-350
Breech delivery, 876
Breech position, labor in, 878
Breech presentation, 367, 369, 371
complete, 368, 369, 876
emergency birth of fetus in, 449
frank, 367, 368, 369, 876
fetal heart rate in, 384
footling, 367, 369
by hydrocephalic child, 975
incomplete, 368, 876
and prolonged labor, 876-878
Briefs—Footnotes on Maternity Care, 1011
Brightening response of neonate, 606
Brim, pelvic, 70, 371
Brittle diabetes, 850
Broad ligament, 60, 65
mesovarian portion of, 68
Bromides
and breast feeding, 663
effect of, on fetus or neonate, 1024
Bromocriptine mesylate to suppress lactation, 705
Bromo-Seltzer; *see* Sodium bromide
Brompheniramine in breast milk, 1032
Bronchial asthma complicating pregnancy, 985-986
Bronchopulmonary dysplasia from oxygen therapy, 636, 926
Bronze baby syndrome, 643
Brow presentation, 369
molding in, 365
Brown fat of neonate, 566
Brudzinski's sign, 601
Bruises on neonate, 564
assessment for, 612
Bruit, uterine, 225
as probable sign of pregnancy, 274
Bubble test, 282
Buds, mammary, 76
Bulb
of urethra, 77, 78
vestibular, 56, 59
Bulbocavernosus muscle, 56, 57, 59
Bulbourethral glands, 82
duct of, 78
Bulbous urethra, 78
Bulging of fontanels, 611-612
Bulk-forming laxatives in breast milk, 1033
Bupivacaine hydrochloride for regional anesthesia, 511
Burp, 601
Burping
of bottle-fed infant, 672
of infant, 665, 666
"Burping" position for neonate, 618
Busulfan, effect of, on fetus or neonate, 1023
Butazolidin; *see* Phenylbutazone
Buttocks of neonate, bruising and swelling of, 612

C

Cafergot; *see* Ergot
Caffeine, 215
in breast milk, 662, 1037
Calcium
in human milk, 661
for infant, 656-657
needs for, during pregnancy, 321-322
supplementation of, during pregnancy, 322
Calcium gluconate
as antidote to magnesium sulfate, 819, 911
in exhange transfusion for hyperbilirubinemia, 964
to prevent convulsions of eclampsia, 822
Calendar method of contraception, 188-189
Calluses, sucking, 560, 612
Calomel in breast milk, 1033
Calories for infant, 654
Cambodian women
labor and delivery in, 120
postpartal behavior of, 121
Camper's fascia, 58
Canadian Nurse, 1011
Canal
alimentary, functional alterations in, during pregnancy, 316
cervical, 65
endocervical, 60, 63, 65
uterine, 65
vaginal, examination of, after delivery, 452
Canal system of testes, 81-82
Canalicular period of fetal lung development, 217
Cancer
and circumcision, 625
ovarian, and oral contraceptives, 192
Cancer chemotherapeutic agents, effects of, on fetus or neonate, 1023

Candida albicans
causing neonatal sepsis, 837
causing oral thrush, 842
causing vaginitis, 834
Candidiasis, oral, 612
Cannabis; see Marijuana
Cannula, Rubin's, 177
Cantil; *see* Mepenzolate bromide
Cap
acrosome, 207
cervical, for contraception, 199
Capacitation of sperm, 81, 178, 206
Caput succedaneum in neonate, 433, 563, 564, 906
Carbamazepine in breast milk, 1031
Carbenicillin in breast milk, 1030
Carbimazole in breast milk, 1035, 1037
Carbocaine; *see* Mepivacaine hydrochloride
Carbohydrates for infants, 655
Carbon monoxide, 215
effect of, on fetus or neonate, 1024
Carcinoma
of breast complicating pregnancy, 989
of cervix, elective abortion in, 990
endometrial, and oral contraceptives, 192
hepatocellular, and oral contraceptives, 194
Cardiac decompensation, 869-870
symptoms of, 867
Cardiac massage, external, 635-636
Cardiac output
changes in, during pregnancy, 230, 231, 233
fetal, 217
Cardinal ligament, 59, 60, 62, 65-66
Cardiopulmonary resuscitation, 635-636
classes on, 629-630
Cardiorespiratory determinations, values for, in neonate, 1027
Cardiovascular agents, effect of, on fetus or neonate, 1023
Cardiovascular determinations, standard values for, pregnant and nonpregnant, 1019
Cardiovascular disease, hypertensive, 823-824
Cardiovascular drugs in breast milk, 1032-1033
Cardiovascular system
congenital anomalies of, screening for, 967-970
discomforts of pregnancy related to, 304-305
embryonic development of, 216-217
of neonate, 555-557
assessment of, 611
during pregnancy, 228-233
Carditis, rheumatic, and pregnancy, 867
Care
child, 717-718
continuity of, and childbearing, 9
contract for, establishing, 36
family-centered, 3, 531-532
and parent-child attachment, 711
health, consumers of, as change agents, 5
of infant
after cesarean delivery, 901-902
cultural differences in, 123-124
at risk, 747-763
maternity; *see* Maternity care; Maternity nursing
of neonate
general, 616-625
planning, implementing, and evaluating, 615-649
in postpartum period, 695, 701
nursing; *see* Maternity nursing; Nursing care
of parents after birth of child with disorder, psychosocial role of nurse in, 767-769
perineal, in postpartum period, 701
postpartal, cultural differences in, 120-122
during pregnancy, protocols for, 9
prenatal
cultural views of, 116-119
delay in, 12
early, 112
psychosocial, maternal and family need for, 283-284
request for, by client, 18
standards of, 40
Care taking, sibling, 116
Career pattern and adolescent, 107, 108
Caretakers, community, as support system, 138
Carisoprodol in breast milk, 1032
Carpal tunnel syndrome, 240
treatment of, 306
Caruncles, hymenal, 56, 687
Carunculae myrtiformes, 56
Cascara in breast milk, 1033
Catecholamines causing increased uterine activity, 490
Categorization of data, 20
Cathartics in breast milk, 663, 1033
Catheter(s)
DeLee mucous-trap, suctioning with, 633, 634
French, size equivalents for, 1016
intermittent or indwelling, for feeding, 755-756
internal, checklist for, 495
intrauterine, to monitor uterine activity, 471, 476, 477, 478-479, 490
nasopharyngeal, with mechanical suction apparatus, 633
suction (vacuum), 993
sictioning with, 632-633
Catheterization
after delivery, 456, 702
during labor, 410-411
umbilical, for hyperbilirubinemia, 966
Catholic Church and contraception, 124
Cathomycin; *see* Novobiocin
Caudal anesthesia, 524
care after, 703
Caudal block, 516
Caudal regression syndrome, 861
Caudal tray, 524
Caution and daring in child, balance of, 136
Cavernous venous plexus, 56
Cavity
intrauterine, 212
pelvic, 371, 374
female and male, contrast of, 72
uterine, manual examination of, after delivery, 452
CCES; *see* Council of Childbirth Education Specialists, Inc.
Cedilanid-D; *see* Deslanoside
Cefazolin in breast milk, 1030
Cell(s)
exfoliated, fetal lipid-containing, staining of, and gestational age, 282
germ, 143-144
glandular, endocervical, effects of estrogens and progesterone on, 89
immune, in human milk, 662
interstitial, of testes, 80
Leydig's, 80
red blood; *see* Red blood cells
Sertoli's, 80
sex, 206
smooth muscle, of uterus, growth of, during pregnancy, 223
somatic, 142-143; *see also* Chromosome(s)
squamous, fetal, in amniotic fluid, 401
of stomach, 560
Cell division in chromosomes, 142, 143-145
disorders of, 148-149
Cellular dysplasia, smear to detect, 160
Center for Family Growth, 1007
Centers
Alternative Birth, 532, 534-536
high-risk factors excluding admission to, 536, 538
birth, freestanding, 538-541
Centimeters, conversion of, to inches, 1016
Central axillary nodes, 74
Central nervous system
effects of estrogen and progesterone on, 89
injuries of, to neonate during delivery, 909
maturity of
and behavior of neonate, 610
and initial oral feeding, 677
Central placenta previa, 793
Central tendon of perineum, 58
Central venous pressure in shock, 801, 802
Cephalexin
in breast milk, 1030
effect of, on glucose determination, 1021
Cephalhematoma in neonate, 563-564, 906
for vacuum extractor, 892
Cephalic presentation, 367
Cephalic prominence, palpation of, 383
Cephalic version, external, to convert breech presentation, 877
Cephalocaudal assessment, 19
Cephalocaudal malformations and hydramnios, 967
Cephalopelvic disproportion as indication for cesarean delivery, 893
Cephaloridine, effect of
on fetus or neonate, 1022
on glucose determinations, 1021
Cephalosporin for mastitis, 833
Cephalothin
in breast milk, 1030
effect of, on glucose determinations, 1021
Cereal, introduction of, 673
Cerebral palsy, choreoathetoid, 959, 962
Cerebrospinal fluid values for neonate, 1027
Certification
of neonatal nurse clinician/practitioner, 13
of nurse-midwife, 13-14
of obstetric-gynecologic nurse practitioner, 13
Certified nurse-midwife, 6, 14, 541
Cervical branch of uterine artery, 67
Cervical canal, 65
sperm migration through, 170
Cervical cap for contraception, 199
Cervical mucus, 65
alkalinity of, 179-180
assessment of, 166, 169, 171-172
changes in, 88
during menstrual cycle, 190
characteristics of, 169
fern patterns of, 169
and sperm, 81, 180
sperm passage through, 169
Cervical mucus method of contraception, 190
Cervical os; *see also* Cervix
abnormalities of, 180
external, 60, 63, 65
internal, 60, 63
incompetent, 63
nonparous, 272
parous, 272
stretching of, 66
Cervical-vaginal factors in female fertility, 179-180
Cervicitis, 180
Cervix, 61, 63-65
abnormalities of, and fertility, 180
canals of, 65
carcinoma of, elective abortion in, 990
cautery of, 180
changes in
during labor, 379
during menstrual cycle, 88, 159, 161
during pregnancy, 226, 227
"cock's comb," 981
color of, 65
columnar epithelium of, 64, 65
conization of, 180
cryosurgery of, 180
after delivery, 687
dilatation of, 385, 386, 387
and descent during first stage of labor, 398, 399
assessment sheet for, 400
edema of
from bearing down, 382
and dystocia, 875
effacement of, 385, 386
elasticity of, 65
function of, 179-180
incompetent, 63, 781

Cervix—cont'd
infections, 180
lacerations of, examination for, after delivery, 452
manipulation of, vagal response to, 196
nonparous, 63
packing of, to induce labor, 890
parous, 63
in postpartum period, evaluative criteria for, 698
softening of, 226
squamous epithelium of, 64, 65
supravaginal portion of, 60
tears in, after delivery, 449
Cesarean Birth Council, 1007
Cesarean delivery, 893-895
alternatives available for, 541-542
antacid before, 987
anesthesia level for, 515
for breech presentation, 877
care after, 901, 904-905
care of neonate after, 901, 902
combination anesthesia for, 524
for dystocia, 886
family-centered, 541-542
fetal indications for, 893
goal of, 893
incidence of vaginal delivery following, 746
maternal indications for, 893
maternal mortality for, 746
for mother with herpes simplex virus, 402
number of, 893
nursing care for, 895-905
patient instructions after, 905
for placenta previa, 794, 796
postmortem, 895
preparation for, 899-901
in prenatal period, 896-899
procedures for, 893-895
prognosis after, 895
for prolapsed cord, 407
psychologic reactions to, 895-896
vaginal delivery following, 895, 898-899
vascular changes after, 687
Cesarean hysterectomy, 895
Cesarean/Support, Education, and Concern (C/SEC), 1007
Cetyltrimethyl ammonium bromide test, 1027
Chadwick's sign, 226, 227, 273
Chairs, birthing, 437, 438, 439
Channing L. Bete Co., Inc., 1007
Charting, 41
checklist for, 495
and fetal monitoring, 493, 494
Chemical agents, fetotoxic, human, 1022-1024
Chemical irritation of peritoneal surfaces, 66
Chemical vaginitis from spermicide, 199
Chemocautery, radial, of cervix, 180
Chemotherapeutic agents, cancer, effects of, on fetus or neonate, 1023
Chemotherapy after hydatidiform mole, 788-789
Chest of neonate, assessment of, 588
Chest breathing, slow, 348, 349
Chest circumference of neonate, 558, 580
measuring, 579, 580
Chest pain and oral contraceptives, 193
Chicago Maternity Center, 542
Chickenpox during pregnancy, 828
Chief cells of stomach, 560
Child(ren); *see also* Infant; Neonate
abuse of, 710
and premature infant, 928-929
active immunization of, recommended schedules for, 1038
anxiety over, 258
with disorder
birth of, care of parents after, 767-769
clinical evaluation and diagnosis of causes of, 768
immediate diagnosis and management of, 768
long-term management of, 768
importance of, among various cultures, 116
Child(ren)—cont'd
male, preference for, cultural views of, 123
naming of, 260
at nutritional risk, 679-681
older, caring for younger siblings, 116
parent attachment to; *see* Parent-child attachment
perfect, mourning loss of, 767-768
response of, to birth of sibling, 135
right of, to be "well-born," 9
sex of, preference for, 260-261
view of, in American family, 122
young, "loss" of mother for, 135
Child care
for infant, 717-718
in postpartum period, evaluative criteria for, 699
Child Study Association of America, 1007
Child Welfare League of America, Inc., 1007
Childbearing; *see also* Childbirth
adverse reactions to, stresses causing, 284
concepts regarding, and culture, 114
continuity of care and, 9
family-centered, 8-9
as normal physiologic function, 8
rational, decisions about, 110
sexual dysfunction after, 112
Child-bearing Center of Maternity Center Association, 538, 540
Childbearing family, goals for, 17
Childbearing psychosis, 950-951
"Childbed fever"; *see* Puerperal infection
Childbirth; *see also* Childbearing
alternative settings for, 529-549
education for, 299
without fear, 347
pain in, 352-353
preparation for, 344-352
prepared
and fetal monitoring, 492-493
movement for, 531
Childbirth education classes, 341-357
cesarean delivery information as part of, 896-898
Childbirth exercises, 350-352
Childbirth practices throughout history, 2-3
Childbirth Without Fear, 345
Childbirth Without Pain Education Association, 1008
Childbirth Without Pain Education League, Inc., 346
Childhood
development of identity in, 102-105
preparation for parenthood during, 116
sexual development in, 104
Child-parent relationships, 446-447; see also Parent-child attachment
Children's Bureau, 1010
Chilling after delivery, 457
Chin presentation, 369, 371
Chinese food pattern, 330
Chinese women
labor and delivery of, 119
postpartal behavior of, 121
postpartal care of, 120, 121
Chinese-American women, pregnancy diet for, 117, 118
Chlamydia trachomatis infection, 828
in neonate, 841
smears to detect, 160
Chlamydial disease in neonate, 841
Chloasma, 238, 271, 273, 987
Chloral hydrate
in breast milk, 1031
effect of, on glucose determination, 1021
Chloramphenicol
in breast milk, 663, 1030
effect of
on fetus or neonate, 1022
on glucose determination, 1021
Chlordiazepoxide
in breast milk, 1036
for epilepsy, 988
to prevent convulsions of eclampsia, 822
Chloromycetin; *see* Chloramphenicol
Chloropyramine, effect of, on fetus or neonate, 1024
Chloroquine
in breast milk, 1030
effect of, on fetus or neonate, 1022
Chlorothiazide, effect of, on fetus or neonate, 1023
Chlorotrianisene in breast milk, 1034
Chlorpromazine
in breast milk, 1036
and neonatal platelets, 558
for schizophrenia, 951
Chlorpropamide, 846
effect of, on fetus or neonate, 1024
Choanal atresia, 677, 967
Choice, informed, in alternative settings for childbirth, 531
Choking, treatment of, 616
Cholecystectomy, 987
Cholecystitis complicating pregnancy, 987
Cholelithiasis complicating pregnancy, 987
Cholelithotomy, 987
Cholesterol for infants, 655, 676
Cholinesterase inhibitors, effect of, on fetus or neonate, 1023
Choosing and values clarification, 32
Chordee and infertility, 181
therapy for, 182
Choreoathetoid cerebral palsy, 959, 962
Chorioamnionitis
antibiotic therapy for, 402
after rupture of membranes, 402
Choriocarcinoma, 788-789
Chorion
and amnion, fusion of, and placenta, 214
development of, 212
Chorion frondosum, 212
Chorionic gonadotropic hormone, 211
Chorionic somatomammotropin, human
and insulin resistance, 845
and lactation, 228
and sodium balance, 236
Chorionic villi, 211, 212
Christmas disease, 800
Chromatin, sex, 149, 151
Chromatography, amino acid, 1027
Chromosomal aberrations, 147-150
disorders caused by, 142, 149
Chromosome(s), 141-143
cell division of, 142, 143-145
definition of, 141
diploid number of, 207
genes on, 142
haploid number of, 206, 207
maldistribution of, during meiosis, 148
numbers of
abnormalities in, 147
normal, 142-143
sex, 132
aberration of, 149
abnormalities of, common, characteristics of, 151
structural defect of, 147
translocated, 148-149
X, 143, 207
inactivated, 149
nondisjunction of, 150
Y, 143, 207
Chronic systemic diseases as nutrition risk factor, 326
Cigarette smoke and placenta, 215
Cigarette smoking, effect of, on fetus or neonate, 1023
Circulation
fetal, 556
maternal, and placenta, 213-214
of newborn, timing of clamping of cord and, 557
pulmonary, changes in, at birth, 557
systemic, changes in, at birth, 557
uteroplacental and fetal, 470-471
Circulation time, changes in, during pregnancy, 233

Circulatory overload from intravenous therapy, 405
Circulatory pattern of fetus, 216
Circumcised penis
  assessment of, 612
  care of, 628
  evaluative criteria for, 647
Circumcision, 625-628
Circumstraint, positioning of infant in, 626
Citrate causing hypocalcemia, 864
Claiming process by parent, 723-724
Clamp
  cord, 440
    removal of, 621
  Yellen, circumcision with, 627
Clamping of umbilical cord, 440
  timing of, and newborn's circulation, 557
"Clap"; *see* Gonorrhea
Clarification
  in communication, 26
  values, 31-32
Classes
  after-birth, 342
  childbirth preparation, cesarean delivery information as part of, 896-898
  early pregnancy, 341
  grandparent, 356-357
  late pregnancy, 342
  midpregnancy, 342
Classic cesarean procedures, 893, 894
Classification
  of birth trauma, 906
  of dystocia, 874
  of heart disease, 868
  of preterm infant, 915
Clavicle of neonate, fracture of, during delivery, 907
Clay, eating of, during pregnancy, 118; *see also* Pica
Clean-catch urine specimen, 285
Cleanliness after delivery, maintaining, 456-457
Cleansing
  of neonate; *see* Bathing of neonate
  perineal, 430
  in postpartum period, 701
Cleavage, 210
Cleft lip, 151, 976-977
Cleft palate, 151, 976-977
  and hydramnios, 967
Client; *see also* Mother
  biographic data on, 18
  biopsychosocial status of
    assessment of, 18-19
    review of, 19
  decision making by, nurses' assistance in, 33-34
  dependency of, 36
  interview of, 18-19
  maternity, 10-12
  and maternity nurse, relationship between, 25-37
    trusting, 19
  noncompliance of, 35
  observation of, 19
  as partner in care, 297
  preconceptional, legal and ethical concepts for, 42-44
  questions asked by, 299-301
  request for care by, 18
  understanding of therapy by, 35
Client advocates, maternity nurses as, 5-6, 7, 30
Clinical nurse specialist, 6
Clinical practice, nutritional intervention in, 681-683
Clinician/practitioner, neonatal nurse, 13
Clinics, adolescent, 943
Clips for sterilization, 997
Clitoral vs. vaginal orgasm, 100
Clitoris, 52, 54, 55, 58
  artery of, 67
  crus of, 59
  response of, to sexual stimulation, 93, 94
Clomid; *see* Clomiphene citrate
Clomiphene, hydatidiform mole after use of, 787
Clomiphene citrate for anovulation, 177, 181
Clonic muscular contractions, reflex, in response to sexual stimulation, 100
Clonus response at ankle joint, 819
Closed chest massage in infant, 635-636
Closed questions, 26
Clostridia causing puerperal infection, 832
Clostridium botulinum in honey, 655
Clot(s), blood
  chemical irritation from, 66
  menstrual, 87
Clothing
  for neonate, 621-624
    care of, 624-625
  during pregnancy, 299
    cultural views of, 118
Clotrimazole for monilial vaginitis, 834
Clotting
  normal, 796-797
  problems with, 797-799
    in pregnancy, 796-800
Clove-hitch restraint for neonate, 644, 645
Clubfoot, 978
CNM; *see* Certified nurse-midwife
Coach, support for, 425
Coaching during second stage of labor, 425
Coagulation
  blood, standard values for, pregnant and nonpregnant, 1018
  intravascular, disseminated, 797-799
    and adult respiratory distress syndrome, 986
  process of, 796-797
  tendency to, during pregnancy, 232
Coagulation tests, 798
Coagulopathy, defibrination; *see* Disseminated intravascular coagulation
Coalition for the Medical Rights of Women, 1008
Coarctation of aorta, 969
Cobalamin
  need for, during pregnancy, 323
  and oral contraceptives, 194
Coccygeus muscles, 57
Coccyx, 58, 70
"Cock's comb" cervix, 981
Codeine in breast milk, 663, 1035
Cognition, 134
Cognitive development, 134-135
Coital play in childhood, 105
Coital position, variation in, during pregnancy, 308-309
Coitus
  abstention from, 162
  and adolescent, 109
  difficulties with, and male infertility, 181
    therapy for, 182
  during pregnancy, 308
  timing and frequency of, and infertility, 181
    therapy for, 182
Coitus interruptus, 199
Cold
  avoidance of, after delivery, cultural views of, 120-121
  treatment of, 629
Cold stress in neonate, 566-567
  with respiratory distress, 749
  signs of, 751
Colicky uterus, 881
Coliform bacteria
  causing puerperal infection, 832
  causing urinary tract infections, 833
Colistin in breast milk, 1030
Colitis, ulcerative, complicating pregnancy, 987
Collection
  of blood specimen from neonate, 645
  of data, 18-19
  of specimens at initial contact with pregnant woman, 291
Collectors, urine specimen, for neonate, 645-646
College of Medicine and Dentistry of New Jersey, ACNM-approved basic education in, 1013
Colles' fascia, 58, 59
Colon, changes in, during pregnancy, 241
Color of neonate, 582
Colostrum, 228, 273, 663
Columbia University Graduate Program in Maternity Nursing and Nurse-Midwifery, ACNM-approved basic education in, 1013
Columnar epithelium of cervix, 64, 65
Colymycin; *see* Colistin
Coma, hyperglycemic hyperosmolar nonketotic, differentiation of, from hypoglycemia and ketoacidosis, 851
Combination anesthesia for cesarean birth, 524
Combined oral hormone therapy for contraception, 192-195
Comfort after delivery, maintaining, 457-458
Comfort measures during labor, 411-414
Commercial formulas
  concentrated, dilution of, 671
  preparation of, 672
  soy-based, 671-672
  supplements for infant receiving, 656
  types of, 671
Commissure, anterior and posterior, 54
Common iliac artery, 67
Common law of torts, 40
Communal family, 132
Communication
  and common violations, 28-29
  in family, 133
  among health team members, importance of, 22
  nonverbal
    time as, 29
    touch as, 28
  in nurse-client relationship, 25-29
  techniques for, 26-27
Community caretakers as support system, 138
Community nutrition, guidelines for population groups in, 682
Community resources
  for child with disorder, 768
  listing of, 1007-1010
Community trends in maternity nursing, 5
Compact layer of endometrium, 87
Complement fixation tests for syphilis, 827
Complementary roles in family, 133
Complete abortion, 782, 783
Complete blood count and differential, 160
  standard values for, pregnant and nonpregnant, 1018
Complete breech presentation, 368, 369
Complete placenta previa, 793, 794
Complete transposition of great vessels, 968
Complex carbohydrates for infant, 655
Compliance with therapy, 35
Complicated labor, comparison of, with true and false labors, 396
Complications
  during birth, 873-934
  coincident with pregnancy, major, 826-871
Comprehensive physical examination, 292-293, 295-296
Compression
  cardiac, 635-636
  cord, variable deceleration caused by, 489
  of fetal head, early deceleration caused by, 488
Compromise, fetal, 280
Computed tomography to determine fetal presentation, position, and descent, 386, 388
Concentrated formulas, dilution of, 671
Conception, 206-216
  to birth, period from, 206-220
  "wrongful," 42
Concrete operational stage of adolescence, 107
Concrete operations stage of cognitive development, 135
Condition
  of infant, physical, and parental response, 720
  of mother, physical, and response to newborn, 719-720
Condom as contraceptive, 199-200
Conduction causing heat loss in neonate, 566

Conduction anesthesia, 508, 511, 513, 516
Condylomas of congenital syphilis, 839
Condylomata acuminata, 238, 987
Confidentiality, 36
Confinement, 268
expected date of, 268, 277-281
Conflict between nurses and physicians, 3
Congenital anomalies
and adolescent pregnancy, 938
assessment of perinatal signs and factors indicating, 967-970
of cardiovascular system, screening for, 967-970
in DES-exposed children, 981
of gastrointestinal tract, screening for, 970
general preoperative and postoperative care of infant with, 970-971
in infants of diabetic mother, 861
and initial oral feeding, 677
neonates with, 966-981
of neurologic system, screening for, 967
not apparent at birth, 980-981
of respiratory tract, screening for, 967
of urogenital tract, screening for, 970
of uterus, infertility from, 179
Congenital dislocated hip, 151
Congenital dysplasia of hip, 977
Congenital disorder, 142; *see also* Congenital anomalies
Congenital factors causing female infertility, 177
Congenital heart disease, 151
and hydramnios, 967
and pregnancy, 867
Congenital hydrocephalus, 975-976
Congenital malformations; *see also* Congenital anomalies
common, 975-980
in twins, 933
Congenital rubella syndrome, 838
Congenital syphilis, 839-841
Congestion, respiratory tract, during pregnancy, 233
Conization of cervix, 180
Conjugata vera, diameter of, 373
Conjugates, obstetric, diameter of, 373
Conjunctiva, neonatal treatment of, 442-445
recommendations for, 445-446
Conjunctivitis, neonatal, 841
Connecting stalk, 212
"Conscience clauses"
for abortions, 45
and sterilization, 42
Consciousness
level of
after delivery, 452
in shock, 801-802
state of, of neonate, 569
Consent, informed, 41
for anesthesia and analgesia, 501
for sterilization, 42
Consent form
English, 502
Spanish, 503
Consolability of neonate, 609
Consolidation and growth phase of nurse-client relationship, 36-37
Consolidation phase of parent-child relationship
assessment of, 724
nursing actions in, 730
Constipation
during pregnancy, 241
prevention and treatment of, 303
as presumptive symptom of pregnancy, 270
Consumer movement, 4
Consumer Product Safety Commission, 1010
Consumerism and alternative childbirth settings, 531
Consumers
as change agents in maternity care, 5
role of, 10
Contact, eye
as communication, 29
in parent-child attachment, 709-711
Contact lenses and oral contraceptives, 195
"Contaminants" in human milk, 662
Continuous insulin infusion, 850-851
Continuous positive airway pressure for neonate with respiratory distress, 749, 750
Contraception, 186
cultural views on, 124-125
after delivery, 704, 717
for diabetic women, 853
effectiveness of, 187
male, 199-201
myths about, 11
in postpartum period, 704, 717
religion and, 124
sterilization as means of, 996-1000
use of, counseling on, nursing action in, 201-203
Contraceptive methods and future fertility, 162
Contraceptive services, 11
Contraceptives
48-hour, 199
oral; *see* Oral contraceptives
2-day, 199
Contract for care, establishing, 36
Contractility, uterine, 225
Contraction(s)
Braxton Hicks, 214, 225
treatment of, 307
in first stage of labor, character of, 395, 397
muscular, clonic, reflex, in response to sexual stimulation, 100
pelvic, 874
during second stage of labor, 418
amnesia between, 425
uterine; *see* Uterine contractions
Contraction stress testing, 5
Contracture
midpelvis, 875
pelvic, 874
of pelvic inlet, 875
pelvic outlet, 875
Conus medullaris of spinal cord, 512
Convection causing heat loss in neonate, 566
Conventional x-ray films to determine fetal presentation, position, and descent, 386
Conversion tables and equivalents, 1015-1018
Convulsions
in eclampsia, 815
prevention and control of, 815, 819-820
emergency care of, 821-822
Cooley's anemia, 984
Coombs' test, 962-963
Cooperative Birth Center Network, 1008
Cooper's ligaments, 74
Coping activities of father during pregnancy, 262-263
Coping mechanisms, 138
of parents, 716-717
Copper in breast milk, 1034
Copper-7 IUD, 197
Copper-T IUD, 197
Cord
nuchal, 471
spermatic, 81
spinal, injuries to, in neonate during birth, 909
umbilical; *see* Umbilical cord
Cord clamp, 440
removal of, 621
Corometrics fetal monitor, 469
Corometrics spiral electrode, 477
Corona radiata, 80, 207
Coronal suture of fetal skull, 363, 364
Corpus of uterus, 60-62
Corpus albicans, 69
Corpus cavernosum, 77, 78, 79
Corpus cavernosum penis, 77
Corpus hemorrhagicum, 69
Corpus luteum, 69, 86-87
changes in, with pregnancy, 246
cystic, of pregnancy, 989
degeneration of, 88
physiology of, during pregnancy, 223
Corpus spongiosum, 77, 78
Cortex, adrenal
fetal, 219
during pregnancy, 247
Corticosteroids
effect of, on fetus or neonate, 1023
for idiopathic thrombocytopenic purpura, 800
Corticotropin in breast milk, 1035
Cortisol
fetal production of, 219
and insulin production, 247
and insulin resistance, 845
and sodium balance, 236
Cortisone
in breast milk, 1035
for disseminated lupus erythematosus, 988
for Sheehan's syndrome, 807
Corynebacterium vaginale vaginitis during pregnancy, 828
Costal border, 69
Cotyledons of placenta, 213, 214
Coumarin derivatives in breast milk, 1031
Coumarins, effect of, on fetus or neonate, 1022
Council of Childbirth Education Specialists, Inc., 346, 357, 1008
Counseling, 155
abortion, 112
of breast-feeding mother, 662-667
on contraceptive use, nursing action in, 201-203
for emotional tension, 298
genetic, 42, 155-156
nutrition, 299, 331, 335-336
pregnancy protocol for, 339
on oral contraceptive use, 195
of pregnant adolescent, 943
sexual, 42
during pregnancy, 302, 308-309
on sterilization methods, 1000
about therapeutic abortion, 996
Counseling services, 155
Counselors, maternity nurses as, 6, 12
Count
daily fetal movement, 498
platelet, 798
white cell, during pregnancy, 232
Counterpressure on sacrum during contraction, 414
Couple, infertile, nursing care of, 183-184
"Couple nursing," 695
Court cases involving abortions, 45
Couvade, 258
Couvelaire uterus, 789, 791, 792
Cowper's glands, 77-78
changes in, in response to sexual stimulation, 93, 96
and formation of semen, 82
Cow's milk, nutrient content of, 662
Coxsackie B virus during pregnancy, 828
CPAP; *see* Continuous positive airway pressure
CPD; *see* Cephalopelvic disproportion
Cradle cap, 620
Cradling hold for neonate, 619
Cramping during ovulatory periods, 89
Cramps
leg, during pregnancy, 305
muscle, during pregnancy, 240
Cranial vault, external, of fetal head, 363
Cravings, food, during pregnancy
cultural views of, 118
treatment of, 303
Crawford needle, 517
Crawling reflex, 601
Creases
of neonate, cleansing of, 620
palm, to detect genetic disorders, 154
sole, of neonate, 917
Creatinine, values of, and gestational age, 282
Creative drive of father during pregnancy, 262
Cremaster muscle, 78
Crest
iliac, 69-70
neural, 218
pubic, 69

Cribriform hymen, 57
Cri-du-chat syndrome, 142, 147, 149, 150
Crisis, 136
  after birth of child with disorder, 767-769
  family and, 136-138
Crisis intervention, 136-138
Critical periods in human development, 208
Crossed extension reflex, 598, 599
Crus of clitoris, 59
Crying behavior of neonate, 569, 571
Cryoprecipitate for disseminated intravascular coagulation, 799
Cryosurgery of cervix, 180
Cryptorchidism, 79
  and fertility, 161
  and male infertility, 181
CT; *see* Computed tomography
Cu 200 IUD, 197
Cubans, view of menstruation of, 124
Cuddliness, infant's response to, 606-607, 608
Cul-de-sac of Douglas, 66
  posterior, 61
Culdocentesis, 66
Culdotomy, 66
Cullen's sign, 785
Cultural aspects of maternity nursing, 114-126
Cultural connotation of space, 27
Cultural food patterns, 329-331, 335
Cultural knowledge, 115
Cultural relativism, 115
  attitude of, by nurse, 125
Cultural views of prenatal care, 116-119
Culturally determined rhythms of speech in infant, 710
Culture
  childbearing concepts and, 114
  and communication patterns, 26
  definition of, 115
  eye contact and, 29
  and father's involvement during labor and delivery, 415
  gonorrheal, 287
  for herpes simplex, types 1 and 2, 287
  influencing behavior of newborn, 610
  languages of, 27
  and postpartum care, 692
  reproduction in, 115-116
  role expectations and, 30
  subgroups of, 27
  and time, 29
  touch and, 28
  use of space and, 27
Cumulus, 80
Cunnilingus during pregnancy, 308
Cup, breast, for inverted or retracted nipple, 300
Curare, effect of, on fetus or neonate, 1024
Curative activities of maternity nursing, 9-10
Curettage
  dilatation and; *see* Dilatation and curettage
  vacuum (suction) for therapeutic abortion, 991, 992, 993, 994
Custom and cultural differences, 125
Cuyahoga County Hospital, ACNM-approved basic education in, 1013
CWPL; *see* Childbirth Without Pain Education League, Inc.
Cyanosis
  "mitten and bootie," 611
  in neonate, 611, 906
  treatment of, 636
  of vagina as presumptive sign of pregnancy, 273
Cyanotic heart disease, 967, 968-969
Cybele Society, 1008
Cyclic fluctuations in fetal heart rate, 480
Cyclic trends in behavior of child, 135
Cyclophosphamide
  in breast milk, 1037
  effect of, on fetus or neonate, 1023
Cystic corpus luteum of pregnancy, 989
Cystic fibrosis, 142, 146
  and meconium ileus, 155
Cystic glandular hyperplasia, infertility after, 179
Cysts
  ovarian
    and oral contraceptives, 192
    during pregnancy, 989
  retention, of neonate, 560
Cytologic enzymes of trophoblast, 210
Cytologic studies to detect genetic disorders, 154
Cytomegalic viral inclusion disease, 563, 976
Cytomegalovirus
  causing neonatal sepsis, 837
  during pregnancy, 828
Cytomegalovirus infection in neonate, 841
Cytomel; *see* Liothyronine
Cytoplasm of ovum, 207
Cytoplasmic membrane around sperm, 80
Cytoplasmic sheath of sperm, 207

D

D and C; *see* Dilatation and curettage
D and E; *see* Dilatation and evacuation
D^u test, 695
Daily fetal movement count, 498
Daily food guide, 331, 332, 335
Danazol for endometriosis, 179
Danger signals for pregnant woman, 298
Danish food pattern, 331
Daraprim; *see* Pyrimethamine
Daring and caution in child, balance of, 136
Darvon; *see* Propoxyphene
Data
  categorizing, 20
  collection of, 18-19
  objective, in problem-oriented record, 23
  recording, 22-24
  subjective, in problem-oriented record, 23
Data base, 23
Data-recording system for amniocentesis, 290
Datril; *see* Acetaminophen
Day 1 of endometrial cycle, 87
Day-care centers, 717-718
Daydreams of fatherhood, 261
DDE in breast milk, 1034
DDT in breast milk, 1034
Deaf mother, response of, to infant, 723
Death
  fetal, 46, 746
    definition of, 762
    and estriol levels, 282
    nursing care of parents experiencing, 774-775
    psychologic aspects of, 774
  of infant, reaction of siblings to, 778
  maternal, 11
  neonatal, 746
Death certificate, 104-106
  filing, legal requirements for, 763
Death rate
  infant, 746
  maternal, 186-187
  perinatal, 746
Deceleration phase of cervical dilatation, 398
Decelerations in fetal heart rate
  early, 485, 486, 488
  late, 486, 487, 489
  prolonged, 485
  variable, 487, 488, 489
Decidua, 211
Decidua basalis, 211, 212
  placentation on, 806
Decidua capsularis, 211, 212
Decidua parietalis, 211
Decidua vera, 211, 212
Decidual stage of spontaneous abortion, 782
Decision making
  accountability and, 34
  by client, nurses' assistance in, 33-34
  in family, 133
  and values, 31-33
Decision-making process, 33-34
Declomycin; *see* Demeclocycline
Decompensation, cardiac, 869-870
  symptoms of, 867
Decreased variability in fetal heart rate, 482-483
Deep tendon reflexes, 601
  assessment of, 819, 820
Deep transverse perineal muscle, 57, 59
Defecation; *see* Bowel movement
Defense activities of father during pregnancy, 262-263
Defense mechanism, language as, 27
Defensive movements of neonate, 608
Defibrination syndrome; *see* Disseminated intravascular coagulation
Deficiency
  folate, 983-984
  folic acid
    anemia from, 983-984
    tests to measure, 327
Deformed extremities and hydramnios, 967
Dehydration
  in infant, formulas and, 655
  in neonate, 611
DeLee mucous-trap catheter, 634
  suctioning with, 633
DeLee-Hillis maneuver, 875
DeLee-Hillis stethoscope, 468, 469
Delivery
  anterior pituitary necrosis after, 807
  of body and extremities, 420
  breech, 876
  care during, 425-439
  care of adolescent mother after, 945
  cesarean; *see* Cesarean delivery
  cleanliness after, maintaining, 456-457
  comfort after, maintaining, 457-458
  depressive state after, 715
  forceps, 890-892
  of head, 419-420
  hemorrhage after, 802-807
    prevention of, 456
  hospitalization after, duration of, 705
  infections after, legal claims in, 47
  instrument table for, 430
  labor and; *see* Labor and delivery
  lateral Sims' position for, 448
  lithotomy position for, culture and, 119-120
  manic-depressive reactions after, 950-951
  maternal hemorrhage after, 449
  maternal position following, 454-456
  maternal position for, 430-431
  mechanism of, 419-420
  of placenta, 450-451
    pharmacologic stimulation of, uterine contractions after, 452-453
  position for, cultural views of, 120
  of preeclamptic woman, 820, 822-823
  premature, reactions to, 769-770
  preparation for, 416-417
  of preterm infant, psychologic aspects of, 928-929
  return visit after, 705
  of shoulders, 420
  side-lying position for, 890
  uterine contractions after, 688
  vaginal, anesthesia level for, 515
Delivery date, determination of, for diabetic pregnant woman, 852
Delivery pack, 424
Delivery room, equipment in, 422-424
Delivery table, 422-424, 425
  transfer to, from labor bed, 425
Delta optical density analysis, 962, 963
Demand feeding of infant, 5
Demeclocycline in breast milk, 1030
Demerol; *see* Meperidine
Dental problems during pregnancy, 301
Deoxyribonucleic acid, 141
Dependence
  drug
    narcotic, and pregnancy, 953-956
    and pregnancy, 951-956

Dependence—cont'd
vs. independence and pregnant woman, 256-257
Dependent behavior by mother, 36, 713-714
Depo-Provera; *see* Medroxyprogesterone acetate
Depressive state after delivery, 715, 950-951
Dermal rash in congenital syphilis, 839
Dermatitis
atopic, 238, 987
"fleabite," 565
herpetiform, 238, 987
seborrheic, 238, 987
Dermatoglyphics to detect genetic disorders, 154
Dermatologic problems, pregnancy-induced, 987
DES; *see* Diethylstilbestrol
"DES daughter," 51, 981
"DES sons," 981
Descent
through birth canal, 378
cervical dilatation and, during first stage of labor, 398, 399
assessment sheet for, 400
in labor in vertex presentation, 388-389
of presenting part during second stage of labor, 421
Desipramine hydrochloride in breast milk, 1036
Deslanoside for cardiac decompensation, 870
Despair vs. ego integrity in personality development, 136
Desquamation of skin of neonate, 564
Developing awareness phase of grieving, 766
Development
cognitive, 134-135
critical periods in, 208
embryonic, and fetal maturation, 216-220
infant, and relationship to feeding, 651-652
neuromuscular, and feeding behavior, 651, 653
personality, 134, 135-136
physiologic, and feeding behavior, 651
prenatal, timetable for, 209-210
psychosocial
within family, 133-136
and feeding behavior, 652, 653
sexual
adult, 109-112
childhood, 104
stages of, 91
Developmental factors causing female infertility, 177
Developmental stages in prenatal growth, 207-208
Developmental tasks of adolescent, 939-940
of parenthood, 942-943
during pregnancy, 940-942
DFMC; *see* Daily fetal movement count
Diabetes
brittle, 850
gestational, 280, 844
overt, 844
secondary, 844
Diabetes mellitus, 142, 844-863
definition of, 844
effects of
on embryo-fetus-neonate, 853, 859-863
on pregnancy, 846-847
estriol levels and, 282
gestational, 845-846
insulin-dependent, 846
juvenile, 151
and oral contraceptives, 193, 194
in pregnancy, 844-863
classification of, 845
diagnosis of, 848-850
incidence of, 844
management of, 848-853
pathogenesis of, 844-845
prognosis for, 847-848
significance of, 844
tests to diagnose, 848-850
tests for, 329
type I, 844
type II, 844
Diabetic mother, 859-863; *see also* Diabetes mellitus
infants of, 219, 280, 859-863
and hydramnios, 967
Diabetic woman, teaching of, 856-859
Diabinese; *see* Chlorpropamide
Diagnosis
nursing
formulating, 20-21
validation of, 21
of pregnancy, 269-281
prenatal, legal aspects of, 43-44
Diagnostic materials and procedures affecting breast milk, 1033
Diagnostic tests for phenylketonuria, 1028
Diagonal conjugate, diameter of, 373
Diameter, biparietal, and fetal weight, correlation of, 297
Diamox; *see* Acetazolamide
Diaper rash, 612, 621
Diaper test for phenylketonuria, 1028
Diapering of neonate, 623-624, 625
Diaphoresis after delivery, 692
Diaphragm
changes in, during pregnancy, 234
pelvic, 56-57
with spermicide for contraception, 198
urogenital, 56, 57, 61
muscles and fascia of, 58
Diaphragmatic hernia, 970, 971
Diaphragmatic paralysis in neonate, 908
Diary, food, for infants, 681
Diastasis of recti abdominis, 69
Diazepam
for analgesia, 523
in breast milk, 663, 1036
causing decreased variability in fetal heart rate, 483
effect of, on fetus or neonate, 1024
for epilepsy, 988
and oral contraceptives, 195
for pregnancy-induced hypertension, 816
to prevent convulsions of eclampsia, 822
Diazoxide
in breast milk, 1032
effect of, on fetus or neonate, 1023
Dibenzyline in breast milk, 1032
DIC; *see* Disseminated intravascular coagulation
Dichlorodiphenyltrichloroethane in breast milk, 1034
Dick-Read, G., 345-346
Dick-Read method of childbirth preparation, 347
Dicumarol
in breast milk, 1031
during pregnancy, 869
Dicurin; *see* Mercurial diuretics
Dieldrin in breast milk, 1034
Diet
and diabetes mellitus in pregnancy, 850
fruitarian, 336
lactoovovegetarian, 335, 336
maternal, impact of, on milk composition, 660
during pregnancy, cultural views of, 117-118
secondary amenorrhea from, 177
vegan, 336
vegetarian, 335-336
food guide for, 336, 337
as nutrition risk factor, 326
Diet history and analysis, 331
Dietary allowances, recommended
for infants, 653
during pregnancy and nutrition, 320-321
Dietary assessment during pregnancy, 329, 331
Diethylstilbestrol
abnormalities caused by, in children, 981
and embryonic tissues, 51
and male infertility, 182
as morning-after pill, 195
as teratogen, 951
and uterine anomalies, 179
Diffusion across placenta, 215
Digestion in infancy, 652
Digestive system
fetal development of, 218-219
of neonate, 560-561
Digitoxin, effect of, on fetus or neonate, 1023
Digits, supernumerary, 978
Digoxin in breast milk, 1032
Dihydrotachysterol in breast milk, 663, 1035
Dihydroxyanthraquinone in breast milk, 1033
Dilantin; *see* Phenytoin
Dilatation
of cervix, 385, 386, 387
and descent during first stage of labor, 398, 399
assessment sheet for, 400
and curettage for therapeutic abortion, 991, 992
and evacuation for therapeutic abortion, 992
Dimetane; *see* Brompheniramine
Dindevan; *see* Phenindione
Dinitrophenylhydrazine test, 1027
for phenylketonuria, 1028
Dinoprost; *see* Prostaglandin F_2 alpha
Diphenhydramine in breast milk, 1032
2,3-Diphosphoglycerate levels during pregnancy, 232
Diploid number of chromosomes, 207
Direct Coombs' test, 962-963
Dirt, eating of, during pregnancy, 118; *see also* Pica
Disbelief and shock phase of grieving, 766
Discharge
early, after delivery, 705
from eyes of neonate, 620-621
from hospital, anticipatory guidance of parents before, 628-630
vaginal, in neonate, 567
Discharge summary, 22
Discomfort
during birth period, nonpharmacologic, noninvasive relief of, 528
during labor, origin of, 501
pharmacologic control of, during birth period, 500-528
in postpartum period, evaluative criteria for, 699
of pregnancy, 301-302, 303-307
Disease
cardiovascular, hypertensive, 823-824
caused by single gene, 142, 145-147
chlamydial, in neonate, 841
Christmas, 800
cytomegalic viral inclusion, 563, 976
gallbladder, and oral contraceptives, 195
genetic, 141-142
detection of, 152-155
heart; *see* Heart disease
Hodgkin's, elective abortion in, 990
hyaline membrane, 217
and cold stress, 566
isoimmune hemolytic, of newborn, 960-964
macrovascular, 844
metabolic, of late pregnancy; 395; *see also* Pregnancy-induced hypertension
microvascular, 844
neoplastic, and oral contraceptives, 194
pelvic inflammatory, 162
and IUD, 196
and oral contraceptives, 192
sexually transmitted, 109
circumcision and, 625
sickle cell, 984
preconceptional detection of, 152
systemic, chronic, as nutrition risk factor, 326
Tay-Sachs, 146, 219
preconceptional detection of, 152
thromboembolic, and oral contraceptives, 193
vascular, hypertensive, 823
von Recklinghausen's, 987
von Willebrand's, 800
Disease states, prevention of, 9
Dislocated hip, congenital, 151, 977
Disorders
autoimmune, 800

Disorders—cont'd
autosomal-dominant, 146
autosomal-recessive, 146
of cell division, 148-149
child with, 767-769
caused by chromosomal aberrations, 142, 149
clotting, in pregnancy, 796-800
congenital; *see* Congenital anomalies
endocrine and metabolic, 844-865
genetic or hereditary, 141-142
and male infertility, 182
hemorrhagic, in pregnancy, 780
of late pregnancy, 789-802
multifactorial, 142
in parenting, signs indicating potential for, 284
polygenic, 150
psychologic, and male infertility, 182
sex-linked, amniocentesis to determine, 288
X-linked, 146
X-linked dominant, 146-147
X-linked recessive, 147
Disproportion
cephalopelvic, as indication for cesarean delivery, 893
fetopelvic, 876-879
Disseminated intravascular coagulation, 797-799
and adult respiratory distress syndrome, 986
Disseminated lupus erythematosus complicating pregnancy, 988
Distention
abdominal, sudden, while feeding, 754
of bladder after delivery, 456, 693
prevention of, 456
Distress, fetal, 46, 407, 491
from decreased fetal circulation, 470
monitoring of, 402-403
treatment of, 407
Diuretics
in breast milk, 663, 1033-1034
for cardiac decompensation, 870
effect of, on fetus or neonate, 1023
during pregnancy, 237, 322
for pregnancy-induced hypertension, 817
Diuril; *see* Thiazides
Diverticular process of labium majus, 59
Dizygotic twins, 930, 932
DNA; *see* Deoxyribonucleic acid
Documentation of observations by nurse, 6
Dominance, principle of, 145
Dominant gene, 145
Donnatal in breast milk, 1029
L-Dopa; *see* Levodopa
Dopar; *see* Levodopa
Doppler ultrasound to pick up fetal heartbeat, 275-276
Dorbane; *see* Anthraquinone laxatives
Dorbantyl; *see* Anthraquinone laxatives
Dorsal recumbent position for labor, 411
Dorsiflexion ankle, in neonate, 918
Dorsolumbar lordosis, 225, 240
Double footling breech presentation, 369
"Double standard" regarding sex, 109
Double-setup procedure for placenta previa, 793
Doubt and shame vs. autonomy in personality development, 135-136
Douche, vaginal, 835
Douching during pregnancy, 227
Douglas, cul-de-sac of, 66
posterior, 61
Down's syndrome, 19, 142, 149, 150
dermatoglyphics and, 154
and hydramnios, 967
Doyle spoon, 182
DPG; *see* 2,3-Diphosphoglycerate
DPT in breast milk, 1037
Drainage from mouth of neonate, position to facilitate, 616, 617
Dreams, sexual, of adolescent, 108
Dressing of neonate, 622, 623
"Drip"; *see* Gonorrhea
Drooling by neonate, 560
"Dropping," 224
Drowsiness in neonate, 569
Drug(s)
of abuse, effect of, on fetus or neonate, 1023
in breast milk, effect of, on infant, 1029-1037
fertility, 177
in human milk, 662, 663
and male infertility, 182
placental transfer of, 215
during pregnancy, 301
to suppress labor, 5
tocolytic, 910
affecting urine glucose determinations, 1021
Drug addiction as nutrition risk factor, 326
Drug dependence
narcotic, and pregnancy, 953-956
and pregnancy, 951-956
Drug interactions and oral contraceptives, 195
Drug therapy in nursing mothers, abbreviated guide to, 663
Drug tray, infant, 443
"Drumstick" in polymorphonuclear leukocyte of female, 151
Duchenne muscular dystrophy, 147
Duct
Bartholin's, opening of, 54
of breast, 72
of bulbourethral gland, 78
ejaculatory, 77, 78, 81
lactiferous, 73, 74, 659
milk, plugged, 668
paraurethral, orifice of, 56
seminal, 78
Skene's, 56
Ductus arteriosus
changes in, at birth, 557
closure of, 555
patent, 969
Ductus deferens; *see* Vas deferens
Ductus venosus, 216
changes in, at birth, 557
closure of, 555
Duncan mechanism, 451
Dura mater in spinal cord, 512
Duration of uterine contractions, 380
Duty, breach of, 40
Dwarfism, achondroplastic, 142
Dynamic ileus; *see* Intestinal obstruction
Dysmature infants, 278
Dysmaturity and estriol levels, 282
Dysmenorrhea, 89
from endometriosis, 179
membranous, 782
oral contraceptives for, 192
primary, 92
Dyspareunia
from endometriosis, 179
during pregnancy, 257
Dysplasia
bronchopulmonary, from oxygen therapy, 636, 926
cellular, smear to detect, 160
of hip, congenital, 977
Dyspnea during pregnancy, 234
treatment of, 305
Dystocia, 362, 874-892
classification of, 874
definition and classification of, 874
with diabetic pregnancies, 847
of fetal origin, 875-879
fetopelvic, 876-879
nursing care of, 884-886
outlet, 378
pelvic, 874-875
shoulder, 448
soft tissue, 875
therapies for, 886-890
uterine, 879-884
Dystonia uterine contractions, 881
Dystrophy, muscular, Duchenne, 147

E

Earlobes, anomalies of, 967
Early adolescence, sexual development in, 106, 107
"Early bird" classes, 341
Early deceleration in fetal heart rate, 485, 486, 488
Early pregnancy, disorders of, 780-789
Early pregnancy classes, 341
Early proliferative phase of endometrial cycle, 87
Early puerperium, 686
Early spontaneous abortion, 782
Early stage of spontaneous abortion, 782
Ears of neonate
anomalies of, 979
assessment of, 586
cleansing of, 621
low-set, 979
Eating habits; *see* Nutrition
Ecchymosis on newborn, 564, 906
with vacuum extractor, 892
Echography; *see* Ultrasonography
Eclampsia, 811
convulsions in, 815
prevention and control of, 815, 819-820
and epilepsy, differentiation of, 987
Economic conditions and parental responses, 722
Economic deprivation as nutrition risk factor, 325-326
Economics and maternity care, 4
Ectocervix, 65
Ectodermal germ layer, 216
Ectopic pregnancy, 158, 784-787
and blocked fallopian tube, 62
and IUD, 196
nursing care of parents experiencing, 773
and oral contraceptives, 192
symptoms of, 782
EDC; *see* Estimated date of confinement
Edecrin; *see* Ethacrynic acid
Edema
cervical
from bearing down, 382
and dystocia, 875
gestational, 810-811
in neonate, 906
and oral contraceptives, 194
physiologic, 237
during pregnancy, 304
in pregnancy-induced hypertension, 809
Education
childbirth and parenthood, 299
of maternity nurses, 4-5
nurse-midwife, 1013-1014
parent, 341-343
organizations involved in, 357
sex, 112
Educational role of nurse, 6-7
Educational measures, 21
Educational and Scientific Plastics, Ltd., 1008
Ed-U-Press, 1008
Edwards' syndrome, 150
Effacement of cervix, 385, 386
Effleurage, 353
during labor, 414
to relieve pain, 528
Egg nest of ovary, 69
Eggs, introduction of, 674
Ego integrity vs. despair in personality development, 136
Egyptian Arab women, view on pregnancy of, 117
Ejaculate, 80-81
split, for artificial insemination, 183
Ejaculation, 93, 100
premature, and circumcision, 625
Ejaculatory duct, 77, 78, 81
Ejaculatory inevitability, 100
Ejection murmurs, systolic, during pregnancy, 230
Elastic hose during pregnancy, 299
Elavil; *see* Amitriptyline hydrochloride

Elective abortion; *see* Therapeutic abortion
Electric breast pump, 670
Electrical nerve stimulation, transcutaneous, for relief of discomfort, 528
Electrocardiograph, abdominal, for fetal heart rate monitoring, 471, 475
Electrode, spiral
  application of, 478
  checklist for, 494
  for fetal heart rate monitoring, 471, 476-478
  to monitor uterine activity, 490
Electrolyte and fluid balance during pregnancy, 236-237
Electronic fetal monitoring, 5, 403
Electroshock therapy after delivery, 950, 951
Elimination; *see* Bowel movement
Elimination behaviors of neonate, 572
  assessment of, 603
Elliott forceps, 891
Emboli, pulmonary
  after delivery, 452
  during pregnancy, 986
Embryo
  effects of diabetes mellitus on, 853, 859
  transplantation of, in vitro fertilization and, 42-43
Embryo stage of development, 207
Embryogenesis, critical periods in, 951
Embryonic development and fetal maturation, 216-220
Embryonic tissue, 51
Emergencies, surgical, most common, 971-975
Emergency childbirth, 447-449
Emergency procedures during first stage of labor, 407
Emergency resuscitation of depressed neonate, equipment and supplies for, 443
Emission in male orgasm, 100
Emory University, ACNM-approved basic education in, 1013
Emotional crisis of infertility, 183-184
Emotional independence, achieving, 106-107
Emotional needs
  of high-risk neonate, 761
  of parents after delivery, support of, 458-461
Emotional response
  in postpartum period, evaluative criteria for, 699
  to pregnancy, 119
  to second stage of labor, 418
  following therapeutic abortion, 990
Emotional tension, counseling for, 298
Empathy in nurse-client relationship, 34-35
Employment during pregnancy, 299-300
E-Mycin; *see* Erythromycin
End piece of sperm, 207
Endocervical canal, 60, 63, 65
Endocervical glandular cells, effects of estrogens and progesterone on, 89
Endocervix during pregnancy, 226
Endocrine changes during pregnancy, 242-247
Endocrine disorders, 844-865
Endocrine system
  changes in, in postpartum period, 689
  embryonic development of, 219
Endocrine therapy for anovulation, 177
Endogenous insulin, 844
Endometrial biopsy as fertility test, 172
Endometrial carcinoma and oral contraceptives, 192
Endometrial cycle, 87-88
Endometrial tuberculosis, infertility from, 179
Endometrial tumors, infertility from, 179
Endometriosis causing female infertility, 178-179
Endometritis and IUD, 196
Endometrium, 60
  changes in, with pregnancy, 246
  characteristics of, during endometrial cycle, 87
  effects of estrogen and progesterone on, 89
  levels of, 87
  regeneration of, in postpartum period, 688
  tumors of, removal of, 179
  of uterine wall, 62-63
Endorphins, 86
Enduron; *see* Thiazides
Enemas, 405
Energy intake, 654
Energy level and initial oral feeding, 677
Energy needs during pregnancy, 320
Engaged fetal head, 365, 367
Engagement in labor in vertex presentation, 388
English lock, 891
Engorged breasts, 667
Engorgement, 663-664
  splanchnic, 454
Enkephalins, 86
Enovid, 192
  in breast milk, 1035
Ensiform process, 69
Enterocolitis, neonatal necrotizing, 636
  and early feeding, 752
  in preterm infant, 927
Entodermal germ layer, 216
Entrainment and parent-child attachment, 710
Environmental agents in breast milk, 1034
Environmental factors in nurseries, 575
Environmental pollutants in human milk, 662
Environmental support of preterm infant, 915
Enzymes
  biochemical tests for, 329
  liver, fetal production of, 219
  of trophoblast, 210
Epidemic parotitis, immunization against, 301
Epididymis, 78, 79, 81
  abnormalities of, and male infertility, 181
  appendix, 79
  and formation of semen, 82
Epidural anesthesia, 518-522
  care after, 703
Epidural block, 513, 516
  lumbar, 512
Epidural blood-patch of post-spinal-puncture headache, 905
Epidural morphine, 524-527
Epidural space in spinal cord, 512
Epidural tray, 517
Epilepsy
  and eclampsia, differentiation of, 987
  and oral contraceptives, 195
  complicating pregnancy, 987-988
Epinephrine
  in breast milk, 663, 1035
  for bronchial asthma, 985
  to prevent convulsions of eclampsia, 822
Episiotomy, 56, 59, 890
  assessment of, 692
  care of, 701
  indications for, 890
  infection of, 693
  lateral, 891
  median, 890, 891
  mediolateral, 890, 891
  types of, 890, 891
  use of, proponents of, 890
Episiotomy area, care of, 457
Epispadias, 77, 980
Epithelium
  columnar, of cervix, 64, 65
  squamous, of cervix, 64, 65
  vaginal, effect of estrogens on, 89
Epoophoron, 60
Epulis (epulides), 238-239, 987
  during pregnancy, 303
  as presumptive sign of pregnancy, 273
Equanil; *see* Meprobamate
Equational division, 143
Equipment; *see* also Instrumentation
  in delivery room, 422-423
  fetal monitoring, checklist for, 494-495
  used for pelvic examination, 286
Erb-Duchenne paralysis, 907, 908
Erection, 93, 100
Ergonovine maleate
  after delivery, lochia and, 692
  for inversion of uterus, 807
  after multiple births, 934
  after spontaneous abortion, 783
  to stimulate uterine contractions, 452
  for subinvolution of uterus, 807
  for uterine bleeding, 803
Ergot in breast milk, 1032
Ergot preparations
  and breast feeding, 663
  after delivery, 688
  and retained placenta, 805
  to stimulate uterine contractions, 452-453
Ergotrate; *see* Ergonovine maleate
Erikson's theory of personality development, 135-136
Erythema, palmar, 238, 987
  treatment of, 305
Erythema multiforme, 238, 987
Erythema neonatorum, 565
Erythema toxicum, 565
Erythroblastosis fetalis, 960-964
Erythrocin; *see* Erythromycin
Erythrocytes; *see* Red blood cells
Erythromycin
  in breast milk, 1030
  effect of, on fetus or neonate, 1022
Erythromycin drops for prophylactic eye care of newborn, 445
Erythromycin solution for cord care, 621
Escherichia coli
  causing neonatal sepsis, 837
  causing vaginitis, 834
Escutcheon, 54
Esidrix; *see* Thiazides
Eskalith; *see* Lithium carbonate
Esophageal atresia, 560, 970, 971, 972
  feeding of infant with, 677
  and hydramnios, 967
Esophagus, changes in, during pregnancy, 241
Essential hypertension, 823-824
  differential diagnosis of, 810
Estimated date of confinement, 268, 277-281
Estradiol, fetoplacental production of, 245
Estriol
  fetoplacental production of, 245-246
  levels of, in maternal urine
    biochemical monitoring of, 283
    determination of, 287
    to determine gestational age, 282
  urinary excretion of, as index of fetal well-being, 246
Estrogen
  and breast development, 75, 76
  in breast milk, 1035
  deficiency of, side effects of, 193
  effect of
    on fetus or neonate, 1023
    on target organs and tissues, 89
  excess of, side effects of, 193
  fetoplacental production of, 242-243, 245
  and fetus, 219
  and gastrointestinal changes during pregnancy, 241
  and insulin production, 247
  and insulin resistance, 845
  levels of
    in menstrual cycle, 86
    during pregnancy, 223
  and onset of labor, 388
  in oral contraceptives, 192
  ovaries and, 68
  for Sheehan's syndrome, 807
  and sodium balance, 236
  and suppression of lactation, 705
  and urinary system changes during pregnancy, 235
  and uterine enlargement, 223
Estrone, fetoplacental production of, 245

Ethacrynic acid for pregnancy-induced hypertension, 817
Ether, effect of, on fetus or neonate, 1022
Ethical issues in maternity care, 4
Ethical and legal aspects of maternity nursing, 39-47
Ethical system, establishing, in adolescence, 107
Ethinyl estradinol in breast milk, 1035
Ethiodol, 174
Ethnic groups; *see also* Culture
  eye contact and, 29
  language of, and communication, 27
  meaning of time for, 29
Ethnic influences on dietary practices, 335
Ethnocentrism, 115
Ethyl biscoumacetate in breast milk, 1031
Euglycemia as goal of management of diabetes mellitus in pregnancy, 848
Eutocia, 362, 392, 398
Eutonyl; *see* Monoamine oxidase inhibitors
Evaluating, planning, and implementing care of newborn, 615-649
Evaluation, 22
  behavioral, Brazelton, 603, 1039-1044
  in cognition, 134
  during prenatal period, 310-312
    as curative activity, 9
Evaluative criteria
  for care during labor, 463-464
  for nursing actions with newborn, 647-649
Evaporated milk formula, 671
  supplements for infant receiving, 656, 671
Evaporation causing heat loss in neonate, 566
Examination
  breast, positions of client for, 694
  for female fertility, 166-176
  for gestational age, 917, 918-919
  manual, of uterine cavity after delivery, 452
  microscopic, of vaginal fluid, 401
  pelvic
    anxiety during, 164
    equipment used for, 286
    procedure for, 285
  physical, 19-20
    of fertile man, 161
    of fertile woman, 159-160
    initial, 19
    and nutrition assessment, 327
  speculum, bivalve, 286
  vaginal
    and bleeding, 384
    to determine fetal presentation, position, and descent, 384-386
    in placenta previa, 793
    of vaginal canal after delivery, 452
Excessive weight gain during pregnancy, 326-327
Exchange transfusion for hyperbilirubinemia, 641, 964-966
Excitement phase of sexual response cycle, 93, 97
Excretion, nutrient, by kidneys during pregnancy, 237
Excursion, 844
Executive behaviors of infant, 708
Exercise(s)
  after cesarean delivery, 905
  childbirth, 350-352
  in diabetes mellitus in pregnancy, 850
  Kegel, 57, 309, 350, 704
  maternal, and fetal circulation, 470
  for pelvic floor, 350
  in postpartum period, 702-704
  during pregnancy, 300
Exercise program, postpartum, 703
Exfoliated cells, fetal lipid-containing, staining of, and gestational age, 282
Exhibitionism in childhood, 105
Exogenous insulin, 844
Expanded family, 132
Expanded role of maternity nurse, 6-7
Expectations, parental, and response to infant, 720
Expiratory grunt, 749
Expression
  of human milk, manual, 667
  sexual, 110
Expulsion of fetus and placenta, forces causing, 379-382
Expulsion breathing, 349-350
Exstrophy of bladder, 978-980
Extended family, 131-132
  cultural views of, 123-124
Extension in labor in vertex presentation, 390-391
External anal sphincter, 58, 61
External cardiac massage, 635-636
External cephalic version to convert breech presentation, 877
External cervical os, 63, 65
External fetal monitoring, 471-476
External genitalia
  female, during pregnancy, 222-223
  female and male homologues of, 51, 52
  of male, 77-78
External hemorrhoidal vein, 68
External hydrocephalus, 975
External iliac artery, 67
External iliac nodes, 68
External iliac vessels, 61
External os of vaginal cervix, 60
External rotation in labor in vertex presentation, 391-392
Extracellular fluid of neonate, 559
Extraction
  menstrual, for therapeutic abortion, 991, 992
  vacuum, 892
Extractor, Malmstroöm, 892
Extraperitoneal cesarean delivery, 895
Extrauterine pregnancy, ruptured, 785
Extravasation of blood into myometrium with premature separation of placenta, 791-792
Extremities
  and body, delivery of, 420
  deformed, and hydramnios, 967
  of neonate, assessment of, 591, 593
  ''seal-like,'' 978
Extremity restraints for neonate, 645
Extrusion reflex, 595
Eye contact
  as communication, 29
  with infant, 568
  in parent-child attachment, 709-710
Eye patches during phototherapy, 641, 642
Eye problems and oral contraceptives, 193
Eyes of neonates
  assessment of, 586, 587
  care of, 442-445
  cleansing of, 620, 621
  discharge from, 620-621

F

Face of neonate
  bruises and petechiae on, 612
  paralysis of, from delivery, 908
  rash on, 621
Face presentation, 369, 371
  molding in, 365
Facial asymmetry in neonate, 577
Facies of neonate, assessment of, 586
Facilitated transfer across placenta, 215
Facilities
  for care of neonate, 574-576
  in postpartum period, 701
Factor VIII antihemophilic factor, deficiency of, 800
Factor assays, 798
Factor IX deficiency, 800
FAD; *see* Fetal activity, determination of
Failure to thrive in breast-feeding infant, 668-669
Faintness during pregnancy, 304
Fallopian tube, 59-62
  abdominal orifice of, 60
  adhesions of, 178
  ampulla of, 60, 61
  blockage of, by IUD, 196
  changes in, during menstrual cycle, 160
Fallopian tube—cont'd
  function of, 178
  gonorrheal infection of, 62
  infertility and, 61, 62
  inflammation of, infertility from, 178
  infundibulum of, 61
  interstitial portion of, 60, 61
  isthmus of, 60, 61
  mucosa of, 61-62
  pain from, 66
  peristaltic activity of, 61
  during pregnancy, 223
  segments of, 61
  special clinical significance of, 61-62
Fallot, tetralogy of, 969
Falope ring for sterilization, 997
False labor, 225, 395, 396
False pelvis, 70, 71, 371
Family, 128-138
  adjustment of, to birth of infant, 4-5
  and adolescent, 107, 108
  American, 122
  boundaries of, 133
  care for, goals of, 17
  childbearing, goals for, 17
  communal, 132
  communication in, 133
  and crisis, 136-138
  definition of, 128
  dynamics and function of, 133
  expanded, 132
  expected behavior of, among various cultures, 116-119
  extended, 131-132
    cultural views of, 123-124
  genes in, 145-147
  grief reactions from, at birth of child with disorder, 768
  initial contact with, 291
  life cycle of, 133
  as major support system, 8
  need of, for psychosocial care, 283-284
  nuclear, 129-131
    American, 122
    Japanese, 123
  preparation of, for home birth, 548-549
  psychosocial development within, 133-136
  reactions of, to childbearing, cultural differences in, 122-124
  responses of
    to birth of child, 707-723
    to birth of high-risk infant, 778
    to pregnancy, 252-265
  roles in, 133
  single-parent, 132-133
  social and economic issues involving, 4
  and social roles, 133
  of stillborn child, care of, 762-763
  stressors on, caused by birth of baby, 3
  structure of, 129-133
Family assessment tool, 293
Family configurations, 129
Family history, 19
Family nurse-practitioner, 6
Family planning, 186
  cultural views on, 124-125
  for diabetic women, 853
  natural, 188-192
Family planning clinic, 112
Family Planning Service and Population Research Act of 1970, 11
Family planning services, 11
Family relationships, initiation of, 700
Family Service Association of America, Inc., 1008
Family therapy, 302
Family-centered care, 3, 531-532
  and parent-child attachment, 711
Family-centered cesarean birth, 541-542
Family-centered childbearing, 8-9
Fantasies, sexual, in adolescent, 108
FAS; *see* Fetal alcohol syndrome

Fascia
of bulbocavernosus muscle, 59
Camper's, 58
Colles', 58, 59
of levator ani, 58, 59
midline, of abdomen, 69
obturator internus, 59
rectal, 58
Scarpa's, 58
urethrovesical, 58
of urogenital diaphragm, 58
uterovaginal, 59
vaginouterine, 58
Fascial planes of male lower genitourinary tract, 78
Fascial sheaths, round ligaments within, 59
Fasting blood sugar, 848, 849
Fat
brown, of neonate, 566
in human milk, 661
for infants, 654-655
subcutaneous, of neonate, 564
necrosis of, 906
Fat content of infant, 651
Fat deposits during pregnancy, 320
Fat stores and lactation, 327
Father, 258
adolescent, 947
in labor suite, 415-416
role of
in birth process, 6
during labor and delivery, 263
cultural views on, 119
support of, during labor, 416
view of birth process by, 415
Father-child relationship, beginning of, 260-261, 263
Fatherhood
with dignity, 414-416
rehearsing for, 261
Father-to-be
responses of, to pregnancy, 258-263
self-concept of, during pregnancy, 261
Fatigue
during pregnancy, 307
as presumptive symptom of pregnancy, 269-270
Fat-soluble vitamins
biochemical tests for, 329
need for, during pregnancy, 322
Fear(s), 136
childbirth without, 347
Fecundation, 207
Feeding
breast; *see* Breast feeding
early, of high-risk infant, 751-752
formula, 671-673
gavage
for neonate with respiratory distress, 749
nursing care after, 756
of infant
demand, 5
method of, selection of, 261
theories of, 5
nasogastric tube, for high-risk infant, 754-756
of newborn, 650-683
evaluative criteria for, 647
questions about, 300-301
of normal infant, general guidelines for, 676-677
oral
for high-risk infant, 753
initial, 676-677
relationship of infant development to, 651-652
right side-lying position after, 620
stooling during, 561
Feeding behavior
assessment of, 603
of neonate, 571-572
Feeding intolerance in tracheoesophageal fistula, 971
Feeding schedule
for high-risk infant, 753
for twins, 934
Female
genitals of
development and function of, 219
internal, 59-71
of neonate, 590
assessment of, 589, 591
gonads of, 68; *see also* Ovaries
hypothalamic-pituitary-gonadal axis in, 88
infertility in
factors implicated in, 165-166
from impaired tubal function, 178
investigation of, 165-181
prognosis for, 180
tests and examinations for, 166-176
therapy for, 177-181
treatment of, 180-181
vaginal-cervical factors in, 179-180
pelvic organs of, 61
pelvis of; *see* Pelvis, female
reproductive system of, 54-76
changes in, 90
external structures of, 54-59
during pregnancy, 222-223
homologues in, of male reproductive system, 51-53
internal structures of, 59-71
during pregnancy, 223-228
supporting structures and, 59
stages of sexual development in, 91
sterilization of, 997-999
urethra of, 56
Feminine social role, achieving, 105-106
Feminist Women's Health Centers, 1008
Femoral nodes, 66
Femoral pulses in neonate, 580, 581
Femur of neonate, fracture of, during delivery, 907
"Fencing" position, 595
Fenestrated blades, 891
Fentanyl for analgesia, 509-510
Ferguson's reflex, 910
Fern patterns of cervical mucus, 169
Fern test, positive, on amniotic fluid, 401
Ferric chloride test, 1027
Ferrous sulfate during pregnancy, 983
Fertile man, assessment data for, 161
Fertile woman, assessment data for, 159-160
Fertility
control of, 186-203
methods of, 187-201
cultural views on, 124
definition of, 158
female; *see* Female, fertility of
fertility test findings favorable to, 170
male, 83
normal, factors essential to, 158
other factors contributing to, 161-162
peak time for, 162
surgical termination of, 996-1000
Fertility awareness method of contraception, 192
Fertility clinic, 112
Fertility drugs, 177
Fertility rate, 11
Fertility test findings favorable to fertility, 170
Fertilization, 144, 206-220
in vitro, 180-181
and embryo transplantation, 42-43
Fertilized ovum; *see* Zygote
Fetal alcohol syndrome, 301, 952-953
Fetal compromise, 280
Fetal distress, 46, 407, 491
from decreased fetal circulation, 470
monitoring of, 402-403
treatment of, 407
Fetal electrocardiography, 275, 276
Fetal factors causing high-risk pregnancy, 740, 741, 742, 746
Fetal heart rate, 217, 225, 282-283
acceleration in, 485, 486
average, 471
base-line, 480-484
Fetal heart rate—cont'd
counting, 275, 276
decelerations in, 485-489
display of, on chart paper, 480
and fetal distress, 491
instrumentation for monitoring
external, 471-475
internal, 471, 476-478
during labor, 402
maximal intensity of, to determine fetal position, 384
monitoring of; *see* Fetal monitoring
nonreassuring patterns of, 491
nonstress test and, 282
ominous patterns of, 492
oxytocin stress test and, 282-283
patterns of
abnormal, 407
pattern of, recognition of, 479-491
periodic changes in, 485-489
reassuring patterns of, 491
regulation of, 471
during second stage of labor, 421, 425
Fetal lie and position, 371
Fetal malformations, 208; *see also* Congenital anomalies
abortions in cases of, 45
and maternal alcoholism, 952; *see also* Fetal alcohol syndrome
Fetal and maternal malnutrition, presumptive signs of, 326
Fetal and maternal nutrition, 314-340
summary of nursing care in, 336-340
Fetal membranes, development of, 212
Fetal monitor
alarm system on, legal aspects of, 46
care of, 493
Corometrics, 469
legal concepts regarding, 46
Fetal monitoring, 468-498
charting and, 493, 494
electronic, 5, 403
equipment for, checklist for, 494-495
external mode of, 471-476
history of, 468, 470
instrumentation for, 471-479
internal mode of, 471, 476-479
legal aspects of, 493-494
legal concepts regarding, 46
legal importance of, 41
nursing care of woman with, 491-495
objectives of, 470
physiologic basis of, 470-471
Fetal movement count, daily, 498
Fetal origin, dystocia of, 875-879
Fetal research, legal aspects of, 44
Fetal stage of development, 208
Fetal stethoscope to hear intrauterine sounds, 225
Fetal stress during labor, 402-403
Fetography, 152-153
Fetopelvic disproportion, 876-879
Fetoplacental unit, hormone production by, 242-244, 245-246
Fetoscope
to detect fetal heartbeat, 276
ultrasound, 469
Fetoscope monitoring, 402-403
Fetoscopy to detect fetal disorders, 153
Fetotoxic chemical agents, human, 1022-1024
Fetus, 207
abnormalities causing premature birth, 909
activity of, determination of, 496
anemia in, sinusoidal pattern in, 483
anomalies of, and dystocia, 875; *see also* Congenital anomalies
attitude of, 367-369
back and small parts of, palpation of, 383
biparietal diameter of, to determine gestational age of fetus, 280, 281, 282
blood sampling of, 491

Fetus—cont'd
circulation of, 556
uteroplacental and
factors affecting, 470-471
monitoring of, 470-471
circulatory pattern of, 216
death of, 46, 746
definition of, 762
estriol levels and, 282
impending
nursing care of parents experiencing, 777
psychologic aspects of, 776-778
nursing care of parents experiencing, 774-775
psychologic aspects of, 774
effects of, after discontinuing oral contraceptives, 194
effects of diabetes mellitus on, 853, 859
emergency birth of, in breech presentation, 449
expulsion of, forces causing, 379-382
gestational age of
amniocentesis to determine, 44
correlation of data in determining, 278
determining, 280-281
and health status, 281-283
growth and development of, by calendar months, 247-251
head
compression of, early deceleration caused by, 488
engaged, 365, 387
and labor, 363-366
at term, diameters of, 365
heartbeat of, as positive sign of pregnancy, 275-276
hemoglobin of, 217
hemolytic anemia of, from Rh incompatibility, sequelae of, 962
hiccough of, periodic, 217
hypoxia in, monitoring of, 491
large, dystocia and, 875
lie of, 366-367
lipid-containing exfoliated cells of, staining of, and gestational age, 282
live-born, legal views of, 45
lung maturity of, 217
pharmacologic stimulation of, 912
malpresentation or position of, and dystocia, 875-876
maturation of, embryonic development and, 216-220
metabolism of, 218-219
and mother, nursing care of, during second stage of labor, 421-439
movement of
cessation of, 774
and fetal health, 283
palpation of, as positive sign of pregnancy, 276
multiple, ultrasonography to detect, 52
neuromuscular behavior of, 218
outline of, palpation of, as positive sign of pregnancy, 276
passage of, during labor, 363-369
periodic auscultation of, 402
pH of, assessment of, 491
position of, 369
presentation of, 367
radiographic demonstration of, as positive sign of pregnancy, 276-277
reflex responses of, 218
rights of, 46
scalp pH of, testing of, 5
shoulder and pelvic girdle of, during labor, 366
skull of, 363-365
squamous cells of, in amniotic fluid, 401
stresses on, 9
superior pole of, palpation of, 383
tachycardia and bradycardia in, 480, 481
transfusion of, for hyperbilirubinemia, 966
ultrasonographic demonstration of, as positive sign of pregnancy, 276

Fetus—cont'd
in vertex position
emergency birth of, 447-448
prebirth passage of meconium with, 448-449
weight of, and biparietal diameter, correlation of, 297
well-being of, estriol excretion as measure of, 246
Fever, childbed, causing maternal mortality, 746
Fibers, muscle
anal sphincter, 57
of myometrium, 62
of uterus, arrangement of, and labor, 224
Fibrin and clotting, 797
Fibrinogen and clotting, 797
Fibrinolytic activity, standard values for, pregnant and nonpregnant, 1018
Fibrinolytic system and clotting, 797
Fibroplasia, retrolental, from oxygen therapy, 636, 926-927
Fibrosis, cystic, 142, 146
and meconium ileus, 155
Filipino women
postpartal behavior of, 121
pregnancy diet of, 117, 118
role of motherhood for, 116
Filipinos
food pattern of, 330
infant care among, 123
use of contraceptives by, 124
welcoming of newborn by, 123
Filshie clip for sterilization, 997
Filtration rate, glomerular
of neonate, 559-560
during pregnancy, 236
functional alterations in, 316
Filum terminale of spinal cord, 512
Fimbria(e), 60, 61
Fingernails
changes in
during pregnancy, 239
as presumptive symptom of pregnancy, 270
of neonate, care of, 621
Fingers, numbness of, during pregnancy, 306
Finnish food pattern, 331
First breath, 558
First polar body, 145
First prenatal visit, 292-293, 295-296
First stage of labor, 394-417
assessment in, 395-397
complications in, 397
contractions in, character of, 395, 397
duration of, 392
emergency procedures during, 407
maternal stress during, 403
paternal stress during, 403-404
progression of, 395-397
minimal reassessment of, 399
review of client's history in, 395
vaginal examination during, 406-407
woman's psychologic response to, 397
Fistula
fourchet, 974
tracheoesophageal, 971-972
feeding of infant with, 677
H-type, 970
Flagyl; *see* Metronidazole
"Fleabite" dermatitis, 565
Flexion in labor in vertex presentation, 389-390
"Floating," legal aspects of, 40
Flocculation tests for syphilis, 827
Floor, pelvic, 222
and perineum, 56-59
Florence Crittenton Association of Mothers, 1008
Flow sheets, 22
Fluctuations in fetal heart rate, cyclic, 480
Flufenamic acid in breast milk, 1029
Fluid(s)
amniotic, 212, 215-216
body, of neonate, composition of, 559
intravenous, effect of, on fetus and neonate, 1024

Fluid(s)—cont'd
parenteral
for high-risk infant, 753
for neonate with respiratory distress, 749
parenteral administration of, monitoring, 757-759
seminal, 82
vaginal, 68
pH of, determining, 401
Fluid balance after delivery, maintaining, 458
Fluid and electrolyte balance during pregnancy, 236-237
Fluid loss in high-risk neonate, 752-753
Fluid overload from shock therapy, 802
Fluid volume, equivalents in, 1015
Fluoride
in human milk, 662
for infant, 657
Fluorine
in breast milk, 1034
effect of, on fetus or neonate, 1023
need for, during pregnancy, 323
supplemental, dosage schedule for, 657
Fluothane; *see* Halothane
Fluoxymesterone in breast milk, 1035
"Flying squad service," 542
FNP; *see* Family nurse-practitioner
Focusing in communication, 26
Folacin
for infant, 656
need for, during pregnancy, 322
supplements of, 335
Folate deficiency, 983-984
Folic acid
deficiency of
and oral contraceptives, 194
tests to measure, 327
need for, during pregnancy, 322
Folic acid deficiency anemia, 983-984
Folic acid supplementation during pregnancy, 322
Follicles, graafian, 86
Follicle-stimulating hormone, 80, 86
and menstrual cycle, 85, 86
during pregnancy, 242, 245
suppression of, 223
Follicular maturation in ovary, 69
Follicular phase of menstrual cycle, 86
Fontanels
bulging of, 611-612
of fetal skull, 363, 364
Food(s)
baby, 675
after delivery, cultural views on, 120
during labor and delivery, cultural views of, 120
protein, 333
semisolid, introduction of, 673-674
Food cravings or aversions during pregnancy, 241
cultural views of, 118
treatment of, 303
Food diary for infants, 681
Food groups, list of, 331, 333-334
Food guide
daily, 331, 332, 335
for vegetarian diets, 336, 337
Food patterns
bizarre, nutrition risk factor in, 326
cultural, 335
characteristics of, 329-331
Food taboos during pregnancy, 117-118
Foot, arch of, in newborn, absence of, 592
Foot massage during labor, 414
"Football" hold
for breast feeding, 664, 665
for neonate, 619
Footling breech, 367
Foramen, obturator, 70
Foramen ovale
changes in, at birth, 557
closure of, 555
Forceps
sterile, unwrapped, 429
types of, 891

Forceps delivery, 890-892
Forceps designation relative to station of head, 892
Forceps locks, types of, 891
Foreskin, 77, 78
Form, consent
  English, 502
  Spanish, 503
Formal operational stage of adolescence, 107
Formal operations stage of cognitive development, 135
Formal thinking, 135
Formula(s)
  commercial; *see* Commercial formulas
  and dehydration in infant, 655
  evaporated milk, 671
    supplementation with, 656, 671
  for high-risk infant, 753
  special, 672
Formula feeding, 671-673
Fornix of vagina, 60, 61, 68
Forty-eight hour contraceptive sponge, 199
Fossa, ischiorectal, extension of, 59
Fossa navicularis, 54, 56, 77
Fourchet, 54, 56
  fistula of, 974
Four-phase response cycle to sexual stimulation, 93-100
Fourth stage of labor, 453-462
  assessment of mother during, 454
  duration of, 392-393
Fourth trimester, 686
Fowler's position during second stage of labor, 421
Fracture
  of clavicle of neonate during delivery, 907
  of humerus or femur in neonate during delivery, 907
  skull, of neonate during delivery, 906-907
Fragments, placental, retained, removal of, 452
Frank breech presentation, 367, 368, 369
Fraternal twins, 930
Free T_4 index, 867
Freestanding birth centers, 538-541
Frejka pillow for congenital hip dysplasia, 977
French lock, 891
French size catheters, equivalents for, 1016
Frenulum of clitoris, 54, 55
Frequency
  urinary, 305
    during pregnancy, 235
    as presumptive symptom of pregnancy, 269
  of uterine contractions, 380
Frondosum, 211
Frontal eminence of fetal skull, 363, 364
Frontier Nursing Service, 542
Frontier School of Midwifery and Family Nursing, ACNM-approved basic education in, 1013
Fructose in seminal fluid, 82
Fruitarian diet, 336
Fruits, 334
  introduction of, 673-674
  vitamin C–rich, 334
FSH; *see* Follicle-stimulating hormone
FTA-ABS IgM test, 827, 832
FTA-ABS test, 827
Fulguration, tubal, for sterilization, 997-999
Functional residual capacity, changes in, during pregnancy, 234
Functioning, neurologic, assessment of, 563
Fundus, 60, 62
  assessment of, in postpartum period, 690, 691, 693
  changes in, after delivery, 687, 688
  height of
    and duration of pregnancy, 277-278
    measurement of, 277-278, 279
    by week of gestation, 224
  palpation of, after delivery, 455, 456
Funic souffle, 225
Funis; *see* Umbilical cord
Furadantin; *see* Nitrofurantoin
Furazolidone for *Trichomonas* vaginitis, 834
Furosemide
  in breast milk, 1033
  for cardiac decompensation, 870
  for pregnancy-induced hypertension, 817

G

^{67}Ga citrate in breast milk, 1033
Gadsup, views of family of, 123
Gadsup women, food cravings of, 118
Gagging, 616
Galactosemia, 146
  heel stick for, 637
  screening for, 154
Galant reflex, 599
Gallbladder
  changes in, during pregnancy, 241
  disease of, and oral contraceptives, 195
Gallstones, 241, 987
Gametes, 206
  cell division in, 143-144
Gametogenesis, 143, 144-145, 206
Gantanol; *see* Sulfonamides
Gantrisin; *see* Sulfisoxazole; Sulfonamides
"Gas tank" theory of infant feeding, 5
Gastric acidity of neonate, 560
Gastric capacity and initial oral feeding, 677
Gastrocnemius spasm during pregnancy, 305
Gastrocolic reflex, 572, 612
  and stooling, 561
Gastrointestinal changes during pregnancy, 240-242
Gastrointestinal problems complicating pregnancy, 987
Gastrointestinal tract
  assessment of, in postpartum period, 693
  blood flow to, during pregnancy, 230
  changes in, in postpartum period, 689
  congenital anomalies of, screening for, 970
  discomforts of pregnancy related to, 303-304
  embryonic development of, 218-219
  of neonate, 560
  in postpartum period, evaluative criteria for, 699
Gate control theory of pain, 353
Gauge, strain, checklist for, 495
Gavage feeding for neonate with respiratory distress, 749
Gender identity, development of, 103
Gender preference, 103
Gene(s), 141
  on chromosomes, 142
  dominant, 145
  in families, 145-147
  heterozygous, 141, 142
  homozygous, 141, 142
  recessive, 145
  single, disorder caused by, 142, 145-147
Gene pairs, 142
General anesthesia, 508, 511
General anesthetics causing decreased variability in fetal heart rate, 483
General arteriolar spasm in preeclampsia-eclampsia, 812
General assessment of mother following delivery, 451-452
General care of neonate, 616-625
General flexion, fetal attitude of, 368
General hygiene during labor, 414
General surgical client and obstetric client, comparison of, 504
Generativity vs. self-absorption in personality development, 136
Genetic counseling, 42, 155-156
Genetic defects, screening for, 43-44
Genetic disorders, 141-142
  detection of, 152-155
  and male infertility, 182
Genetics, 141-156
  principle of, 145
Genital abnormalities in DES-exposed children, 981
Genital herpes, 829
  management of, 827
Genitalia
  ambiguous, 970, 980
  external
    female, during pregnancy, 222-223
    female and male homologues of, 51, 52
  female
    development and function of, 219
    internal, 59-71
      changes in, as presumptive sign of pregnancy, 273-274
      during pregnancy, 223-228
  internal
    female and male homologues of, 51, 53
    innervation of, 66, 68
  male
    development and function of, 219
    external, 77-78
    internal, 79-83
  of neonate
    assessment of, 589-591
    bruising and swelling of, 612
    cleansing of, 621
Genitourinary tract
  anomalies of, in neonate, 978-980
  lower, of male, 78, 79
Genotypes, Rh, 961
Gentamicin in breast milk, 1030
Gentian violet
  for monilial vaginitis, 834
  for oral thrush, 842
Geopen; *see* Carbenicillin
Georgetown University School of Nursing, ACNM-approved basic education in, 1013
Germ cells
  cell division in, 143-144
  formation of, 143-144
Germ layers, organ systems developed from, 216
German lock, 891
German measles
  immunization against, 301
  during pregnancy, 830
Gestational age, 208
  amniocentesis to determine, 44
  and behavior of newborn, 610
  correlation of data in determining, 278
  determining, 280-281
  examination for, 917, 918-919
  and health status, 281-283
  maternal estriol levels to determine, 282
  tests for, 282
Gestational diabetes, 280, 844
Gestational diabetes mellitus, 845-846
Gestational diabetic mother, infant of, 859-863
Gestational edema, 810-811
Gestational glycosuria, tests for, 329
Gestational hypertension, 810; *see also* Pregnancy-induced hypertension
Gestational proteinuria, 810
Gestational time units, 208
GFR; *see* Glomerular filtration rate
GH; *see* Growth hormone
Gingival granuloma gravidarum, 238-239, 273
Gingivitis, 303
Girdle, maternity, 299
Glabellar reflex, 595
Gland(s)
  adrenal, changes in, during pregnancy, 247
  Bartholin's, 54, 56
    changes in, in response to sexual stimulation, 95
  bulbourethral, 82
    duct of, 78
    formation of semen and, 82
  Cowper's, 77-78, 82
    changes in, in response to sexual stimulation, 93, 96
    and formation of semen, 82
  of Littre, 77, 78
  mammary; *see* Breast(s)
  of Montgomery, 74
  parathyroid, changes in, during pregnancy, 246

Gland(s)—cont'd
paraurethral, 54, 55
periurethral, orifice of, 56
pituitary
and menstrual cycle, 84, 85
during pregnancy, 242, 244-245
prostate; *see* Prostate gland
reproductive tract, accessory, of male, 82
sebaceous, hyperplasia of, in neonate, 564
Skene's, 54, 55
sweat, of neonate, 564
thyroid
changes in, during pregnancy, 246
fetal development of, 219
vestibular
greater, 54, 56
lesser, 54, 55, 56
vulvovaginal, 54, 56
Glandular cells, endocervical, effects of estrogens and progesterone on, 89
Glandular hyperplasia, cystic, infertility after, 179
Glans of clitoris, 54, 55, 61
Glans penis, 77-78
Glomerular filtration rate
of neonate, 559-560
during pregnancy, 236
alterations in, 316
Glomerulonephritis, 985
Gloving procedure, 428
Glucocorticoids for respiratory distress syndrome, 912
Glucose
biochemical tests for, 329
blood, monitoring of, with diabetes mellitus during pregnancy, 850
determinations of, urine, drugs affecting, 1021
excretion of, by kidney during pregnancy, 237
for fetus, 219
levels of, during pregnancy, 247
Glucose intolerance, 844
pregnancy-induced, 845
Glucose reflectance meter, 850
Glucose screen, 1-hr, 848
Glucose tolerance
changes in, with oral contraceptives, 194
impaired, 844
Glucose tolerance test, 844, 848, 849
Glucosuria, 237
Glutethimide, effect of, on fetus or neonate, 1023
Glycohemoglobin, 844
Glycohemoglobin test, 848, 850
Glycosuria, gestational, tests for, 329
GnRH; *see* Gonadotropin-releasing hormone
Goat's milk for infant, 671
Gold thiomalate in breast milk, 1034
Gonadotropic hormone, chorionic, 211
Gonadotropin-releasing hormone, 85
and menstrual cycle, 86
Gonads
female; *see* Ovary(ies)
male; *see* Testes
pituitary, and hypothalamus, interaction between, 85, 88
Gonococcal infection causing infertility, 178
Gonococci causing puerperal infection, 832
Gonorrhea, 62, 109
in neonate, 839
during pregnancy, 828
smears to detect, 160
Gonorrheal culture, 287
Gonorrheal infection of fallopian tubes, 62
Goodell's sign, 226
Gossypol to inhibit spermatogenesis, 200-201
Graafian follicles, 86
Grain products, 333-334
Grams, conversion of pounds and ounces to, 1017
Grandparenthood, reverence for, in various cultures, 116
Grandparents, 719, 720
grief reactions from, at birth of child with disorder, 768
Grandparents—cont'd
preparation for becoming, 355-357
reaction of, to birth of high-risk infant, 778
responses of, to pregnancy, 265
role of, cultural views of, 123
Grandparent class, 356-357
Granuloma(s)
gingival, during pregnancy, 273
pregnancy, 238, 987
Granuloma gravidarum, gingival, 238-239
Granuloma inguinale, 238, 987
Grasp
palmar, 596
plantar, 596
Grasp reflex, 596, 919
and parent-child attachment, 709
Gravida, 268
Gravidity and parity, coding of, 268, 269
Great vessels, complete transposition of, 968
Greater sacrosciatic notch, female and male, contrast of, 72
Greater vestibular glands, 54, 56
Greek-American women, postpartal behavior of, 121
Grief
after birth of child with disorder, 767
at fetal death, 776, 778
at giving baby up for adoption, 945
and loss, 765-778
Grief reactions of family at birth of child with disorder, 768
Grieving, anticipatory, for premature child, 769
Grieving process, 765-766
Group B streptococcus infection, 828
Growth
intrauterine, classification of newborn based on, 913, 914
physical, and feeding behavior, 651
tissue, during pregnancy, 315-316
Growth hormone, 86
and nutrition, 316
during pregnancy, 242, 244
Growth phase of parent-child relationship
assessment of, 724
nursing actions in, 730-731
Growth retardation, intrauterine, 280
and maternal weight gain, 326
Growth status, intrauterine, 578
Grunt, expiratory, 749
Guanethidine in breast milk, 1032
Guatemalan women, labor and delivery in, 119
Guidance of parents, anticipatory
before discharge from hospital, 628-630
at first well-baby visit, 630
Guidelines for Childbirth Education, 341
Guilt vs. initiative in personality development, 135-136
Gums
bleeding
during pregnancy, 238-239
as presumptive sign of pregnancy, 273
changes in, during pregnancy, 240
Guthrie inhibition assay methods for phenylketonuria, 1028
Gynecoid pelvis, 372, 378-379
Gynecologic problems complicating pregnancy, 989
Gyne-Lotrimin; *see* Clotrimazole

H

Haase's rule, 251
Habitual abortion from small uterus, 179
Habituation in neonate, 570
Hair
changes in, during pregnancy, 273
lanugo, 564
pubic, 54
of female, 54
of male, 76, 77
Haitians, view on menstruation of, 124
Haldol; *see* Haloperidol
Haloperidol in breast milk, 1036
Halotestin; *see* Fluoxymesterone
Halothane
in breast milk, 1034
effect of, on fetus or neonate, 1022
for general anesthesia, 508, 511
Handicapped infant
birth of, sibling's response to, 135
incidence of, 739
Hand-knees position during second stage of labor, 421
Hands, numbness of, during pregnancy, 240
Hand-washing technique in nursery, 575
Haploid number of chromosomes, 206, 207
Harbor Medical Group Childbirth education classes, 344-345
Harmony
after pregnancy, returning to, 120-121
during pregnancy, 116
balance and, 116
cultural views on, 119
HbA_{1c}; *see* Glycohemoglobin
HbA_{1c} test, 848, 850
HCB; *see* Hexachlorobenzene
HBS; *see* Human chorionic somatomammotropin
Head
fetal
compression of, early deceleration caused by, 488
delivery of, 419, 420
engaged, 365, 387
and labor, 363-366
relation of, to spinal column before and after flexion, 391
station of, forceps designation relative to, 892
of neonate
assessment of, 584
circumference of, 580
measurement of, 579
molding of, during delivery, 906
of sperm, 80, 81, 207
Headache(s)
migraine, and oral contraceptives, 195
and oral contraceptives, 193
post-spinal-puncture, 904-905
during pregnancy, 240, 306
and pregnancy-induced hypertension, 689
vascular, during pregnancy, 232
Health assessment by nurses, 4
Health care
consumers of, as change agents, 5
reproductive, responsible, 110
Health care services, regionalization of, 745
Health care specialists, women's, 6
Health maintenance in postpartum period, evaluative criteria for, 700
Health promotion, 9
Hearing of neonate, 568
assessment of, 603
Heart
changes in, during pregnancy, 229
fetal, periodic auscultation of, 402
fetal development of, 216-217
growth of, 555
Heart disease
classification of, 868
congenital, 151
and hydramnios, 967
cyanotic, 967, 968-969
diagnosis of, 867-868
effects of, on pregnancy, 867
effects of pregnancy on, 867
elective abortion in, 990
ischemic, 151
medical management of, 868
nursing care of, 868-871
and pregnancy, 867-871
symptoms of, 867
Heart function in shock, 802
Heart murmurs in neonate, 555
Heart rate
changes in, during pregnancy, 232, 233

Heart rate—cont'd
fetal; *see* Fetal heart rate
of neonate, 555, 580
evaluative criteria for, 647
Heart sounds
of neonate, 555
during pregnancy, 229
Heart surgery during pregnancy, 867
Heartbeat, fetal, as positive sign of pregnancy, 275-276
Heartburn, 241, 303
Heat lamp in care of episiotomy, 701
Heat loss by neonate, 566
preventing, 620
Heat production by neonate, 566
Heat support for neonate, 630-632
Heater, overhead radiant, 630-631
Heavy metals
in breast milk, 1034
effect of, on fetus or neonate, 1024
Hedulin; *see* Phenindione
Heel stick, 637, 638
puncture sites for, 637
Hegar's sign, 225, 226, 272, 273
Height, fundal
and duration of pregnancy, 277-278
measurement of, 277-278, 279
Hemantigen test, 962
Hematocrit values during pregnancy, 232, 983
Hematologic changes during pregnancy, 232
Hematologic conditions, neonatal, 807-808
Hematologic system, effects of estrogens on, 89
Hematologic values
for neonate, 1025
standard, pregnant and nonpregnant, 1018-1019
Hematoma(s)
of labia, 55
subdural, from delivery, 909
vaginal, postdelivery hemorrhage from, 804-805
Hematopoiesis, fetal, 219
Hematopoietic system
embryonic development of, 217
of neonate, 558
Hematuria after delivery, 688
Hemodynamic monitoring, 5
Hemodynamics, changes in, during pregnancy, 230
Hemoglobin, fetal, 217
Hemoglobin values
of neonate, 558
during pregnancy, 232, 983
Hemoglobinopathy, sickle cell, 984
Hemolytic anemia, fetal, sequelae of, 962
Hemolytic disease of newborn, isoimmune, 960-964
Hemophilia, 142, 147, 800
Hemophilia A, 800
Hemophilia B, 800
Hemiphilus vaginalis vaginitis during pregnancy, 828
Hemorrhage
into abdominal organs of neonate, 906
intracranial
from birth trauma, 909
suspected, 630, 633
causing maternal mortality, 746
physiologic mechanisms to respond to, 800-801
postdelivery, 449, 802-807
from adult respiratory distress syndrome complicating pregnancy, 986
assessment for, 692
in diabetic women, 853
prevention of, 456
from spontaneous abortion, 781
subconjunctival and retinal, in neonate, 906
Hemorrhagic disorders in pregnancy, 780
Hemorrhagic shock, 800-802
Hemorrhoidal artery, middle, 68
Hemorrhoidal nerves, 68
Hemorrhoidal vein, external, 68
Hemorrhoids
after delivery
assessment for, 692
Hemorrhoids—cont'd
after delivery—cont'd
care of, 457, 701-702
during pregnancy, 241, 303
Hemostatic system and clotting, 796-797
Heparin
in breast milk, 1031
for disseminated intravascular coagulation, 799
during pregnancy, 867, 869
Heparin sodium to prevent convulsions of eclampsia, 822
Heparinized solution, discontinuance of, in umbilical catheterization, 966
Hepatic adenomas and oral contraceptives, 194
Hepatic system
embryonic development of, 219
of neonate, 561-562
Hepatic values, standard, pregnant and nonpregnant, 1020
Hepatitis A during pregnancy, 828
Hepatitis B during pregnancy, 828
Hepatocellular carcinoma and oral contraceptives, 194
Heptachlorepoxide in breast milk, 1034
Hereditary disorders, 142
Hernia(s)
abdominal, complicating pregnancy, 989
diaphragmatic, 970, 971
hiatal, 241
Heroin
in breast milk, 1035
effect of, on fetus or neonate, 1023
Herpes
genital, 827, 829
smears to detect, 160
Herpes gestationis, 238, 987
Herpes simplex virus, 109, 563
cesarean birth for mother with, 402
causing infection in neonate, 838-839
causing neonatal sepsis, 837
during pregnancy, 238
types 1 and 2, culture for, 287
Herpetic infection, 162
Herpetiform dermatitis, 238, 987
Hesseltine cord clamp, 440
Heterologous insemination, 182
Heterosexuality, 110
Heterozygous genes, 141, 142
Hexachlorobenzene in breast milk, 1034
Hexamethonium, effect of, on fetus or neonate, 1024
Hexamine; *see* Methenamine
HgF; *see* Fetal hemoglobin
Hiatal hernia, 241
Hiccup, 601
fetal, periodic, 2[illegible]
High forceps delivery, 892
High-risk infant
birth of, response of family members to, 778
care of, general, 747-763
High-risk mother and neonate, 736-1000
High-risk neonate
emotional needs of, 761
nursing care of, emotional aspects of, 761-762
nutrition and elimination in, 751-761
supportive care of, 761-762
temperature support and regulation for, 750-751
High-risk parenting behaviors, 724
High-risk pregnancy, 738-739
care of, goals for, 743, 744
categories of, 741
Hip
congenital dysplasia of, 977
dislocated, congenital, 151, 977
Hip bones, 70
Hirsutism during pregnancy, 239
History
client's review of, in first stage of labor, 395
diet, 331
family, 19
of infertile male, 182
History—cont'd
medical, 18
and nutrition assessment, 327
reproductive, 18-19
poor, as nutrition risk factor, 325
of twins, 19
History taking, psychosocial, 4
HMD; *see* Hyaline membrane disease
HMG; *see* Human menopausal gonadotropin
Hodgkin's disease, elective abortion in, 990
Holding
infant's response to, 606-607, 608
of neonate, 618, 619-620
for breast feeding, 664, 665
Holistic approach to nursing care, 3
Holistic Childbirth Institute, 1008
Holistic view of nursing, 8
Hollister cord clamp, 440
Hollister U-bag, 645-646
Hollow viscera, pain from, 66
Homan's sign, 233, 692
Home births, 542-549
legal aspects of, 44
Home Oriented Maternity Experience, 542, 1008
Homologous insemination, 182
Homosexual behaviors, prepubescent, 104-105
Homosexuality, 110
and adolescent, 108
Homozygous genes, 141, 142
Honey as sweetener, 655
Hood, plastic, for oxygen administration, 637
Hormonal control of menstrual cycle, 84
Hormonal factors in pregnancy, 242-245
Hormonal reduction after delivery, 689
Hormonal therapy, oral, for contraception, 192-195
Hormone(s)
adrenocorticotropic, 86
alpha-lipotropin, 86
alpha-melanocyte–stimulating, 86
androgenic, and male development, 219-220
antidiuretic, storage of, 86; *see also* Vasopressin
beta-lipotropin, 86
beta-melanocyte–stimulating, 86
in breast milk, 1035
chorionic gonadotropic, 211
effect of, on fetus or neonate, 1023
fetoplacental, production of, 242-244, 245-246
follicle-stimulating, 80
and menstrual cycle, 85, 86
during pregnancy, 242, 245
suppression of, during pregnancy, 223
gonadotropin-releasing, 85
and menstrual cycle, 86
growth, 86
and nutrition, 316
during pregnancy, 242, 244
increase in, during pregnancy, nutrition and, 316
interstitial cell–stimulating, 80
luteinizing, 80
and menstrual cycle, 85, 86
during pregnancy, 242
suppression of, 223
parathyroid, and nutrition, 316
pituitary, causing increased uterine activity, 490
produced by adenohypophysis, 86
sex
ovaries and, 68
steroid
secretion of, testosterone and, 80
and skeletal changes during pregnancy, 239
thyroid, for Sheehan's syndrome, 807
thyroid-stimulating, 86
Hormone analysis as fertility test, 171
Hose, elastic, during pregnancy, 299
Hospital, discharge from, anticipatory guidance of parents before, 628-630
Hospitalization
after delivery, duration of, 705
of diabetic pregnant woman, 852
HPL; *see* Human chorionic somatomammotropin
Hulka-Clemens clip for sterilization, 997

Human chorionic gonadotropin, 211
fetoplacental production of, 243, 246
immunologic assays for, as pregnancy test, 277
and morning sickness, 241
Human chorionic somatomammotropin
fetoplacental production of, 244, 246
and insulin production, 247
and insulin resistance, 845
and lactation, 228
and nutrition, 316
and sodium balance, 236
Human development, critical periods in, 208
Human fetotoxic chemical agents, 1022-1024
Human menopausal gonadotropin for anovulation, 177, 181
Human milk
composition of, 660-662
impact of maternal diet on, 660
drugs in, and effect of, on infant, 1029-1037
energy intake from, 654
manual expression of, 667
nutrient content of, 662
pollutants in, 301
production of, physiological features of, 659
Human placental lactogen; *see* Human chorionic somatomammotropin
Human sexuality, fallacies about, 111
Humerus of neonate, fractures of, during delivery, 907
Humoral antibodies, 562
Humoral pathology, 116
Husband
artificial insemination by, 182
and wife, relationship of, after birth of baby, 717
Husband-Coached Childbirth, 346
Hyaline membrane disease, 217
and cold stress, 566
Hyaluronidase
and acrosome reaction, 206
and fertilization, 178
in sperm, 80
Hydantoin homologue of mephobarbital; *see* Mephenytoin
Hydatid of Morgagni, 60
Hydatidiform mole, 787-789
Hydatoci lualba and preeclampsia-eclampsia, 812
Hyde Amendment, 45
Hydralazine
in breast milk, 1032
for pregnancy-induced hypertension, 817
to prevent convulsions of eclampsia, 822
Hydramnios, 216, 280
and congenital anomalies, 967
with diabetic pregnancies, 847
Hydration of neonate, 583
adequate, evidence of, 611
Hydrocephalus, 151, 975-976
and hydramnios, 967
Hydrocephaly, 152
Hydrochloric acid and infant digestion, 652
Hydrocortisone sodium succinate for acute bronchial asthma, 985
Hydrodiuril; *see* Thiazides
Hydrogen cyanide across placenta, 215
Hypoglycemic agents, effect of, on fetus or neonate, 1024
Hydrops fetalis, 961
Hydroxyzine pamoate
for analgesia, 510, 523
causing decreased variability in fetal heart rate, 483
causing fetal tachycardia, 481
Hygiene
general, during labor, 414
personal, in postpartum period, 701
Hymen, 54, 55-57, 59
tags of, 223
Hymenal caruncles, 56, 687
Hymenotomy, 56
Hyoscine; *see* Scopolamine
Hyoscine hydrobromide; *see* Donnatal
Hyoscyamine sulfate; *see* Donnatal
Hyperalimentation; *see* Total parenteral nutrition
Hyperbilirubinemia
causes of, 959
with cephalhematoma, 564
definitions of, 958-959
in infants of diabetic mothers, 860
in neonate, 561, 611, 958-966
nursing care for, 959, 960
pathologic, 959
physiologic, 561-562, 958-959
therapy for, 641-643, 964-966
Hypercalcemia, 322
Hyperemesis gravidarum, 241, 865-866
Hyperesthesia during labor, 414
Hyperestrogenism of pregnancy and breast tissue swelling in neonate, 567
Hyperglycemic hyperosmolar nonketotic coma, differentiation of, from hypoglycemia and ketoacidosis, 851
Hypernatremia from concentrated formulas, 655
Hyperosmolar nonketotic coma, hyperglycemia, differentiation of, from hypoglycemia and ketoacidosis, 851
Hyperparathyroidism, 246
Hyperplasia
glandular, cystic, infertility after, 179
sebaceous gland, in neonate, 564
Hyperstat; *see* Diazoxide
Hyperstimulation oxytocin challenge test, 497, 498
Hypertension, 151
after delivery, assessment for, 692
differential diagnosis of, 824
essential, 823-824
differential diagnosis of, 810
gestational, 810
and infant feeding, 676
maternal, and fetal circulation, 470
and oral contraceptives, 194
pregnancy-induced; *see* Pregnancy-induced hypertension
primary, 823
Hypertensive cardiovascular disease, 823-824
Hypertensive disorders of pregnancy causing maternal mortality, 746
Hypertensive states in pregnancy, 809-823
Hypertensive vascular disease, 823
Hyperthyroidism, 866-867
Hypertonic sodium chloride, intraamniotic injection of, 890
Hypertonic uterine contractions, 881-882
Hyperventilation
from breathing methods, 348, 349
during pregnancy, 234
Hypervitaminosis A, 322
Hypervitaminosis C, 323
Hypervitaminosis D, 322
Hypnosis
for analgesia, 523
and childbirth, 346
effect of, on fetus or neonate, 1022
Hypocalcemia
in infants of diabetic mothers, 860, 861
neonatal, 863-865
during pregnancy, 240
Hypogastric artery, 66, 67
Hypogastric nodes, 66, 68
Hypoglycemia
differentiation of, from ketoacidosis and hyperglycemic hyperosmolar nonketotic coma, 851
in infants of diabetic mothers, 860
neonatal, 863, 865
Hypophosphatemic rickets, 147
Hypospadias, 77, 980
and fertility, 161
and male infertility, 181
Hypotension
after delivery, assessment for, 692
orthostatic
following delivery, 454, 701
Hypotension—cont'd
orthostatic—cont'd
during pregnancy, prevention of, 304
supine, 470
during pelvic examination, 379
from recumbent position for labor, 411
Hypotension syndrome, supine, 285, 379, 411, 470
Hypotensive agents, effect of, on fetus or neonate, 1024
Hypotensive syndrome, 236
Hypothalamic-pituitary cycle, 85, 86
Hypothalamic-pituitary-gonadal axis, 88
Hypothalamus
effect of estrogens and progesterone on, 89
and menstrual cycle, 84, 85
Hypothermic infant, warming of, 632
Hypothyroidism, 867
heel stick for, 637
screening for, 153
Hypotonia, uterine, after delivery, 452
Hypotonic uterine contractions, 882
Hypovolemia
causing intracranial hemorrhage in neonate, 909
from sodium imbalance, 236
Hypovolemic shock in neonate, 808-809
Hypoxemia, 636
Hypoxia
fetal, monitoring for, 491
in infant, 218
causing intracranial hemorrhage in neonate, 909
Hysterectomy
cesarean, 895
for endometriosis, 179
for sterilization, 999
for therapeutic abortion, 992
Hysterosalpingogram, 175
Hysterosalpingography
to diagnose uterine anomalies, 179
as fertility test, 174
for tubal obstruction, 178
Hysterotomy for therapeutic abortion, 992, 995
Hytakerol; *see* Dihydrotachysterol

I

^{125}I in breast milk, 1033, 1037
^{131}I
in breast milk, 1033, 1037
effect of, on fetus or neonate, 1024
Iatrogenic prematurity, 909
Ibuprofen for primary dysmenorrhea, 92
ICSH; *see* Interstitial cell–stimulating hormone
Icterus gravis, 961, 962
Icterus neonatorum, 648
Ideas, generation of, in cognition, 134
Identical twins, 930
Identification
of newborn in delivery room, 443
with parent of same sex, 103
Identity
gender, development of, 103
vs. identity confusion in personality development, 136
sexual, 102
development of, 103
Idiopathic thrombocytopenic purpura, 800
IgA, 562-563
IgG, 562
IgM, 562
Ileal obstruction, congenital, 973
Ileus
dynamic; *see* Intestinal obstruction
meconium, 970
and cystic fibrosis, 155
Iliac artery, 66, 67
Iliac crest, 69, 70
Iliac nodes, 66, 68
Iliac spines, 70
Iliac veins, internal, 66
Iliac vessels, 59, 61
Iliococcygeus muscles, 57
Ilium, 70

Illegitimacy and artificial insemination, 43
Ilosone; *see* Erythromycin
Image, body, 31
and pregnancy, 255-256, 300
Imferon; *see* Iron-dextran complex
Imipramine
in breast milk, 1036
effect of, on fetus or neonate, 1024
causing phocomelia, 978
Immaturity, neonatal, and resultant problems, 741
Immediate puerperium, 686
Immune cells in human milk, 662
Immune deficiency syndrome, acquired, 841-842
Immune system, assessment of, in postpartum period, 693, 695
Immunity
of neonate, 562-563
nonspecific, 563
Immunization
active, of normal infants and children, recommended schedule for, 1038
during pregnancy, 301
sequential, in infants, 563
Immunoglobulin(s), 562-563
in human milk, 662
Rh, for Rh-negative mother, 964
Immunologic assays for HCG as pregnancy test, 277
Immunologic reactions to spermatozoa, 180
Impaired glucose tolerance, 844
Impairment, sensory, of parent and response to infant, 722-723
Impending fetal death, 776-778
Imperforate anus, 970, 974-975
and hydramnios, 967
Imperforate hymen, 56
Imperial equivalents, 1015
Imperial system, units of, 1015
Impersonal space range, 27
Implantation, 207, 210-211
low-lying, 793, 794
Implantation bleeding, 210
Implementation, 21-22
of goals during prenatal period, 297-310
planning, and evaluating care of newborn, 615-649
Impregnation, 207
In vitro fertilization, 180-181
and embryo transplantation, 42-43
Inactivation, X, 149
Inborn errors of metabolism, 219
amniocentesis to determine, 288
urine screening tests for, 1027
Inches, conversion of, to centimeters, 1016
Inclination, pelvic, 374
Incompatibility
ABO, 960
Rh, 960-964
Incompetent cervix, 63, 781
Incomplete abortion, 782, 783
Incomplete breech presentation, 368
Increased intracranial pressure in neonate, 611-612
Increased variability in fetal heart rate, 482, 483
Incubator
for oxygen administration, 637
Servo-Control, 631-632
transport, 970
Independence vs. dependence and pregnant woman, 256-257
Independent assortment, principle of, 145
Inderal; *see* Propranolol
Index, free T_4, 867
India, labor and delivery in, 119
Indians, American; *see* American Indians
Indigestion, acid, 241, 303
Indirect Coombs' test, 962
Indochinese women, labor and delivery in, 120
Indocin; *see* Indomethacin
Indomethacin
in breast milk, 1029
effect of, on fetus or neonate, 1022
for primary dysmenorrhea, 92
Induced lactation, 669-671
Induction of labor
Bishop's scale for assessing candidates for, 886, 887
indications for, 887
Industry vs. inferiority in personality development, 136
Indwelling catheter for feeding, 755-756
Inertia, uterine, 879-882
Inevitable abortion, 782-783
Infancy, digestion in, 652
Infant; *see also* Child; Neonate
accomplishment of specific behaviors by, mothers' expectation of, 946
active immunization of, recommended schedule for, 1038
addicted, nursing care of, 953-955
aggressive behavior by siblings toward, 719
appropriate for gestational age, 915
assessment of, nutritional screening and, 677-681
birth of, family adjustment to, 4-5
birth trauma to, 905-909
birth weight of, and maternal nutrition, 318
bottle-fed, stools of, 673
breast-feeding, failure to thrive in, 668-669
burping, 665, 666
care of
cultural differences in, 123-124
goals of, 17
condition of, at birth, and prenatal diet of mother, 319
cultural views of, 123
demand feeding of, 5
development of, and relationship to feeding, 651-652
dysmature, 278
of diabetic mothers, 219, 280, 859-863
and hydramnios, 967
effect of drugs in breast milk on, 1029-1037
feeding of, theories of, 5
food diary for, 681
of gestational diabetic mother, 859-863
handicapped, birth of, response of siblings to, 135
hypothermic, warming of, 632
hypoxia in, 218
large for gestational age, 913, 915
low–birth weight, 12
and adolescent pregnancy, 938
normal, feeding of, general guidelines for, 676-677
nutrient needs of, 652-657
nutritional screening questionnaire for, 678
physical condition of, and parental response, 720
placing of, for adoption, 945
postterm, 912
premature; *see* Premature infant
preterm; *see* Premature infant
recommended dietary allowances for, 653
removing, from breast, 665
at risk, care of, general, 747-763
sex of, disappointment over, 720
small for gestational age, 913, 915
stillborn
care of, 763
legal concepts regarding, 46
sucking behavior of, 665
suggested supplements for, 656
term, 912
touching of, by mother, 28
Infant drug tray, 443
Infant Kresselmann resuscitator, 442
Infant mortality, 11, 746
Infarction, myocardial, and oral contraceptives, 193
Infection
bladder, 702
breast, 833
treatment of, 668
cervical, 180
Chlamydia trachomatis, 828
cytomegalovirus, in neonate, 841
Infection—cont'd
after delivery, legal claims in, 47
with diabetic pregnancies, 847
in diabetic women after delivery, 853
of episiotomy site, 693
gonococcal, causing infertility, 178
gonorrheal, of fallopian tubes, 62
herpesvirus type 2, in neonate, 838-839
herpetic, 162
from intravenous therapy, 405
from IUD, 196
monilial, during pregnancy, 227
nursing care for, 836-837
postnatal, 832-833
during pregnancy, 827-837
causing premature labor, 910
prenatal, 827, 832
puerperal, 832-833
causing maternal mortality, 746
resistance to, in newborn, 562-563
from retained placental fragments, 452
after rupture of membranes, 402
and stress, 162
tubal, bacterial, 178
tubercular, causing infertility, 178
urinary tract
after delivery, 833
during pregnancy, 984-985
vaginal, 180
after delivery, 833-835
and fertility, 161-162
Infection control measures in nurseries, 575
Inferior fascia
of levator ani, 58-59
of urogenital diaphragm, 58
Inferior vena cava, 67
Inferior vesical artery, 67
Inferiority vs. industry in personality development, 136
Infertile couple, nursing care of, 183-184
Infertility, 163-185
behavior associated with, 184
cultural views on, 124
definition of, 163
from development of antibodies to man's sperm, 80
emotional crisis of, 183-184
and fallopian tubes, 61, 62
female; *see* Female, infertility in
history of, before pregnancy, 183
incidence of, 163
investigation of, 163-165
from IUD, 196
male; *see* Male, infertility in
and marijuana, 164
primary, 163
progesterone and, 81
religious factors leading to, 164
secondary, 163
causing sense of loss, 183
and sperm count, 83
Infiltration, intravenous, in small infant, ischemia from, 758
Infiltration anesthesia, local, tray for, 515
Influenza
immunization against, during pregnancy, 301
during pregnancy, 829
Information
privileged, 42
sources of, 18-19
Informed choice in alternative settings for childbirth, 531
Informed consent, 41
for anesthesia and analgesia, 501
for sterilization, 42
Infundibulopelvic ligament, 59-61
Infundibulum of fallopian tube, 61
Infusion
insulin, continuous, 850-851
intraamniotic, for therapeutic abortion, 991
Inguinal nodes, superficial, 68

Inguinal ring, internal, 79
INH; *see* Isoniazid
Inhalation analgesia, 508, 510-511
Inheritance
  autosomal-dominant, 146
  autosomal-recessive, 146
  biologic basis of, 141-145
  multifactorial, 150-151
  patterns of, 146-147
  X-linked, 146-147
Initial contact with woman and family, 291
Initial plan, 23
Initiating phase of parent-child interaction, assessment of, 724
Initiation phase of nurse-client relationship, 36
Initiative vs. guilt in personality development, 135-136
Injectable medication for contraception, 195-196
Injection
  intraamniotic, of hypertonic sodium chloride, 890
  intramuscular, for neonate, 637, 639, 640, 641
  intrauterine; *see* Intrauterine injection
  transabdominal intrauterine, of hypertonic sodium chloride for therapeutic abortion, 991, 994-995
  of urea solution after amniocentesis for therapeutic abortion, 995
Injury(ies) to neonate during delivery
  central nervous system, 909
  nervous system, 907-909
  peripheral nerve, 907-908
  phrenic nerve, to neonate at birth, 908
  skeletal, 906-907
  soft tissue, 906
  spinal cord, 909
Inlet, pelvic; *see* Pelvic inlet
Innervation of vagina, 68
Innominate bones, 70
Insecticide, effect of, on fetus or neonate, 1024
Insemination
  artificial; *see* Artificial insemination
  heterologous, 182
  homologous, 182
Insensible water loss
  in high-risk neonate, 752
  in neonate, 566
Insomnia during pregnancy, 307
Instrument table for delivery, 430
Instrumentation for fetal monitoring, 471-479
Instruments, sterile, lifting, 425
Insufficiency, uteroplacental, 470
  late deceleration caused by, 489
Insulin
  and breast feeding, 663, 1035
  changing needs for, during pregnancy, 845, 846, 847
  in diabetes mellitus in pregnancy, 850
    continuous infusion of, 850-851
  effect of, on fetus or neonate, 1024
  endogenous, 844
  exogenous, 844
  fetal production of, 219
  production of, during pregnancy, 247
Insulin reserve, 844
Insulin resistance in pregnancy, 845
Insulinase, 247
  and insulin resistance, 845
Insulin-dependent diabetes mellitus, 846
Insurance, nurses, 41-42
Intake and output during labor, 410-411
Integument of neonate, assessment of, 582-584
Integumentary system
  discomforts of pregnancy related to, 306
  of neonate, 563-565
    assessment of, 611-612
  during pregnancy, 238-239
Intellectual components of childbirth preparation, 346
Intensity of uterine contractions, 380-381
Intensive care nursing, 926
Intercapillary nephrosclerosis, Kimmelstiel-Wilson, 845
Intercostal retractions, 748
Intercourse
  abstinence from, in natural family planning, 188
  forms of, 110
  frequency and timing of, and fertility, 161
  penile-vaginal, alternatives to, during pregnancy, 308
  resumption of, after delivery, 704, 717
Interdependent behavior by family, 717-718
Interferon in human milk, 662
Intermediate stage of spontaneous abortion, 782
Intermittent catheter for feeding, 755-756
Internal ballottement, 274
Internal catheter, checklist for, 495
Internal cervical os, 63
  incompetent, 63
Internal female reproductive tract and supporting structures, 59
Internal fetal monitoring, 471, 476-479
Internal genitalia
  female, 59-71
    changes in, as presumptive signs of pregnancy, 273-274
    innervation of, 66, 68
    during pregnancy, 223-228
  female and male homologues of, 51, 53
  male, 79-83
Internal hydrocephalus, 975
Internal iliac veins, 66
Internal inguinal ring, 79
Internal mammary nodes, 74
Internal os of cervix, 60
Internal pudendal artery, 67, 68
Internal rotation in labor in vertex presentation, 390
International Childbirth Education Association, 346, 357, 531, 1008
Interprofessional Task Force on Health Care of Women and Children, 531
Interspinous diameter, measurement of, 374
Interstitial cells of testes, 80
Interstitial cell–stimulating hormone, 80
Interstitial portion of fallopian tube, 60, 61
Intertuberous diameter
  measurement of, 375
  of pelvic outlet, 375
Intervention, crisis, 136-138
Interview
  client, 18-19
  format for, 18
  of pregnant woman, initial, 291
Interview questions, sample, for pregnant adolescent, 946-947
Intestinal obstruction, 973
  complicating pregnancy, 990
Intestine(s)
  fetal development of, 218
  small, changes in, during pregnancy, 241
Intimacy vs. isolation in personality development, 136
Intimate space range, 27
Intolerance
  glucose, 844
  pregnancy-induced, 845
  lactose, 329
Intoxication, water, in infant, 655
Intraamniotic infusion for therapeutic abortion, 991
Intraamniotic injection of hypertonic sodium chloride, 890
Intracellular fluid of neonate, 559
Intracranial hemorrhage
  from birth trauma, 909
  suspected, 630, 633
Intracranial pressure, increased, in neonate, 611-612
Intrafamily relationships, "prying" into, 4-5
Intramuscular injection for neonate, 637, 639, 640, 641
Intramuscular oxytocin, 890
Intramuscular route of administration of medication, 504
Intranasal oxytocin, 890
Intrapartum, 268
Intraspinal narcotic method to block pain, 524-527
Intrathecal subarachnoid spinal anesthesia, care after, 702
Intratubal infection and IUD, 196
Intrauterine catheter to monitor uterine activity, 471, 476, 477, 478-479, 490
Intrauterine cavity, 212
Intrauterine device
  for contraception, 196-198
  endometrial infection from, 179
  expulsion of, 197
  and future fertility, 162
  types of, 197
Intrauterine fetal transfusion for hyperbilirubinemia, 966
Intrauterine growth, classification of newborns based on, 913, 914
Intrauterine growth retardation, 280
  and maternal weight gain, 326
Intrauterine growth status, 578
Intrauterine infection and IUD, 196
Intrauterine injection
  of hypertonic sodium chloride, transabdominal, for therapeutic abortion, 991, 994-995
  of PGF_2 alpha, transabdominal, for therapeutic abortion, 991, 995
Intrauterine sounds, auscultation of, 225
Intravascular coagulation, disseminated, 797-799
  and adult respiratory distress syndrome, 986
Intravenous fluids, effect of, on fetus or neonate, 1024
Intravenous infiltration in small infant, ischemia from, 758
Intravenous route of administration of medication, 504, 505
Intravenous therapy
  circulatory overload from, 405
  infection from, 405
  during labor, 405
Introitus
  changes in shape of, before delivery, 419
  parous, 57
  vaginal, 54, 55-56
Introspection
  by father-to-be, 261
  during pregnancy, 254
    husband's reaction to, 260
Introversion during pregnancy and employment, 299-300
Inversion of uterus, postdelivery hemorrhage from, 806-807
Inverted nipple, breast cup for, 300
Involution, uterine, 686, 687-688
Iodides and breast feeding, 663
Iodine
  allergy to, 384
  effect of, on fetus or neonate, 1024
  for hyperthyroidism, 867
  for infant, 657
  metabolism of, during pregnancy, 246
  radioactive, 867
Iopanoic acid in breast milk, 1033
"Iowa trumpet," 514
Iranian women, views on pregnancy of, 117
Iron
  in human milk, 661-664, 1034
  for infant, 656
  needs for, during pregnancy, 321, 326
Iron deficiency anemia, 983
Iron supplementation during pregnancy, 87, 232, 321, 326
Iron supplements, 335
Iron therapy during pregnancy, 983
Iron-dextran complex during pregnancy, 983
Irregular sleep state of neonate, 569
Irreversible preterm labor and delivery, care during, 912
Irritability, paradoxic, 601
Irritation, chemical, of peritoneal surfaces, 66

Ischemia
of hollow viscera, 66
from intravenous infiltration in small infant, 758
Ischemic heart disease, 151
Ischemic phase of endometrial cycle, 87
Ischial spines, 70
female and male, contrast of, 72
and pelvic measurements, 374
Ischial tuberosities, 70
Ischiocavernosus muscles, 57, 59
Ischiopubic ramus, 59
Ischiorectal fossa, extension of, 59
Ischium, 70
Ismelin; *see* Guanethidine
Isoimmune hemolytic disease of newborn, 960-964
Isoimmunization, Rh, 961
prevention of, 695
prophylaxis for, 963-964
treatment of, 180
Isolation vs. intimacy in personality development, 136
Isolation room, leaving, procedure for, 842
Isoniazid
in breast milk, 1030
effect of
on fetus or neonate, 1023
on glucose determination, 1021
Isoproterenol inhalation for bronchial asthma, 985
Isoxsuprine causing fetal tachycardia, 481
Isthmus
of fallopian tube, 60, 61
of uterus, 62
during pregnancy, 225
Italian food pattern, 330
ITP; *see* Idiopathic thrombocytopenic purpura
IUD; *see* Intrauterine device

J

Jacquemier's sign, 273
Japanese
handling of umbilical cord by, 123
infant care among, 123
use of contraceptives by, 124
welcoming of newborn by, 123
Japanese food pattern, 330
Japanese women
modesty of, 117
pregnancy diet for, 117
Jaundice
breast milk, 562
with cephalhematoma, 564
in neonate, 561, 611
Jealousy
by new father, 717
by siblings, 719
Jelly, Wharton's 213
Jejunal obstruction, congenital, 973
Jogging, secondary amenorrhea from, 177
Johns Hopkins University, ACNM-approved basic education in, 1013
Joint(s)
pain in, during pregnancy, 305
pelvic, and labor, 371-372
sacrococcygeal, and labor, 371
sacroiliac, and labor, 371
Journal of California Perinatal Association, 1011
Journal of Nurse-Midwifery, 1011
Journal of Obstetric, Gynecologic and Neonatal Nursing, 1011
Juices, introduction of, 673-674
Junction, squamocolumnar, 64, 65

K

Kahn test, 827
Kanamycin in breast milk, 1030
Kantrex; *see* Kanamycin
Kaplan's theory of sexual response, 100
Karmel, M., 346
Karyotypes, 141, 142
amniocentesis to determine, 287
of trisomy 21(G), 149
Keflex; *see* Cephalexin
Keflin; *see* Cephalothin
Kefzol; *see* Cefazolin
Kegel exercises, 57, 309, 350, 704
Kernicterus, 959-960
as complication of neonatal hyperbilirubinemia, 562
Kernig's sign, 601
Ketoacidosis, differentiation of, from hypoglycemia and hyperglycemic hyperosmolar nonketotic, coma, 851
Kidney(s)
blood flow to, during pregnancy, 230
changes in, during pregnancy, 235
development of, in infant, 651
fetal development of, 218
of neonate, 559-560
and renal function, overview of, 235
Kielland forceps, 891
Kielland sliding lock, 891
Kimmelstiel-Wilson intercapillary nephrosclerosis, 845
Kitzinger method, 346
Kleihauer-Betke smear, 695
Klinefelter's syndrome, 142, 151
and male infertility, 181, 182
Klumpke's palsy, 907-908
Knee-chest position with prolapsed cord, 407, 408, 409
Knowledge
cultural, 115
nursing, sharing, 3
Kolmer test, 827
Kreisselmann resuscitator, infant, 442
Kübler-Ross' five stages of the grieving process, 766
Kwashiorkor, 654

L

La Cuarentina, 121
La Leche League International, Inc., 1008
Labeling, gender, 103
Labia
hematomas of, 55
innervation of, 55
lacerations of, postdelivery hemorrhage from, 804
varicose veins of, 55
Labia majora, 52, 54-55, 59, 61
changes in
after pregnancy, 222-223
in response to sexual stimulation, 94
diverticular process of, 59
Labia minora, 52, 54, 55, 56, 59, 61
changes in, in response to sexual stimulation, 94
Labium; *see* Labia
Labor
birth canal during, 369-379
in breech position, 878
care of pregnant adolescent in, 945
cervical changes during, 379
comfort measures during, 411-414
complicated, comparison of, with true and false labors, 396
definition of, 362
and delivery
breathing techniques during, 348-350
cultural views of, 119-120
father's role during, 263
food during, cultural views of, 120
legal concepts during, 46
premature
irreversible or acceptable, care during, 912
nursing care of parents after, 771-772
psychologic aspects of, 769-772
discomfort during, origin of, 501
drugs to suppress, 5
duration of, 392-393
essential factors of, 362-393
false, 225, 395
comparison of, with true labor, 396
first stage of; *see* First stage of labor
Labor—cont'd
five P's in, 363
fourth stage of, 453-462
duration of, 392-393
general hygiene during, 414
impending, symptomatology of, 309-310
induction of
Bishop's scale for assessing candidates for, 886, 887
with chorioamnionitis, 402
indications for, 887
intravenous therapy during, 405
maternal position during, 411
mechanism of, 388-392
in left occiput anterior presentation, 389
steps in, 390
in vertex presentation, 388-392
normal, progress of, 398
nursing actions during, 353-355
evaluative criteria for, 463-464
onset of, 388
pain in, 352
pelvis during, 370-379
placenta during, 382
premature, 770
obstetric management of, 910-912
suppression of, 910-912
process of, 388-393
prodromal, 388
progress in, 398-402
prolonged, nursing care for, 884
psychologic response of woman to, 382
rapid, client with, 18-19
records of woman during, 416
second stage of, 418-449
duration of, 392
"silent," 398
stages of, and mean durations for nulliparas and multiparas, 392
stimulation of
in dystocia, 886-888
methods not recommended for, 890
stress in, 402-404
supporting father during, 416
third stage of, 450-453
duration of, 392
touch during, 414
trial of, for dystocia, 886
true, comparison of, with false or complicated labor, 396
uterine changes during, 379, 380
uterine muscle fibers and, 224
vaginal changes during, 379
Labor admission record, 507
Labor bed, transfer to delivery table from, 425
Labor and delivery area, atmosphere of, 414
Labor rooms, 414, 874
Labor suite, fathers in, 415-416
Labor unit, admission to, 409-410
Laboratory tests, 20
using amniotic fluid aspiration, 289
of fertile woman, 160
for pregnancy, 277
as probable sign of pregnancy, 275
in prenatal period, summary of, 296
Laboratory values
alterations in, with oral contraceptives, 194-195
standard
in neonatal period, 1025-1027
pregnant and nonpregnant, 1018-1020
Laceration(s)
of birth canal, postdelivery hemorrhage from, 803-805
cervical and vaginal, examination for, after delivery, 452
perineal, after delivery, 449
Lact-Aid Nursing Trainer, 669-670
Lactating women, milk loss in, during sexual stimulation, 309
Lactation; *see also* Breast feeding
daily food plan for, 333

Lactation—cont'd
induced, 669-671
initiation of, 228
nutritional demands of, 327
onset of, 658
recommended daily dietary allowances of nutrients for, 320-321
suppression of, 704-705
Lactiferous ducts, 73, 74, 659
Lactiferous sinuses, 72, 73, 659
Lactoferrin in human milk, 662
Lactogen, placental, human; *see* Human chorionic somatomammotropin
Lactoovovegetarian, 326
Lactoovovegetarian diet, 335
Lactoperoxidase in human milk, 662
Lactose
in human milk, 662
for infant, 655
and infant digestion, 652
Lactose intolerance, 329
Lactovegetarian diet, 336
Lacunae of Morgagni, 77, 78
LAC/USC Medical Center, ACNM-approved basic education in, 1013
Ladin's sign, 272, 273
LaDu-Michael method for phenylketonuria, 1028
Lamaze method, 346, 347-348
classes in, 299
Lambdoidal suture of fetal skull, 363, 364
Laminaria, 162, 172
Laminaria tent for therapeutic abortion, 992
Lamp, heat, in care of episiotomy, 701
Landau reflex, 601
Language
and communication, 27
and cultural differences, 125
as defense mechanism, 27
professional, 27
sign, by deaf parent, 723
social, 27
Language differences and informed consent, 41
Lanugo hair, 564, 584
Laparoscopy
as fertility test, 172-173, 176, 177
to investigate infertility, 173
surgical procedures via, 173
for tubal obstruction, 178
Laparotomy
for ectopic pregnancy, 786-787
for tubal obstruction, 178
Large for dates, 913
Large for gestational age, 913, 915
Largon; *see* Propiomazine hydrochloride
Larodopa; *see* Levodopa
Laryngeal web, congenital, 967
Lasix; *see* Furosemide
Lassitude as presumptive symptom of pregnancy, 269-270
Last menstrual period and diagnosis of prolonged pregnancy, 280
Late adolescence, sexual development in, 106, 108
Late adulthood, sexual development in, 110, 111
Late decelerations in fetal heart rate, 486, 487, 489
Late pregnancy, disorders of, 789-802
Late pregnancy classes, 342
Late puerperium, 686
Late spontaneous abortion, 782
Latent phase
of cervical dilatation, 398
of labor, 392
Lateral episiotomy, 891
Lateral sacral nodes, 66
Lateral Sims' position for delivery, 448
Lateral tubal branch of ovarian artery, 67
Lateral vesicoumbilical ligaments, 557
Latin American women, pregnancy diets among, 117
Latin American views of health and illness, 116
Law(s)
common, of torts, 40
Law(s)—cont'd
Mendel's, 145
statutory, 40
on voluntary sterilization, 996-997
Lawsuit, malpractice, 39, 40, 41
insurance to cover, 41-42
Laxatives
in breast milk, 1033
after delivery, 702
Lay midwives, 541
Lead
in breast milk, 1034
effect of, on fetus or neonate, 1024
Leafy green vegetables, 334
Leakage across placenta, 215
Leaking from breasts, 668
Learning processes in neonate, 570
Lecithin in amniotic fluid, 215
Lecithin/sphingomyelin ratio, 44, 282
and fetal lung maturity, 217
Leffscope, 469
Left fornix, 68
Left-to-right shunt in neonate, 555
Legal aspects of fetal monitoring, 493-494
Legal concepts, general, 39-42
Legal and ethical aspects of maternity nursing, 39-47
Legal requirements for filing certificate of death, 763
Legislative process, nurses' involvement in, 7
Legitimacy of child and artificial insemination, 43
Leg(s)
cramps in, during pregnancy, 305
of neonate, assessment of, 593
pain in, and oral contraceptives, 193
sensory changes in, during pregnancy, 240
Length of neonate, 577
measurement of, 579
Lenses, contact, and oral contraceptives, 195
Leocillin; *see* Penethamate
Leopold's maneuvers, 382, 383-384
Lesions, neuroocular, in oral contraceptives, 195
Lesser vestibular glands, 54, 55, 56
Let-down reflex, 660, 665
Leukemia, palm creases and, 154
Leukocytosis in neonate, 558
Leukorrhea during pregnancy, 227, 273, 834
treatment of, 307
Levallorphan, effect of, on fetus or neonate, 1024
Levallorphan tartrate, 510, 523
Levarterenol; *see* Norepinephrine
Levator ani muscle, 56, 57, 58, 61, 67
fascia of, 58, 59
Levodopa, effect of, on glucose determinations, 1021
Leydig's cells, 80
LGA; *see* Large for gestational age
LH; *see* Luteinizing hormone
Liability insurance, 41-42
Librium; *see* Chlordiazepoxide
Lidocaine for regional anesthesia, 511
Lie
fetal, 366-367, 371
longitudinal, 371
transverse, 369, 371
Life cycle of family, 133
Life role, concept of, 30
Life-style
of adolescent, 108
establishment of, in adolescence, 107
Ligament
anterior, 62, 65
broad, 60, 65
mesovarian portion of, 68
cardinal, 59, 62, 65-66
Cooper's, 74
infundibulopelvic, 59-61
Mackenrodt's (cardinal), 60, 65-66
ovarian, 60, 62, 68
posterior, 66
pubocervical, 65
Ligament—cont'd
rectovaginal, 66
round, 59, 61, 62, 65, 67
within fascial sheaths, 59
supporting uterus, 65-66
transverse, 65-66
uterosacral, 60-62, 66
uterovesical, 65
vesicoumbilical, lateral, 557
Ligamentum arteriosum, 557
Ligamentum flavum of spinal cord, 512
Ligamentum teres hepatis, 557
Ligamentum venosus, 557
Ligation, tubal, for sterilization, 997-999
Light, response decrement to, 604
Lightening, 224, 225, 388
"Lightheadedness" during pregnancy, 240
Lincocin; *see* Lincomycin
Lincomycin in breast milk, 1030
Lindemann's three phases of grieving process, 766
Line, sagittal suture, vaginal palpation of, 385
Linea alba, 69
Linea nigra, 238, 272
Linea terminalis, 70
Linear fracture of skull of neonate during delivery, 906
Linens of neonate, care of, 624-625
Linoleic acid, need for, by infant, 655
Liothyronine in breast milk, 1035
Lip, cleft, 151, 976-977
repair of, 976-977
Lipase and neonatal digestion, 560
Lipid fractions, plasma, during pregnancy, 316
Lipid-containing exfoliated cells, fetal, staining of, and gestational age, 282
Lipids, blood, biochemical tests for, 329
Lippes loop, 197
Listening as communication, 26
Listeria causing neonatal sepsis, 837
Listeria monocytogenes infection during pregnancy, 829
Listeriosis during pregnancy, 829
Lithane; *see* Lithium carbonate
Lithium carbonate
in breast milk, 663, 1036
effect of, on fetus or neonate, 1024
for manic reactions after delivery, 950
Lithonate; *see* Lithium carbonate
Lithopedion, uterine, 781
Lithotomy position for delivery, 430-431
culture and, 119-120
Littre, glands of, 77, 78
Live-born fetus, legal views of, 45
Liver
changes in, during pregnancy, 241-242
enzymes of, fetal production of, 219
fetal development of, 217, 219
of neonate, 561
"Living ligature," 802
uterine muscle fibers as, 63
Lobe(s)
of breast, 72
of placenta, 215
Lobules
of breast, 72
of testes, 80
Local infiltration anesthesia, tray for, 515
Lochia, 211, 456
in postpartum period
assessment of, 690, 692, 693
evaluative criteria for, 698
Lochia alba, 688
Lochia rubra, 688
Lochia serosa, 688
Locks, forceps, types of, 891
Loestrin 1/20, 192
Logic, propositional, 135
Longitudinal lie, 366-367, 371
Long-term variability in fetal heart rate, 482-483
Lordosis, dorsolumbar, 225, 240
Lorfan; *see* Levallorphan tartrate

Loridine; *see* Cephaloridine
Loss
"adopting out," 945
and grief, 765-778
of mother, young child's view of, 135
of mother-fetal relationship, 715
of perfect child, mourning, 767-768
sense of, infertility causing, 183
weight and fluid, in high-risk neonate, 752-753
Low cervical cesarean delivery, 893, 894
Low forceps delivery, 892
Low–birth weight infants, 12
and adolescent pregnancy, 938
Lower arm, paralysis of, from delivery, 907-908
Lower pelvic diaphragm, 57
Lower segment cesarean delivery, 893, 894
Lower sternal border, 69
Lower uterine segment, 62
Low-income mothers, 956-957
Low-lying implantation, 793, 794
Low-set ears, 979
LPH; *see* Alpha-lipotropin hormone; Beta-lipotropin hormone
L/S ratio; *see* Lecithin/sphingomyelin ratio
LSD, effect of, on fetus or neonate, 1023
Lubrication, vaginal, in response to sexual stimulation, 93, 100
Lues; *see* Syphilis
Lumbar epidural block, 512
Lumbar sympathetic block, 512
Luminal; *see* Phenobarbital
Luminal Sodium; *see* Phenobarbital sodium
Lung(s)
changes in, during pregnancy, 233
fetal development of, 217
immaturity of, in infants of diabetic mothers, 860
maturity of, fetal, 217
pharmacologic stimulation of, 912
of neonate, 558
shock, 802; *see also* Adult respiratory distress syndrome
Lupus erythematosus, 238, 987
disseminated, complicating pregnancy, 988
Luteal phase of menstrual cycle, 86-87
Luteinizing hormone, 80
and menstrual cycle, 85, 86
during pregnancy, 242
suppression of, 223
Lymphatic system of pelvic area of female, 55
Lymphatics
of breast, 74
of ovaries, 68
uterine, 66
of vagina, 68
Lysergic acid; *see* LSD
Lysozyme in human milk, 662

M

Mackenrodt's ligament, 60, 65-66
Macroglossia of neonate, 559
Macrophages in human milk, 662
Macrosomia
with diabetic pregnancies, 847
in infants of diabetic mother, 859
Macrovascular disease, 844
Magazines, nursing, 1011-1012
Magnesium in breast milk, 1034
Magnesium sulfate
effect of, on fetus or neonate, 1024
for epilepsy, 988
monitoring of, 819
for preeclampsia, 822
to prevent convulsions of eclampsia, 815-820, 822
to suppress preterm labor, 910-911
toxicity from, 911
Magnet reflex, 598, 599
Malaria, 829
Male
accessory reproductive tract glands of, 82
contraception for, 199-201
Male—cont'd
fertile, assessment data for, 161
genitals of
development and function of, 219-220
external, 77-78
internal, 79-83
of neonate, 590, 591
genitourinary tract of, lower, 78, 79
gonads of; *see* Testes
hypothalamic-pituitary-gonad interaction in, 85, 88
"independent qualities" of, 103
infertility of, factors implicated in, 181-183
pelvis of, and female, contrast of, 72
reproductive system of, 76-83
homologues in, of female reproductive system, 51-53
sexual response cycle in, 93-100
stages of sexual development in, 91
sterilization of, 999
XYY, 151
Male child, preference for, cultural views of, 123
Malformations; *see also* Congenital anomalies
cephalocaudal, and hydramnios, 967
congenital, in twins, 933
fetal, 208
abortions in cases of, 45
and maternal alcoholism, 952; *see also* Fetal alcohol syndrome
Malmstroöm extractor, 892
Malnutrition, maternal and fetal, presumptive signs of, 326
Malpractice lawsuit, 39, 40, 41
insurance to cover, 41-42
Malpresentation, fetal, and dystocia, 875-876
Mammary buds, 76
Mammary glands; *see* Breast(s)
Mammary nodes, internal, 74
Mammary papilla; *see* Nipple
Manager, maternity nurse as, 12
Mandelic acid in breast milk, 1030
Manic reactions after delivery, 950
Manic-depressive psychosis, pregnancy-related, 950-951
Mannitol for pregnancy-induced hypertension, 817
Manual examination of uterine cavity after delivery, 452
Manual expression of human milk, 667
Manual separation of placenta, 805
Maproxen for primary dysmenorrhea, 92
Marcaine; *see* Bupivacaine
Marfan's syndrome, 146
elective abortion in, 990
Marginal placenta previa, 793, 794
Marijuana
in breast milk, 622, 1035
and infertility, 164
Marriage, 109-110
Masculine social role, achieving, 105-106
Mask of pregnancy, 238, 271
Mass screening, 43-44
preconceptional, 152
Massage
cardiac, external, 635-636
closed chest, in infant, 635-636
during labor, 414
sacral, to relieve pain, 528
Mastalgia, 269
Masters and Johnson theory of sexual response, 93-100
Mastery roles, 30
Mastitis, 833
after delivery, 693
Mastodynia, 269
Mastoid fontanel of fetal skull, 364
Masturbation
in adolescence, 108-109
mutual, 110
during pregnancy, 308
Mate, role of, 4-5
Maternal and Child Health Service, 11
Maternal-child nursing, standards of care for, 1047
Maternal/Newborn Advocate, 1011
Maternity care
community trends in, 5
consumers as change agents in, 5
economics and, 4
ethical issues in, 4
introduction to, 1-47
political climate and, 4
statements on, 1005-1006
Maternity Center Association, 538, 540, 1008
ACNM-approved basic education in, 1013
childbirth education classes of, 345
Maternity client, 10-12
Maternity girdle, 299
Maternity nurse(s)
beliefs held by, 8-9
client advocacy by, 5-6, 7, 30
education of, 4-5
expanded role of, 6-7
health assessment by, 4
practice of, 3
responsibility of, 4
role of, 3-4, 12-13
expanding, 13-14
sex counseling by, 302
support provided by, 6
support of profession by, 3-4, 7
as teachers and counselors, 6
working with adolescents, 943
Maternity nurse–client relationships, 25-37
Maternity nursing
cultural aspects of, 114-126
curative activities of, 9-10
goals of, implementation of, during prenatal period, 297-298
issues and trends in, 2-7
legal and ethical aspects of, 39-47
loss and grief and, 766-767
nature and scope of, 9-10
practice of, 5-6
preventive activities of, 9
process of, 16-24
rehabilitative activities of, 10
science and art of, 5
today, 8-15
Matings, types of, results of, 145
Maturation
fetal, embryonic development and, 216-220
fetal lung, pharmacologic stimulation of, 912
follicular, in ovary, stages of, 69
Maturity rating and classification, newborn, 916
Maturity scales, neuromuscular, 920-921
Maximal breathing capacity during pregnancy, 234
Maximal slope, phase of, in cervical dilatation, 398
McCaman and Robins fluorometric method for phenylketonuria, 1028
McDonald operation for incompetent cervix, 781
McDonald's rule, 251, 278
McDonald's sign, 272, 274
MCN: The American Journal of Maternal Child Nursing, 1011
Meal pattern, sample, 335
Measles
German, 830
immunization against, 301
Meat, strained, introduction of, 674
Meatus
urethral
of female, 55, 56
of male, 77
urinary
of female, 55, 56
of male, 77
Mechanical suction apparatus, nasopharyngeal catheter with, 633
Mechanical suppression of lactation, 705
Meconium, 219, 560-561
in amniotic fluid and fetal distress, 283

Meconium—cont'd
passage of, 612
prebirth, with fetus in vertex presentation, 448-449
Meconium ileus, 970
and cystic fibrosis, 155
with midgut volvulus, 973
Meconium-stained amniotic fluid, 401-402
Medial tubal branch of ovarian artery, 67
Median episiotomy, 890, 891
Mediastinum testes, 79
Medical history, 18
Medical problems complicating pregnancy, 983-988
Medical University of South Carolina, ACNM-approved basic education in, 1013
Medicated IUD, 197
Medicine dropper, administering medication by, 842
Mediolateral episiotomy, 890, 891
Mediterranean anemia, 984
Medroxyprogesterone acetate
in breast milk, 1035
as contraceptive, 195-196
Mefenamic acid
in breast milk, 1035
for primary dysmenorrhea, 92
Megavitamin supplementation as risk factor, 326
Meharry Medical College, ACNM-approved basic education in, 1013
Meiosis, 143-144, 206
maldistribution of chromosomes during, 148
in spermatogonia, 80
Meiosis I, 143
Meiosis II, 143
Melanocyte-stimulating hormone, 86
Melasma, 987
facial, 238, 271
Mellaril; *see* Thioridazine
Membrane(s)
artificial rupture of, 888, 890
cytoplasmic, around sperm, 80
fetal, development of, 212
obturator, 59
rupture of, 397, 401-402
and spaces of spinal cord, 512
"stripping of," to induce labor, 890
Membranous dysmenorrhea, 782
Membranous urethra, 77
Memory in cognition, 134
Menarche, 54, 88
triggering of, 88
Mendel's laws, 145
Meningitis after septicemia, 837
Meningocele, 975
Meningomyelocele, 975
Menses, 88
Menstrual abnormalities from endometriosis, 179
Menstrual age, 208
Menstrual blood clots, 87
Menstrual changes and breasts, 76
Menstrual cycle, 83-85
cervical changes during, 88
history of, and fertility, 159
hormonal control of, 84
knowledge of, historical perspective on, 83, 85
length of, 86-87
phases of, 86-87
markers for, 159-160
regulation of, with oral contraceptives, 192
Menstrual extraction for therapeutic abortion, 991, 992
Menstrual period, last, and diagnosis of prolonged pregnancy, 280
Menstrual phase of endometrial cycle, 87
Menstruation, 88
blood loss from, 87
cultural views of, 124-125
duration of, 87
and endometrium, 62-63
as indication of puberty, 105
iron loss from, 87
myths about, 83
Menstruation—cont'd
painful; *see* Dysmenorrhea
retrograde, 178
Menus, sample, 335
Mepenzolate bromide in breast milk, 1032
Meperidine
for analgesia, 509, 523
in breast milk, 1035
for bronchial asthma, 985
for cholelithiasis, 987
checking for allergy to, 397
causing decreased variability in fetal heart rate, 483
causing increased uterine activity, 490
Mephenytoin in breast milk, 1031
Mepivacaine hydrochloride
checking for allergy to, 397
for regional anesthesia, 511
Meprobamate in breast milk, 1036
Meralgia paresthetica, 240
6-Mercaptopurine, effect of, on fetus or neonate, 1023
Mercurial diuretics in breast milk, 1033
Mercury
in breast milk, 1034
effect of, on fetus or neonate, 1024
Mesantoin; *see* Mephenytoin
Mesodermal germ layer, 216
Mesonephric embryonic tissue, 51
Mesoridazine in breast milk, 1036
Mesovarian portion of uterine broad ligament, 68
Mestranol
in breast milk, 1035
in oral contraceptives, 192
Metabolic adaptations to pregnancy, normal, 845
Metabolic disease of late pregnancy, 395; *see also* Pregnancy-induced hypertension
Metabolic disorders, 844-865
Metabolic needs during pregnancy, 320
Metabolic support of preterm infant, 915
Metabolism
alterations in, and oral contraceptives, 194
basal, rate of, during pregnancy, 234, 320
changes in, 246
effect of estrogens and progesterone on, 89
fetal, 218-219
inborn errors of, 219
amniocentesis to determine, 288
urine screening tests for, 1027
water, of pregnancy, reversal of, 688, 692
Metachromatic stain of urine sediment, 1027
Metaclopramide for itching, 524
Metal wall scale used to measure pelvic inlet, 373
Metals, heavy, in breast milk, 1034
Metaxalone, effect of, on glucose determination, 1021
Methacycline in breast milk, 1030
Methadone
in breast milk, 1035
effect of, on fetus or neonate, 1023
Methadone-dependent neonate, 955
Methdilazine in breast milk, 1032
Methenamine in breast milk, 1030
Methergine; *see* Methylergonovine
Methimazole in breast milk, 1037
Methocarbamol in breast milk, 1032
Methotrexate
in breast milk, 1037
effect of, on fetus or neonate, 1023
Methoxyflurane for analgesia, 508, 510
Methyl mercury in breast milk, 1034
Methyldopa
in breast milk, 1032
effect of, on glucose determination, 1021
for pregnancy-induced hypertension, 817
Methylergonovine to stimulate uterine contractions, 452
Metric system, units of, 1015
Metric system equivalents, 1015
Metronidazole
in breast milk, 663, 1031
Metronidazole—cont'd
for *Trichomonas* vaginitis, 834
Mexican women
labor and delivery practices of, 119
modesty of, 117
pica among, 118
proscriptions during pregnancy for, 119
Mexican-American families
child care in, 124
views of, regarding sexual activity during pregnancy, 118-119
views of family by, 123
welcoming of newborn by, 123
Mexican-American women
infertility in, 124
postpartal behavior of, 121
Mexican-Spanish food pattern, 331
Mexicans, pregnancy diets among, 117
Microcephaly, 152, 976
and hydramnios, 967
Microorganisms, transfer of, across placenta, 215
Microscopic examination of vaginal fluid, 401
Microvascular disease, 844
Midairway aspiration, 632-633
Midcycle bleeding, 87
Middle adolescence, sexual development in, 106, 107-108
Middle adulthood, sexual development in, 110, 111
Middle Eastern food patterns, 329
Middle hemorrhoidal artery, 68
Middle piece of sperm, 80, 207
Middle tubal branch of ovarian artery, 67
Midforceps delivery, 892
Midgut volvulus, meconium ileus with, 973
Midpelvis, 71, 371
contracture of, 875
Midplane of pelvis, dimension of, 374
Midpregnancy classes, 342
Midtract bladder, 79
Midwife
cultural views of, 117
for home birth, 542-543
lay, 541
role of, 14; *see also* Nurse-midwife
Migraine headaches and oral contraceptives, 195
Mikvah, 164
Mild preeclampsia, 813-814
Mild uterine contractions, 400, 485
Milia on neonate, 564
Military attitude of fetus, 368, 369
Milk
breast; *see* Human milk
cow's, nutrient content of, 662
goat's, for infant, 671
human; *see* Human milk
of magnesia in breast milk, 1033
and milk products, 333
skim, for infants, 672
"witch's," 76, 567
Milk blisters; *see* Sucking calluses
Milk cup, Swedish, 228
Milk duct, plugged, 668
"Milk leg," 832
"Milking" of trachea, 633
Milk-producing structures, 73
Milontin; *see* Phensuximide
Miltown; *see* Meprobamate
Mineral oil in breast milk, 1033
Minerals
concentration of, standard values for, pregnant and nonpregnant, 1019
in human milk, 661-662
for infants, 656-657
major, need for, during pregnancy, 321-322
trace
biochemical tests for, 329
need for, during pregnancy, 323
Minilaparotomy, tubal ligation by, 999
Minipill, 195
"Mini-prep," 405
Minors, abortions for, 45

Minute oxygen uptake, changes in, during pregnancy, 234
Minute ventilation, changes in, during pregnancy, 234
Miscarriage, 780; *see also* Spontaneous abortion
Missed abortion, 782, 783
Mistrust vs. trust in personality development, 135
Mitleiden, 259-260
Mitochondria of sperm, 80
Mitosis, 143-145, 210
"Mitten and bootie" cyanosis, 611
Moderate preeclampsia, 814-823
Moderate uterine contractions, 400, 485
Modesty and prenatal care, 117
Modified Ritgen maneuver, 420
Molding, 363, 364, 365, 433, 585, 906
Mole, hydatidiform, 787-789
Mongolian spots, 564-565
Mongolism; *see* Down's syndrome
Monilial infections during pregnancy, 227
Monilial vaginitis, 834
Moniliasis, oral, 612
Monitor
  fetal; *see* Fetal monitor
  transcutaneous oxygen tension, 926
Monitoring
  of blood glucose with diabetes mellitus during pregnancy, 850
  fetal; *see* Fetal monitoring
  of fetal heart rate, legal concepts regarding, 46
  fetoscope, 402-403
  hemodynamic, 5
  of infant responses, 630
  of magnesium sulfate, 819
  oxygen tension, transcutaneous, for neonate with respiratory distress, 749-750
  of parenteral fluid administration, 757-759
  of uterine activity, 485, 490-491
  of women taking ritodrine to suppress labor, 911
Monitoring techniques for fetal distress, 402-403
Monitrices and birthing rooms, 532
Monoamine oxidase inhibitors in breast milk, 1036
Monogamy, serial, 110
Monophasic temperature curve, 168
Monosomy, 147
  XO, 149, 150; *see also* Turner's syndrome
Monozygotic twinning, 930, 931
Mons pubis
  of female, 54
  of male, 77
Mons veneris, 54
Montevideo units to measure uterine contractions, 381
Montgomery, glands of, 74
Montgomery's tubercle, 73, 228, 273
Mood swings during pregnancy, 256, 306
Mood-changing drugs in breast milk, 1036
Morgagni
  hydatid of, 60
  lacunae of, 77, 78
Mormons
  parenting by, 122
  views on contraception of, 124
  views on pain of, 120
"Morning sickness," 241
  as presumptive symptoms of pregnancy, 269
  prevention and treatment of, 303
Morning-after pill, 195
Moro reflex, 596, 597
  in addicted infant, 954, 955
  during bath, 620
Morphine
  for analgesia, 509, 523
  in breast milk, 1035
  for cholelithiasis, 987
  epidural, 524-527
Morphine sulfate
  causing decreased variability in fetal heart rate, 483
  for intraspinal block, 524-527
Mortality
  infant, 11, 746
  maternal, 11-12, 745-746
  perinatal, in diabetic pregnancy, 848
Morula, 210
Mosaicism, 148
Mother
  adolescent, 937-947
  anesthetics for, causing fetal bradycardia, 481
  blind, response of, to infant, 722-723
  blood of, biochemical monitoring of, 283
  breast-feeding, counseling of, 662-667
  care for, goals of, 17; *see also* Maternity nursing
  circulation of, and placenta, 213-214
  complications of, during labor and delivery, legal concepts regarding, 46
  deaf, response of, to infant, 723
  death of, 11
  death rates for, 186-187
  dependent behavior by, 713-714
  diabetic; *see* Diabetic mother
  diet of, impact of, on milk composition, 660
  estriol levels in, to determine gestational age, 282
  exercise by, and fetal circulation, 470
  factors related to, causing high-risk pregnancy, 740, 741, 742, 745-746
  and fetal malnutrition, presumptive signs of, 326
  and fetal nutrition, 314-320
    summary of nursing care in, 336-340
  general assessment of, following delivery, 451-452
  high-risk, 736-1000
  hypertension in, and fetal circulation, 470
  immediate care of, in third stage of labor, 451-453
  Japanese, 123
  loss of, young child's view of, 135
  low-income, 956-957
  mortality of, 11-12, 745-746
  need of, for psychosocial care, 283-284
  nursing of, drug therapy in, abbreviated guide to, 663; *see also* Maternity nursing
  nursing care of; *see* Maternity nursing
  nutrition of, and condition of infants at birth, 319
  nutritional needs of, during lactation, 660, 661
  physical condition of, and response to newborn, 719-720
  physiology of, and nursing care, 686-705
  position of
    for delivery, 430-431
    following delivery, 454-456
    and fetal circulation, 470
    during labor, 411
    during second stage of labor, 421, 431
  postdelivery hemorrhage in, 449
  problems in, causing premature birth, 909
  psychologic adaptation of, to pregnancy and parenting, assessment of, 294-295
  recovery of, 453-462
  return to work by, 717-718
  rights of, 41
  role of, "classic model" of, 253
  sensitization of, to Rh factor, 961-962
  stress of, during first stage of labor, 403
  supportive care of, 297-298
  tasks of, during pregnancy, 253-255
  teaching of, about child care, 714-715
  traditional role of, 30
  transfer of, to postdelivery area, 461-462
  urinary estriol determinations in
    biochemical monitoring of, 283
    procedure for, 287
  weight of
    standard and deviations from, 318
    at term, distribution of, 317
  weight gain grid for, 319
Mother-child relationship
  beginning of, 254
  and child with disorder, 767-768
  and premature child, 770
  with twins, 934
Motherhood with dignity, 409-414
Mother-fetal relationship, loss of, 715
"Mothering," 103
"Mothering function," 707
Mother-infant unit, assessment for, 723
"Motherliness," 708
  assessment for, 723
Mother-to-be, response of, to pregnancy, 252-258
Motor nerves of uterus, 66
Motor response of neonate, assessment of, 603
Motrin; *see* Ibuprofen
Mottling of skin of neonate, 583
Mourning
  acute, 766
  of loss of perfect child, 767-768
  pathologic, 766
Mouth
  changes in, during pregnancy, 240
  of neonate, 560
    assessment of, 586-587, 612
  suctioning of secretions from, 632
Mouth-to-mouth resuscitation, 633-635
Movement
  fetal; *see* Fetus, movement of
  prepared childbirth, 531
  response of neonate to, 568
MSH; *see* Melanocyte-stimulating hormone
Muckleshoot
  view of harmony during pregnancy by, 119
  views on pregnancy of, 117
Mucosa
  of fallopian tubes, 61-62
  vaginal, 68
Mucous plug, 212
  formation of, 226
Mucous-trap catheter, DeLee, 634
  suctioning with, 633
Mucus
  cervical; *see* Cervical mucus
  in mouth of neonate, 616
  from mouth and nose, suctioning, 632
Mucus sign, peak, 171-172, 190
Müllerian embryonic tissue, 51
Multifactorial disorders, 142
Multifactorial inheritance, 150-151
Multigravida, 268
Multipara, 268
Multiple abortions, 110
Multiple fetuses, ultrasonography to detect, 152
Multiple orgasm, 100
Multiple ovulation, 19
Multiple pregnancy, 930-934
Multiple sclerosis complicating pregnancy, 988
Mummy restraint of neonate, 643-644
Mumps
  immunization against, 301
  during pregnancy, 829
Mumps orchitis, 162
Muneco, 118
Murmurs
  ejection, systolic, during pregnancy, 230
  heart, in neonate, 555
Muscle
  bladder, 56
  bulbocavernosus, 56, 57, 59
  coccygeus, 57
  cremaster, 78
  ileococcygeus, 57
  ischiocavernosus, 57, 59
  levator ani, 56, 57, 58, 61, 67
  obturator internus, 59
  pectoralis major, 71, 73
  perineal, transverse, 57, 59
  pubococcygeal, exercise of, 704
  pubococcygeus, 57, 58
  puborectalis, 57
  rectus abdominis, 58, 69
  serratus anterior, 71
  smooth cells of, of uterus, growth of, during pregnancy, 223
  of urogenital diaphragm, 58

Muscle cramps during pregnancy, 240
Muscle fibers
anal sphincter, 57
of myometrium, 62
of uterus, arrangement of, and labor, 224
Muscle relaxants, effect of, on fetus or neonate, 1024
Muscular contractions, clonic, reflex, in response to sexual stimulation, 100
Muscular dystrophy, Duchenne, 147
Muscular layers of abdominal wall, 68-69
Musculature, abdominal, changes in, in postpartum period, 689
Musculoskeletal system
changes in, during pregnancy, 239-240
discomforts of pregnancy related to, 305
Musculoskeletal problems in neonate, 977-978
Mutation, gene, 141
Mutual goals, setting, in nurse-client relationship, 35
Mutual masturbation, 110
Mutuality in parent-child attachment, 708
Myasthenia gravis complicating pregnancy, 988
Mycostatin; *see* Nystatin
Mycotic stomatitis in neonate, 842
Myelomeningocele, 151
Myerson's reflex, 595
Myocardial infarction and oral contraceptives, 193
Myocrisin; *see* Gold thiomalate
Myometrial tumors, infertility from, 179
Myometrium, 60
changes in, during menstrual cycle, 160
effects of estrogen and progesterone on, 89
extravasation of blood into, with premature separation of placenta, 791-792
of uterine wall, 62, 63
Myotonia from sexual stimulation, 93
Mysoline; *see* Primidone

N

NAACOG; *see* Nurses' Association of the American College of Obstetricians and Gynecologists
NAACOG Certification Cooperation, 13
NACE; *see* National Association of Childbirth Education, Inc.
Naegele's rule, 277
Nalidixic acid
in breast milk, 663, 1030
effect of, on glucose determination, 1021
Nalline; *see* Nalorphine
Nalorphine, 510, 523
effect of, on fetus or neonate, 1024
Naloxone, 510, 523
for neonate, 740
to reverse morphine, 525
Naming of child, 260
Naphthalene, effect of, on fetus or neonate, 1024
Naprosine; *see* Naproxen
Naprosyn; *see* Naproxen
Naproxen in breast milk, 1029
NAPSAC; *see* National Association of Parents and Professionals for Safe Alternatives in Childbirth
Narcan; *see* Naloxone
Narcotic analgesia, intravenous administration of, 505
Narcotic antagonists, 510, 523
effect of, on fetus or neonate, 1024
Narcotics
for anesthesia and analgesia, 508, 509-510, 523
and breast feeding, 663
in breast milk, 1035
causing decreased variability in fetal heart rate, 483
dependence on, and pregnancy, 953-956
effect of, on fetus or neonate, 1022, 1023
causing increased uterine activity, 490
intraspinal, to block pain, 524-527
and placenta, 215
Nardil; *see* Monoamine oxidase inhibitors
Narrative notes, nurse's, 22
Nasal route for feeding tube, 756
Nasal stuffiness, pregnancy-induced, 233
treatment of, 305
Nasogastric feeding tube, correct placement of, tests for, 755
Nasogastric tube feeding
for high-risk neonate, 754-756
nursing care after, 756
Nasopharyngeal catheter with mechanical suction apparatus, 633
Nasopharynx, aspiration of, 632-633
National Academy of Sciences, 1008
National Association of Childbirth Education, Inc., 346, 357, 1008
National Association of Parents and Professionals for Safe Alternatives in Childbirth, 531, 542, 1008
National Childbirth Trust, 1009
National Clearinghouse for Drug Abuse Information, 1009
National Committee on Homemaker Services, 1009
National Conference of Catholic Charities, 1009
National Dairy Council, 1009
National Foundation-March of Dimes, 1009, 1010
National Genetics Foundation, Inc., 1010
National Organization for NonParents, 184
National SIDS Foundation, 1009
National Society for Crippled Children and Adults, Inc., 1009
National Society for the Prevention of Blindness, Inc., 1009
National Tuberculosis Association, Inc., 1009
National Women's Health Network, 1009
Natural Childbirth, 345
Natural family planning, 188-192
Nausea and vomiting
initial plan for, 23
during pregnancy, 241
as presumptive symptoms of pregnancy, 269
progress notes for, 24
Navajo women
labor and delivery in, 119
role of, 122-123
Naxen; *see* Naproxen
NCC; *see* NAACOG Certification Cooperation
Neck
of neonate, assessment of, 587-588
of sperm, 80, 207
of uterus; *see* Cervix
Neck righting reflex, 599
Necrosis
anterior pituitary, after delivery, 807
subcutaneous fat, in neonate, 906
Necrotizing enterocolitis, 636
and early feeding, 752
neonatal, in preterm infant, 927
Needle
Crawford, 517
Tuohy, 517, 520, 521
Negative clonus response at ankle joint, 819
Negative oxytocin challenge test, 497
NegGram; *see* Nalidixic acid
Neglect, child abuse and, and premature infant, 928-929
Negligence, 40-41
Negotiation of social roles, 133
Neisseria gonorrhoeae causing neonatal sepsis, 837
Neisseria gonorrhoeae infection during pregnancy, 828
Nembutal; *see* Pentobarbital
Neo-mercazole; *see* Carbimazole
Neonatal care center, regional, transfer of preterm infant to, 915, 918
Neonatal necrotizing enterocolitis in preterm infant, 927
Neonatal nurse clinician/practitioner, 13
Neonatal period, standard laboratory values in, 1025-1027
Neonatal sepsis, 837-844
Neonate; *see also* Child; Infant
anemia, 807-808
assessment of; *see* Assessment of neonate
behavioral characteristics of, 567-572
behavioral tasks of, 554
biologic characteristics of, 555-567
breathing of, abnormal, 442
cardiovascular system of, 555-557
care of
after cesarean delivery, 901, 902
general, 616-625
planning, implementing, and evaluating, 615-649
in postpartum period, 695, 701
chlamydial disease in, 841
clearing airway for, 440
with congenital anomalies, 966-981
conjunctivitis of, 841
cytomegalovirus infection in, 841
death of, 746
incidence of, 739
depressed, emergency resuscitation of, equipment and supplies for, 443
digestive system of, 560-561
effect of diabetes mellitus on, 853, 859-863
elimination behaviors of, 572
eye care of, 442-445
factors related to, causing high-risk pregnancy, 740, 742, 746
feeding of, questions about, 300-301
feeding behaviors of, 571-572
goals for care of, 615-616
gonorrhea in, 839
handicapped, 739
hematologic conditions of, 807-808
hematopoietic system of, 558
hepatic system of, 561-562
herpesvirus type 2 infection in, 838-839
high-risk; *see* High-risk noenate
high-risk mother and, 736-1000
with hyperbilirubinemia, 958-966
hypocalcemia in, 863-865
hypoglycemia in, 863, 865
hypovolemic shock in, 808-809
identification of, in delivery room, 443
ill, and parenting disorders, 724
immaturity of, and resultant problems, 741
immunity of, 562-563
integumentary system of, 563-565
isoimmune hemolytic disease of, 960-964
methadone-dependent, 955
mistaken identities of, 41
neurologic system of, 563
normal
assessment strategies and tools for, 610-613
nursing care of, 552-683
nursing assessment and diagnosis of, 574-614
nursing care of, 439-446
nutrition of, feeding and, 650-683
oral thrush in, 842
parental response to, 458-461
physiologic tasks of, 554
polycythemia in, 807-808
positioning of, 618, 619-620, 636
premature; *see* Premature infant
prone position of, 917
renal system and water balance in, 559-560
reproductive system of, 567
with respiratory distress, nursing of, 747-750
respiratory system in, 558-559
responses of, monitoring and recording of, 630
restraining of, 643-645
rubella in, 838
sensory behaviors of, 567-569
sepsis in, nursing care of, 865
skeletal injuries to, during delivery, 906-907
sleeping and waking behavior of, 569-571
small-for-gestational-age, nutrition for, 751
social behaviors of, 571
sole creases in, 917
suctioning of, 632-633

Neonate—cont'd
symptoms of, to report to physician, 629
syphilis in, 839-841
tetany of, 864
thermogenesis in, 566-567
transfer of, to postdelivery area, 461-462
weighing of, 578
weight loss of, 647-648
withdrawal in, signs of, 955
Neonate and parent interaction, statements on, 1006
Neoplastic disease and oral contraceptives, 194
Neopresol; *see* Hydralazine
Neostigmine
in breast milk, 1032
for neonate showing myasthenic signs, 988
Nephrosclerosis, intercapillary, Kimmelstiel-Wilson, 845
Nephroureterolithiasis, 985
Nerve(s)
autonomic, of uterus, 66
hemorrhoidal, 68
motor, of uterus, 66
pelvic, compression of, during pregnancy, 240
peripheral, injury to, in neonate during delivery, 907-908
phrenic, injury to, in neonate at birth, 908
pudendal, 68
sacral, and uterus, 66
sensory, of uterus, 66
Nerve block
peridural, 513, 516
peripheral, 513
Nerve root block, 513
Nerve stimulation, transcutaneous electrical, 528
"Nervous breakdowns" and pregnancy, 950
Nervous system
central, effects of estrogen and progesterone on, 89
fetal development of, 218
injuries of, to neonate during delivery, 907-909
"Nervousness," counseling about, 298
Neural crest, 218
Neural plate, 218
Neural tube defects, 218
amniocentesis to determine, 288
Neurofibromatosis, 238, 987
Neurohypophysis, 86
Neurologic assessment of neonate, 594-601
Neurologic changes during pregnancy, 240
Neurologic disorders complicating pregnancy, 987-988
Neurologic functioning, assessment of, 563
Neurologic system
congenital anomalies of, screening for, 967
discomforts of pregnancy related to, 306
embryonic development of, 218
of neonate, 563
Neuromuscular behavior, fetal, 218
Neuromuscular development and feeding behavior, 651, 653
Neuromuscular maturity scales, 920-921
Neuroocular lesions and oral contraceptives, 195
Nevus(i)
spider, 304
telangiectatic, 565
Nevus flammeus, 565
Nevus vasculosus, 565
New Beginnings, Inc., 539
Newborn; *see* Neonate
Newborn maturity rating and classification, 916
Niacin and oral contraceptives, 194
Nicotine, 215
in breast milk, 662, 1037
and male infertility, 182
Nida state, 164
Nidation, 207, 210-211
Night sweats after delivery, 692
Nipple, 72, 73, 74
changes in, during pregnancy, 228
discharge from, 272
inverted or retracted, breast cup for, 300
Nipple—cont'd
preparation of, for breast feeding, 300
sore, 667-668
Nipple rolling to prepare for breast feeding, 668
Nisentil; *see* Alphaprodine
Nitrazine paper; *see* Phenaphthazine paper
Nitrites in infant food, 674
Nitrofurantoin
in breast milk, 1030
effect of, on fetus or neonate, 1022
for urinary tract infection during pregnancy, 985
Nitrous oxide
for analgesia, 508, 511
for cesarean birth, 524
Noctec; *see* Chloral hydrate
Nocturia during pregnancy, 237
Nodes, lymphatics to
from breast, 74
from ovaries, 68
from uterus, 66
from vagina, 68
Nodules, breast, and menstrual cycle, 76
Nonadherent placenta, postdelivery hemorrhage from, 805
Noncompliance, client, 35
Nondisjunction, 148
Noninflammatory pruritus of pregnancy, 238, 987
Noninvasive nonpharmacologic relief of discomfort, 528
Nonmedicated IUD, 197
Nonparous cervix, 63
Nonpharmacologic noninvasive relief of discomfort, 528
Nonreactive nonstress test, 496
Nonshivering thermogenesis, 566
Nonspecific immunity, 563
Nonstress test
in diabetic pregnant woman, 852
and fetal heart rate, 282
Nonstress testing, 5, 496, 497
Nonverbal communication
time as, 29
touch as, 28
Noradrenalin; *see* Norepinephrine
Norepinephrine causing increased uterine activity, 490
Norethindrone in breast milk, 1035
Norethynodrel
in breast milk, 1035
in oral contraceptives, 192
Norlutin; see Norethindrone
Normal labor, progress of, 398
Norpramin; *see* Desipramine
19-Nortestosterone in breast milk, 1035
Nortriptyline, effect of, on fetus or neonate, 1024
Norwegian food patterns, 331
Nose of neonate
assessment of, 586
cleansing of, 621
suctioning of secretions from, 632
Notch, sciatic, sacral, 70
Notes
narrative, nurse's, 22
progress, nursing, legal importance of, 41
Novobiocin
in breast milk, 1030
effect of, on fetus or neonate, 1022
Novocain; *see* Procaine
NST; *see* Nonstress testing
Nuchal cord, 471
tight, 449
Nuclear family, 129-131
American, 122
Japanese, 123
Nucleus
of ovum, 207
of sperm, 207
Nulligravida, 268
Nullipara, 55, 268
Numbness
of fingers during pregnancy, 306
Numbness—cont'd
of hands during pregnancy, 240
Nurse; *see also* Maternity nurse
and alternative settings for childbirth, 549
assistance to client with decision making by, 33-34
and client, trusting relationship between, 19
and infertile client, 164-165
and infertility, 183-184
involvement of, in legislative process, 7
liability insurance, 41-42
narrative notes of, 22
options for, 6-7
psychosocial role of, in care of parents after birth of child with disorder, 767-769
reasonably prudent, 40
and fetal monitoring, 494
role of
in client decision making, 33
in genetic counseling, 155-156
Nurse practitioner
family, 6
obstetric-gynecologic, 13, 14
Nurse Practitioner: A Journal of Primary Nursing Care, 1011
Nurse specialists, clinical, 6
Nurse-client relationship, 297, 298
Nurse-midwife, 13-14
certified, 6, 541
education of, 1013-1014
legal view of, 42
Nurse-midwifery, 541
Nurse-physician relationship, 3
Nurses' Association of the American College of Obstetricians and Gynecologists, 13, 14, 40, 341, 357, 531, 1009
on nurses' role with abortion client, 990
Nursery
admission of preterm infant to, 915
intensive care, 926
standards for, 575
transitional, 574-575
Nursing
"couple," 695
holistic view of, 8
maternity; *see* Maternity nursing
Nursing actions
toward client during prenatal period, 298-310
goal for, 21
for normal newborn, evaluative criteria for, 647-649
priority in, 22
selection of, 22
Nursing assessment and diagnosis of newborn, 574-614
Nursing bottle syndrome, 675
Nursing care
of addicted infant, 953-955
after cesarean delivery, 901, 904-905
for cesarean delivery, 895-905
culturally sensitive, 114-126
of diabetic mother, 853, 854-855
for dystocia, 884-886
after gavage tube feeding, 756
for heart disease, 868-871
of high-risk neonate, emotional aspects of, 761-762
for hyperemesis gravidarum, 866
in induction of labor, 888
of infant with congenital anomalies, 970-971
for infant birth trauma, 906-909
for infections, 836-837
during labor, evaluative criteria for, 463-464
maternal physiology and, 686-705
for medical complications during pregnancy, 988
of mother and fetus during second stage of labor, 421-439
for neonatal hypocalcemia, 864
in neonatal sepsis, 837-838, 842-844
of neonate with respiratory distress, 747-750
of newborn, 439-446

Nursing care—cont'd
of normal newborn, 552-683
of parents
experiencing ectopic pregnancy, 773
experiencing premature labor and delivery, 771-772
experiencing spontaneous abortion, 773
related to pharmacologic control of discomfort during birth period, 500-501, 504-508
postpartum; *see* Postpartum nursing care
for preeclampsia and eclampsia, 820-823
of pregnant adolescent, 943-945
during prenatal period, 267-312
of preterm infant, 915-925
for surgical conditions coincident with pregnancy, 990
in voluntary sterilization, 999-1000
of woman with fetal monitoring, 491-495
Nursing care plan, 22
chart for, 696
Nursing diagnosis
and assessment of newborn, 574-614
during first stage of labor, 404
formulating, 20-21
during fourth stage of labor, 454
in newborn care, 439
regarding parental behavior, 729-730
in postpartum period, 695
in prenatal period, 291
during second stage of labor, 421
validation of, 21
Nursing knowledge, sharing, 3
Nursing magazines and publications, 1011-1012
Nursing mothers, drug therapy in, abbreviated guide to, 663; *see also* Breast feeding
Nursing practice, legislated definition of, 40
Nursing process, 16, 17
Nursing progress notes, legal importance of, 41
Nursing Research, 1011
Nursing skills, sharing, 3
Nurturing in family, 133
Nutrient(s)
blood-forming, tests to measure, 327
excretion of, by kidneys during pregnancy, 237
transfer of, across placenta, 215
Nutrient content of human milk and cow's milk, 662
Nutrient needs
of infants, 652-657
during pregnancy, 320-325
Nutrition
community, guidelines for population groups in, 682
for high-risk neonate, 751-761
and male infertility, 182
maternal
and condition of infant at birth, 319
and fetal, 314-340
in neonate with respiratory distress, 749
newborn, 650-683
and oral contraceptives, 194
in postpartum period, 702
and preeclampsia-eclampsia, 812
total parenteral; *see* Total parenteral nutrition
Nutrition assessment, 327-331
Nutrition guidelines for pregnancy, 327-336
Nutrition questionnaire, 329, 332
Nutrition risk factors in pregnancy, 325-327
Nutritional counseling, 299, 331, 335-336, 339
Nutritional intervention in clinical practice, 681-683
Nutritional needs
after delivery, maintaining, 458
for high-risk neonate, 752
maternal
during lactation, 660, 661
in pregnancy, basis for, 315-320
of pregnant adolescent, 944-945
Nutritional risk, children at, 679-681
Nutritional screening and assessment of infants, 677-681
Nutritional screening questionnaire for infants, 678
Nutritional status, physical assessment of, 328
Nutritional supplements during pregnancy, 323
Nydrazid; *see* Isoniazid
Nystatin
in breast milk, 1030
for monilial vaginitis, 834
for oral thrush, 842

O

Obesity
development of, 655
and infant feeding, 675-676
and male infertility, 181, 182
and pregnancy, 318, 320
Objective data in problem-oriented record, 23
Observation of client, 19
Observer role of father, 263
Obstetric client and general surgical client, comparison of, 504
Obstetric conjugate, diameter of, 373
Obstetric labor admission record, 507
Obstetric measurements, 373-378
Obstetric operations, 890-892
Obstetric-gynecologic nurse practitioner, 13, 14
Obstruction, intestinal, 973, 990
Obturator artery, 67
Obturator foramen, 70
Obturator internus fascia, 59
Obturator internus muscle, 59
Obturator membrane, 59
Occipital presentation, 368, 369, 370
Occipitoanterior presentation, molding in, 365
Occipitofrontal diameter of fetal skull, 365
Occipitomental diameter of fetal skull, 365
Occipitoposterior presentation, molding in, 365
Occiput anterior position, abdominal contours in, 879
Occiput posterior position, 878-879
persistent, 392
Occiput transverse position, persistent, 392
Occlusion
tubal, for sterilization, 997-999
umbilical cord, 470-471
OCT; *see* Oxytocin challenge test
ΔOD analysis, 962, 963
Odor and parent-child attachment, 710
Office of Economic Opportunity, 11
Oily skin during pregnancy, 239, 273
Old age
personality development in, 136
sexual fulfillment in, 111
Older woman, response of, to pregnancy, 721
Oligohydramnios, 216, 402
and congenital anomalies, 967
Oligospermia from autoimmunity, 181
Oliguria, 236
Omnipen; *see* Polycillin
Omphalocele, 218, 972-973
One-stage prothrombin time, 798
Oocytes, 86
primary, 144
secondary, 144, 145
Oogenesis, 144, 206
Oogonium, 144
Open marriage, 110
Opening statements, broad, and communication, 26
Openness during pregnancy, 256
Operation; *see also* Surgery
McDonald, for incompetent cervix, 781
obstetric, 890-892
Operculum, 212
formation of, 226
Ophthalmia neonatorum, eye care to prevent, 442, 444-445
Opium, tincture of, for addicted infant during withdrawal, 955
Oral contraceptives, 192-195
and breast feeding, 663
and drug interactions, 195
and future fertility, 162
Oral contraceptives—cont'd
and lactation, 660
for primary dysmenorrhea, 92
Oral feedings
for high-risk infant, 753
initial, 676-677
Oral hormonal therapy for contraception, 192-195
Oral insertion of feeding tube, 755-756
Oral thrush in neonate, 842
Oral-genital intercourse, 110
during pregnancy, 308
Ora-Testryl; *see* Fluoxymesterone
Orchiopexy, 79
Orchitis
and fertility, 161
and male infertility, 181
mumps, 162
Oretic; *see* Thiazides
Organization in cognitive development, 134
Organochlorine, effect of, on fetus or neonate, 1024
Organs
abdominal, of neonate, hemorrhage into, 906
pelvic, female, midsagittal view of, 61
Orgasm, 100-101
Orgasmic phase of sexual response cycle, 93, 98
"Orgasmic platform," 93, 100
Orientation, sexual, 110
Orientation response of neonate, 606
Orifice
urethral, 56
vaginal, 61
Orinase; *see* Tolbutamide
Oropharynx, aspiration of, 632-633
Orthostatic hypotension
in postpartum period, 454, 701
during pregnancy, prevention of, 304
Ortolani's sign, 977
assessing for, 592
Os, cervical; *see* Cervical os
Osteogenesis imperfecta, 146
Osteoporosis, 177
Otitis media from propping of bottle, 672
Otolith righting reflex, 601
OURS, Inc., 184
Outlet, pelvic, 71, 371, 372
Output and intake during labor, 410-411
Ovarian artery, 66, 67, 68
Ovarian branch of uterine artery, 67
Ovarian cycle, 86-87
Ovarian ligament, 60, 62, 68
Ovarian veins, 68
Ovarian vessels, 67
Ovary(ies), 59, 60, 61, 68
blood supply to, 68
cancer of, and oral contraceptives, 192
changes in
during menstrual cycle, 160
during pregnancy, 246
cross section of, 69
cysts of
and oral contraceptives, 192
during pregnancy, 989
development of, 219
and follicle-stimulating hormone, 86
functions of, 68
innervation of, 68
location of, 68
luteinizing hormone and, 86
lymphatics of, 68
of neonate, 567
during pregnancy, 223
structure of, 68
support of, 68
tumors of, excision of, 177
twisted or blocked, from IUD, 196
Overdosage, oxygen, 636
Overhead radiant heater, 630-631
Overt diabetes, 844
Over-the-shoulder technique for breast feeding, 666

Overweight and infant feeding, 675-676
Ovulation, 68, 86
 and fertility, 177-178
 induction of, for in vitro fertilization, 181
 multiple, 19
Ovulation method of contraception, 190
Ovulatory agents, effect of, on fetus or neonate, 1023
Ovulatory periods, establishing, 89
Ovum(a)
 diagram of, 207
 fertilized; *see* Zygote
 primordial, 69
 and sperm, union of, 206
Ovum stage of development, 207
Oxacillin in breast milk, 1030
Oxycodone
 in breast milk, 1035
 for relief of pain of episiotomy, 701
Oxycodone aspirin; *see* Percodan
Oxygen
 administration of, methods of, 637
 for cardiac decompensation, 870
 dosage of, regulating, 636-637
 needs and administration of, to neonate with respiratory distress, 749-750
 overdosage of, 636
 for respiratory distress syndrome, 926
 supply of, to neonate, maintaining, 616
 transfer of, across placenta, 215
Oxygen consumption in cold stress, 566
Oxygen tension monitor, transcutaneous, 926
Oxygen tension monitoring, transcutaneous, for neonate with respiratory distress, 749-750
Oxygen therapy, 636-637
 weaning from, 750
Oxygen toxicity
 and prematurity, 926-927
 from shock therapy, 802
Oxygen uptake, minute, changes in, during pregnancy, 234
Oxyphenbutazone in breast milk, 1029
Oxytocin
 and breast feeding, 658, 660
 after cesarean delivery, 904
 after delivery, 688
  lochia and, 692
 effect of, on fetus and neonate, 1024
 function of, 86
 intramuscular, 890
 intranasal, 890
 for inversion of uterus, 806
 and labor and delivery, 245
 after multiple births, 934
 in preterm labor, 912
 for secondary uterine inertia, 882
 for shock after delivery, 456
 for spontaneous abortion, 783
 stimulation of labor with, 887-888
  in dystocia, 887–888
 to stimulate uterine contractions following delivery, 453
 storage of, 86
 for uterine bleeding, 803
 and uterine contractions, 381
 causing uterine hyperstimulation, 491
Oxytocin challenge test, 496-498
 and fetal heart rate, 282-283

P

Pads, perineal, 701
Pain
 abdominal, during pregnancy, 242
 in childbirth, 352-353
 from endometriosis, 179
 expression of, cultural variations in, 120
 gate control theory of, 353
 joint, during pregnancy, 305
 in labor, 352
  relief of, 414
Pain—cont'd
 and oral contraceptives, 193
 pathways of, and sites of interruption, 512
 in postpartum period, evaluative criteria for, 699
 round ligament, during pregnancy, 307
 sciatic, during pregnancy, 240
 shoulder
  referred, from ruptured extrauterine pregnancy, 785
  from subphrenic irritation, 174
 from uterus and tubes, 66
Pain sensations, unexpected, during labor, 884, 886
Pairs, gene, 142
Palate, cleft, 151, 976-977
 and hydramnios, 967
 repair of, 977
Paleness in neonate, 611
Palm creases to detect genetic disorders, 154
Palmar erythema, 238, 987
 treatment of, 305
Palmar grasp, 596
Palpation, 19-20
 abdominal, to determine fetal presentation, position, and descent, 382-384
 of cephalic prominence, 383
 of fetal back and small parts, 383
 of fetal movements as positive sign of pregnancy, 276
 of fetal outline as positive sign of pregnancy, 276
 of fundus of uterus after delivery, 455, 456
 of superior pole of fetus, 383
 of vaginal, or sagittal suture line, 385
Palpitations during pregnancy, 304
Palsy
 cerebral, choreoathetoid, 959, 962
 Klumpke's, 907-908
Pancreas
 changes in, during pregnancy, 247
 fetal development of, 219
Panmycin; *see* Tetracycline
Panting breaths, 349
 to control urge to push, 382
Panwarfin; *see* Warfarin
Papanicolaou smear, 65, 68, 110, 160, 285, 287
Papilla, mammary; *see* Nipple
Para-aminosalicylic acid in breast milk, 1030
Paracervical block, 512, 513
Paradione; *see* Paramethadione
Paradoxic irritability, 601
Paraldehyde, effect of, on fetus or neonate, 1024
Paralysis
 of arm from delivery, 907-908
 brachial, from delivery, 907-908
 diaphragmatic, in neonate, 908
 Erb-Duchenne, 907, 908
 facial, from delivery, 908
Paramethadione, effect of, on fetus or neonate, 1022
Parasympatholytics causing decreased variability in fetal heart rate, 483
Parathormone levels during pregnancy, 246
Parathyroid glands, changes in, during pregnancy, 246
Parathyroid hormone and nutrition, 316
Paraurethral duct, orifice of, 56
Paraurethral glands, 54, 55
Paregoric for addicted infant during withdrawal, 955
Parenchyma of breast, 72
Parent(s)
 age of, and response to infant, 720-722
 in American family, 122
 anticipatory guidance of, 628-630
 care of, after birth of child with disorder, 767-769
 coping mechanisms of, 716-717
 emotional needs of, after delivery, support of, 458-461
 expectations of, and response to infant, 720
 expected behavior of, among various cultures, 116-119
 goals for, in care of neonate, 615-616
Parent(s)—cont'd
 identification of child with, and sexual development, 103
 and newborn, interaction between, 1006
 in nuclear family, 129
 of premature infant, postpartum care of, 912
 psychosocial stress of, 9
 reactions of, to childbearing, cultural differences in, 122-124
 responses of
  assessment of, 723-729
  factors influencing, 719-723
  to newborn, 458-461
 role of
  adjustment to, 714-718
  assumption of, 31
   reality phase of, 711-718
  development of, stages of, 713-718
  perception of, 714-715
  redefinition of, after birth of child with disorder, 769
  situational supports of, 715-716
 of stillborn child, care of, 762-763
 tasks of, 713
 views of, cultural variations in, 122-124
Parent education, 341-343
 organizations involved in, 357
Parent-baby interaction, assessment tool for, 725-729
Parent-child attachment, 708-710
 contact and, 710-711
 in postpartum period, 695, 701
Parent-child relationship, 133
 assessment of, 724-729
 and child with disorder, 767-768
 after delivery, 446-447
 evaluative criteria for, 732
 psychologic components of, 708
Parenteral fluids
 administration of, monitoring of, 757-759
 for high-risk infant, 753
 for neonate with respiratory distress, 749
Parenteral therapy, weaning from, 753
Parenthood, 707-708
 adolescent, 937-947
 after age 30, 722
 and childbirth education, 299
 cultural views of, 122-123
 developmental tasks of, during adolescence, 942-943
 maternal psychologic adaptation to, assessment of, 294-295
 in persons over 30 years, 720-722
 preparation for, during childhood, 116
 responsibilities of, 9
 reverence for, in various cultures, 116
Parenthood tasks with newborn, 647, 648, 649
Parenting; *see also* Parent(s); Parenthood
 alterations in, 20
 difficulties in, 724
 disorders in, 724
  signs indicating potential for, 284
 preparation for, 341-357
 quality of, indicators of, 725
Parenting behaviors, high-risk, 724
Parents clubs for parents of infants in intensive care nurseries, 928
Parents Without Partners, Inc., 1009
Parietal cells of stomach, 560
Parietal eminence of fetal skull, 363, 364
Parietal peritoneum of uterine wall, 63
Parity, 268
 and gravidity, coding of, 268, 269
Parlodel; *see* Bromocriptine mesylate
Parotitis, epidemic, immunization against, 301
Parous cervix, 63
Parous introitus, 57
Partial placenta previa, 793, 794
Partial separation of placenta, estriol levels and, 282

Partial thyroidectomy for hyperthyroidism, 867
Partogram of time in labor, 883
Parturient, 268, 362
Parturition, 268, 362
Passive immunity of neonate, 562
Patau's syndrome, 150
Patches, eye, during phototherapy, 641, 642
Patellar reflex, elicitation of, 818
Patent ductus arteriosus, 969
Pathologic hyperbilirubinemia, 959
Pathologic mourning, 766
Pathologic retraction ring, 380, 882
Pathology, humoral, 116
Patient Counseling Library, 1009
Patterns
food, cultural, 329-331, 335
fetal heart rate
abnormal, 407
recognition of, 479-491
meal, sample, 335
pseudosinusoidal, in fetal heart rate, 483
sinusoidal, in fetal heart rate, 483, 484
PBB; *see* Polybrominated biphenyl
PCBs; *see* Polychlorinated biphenyls
Peak mucus sign, 171-172, 190
Pectoral nodes, anterior, 74
Pectoralis major muscle, 71, 73
Peer group influence during adolescence, 105, 107, 108
Pelvic area of female, lymphatic system of, 55
Pelvic brim, 70, 371
Pelvic cavity, 371, 374
female and male, contrast of, 72
Pelvic congestion syndrome, 224
Pelvic contraction, 874
Pelvic diaphragm, 56-57
Pelvic dystocia, 874-875
Pelvic floor, 222
exercises for, 350
and perineum, 56-59
Pelvic girdle of fetus during labor, 366
Pelvic inclination, 374
Pelvic inflammatory disease, 162
and IUD, 196
and oral contraceptives, 192
Pelvic inlet, 70, 71, 371
anteroposterior diameters of, 373
contracture of, 875
female and male, contrast of, 72
oblique diameter of, 374
plane of, measurement of, 373-374
transverse diameter of, 374
Pelvic joints and labor, 371-372
Pelvic nerves, compression of, during pregnancy, 240
Pelvic organs, female, midsagittal view of, 61
Pelvic outlet, 71, 371, 372
contracture of, 875
dystocia of, 378
plane of, 374-375, 378
Pelvic rocking, 351
Pelvic tilt, 374
Pelvimeter, Thom's, to measure intertuberous diameter, 375
Pelvimetry, computed tomography; *see* Computed tomography
Pelvimetry chart, x-ray, 377
Pelvis, 59
adequacy of, diagnosis of, 875
android, 372, 378, 875
anthropoid, 372, 378
blood supply of, 67
bony, 69-71
assessment of, 370-373
measurement of, methods of taking, 371
relaxation of joints and ligaments of, 274
classification of, 378-379
diameters of, measurement of, to anticipate dystocia, 875
examination of
anxiety during, 164
Pelvis—cont'd
equipment used for, 286
procedure for, 285
false, 70, 71, 371
female, 71
adult, showing origin of parts, 70
pure and mixed types of, 378
gynecoid, 372, 378-379
inadequacy of, diagnosis of, 875
during labor, 370-379
landmarks of, 71
male and female, contrast of, 72
mid, 71
midplane of, dimensions of, 374
platypelloid, 378
renal, changes in, during pregnancy, 235
true, 70-71, 371
cavity of, 374
planes of, 372
types of, 378, 379
and woman's body build, 372-373
variations in, 71
Pemphigus, 238, 987
Penbritin; *see* Polycillin
Penethamate in breast milk, 1030
Penfluridol in breast milk, 1036
Penicillin, prophylactic use of, for cardiac disease, 868
Penicillin G, benzathine, in breast milk, 1031
Penicillin G, potassium, in breast milk, 1031
Penicillin ointment in eyes of newborn, 902
Penile urethra, 78
Penile-vaginal intercourse, alternatives to, during pregnancy, 308
Penis, 77-78
abnormalities of, and male infertility, 181
changes in, in response to sexual stimulation, 96
circumcised; *see* Circumcised penis
transverse section of, 78
uncircumcised, care of, 628
Pentazocine
for analgesia, 509
in breast milk, 1029
causing decreased variability in fetal heart rate, 483
Penthrane; *see* Methoxyflurane
Pentobarbital
for analgesia, 509
in breast milk, 1032
Pentobarbital sodium
for analgesia, 523
causing decreased variability in fetal heart rate, 483
Pentothal; *see* Thiopental sodium
Peppermint, spirits of, to aid voiding, 456, 702
Pepsin and neonatal digestion, 560
Peptic ulcers, 151, 241, 987
Perception
in cognition, 134
of parental role, 714-715
Percodan; *see* Oxycodone
Percussion, 20
Perfect child, mourning loss of, 767-768
Perforation of uterus from IUD, 196
Perfusion, placental, reduced, from sodium imbalance, 236
Pergonal; *see* Human menopausal gonadotropin
Periaortic nodes, 68
Peridural nerve block, 513, 516
Perinatal asphyxia in infants of diabetic mothers, 861
Perinatal mortality, 11, 746
in diabetic pregnancy, 848
Perinatal period, 268
Perinatal Press, 1011
Perinatal signs and factors indicating congenital anomalies, 967-970
Perinatology, development of, 574
Perineal artery, 59, 67
Perineal body, 57, 59
Perineal muscles, transverse, 57, 59
Perineal pads, 162, 701
Perineal tightening, 309
Perineum, 54, 56, 57, 59
assessment of, after delivery, 693
blood supply of, 67
care of, in postpartum period, 701
central tendon of, 58
changes in, during pregnancy, 222
cleansing of, 430
lacerations of, after delivery, 449
hemorrhage from, 804
pelvic floor and, 56-59
Periodic auscultation of fetal heart, 402
Periodic fetal hiccough, 217
Peripheral nerve block, 513
Peripheral nerves, injury to, in neonate during delivery, 907-908
Peristaltic activity of fallopian tubes, 61
Peritoneal exclusion cesarean delivery, 893, 895
Peritoneum, 58, 59
factors related to, in female infertility, 178
parietal, of uterine wall, 63
surfaces of, stretching of, 66
Peritonitis, 989
Periurethral gland, orifice of, 56
Pernicious vomiting of pregnancy; *see* Hyperemesis gravidarum
Persistent occiput posterior or occiput transverse position, 392
Personal aspirations, interference with, and parental responses, 722
Personal characteristics and nurse-client relationship, 34-35
Personal hygiene in postpartum period, 701
Personal space, 28
Personal values, 31
Personality(ies)
androgynous, 103
development of, 134, 135-136
Personnel
for care of neonate, 574-576
in postpartum unit, 701
Pertofrane; *see* Desipramine
Pesticides
effect of, on fetus or neonate, 1024
in human milk, 662
Petechiae on neonate, 612, 906
PG; *see* Prostaglandin(s)
PGE, 92
PGE_1, 92
PGE_2, 92
PGF, 92
$PGF_2\alpha$; *see* Prostaglandin F_2 alpha
pH
fetal
assessment of, 491
scalp, testing of, 5
and sperm motility, 82
of vaginal fluid, 401
Pharmacologic analgesia and anesthesia, 508-509
Pharmacologic control
of discomfort during birth period, 500-528
of pregnancy-induced hypertension, 816-817
Pharmacologic stimulation
of fetal lung maturity, 912
of uterine contractions after delivery of placenta, 452-453
Phenaphthazine paper
to test amniotic fluid, 401
to test vaginal discharge, 397
Phenergan; *see* Promethazine
Phenformin in breast milk, 1035
Phenindione in breast milk, 1031
Phenistix test for phenylketonuria, 1028
Phenobarbital; *see also* Donnatal
for addicted infants during withdrawal, 955
in breast milk, 1032
for bronchial asthma, 985
for preeclampsia, 822
Phenobarbital sodium for analgesia, 509
Phenolphthalein in breast milk, 1033

Phenothiazine(s)
in breast milk, 1036
effect of, on fetus or neonate, 1024
Phenothiazine tranquilizers for schizophrenia, 951
Phensuximide in breast milk, 1032
Phenylbutazone
in breast milk, 1029
and oral contraceptives, 195
Phenylketonuria, 146, 219
diagnostic tests for, 1028
heel stick for, 637
screening for, 152, 153
Phenytoin
in breast milk, 663, 1031
effects of, on fetus or neonate, 1022
for epilepsy, 988
and oral contraceptives, 195
to prevent convulsions of eclampsia, 822
as teratogen, 951
Pheromone, 55
Phimosis, 625
pHisoHex for infant bathing, 620
Phobias, 136
Phocomelia, 978
Phonotransducer for fetal heart rate monitoring, 471, 474
Phototherapy for hyperbilirubinemia, 641-643
Phrenic nerve injury to neonate at birth, 908
Physical activity during pregnancy, 300
Physical assessment
of neonate, 576-593, 613
of nutritional status, 328
Physical condition
of infant and parental response, 720
of mother and response to newborn, 719-720
Physical examination, 19-20
comprehensive, 292-293, 295-296
of fertile man, 161
of fertile woman, 159-160
of infertile male, 182
initial, 19
of pregnant woman, 291
and nutrition assessment, 327
Physical growth and feeding behavior, 651
Physical symptoms, 19
Physician, symptoms of neonate to report to, 629
Physician-nurse relationship, 3
Pysiologic adjustments and basis for nutrition needs in pregnancy, 315-320
Physiologic and anatomic adaptations to pregnancy, 221-251
Physiologic anemia of pregnancy, 315, 983
Physiologic basis of fetal monitoring, 470-471
Physiologic changes in postpartum period, 686-689
Physiologic development and feeding behavior, 651
Physiologic edema, 237
Physiologic features of milk production, 659
Physiologic function, normal, childbearing as, 8
Physiologic hyperbilirubinemia, 561-562, 958-959
Physiologic response to sexual stimulation, 93-101
Physiologic retraction ring during labor, 380
Physiologic S_3, 230
Physiologic tasks of neonate, 554
Physiology
anatomy and, of reproduction, 50-101
maternal, and nursing care, 686-705
placental, 213-215
Pia mater in spinal cord, 512
Piaget, J., theories of, 134-135
Pica, 118, 241, 326
and stretch marks, 239
Pigmentation
during pregnancy, 238, 306
as presumptive sign of pregnancy, 272
Pigments, bilirubinoid, test for, and gestational age, 282
PIH; *see* Pregnancy-induced hypertension
"Pill"; *see* Oral contraceptives
Pillow, Frejka, for congenital hip dysplasia, 977
Pinch test on nipples, 228, 300
Pineazepam in breast milk, 1036
"Ping-Pong ball" indentations of head of neonate from delivery, 907
Pinhole os, 180
Pinocytosis and placenta, 215
Pinprick, response decrement to, 605
Piper forceps, 891
Piperacetazine in breast milk, 1036
Piskacek's sign, 274
Pitocin; *see* Oxytocin
Pitressin; *see* Vasopressin
Pituitary
anterior, necrosis of, postdelivery, 807
anterior and middle lobes of, 86
gonads, and hypothalamus, interaction between, 85, 88
and menstrual cycle, 84, 85
posterior, 86
during pregnancy, 242, 244-245
Pituitary hormones causing increased uterine activity, 490
PKU; *see* Phenylketonuria
"Placebo effect" with TENS, 528
Placenta, 213-215
adherent, postdelivery hemorrhage from, 805-806
battledore, 214
and chorion and amnion, 214
delivery of, 450-451
pharmacologic stimulation of uterine contractions after, 452-453
development of, 212
by calendar months, 247-251
expulsion of, forces causing, 379-382
fetal surface of, 213, 214
during labor, 382
maternal circulation and, 213-214
maternal surface of, 213, 214
nonadherent, postdelivery hemorrhage from, 805
nutrition and, 315
nutrient transfer via, 215
partial separation of, estriol levels and, 282
premature separation of, 789-792
physiology of, 213-215
reduced surface area of, and fetal circulation, 470
retained, causing postdelivery hemorrhage, 805-806
separation of, 450-451
bleeding from, 805
size and weight of, 213
variations in, 215
Placenta accreta, 806
Placentra destruans, 806
Placenta increta, 806
Placenta percreta, 806
Placenta previa, 210, 382, 792-796
in multiple pregnancies, 932-933
symptoms of, 790, 793
Placenta vera, 806
Placental barrier, 215
Placental disorders causing premature birth, 909
Placental fragments, retained, removal of, 452
Placental lactogen, human; *see* Human chorionic somatomammotropin
Placental lakes, blood in, 214-215
Placental perfusion, reduced, from sodium imbalance, 236
Placental separation, 448
Placental site
healing of, 688
subinvolution of, 688
Placental stage of spontaneous abortion, 782
Placental transfer, 215
of immunoglobulins, 562
Placentation, 212
Placentitis, 215
Plan
initial, 23
nursing care, 22
in problem-oriented record, 23
Plane(s)
fascial, of male lower genitourinary tract, 78
of pelvic outlet, 374-375, 378
Plane(s)—cont'd
of true pelvis, 372
Planned Parenthood Federation of America, Inc., 1010
Planning, 21
family, 186
cultural views on, 124-125
implementing, and evaluating care of newborn, 615-649
during prenatal period, 291-297
Plantar grasp, 596
Plantar reflex, 599
Plasma flow, renal, during pregnancy, 236
Plasma lipid fractions during pregnancy, 316
Plasma progesterone level, assessment of, and fertility, 171
Plasmin and clotting, 797
Plasminogen and clotting, 797
Plasmodium falciparum infection during pregnancy, 829
Plastic bell for circumcision, 628
Plastic hood for oxygen administration, 637
Plateau phase of sexual response cycle, 93, 97, 98
Platelet(s)
for disseminated intravascular coagulation, 799
for idiopathic thrombocytopenic purpura, 800
Platelet aggregation in neonate, 558
Platelet count, 798
in neonate, 558
Platypelloid pelvis, 378
Play
coital, in childhood, 105
sex, 104-105
Plethora in neonate, 611
Plexus, venous, cavernous, 56
Plug, mucous, 212
Plugged milk ducts, 668
Pneumonia, aspiration, complicating pregnancy, 986-987
Polar body, 145, 207
Polio vaccine for neonate, 562-563
Poliomyelitis
immunization against, during pregnancy, 301
during pregnancy, 829
Poliovirus vaccine in breast milk, 1037
Polish food pattern, 331
Political climate and maternity care, 4
Pollutants in breast milk, 301
environmental, 662
Pollution state, postpartal, cultural views of, 121-122
Polybrominated biphenyl in breast milk, 301, 662, 1034
Polychlorinated biphenyl in breast milk, 662, 1034
Polycillin; *see* Ampicillin
Polycythemia, neonatal, 807-808
Polydactyly, 146, 978
Polydipsia in diabetes mellitus, 845
Polyethylene splint to open blocked fallopian tubes, 178
Polygenic disorders, 142, 150
Polyhydramnios, 402
with diabetic pregnancies, 847
Polymyxin for meningitis, 837
Polyuria in diabetes mellitus, 845
Ponstel; *see* Mefamic acid
Pontocaine; *see* Tetracaine
POR; *see* Problem-oriented record
Port-wine stain, 565
Port-wine–colored amniotic fluid, 402
Position(s)
for breast feeding, 664-665
of client for breast examination, 694
for delivery, cultural views of, 120
fetal, 369, 371
and dystocia, 875-876
lateral Sims', for delivery, 448
lithotomy, for delivery, 430-431
culture and, 119-120
maternal; *see* Mother, position of
of neonate after feeding, right side-lying, 620

Position(s)—cont'd
occiput posterior, 878-879
persistent, 392
occiput transverse, persistent, 392
for pushing, 351
for rest and relaxation, 350, 351
side-lying, for delivery, 890
tailor sitting, to relax muscles, 351
uterine, 64, 65
vertex, fetus in, emergency birth of, 447-448
Positioning of neonate, 618, 619-620, 636
with respiratory distress, 747, 749
Positive clonus response at ankle joint, 819
Positive fern test on amniotic fluid, 401
Positive oxytocin challenge test, 497, 498
Positive signs of pregnancy, 275-277
summary of, 270
Postabortal sepsis causing infertility, 178
Postcoital test as fertility test, 173
Postdate pregnancy, 278, 280-281
Postdelivery area, transfer of mother and neonate to, 461-462
Postdelivery detection of genetic disease, 153-155
Postdelivery hemorrhage, 802-807
from adult respiratory distress syndrome complicating pregnancy, 986
Postdelivery period, care of adolescent in, 945
Posterior commissure, 54
Posterior cul-de-sac of Douglas, 61
Posterior fontanel of fetal skull, 363, 364
Posterior fornix, 68
Posterior ligament, 66
Posterior pituitary gland, 86
Posterior sagittal diameter of pelvic outlet, 375
Postmortem cesarean delivery, 895
Postnatal, 268
Postnatal infection, 832-833
Postovulatory phase of menstrual cycle, 86-87
Postpartum, 268
Postpartum care, 689-705
of adolescent, 945
cultural differences in, 120-122
goals of, 695
implementation of, 695, 701-705
nursing actions in, 695, 701-705
Postpartum exercise program, 703
Postpartum period
assessment of woman in, 690-695
divisions of, 686
nursing care during, 684-733
nursing diagnosis in, 695
physiologic changes in, 686-689
planning for nursing care in, 695
Postpartum teaching, 697
Postpartum unit
admission to, 690
legal issues in, 47
Postterm, 912
Posture
of newborn, assessment of, 576
during pregnancy, 225, 239
Potter's syndrome, 967, 979
Potassium iodide in breast milk, 1037
Pouch, rectouterine, 66
Pounds and ounces, conversion of, to grams, 1017
Poverty and pregnancy, 956-957
PPM; *see* Psychoprophylactic method
Practice
of maternity nurses, 3, 5-6
nursing, legislated definition of, 40
Prebirth passage of meconium with fetus in vertex presentation, 448-449
Precolostrum, 228
Preconceptional clients, legal and ethical concepts for, 42-44
Preconceptional detection of genetic disease, 152
Prednisone in breast milk, 1035
Preeclampsia; *see* Pregnancy-induced hypertension
Preeclampsia-eclampsia, 809, 811-813; *see also* Pregnancy-induced hypertension
Pregnancy
abdominal hernias complicating, 989
abnormal, and parenting disorders, 724
acceptance of, 256
activity and rest during, cultural views of, 118
adolescent, 937-947
adolescent adjustment to, 135
age-related problems in, 721
ambivalence about, 256
anatomic and physiologic, adaptations to, 221-251
anemia during, 326, 983-984
assessment during with evaluative criteria, 310-312
balance and harmony during, 116
body image and, 255-256
carcinoma of breast complicating, 989
chronology of, 208
clothing worn during, cultural views of, 118
clotting disorders in, 796-800
complications of, 779-824
daily food plan for, 333
dermatologic problems associated with, 987
developmental tasks of, for adolescent, 940-942
deviation of body systems during, 9
diagnosis of, 269-281
woman's response to, 254
discomforts of, 301-302, 303-307
douching during, 227
drug dependence and, 951-956
duration of, 277-281
early, disorders of, 780-789
early detection of, 112
ectopic; *see* Ectopic pregnancy
effects of, on heart disease, 867
effects of diabetes on, 846-847
effects of heart disease on, 867
emotional response to, and culture, 119
extrauterine, ruptured, 785
factors affecting, 315
failing, and estriol levels, 282
false diagnosis of, 224
family response to, 252-265
father-to-be's response to, 258-263
frequent, as nutrition risk factor, 325
gastrointestinal problems complicating, 987
gynecologic problems complicating, 989
hemorrhagic disorders in, 780
high-risk, 738-739
care of, goals for, 743, 744
history of infertility before, 183
hormonal factors in, 242-245
hypertensive disorders of, causing maternal mortality, 746
hypertensive states in, 809-823
infection during, 827-837
intestinal obstruction complicating, 990
with IUD, 196
laboratory tests for, 275, 277
laboratory values during, 989
late
disorders of, 789-802
metabolic disease of, 395; *see also* Pregnancy-induced hypertension
major complications coincident with, 826-871
manic-depressive psychosis related to, 950-951
mask of, 238, 271
maternal psychologic adaptation to, assessment of, 294-295
maternal sensitization to Rh factor during, 961-962
maternal tasks during, 253-255
medical problems complicating, 983-988
monilial infections during, 227
multiple, 930-934
narcotic drug dependence and, 953-956
neurologic disorders complicating, 987-988
nonacceptance of, 254
normal metabolic adaptations to, 845
nutrient needs during, 320-325
nutrition guidelines for, 327-336
Pregnancy—cont'd
nutrition needs in, basis for, 315-320
nutrition risk factors in, 325-327
outcome of, risk factors affecting, 743
paternal tasks during, 258-263
pernicious vomiting of; *see* Hyperemesis gravidarum
physiologic anemia of, 315
posture during, 225
poverty and, 956-957
"pride of," 225, 239
prolonged, 278, 280-281
protocols for care during, 9
psychosocial risk factors and, 950-957
pulmonary complications during, 985-987
recommended daily dietary allowances of nutrients for, 320-321
response of older woman to, 721
risk factors in, 739-743
risks of, 186-187
schizophrenia related to, 951
sexual activity during, cultural views of, 118-119
sexual concerns during, 257
signs and symptoms of; *see* Signs and symptoms of pregnancy
stress and anxiety during, 256-258
surgical conditions coincident with, 988-990
surgical interruption of, 990-996; *see also* Therapeutic abortion
term, 277-278
test-tube, 180-181
unwanted, 110
urinary problems complicating, 984-985
water metabolism of, reversal of, 688, 692
weight gain during, 237, 316-320
Pregnancy granulomas, 238, 987
Pregnancy tests, results of, and responsible sexuality, 112
Pregnancy-induced glucose intolerance, 845
Pregnancy-induced hypertension, 19, 237, 240, 326, 689, 692, 809, 811
clinical assessment guide for, 821
controversy over, 395
in diabetic women after delivery, 853
differential diagnosis of, 810
and estriol levels, 282
incidence of, 809-810
management of, 813-823
maternal and fetal morbidity and mortality in, 810
causing maternal mortality, 746
mons veneris in, 54
mild, 811, 813-814
moderate to severe, 814-823
pharmacologic control of, 816-817
severe, 811
Pregnancy-induced nasal stuffiness, 233
Pregnanediol in breast milk, 1035
Pregnant adolescent
nursing care of, 10, 943-945
nutritional needs of, 944-945
prenatal classes for, 943-944
postdelivery care of, 945
sample interview questions for, 946-947
Pregnant Patient's Bill of Rights, 41, 1003-1004
Pregnant state, "loss" of, 715
Pregnant woman
changes in, by calendar month, 247-251
danger signals for, 298
egocentric needs of, 254
initial contact with, 291
initial interview with, 291
physical examination of, initial, 291
response of, to pregnancy, 252-258
subsequent visits of, 296-297
Premature, 912
Premature delivery, reactions to, 769-770
Premature ejaculation and circumcision, 625
Premature infant
admission of, to nursery, 915
age of, correction of, 928
baptism of, 929

Premature infant—cont'd
birth and management of, 449
care of, 912-930
child abuse and neglect and, 928-929
classification of, 915
delivery of, psychologic aspects of, 928-929
favorable evaluative criteria for, 928
mother-child relationship and, 770
nursing care of, 915-925
nutrition for, 751
and parenting disorders, 724
physiologic basis for problems in, 915
parents of, postpartum care of, 912
prognosis for, 909, 927-928
transfer of, to regional neonatal care center, 915, 918
Premature labor, 770, 910-912
and delivery
irreversible or acceptable, care during, 912
nursing care of patients after, 771-772
psychologic aspects of, 769-772, 928-929
Premature rupture of membranes, 397
Premature separation of placenta, 789-792
Prematurity, 909
and adolescent pregnancy, 938
complications of, 925-927
and hydramnios, 967
and oxygen toxicity, 926-927
Premenstrual tension, oral contraceptives for, 192
Prenatal, 268
Prenatal care
cultural views of, 116-119
delay in, 12
early, 112
of low-income mothers, 956-957
Prenatal classes for pregnant adolescent, 943-944
Prenatal detection of genetic disease, 152-153
Prenatal development, timetable for, 209-210
Prenatal developmental stages, 207-208
Prenatal diagnosis, legal aspects of, 43-44
Prenatal evaluation as curative activity, 9
Prenatal examination procedures, 285-291
Prenatal infection, 827, 832
Prenatal management, phases of, 268
Prenatal period, 204-357
assessment during, 269-291
evaluation during, 310-312
laboratory tests in, 296
nursing care during, 267-312
nursing diagnosis in, 291
planning during, 291-297
Prenatal teaching guide, 342-343
Prenatal visit
first, 292-293, 295-296
with multiple pregnancy, 933
Preoperational stage of cognitive development, 135
Preovulatory phase of menstrual cycle, 86
Preparatory phase of nurse-client relationship, 35-36
Prepared childbirth and fetal monitoring, 492-493
Prepared childbirth movement, 531
Prepartum, 268
Prepregnant weight as nutrition risk factor, 326
Prepubescent homosexual behaviors, 104-105
Prepuce, 54, 55, 77, 78
of neonate, 567
Presacral nodes, 68
Presentation
breech; *see* Breech presentation
brow, 369
molding in, 365
chin, 369, 371
face, 369, 371
molding in, 365
fetal, 367
left occiput anterior, mechanism of labor in, 389
occipital, 368, 369, 370
occipitoanterior, molding in, 365
occipitoposterior, molding in, 365
shoulder, 368, 369
sinciput, 368, 369
vertex; *see* Vertex presentation
Presenting part, 367
assessment of, 383
descent of, during second stage of labor, 421
Pressure
blood; *see* Blood pressure
continuous positive airway, for neonate with respiratory distress, 749, 750
intracranial, increased, in neonate, 611-612
sacral, to relieve pain, 528
venous, central, in shock, 801, 802
Pressure-type douches, 227
Presumptive signs and symptoms of pregnancy, 269-274
Preterm, 912
Preterm birth, 909-912
Preterm labor; *see* Premature labor
Preventive activities in maternity nursing, 9
Pride of pregnancy, 225, 239
Primary anovulation, 177
Primary dysmenorrhea, 92
Primary hypertension, 823
Primary infertility, 163
Primary oocyte, 144
Primary spermatocyte, 144
Primary uterine inertia, 879-882
Primary villi, 211
Primidone in breast milk, 1032
Primigravida, 268
Primipara, 268
Primordial ova, 69
Principal piece of sperm, 207
Principles of genetics, 145
Privacy, right to, and genetic counseling, 42
Privileged information, 42
Prizing and values clarification, 32
PRL; *see* Prolactin
Probable signs and symptoms of pregnancy, 274-275
summary of, 270
Pro-Banthine; *see* Propantheline bromide
Probenecid, effect of, on glucose determinations, 1021
Problem list, 23
Problem solving, 16
in family, 133
Problem-oriented record, 22-24
Procaine for regional anesthesia, 511
Procedures, 630-646
Process
decision-making, 33-34
diverticular, of labium majus, 59
ensiform, 69
maternity nursing as, 16-24
of nurse-client relationship, 35-37
nursing, 16, 17
xiphoid, 69
Professional language, 27
Professional values, 31
Progestasert-T intrauterine device, 197
Progesterone
and breast development, 75, 76
and development of decidua, 211
effects of, on target organs and tissues, 89
in endometrial cycle, 87
fetoplacental production of, 243, 245
and gastrointestinal changes during pregnancy, 241
and hemodynamic changes during pregnancy, 230
and infertility, 81
and insulin production, 247
and insulin resistance, 845
levels of, during pregnancy, 223
in minipill, 195
and onset of labor, 388
in oral contraceptives, 192
ovaries and, 68
in Progestasert-T, 197
role of, during pregnancy, 316
and urinary system changes during pregnancy, 235
and uterine enlargement, 223
Progesterone level, plasma, assessment of, 171
Progestin
deficiency of, 194
effect of, on fetus or neonate, 1023
excess of, 193-194
Progress notes, 23-24
nursing, legal importance of, 41
Prolactin, 86
and breast feeding, 658, 660, 704
effects of, on target organs and tissues, 90
and lactation, 228
during pregnancy, 242, 244, 245
and sodium balance, 236
Prolapse
of umbilical cord, 406, 407
treatment of, 408, 409
of uterus, 66
Proliferative phase of endometrial cycle, 87
Prolonged decelerations in fetal heart rate, 485
Prolonged labor, nursing care for, 884
Prolonged pregnancy, 278, 280-281
Prolonged rupture of membranes, 397
PROM; *see* Premature rupture of membranes; Prolonged rupture of membranes
Promazine
for analgesia, 510, 523
causing decreased variability in fetal heart rate, 483
Promethazine
for analgesia, 510, 523
causing decreased variability in fetal heart rate, 483
for itching, 524
for manic reactions after delivery, 950
Prominence, cephalic, palpation of, 383
Promontory, sacral, 70
female and male, contrast of, 72
nodes of, 66
Prone position of neonate, 917
Propantheline bromide in breast milk, 1032
Prophylactic eye care of newborn, 442-445
Propiomazine
for analgesia, 510
causing decreased variability in fetal heart rate, 483
Propositional logic, 135
Propoxyphene
in breast milk, 1030
after cesarean delivery, 905
"Propping" of bottle, 672
Propranolol
as antidote to ritodrine, 911-912
in breast milk, 1033
effect of, on fetus or neonate, 1023
causing fetal bradycardia, 481
causing increased uterine activity, 491
to prevent convulsions of eclampsia, 822
Propylthiouracil in breast milk, 663, 1037
Prostaglandin(s), 92
effects of, 92
causing increased uterine activity, 490
and onset of labor, 388
and ovulation, 92
during pregnancy, 244
and primary dysmenorrhea, 92
role of, in reproductive functions, 92
in semen, 92
in seminal fluid, 82
stimulation of labor in dystocia with, 886-887
for therapeutic abortion, 991
in Wharton's jelly, 213
Prostaglandin F_2 alpha, 92
causing increased uterine activity, 490
and primary dysmenorrhea, 92
transabdominal intrauterine injection of, for therapeutic abortion, 991, 995
Prostaphlin; *see* Oxacillin
Prostate gland, 77-79, 82
abnormalities of, and male infertility, 182
effects of estrogens on, 89
enlargement of, 82

Prostate gland—cont'd
and formation of semen, 82
Prostatectomy, 82
Prostatic secretion, 82
Prostatic urethra, 77, 81
Protein
in human milk, 661
for infant, 654
intake of
inadequate, 654
in pregnancy-induced hypertension, 813
urine test for, in pregnant woman, 237
Protein concentration, total, during pregnancy, 315-316
Protein deposits during pregnancy, 320
Protein foods, 333
Protein needs during pregnancy, 320-321
Proteinuria
after delivery, 688
during pregnancy, 237-238, 810, 811
in pregnancy-induced hypertension, 809
Proteolytic enzymes of trophoblast, 210
Prothrombin and clotting, 797
Prothrombin activator and clotting, 797
Prothrombin time, one-stage, 798
Protocols for care during pregnancy, 9
Provera; *see* Medroxyprogesterone acetate
Proxen; *see* Naproxen
Pruritus of pregnancy, 241-242, 306
noninflammatory, 238, 987
Pruritus gravidarum, 241-242
"Prying" into intrafamily relationships, 4-5
Pseudoanemia of pregnancy, 315
Pseudoglandular period of fetal lung development, 217
Pseudosinusoidal pattern in fetal heart rate, 483
Pseudostrabismus, 587
Psoriasis, 151, 238, 987
Psychologic adaptation to pregnancy and parenting, maternal, assessment for, 294-295
Psychologic aspects of preterm labor and delivery of preterm infant, 928-929
Psychologic components of childbirth preparation, 346
Psychologic disorders and male infertility, 182
Psychologic response of woman to labor, 382, 397
Psychophysical components of childbirth preparation, 346
Psychoprophylactic method, 346, 347-348
Psychoprophylaxis for analgesia, 523
Psychosis
childbearing, 950-951
manic-depressive, pregnancy-related, 950-951
Psychosocial aspects of reproduction, 102-112
Psychosocial care, maternal and family need for, 283-284
Psychosocial development
within family, 133-136
and feeding behavior, 652, 653
Psychosocial factors that place the mother-infant dyad at risk, 740
Psychosocial history taking, 4
Psychosocial risk factors and pregnancy, 950-957
Psychosocial role of nurse in care of parents after birth of child with disorder, 767-769
Psychosocial stress of parents, 9
Psychosocial system, 19
Psychotherapy after delivery, 950, 951
Psychotropic drugs
in breast milk, 1036
effect of, on fetus or neonate, 1024
Ptyalin and infant digestion, 652
Ptyalism, 240, 303
Pubarche, 54
Puberty, 88-89
onset of, 105
Pubic bone, 58, 70
Pubic crest, 69
Pubic hair
of female, 54
of male, 76, 77
Pubis, 70
Public Documents Distribution Center, 1010
Pubocervical ligament, 65
Pubococcygeus muscles, 57, 58
exercise of, 704
Puborectalis muscle, 57
Pudendal artery, internal, 67, 68
Pudendal block, 512, 513, 514
Pudendal nerves, 68
Pudendal vein, 68
Puerperal infection, 832-833
causing maternal mortality, 746
Puerperal sepsis, 452
Puerperium, 686; *see also* Postpartum period
Puerto Rican women, modesty of, 117
Puerto Ricans
food pattern of, 331
views of family on, 123
view on menstruation of, 124
Pull-to-sit with neonate, 607
Pulmonary circulation, changes in, at birth, 557
Pulmonary complications during pregnancy, 985-987
Pulmonary emboli
after delivery, 452
during pregnancy, 986
Pulmonary function during pregnancy, 234
Pulmonary surfactants, 217
Pulsations, cord, after birth, 440
Pulse(s)
apical, in neonate, location of, 579
of neonate, 580
in postpartum period, evaluative criteria, for, 698
in shock, 801
Pumps, breast, 670, 671
Puncture, spinal, headache following, 904-905
Puncture sites for heel-stick samples of capillary blood, 637
Purpura, thrombocytopenic, idiopathic, 800
Push, controlling urge to, 349
Pushing
breathing while, 349-350
position for, 351
during second stage of labor, 421, 425
Pyarthrosis after septicemia, 837
Pyelonephritis, 829, 984, 985
Pyloric stenosis, 142, 151
and hydramnios, 967
Pyopen; *see* Carbenicillin
Pyribenzamine; *see* Tripelennamine
Pyridoxine
deficiency of, and oral contraceptives, 194
effect of, on fetus or neonate, 1023, 1024
need for, during pregnancy, 322
Pyrimethamine in breast milk, 1031
Pyrosis, 241, 303

Q

Quadrants of mother's abdomen and fetal position, 369
Quadruplets, 930-934
Quality
of human milk and maternal diet, 660
of parenting, indicators of, 725
Quantity of human milk and maternal diet, 660
Questionnaire
nutrition, 329, 332
nutritional screening, for infant, 678
Questions
asked by clients, 299-301
and communication, 26
interview, sample, for pregnant adolescent, 946-947
Quickening as presumptive symptom of pregnancy, 270
Quide; *see* Piperacetazine
Quinidine
in breast milk, 1033
effect of, on fetus or neonate, 1022
Quinine, effect of, on fetus or neonate, 1022
Quinine sulfate in breast milk, 1031

R

Radial chemocautery of cervix, 180
Radiant heater, overhead, 630-631
Radiation
effect of, on fetus and neonate, 1024
causing heat loss in neonate, 566
Radioactive compounds in breast milk, 662, 663, 1033
Radioactive iodine, 867
in breast milk, 1037
Radioactive sodium in breast milk, 1033
Radiographic demonstration of fetus as positive sign of pregnancy, 276-277
Radiography to determine gestational age, 283
Radioimmunoassay test for HCG as pregnancy test, 277
Radiologic studies to detect genetic disorders, 155
Radiopaque media, effect of, on fetus or neonate, 1024
Ramus, ischiopubic, 59
Rape and artificial insemination, 43
Rapid labor, 18-19
Rapid surfactant test, 282
Rash
dermal, in congenital syphilis, 839
diaper, 612, 621
on face of neonate, 621
on neonate, assessment for, 612
during pregnancy, 306
Ratio, lecithin/sphingomyelin, 44, 282
Rattle, response decrement to, 604
RDS; *see* Respiratory distress syndrome
Reaction(s)
acrosome, 206
to childbearing, adverse, stresses causing, 284
depressive, after delivery, 715, 950-951
of family members to birth of high-risk infant, 778
grief, of family at birth of child with disorder, 768
immunologic, to spermatozoa, 180
manic, after delivery, 950-951
to pain in childbirth, 352-353
to premature delivery, 769-770
sperm immobilization antigen-antibody, 172
vasocongestive, to sexual stimulation, 100
Reactive nonstress test, 496
Reactivity
periods of, in neonate, 571
reflex, of neonate on BNBAS, 602
Real-time scanner, 281; *see also* Ultrasonography
Reasonably prudent nurse, 40
and fetal monitoring, 494
Rebellion in adolescents, 107
Recessive gene, 145
Recommended dietary allowances
for infants, 653
during pregnancy and lactation, 320-321
Record
basal temperature, 168
obstetric labor admission, 507
in postpartum period, evaluative criteria for, 700
problem-oriented, 22-24
of woman during labor, 416
Recording
of data, 22-24
of infant responses, 630
Recovery, maternal, 453-462
Rectal fascia, 58
Rectal temperature in neonate, 580, 611, 617
Rectouterine pouch, 66
Rectovaginal ligament, 66
Rectovaginal septal nodes, 68
Rectum, 58, 61
varicose veins of, 241
Rectus abdominis muscle, 58, 69
diastasis of, 69
Rectus femoris muscle, injection in, 637
Rectus sheath, 58
Recurrent abortion, 780-781
Red blood cell count in neonate, 558

Red blood cells
agglutination of, and Rh factor, 960
antigenicity of, 960
increase in, during pregnancy, 232, 233
production of, during pregnancy, 315
Reduction division, 143
Referred shoulder pain from ruptured extrauterine pregnancy, 785
Reflectance meter, glucose, 850
Reflex
automatic walking, 600
Babinski, 599
biceps, 818
breathing, 558
crawling, 601
crossed extension, 598, 599
deep tendon, 601, 819, 820
extrusion, 595
Ferguson's, 910
Galant, 599
gastrocolic, 572, 612
and stooling, 561
glabellar, 595
grasp, 596, 919
and parent-child attachment, 709
Landau, 601
let-down, 660, 665
magnet, 598, 599
Moro, 596, 597
in addicted infant, 954, 955
during birth, 620
Myerson's, 595
neck righting, 599
neonatal, assessment of, 594-601
otolith righting, 601
patellar, 818
plantar, 599
response to, assessment of, 603
rooting, 594, 665
startle, 597
stepping, 599, 600
sucking, 594
swallowing, 595
tonic neck, 595
traction, 597
trunk incurvation, 598, 599
vagal; *see* Vagal reflex response
"walking," 599, 600
"wink," of anal sphincter, 593
Reflex clonic muscular contractions in response to sexual stimulation, 100
Reflex activity of neonate on BNBAS, 602
Reflex response(s)
assessment of, 603
fetal, 218
vagal; *see* Vagal reflex response
Refractory period, 100, 101
Refusal of therapy, 41
Regeneration, endometrial, in postpartum period, 688
Regional anesthesia, 508, 511, 513, 516
Regional neonatal care center, transfer of preterm infant to, 915, 918
Regionalization of health care services, 745
Registered nurse certified, 13
Regression in behavior by siblings, 719
Regular sleep state of neonate, 569
Regularity of uterine contractions, 380
Rehabilitative activities of maternity nursing, 10
Rejection of infant and manic-depressive psychosis, 950
Rela; *see* Carisoprodol
Relactation, 669-671
Relationship
family, initiation of, 700
of husband and wife after birth of baby, 717
intrafamily, "prying" into, 4-5
maternity nurse-client, 25-37
mother-fetal, loss of, 715
nurse-client, 297-298
trusting, 19
Relationship—cont'd
nurse-physician, 3
parent-child; *see* Parent-child relationships
sexual, commitment to, 109-110
Relativism, cultural, 115
attitude of, by nurse, 125
Relaxation
in Bradley method, 348
in Dick-Read method, 347
in Lamaze method, 347
positions for, 350, 351
uterine
between contractions, 881
inadequate, 407
Relaxin
and musculoskeletal system changes in pregnancy, 239
role of, during pregnancy, 224, 244, 246
Religion and contraception, 124
Religious factors leading to infertility problems, 164
Renal agenesis and oligohydramnios, 967
Renal blood flow, functional alterations in, during pregnancy, 316
Renal dysplasia and oligohydramnios, 967
Renal function, changes in, during pregnancy, 236-238, 316
Renal pelves, changes in, during pregnancy, 235
Renal plasma flow during pregnancy, 236
Renal system
discomforts of pregnancy related to, 305
embryonic development of, 217-218
of neonate, 559-560
Renal values, standard, pregnant and nonpregnant, 1020
Renin-angiotensin-aldosterone system and pregnancy, 236
Repair phase of endometrial cycle, 87
Reproduction
anatomy and physiology of, 50-101
basic concepts of, 48-203
myths about, 111
psychosocial aspects of, 102-112
in various cultures, 115-116
Reproductive health care, responsible, 110
Reproductive history, 18-19
poor, as nutrition risk factor, 325
Reproductive system
assessment of, in postpartum period, 693
changes in, in postpartum period, 687-688
embryonic development of, 219-220
female; *see* Female, reproductive system of
male, 76-83
and female, homologues of, 51-53
of neonate, 567
principal components of, 51
Request for care, client's reason for, 18
Research, fetal, legal aspects of, 44
Research role of nurse, 7
Researcher, maternity nurse as, 12-13
Reserpine
in breast milk, 663-1033
effect of, on fetus or neonate, 1024
Residual capacity, functional, changes in, during pregnancy, 234
Residual volume, changes in, during pregnancy, 234
Resistance
to infection in newborn, 562-563
insulin, in pregnancy, 845
Resolution of grief, 766
Resolution phase of sexual response cycle, 93, 99, 100
RESOLVE, Inc., 184
Respiration(s)
of neonate, 558, 559
assessment of, 610-611
evaluative criteria for, 647, 648
maintenance of, 616
parental guidance concerning, 629
in postpartum period, evaluative criteria for, 698
in shock, 801
Respiratory distress
neonate with, nursing of, 747-750
sequence of development of, 747
Silverman-Anderson index of, 748
Respiratory distress syndrome, 44, 217, 925-926
adult, complicating pregnancy, 986
and cold stress, 566
drugs to combat, 912
in infants of diabetic mothers, 860
in preterm infant, 925-926
Respiratory rate
changes in, during pregnancy, 234
and effort in neonate, 582
Respiratory system
congenital anomalies of, screening for, 967
discomforts of pregnancy related to, 305
embryonic development of, 217
functional alterations in, during pregnancy, 316
in neonate, 558-559
during pregnancy, 233-235
Response
clonus, at ankle joint, 819
emotional; *see* Emotional response(s)
of family
to birth of child, 707-723
to pregnancy, 252-265
to movement by neonate, 568
of neonate, monitoring and recording of, 630
parental
assessment of, 723-729
factors influencing, 719-723
physiologic, to sexual stimulation, 93-101
to pregnancy, emotional, and culture, 119
psychologic, of woman to labor, 382, 397
reflex; *see* Reflex; Reflex response(s)
sexual, biphasic, 100
shiver, in neonate, 601
sweat, in neonate, 601
vagal; *see* Vagal reflex response
Response cycle, four-phase, to sexual stimulation, 93-100
Responsibility
of maternity nurses, 4
of parenthood, 9
Rest
in postpartum period, 702
during pregnancy, cultural views of, 118
and relaxation, positions for, 350, 351
Restating in communication, 26
Resting phase of endometrial cycle, 87
Restitution in labor, 391
Restraining of neonate, 643-645
Resuscitation
cardiopulmonary, classes on, 629-630
emergency, of depressed neonate, 443
Kreisselmann, infant, 442
mouth-to-mouth, 633-635
Retained placenta causing postdelivery hemorrhage, 805-806
Retained placental fragments, removal of, 452
Retardation, growth, intrauterine, 280
and maternal weight gain, 326
Retention cysts of neonate, 560
Retinal hemorrhage in neonate, 906
Retracted nipple, breast cup for, 300
Retraction ring
pathologic, 380, 882
physiologic, during labor, 380
Retractions, observation of, 748
Retrocession of uterus, 64
Retroflexion of uterus, 64, 65
Retrograde menstruation, 178
Retrolental fibroplasia from oxygen therapy, 636, 926-927
Retroversion of uterus, 64, 65
Return visit after delivery, 705
Reverse polarity in uterine contractions, 881-882
Rh antibodies in breast milk, 1037
Rh antigens, 960-961
Rh factor, discovery of, 960-961
Rh genotypes, 961

Rh immunoglobulin for Rh-negative mother, 964
Rh incompatibility, 960-964
Rh isoimmunization, 961
  prevention of, 695
  prophylaxis for, 963-964
Rh typing of mother, 962
Rhagades in congenital syphilis, 840
Rheumatic carditis and pregnancy, 867
RhIG; *see* Rh immunoglobulin
Rh-negative cells, 960
Rh-negative woman, 217
Rh_o (D) human immune globulin, 960, 963-964
  after delivery, 695
  for spontaneous abortion, 783
  after therapeutic abortion, 990
Rh_o D^u group incompatibility, 960
RhoGAM; *see* Rh_o (D) human immune globulin
Rh-positive cells, 960
Rhubarb in breast milk, 1033
Rhythm method of contraception, 188-189
Rhythms of speech, culturally determined, in infant, 710
RIA; *see* Radioimmunoassay test
Rib cage, changes in, during pregnancy, 233-234
Riboflavin, need for, during pregnancy, 323
Rickets, 657
  hypophosphatemic (viatmin D–resistant), 147
  vitamin D–deficiency, 147, 662
Rifampin and oral contraceptives, 195
Right(s)
  fetal, 46
  maternal, 41
  to privacy and genetic counseling, 42
Right fornix, 68
Right side-lying position after feeding, 620
Right-to-left shunt in neonate, 555
Ring
  Bandl's, 380, 882, 884
  Falope, for sterilization, 997
  inguinal, internal, 79
  retraction
    pathologic, 380, 882
    physiologic, 380
Risk factors
  at onset of pregnancy, 325-326
  in pregnancy, 326-327
  affecting pregnancy outcome, 743
  psychosocial, and pregnancy, 950-957
Ritgen maneuver, modified, 420
Ritodrine
  causing fetal tachycardia, 481
  to suppress preterm labor, 911-912
Rivalry, feeling of, of expectant father, 260
RNC; *see* Registered nurse certified
Robaxin; *see* Methocarbamol
Rocking, pelvic, 351
Roentgenography to detect fetal disorders, 152-153
Role(s)
  complementary, in family, 133
  life concept of, 30
  mastery, 30
  of maternity nurse, expanded, 6-7
  of mother, traditional, 30
  parental; *see* Parental role
  sex, stereotyped, in various cultures, 116
  sexual, 30
  social; *see* Social role
Role expectations, 30
  and father's involvement during labor and delivery, 415
Role playing after birth of child with disorder, 769
Role taking, 31
Roller to move woman, 453
Rolling by neonate, preventing, 619
Roll-over test in preeclampsia-eclampsia, 812-813
Rondomycin; *see* Methacycline
Rooming-in, 5
  and parent-child attachment, 711
Rooming-in unit, 575
Rooms
  birthing, 532-534
Rooms—cont'd
  labor, 874
Rooting reflex, 594, 665
Rotation in labor in vertex presentation
  external, 391-392
  internal, 390
Rotter's nodes, 74
Round ligament, 59, 61, 62, 65, 67
  within fascial sheaths, 59
  pain of, during pregnancy, 307
RPF; *see* Renal plasma flow
RPR test, 827
Rubella
  immunization against, 301
  in neonate, 838
  during pregnancy, 830
Rubella syndrome
  congenital, 838
  palm creases and, 154
Rubella vaccination after delivery, 693, 695
Rubella virus vaccine in breast milk, 1037
Rubeola
  immunization against, 301
  during pregnancy, 830
Rubin's cannula, 177
Rubin's test and fertility, 174, 175
Rugae of vagina, 68
Rule
  Haase's, 251
  McDonald's, 251
  Naegele's, 277
Running away by adolescents, 107
Rupture
  of membranes
    and amniotic fluid, 401-402
    artificial, 888, 890
    complications associated with, 402
    premature or prolonged, 397
    spontaneous, 397
  uterine, with hydatidiform mole, 787
Ruptured extrauterine pregnancy, 785

S

SA hemoglobin pattern, 984
Sacral agenesis, 861
Sacral backache from endometriosis, 179
Sacral nerves and uterus, 66
Sacral nodes, lateral, 66
Sacral pressure to relieve pain, 528
Sacral promontory, 61, 70
  female and male, contrast of, 72
  nodes of, 66
Sacral sciatic notch, 70
Sacrococcygeal joint and labor, 371
Sacrococcygeal teratoma, 980
Sacroiliac joints and labor, 371
Sacrosciatic notch, greater, female and male, contrast of, 72
Sacrum, 70
  counterpressure on, during contraction, 414
  female and male, contrast of, 72
Saf-T-Coil, 197
Sagittal fontanel of fetal skull, 363
Sagittal suture of fetal skull, 363, 364
Sagittal suture line, vaginal palpation of, 385
St. Kitt, women of, views on pregnancy of, 117
St. Louis University, ACNM-approved basic education in, 1013
Salicylates, effect of
  on fetus or neonate, 1022
  on glucose determination, 1021
"Saline abortion," 991, 994-995
Saline cathartics in breast milk, 1033
Salivation, excessive, during pregnancy, 240, 303
Salmonella kottbus organisms in breast milk, 301
Salpingectomy and IUD use, 196
Salpingitis, tubal surgery after, 178
Salpix; *see* Sodium acetrizoate
Salt and preeclampsia-eclampsia, 811-812, 813
Salting of infant foods, 657
Same-sex comparisons in children, 104-105
Samoans
  contraceptive practices of, 124
  views on sterility in, 124
Sample interview questions for pregnant adolescent, 946-947
Sampling, fetal blood, 491
Save the Children Federation, Inc., 1010
SC hemoglobin pattern, 984
Scalp
  bruises on, in neonate, 612
  fetal, pH of, testing of, 5
  of neonate, cleansing of, 620
Scalp vein, venipuncture of, 757
Scandinavian food pattern, 331
Scanners; *see also* Ultrasonography
  beta, 281
  real-time, 281
Scaphoid abdomen, 970
Scar tissue, uterine, causing infertility, 179
Scarf sign, 918
Scarpa's fascia, 58
Schistosomiasis, infertility from, 179
Schizophrenia, 151
  pregnancy-related, 951
Schultze mechanism, 451
Sciatic notch, sacral, 70
Sciatic pain during pregnancy, 240
Science and art of nursing, 5
Scientific method, 16
Scleral hemorrhages in neonate, 906
Sclerosis, multiple, 988
Scopolamine
  for analgesia during birth period, 510
  in breast milk, 1032
  effect of, on fetus or neonate, 1023
Scopolamine hydrobromide for analgesia, 523
Score
  Apgar, 441-442
  Bishop's, 886, 887
Screening
  mass, 43-44
    preconceptional, 152
  nutritional, and assessment of infants, 677-681
Screening tests, urine, for inborn errors of metabolism, 1027
Scrotum, 78
  changes in, in response to sexual stimulation, 96
"Seal-like" limbs, 978
Sebaceous gland hyperplasia in neonate, 564
Seborrhea dermatitis, 987
Seborrheic dermatitis, 238
Sebum, secretion of, in neonate, 564
Secobarbital sodium
  for analgesia, 523
  causing decreased variability in fetal heart rate, 483
Seconal; *see* Secobarbital sodium
Second polar body, 145
Second stage of labor, 418-449
  duration of, 392, 418
  emotional responses to, 418
  forces at work in, 418
Secondary amenorrhea in young women, 177
Secondary anovulation, 177
Secondary diabetes, 844
Secondary infertility, 163
Secondary oocyte, 144, 145
Secondary spermatocyte, 144
Secondary uterine inertia, 882
Secretion, prostatic, 82
Secretory IgA, 562
Secretory phase of endometrial cycle, 87
Sedatives
  for anesthesia and analgesia, 508, 509
  in breast milk, 1031-1032
  effect of, on fetus or neonate, 1024
  and placenta, 215
Sedatives-hypnotics for analgesia, 523
Seesaw respirations of neonate, 559
Segregation, principle of, 145
Self, 30, 31

Self-absorption vs. generativity in personality development, 136
Self-awareness and nurse-client relationship, 29-33
Self-concept, 30-31
of father-to-be during pregnancy, 261
Self-esteem, 31
Self-exploration in childhood, 105
Self-image, changes in, counseling about, 298
Self-manipulation in childhood, 105
Self-stimulation in adults, 110
Semen, 82-83
abnormalities of, and male infertility, 181
composition of, 82
liquefaction of, 83
production of, by epididymis, 81
Seminal duct, 78
Seminal fluid, 82
Seminal vesicles, 77-79, 82
abnormalities of, and male infertility, 182
Seminiferous tubules, 80, 81
Semirecumbent position for labor, 411
Semisolid foods, introduction of, 673-674
Senna in breast milk, 1033
Sensations, pain, unexpected, during labor, 884, 886
Sensitive periods in human development, 208
Sensitization, maternal, to Rh factor, 961-962
Sensorimotor stage of cognitive development, 134-135
Sensory behaviors of neonate, 567-569
Sensory capability of neonate, assessment of, 603
Sensory impairment of parent and response to infant, 722-723
Sensory nerves of uterus, 66
Separation
of placenta, 450-451
bleeding from, 805
partial, estriol levels and, 282
premature, 789-792
signs of, 448
of sutures from increased intracranial pressure, 611
Separation anxiety, 135
Sepsis
neonatal, 837-844
nursing care of, 865
postabortal, causing infertility, 178
puerperal, 452, 832-833
from spontaneous abortion, 781
Septal defect
atrial, 968
ventricular, 969
Septal nodes, rectovaginal, 68
Septate hymen, 57
Septic abortion, 782, 783
Septic shock, 837
Sequential immunization in infants, 563
Serentil; *see* Mesoridazine
Serial monogamy, 110
Serotonin and clotting, 66
Serpasil; *see* Reserpine
Serratus anterior muscle, 71
Sertoli's cells, 80
Serum albumin, tests to measure, 329
Serum hepatitis during pregnancy, 828
Servo-Control incubators, 631-632
Severe preeclampsia, 814-823
Sex
attitudes toward, changes in, 109
of child, preferences for, 260-261
determination of, 207
of infant, disappointment over, 720
Sex cells, 206
Sex chromatin, 149, 151
Sex chromosomes, 143
aberrations of, 149
abnormalities of, common, 151
Sex education, 112
Sex hormones
ovaries and, 68
Sex hormones—cont'd
steroid
secretion of, testosterone and, 80
and skeletal changes during pregnancy, 239
Sex play, 104-105
Sex role standards, 103-104
Sex roles, stereotyped, in various cultures, 116
Sex therapy, 302
Sex-linked disorder, amniocentesis to determine, 288
Sex-linked trait, 145-146
Sexual activities during pregnancy, cultural views of, 118-119
Sexual ambiguity, 980
Sexual concerns during pregnancy, 257
Sexual counseling, 42, 302, 308-309
Sexual development
adult, 109-112
childhood, 104
stages of, 91
Sexual drives during pregnancy, 257
Sexual dysfunctional problems, 112
Sexual experience of adolescents, 109
Sexual expression, 110
Sexual fantasies in adolescent, 108
Sexual orientation, 110
Sexual relationship
commitment to, 109-110
counseling about, 298
Sexual response, biphasic, 100
Sexual response cycle
female, 94-95
male, 96
Sexual roles, 30
Sexual stimulation, physiologic response to, 93-101
Sexual identity, 102, 103
Sexual taboos, postpartal, 124
Sexuality
human, fallacies about, 111
male, during pregnancy, 260
Sexually transmitted diseases, 109
circumcision and, 625
SGA; *see* Small for gestational age
Shaft
of clitoris, 54, 55
of penis, 77
Shake test, 282
Shame and doubt vs. autonomy in personality development, 135-136
Shaving of vulva, 405
Sheath
cytoplasmic, of sperm, 207
fascial, round ligaments within, 59
rectus, 58
Sheehan's syndrome, 790, 799, 807
Shiver response in neonate, 601
Shock
bacteremic, 835-836
after delivery, 456
hemorrhagic, 800-802
hypovolemic, in neonate, 808-809
septic, 837
symptoms of, 801
therapy for, hazards of, 802
Shock and disbelief phase of grieving, 766
Shock lung; *see* Adult respiratory distress syndrome
Shoes during pregnancy, 299
Short-term variability in fetal heart rate, 482-483
Shoulder dystocia, 448
Shoulder presentation, 367, 368, 369
Shoulders
delivery of, 420
of fetus during labor, 366
pain in, referred
from ruptured extrauterine pregnancy, 785
from subphrenic irritation, 174
"Show," bloody, 309, 388
in first stage of labor, 397
Shunts, left-to-right and right-to-left, in neonate, 555
Shut-down responses of neonate on BNBAS, 602, 604
Siblings, 718-719
adjustment to infant by, 5
and adolescent, 107
aggressive behavior by, toward baby, 719
birth of
and "loss" of mother, 135
response of child to, 135
focusing on, 731
reaction of, to birth of high-risk infant, 778
regression in behavior by, 719
response of
to birth of handicapped infant, 135
to pregnancy, 263-265
Sibling care taking, 116
Sibling visitation, 5
Sick role, 10
Sickle cell anemia, 146
screening for, 43
Sickle cell disease, preconceptional detection of, 152
Sickle cell hemoglobinopathy, 984
Sickle cell test, 984
Sickle cell trait, 984
Sickness, morning, 241
Side-lying position
for breast feeding, 664
for delivery, 890
after feeding, 620
during second stage of labor, 421, 431
SIECUS, 1010
Sign
Babinski's, 599
Braun von Fernwald's, 272, 274
Braxton Hicks', 275
Brudzinski's, 601
Chadwick's, 226, 227, 273
Cullen's, 785
Goodell's, 226
Hegar's, 225, 226, 272, 273
Homan's, 233, 692
Jacquemier's, 273
Kernig's, 601
Ladin's, 272, 273
McDonald's, 272, 274
Ortolani's, 977
assessing for, 592
peak mucus, 171-172, 190
Piskacek's, 274
of pregnancy
positive, 275-277
summary of, 270
presumptive, 269-274
summary of, 270
probable, 274-275
summary of, 270
scarf, 918
vital; *see* Vital signs
Sign language by deaf parent, 723
Signaling behavior by infant, 708
Significant others
family as, 133
mother as, 708
and self-esteem, 31
"Silent" labor, 398
Silver nitrate for prophylactic eye care of newborn, 444
Silverman-Anderson index of respiratory distress, 748
Simian line, 154
Simple vaginitis, 834-835
Simpson forceps, 891
Sims' position
lateral, for delivery, 448
for prolapsed umbilical cord, 409
Simultaneous orgasm, 100
Sinciput presentation, 368, 369
Single footling breech presentation, 369
Single-parent family, 132-133
Sinhalase women, food cravings of, 118

Sinus arrhythmia in neonate, 555
Sinuses, lactiferous, 72, 73, 659
Sinusoidal pattern in fetal heart rate, 483, 484
Sitting technique for breast feeding, 666
Situational supports of parental role, 715-716
Sitz bath in care of episiotomy, 701
Skelaxin; *see* Metaxalone
Skeletal injuries in neonate during delivery, 906-907
Skene's duct, 56
Skene's glands, 54, 55
Skim milk for infants, 672
Skin; *see also* Integumentary system
  blood flow to, during pregnancy, 230
  changes in
    during pregnancy, 238-239
    as presumptive sign of pregnancy, 272-273
    in response to sexual stimulation, 94, 96
  of neonate, 563
    color of, assessment of, 611
  in shock, 801
Skull
  fetal, 363-365
  of neonate, fractures of, during delivery, 906-907
Sleep, "twilight," 529
Sleep states of neonate, 569
Sleeping and waking behaviors of neonate, 569-571
Sleep-wake cycles in neonate, 570-571
Sleep-wakefulness, assessment of, 603
Slow chest breathing, 348, 349
Small for dates, 913
Small for gestational age, 913, 915
Small for gestational age neonate, nutrition for, 751
Small intestine, changes in, during pregnancy, 241
Smallpox vaccine in breast milk, 1037
Smear
  Kleihauer-Betke, 695
  Papanicolaou, 65, 68, 110, 160
    procedure for, 285, 287
Smegma, 55
Smell, neonate's sense of, 568-569
Smell response of neonate, assessment of, 603
Smiling by neonate, 571
Smoking
  effect of, on fetus or neonate, 1023
  as nutrition risk factor, 326
  and placenta, 215
  during pregnancy, 301
Smooth muscle cells of uterus, growth of, during pregnancy, 223
Sneeze, 601
Snuffles with congenital syphilis, 839
SOAP, 23
Soupsuds enema, 405
Social adjustment during adolescence, 105
Social behaviors of neonate, 571
  assessment of, 603
Social conditions and parental responses, 722
Social language, 27
Social network after birth of child with disorder, 769
Social roles, 30-31
  achieving, 105-106
  concept of, 30
  family and, 133
Socialization within family, 133
Societal reactions to childbearing, cultural differences in, 122-124
Sodium for infant, 657, 676
Sodium acetrizoate, 174
Sodium amobarbital
  for epilepsy, 988
  for pregnancy-induced hypertension, 816
Sodium balance during pregnancy, 236
Sodium bicarbonate
  in exchange transfusion for hyperbilirubinemia, 964
  to prevent convulsions of eclampsia, 822
Sodium bromide in breast milk, 1032
Sodium chloride, hypertonic
  intraamniotic injection of, 890
Sodium chloride—cont'd
  transabdominal intrauterine injection of, for therapeutic abortion, 991, 994-995
Sodium depletion during pregnancy, 236
Sodium fisidate in breast milk, 1031
Sodium needs during pregnancy, 322
Sodium phenobarbital for pregnancy-induced hypertension, 816
Sodium sulfacetamide for neonatal conjunctivitis, 841
"Soft spots"; *see* Fontanel(s)
Soft tissue dystocia, 875
Soft tissue injuries to infant at birth, 906
Soft tissues of birth canal, 379
Softening
  of cervix, 226
  of uterus, 272
    as presumptive sign of pregnancy, 273-274
Sole creases of neonate, 917
Solids, introduction of, 673-675
Soma; *see* Carisoprodol
Somatic cells, 142-143; *see also* Chromosome(s)
Somatic pain during labor, 501
Somatomammotropin, chorionic, human
  and insulin resistance, 845
  and lactation, 228
  and sodium balance, 236
Somnos; *see* Chloral hydrate
Sore nipples, 667-668
Souffle
  funic, 225
  uterine, 225
    as probable sign of pregnancy, 274
Sounds
  bowel, in neonate, 560
  breath, of neonate, 558
  heart
    of neonate, 555
    during pregnancy, 229
  intrauterine, auscultation of, 225
  during labor, 414
Southeast Asian women
  labor and delivery of, 119
  pregnancy diet of, 117
Southeast Asians
  infant care among, 123
  male progeny of, 123
  value of children to, 116
Soy formulas, 671-672
Space(s)
  and communication, 27-28
  and membranes of spinal cord, 512
  personal, 28
  utilization of, 28
Spanish-Mexican food pattern, 331
Spanish-speaking groups, value of children in, 116
Sparine; *see* Promazine
Spasm
  arteriolar, general, in preeclampsia-eclampsia, 812
  gastrocnemius, during pregnancy, 305
Specialist
  health care, women's, 6
  nurse, clinical, 6
Specimen
  blood, collection of, from neonate, 645
  care of, following collection, 842
  collection of, at initial contact with pregnant woman, 291
  urine, collection of, from neonate, 645-646
Speculum examination, bivalve, 286
Speech, rhythms of, culturally determined, in infant, 710
Spence, tail of, 71
Sperm, 80-81
  abnormalities of, and male infertility, 181
  analysis of, in infertile male, 182
  antibodies to, 172
    and male infertility, 181
  autoantibodies to, reduction in, 182
  autoimmunization to, 172
Sperm—cont'd
  cervical mucus and, 81, 180
  diagram of, 207
  formation of, 144
  immunologic reactions to, 180
  maturation of, 80, 81
  migration of, through cervical canal, 170
  motility of, 80
    pH and, 82
  and ovum, union of, 206
  passage of, through cervical mucus, 169
  temperature and, 78
Sperm count, 83
Sperm immobilization antigen-antibody reaction, 172
Spermatic cord, 81
Spermatic vessels, 79
Spermatids, 80, 144
Spermatocyte, 80, 144
Spermatogenesis, 80, 144, 206
  marijuana, 164
  suppression of, by steroid hormones, 200
Spermatogonia, 80
  in gametogenesis, 144
Spermatozoa; *see* Sperm
Spermicide
  diaphragm with, for contraception, 198
  vaginal, for contraception, 199
Sphenoid fontanel of fetal skull, 364
Sphincter; *see* Anal sphincter
Sphincter action of myometrial fibers of uterine wall, 63
Sphincter vaginae, 57
Sphingomyelin
  in amniotic fluid, 215
  and lecithin, ratio of, and fetal lung maturity, 217
Spider angiomas, 238
Spiders, vascular, during pregnancy, 304
Spina bifida, 975
  and hydramnios, 967
Spinal anesthesia, intrathecal subarachnoid, care after, 702
Spinal column, relation of head to, before and after flexion, 391
Spinal cord
  injuries to, in neonate during delivery, 909
  membranes and spaces of, 512
Spinal puncture, headache following, 904-905
Spinal tray, 525
Spines
  iliac, 70
  ischial, 70
    female and male, contrast of, 72
    and pelvic measurements, 374
Spinnbarkheit, 171, 190
Spiral electrode
  application of, 478
  checklist for, 494
  for fetal heart rate monitoring, 471, 476-478
  to monitor uterine activity, 490
Spirits of peppermint to aid voiding, 456
Spironolactone in breast milk, 1034
Splanchnic engorgement, 454
Splint, polyethylene, to open blocked fallopian tubes, 178
Split ejaculates for artificial insemination, 183
Spondylolisthesis, 240
Spongy layer of endometrium, 87, 88
Spontaneous abortion, 780-784
  incidence of, 739
  and IUD, 196
Spontaneous rupture of membranes, 397
Spots, Mongolian, 564-565
Squamous cells, fetal, in amniotic fluid, 401
Squamocolumnar junction, 64, 65
Squamous epithelium of cervix, 64, 65
Squatting position
  for labor, 411
  during second stage of labor, 421
^{89}Sr in breast milk, 1034
^{90}Sr in breast milk, 1033, 1034

SRM; *see* Spontaneous rupture of membranes
SS hemoglobin pattern, 984
Stagnated urine during pregnancy, 235
Stain
metachromatic, of urine sediment, 1027
port-wine, 565
Stalk, connecting, 212
Standard laboratory values
in neonatal period, 1025-1027
pregnant and nonpregnant, 1018-1020
Standards
of care, 40
sex role, 103-104
Staphylococci causing vaginitis, 834
Staphylococcus aureus
causing mastitis, 833
causing puerperal infection, 832
Starch, laundry, eating of, during pregnancy, 118; *see also* Pica
Startle reflex, 597
Stasis, urinary, during pregnancy, 235
State University of New York, ACNM-approved basic education in, 1013
Statements, opening, broad, and communication, 26
Station, 386, 387
of head, forceps designation relative to, 892
Station 0, 386
Statutory law, 40
Stelazine; *see* Trifluoperazine
Stenosis
pyloric, 142, 151
and hydramnios, 967
subaortic, 969
urethral, and oligohydramnios, 967
Stepping reflex, 599, 600
Stercobilin, 561
Stereotyped sex roles, 116
Sterile instruments, lifting, 425
Sterile forceps, unwrapping, 429
Sterile packages, opening, 426-427
Sterile techniques in delivery room, 425-431
Sterile water for initial oral feeding, 677
Sterility
and blocked fallopian tube, 62
from IUD, 196
Sterilization, voluntary, 42, 996-1000
Sterilizing of bottles, 672
Sternal border, lower, 69
Steroid sex hormones
secretion of, testosterone and, 80
and skeletal changes during pregnancy, 239
Steroids and breast feeding, 663
Stethoscope
DeLee-Hillis, 468, 469
to detect fetal heartbeat, 276
fetal, to hear intrauterine sounds, 225
ultrasound, 469
Stillbirth, 762-763
Stillborn child
care of, 763
legal concepts regarding, 46
Stimulants in breast milk, 1037
Stimulation
of fetal lung maturity, pharmacologic, 912
of labor
in dystocia, 886-888
methods not recommended for, 890
sexual, physiologic response to, 93-101
transcutaneous electrical nerve, 528
of uterine contractions, pharmacologic, after delivery of placenta, 452-453
Stimuli influencing behavior of newborn, 610
Stomach
aspiration of, 632-633
cells of, 560
changes in, during pregnancy, 241
Stomatitis, mycotic, in neonate, 842
Stones, urinary, during pregnancy, 985
Stool softners in breast milk, 1033
Stooling during feeding, 561; *see also* Gastrocolic reflex
Stools
of bottle-fed infant, 673
of breast-fed infant, 665
of neonate, 561
"Stork bites," 565
Strain guage, checklist for, 495
Strawberry mark, 565
Streptococcus(i)
group B, infection with, during pregnancy, 828
β-hemolytic, causing neonatal sepsis, 837
causing puerperal infection, 832
causing vaginitis, 834
Streptomycin
in breast milk, 1031
effect of, on fetus or neonate, 1022
Stress(es)
causing adverse reactions to childbearing, 284
causing amenorrhea, 84
cold, 751
in neonate, 566-567
with respiratory distress, 749
family and, 136-138
on fetus, 9
during labor, 402-403
and infections, 162
in labor, 402-404
maternal, during first stage of labor, 403
paternal, during first stage of labor, 403-404
during pregnancy, 256-258
psychosocial, of parents, 9
and vaginitis, 180
Stress test, oxytocin, and fetal heart rate, 282-283
Stress testing, contraction, 5
Stressors caused by birth of baby, 3
Stretch, 601
Stretch marks, 238, 273
Stretching
of cervical os, 66
of hollow viscera, 66
of peritoneal surfaces, 66
Striae gravidarum, 238, 273
Stricture
urethral, and male infertility, 181
uterine, annular, from obstructed labor, 882
"Stripping"
of membranes to induce labor, 890
of umbilical cord toward neonate, 441
Stroma of breast, 72
Strong uterine contractions, 400, 485
Strontium; *see* ^{89}Sr; ^{90}Sr
Structural defect of chromosome, 147
Stuffiness, nasal, pregnancy-induced, 233, 305
Subaortic stenosis, 969
Subarachnoid block, 516
Subarachnoid space in spinal cord, 512
Subclavian nodes, 74
Subconjunctival hemorrhages in neonate, 906
Subcostal retractions, 748
Subculture, 115
Subcutaneous fat of neonate, 564
necrosis of, 906
Subdural hematoma from delivery, 909
Subdural space in spinal cord, 512
Subgroups, cultural, 27
Subinvolution
of placental site, 688
of uterus, postdelivery hemorrhage from, 807
Subjective data in problem-oriented record, 23
Suboccipitobregmatic diameter of fetal skull, 365
Subpubic arch, 70
angle of, estimation of, 375, 376, 378
female and male, contrast of, 72
measurement of, 375, 376, 378
Subscapular nodes, 74
Substernal retractions, 748
Subtotal hysterectomy after cesarean section, 895
Succinylcholine chloride for cesarean birth, 524
Sucking of neonate, 560
Sucking behavior of infant, 665
Sucking calluses, 560, 612
Sucking pads of cheeks, 560
Sucking reflex, 594
in fetus, 218
Suction apparatus, mechanical, nasophagyngeal catheter with, 633
Suction catheters, 993
Suction curettage for therapeutic abortion, 991, 992, 993, 994
Suction curettage machine, 993
Suctioning
with DeLee mucous-trap catheter, 633
of newborn, 632-633
with respiratory distress, 749
Sugar, urine test for, in pregnant woman, 237
Sulfamoylanthranilic acid; *see* Furosemide
Sulfanilamide in breast milk, 1031
Sulfapyridine in breast milk, 1031
Sulfathiazole in breast milk, 1031
Sulfisoxazole
in breast milk, 1031
for urinary tract infections during pregnancy, 985
Sulfonamides
and breast feeding, 663
effect of
on fetus or neonate, 1022
on glucose determination, 1021
Summary, discharge, 22
Sumner, P., 532
Sumycin; *see* Tetracycline
Super female syndrome, 151
Superficial inguinal nodes, 68
Superior fascia
of levator ani, 58, 59
of urogenital diaphragm, 58
Superior pole of fetus, palpation of, 383
Superior vesical artery, 67, 557
Supernumerary digits, 978
Supine hypotension, 470
during pelvic examination, 379
from recumbent position for labor, 411
Supine hypotension syndrome, 285
Supplemental bottles, 666
Supplemental fluorine dosage schedule, 657
Supplemental Food Program for Women, Infants, and Children, 681
Supplementation during pregnancy
calcium, 322
folic acid, 322
iron, 232, 321, 326
megavitamin, as nutrition risk factor, 326
Supplements
ascorbic acid, 323
folacin, 335
for infants, suggested, 656
iron, 335
nutritional, during pregnancy, 323
Supplies in postpartum unit, 701
Support(s)
provided by maternity nurses, 6
situational, of parental role, 715-716
towel, to restrain neonate, 645
Support persons, role of, 36
Support system, 136, 138
Supporting structures of female reproductive tract, 59
Supportive care
of client, 297-298
of high-risk neonate, 761-762
Suppositories and breast milk, 1033
Suppression
of labor, 910-912
of lactation, 704-705
Surfactant test, rapid, 282
Surfactants, pulmonary, 217
Surgery; *see also* Operation
for endometriosis, 179
heart, during pregnancy, 867
for tubal blockage, 178
Surgical conditions coincident with pregnancy, 988-990
Surgical emergencies, most common, 971-975
Surgical interruption of pregnancy, 990-996

Surgical termination of fertility, 996-1000
Surgical transfer system, 530
Suspicious oxytocin challenge test, 497, 498
Suture(s)
of fetal skull, 363, 364
sagittal, line of, vaginal palpation of, 385
separation of, from increased intracranial pressure, 611
Swallowing reflex, 595
Sweat glands of neonate, 564
Sweat response in neonate, 601
Sweats, night, after delivery, 692
Swedish breast pump, 670
Swedish food pattern, 331
Swedish milk cup, 228
Swimming during pregnancy, 299
Sydney line and rubella syndrome, 154
Symmetrel; *see* Amantadine
Sympathetic block, lumbar, 512
Sympathy, 34
Symphysis pubis, 58, 61, 70, 78
and labor, 371
length and inclination of, estimation of, 373
Symptoms(s)
of impending labor, 309-310
of neonate to report to physician, 629
physical, 19
Sympto-thermal method of contraception, 190-192
Synaxsyn; *see* Naproxen
Synchrony by neonate, 571
Synclitism, 389, 391
Syncope, 240, 304
Syndrome
acquired immune deficiency, 109, 841-842
adult respiratory distress, 986
Arnold-Chiari, 975
bronze baby, 643
carpal tunnel, 240, 306
caudal regression, 861
congenital rubella, 838
cri du chat, 142, 147, 149, 150
defibrination; *see* Disseminated intravascular coagulation
Down's, 19, 142, 149, 150
and hydramnios, 967
Edwards', 150
fetal alcohol, 301, 952-953
hypotensive, 236
Klinefelter's, 142, 151
and male infertility, 181, 182
Marfan's, 146
elective abortion in, 990
nursing bottle, 675
Patau's, 150
"pelvic congestion," 224
Potter's, 967, 979
respiratory distress; *see* Respiratory distress syndrome
rubella, palm creases and, 154
Sheehan's, 790, 799, 807
supine hypotension, 285
triple X, 151
Turner's, 142, 149, 150, 151
dermatoglyphics and, 154
vena cava, 214, 236, 411, 412, 470
prevention of, 304
in woman with heart disease, 869, 870
Syntocin; *see* Oxytocin
Syphilis, 109, 830-831
assessment for, 827, 832
congenital and neonatal, 839-841
test for, 827, 832
VDRL test to detect, 160
Syringe breast pump, 670
Systemic circulation, changes in, at birth, 557
Systemic diseases, chronic, as nutrition risk factor, 326
Systemic medication for anesthesia and analgesia, 508, 509-510
Systolic ejection murmurs during pregnancy, 230

T

T_4 index, free, 867
Table
delivery; *see* Delivery table
instrument, for delivery, 430
Taboos
food, during pregnancy, 117-118
sexual, postpartal, 124
Tacaryl; *see* Methdilazine
Tace; *see* Chlorotrianisene
Tachycardia, fetal, 402, 480, 481
Tail
of Spence, 71
of sperm, 80, 207
Tailbone, 70
Tailor sitting position to relax muscles, 351
Taking-hold phase of parental role, 717
Taking-in phase of parenthood, 714
Talipes equinovarus, 978
Talwin; *see* Pentazocine
Tampons, 162
Tandearil; *see* Oxyphenbutazone
Tapazole; *see* Methimazole
Taste, sense of
by neonate, 568
during pregnancy, 241
Taste response of neonate, assessment of, 603
Tatum copper-bearing IUD, 197
Tay-Sachs disease, 146, 219
preconceptional detection of, 152
Tay-Sachs gene, screening for, 43
^{99m}Tc in breast milk, 1033
T-Cu 200, 197
Teaching
of care of child, 714-715
with disorder, 768
diabetic, 856-859
postpartum, 697
of pregnant adolescent, 943
Teaching guide, prenatal, 342-343
Teachers, maternity nurses as, 6, 12
Tears, cervical or vaginal, after delivery, 449
Technician, maternity nurse as, 12
Technology related to birth process, 4, 5
Teenager, pregnant; *see* Pregnant adolescent
Teeth, changes in, during pregnancy, 240-241
Tegretol; *see* Carbamazepine
Telangiectasia, 238, 273, 304
Telangiectatic nevi, 565
Telepaque; *see* Iopanoic acid
Temperature
axillary, taking, 617
basal body; *see* Basal body temperature
after delivery, 689, 691
of neonate, 580-581
assessment of, 611
evaluative criteria for, 647, 648
maintenance of, 616, 618, 619
parental guidance concerning, 629, 630
predisposed, 570
rectal, 581, 611, 617
in postpartum period, evaluative criteria for, 698
Temperature equivalents, 1016
regulation of, 566
Temperature support and regulation for high-risk neonate, 750-751
Tendon of perineum central, 58
Tendon reflexes, deep, assessment of, 819, 820
TENS; *see* Transcutaneous electrical nerve stimulation
Tension
emotional, counseling for, 298
premenstrual, oral contraceptives for, 192
Tension headache, 240
Teratogenicity of drugs, 301
Teratogens, sensitivity to, periods of, 208
Teratoma, 980
Term, 912
Term pregnancy, 277-278
Terminal sac period of fetal lung development, 217
Termination phase of nurse-client relationship, 37
Territoriality, 27-28
Test
Benedict's, 1027
for bilirubinoid pigments, gestational age and, 282
biochemical
to detect genetic disorders, 153-154
and nutrition assessment, 327, 329
blood serum phenylalanine, for phenylketonuria, 1028
bubble, 282
cetyltrimethylammonium bromide, 1027
coagulation, 798
Coombs', 962-963
D^u, 695
diagnostic
for diabetes mellitus, 848-850
for phenylketonuria, 1028
diaper, for phenylketonuria, 1028
dinitrophenylhydrazine, 1027, 1028
for female fertility, 166-176
fern, positive, on amniotic fluid, 401
ferric chloride, 1027
fertility, findings of, favorable to fertility, 170
FTA-ABS, 827
FTA-ABS IgM, 827, 832
glucose tolerance, 844, 848, 849
HbA_{lc}, 848, 850
Hemantigen, 962
Kahn, 827
Kolmer, 827
laboratory; *see* Laboratory tests
nonstress
in diabetic pregnant woman, 852
and fetal heart rate, 282
oxytocin challenge, 496-498
and fetal heart rate, 282-283
Phenistix, for phenylketonuria, 1028
pinch, on nipples, 228, 300
postcoital, as fertility test, 173
for pregnancy, 275
results of, and responsible sexuality, 112
radioimmunoassay, for HCG, 277
rapid surfactant, 282
roll-over, in preeclampsia-eclampsia, 812-813
RPR, 827
Rubin's, and fertility, 174, 175
for rupture of membrane, 401
shake, 282
sickle cell, 984
for syphilis, 827, 832
tolbutamide response, 849
TPI, 827
urine
for phenylketonuria, 1028
for sugar and protein in pregnant woman, 237
urine screening, for inborn errors of metabolism, 1027
VDRL, 160, 827
for virginity, 56
Wasserman, 827
Testes, 78-81
abnormalities of, and male infertility, 181
agenesis or dysgenesis of, and male infertility, 181
development of, 219
elevation of, in response to sexual stimulation, 93, 96
and follicle-stimulating hormone, 86
and formation of semen, 82
and luteinizing hormone, 86
of neonate, 567
undescended, and fertility, 161
Testicle, 79
Testing
antepartum, 496-498
of fetal scalp pH, 5
nonstress, 5, 496, 497
of nurse's teaching, 716
stress, contraction, 5

Testosterone, 80
and male development, 220
and prostatic function, 82
"Test-tube babies," 43
Test-tube pregnancy, 180-181
Tetany
of newborn, 864
during pregnancy, 240
Tetracaine for regional anesthesia, 511
Tetracycline
and breast feeding, 663, 1031
for *Chlamydia trachomatis* infection, 841
effect of
on fetus or neonate, 1022
on glucose determination, 1021
and oral contraceptives, 195
as teratogen, 951
Tetralogy of Fallot, 969
Thai women
binding of wrists of, during labor, 121
views on pregnancy of, 116
Thalassemia, 984
β-Thalassemia, 984
Thalassemia major, 984
Thalassemia minor, 984
Thalidomide
effect of, on fetus or neonate, 1024
causing phocomelia, 978
as teratogen, 951
Thank You, Dr. Lamaze, 346
Theobromine in breast milk, 1037
Theophylline and breast feeding, 663, 1037
Therapeutic abortion, 990-996
counseling about, 996
early, 991, 992-994
legalization of, 990
nurse's role in, 995-996
"saline," 991, 994-995
second- and third-trimester, 991-992, 994-995
for woman with heart disease, 868
Therapeutic measures, 21
Therapeutic touch, 28
Therapy
antibiotic, for chorioamnionitis, 402
client understanding of, 35
compliance with, 35
drug, in nursing mothers, 663
for dystocia, 886-890
family, 302
for female infertility, 177-181
goal for, 21
for hyperbilirubinemia, 641-643
intravenous; *see* Intravenous therapy
iron, during pregnancy, 983
oxygen, 636-637
for neonate with respiratory distress, 749-750
weaning from, 750
parenteral, weaning from, 753
refusal of, 41
sex, 302
Thermal shift, 190
Thermistor probe of overhead radiant heater, positioning of, 631
Thermocautery of cervix, 180
Thermogenesis in neonate, 566-567
Thermometer for recording basal body temperature, 167
Thiamin, need for, during pregnancy, 322-323
Thiazide(s)
in breast milk, 1034
effect of, on fetus or neonate, 1023
for pregnancy-induced hypertension, 817
Thinking, formal, 135
5-Thio-D-glucose to inhibit spermatogenesis, 200
Thiomerin; *see* Mercurial diuretics
Thiopental
for cesarean birth, 524
for general anesthesia, 508, 511
Thioridazine in breast milk, 1036
Thiouracil
in breast milk, 662, 1037
Thiouracil—cont'd
for hyperthyroidism, 867
Thioureas, effect of, on fetus or neonate, 1024
Third stage of labor, 450-453
duration of, 392
Thiuretic tablets; *see* Thiazide(s)
Thom's pelvimeter to measure intertuberous diameter, 375
Thorazine; *see* Chlorpromazine
Threatened abortion, 782, 783
Thrombin, formation of, and clotting, 797
Thrombin time, 798
Thrombocytopenic purpura, idiopathic, 800
Thromboembolic disease and oral contraceptives, 193
Thromboembolism
assessment for, 692
and oral contraceptives, 192, 193
during pregnancy, 232, 233
susceptibility to, 702-703
Thrombophlebitis from adult respiratory distress syndrome during pregnancy, 986
Thromboplastin time, activated partial, 798
Thrombosis
exercise for prevention of, 702
signs of, 692
Thrush, 612
oral, in neonate, 842
Thyroid in breast milk, 1037
Thyroid gland
changes in, during pregnancy, 246
fetal development of, 219
Thyroid hormone for Sheehan's syndrome, 807
Thyroid medications
in breast milk, 1037
effect of, on fetus or neonate, 1024
Thyroidectomy, partial, for hyperthyroidism, 867
Thyroid-stimulating hormone, 86
Thyrotropin, 86
Thyroxine
in breast milk, 1037
and nutrition, 316
Tidal volume, changes in, during pregnancy, 234
Tilt, pelvic, 374
Time
activated partial thromboplastin, 798
of birth, 391-392
bleeding, 798
circulation, changes in, during pregnancy, 233
and communication, 29
one-stage prothrombin, 798
thrombin, 798
Time units, gestational, 208
Timetable of human prenatal development, 209-210
Timing
for assessing neonate
with Brazelton Scale, 602
with physical assessment, 613
with reflex assessment, 594
influencing behavior of newborn, 610
Tissue
deposition of, during pregnancy, 320
embryonic, 51
growth of, during pregnancy, 315-316
soft
of birth canal, 379
dystocia of, 875
injuries to, in infant at birth, 906
Tocolytic drugs, 910
Tocopherol, need for, during pregnancy, 322
Tocotransducer
checklist for, 494
for monitoring uterine activity, 471, 472, 473, 475-476, 490
Toddler, alienation felt by, 135
Toenails of neonate, care of, 621
Tofranil; *see* Imipramine
Tofu, 329
Tolbutamide, 846
in breast milk, 1035
effect of, on fetus or neonate, 1024
Tolbutamide response test, 849
Tolerance, glucose
changes in, with oral contraceptives, 194
impaired, 844
Tomography, computed, to determine fetal presentation, position, and descent, 386, 388
Tone of voice and communication, 28-29
Tongue of neonate, 612
Tongue-tie, 612
Tonic neck reflex, 595
Tools, assessment, for normal newborn, 610-613
Tort, 40
Total body water during pregnancy, 316
changes in, 233
Total hysterectomy after cesarean section, 895
Total parenteral nutrition
for high-risk infant, 753, 759-761
for neonatal necrotizing enterocolitis, 927
for neonate with respiratory distress, 749
Total placenta previa, 793, 794
Total protein concentration during pregnancy, 315-316
Touch
in communication, 28
of infant by mother, 28
during labor, 414
and neonate, 568
assessment of, 603
as nonverbal communication, 28
in parent-child attachment, 709
therapeutic, 28
Towel support to restrain neonate, 645
Toxemia, 809, 811; *see also* Pregnancy-induced hypertension
Toxicity
magnesium sulfate, 911
oxygen
and prematurity, 926-927
from shock therapy, 802
Toxins, effect of, on fetus or neonate, 1024
Toxoplasmosis, 831, 976
TPI test, 827
Trace minerals
biochemical tests for, 329
need for, during pregnancy, 323
Trachea, "milking" of, 633
Trachelorrhaphy, 180
wedge, for weakened cervix, 781
Tracheoesophageal anomalies, 971-972
Tracheoesophageal fistula, 971-972
feeding of infant with, 677
H-type, 970
Traction reflex, 597
Traditional role of mother, 30
Traditions, cultural, 115
Trainex Corporation, 1010
Trait
autosomal, 145
sex-linked, 145-146
sickle cell, 984
Tranquilizers
for analgesia, 508, 510, 523
for anesthesia, 508, 510
causing decreased variability in fetal heart rate, 483
Transabdominal amniocentesis in erythroblastosis, 963
Transabdominal intrauterine injection
of hypertonic sodium chloride for therapeutic abortion, 991, 994-995
of prostaglandin F_2 alpha for therapeutic abortion, 991, 995
Transcervical amniotomy, 888, 890
Transcutaneous electrical nerve stimulation for relief of discomfort, 528
Transcutaneous oxygen tension monitor, 926
for neonate with respiratory distress, 749-750
Transducer, ultrasound
checklist for, 494
for fetal heart rate monitoring, 471-474

Transfer
from labor bed to delivery room, 425
of mother and neonate to postdelivery area, 461-462
placental, 215
of preterm infant to regional neonatal care center, 915, 918
Transfusion
exchange, for hyperbilirubinemia, 641, 964-966
intrauterine fetal, for hyperbilirubinemia, 966
maternal sensitization to Rh factor after, 961, 962
twin-to-twin, 933
Transition, breathing during, 348-349
Transitional nursery, 574-575
Transitional period between intrauterine and extrauterine existence, 570-571, 575
Transitional stools of neonate, 561
Translocation, 148-149
Translocation phenomenon, 147
Transplantation, embryo, in vitro fertilization and, 42-43
Transport incubator, 970
Transposition of great vessels, complete, 968
Transverse diameter of pelvic outlet, 375
Transverse lie, 367, 369, 371
Transverse ligament, 65-66
Transverse perineal muscle, 57, 59
Trauma
birth, 905-909
in infants of diabetic mother, 861
and male infertility, 181
Travel during pregnancy, 300
Travelers Aid and International Social Services Association, 1010
Tray
caudal, 524
epidural, 517
for local infiltration anesthesia, 515
spinal, 525
Tremors
after delivery, 457
in newborn, 563
Trendelenburg's position with prolapsed cord, 407, 408
Treponema pallidum immobilization test, 827
Trial of labor for dystocia, 886
Trichloroethylene
effect of, on fetus or neonate, 1022
for inhalation analgesia, 510-511
Trichomonas vaginalis causing vaginitis, 834
Trichomonas vaginitis, 180, 834
Tricofuron; *see* Furazolidone
Tricuspid atresia, 968
Tricyclic antidepressants in breast milk, 1036
Tridione; *see* Trimethadione
Trifluoperazine
in breast milk, 1036
for depressive reactions after delivery, 951
Trigone, 79
Trilene; *see* Trichloroethylene
Trimester, fourth, 686
Trimethadione
in breast milk, 1032
effect of, on fetus or neonate, 1022
Tripelennamine in breast milk, 1032
Triple Blue for cord care, 621
Triple X syndrome, 151
Triplets, 930-934
Trisomy, 147, 148, 149
Trisomy 13, 149, 150
dermatoglyphics and, 154
Trisomy 18, 149, 150
Trisomy 21, 149, 150; *see also* Down's syndrome
Trisomy 21(G), 149
Tromexan; *see* Ethyl biscoumacetate
Trophoblast, 210, 211
True conjugate, diameter of, 373
True labor, comparison of, with false or complicated labor, 396
True pelvis, 70-71, 371
cavity of, 374
True pelvis—cont'd
planes of, 372
Truncus arteriosus, 969
Trunk incurvation reflex, 598, 599
Trunk incurvation reflex, 598, 599
Trust, 34
vs. mistrust in personality development, 135
in nurse-client relationship, 19, 34
TSH; *see* Thyroid-stimulating hormone
T-shaped uterus, 981
Tub baths during pregnancy, 299
Tubal branch(es)
of ovarian artery, 67
of uterine artery, 67
Tubal factors in female infertility, 178
Tubal occlusion for sterilization, 997-999
Tubal reanastomosis after ligation, 997, 999
Tubercle, Montgomery's, 73, 228, 273
Tubercular infection causing infertility, 178
Tuberculin test in breast milk, 1033
Tuberculosis
endometrial, infertility from, 179
during pregnancy, 831
Tuberosities, ischial, 70
Tube(s)
fallopian; *see* Fallopian tubes
nasogastric, feeding via, for high-risk infant, 754-756
neural, 218
Tuboovarian abscess and IUD, 196
Tubules, seminiferous, 80, 81
Tucker-McLean forceps, 891
Tumors
endometrial and myometrial
infertility from, 179
removal of, 179
ovarian, excision of, 177
uterine, removal of, 179
Tuohy needle, 517, 520, 521
Turner's syndrome, 142, 149, 150, 151
dermatoglyphics and, 154
"Twilight sleep," 529
Twins, 930-934
dizygotic or fraternal, 930, 932
history of, 19
monozygotic or identical, 930, 931
Twin-to-twin transfusion, 933
Two-day contraceptive sponge, 199
Tylenol; *see* Acetaminophen
Typhoid fever during pregnancy, 831
Typing of mother
blood, 962
Rh and ABO, 962

U

U-Bag, Hollister, 645-646
Ulcerative colitis complicating pregnancy, 987
Ulcers, peptic, 151, 241
complicating pregnancy, 987
Ultandren; *see* Fluocymesterone
Ultrasonographic demonstration of fetus as positive sign of pregnancy, 276
Ultrasonography, 281
to detect fetal disorders, 152
for placenta previa, 793
Ultrasound, 5
Ultrasound device to hear intrauterine sounds, 225
Ultrasound examinations to determine gestational age of fetus, 280, 281
Ultrasound fetoscope, 469
Ultrasound stethoscope, 469
Ultrasound transducer
checklist for, 494
for fetal heart rate monitoring, 471-474
Umbilical arteries, 67, 213
changes in, at birth, 557
and fetal development, 216
Umbilical catheterization for hyperbilirubinemia, 966
Umbilical cord, 212-213
assessment of, 612
Umbilical cord—cont'd
care of, 621
clamping of, 440
timing of, and newborn's circulation, 557
compression of, variable deceleration caused by, 489
cross section of, 213
cultural views of, 123
evaluative criteria for, 647, 648
flow through, disruption of, 470-471
around neck of fetus, 449
prolapse of, 406, 407
treatment of, 408, 409
pulsations of, after birth, 440
tying off of, 441
Umbilical cord blood, studies using, 962-963
Umbilical vein, 213
changes in, at birth, 557
closure of, 555
and fetal development, 216
Umbilical vessels, 212, 214
Umbilicus, 69
Uncircumcised penis, care of, 628
Understanding of therapy by client, 35
Undescended testes and fertility, 161
United Cerebral Palsy Association, Inc., 1010
United States Air Force, ACNM-approved basic education in, 1014
United States Government Printing Office, 1010
University of California at San Diego, ACNM-approved basic education in, 1014
University of California at San Francisco, ACNM-approved basic education in, 1014
University of Illinois at the Medical Center, ACNM-approved basic education in, 1014
University of Kentucky, ACNM-approved basic education in, 1014
University of Miami, ACNM-approved basic education in, 1014
University of Minnesota, ACNM-approved basic education in, 1014
University of Mississippi, ACNM-approved basic education in, 1014
University of Utah, ACNM-approved basic education in, 1014
Unmarried women, births to, 11
Unsatisfactory nonstress test, 496
Unsatisfactory oxytocin challenge test, 497, 498
Unwanted pregnancy, 110
Upper airway aspiration of neonate, 632
Upper arm, paralysis of, from delivery, 907
Upper pelvic diaphragm, 56-57
Upright position for labor, 411
Urachus, 67
Urea solution, injection of, after amniocentesis for therapeutic abortion, 995
Ureter, 59, 60, 61, 62, 67, 79
changes in, during pregnancy, 235
Ureteral nodes, 66
Urethra, 56, 61
abnormalities of, and male infertility, 181
female, 56
male, 77-79
during pregnancy, 235-236
prostatic, 81
Urethral meatus
of female, 55, 56
of male, 77
Urethral orifice, 56
Urethral stenosis and oligohydramnios, 967
Urethritis in male, 78
Urethrovesical fascia, 58
Urinalysis, 160
values for, for neonate, 1027
Urinary bladder, 78
Urinary frequency
during pregnancy, 235
and urgency, 305
as presumptive symptoms of pregnancy, 269
Urinary meatus
in female, 55, 56

Urinary meatus—cont'd
in male, 77
Urinary output in shock, 801
Urinary problems complicating pregnancy, 984-985
Urinary retention after delivery, 456
Urinary stasis during pregnancy, 235
Urinary stones during pregnancy, 985
Urinary system
assessment of, in postpartum period, 693
changes in, in postpartum period, 688-689
in postpartum period, evaluative criteria for, 699
during pregnancy, 235-238
Urinary tract infections
after delivery, 833
during pregnancy, 984-985
Urination by neonate, 572
assessment of, 612
evaluative criteria for, 647, 648
Urine
maternal, estriol level in
biochemical monitoring of, 283
determination of, 287
of neonate, 560
Urine glucose determinations, drugs affecting, 1021
Urine screening tests for inborn errors of metabolism, 1027
Urine specimen, clean-catch, 285
Urine specimen collectors for neonate, 645-646
Urine tests
for phenylketonuria, 1028
for protein and sugar in pregnant women, 237
Urobilinogen, 561
Urogenital diaphragm, 56, 57, 61
muscles and fascia of, 58
Urogenital tract, congenital anomalies of, screening for, 970
Uterine activity
display of, on chart paper, 480
increased, 490-491
information on, and signal source, 490
instrumentation for monitoring, 475-476
internal, 471, 478-479
monitoring of, 485, 490-491
suppression of, 910
Uterine artery, 67, 68
Uterine aspiration for therapeutic abortion, 992
Uterine atony
causes of, 803
factors associated with, 452
postdelivery hemorrhage caused by, 803
Uterine canal, 65
Uterine cavity, manual examination of, after delivery, 452
Uterine contractions, 380-382
after delivery, 688
dystonic, 881
and fetal circulation, 470
and fetal jeopardy, 407
in first stage of labor, 398, 400-401
hypertonic, 881-882
hypotonic, 882
ineffectual, 882
inefficient, 880, 881
intensity of, 398, 400, 485
causing intermittent cord occlusion, 470-471
mild, 400
moderate, 400
Montevideo units to measure, 381
normal, 881
pharmacologic stimulation of, after delivery of placenta, 452-453
as probable sign of pregnancy, 275
reverse polarity in, 881-882
strong, 400
as symptom of impending labor, 309
uterine relaxation between, 881
Uterine isthmus during pregnancy, 225
Uterine lithopedion, 781
Uterine segment, lower, 62
Uterine souffle, 225
as probable sign of pregnancy, 274
Uterine tubes; *see* Fallopian tubes
Uterine veins, 66
Uterine vessels, 59, 60
Uteroplacental and fetal circulation
factors affecting, 470-471
monitoring of, 470-471
Uteroplacental insufficiency, 470
late decelerations caused by, 489
Uterosacral ligament, 60, 61, 62, 66
Uterovaginal fascia, 59
Uterovesical ligament, 65
Uterus, 58, 59, 62-68
abnormalities of, and IUD, 196
anomalies of, surgical repair of, fertility following, 177
assessment of, after delivery, 690, 692, 693
atony of, 456
autonomic nerves of, 66
blood flow to, during pregnancy, 225, 230
blood supply to, 66, 67
changes in
during labor, 379, 380
during pregnancy, 223-226
in response to sexual stimulation, 95
colicky, 881
congenital abnormalities of, infertility from, 179
contractility of, 225
corpus of, 60-62
Couvelaire, 789, 791, 792
cross section of, 60
after delivery, 687
divisions of, 62
dysfunction of, 879
complications of, 882-884
dystocia of, 879-884
enlargement of, 223-224
as probable sign of pregnancy, 274
factors related to, causing female infertility, 179
function of, 66, 68, 179
fundus of; *see* Fundus
hypotonia of, after delivery, 452
inertia of, 879-882
innervation of, 66, 68
inversion of, postdelivery hemorrhage from, 806-807
involution of, 687-688
isthmus of, 62
ligaments supporting, 65-66
location of, 65
lymphatics of, 66
malposition of, 64, 65
mobility of, 65
motility of, and innervation, 66
motor nerves of, 66
muscle fibers of, arrangement of, and labor, 224
neck of; *see* Cervix
pain from, 66
perforation of, from IUD, 196
position of, 64, 65
during pregnancy, 224-225
posterior view of, 60
in postpartum period, evaluative criteria for, 698
prolapse of, 66
relaxation of
between contractions, 881
inadequate, 407
rupture of, with hydatidiform mole, 787
scar tissue in, causing infertility, 179
sensory nerves of, 66
shape of, 62
and consistency of, during pregnancy, 224
size of, 62
and IUD, 196
small, spontaneous abortion due to, 179
smooth muscle cells of, growth of, during pregnancy, 223
softening of, 272
as presumptive sign of pregnancy, 273-274
structure of, 62-65
stricture of, annular, from obstructed labor, 882
Uterus—cont'd
subinvolution of, postdelivery hemorrhage from, 807
support for, 65-66
T-shaped, 981
tumors of, removal of, 179
wall of, 62-63

V

Vaccination, rubella, after delivery, 693, 695
Vaccine, polio, for neonate, 562-563
Vacuum catheters, 993
Vacuum curettage for therapeutic abortion, 991, 992, 993, 994
Vacuum curettage machine, 993
Vacuum extraction, 892
Vagal reflex response, 285
to cervical manipulation, 196
during pelvic examination, 379
while suctioning neonate, 633
Vagina, 58-61, 68
anomalies of, surgical repair of, fertility following, 177
blood supply of, 68
changes in
during labor, 379
during menstrual cycle, 160
during pregnancy, 227-228
cyanosis of, as presumptive sign of pregnancy, 273
after delivery, 687
discharge from, in neonate, 567
epithelium of, effect of estrogens on, 89
examination of
and bleeding, 384
to determine fetal presentation, position, and descent, 384-386
during first stage of labor, 406-407
in placenta previa, 793
fornix of, 60, 61
function of, 179-180
infections of, 180
after delivery, 833-835
and fertility, 161-162
innervation of, 68
lacerations of
examination for, after delivery, 452
and hematomas of, postdelivery hemorrhage from, 804-805
lymphatics of, 68
mucosa of, 68
palpation of sagittal suture line via, 385
in postpartum period, evaluative criteria for, 699
response of, to sexual stimulation, 93, 95
support for, 68
tears of, after delivery, 449
upper, 60
Vaginal artery, 59, 67
Vaginal canal, examination of, after delivery, 452
Vaginal cesarean delivery, 895
Vaginal cervix, external os of, 60
Vaginal vs. clitoral orgasm, 100
Vaginal delivery
anesthesia level for, 515
following cesarean delivery, 746, 898-899
vascular changes after, 687
Vaginal douche, 835
Vaginal fluid, 68
pH of, determining, 401
Vaginal hysterotomy for therapeutic abortion, 992, 995
Vaginal introitus, 54, 55-56
Vaginal lubrication in response to sexual stimulation, 93, 100
Vaginal orifice, 61
Vaginal spermicides for contraception, 199
Vaginal tags in neonate, 567
Vaginal-cervical factors in female infertility, 179-180
Vaginal-penile intercourse, 110

Vaginitis
chemical, from spermicide, 199
Corynebacterium vaginale, during pregnancy, 828
Hemophilus vaginalis, during pregnancy, 828
monilial, 834
simple, 834-835
and stress, 180
Trichomonas, 180, 834
Vaginouterine fascia, 58
Vagisec for *Trichomonas* vaginitis, 834
Validation
in communication, 26
of nursing diagnosis, 21
Valium; *see* Diazepam
Value conflict, 31
Values, 29
clarification of, 31-33
effect of, on actions, 29-33
establishing, in adolescence, 107
Vancomycin for mastitis, 833
Variability in fetal heart rate, 480, 482-483
Variable decelerations in fetal heart rate, 487, 488, 489
Varicella during pregnancy, 828
Varices, anal and vulvar, 223
Varicocele
and male infertility, 182
surgical repair of, 182
Varicose veins
of labia, 55
during pregnancy, 304
of rectum and anus, 241
Vas deferens, 78, 79, 81
abnormalities of, and male infertility, 181
Vascular disease, hypertensive, 823
Vascular damage in diabetic pregnancies, 847
Vascular headache during pregnancy, 232
Vascular spiders, 238, 273, 987
Vascular system after delivery
assessment of, 692
changes in, 686-687
evaluative criteria for, 699
Vasectomy, 82, 998, 999
and autoimmunization, 181
Vasocongestion from sexual stimulation, 93
Vasocongestive reactions to sexual stimulation, 100
Vasopressin, 86; *see also* Antidiuretic hormone
causing increased uterine activity, 490
Vastus lateralis muscle, injection of, 637, 640
VDRL test, 160, 827
Vegan, 326
Vegan diet, 336
Vegetables, 334
introduction of, 673-674
leafy green, 334
vitamin C–rich, 334
Vegetarian diet, 335-336
food guide for, 336, 337
as nutrition risk factor, 326
Vein
hemorrhoidal, external, 68
iliac, internal, 66
ovarian, 68
pudendal, 68
scalp, venipuncture of, 757
umbilical; *see* Umbilical vein
uterine, 66
varicose; *see* Varicose veins
Vena cava
fetal, 216
inferior, 67
Vena cava syndrome, 214, 236, 411, 412, 470
prevention of, 304
in woman with heart disease, 869, 870
Venipuncture
of neonate, 645
of scalp vein, 757
Venous blood pressure, changes in, during pregnancy, 233
Venous plexus, cavernous, 56
Venous pressure, central, in shock, 801, 802
Venous return, anomalous, 968
Ventilation
alveolar, changes in, during pregnancy, 234
minute, changes in, during pregnancy, 234
Ventouse, 892
Ventricular septal defects, 969
Vernix caseosa of neonate, 563, 564
assessment of, 583-584
Veronal; *see* Barbital
Version, external cephalic, to convert breech presentation, 877
Vertex position, fetus in, emergency birth of, 447-448
Vertex presentation, 368, 369, 370, 371
delivery in, 419
fetal heart rate in, 384
fetus in, prebirth passage of meconium with, 448-449
mechanism of labor in, 388-392
Veromontanum, 79
Vesicles, seminal, 77-79, 82
abnormalities of, and male infertility, 182
Vesical artery, 67
superior, 67, 557
Vesicoumbilical ligaments, lateral, 557
Vessels
iliac, 59
external, 61
ovarian, 67
spermatic, 79
umbilical, 212, 214
uterine, 59, 60
Vestibular bulb, 56, 59
Vestibular glands
greater, 54, 56
lesser, 54, 55, 56
Vestibule, 54, 55, 59
Viability, 220
legal definition of, 45
Vietnamese families, child care in, 123
Vietnamese women, pregnant, food taboos for, 117
Vietnamese views
regarding sexual activity during pregnancy, 118-119
on sterility, 124
Villi
chorionic, 211
in placentation, 212
primary, 211
Virginity, "test" for, 56
Virus
Coxsackie B, during pregnancy, 828
herpes simplex, 563
cesarean birth of mother with, 402
placental transfer of, 215
Viscera, hollow, pain from, 66
Visceral discomfort during labor, 501
Vision of neonate, 568
assessment of, 603
Visit, prenatal
first, 292-293, 295-296
with multiple pregnancy, 933
Visitation, sibling, 5
Visiting hours, 5
Visiting policies, liberalization of, 5
Vistaril; *see* Hydroxyzine pamoate
Visual acuity of neonate, 568
Visual disorders and oral contraceptives, 195
Vital capacity, changes in, during pregnancy, 234
Vital signs
changes in, in postpartum period, 689
of neonate, assessment of, 580-582
in postpartum period, 691, 692
Vitamin A
effect of, on fetus or neonate, 1024
need for, during pregnancy, 322
and oral contraceptives, 194
transfer of, by placenta, 215
Vitamin B complex transfer by placenta, 215
Vitamin B_1, need for, during pregnancy, 322-323
Vitamin B_2
need for, during pregnancy, 323
and oral contraceptives, 194
Vitamin B_6
deficiency of, and oral contraceptives, 194
need for, during pregnancy, 322
Vitamin B_{12}
need for, during pregnancy, 323
and oral contraceptives, 194
Vitamin C
need for, during pregnancy, 323
and oral contraceptives, 194
transfer of, by placenta, 215
Vitamin C–rich fruits and vegetables, 334
Vitamin concentrations, standard values for, pregnant and nonpregnant, 1019
Vitamin D
effect of, on fetus or neonate, 1024
and fetus, 215
in human milk, 662
for infant, 656
need for, during pregnancy, 322
Vitamin D–deficiency rickets, 662
Vitamin D–resistant rickets, 147
Vitamin E
need for, during pregnancy, 322
transfer of, by placenta, 215
Vitamin K
effect of, on fetus or neonate, 1024
for infant, 656
transfer of, by placenta, 215
Vitamin K_1 for neonate, 628, 637-641
Vitamins
administering, by medicine dropper, 842
effect of, on fetus or neonate, 1024
fat-soluble, 322
biochemical tests for, 329
in human milk, 662
for infants, 656
needs for, during pregnancy, 322-323
water-soluble, 322-323
biochemical tests for, 329
Vocalizing by neonate, 571
Vocational choice of adolescent, 107, 108
Voice
and communication, 28-29
and parent-child attachment, 710
Voiding
during labor, 410
by neonate, 572
in postpartum period, 702
Volume
blood; *see* Blood volume
fluid equivalents in, 1015
minute, changes in, during pregnancy, 234
residual, changes in, during pregnancy, 234
tidal, changes in, during pregnancy, 234
Voluntary bearing-down efforts and expulsion of fetus, 382
Voluntary sterilization, 42, 996-1000
of female, 997-999
of male, 999
nurse's role in, 999-1000
procedures for, 997-999
Volvulus
and hydramnios, 967
midgut, meconium illeus with, 973
Vomiting
nausea and; *see* Nausea and vomiting
pernicious, of pregnancy; *see* Hyperemesis gravidarum
von Recklinghausen's disease, 987
von Willebrand's disease, 800
Vulva, 56
changes in, during pregnancy, 227-228
preparation of, during labor, 405
varices of, 223
Vulvovaginal glands, 54, 56

W

Wake states of neonate, 569
Waking and sleeping behaviors of neonate, 569-571
Waking activity of neonate, 569
"Walking" reflex, 599, 600
Wall
  abdominal, 68-69
  uterine, 62-63
Warfarin
  in breast milk, 1031
  during pregnancy, 867
Warming of hypothermic infant, 632
Warmth
  body, and parent-child attachment, 710
  for neonate with respiratory distress, 749
Wasserman test, 827
Water
  body, total, during pregnancy, 316
    changes in, 233
  for infants, 655
  insensible loss of, in neonate, 566
  sterile, for initial oral feeding, 677
Water balance
  in neonate, 559-560
  during pregnancy, 236-237
Water intoxication in infant, 655
Water loss in high-risk neonate, 752
Water metabolism of pregnancy, reversal of, 688, 692
"Water pills"; *see* Diuretics
Water-soluble vitamins
  biochemical tests for, 329
  need for, during pregnancy, 322-323
Weaning
  from breast, 666
  from oxygen therapy, 750
  from parenteral therapy, 753
Wedge trachelorrhaphy for weakened cervix, 781
Weighing of infant, 578
Weight
  birth, infant, and maternal nutrition, 318
  equivalents for, 1017
  fetal, and biparietal diameter, correlation of, 297
  maternal
    standards and deviations from, 318
    at term, distribution of, 317
  of neonate, 577
  in postpartum period, evaluative criteria for, 699
  prepregnant, as nutrition risk factor, 326
Weight gain
  excessive, during pregnancy, 326-327
  during first year, 651
  inadequate, during pregnancy, 326
  maternal, grid for, 319
Weight gain—cont'd
  during pregnancy, 237, 316-320
  as presumptive symptom of pregnancy, 270
Weight loss
  in high-risk neonate, 752-753
  neonatal, 611, 647-648
  secondary amenorrhea from, 177
Well-baby visit, first, anticipatory guidance of parents at, 630
Well-being, fetal, estriol excretion as measure of, 246
"Well-born," right of child to be, 9
Wharton's jelly, 213
"What" questions, 26
White blood cell count
  in neonate, 558
  during pregnancy, 232
White infants, mortality for, 11
Whites, maternal mortality among, 12
White's classification of pregnant diabetics, 845
"Why" questions, 26
WIC program, 326, 336
Wife and husband, relationship of, after birth of baby, 717
Windows in labor room, 414
"Wink" reflex of anal sphincter, 593
"Witch's milk," 76, 567
Withdrawal, signs of, in neonate, 955
Withdrawal bleeding, 87
  from oral contraceptives, 192
Woman
  diabetic; *see* Diabetic mother
  eliciting attitudes and feelings of, about parenting, 4
  fertile, assessment data for, 159-160
  four-phase sexual response cycle in, 93-100
  "mothering qualities" of, 103
  nulliparous, 55
  older, response of, to pregnancy, 721
  pregnant, rights of, 41
  preparation of, for activities of parenting, 4
  records of, during labor, 416
  Rh-negative, 217
  sexual response cycle in, 94-95
  unmarried, births to, 11
"Womb stone," 781
Women's health care specialist, 6
Women's Health Forum (Healthright), 1010
Work, return to, by mother, 717-718
Working Party on Midwifery Training in European Countries, 14
World Health Organization definition of midwife, 14
Wright method, 346
"Wrongful conception," 42

X

45, X, 151
X chromosomes, 143, 207
  inactivated, 149
  nondisjunction of, 150
X inactivation, 149
Xiphoid process, 69
X-linked disorders, 146
X-linked dominant disorders, 146-147
X-linked inheritance, 146-147
X-linked recessive disorders, 147
XO monosomy, 149, 150; *see also* Turner's syndrome
X-ray films
  and breast milk, 1033
  conventional, to determine fetal presentation, position, and descent, 386
X-ray pelvimetry chart, 377
47, XXX, 151
XXX syndrome, 151
48, XXXX, 151
49, XXXXX, 151
49, XXXXY, 151
48, XXXY, 151
47, XXY, 151
48, XXYY, 151
46, XY, D−G−, 150
46, XY, 5p−, 150
46, XY/47, XY, 21+, 150
47, XY, 13+, 150
47, XY, 18+, 150
47, XY, 21+, 150
Xylocaine; *see* Lidocaine
47, XYY, 151
XYY male syndrome, 151
48, XYYY, 151

Y

Y chromosomes, 143, 207
Yale University School of Nursing, ACNM-approved basic education in, 1014
Yawn, 601
Yellen clamp, circumcision with, 627
Yellow-stained amniotic fluid, 401
Yin and yang, 116
Yogurt to maintain vaginal-cervical pH, 180
Young adulthood, sexual development in, 109-111
Yutopar; *see* Ritodrine

Z

Zinc
  in human milk, 661
  for infant, 657
  need for, during pregnancy, 323
Zona pellucida, 207
Zygote, 145, 206, 207